EVIDENCE-BASED PRACTICE

FOCUS ON DIVERSITY AND CULTURE

FOCUS ON INTEGRATIVE HEALTH

MEDICATIONS

MULTISYSTEM EFFECTS OF

NURSING CARE PLAN

A Patient with:

PATIENT TEACHING

VOLUME 2

NURSING

A Concept-Based Approach to Learning

Fourth Edition

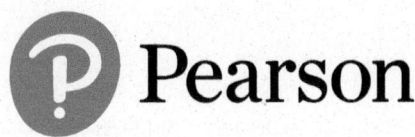

Content Development: Adelaide R. McCulloch and Laura S. Horowitz
Content Management: Kevin Wilson and Jeanne Zalesky
Content Production: Melissa Bashe, Jeff Henn, William Johnson, Amy Peltier, and Brian Prybella
Product Management: Katrin Beacom
Product Marketing: Kelly Galli and Rachele Strober
Rights and Permissions: Ben Ferrini, Angelica Aranas, and Regine Diaz

Please contact https://support.pearson.com/getsupport/s/ with any queries on this content
Cover Image by Shutterstock

CIP Available at the Library of Congress

4 2022

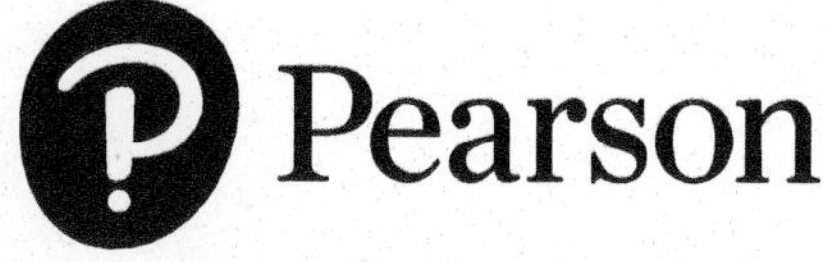

ISBN-13: 978-0-13-688339-5
ISBN-10: 0-13-688339-7

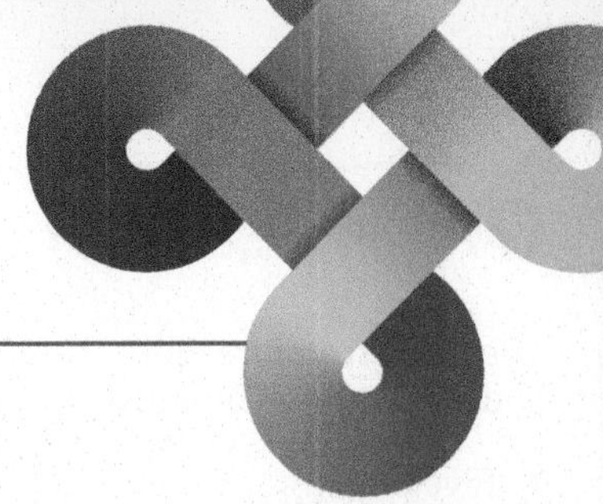

Pearson's Concepts Solution

Nursing: A Concept-Based Approach to Learning is the #1 choice for schools of nursing that use a concept-based curriculum. It is the ONLY true concept-based learning solution and the ONLY concepts curriculum developed from the ground up as a cohesive, comprehensive learning system. The three-volume series, along with MyLab Nursing, provides everything you need to deliver an effective concept-based program that teaches students to think like a nurse and develops practice-ready nurses.

Nursing: A Concept-Based Approach to Learning, Fourth Edition, represents the cutting edge in nursing education. This uniquely integrated solution provides students with a consistent design of content and assessment that specifically supports a concept-based curriculum. Available as a fully integrated digital experience or in print format, this solution meets the needs of today's nursing student. The goal of this program is to help students learn the essential knowledge they will need for patient care.

Starting with the cover, our goal for the Fourth Edition is to help students learn the essential knowledge they will need for patient care. The cover, a Möbius strip, represents the relationships among the concepts and how they are all interconnected. By understanding important connections of concepts, students are able to relate topics to broader contexts.

What Makes Pearson's Solution Different?

As demonstrated with the previous three editions of *Nursing: A Concept-Based Approach to Learning*, Pearson's program has the ability to meet the needs of students and instructors in a concept-based education program. The Fourth Edition builds on our commitment to excellence: Every page, every word, every feature has been examined—all to help enhance the learning and teaching process. The result is an integration of content and features that you, our customer, have asked for and that you will not find in other concept-based nursing learning materials. Pearson's program includes:

- Everything instructors and students need in one solution: all concepts, all exemplars, all assessment tools.
- Content designed by instructional designers for conceptual learning, including learning and enabling objectives for every main section and measurable outcomes for each.
- Content that covers the lifespan from pregnancy and birth, through childhood and adolescence, and into young, middle, and old age.

Why Teach Concept-Based Learning?

Nursing education is evolving. As the nursing profession has developed to encompass a variety of roles at all levels of society—including direct client care, advocacy, and leadership at the local, state, and national levels—nursing education is changing to help nursing students prepare to enter a more robust, demanding, and rewarding profession. Societal forces that have created the climate for transforming nursing education include, but are not limited to, the global economy, technological advances, and changes in healthcare delivery systems. Tried and true teaching methods now seem antiquated as faculty compete for students' attention with a variety of new and engaging sources of information and entertainment. In addition, the overwhelming discovery of new knowledge in the "information age" has resulted in nursing students feeling overwhelmed by the quantity of knowledge and skills they must gain in order to become practicing nurses.

University and college nursing programs across the United States have begun evaluating how their programs can meet the needs of today's nursing students. Many are moving to the model of concept-based learning in an effort to meet the challenges facing nursing students and nurses today. This model provides the impetus for educators to transition away from traditional methods of faculty-centered teaching and passive learning toward active, focused, participative, and collaborative teaching and learning. Pearson's *Nursing: A Concept-Based Approach to Learning*, Fourth Edition, is designed to assist nursing faculty to provide students with a broader perspective while promoting a deeper understanding of content across the lifespan in a focused, participative, and collaborative learning environment.

Organization and Structure of the Fourth Edition

The basic structure of the Third Edition was retained for the Fourth Edition. There are:

- Five parts:
  - I: The Biophysical Modules (in the Individual Domain)
  - II: The Psychosocial Modules (in the Individual Domain)
  - III: Reproduction (in the Individual Domain)
  - IV: The Nursing Domain
  - V: The Healthcare Domain
- Fifty-one concepts
- One hundred sixty-one exemplars

The Concepts were chosen after surveying numerous concept-based curricula and finding the common elements. Some Concepts were added after requests by users. The result is a comprehensive set of Concepts that cover the essentials of nursing education.

The Exemplars were chosen based on selected national initiatives such as the Institute of Medicine, *Healthy People 2030*, HIPAA, the Centers for Medicare and Medicaid, OSHA, and QSEN. Prevalence rates were considered for the biophysical and psychosocial exemplars with the more common disorders prioritized over less common ones. Certain exemplars were chosen because they lend themselves to teaching across concepts or across the lifespan.

For the Fourth Edition, as shown in the Module Outline and Learning Outcomes listed at the beginning of each module, each main section has a dedicated learning outcome. Our editorial and instructional design teams worked to create consistent, accurate, challenging, achievable, and measurable objective statements based on objective-driven design practices to better engage students, improve performance, increase student gains, and promote deep learning.

Module 2

Cellular Regulation

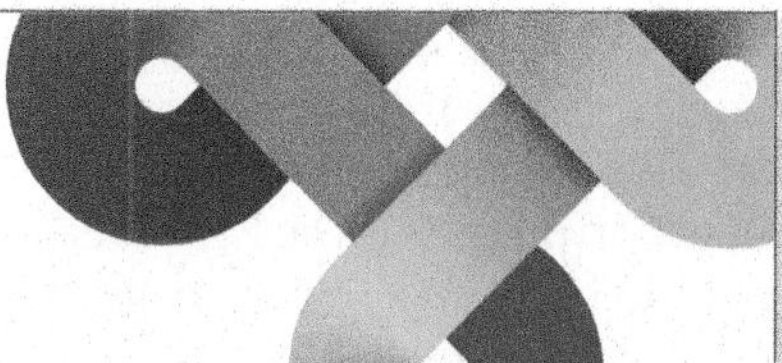

Module Outline and Learning Outcomes

The Concept of Cellular Regulation

Normal Cellular Regulation

2.1 Analyze the physiology of cellular regulation in the body.

Alterations to Cellular Regulation

2.2 Differentiate alterations in cellular regulation.

Concepts Related to Cellular Regulation

2.3 Outline the relationship between cellular regulation and other concepts.

Health Promotion

2.4 Explain the promotion of healthy cellular regulation.

Nursing Assessment

2.5 Differentiate common assessment procedures and tests used to examine cellular regulation.

Independent Interventions

2.6 Analyze independent interventions nurses can implement for patients with alterations in cellular regulation.

Collaborative Therapies

2.7 Summarize collaborative therapies used by interprofessional teams for patients with alterations in cellular regulation.

Lifespan Considerations

2.8 Differentiate considerations related to the care of patients with alterations in cellular regulation throughout the lifespan.

Cellular Regulation Exemplars

Exemplar 2.A Cancer

2.A Analyze cancer as it relates to cellular regulation.

Exemplar 2.B Anemia

2.B Analyze anemia as it relates to cellular regulation.

Exemplar 2.C Breast Cancer

2.C Analyze breast cancer as it relates to cellular regulation.

Exemplar 2.D Colorectal Cancer

2.D Analyze colorectal cancer as it relates to cellular regulation.

Exemplar 2.E Leukemia

2.E Analyze leukemia as it relates to cellular regulation.

Exemplar 2.F Lung Cancer

2.F Analyze lung cancer as it relates to cellular regulation.

Exemplar 2.G Prostate Cancer

2.G Analyze prostate cancer as it relates to cellular regulation.

Exemplar 2.H Sickle Cell Disease

2.H Analyze sickle cell disease as it relates to cellular regulation.

Exemplar 2.I Skin Cancer

2.I Analyze skin cancer as it relates to cellular regulation.

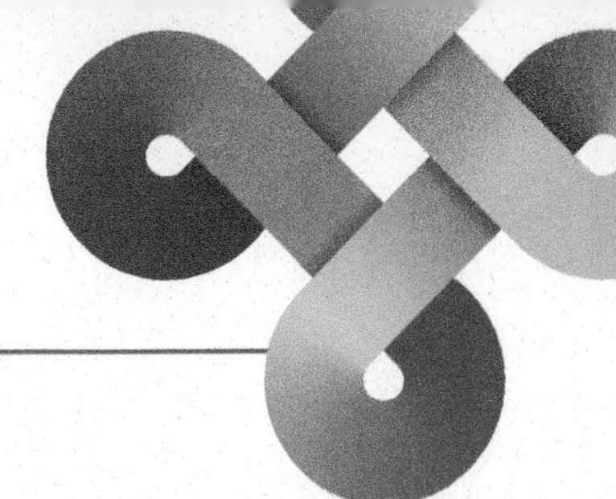

What's New in the Fourth Edition?

All content in the Fourth Edition has been reviewed and updated or revised by experienced nurse educators working with the editorial team. Notable additions include:

Changes to Exemplars

In the Fourth Edition, changes to exemplars include:

- Ménière Disease has been added to Module 18, Sensory Perception
- Medication Safety has been added to Module 51, Safety
- Professional Development has been moved from Module 42, Accountability, to Module 40, Professionalism
- Sexual Violence has replaced Rape and Rape-Trauma Syndrome in Module 32, Trauma
- Spirituality and Religion have been folded into Module 30, Spirituality, and are no longer separate exemplars.

Expanded Medication Coverage

Based on user feedback, the Fourth Edition includes updated and expanded coverage of medications in each Pharmacologic Therapy section and in over 70 Medications features. For example, instead of a single table on medications in Module 16 in The Concept of Perfusion, in that module Fourth Edition users will find:

- Medications 16.1, Drugs Used to Improve Perfusion
- Medications 16.2, Drugs Used to Lower Cholesterol
- Medications 16.3, Antiplatelet Drugs
- Medications 16.4, Anticoagulants
- Medications 16.5, Drugs Used to Treat Heart Failure
- Medications 16.6, Antihypertensive Drugs
- Medications 16.7, Antidysrhythmic Drugs
- Medications 16.8, Drugs Used to Treat Shock

New Communication Feature

For the Fourth Edition, Pearson has introduced a new feature, *Communicating with Patients*. This feature was written to help new nurses learn what to say to patients. Some are written for the Introductory Phase of the nurse–patient relationship, and others are written for the Working Phase. These features are designed to help new nurses learn how to start conversations, broach difficult subjects, and connect with patients.

Communicating with Patients

Introductory Phase

Being obese puts your patient at risk for many preventable health problems. But how do you tactfully discuss obesity without being judgmental or making your patient feel uncomfortable? Research suggests that having a discussion with a patient about weight loss can have a positive impact on lifestyle changes. Studies also advise using the terms "weight" or "BMI" rather than "fat," "excess fat," or "obesity" (NIDDK, 2017d). Above all, be respectful and be nonjudgmental. The following suggestions can help to introduce the topic:

- Let's talk about the effects of your weight on your health.
- Tell me how you feel about your weight.

Once you determine that your patient is ready to take positive actions to improve health, here are some ways to open the discussion about lifestyle changes:

- What are your favorite foods?
- Tell me who shops for food and cooks in your home.
- What types of activities do you like to do?

COVID-19 Coverage

The COVID-19 virus emerged during the writing and editing of this text. The variable reporting of constantly changing data made it difficult to accurately reflect information about the virus and its treatment parameters.

Where possible, we have made every effort to reflect new, relevant information related to COVID-19, but we acknowledge the impermanence of data given the ongoing emergence of new research in this area. However, readers will still find relevant content related to:

- Effects of COVID-19 on healthcare systems and personnel, specifically nurses
- Strategies for dealing with losses of routine associated with long-term crises
- Nurse self-care and COVID-19
- Disparities in healthcare exacerbated by the pandemic
- Impact of the pandemic on stress levels in the United States
- Strategies for providing care to patients and families directly affected by COVID-19.

New and Increased Coverage of Selected Topics

- ***Autoimmune diseases.*** A six-page illustrated table on Additional Autoimmune Disorders (Table 8.2) has been added to Module 8, Immunity. It features disorders such as Addison disease, GVHD, Lyme disease, myasthenia gravis, and Rh incompatibility.
- ***Care settings.*** Content on medical and mental health care settings has been added to Module 7, Health, Wellness, Illness, and Injury.
- ***Diabetes insipidus and SIADH.*** Content on these two disorders has been added to Module 6, Fluids and Electrolytes.
- ***Enteral and total parenteral nutrition.*** Per requests from users, content on enteral nutrition and TPN has been moved from Module 4, Digestion, to Module 14, Nutrition.
- ***Food allergies and food intolerances.*** A new section on food allergies and food intolerances has been added to Module 14, Nutrition, along with expanded coverage of plant-based diets.
- ***Gene editing.*** A section on gene editing to treat sickle cell disease has been added to Module 2, Cellular Regulation.
- ***Healthy People 2030.*** The objectives and leading health indicators from *Healthy People 2030* have been incorporated throughout, with a particular emphasis on the social determinants of health.
- ***Maternal morbidity and epidural analgesia.*** Module 33 includes expanded coverage on issues related to maternal mortality and morbidity, including new information on nursing assessment to reduce risk and nursing interventions in response to complications, such as obstetric hemorrhage. In addition, a new section on epidural analgesia will be available to users online.
- ***Plain language for patient problems.*** In keeping with the shift to the use of electronic health records, the Fourth Edition uses plain language to describe patient problems and the nursing care that will be needed. In the Nursing Process sections and Nursing Care Plan features, the ADPIE format has been retained, but in the Diagnosis section, instead of formal NANDA-I nursing diagnoses, priorities for care are listed as they would be seen in an electronic health record.
- ***Volume 3: Clinical Nursing Skills.*** Links to the Skills in Volume 3 are incorporated within the text in the Fourth Edition rather than being listed in the Review sections.

Pearson's Commitment to Diversity, Equity, and Inclusion

Pearson is dedicated to creating bias-free content that reflects the diversity of all learners. We embrace the many dimensions of diversity, including but not limited to race, ethnicity, gender, socioeconomic status, ability, age, sexual orientation, and religious or political beliefs.

Education is a powerful force for equity and change in our world. It has the potential to deliver opportunities that improve lives and enable economic mobility. As we work with authors to create content for every product and service, we acknowledge our responsibility to demonstrate inclusivity and incorporate diverse scholarship so that everyone can achieve their potential through learning. As the world's leading learning company, we have a duty to help drive change and live up to our purpose to help more people create a better life for themselves and to create a better world.

Our ambition is to purposefully contribute to a world where:

- Everyone has an equitable and lifelong opportunity to succeed through learning.
- Our educational products and services are inclusive and represent the rich diversity of learners.
- Our educational content accurately reflects the histories and experiences of the learners we serve.
- Our educational content prompts deeper discussions with students and motivates them to expand their own learning (and worldview).

We are also committed to providing products that are fully accessible to all learners. As per Pearson's guidelines for accessible educational Web media, we test and retest the capabilities of our products against the highest standards for every release, following the WCAG guidelines in developing new products for copyright year 2022 and beyond. You can learn more about Pearson's commitment to accessibility at https://www.pearson.com/us/accessibility.html.

While we work hard to present unbiased, fully accessible content, we want to hear from you about any concerns or needs with this Pearson product so that we can investigate and address them.

- Please contact us with concerns about any potential bias at https://www.pearson.com/report-bias.html.
- For accessibility-related issues, such as using assistive technology with Pearson products, alternative text requests, or accessibility documentation, email the Pearson Disability Support team at disability.support@pearson.com.

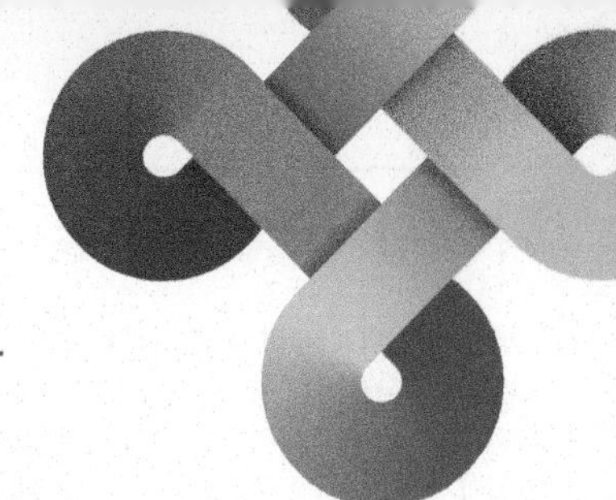

Structure and Features of the Concepts

The opening "Concept" sections of each module are set up consistently throughout the program. This allows students to anticipate the learning they will experience. Special features recur in each Concept as well, which students can use for learning and review. The basic structure of the Concepts is shown below with visuals and annotations describing the content. Note that each red heading has a corresponding learning outcome. Concepts begin with a list of Concept Key Terms, the definitions of which can be found in the Glossary.

›› The Concept of Cellular Regulation

Concept Key Terms

Anaplasia, **36**	Deoxyribonucleic acid (DNA), **34**	Genome, **35**	Meiosis, **35**	Ribonucleic acid (RNA), **34**
Autosomes, **35**	Differentiation, **36**	Homologous chromosomes, **35**	Metaplasia, **36**	Sex chromosomes, **35**
Cell cycle, **35**	Dysplasia, **36**	Hyperplasia, **36**	Mitosis, **35**	Somatic cells, **35**
Chromosomes, **35**				

The cell is the basic unit of all living systems. Humans are complex organisms made up of an estimated 30 trillion cells working together to carry out the basic functions needed for survival (Cafasso, 2018). The many types of specialized cells in the body function differently depending on their location. For example, pancreatic cells have a very different function from that of nerve cells. However, all cells have common features, such as a nucleus and mitochondria.

Cell reproduction, proliferation, and growth are regulated by the body. Alterations in cellular regulation can have devastating consequences for body tissues and functions.

Normal Cellular Regulation

Almost all of the cells in the human body are microscopic. Although they vary greatly in size, shape, and function, they all share certain features. Any change in or disturbance to one

Normal Presentation Each Concept starts with a review of normal, healthy function, including subsections on Physiology Review and Genetic Considerations where appropriate.

Physiology Review

Genetic Considerations

Alterations The second section of each Concept focuses on alterations, including subheads on Alterations and Manifestations, Prevalence, Genetic Considerations, and Risk Factors. A standard feature in this section is the Alterations and Therapies table.

Alterations and Manifestations

Prevalence

Genetic Considerations and Risk Factors

Alterations and Manifestations

Cellular Regulation

ALTERATION	DESCRIPTION	MANIFESTATIONS	INTERVENTIONS AND THERAPIES
Cancer (e.g., breast, colorectal, lung, ovarian, uterine, bladder, prostate, testicular, skin, and leukemia)	Abnormal and rapid growth of body cells that may invade surrounding body tissues and spread (metastasize) to other sites	▪ Manifestations are variable, depending on the location and size of the growth, as well as on whether other tissues and organs are affected. ▪ Surrounding blood vessels and organs may also be affected, producing varying effects. ▪ General signs and symptoms may include fatigue, fever, weight changes, and persistent, unexplained pain (Mayo Clinic, 2018b).	▪ Identify and treat the affected organ(s) and/or tissue(s). Conventional treatments may include chemotherapy, radiation, and surgical removal of the affected organ/tissue. Alternative treatments may include relaxation therapy, guided imagery, and certain homeopathic supplements.
Anemia (e.g., aplastic, hemolytic, and iron deficiency)	Deficiency of hemoglobin or reduction of number of RBCs that leads to inadequate delivery of oxygen to cells, tissues, and organs; may also be caused by blood loss, impaired RBC production, or excessive RBC destruction	▪ Manifestations are variable, depending on the underlying cause. ▪ General signs and symptoms may include lethargy, pallor, dyspnea, dizziness, and confusion.	▪ Identify and treat the underlying cause. Medical interventions may include blood transfusions and surgical measures to stop internal bleeding. Nutritional supplements may include iron (for treatment of iron deficiency anemia) and folate or vitamin B_{12} (for treatment of anemia due to vitamin deficiency). ▪ When possible, aplastic anemia is treated through elimination of the known cause. Pharmacologic treatments may include medications that induce RBC production, such as erythropoietin and colony-stimulating factors. Other treatments include blood transfusions and stem cell transplants (also known as bone marrow transplants) (Mayo Clinic, 2020a).

Case Studies

Most Concept sections contain a three-part unfolding case study to help students apply what they are learning to a patient. Each section of the case study ends with two sets of questions. Clinical Reasoning Questions Level 1 can be answered by students after reading the content in the Concept. Clinical Reason Questions Level 2 require students to integrate content from other modules in order to answer the questions.

Case Study » Part 1

Andrew Ladeaux, an 8-year-old boy, is brought to the emergency department by his mother. On arrival, Andrew is pressing a bloody towel against his nose. As the triage nurse, you direct the boy and his mother to the assessment station. Andrew's mother explains that his nose began bleeding "about an hour ago" during a baseball tournament. Andrew denies any traumatic injury, and his mother reports that her son's game had not yet begun when the bleeding started. He appears to be in no acute distress. His respiratory rate is 28/min, and his respirations are regular and not labored. Andrew's pulse rate is 136 bpm, which is elevated. As you apply a blood pressure cuff to his arm, you notice light, scattered bruising along his forearm. His blood pressure is 118/71 mmHg, which is slightly elevated.

Although Andrew denies any additional symptoms, during further exploration of his health status, his mother reports that her son has seemed "really tired lately" and that he "seems like he's been bruising very easily."

Clinical Reasoning Questions Level I

1. Considering your assessment of Andrew, which cues might suggest an alteration in cellular regulation?
2. Why might Andrew's blood pressure and pulse rate be elevated?
3. What is the relationship between bleeding and bruising?

Clinical Reasoning Questions Level II

4. At this time, presuming that Andrew has lost a significant amount of blood, what is the priority for care of this patient?
5. *Refer to Exemplar 2.E on Leukemia.* Which blood test do you expect to be ordered for further assessment of Andrew's condition?

Case Study » Part 2

Andrew Ladeaux is admitted to the emergency department. During the emergency department physician's assessment, he tells the physician he feels "a little short of breath," especially when he runs. Andrew's mother reports that he has been treated for strep throat three times and has had several ear infections within the past 6 months. The healthcare provider (HCP) orders a CBC with differential for Andrew. After the phlebotomist draws his blood, she has to apply pressure to the puncture site for nearly 2 minutes before the site stops bleeding. You return to check on Andrew's status. The HCP tells you he suspects that Andrew may have developed leukemia.

Case Study » Part 3

Andrew Ladeaux's laboratory results are available. His CBC results include the following:

WBC: 37.8 (normal = 4.5–10 K/μL)
RBC: 3.2 (normal = 4.6–6 M/μL)
PLT (platelets): 90 (normal = 150–400 K/μL)
Lymphocytes: 70 (normal = 25–35%)

Concepts Related to

Cellular Regulation

CONCEPT	RELATIONSHIP TO CELLULAR REGULATION	NURSING IMPLICATIONS
Advocacy	The nurse should ensure that patients receive sufficient information on which to base their consent for care and related treatment. The nurse provides an environment favorable for patients to make their own care decisions, as appropriate.	■ Assess the patient's level of understanding related to care and treatment options. ■ Discuss the plan of care with the patient and allow for self-determination such as which treatment may be the best option, as appropriate. ■ Assess your own values and beliefs related to refusal of treatment/procedures. ■ Recognize the patient's right to refuse treatment/procedures.
Infection	Introduction of bacteria, viruses, fungi, or foreign substances → activation of immune response → increased production of WBCs	■ Assess for signs and symptoms of infection, including redness, swelling, and draining from the injured site. Be aware that fever often accompanies infectious processes. ■ Anticipate potential need for blood and/or wound cultures and administration of antibiotics. ■ Antipyretics may be indicated. ■ Be aware that increased WBC count may indicate an inflammatory process, infection, or a combination of both.
Inflammation	Trauma → activation of inflammatory response → recruitment of WBCs to site of injury and increased WBC production	■ Assess for signs and symptoms of inflammation, including redness and swelling. Be aware that fever may accompany inflammatory processes even in the absence of infection. ■ Anticipate administration of anti-inflammatory medications, possible application of ice to inflamed area, and, if possible, elevation of injured site. ■ Be aware that an increased WBC count may indicate an inflammatory process, infection, or a combination of both.
Managing Care	Patients with alterations in cellular regulation can greatly benefit from participating in managed care and have more positive health outcomes.	■ Assess the needs of the patient to identify actual or potential problems related to care. ■ Advocate for the patient in relation to care needs. ■ Participate in coordination of care to secure the patient's well-being.
Stress and Coping	Physical and/or emotional stress → OS → production of free radicals → increased risk for development of diseases and disorders	■ Assess psychosocial factors that affect the patient. ■ Recognize the potential health effects of physical and emotional stressors. ■ Anticipate the need for patient teaching related to coping and relaxation. When indicated, referral to other healthcare professionals may be appropriate for both disease prevention and health promotion.

Concepts Related to This section encourages students to look beyond the concept being studied to see how it relates to other concepts that apply to patients in real life. No patient has an alteration to just one concept; nurses must learn to look beyond the reported problem to see how their patients are affected in all domains.

Patient Teaching

Health Promotion for Cancer Prevention: Modifiable Risk Factors

- ***Discourage smoking or use of other tobacco products.*** Emphasize the importance of patients protecting children and themselves from exposure to tobacco smoke. This is one of the most important health decisions an individual can make.
- ***Encourage patients, especially children, to consume a healthy diet.*** This should include a minimum of five servings of fruits and vegetables daily as well as whole grains, iron-rich foods, and foods that are rich in vitamin B_{12}. Teach patients to limit their consumption of processed meats; drink alcohol in moderation; and choose fewer high-calorie foods.
- ***Explain the importance of maintaining a healthy weight and being physically active.*** Physical activity helps to control weight. Together, these factors may lower the risk for various types of cancer.
- ***Teach patients effective ways to protect themselves from ultraviolet radiation.*** Early excessive sun exposure and one or more severe sunburns during childhood increase the chances of skin cancers developing in adulthood. Patients who work outdoors, athletes, coaches, and others who spend time outside should regularly use sunscreen daily (sun protection factor [SPF] 15 or greater), regardless of the climate in which they live. Emphasize the importance of avoiding midday sun, when the sun's rays are strongest. Instruct patients to cover exposed skin and wear a hat with a wide brim. Tanning beds and sunlamps should be avoided.
- ***Explain the importance of avoiding risky behaviors.*** Practicing risky behaviors such as needle sharing or unsafe sexual contact can increase the risk of developing certain cancers.
- ***Suggest that patients have their homes tested for radon and explore their exposure to harmful chemicals.*** Patients may be exposed to hazardous substances in the home or in the workplace.
- ***Stress the importance of getting immunizations, receiving regular medical care, and doing self-examinations.*** By protecting against certain viral infections, immunizations can decrease the risk of some cancers. Regular screenings and self-examinations increase the chances of early detection of cancer, allowing for a better chance of successful treatment (Mayo Clinic, 2018c).

Health Promotion

This section covers modifiable risk factors, screenings, general health information for nurses to share with patients, and care in the community. Many Health Promotion sections include a Patient Teaching feature.

Modifiable Risk Factors

Screenings

Nursing Assessment

The Nursing Assessment section covers everything the new nurse needs to know about assessing patients. It includes sections on Observation and Patient Interview, Physical Examination, and Diagnostic Tests and a feature on Assessment.

Observation and Patient Interview

Physical Examination

Diagnostic Tests

Digestion Assessment

ASSESSMENT/ METHOD	NORMAL FINDINGS	ABNORMAL FINDINGS	LIFESPAN OR DEVELOPMENTAL CONSIDERATIONS
Inspection	The abdomen is symmetrical, and its contours are flat, rounded, or scaphoid. The abdomen is free of masses. The umbilicus is centered and may be protruding or inverted. A consistent skin color with macules and moles is considered to be normal (Fenske et al., 2019).	▪ Asymmetrical contours ▪ Marked pulsations ▪ Engorged veins ▪ Marked distention ▪ Bruising around the umbilicus (Cullen sign) or bruising of the flanks (Grey Turner sign) indicative of pancreatic necrosis with retroperitoneal or intra-abdominal bleeding	▪ Inspection of a pediatric patient: a sunken abdomen is abnormal and may indicate dehydration. ▪ Assess the midline of the abdomen for depression or bulging, which could indicate separation of the rectus abdominis muscle. As growth occurs, the separation usually becomes less prominent. ▪ Infants and children up to age 6 breathe with the diaphragm, causing the abdomen to rise in inspiration and fall with expiration. ▪ Abdominal movements such as peristaltic waves are considered abnormal and may indicate intestinal obstruction or pyloric stenosis (Ball, Bindler, Cowen, & Shaw, 2022).
Auscultation	Normal bowel sounds are irregular, high-pitched gurgling sounds that occur 5–30 times a minute.	▪ Hyperactive bowel sounds (may be loud, higher pitched, and rushing) ▪ Hypoactive bowel sounds (slow and sluggish) ▪ Absent bowel sounds ▪ Bruits and venous hums ▪ Friction rubs over the liver and spleen	▪ For infants, take advantage of opportunities presented when the infant is sleeping or quiet to listen to abdomen (Ball et al., 2022). ▪ Toddlers and preschoolers should be allowed to touch and play with the stethoscope.

Independent Interventions

In this section, we cover those interventions that nurses can perform on their own, without a prescription from the healthcare provider. Examples of subsections include:

Prevent Infection

Promote Safety

Sleep Hygiene

Communicating with Patients

Introductory Phase

Patients with alterations in cellular regulation may be angry, depressed, afraid, or sad. After introducing yourself, you can break the ice by talking about small things that may help you find commonalities with the patient. Be observant by noticing items in the room such as books, greeting cards, photographs, magazines, or the television show they are currently watching to assist you with conversation starters:

- I see you are watching ______, do you like ______?
- I noticed you are reading a book about ______, do you like ______?
- You have a beautiful bouquet of roses on the table, are they your favorite flower?

Many Independent Intervention sections include a new feature, Communicating with Patients. This feature was written to help new nurses learn what to say to patients. Some are written for the Introductory Phase of therapeutic communication, and others are written for the Working Phase. These features are designed to help new nurses learn how to start conversations, broach difficult subjects, and connect with patients.

Medications 2.1

Drugs Used to Treat Cancer

CLASSIFICATION AND DRUG EXAMPLES	MECHANISMS OF ACTION	NURSING CONSIDERATIONS
Alkylating Agents ***Drug examples:*** bendamustine (Treanda) busulfan (Busulfex, Myleran) carboplatin (Paraplatin) carmustine (BiCNU, Gliadel) chlorambucil (Leukeran) cisplatin cyclophosphamide ifosfamide (Ifex) lomustine (CCNU, Gleostine) mechlorethamine melphalan (Alkeran) streptozocin (Zanosar)	Interfere with DNA replication and the transcription of RNA, causing cellular death. They are not cell specific, so both cancerous and noncancerous cells are destroyed.	▪ Monitor CBC with differential, platelet count, uric acid levels, and kidney and liver function studies. ▪ Monitor temperature; avoid rectal temperature assessment. ▪ Assess mentation and neurologic status. ▪ Monitor nutritional and fluid intake. ▪ Monitor respiratory status, cardiovascular status, and skin. ▪ Concurrent administration with drugs that are toxic to kidneys or liver is contraindicated. ▪ Use in patients with liver, kidney, or GI disorders is contraindicated.
Antimetabolites ***Drug examples:*** capecitabine (Xeloda) cytarabine fludarabine fluorouracil (Adrucil) gemcitabine (Gemzar) mercaptopurine (Purixan) methotrexate (MTX, Trexall) pentostatin (Nipent) pemetrexed (Alimta) pralatrexate (Folotyn) thioguanine (Tabloid)	Interfere with the use of either folate, purine, or pyrimidine that help form amino acids in the DNA of the cell.	▪ Monitor CBC with differential, electrolytes, and kidney and liver function studies. ▪ Monitor for bleeding and protect the patient from traumatic injury. ▪ Monitor for signs of infection. ▪ Monitor nutritional and fluid intake. ▪ Monitor for dyspnea and cough.

Collaborative Therapies

Collaborative Therapies This section covers interventions that require the interprofessional team. Team members are listed and the therapies the team may deliver are introduced. Revised and updated Medications features cover the most common drugs used to treat alterations.

Surgery

Pharmacologic Therapy

Nonpharmacologic Therapy

Complementary Health Approaches

Lifespan Considerations

Lifespan Considerations This section presents content specific to patients of selected age groups. Sections may include those for newborns to infants, school-age children to adolescents, young adults through middle age, pregnant women, and older adults. These sections may include Communicating with Patients and Patient Teaching features.

Considerations for Infants

Considerations for Children and Adolescents

Considerations for Pregnant Women

Considerations for Older Adults

REVIEW Each Concept ends with a review that includes linking questions, a link to Volume 3, and a short case study with questions so students can apply their knowledge.

REVIEW The Concept of Cellular Regulation

RELATE Link the Concepts

Linking the concept of cellular regulation with the concept of infection:

1. How does impaired cellular regulation influence a patient's susceptibility to infection?
2. What can the nurse do to help reduce the likelihood of infection in patients with disorders related to impaired cellular regulation?

Linking the concept of cellular regulation with the concept of stress and coping:

3. What is the relationship between poor coping abilities and disorders of cellular regulation?
4. Which personality types are most often correlated with a risk for ineffective coping?
5. Is there a relationship between personality and impaired cellular regulation? Explain your answer.

Linking the concept of cellular regulation with the concept of safety:

6. Identify three safety concerns specific to the patient with a disorder related to impaired cellular regulation.
7. Based on QSEN competencies, how can the nurse promote safety for the patient with a disorder of cellular regulation?

READY Go to Volume 3: Clinical Nursing Skills

REFER Go to Pearson MyLab Nursing and eText

REFLECT Apply Your Knowledge

Jason Marchetti is a 25-year-old man who has been going to the gym daily after work for the past 8 months. Approximately 4 months ago, he noticed a small nodule on the left side of his chest. Now the nodule is somewhat larger, and the nipple has an odd shape. The area is not painful, but Mr. Marchetti is worried that he may have injured a muscle at the gym and decides to go to his primary HCP to have the area evaluated. Upon examination, the provider finds a 2.5 cm, nontender, movable nodule in Mr. Marchetti's left breast area. There are no risk factors for breast cancer in Mr. Marchetti's previous medical or family history. The provider tells him that he is concerned about the nodule and a biopsy is needed to determine whether it is benign or cancerous. The biopsy is performed, and Mr. Marchetti returns the next week to get the results. The provider informs him that he has invasive ductal carcinoma of the breast and that they should discuss options for treatment. Mr. Marchetti sits in the examination room in disbelief, saying, "I don't understand how I can have breast cancer. I thought only women got that."

1. What treatment options are available for Mr. Marchetti and could be recommended by the provider?
2. What patient problems might the nurse address when writing out the plan of care?
3. What would be appropriate primary nursing interventions for the nurse to implement for Mr. Marchetti at this time?

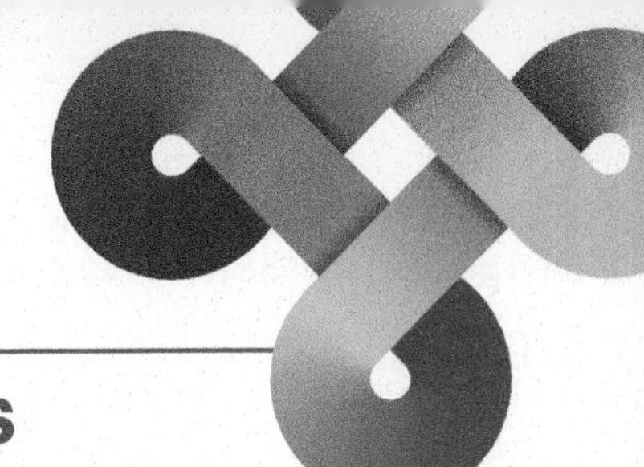

Structure and Features of the Exemplars

Note that each Exemplar has one main learning outcome with multiple enabling objectives.

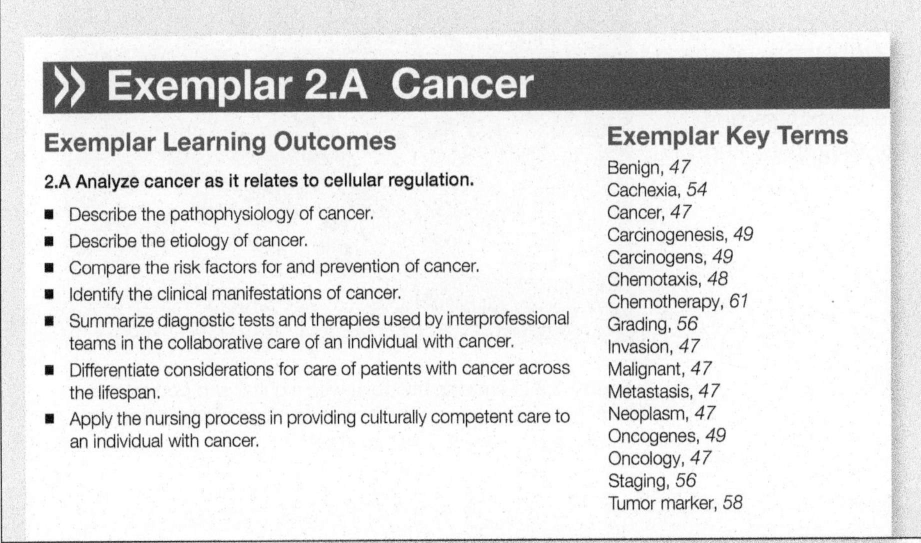

Exemplar 2.A Cancer

Exemplar Learning Outcomes

2.A Analyze cancer as it relates to cellular regulation.

- Describe the pathophysiology of cancer.
- Describe the etiology of cancer.
- Compare the risk factors for and prevention of cancer.
- Identify the clinical manifestations of cancer.
- Summarize diagnostic tests and therapies used by interprofessional teams in the collaborative care of an individual with cancer.
- Differentiate considerations for care of patients with cancer across the lifespan.
- Apply the nursing process in providing culturally competent care to an individual with cancer.

Exemplar Key Terms

Benign, *47*
Cachexia, *54*
Cancer, *47*
Carcinogenesis, *49*
Carcinogens, *49*
Chemotaxis, *48*
Chemotherapy, *61*
Grading, *56*
Invasion, *47*
Malignant, *47*
Metastasis, *47*
Neoplasm, *47*
Oncogenes, *49*
Oncology, *47*
Staging, *56*
Tumor marker, *58*

Overview The Overview sets the stage for the Exemplar and often includes information on the prevalence of the disorder. It also includes the pathophysiology and etiology of the alteration, and risk factors and prevention where appropriate.

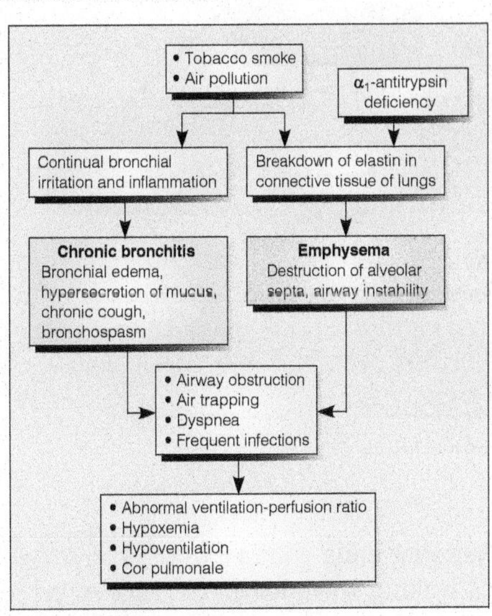

Clinical Manifestations and Therapies

Cellulitis

CUES	CLINICAL MANIFESTATIONS	CLINICAL THERAPIES
Fever	Tachycardia, tachypnea, elevated temperature, lethargy, chills	■ Maintain adequate hydration. ■ Administer antipyretics. ■ Treat underlying cause.
Skin inflammation	Redness, pain, warmth, edema	■ Administer antibiotics. ■ Provide adequate nutrition to promote healing. ■ Manage pain using both pharmacologic and nonpharmacologic therapies.
Septicemia	Whole-body inflammation manifested by fever, altered WBC count (may be high or low), and hemodynamic alterations (tachycardia, tachypnea, decreased cardiac output); elevated lactic acid level	■ Monitor hemodynamic status. ■ Administer antibiotic therapy. ■ Provide fluid management. ■ Provide supportive care based on symptoms. ■ Measure vital signs frequently.

Clinical Manifestations The Clinical Manifestations section describes what the nurse might see in a patient with the alteration. The Clinical Manifestations and Therapies feature is an excellent tool for review.

Collaboration

This section covers the work of the interprofessional healthcare team.

Diagnostic Tests

Surgery

Pharmacologic Therapy

Nonpharmacologic Therapy

Complementary Health Approaches

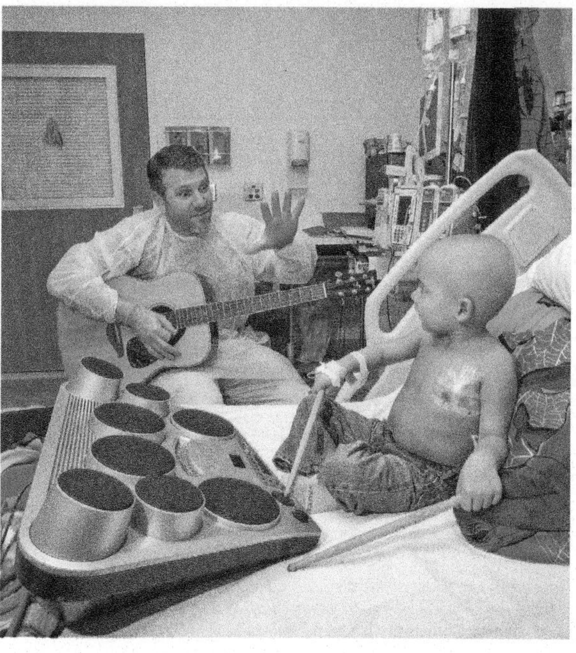

Figure 2.5 » A music therapist with a guitar and portable drum kit engages a young child with cancer at a children's hospital.
Source: Spencer Grant/Alamy Stock Photo.

Lifespan Considerations

The lifespan section covers the etiology, clinical manifestations, diagnosis, and interventions unique to specific age groups.

Considerations for Infants

Considerations for Children and Adolescents

Considerations for Pregnant Women

Considerations for Older Adults

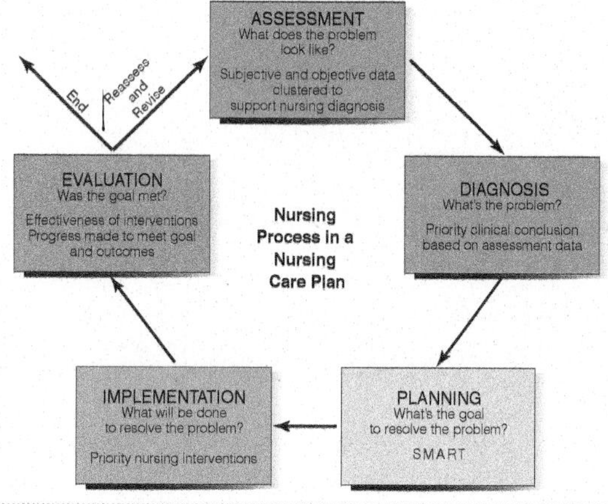

Figure 36.10 » Using the nursing process in a nursing plan of care.

Nursing Process

A detailed look at the nursing process helps students put together all of the content in the exemplar and see the care of patients with the disorder.

Assessment

Diagnosis

Planning

Implementation

Evaluation

REVIEW

Each exemplar ends with a Review that includes linking questions and a short case study with questions so students can apply their knowledge.

RELATE Link the Concepts and Exemplars

READY Go to Volume 3: Clinical Nursing Skills

REFER Go to Pearson MyLab Nursing and eText

REFLECT Apply Your Knowledge

REVIEW Cancer

RELATE Link the Concepts and Exemplars

Linking the exemplar of cancer with the concept of evidence-based practice:

1. How does evidence-based practice affect cancer screening guidelines?
2. In what ways can the nurse ensure that he or she is adhering to current principles of evidenced-based practice?

Linking the exemplar of cancer with the concept of comfort.

3. Describe pharmacologic and nonpharmacologic comfort measures that can be used by a patient with a cancer diagnosis.
4. Describe barriers related to adequate pain relief that patients with a cancer diagnosis may encounter.

Linking the exemplar of cancer with the concept of development.

5. Using Erikson's "Eight Stages of Development," describe how the development of a school-age child might be affected by a cancer diagnosis.
6. Describe how the normal developmental tasks of an adolescent could be affected by a diagnosis of cancer.

READY Go to Volume 3: Clinical Nursing Skills

REFER Go to Pearson MyLab Nursing and eText

REFLECT Apply Your Knowledge

Mandy Leno, 63 years old, has lived with bipolar disorder since young adulthood. She has recently been diagnosed with pancreatic cancer. Following her diagnosis of cancer, Ms. Leno experiences an acute manic episode and is admitted to an inpatient psychiatric unit for evaluation and treatment. She is currently pacing up and down the hall, stating that she will conquer her cancer without drugs or surgery. Ms. Leno is refusing all medications. She has barely slept and has deep circles under her eyes. She has eaten very little in the past few days. Her urine output is low, she is disheveled, and her clothes are dirty. Ms. Leno is divorced and has no family nearby. Her only daughter lives across the country and has three small children.

1. What are the priorities of care for Ms. Leno?
2. Is Ms. Leno capable of giving consent for surgery? Is surgical consent needed? Why or why not?
3. Should Ms. Leno's daughter be contacted? Explain your answer.

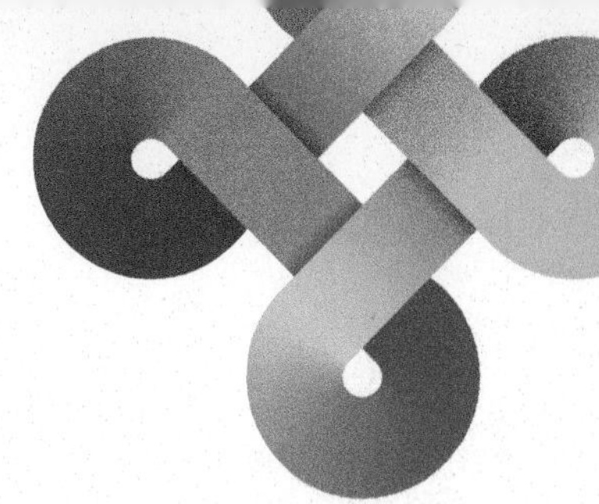

Additional Features

Additional features found throughout the program include numbered tables, figures, boxes that contain content presented in visual formats, and the following highlighted content: Multisystem Effects, Safety Alert, Stay Current, Evidence-Based Practice, Nursing Care Plan, Focus on Integrative Health, and Focus on Diversity and Culture. New to the Fourth Edition is Communicating with Patients.

The **Multisystem Effects** features highlight for the students the effects that disorders have on various systems of the body.

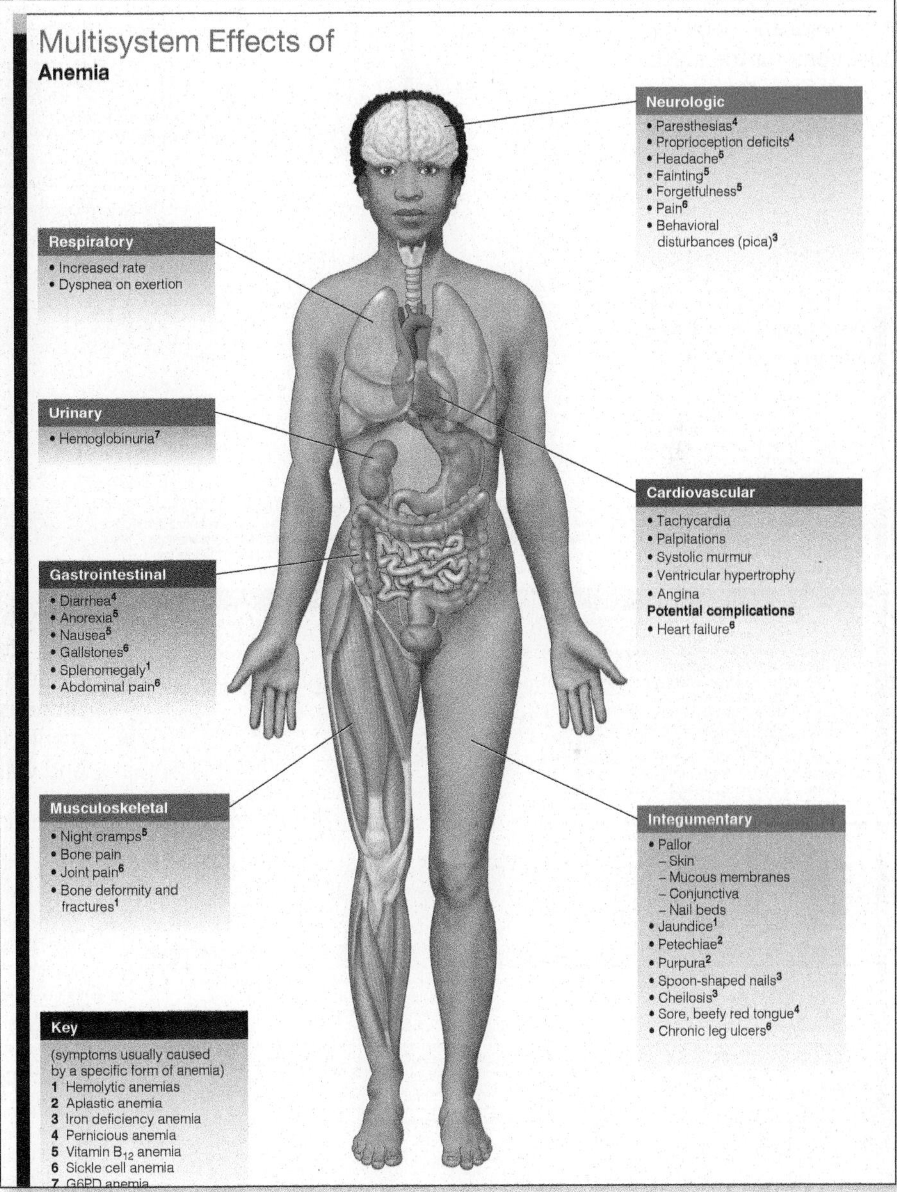

SAFETY ALERT Often the earliest manifestations of a change in ICP are alterations in LOC and respirations. Therefore, the importance of assessing a patient's neurologic status cannot be overemphasized. Reduce environmental stimuli (including the number of visitors) and follow all safety protocols (e.g., keeping bedrails up, placing call lights within reach).

Each **Safety Alert** provides critical information the nurse needs to know to keep patients and staff safe.

>> **Stay Current:** Visit the Safe to Sleep website at https://safetosleep.nichd.nih.gov for more information, including free brochures for HCPs and patients and information on continuing education for nurses.

Each **Stay Current** provides a weblink to a website that will keep students informed on the most recent updates.

The goal of the **Evidence-Based Practice** features is to show students the need for evidence to drive practice. Each starts with a problem, delves into the research, presents implications for the nurse, and ends with critical thinking questions for the student.

Evidence-Based Practice

How Many Steps Are Enough to Walk Each Day?

Problem

The specific, common, physical fitness goal of reaching 10,000 steps/day has little supportive evidence. How many daily steps are needed to significantly improve well-being?

Evidence

- A study of more than 16,000 older women found that they were 40% less likely to die over a 4-year timeframe if they walked 4400 steps a day, even if those steps were taken with low to moderate intensity (Lee et al., 2019). Their longevity continued to improve with increased steps, up to 7500 steps a day; surprisingly, walking 7500 to 10,000 steps a day did not correlate with changes in mortality (Lee et al., 2019).
- For 21- to 40-year-olds, a moderate to vigorous walking cadence or pace of 100 to 130 steps/minute may have greater health benefit than the total number of steps taken in a day; 150 minutes of moderate physical activity weekly is the measure that is most highly correlated with improvements in physical wellness (Tudor-Locke et al., 2019).
- Studies have found that individuals at risk for heart disease or diabetes may significantly decrease those risks by walking. Every 1000 additional steps taken daily above baseline are correlated with improved lab values and risk reduction; evidence suggests that 7000 steps/day may be sufficient to achieve wellness guidelines (Lee et al., 2019).

Implications

The evidence suggests that health benefits from walking can be accrued at less than 10,000 daily steps; individuals who track their daily step count with wearable fitness trackers may want to reconsider and individualize their activity goals.

Critical Thinking Application

1. How might the evidence about the benefits of walking impact physical activity recommendations for older women?
2. For the individual patient who has been sedentary and wants to start increasing physical activity, how would you explain the evidence about the health benefits of walking?
3. What are the pros and cons of monitoring daily step count?

Nursing Care Plan

A Patient with T1D

Jim Meligrito, age 24, is a third-year nursing student at a large midwestern university. He also works 20 hours a week as a campus student security guard. His working hours are 8:00 p.m. to midnight, five nights a week. Mr. Meligrito lives off campus with another nursing student. Neither of them likes to cook, and they usually eat "whatever is handy." Mr. Meligrito has smoked 8–10 cigarettes a day for 5 years.

Mr. Meligrito was diagnosed with T1D at age 12. Although his insulin dosage has varied, he currently takes a total of 32 units of insulin each day, 10 units of NPH, and 6 units of regular insulin each morning and evening. He monitors his blood glucose about three times a week. Mr. Meligrito feels that he is too busy for a regular exercise program and that he gets enough exercise in clinicals and in weekend sports activities. He skipped his last appointment with his HCP.

One day during a 6-hour clinical laboratory in pediatrics, Mr. Meligrito notices that he is urinating frequently, is thirsty, and has blurred vision. He also is very tired, but he blames his symptoms on drinking a couple of beers and having had only 4 hours of sleep the night before while studying for an exam and on the stress he has been under lately from school and work. When Mr. Meligrito remembers that he forgot to take his insulin that morning, he realizes he must have hyperglycemia but decides that he will be all right until he gets home in the afternoon. Around noon, he begins having abdominal pain, feels weak, has a rapid pulse, and vomits. When he reports his physical symptoms to his clinical instructor, she immediately sends him, accompanied by another student, to the hospital emergency department.

ASSESSMENT	DIAGNOSES	PLANNING
As soon as Mr. Meligrito arrives at the emergency department, his blood glucose level is measured at 300 mg/dL. Urine samples and additional blood samples are sent to the laboratory for analysis. Hemoglobin A1C is 9.5%, urine shows the presence of ketones, electrolytes are normal, and pH is 7.1. His vital signs are as follows: T 37.2°C (99°F); P 140 bpm; R 28/min; BP 102/52 mmHg. An IV infusion of 1000 mL of normal (0.9%) saline with 40 mEq of KCl is started at a rate of 400 mL/hr. After 800 mL is infused, IV regular insulin at 5 U/hr (diluted in 0.9% saline) is begun. Hourly blood glucose monitoring also is initiated. Mr. Meligrito is nauseated and lethargic but remains oriented. Three hours later, he has a blood glucose level of 220 mg/dL. The pH is 7.3 and the serum potassium 3 mEq/L. There are trace ketones in the urine, and his pulse and blood pressure are normal. He is admitted to the intensive care unit until his blood glucose, pH, and serum potassium levels are within normal range and then transferred to a medical unit to prepare for discharge. When the diabetes nurse educator visits Mr. Meligrito, he says that he no longer feels in control of his diabetes or his future goal of becoming a nurse anesthetist.	Problems that Mr. Meligrito have include the following: ■ Powerlessness related to a perceived lack of control of diabetes because of present demands on time ■ Lack of knowledge of self-management of diabetes ■ Compromised self-image related to uncertainty about his capacity to achieve the desired role as a registered nurse.	The expected outcomes for the plan of care specify that Mr. Meligrito will: ■ Identify those aspects of diabetes that can be controlled and participate in making decisions about self-managing his care. ■ Demonstrate an understanding of diabetes self-management through planned medication, diet, exercise, and blood glucose self-monitoring activities. ■ Explore and clarify his perceptions of his role as a student nurse and verbalize his ability to meet his expectations.

IMPLEMENTATION

The following interventions may be appropriate for Mr. Meligrito:

- Mutually establish individualized short-term and long-term goals for self-management to control blood glucose.
- Provide opportunities to express his feelings about himself and his illness.
- Explore perceptions of his own ability to control his illness and his future and clarify these perceptions by providing information about resources and support groups.
- Facilitate his decision-making abilities in self-managing his prescribed treatment regimen.
- Provide positive reinforcement for increasing his involvement in self-care activities.
- Provide education about insulin administration, dietary management, exercise, SMBG, and healthy lifestyle.
- Encourage enrollment in weekly education program for individuals with diabetes.

Many exemplars contain **Nursing Care Plans** to help students examine aspects of patient care in context. The Nursing Care Plans follow the nursing process, with sections on assessment, diagnosis, planning, implementation, and evaluation. They end with a series of Critical Thinking questions.

Focus on Integrative Health

Acupuncture

Acupuncture is an alternative health approach that involves the placement of special needles at certain points in the skin. Needle placement can be followed by manual manipulation or the application of heat or electrical impulses that stimulate nervous system activity. Clinical trials have indicated that acupuncture is both safe and effective in relieving numerous symptoms experienced by both adults and children with cancer. The scientific evidence provides the most

For the most part, care of all patients from all cultures is covered in the main text. **Focus on Diversity and Culture** features are used only for unique situations of which the nurse should be aware.

Focus on Integrative Health boxes highlight the use of complementary healing in addition to traditional nursing practice.

Focus on Diversity and Culture

African Americans and Kidney Disease

Chronic kidney disease is a major public health problem that disproportionately affects African Americans and people with low income. In the United States, African Americans experience some of the highest rates of ESRD in comparison to other racial and ethnic groups. This appears to be related to multiple factors, including the number of and degree of control of CKD risk factors, access to and receipt of high-quality care, health beliefs and health behaviors, social determinants of health, and other factors that combine to cre-

MyLab Nursing

MyLab Nursing is an online learning and practice environment that works with the text to help students master key concepts, prepare for the NCLEX-RN® exam, and develop clinical reasoning skills. Through a new mobile experience, students can study *Nursing: A Concept-Based Approach to Learning* anytime, anywhere. New adaptive technology with remediation personalizes learning, moving students beyond memorization to true understanding and application of the content. MyLab Nursing contains the following features:

Dynamic Study Modules

New adaptive learning modules with remediation that personalize the learning experience by allowing students to increase both their confidence and their performance while being assessed in real time.

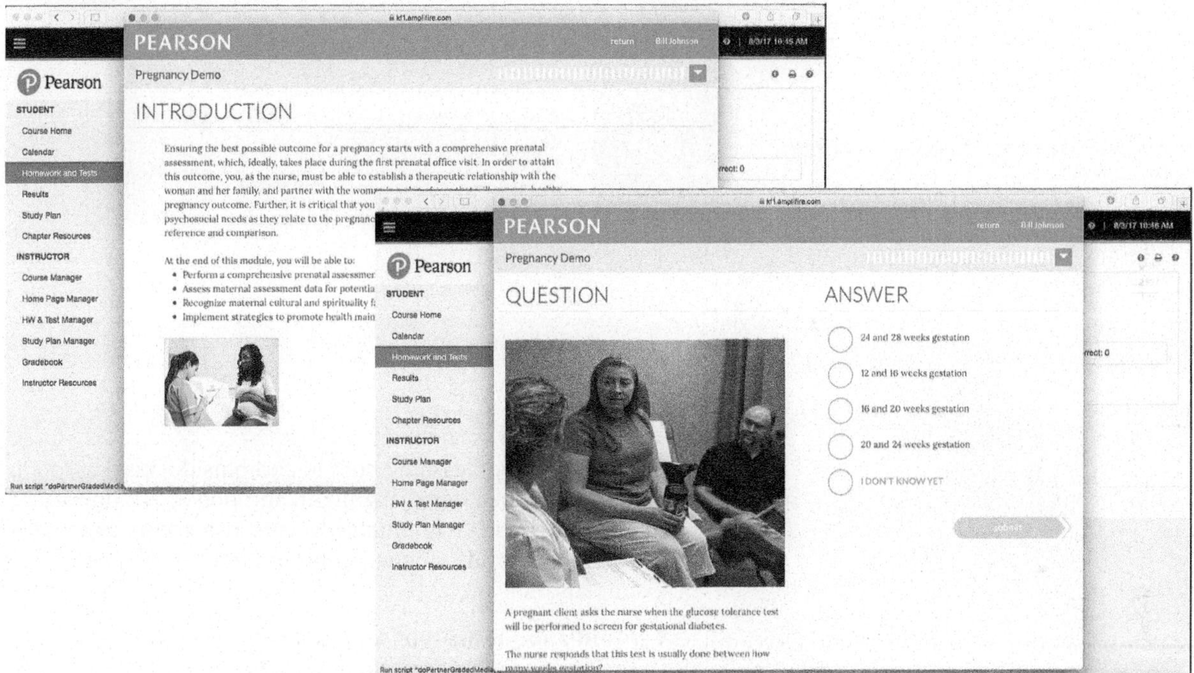

NCLEX-Style Questions

Practice tests with more than 4000 NCLEX-style questions of various types, including Next Gen, build students' confidence and prepare them for success on the NCLEX-RN® exam. Questions are organized by Concept and Exemplar.

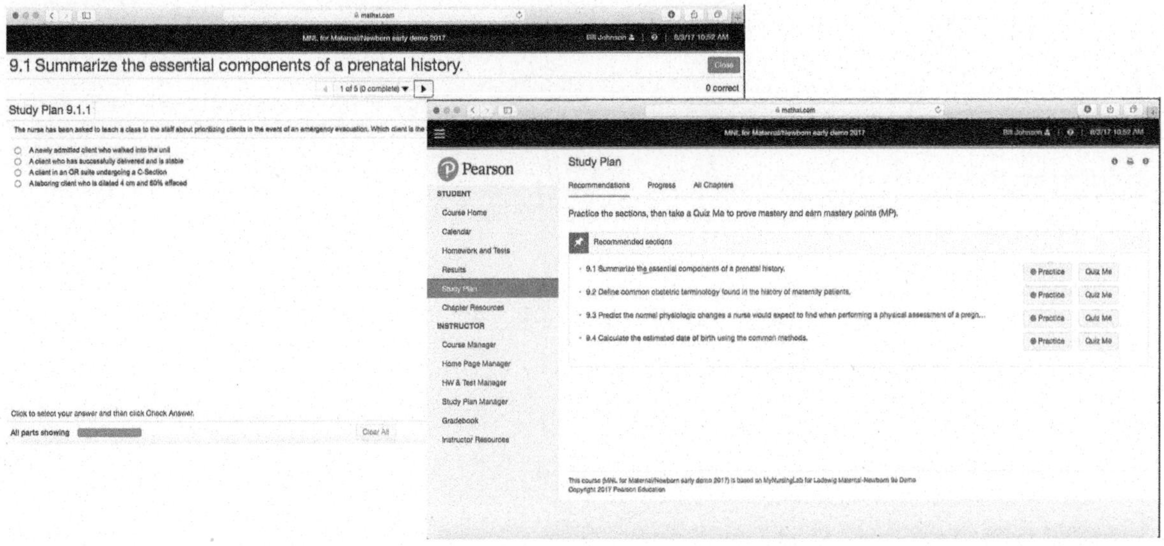

Decision-Making Cases

Clinical case studies that provide opportunities for students to practice analyzing information and making important decisions at key moments in patient care scenarios. These case studies are designed to help prepare students for clinical practice.

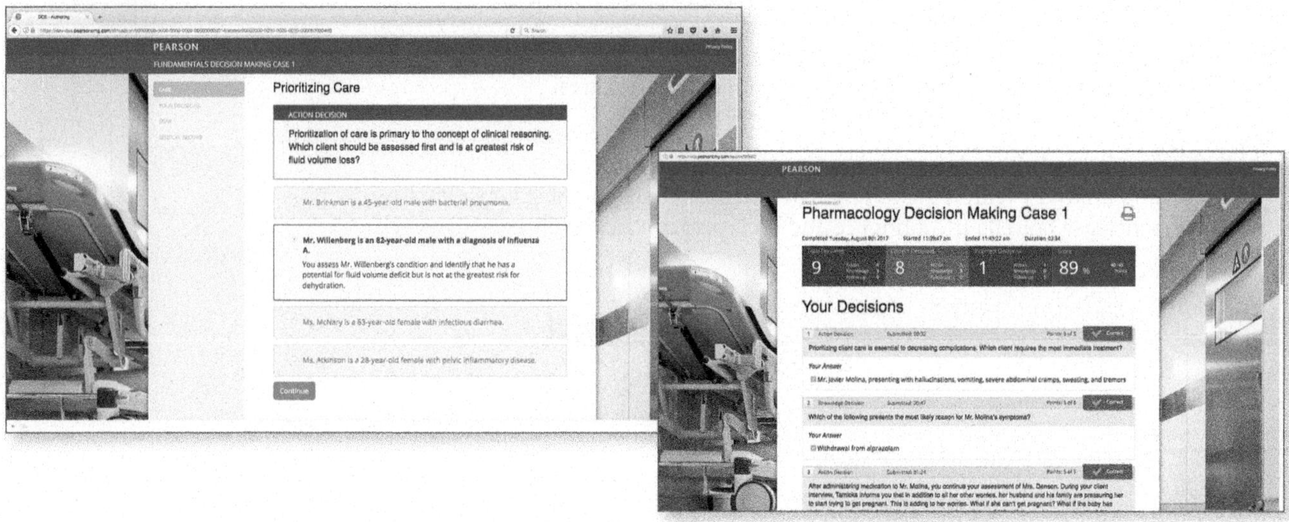

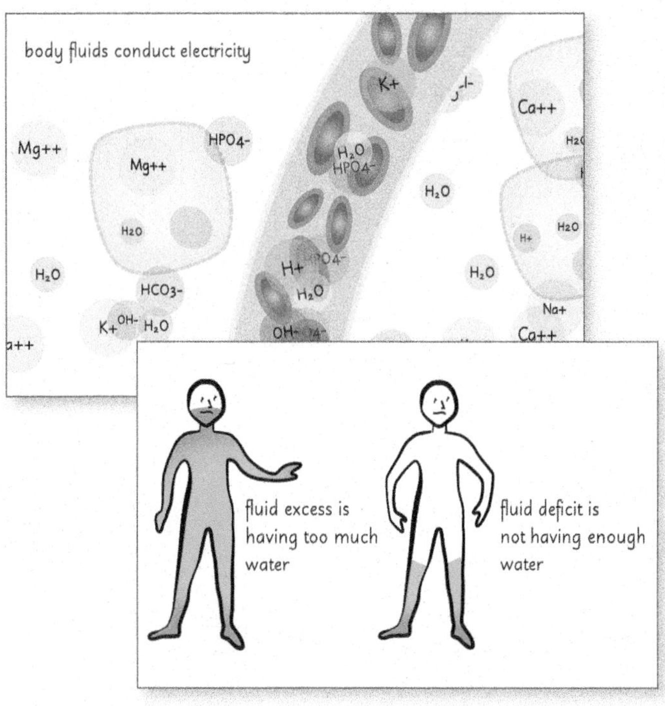

Pearson eText

Enhances student learning both in and outside the classroom. Students can take notes, highlight, and bookmark important content, or engage with interactive and rich media to achieve greater conceptual understanding of the Concepts and their Exemplars.

- **Fluid and Electrolyte Animations** provide students with the necessary information about the balance and imbalance of fluids and electrolytes to think, reason, and make clinical judgments.

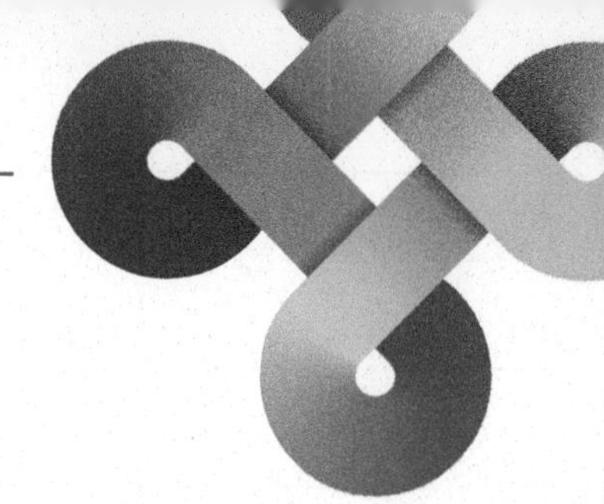

Resources

Instructor Resources

Instructor Resource Manual—with lecture outlines and large/small group, individual, and clinical activities

Lecture Note PowerPoint slides

Image Bank

Test Bank

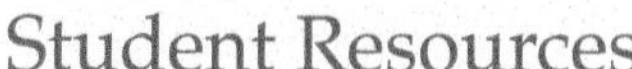

Student Resources

The following resources are available for course adoption or student purchase:

Pearson *Reviews & Rationales: Comprehensive Review for NCLEX-RN®*

The Ultimate NCLEX-RN® Exam Preparation Guide! New and updated, the best-selling Pearson *Reviews & Rationales: Comprehensive Review for NCLEX-RN®* offers a comprehensive outline review of the essential content areas tested on the NCLEX-RN® exam, including critical areas such as management, delegation, leadership, decision-making, pharmacology, and emergency care. This edition provides access to Pearson Test Prep—a new web-based application that enables students to practice for the NCLEX anytime and anywhere using their smartphone, tablet, or computer. Pearson Test Prep includes all 1600 questions from the book, plus an additional 4000 questions, and features all NCLEX-style question formats.

Neighborhood 3.0

Foster clinical decision making with *The Neighborhood*, version 3. This redesigned online community tells the story of virtual patients from diverse cultural, socioeconomic, and family backgrounds and with various medical conditions. Through assignable, interactive learning tools, students practice making clinical decisions that weigh the impact of each patient's background and circumstances. Easy to incorporate into your class, *The Neighborhood* can be used as a course-specific supplement or across an entire curriculum. Now delivered with a companion eText, version 3 has new Clinical Care Sims that challenge students to care for patients virtually in a clinic or hospital setting.

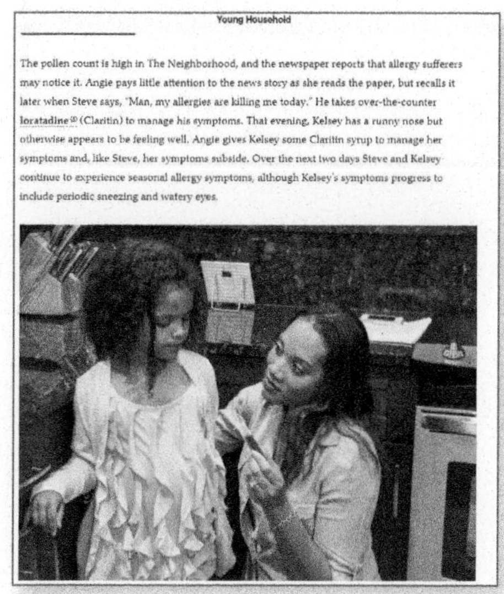

Young Household

The pollen count is high in The Neighborhood, and the newspaper reports that allergy sufferers may notice it. Angie pays little attention to the news story as she reads the paper, but recalls it later when Steve says, "Man, my allergies are killing me today." He takes over-the-counter loratadine® (Claritin) to manage his symptoms. That evening, Kelsey has a runny nose but otherwise appears to be feeling well. Angie gives Kelsey some Claritin syrup to manage her symptoms and, like Steve, her symptoms subside. Over the next two days Steve and Kelsey continue to experience seasonal allergy symptoms, although Kelsey's symptoms progress to include periodic sneezing and watery eyes.

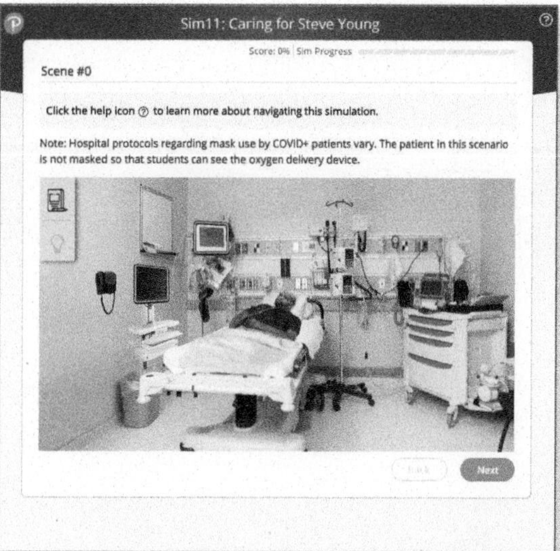

NEW Digital Skills Lab

Clinical Nursing Skills: Practice for Mastery

One of Pearson's newest products, *Clinical Nursing Skills: Practice for Mastery* provides an online review of common clinical nursing skills, including animated demonstrations of some of the most challenging skills that student nurses must learn to practice nursing across the continuum of healthcare. In addition to animations, this digital skills lab offers:

- The opportunity for students to upload and evaluate their own videos of them demonstrating skill performance
- Decision-Making Cases that take students through a series of critical thinking questions to learn more about how skills are performed in context
- Reflection questions to help students make important relevance connections between skill performance and patient care
- NCLEX-RN® questions to provide students additional opportunities to think critically about skill performance and prepare for the NCLEX-RN® examination.

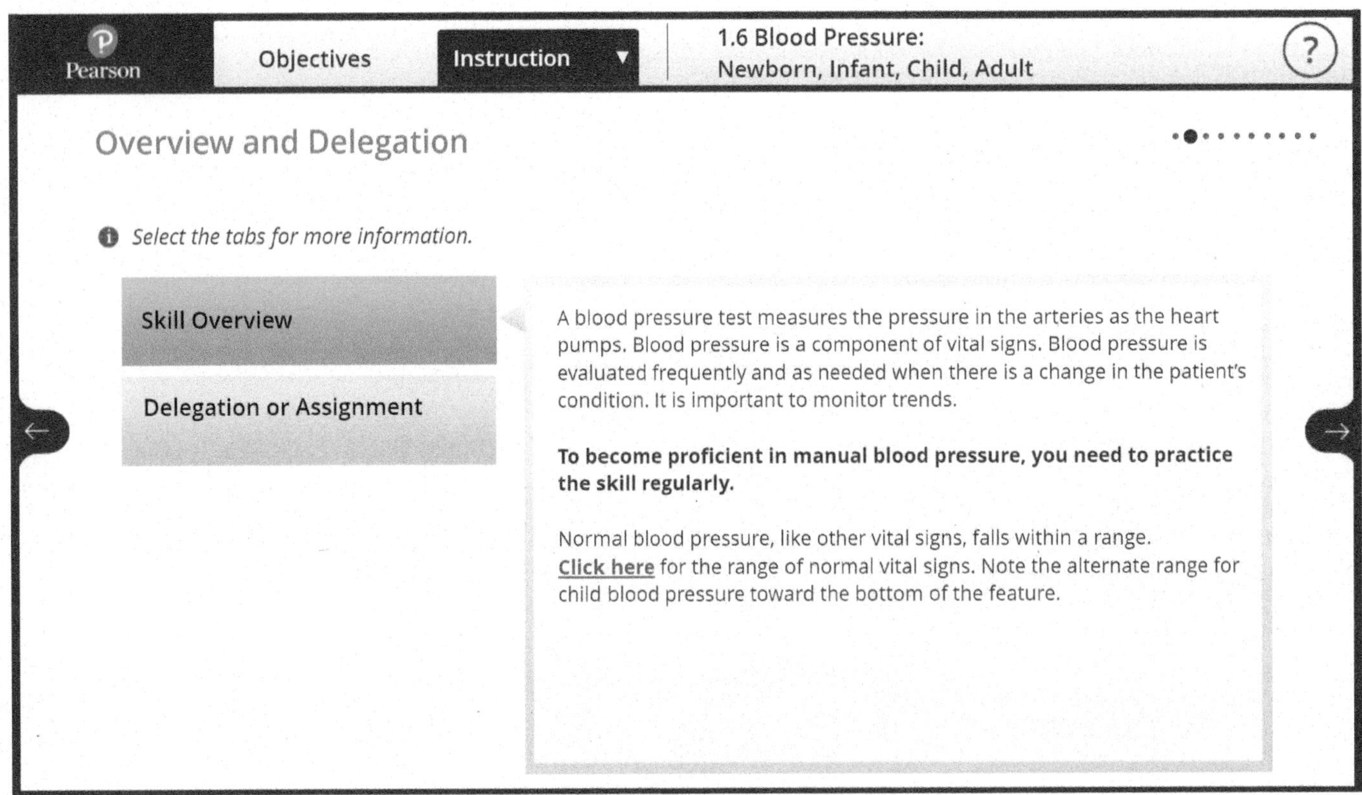

Acknowledgments

We would like to extend our heartfelt thanks to more than 80 instructors from schools of nursing across the country who have given their time generously during the past few years to help us create this concept-based learning package. The talented faculty on our Concepts Editorial Board and all of the Contributors and Reviewers helped us to develop this Fourth Edition through a variety of contributions and by answering myriad questions right up to the time of publication. *Nursing: A Concept-Based Approach to Learning*, Fourth Edition, has benefited immeasurably from their efforts, insights, suggestions, objections, encouragement, and inspiration, as well as from their vast experience as faculty and practicing nurses.

We would like to thank the editorial team, Katrin Beacom, Director, Product Management, Health Sciences, for championing this project; Kevin Wilson, Content Manager, Health Sciences, for managing multiple contributors, editors, and reviewers; Melissa Bashe, Managing Producer, Health Sciences, for keeping us organized and putting together all of the components of the concepts program; Susan Turley, for reviewing and updating all of the Pharmacologic Therapy sections and Medications charts; and most of all, Laura Horowitz and Addy McCulloch, development editors, for their dedication and attention to detail that promoted an excellent outcome once again.

Concepts Editorial Review Board

Barbara Callahan, MEd, RN, NCC, CHSE
Lenoir Community College (Emerita)
La Grange, NC

Mark C. Hand, PhD, RN, CNE
Clinical Associate Professor
East Carolina University
Greenville, NC

Nora F. Steele, DNS, RN, CNE
Charity School of Nursing
Delgado Community College
New Orleans, LA

Contributors, Volume 2

Michelle Aebersold, PhD, RN, CHSE, FAAN
Clinical Professor
University of Michigan School of Nursing
Module 48, Informatics
Module 50, Quality Improvement

Barbara Arnoldussen, DBA, RN
International Technological University
Santa Clara, CA
Module 34, Assessment
Module 46, Healthcare Systems

Jennifer Atzen, DNP, RN, CNM, CNE, CHSE
Western Governors University
Eldridge, IA
The Concept of Reproduction
Exemplar 33.A, Antepartum Care

Ashley Bear, DNP, RN, CNS
Associate Professor of Nursing
Harrisburg Area Community College
Gettysburg, PA
Module 28, Mood and Affect
Module 29, Self

Eleisa Bennett, RN, MSN
James Sprunt Community College (Retired)
Kenansville, NC
Module 38, Communication

Shelley Lynne Blackwood, EdD, MSN, RN, CCRN-K, PCCN, CHSE
Liberty University
McLennan Community College
Module 36, Clinical Decision Making

Katrina Browning, DNP, RN, CNE
St. Ambrose University
Davenport, IA
Module 26, Family
Module 35, Caring Interventions

Barbara Callahan, MEd, RN, NCC, CHSE
Lenoir Community College (Emerita)
La Grange, NC
Module 30, Spirituality
Module 45, Evidence-Based Practice
Module 51, Safety

Marcy Caplin, PhD, RN, CNE
Associate Professor
Kent State University
Kent, OH
Module 25, Development
Module 31, Stress and Coping
Module 37, Collaboration

Linda S. K. Daley, PhD, RN, ANEF
Clinical Professor Emeritus
The Ohio State University
College of Nursing
Nurse Scientist, Professional Development
Nationwide Children's Hospital
Columbus, OH
Module 42, Accountability

Danielle Hoffman, DNP, RN, TNS, EMT-P, CNE
Assistant Professor and Assistant Chair
St. Ambrose University
Department of Nursing
Davenport, IA
Module 32, Trauma

Christine Kleckner, MA, MAN, RN, PHN
Director of Nursing
Hennepin Technical College
Brooklyn Park, MN
Module 24, Culture and Diversity
Module 27, Grief and Loss

Jacqueline M. Loversidge, PhD, RNC-AWHC
Associate Professor of Clinical Nursing
The Ohio State University College of Nursing
Columbus, OH
Module 43, Advocacy
Module 47, Health Policy

Dawna Martich, MSN, RN
Nursing – Subject Matter Expert
Pittsburgh, PA
Module 40, Professionalism
Module 41, Teaching and Learning

Amy McCormick, DNP, ARNP, CPNP-PC
St. Ambrose University
Davenport, IA
Exemplar 33.E, Prematurity

Sharon Norris, DNP, RN, IBCLC
ADN Instructor
Cape Fear Community College
Wilmington, NC
Exemplar 33.B, Intrapartum Care
Exemplar 33.C, Postpartum Care

Pamela Phillips, PhD, RN, CARN
Adjunct Faculty
University of South Carolina
Beaufort, SC
Module 22, Addiction
Module 23, Cognition

Christine Sayre, DNP, RN
Assistant Professor of Clinical Practice
The Ohio State University
College of Nursing
Columbus, OH
Exemplar 33.D, Newborn Care

Reviewers

Lynn Acierno, BSN, RN-BC, OCN
UPMC Shadyside School of Nursing
Pittsburgh, PA

Barbara Arnoldussen, MBA, BSN, RN, CPHQ
International Technological University
San Jose, CA

Jennifer Atzen, DNP, RN, CNM, CNE, CHSE
Western Governor's University
Eldridge, IA

Mary Barrow, PhD, RN
Delgado Community College
New Orleans, LA

Trudy L. Bauer, DNP, FNP-BC, CNE
Harrisburg Area Community College
Lancaster, PA

Ashley Bear, DNP, RN, CNS
Harrisburg Area Community College
Gettysburg, PA

Barbara Blackwell, EdD, MSN, RN
Hampton University
Hampton, VA

Christy Bowen, DNP, RN
Midwestern State University
Wichita Falls, TX

Bobbie Brown,
North Carolina A&T University
Greensboro, NC

Katrina Browning, DNP, RN, CNE
St. Ambrose University
Davenport, IA

Valerie J. Bugosh, MSN, RN, CNE
Harrisburg Area Community College
Gettysburg, PA

Schvon Bussey, RN, FNP-C, PMHNP-BC
Albany State University
Albany, GA

Marcy Caplin, PhD, RN, CNE
Kent State University
Kent, OH

Margaret-Ann Carno, RN, MBA, MJ, PhD, CPNP, D,ABSM, FAAN
University of Rochester
Rochester, NY

Stephanie Cassone, MSN, FNP-BC, ACHPN
Simmons University
Boston, MA

Patricia Catlin, DNP, APRN, NP-C
Martin Methodist College
Pulaski, TN

Donyale Childs, PhD, MSN, RN
Albany State University
Albany, GA

Connie Dagen, MSN, RN
Harrisburg Area Community College
Lancaster, PA

Abimbola Farinde, PhD, PharmD
Columbia Southern University
Phoenix, AZ

Melissa M. Gomes, PhD, APRN, PMHNP-BC, FNAP
Hampton University
Hampton, VA

Wanda Goodwyn, MSN, RN
Fayetteville State University
Fayetteville, NC

Annette Griffin, MSN, RN
Rhode Island College
Providence, RI

Sharon L. Haas, MSN, RN, CNEs
Cardinal Stritch University
Milwaukee, WI

Susan Hall, EdD, MSN, RNC-OB, CCE
Winston-Salem State University
Winston-Salem, NC

Deborah Henry, PhD, RN
Blue Ridge Community College
Henderson, NC

Veela Hughes, DNP, MSN ED, RN
Albany State University
Cordele, GA

Alnita Jackson, DNP, APRN, FNP-BC, CNE
Fayetteville State University
Fayetteville, NC

Koretta King, RN-BSN
Northwell Health Long Island Jewish
Forest Hills Hospital
Forest Hills, NY

Christine Kleckner, MA, MAN, RN, PHN
Hennepin Technical College
Brooklyn Park, MN

Lisa Lehmann, RN, MA, MSN
Alcorn School of Nursing
Natchez, MS

Dawna Martich, MSN, RN
Nursing Education Consultant
Pittsburgh, PA

Juleann H. Miller, RN, PhD., CNE
St. Ambrose University
Davenport, IA

Zelda Peters, RN, DNP, FNP-C
Albany State University
Albany, GA

Judith Pulito, EdD, MSN, RN
Lorain County Community College
Elyria, OH

Rhonda Schoville, PhD, MSBA, RN
University of Michigan
Ann Arbor, MI

Jeremiah Underwood, MHS, CCP, NC-P
Guilford Technical Community College
Jamestown, NC

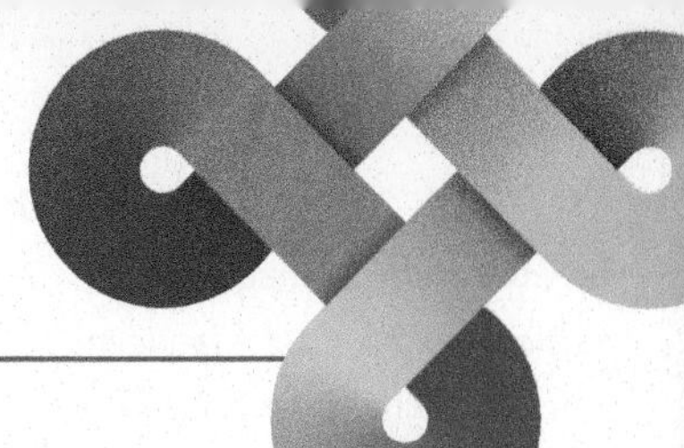

Contents

Part II

Psychosocial Modules

Part II consists of the psychosocial modules within the individual domain. Each module presents a concept that directly relates to sociologic or psychologic domains that impact patient health and well-being—such as cognition, family, and stress and coping—and selected alterations of that concept presented as exemplars. In the concept of cognition, for example, exemplars include Alzheimer disease, delirium, and schizophrenia. Each module addresses the impact of that concept and selected alterations on individuals across the lifespan, inclusive of cultural, gender, and developmental considerations.

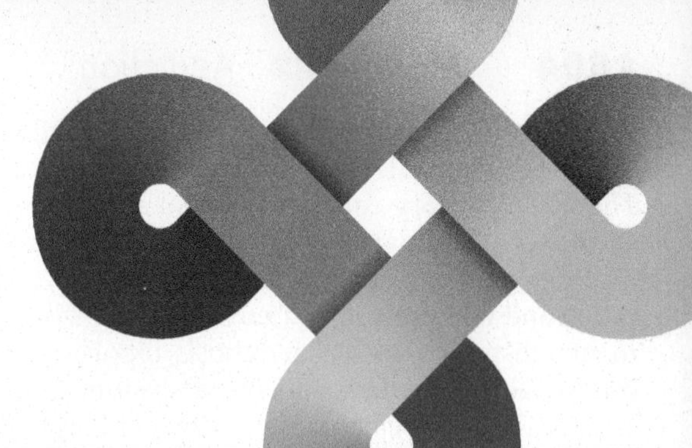

Module 22
Addiction

Module Outline and Learning Outcomes

The Concept of Addiction

Addiction

22.1 Summarize the processes involved in addiction.

Manifestations of Substance Use Disorders

22.2 Summarize manifestations of substance use disorders.

Concepts Related to Addiction

22.3 Outline the relationship between addiction and other concepts.

Harm Reduction and Health Promotion

22.4 Outline harm reduction and health promotion activities to reduce the risk for substance abuse and consequences of addictive behaviors.

Nursing Assessment

22.5 Differentiate common assessment procedures and tests used to examine individuals suspected of abusing a substance.

Independent Interventions

22.6 Analyze independent interventions nurses can implement for patients with substance use disorders.

Collaborative Therapies

22.7 Summarize collaborative therapies used by interprofessional teams for patients with substance use disorders.

Lifespan Considerations

22.8 Differentiate considerations related to the assessment and care of patients throughout the lifespan who abuse substances.

Addiction Exemplars

Exemplar 22.A Alcohol Use Disorder

22.A Analyze manifestations and treatment considerations for patients with an addiction to alcohol.

Exemplar 22.B Nicotine Use Disorder

22.B Analyze manifestations and treatment considerations for patients with an addiction to nicotine.

Exemplar 22.C Substance Use Disorders

22.C Analyze manifestations and treatment considerations for patients with an addiction to substances.

» The Concept of Addiction

Concept Key Terms

Abstinence, **1697**
Addiction, **1693**
Behavioral therapy, **1706**
Binge drinking, **1695**
Boundaries, **1697**
Brief strategic family therapy (BSFT), **1708**
Codependence, **1697**
Cognitive-behavioral therapy (CBT), **1706**
Co-occurring disorders, **1697**
Delirium tremens (DTs), **1697**
Dependence, **1694**
Dialectical behavior therapy (DBT), **1706**
Enabling behavior, **1697**
Family behavior therapy (FBT), **1707**
Functional family therapy (FFT), **1708**
Gambling disorder, **1698**
Group therapy, **1706**
Internet gaming disorder (IGD), **1699**
Intervention, **1705**
Milieu therapy, **1706**
Online shopping addiction (OSA), **1699**
Polysubstance abuse, **1697**
Rational emotive behavior therapy (REBT), **1706**
Recovery, **1703**
Reinforcement, **1706**
SBIRT, **1701**
Sex addiction, **1699**
Sobriety, **1697**
Substance use disorder, **1693**
Teratogen, **1710**
Tolerance, **1694**

Addiction

Addiction is defined as a psychologic or physical need for a substance (such as alcohol) or a process (such as gambling) to the extent that the individual will risk negative consequences to meet the need. Many individuals use substances recreationally to modify mood or behavior, and there are wide sociocultural variations in the acceptability of chemical use. For example, marijuana/hashish use is legal in some states, such as Colorado, but not in others. Although misuse and abuse of prescription medications is illegal throughout the United States, some narcotics, sedatives, and stimulants are popular drugs of abuse. Illegal drugs include forms of cocaine, heroin, hallucinogens, and inhalants. An individual may abuse any of these substances to the point of becoming addicted and unable to stop, despite dangerous, often life-threatening consequences. An individual who uses one or more substances to this extent may be diagnosed with a **substance use disorder**.

Substance use disorders (SUDs) are divided into two categories: the SUD itself and substance-*induced* disorders. The SUD category covers the actual addictive process to a substance, such as alcohol or opiates. The substance-induced disorder grouping includes related conditions, such as intoxication and withdrawal, and substance- or medication-related mental disorders, such as psychosis, bipolar and related disorders, sleep disorders, and sexual dysfunction, among others (American Psychiatric Association [APA], 2013). Nursing interventions include providing acute care for patients with substance-induced disorders who are experiencing intoxication or withdrawal, educating patients and their family members about the disorder, and supporting patients' recovery and abstinence in community-based programs.

The etiology of addiction is multifaceted. Childhood trauma, genetic variabilities, and other considerations are thought to play a role. Regardless of the reasons or etiology behind addiction, it can have grave consequences for both individuals, families, and those who care for them, especially because affordable, effective treatment is often hard to access due to cost, availability, or both.

Addictive processes create cognitive, behavioral, and physiologic symptoms. The term *addiction* needs to be differentiated from dependence. **Dependence** is a physiologic need for a substance that the patient cannot control and that results in withdrawal symptoms if the drug or substance is stopped or withheld. Dependence on a substance also causes the user to develop a physiologic **tolerance** for the substance, requiring greater quantities of the substance to achieve the same pleasurable effects. In addition to physiologic symptoms of dependence, addiction also includes a psychologic need that causes affected individuals to seek the substance to which they are addicted—at any cost. Individuals with SUDs may neglect their children, their work, or other responsibilities to meet their physiologic and psychologic needs.

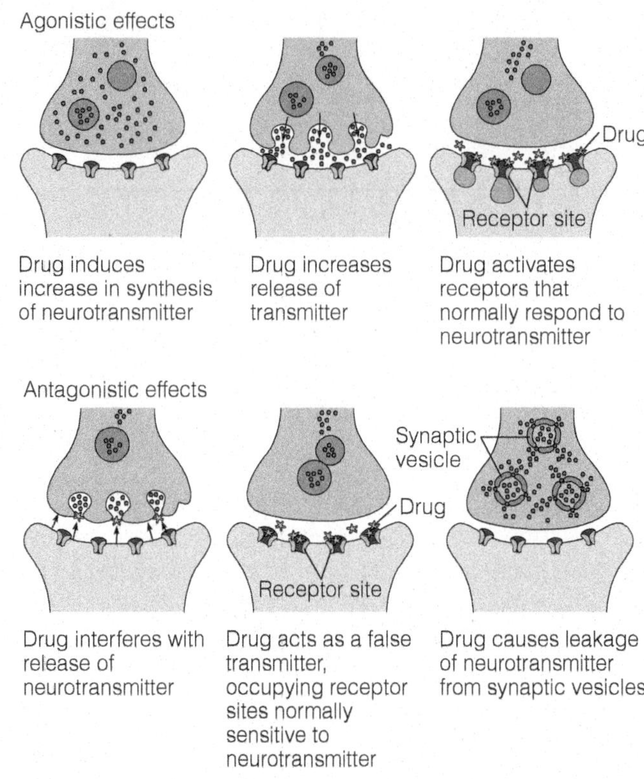
Agonistic effects
Drug
Receptor site
Drug induces increase in synthesis of neurotransmitter
Drug increases release of transmitter
Drug activates receptors that normally respond to neurotransmitter
Antagonistic effects
Synaptic vesicle
Drug
Receptor site
Drug interferes with release of neurotransmitter
Drug acts as a false transmitter, occupying receptor sites normally sensitive to neurotransmitter
Drug causes leakage of neurotransmitter from synaptic vesicles

Figure 22.1 >> Action of abused substances at brain receptor sites.

Physiology and Psychology of Addiction

Various factors help explain why one person becomes addicted, but another does not. The biopsychosocial model theorized by psychiatrist George L. Engel (1978) has been generally accepted as the most comprehensive theory for the process of addiction. Clinicians use his model as a foundation to link biological, genetic, psychologic, and sociocultural factors contributing to the development of addiction.

Biological Factors

E. Morton Jellinek (1946) first identified biological factors in his disease model of alcoholism. He hypothesized that addiction to alcohol had a biochemical basis and identified specific phases of the disease. Expanding on Jellinek's early work, later researchers implicated low levels of dopamine and serotonin in the development of alcohol dependence (Czermak et al., 2004; Nellissery et al., 2003). More recent clinical studies have continued to confirm this finding (Cross, Lotfipour, & Leslie, 2017).

Dopamine, dopamine receptor sites, and transporters, which recycle the neurotransmitter and cut off communication between neurons, are all intricately involved in the complex interactions between the nervous system and substances of abuse (National Institute on Drug Abuse [NIDA], 2018a). Dopamine is a neurotransmitter present in regions of the brain that regulate movement, emotion, motivation, and feelings of pleasure. The limbic system, which links together a number of brain structures, contains the brain's reward circuit. The limbic system controls and regulates the ability to feel pleasure and mediates perception of other emotions, which helps to explain the mood-altering properties of many substances (NIDA, 2018a). When activated at normal levels, this system rewards natural human behaviors.

Overstimulating the reward system with drugs produces euphoric effects, which strongly reinforce the behavior of drug use (NIDA, 2018a). Most drugs that impact the biochemical mechanism of the brain affect one or more receptor sites (**Figure 22.1** >>). Most abused substances mimic or block the brain's most important neurotransmitters at these respective receptor sites. For example, heroin and other opiates mimic natural opiate-like neurotransmitters, such as endorphins. Cocaine and other stimulants bind to the transporters that would normally remove excess dopamine, serotonin, and norepinephrine from the synaptic gap to undergo reabsorption. When these neurotransmitters are not reabsorbed, they continue as abnormally large amounts in the synapses and their effects are multiplied. These imbalances produce greatly amplified signals in the brain, ultimately permanently altering or disrupting neurons and neural pathways (NIDA, 2018a).

Whenever the reward circuit is activated, the brain encodes a memory, which encourages the individual to perform the same pleasurable act—or take the pleasurable substance—again and again. The reward experienced can be significant: For instance, cocaine can cause the release of 2 to 10 times the amount of dopamine released by eating or sexual intercourse (NIDA, 2018a). Neurobiological research into addiction postulates that addiction is the result of an increase in focus on a particular addictive behavior with a corresponding gradual loss of interest in other activities. When the reward circuit is stimulated as a result of addiction, the level of need for the substance or behavior increases.

In some individuals, substance abuse may be related to another medical condition. Mental disorders such as anxiety, depression, and schizophrenia may precede addiction. In other cases, drug abuse may trigger or exacerbate those mental disorders, particularly in people with specific vulnerabilities (NIDA, 2018a).

Genetic Factors

As stated earlier, addiction is strongly linked to the dopaminergic activity of the brain's reward system. The speed with which someone becomes addicted depends on the substance, the frequency of use, the means of ingestion, the intensity of the high the person obtains, and the person's genetic and psychologic susceptibility. Adequate proof exists that addiction is, at least in part, genetically moderated. Researchers estimate that genetic factors account for between 40 and 60% of an individual's vulnerability to addiction, a statistic that also accounts for the effects of environmental factors on the function and expression of a person's genes (NIDA, 2018a). Several genes have been identified that seem to influence the risk for alcohol dependence (Walker & Nestler, 2018).

Psychologic Factors

Research indicates a high correlation among substance use and childhood and adolescent trauma, such as emotional, physical, or sexual abuse (Center for the Application of Prevention Technologies [CAPT], 2018; NIDA, 2018a). Substance abuse often co-occurs with psychiatric disorders such as anxiety and depression, as some individuals use a substance as a coping strategy and, over time, develop an addiction.

Sociocultural Factors

Sociocultural factors are thought to play a strong role in the development of and tolerance for an addiction. Sociocultural factors often influence individuals' decisions as to when, what, and how they use substances. The way drugs are processed, the degree of acceptance or rejection of drug use, and an individual's financial resources influence what substance is used, how much is used, and what peer pressure the individual will face in their culture or peer group as the abuse becomes evident.

Family environment can increase a child's risk for developing addictive behaviors as an adolescent or adult. Parents or older family members who abuse alcohol or drugs or engage in criminal behavior can increase adolescents' risks of developing drug problems. Violence, physical and emotional abuse, and mental illness in the household also increase this risk (CAPT, 2018; NIDA, 2018a). Other factors include the availability of drugs within the neighborhood, community, and school and whether the adolescent's friends are using them (CAPT, 2018). Academic failure or poor social skills can put a child at further risk for using or becoming addicted to drugs. Other factors predicting addiction are early use of substances and smoking a drug or injecting the substance into a vein, which increases its addictive potential. Smoked or injected drugs enter the brain within seconds and produce a powerful pleasure effect (NIDA, 2018a).

Many factors place an individual at risk for substance use, abuse, and dependence. No single cause can explain why one individual develops a pattern of drug use and another person does not.

Manifestations of Substance Use Disorders

Specific behavioral and physiologic manifestations of substance use vary by substance. An overview of these manifestations and treatment options is provided in the Alterations and Therapies feature; further details can be found in the exemplars for this module. Most individuals who abuse substances for more than a few weeks begin to experience an array of health and emotional problems. They face increased risk for comorbid illness and family complications. It is helpful to nurses and practitioners working with this patient population to understand the prevalence of substance use in this country as well as the language of addiction and recovery.

Prevalence

Substance abuse in the United States is so common that very few people are unaffected by it. In 2018 (Center for Behavioral Health Statistics and Quality [CBHSQ], 2019):

- More than 31.9 million people reported the current use of illicit drugs or misuse of prescription drugs.
- An estimated 51.1% of the population age 12 and older (139.8 million people) used alcohol, with more than 67 million engaging in **binge drinking** (consumption of five or more drinks on one occasion) within the past month.
- 5.5 million people (2.0% of the population) age 12 and older were current users of cocaine; this figure included about 757,000 current users of crack.
- An estimated 43.5 million people (15.9% of the population) age 12 and older were current users of marijuana. This represents increased use in 2018 for young adults and adults, likely due to the decriminalization and commercial sale of marijuana in several states.

Abuse of tobacco, alcohol, opioids, and illicit drugs is costly. In the United States, the costs related to crime, lost work productivity, and healthcare are estimated to exceed $249 billion annually for alcohol misuse and $193 billion annually for illicit drug use (Office of the Surgeon General, 2016). These statistics only scratch the surface of the number of people dealing with addiction. These figures in combination with the number of people with process addictions demonstrate the need for nurses to understand, recognize, and be able to screen patients for past and present addictions and behaviors.

The Language of Addiction and Recovery

Healthcare professionals who care for patients who use or abuse substances use a number of specific terms, many of which are appropriate regardless of the substance used.

Alterations and Therapies

Addictions

ALTERATION	DESCRIPTION	TREATMENT
Nicotine addiction	Addiction to nicotine can result from smoking tobacco in the form of cigarettes, cigars, or pipes as well as from chewing tobacco and vaping nicotine products.	▪ Medications (e.g., bupropion and varenicline [Chantix]) ▪ Nicotine replacement treatments (e.g., nicotine gum/ lozenge, nasal spray, inhaler, and the transdermal patch as the trade names of NicoDerm CQ, Nicorette, and Nicotrol) ▪ Behavioral therapy ▪ Support groups
Alcohol addiction	Chronic use of alcohol can lead to addiction, resulting in delirium tremens (DTs) if alcohol is not consumed.	▪ Medications (e.g., disulfiram [Antabuse], naltrexone [Depade, Vivitrol]) ▪ Behavioral therapy ▪ Support groups ▪ 12-step program (e.g., Alcoholics Anonymous [AA]) ▪ Detoxification ▪ Milieu therapy ▪ Family therapy
Substance addiction	Substance addiction may include abuse of heroin, cocaine, marijuana, crack, narcotics, barbiturates, inhalants, or any chemical substance that leads to addiction.	▪ Behavior therapy ▪ Support groups ▪ Detoxification ▪ Pharmacologic therapy (if needed to minimize complications from withdrawal) ▪ Milieu therapy ▪ 12-step programs (e.g., Narcotics Anonymous [NA]) ▪ Family therapy
Process addictions (sex, gambling, shopping, work)	Process addictions are those behaviors compulsively performed to reduce anxiety; they are considered by some to be a form of obsessive–compulsive disorder.	▪ Psychotherapy ▪ Behavior therapy ▪ Milieu therapy ▪ Support groups ▪ 12-step programs (e.g., Gamblers Anonymous) ▪ Family therapy

Nurses working in all settings should be familiar with these terms, which are defined in **Table 22.1** ».

Comorbidities

Substance abuse has a high rate of morbidity with both physical and mental illness (see the Concepts Related to Addiction feature). Imaging scans, chest x-rays, and blood tests show the damaging effects of drug abuse throughout the body. For example, tests show that tobacco smoke causes cancer of the mouth, throat, larynx, blood, lungs, stomach, pancreas, kidney, bladder, and cervix.

Patients who abuse substances often neglect their physical health at the expense of their addiction. Their immunity is often compromised by malnutrition, poor hygiene, and risky behaviors related to addiction. Some infectious diseases, such as hepatitis A, B, and C, HIV and AIDS, and tuberculosis, are transmitted by substance abuse, either directly or indirectly. Adverse central nervous system (CNS) effects are seen in manifestations of substance dependence, tolerance, craving, and withdrawal. Addiction behaviors affect the mental health and physical health of both the addicted patient and the patient's family.

Individuals who abuse substances have a higher incidence of mental health disorders than the general population. In 2018, 9.2 million adults had both a mental illness and an SUD, which corresponded to 3.7% of all adults age 18 and older (CBHSQ, 2019). Because SUD often co-occurs with other mental illnesses, patients presenting with one condition should be assessed for the other.

Because of the scope of problems associated with chronic substance abuse and the staggering impact of untreated behavioral health conditions on individuals' lives and the cost of healthcare delivery, the Substance Abuse and Mental Health Services Administration (SAMHSA) and the National Council for Behavioral Health, the federal agencies that spearhead the nation's public health efforts related to substance abuse treatment and behavioral health, support *integrative* care of co-occurring mental health and substance use disorders. Integration extends beyond health (including primary, specialty, emergency, and rehabilitative care) and behavioral healthcare systems. It also requires addressing patients' social needs, such as housing, employment, and transportation (Center of Excellence for Integrated Health Solutions, 2020).

TABLE 22.1 Terminology Associated with Substance Abuse

Term	Definition
Abstinence	Voluntarily refraining from use of drugs or alcohol
Codependence	A cluster of maladaptive behaviors used by family members or significant others to enable and protect a loved one at the expense of their own well-being
Co-occurring disorder	Comorbid or concurrent diagnosis of a mental illness and an SUD (*dual diagnosis* is an older term)
Craving	Compelling desire for previously experienced positive effects of a substance
Cross-tolerance	Tolerance to one substance conferring tolerance to another substance
Delirium tremens (DTs)	A medical emergency associated with alcohol withdrawal, usually occurring 3–5 days following cessation and lasting for up to 3 days. Symptoms include disorientation, delusions, visual hallucinations, and paranoia. Objective signs include elevated vital signs, diaphoresis, vomiting, and diarrhea.
Dependence	A physical need for a specific substance to the degree that cessation may result in withdrawal syndrome.
Detoxification	Safe, effective withdrawal from an addictive substance. Commonly referred to as "detox."
Dual diagnosis	Co-occurring psychiatric disorder and substance abuse disorder
Korsakoff psychosis	Altered cognition resulting from thiamine (B_1) deficiency as a result of chronic alcohol use. Characterized by progressive deterioration of cognitive abilities, confabulation, and peripheral neuropathy.
Polysubstance abuse	Concurrent use of multiple substances
Recovery	Voluntarily refraining (or working toward refraining) from substance use and addictive behaviors
Relapse	Return of symptoms after stabilization (including return of drug-seeking behaviors after individual has been abstaining)
Self-medicating	Use of substances to alleviate symptoms of an untreated or undertreated medical or psychiatric illness
Sobriety	Persistent abstinence from substance use characterized by improved quality of life
Tolerance	Need for increased amount of a particular drug to achieve the same effect as a lower, previous dose
Wernicke encephalopathy	Neurologic symptoms resulting from vitamin B depletion associated with chronic alcohol use. Characterized by abnormal eye movements, ataxia, and confusion.
Withdrawal	A constellation of signs and symptoms associated with rapid discontinuation or decrease in substance use in individual who is physically dependent

Effects of Addiction on Families

Substance abuse can have particularly devastating consequences for families because it increases the family members' risk for social isolation and decreases their access to social supports that can be helpful to those experiencing addiction and their families. Typically, defensive coping mechanisms (particularly denial) arise as family members find themselves unable to cope with the addiction in a healthy way. Substance abuse can also interfere with normal family processes, from day-to-day activities related to parenting (such as not being able to drive the carpool in the morning) to long-term changes such as role reversals, with older children taking on caregiving responsibilities.

Addiction within the family is often cloaked in secrecy and shame. Family members, in an effort to protect the family and the addicted member from discovery, often close family ranks to the outside world.

Often, the term **boundaries** is used when talking about interpersonal relationships and addiction. Boundaries represent a type of relationship safety zone around a family and its members. Normally, boundaries around families are flexible, allowing members to interact with those outside of the family and with the community as needed and desired. Clear boundaries keep people safe within functional relationships. When addiction is present in a family, these boundaries often become rigid and inflexible. Such boundaries do not let information about the family needs or requests for needed assistance out and do not allow input or assistance from individuals or community agencies outside of the family. This increases the family's isolation and can further impede participation in treatment.

Family members often inadvertently support the addictive behaviors. **Enabling behavior** is any action an individual takes that consciously or unconsciously facilitates substance dependence. Examples of enabling include family members making excuses to employers or teachers or discontinuing their own social relationships with friends or neighbors in order to preserve the "healthy image" of the family in the community.

In families where addiction is present, communication is poor within and outside of the family system. Isolation results in an escalating cycle of addiction and dysfunction for the entire family. It is important for healthcare providers (HCPs) to recognize that shame and fear often lead to this isolation. A nonjudgmental approach to assessment and intervention, coupled with empathy and respect, is essential when working with those who are addicted to substances and their families. Substance abuse sometimes correlates with a history of abuse, economic instability, criminal behavior, and educational upheaval.

The longer the addiction continues, the more entrenched family members become in behaviors that further the addiction, such as denial and enabling. This codependency, in which the behaviors of the addict and those of the family revolve around the addiction and their shared behaviors in service of the addiction, harms the family. Children may carry these behaviors into adulthood, taking on specific characteristics beyond the family relationship. Characteristics of

Box 22.1
Characteristics of Codependent Individuals

- Have low self-esteem.
- Have an exaggerated sense of responsibility for others' actions.
- Feel guilty when they assert themselves.
- Deny that they have a problem; think the problem is someone else or the situation.
- Tend to become hurt when their efforts aren't recognized.
- Do more than their share of work all of the time; have trouble saying "no" to anyone.
- Need approval and recognition.
- Fear being abandoned or alone.
- Have difficulty identifying their feelings despite experiencing painful emotions.
- Have difficulty adjusting to change.
- Struggle with intimacy and boundaries.
- Have poor communication skills.
- Have difficulty making decisions.
- Offer advice whether it has been asked for or not.
- Feel like a victim.
- Use manipulation, shame, or guilt to control others' behavior.

codependent individuals are described in **Box 22.1** ». A number of support networks and groups, including Adult Children of Alcoholics and Al-Anon, exist to help family members learn about and recover from the effects of addiction.

Approximately 7.5 million children younger than the age of 18 (10.5% of all children) live with a parent or caregiver who had an alcohol use disorder in the past year (Lipari & Van Horn, 2017). These children are at a greater risk for depression, anxiety disorders, problems with cognitive and verbal skills, and parental abuse or neglect. Moreover, they are four times more likely than other children to develop alcohol problems themselves (Lipari & Van Horn, 2017). Similar issues exist with parents who abuse other substances or combine other substances with alcohol.

Children whose parents abuse substances also are at risk for disruptive behavioral problems and are more likely to be sensation seeking, aggressive, and impulsive. Because of the secrecy and shame associated with substance abuse, many are hesitant to talk about their own feelings, needs, and wants.

While some children growing up in families with addiction have obvious and apparent problems, others cope quite well. The level of dysfunction or resiliency of the nonabusing spouse is a key factor in the impact of the addiction on the children (Shank, Petrarca, & Barry, 2019). However, longitudinal research has confirmed the adverse lifelong psychosocial, behavioral, and developmental effects of growing up in a household headed by a parent with addiction. Of particular concern is the increased lifetime risk of major depressive disorder and persistent depressive disorder among children of alcoholics (Thapa, Selya, & Jonk, 2017).

Case Study » Part 1

Paul is the 19-year-old son of Mark and Susan John. The Johns have been married for 20 years. Ms. John is a full-time stay-at-home mom. Paul's dad is a corporate attorney who has always been somewhat demanding of his wife and children. He drinks alcohol daily but has always been employed and has maintained a middle-class lifestyle for his family. Paul has two younger sisters. Mara, the younger of the two, has been treated for anorexia since the age of 12. His 15-year-old sister, Jess, is doing well in high school. Paul did well in high school, where he played varsity soccer and did fairly well academically.

Paul has just returned home from his first full year at college. His mother is concerned because he doesn't seem like his old self; he shows no interest in his old friends or in getting a summer job. On the other hand, he seems secretive and has left the house on many occasions claiming that he has new friends who "get it." He is very short-tempered with his sisters, constantly irritable and discontented. He is very evasive when asked about his grades or any college activities. He has noticeable weight loss and appears unkempt. His father is intolerant of his behavior. His mother is concerned and has arranged to accompany him on a visit to his primary care provider. She is hoping to find out what his problem is so it can be treated before his father becomes angrier with him and his behavior. You are the nurse who is assessing Paul.

Clinical Reasoning Questions Level I

1. Describe the elements of the interview/assessment environment that you should consider before beginning Paul's patient assessment.
2. What questions would be appropriate in assessing Paul's physiologic, emotional, and psychologic status?
3. What cues in the family history might indicate a potential for substance use or abuse in Paul?

Clinical Reasoning Questions Level II

4. If substance abuse is suspected, how should you proceed to address any defense mechanisms displayed?
5. What diagnostic measures might be needed based on your assessment?
6. If depression is suspected, what further assessments would you perform?

Process Disorders

Although this chapter focuses on the care of patients with SUDs, it is important for nurses to also be able to recognize that individuals can become addicted to certain behaviors. Process disorders, also known as behavioral addictions, are groups of repetitive behaviors (e.g., gambling, shopping, internet gaming, exercise, sex) that activate biochemical reward systems similar to those activated by drugs of abuse. Process addictions produce behavioral symptoms comparable to those seen in SUDs (APA, 2013). One significant difference, however, is that the individual may not be addicted to a substance, but rather to the behavior or the feeling brought about by the relevant action. However, many people with behavioral addictions may also have substance addictions (Hajela, 2017).

Gambling disorder is the only one of the repetitive processes with sufficient data to be included in the fifth edition of the *Diagnostic and Statistical Manual of Mental Disorders* (DSM-5; APA, 2013) as a diagnosable mental disorder (**Figure 22.2** »). The essential feature of gambling is the individual's willingness to risk something of value in the hope of obtaining something of greater value. The diagnostic criteria for gambling disorder highlight the similarities between a process addiction and an SUD. To be diagnosed with gambling disorder, an individual must experience clinically significant impairment or distress related to the gambling; experience distress when trying to reduce or quit gambling; be preoccupied with gambling to the extent of jeopardizing income, employment, or

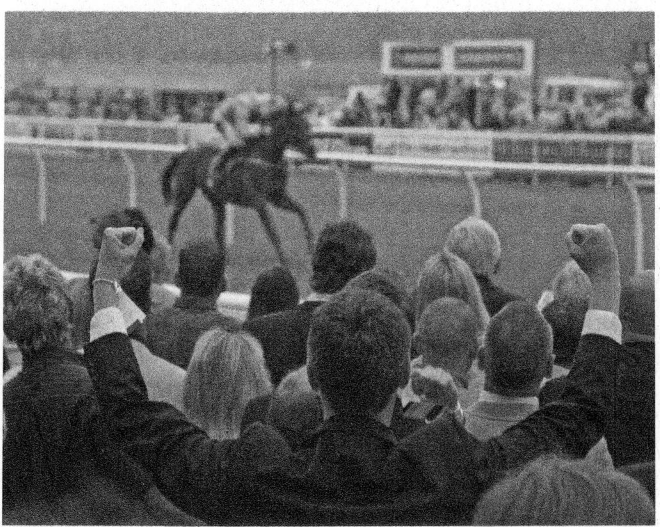

Figure 22.2 ›› Gambling disorder, one of the process disorders, produces behavioral symptoms comparable to those seen in substance use disorders.

Source: Mikedabell/E+/Getty Images.

significant relationships; and have a history of unsuccessful attempts to control or stop gambling (APA, 2013).

Other process addictions, which do not yet appear in the DSM-5 as diagnosable mental health disorders, also cause severe stress and strain to individuals and families. For example, excessive online shopping comprises compulsive and addictive forms of consumption and buying behavior. Review of the literature has shown that attributes associated with **online shopping addiction (OSA)** include low self-esteem, low self-regulation, negative emotional state, social anonymity, and cognitive overload (Müller et al., 2019). While compulsive shopping has been documented in the literature for more than 100 years, the internet has added increased accessibility, stimulating marketing techniques, a loss of the protective delay between impulse and purchase, and overvaluing of the shopping process and objects purchased—all factors that contribute to the potentially addictive nature of shopping (Uzarska, Czerwiński, & Atroszko, 2019). Shopping addiction can adversely affect the individual's family, social, and occupational life. It is associated with high rates of psychiatric comorbidity (e.g., substance addiction, depression, and obsessive–compulsive disorder, as well as hoarding), but some research has found that one salient feature of excessive shopping is an increased sensitivity to reward (Müller et al., 2019).

Internet gaming disorder (IGD) is the persistent use of the internet to engage in games, often with other players, leading to clinically significant impairment or distress. Proposed criteria for diagnosis of IGD include preoccupation with gaming; withdrawal symptoms when gaming is taken away; tolerance (the need to spend increasing amounts of time in gaming or gaming-related activities); unsuccessful attempts to control use and participation; continued gaming despite distress or interference with other activities or interference with relationships; lying about time spent gaming; and using gaming to relieve a negative mood (APA, 2013).

There have been several proposed diagnostic labels for persistent, excessive sexual behaviors, often referred to as **sex addiction** or *compulsive sexual behavior (CSB)*. Typical activities may include engaging in risky sexual practices with a number of partners; preoccupation with recurrent, intense, sexually arousing fantasies, sexual urges, or behaviors; visiting strip clubs; and engaging in phone sex. With the advent of the internet, sexual behavior has expanded to include compulsive viewing of online pornography and contact with online services, also known as cybersex (Wéry & Billieux, 2017). These behaviors are distinguishable from paraphilias, which are abnormal sexual desires that involve dangerous behaviors. CSB is estimated to affect up to 10.3% of males and 7.0% of females in the United States (Dickenson, Gleason, Coleman, & Miner, 2018).

Concepts Related to Addiction

Substance use disorder is not a self-contained disorder. Substance use and abuse can affect the physical, psychologic, and spiritual health of both the individual and the family. A few examples of systems and concepts that are related to substance abuse are outlined here.

Substance use impacts cognitive ability, including slowing reaction times, decreasing inhibitions, and impairing judgment and memory (SAMHSA, 2015b). Substance use also negatively impacts intellectual development in the children of abusing parents. Alcohol abuse is the primary factor contributing to the neurocognitive deficits and intellectual disabilities exhibited by children who have fetal alcohol spectrum disorders (FASD) because of in utero exposure to alcohol (Popova, Lange, Probst, Gmel, & Rehm, 2018).

Gastrointestinal (GI) disorders (including the GI tract, liver, and pancreas) occur frequently with long-term substance use. For example, cocaine abuse can result in various GI complications, including gastric ulcerations, retroperitoneal fibrosis, visceral infarction, intestinal ischemia, and GI tract perforations (SAMHSA, 2015b). Long-term alcohol use often leads to cirrhosis of the liver, which impairs digestion of food and absorption of key nutrients.

Infectious diseases are common in individuals who abuse substances. At least 76% of patients who have used injectable drugs for less than 7 years are positive for hepatitis C, while 25% of patients who abuse alcohol and those who do not inject drugs also show serologic evidence of infection (SAMHSA, 2015b). Other infectious diseases associated with SUD are endocarditis, bacterial pneumonia, tuberculosis, skin infections resulting from administration of intravenous drugs (e.g., *Staphylococcus aureus* and *Streptococcus pyogenes*), and HIV/AIDS.

Individuals with SUD are prone to accidents of all kinds, with complications ranging from head trauma to falls with fractures. Chronic pain frequently is seen in patients as a result of trauma, poor health maintenance, or an inability to deal with pain without opioid drug use (SAMHSA, 2015b). Also, clinicians should also consider traumatic brain injury (TBI) when individuals with SUD present with neurologic impairment. People who abuse substances have a high risk of falls, motor-vehicle accidents, gang violence, domestic violence, and so on, all of which may result in head injury (SAMHSA, 2015b).

Posttraumatic stress disorder (PTSD) has been found in 14–22% of veterans returning from recent wars in Afghanistan and Iraq and has been linked to increased risk for alcohol abuse and dependence (National Center for PTSD, 2018; Norman, Haller, Hamblen, Southwick, & Pietrzak, 2018). Individuals who abuse substances and have experienced trauma have worse treatment outcomes for substance abuse than those without histories of trauma. Because traumatic experiences and their sequelae are closely tied to behavioral health problems, many clinicians have integrated trauma-informed care into addiction recovery programs (Shier & Turpin, 2017).

The Concepts Related to Addiction feature links some, but not all, of the concepts integral to addiction. They are presented in alphabetical order.

Harm Reduction and Health Promotion

Harm reduction refers to interventions aimed at reducing the negative consequences related to unhealthy behaviors, such as alcohol and drug abuse. One of the first successful harm reduction programs was needle exchange to minimize the spread of HIV and hepatitis C. The harm reduction approach has aided in the development of medications such as methadone and buprenorphine to help treat opiate use disorders (Des Jarlais, 2017). There has been political resistance to implementation of harm reduction measures because some public officials contend that harm reduction enables or excuses addictive behaviors and does not advance sobriety (Des Jarlais, 2017). Goals of harm reduction programs include reduced use, having an opioid-reversal agent such as naloxone (Narcan) on hand, and using test strips to detect fentanyl in street drugs (Harm Reduction Coalitition, 2020). Evidence shows that harm reduction does not increase or encourage substance use (HealthLink BC, 2020). Nurses play a valuable role as harm-reduction educators.

Health promotion efforts related to substance abuse also generally revolve around education. Federal initiatives include prevention efforts by SAMHSA and other federal organizations. Community and local initiatives, often sponsored as collaborations among law enforcement and local health and mental health professionals, may be developed to

Concepts Related to Addiction

CONCEPT	RELATIONSHIP TO ADDICTION	NURSING IMPLICATIONS
Cognition	↓ B_1 (thiamine) in the brain can cause changes in cognition, specifically confusion ↓ Memory, judgment, reaction times, cognitive ability	■ Assess for Wernicke encephalopathy, Korsakoff psychosis, and dementia. ■ Provide for patient safety. ■ Anticipate provision of thiamine therapy.
Family	↑ Substance use and abuse of family member → ↑ family secrecy → ↑ family isolation → ↓ supportive resources available	■ Determine family understanding of substance abuse and addiction. ■ Communicate clearly, honestly, openly, and without judgment. ■ Anticipate involving the entire family in all aspects of the treatment process.
Infection	↑ Spread of infection through intravenous use of drugs (e.g., needle sharing) ↑ Risk of sexually transmitted infections	■ Assess for hepatitis C, endocarditis, bacterial pneumonia, tuberculosis, skin infections resulting from administration of intravenous drugs. ■ Assess for sexually transmitted infections such as HIV/AIDS.
Nutrition	↓ Nutritional status → ↓ body's ability to synthesize antibodies	■ Be alert to cues that indicate malnutrition and opportunistic infection. ■ Anticipate the need for a nutritional assessment, balanced diet, vitamin and mineral supplements. ■ Provide discharge planning that promotes patient's ability to meet nutritional needs.
Safety	↑ Risk-taking behaviors leads to ↑ risk for injury, violence, and HIV	■ Assess for risky behaviors, including driving under the influence, unprotected sex, or sharing needles. ■ Provide education related to safety. ■ Anticipate denial, family interference, or enabling.
Trauma	Substance abuse as coping mechanism → poorer outcomes Combat, TBI ↑ risk for PTSD → ↑ risk for substance abuse	■ Assess for patient and family safety. ■ Identify and refer to recovery programs that provide integrative, trauma-informed care. ■ Support family during recovery process.

target needs in a specific community. At the individual level, nurses and other healthcare professionals assess patients' risk for substance abuse and provide education related to prevention, especially related to using healthy coping mechanisms and obtaining appropriate treatment for existing mental health disorders, such as depression.

Health promotion activities can be particularly important for patients who are in recovery from an addiction. Generally speaking, health promotion activities help prevent patients from experiencing relapse. They often include reviewing with patients the situations or feelings that triggered use in the past and helping patients recall and maintain healthy coping strategies that have been successful in helping them maintain sobriety. Nurses working with sober patients may need to help identify additional resources for patients during challenging times such as childbirth and illness. For example, a mother with a history of substance use who gives birth to a premature newborn may need the nurse or case worker to set up early childhood intervention services. A nurse or early childhood intervention specialist will then make weekly home visits to see how mother and baby are doing and provide supportive interventions that may include teaching feeding and parenting strategies. By reducing the stress level of the mother and promoting mother–child bonding, the mother will be at less risk for resuming addictive behaviors.

» **Stay Current:** SAMHSA offers free downloadable information on evidence-based prevention and treatment at https://www.samhsa.gov/ebp-resource-center.

Nursing Assessment

A trusting nurse–patient relationship, along with the nurse's ethical obligation to maintain confidentiality, may help the patient share information more freely. By including family members in the assessment process, nurses may uncover addictions or behaviors the patient is hiding or fails to recognize. Nurses must help patients understand that full disclosure of any addictions helps protect them from potential treatment complications. All too often patients fail to admit addiction until permanent damage has already occurred. The nurse's responsibility is to recognize cues while complications are still preventable.

SAMHSA recommends that HCPs at all levels of treatment use **SBIRT** (screening, brief intervention, and referral to treatment) to identify patients with substance abuse issues (U.S. Preventive Services Task Force [USPSTF], 2018). The goal is early intervention and treatment services for persons with SUDs, as well as those who are at risk of developing these disorders. *Screening* quickly assesses the severity of substance use and identifies the appropriate level of treatment. *Brief intervention* focuses on increasing insight and awareness regarding substance use and motivation toward behavioral change. *Referral to treatment* helps direct those who need more extensive treatment toward access to specialty care (SAMHSA, 2015a).

Holistic assessment includes determining patient considerations beyond the addiction itself. SAMHSA has researched and recommended some sex-based treatment considerations. These include recommendations that treatment programs include provisions for child care or assistance with services for children. Women who have children often fear that admitting a substance use problem will cause them to lose custody of their children. Nurses and clinicians need to be sensitive to this barrier, explore resources in the community, and help female patients deal with this issue. For men, employment-related issues can strongly affect their substance use/abuse, and men with SUDs are at greater risk for unemployment (SAMHSA, 2014). For men who are employed, their type of profession may affect the pattern and extent of their substance use. Employment-related issues can strongly affect men's substance use/abuse, and men with SUDs are at greater risk for unemployment (SAMHSA, 2014). Nurses and clinicians working to assess patients' need for treatment should be aware of considerations related to employment, child care, and related issues.

Determining Level of Care

Most clinicians use multidimensional assessment criteria developed by the American Society of Addiction Medicine (ASAM; 2020a, 2020b) when determining the most appropriate facility and level of care for initial placement, continued stay, and transfer/discharge of patients who abuse substances. Assessment criteria include acute intoxication or withdrawal potential; biomedical conditions and complications; emotional, behavioral, or cognitive conditions and complications; readiness to change; relapse, continued use, or continued problem potential; and recovery/living environment. The levels of care typically used in the United States range from ambulatory (outpatient) detoxification without extended onsite monitoring to medically managed, intensive inpatient detoxification (ASAM, 2020a).

For individuals withdrawing from alcohol, sedative-hypnotics, or opioids, hospitalization (or some form of 24-hour medical care) is the preferred setting for detoxification, based on safety and symptom-relief concerns (SAMHSA, 2015b). Concurrent mental health issues, such as exacerbation of schizophrenia or bipolar disorder, may also require hospitalization for stabilization. Significant physiologic cues (such as a change in mental status, GI pain or bleeding, seizures, or suspected infection) also indicate the need for immediate hospitalization (SAMHSA, 2015b). Young individuals in good health, with no history of previous withdrawal reactions, may be able to manage withdrawal without medication. Nonmedical detoxification is a current trend because of cost effectiveness and inexpensive access to treatment for certain individuals seeking treatment (SAMHSA, 2015b).

SAFETY ALERT! Assess for suicidality in individuals with substance use issues. Individuals with alcohol dependence and persons who use drugs have a 10 to 14 times greater risk of death by suicide, and approximately 22% of deaths by suicide involve alcohol intoxication (Esang & Ahmed, 2018).

Observation and Patient Interview

Nurses who work with individuals with addiction issues often note observable manifestations at the first patient encounter. Familiar manifestations include unsteady gait and poor balance, lack of coordination, slurred speech, tremors, and unusual smells on the breath, body, or clothes. Other common manifestations include:

- Loss of interest in personal hygiene and grooming
- Watering or bloodshot eyes; large or small pupils
- Rhinorrhea (runny nose)
- Obvious weight loss or gain
- Inability to concentrate; hyperactivity, agitation, or giddiness
- Anger, frustration, or mood swings
- Appearing fearful, anxious, or paranoid with no reason
- Appearing lethargic or "spaced out."

These are only a few observable manifestations of substance use. Symptoms specific to certain substance addictions are described in more detail in the following sections.

Patients also may need to be assessed regarding the extent of crisis they are facing in their lives as the result of their SUD, particularly if a crisis event or behavior motivates them to seek healthcare. The following list of questions provides a general crisis assessment that can be used in any problem-solving situation. It is of particular use for the patient whose crisis is the result of addiction behavior.

Individual Assessment

1. What is the most significant stress/problem occurring in your life right now?
2. Has this problem increased the frequency of substance use? (Quantify change in frequency or amount of substance used.)
3. Is your addiction behavior causing or contributing to the problem?
4. Who is the problem impacting? You? Your family? Your employer?
5. How long has this been a problem?
6. What does this problem mean to you?
7. What are the factors that cause this problem to continue?
8. Would the problem resolve if you stopped abusing the substance?
9. Have you had similar stresses/problems in the past?
10. What other stresses do you have in your life?
11. How are you managing your usual life roles (partner, parent, homemaker, worker, student, and so on)?
12. In what way has your life changed as a result of this problem?
13. Are you feeling as though you want to harm yourself or anyone else?
14. Describe how you have managed problems in the past.
15. What have you done to try to solve the problem so far? What happened when you tried this?
16. Describe possible resources (e.g., family, friends, employer, teacher; financial, spiritual).
17. Are you interested in abstaining from substance abuse? Are you considering a rehabilitation program?
18. What part of the overall problem is most important to deal with first?

Family Assessment

1. How do you perceive the current problem and the patient's addiction behavior?
2. In what way has the problem and the patient's addiction behavior affected your roles in the family?
3. How has your lifestyle changed since this problem began?
4. Describe communication within the family before and since this current problem began.
5. How does the family typically manage problems?
6. What has the family done to try to solve the problem so far?
7. What happened when you tried this?
8. How well do you believe the family is coping at this time?
9. Describe possible resources (e.g., extended family, friends; financial).
10. What are your expectations and hopes concerning this problem and the patient's addiction behavior?
11. Which part of the overall problem is most important to deal with first?
12. Can the problem be resolved without resolution of the addiction behavior?

Community Assessment

1. What are the living conditions of the neighborhood?
2. Are affordable child care services available?
3. Is there a community mental health center or rehabilitation center?
4. What support groups are available in the community?
5. Are there any possible funding resources?

Physical Examination

Physical assessment findings depend on the nature of the addiction and the substance being used. When performing a physical assessment, nurses must be alert for symptoms that are abnormal or not within expected boundaries and assess patient explanations for inconsistencies. Unless the patient comes to the HCP under the influence or is referred by an employer, the physical examination may provide the first indications that an addiction is involved.

Diagnostic Tests

Diagnostic tests required for patients with addiction will be ordered based on the type of addiction they display. Specific diagnostic tests will be ordered for each type of addiction and may include serum drug levels; toxicology; chest x-rays for inhaled substances; organ biopsies related to damage caused by a substance; and urine, saliva, and serum testing for substance metabolites. Hair testing may be done to determine substance use within a period of 90 days.

Case Study » Part 2

Paul is admitted to the emergency department (ED) at 2:00 a.m. on a Sunday morning in August as the result of a motor-vehicle crash. His speech is slurred and his gate is ataxic. He is bleeding from a laceration on his left forehead, and he is complaining that his left arm is extremely painful and "falling off." A decision is made to admit Paul to the trauma unit. His father, as next of kin, is notified of the admission. His father states, "I knew this would happen. Let him rot." Paul becomes combative as you attempt to assess his state of consciousness and physical injuries.

Clinical Reasoning Questions Level I

1. You suspect substance use. What are your immediate concerns?
2. How will you promote Paul's cooperation with your assessment and eventual treatment?
3. What specific diagnostic tests will be appropriate related to both his suspected substance use and his physical injuries?

Clinical Reasoning Questions Level II

4. *Refer to Module 49, Legal Issues:* Are you able to begin assessment and treatment of Paul without consent from next of kin? What are the legal implications in this situation?
5. Paul's mother arrives in the ED. She is very upset and demanding to see him. Will you involve Paul's mother in his care? Why or why not?

Independent Interventions

Nurses may use a number of independent and collaborative caring interventions with patients who are addicted or who exhibit addiction behaviors. **Recovery** is generally defined as a state of voluntary sobriety in which the individual maintains personal health and functions normally within society without the use of the addictive substance or behavior. The goal of all interventions is to move the patient toward treatment and into recovery. Recovery is a lifelong process. Nurses must remember that no single intervention is sufficient to ensure permanent recovery, which requires substantial and continual work on the part of the individual.

Independent nursing interventions for patients with SUDs primarily focus around nursing care for any specific presenting symptoms, developing and maintaining the therapeutic nurse–patient relationship (including establishing and maintaining appropriate boundaries), and promoting healthy patient communication and coping skills. See Module 31, Stress and Coping, for a discussion about defense mechanisms and nursing interventions to help patients develop healthy coping skills. As always, providing culturally competent care is critical to reducing barriers and improving outcomes.

Promote Communication

Respect, empathy, and caring are essential components of caring for those with SUDs. Establishing a therapeutic nurse–patient relationship that places the patient at the center of all communication is essential because patients with SUDs have poor communication skills and are experienced at hiding their addictions and avoiding their addiction as the topic of discussion.

Because many individuals who abuse substances come from families with impaired communication, it is important that communication be simple, direct, and powerful (Hazelden Betty Ford Foundation, 2020). Many student and new nurses will use euphemisms or talk too much when communicating with a substance abuser. This is counterproductive, as many of these patients do not want to hear the message being conveyed and are often skilled at manipulating words and phrases as well as people (Hazelden Betty Ford Foundation, 2020). Recommended strategies for communicating with individuals who abuse substances include:

- Express concerns or pass along information without judgment. Correct any false ideas and fill in information gaps.
- Use "I" statements to describe concerns without singling out the individual.
- Remain calm without arguing or getting angry.
- Listen for contingency words such as "probably," "possibly," or "maybe" in conversations with individuals who abuse substances. These adverbs usually mean that the individual is not going to follow through on the topics being discussed.
- Hold patients accountable. If they agree to follow through on a task or plan, make a specific plan with them to encourage completion.
- Practice active listening skills. Notice when patients with SUDs are using defense mechanisms such as *deflecting* (turning the topic back on the speaker, changing the subject, or using humor to lighten the mood), *rationalizing* (explaining why a behavior or action that is clearly not acceptable is acceptable), *minimizing* (downplaying the extent of the addiction and its consequences), and *avoiding* (pretending not to hear or refusing to engage in discussion).
- Notice body language. Eye contact may indicate interest, while staring at the floor or other spots may indicate shame, exasperation, or refusal to engage. Other nonverbal indicators are muscle tension, indicating stress and fear; hand wringing, indicating anxiety and worry; and turning away, indicating termination of the conversation (Kelly, Saitz, & Wakeman, 2016).

Examples of some of these strategies are provided in the *Communicating with Patients* features in this module.

To promote successful therapeutic communication with patients with SUDs, it is important for nurses to examine their own biases and feelings regarding substance use and abuse. Nurses are not immune to societal stigma surrounding drug use. Self-examination, education, and mentorship are some strategies to promote greater empathy and understanding toward patients with SUDs (see the Evidence-Based Practice feature).

Limit Setting and Boundary Violations

Limit setting refers to establishing parameters of desirable and acceptable patient behavior. Limit setting helps patients feel safe, advances therapeutic goals by eliminating nonproductive behaviors, promotes positive behavior change, and protects significant others and children of individuals who abuse substances from unacceptable behaviors (Suchman, Borelli, & DeCoste, 2020). Limit setting teaches the individual that there are choices, but there are also consequences for making poor decisions. The goal of setting limits is to teach patients how to consistently make good decisions. Unfortunately, setting limits can be challenging for both clinicians and family members, as patients often respond with anger and resentment, with some even threatening to terminate the therapeutic or personal relationship. Clinicians and family members may feel defeated, angry, and frustrated when limits are breached (Suchman et al., 2020).

Many people who abuse substances have an unhealthy sense of personal boundaries and frequently cross them, such as by appropriating and selling or pawning a family member's property to pursue an addiction. Clinicians should encourage family members to set and enforce clear

Evidence-Based Practice

Patients with Substance Use Disorders and Nursing Stigma

Problem

Nurses are crucial players in identifying and addressing substance use problems, but traditionally often report negative attitudes, poor motivation, and insufficient training for working with these patients. One approach to reducing nursing stigma is to integrate more extensive SUD learning and clinical opportunities into nursing student education.

Evidence

One college used a combined a 120-hour mentorship practicum with focus groups for nursing students. This study examined nursing students' attitudes toward and empathy for patients with SUD before and after mentorship to determine whether there were differences across practice settings (Schuler & Horowitz, 2020). Students' empathy scores improved significantly across all practice settings, and students' attitudes improved significantly after mentorship. Qualitative research analysis revealed student issues relating to stigma, such as perceived lack of educational preparation, observing generational differences in nursing care, transitioning from fear to empathy, familial exposure, and feelings of helplessness and blame (Schuler & Horowitz, 2020).

Another nursing program used an educational intervention based on SBIRT (Mahmoud et al., 2019). The students had a 1.5-hour SBIRT education session and a 12-week clinical experience with patients who had alcohol and/or opioid use problems. The sample showed that pretest–posttest scores indicated students' stigma perceptions improved toward patients who had alcohol and/or opioid use problems (Mahmoud et al., 2019).

Yet another university developed an educational experience that integrated alcohol use disorder curriculum into a community/public health nursing clinical practicum (Nash, Marcus, et al., 2017). To prepare students to apply their skills working directly with a population affected by SUDs, the instructor integrated into the practicum up to 30 hours of educational experiences (e.g., agency visits, media, expert speakers, skills workshops, observational experiences, and reflective activities). Students participated in reflective exercises, including writing essays on their reactions to observational experiences and plans to implement (or not) the new knowledge in their professional nursing practice. Students also participated in weekly group reflections on issues that arose throughout the clinical experience. After the practicum, qualitative analysis showed student growth in the professional role; a new understanding of the complex health determinants of addiction; and growth in empathy and respect for patients affected by SUDs (Nash, Marcus, et al., 2017).

Implications for Nursing

These studies indicate that student perceptions of and empathy toward individuals with SUDs can be changed with greater education, mentorship, and/or reflective practice in conjunction with clinical experience, which may improve the delivery of healthcare to this vulnerable population (Lanzillotta-Rangeley et al., 2020).

Critical Thinking

1. Many nursing students report having had experience in their personal life with someone who had an SUD. How do you think this experience affects your perception of patients who have an SUD?
2. What are some measures you can take to avoid countertransference issues when dealing with patients with SUDs?

boundaries with defined consequences. Reluctance by family members to enforce personal boundaries is often related to poor communication and enmeshed, codependent behavior (National Alliance on Mental Illness, 2020).

Likewise, nurses and other clinicians need to be aware of professional boundaries, which the patient can violate or exploit. Boundary crossing can involve inappropriate physical contact, giving and receiving gifts, contact outside of the normal therapy session, use of provocative language and clothing, and proximity of the therapist and patient during sessions (Hook & Devereux, 2018). The nurse also needs to guard against ambiguous relationships where multiple roles exist between a therapist and a patient, such as if the patient is also a student, friend, family member, employee, or an associate of the nurse.

Promote Patient Safety During Acute Withdrawal

Acute withdrawal from alcohol and benzodiazepines can be a medical emergency. Withdrawal from some substances can increase suicide risk. Nurses promote patient safety following agency protocols and through close observation and monitoring.

- Observe the patient for withdrawal symptoms. Monitor vital signs frequently per protocol until the patient has stabilized. Provide adequate nutrition and hydration. Take seizure precautions. These actions provide supportive physical care during detoxification.
- Assess blood alcohol or substance level routinely and look for escalating signs of withdrawal, using an instrument such as the Clinical Institute Withdrawal Assessment for Alcoho (CIWA-Ar). Reliable information about withdrawal symptoms comes from blood levels and vital signs; these measurements provide information about the need for additional medications to prevent severe complications. See Table 22.4 in Exemplar 22.C for an overview of substance overdose and withdrawal.
- Administer scheduled medications according to the detoxification protocol. For example, in the case of alcohol withdrawal, benzodiazepines reduce the severity of withdrawal symptoms, anticonvulsants (especially carbamazepine) help prevent seizures and delirium, and vitamins and nutritional supplements support neurologic health (ASAM, 2020a).
- Assess the patient's level of orientation frequently. Orient and reassure the patient of safety in the presence of hallucinations, delusions, or illusions.
- Explain all interventions before approaching the patient. Use simple step-by-step instructions and face-to-face interaction. Minimize environmental distractions and talk softly to the patient. Excessive stimuli increase agitation.

- Provide positive reinforcement when thinking and behavior are appropriate or when the patient recognizes that delusions are not based in reality. Alcohol and other substances can interfere with the patient's perception of reality.
- Express reasonable doubt if the patient relays suspicious or paranoid beliefs. Reinforce accurate perception of people or situations. It is important to communicate that you do not share the false belief as reality.
- Do not argue with the patient who is experiencing delusions or hallucinations. Convey acceptance that the patient believes a situation to be true, but that you do not see or hear what is not there. Arguing with the patient or denying the belief serves no useful purpose because it does not eliminate the delusions.
- Talk to the patient about real events and real people. Respond to feelings and reassure the patient about being safe from harm. Discussions that focus on the delusions may aggravate the condition. Verbalization of feelings in a nonthreatening environment may help the patient develop insight.

Promote Adequate Nutrition

Patients who engage in any type of substance abuse are at risk for deficiencies in key nutrients. In the case of alcoholism, for example, thiamine deficiency can cause complications such as Wernicke syndrome. Nurses administer vitamins and dietary substances as ordered and monitor labwork (e.g., total albumin, complete blood count, urinalysis, electrolytes, and liver enzymes) and report significant changes to the HCP. Nurses also collaborate with dietitians to determine the number of calories necessary for patients to maintain adequate nutrition and weight. In inpatient settings, nurses document intake and output and calorie count and weigh patients daily, if necessary. Nurses also teach patients with substance abuse about the importance of adequate nutrition and the physical effects of alcohol or substance abuse and related malnutrition on body systems. Nurses provide information about adequate nutrition using U.S. Department of Agriculture recommendations.

Promote Participation in Treatment

Patients are more likely to participate in treatment when nurses and other clinicians are genuine, honest, and respectful of patients. Keep all promises and convey an attitude of acceptance. Do not accept the use of defense mechanisms such as rationalization or projection as patients attempt to blame others or make excuses for their behavior. Encourage patients to examine how unhealthy coping mechanisms and maladaptive behaviors are impacting their lives and those they care about and help them learn more healthy ways of coping and responding to stressful situations. Encourage patient participation in therapeutic group activities such as 12-step and support-group meetings with other people who are experiencing or have experienced similar problems. Patients often are more accepting of peer feedback than feedback from authority figures.

Collaborative Therapies

Treatment for addiction may be determined by level of severity and how the individual comes to seek treatment. Some patients are adjudicated to treatment by the judicial system. Patients with severe impairment of function may be involuntarily admitted or may be admitted for medical care associated with an injury. Other factors include access to affordable treatment, stigma, and cultural barriers (see Focus on Diversity and Culture: Substance Abuse Treatment). These are some of the many factors that influence individual patient plans of care.

Many HCPs routinely use the 5A's to help identify users and appropriate interventions based on the patient's willingness to quit (Kastaun et al., 2020). The steps are described below.

1. **Ask:** Identify and document substance use status for every patient at every visit.
2. **Advise:** In a clear, strong, and personalized manner, urge every patient who is using to quit.
3. **Assess:** Is the patient willing to make a quit attempt at this time?
4. **Assist:** For the patient willing to make a quit attempt, use counseling and pharmacotherapy to help in quitting. For those who need a higher level of care, for example, inpatient detoxification, make arrangements for admission.
5. **Arrange:** Schedule follow-up contact, in person or by telephone, preferably within the first week after the quit date.

In some cases, individuals seek care after being persuaded they need care through a process of confrontation called **intervention**. The goal of intervention is to prevent individuals who are abusing substances from denying the problem and force them to face the negative aspects of behavior and enroll in treatment, typically in a residential treatment facility. In *family intervention*, the family enlists the help of a professional clinician to conduct the intervention with the participation of the family. The clinician and family meet with the individual together, with family members stating how the individual's addiction affects the family.

Frequently, individuals enter treatment because their inability to manage life skills and events results in a crisis, such as an impaired driving citation or a child custody dispute. Other challenges such as job loss, financial difficulties, ruptured relationships, and distressing medical symptoms can also lead a patient with SUD to seek treatment. It is during crisis situations that patients with SUDs are most likely to be motivated to seek help. The inability to maintain emotional equilibrium is an important but short-lived feature of crisis. Typically, the high level of anxiety created by a crisis forces the individual to return to the previous level of addiction; develop more constructive coping skills and seek help; or decompensate to a lower level of functioning.

While the process of detoxification, stabilization, and recovery frequently contains significant medical and pharmaceutical components, the motivation for long-term change often comes from psychosocial interventions. Psychosocial interventions for SUDs can be defined as interpersonal or informational activities, techniques, or strategies that target biological, behavioral, cognitive, emotional, interpersonal, social, or environmental factors with the aim of improving health functioning and well-being (Verdejo-García, Alcázar-Córcoles, & Albein-Urios, 2019).

Focus on Diversity and Culture

Substance Abuse Treatment

Although there is growing interest in culturally sensitive treatment for SUDs, evidence regarding outcomes, especially among young people, is lacking (Steinka-Fry, Tanner-Smith, Dakof, & Henderson, 2017). However, nursing as a profession recognizes the importance of providing culturally sensitive care, acknowledging that "when people feel understood and supported within the context of their values and beliefs, treatment outcomes are better" ("Culturally Competent," 2013). This includes awareness of culturally informed behaviors and cues. The lack of cultural awareness in treatment is thought to be partially responsible for lower rates of treatment seeking and treatment success among people of color and other diverse populations (Gainsbury, 2017). Other barriers to treatment include cultural stigma, issues of access (such as inadequate health insurance and financial means) and language barriers (Giger & Haddad, 2021).

The efficacy of psychosocial interventions, by themselves or combined with medication, has been well documented. Psychosocial interventions can address psychosocial problems that negatively impact adherence to medical treatments or can help the patient deal with the interpersonal and social challenges present during recovery. Not only are psychosocial interventions effective, but patients often prefer them to medications for SUD (Capone et al., 2018). Psychosocial interventions also can be important to provide an alternative for those for whom medication is inadvisable (such as pregnant women, children, or those with complex medical conditions); to enhance medication adherence; or to deal with the social and interpersonal issues that complicate recovery from mental health and substance use disorders (Institute of Medicine, 2015). One such intervention is the incorporation of trauma-informed care into the overall treatment plan for individuals with alcohol or substance use disorders who have a history of trauma. Implementing trauma-informed services can improve screening and assessment, treatment planning, and placement while also decreasing the risk for retraumatization (Hazelden Betty Ford Foundation, 2018). For more information on trauma-informed care, see Module 32, Trauma.

Behavior-Related Therapies

In **behavioral therapy**, patients learn techniques to modify or change their addictive behaviors. Classic *behavioral modification* therapy is typically used with adolescents. It is based on the principle that all behavior has specific consequences and can be changed by conditioning—a process of **reinforcement**. *Positive reinforcement* provides a reward for the desired behavior or treatment compliance (such as a favorite activity at the end of the week as a reward for improved behavior in class that week). *Negative reinforcement* removes a negative stimulus to increase the chances that the desired behavior will occur (such as removing a chore a child hates if all the other assigned chores are completed) (Letourneau, McCart, Sheidow, & Mauro, 2017).

Cognitive-behavioral therapy (CBT) is often used for a wide array of mental health and substance use disorders. It combines behavioral techniques with cognitive psychology. The goal is to replace maladaptive or inappropriate behaviors and faulty cognitions with thoughts and self-statements that promote adaptive behavior. Variants of CBT include **rational emotive behavior therapy (REBT)**, an active, solution-oriented therapy that focuses on resolving emotional, cognitive, and behavioral problems resulting from faulty evaluation of negative life events (Ellis, 2020), and **dialectical behavior therapy (DBT)**. During DBT, patients are taught how to regulate destructive emotions, practice mindfulness, and better tolerate distress (Behavioral Tech, 2019).

Motivational Interviewing

Many patients have contradictory or ambivalent feelings about their alcohol or other substance use, which may contribute to lack of a desire or will to change. *Motivational interviewing (MI)* is a structured approach to engaging patients by promoting change talk and helping patients become motivated to make change without the nurse or other provider directly giving advice (Miller & Rollnick, 2004). MI is person-centered, using guided conversation without attempting to control the patient. Nurses may use MI to help assess patient readiness for change. In patients with SUDs, therapists and clinicians may use MI more extensively to help patients move through the stages of change. Motivational interviewing and stages of change are covered further in Module 35, Caring Interventions.

Milieu Therapy

A successful recovery environment supports behavior changes, teaches new coping strategies, and helps the patient move from addiction to a sober life. This supportive environment is often referred to as **milieu therapy**. The milieu is a supportive inpatient or outpatient environment where clinicians and staff work with patients to provide safety and structure while assessing the patient's relationships and behavior (Smith & Spitzmueller, 2016). Patients benefit from a consistent routine that fosters predictability and trust. A milieu is considered therapeutic when the program's community provides a sense of civility, membership, belonging, care, and accountability (Smith & Spitzmueller, 2016). A therapeutic milieu can be provided in a variety of inpatient and outpatient settings, and nurses play a pivotal role by modeling and teaching desirable behaviors. An overview of mental healthcare settings and nurses' roles in these environments can be found in Table 7.1 in Module 7, Health, Wellness, Illness, and Injury.

Group Therapy

Therapeutic groups provide support to individual members as they work through problems. During **group therapy**, which is facilitated by a professional group therapist, the group navigates psychologic, cognitive, behavioral, and spiritual dysfunctions.

Groups can be held in the inpatient or outpatient setting, community mental health centers, or other locations. Therapeutic factors of group therapy provide a rationale for a variety of group interventions. **Table 22.2** » describes these factors. See Exemplar 38.A, Groups and Group Communication, in Module 38, Communication, for more information.

TABLE 22.2 Therapeutic Factors of Group Therapy

Factor	Description
Instillation of hope	As patients observe other members further along in the therapeutic process, they begin to feel a sense of hope for themselves.
Universality	Through interaction with other group members, patients realize they are not alone in their problems or pain.
Imparting of information	Teaching and suggestions usually come from the group leader but may also be generated by the group members.
Altruism	Through the group process, patients recognize that they have something to give to the other group members.
Corrective recapitulation of the primary family group	Many patients have a history of dysfunctional family relationships. The therapy group is often like a family, and patients can learn more functional patterns of communication, interaction, and behavior.
Development of socializing techniques	Development of social skills takes place in groups. Group members give feedback about maladaptive social behavior. Patients learn more appropriate ways of socializing with others.
Imitative behavior	Patients often model their behavior after the leader or other group members. This trial process enables them to discover what behaviors work well for them as individuals.
Interpersonal learning	Through the group process, patients learn the positive benefits of good interpersonal relationships. Emotional healing takes place through this process.
Existential factors	The group provides opportunities for patients to explore the meaning of their life and their place in the world.
Catharsis	Patients learn how to express their own feelings in a goal-directed way, speak openly about what is bothering them, and express strong feelings about other members in a responsible way.
Group cohesiveness	Cohesiveness occurs when members feel a sense of belonging.

Source: Based on Yalom and Leszcz (2005).

Support Groups

Because individuals with addictions typically have inadequate social networks, often restricted to fellow substance users, it is important for them to develop more functional support networks that can contribute to increased self-esteem and dignity, a sense of identity, and improved self-responsibility. Nurses frequently refer patients and their families to support groups that allow peers to share their thoughts and feelings and help one another examine issues and concerns. In support groups, members define their own needs, have equal power, and usually participate voluntarily. They may or may not be assisted by a mental health professional. For individuals with substance use issues, group recovery support generally consists of peer-based mentoring, education, and support services provided by individuals in recovery to individuals with SUDs or co-occurring substance use and mental disorders (Smith et al., 2020).

The support group SMART Recovery (Self-Management and Recovery Training) is a global community of mutual-support groups. Participants help one another resolve problems with substance and/or process addictions. The SMART program emphasizes teaching how to increase self-empowerment and self-reliance. SMART features both face-to-face and online support. SMART's recovery program focuses on enhancing and maintaining motivation to abstain; coping with urges; managing thoughts, feelings, and behaviors; and balancing momentary and enduring satisfactions (SMART Recovery, 2020).

Twelve-Step Programs

Twelve-step programs are support groups that offer a spiritual plan for recovery. These include Al-Anon, Narcotics Anonymous, Cocaine Anonymous, Adult Children of Alcoholics, Emotions Anonymous, Gamblers Anonymous, Overeaters Anonymous, and Sex and Love Addicts Anonymous.

The 12-step program consists of prescribed beliefs, values, and behaviors. The sequential plan for recovery is stated in 12 steps. It begins with the individual admitting powerlessness over the substance and continues through steps that help individuals take responsibility for addictive behaviors and seek spiritual awakening in community with others. Step work is considered to be a lifelong process, usually facilitated by a peer sponsor. Twelve-step fellowship includes activities such as helping others, building relationships among members, and sharing joys and hardships. The only requirement for membership in 12-step programs is the sincere desire to change the target behavior.

>> **Stay Current:** The 12 Steps of Alcoholics Anonymous can be found at https://www.aa.org/assets/en_US/smf-121_en.pdf.

Evidence is mixed regarding the effectiveness of 12-step programs, primarily because it is difficult to separate the effects of the program from other concurrent recovery support activities (Smith et al., 2020). Historically, however, AA and similar programs have been mainstays of successful addictions treatment.

Family Therapy

Family behavior therapy (FBT), which has demonstrated positive results in both adults and adolescents, addresses not only substance use problems but other co-occurring problems as well, including conduct disorders, mistreatment of children, depression, family conflict, and unemployment (NIDA, 2018d). In FBT, the patient and at least one significant other, such as a cohabiting partner or a parent (in the case of adolescents), try to apply the behavioral strategies taught in sessions and acquire new skills to improve the home environment.

In the treatment of adolescents, family involvement can be particularly important, since the adolescent will often be living with at least one parent and be subject to the parent's controls, rules, and/or supports (NIDA, 2014, 2018d). Family-based approaches generally address a wide array of problems in addition to the substance problems, including family communication and conflict; co-occurring behavioral, mental health, and learning disorders; problems with school or work attendance; and peer networks. Research shows that family-based treatments are highly effective; some studies even suggest they are superior to other individual and group treatment approaches (NIDA, 2014).

Family-based treatments can be adapted to various settings (e.g., mental health clinics, drug abuse treatment programs, social service settings, families' homes) and treatment modalities. One example is **brief strategic family therapy (BSFT)**. BSFT is based on a family systems approach to treatment, in which one member's problem behaviors appear to stem from unhealthy family interactions. Over the course of 12 to 16 sessions, the BSFT counselor establishes a relationship with each family member, observes how the members behave with one another, and assists the family in changing negative interaction patterns (Brewer, Godley, & Hulvershorn, 2017). Another example is **functional family therapy (FFT)**, which combines a family systems view of family functioning (e.g., unhealthy family interactions underlie an individual's problem behaviors) with behavioral techniques to improve communication, problem-solving, conflict-resolution, and parenting skills. Principal treatment strategies include engaging families in the treatment process and enhancing their motivation for change, as well as modifying family members' behavior using communication and problem solving, behavioral contracts, and other methods (Brewer et al., 2017).

Pharmacologic Therapy

Pharmacologic therapies are available to treat and prevent symptoms of withdrawal and to treat overdose. Treating symptoms of withdrawal may involve reducing physiologic cravings for the drug of choice, but it may also involve reducing anxiety that serves as a stimulus for using a substance or to prevent dangerous symptoms associated with sudden withdrawal from powerful substances such as sedatives and hypnotics. A number of pharmacologic therapies are available. Many of these, however, have multiple drug interactions and should be used with caution. For example, disulfiram (Antabuse) should never be used during pregnancy and should be used with caution in patients taking phenytoin. See **Medications 22.1** for an overview of drugs used to treat addiction and withdrawal manifestations. For more information on benzodiazepines, see Medications 31.1 in Module 31, Stress and Coping.

Medications 22.1

Drugs Used to Treat Addiction and Withdrawal Manifestations

CLASSIFICATION AND DRUG EXAMPLES	MECHANISMS OF ACTION	NURSING CONSIDERATIONS
Drugs for Alcohol Use Disorder ***Drug examples:*** acamprosate disulfiram (Antabuse) naltrexone (Depade, Vivitrol) clorazepate (Tranxene-T) oxazepam	Acamprosate restores the normal balance of gamma-aminobutyric acid (GABA) and glutamate that are disrupted by drinking alcohol and decreases cravings and emotional distress from discontinuing alcohol. Disulfiram blocks the oxidation of any alcohol that is consumed. Naltrexone is also indicated for alcohol use disorder. These benzodiazepine anti-anxiety drugs are specifically indicated to treat alcohol withdrawal.	▪ Disulfiram can cause flushing of the face, headache, vomiting, and other unpleasant sensations if alcohol is consumed. ▪ Disulfiram can cause an adverse drug interaction if taken with: anticonvulsant drug (phenytoin [Dilantin]) antipsychotic drug (clozapine [Clozaril]); antiretroviral drugs (atazanavir [Reyataz], tipranavir [Aptivus]); benzodiazepine drugs (chlordiazepoxide, diazepam [Valium]); muscle relaxant drugs (chlorzoxazone [Lorzone], tizanidine [Zanaflex]); phosphodiesterase (PDE) inhibitor drug (theophylline [Elixophyllin]) ▪ Naltrexone will cause opioid withdrawal if given to an individual who has not detoxed.
Nicotine Replacement Drugs ***Drug examples:*** NicoDerm CQ (transdermal patch) Nicorette (gum or lozenge) Nicotrol (inhaler, nasal spray)	Supply the body with nicotine to support a gradual smoking cessation therapy.	▪ Patient support is an important element of smoking cessation, and patients benefit from cognitive-behavioral therapy in addition to pharmacotherapy.
varenicline (Chantix)	Stimulates nicotine receptors to a lesser degree than nicotine itself does, reducing cravings for and decreasing the pleasurable effects of nicotine.	▪ Assess for nicotine withdrawal symptoms such as depression, agitation, and exacerbation of preexisting mental health disorders. ▪ Suicide and suicidal ideation have been associated with use of varenicline. Assess patients for thoughts of suicide or changes in mood and affect.

Medications 22.1 *(continued)*

CLASSIFICATION AND DRUG EXAMPLES	MECHANISMS OF ACTION	NURSING CONSIDERATIONS
Antidepressants ***Drug examples:*** bupropion (Aplenzin, Wellbutrin SL)	Block dopamine and norepinephrine uptake in the brain to reduce the craving for nicotine. Also help to reduce depression occurring as the result of substance withdrawal.	■ Monitor and assess for suicidal ideation. ■ Assess for drug side effects, including drowsiness, insomnia, and blurred vision. ■ Teach patient about self-administration of medications and symptoms to report. ■ Teach patient not to mix drug with alcohol because of increased risk of seizures and sedation. ■ Teach patient that antidepressants can take 3–4 weeks to become effective and not to discontinue abruptly; medication should be tapered off.
Benzodiazepines ***Drug examples:*** alprazolam (Xanax) chlordiazepoxide clorazepate (Tranxene-T) diazepam (Diastat, Valium) lorazepam (Ativan) oxazepam *Note:* Greater clinical benefits are observed in longer-acting forms of benzodiazepines (ASAM, 2020a).	Diminish anxiety associated with withdrawal; anticonvulsant qualities help provide safe withdrawal. May be ordered every 4 hr or as needed to manage effects from withdrawal; then dose is tapered to zero.	■ Monitor for oversedation. ■ Caution patients not to mix with alcohol or other CNS depressants; can cause respiratory depression. ■ Potential for addiction; should be used for short term only. ■ Taper dosage; stopping abruptly may trigger seizures.
Opioid Antagonists ***Drug example:*** naloxone (Evzio, Narcan)	Block opioid receptor sites and quickly reverse the effect of an opioid drug. Can be used for opioid overdose if administered intravenously.	■ Monitor patient condition, including respiratory rate, and anticipate the need for pain management as narcotic effects are reversed.
Opioid Drugs ***Drug examples:*** methadone (Methadose) naltrexone (Depade, Vivitrol)	Bind to opiate receptors in the CNS. Used during supervised withdrawal for patient with opioid use disorder. Naltrexone blocks any opioid drugs the patient may try to self-administer.	■ Methadone is addictive (Schedule II) and can be abused. Monitor for cardiac arrhythmias. Overdose can cause respiratory depression, especially if mixed with alcohol. ■ Naltrexone will cause opioid withdrawal if given to an individual who has not detoxed.
Opioid Agonist–Antagonists buprenorphine (Buprenex, Suboxone)	Approximately 30× greater agonist activity than morphine and up to 3× antagonist activity of naloxone.	■ Contraindicated in cases of significant respiratory depression or asthma without resuscitative equipment. ■ Prolonged use during pregnancy can cause life-threatening neonatal abstinence syndrome (NAS). ■ Monitor respiratory status ■ Monitor intake and output as urinary retention is a potential adverse effect. ■ Monitor liver function tests and renal function tests.
Vitamins ***Drug examples:*** folic acid multivitamins thiamine (vitamin B_1)	Prevent alcohol-related Wernicke encephalopathy. Correct vitamin deficiency caused by heavy, long-term alcohol abuse.	■ May not be absorbed properly in patients with impaired liver function. ■ High-dose folic acid may increase risk of heart attack in some patients. ■ Water-soluble vitamin overdoses can cause nausea and diarrhea.

SAFETY ALERT! Drugs of abuse alter the brain's structure and function, resulting in changes that persist long after drug use has ceased. This may explain why individuals with SUDs are at risk for relapse even after long periods of abstinence and despite the potentially devastating consequences (NIDA, 2018a).

Lifespan Considerations

Addiction in Children and Adolescents

As stated earlier, addiction can have wide-ranging effects on the family. Children of parents or caregivers who abuse substances are at greater risk for abuse, neglect, or other trauma. Poor communication and family systems may impact children well into adulthood. Unfortunately, children exposed to substance abuse at home are at greater risk for using substances as adolescents.

During adolescence, the prefrontal cortex—the part of the brain that helps individuals to assess situations, make sound decisions, and moderate emotions and impulses—is still developing. Thus, adolescents are at risk for making poor decisions about trying drugs or continuing to take them. Unfortunately, introducing drugs during this period of development may cause brain changes that have profound and long-lasting consequences (NIDA, 2018a). Abusing drugs during adolescence can interfere with meeting crucial social and developmental milestones and also compromise cognitive development. For example, heavy marijuana use in the teen years may cause a loss of several IQ points that are not regained even if users later quit in adulthood (Levine, Clemenza, Rynn, & Lieberman, 2017).

Among adolescents, alcohol appears to be a preferred substance. In 2018, 2.2 million adolescents ages 12 to 17 surveyed reported drinking alcohol, and 1.2 million of them reported binge drinking (CBHSQ, 2019). In the same year, an estimated 2.1% of adolescents reported having a marijuana use disorder (CBHSQ, 2019).

Although cigarette smoking among adolescents has decreased since 2011, current (past 30 days) use of e-cigarettes has increased among both middle and high school students. In 2019, one of every 10 middle school students (10.5%) reported that they used electronic cigarettes in the past 30 days—an increase from 0.6% in 2011 (Centers for Disease Control and Prevention [CDC], 2019e).

Addiction in Pregnant Women

Since 2017, there has been an increase of substance use in pregnancy, particularly marijuana use (CBHSQ, 2019). Tobacco is the substance used most often by pregnant women (11.6%), followed by alcohol (9.9%) and marijuana (CBHSQ, 2019).

Alcohol, nicotine, illicit drugs, and some prescription drugs are considered **teratogens**—agents that interrupt development or cause malformation in an embryo or fetus. Alcohol use during pregnancy can lead to FASDs and other adverse birth outcomes, while substance use or abuse can cause neonates to experience substance dependence and withdrawal symptoms, low birth weight, neurologic issues, developmental delays, and other issues (CBHSQ, 2019; National Center on Substance Abuse and Child Welfare, 2018). It is generally assumed that pregnant women who use alcohol or illicit drugs during pregnancy are continuing behaviors started prior to pregnancy. For this reason, health promotion related to substance use and abuse is important for all women seeking to become pregnant and at each healthcare interaction with the pregnant woman.

Addiction in Older Adults

Substance abuse in older adults is believed to be underestimated, underidentified, underdiagnosed, and undertreated. Until relatively recently, alcohol and prescription drug misuse, which affects a growing number of older adults, was not discussed in either the substance abuse or the gerontologic literature. By 2020, it has been estimated that SUDs among adults over age 50 will increase to 5.7 million, up from 2.8 million in 2006 (Minkove, 2019).

Insufficient knowledge, limited research data, and hurried office visits are cited as causes for why HCPs often overlook substance abuse and misuse in this population. Diagnosis is often difficult because symptoms of substance abuse in older individuals sometimes mimic symptoms of other disorders common among this population, such as diabetes, dementia, and depression. In addition, many older adults do not seek treatment for substance abuse because they do not feel they need it or because they feel hopeless about positive outcomes (SAMHSA, 2020b).

Impaired Nurses

Since 1982, the American Nurses Association (ANA) has stressed the need for peer assistance programs to support nurses who engage in substance use or abuse. In 2016, the ANA joined with the International Nurses Society on Addictions and the Emergency Nurse Association in their commitment to peer assistance programs offered by most—but not all—of the state boards of nursing. These programs offer comprehensive monitoring and support services to reasonably ensure the safe rehabilitation and return of the nurse to the professional community (ANA, 2020b).

Nurses and other HCPs are as susceptible as any other individuals to developing an SUD. They often work in highly stressful work settings with easy access to drugs. Prevalence of impairment or recovery from alcohol or drug addiction among nurses is estimated at between 10 and 20% of all nurses (Foli, Reddick, Zhang, & Edwards, 2019; Starr, 2015). Length of treatment and motivation are associated with successful recovery, with nurses who remain in treatment for at least a year being twice as likely to achieve long-term sobriety.

Nurses are expected to act when they suspect another nurse is working under the influence of a substance. The ANA Code of Ethics for Nurses (2020a) provides a framework for patient safety. Suggestions for implementing its philosophy include:

- Do not ignore poor performance.
- Do not lighten or change the nurse's patient assignment.
- Do not accept excuses.
- Do not allow yourself to be manipulated or fear confronting a nurse if patient safety is in jeopardy.

State boards of nursing provide information about impaired nurse programs, including drug diversion (the transfer of a legally controlled substance to a person other

TABLE 22.3 Warning Signs of Impaired Nurses in the Workplace

At-Risk Situations	Observable Warning Signs
Easy access to prescription drugs	Inaccurate narcotic counts or drugs frequently missing
	Patient complaints of ineffective pain control; denial of having received pain meds
	Excessive "wasting" of drugs
	Likelihood of volunteering to give medications to patients
	Frequent trips to the bathroom
Role strain	Frequent tardiness or absenteeism, especially before and after scheduled days off
	Haphazard, shoddy charting
	Judgment errors in patient care
	Unorganized, erratic behavior; unkempt appearance
Depression	Irritability; unable to focus or concentrate
	Abrupt mood swings
	Isolating self; taking long breaks
	Apathetic, depressed, lethargic
	Unexplained absences from assigned unit
Signs of alcohol or drug use	Smell of alcohol on breath
	Excessive use of perfumes, mouthwash, or mints
	Slurred speech, flushed face, reddened eyes, unsteady gait
	Long sleeves worn in hot weather to cover up arms
Signs of withdrawal	Tremors, restlessness, sweating
	Watery eyes, runny nose, stomachaches

Source: From Bauldoff, Gubrud, and Carno (2020). Pearson Education, Inc., Hoboken, NJ.

than for whom it was prescribed). Warning signs of impaired nurses in the workplace are listed in **Table 22.3** ».

The ANA (2020b) has stated that nurses with substance abuse problems not only pose a potential threat to their patients, but they also tend to neglect their own health and well-being. Nurses with addiction issues may be reluctant to report themselves because of shame, guilt, or fear of job loss. The ANA encourages nurses to self-report and contact peer assistance programs offered by their state nursing organization or state board of nursing. Resources vary by state but are generally accessible through each state association's website. Many state boards of nursing offer programs designed to guide nurses to sobriety, rather than instituting immediate disciplinary consequences. Nurses who feel they are developing a substance abuse problem are ethically required to seek help in order to prevent mistakes in the workplace.

SAFETY ALERT! Student nurses may believe that CBD oils (cannabidiol), used as medical marijuana for anxiety, depression, pain, nausea, seizures, and other health problems, cannot be detected by a drug test. Unfortunately, trace amounts of THC (tetrahydrocannabinol, a compound that is the main active ingredient of cannabis) can be detected in some oils, depending on how they have been manufactured (Bonn-Miller et al., 2017).

Case Study » Part 3

It is 36 hours post-ED admission, and Paul is being transferred from the trauma unit to a semiprivate room on a general medical–surgical unit. His scalp laceration is healing; there is no evidence of further head injury. Paul's right humerus was fractured in the crash and a cast applied following a closed reduction. Laboratory studies revealed a blood alcohol level of 0.28 on admission. Paul now appears mildly anxious and has a mild visible hand tremor. He is being prepared for discharge tomorrow. Admission to a substance abuse treatment program is being considered.

Clinical Reasoning Questions Level I

1. List at least three nursing care priorities that would apply to Paul.
2. What members of the interprofessional (IP) healthcare team should be involved in Paul's care and discharge planning? Delineate the role of each team member.
3. Consider the impact of Paul's addiction on him and on his entire family.
4. Can Paul be treated independently of his family?
5. Give some specific examples of how family involvement could be planned by members of the IP team.

Clinical Reasoning Questions Level II

6. Identify comprehensive, measurable long-term treatment goals for Paul and his family.
7. Discuss inpatient, outpatient, and community treatment options for Paul and his family. Consider the advantages and disadvantages of each.
8. Consider the impact of cognition (both Paul's and his family's) in Paul's long-term treatment plan.
9. What lifestyle changes may be necessary for Paul and his family?

REVIEW The Concept of Addiction

RELATE Link the Concepts

Linking the concept of addiction with the concept of family:

1. In a family with rigid boundaries—those in which rules and roles remain fixed under all circumstances—what approach(s) might be optimal for gaining trust in and building a therapeutic relationship?
2. Considering the many treatment options for those with addictions, design a comprehensive treatment plan to meet the needs of a family such as the one that we have been exploring through our case study, the John family.

Linking the concept of addiction with the concept of immunity:

3. Dietary support is an essential component of recovery. Describe the diagnostic assessment for deficiencies in the B-complex vitamins, particularly thiamin, folate, and B_{12}, and the fat-soluble vitamins, A, D, and E.
4. Why are individuals with addictions prone to opportunistic infection?

READY Go to Volume 3: Clinical Nursing Skills

REFER Go to Pearson MyLab Nursing and eText

REFLECT Apply Your Knowledge

Max Brown is a 68-year-old man, in apparent good health with unremarkable labwork, who came to the ambulatory surgery center for elective gallbladder surgery. During the laparoscopic surgery, which started at 1:00 p.m., the surgeon noted some inflammation that made visualization of the gallbladder difficult. There was also more bleeding than expected. The surgeon converted the surgery into an open cholecystectomy, and the procedure was finished without any further issues.

After recovery in the perianesthesia unit, Mr. Brown is sent to the medical–surgical floor and arrives on the floor at 7:30 p.m. His wife joins him and remains at the bedside until 11:00 p.m. Aside from some occasional pain at the incision site, which is treated successfully with oral oxycodone/acetaminophen, Mr. Brown spends most of the night resting. On postoperative day 1, he is to ambulate. He receives two remaining doses of intravenous antibiotics because of the open surgery. If Mr. Brown progresses as anticipated, the surgeon expects to discharge him in the early evening.

When the day-shift nurse makes her initial morning assessment, Mr. Brown is restless but alert and oriented × 4. At noon, he is extremely restless, but knows he is in the hospital and reports some pain at the incision site. At 4:00 p.m., Mr. Brown is trying to get out of bed and leave the hospital; he knows who he is but thinks he is in the men's room at a local sports arena. By the time Ms. Brown arrives at 6:30 p.m., Mr. Brown is agitated and aggressive, trying to hit anyone approaching his bed. The attending physician is notified, and her adult nurse practitioner (ANP), who is rounding in the hospital, comes to Mr. Brown's room. After looking at recent vital signs of T 99.9°F, HR 110, and BP 165/98 mmHg, the ANP orders a dose of intramuscular ziprasidone for agitation. After vigorously objecting to the shot, Mr. Brown eventually calms somewhat, but his eyes dart around the room and he hisses and startles occasionally, throwing his hands over his head. When asked, he reports seeing buzzards in the room. The ANP asks the night-shift nurse (who requests the CNA to stay with Mr. Brown while she left the room) and Ms. Brown to join her in a small family meeting room.

During the conference, the ANP states that she suspects Mr. Brown was going into alcohol withdrawal delirium. She asks Ms. Brown about his social history. Ms. Brown reports that she and her husband moved to a nearby upscale retirement community 6 or 7 years ago. Mr. Brown had been suddenly retired from the investment firm he worked, when the company collapsed because of poor management and was acquired by a competitor. Ms. Brown shares that they moved to another state, stabilized their living expenses, and they are now "comfortable." Mr. Brown had worked at his job for 35 years, was devoted to the company, and enjoyed his job. He was "devastated" when his job ended and was "anguished" when executives of his former company were vilified online for bad business decisions. Since his move, Mr. Brown has been a "little down," but he has thrown himself into charitable endeavors, serving on a number of boards and committees. Ms. Brown says that her husband is a "moderate" social drinker, who drinks four large vodka tonics every night and never appears to be drunk. She seems surprised that the ANP thinks her husband is withdrawing from alcohol.

1. Why do you think the ANP immediately suspected alcohol withdrawal? What were the clues that led her in that direction?
2. Do you think Mr. Brown has some unresolved psychosocial issues from his forced retirement? Are there any underlying mental health issues that may need treatment?
3. What will likely happen to Mr. Brown now? How will his hospital plan of care change? What orders are commonly on a detox protocol?
4. What will be Mr. Brown's discharge plan after he has been stabilized in the hospital? What will be Ms. Brown's role?

Exemplar 22.A Alcohol Use Disorder

Exemplar Learning Outcomes

22.A Analyze the manifestations and treatment considerations for patients with an addiction to alcohol.

- Describe the pathophysiology of alcohol abuse.
- Describe the etiology of alcohol abuse.
- Compare the risk factors and prevention of alcohol abuse.
- Identify the clinical manifestations of alcohol abuse.
- Identify the clinical manifestations of alcohol withdrawal.
- Summarize diagnostic tests and therapies used by interprofessional teams in the collaborative care of an individual with an alcohol use disorder.
- Differentiate the care of patients across the lifespan who abuse alcohol.
- Apply the nursing process to promote patient safety during withdrawal and detoxification.
- Apply the nursing process in providing culturally competent care to an individual with alcohol use disorder.

Exemplar Key Terms

Alcohol dependence, *1713*
Alcohol intoxication, *1716*
Alcohol overdose, *1716*
Alcohol use disorder, *1713*
Alcohol withdrawal delirium, *1717*
Alcohol withdrawal syndrome, *1717*
Alcoholism, *1713*
Binge drinking, *1713*
Blackouts, *1717*
Confabulation, *1716*
Craving, *1714*
Fetal alcohol syndrome (FAS), *1719*

Overview

Alcohol includes liquor, beer, and wine. While much of society sees the use of nicotine and drugs as inappropriate, use of alcohol is still socially acceptable and often encouraged. Alcohol is frequently offered at family events, beer is the favorite drink at sports venues across the country, and many grocery stores and restaurants offer wine tastings. Alcohol's availability may be the primary reason it is the most commonly used and abused substance in the United States, with 70% of adults reporting that they drink alcohol at least once each year (National Institute on Alcohol Abuse and Alcoholism [NIAAA], 2020a). The most recent estimate of the economic costs of alcohol abuse in the United States is $249 billion annually (CDC, 2020e). These costs result from losses in workplace productivity, healthcare expenses for problems caused by excessive drinking, law enforcement and other criminal justice expenses related to excessive alcohol consumption, and motor-vehicle crash costs from impaired driving (CDC, 2020e).

In 1992, the Joint Committee of the National Council on Alcoholism and Drug Dependence and the American Society of Addiction Medicine defined **alcoholism** as a "primary, chronic disease with genetic, psychosocial, and environmental factors influencing its development and manifestations" (Morse & Flavin, 1992). It is characterized by the behaviors discussed in the Concepts section of this module: inability to control the primary addictive behavior (drinking), fixation with the drug and continued use of it regardless of consequences, and impaired thought processes. The terms *alcoholism, alcohol abuse,* and *alcohol use disorder* are often used interchangeably. However, it should be noted that an individual can abuse alcohol to the extent that it impairs function and results in life-threatening symptoms without developing addiction behaviors or dependency. Alcoholism and **alcohol use disorder** (AUD) more specifically refer to a chronic disease process with specific, identifiable manifestations and patterns. Clinicians following the guidelines of the ASAM may be more likely to use the term *alcoholism*, whereas those adhering to the DSM-5 may be more likely to use the term *alcohol use disorder*. Nurses working in all settings should be able to identify acute manifestations of both abuse and withdrawal, as well as patterns of dependence.

The pattern of **alcohol dependence** varies from person to person. Moderate drinking is defined as up to one drink per day for women and up to two drinks per day for men—and only by adults of legal drinking age (U.S. Department of Health and Human Services & U.S. Department of Agriculture, 2020). The measurement of a standard drink is shown in **Figure 22.3** ».

Some people regularly drink large amounts of alcohol daily. Others restrict their use to heavy drinking on weekends or days off from work, often drinking copious amounts in a single session, a pattern of consumption known as **binge drinking**. Binge alcohol use is defined as drinking five or more drinks on the same occasion on at least 1 day in the past 30 days. *Heavy alcohol use* is defined as drinking five or more drinks on the same occasion on 5 or more days in the past 30 days (CBHSQ, 2019). Many individuals who engage in binge drinking begin doing so in college. College alcohol consumption has been linked with adverse consequences such as alcohol poisoning, drug overdoses, sexual assaults, and alcohol-impaired driving, which accounts for the majority of alcohol-related deaths among college students nationwide (NIAAA, 2020b).

Some people are able to abstain for long periods of time and then begin dysfunctional drinking patterns again. At times, individuals with alcohol dependence can drink with control; at other times, they cannot control their drinking behavior. As the course of alcoholism continues, addiction behaviors appear with increasing frequency. These may include starting the day off with a drink, sneaking drinks throughout the day, shifting from one alcoholic beverage to another, and hiding bottles at work and at home. An individual with alcoholism may find that drinking—or being sick from drinking—has often interfered with home or family duties, caused trouble at school or work, and created legal difficulties resulting from impaired driving (SAMHSA, 2018a).

» **Stay Current:** Visit the website of the National Institute on Alcohol Abuse and Alcoholism to see current research on alcohol dependence: http://www.niaaa.nih.gov/research.

Pathophysiology

As a CNS depressant, alcohol acts on neurotransmitters such as GABA. GABA plays a role in the inhibiting and depressing action of the autonomic nervous system. Alcohol interacts with GABA to further depress the autonomic nervous system, further inhibiting arousal. Because of this interaction, the combination of alcohol with one or more additional CNS depressants can be particularly dangerous, increasing risk for respiratory depression and death. Long-term, excessive use of alcohol can lead to damage in the cerebral cortex, hippocampus, and cerebellum.

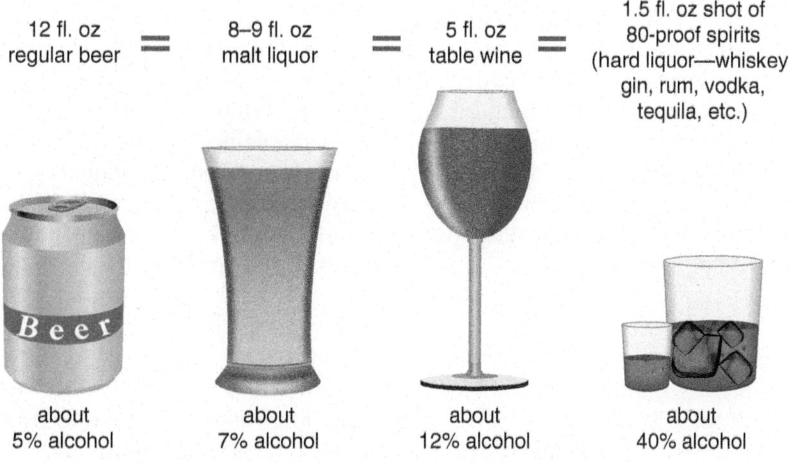

Figure 22.3 » One standard drink = $\frac{1}{2}$ oz of ethyl alcohol.

Following absorption through the mouth, stomach, and digestive tract, alcohol enters the bloodstream. Approximately 95% of alcohol reaches the liver, where it is metabolized by the antidiuretic hormone–aldehyde dehydrogenase enzymatic system. The rest is excreted through the kidneys, lungs, and skin. Typically, it takes approximately 90 minutes for the body to break down one standard drink—1.5 ounces of distilled spirits or liquor, 5 ounces of wine, or 12 ounces of beer. Factors that affect this rate are varied but include height, weight, sex, liver function, and food consumption.

Etiology and Epidemiology

Alcoholism is a complex disorder with many pathways leading to its development. Research has long suggested that certain people develop a different, more powerful relationship with alcohol than others. Researchers believe that genetics, epigenetics (changes in the body caused by modification of gene expression rather than alteration of the genetic code itself), and other biological factors significantly influence the development of alcohol dependence, along with cognitive, behavioral, temperament, psychologic, and sociocultural factors. Alcohol use patterns, including alcohol abuse and alcohol dependence, are familial in nature, with genetics making up 50% of the risk for alcohol and drug dependence (Edenberg, Gelernter, & Agrawal, 2019; Lovallo et al., 2019). Similar styles of alcohol use and the presence of alcoholism are often found within the same family, running from parent to child and across multiple generations of biologically related individuals (Alvanzo et al., 2017).

There are some cultural differences in alcohol use. In 2018, white populations were more likely than other racial/ethnic groups to report current use of alcohol (56.7%). The rates were 46% for persons reporting two or more races, 43% for Black populations, 41.7% for Hispanics, 35.4% for Native Hawaiians or other Pacific Islanders, 35.9% for American Indians or Alaska Natives, and 39.3% for Asians (CBHSQ, 2019). Researchers have examined biological differences among groups, including the effect of alcohol-metabolizing genes on drinking behaviors and the effects of alcohol consumption in populations with health disparities, with no findings that have translated into treatment interventions (NIAAA, 2020a).

Mood and substance use disorders commonly co-occur with alcoholism (Schoenthaler et al., 2017). *Dual diagnosis* and *dual disorder* are older terms used to describe an individual who has both a diagnosis of substance abuse and a mental illness. For example, an individual with a depressive disorder may self-medicate with alcohol to treat the depression, or someone with alcoholism may become depressed. Research has found that medications for managing mood symptoms can be effective in individuals with substance abuse; however, these medications do not necessarily impact the SUD, further strengthening the argument for integrative treatment of co-occurring substance abuse and mental illness (Vitali et al., 2018).

Prevalence

In 2018, a total of 139.8 million Americans aged 12 and older reported current use of alcohol, 67.1 million reported binge alcohol use in the past month, and 16.6 million reported heavy alcohol use in the past month (CBHSQ, 2019). Worldwide, 3 million deaths every year result from harmful use of alcohol, which represents 5.3 % of all deaths (World Health Organization [WHO], 2020a).

In the United States, approximately one of every 11 adolescents reported using alcohol in the past month (CBHSQ, 2019). In younger users, negative outcomes from alcohol use include interference with normal adolescent brain development, increased risk of developing AUD, sexual assaults, and injuries (NIAAA, 2020a). Among college-age alcohol users, adverse consequences related to alcohol use include motor-vehicle crashes, assault by another student who has been drinking, alcohol-related sexual assault or date rape, and potential for developing an AUD (NIAAA, 2020b). About one in four college students report academic consequences from drinking (NIAAA, 2020b).

Risk Factors and Prevention

In the past, American Indians experienced alcoholism at higher rates than other populations. Genetics is believed to be a contributing factor to risk for alcohol abuse in American Indians. Although definitive results have not yet been discovered, researchers have found an overlap in the gene location for addiction with that for body mass index. Some American Indians do not have the genes that alter alcohol-metabolizing enzymes and may lack protective variants found in other groups. Some research has implicated genes found in American Indians associated with risk factors for drug sensitivity or tolerance, but more recent research has argued that the incidence of alcoholism among American Indians is not significantly different than other segments of the population (Vaswani, 2019). Specific environmental factors may play a greater role in the elevated risk for addiction among American Indians. These include trauma exposure, early-onset substance use, and environmental hardship (Fish, Osberg, & Syed, 2017).

Sociocultural factors influence risk for alcohol abuse. Demographic characteristics that have been associated with higher rates of substance use include lower educational levels and lack of meaningful familial relationships. There is some evidence that systemic stigma or discrimination against some groups, such as American Indians, may contribute to increased risk for alcohol abuse (Skewes & Blume, 2019).

Stigma and discrimination may also play a role in substance abuse risk among the LGBTQ (lesbian, gay, bisexual, transgender, and queer/questioning) population. Research has indicated that, when compared with the general population, LGBTQ individuals are more likely to use alcohol and drugs, have higher rates of substance abuse, are less likely to abstain from use, and are more likely to continue heavy drinking into later life (NIDA, 2017; Wallace & Santacruz, 2017). Although strides have been made toward validating and normalizing LGBTQ sexual and emotional expression, LGBTQ individuals experience stigma, internalized homophobia, skewed social norms, lack of access to care, and trauma at higher rates than other populations (Kerr & Oglesby, 2017).

Clinical Manifestations of Alcohol Abuse

Occasional use of alcohol may produce mild euphoric effects. However, excessive use of alcohol can lead to serious clinical manifestations and consequences, including diminished function and life-threatening conditions (see the Clinical Manifestations and Therapies feature). **Craving**, a compelling

Clinical Manifestations and Therapies

Alcohol Abuse

CUES	CLINICAL MANIFESTATIONS	CLINICAL THERAPIES
Delirium tremens as a result of sudden withdrawal of alcohol	▪ Confusion ▪ Disorientation ▪ Agitation ▪ Severe autonomic instability ▪ Perceptual disturbances ▪ Hallucinations (primarily visual but may be tactile) ▪ Tremors of extremities ▪ Anxiety, panic, and paranoia	▪ Prescribe benzodiazepines, specifically clorazepate (Tranxene-T) and oxazepam, that are indicated for alcohol withdrawal. ▪ Reduce stimuli but keep well lit to minimize visual misinterpretations. ▪ If present, treat with antiseizure medications.
Cirrhosis of the liver resulting from damage done by chronic alcoholism	▪ Spider angiomata ▪ Palmar erythema ▪ Muehrcke nails, Terry nails, or clubbing ▪ Hypertrophic osteoarthropathy ▪ Dupuytren contracture ▪ Gynecomastia ▪ Hypogonadism ▪ Hepatomegaly ▪ Ascites ▪ Splenomegaly ▪ Jaundice ▪ Asterixis ▪ Weakness, fatigue, anorexia, weight loss	▪ Explain that cirrhosis cannot be reversed but abstaining from alcohol can delay or prevent further damage. ▪ Emphasize abstaining from alcohol. ▪ Stop any medications that are potentially damaging to the liver, such as acetaminophen. ▪ Consider abdominocentesis to reduce ascites. ▪ Monitor ammonia levels. ▪ Prevent complications such as esophageal varices, hepatic encephalopathy, and hepatorenal syndrome. ▪ Monitor for delayed coagulation times and apply pressure to punctures for 10 minutes.
Assaultive behaviors	▪ Sexual assault in adolescents and young adults is commonly related to alcohol use. ▪ Because of the release of inhibitions, control of emotions such as anger is reduced. ▪ Access to weapons increases the risk of assaultive behavior becoming homicide. ▪ Spousal or child abuse has strong link to alcohol ingestion.	▪ Promote sobriety. ▪ Encourage management classes. ▪ Provide crisis intervention for family members who have been assaulted. ▪ Provide follow-up counseling to reduce posttraumatic stress response.
Esophageal varices, which may result from portal hypertension due to cirrhosis	▪ Hematemesis ranging from mild to severe ▪ Heartburn ▪ Black or tarry stools ▪ Decreased urination secondary to hypotension ▪ Light-headedness ▪ Shock ▪ Weight loss ▪ Weakness, fatigue, jaundice ▪ Pruritus of hands and feet ▪ Edema of lower extremities ▪ Mental confusion	▪ Encourage abstinence from alcohol. ▪ Perform emergency surgery to stop bleeding, involving removal of part of the esophagus or cauterization of varicosities. ▪ Perform therapeutic endoscopy. ▪ Monitor intake and output. ▪ Take vital signs frequently during bleeding episodes to monitor for shock. ▪ Administer fluids via IV therapy. ▪ Administer beta adrenergic blockers, if necessary, to reduce incidence of bleeding.
Gastritis	▪ Esophageal reflux ▪ Decreased appetite ▪ Recurrent diarrhea	▪ Provide foods that will not exacerbate GI symptoms while meeting nutritional requirements. ▪ Teach patient to remain upright for 3–4 hours following meals; eat small, frequent meals; and avoid gas-producing foods. ▪ Antidiarrheals, antacids, and H_2 blockers may be appropriate medications to reduce symptoms.

(continued on next page)

Clinical Manifestations and Therapies *(continued)*

CUES	CLINICAL MANIFESTATIONS	CLINICAL THERAPIES
Wernicke encephalopathy	▪ Ataxia ▪ Abnormal eye movements ▪ Mental confusion ▪ Short-term memory loss	▪ Provide for patient safety. ▪ Place clocks and calendars to reduce mental confusion. ▪ Assess cognition and document findings. ▪ Administer IV or IM thiamine. ▪ Avoid glucose administration until after thiamine administration. ▪ Hydrate patient.

urge to consume alcohol, is a potent, distracting symptom that many individuals who abuse alcohol find particularly challenging.

Behavioral signs of alcohol abuse include focus on the acquisition of alcohol, its overuse, and inability to reduce or stop drinking (Mayo Clinic, 2020a). Other negative behaviors include impairment in role function, risky consumption, and strong cravings to drink. As AUD progresses, it takes over most aspects of an individual's life.

Some physiologic symptoms are developing a tolerance to alcohol so that the individual needs more alcohol to feel its effect or having a reduced effect from the same amount and experiencing withdrawal symptoms—such as nausea, sweating, and shaking—when not consuming alcohol or drinking to avoid these symptoms (APA, 2013; Mayo Clinic, 2020a).

Alcohol Intoxication and Overdose

Alcohol intoxication is the presence of clinically significant behavioral or psychologic changes due to alcohol use. Changes may include any combination of inappropriate sexual or aggressive behavior, mood lability, impaired judgment, and impaired social or occupational functioning (APA, 2013). Signs of alcohol intoxication include nausea and vomiting, lack of coordination, slurred speech, staggering, disorientation, irritability, short attention span, loud and frequent talking, poor judgment, lack of inhibition, and (for some) violent behavior. Alcohol intoxication may result in accidents or falls that cause contusions, sprains, fractures, and facial or head trauma. Evidence of mild intoxication can be seen after two drinks, with signs and symptoms of intoxication becoming more intense as the blood alcohol level (BAL or EtOH) increases (APA, 2013). High BALs may result in unconsciousness, coma, respiratory depression, and death.

Alcohol overdose (also known as *alcohol poisoning*) is a toxic condition that results from excessive consumption of large amounts of alcohol in a very short period of time. At BALs greater than 300 mg/dL, the symptoms of intoxication become greatly intensified. Signs and symptoms of alcohol overdose include excessive sleepiness; amnesia; difficulty waking the patient; coma; serious decreases in pulse, temperature, blood pressure, and rate of breathing; urinary and bowel incontinence; and, eventually, death (APA, 2013). Advanced states of intoxication and alcohol poisoning are critical situations in the ED and necessitate careful triage and monitoring to prevent death or permanent disability.

BALs are highly predictive of CNS effects. At 0.10%, ataxia and dysarthria occur. From 0.20 to 0.25%, the person is unable to sit or stand upright without support. Between 0.3 and 0.4%, slipping into a coma is possible. Toxic levels in excess of 0.5% can cause death. Note that individuals with chronic alcoholism might have BALs in these ranges, but not have the same consequences because of their developed tolerance to the effect of drinking (Medline Plus, 2020a). In the United States, the legal threshold of intoxication is typically 0.08%.

Consequences of Chronic Use

Long-term alcohol use contributes to more than 200 diseases and injury-related health conditions, including alcohol dependence, liver cirrhosis, cancers, pancreatitis, myocardial disease, erosive gastritis, and injuries. In 2018, 5.1% of the global burden of disease and injury (139 million disability-adjusted life years) was attributable to alcohol consumption (WHO, 2020a).

Malnutrition is another serious complication of chronic alcoholism. Thiamine (B_1) deficiency in particular can result in neurologic impairments, such as Wernicke-Korsakoff syndrome (WKS). WKS typically consists of two components, a short-lived and severe condition called Wernicke encephalopathy (WE) and a long-lasting and debilitating condition known as Korsakoff psychosis (Arts, Walvoort, & Kessels, 2017). WE is an acute, life-threatening neurocognitive disorder with symptoms that include mental confusion, paralysis of the nerves that move the eyes, and impaired coordination (e.g., ataxia). Approximately 80–90% of individuals with WE develop Korsakoff psychosis, a chronic neuropsychiatric syndrome characterized by behavioral abnormalities and memory impairments. Patients with Korsakoff psychosis have difficulties remembering old information; they are also unable to acquire new information (Arts et al., 2017; National Institute on Neurological Disorders and Stroke, 2020). They also frequently use **confabulation**, making up information to fill in memory blanks.

Another common consequence of thiamine deficiency and long-term alcohol consumption is cerebellar degeneration, caused by atrophy of certain regions of the cerebellum, the brain area involved in muscle coordination. Cerebellar degeneration is associated with difficulties in movement coordination and involuntary eye movements, such as nystagmus. Cerebellar degeneration is found both in those abusing alcohol with WKS and in those without it (Arts et al., 2017; Zahr & Pfefferbaum, 2017).

Chronic consumption of alcohol not only produces tolerance, but it creates cross-tolerance to general anesthetics, barbiturates, benzodiazepines, and other CNS depressants. If alcohol is withdrawn abruptly, the brain becomes overly excited because previously inhibited receptors are no longer inhibited. This hyperexcitability manifests clinically as anxiety, tachycardia, hypertension (HTN), diaphoresis, nausea and vomiting, tremors, sleeplessness, and irritability. Severe manifestations of alcohol withdrawal include seizures, convulsions, and DTs. Complications of DTs include respiratory failure, aspiration pneumonitis, and cardiac arrhythmias.

Alcohol Abuse and Memory

Alcohol primarily interferes with the ability to form new long-term memories. Large amounts of alcohol, particularly if consumed rapidly, can produce partial or complete **blackouts**, periods of memory loss for events that occurred while a person was drinking. Blackouts are much more common among social drinkers—including college drinkers—than was previously assumed, and blackouts have been found to encompass events ranging from conversations to sexual intercourse (Miller et al., 2019). Mechanisms underlying alcohol-induced memory impairments include disruption of activity in the hippocampus, a brain region that plays a central role in the formation of new memories (Van Skike, Goodlett, & Matthews, 2019). A more advanced CNS problem is Wernicke-Korsakoff syndrome, described previously.

Some research has indicated that dementia occurs as much as five times more often in older adults with alcoholism than in nondrinkers, but the exact underlying biochemical mechanism has not yet been discovered (Wiegmann, Mick, Brandl, Heinz, & Gutwinski, 2020). The issue of the effects of alcohol consumption have on dementia is confusing because modest consumption appears actually to reduce the risk of dementia (Koch et al., 2019).

Alcohol Withdrawal

Mild alcohol withdrawal generally consists of anxiety, irritability, difficulty sleeping, and decreased appetite. The signs and symptoms of acute alcohol withdrawal generally start 6 to 24 hours after the individual takes the last drink. Alcohol withdrawal may begin when the patient still has significant blood alcohol concentrations. The signs and symptoms of acute alcohol withdrawal (**alcohol withdrawal syndrome**) may include the following: agitation; anorexia (lack of appetite); nausea and vomiting; tremor (shakiness), elevated heart rate, and increased blood pressure; insomnia, intense dreaming, and nightmares; poor concentration and impaired memory and judgment; increased sensitivity to sound, light, and tactile sensations; hallucinations (auditory, visual, or tactile); delusions, usually paranoid or persecutory; grand mal seizures resulting in loss of consciousness, brief cessation of breathing, and muscle rigidity; hyperthermia; delirium with disorientation; and fluctuation in level of consciousness (LOC) (Harvard Health Online, 2019; SAMHSA, 2015a).

Alcohol withdrawal delirium, sometimes referred to as delirium tremens, usually occurs on days 2 and 3 but may appear as late as 14 days after the last drink consumed. The major goal of medical management is to avoid seizures and DTs, typically with aggressive use of higher doses of benzodiazepines coupled with antiseizure medications (Harvard Health Online, 2019). DTs do not develop suddenly, but instead progress from earlier withdrawal symptoms. Properly administered medication and adherence to detoxification protocols will prevent DTs and limit possible overmedication. During acute withdrawal, the individual experiences confusion, disorientation, hallucinations, tachycardia, hypertension or hypotension, extreme tremors, agitation, diaphoresis, and fever. Death may result from cardiovascular collapse or hyperthermia (SAMHSA, 2015a). Alcohol withdrawal delirium occurs in about 8% of hospitalized patients with AUD; with early detection and appropriate treatment, the expected mortality is in the range of 1% or less (Jesse et al., 2017).

Collaboration

When caring for a patient who abuses alcohol, the nurse works as a collaborative member of a team that may include physicians, psychologists, counselors, nutritionists, and assistive personnel who share the goal of helping the patient achieve sobriety. Individuals may also work with a peer counselor or specialist through recovery programs such as AA or other 12-step programs. If the recovery program is associated with a treatment facility, the peer specialist may be part of the interprofessional team.

Diagnostic Tests

The simplest method of detecting blood alcohol content is by using a breathalyzer. BALs are the main biologic measures for assessment purposes. Knowledge of the symptoms associated with a range of BALs is helpful in ascertaining level of intoxication, level of tolerance, and whether the individual accurately reported recent drinking. At 0.10% (after 5 to 6 drinks in 1 to 2 hours), voluntary motor action becomes clumsy, resulting in ataxia and dysarthria. The degree of impairment varies with sex, weight, and food ingestion. Small women who drink alcohol on an empty stomach achieve intoxication more quickly than large men who have eaten a full meal. At 0.20–0.25% (after 10 to 12 drinks in 2 to 4 hours), function of the motor area in the brain is depressed, causing an inability to remain upright (Medline Plus, 2020a). A level above 0.10% without associated behavioral symptoms indicates the presence of tolerance. High tolerance is a sign of physical dependence.

Assessing for withdrawal symptoms is important when the BAL is high. Medications given for treatment of withdrawal from alcohol are usually not started until the BAL is below a set norm (usually below 0.10%) unless withdrawal symptoms become severe. Measurement of BAL may be repeated several times, several hours apart, to determine the body's metabolism of alcohol and at what time it is safe to give the patient medication to minimize the withdrawal symptoms.

Biomarkers are lab tests that suggest heavy alcohol consumption by detecting the toxic effects that alcohol may have had on organ systems or body chemistry. Included in this class are the serum measures of gamma glutamyl transferase (GGT), aspartate amino transferase (AST), alanine amino transferase (ALT), mean corpuscular volume (MCV), high-sensitivity C-reactive protein (hs-CRP), and interleukin-6 (IL-6) (Archer et al., 2019). Another indirect alcohol biomarker is carbohydrate-deficient transferrin (CDT); an elevation in

CDT can indicate heavy alcohol consumption. Other biomarker laboratory tests include ethyl glucuronide (EtG) and ethyl sulfate (EtS), usually measured in urine. EtG and EtS are often used to monitor abstinence in clinical and justice system settings (Reisfield et al., 2020).

Treatment of Withdrawal

All CNS depressants can cause potentially dangerous withdrawal symptoms. In managing any substance withdrawal, the goal is to minimize adverse outcomes to the patient, regardless of severity, and to prevent adverse effects resulting from the use of withdrawal medications. Close monitoring is essential, and patients experiencing alcohol withdrawal may require critical care if co-occurring medical conditions (such as liver cirrhosis or diabetes) are present or if high doses of benzodiazepines are needed as part of the treatment protocol. Medications such as the benzodiazepines clorazepate (Tranxene-T) and oxazepam are a first-line therapy used to minimize the discomfort associated with alcohol withdrawal and to prevent serious adverse effects, particularly seizures (Long, Long, & Koyfman, 2017).

Healthcare providers may order one of several treatment approaches, including fixed-schedule dosing, symptom-triggered dosing, or a combination of the two. The CIWA-Ar scale has traditionally been used by many facilities to assess the severity of symptoms of acute alcohol withdrawal (Chen et al., 2017). However, clinicians have criticized the scale because it requires subjective assessment of withdrawal symptoms, takes up to 5 minutes to administer, and may not be appropriate for patients with more severe alcohol withdrawal symptoms who cannot participate in reporting (Chen et al., 2017). As a result, there has been increased interest in more brief and objective instruments to assess alcohol withdrawal symptoms, such as the Prediction of Alcohol Withdrawal Severity Scale (PAWSS) and Luebeck Alcohol-Withdrawal Risk Scale (LARS) that use different criteria to identify patients at risk of developing severe alcohol withdrawal syndrome (Wood et al., 2018). For example, the PAWSS uses a combination of patient-reported criteria along with BAL>200 mg/dL and signs of increased autonomic activity (such as a heart rate greater than 120, tremors, nausea, and agitation) to gauge the likelihood of severe withdrawal. Interactive versions of the CIWA-Ar and the PAWSS are available at mdcalc.com.

SAFETY ALERT! Close attention to vital signs and presence of withdrawal symptoms is essential when a patient is withdrawing from alcohol. Trending the vital signs and CIWA-Ar, PAWSS, or LARS scores over time can often show when an individual may be heading into DTs. Preventive steps, such as aggressive use of prn medications and application of protocols, should be used to prevent DTs from occurring.

Pharmacologic therapies used in the treatment of alcohol abuse include acamprosate, disulfiram (Antabuse), and naltrexone (Depade, extended-release Vivitrol). (See Medications 22.1.) Disulfiram prevents the breakdown of alcohol, causing intense vomiting if taken while drinking any form of alcohol, including over-the-counter cough medicines. Naltrexone blocks the pathways to the brain that cause euphoria when a substance is used; it helps reduce cravings. Patients should avoid taking any type of narcotic, such as codeine, morphine, or heroin, while on naltrexone. Because naltrexone taken while the individual is still on opioids will trigger withdrawal, it should not be used until a patient has been off all narcotics for 7 to 10 days. Patients taking naltrexone should wear a medical alert bracelet to prevent administration of contraindicated medications in the event of an emergency.

Disulfiram and naltrexone are not stand-alone treatments. Patients taking them should also participate in nonpharmacologic therapies such as AA meetings, individual counseling, or group therapy to prevent relapse. AA meetings and therapy provide support and reinforce patients' efforts to continue treatment. Peer connections made through AA can help encourage sobriety.

Complementary Health Approaches

Alternative and complementary therapies are not usually employed by themselves to treat alcohol withdrawal. They are, however, generally used in a comprehensive, integrated substance abuse treatment system that promotes health and well-being, provides palliative symptom relief, and improves treatment retention. Acupuncture has been used to reduce the craving for a variety of substances, including alcohol, and appears to contribute to improved treatment retention rates. If used correctly, acupuncture may effectively reduce alcohol intake, attenuate alcohol withdrawal syndrome, and rebalance alcohol-induced changes in neurotransmitters and hormones in related brain areas (Chen et al., 2018).

There has been renewed interested in electroencephalographic neurofeedback (EEG-NF), also called *neurotherapy*, as an add-on therapy to the cognitive therapy used to maintain abstinence (Dousset et al., 2020). Traditional Chinese medicine supports administration of herbal products such as *Pueraria lobata* to provide some benefit in the treatment of alcoholism; however, their use has not been supported by controlled studies in the United States (Liu, Shi, & Lee, 2019).

Lifespan Considerations

In recent years, research has focused on discovering the differences in how alcohol affects individuals at different ages, using subsequent findings to determine appropriate interventions and treatment protocols. Some of the characteristics of various ages and gender differences throughout the lifespan are detailed in this section.

Alcohol Use Among Adolescents

More youth in the United States drink alcohol than smoke tobacco or marijuana, making it the drug most used by American young people. Nationally, 9% of adolescents (or one in 11) reported using alcohol in 2018, and one in 21 adolescents (1.2 million, or 4.7%) reported binge drinking during the past month (CBHSQ, 2019).

Many adolescents start to drink at very young ages. In the United States, by age 15, about 29.8% of all teens have had at least one drink; by age 18, about 58% of all teens have had at least one drink (NIAAA, 2019, 2020c). Individuals who reported starting to drink before the age of 15 were four times more likely to also report meeting the criteria for alcohol dependence at some point in their lives (NIAAA, 2020c). The younger children and adolescents are when they start to drink, the more likely they will be to engage in risky behaviors. Adolescents who engage in binge drinking are more likely to use illicit substances, have sex with more partners, and earn poor grades in school (NIAAA, 2020c).

Factors implicated in adolescent use of alcohol include:

- ***Sensitivity and tolerance to alcohol.*** Differences between the adult brain and the brain of the maturing adolescent also may help to explain why many young drinkers are able to consume much larger amounts of alcohol than adults before experiencing the negative consequences of drinking, such as drowsiness, lack of coordination, and withdrawal/hangover effects. This unusual tolerance may help to explain the high rates of binge drinking among young adults. At the same time, adolescents appear to be particularly sensitive to the positive effects of drinking, such as feeling more at ease in social situations, and they may drink more than adults because of these positive social experiences (Taylor & Miloh, 2018).
- ***Personality characteristics and psychiatric comorbidity.*** Children who begin to drink at a very early age (before age 12) often share similar personality characteristics, such as hyperactivity and aggression. These young people, as well as those who are depressive or anxious, may be at greatest risk for alcohol problems. Other behavior problems associated with alcohol use include rebelliousness, difficulty avoiding harmful situations, and acting out without regard for rules or the feelings of others (Li et al., 2017).
- ***Environmental aspects.*** Parental and peer consumption of alcohol play a role in how adolescents view and use alcohol. The impact of the media also is believed to be a significant influence. Greater exposure to alcohol advertising contributes to an increase in drinking among underage youth (NIAAA, 2020c).
- ***Exposure to adverse childhood experiences.*** Exposure to adverse childhood experiences (such as abuse or other trauma) is a known risk factor for adolescent alcohol and substance use (Zarse et al., 2019).

Communicating with Patients

Working Phase

Teens often minimize the impact of problem drinking behaviors and resist being referred to treatment or support organizations. To counter this resistance, nurses may need to reinforce reality with direct, yet nonconfrontative, questions and statements. A nurse in an acute care setting where teens are treated with alcohol-related injuries may discuss these issues:

- I am concerned that you were driving, wrecked your mother's car, and your BAL (blood alcohol level) is twice the legal limit.
- Do not yell at me or the phlebotomist. We are trying to help you.
- I heard you say that you are "maybe" interested in attending AA. Can I get some materials to share with you?

Alcohol Use Among Women

Research has supported the concept that women are more vulnerable to the adverse consequences of alcohol abuse than men. No sex difference has been noted for age at onset of regular use, but women use alcohol for fewer years than men before entering treatment. The severity of drug and alcohol dependence has not been shown to differ by sex, but women have reported more severe psychiatric, medical, and employment complications than men (SAMHSA, 2015c).

Compared with men, women experience greater cognitive impairment by alcohol and are more susceptible to alcohol-related organ damage. Women develop alcohol abuse and dependence in less time than do men, a phenomenon known as *telescoping*; women also develop damage at lower levels of consumption over a shorter period of time (SAMHSA, 2015c). Women who drink the same amount as men will have higher blood alcohol concentrations because women have proportionately more body fat and a lower volume of body water to dilute the alcohol. In comparison with men, women have a lower first-pass metabolism of alcohol in the stomach and upper small intestine before it enters the bloodstream and reaches other body organs, including the liver (SAMHSA, 2015c).

Women develop alcohol-induced liver disease over a shorter period of time and after consuming less alcohol, and they are more likely than men to develop alcoholic hepatitis and to die from cirrhosis. Women who are dependent on alcohol or consume greater amounts are more likely to die prematurely from cardiac-related conditions and have an increased risk of HTN (SAMHSA, 2015c; Wilsnack, Wilsnack, Gmel, & Kantor, 2018). Numerous studies have documented associations and suggested causal relationships between alcohol consumption and breast cancer risk, especially among postmenopausal women who are moderate alcohol drinkers and who are using menopausal hormone therapy. Other negative side effects of alcohol abuse for women include osteoporosis, increased cognitive decline and brain atrophy, memory deficits, and an increased risk for Alzheimer disease (SAMHSA, 2015c; Wilsnack et al., 2018).

Alcohol Use Among Pregnant Women

Alcohol use can result in obstetric complications, miscarriage, or significant problems for the fetus. It is difficult to isolate the effects related solely to alcohol on fetal and infant development because women who abuse alcohol may be abusing other substances (Popova, 2017; SAMHSA, 2015c).

Above all other drugs, alcohol is the most common teratogen in pregnancy. Alcohol use during pregnancy is associated with an increased risk of spontaneous abortion, as well as increased rates of prematurity and *abruptio placentae* (premature separation of the placenta from the uterus). Women who consumed five or more drinks per week were three times more likely to deliver a stillborn baby compared with those who had fewer than one drink per week (SAMHSA, 2015c).

Alcohol contributes to a wide range of effects on exposed offspring, known as fetal alcohol spectrum disorders (FASDs). The most serious consequence is **fetal alcohol syndrome (FAS)**, characterized by abnormal facial features, growth deficiencies, and CNS problems (see Module 23, Cognition, for more information on FAS). Women who drink during breastfeeding pass alcohol on to the baby (Popova, 2017). Patient teaching must emphasize that the ***only*** way to prevent FAS is to abstain from all alcohol of all types for the entire duration of pregnancy. This message should be communicated to all female patients of childbearing age, including teenagers, so they understand how important it is to stop drinking immediately if they become pregnant. Nurses should also explain that the most dangerous time for fetal alcohol exposure may be early in pregnancy—often before a woman even knows she's expecting.

Alcohol Use Among Older Adults

Nearly 16.2 million older adults over the age of 65 drank alcohol in the past month, with 3.4 million reporting binge alcohol use and 772,000 reporting heavy alcohol use (CBHSQ, 2017; Solomon, 2019). About 55.2% of adults age 65 and over drink alcohol (Grant et al., 2017). Older adults who abuse alcohol have a greater risk for numerous physical problems and premature death. Public health clinicians have suggested that people over age 65 should have no more than 7 drinks a week and no more than 3 drinks on any one day (Kaiser Permanente, 2020).

Alcohol interacts negatively with the natural aging process to increase risks for HTN, certain cancers, liver damage and cirrhosis, immune system disorders, and brain damage (Kaiser Permanente, 2020). Alcohol can worsen some health conditions such as osteoporosis, diabetes, HTN, and ulcers. It can also cause changes in the heart and blood vessels, which can dull cardiac pain, leading to delayed diagnosis of impending heart attacks (Kaiser Permanente, 2020). Alcohol can cause older adults to be forgetful and confused, symptoms that could be mistaken for signs of Alzheimer disease, other dementias, and depression (Koch et al., 2019).

Mixing prescription and over-the-counter medicines or herbal remedies with alcohol can be dangerous or even deadly for older adults, who routinely take medications for chronic health issues. Medications that cause problems when mixed with alcohol include aspirin, which increases the risk of stomach or intestinal bleeding; cold and allergy medicines containing antihistamines, which can cause drowsiness or sleepiness; and acetaminophen, which can cause liver damage (Holton, Gallagher, Ryan, Fahey, & Cousins, 2017). Cough syrups and laxatives that have a high alcohol content will create an additive effect with alcohol, causing the blood alcohol level to increase, and may cause intoxication. Alcohol combined with some sleeping pills, opioid pain pills, or antianxiety/antidepressant medications can cause respiratory difficulties leading to death (Holton et al., 2017).

Because depression and alcohol abuse are the most frequently found disorders in completed suicides, nurses should routinely screen older adults for concurrent substance abuse and mental disorders. Prevention of drinking relapse in older adults who abuse alcohol can be equivalent to and often more successful than in younger patients (Sacco, Kuerbis, & Harris, 2020).

NURSING PROCESS

Patients who abuse alcohol may present in any setting. The sensory impairments and increased risk-taking behaviors associated with alcohol use can lead to injuries that require medical attention, so nurses will encounter these patients in primary care offices, emergency departments and urgent care settings, and medical–surgical units. Occupational nurses may encounter these patients in employee assistance programs, and school nurses may encounter adolescents who abuse alcohol. Alcohol abuse treatment programs also employ nurses. Many programs are provided through outpatient settings, but inpatient detoxification (short-term) and therapeutic settings (10 to 28 days) are also available in many communities. While many patients participate in treatment voluntarily, those that have had a charge of driving under the influence or a finding of child abuse or neglect may be participating under a court order.

Assessment

There have been many research studies that have shown that a high number of patients presenting in primary or acute care settings are at risk for alcohol abuse. The USPSTF (2018) recommends screening for unhealthy alcohol use in primary care settings in all adults 18 years or older, including pregnant women, and providing persons engaged in risky or hazardous drinking with brief behavioral counseling interventions to reduce unhealthy alcohol use.

The USPSTF (2018) determined that brief one- to three-item screening instruments have the best accuracy for assessing unhealthy alcohol use in adults. The recommended instruments include the abbreviated Alcohol Use Disorders Identification Test–Consumption (AUDIT-C) and the NIAAA-recommended Single Alcohol Screening Question (SASQ). The Cutdown, Annoyed, Guilty, Eye opener (CAGE) tool is well known, but primarily detects alcohol dependence rather than the full spectrum of unhealthy alcohol use (USPSTF, 2018).

Many providers discover unhealthy alcohol behaviors in patients by using DSM-5 criteria. Discussion includes the following topics (APA, 2013; National Council for Behavioral Health [NCBH], 2018):

- Amounts of alcohol consumed, frequency, time spent acquiring alcohol, time spent thinking about alcohol use, previous efforts to stop using
- Cravings, tolerance, and withdrawal symptoms
- Effects of alcohol use on family, work, school, or recreational obligations and activities
- If use is continuing despite persistent or recurrent effects of relationships or despite potentially hazardous outcomes (such as driving under the influence)
- Awareness of the persistent and recurring physical and psychological problems caused by alcohol.

When unhealthy alcohol use is detected, behavioral counseling interventions vary. Primary care settings often use the SBIRT approach, which involves the provider giving general feedback to patients on how their drinking fits within recommended limits and how their alcohol use compares with that of others (USPSTF, 2018). Patients who are willing are then referred to an appropriate level of treatment. Screening and behavioral counseling interventions in the primary care setting can reduce unhealthy drinking behaviors in adults, including heavy episodic drinking, high daily or weekly levels of alcohol consumption, and exceeding recommended drinking limits (USPSTF, 2018).

When screening reveals unhealthy use of alcohol, nurses should inquire further about trauma history and screen for comorbid psychiatric disorders (NCBH, 2018). In the absence of a history of trauma or previously diagnosed psychiatric disorders, screening for symptoms of depression and anxiety is a good starting point.

Observation and Physical Assessment

Signs and symptoms of alcohol use may present when a patient is actively drinking or when withdrawing from alcohol.

The signs and symptoms of *alcohol withdrawal* include nausea and vomiting, diaphoresis, agitation and anxiety, headache, tremor, seizures, and visual and auditory hallucinations (many patients who are not disoriented can have hallucinations) (Thompson, Lande, Kalapatapu, Talavera, & Xiong, 2020).

>> **Skills:** See Skills 1.1 Appearance and Mental Status Assessment and 1.22 Neurologic System: Assessing in Volume 3.

The signs and symptoms of *alcohol withdrawal delirium* include tachycardia and HTN, temperature elevation, and delirium (e.g., auditory and visual hallucinations) (Thompson et al., 2020). Alcohol withdrawal delirium is a medical emergency.

SAFETY ALERT! Alcohol withdrawal symptoms present within 8 hours after the last drink and usually peak within 24 to 72 hours. Patients with severe liver impairment and other physical complications may exhibit withdrawal symptoms for as long as a week after the last drink.

Diagnosis

Nursing care priorities are individualized to specific patient needs and may include the following:

- Risk of injury
- Potential for violence against self or others
- Denial
- Inadequate or poor coping
- Undernutrition
- Lack of knowledge about disease or its effect on others
- Potential for impaired liver function
- Impaired family functioning
- Confusion.

Planning

Goals for patient care depend on patient needs. The patient who denies a problem with alcohol will have far different needs than the patient experiencing withdrawal, participating in an alcohol abuse program, or facing serious complications from years of abuse. Possible goals may include the following:

- The patient will admit alcohol is controlling their life.
- The patient will agree to enter an alcohol treatment facility or outpatient program.
- The patient will experience no complications (or no further complications) as a result of alcohol abuse or alcohol withdrawal.
- The patient will achieve optimal nutritional status.
- The patient will remain sober.
- The patient will participate in a support group, such as AA.

Implementation

During recent years, addiction specialists have sought to develop an efficient system of care that matches patients' clinical needs with an appropriate care setting in the least confining and most cost-effective manner, a practice known as *least restrictive care* (NIDA, 2018d).

Unlike in the past, when patients in active withdrawal were always monitored in acute care settings, today's patients are more likely to withdraw from alcohol in community-based *social detoxification* programs with limited medical oversight (SAMHSA, 2015b). Care settings include residential rehabilitation programs, halfway houses, and partial hospitalization programs. Community and faith groups often operate social detoxification programs that may or may not have clear procedures for pursuing appropriate medical referral and emergency care. An advantage of these outpatient programs is that they provide structured environments while allowing the patient to maintain a viable presence in the community.

Another trend is *home detoxification*. ED and family physicians are now implementing outpatient alcohol detoxification guidelines with pharmacotherapy for individuals with mild to moderate alcohol withdrawal symptoms and no serious psychiatric or medical comorbidities (Nadkarni et al., 2017). Many of these protocols advocate daily office, home, or telehealth visits.

Unsupervised withdrawal is often accompanied by poor physiologic and psychologic outcomes. As described earlier, withdrawal is a particularly high-risk event, when potentially dangerous withdrawal symptoms—confusion; seizures accompanied by rapid heartbeat, high blood pressure, and hyperthermia; DTs; and coma leading to death—occur. Safety is a paramount concern. Equally important after detoxification are promoting physical recovery from alcohol addiction, enhancing coping skills, and providing referrals to services that prepare the patient for long-term abstinence from alcohol use. Among these necessary referrals are vocational counseling, self-help groups such as AA, and individual, group, and family therapy.

Patients with trauma histories may perceive themselves as having fewer options (Grasser et al., 2020). In addition, they may avoid engaging in treatment because it is one step closer to addressing their trauma. These patients may exhibit challenging behaviors and need a longer course of treatment.

Caring interventions are based on the patient's need, individualized plan of care, and goals set for care throughout the course of treatment. For all patients, nurses will work to promote healthy coping skills (see Module 31, Stress and Coping) to help patients reduce the need to use alcohol as a coping mechanism. In addition, patients who abuse alcohol require health promotion related to maintaining adequate nutrition, and in particular should take thiamine supplements as necessary to prevent complications from chronic alcoholism. Specific interventions to help patients begin the path to recovery from alcohol abuse follow.

Promote Patient Safety During Acute Withdrawal

As stated earlier in the Concept, close monitoring and following of agency protocols is necessary to ensure patient safety during acute withdrawal. BAL and vital signs provide the most reliable information about withdrawal symptoms and may signal the need for medication to prevent DTs or other severe complications. The benzodiazepines clorazepate (Tranxene-T) and oxazepam help minimize the discomfort of withdrawal symptoms by binding to receptors in the limbic system and reticular formation in the brain to enhance the effect of GABA, a neurotransmitter that helps inhibit neuron activity. Vitamins and nutritional supplements also support neurologic health. Administer medications as ordered and assess patient level of orientation frequently.

Promote Safety in Outpatient and Home Settings

When an individual initiates outpatient or home care, obtain a drug history as well as urine and blood samples for laboratory analysis of substance content. Subjective history often is not accurate, and knowledge regarding substance use is important for accurate assessment and determining the appropriate care setting.

- Assess orientation and cognition. If the patient's level of cognitive functioning is not sufficient to implement the outpatient or home plan of care, contact an HCP who can evaluate the patient, and assist in transfer to a higher level of care, if needed.
- Have the patient (if able) or others in the home or community setting monitor vital signs frequently during the first day of detox using reliable home equipment, and several times per day subsequently. Teach the patient and lay personnel about the signs and symptoms of severe withdrawal and make sure they understand when they should notify the HCP or seek emergency care.
- Administer or teach the patient/others to administer scheduled medications according to the detoxification protocol. Monitor vital signs and symptoms such as increasing agitation and a change in LOC to determine whether the patient should remain in outpatient or home care. Use vital signs to determine whether prn medications are indicated.
- Monitor for signs of alcohol intoxication. Some patients will start drinking again when withdrawal symptoms become too distressing.
- Suggest that the patient remain in a quiet room to decrease excessive stimuli. Monitor for excessive hyperactivity or agitation, which may indicate severe withdrawal symptoms, and suicidal ideation. These symptoms indicate that the patient may need emergency care.
- Determine specific risks to patient safety. Make sure that the patient is oriented to reality and the environment. Ensure that potentially harmful objects are stored outside the patient's immediate area, so that the patient cannot harm self or others if disoriented and confused.

Promote Healthy Self-Esteem

Research has long documented a relationship between addiction and poor self-esteem. Steps that patients may take to boost self-esteem include the following (Hartney, 2020; Nakhaee, Vagharseyyedin, Afkir, & Mood, 2017):

- Expressing appreciation for and showing kindness to others.
- Making and recognizing positive changes, even incremental progress and small gains.
- Engaging in assertive communication to express needs in a healthy way.
- Refusing to let others misuse them.

Provide Patient Education

Patient education begins with assessment of patient's level of knowledge, readiness to learn, and motivation to learn and begin the recovery process. Begin by teaching simple concepts and progress to more complex issues as the patient responds. Include physiologic effects of alcohol, process of physical and psychologic dependence, and increased risks associated with alcohol consumption. For pregnant women, provide patient teaching about the risks to the fetus.

Patients are at highest risk for relapse within the first few months of stopping use of alcohol. An acronym that many therapists use to assist the patient in recognizing some behaviors that lead to relapse is HALT:

Hungry
Angry
Lonely
Tired.

Nurses should also emphasize the importance of a balanced diet, adequate sleep, healthy recreational activities, and a caring support system to prevent relapse.

Evaluation

The patient is evaluated on the ability to meet goals set during the planning stage of the nursing process. Potential expected outcomes include the following:

- The patient in the acute, community, or home setting undergoes withdrawal without physiologic complications.
- The patient controls anxiety to the extent the patient refrains from drinking when anxiety levels rise.
- The patient displays new coping mechanisms.
- The patient does not start using alcohol again.
- The patient does not experience any new physiologic or psychologic complications as a result of sobriety.
- The patient accepts responsibility for how their behavior impacts the family unit.

New nurses may be surprised to see how often patients with an AUD return to drinking. Between 40 and 60% of people who have been treated for addiction or alcoholism relapse within a year (NIDA, 2018a). There are many factors associated with maintenance of sobriety, including psychiatric comorbidity, AUD severity, craving, use of other substances, health, and social factors (Sliedrecht, de Waart, Witkiewitz, & Roozen, 2019). In contrast, a supportive social network, self-efficacy, and purpose and meaning in life seem to be protective factors against AUD relapse.

When revaluating the plan of care, nurses should consider factors such as the patient's physiologic health, mental health, coping responses, legal involvement, vocational involvement, housing, peers, and social and spiritual support. Other factors hindering sobriety include the success of the transition from rehab to home, engagement with aftercare, motivation and ambivalence toward recovery, and unrealistic expectations. After considering all of these factors, the clinician should work with the patient to modify the plan of care to accommodate these new circumstances.

Nursing Care Plan

A Patient Experiencing Withdrawal from Alcohol

George Russell, age 58, fell at home, landing on his wrist. His wife took him to the ED, where an open reduction and internal fixation of his right wrist was performed under general anesthesia in the operating room. He was admitted to the postoperative unit for observation following surgery because he required large amounts of anesthesia during the procedure.

Mr. Russell has a ruddy complexion and looks older than his stated age. He discloses that he was laid off from his factory job 2 years ago and has been working odd jobs until last week, when he was hired by a local assembly plant. His father was a recovering alcoholic, and his 30-year-old son has been treated for alcohol abuse in the past. Mr. Russell states that he knows alcoholism runs in the family, but he believes that he has his drinking under control. However, he cannot remember the events that led up to his fall and how he might have broken his wrist.

ASSESSMENT	DIAGNOSES	PLANNING
During the nursing assessment, Mr. Russell is hesitant to provide information and refuses to make eye contact. Prior to his operation, a BAL was drawn because the ED nurse detected alcohol on his breath. His BAL was 0.40%, which is five times the legal limit for intoxication. His vital signs are within the upper limits of normal, but he is confused and disoriented with slurred speech and a slight tremor of the hands. He is 6 feet tall and weighs 140 pounds. His total albumin is 2.9 mg, and he has elevated liver enzymes. His wife states that he rarely eats the meals she prepares because he is usually drinking and has no appetite for food.	■ Poor coping skills ■ Potential for injury ■ Poor nutrition related to drinking and poor appetite	■ The patient will express his true feelings associated with using alcohol as a method of coping with stressful situations. ■ The patient will identify three adaptive coping mechanisms he can use as alternatives to alcohol in response to stress. ■ The patient will verbalize the negative effects of alcohol and agree to seek professional help with his drinking. ■ The patient will be free of injury as evidenced by steady gait and absence of subsequent falls. ■ The patient will gain 1 lb (0.45 kg) per week without evidence of increased fluid retention. Serum albumin levels will return to normal range.

IMPLEMENTATION

- Establish a trusting relationship with the patient and spend time with him discussing his feelings, fears, and anxieties.
- Consult with a physician regarding a schedule for medications during detoxification and observe the patient for signs of withdrawal syndrome.
- Explain the effects of alcohol abuse on the body and emphasize that prognosis is closely associated with abstinence.
- Teach a relaxation technique that the patient believes is useful.
- Provide community resource information about self-help groups and, if the patient is receptive, a list of meeting times and phone numbers.
- Consult with a dietitian to determine the number of calories needed to provide adequate nutrition and a realistic weight. Document intake and output and calorie count.
- Consult with a physician to begin vitamin B_1 (thiamine) and dietary supplements.

EVALUATION

Mr. Russell is discharged from the postoperative unit without complications. He successfully undergoes detoxification and contacts the employee assistance program at his new place of employment. He is on medical leave while his arm completely heals and now attends AA meetings 5 days a week. He reports that he enjoys taking long walks with his wife in the warm weather and that his appetite has returned. He has gained 10 pounds in the past 6 weeks and feels better physically than he has in many years.

CRITICAL THINKING

1. Explain why, during the initial nursing assessment, it would be important to ask questions about Mr. Russell's medication history and his use of other medications.
2. Mr. Russell asks you to explain the risks of taking disulfiram (Antabuse). What should you tell him?
3. Develop a care plan for Mr. Russell to address the nursing problem of poor nutrition. Why is this care plan necessary?

REVIEW Alcohol Use Disorder

RELATE Link the Concepts and Exemplars

Linking the exemplar of alcohol use disorder with the concept of comfort:

1. Why might the patient who has detoxified from alcohol have trouble sleeping?
2. What nursing care might you provide to improve the patient's ability to sleep?

Linking the exemplar of alcohol use disorder with the concept of infection:

3. What pathophysiology would increase the risk for infection in the patient who chronically abuses alcohol?
4. What nursing care would you provide this patient to reduce the risk of infection?

Linking the exemplar of alcohol use disorder with the concept of legal issues:

5. The nurse, working in an ED, admits a patient accompanied by a police officer who requests that a serum BAL be drawn and tested for use in a court case related to the patient's driving while intoxicated. What are the patient's legal rights, and what legal obligations does the nurse have regarding this patient's right of privacy?

Linking the exemplar of alcohol use disorder with the concept of safety:

6. The nurse is caring for a patient who was brought to the ED with a BAL of 0.32%. The patient is somnolent, is speaking in incomplete sentences that are garbled and difficult to understand, and has a laceration on his forehead. He is admitted to the acute care facility for observation. How will you assess this patient's neurologic status to determine whether there is an alteration in LOC reflecting a brain injury or alcohol intoxication?

READY Go to Volume 3: Clinical Nursing Skills

REFER Go to Pearson MyLab Nursing and eText

REFLECT Apply Your Knowledge

Candy Collins, a 46-year-old wife and mother of two, comes to her primary care provider's office seeking help for alcohol abuse. She says her husband has threatened to leave her and take her children with him if she doesn't stop. The nurse determines that Mrs. Collins drinks at least five or six alcoholic beverages daily, usually starting after dinner, although sometimes she begins drinking after the children leave for school. The nurse learns that Mrs. Collins's behavior began 5 years ago, shortly after her youngest child began preschool. She denies having blackouts, although she reports occasionally waking in the morning with no memory of the night before.

1. What other data would you want to collect from Mrs. Collins related to her abuse of alcohol?
2. What treatment would you anticipate as appropriate for this patient?
3. What teaching would you provide both Mrs. Collins and her husband?

Exemplar 22.B Nicotine Use Disorder

Exemplar Learning Outcomes

22.B Analyze manifestations and treatment considerations for patients with an addiction to nicotine.

- Describe the pathophysiology of nicotine abuse.
- Describe the etiology of nicotine abuse.
- Compare the risk factors and prevention of nicotine abuse.
- Identify the clinical manifestations of nicotine abuse.
- Summarize diagnostic tests and therapies used by interprofessional teams in the collaborative care of an individual who abuses nicotine.
- Differentiate care of patients across the lifespan who abuse nicotine.
- Apply the nursing process in providing culturally competent care to an individual with a nicotine use disorder.

Exemplar Key Terms

Nicotine, *1724*
Nicotine replacement therapy (NRT), *1727*

Overview

Cigarette smoking is the single most preventable cause of disease and death in the United States. The CDC (2020c) estimates that 480,000 deaths each year are attributable to cigarette smoking. This estimate does not include patients exposed to secondhand smoke or patients who consume nicotine by using chewing tobacco.

Nicotine, a highly addictive chemical found in tobacco, is used worldwide and results in many complications. Nicotine enters the body via the lungs (cigarettes, pipes, and cigars) and oral mucous membranes (chewing tobacco as well as smoking). Although smoking is legal, it has become increasingly socially unacceptable, as evidence of the danger of both smoking and breathing in others' secondhand smoke has been demonstrated. Burning of tobacco releases the active substances in the plant, making it available for absorption via the lungs into the bloodstream.

Commercial tobacco contains more than 7000 chemicals. Among these are nicotine (one of the most addictive substances known to humans), arsenic and hydrogen cyanide (poisons), acetone (a simple ketone that can irritate tissues and is a CNS depressant), and tar (which deposits on the lungs via cigarette smoke and reduces the elasticity of the alveoli, slowing air exchange). Cancer-causing agents in commercial tobacco include nitrosamines, cadmium, benzopyrene, polonium-210, nickel, urethane, and toluidine. As a result of the combination of chemicals entering the bloodstream, smoking has profound effects on virtually every organ system, ranging from HTN due to vasoconstriction to suppression of the immune system.

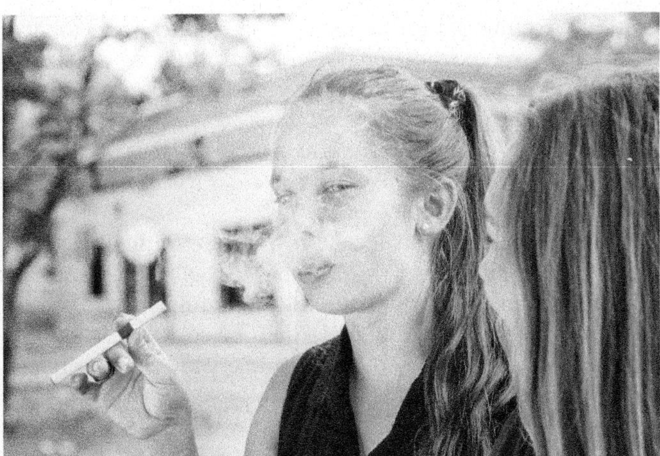

Figure 22.4 ››› At least 2 million teens and young adults are using e-cigarettes. Researchers have yet to determine whether e-cigarettes are actually safe or are simply less harmful than tobacco.

Source: Nicolas McComber/E+/Getty Images.

One public health concern is *vaping* (sometimes called juuling), which uses battery-powered electronic cigarettes (e-cigarettes) that aerosolize liquid (consisting of propylene glycol, glycerol, distilled water, flavorings that may or may not be approved for food use, and preservatives) for inhalation (CDC, 2020a). E-cigarettes often contain nicotine. Consumers, known as *vapers*, may choose from several nicotine strengths, as well as non-nicotine liquids and flavorings. In 2016, the U.S. Food and Drug Administration (FDA) started regulating e-cigarettes as a tobacco product. In 2019, the federal Food, Drug, and Cosmetic Act was amended to raise the federal minimum age of sale of all tobacco products, including e-cigarettes, from 18 to 21 years (FDA, 2020b).

Of particular concern has been the exploding popularity of e-cigarettes among teens and young adults (**Figure 22.4 ›››**). According to the CDC (2020a), in 2019 some 5 million U.S. middle and high school students used e-cigarettes in the past 30 days, including 10.5% of middle school students and 27.5% of high school students.

Originally, e-cigarettes were introduced as a method of helping adults quit smoking traditional nicotine products. While vaping has helped some smokers quit, most adult e-cigarette users do not stop smoking cigarettes and are instead continuing to use both products (known as "dual use") (CDC, 2020a). Other health concerns include defective e-cigarette batteries causing fires and explosions and lung injuries associated with vaping (CDC, 2020i). In summary, the CDC (2020a) has taken the position that e-cigarettes are not safe for youth, young adults, and pregnant women, as well as adults who do not currently use tobacco products.

Pathophysiology

By stimulating nicotinic receptors in the brain, nicotine effects the release of dopamine and epinephrine, causing vasoconstriction. This, in turn, increases blood pressure and heart rate, as well as peripheral vascular resistance, thereby increasing cardiac workload. GI symptoms can result, including increased gastric acid secretion, nausea, and sometimes vomiting. Nicotine can interfere with gas exchanges, reducing the capacity of breathing and increasing risk for respiratory infections and cyanosis.

As mentioned before, researchers have also found an association between ingredients in vaping liquids and lung disease. E-cigarette product use–associated lung injury (EVALI) has been linked with e-cigarette (vaping) products containing vitamin E acetate or tetrahydrocannabinol (THC) (CDC, 2020i). Signs and symptoms of EVALI include respiratory symptoms, such as cough, shortness of breath, or chest pain; GI symptoms, including nausea and vomiting, stomach pain, or diarrhea; and nonspecific body symptoms, such as fever, chills, or weight loss (CDC, 2020j).

Dependence can occur from chronic use, brought on by the dopaminergic processes that reinforce the effects of nicotine. Withdrawal symptoms include craving, restlessness and irritability, sleep disturbance, impaired concentration, increased appetite, and weight gain. Chronic use can lead to chronic obstructive pulmonary disease (COPD), cancer, and high blood pressure.

Etiology and Epidemiology

Some of the most common factors that influence people to smoke are emotions, social pressure, alcohol use, lack of education, and age. Young people are more likely to use tobacco if they have friends, brothers, or sisters who use tobacco; watch movies that have smoking in them; are not doing well in school or have friends who are not doing well in school; are not engaged in school or religious activities; and use other substances, such as alcohol or marijuana (CDC, 2019e). People of lower socioeconomic status (SES) are more likely to smoke than those of higher SES and are more likely to smoke more heavily and for longer periods of time. Furthermore, people with fewer resources are less successful in quitting smoking because they lack high-quality health education, lack support for quitting and access to workplace smoking cessation programs, and are exposed to smoking more often.

In the United States, an estimated 47.0 million people age 12 and older (approximately 17.2% of the population) smoke cigarettes (CBHSQ, 2019). Approximately 571,000 adolescents try cigarette smoking for the first time each year, averaging approximately 1600 adolescents a day (CBHSQ, 2019). In general, teen smoking has been declining slightly in recent years.

On a global scale, nicotine use remains epidemic. Worldwide, tobacco kills more than 8 million people each year, with more than 7 million of those deaths resulting from direct tobacco use and another 1.2 million attributed to secondhand smoke exposure (WHO, 2019). Around 80% of the 1.1 billion smokers worldwide live in low- and middle-income countries, where the burden of tobacco-related illness and death is heaviest (WHO, 2019). Tobacco use contributes to poverty by diverting household spending from basic needs such as food and shelter to tobacco.

Risk Factors

As stated above, young age, low SES, and lack of engagement in activities are among the risk factors for smoking. Smoking itself is a risk factor for a number of diseases. It harms nearly every organ in the body and is a main cause of lung cancer and COPD. Smoking is also a cause of coronary heart disease, stroke, and a host of other cancers and diseases (American Lung Association, 2020). Graves' disease, infertility, early menopause, dysmenorrhea, impotence, osteoporosis, and degenerative disc disease have also been associated with smoking. Other, less serious consequences include discolored teeth and fingernails, premature aging and wrinkling, bad breath, reduced sense of smell and taste, strong smell of smoke clinging to hair and clothing, and gum disease (CDC, 2020k). Smoking during pregnancy has been associated with preterm labor, spontaneous abortion, low-birth-weight infants, sudden infant death syndrome (SIDS), and learning disorders (CDC, 2020m).

Nonsmokers who are exposed to secondhand smoke at home or at work increase their lung cancer risk by 20–30%. Concentrations of many cancer-causing and toxic chemicals are higher in secondhand smoke than in the smoke inhaled by smokers (CDC, 2018). Risks from secondhand smoke include cardiovascular disease and lung cancer. In children, secondhand smoke increases risk for SIDS, respiratory illnesses such as asthma, and otitis media. In addition, mothers who smoke and mothers who are exposed to secondhand smoke are more likely to have lower-birth-weight babies (CDC, 2018). *Thirdhand smoke* is a term referring to residual nicotine and other chemicals left on indoor surfaces by tobacco smoke. Research about the dangers of thirdhand smoke is still inconclusive.

Prevention

Smoking and smokeless tobacco use are initiated and established primarily during adolescence, with nearly 9 out of 10 cigarette smokers first trying cigarette smoking by age 18, and 98% first trying smoking by age 26 (CDC, 2019e). Adolescents and young adults are uniquely susceptible to social and environmental influences to use tobacco, and tobacco companies have traditionally spent billions of dollars on cigarette and smokeless tobacco marketing. However, from 2011 to 2019, use of smokeless tobacco went down among middle and high school students, with fewer than 5 of every 100 students reporting use of smokeless tobacco within the past 30 days (CDC, 2019e).

National, state, and local program activities that have reduced and prevented youth tobacco use in the past have included combinations of the following: mass media campaigns (such as TV, radio, and YouTube commercials), comprehensive school-based tobacco-use prevention policies and programs, and higher costs of tobacco products through increased excise taxes (CDC, 2019e).

Clinical Manifestations

Adverse effects of nicotine use may not manifest until complications (such as COPD, cancer, or heart disease) develop (see the Clinical Manifestations and Therapies feature). Vocal-cord trauma, manifested by a deepening voice, may occur. This is caused by the heat of smoke and the chronic cough often experienced by smokers. See Exemplar 2.F, Lung Cancer, in Module 2, Cellular Regulation, for manifestations of cancers associated with nicotine use; Exemplar 15.C, Chronic Obstructive Pulmonary Disease, in Module 15, Oxygenation, for the impact of smoking on lung function; and Exemplar 16.C, Coronary Artery Disease, and Exemplar 16.J, Peripheral Vascular Disease, in Module 16, Perfusion, for information related to heart disease and peripheral vascular disease.

Clinical Manifestations and Therapies

Nicotine Addiction

ROUTES OF ADMINISTRATION	CLINICAL MANIFESTATIONS	CLINICAL THERAPIES
Smoking cigarettes, cigars, pipes	*Early manifestations* ↑ Wrinkles in the skin, yellowing of fingers and fingernails due to impact on cellular radiation ↓ Sense of smell → smell of smoke in hair, clothing ↑ Restlessness when cigarettes or smoking time curtailed *Late manifestations* ■ Chronic cough ■ COPD ■ Increased mucus production ■ Lung, stomach, bladder, oral, or laryngeal cancers	■ Bronchodilators ■ Expectorants ■ Oxygen therapy ■ Coughing and deep breathing ■ Positioning ■ Smoking cessation ■ Nicotine replacement therapy ■ Chemotherapy ■ Radiation therapy ■ Supportive care (group and individual support and/or therapy, motivational strategies) ■ Pain management
Chewing tobacco	■ Gum disease and gum recession ■ Staining and wearing down of teeth ■ Tooth decay, tooth loss ■ ↑ Risk for cardiovascular disorders ■ Oral cancers (gums, lips, tongue, floor and roof of mouth)	■ Tobacco cessation programs ■ Nicotine replacement therapy ■ Daily dental hygiene and regular professional dental care ■ Supportive care (group and individual support and/or therapy, motivational strategies) ■ Cancer treatment as necessary ■ Pain management as necessary

Collaboration

Individuals who are addicted to nicotine and attempting to quit need the support of family and friends, especially during the first week or so of quitting, when they are unusually irritable. Most pharmacologic products are available over the counter, but patients will cope with tobacco withdrawal better if they have talked with HCPs about approaches to minimize symptoms of withdrawal and are aware of possible side effects from the medications. Internet and in-person support groups are available to help patients in their recovery. Some patients may also choose complementary health approaches such as acupuncture to help them quit.

Nicotine Replacement Therapy

Nicotine replacement therapy (NRT) is available over the counter in the form of chewing gum, lozenges, nasal spray, inhalers, and transdermal patches (see Medications 22.1). Inhalers and nasal sprays are available by prescription only. NRT relieves some of the physiologic effects of withdrawal, including cravings, for patients trying to quit smoking or using tobacco. Keep in mind that nicotine substitution products do not treat underlying psychologic needs or address other addictive behaviors associated with tobacco use. Nurses should caution patients about the contraindications and warnings about NRT before they initiate therapy. Nicotine therapy works best when combined with a smoking cessation program that addresses psychologic issues related to nicotine abuse.

Smoking Cessation Programs

Most smoking cessation programs use a combination of peer support, group therapy, and behavior therapy. The websites of the CDC, the American Heart Association, and the American Lung Association all provide information about smoking cessation programs and other means of quitting smoking.

>> **Stay Current:** The U.S. Department of Health and Human Services provides information and resources to help individuals quit smoking at its website at http://betobaccofree.hhs.gov.

Complementary Health Approaches

A number of complementary therapies, including acupuncture, may be used as stand-alone or adjunct therapies to help people quit using nicotine. Almost any therapy that helps reduce anxiety levels, such as meditation and yoga, will help decrease feelings of anxiety that may trigger the desire to smoke (Jang et al., 2019). In many communities, hypnotherapy is available. However, there is conflicting evidence about the efficacy of hypnotherapy as a smoking cessation strategy. Nurses working with patients who are interested in hypnotherapy should encourage them to also participate in more proven smoking cessation programs even if they decide to try hypnotherapy (Barnes, McRobbie, Dong, Walker, & Hartmann-Boyce, 2019).

> **Patient Teaching**
>
> **What Is Too Much Nicotine?**
>
> A potential issue with NRT is that some products are designed for heavy smokers and may contain too large a dose of nicotine. Depending on weight and customary nicotine usage, patients may experience unpleasant side effects from ingesting too much nicotine. Some of these signs include abdominal cramps, nausea and/or vomiting, chest pain or difficulty breathing, rapid heart rate, panic attacks, dizziness, ringing in the ears, anxiety or agitation, headache, and muscle twitching.
>
> Keep in mind that there is the possibility of nicotine poisoning with children who chew on patches or gum. This may present a medical emergency. Because of this risk, teach consumers to store NRT products out of the reach of children.

Lifespan Considerations

Nicotine and Adolescents

In 2018, an estimated 672,000 adolescents ages 12 to 17 (2.7%) smoked cigarettes, a significant decline from the 13% who reported smoking in 2002 (CBHSQ, 2019). However, nicotine use reports have not yet included vaping use, which has exploded. In 2018, among adolescents ages 12 to 17 who reported nicotine use, 65.5% smoked cigarettes but did not use other tobacco products, 14.4% smoked cigarettes and used some other type of tobacco product, and 20.1% used other tobacco products but not cigarettes (CBHSQ, 2019).

As with other substances, the teen years seem to be the gateway for nicotine use. Early research studies of the psychosocial risk factors for smoking indicated that stress, peer and family influences (such as whether or not family members smoke at home), and depression all serve as risk factors for the development and maintenance of smoking in adolescents (Sylvestre, Wellman, O'Loughlin, Dugas, & O'Loughlin, 2017). Protective factors include adolescent connectedness, parental expectations and monitoring, parental engagement in schools, religious activity, and prevention strategies such as tobacco-related marketing bans and higher cigarette taxes.

Among young people, the short-term health consequences of smoking include respiratory and nonrespiratory effects, addiction to nicotine, and associated use of other drugs (WHO, 2020c). Significantly, most young people who smoke regularly continue to smoke throughout adulthood. Smoking harms both performance and endurance in teen sports. Smoking reduces the rate of lung growth and reduces lung function: Teenage smokers experience shortness of breath almost three times more often than teens who do not smoke and produce phlegm more than twice as often as teens who do not smoke. Young adult smokers also show early vascular signs of heart disease and stroke and are at increased risk of lung cancer. The resting heart rates of young adult smokers are two to three beats per minute faster than those of nonsmokers. On average, someone who smokes a pack or more of cigarettes each day lives 7 years less than someone who never smoked (WHO, 2020c).

Smoking among adolescents is associated with increased risk for use of other substances. Teens who smoke are 3 times more likely than nonsmokers to use alcohol, 8 times more likely to use marijuana, and 22 times more likely to use cocaine. Smoking is associated with a host of other risky behaviors, such as fighting and engaging in unprotected sex (WHO, 2020c).

Nicotine and Pregnant Women

Generally speaking, pregnant women smoke at lower rates than women who are not pregnant, and this seems to hold true across all age groups. While there is some evidence of decline in smoking in pregnancy, it is not enough: in 2018, 11.4% of pregnant women used tobacco products (CBHSQ, 2019).

There is a substantial body of literature documenting the dangers of maternal nicotine use for the fetus. More than 40 of the 7000 chemicals released in cigarette smoke are known carcinogens. Nicotine crosses the placenta, and fetal concentrations of nicotine can be 15% higher than maternal concentrations (CDC, 2020m). Maternal cigarette smoking during pregnancy is associated with increased risk for:

- Spontaneous abortion
- Preterm delivery
- Respiratory disease
- Immune system difficulties such as asthma and allergies
- Cancer later in life.

Various studies link placental complications due to prenatal exposure to cigarette smoke, including alterations to the development and function of the placenta. A body of research has suggested that prenatal tobacco exposure has been associated with serious neurodevelopmental and behavioral consequences in infants, children, and adolescents, including delayed psychomotor and mental development, increased physical aggression during early childhood, attention deficits, issues with learning and memory, increased impulsivity, and speech and language impairments (Alkam & Nabeshima, 2019; CDC, 2020m).

Nicotine and Older Adults

In 2018, 8.4% of adults age 65 and older were current smokers (CDC, 2019b). Older smokers had lower SES, were more socially isolated, and had higher depressive symptoms than older adults who never smoked. Two-thirds of older adults said that a HCP had advised them to quit smoking, but just over one-third who tried to quit used evidence-based tobacco cessation treatments and only one in 20 successfully quit in the past year (Henley et al., 2019). The odds of successful smoking cessation increased if the individual received a new diagnosis of chronic illness (Nash, Liao, Harris, & Freedman, 2017). Even participants who quit during their 60s were at substantially decreased risk of death, relative to participants who continued to smoke (National Institute on Aging [NIA], 2019). However, the odds of quitting decrease in those who are heavy smokers; these patients may require extended pharmacotherapy and counseling to be successful in smoking cessation.

Among people age 50 and older, smokers are more likely to report health problems such as coughing, trouble breathing, and getting tired more easily than nonsmokers. Smoking often worsens existing medical conditions. Smoking increases the risk of many types of cancer, especially cancers along the respiratory and GI tracts (NIA, 2019). Smoking has also been linked to diseases other than cancer in seniors, including pulmonary and cardiovascular diseases, diabetes complications, bone disease, bone density loss, cataracts, and stomach ulcers. Smokers are up to 10 times more likely to get cancer than a person who has never smoked (NIA, 2019).

NURSING PROCESS

Nurses may interact with patients addicted to nicotine in a variety of settings ranging from acute care to outpatient centers. Nurses often note the smell of smoke on a nicotine user and can implement a plan of care aimed at helping the patient make healthier lifestyle choices. Because of the high rate of smoking among patients with mental health disorders, psychiatric facilities are a common place to meet patients with nicotine addictions. It is not uncommon for patients to have addictions to multiple substances, and nurses should assess for other substance abuse problems. A nonjudgmental approach is important when caring for patients addicted to nicotine. Health promotion efforts are directed toward education about making healthy life choices and strategies to support the patient in abstaining from nicotine. Through school programs, nurses can provide adolescents with ways to avoid peer pressure, thereby preventing nicotine use.

Assessment

When assessing patients who use nicotine, it is important to assess for amount and frequency of use, length of time nicotine has been used, and the presence of any symptoms indicating possible complications, such as a chronic cough, shortness of breath, hypertension, chest pain, or unexpected symptoms. When assessing, keep in mind that about 50% of people with behavioral health disorders smoke, compared to 23% of the general population, so always be sure to screen for tobacco use in patients with behavioral disorders or other substance use (SAMHSA-HRSA Center for Integrated Health Solutions, 2020). Often, there are no physical symptoms yet present in younger adults.

The USPSTF (2020) recommends that primary care clinicians provide interventions, including education or brief counseling, to prevent initiation of tobacco use among school-age children and adolescents. Primary care providers should assess adults annually—and pregnant women upon initiation of care—about nicotine use (USPSTF, 2016). Since there may be no physical symptoms present, clinicians rely on instruments to determine nicotine use.

Two approaches nurses can use to assess patients and help guide them toward smoking cessation are the 5As and Ask, Advise, and Refer (USPSTF, 2016). The 5As are:

Ask about smoking

Advise to quit through clear, personalized message

Assess willingness to quit

Assist in quitting

Arrange follow-up and support.

Using the Ask, Advise, and Refer model, nurses can ask patients about tobacco use, advise them to quit, and refer them to telephone quit lines and/or other evidence-based cessation interventions (USPSTF, 2016).

Many primary care and acute care institutions will use their own rating scales to assess tobacco use. Regardless of assessment method used, HCPs are encouraged to provide positive feedback to patients who screen negative and support their choice to abstain from substances.

Communicating with Patients

Working Phase

Women who are pregnant are often highly motivated to quit smoking. However, the nurse should not assume their motivations and should provide appropriate assessment as with any patient. Use open-ended statements or questions to explore further what the patient said and seek clarification:

- Tell me more about your cigarette use.
- The doctor explained the potential harm of cigarette use to you and your baby. What are your concerns or questions about that?
- What are your thoughts about quitting?
- I would be happy to give you some information on smoking cessation and refer you to a support group.

Diagnosis

Every patient is unique, and identifying patient care needs will depend on the type of complications the patient may be experiencing as a result of nicotine use. The needs of a patient being treated for lung cancer or heart disease after years of smoking will differ from the needs of the adolescent patient who may not yet be experiencing adverse effects from the newly begun habit. Nursing care priorities are individualized to specific patient needs and may include the following:

- Risk of injury
- Denial
- Inadequate coping skills
- Impaired airway clearance
- Anxiety.

Planning

When setting goals with patients, keep in mind that quitting smoking and use of other tobacco products may be a lengthy process. Research has suggested that a current smoker tries to quit on average 30 times or more before successfully quitting for 1 year or longer (Chaiton et al., 2016).

Patient education should address nicotine withdrawal symptoms. These include an intense craving for nicotine; anxiety, tension, restlessness, frustration, or impatience; difficulty concentrating; drowsiness or trouble sleeping; headaches; increased appetite and weight gain; and irritability or depression (Medline Plus, 2020b).

Goals for patient care must be measurable and may include the following:

- The patient will verbalize the harmful effects of smoking following patient education.
- The patient will verbalize strategies for quitting smoking that the individual would consider using when ready to quit.
- The patient will not experience any complications as a result of nicotine use.

Implementation

In every setting, the nurse engages in health promotion by not smoking, offering resources (such as lifestyle training), and providing patient education. The nurse also maintains awareness of marketing campaigns that encourage smoking among young adults by advertising and sponsoring entertainment events.

Provide Resources

Nurses often reinforce teaching to patients about the risks of continued nicotine use and the benefits of quitting. The nurse should always use judgment-free language and support the patient's decisions. After helping patients select their best approach for quitting nicotine use, nurses should help them investigate financial resources for NRT; Medicare and many Medicaid and private insurers will help pay for NRT.

Nurses should make sure that the patient has contacts for continued support (often free) during the process. Smokefree.gov (https://smokefree.gov/tools-tips/how-to-quit/using-nicotine-replacement-therapy) has some excellent tips for constructing and maintaining a successful plan for quitting. Government websites, social media, and smartphone apps may help during the often painful quitting process. Smokefree.gov suggests the following ideas for receiving support:

- Signing up for smartphone quit programs such as SmokefreeTXT (sign up online at https://smokefree.gov/tools-tips/text-programs/quit-for-good/smokefreetxt or text QUIT to 47848). Note that there are free and paid smartphone apps to support quitting smoking.
- Calling a quitline (https://smokefree.gov/tools-tips/get-extra-help/speak-to-an-expert) and talking to a counselor.
- Using the QuitGuide app (https://smokefree.gov/tools-tips/apps/quitguide) for tips and inspiration to help to support nicotine withdrawal.

Additional strategies for assisting patients to quit tobacco use can be found in **Box 22.2** ».

Evaluation

Expected outcomes for patients trying to eliminate nicotine use include:

- The patient refrains from using products that contain tobacco or nicotine.
- The patient remains free of complications related to nicotine or tobacco use.
- The patient verbalizes strategies for refraining from nicotine or tobacco use.
- The patient verbalizes an understanding of the negative effects of nicotine or tobacco use on the individual's own life and on the lives of others.

Nurses should not be surprised when patients have difficulty quitting. Government research has shown (Henley et al., 2019) that smoking cessation programs, like other programs that treat addictions, often have a fairly low success rate. According to the CDC, fewer than one in 10 adult cigarette smokers succeed in quitting each year; in 2018, 7.5%

Box 22.2

Guidelines for Assisting with Tobacco Cessation

- Assess and document tobacco use, history of attempts to quit, and willingness to quit on admission (in inpatient settings) or at each healthcare interaction (in community-based settings).
- Seek NRT or other tobacco cessation medication order from the HCP.
- Suggest to individuals who are participating in NRT or other therapies that they are on their way to quitting.
- Provide tobacco cessation publications and materials (e.g., quit guides or videos) and teach about physiologic consequences of tobacco use. Whenever possible, materials should be tailored to the individual (e.g., written for pregnant women or in the patient's first language).
- Reinforce strategies for quitting offered in quit guides and other resources. For example, identifying reasons to quit; planning activities during the times the patient is most likely to use tobacco; getting rid of all cigarettes, e-cigarettes, or tobacco; engaging in physical exercise; and rewards for short-term goals, such as making it through the first week.
- Provide resources and referrals for psychotherapy (e.g., cognitive-behavioral therapy), support groups, and social media or text-based interventions for the individual willing to attempt to quit tobacco use. In other words, "assist in the quit."
- Establish a plan for follow-up contact for the individual willing to attempt to quit tobacco use within 1 week of the quit date.
- Continue to ask tobacco users about quitting tobacco use at each visit.

Sources: From Medline Plus (2020b); Naslund et al. (2017); U.S. Department of Health and Human Services (2020).

of adult smokers (2.9 million) had successfully quit smoking in the past year (CDC, 2020l). However, the success rate increases for patients who use adjunct therapies with NRT. When used properly, NRT is a safe and effective cessation method and can double a smoker's chances of quitting cigarettes successfully (FDA, 2020a). Moreover, combining NRT with telephone counseling or other support can be more successful for quitting smoking than NRT alone (FDA, 2020a).

REVIEW Nicotine Use Disorder

RELATE Link the Concepts and Exemplars

Linking the exemplar of nicotine use disorder with the concept of oxygenation:

1. Describe the pathophysiology of the respiratory system and the ability of the alveoli to oxygenate the tissues when a patient smokes.
2. While caring for a patient who is known to have smoked for more than 30 years, how would you amend your nursing plan of care as related to oxygenation?

Linking the exemplar of nicotine use disorder with the concept of grief and loss:

3. The nurse is caring for a patient with terminal lung cancer and is talking with the family. The patient's daughter says, "If Dad wanted to stay around and be with us, he wouldn't have made the choice to smoke." How would you respond to this statement and help the family members deal with their anger over the patient's lifestyle choices?
4. Why might a patient with acute COPD who continues to smoke be denied a lung transplant? How can you help this patient (and family) deal with the grief and loss they experience as a result of this decision?

READY Go to Volume 3: Clinical Nursing Skills

REFER Go to Pearson MyLab Nursing and eText

REFLECT Apply Your Knowledge

Ronald Kohler, age 32, began smoking when he was a junior in high school. His parents tried to discourage his smoking, but they never actually forbade it in their home because both of them smoked and believed it would be hypocritical to hold him to different standards than they practiced. Mr. Kohler now says he wishes his parents had told him all of the negatives and enforced a strict no-smoking rule because, he says, "It would have been easier not to start than it is to quit." Recently, during an annual health exam required by his employer, the physician pointed out early pulmonary changes associated with emphysema. Mr. Kohler denies any symptoms other than a productive cough in the morning upon awakening. He lives with his wife and two daughters, age 8 and 5. His wife strictly forbids smoking in the house and wishes her children did not see their father smoking for fear that they will eventually smoke as adults because of the poor role model he portrays.

The nursing assessment reveals that Mr. Kohler's vital signs are T 37°C (98.6°F, oral), P 80 bpm, R 16/min, BP 138/86 mmHg. Breath sounds are clear and equal except for mild crackles in the lowest part of the lung bases. He has an intermittent moist, often productive cough, and his oxygen saturation is 91%. Peak flow readings are 480 mL, but he has no baseline for comparison purposes. When questioned, Mr. Kohler reports that he has smoked 1 pack of filtered low-tar cigarettes a day on most days but when under stress he may smoke as much as 2 packs (or 50 cigarettes) per day. He has tried quitting twice, but both times he lasted less than 24 hours before smoking again. Mr. Kohler says he knows he should quit for his girls, because his wife would be much happier if he didn't smell like cigarettes when he got close to her, and because it would be better for his health, but he reports he is just not interested in quitting because he enjoys the habit and finds that it calms him during times of stress.

1. Explain why it would be important during the initial nursing assessment to include questions about Mr. Kohler's medication history and his use of other medications.
2. Mr. Kohler asks you to explain the risks of taking Chantix (varenicline). What do you tell him?
3. On the basis of this visit, develop a nursing care plan for Mr. Kohler.

» Exemplar 22.C Substance Use Disorders

Exemplar Learning Outcomes

22.C Analyze manifestations and treatment considerations for patients with an addiction to substances.

- Describe the pathophysiology of substance abuse.
- Describe the etiology of substance abuse.
- Compare the risk factors and prevention of substance abuse.
- Identify clinical manifestations of substance abuse.
- Summarize diagnostic tests and therapies used by interprofessional teams in the collaborative care of an individual who abuses substances.
- Differentiate care of patients across the lifespan who abuse substances.
- Apply the nursing process in providing culturally competent care to an individual with a substance use disorder.

Exemplar Key Terms

Overview

Substance abuse is a pattern of using a chemical outside of medically or culturally defined norms despite harmful physical, psychologic, or social effects. *A substance use disorder* is a cluster of cognitive, behavioral, and physiologic symptoms that indicate continued use of a substance despite significant negative consequences such as illness, functional impairment, or disruption of relationships (APA, 2013). Although all SUDs have common psychologic symptoms, researchers have been focusing on the underlying physiologic changes in brain circuitry that often persist even after detoxification, especially in individuals with severe disorders. It is believed that these permanent brain changes cause the behavioral effects characteristic of individuals with SUD, such as repeated relapses and intense substance craving (APA, 2013).

To be diagnosed with an SUD, an individual must exhibit a problematic pattern of substance use and a pathologic pattern of behaviors related to substance use. Patterns of symptoms recognized as part of the diagnostic criteria for SUD from the DSM-5 include symptoms related to impaired control, social impairment, and risky use, as well as pharmacologic criteria (APA, 2013).

Symptoms of **impaired control** include taking a substance in larger amounts over a longer period of time; wanting to reduce use and reporting multiple unsuccessful attempts to cut down or quit; spending a lot of time obtaining, using, or recovering from the effects of the substance; and having daily activities that revolve around the substance. **Craving**, an intense desire for the substance, where it is difficult to think of anything else, also falls in the category of impaired control (APA, 2013). Craving often causes individuals to start using substances again.

Social impairment or dysfunction due to substance use may exhibit as failure to fulfill major roles at work, school, or home; continued substance use despite ongoing or recurrent social or interpersonal problems caused by the substance; and leaving or withdrawing from family, occupational, social, and/or recreational obligations and activities (APA, 2013).

Risky use is defined as repeated use of substances in situations in which it is physically hazardous and despite knowledge that the individual has a persistent physical or psychologic problem caused or worsened by substance use (APA, 2013). Pharmacologic criteria or symptoms include **tolerance**, needing a markedly larger dose of substance to achieve its desired effect. When attempting **withdrawal**, that is, abstinence from substances, the individual experiences uncomfortable withdrawal symptoms that often prompt resumed consumption of the substance (APA, 2013). Withdrawal occurs when an individual reduces or stops a drug that has been used heavily over a long period of time; it consists of a cluster of substance-specific behavioral symptoms with physiologic and cognitive components. Withdrawal causes clinically significant distress or impairment in social, occupational, or other important areas of function (APA, 2013). When an individual stops using a substance, uncomfortable, distressing, or even dangerous withdrawal symptoms can occur within hours. Severity of withdrawal varies depending on the amount of drug(s) consumed. In some cases, withdrawal symptoms may result in a medical emergency and/or last up to several days.

The DSM-5 includes 10 separate classes of substances, ranging from alcohol, caffeine, and tobacco to cannabis, hallucinogens, opioids, sedatives, and stimulants (APA, 2013). For the purpose of this exemplar, the term *substance abuse* refers specifically to drugs, both legal and illegal, that lead to addiction and dependence. Because alcohol and nicotine are often abused, they are covered in separate exemplars in this concept. Three other commonly abused substances are cannabis (marijuana), opioids, and stimulants, which are discussed later in this exemplar.

Substance use disorders can range in severity from mild to severe, depending on the number of symptoms displayed by the individual. Substances can also induce disorders, such as psychosis experienced from taking hallucinogens. Substance use or abuse may co-occur with other mental health disorders. Approximately 20% of Americans with an anxiety or mood disorder such as depression also have alcohol use disorder or another SUD (Anxiety and Depression Association of America, 2018). SUDs by themselves are second only to mood disorders as the most frequent risk factors for suicidal behaviors (National Action Alliance for Suicide Prevention, 2018).

Pathophysiology

The pathophysiology of substance abuse was discussed earlier in the module. In summary, it is a complicated, multifactorial process that involves a combination of biological, genetic, psychologic, and sociocultural factors. Both short-term and long-term use can affect patient physiology. For example, long-term changes in neurotransmission called **kindling** can occur after repeated recurrences of use followed by detoxification (Post & Kegan, 2017). Kindling, in turn, can heighten cravings, which may explain why multiple cycles of use and withdrawal seem to make long-term abstinence and recovery progressively difficult (Ooms et al., 2020).

Etiology and Epidemiology

As stated earlier in this module, the etiology of substance use is multifactorial, and it varies among individuals. Adolescents, for example, may begin to use if friends or peers are using and then continue to use when they find that the drug activates the brain's reward center and results in a desired effect. In contrast, an adult who experiences a severe injury may initially take an opiate, such as oxycodone, for pain relief and find that they need more of the drug to continue to cope with psychologic consequences of the injury well after it has physically healed. Regardless of the initial reasons for use, however, most individuals experience similar patterns of tolerance and dependency the longer they continue to use a substance. Individuals who use substances within the context of social groups that encourage or celebrate use may be more resistant to treatment and are at greater risk for relapse.

As stated earlier, in 2018, nearly 1 in 5 people aged 12 and older (19.4%) used an illicit drug in the past year, more than in 2015 and 2016 (CBHSQ, 2019). Past-year illicit drug use for 2018 was driven primarily by marijuana use, with 43.5 million past-year marijuana users. An estimated 1.3 million adolescents ages 12 to 17 use marijuana for the first time each year, which translates to approximately 3700 adolescents a day (CBHSQ, 2019).

Prescription pain reliever misuse was the second most common form of illicit drug use in the United States. Approximately 16.9 million Americans (6.2%) misuse psychotherapeutic drugs (stimulants, tranquilizers, and sedatives) and pain relievers each year (CBHSQ, 2019).

In 2018, prescription opioid use declined, primarily because of tightened prescriber regulation (CBHSQ, 2019). The overall national opioid prescribing rate declined from 2012 to 2018, when it reached its lowest rate in 13 years (CDC, 2020h). Unfortunately, the decrease in prescribed opioids has resulted in an increase in users who have switched from prescription opiates to potent synthetic opioids such as fentanyl, fentanyl analogs, and heroin, a semi-synthetic opioid (Armenian, Vo, Barr-Walker, & Lynch, 2018). Despite a 4% decrease from 2017 to 2018, more than 67,000 people died from drug overdoses in 2018, making it one of the leading causes of injury-related death in the United States (CDC, 2020g). The decline was decimated by a 5% increase in drug overdose deaths in 2019 and a 29% increase in 2020. More than 93,000 people in the United States died from drug overdose in 2020, 69,710 from opioid overdose, reflecting the psychosocial effects of COVID-19 and disruptions in access to addiction treatment and other resources (Ahmad, Rossen & Sutton, 2021).

Substance use disorders in the United States cost over $700 billion a year, including the costs of treatment, related health problems, absenteeism, lost productivity, drug-related crime and incarceration, and education and prevention (NIDA, 2020b). The relapse rates for drug addiction are 40–60%, comparable to rates of exacerbations seen in other chronic illnesses, such as diabetes, HTN, and asthma (NIDA, 2020b). Although cocaine, hallucinogens, inhalants, and heroin continue to be popular, marijuana use has experienced the greatest increase (CBHSQ, 2019).

Increasing regulation of opioid prescriptions has resulted in increased use of heroin, which is cheaper and often easier to obtain than prescription opioids (NIDA, 2018c). Heroin abuse is dangerous because of the drug's addictiveness and its high risk for overdosing. With heroin, this danger is compounded by the lack of control over the purity of the injected drug and its possible contamination with other drugs. Heroin use has increased across the United States among men and women, most age groups, and all income levels. Some of the greatest increases occurred in demographic groups with historically low rates of heroin use: women, the privately insured, and people of higher SES. Despite an increase in heroin use from 2017 to 2018, heroin-involved overdose death rates for that year actually declined by 4.1% (CDC, 2020f). This decrease was not related to a decline in use but to the increased availability of naloxone, an opioid reversal medication (CDC, 2019c). In contrast, the increase in overdose deaths seen in 2020 was largely fueled by a national surge in the use of fentanyl, a high potency synthetic opioid.

SAFETY ALERT! Naloxone (Evzio, Narcan) is a lifesaving medication that can stop or reverse the effects of an opioid or heroin overdose. Drug overdose deaths, driven largely by prescription drug overdoses, are among the leading causes of injury and death in the United States. Naloxone is available in a nasal spray and self-injectable forms over the counter, can be used in adults or children, and is easily administered by anyone, even those without medical training (CDC, 2019c). Many states have laws that allow pharmacists to dispense naloxone without a prescription, and this has contributed to lowering death rates. Dispensing of naloxone has increased in recent years, but more work needs to be done, particularly in rural counties. Family members and support persons of individuals with known addiction problems should acquire these rescue medications and prepare themselves to administer them in case of an overdose.

Risk Factors

Risk factors for drug abuse are multifactorial and can affect individuals of any age, sex, or SES. Some factors that affect the likelihood and speed of developing an addiction include a family history of addiction, the presence of another mental disorder, the use of drugs as a coping mechanism to manage anxiety or depression, peer pressure, and lack of family involvement. Although men are more likely to experience problems with drugs than women, progression of addiction is faster among women than among men (McHugh, Votaw, Sugarman, & Greenfield, 2018; Webster, 2017).

Clinical Manifestations

Clinical manifestations, and their severity, depend on amount, frequency, and specific combination of substances used. Combining two CNS depressants, for example, will produce far more significant manifestations than using only one CNS depressant. Some symptoms can be alarming or even fatal. For example, long-term crack use can result in sensory hallucinations, and even the first use of cocaine can result in death for individuals with undiagnosed cardiac disorders. Clinical manifestations are linked to specific substances in the following sections.

Caffeine

Caffeine is a commonly used stimulant that increases the heart rate and acts as a diuretic. Found in soft drinks, coffee, tea, chocolate, and some pain relievers, caffeine can cause negative physiologic effects when used in excess. Up to 400 mg of caffeine per day (roughly three 8-ounce cups) is safe for most adults, with higher quantities not recommended, particularly for adolescents (Mayo Clinic, 2020b). Individuals with a history of cardiovascular disease should be advised to cut back or eliminate caffeine consumption completely. Side effects that indicate a need for reducing consumption include headaches, insomnia, nervousness and irritability, stomach upset, and tachycardia. Abrupt withdrawal will likely cause headaches and irritability. Because of its withdrawal symptoms, some clinicians do consider caffeine as addicting, even though it does not have a major action on the mesolimbic dopamine system (Uddin et al., 2017).

A rising number of adolescents are developing symptoms of caffeine dependence from consuming sizable quantities of caffeinated energy drinks (CEDs). Energy drinks contain caffeine that ranges from 50 mg to 500 mg per can or bottle, compared with the average can of cola that has 35 mg (CDC, 2019a). Researchers report an increase in caffeine intoxication and problems with caffeine dependence and withdrawal, dehydration, heart complications (such as irregular heartbeat and heart failure), anxiety, and insomnia from CEDs (CDC, 2019a). Genetic factors may also play a role in these clinical manifestations (De Sanctis et al., 2017).

Young people who ingest energy drinks are more likely to participate in unhealthy behaviors, including alcohol use. Of particular concern are alcoholic beverages mixed with energy drinks because the caffeine in these drinks can mask the depressant effects of alcohol. Individuals who consume alcohol mixed with energy drinks are three times more likely to binge drink and are twice as likely to report being taken advantage of sexually, to report taking advantage of someone else sexually, and to report riding with a driver who was under the influence of alcohol than drinkers who do not mix caffeine with alcohol (CDC, 2020d). Furthermore, researchers have found that recent TBI is more strongly related to consuming alcohol, energy drinks, and energy drinks and alcohol mixed (Yamakawa, Lengkeek, Salberg, Spanswick, & Mychasiuk, 2017).

Cannabis

Marijuana (known as grass, weed, pot, and reefer, among others) comes from the **cannabis sativa** plant. Its psychoactive component is THC (delta-9-tetrahydrocannabinol). THC activates certain cannabinoid receptors in the brain, inducing euphoria. Physiologic effects of use are dose related and may include increased heart rate and bronchodilation with short-term use, airway constriction and inflammation and respiratory illness with long-term use (WHO, 2020b) Marijuana use affects endocrine hormones, particularly decreasing spermatogenesis and testosterone levels in men, and suppressing follicle-stimulating, luteinizing, and prolactin hormones in women. New mothers should avoid cannabis use while breastfeeding, as marijuana crosses the placental barrier.

Marijuana is the most commonly used illicit substance (CBHSQ, 2019). In addition to euphoria (which can last as long as 3 hours and is the pleasurable effect associated with marijuana use), sedation is also possible. Hallucinations and paranoia may present when large amounts are used. Increased use may result in apathy, poor hygiene, and disinterest. Short-term memory impairment is common due to marijuana's effect on the hippocampus.

It is estimated that up to a third of people who use marijuana will become dependent on it. People who begin using marijuana before age 18 are four to seven times more likely than adults to develop a marijuana use disorder (NIDA, 2019d). Marijuana addiction is linked to a mild withdrawal syndrome, with frequent users reporting irritability, mood and sleep difficulties, decreased appetite, cravings, restlessness, and/or various forms of physical discomfort that peak within the first week after quitting and last up to 2 weeks (NIDA, 2019d).

The potency of cannabis has increased significantly over the past few decades in response to consumer demand and policies in some states that have legalized marijuana for medicinal and recreational purposes. The THC content of "street" marijuana was less than 1% in the 1970s and 4% in the 1990s. By 2012, analyses of cannabis samples seized by law enforcement agencies documented a rise in average THC potency to more than 12% (Pierre, 2017). Also, new methods of smoking or eating THC-rich oil extracted from the marijuana plant may deliver very high levels of THC to the user. Ultra-high-potency hash oil extracts are also known as "wax," "dabs," or "crumble," among other names (Pierre, 2017). The average marijuana extract contains over 50% THC, with some samples exceeding 90% (NIDA, 2019d). These trends raise concerns that the consequences of marijuana use could be worse than in the past, particularly among new users or in young people, whose brains are still developing.

In 2018, there were 43.5 million current users age 12 and older (15.9%). In 2019, as many as 11.8% of 8th-graders reported marijuana use in the past year. By 12th grade, 35.7% had used marijuana during the year prior to the survey and 22.3% were current users, with 6.4% saying they used marijuana daily or near daily (NIDA, 2019d).

Central Nervous System Depressants

Central nervous system depressants commonly used as drugs of abuse include tranquilizers and sedatives. Examples of CNS depressants include the antianxiety tranquilizers benzodiazepines (e.g., alprazolam [Xanax], clonazepam [Klonopin], diazepam [Valium], and lorazepam [Ativan]) and some muscle relaxants (for example, carisoprodol [Soma]) that are Schedule IV drugs. Prescription sedatives include zolpidem (Ambien), eszopiclone (Lunesta), zaleplon (Sonata), barbiturates (for example, secobarbital [Seconal]), among others (CBHSQ, 2019). An estimated 6.4 million people (2.4%) age 12 and older in 2018 misused prescription tranquilizers or sedatives, which is roughly comparable to past-years' use (CBHSQ, 2019).

Benzodiazepines (BZDs) are often abused because they have anxiolytic, hypnotic, muscle-relaxant, anticonvulsant, and amnesic effects. They are used as sedatives and some are used specifically to treat withdrawal symptoms, including alcohol withdrawal delirium (Soyka, 2017). Benzodiazepines are relatively safe for short-term use for anxiety or withdrawal symptoms (2 to 4 weeks). Dependence develops in approximately half of patients who use BZDs for longer than 1 month (Soyka, 2017). These drugs cause drowsiness and may impair motor skills, such as operating a motor vehicle or machinery, and cause falls and fractures. Sudden withdrawal from benzodiazepines can result in seizures, delirium, and psychosis (Soyka, 2017).

Benzodiazepines, when combined with other substances, can cause cross-tolerance, where tolerance to the effects of a certain drug produces tolerance to a similar drug, usually other CNS depressants, and create synergistic effects (an increased interaction between two or more drugs) (Ogawa et al., 2019). Drug fatality rates rise when BZDs are used to enhance the euphoric effects of opioids, a synergistic effect between two respiratory depressants that causes overdose, respiratory arrest, and death (Platt, 2020; Smith et al., 2019). Alcohol consumption combined with BZDs and related medications enhance CNS depressant effects, often leading to respiratory arrest (Holton et al., 2017). Some research points to a significantly increased risk of a diagnosis of dementia in people who have taken BZDs for a long time, alone or with other sedatives (DeKosky & Williamson, 2020).

Psychostimulants

Psychostimulants include cocaine (also crack), methamphetamine, and prescription stimulants (such as methylphenidate [Concerta, Ritalin] and amphetamine/dextroamphetamine [Adderall]), which are often used to treat attention-deficit/hyperactivity disorder and certain sleep disorders. Psychostimulants with abuse potential include drugs such as methamphetamine (3,4-methylenedioxy-methamphetamine, or MDMA), dextroamphetamine, levoamphetamine, methylphenidate, and caffeine (Kariisa, Scholl, Wilson, Seth, & Hoots, 2019). Many psychostimulants are Schedule II drugs with a high potential for abuse and addiction. SUD occurs when an individual experiences clinically significant impairment caused by the recurrent use, including health problems, persistent or increasing use, and failure to meet major responsibilities at work, school, or home (CBHSQ, 2019). Rates of use vary by type of stimulant, and while use of these is comparatively low, overdose rates are fairly high. Among all 2017 drug-overdose deaths, 13,942 (19.8%) involved cocaine and 10,333 (14.7%) involved psychostimulants (Kariisa et al., 2019). Nearly three-fourths (72.7%) of cocaine-involved deaths in 2017 also involved opioids.

Prescription stimulants increase alertness, attention, and energy. Popular slang terms for prescription stimulants include speed, uppers, and vitamin R (NIDA, 2018e). At high doses, prescription stimulants can lead to a dangerously high body temperature, an irregular heartbeat, heart failure, and seizures.

Cocaine is a powerfully addictive stimulant made from the leaves of the coca plant native to South America; popular nicknames for cocaine include blow, coke, crack, rock, and snow (NIDA, 2018f). Cocaine is usually snorted or smoked. Street dealers often add amphetamine or synthetic opioids, including fentanyl, to cocaine, which has increased death rates. Cocaine use is associated with increased stroke risk, incidence of hemorrhagic stroke, and fatal stroke, particularly among young adults with no prior medical history (Darke, Duflou, Kaye, Farrell, & Lappin, 2019). Cocaine may cause sudden death by creating arrhythmias, status epilepticus, respiratory arrest, and intracerebral hemorrhage, as well as interacting with congenital and coronary artery anomalies (Mehdi, Mehdi, Siddique, & Ahmad, 2017).

Methamphetamine causes increased activity and talkativeness, decreased appetite, and a pleasurable sense of well-being or euphoria and is a potent stimulant, with long-lasting and harmful effects on the CNS (NIDA, 2019e). Methamphetamine can be smoked, swallowed as a pill, snorted as a powder, or injected when the powder has been dissolved in water/alcohol.

Methamphetamine deaths are usually caused by hemorrhagic stroke and occasional ruptured aneurysms, especially when the person has underlying systemic HTN (Darke, Lappin, Kaye, & Duflou, 2018).

Opiates

Opiates are a natural substance derived from the poppy plant. Common drugs derived directly from poppy plants include opium and morphine. **Opioids** are synthetic or partly synthetic substances that act like opiates, and include some narcotic analgesics (such as oxycodone, hydromorphone, meperidine, and prescription fentanyl), as well as illicitly manufactured forms of fentanyl and heroin. Prescription opiates and opioids are used to relieve moderate to severe pain. For the purposes of this text, the term *opiate* is used to refer to both naturally derived opioids and their opiate counterparts.

Opiate abuse in the United States is an epidemic. In 2020, approximately 190 people in the United States died every day from overdosing on opioids—a total of 69,710 people in that year alone (Ahmad et al., 2021). An estimated 1.7 million people in the United States suffer from SUDs related to prescription opioid pain relievers, and 526,000 suffer from a heroin use disorder (NIDA, 2020a). The consequences of this abuse are devastating.

Long-term use and misuse can result in physiologic effects such as hyperalgesia, hypogonadism, and sexual dysfunction, as well as depressing respirations and increasing risk for infectious disease.

The resurgence of heroin and insurgence of fentanyl use have become epidemic. The illegal drug heroin is usually administered intravenously, whereas the Schedule II drug fentanyl may be taken orally in tablet form or snorted as a liquid, or the gel in the transdermal patch can be placed sublingually or injected intravenously. Physical dependence can occur quickly or through long-term use (**Figure 22.5** »).

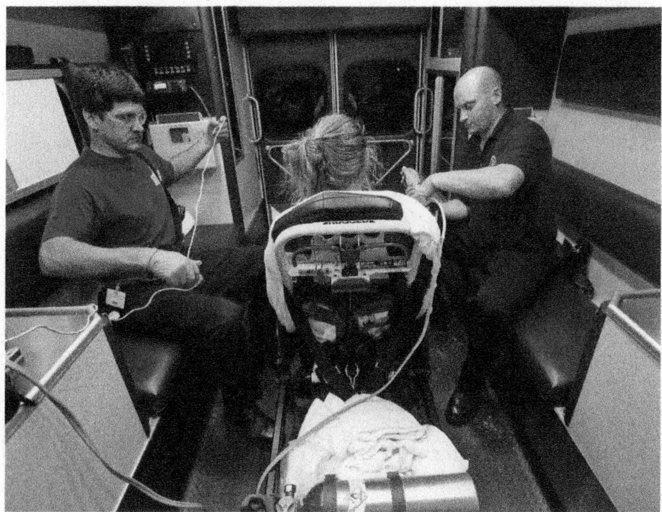

Figure 22.5 » Paramedics monitor a 29-year-old woman after she was found unconscious from a heroin overdose. The woman thanked the paramedics, one of whom recognized her from an overdose about a month ago. "At least I still have my shoes this time," said the woman, who told the paramedics that she normally uses $^1/_2$ gram of heroin twice a day but had cut her dose to $^1/_4$ gram that night because she had heard that it was stronger than usual.

Source: Derek Davis/Portland Press Herald/Getty Images.

Symptoms of opiate intoxication include slurred speech, drowsiness, pupillary constriction, and psychomotor agitation (Potter & Moller, 2020). Initial withdrawal symptoms including cravings, runny nose, and sweating and can take up to 10 days to recede. Especially with long-term use, a second phase of withdrawal may occur for months, with symptoms including insomnia, irritability, fatigue, and abdominal cramping, among others.

In the past, treatment of opiate use disorder typically included methadone, a synthetic opiate that when used as prescribed does not hinder function or productivity. More recently, clinicians are using buprenorphine, a partial opioid agonist, and naltrexone, an opioid antagonist. All can assist in reducing symptoms of withdrawal, particularly cravings (ASAM, 2020b; NIDA, 2018b). Pharmacologic management of withdrawal is recommended over stopping abruptly, which can result in life-threatening withdrawal or overdose. Ongoing pharmacologic therapy combined with psychotherapy is recommended (ASAM, 2020b).

Hallucinogens

Hallucinogens are typically used by the young. In 2018, 2.3 million (6.9%) young adults ages 18 to 25 in 2018 were past-year users of hallucinogens (CBHSQ, 2019). Drugs under the category of hallucinogens include:

- LSD (*lysergic acid diethylamide*; also known as acid, yellow sunshine, tab, and blotter)
- PCP (*phencyclidine*; angel dust, peace pill, dippers, greens)
- Peyote (cactus, buttons)
- Psilocybin mushrooms (little smoke, magic mushrooms)
- "Ecstasy" (MDMA, *3,4-methylenedioxy-methamphetamine*, or "Molly")
- Ketamine
- DMT (*N,N-dimethyltryptamine*/AMT (*α-Methyltryptamine*).

The over-the-counter cough suppressant dextromethorphan (DXM) also can potentiate hallucinations if taken in large quantities (CBHSQ, 2019; NIDA, 2019c).

Hallucinogens alter awareness of surroundings, thoughts, and feelings and can cause visual and tactile hallucinations. Some hallucinogens cause *dissociation*, a sensation of being out of control or disconnected from the body and environment. Hallucinogens affect the neurotransmitters serotonin, which regulates sleep, muscle control, and mood, and glutamate, which regulates pain perception, learning, memory, and other areas. Because of their impact on the brain, hallucinogens can cause lasting consequences for a user, such as psychosis or mental disorders (SAMHSA, 2020d). The results of hallucinogens are unpredictable, showing up as soon as 20 minutes after ingestion; the effects can last as long as 12 hours (SAMHSA, 2020d). Hallucinogen users often refer to unpleasant experiences brought on by these drugs as a "bad trip."

Regular users of hallucinogens can develop tolerance and addiction. For example, while LSD is not considered addictive, regular use can lead to tolerance and higher doses, which can result in death or injury from dangerously altered perceptions (NIDA, 2019c). On the other hand, PCP is a hallucinogen that can be addictive; common withdrawal symptoms include drug cravings, headaches, and sweating (NIDA, 2019c).

Potential side effects and symptoms of hallucinogen use include the following: nausea and vomiting, loss of appetite, impaired muscle movement, mixed senses (e.g., "seeing" sounds or "hearing" colors), excessive sweating, paranoia, weight loss, and possibly seizures when mixed with medications or other illicit drugs. Other symptoms, especially with long-term use of hallucinogens, are memory loss, anxiety, depression and suicidal thoughts, persistent psychosis/ hallucinations, speech problems, and social withdrawal and disorganization (SAMHSA, 2020d). Hallucinogen-persisting perception disorder (HPPD) is a syndrome characterized by prolonged or recurring perceptual symptoms, reminiscent of acute hallucinogen effects; HPPD is potentially permanent (Orsolini et al., 2017).

Inhalants

Inhalants include a variety of substances and products, such as nitrous oxide, amyl nitrite, cleaning fluids, gasoline, spray paint, computer keyboard cleaner, other aerosol sprays, felt-tip pens, and glue. In 2018, approximately 2.0 million (0.7%) of people age 12 and older were past-year users of inhalants (CBHSQ, 2019). Inhalants are mostly used by young preteens and adolescents and are the only class of substance used more by younger than by older teens (CBHSQ, 2019).

Inhalants include solvents (liquids that become gas at room temperature), aerosol sprays, gases, and nitrites. Nitrites are prescription medicines for chest pain, and amyl nitrate is available as a liquid that can be inhaled and used illicitly to improve sexual pleasure by producing vasodilation of the blood vessels in the genital area. People who use inhalants breathe in the fumes through their nose or mouth, usually by sniffing, snorting, bagging, or huffing. Although the high that inhalants produce usually lasts just a few minutes, many users often try to make it last by continuing to inhale again and again over several hours (NIDA, 2020c). Most inhalants affect the CNS and slow down brain activity. Short-term effects are similar to alcohol and include slurred or distorted speech, nausea and vomiting, headache, lack of coordination, euphoria, and dizziness. Users may also have hallucinations or delusions (NIDA, 2020c).

Long-term effects of inhalant use may include liver and kidney damage; damage to the sense of smell; loss of muscle control; increased risk of cancer; liver, lung, and kidney problems; hearing loss; bone marrow damage; loss of coordination and limb spasms from nerve damage; delayed behavioral development; and brain damage from constricted oxygen flow to the brain (NIDA, 2020c; SAMHSA, 2018d). Because nitrites are misused for sexual pleasure and performance, they can lead to unsafe sexual practices or other risky behavior, leading to increased risk of acquiring sexually transmitted infections and infectious diseases such as HIV/AIDS or hepatitis (NIDA, 2020c).

Inhalant overdose can result in serious symptoms, such as seizures, coma, or death. Many solvents and aerosol sprays are highly concentrated and, if sniffed, these products can cause immediate heart failure and death within minutes, a condition known as sudden sniffing death (SSD; NIDA, 2020c).

Treatment for inhalant use most commonly occurs in emergency departments if a cardiac condition, seizures, coma, or other adverse effect has occurred. Inhalant addiction is not common, but repeated use of inhalants can lead to addiction. Withdrawal symptoms may include nausea, loss of appetite, sweating, problems sleeping, and mood changes (NIDA, 2020c).

Collaboration

Effective treatment of SUDs and related dependence and addictive behaviors requires interprofessional care that targets both the substance abuse and any underlying psychiatric illness. Team members may include physicians, psychiatrists, advanced practice and registered nurses, psychologists or other licensed therapists, vocational specialists, and peer counselors. Treatments may include detoxification, medications for side effects, individual or group psychotherapy, cognitive-behavioral strategies, family counseling, and self-help groups. Treatment setting may be inpatient, outpatient, or a combination, depending on the severity of the SUD, medical comorbidities, and other factors, ranging from health insurance to child care. A substance overdose is a life-threatening condition that requires inpatient medical stabilization before any other interventions can be attempted. Several diagnostic tests can identify helpful information about the patient's condition and issues to be included in the treatment plan.

Diagnostic Tests

Common laboratory tests for drug use include blood, urine, saliva, perspiration, and hair. Urine drug screening is often the preferred method and is noninvasive. Serum drug levels may be taken in hospital settings to identify drug overdoses and complications. The length of time a drug can be found in blood or urine varies depending on the property of the drug and other factors. Heroin is eliminated within 1 to 3 days, but barbiturates can show up in drug tests for up to 3 weeks (FDA, 2018). For patients who smoke marijuana regularly, THC may linger in their system for 30 days or more (Villines, 2019).

Pharmacologic Therapy

Common drugs used in the treatment of substance abuse and withdrawal are presented in Medications 22.1 in the sections on Opioid Antagonists and Opioid Drugs.

Emergency Care for Overdose

As stated earlier, overdose is a medical emergency. Patients experiencing cardiac arrest, asphyxiation from toxic fumes, suffocation, convulsions or seizures, coma, choking from aspirated vomit, and other harmful events may exhibit respiratory depression and require mechanical ventilation. Nurses should try to actively monitor the patient if delirious, psychotic, suicidal, homicidal, or gravely disabled. Medications (e.g., haloperidol, risperidone, carbamazepine) may be needed to relieve any psychosis (Medscape, 2019). Patient safety is the care priority.

If the overdose was intentional or the patient is unable or unwilling to report intention, suicide precautions should be implemented until the patient's risk for suicide decreases per agency protocol.

Table 22.4 >> summarizes signs of overdose and withdrawal and recommended treatments for several common substances.

Complementary Health Approaches

Auricular (ear) acupuncture has been used throughout the world as an adjunctive treatment during opioid detoxification for about 30 years. However, research has found no consistent differences between acupuncture and comparative treatments for substance use. There have been some findings in favor of acupuncture for withdrawal/craving and anxiety symptoms, however, those findings were limited by low-quality evidence (National Center for Complementary and Integrative Health [NCCIH], 2018). A randomized controlled trial of military veterans in recovery from SUD found that participants' craving and anxiety levels decreased significantly after a single session of acupuncture or relaxation response intervention, suggesting there may be some value in attending regular acupuncture or relaxation response intervention sessions (NCCIH, 2018).

Mindfulness-based interventions may help significantly reduce the consumption of several substances including alcohol, cigarettes, opiates, and other substances. Mindfulness-based interventions have also proved useful in addressing cravings that trigger relapse (NCCIH, 2018).

Lifespan Considerations

At various stages of life, individuals become involved with substances for an assortment of reasons. Some of the salient lifespan factors associated with SUD are discussed in the following sections.

TABLE 22.4 Signs and Treatment of Overdose and Withdrawal

	Overdose		Withdrawal	
Drug	**Signs**	**Treatment**	**Signs**	**Treatment**
CNS Depressants				
Alcohol Barbiturates Benzodiazepines	Cardiovascular or respiratory depression or arrest (mostly with barbiturates) Coma Shock Convulsions Death	*If awake:* 1. Keep awake. 2. Induce vomiting. 3. Use activated charcoal to absorb drug. 4. Vital signs (VS) every 15 minutes. *Coma:* 1. Clear airway, intubate, IV fluids. 2. Perform gastric lavage. 3. Take seizure precautions. 4. Administer hemodialysis or peritoneal dialysis, if ordered. 5. Assess VS as ordered. 6. Assess for shock and cardiac arrest.	Nausea and vomiting Tachycardia Diaphoresis Anxiety or agitation Tremors Marked insomnia Grand mal seizures Delirium (after 5–15 years of heavy use)	Carefully titrated detoxification with similar drug *Note:* Abrupt withdrawal can lead to death.
Hallucinogens				
LSD	Psychosis Brain damage Death	1. Reduce environmental stimuli. 2. Have one person "talk down patient"; reassure. 3. Speak slowly and clearly. 4. Administer diazepam or chloral hydrate for anxiety as ordered.	No pattern of withdrawal	
PCP	Possible hypertensive crisis Respiratory arrest Hyperthermia Seizures	1. Acidify urine to help excrete drug (cranberry juice, ascorbic acid); in acute stage: ammonium chloride. 2. Minimize stimuli. 3. Do *not* attempt to talk down; speak slowly in low voice. 4. Administer diazepam or Haldol as ordered.	Cravings Headaches Sweating	
Inhalants				
Volatile solvents (such as butane, paint thinner, airplane glue, nail polish remover)	Intoxication Agitation Drowsiness Disinhibition Staggering Light-headedness Death	Support affected systems.	No pattern of withdrawal	
Nitrites	Enhanced sexual pleasure	Neurologic symptoms may respond to vitamin B_{12} and folate.	No pattern of withdrawal	
Anesthetics such as nitrous oxide	Giggling, laughter Euphoria	Chronic users may experience polyneuropathy and myelopathy.	No pattern of withdrawal	

(continued on next page)

TABLE 22.4 *(continued)*

	Overdose		Withdrawal	
Drug	**Signs**	**Treatment**	**Signs**	**Treatment**
Opiates				
Heroin Meperidine Morphine Methadone	Pinpoint pupils Respiratory depression/arrest Unconsciousness/coma Shock Convulsions Death	Narcotic antagonist (Narcan) quickly reverses CNS depression.	Yawning, insomnia Irritability Rhinorrhea Panic Diaphoresis Cramps Nausea and vomiting Muscle aches Chills and fever Lacrimation Diarrhea	Methadone tapering Clonidine-naltrexone detoxification Buprenorphine
Stimulants				
Cocaine/crack Amphetamines	Respiratory distress Ataxia Hyperpyrexia Convulsions Coma Stroke Myocardial infarction Rhabdomyolysis Death	*Management for:* 1. Hyperpyrexia 2. Convulsions 3. Respiratory distress 4. Cardiovascular shock 5. Acidic urine (ammonium chloride for amphetamine).	Fatigue Depression Agitation Apathy Anxiety Sleepiness Disorientation Lethargy Craving	Antidepressants (desipramine) Dopamine agonist Bromocriptine

Source: Adapted from Bauldoff et al. (2020).

Newborns Exposed to Substances

Common complications of newborns exposed to substances in the womb including respiratory distress, neonatal jaundice, congenital anomalies, growth restriction, neurobehavioral deficits and delays, and withdrawal. Onset of withdrawal may begin as soon as 24 hours after life and may take up to 21 days. Care of the newborn experiencing withdrawal from a substance usually follows agency protocols. Selected clinical manifestations are summarized in **Table 22.5** ›. Note that fetal abstinence syndrome is discussed in Module 25, Development.

Use of opiates during pregnancy can result in a drug withdrawal syndrome in newborns called **neonatal abstinence syndrome (NAS)** or **neonatal opioid withdrawal syndrome (NOWS)**. NAS/NOWS is occurring in epidemic numbers: There was a fivefold increase in the number of babies born with opioid side effects from 2004 to 2014, when an estimated 32,000 infants were born with NAS/NOWS—equivalent to one baby suffering from opioid withdrawal born approximately every 15 minutes (NIDA, 2019a). Newborns with NAS/NOWS are more likely than other babies to also have low birth weight and respiratory complications and require lengthy, costly hospital care. In 2014, \$563 million was spent on costs for treatment of NAS/NOWS; the majority of these charges (82%) were paid by state Medicaid programs, reflecting the tendency of mothers using opioids during pregnancy to be from lower-income communities (NIDA, 2019a).

Substance Abuse in Adolescents

Approximately 4.2 million adolescents (16.7%) aged 12 to 17 in 2018 were past-year illicit drug users, which corresponds to about 1 in 6 adolescents; among the same group of adolescents, 699,000 (2.8%) misused opioids (CBHSQ, 2019). Percentages have been comparable in previous years. By the time they are seniors, 50% of high school students will have taken an illegal drug and more than 20% will have used a prescription drug for nonmedical reasons (CDC, 2020n). Substance use during adolescence has many negative consequences: It can affect the growth and development of teens, especially brain development; trigger other risky behaviors, such as unprotected sex and dangerous driving; and contribute to the development of adult health problems, such as heart disease, high blood pressure, and sleep disorders (CDC, 2020n). Adolescents use illicit substances for a variety of reasons, including the desire for new experiences, an attempt to deal with problems or perform better in school, and peer pressure. Many factors influence adolescent drug use, including the availability of drugs within the neighborhood, community, and school and whether the adolescent's friends are using drugs (U.S. Drug Enforcement Administration, 2018). Factors such as violence, physical or emotional abuse, mental illness, or drug use in the home increase the likelihood that an adolescent will use drugs. Adolescents who use drugs may have an inherited genetic vulnerability. Personality traits such as poor impulse control, a heightened need for excitement, and mental health conditions such as depression, anxiety, or

TABLE 22.5 Clinical Manifestations of Newborn Withdrawal

Body System	Clinical Manifestations
Central nervous system signs	High-pitched cry Hyperirritability (difficult to console, restless) Increased muscle tone Exaggerated reflexes Tremors, myoclonic jerks Seizures Sneezing, hiccups, yawning Short, restless sleep
Gastrointestinal signs	Disorganized, vigorous suck Excessive sucking Vomiting Poor weight gain Sensitive gag reflex Diarrhea Poor feeding (less than 15 mL on first day of life; feedings take more than 30 minutes each)
Autonomic signs	Stuffy nose, sneezing Yawning Mottled skin Tachypnea (greater than 60 breaths/minute when quiet) Sweating Hyperthermia
Cutaneous signs	Excoriated buttocks, knees, elbows Facial scratches Pressure-point abrasions

Source: From London, Ladewig, Ball, Bindler, and Cowen (2017). Pearson Education, Inc., Hoboken, NJ.

ADHD make substance use more likely (Volkow et al., 2018). Drug use at an early age is an important predictor of development of an SUD later.

Substance Abuse in Pregnant Women

During pregnancy, the fetus is exposed to chemicals or substances that have the potential to harm the fetus. These teratogens can cause the fetus to experience alterations ranging from developmental delays to death. Substances commonly misused include cocaine, amphetamines, barbiturates, hallucinogens, club drugs, heroin, and other narcotics. Polysubstance use, which involves combining multiple substances with alcohol, tobacco, and illicit drugs, is common. Of pregnant women ages 15 to 44, an estimated 5.4% in 2018 were illicit drug users (CBHSQ, 2019). An overview of the potential effects of selected drugs is provided in **Table 22.6** ».

In some states, prenatal substance abuse constitutes criminal child abuse. Other states have expanded civil child welfare requirements to include prenatal substance abuse, so that prenatal drug exposure can provide grounds for forcing treatment and even terminating parental rights because of child abuse or neglect. To protect the fetus, some states have authorized civil commitment, such as forced admission to an inpatient treatment program, of pregnant women who use drugs and alcohol. Some states require healthcare professionals to report or test for prenatal drug exposure, which can be used as evidence in child-welfare proceedings. In order to receive federal child abuse prevention funds, states must require HCPs to notify child protective services when a provider who cares for an infant is affected by illegal substance abuse (Guttmacher Institute, 2020). Nurses working with women of childbearing age should know the laws in their own state.

TABLE 22.6 Potential Effects of Selected Drugs on Fetus/Newborn

Maternal Drug	Effects on Fetus/Newborn
CNS Depressants	
Alcohol	Drinking alcohol during pregnancy can cause miscarriage, stillbirth, and a range of lifelong physical, behavioral, and intellectual disabilities, known fetal alcohol spectrum disorders (FASDs). These include: ■ Abnormal facial features, such as a smooth ridge between the nose and upper lip (the philtrum) ■ Small stature ■ Poor coordination ■ Hyperactivity, inattention, memory problems ■ Learning disabilities, speech and language delays ■ Poor reasoning and judgment skills ■ Sleep and sucking problems as a baby ■ Vision or hearing problems ■ Problems with the heart, kidney, or bones
Benzodiazepines and sedative/hypnotics (e.g., Ambien)	■ Motor deficits ■ Communication deficits ■ Low birth weight ■ Short-term neonatal effects of hypotonia, depression, and withdrawal
Opioids/opiates	■ Congenital heart defects ■ Gastroschisis ■ Glaucoma ■ Neural tube defects (also called NTDs), birth defects of the brain, spine, and spinal cord. Spina bifida is the most common NTD. ■ Fetal growth restriction (also called growth-restricted, small for gestational age [SGA]). ■ Low birth weight (< 5 pounds, 8 ounces) ■ Sudden infant death syndrome (SIDS), unexplained death of a baby younger than 1 year old. SIDS usually occurs when a baby is sleeping; babies born to mothers who use opioids are at increased risk for SIDS.

(continued on next page)

TABLE 22.6 *(continued)*

Maternal Drug	Effects on Fetus/Newborn
Stimulants	
Amphetamine sulfate	■ Risk of low birth weight/SGA infants ■ Defects of the fetal CNS, cardiovascular system, and gastrointestinal system ■ Neurodevelopmental defects: lower attention, visual-motor integration, verbal memory, and long-term spatial memory ■ Oral cleft defects ■ Limb defects
Nicotine	■ Preterm birth ■ Low birth weight ■ Birth defects of the mouth and lip (cleft lip/palate) ■ Increased risk of SIDS
Cocaine	■ Placental abruption, where the placenta separates from the wall of the uterus before birth ■ Premature birth (<37 weeks of pregnancy) ■ Low birth weight (<5 pounds, 8 ounces) ■ Miscarriage (fetal demise in utero at <20 weeks of pregnancy) ■ Neonatal abstinence syndrome (NAS). The infant will abruptly withdraw from cocaine after birth and will need treatment for symptoms.
LSD	■ Increased risk for microcephaly and alterations in facial features ■ Decreased attention, high-pitched cry, poor visual tracking, tremors, lethargy, nystagmus, poor feeding, and altered reflexes
Other	
Marijuana	■ Fetal growth restriction, stillbirth, and preterm birth ■ Issues with neurologic development, resulting in hyperactivity and poor cognitive function

Sources: From American College of Obstetricians and Gynecologists (2017); Bailey and Diaz-Barbosa (2018); Center for Behavioral Health Statistics and Quality (2019); Centers for Disease Control and Prevention (2019d, 2020b); March of Dimes (2019, 2020); Poels, Bijma, Galbally, and Bergink (2018); Shyken, Babbar, Babbar, and Forinash (2019); Substance Abuse and Mental Health Services Administration (2018c, 2018e); Vigod and Dennis (2019).

Substance Abuse in Older Adults

Accurate data on substance abuse in older adults is difficult to determine due to failure to adequately screen by some HCPs and underreporting by patients themselves. Generally, however, researchers agree that it is a growing problem (Chhatre, Cook, Mallik, & Jayadevappa, 2017; Cho et al., 2018).

More than 80% of older patients (ages 57 to 85) use at least one prescription medication on a daily basis, with more than 50% taking more than five medications or supplements daily (NIDA, 2018g). Older patients are more likely to be prescribed long-term and multiple prescriptions, and some experience cognitive decline, which may lead to improper use of medications. High rates of comorbid illnesses in older populations, age-related changes in drug metabolism, and the potential for drug interactions make these practices more dangerous than in younger populations.

The negative consequences of substance use are more critical in older adults. Substance abuse increases the risk of falls by affecting alertness, judgment, coordination, and reaction time. Substance abuse and dependence are less likely to be recognized in older adults because many of the symptoms of abuse (e.g., insomnia, depression, loss of memory, anxiety, musculoskeletal pain) may be confused with conditions commonly seen in older patients. This results in treating the symptoms of abuse rather than diagnosing and treating the abuse itself. Research has shown that adults age 50 and older who misuse prescription opioids and benzodiazepines are at increased risk for suicidal thoughts (NIDA, 2019b).

Older adults often have individual, family, peer, school, community, and societal protective factors that help prevent illicit and nonmedical drug use: being married, never using alcohol or tobacco, and regularly attending religious services (Lipari, Ahrnsbrak, Pemberton, & Porter, 2017).

Communicating with Patients

Working Phase

Healthcare providers often neglect to screen older adults properly for substance abuse. Many older adults will present with signs of injury, and the HCP may not realize that the underlying problem is misuse or overuse of prescription medications, often coupled with alcohol abuse. Older adults may be resistant to providing information about their substance use and refuse to accept that it is dangerous. Nurses need to confront resistive behaviors and cognitive distortions in patients and family members using the following approaches:

- I know you say that your father has been taking pain medicine most of his adult life and is too old to change. However, he will realize immediate benefit from stopping opioids, and his pain may actually lessen.
- I hear you are interested in stopping your "nerve pills." Can I tell you about a schedule that will help you slowly taper off of your lorazepam? It may take a while, but you can do it.
- Despite being filled a week ago, your container of Vicodin (hydrocodone) is almost empty. Are you not using your medminder box as you agreed to last visit?
- Mr. Smith, are you aware that you stare out the window when I try to talk to you about the danger of using your pain medication and driving?

NURSING PROCESS

Due to the prevalence of psychiatric and medical comorbidities, nurses can expect to encounter patients who use or abuse substances in any setting. Nursing care of patients with substance abuse and dependence issues is challenging at best and requires a nonjudgmental attitude that promotes trust and respect. For adults, nurses should provide:

- Information on healthy coping mechanisms and stress-reduction techniques
- Education on the physiologic effects of substances on the body
- Support during periods of abstinence and when making lifestyle changes.

For children and adolescents:

- Health promotion activities that address the prevention of drug use: healthy lifestyle choices, stress-management strategies, healthy coping, good nutrition, and how to deal with peer pressure.

Because adolescents are still forming cognitive pathways for critical thinking and judgment and because of the risk-taking behaviors associated with their stage of development, adolescents are particularly vulnerable to experimenting with drugs. Adolescents and adults of any age may turn to substances for stress relief or to self-medicate for undertreated medical or psychiatric illness.

Assessment

Observation and Patient Interview

Many high-functioning substance abusers do not fit the stereotypical picture of someone who abuses drugs or alcohol. They are often members of the community, functioning in many responsible roles. They may not drink or use drugs every day. They may avoid the serious consequences that befall most individuals with addictions and their families. High-functioning individuals with SUDs can spend years, even decades, in denial. The high-functioning substance abuser's denial may be compounded by family and friends who fail to recognize or confront the problem.

A comprehensive approach to the assessment of all patients for substance use is essential to ensure adequate and appropriate intervention. Patients with substance use and dependency issues often have difficulty communicating, and nurses may need to try different therapeutic communication strategies to keep the patient engaged and build the therapeutic relationship. Open-ended questions will be more likely to elicit accurate information than questions that prompt a yes or no answer. Examples of open-ended questions include:

- On average, how many days a week do you use substances? How many times a week?
- On a typical day, how much of the substance do you use?
- How long have you been using substances?
- What specific substance(s) did you take before coming here today? How much?
- When was the last time you used substances?
- What problems has substance use caused for you? Your family?

History of Past Substance Use

A thorough assessment of past substance use includes a detailed record of the age at first use; drugs used, including type, amount, frequency; routes of administration (e.g., injection) and ingestion; length of use; comorbid alcohol and tobacco use; history of tolerance, withdrawal, drug mixing, and overdose; and consequences (e.g., legal changes or incarceration) of the patient's substance use (SAMHSA, 2020c). The history should also include patients' perception of use and readiness to change. Assess for family history of substance abuse as well as social determinants of health that may contribute to substance use or affect treatment (e.g., homelessness, lack of health insurance) (Dugosh & Cacciola, 2019). Assess for previous attempts to quit using and treatment and admission history.

Many times, patients do not remember or cannot provide their history. Additional information about risk factors can be obtained by interviewing family, friends, and caregivers about a patient's history of withdrawal, seizures, and delirium as well as attempts at stopping illicit substances such as opioids or cocaine. Whenever possible in nonemergent situations, obtain written or verbal consent from the patient before speaking with or consulting collateral sources (ASAM, 2020c).

Medical and Psychiatric History

The patient's medical history should include screening for medical comorbidities and identification or medications, allergies, pregnancy, family medical history, and more. Specific questions should focus on infectious diseases such as hepatitis, HIV, and tuberculosis; and current and past acute trauma (ASAM, 2020a, 2020b). A current physical examination should be contained within the medical record before a patient is started on a new medication for substance use. The exam should include objective signs of intoxication and withdrawal with notation of new and older puncture marks (for injectable drugs) (ASAM, 2020a, 2020b).

Physical and Psychiatric Examinations

Objective physical signs of SUDs include the following (ASAM, 2020a, 2020b):

Dermatologic: Abscesses, rashes, cellulitis, thrombosed veins, jaundice, scars, track marks, pock marks from skin popping

Ear, nose, throat, and eyes: Pupils pinpoint or dilated, yellow sclera, conjunctivitis, ruptured eardrums, otitis media, discharge from ears, rhinorrhea, rhinitis, excoriation or perforation of nasal septum, epistaxis, sinusitis, hoarseness, or laryngitis

Mouth: Poor dentition, gum disease, abscesses

Cardiovascular: Murmurs, arrhythmias

Respiratory: Asthma, dyspnea, rales, chronic cough, hematemesis

Musculoskeletal and extremities: Pitting edema, broken bones, traumatic amputations, burns on fingers

Gastrointestinal: Hepatomegaly, hernias.

A thorough psychiatric evaluation is needed for all individuals with SUDs. Nearly one in four adults with any mental illness had a perceived unmet need for mental health services in the past year; of adults with a serious mental illness, more than two out of every five adults had a perceived unmet need for mental health services in the previous year (SAMHSA, 2020a).

Psychosocial Issues

Psychosocial concerns can worsen or alleviate substance abuse problems. They also have implications for treatment. Ask how the patient's substance abuse has affected relationships with family and friends and at work. Assess anxiety level and coping mechanisms and issues related to treatment adherence, such as health insurance, financial resources, sick or vacation leave from work, and child care. Always assess for homelessness and the presence of family and social supports.

Screening Tools

Nurses working with patients who experience opiate withdrawal find several scales useful for assessing symptoms. First, the *Objective Opiate Withdrawal Scale (OOWS)* has the nurse rate 13 common, physically observable signs of opiate withdrawal as being either absent or present. These include hand tremors, shivering or huddling for warmth, vomiting, muscle twitches, and hand tremors. Second, the *Subjective Opiate Withdrawal Scale (SOWS)* asks the patient to rate 16 symptoms (including restlessness, twitching, vomiting, and an urge to use "now") on a scale of 0 (not at all) to 4 (extremely). In either case, the total score can be used to assess the intensity of opiate withdrawal and determine the extent of a patient's physical dependence on opioids. Higher scores mean a more intense withdrawal and more physical dependence (Handelsman et al., 1987). Another scale being used is the *Clinical Opiate Withdrawal Scale (COWS)*, an 11-item nurse-administered scale assessing opioid withdrawal. It can be used in an outpatient or office setting as well (ASAM, 2020b).

>> **Stay Current:** SAMHSA offers free downloadable information about suggested medication-assisted treatment for opioid addiction, as well as detailed discussion with examples of common instruments used in assessing and managing the care of a patient with a SUD. Download *TIP 63: Medications for Opioid Use Disorder* at https://store.samhsa.gov/product/TIP-63-Medications-for-Opioid-Use-Disorder-Full-Document/PEP20-02-01-006.

Diagnosis

Nursing care for patients with substance abuse problems are highly individualized depending on the substance abused, the length of time the patient has abused the chemical, and the sources of support available to the patient. Nursing care priorities are individualized to specific patient needs and may include the following:

- Potential for injury
- Difficulty adhering to the treatment plan
- Denial
- Inadequate family coping skills/resources
- Impaired family functioning
- Anxiety
- Depressed mood.

Planning

When planning care for a patient who is abusing substances, it is important to keep goals and expectations reasonable. Substance abuse recovery takes many months and often requires multiple attempts before abstinence is achieved and maintained. As a result, setting both short- and long-term goals for the patient is often most effective.

Short-term goals may include the following:

- The patient will admit having a substance abuse problem and having lost control of the individual's life as a result.
- The patient will seek help to stop using the substance.
- The patient will experience no complications as a result of drug withdrawal symptoms.
- The patient will enter a substance abuse program to change the behavior.

Long-term goals may include the following:

- The patient will explore the impact of the substance addiction on family, job, and friends.
- The patient will change thinking and behavior as a result of understanding the negative consequences of substance abuse.
- The patient will regularly attend a support group to maintain sobriety.
- The patient will remain free of the substance and maintain sobriety.

Implementation

Because patients with SUDs have difficulty communicating and maintaining relationships, it is important that the nurse convey an attitude of acceptance and promote healthy coping and appropriate behaviors. Teach and model assertive communication, as patients may have become dependent on unhealthy and less successful communication techniques. Set limits on manipulative behaviors and maintain consistency in responses. Encourage patients to focus on strengths and accomplishments rather than ruminating on weaknesses and failures. Minimize attention to any such ruminations. Help patients explore dealing with stressful situations rather than resorting to substance use, and teach healthy coping mechanisms such as physical exercise, deep breathing, meditation, and progressive muscle relaxation. Encourage participation in therapeutic group activities.

Other specific interventions for patients with substance abuse and addiction address patient safety related to abuse and withdrawal and adherence to treatment. The following interventions have implications for nursing care in both acute and home care settings.

Promote Safety

- Assess LOC, suicide risk, and risk for harm to self or others.
- If the patient is disoriented, provide orientation to reality and the environment. Remove any potentially harmful items.
- If patient cannot safely withdraw from a substance at home or in an outpatient setting, consider inpatient detoxification and treatment.

Patient Teaching

Substance Abuse

When planning education for patients with SUDs, always keep in mind that patients who are still intoxicated have impaired memory and limited ability to focus. Therefore, education should not be in a single session but take place over several sessions (Potter & Moller, 2020). Remember that the goal of treatment for SUD is remission of the disorder leading to lasting recovery and sobriety.

- Teach patients about the harmful effects of substance use.
- Patients on medication-assisted therapy (MAT) always need specific teaching and information about the drugs they are taking, including side effects.
- Discuss the benefits of counseling and recovery programs: improved problem solving and interpersonal skills
- Help patients identify constructive activities that can take the place of drug use and time spent using
- Teach patients how to access resources for recovery; this includes how to obtain and pay for needed medications, access to transportation, and other services
- Reinforce the need to adhere to the recommended treatment regimen in order to maintain sobriety
- Teach mindfulness and other coping strategies to help patients reduce stress and the potential impact of triggers that might cause them to relapse.

When a person has decided to use MAT, the nurse should facilitate rapid assessment and treatment initiation while the patient is motivated. The nurse should also discuss strategies with the patient on how to return to treatment when the individual has discontinued treatment prematurely and is thinking about using or has started using illicit drugs again (SAMHSA, 2020c).

For the patient with an opiate use disorder, the patient, family members, and significant others should receive opioid overdose prevention education and a naloxone prescription for injectable or intranasal naloxone, an opioid antagonist; in many states, these rescue medications can be bought over the counter. Persons who have high risk of overdose often have recently completed opioid detoxification, been recently released from incarceration, or have been abstinent for a period of time and have a reduced opioid tolerance (SAMHSA, 2018b). If they return to opioid use using their prior high doses, they may overdose.

- Obtain urine and blood samples. Patients do not always admit to drug use or may not fully discuss the extent of their abuse.
- Decrease environmental stimuli. Place patient in a quiet room, but do not leave patient alone if the individual reports suicidal ideation or intent or exhibits hyperactivity.
- Monitor vital signs every 15 minutes until stable or per agency protocol.

Promote Patient Safety During Withdrawal

Interventions to ensure patient safety vary on the type of substance used. Nurses will monitor vital signs and neurologic signs and symptoms and provide nutrition and hydration according to protocol or provider orders. A calm environment and frequent reorientation as well as a nonjudgmental manner will help ensure patients that they are safe. Other interventions are listed in the Independent Interventions section earlier in this module.

Evaluation

Patients with substance abuse issues often struggle to meet treatment goals. It is essential to provide positive reinforcement for sincere efforts to reach goals and for even incremental improvements. Evaluation may include:

- The patient admits struggling with substance abuse and seeks help.
- The patient remains free of withdrawal complication.
- The patient enters recommended treatment.
- The patient attends treatment sessions.
- The patient remains free of substances for __________ (time period).

The National Institute on Drug Abuse (2020a) estimated that the relapse rate of 40–60% for substance abuse is similar to that for other chronic illnesses, such as diabetes, HTN, or asthma. NIDA has recommended that clinicians treat substance addiction like any other chronic illness for which relapse serves as a trigger for renewed intervention.

Nursing Care Plan

A Patient with Substance Use Disorder

Donna Smith is brought to the ED by her husband. She is agitated and can't stand still. Her husband tells the nurse that she has been getting high on crack cocaine on a regular basis. When Donna didn't come home last night, he called their cell phone company to activate her GPS and found her outside a motel on the highway. He took her home, where she began shouting, yelling, and throwing things and talking about the "men in the trees" who are after her. The nurse conducting the assessment determines that they have two children, ages 11 and 15, living at home.

(continued on next page)

Nursing Care Plan *(continued)*

ASSESSMENT	DIAGNOSES	PLANNING
The nurse collects the following data during assessment: Temperature 99.4°F axillary; P 114 bpm; R 20/min; BP 168/92 mmHg Pupils constricted and equally responsive to light Patient is muttering to herself in mostly unintelligible sentences, with phrases such as "men in trees," "gonna get me," and "don't worry" understood among gibberish words. Patient says she hears voices and points out things that are not there, apparently having both visual and auditory hallucinations. Peripheral pulses are 3+ and bounding, sinus tachycardia is noted on ECG with frequent premature ventricular contractions, and hyperreactive reflexes. Patient is admitted to monitored unit (telemetry) for observation until cardiac and neurologic systems are stable.	■ Potential for injury ■ Impaired family functioning ■ Inadequate coping skills ■ Confusion ■ Potential for violence against self or others	Goals of care include the following: ■ Experience no adverse cardiac event. ■ Orient to time and place. ■ ECG will return to normal sinus rhythm. ■ Neurologic assessment will return to pre–substance use baseline. ■ Agree to psychosocial intervention to assist in substance avoidance.

IMPLEMENTATION

- Monitor cardiorespiratory function.
- Assess orientation and maintain safety while hallucinating.
- Maintain low-stimulation environment until effects of drug subside.
- Maintain hydration to promote excretion of drug from system.
- Obtain complete history of substance use when patient's cognitive function returns.
- Administer sedatives and antiarrhythmics as required per orders.
- Refer Mr. Smith to a support program for spouses and children.
- Refer to substance abuse program to assist in abstinence once drugs have been cleared from system if patient is willing to participate.

EVALUATION

Evaluation of patient response may be based on the following expected outcomes:

- The patient experiences no cardiac event as the result of cocaine use.
- The patient's cognition returns to prior baseline.
- The patient admits to having a problem and agrees to seek treatment.

CRITICAL THINKING

1. While the patient is experiencing both auditory and visual hallucinations, how will the nurse respond if the patient insists there is something in the room that is not seen by the nurse?
2. What actions will the nurse implement to maintain the patient's safety?
3. After detoxification, the patient regains normal cognitive function and informs the nurse she is leaving the facility because she wants to "get high again." What is the nurse's legal obligation to this patient?

REVIEW Substance Use Disorders

RELATE Link the Concepts and Exemplars

Linking the exemplar of substance use disorders with the concept of safety:

1. The nurse had surgery a few days ago and is taking a narcotic analgesic to control pain. Is it safe for the nurse to work assigned shifts while taking this medication? Why or why not?

2. You suspect that a coworker whom you admire for his experience and knowledge may be using an illegal drug. What is your best action to maintain patient safety? How would you handle this issue?

Linking the exemplar of substance use disorders with the concept of trauma:

3. How does the abuse of substances affect the risk for violence committed by the patient?

4. When working in a substance abuse treatment facility, how can you, as the nurse, encourage spouses at risk for acts of domestic violence by your patients seek support for their own health?

READY Go to Volume 3: Clinical Nursing Skills

REFER Go to Pearson MyLab Nursing and eText

REFLECT Apply Your Knowledge

Jacob is a 23-year-old male who works in the shipping department at a large factory in his rural community. A high-school dropout who discovered beer and marijuana in his mid-teens, Jacob moved through a series of minimum-wage jobs before getting his GED at a local community college. He was then able to secure an entry-level job at the factory and has worked there for the past 2 years.

Jacob is able to curtail his beer drinking during the work week, but he smokes a large joint two to three times a week for his "nerves." On the weekend, he often buys two 12-packs of beer and drinks all of it while hanging out with his friends, watching sports on TV.

One Monday, Jacob shows up for work unkempt and unable to concentrate. His hands shake and his eyes are bloodshot. He fell during the weekend and gouged his scalp, which is now bandaged, and he has facial bruising. His supervisor pulls him aside and asks him about drinking. Jacob admits to drinking too much over the weekend. Concerned, his boss refers him to the company's employee assistance program (EAP). Jacob is suspended from his job until he reports to the EAP counselor.

Alarmed, Jacob immediately visits the counselor, who assures him that his visit and subsequent actions are confidential. She refers Jacob to a local community drug treatment center, where he is assessed by a psychiatric–mental health nurse practitioner (PMH-NP), who specializes in addictions. After assessment, the PMH-NP refers Jacob to an outpatient treatment program of education, counseling, support groups, and Alcoholics Anonymous meetings. She tells him that treatment and counseling are 80% covered by his employer. Jacob follows the plan of care exactly as outlined. Two weeks later, contingent on remaining engaged in treatment, he is allowed to return to work. He is required to maintain contact with the treatment center for the next 6 months.

1. What were the priority nursing interventions after the initial assessment and confirmation of Jacob's substance use?
2. What were Jacob's motivations for treatment?
3. What are Jacob's risks for relapse?

References

Ahmad, F. B., Rossen, L. M., & Sutton, P. *Provisional drug overdose death counts.* https://www.cdc.gov/nchs/nvss/vsrr/drug-overdose-data.htm#citation

Alkam, T., & Nabeshima, T. (2019). Prenatal nicotine exposure and impact on the behaviors of offspring. In V. R. Preedy (Ed.), *Neuroscience of nicotine* (pp. 191–197). Academic Press.

Alvanzo, A. A., Wand, G. S., Kuwabara, H., Wong, D. F., Xu, X., & McCaul, M. E. (2017). Family history of alcoholism is related to increased D2/D3 receptor binding potential: A marker of resilience or risk? *Addiction Biology, 43*(17), 218–228. https://doi.org/10.1111/acer.14079

American Cancer Society. (2020). *Great American Smokeout.* https://www.cancer.org/healthy/stay-away-from-tobacco/great-american-smokeout.html

American College of Obstetricians and Gynecologists. (2017). *Methamphetamine abuse in women of reproductive age* [Committee Opinion No. 479]. https://www.acog.org/clinical/clinical-guidance/committee-opinion/articles/2011/03/methamphetamine-abuse-in-women-of-reproductive-age

American Lung Association. (2020). *Health effects of smoking and tobacco products.* https://www.lung.org/quit-smoking/smoking-facts/health-effects

American Nurses Association. (2020a). *Healthy work environment.* https://www.nursingworld.org/practice-policy/work-environment/

American Nurses Association. (2020b). *Substance use among nurses and nursing students.* https://www.nursingworld.org/practice-policy/nursing-excellence/official-position-statements/id/substance-use-among-nurses-and-nursing-students/

American Psychiatric Association. (2013). *Diagnostic and statistical manual of mental disorders* (5th ed.). Author.

American Society of Addiction Medicine (ASAM). (2020a). *ASAM clinical practice guideline on alcohol withdrawal management.* Author.

American Society of Addiction Medicine (ASAM). (2020b). *The ASAM national practice guideline for the use of medications in the treatment of addiction involving opioid use: 2020 focused update.* Author.

American Society of Addiction Medicine (ASAM). (2020c). *What is the ASAM criteria?* https://www.asam.org/asam-criteria/about

Anxiety and Depression Association of America. (2018). *Substance use disorders.* https://adaa.org/understanding-anxiety/related-illnesses/substance-abuse

Archer, M., Kampman, O., Bloigu, A., Bloigu, R., Luoto, K., Kultti, J., et al.. (2019). Assessment of alcohol consumption in depression follow-up using self-reports and blood measures including inflammatory biomarkers. *Alcohol and Alcoholism, 54*(3), 243–250. https://doi.org/10.1093/alcalc/agz002

Armenian, P., Vo, K. T., Barr-Walker, J., & Lynch, K. L. (2018). Fentanyl, fentanyl analogs and novel synthetic opioids: A comprehensive review. *Neuropharmacology, 134*, 121–132. https://doi.org/10.1016/j.neuropharm.2017.10.016

Arts, N. J. M., Walvoort, S. J. W., & Kessels, R. P. C. (2017). Korsakoff's syndrome: A critical review. *Neuropsychiatric Disease and Treatment, 13*, 2875–2890. https://doi.org/10.2147/NDT.S130078

Bailey, N. A., & Diaz-Barbosa, M. (2018). Effect of maternal substance abuse on the fetus, neonate, and child. *Pediatrics in Review, 39*(11), 551–559. https://doi.org/10.1542/pir.2017-0201

Barnes, J., McRobbie, H., Dong, C. Y., Walker, N., & Hartmann-Boyce, J. (2019). Hypnotherapy for smoking cessation. *Cochrane Database of Systematic Reviews*, Issue 6, Article No. CD001008. https://doi.org/10.1002/14651858.CD001008.pub3

Bauldoff, G., Gubrud, P., & Carno, M. (2020). *LeMone & Burke's medical-surgical nursing* (7th ed.). Pearson.

Behavioral Tech. (2019). *What is dialetical behavior therapy (DBT)?* https://behavioraltech.org/resources/faqs/dialectical-behavior-therapy-dbt/

Bonn-Miller, M. O., Loflin, M. J. E., Thomas, B. F., Marcu, J. P., Hyke, T., & Vandrey, R. (2017). Labeling accuracy of cannabidiol extracts sold online. *Journal of the American Medical Association, 318*(17), 1708–1709. https://doi.org/10.1001/jama.2017.11909

Brewer, S., Godley, M. D., & Hulvershorn, L. A. (2017). Treating mental health and substance use disorders in adolescents: What is on the menu? *Current Psychiatry Reports, 19*(1), 5. https://doi.org/10.1007/s11920-017-0755-0

Capone, C., Presseau, C., Saunders, E., Eaton, E., Hamblen, J., & McGovern, M. (2018). Is integrated CBT effective in reducing PTSD symptoms and substance use in Iraq and Afghanistan veterans?: Results from a randomized clinical trial. *Cognitive Therapy and Research, 42*(6), 735–746. https://doi.org/10.1007/s10608-018-9931-8

Center for Behavioral Health Statistics and Quality (CBHSQ). (2017). *A day in the life of older adults: Substance use facts.* Substance Abuse and Mental Health Services Administration. https://www.samhsa.gov/data/sites/default/files/report_2792/ShortReport-2792.pdf

Center for Behavioral Health Statistics and Quality (CBHSQ). (2019). *Key substance use and mental health indicators in the United States: Results from the 2018 National Survey on Drug Use and Health* (HHS Publication No. PEP19-5068, NSDUH Series H-54). Substance Abuse and Mental Health Services Administration. https://www.samhsa.gov/data/sites/default/files/cbhsq-reports/NSDUHNationalFindingsReport2018/NSDUHNationalFindingsReport2018.pdf

Center for the Application of Prevention Technologies (CAPT). (2018). *The role of adverse childhood xxperiences in substance misuse and related behavioral health problems.* Substance Abuse and Mental Health Services Administration. https://mnprc.org/wp-content/uploads/2019/01/aces-behavioral-health-problems.pdf

Center of Excellence for Integrated Health Solutions. (2020). *Center of Excellence on-demand tools and resources now available to help you improve your integrated health.* https://www.thenationalcouncil.org/integrated-health-coe/

Centers for Disease Control and Prevention (CDC). (2018). *Secondhand smoke (SHS) facts.* https://www.cdc.gov/tobacco/data_statistics/fact_sheets/secondhand_smoke/general_facts/index.htm

Centers for Disease Control and Prevention (CDC). (2019a). *The buzz on energy drinks.* https://www.cdc.gov/healthyschools/nutrition/energy.htm

Centers for Disease Control and Prevention (CDC). (2019b). *Current cigarette smoking among adults in the United States.* https://www.cdc.gov/tobacco/data_statistics/fact_sheets/adult_data/cig_smoking/index.htm

Centers for Disease Control and Prevention (CDC). (2019c). *Life-saving naloxone from pharmacies: More dispensing needed despite progress.* https://www.cdc.gov/vitalsigns/naloxone/

Centers for Disease Control and Prevention (CDC). (2019d). *Substance use during pregnancy.* https://www.cdc.gov/reproductivehealth/maternalinfanthealth/substance-abuse/substance-abuse-during-pregnancy.htm

Centers for Disease Control and Prevention (CDC). (2019e). *Youth and tobacco use.* https://www.cdc.gov/tobacco/data_statistics/fact_sheets/youth_data/tobacco_use/index.htm#current-estimates

Centers for Disease Control and Prevention (CDC). (2020a). *About electronic cigarettes (e-cigarettes): What's the bottom line?* https://www.cdc.gov/tobacco/basic_information/e-cigarettes/about-e-cigarettes.html

Centers for Disease Control and Prevention (CDC). (2020b). *Alcohol use in pregnancy.* https://www.cdc.gov/ncbddd/fasd/alcohol-use.html

Centers for Disease Control and Prevention (CDC). (2020c). *Burden of cigarette use in the U.S.* https://www.cdc.gov/tobacco/campaign/tips/resources/data/cigarette-smoking-in-united-states.html

Centers for Disease Control and Prevention (CDC). (2020d). *Caffeine and alcohol: Dangers of mixing alcohol and caffeine.* https://www.cdc.gov/alcohol/fact-sheets/caffeine-and-alcohol.htm

Centers for Disease Control and Prevention (CDC). (2020e). *Data on excessive drinking.* https://www.cdc.gov/alcohol/data-stats.htm#economicCosts

Centers for Disease Control and Prevention (CDC). (2020f). *Heroin overdose.* https://www.cdc.gov/drugoverdose/data/heroin.html

Centers for Disease Control and Prevention (CDC). (2020g). *Opioid overdose*. https://www.cdc.gov/drugoverdose/index.html

Centers for Disease Control and Prevention (CDC). (2020h). *Opioid overdose: U.S. opioid prescribing rate maps*. https://www.cdc.gov/drugoverdose/maps/rxrate-maps.html

Centers for Disease Control and Prevention (CDC). (2020i). *Outbreak of lung injury associated with the use of e-cigarette, or vaping, products*. https://www.cdc.gov/tobacco/basic_information/e-cigarettes/severe-lung-disease.html

Centers for Disease Control and Prevention (CDC). (2020j). *Questions about symptoms of EVALI*. https://www.cdc.gov/tobacco/basic_information/e-cigarettes/severe-lung-disease/faq/index.html

Centers for Disease Control and Prevention (CDC). (2020k). *Smoking and tobacco use: Health effects*. https://www.cdc.gov/tobacco/basic_information/health_effects/index.htm

Centers for Disease Control and Prevention (CDC). (2020l). *Smoking cessation: Fast facts*. https://www.cdc.gov/tobacco/data_statistics/fact_sheets/cessation/smoking-cessation-fast-facts/index.html

Centers for Disease Control and Prevention (CDC). (2020m). *Smoking during pregnancy*. https://www.cdc.gov/tobacco/basic_information/health_effects/pregnancy/index.htm

Centers for Disease Control and Prevention (CDC). (2020n). *Teen substance use and risks*. https://www.cdc.gov/ncbddd/fasd/features/teen-substance-use.html

Chaiton, M., Diemert, L., Cohen, J. E., Bondy, S. J., Selby, P., Philipneri, A., & Schwartz, R. (2016). Estimating the number of quit attempts it takes to quit smoking successfully in a longitudinal cohort of smokers. *BMJ Open*, *6*(6), e011045. https://doi.org/10.1136/bmjopen-2016-011045

Chen, E. S., Applewhite, D., Alvanzo, A. A. H., Welsh, C., Niessen, T., & Rastegar, D. A. (2017). C51 Critical Care: More non-pulmonary critical care problems: Development and implementation of an alcohol withdrawal protocol using the 5-item Brief Alcohol Withdrawal Scale (BAWS). *American Journal of Respiratory and Critical Care Medicine*, *195*, A5782. https://search.proquest.com/openview/16d63dfef8017f56ee740aa76d5c6afd/1?pq-origsite=gscholar&cbl=40575

Chen, P., Li, J., Han, X., Grech, D., Xiong, M., Bekker, A., & Ye, J.-H. (2018). Acupuncture for alcohol use disorder. *International Journal of Physiology, Pathophysiology and Pharmacology*, *10*(1), 60–69.

Chhatre, S., Cook, R., Mallik, E., & Jayadevappa, R. (2017). Trends in substance use admissions among older adults. *BMC Health Services Research*, *17*(1), 584. https://doi.org/10.1186/s12913-017-2538-z

Cho, J., Bhimani, J., Patel, M., & Thomas, M. N. (2018). Substance abuse among older adults: A growing problem. *Current Psychiatry*, *17*(3), 14–20.

Cross, S. J., Lotfipour, S., & Leslie, F. M. (2017). Mechanisms and genetic factors underlying co-use of nicotine and alcohol or other drugs of abuse. *American Journal of Drug and Alcohol Abuse*, *43*(2), 171–185. https://doi.org/10.1080/00952990.2016.1209512

Culturally competent substance abuse nursing. (2013). *Minority Nurse*. https://minoritynurse.com/culturally-competent-substance-abuse-nursing/

Czermak, C., Lehofer, M., Wagner, E. M., Prietl, B., Lemonis, L., Rohrhofer, A., & Liebmann, P. M. (2004). Reduced dopamine D4 receptor mRNA expression in lymphocytes of long-term abstinent alcohol and heroin addicts. *Addiction*, *99*(2), 251–257.

Darke, S., Duflou, J., Kaye, S., Farrell, M., & Lappin, J. (2019). Psychostimulant use and fatal stroke in young adults. *Journal of Forensic Sciences*, *64*(5), 1421–1426. https://doi.org/10.1111/1556-4029.14056

Darke, S., Lappin, J., Kaye, S., & Duflou, J. (2018). Clinical characteristics of fatal methamphetamine-related stroke: A national study. *Journal of Forensic Sciences*, *63*(3), 735–739. https://doi.org/10.1111/1556-4029.13620

De Sanctis, V., Soliman, N., Soliman, A. T., Elsedfy, H., Di Maio, S., El Kholy, M., & Fiscina, B. (2017). Caffeinated energy drink consumption among adolescents and potential health consequences associated with their use: A significant public health hazard. *Acta Bio-Medica: Atenei Parmensis*, *88*(2), 222–231. https://doi.org/10.23750/abm.v88i2.6664

DeKosky, S. T., & Williamson, J. B. (2020). The long and the short of benzodiazepines and sleep medications: Short-term benefits, long-term harms? *Neurotherapeutics*, *17*(1), 153–155. https://doi.org/10.1007/s13311-019-00827-z

Des Jarlais, D. C. (2017). Harm reduction in the USA: The research perspective and an archive to David Purchase. *Harm Reduction Journal*, *14*(1), 51. https://doi.org/10.1186/s12954-017-0178-6

Dickenson, J. A., Gleason, N., Coleman, E., & Miner, M. H. (2018). Prevalence of distress associated with difficulty controlling sexual urges, feelings, and behaviors in the United States. *JAMA Network Open*, *1*(7), e184468. https://doi.org/10.1001/jamanetworkopen.2018.4468

Dousset, C., Kajosch, H., Ingels, A., Schröder, E., Kornreich, C., & Campanella, S. (2020). Preventing relapse in alcohol disorder with EEG-neurofeedback as a neuromodulation technique: A review and new insights regarding its application. *Addictive Behaviors*, *106*, 106391. https://doi.org/10.1016/j.addbeh.2020.106391

Dugosh, K. L., & Cacciola, J. S. (2019). *Clinical assessment of substance use disorders*. UpToDate. https://www.uptodate.com/contents/clinical-assessment-of-substance-use-disorders

Edenberg, H. J., Gelernter, J., & Agrawal, A. (2019). Genetics of alcoholism. *Current Psychiatry Reports*, *21*(4), 26. https://doi.org/10.1007/s11920-019-1008-1

Ellis, A. (2020). *Rational emotive behavior therapy*. https://albertellis.org/rebt-cbt-therapy/

Engel, G. L. (1978). The biopsychosocial model and the education of health professionals. *Annals of the New York Academy of Sciences*, *310*(1), 169–181. https://doi.org/10.1111/j.1749-6632.1978.tb22070.x

Esang, M., & Ahmed, S. (2018). A closer look at substance use and suicide. *American Journal of Psychiatry Residents' Journal*, *13*(6), 6–8. https://doi.org/10.1176/appi.ajp-rj.2018.130603

Fish, J., Osberg, T. M., & Syed, M. (2017). "This is the way we were raised": Alcohol beliefs and acculturation in relation to alcohol consumption among Native Americans. *Journal of Ethnicity in Substance Abuse*, *16*(2), 219–245. https://doi.org/10.1080/15332640.2015.1133362

Foli, K. J., Reddick, B., Zhang, L., & Edwards, N. (2019). Substance use in registered nurses: Where legal, medical, and personal collide. *Journal of Nursing Regulation*, *10*(2), 45–54. https://doi.org/10.1016/S2155-8256(19)30115-2

Gainsbury, S. M. (2017). Cultural competence in the treatment of addictions: Theory, practice and evidence. *Clinical Psychology & Psychotherapy*, *24*(4), 987–1001.

Giger, J. N., & Haddad, L. G. (2021). *Transcultural nursing: Assessment and intervention* (8th ed.). Elsevier.

Grant, B. F., Chou, S. P., Saha, T. D., Pickering, R. P., Kerridge, B. T., Ruan, W. J., et al. (2017). Prevalence of 12-month alcohol use, high-risk drinking, and DSM-IV alcohol use disorder in the United States, 2001–2002 to 2012–2013: Results from the National Epidemiologic Survey on Alcohol and Related Conditions. *JAMA Psychiatry*, *74*(9), 911–923. https://doi.org/10.1001/jamapsychiatry.2017.2161

Grasser, L., Wanna, C., Minton, S., Phillips, K., Dumornay, N., Seligowski, A., et al. (2020). Fear-potentiated startle prospectively predicts alcohol use patterns in individuals exposed to trauma. *Biological Psychiatry*, *87*(9), S393–S394. https://doi.org/10.1016/j.biopsych.2020.02.1007

Guttmacher Institute. (2020). *Substance use during pregnancy*. https://www.guttmacher.org/state-policy/explore/substance-use-during-pregnancy#

Hajela, R. (2017). Addiction is more than a substance use disorder. *Journal of Addiction Medicine*, *11*(4), 331. https://doi.org/10.1097/adm.0000000000000332

Handelsman, L., Cochrane, K. J., Aronson, M. J., Ness, R., Rubinstein, K. J., & Kanof, P. D. (1987). Two new rating scales for opiate withdrawal. *American Journal of Drug and Alcohol Abuse*, *13*(3), 293–308. https://doi.org/10.3109/00952998709001515

Harm Reduction Coalitition. (2020). *Fentanyl*. https://harmreduction.org/issues/fentanyl/

Hartney, E. (2020). *How to build self-esteem during recovery from addiction*. Verywell Mind. https://www.verywellmind.com/five-ways-to-build-self-esteem-22380

Harvard Health Online. (2019). *Alcohol withdrawal*. https://www.health.harvard.edu/a_to_z/alcohol-withdrawal-a-to-z

Hazelden Betty Ford Foundation. (2018). *Trauma informed care for substance abuse counseling: A brief summary*. https://www.hazeldenbettyford.org/education/bcr/addiction-research/trauma-informed-care-ru-118

Hazelden Betty Ford Foundation. (2020). *Addiction communication: Putting CRAFT to work for you*. https://www.hazeldenbettyford.org/articles/addiction-communication

HealthLink BC. (2020). *Understanding harm reduction: Substance use*. https://www.healthlinkbc.ca/healthlinkbc-files/substance-use-harm-reduction

Henley, S. J., Asman, K., Momin, B., Gallaway, M. S., Culp, M. B., Ragan, K. R., et al. (2019). Smoking cessation behaviors among older U.S. adults. *Preventive Medicine Reports*, *16*, 100978. https://doi.org/10.1016/j.pmedr.2019.100978

Holton, A. E., Gallagher, P. J., Ryan, C., Fahey, T., & Cousins, G. (2017). Consensus validation of the POSAMINO (POtentially Serious Alcohol–Medication INteractions in Older adults) criteria. *BMJ Open*, *7*(11), e017453. http://dx.doi.org/10.1136/bmjopen-2017-017453

Hook, J., & Devereux, D. (2018). Boundary violations in therapy: The patient's experience of harm. *BJPsych Advances*, *24*(6), 366–373. https://doi.org/10.1192/bja.2018.26

Institute of Medicine. (2015). *Psychosocial interventions for mental and substance use disorders: A framework for establishing evidence-based standards*. Author.

Jang, S., Lee, J. A., Jang, B.-H., Shin, Y.-C., Ko, S.-G., & Park, S. (2019). Clinical effectiveness of traditional and complementary medicine interventions in combination with nicotine replacement therapy on smoking cessation: A randomized controlled pilot trial. *Journal of Alternative and Complementary Medicine*, *25*(5), 526–534. https://doi.org/10.1089/acm.2019.0009

Jellinek, E. (1946). *Phases in the drinking history of alcoholics*. Hillhouse Press.

Jesse, S., Bråthen, G., Ferrara, M., Keindl, M., Ben-Menachem, E., Tanasescu, R., et al. (2017). Alcohol withdrawal syndrome: Mechanisms, manifestations, and management. *Acta Neurologica Scandinavica*, *135*(1), 4–16. https://doi.org/10.1111/ane.12671

Kaiser Permanente. (2020). *Alcohol use in older adults*. https://wa.kaiserpermanente.org/healthAndWellness/index.jhtml?item=%2Fcommon%2FhealthAndWellness%2FhealthyLiving%2Flifestyle%2Falcohol-seniors.html

Kariisa, M., Scholl, L., Wilson, N., Seth, P., & Hoots, B. (2019). Drug overdose deaths involving cocaine and ssychostimulants with abuse potential—United States, 2003–2017. *Morbidity and Mortality Weekly Report*, *68*(17), 388–395. https://doi.org/10.15585/mmwr.mm6817a3

Kastaun, S., Leve, V., Hildebrandt, J., Funke, C., Klosterhalfen, S., Lubisch, D., et al. (2020). Effectiveness of training general practitioners in the ABC versus 5As method of delivering brief stop-smoking advice: A pragmatic, two-arm cluster randomised controlled trial. *medRxiv*. https://doi.org/10.1101/2020.03.26.20041491

Katz, J., Goodnough, A, & Sanger-Katz, M. (2020). In shadow of pandemic, U.S. drug overdose deaths resurge to record. *New York Times*. https://www.nytimes.com/interactive/2020/07/15/upshot/drug-overdose-deaths.html

Kelly, J. F., Saitz, R., & Wakeman, S. (2016). Language, substance use disorders, and policy: The need to reach consensus on an "addiction-ary." *Alcoholism Treatment Quarterly*, *34*(1), 116–123. https://doi.org/10.1080/07347324.2016.1113103

Kerr, D. L., & Oglesby, W. H. (2017). LGBT populations and substance abuse research: An overview. In J. B. VanGeest, T. P. Johnson, & S. A. Alemagno (Eds.), *Research methods in the study of substance abuse* (pp. 341–355). Springer.

Koch, M., Fitzpatrick, A. L., Rapp, S. R., Nahin, R. L., Williamson, J. D., Lopez, O. L., et al. (2019). Alcohol consumption and risk of dementia and cognitive decline among older adults with or without mild cognitive impairment. *JAMA Network Open*, *2*(9), e1910319. https://doi.org/10.1001/jamanetworkopen.2019.10319

Lanzillotta-Rangeley, J., Leslie, J., Little, M., Stem, J., Asselin, E., & Kurahovic, M. (2020). Educational program to increase substance use disorder knowledge and decrease stigma in first-year nursing students. *Pain Management Nursing*, *21*(5), 435–440. https://doi.org/10.1016/j.pmn.2020.05.002

Letourneau, E. J., McCart, M. R., Sheidow, A. J., & Mauro, P. M. (2017). First evaluation of a contingency management intervention addressing adolescent substance use and sexual risk behaviors: Risk reduction therapy for adolescents. *Journal of Substance Abuse Treatment*, *72*, 56–65. https://doi.org/10.1016/j.jsat.2016.08.019

Levine, A., Clemenza, K., Rynn, M., & Lieberman, J. (2017). Evidence for the risks and consequences of adolescent cannabis exposure. *Journal of the American Academy of Child and Adolescent Psychiatry*, *56*(3), 214–225. https://doi.org/10.1016/j.jaac.2016.12.014

Li, J. L., Savage, J. E., Kendler, K. S., Hickman, M., Mahedy, L., Macleod, J., et al. (2017). Polygenic risk, personality dimensions, and adolescent alcohol use problems: A longitudinal study. *Journal of Studies on Alcohol and Drugs, 78*(3), 442–451. https://doi.org/10.15288/jsad.2017.78.442

Lipari, R. N., Ahrnsbrak, R. D., Pemberton, M. R., & Porter, J. D. (2017). *Risk and protective factors and estimates of substance use initiation: Results from the 2016 National Survey on Drug Use and Health.* Substance Abuse and Mental Health Services Administration. https://www.samhsa.gov/data/sites/default/files/NSDUH-DR-FFR3-2016/NSDUH-DR-FFR3-2016.htm

Lipari, R. N., & Van Horn, S. L. (2017). *Children living with parents who have a substance use disorder.* Substance Abuse and Mental Health Services Administration.

Liu, J., Shi, Y.-C., & Lee, D. Y.-W. (2019). Applications of Pueraria lobata in treating diabetics and reducing alcohol drinking. *Chinese Herbal Medicines, 11*(2), 141–149. https://doi.org/10.1016/j.chmed.2019.04.004

London, M. L., Ladewig, P. W., Ball, J. W., Bindler, R. C., & Cowen, K. J. (2017). *Maternal and child nursing care* (5th ed.). Pearson.

Long, D., Long, B., & Koyfman, A. (2017). The emergency medicine management of severe alcohol withdrawal. *American Journal of Emergency Medicine, 35*(7), 1005–1011. https://doi.org/10.1016/j.ajem.2017.02.002

Lovallo, W. R., Cohoon, A. J., Sorocco, K. H., Vincent, A. S., Acheson, A., Hodgkinson, C. A., & Goldman, D. (2019). Early-life adversity and blunted stress reactivity as predictors of alcohol and drug use in persons with COMT (rs4680) Val158Met genotypes. *Alcoholism: Clinical and Experimental Research, 43*(7), 1519–1527. https://doi.org/10.1111/acer.14079

Mahmoud, K. F., Finnell, D., Lindsay, D., MacFarland, C., Marze, H. D., Scolieri, B. B., & Mitchell, A. M. (2019). Can Screening, Brief Intervention, and Referral to Treatment Education and clinical exposure affect nursing students' stigma perception toward alcohol and opioid use? *Journal of the American Psychiatric Nurses Association, 25*(6), 467–475. https://doi.org/10.1177/1078390318811570

March of Dimes. (2019). *Prescription opioids during pregnancy.* https://www.marchofdimes.org/pregnancy/prescription-opioids-during-pregnancy.aspx

March of Dimes. (2020). *Cocaine and pregnancy.* https://www.marchofdimes.org/pregnancy/cocaine.aspx

Mayo Clinic. (2020a). *Alcohol use disorder.* https://www.mayoclinic.org/diseases-conditions/alcohol-use-disorder/symptoms-causes/syc-20369243

Mayo Clinic. (2020b). *Nutrition and healthy eating.* https://www.mayoclinic.org/healthy-lifestyle/nutrition-and-healthy-eating/in-depth/caffeine/art-20045678

McHugh, R. K., Votaw, V. R., Sugarman, D. E., & Greenfield, S. F. (2018). Sex and gender differences in substance use disorders. *Clinical Psychology Review, 66*, 12–23. https://doi.org/10.1016/j.cpr.2017.10.012

Medline Plus. (2020a). *Blood alcohol level.* https://medlineplus.gov/lab-tests/blood-alcohol-level/

Medline Plus. (2020b). *Tips on how to quit smoking.* https://medlineplus.gov/ency/article/001992.htm

Medscape. (2019). *Inhalant-related psychiatric disorders: Treatment & management.* https://emedicine.medscape.com/article/290344-treatment

Mehdi, S., Mehdi, S., Siddique, R., & Ahmad, A. (2017). The effect of cocaine addiction on humans and its treatment. *Journal of Toxicological & Pharmaceutical Sciences, 1*(2), 115–119.

Miller, M. B., DiBello, A. M., Meier, E., Leavens, E. L. S., Merrill, J. E., Carey, K. B., & Leffingwell, T. R. (2019). Alcohol-induced amnesia and personalized drinking feedback: Blackouts predict intervention response. *Behavior Therapy, 50*(1), 25–35. https://doi.org/10.1016/j.beth.2018.03.008

Miller, W., & Rollnick, S. (2004). Talking oneself into change: Motivational interviewing, stages of change, and therapeutic process. *Journal of Cognitive Psychotherapy, 18*(4), 299–308. https://doi.org/10.1891/jcop.18.4.299.64003

Minkove, J. F. (2019). *Substance use disorders in older adults: A growing threat.* Johns Hopkins Medicine. https://www.hopkinsmedicine.org/news/articles/substance-use-disorders-in-older-adults-a-growing-threat

Morse, R. M., & Flavin, D. K. (1992). The definition of alcoholism. The Joint Committee of the National Council on Alcoholism and Drug Dependence and the American Society of Addiction Medicine to Study the Definition and Criteria for the Diagnosis of Alcoholism. *Journal of the American Medical Association, 268*(8), 1012–1014. https://doi.org/10.1001/jama.268.8.1012

Müller, A., Brand, M., Claes, L., Demetrovics, Z., de Zwaan, M., Fernández-Aranda, F., et al. (2019). Buying-shopping disorder—Is there enough evidence to support its inclusion in ICD-11? *CNS Spectrums, 24*, 1–6. https://doi.org/10.1017/S1092852918001323

Nadkarni, A., Endsley, P., Bhatia, U., Fuhr, D. C., Noorani, A., Naik, A., et al. (2017). Community detoxification for alcohol dependence: A systematic review. *Drug and Alcohol Review, 36*(3), 389–399. https://doi.org/10.1111/dar.12440

Nakhaee, S., Vagharseyyedin, S. A., Afkar, E., & Mood, S. M. (2017). The relationship of family communication pattern with adolescents' assertiveness. *Modern Care Journal, 14*(4), e66696. https://doi.org/10.5812/modernc.66696

Nash, S. H., Liao, L. M., Harris, T. B., & Freedman, N. D. (2017). Cigarette smoking and mortality in adults aged 70 Years and older: Results From the NIH-AARP cohort. *American Journal of Preventive Medicine, 52*(3), 276–283. https://doi.org/10.1016/j.amepre.2016.09.036

Nash, A. J., Marcus, M. T., Cron, S., Scamp, N., Truitt, M., & McKenna, Z. (2017). Preparing nursing students to work with patients with alcohol or drug-related problems. *Journal of Addictions Nursing, 28*(3), 124–130. https://doi.org/10.1097/jan.0000000000000175

Naslund, J. A., Kim S. J., Aschbrenner, K. A., McCulloch, L. J., Brunette, M. F., Dallery, J., et al. (2017). Systematic review of social media interventions for smoking cessation. *Addictive Behaviors, 73*, 81–93.

National Action Alliance for Suicide Prevention. (2018). *Recommended standard care for people with suicide risk: Making health care suicide safe.* https://theactionalliance.org/sites/default/files/action_alliance_recommended_standard_care_final.pdf

National Alliance on Mental Illness. (2020). *Maintaining a health relationship.* https://www.nami.org/Your-Journey/Family-Members-and-Caregivers/Maintaining-a-Healthy-Relationship

National Center for Complementary and Integrative Health (NCCIH). (2018). *Mind and body approaches for substance use disorders: What the science says.* https://www.nccih.nih.gov/health/providers/digest/mind-and-body-approaches-for-substance-use-disorders-science

National Center for PTSD. (2018). *How common is PTSD in veterans?* https://www.ptsd.va.gov/understand/common/common_veterans.asp

National Center on Substance Abuse and Child Welfare. (2018). *Special topic: Understanding prenatal substance exposure and child welfare implications.* Substance Abuse and Mental Health Services Administration. https://ncsacw.samhsa.gov/files/toolkitpackage/topic-prenatal/topic-prenatal-slides-508.pdf

National Council for Behavioral Health. (2018). *Implementing care for alcohol & other drug use in medical settings: An extension of SBIRT (SBIRT Change Guide 1.0).* Substance Abuse and Mental Health Services Administration. https://integration.samhsa.gov/sbirt/Implementing_Care_for_Alcohol_and_Other_Drug_Use_In_Medical_Settings_-_An_Extension_of_SBIRT.pdf

National Institute on Aging (NIA). (2019). *Quitting smoking for older adults.* National Institutes of Health. https://www.nia.nih.gov/health/quitting-smoking-older-adults

National Institute on Alcohol Abuse and Alcoholism (NIAAA). (2019). *Monitoring the Future Survey: High school and youth trends.* https://www.drugabuse.gov/publications/drugfacts/monitoring-future-survey-high-school-youth-trends

National Institute on Alcohol Abuse and Alcoholism (NIAAA). (2020a). *Alcohol facts and statistics.* https://www.niaaa.nih.gov/publications/brochures-and-fact-sheets/alcohol-facts-and-statistics

National Institute on Alcohol Abuse and Alcoholism (NIAAA). (2020b). *College drinking.* https://www.niaaa.nih.gov/publications/brochures-and-fact-sheets/college-drinking

National Institute on Alcohol Abuse and Alcoholism (NIAAA). (2020c). *Underage drinking.* https://pubs.niaaa.nih.gov/publications/underagedrinking/Underage_Fact.pdf

National Institute on Drug Abuse (NIDA). (2014). *Principles of adolescent substance use disorder treatment: A research-based guide.* (NIH Publication No. 14-7953). https://www.drugabuse.gov/publications/principles-adolescent-substance-use-disorder-treatment-research-based-guide/principles-adolescent-substance-use-disorder-treatment

National Institute on Drug Abuse (NIDA). (2017). *Substance use and SUDs in LGBTQ* Populations.* https://www.drugabuse.gov/related-topics/substance-use-suds-in-lgbtq-populations

National Institute on Drug Abuse (NIDA). (2018a). *Drugs, brains, and behavior: The science of addiction* (NIH Publication No. 18-DA-5605). https://www.drugabuse.gov/publications/drugs-brains-behavior-science-addiction/preface

National Institute on Drug Abuse (NIDA). (2018b). *Methadone.* https://www.drugabuse.gov/publications/principles-drug-addiction-treatment-research-based-guide-third-edition/evidence-based-approaches-to-drug-addiction-treatment/pharmacotherapies

National Institute on Drug Abuse (NIDA). (2018c). *Prescription opioids and heroin.* https://www.drugabuse.gov/node/pdf/19774/prescription-opioids-and-heroin

National Institute on Drug Abuse (NIDA). (2018d). *Principles of drug addiction treatment: A research-based guide* (NIH Publication No. 12–4180). https://www.drugabuse.gov/node/pdf/675/principles-of-drug-addiction-treatment-a-research-based-guide-third-edition

National Institute on Drug Abuse (NIDA). (2018e). *What are prescription stimulants?* https://www.drugabuse.gov/publications/drugfacts/prescription-stimulants

National Institute on Drug Abuse (NIDA). (2018f). *What is cocaine?* https://www.drugabuse.gov/publications/drugfacts/cocaine

National Institute on Drug Abuse (NIDA). (2018g). *What is the scope of prescription drug misuse?* https://www.drugabuse.gov/publications/research-reports/misuse-prescription-drugs/what-scope-prescription-drug-misuse

National Institute on Drug Abuse (NIDA). (2019a). *Dramatic increases in maternal opioid use and neonatal abstinence syndrome.* https://www.drugabuse.gov/related-topics/trends-statistics/infographics/dramatic-increases-in-maternal-opioid-use-neonatal-abstinence-syndrome

National Institute on Drug Abuse (NIDA). (2019b). *Drug use and its consequences increase among middle-aged and older adults.* https://www.drugabuse.gov/news-events/nida-notes/2019/07/drug-use-its-consequences-increase-among-middle-aged-older-adults

National Institute on Drug Abuse (NIDA). (2019c). *What are hallucinogens?* https://www.drugabuse.gov/publications/drugfacts/hallucinogens

National Institute on Drug Abuse (NIDA). (2019d). *What is marijuana?* https://www.drugabuse.gov/publications/drugfacts/marijuana

National Institute on Drug Abuse (NIDA). (2019e). *What is methamphetamine?* https://www.drugabuse.gov/publications/research-reports/methamphetamine/what-methamphetamine

National Institute on Drug Abuse (NIDA). (2020a). *Opioid overdose crisis.* https://www.drugabuse.gov/drugs-abuse/opioids/opioid-overdose-crisis

National Institute on Drug Abuse (NIDA). (2020b). *Trends and statistics.* https://www.drugabuse.gov/related-topics/trends-statistics

National Institute on Drug Abuse (NIDA). (2020c). *What are inhalants?* https://www.drugabuse.gov/publications/drugfacts/inhalants

National Institute on Neurological Disorders and Stroke. (2020). *Wernicke-Korsakoff syndrome.* https://www.ninds.nih.gov/Disorders/All-Disorders/Wernicke-Korsakoff-Syndrome Information-Page

Nellissery, M., Feinn, R. S., Covault, J., Gelernter, J., Anton, R. F., Pettinati, H., & Kranzler, H. R. (2003). Alleles of a functional serotonin transporter promoter polymorphism are associated with major depression in alcoholics. *Alcoholism: Clinical and Experimental Research, 29*(9), 1402–1408.

Norman, S. B., Haller, M., Hamblen, J. L., Southwick, S. M., & Pietrzak, R. H. (2018). The burden of co-occurring alcohol use disorder and PTSD in U.S. military veterans: Comorbidities, functioning, and suicidality. *Psychology of Addictive Behaviors, 32*(2), 224–229. https://doi.org/10.1037/adb0000348

Office of the Surgeon General. (2016). *Facing addiction in America: The Surgeon General's report on alcohol, drugs, and health* (DHHS Publication No. [SMA] 16-4991). U.S. Department of Health and Human Services. https://addiction.surgeongeneral.gov/sites/default/files/surgeon-generals-report.pdf

Ogawa, Y., Takeshima, N., Hayasaka, Y., Tajika, A., Watanabe, N., Streiner, D., & Furukawa, T. A. (2019). Antidepressants plus benzodiazepines for adults with major depression. *Cochrane Database of Systematic Reviews*, Issue 6, Article No. CD001026. https://doi.org/10.1002/14651858.CD001026.pub2

Ooms, M., Roozen, H. G., Willering, J. H., Zijlstra, W. P., de Waart, R., & Goudriaan, A. E. (2020). Effects of multiple detoxifications on withdrawal symptoms, psychiatric distress and alcohol-craving in patients with an alcohol use disorder. *Behavioral Medicine*. https://doi.org/10.1080/08964289.2020.1760777

Orsolini, L., Papanti, G. D., De Berardis, D., Guirguis, A., Corkery, J. M., & Schifano, F. (2017). The "endless trip" among the NPS users: Psychopathology and psychopharmacology in the hallucinogen-persisting perception disorder. A systematic review. *Frontiers in Psychiatry, 8*(240). https://doi.org/10.3389/fpsyt.2017.00240

Pierre, J. M. (2017). Risks of increasingly potent cannabis: The joint effects of potency and frequency. *Current Psychiatry, 16*(2), 15–20.

Platt, L. M. (2020). Benzodiazepines: Why nurses must be concerned about their use. *Journal of Psychosocial Nursing and Mental Health Services, 58*(1), 5–6. https://doi.org/10.3928/02793695-20191218-02

Poels, E. M. P., Bijma, H. H., Galbally, M., & Bergink, V. (2018). Lithium during pregnancy and after delivery: A review. *International Journal of Bipolar Disorders, 6*(1), 26. https://doi.org/10.1186/s40345-018-0135-7

Popova, S. (2017). Counting the costs of drinking alcohol during pregnancy. *Bulletin of the World Health Organization, 95*(5), 320–321. http://dx.doi.org/10.2471/BLT.17.030517

Popova, S., Lange, S., Probst, C., Gmel, G., & Rehm, J. (2018). Global prevalence of alcohol use and binge drinking during pregnancy, and fetal alcohol spectrum disorder. *Biochemistry and Cell Biology, 96*(2), 237–240. https://doi.org/10.1139/bcb-2017-0077

Post, R. M., & Kegan, R. (2017). Prevention of recurrent affective episodes using extinction training in the reconsolidation window: A testable psychotherapeutic strategy. *Psychiatry Research, 249*, 327–336. https://doi.org/10.1016/j.psychres.2017.01.034

Potter, M. L., & Moller, M. D. (Eds.). (2020). *Psychiatric-mental health nursing: From suffering to hope* (2nd ed.). Pearson.

Reisfield, G. M., Teitelbaum, S. A., Large, S. O., Jones, J., Morrison, D. G., & Lewis, B. (2020). The roles of phosphatidylethanol (PEth), ethyl glucuronide (EtG), and ethyl sulfate (EtS) in identifying alcohol consumption among participants in professionals' health programs. *Drug Testing and Analysis, 12*(8), 1102–1108. https://doi.org/10.1002/dta.2809

Sacco, P., Kuerbis, A., & Harris, R. (2020). *Older adults and substance misuse*. Routledge.

SAMHSA-HRSA Center for Integrated Health Solutions. (2020). *Tobacco cessation*. https://www.integration.samhsa.gov/health-wellness/wellness-strategies/tobacco-cessation-2#assessments

Schoenthaler, S. J., Blum, K., Fried, L., Oscar-Berman, M., Giordano, J., Modestino, E. J., & Badgaiyan, R. (2017). The effects of residential dual diagnosis treatment on alcohol abuse. *Journal of Systems and Integrative Neuroscience, 33*(44), 1–17. https://dx.doi.org/10.15761%2FJSIN.1000169

Shank, F. A., Petrarca, K., & Barry, C. (2019). Child outcomes of having a parent with an AUD. *Modern Psychological Studies, 25*(1). https://scholar.utc.edu/mps/vol25/iss1/1

Shier, M. L., & Turpin, A. (2017). A multi-dimensional conceptual framework for trauma-informed practice in addictions programming. *Journal of Social Service Research, 43*(5), 609–623. https://doi.org/10.1080/01488376.2017.1364318

Schuler, M. S., & Horowitz, J. A. (2020). Nursing students' attitudes toward and empathy for patients with substance use disorder following mentorship. *Journal of Nursing Education, 59*(3), 149–153. https://doi.org/10.3928/01484834-20200220-05

Shyken, J. M., Babbar, S., Babbar, S., & Forinash, A. (2019). Benzodiazepines in pregnancy. *Clinical Obstetrics and Gynecology, 62*(1), 156–167. https://doi.org/10.1097/grf.0000000000000417

Skewes, M. C., & Blume, A. W. (2019). Understanding the link between racial trauma and substance use among American Indians. *American Psychologist, 74*(1), 88–100. https://doi.org/10.1037/amp0000331

Sliedrecht, W., de Waart, R., Witkiewitz, K., & Roozen, H. G. (2019). Alcohol use disorder relapse factors: A systematic review. *Psychiatry Research, 278*, 97–115. https://doi.org/10.1016/j.psychres.2019.05.038

SMART Recovery. (2020). *SMART Recovery: There's life beyond addiction*. https://www.smartrecovery.org

Smith, L. B., Golberstein, E., Anderson, K., Christiaansen, T., Paterson, N., Short, S., & Neprash, H. T. (2019). The association of EHR drug safety alerts and co-prescribing of opioids and benzodiazepines. *Journal of General Internal Medicine, 34*(8), 1403–1405. https://doi.org/10.1007/s11606-019-04985-w

Smith, N. Z., Vasquez, P. J., Emelogu, N. A., Hayes, A. E., Engebretson, J., & Nash, A. J. (2020). The good, the bad, and recovery: Adolescents describe the advantages and Disadvantages of alternative peer groups. *Substance Abuse: Research and Treatment, 14*, 1178221820909354. https://doi.org/10.1177%2F1178221820909354

Smith, Y., & Spitzmueller, M. C. (2016). Worker perspectives on contemporary milieu therapy: A cross-site ethnographic study. *Social Work Research, 40*(2), 105–116. https://doi.org/10.1093/swr/svw003

Solomon, J. (2019). *Get connected: Linking older adults with resources on medication, alcohol, and mental health can help reduce social isolation and improve health.* National Council for Behavioral Health. https://www.thenationalcouncil.org/?api&do=attachment&name=closing-the-gap-social-isolation-and-older-adults&index=0&type=webinars

Soyka, M. (2017). Treatment of benzodiazepine dependence. *New England Journal of Medicine, 376*(12), 1147–1157. https://doi.org/10.1056/NEJMra1611832

Starr, K. T. (2015). The sneaky prevalence of substance abuse in nursing. *Nursing2020, 45*(3). https://journals.lww.com/nursing/Fulltext/2015/03000/The_sneaky_prevalence_of_substance_abuse_in.6.aspx

Steinka-Fry, K. T., Tanner-Smith, E. E., Dakof, G. A., & Henderson, C. (2017). Culturally sensitive substance use treatment for racial/ethnic minority youth: A meta-analytic review. *Journal of Substance Abuse Treatment, 75*, 22–37.

Substance Abuse and Mental Health Services Administration (SAMHSA). (2014). *Addressing the specific behavioral health needs of men* (DHHS Publication No. [SMA] 13-4736). https://store.samhsa.gov/product/TIP-56-Addressing-the-Specific-Behavioral-Health-Needs-of-Men/SMA14-4736

Substance Abuse and Mental Health Services Administration (SAMHSA). (2015a). *About screening, brief intervention, and referral to treatment (SBIRT)*. http://www.samhsa.gov/sbirt/about

Substance Abuse and Mental Health Services Administration (SAMHSA). (2015b). *Detoxification and substance abuse treatment: A treatment improvement protocol* (DHHS Publication No. [SMA] 15-4131). https://store.samhsa.gov/product/TIP-45-Detoxification-and-Substance-Abuse-Treatment/SMA15-4131

Substance Abuse and Mental Health Services Administration (SAMHSA). (2015c). *Substance abuse treatment: Addressing the specific needs of women* (DHHS Publication No. SMA15-4426). Author.

Substance Abuse and Mental Health Services Administration (SAMHSA). (2018a). *Alcohol use: Facts and resources*. https://www.samhsa.gov/sites/default/files/alcohol-use-facts-resources-fact-sheet.pdf

Substance Abuse and Mental Health Services Administration (SAMHSA). (2018b). *Opioid overdose prevention toolkit* (DHHS Publication No. [SMA] 18-4742). https://store.samhsa.gov/product/Opioid-Overdose-Prevention-Toolkit/SMA18-4742

Substance Abuse and Mental Health Services Administration (SAMHSA). (2018c). *Opioid use disorder and pregnancy* (DHHS Publication No. [SMA] 18-5071FS1). https://store.samhsa.gov/product/Opioid-Use-Disorder-and-Pregnancy/SMA18-5071FS1

Substance Abuse and Mental Health Services Administration (SAMHSA). (2018d). *Tips for teens: The truth about inhalants* (DHHS Publication No. [PEP] 18-04). https://store.samhsa.gov/product/Tips-for-Teens-The-Truth-About-Inhalants/PEP18-04

Substance Abuse and Mental Health Services Administration (SAMHSA). (2018e). *Treating babies who were exposed to opioids before birth* (DHHS Publication No. [SMA] 18-5071FS3). Retrieved from https://store.samhsa.gov/product/Treating-Babies-Who-Were-Exposed-to-Opioids-Before-Birth/SMA18-5071FS3?referer=from_search_result

Substance Abuse and Mental Health Services Administration (SAMHSA). (2020a). *Substance use disorder treatment for people with co-occurring disorders* [DHHS Publication No. [PEP] 20-02-01-004]. Author.

Substance Abuse and Mental Health Services Administration (SAMHSA). (2020b). *Substance use treatment for older adults*. https://www.samhsa.gov/homelessness-programs-resources/hpr-resources/substance-use-treatment-older-adults

Substance Abuse and Mental Health Services Administration (SAMHSA). (2020c). *Tip 63: Medications for opioid use disorder* (DHHS Publication No. [PEP] 20-02-01-006). https://store.samhsa.gov/product/TIP-63-Medications-for-Opioid-Use-Disorder-Full-Document/PEP20-02-01-006?referer=from_search_result

Substance Abuse and Mental Health Services Administration (SAMHSA). (2020d). *Tips for teens: Hallucinogens* (DHHS Publication No. [PEP] 20-03-03-001). https://store.samhsa.gov/product/Tips-for-Teens-The-Truth-About-Hallucinogens/PEP20-03-03-001?referer=from_search_result

Suchman, N. E., Borelli, J. L., & DeCoste, C. L. (2020). Can addiction counselors be trained to deliver Mothering from the Inside Out, a mentalization-based parenting therapy, with fidelity? Results from a community-based randomized efficacy trial. *Attachment & Human Development, 22*(3), 332–351. https://doi.org/10.1080/14616734.2018.1559210

Sylvestre, M.-P., Wellman, R. J., O'Loughlin, E. K., Dugas, E. N., & O'Loughlin, J. (2017). Gender differences in risk factors for cigarette smoking initiation in childhood. *Addictive Behaviors, 72*, 144–150. https://doi.org/10.1016/j.addbeh.2017.04.004

Taylor, S. A., & Miloh, T. (2018). Adolescent alcoholic liver. In N. L. Sussman & M. R. Lucey (Eds.), *Alcoholic liver disease, an issue of clinics in liver disease* (Vol. 23, pp. 51–54). Elsevier.

Thapa, S., Selya, A. S., & Jonk, Y. (2017). Time-varying effects of parental alcoholism on depression. *Preventing Chronic Disease, 14*, 170100. http://dx.doi.org/10.5888/pcd14.170100

Thompson, W., Lande, R. G., Kalapatapu, R. K., Talavera, F., & Xiong, G. L. (2020). *Alcoholism treatment & management*. Medscape. https://emedicine.medscape.com/article/285913-treatment

Uddin, M. S., Sufian, M. A., Hossain, M. F., Kabir, M. T., Islam, M. T., Rahman, M. M., & Rafe, M. R. (2017). Neuropsychological effects of caffeine: Is caffeine addictive? *Journal of Psychology and Psychotherapy, 7*(2). https://doi.org/10.4172/2161-0487.1000295

U.S. Department of Health and Human Services. (2020). *Smoking cessation: A report of the Surgeon General*. https://www.hhs.gov/sites/default/files/2020-cessation-sgr-full-report.pdf#p512.

U.S. Department of Health and Human Services & U.S. Department of Agriculture. (2020). *Dietary guidelines for Americans 2015–2020*. http://health.gov/dietaryguidelines/2015/guidelines/.

U.S. Drug Enforcement Administration. (2018). *Why do teens use drugs?* https://www.getsmartaboutdrugs.gov/contact-us

U.S. Food and Drug Administration (FDA). (2018). *Drugs of abuse home use test*. https://www.fda.gov/medical-devices/drugs-abuse-tests/drugs-abuse-home-use-test

U.S. Food and Drug Administration (FDA). (2020a). *Quitting smoking: Closer with every attempt*. https://www.fda.gov/tobacco-products/health-information/quitting-smoking-closer-every-attempt

U.S. Food and Drug Administration (FDA). (2020b). *Vaporizers, e-cigarettes, and other electronic nicotine delivery systems (ENDS)*. https://www.fda.gov/tobacco-products/products-ingredients-components/vaporizers-e-cigarettes-and-other-electronic-nicotine-delivery-systems-ends

U.S. Preventive Services Task Force (USPSTF). (2016). Behavioral and pharmacotherapy interventions for tobacco smoking cessation in adults, including pregnant women: Recommendation statement. *American Family Physician, 93*(10). https://www.aafp.org/afp/2016/0515/od1.html

U.S. Preventive Services Task Force (USPSTF). (2018). Screening and behavioral counseling interventions to reduce unhealthy alcohol use in adolescents and adults: US Preventive Services Task Force recommendation statement. *Journal of the American Medical Association, 320*(18), 1899–1909. https://doi.org/10.1001/jama.2018.16789

U.S. Preventive Services Task Force (USPSTF). (2020). Primary care interventions for prevention and cessation of tobacco use in children and adolescents: U.S. Preventive Services Task Force recommendation statement. *Journal of the American Medical Association, 323*(16), 1590–1598. https://doi.org/10.1001/jama.2020.4679

Uzarska, A., Czerwiński, S. K., & Atroszko, P. A. (2019). Shopping addiction is driven by personal focus rather than social focus values but to the exclusion of achievement and self-direction. *International Journal of Mental Health and Addiction*. https://doi.org/10.1007/s11469-019-00193-z

Van Skike, C. E., Goodlett, C., & Matthews, D. B. (2019). Acute alcohol and cognition: Remembering what it causes us to forget. *Alcohol, 79*, 105–125. https://doi.org/10.1016/j.alcohol.2019.03.006

Vaswani, M. (2019). ADH and ALDH polymorphisms in alcoholism and alcohol misuse/dependence. In V. R. Preedy (Ed.), *Neuroscience of alcohol* (pp. 29–38). Academic Press.

Verdejo-García, A., Alcázar-Córcoles, M. A., & Albein-Urios, N. (2019). Neuropsychological Interventions for decision-making in addiction: A systematic review. *Neuropsychology Review, 29*(1), 79–92. https://doi.org/10.1007/s11065-018-9384-6

Vigod, S. N., & Dennis, C. L. (2019). Benzodiazepines and the Z-drugs in pregnancy—Reasonably reassuring for neurodevelopment but should we really be using them? *JAMA Network Open, 2*(4), e191430. https://doi.org/10.1001/jamanetworkopen.2019.1430

Villines, Z. (2019). *How long can you detect marijuana in the body?* https://www.medicalnewstoday.com/articles/324315

Vitali, M., Mistretta, M., Alessandrini, G., Coriale, G., Romeo, M., Attilia, F., et al. (2018). Pharmacological treatment for dual diagnosis: A literature update and a proposal of intervention. *Rivista di Psichiatria, 53*(3), 160–169. https://doi.org/10.1708/2925.29419

Volkow, N. D., Koob, G. F., Croyle, R. T., Bianchi, D. W., Gordon, J. A., Koroshetz, W. J., et al. (2018). The conception of the ABCD study: From substance use to a broad NIH collaboration. *Developmental Cognitive Neuroscience, 32*, 4–7. https://doi.org/10.1016/j.dcn.2017.10.002

Walker, D. M., & Nestler, E. J. (2018). Neuroepigenetics and addiction. In D. H. Geschwind, H. L. Paulson, & C. Klein (Eds.), *Handbook of clinical neurology* (Vol. 148, pp. 747–765). Elsevier.

Wallace, B. C., & Santacruz, E. (2017). *Health disparities and LGBT populations*. ABC-CLIO.

Webster, L. R. (2017). Risk factors for opioid-use disorder and overdose. *Anesthesia & Analgesia, 125*(55), 1741–1748. https://doi.org/10.1213/ANE.0000000000002496

Wéry, A., & Billieux, J. (2017). Problematic cybersex: Conceptualization, assessment, and treatment. *Addictive Behaviors, 64*, 238–246. https://doi.org/10.1016/j.addbeh.2015.11.007

Wiegmann, C., Mick, I., Brandl, E. J., Heinz, A., & Gutwinski, S. (2020). Alcohol and dementia–What is the link?: A systematic review. *Neuropsychiatric Disease and Treatment, 16*, 87–99. https://doi.org/10.2147/NDT.S198772

Wilsnack, R. W., Wilsnack, S. C., Gmel, G., & Kantor, L. W. (2018). Gender differences in binge drinking. *Alcohol Research: Current Reviews, 39*(1), 57–76.

Wood, E., Albarqouni, L., Tkachuk, S., Green, C. J., Ahamad, K., Nolan, S., et al. (2018). Will this hospitalized patient develop severe alcohol withdrawal syndrome?: The rational clinical examination systematic review. *Journal of the American Medical Association, 320*(8), 825–833. https://doi.org/10.1001/jama.2018.10574

World Health Organization (WHO). (2019). *Tobacco*. https://www.who.int/news-room/fact-sheets/detail/tobacco

World Health Organization (WHO). (2020a). *Alcohol*. https://www.who.int/news-room/fact-sheets/detail/alcohol

World Health Organization (WHO). (2020b). *Cannabis*. https://www.who.int/substance_abuse/facts/cannabis/en/

World Health Organization (WHO). (2020c). *Health effects of smoking among young people*. https://www.who.int/tobacco/control/populations/youth_health_effects/en/

Yalom, I. D., & Leszcz, M. (2005). *The theory and practice of group psychotherapy* (5th ed.). Basic Books.

Yamakawa, G. R., Lengkeek, C., Salberg, S., Spanswick, S. C., & Mychasiuk, R. (2017). Behavioral and pathophysiological outcomes associated with caffeine consumption and repetitive mild traumatic brain injury (RmTBI) in adolescent rats. *PLoS One, 12*(11), e0187218. https://dx.doi.org/10.1371%2Fjournal.pone.0187218

Zahr, N. M., & Pfefferbaum, A. (2017). Alcohol's effects on the brain: Neuroimaging results in humans and animal models. *Alcohol Research: Current Reviews, 38*(2), e1–e24.

Zarse, E. M., Neff, M. R., Yoder, R., Hulvershorn, L., Chambers, J. E., & Chambers, R. A. (2019). The Adverse Childhood Experiences Questionnaire: Two decades of research on childhood trauma as a primary cause of adult mental illness, addiction, and medical diseases. *Cogent Medicine, 6*(1), 1581447. https://doi.org/10.1080/2331205X.2019.1581447

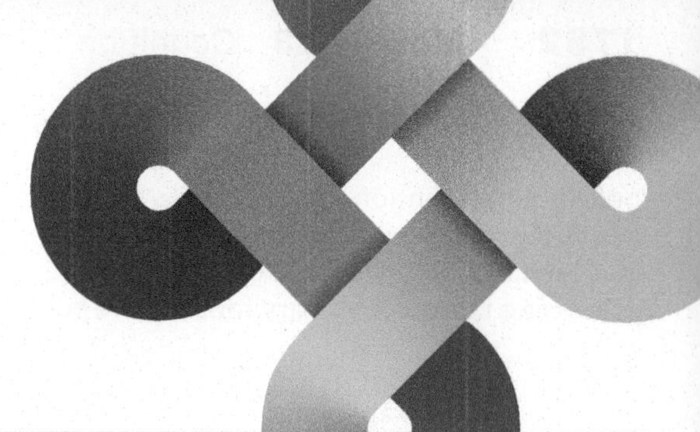

Module 23
Cognition

Module Outline and Learning Outcomes

The Concept of Cognition

Normal Cognition

23.1 Analyze the physiology of normal cognition.

Alterations to Cognition

23.2 Differentiate alterations in cognition.

Concepts Related to Cognition

23.3 Outline the relationship between cognition and other concepts.

Health Promotion

23.4 Explain measures to promote optimal cognition.

Nursing Assessment

23.5 Differentiate common assessment procedures and tests used to examine cognition.

Independent Interventions

23.6 Analyze independent interventions nurses can implement for patients with alterations in cognition.

Collaborative Therapies

23.7 Summarize collaborative therapies used by interprofessional teams for patients with alterations in cognition.

Lifespan Considerations

23.8 Differentiate considerations related to the assessment and care of patients with alterations in cognition throughout the lifespan.

Cognition Exemplars

Exemplar 23.A Alzheimer Disease

23.A Analyze Alzheimer disease as it relates to cognition.

Exemplar 23.B Delirium

23.B Analyze delirium as it relates to cognition.

Exemplar 23.C Schizophrenia

23.C Analyze schizophrenia as it relates to cognition.

›› The Concept of Cognition

Concept Key Terms

Adaptive behavior, **1753**
Agnosia, **1755**
Alogia, **1756**
Amnesia, **1755**
Anomia, **1756**
Aphasia, **1755**
Apraxia, **1756**
Ataxia, **1756**
Avolition, **1756**
Carphologia, **1756**
Cognition, **1751**
Confabulation, **1755**
Confusion, **1754**
Delirium, **1759**
Delusions, **1754**
Dementia, **1759**
Down syndrome, **1757**
Dyspraxia, **1756**
Echolalia, **1756**
Essential tremor, **1756**
Executive function, **1753**
Fetal alcohol spectrum disorders (FASD), **1757**
Fragile X syndrome, **1757**
Hallucinations, **1755**
Intellectual disability, **1757**
Learning disabilities, **1756**
Limbic system, **1753**
Long-term memory, **1752**
Neurons, **1753**
Neurotransmitters, **1753**
Orientation, **1752**
Physiologic tremor, **1756**
Praxis, **1753**
Proprioceptive, **1752**
Psychosis, **1754**
Sensory memory, **1752**
Short-term memory, **1752**
Social cognition, **1753**
Tic, **1756**
Tremor, **1756**
Trisomy 21, **1757**

Normal Cognition

Cognition is the complex set of mental processes by which individuals acquire, store, retrieve, and use information. Cognition primarily involves activities that are controlled by the cerebral hemispheres, including perception, attention, memory, communication, decision making, and problem solving. The ability to think and reason is an essential component of human identity and function.

A definition of normal cognition depends on social and cultural norms and the environment in which the individual operates. In general, the desired and most basic consequences of normal cognition are to obtain a level of survival and adaptation, to function effectively as a social being, and to engage in meaningful and purposeful activity. There is a great deal of variation in cognitive function among healthy individuals. Normal variations in cognition can be better understood by looking at some of the related components and categories associated with this concept. For an overview of cognitive development and related theories, see Module 25, Development.

Key Components and Categories

The key components that make up human cognition include perception, attention, and memory. Communication and social cognition, motor function, and planning, executive, and intellectual functions are broader categories of mental processing that are necessary for adaptive behavior.

Perception

Perception refers to an interpretation of stimuli or inputs that takes place in the brain. The process of perception depends on the sensory reception of internal and external data and is discussed in depth in Module 18, Sensory Perception. External stimuli or inputs include touch, taste, vision, hearing, and smell. Internal stimuli include **proprioceptive** sensations that contribute to motor function and spatial awareness. Perceptual variations are normal among individuals across the lifespan and can be influenced by factors such as genetics and culture. **Orientation** is a component of normal perception that includes four basic elements: person, place, time, and situation. *Orientation to person* is the ability to correctly identify one's own name. *Orientation to place* is the ability to identify one's location. *Orientation to time* is the ability to correctly identify the time of day, the date, and the season. *Orientation to situation* is the ability to describe the global circumstances surrounding a particular event.

Attention

Attention refers to the brain's ability to remain alert and aware while selectively prioritizing concentration on a stimulus (such as something that is seen or heard) or mental event (thinking and problem solving). The reticular activating system (RAS), thalamus, and frontal cortex are the structures that are primarily involved in arousal and attention. The neurotransmitters dopamine and norepinephrine both play a major role in regulating attention.

The human capacity to sustain attention and attend to multiple stimuli is limited. Variations in attention span are typical among healthy individuals and may be impacted by development, genetics, biological rhythms, culture, and other environmental factors (Nitza, Winer, & Zaks, 2017). A change in any individual's level of awareness and attention span often signifies an underlying change or alteration in biophysical or psychosocial status. Individual safety depends on the ability to attend and focus.

Memory

Memory refers to the process by which individuals retain, store, and retrieve information gained from previous experiences. The ability to remember meaningful information provides the foundation for learning and adaptation from birth to death. Alterations in memory have a significant impact on the holistic needs of the individual. Most models of memory classify subtypes according to their sequence and duration. These include sensory, short-term, and long-term memory (see **Figure 23.1** »).

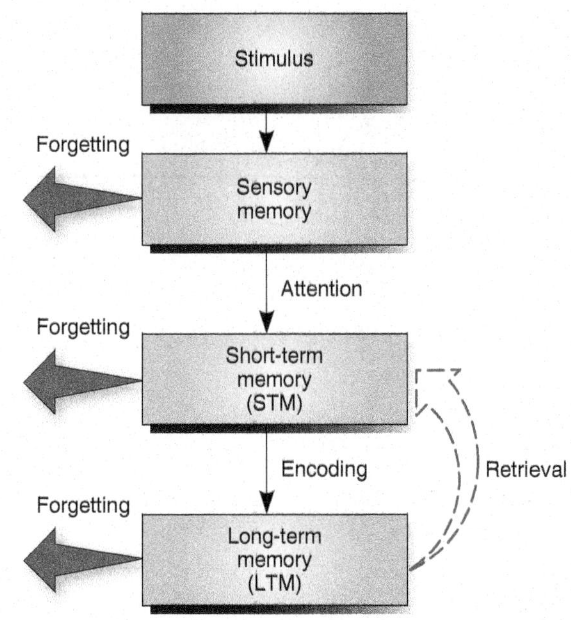

Figure 23.1 » An information-processing model of memory. Many stimuli register in sensory memory. Those that are noticed are briefly stored in short-term memory, and those that are encoded are transferred to long-term memory. As shown, forgetting may be caused by failures of attention, encoding, or retrieval.

Sensory memory refers to the earliest stage of memory, in which visual input and auditory information are retained for less than a few seconds. Sensory information that receives attention from an individual passes into short-term memory.

Short-term memory refers to the active processing and manipulation of information in conscious awareness. Short-term memory only lasts several seconds, but it can be rehearsed or repeated and transferred into long-term memory. The total amount of information that can be managed in short-term memory is also finite. For example, most research has demonstrated that longer strings of information, such as a sequence of numbers exceeding five to nine digits, cannot be retained (Cowan, 2017). An important aspect of short-term memory is working memory. *Working memory* is defined as the capacity to manipulate information stored in short-term memory. Examples include following a sequence of directions and performing mental mathematical calculations (Cowan, 2017).

Long-term memory is used to describe the final sequence or destination of information that can be stored indefinitely. Long-term memory is further broken down into declarative and nondeclarative memories. *Declarative memories* are those that are explicit and can be consciously accessed; they are distinguished as *semantic* (storing facts and verbal information) and *episodic* (composed of personal experiences). *Nondeclarative memories* are characterized by information that is outside of our conscious awareness. *Procedural memories* are a type of implicit memories that enable individuals to perform learned skills and tasks. Examples include such activities as walking, riding a bike, and driving a car (Heyselaar, Segaert, Walvoort, Kessels, & Hagoort, 2017; Steingartner, Novitzká, Bačíková, & Korečko, 2018).

Communication and Social Cognition

The ability to receive, interpret, and express communication is an essential component of cognitive function (see Module 38, Communication). Memory plays a significant role in communication and speech.

Social cognition is the ability to process and apply social information accurately and effectively. It depends on the integrated function of the areas responsible for visual motor processing, language, and executive function. Individuals are normally able to apply an understanding of the needs of others and to interpret both verbal and nonverbal information or social cues with some degree of proficiency (American Speech Language and Hearing Association, 2020). Researchers have demonstrated that social cognition is essential for adaptive functioning across the lifespan (Rutter et al., 2019).

Motor Coordination

Motor coordination refers to the planning, organizing, and execution of complex motor tasks. Cognitive function and motor coordination are carried out by shared neuronal pathways in the brain (Oberer, Gashaj, & Roebers, 2018). Normally the ability to plan and coordinate motor functions progresses through the expected stages of development, with adults exercising **praxis**, the ability to control movement in a deliberate, smooth, and coordinated fashion. Individuals with intact cognition exhibit normal variations in motor function and coordination. Impaired motor function is characteristic of many of the alterations discussed in this module.

Executive Function

Executive function is an umbrella term that is used to describe the mental skills involved in planning and executing complex tasks. It incorporates coordination of the previously mentioned attributes of normal cognition, enabling individuals to selectively focus, control emotions, problem-solve, and organize speech and motor activity. Examples include following multistep directions and prioritizing to manage time on a project.

Intellectual Function

Intelligence is a general term used to describe the mental capacity of an individual in relation to learning, reasoning, and problem solving. It is generally measured through the administration of one or more psychometric tests. The most commonly administered tests are the Stanford-Binet Intelligence Scales and Wechsler Intelligence Scales. Subtest scores for both are used to compare performance in areas such as general knowledge, quantitative and verbal reasoning, visuospatial processing, and working memory. The average of the scores is used to calculate an overall or full-scale intelligence quotient (IQ). Subtest scores are also used to provide insight into individual strengths and weaknesses (Haertel, 2018).

Adaptive Behavior

Adaptive behavior refers to a set of practical skills people need to function in their everyday lives. The three categories of adaptive behavior are conceptual skills (use of language, reading, or telling time), social skills (ability to follow rules and interact appropriately with others), and practical skills (ability to engage in work and perform activities of daily living [ADLs]).

Physiology Review

Cognition largely depends on brain and nervous system functioning. The structural integrity of and complex physiologic processes that occur within the cerebral cortex are responsible for most aspects of the individual's ability to process sensory information. However, the **limbic system**, RAS, and cerebellum also play a role in arousal, motivation, emotional regulation, and balance (see Module 11, Intracranial Regulation, for more information).

The physiologic processes that occur in the brain have particular significance in the maintenance and regulation of cognitive processes. **Neurons** are the specialized cells of the nervous system that have the capacity to carry messages through electrical and chemical signals. Microglia are the resident immune cells of the brain. They play an important role in regulating response to inflammation. **Neurotransmitters** are specialized chemicals that carry nerve impulses across the synaptic gaps between neurons. Research has demonstrated that abnormalities in cellular and neurotransmitter function are associated with many cognitive disorders. Various neurotransmitters are discussed in some detail in Module 28, Mood and Affect, and Module 31, Stress and Coping.

Normal Genetic Variations

Research demonstrates that genetic makeup accounts for as much as 80% of the variations in cognition found in the general population (Grimm, Kranz, & Reif, 2020). Different genes can be linked to particular components of cognitive function, such as attention in working memory in healthy adults (Briley & Tucker-Drob, 2017).

Alterations to Cognition

Although the etiology, presentation, and course of diseases impacting cognitive function vary, the key clinical manifestations of alterations in mental processing all relate to dysregulation of one or more of the key components or categories of normal cognition. The Alterations and Therapies table gives an overview of alterations common across a range of disorders that can impair cognitive function.

General Manifestations of Altered Cognitive Function

Alterations in different aspects of cognition occur to varying degrees and are found in a number of conditions associated with this concept. The pathophysiology of these conditions is generally related to conditions causing abnormalities in the structure and function of the brain. An understanding of the general manifestations of cognitive dysfunction is essential for providing nursing care to individuals presenting with cognitive problems, regardless of the patient's specific medical diagnosis or condition.

Alterations in Perception

Altered perception and thinking are hallmarks of many of the conditions that impact cognition across the lifespan. Perceptual disturbances may be a function of structural and physiologic brain abnormalities in several areas of the cerebral cortex. They may be related to a primary cognitive disorder, such as dementia or schizophrenia or to an underlying medical condition. Illogical thinking may be the result of frontal lobe dysfunction and dopamine imbalance. Distortions in perceptual processing are often the result of abnormalities in the lobes responsible for that aspect of

Alterations and Therapies

Cognition

ALTERATION	DESCRIPTION	MANIFESTATIONS	INTERVENTIONS AND THERAPIES
Perceptual disturbances/ psychosis	Alterations in ability to interpret environmental stimuli, think clearly and logically, and maintain orientation to person, place, time, and situation	▪ Hallucinations ▪ Delusions ▪ Disordered thinking ▪ Disorientation/confusion	▪ Identify and treat underlying cause ▪ Reduce environmental stimulation ▪ Reality orientation and validation therapy
Impaired attention	Difficulty sustaining or directing focus	▪ Easily distracted ▪ Avoids situations requiring sustained focus ▪ Difficulty learning	▪ Identify and treat underlying cause ▪ Reduce distractions
Memory problems	Impairment in ability to recall information	▪ Getting lost ▪ Difficulty with word finding and recognition ▪ Difficulty remembering recent events ▪ Difficulty remembering remote events	▪ Identify and treat underlying cause ▪ Cognitive remediation ▪ Provide compensatory strategies and memory aids
Problems with communication/ social cognition	Impairments in the ability to process social information and communicate with others	▪ Difficulty adhering to social conventions ▪ Receptive and expressive language problems	▪ Refer for speech therapy ▪ Provide accommodations and modifications ▪ Provide social skills training
Problems with motor function/ control	Inability to carry out smooth, purposeful movement	▪ Tics ▪ Tremors ▪ Dyskinesia	▪ Identify and treat underlying cause ▪ Provide environmental modifications ▪ Refer for occupational therapy (OT) and physical therapy (PT)
Problems with executive function	Weaknesses in key mental skills required for adaptive function	▪ Difficulty organizing ▪ Difficulty planning ▪ Poor impulse control ▪ Problems with attention and memory	▪ Provide compensatory strategies (lists, organizers) ▪ Refer for OT ▪ Support safety needs
Problems with intellectual function and learning	Problems with global intellectual function or acquisition of knowledge required for adaptive function	▪ Low IQ ▪ Problems with adaptive function ▪ Academic problems ▪ Social/emotional problems	▪ Provide modifications and accommodations ▪ Provide remediation ▪ Focus on strengths

sensory processing. Terms related to thinking and perception include the following:

- **Confusion** is a general term used to describe increased difficulty in thinking clearly, making judgments, and focusing attention.
- *Disorientation* is an element of confusion in which the individual is unable to correctly identify one or more of the following: person, place, time, and situation.
- **Psychosis** is a general term used to describe an abnormal mental state that alters an individual's thought processes and content in a manner that impacts the individual's perception of reality. Indicators of altered thought processes and content are most often observed through the patient's speech and behaviors. Common indicators of disorganized thinking are outlined in **Table 23.1** ».
- **Delusions** are rigid, false beliefs—for example, believing that members of a healthcare team are actually government spies assigned to gather information that will be used to harm the patient or others. Common types of delusions include *delusions of persecution,* in which an individual believes that others are hostile or trying to harm

TABLE 23.1 Indicators of Disordered Thinking

Indicator	Description
Loose associations	Pattern of speech in which a person's ideas slip off track onto another unrelated or obliquely related topic; also known as *derailment*.
Tangentiality	Occurs when a person digresses from the topic at hand and goes off on a tangent, starting an entirely new train of thought.
Incoherence/word salad/ neologisms	Speaking in meaningless phrases with words that are seemingly randomly chosen, often made up, and not connected.
Illogicality	Refers to speech in which there is an absence of reason and rationality.
Circumstantiality	Occurs when a person goes into excessive detail about an event and has difficulty getting to the point of the conversation.
Pressured/distractible speech	Can be identified when a patient is speaking rapidly and there is an extreme sense of urgency or even frenzy as well as tangentiality, making it is nearly impossible to interrupt the person.
Poverty of speech	The opposite of pressured speech; identified by the absence of spontaneous speech in an ordinary conversation. The person cannot engage in small talk and gives brief or empty responses.

Source: From Potter and Moller (2020). Pearson Education, Inc., Hoboken, NJ.

him; *delusions of reference*, in which an individual falsely believes that public events or people are directly related to her; and *delusions of grandeur*, in which an individual has an inflated sense of self-worth and abilities.

- **Hallucinations** are sensory experiences that do not represent reality, such as hearing, seeing, feeling, or smelling things that are not actually present. Sometimes the type of hallucinations experienced by an individual provides clues to the underlying cause. Types of hallucinations include *auditory*, in which an individual hears voices or sounds that are not there; *visual*, in which an individual sees things that are not there or sees distortions of things that are there; or *tactile* (also known as *somatic* or *haptic*), in which an individual feels things that are not present.

Alterations in Attention

Individuals with attention difficulties demonstrate deficits in the ability to focus, shift, and sustain attention consistently. Attention deficits are characteristic of many of the cognitive disorders discussed in this module and may also occur as a distinct disorder classified as attention-deficit disorder (ADD) or attention-deficit/hyperactivity disorder (ADHD). More information on ADHD can be found in Module 25, Development. Short-term difficulties with attention can also occur under conditions such as acute stress and anxiety and during periods of acute illness. Problems with attention can be related to any conditions that impact the structure and function of the brain. Such problems are manifested by alterations in one or more aspects of attention. For example, deficits in mental energy manifest in the ability to sustain effort required to complete certain tasks. Individuals with altered attention have difficulty determining what information is salient and connecting new information to what they already know. Issues in processing arise from the inability to control output—meaning that an individual may lack the ability to preview and inhibit an inappropriate or unsafe response or action.

Alterations in Memory

Memory impairment may be an initial manifestation of a cognitive disorder, with one or more memory functions impacted at any given time. Imbalances of acetylcholine, dopamine, gamma-aminobutyric acid (GABA), and glutamate have been implicated in memory problems (Marsman et al., 2017; Wideman, Jardine, & Winters, 2018). Memory impairments may be temporary or chronic and may range from mild to severe. They may also be related to an underlying illness or trauma or be caused by a medical treatment or medication. **Amnesia** is a general term that is used to refer to the loss of recent or remote memory. Patients experiencing memory loss may unconsciously attempt to compensate for memory gaps by filling them in with fabricated events through a process known as **confabulation**.

Memory loss may manifest as problems related to short-term or long-term memory. Individuals with *short-term memory loss* may retain the ability to remember events that occurred 15 years ago but have difficulty recalling something that happened several minutes ago. Issues with working memory include difficulty following multistep directions, remembering the sequencing of numbers, or performing simple calculations. Individuals with *long-term memory problems* have difficulty recalling events and learning that occurred in the distant past. Examples include forgetting work skills that were learned 10 years ago or the inability to remember important life events, such as a wedding or the death of a loved one. Deficits in semantic memory can be manifested as **agnosia**, the inability to recognize objects through the use of one or more senses.

Alterations in Communication and Social Cognition

The ability to communicate with others is contingent on adequate perception, attention, and memory. In addition, any injury or insult to the areas of the brain responsible for the use of gestures and written and spoken words can impair communication and social cognition. Alterations in communication are common findings in many neurocognitive disorders. Common related terms include the following:

- **Aphasia** is the inability to use or understand language. Aphasia may be classified as expressive aphasia, receptive aphasia, or mixed (global) aphasia. Aphasia is discussed in greater depth in Module 11, Intracranial Regulation.

- **Anomia** is a type of aphasia where the individual is not able to recall the names of everyday objects. It is often related to the progressive degeneration and loss of semantic memory that occurs with dementia.
- **Alogia** refers to a lack of (sometimes called impoverished) speech.

Frontal-lobe and right-brain dysfunction impact spatial awareness to the extent that affected individuals have difficulty gauging physical aspects of social communication, such as how close to stand to someone else. Impaired visual processing can result in the inability to accurately read and respond to nonverbal cues. Sometimes these individuals are mistakenly believed to be deliberately demonstrating rude or annoying behaviors. The deficits in communication and social function place patients at significant risk for health problems, social isolation, victimization, depression, and anxiety (Cacioppo & Cacioppo, 2014).

Alterations in Motor Coordination

The pathways used for cognitive processing and motor coordination and function are shared. Problems with the speed, fluency, and quality of movement are associated with many cognitive disorders and can also be a side effect of medications that alter neurotransmitter function. **Dyspraxia** is a general term used to describe difficulty with the acquisition of motor learning and coordination through the process of growth and development. **Apraxia** refers to alterations in speech as a result of impaired motor function. **Ataxia** is a term used to describe problems with balance and coordination associated with neurologic dysfunction.

Involuntary movements include those that are not completely purposeful and occur without initiation by the patient, such as tics and tremors (Ganos, Rothwell, & Haggard, 2018). **Tics** are semi-involuntary movements that are sudden, repetitive, and nonrhythmic. They may involve muscle groups or vocalizations (motor or phonic). Suppression of a tic may be possible but results in discomfort or anxiety for the patient (Ganos et al., 2018). Examples of simple tics (brief movements involving one muscle group) include eye blinking and head jerking (motor tics) and throat clearing and humming (phonic tics). Complex tics involve a cluster of movements that appear coordinated and more purposeful and thus may be more difficult to identify. Complex motor tics include pulling at clothing or touching people or objects; *echopraxia*, imitating the movements of others; *copropraxia*, performing obscene or forbidden gestures; and **carphologia**, lint-picking behavior that is often seen in dementia. Examples of complex phonic tics include **echolalia**, the meaningless repetition of phrases spoken by another, and *coprolalia*, obscene language (Martino & Hedderly, 2019; Müller-Vahl, Sambrani, & Jakubovski, 2019).

Tremors are unintentional rhythmic movements manifested in shaking of the affected part of the body. **Essential tremors** are those that are not associated with another condition and may be genetic in origin. **Physiologic tremors** occur normally as a result of physiologic exhaustion or emotional stress. Common tremors include *resting tremors*, a coarse, rhythmic tremor often observed in resting arms and hands that is characteristic of Parkinson disease and sometimes seen as a side effect of certain medications, and *dystonic tremors*, sustained involuntary muscle contractions causing twisting repetitive movements and painful or abnormal postures (Barkmeier-Kraemer, Louis, & Smith, 2020; Crawford & Zimmerman, 2018).

Dyskinesia represents a general category of difficulty with or distortions of movement. It may be associated with acquired disorders such as Parkinson disease or as a side effect of some medications. Types of dyskinesias are:

- *Akathisia:* An internal feeling of restlessness that may lead to rocking, pacing, or other constant movement
- *Akinesia:* Diminished movement as a result of difficulty initiating movement
- *Bradykinesia:* Dyskinesia characterized by slow movement
- *Dystonia:* An acute episode of muscle contractions (may result from a neurodegenerative disease or a reaction to medication)
- *Rigidity:* Resistance to movement; *cogwheel rigidity* refers to ratchet-like resistance when attempting to move the joints.

Alterations in Executive Function

Executive function is significantly affected by structural and physiologic abnormalities impacting the frontal cortex (Han & Chan, 2017; Nguyen et al., 2017). Manifestations of impaired function include emotional dysregulation; poor judgment and decision making; reduced insight; forgetfulness; difficulty in planning, organizing, and concrete thinking; and personality changes. Difficulties can range from mild to severe. **Avolition** is decreased motivation, or the inability to initiate goal-directed activity, and may be in part related to deficits in executive dysfunction (Foti et al., 2020).

Alterations in Intellectual Function and Learning

Alterations in intellectual function and learning may be either developmental or acquired. Nurses should recognize that there are a broad range of issues impacting learning and intellectual function and that many individuals may demonstrate deficits in adaptive function without meeting diagnostic criteria of a specific delay or disorder. For more information on learning and associated problems, refer to Module 25, Development.

Learning disabilities are a group of disorders that impact an individual's ability to process information. The cause of learning disabilities is not entirely understood, but researchers believe that subtle variations in brain structure and function may be responsible. Both genetics and environmental factors probably contribute to these variations. In general, individuals with learning disabilities have average to above-average intelligence but demonstrate a gap between their actual and potential achievement. The impact of learning disabilities goes well beyond difficulty with basic academic skills. Most individuals with specific learning difficulties also experience one or more related problems with social cognition, executive function, memory, processing speed, attention, and motor coordination. As a result, they often face significant challenges with interpersonal relationships and other aspects of adaptive function (Learning Disabilities Association of America, 2020). Nurses are in a key position to assess for variations in development that may suggest an underlying learning issue.

TABLE 23.2 Physical Traits Associated with Three Causes of Intellectual Disability

Down Syndrome (see Figure 23.2)	Fragile X Syndrome (see Figure 23.3)	Fetal Alcohol Syndrome (see Figure 23.4)
Broad hands with a single traverse palmar crease	Crossed eyes	Small eyes
Congenital cataracts	Enlarged testicles	Abnormal joints and bones
Decreased muscle tone	Epicanthic eye folds	CNS abnormalities
Epicanthic eye folds	Excessively flexible joints	Flattened nasal bridge
Flattened nose	High palate	Growth deficits
Hearing impairment	Increased likelihood of middle ear infections	Hearing impairment
Increased likelihood of diabetes, leukemia, and heart defects	Increased seizure risk	Lack of coordination
Protruding tongue	Large ears	Small nose that turns up at the tip
Short, stocky neck	Long head with protruding jaw	Small palpebral fissures
Small ears located low on the head	Scoliosis	Smooth philtrum
Small head		Thin vermillion border
Wide space between first two toes		

Intellectual disabilities are characterized by significant limitations in intellectual functioning and adaptive behavior that begin prior to age 18. An IQ score of 70 to 75 or below is considered indicative of limited intellectual functioning. Intellectual disability can result from prenatal errors in central nervous system (CNS) development, external factors that damage the CNS, or pre- or postnatal changes in an individual's biological environment. Sometimes, these changes produce only mental limitations. Other times, intellectual disability is one of a constellation of symptoms linked to a particular cause (American Association of Intellectual and Developmental Disabilities, 2020).

Selected Alterations in Cognition

The exemplars included in this module represent only a fraction of the disorders that impair cognition. The classification of these disorders in the fifth edition of the *Diagnostic and Statistical Manual of Mental Disorders* (DSM-5; American Psychiatric Association [APA], 2013) provides a context for understanding both similarities and differences in the exemplars and related conditions; however, the nursing care focuses primarily on supporting adaptive function and collaborating with healthcare professionals to provide holistic care that meets the unique needs of affected individuals regardless of medical diagnosis.

Selected Learning Disabilities

The DSM-5 recognizes a number of specific learning disabilities. Two more common ones are *auditory processing disorder (APD)* and *language processing disorder (LPD)*, in which individuals have difficulty processing sounds and recognizing their source. For example, a student with APD may have difficulty processing and acting on verbal instructions and benefit from visual cues, pictorial schedules, and active demonstrations.

For all patients with learning difficulties, nurses support them and their families in seeking appropriate services and accommodations and encourage activities that focus on strengths and build self-esteem.

Selected Intellectual Disabilities

Of the various conditions associated with intellectual disability, three deserve special mention because of the range of physical and cognitive alterations they involve. **Down syndrome**, **fragile X syndrome**, and **fetal alcohol spectrum disorders (FASD)**, including *fetal alcohol syndrome*, are all caused by problems during prenatal development, although the first two conditions involve genetic errors while the third involves alcohol consumption during pregnancy. All three conditions are present at birth and affect individuals for the rest of their lives. See **Table 23.2** » for a summary of physical traits associated with these conditions.

Down Syndrome

Down syndrome occurs when an individual's cells contain a third full or partial copy of the 21st chromosome (National Down Syndrome Society, 2020). Usually, a full copy of the extra chromosome is present, a situation known as **trisomy 21**. In either case, the excess genetic material leads to intellectual disability and physical impairments that can range from mild to severe (**Figure 23.2** »).

Individuals with Down syndrome are at increased risk of several problems not normally seen in childhood. Roughly 50% are born with congenital heart defects. Children with Down syndrome are also more likely to experience hearing

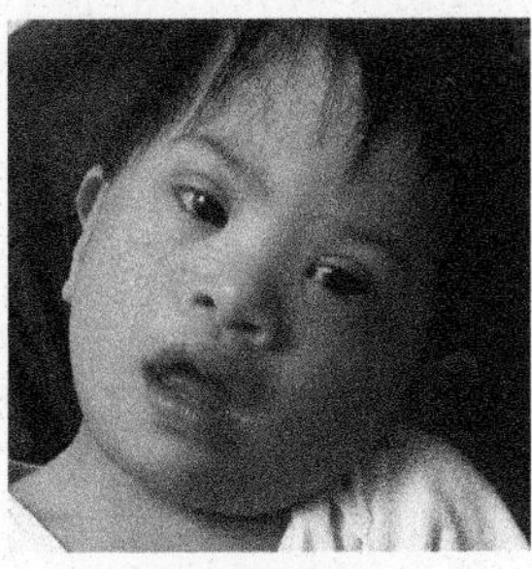

Figure 23.2 » A child with Down syndrome.
Source: George Dodson/Pearson Education, Inc.

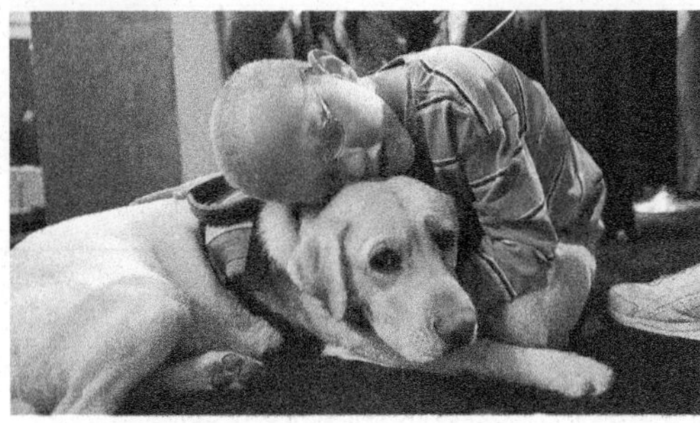

Figure 23.3 ›› A child with fragile X syndrome.
Source: ZUMA Press Inc/Alamy Stock Photo.

loss, gastrointestinal blockages, celiac disease, vision problems, thyroid disease, skeletal abnormalities, orthodontic problems, leukemia, and eventual dementia. With appropriate support, affected individuals can lead healthy lives and sometimes live and work independently. Average life expectancy for individuals with Down syndrome is about 60 years, although some individuals live 10 or even 20 years longer (Centers for Disease Control and Prevention [CDC], 2019c; National Down Syndrome Society, 2020).

Fragile X Syndrome

Fragile X syndrome arises from a single recessive abnormality on the X chromosome. Specifically, a mutation in the *FMR-1* gene causes a small section of DNA to be repeated 200 or more times, rather than the normal 5 to 40 times. This change renders the gene unable to make its associated protein, and absence of the protein leads to errors in brain development and function (U.S. National Library of Medicine, 2020).

A variety of signs and symptoms are associated with fragile X syndrome (**Figure 23.3** ››). The most notable is intellectual disability, typically accompanied by behavioral problems such as ADHD. Affected children may also exhibit autistic behaviors; speech problems; anxiety and mood problems; delays in learning to sit, walk, and talk; and enhanced sensitivity to environmental stimuli. Most individuals with fragile X syndrome are in generally good health and have a normal lifespan. Still, approximately 15% of affected males and 6–8% of females will experience seizures and require anticonvulsant medications (Hagerman et al., 2017; Myers et al., 2019; National Fragile X Foundation, 2020). Interestingly, males usually experience the effects of fragile X syndrome to a much greater degree than females. Because females have two copies of the X chromosome, one X chromosome's *FMR-1* gene is able to produce enough protein to partially compensate for the amount normally produced by the other copy. Males, however, have just one X chromosome, so no compensatory mechanism is available (Hagerman et al., 2017; National Fragile X Foundation, 2020).

Fetal Alcohol Spectrum Disorders

Unlike Down syndrome and fragile X syndrome, FASDs are completely preventable conditions caused by maternal alcohol intake during pregnancy. The *only* way to prevent FASD is for the woman to abstain from consuming alcohol for the duration of the pregnancy. All FASDs involve some degree of physical, intellectual, behavioral, and/or learning disability, with fetal alcohol syndrome (FAS) being the most severe (**Figure 23.4** ››).

FASDs result from the presence of alcohol in a woman's bloodstream. Because alcohol crosses the placenta and the

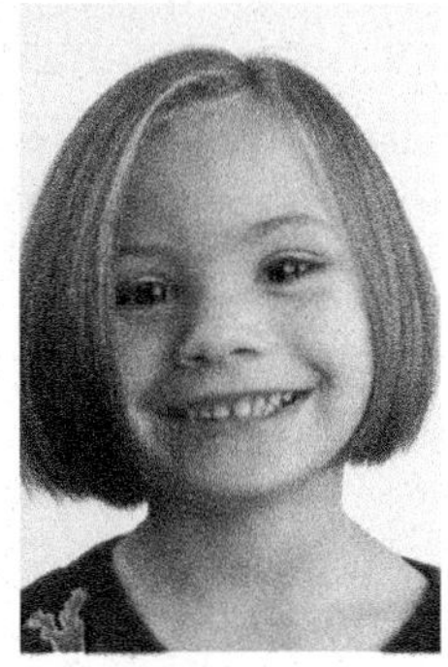

Figure 23.4 ›› A child with fetal alcohol syndrome.
Source: Rick's Photography/Shutterstock.

fetal liver cannot process it, the fetus has the same blood alcohol content as its mother, regardless of the type or amount of alcohol consumed (Denny, Coles, & Blitz, 2017; Mukherjee, Cook, Norgate, & Price, 2019). Even small amounts of alcohol can dramatically disrupt prenatal development, causing facial, skeletal, and organ abnormalities, along with a variety of other problems. However, for a diagnosis of FAS (as opposed to another fetal alcohol spectrum disorder), a child must exhibit all of the following conditions (National Organization on Fetal Alcohol Syndrome, 2020):

- Growth deficits
- Characteristic facial abnormalities, including a smooth philtrum (ridge between the nose and upper lip), thin vermillion border (line between the lips and surrounding skin), and small palpebral fissures (separations between the upper and lower eyelids)
- CNS abnormalities (structural, neurologic, and/or functional).

These nervous system abnormalities almost always result in some degree of mental impairment, such as intellectual disability, learning disability, communication problems, poor memory, or limited attention span. Although the many effects of FAS last a lifetime, early treatment can help lessen some symptoms and improve an affected individual's quality of life.

Other Preventable Causes of Intellectual Disability

- Maternal drug use, smoking, malnutrition, exposure to environmental toxins, and illness during pregnancy.
- Prematurity and low birth weight forecast disability more reliably than any other conditions. Difficulties at delivery, such as oxygen deprivation or birth injury, may also cause problems in intellectual functioning.
- Head injuries, near-drowning, and diseases such as whooping cough, chickenpox, measles, and *Haemophilus influenzae* type B (Hib) can damage the brain in childhood. Childhood exposure to toxins (especially lead) can also cause irreparable damage to the nervous system.
- Malnutrition, childhood diseases, exposure to environmental health hazards, and a lack of intellectual stimulation early in life are also factors that have been linked to intellectual disability.

In the United States and in other countries around the world, prevalence rates of intellectual disability have dropped thanks to public health measures that mandate newborn screening for phenylketonuria and require vaccinations for Hib, measles, encephalitis, and rubella. Comprehensive prenatal care, including testing for diseases and administering folic acid to expectant mothers, also reduces the risk of intellectual disability.

Delirium

Delirium is usually an acute change in mental state that is characterized by confusion; inability to focus, shift, or sustain attention; disorientation; sleep-wake cycle disturbances; disorganized thinking; perceptual abnormalities; mood changes; and both psychomotor retardation and agitation. Delirium typically results from a medical condition, trauma, or chemical/substance exposure or withdrawal and is a common complication observed during stays in acute-care settings. Delirium is presented as an exemplar in this module.

Dementia

Dementia is a general term used to describe the loss of one or more cortical functions or cognitive attributes as a result of degeneration of the neurologic systems of the brain. The DSM-5 uses the term *mild and major neurocognitive disorder (NCD)* to replace the older term *dementia* (APA, 2013). Individuals with mild NCDs are those who demonstrate limited impairment and are able to maintain independent functioning with some modifications (such as medication reminders). They are often in the initial stages of disease progression. NCDs are classified as major when additional cortical functions are lost and the individual can no longer maintain independence (Eramudugolla et al., 2017). Dementia can be caused or exacerbated by other conditions and variables, including metabolic problems, nutritional deficiencies, infections, poisoning, medications, and any conditions that compromise oxygenation and perfusion (National Institute of Neurological Disorders and Stroke, 2019).

Subtypes of NCDs are classified by etiology and are discussed briefly below and in more detail in the exemplar on Alzheimer disease. The terms *major neurocognitive disorder* and *dementia* are both used in clinical practice and are used interchangeably in this module.

Alzheimer disease (Exemplar 23.A) is the most common form of dementia, accounting for about 80% of all cases and affecting more than 5 million adults in the United States (Alzheimer's Association, 2020e). *Vascular dementia* often results from multiple small strokes or infarcts that block major blood vessels in the brain. Low blood pressure (hypoperfusion) from other conditions, such as blood clots, ruptured blood vessels, or narrowing or hardening of blood vessels that supply the brain, can also lead to vascular dementia. The symptoms vary widely, depending on severity of the blood vessel damage and the part of the brain affected. Unlike other dementias, memory loss may or may not be a significant symptom (Alzheimer's Association, 2020j). Often, seizures will follow a stroke, caused by bleeding in the brain (hemorrhagic stroke) or a stroke in the cerebral cortex (American Stroke Association, 2020). Many times, the progression of vascular dementia follows a "sawtooth" or stair-step pattern, where a series of strokes or ministrokes cause cognitive decline followed by periods of stabilization. After each vascular event, changes in thought processes occur in noticeable steps downward from the prior level of function (Mayo Clinic, 2020c).

Vascular dementia can occur alone or in combination with other forms of dementia and is thought to represent at least 10% of all cases of neurocognitive decline (Alzheimer's Association, 2020j). **Table 23.3** » outlines other forms of dementia substance.

TABLE 23.3 Selected Neurocognitive Disorders Resulting in Dementia

Disorder	Etiology	Clinical Manifestations	Onset/Course
Dementia due to HIV	Infection with HIV-1 produces a dementing illness called HIV-1-associated cognitive/motor complex.	Symptoms vary in early stages. Severe cognitive changes, particularly confusion, changes in behavior, and sometimes psychosis, are not uncommon in the later stages.	At first symptoms are subtle and may be overlooked. The severity of symptoms is associated with the extent of the brain pathology.
Dementia due to traumatic brain injury (see Module 11, Intracranial Regulation)	Any type of head trauma.	Amnesia is the most common neurobehavioral symptom following head trauma.	A degree of permanent disturbance may persist.
Dementia due to Parkinson disease	Parkinson disease is a neurologic condition resulting from the death of neurons, including those that produce dopamine, the chemical responsible for movement and coordination. It is characterized by tremor, rigidity, bradykinesia, and postural instability.	Dementia has been reported in approximately 20–60% of people with Parkinson disease and is characterized by cognitive and motor slowing, impaired memory, and impaired executive functioning.	Onset and course are slow and progressive.
Dementia due to Huntington disease	Huntington disease is an inherited, dominant-gene, neurodegenerative disease. The first symptoms are typically movements that involve facial contortions, twisting, turning, and tongue movements.	Cognitive symptoms include memory deficits, both recent and remote, as well as significant problems with frontal executive function, personality changes, and other signs of dementia.	The disease begins in the late 30s or early 40s and may last 10–20 years or more before death.
Lewy body dementia	This disorder is distinguished by the presence of Lewy bodies—eosinophilic inclusion bodies—seen in the cortex and brainstem.	Clinically, Lewy body disease is similar to Alzheimer disease; however, there is an earlier appearance of visual hallucinations and parkinsonian features.	Irreversible and progressive; tends to progress more rapidly than Alzheimer disease.

(continued on next page)

TABLE 23.3 *(continued)*

Disorder	Etiology	Clinical Manifestations	Onset/Course
Vascular dementia	Vascular dementia features strokes or infarcts in the blood vessels of the brain. Also caused by hypoperfusion due to blood clots, ruptured blood vessels, or narrowing or hardening of blood vessels.	Symptoms vary widely, depending on the severity of the blood vessel damage and the part of the brain affected. Seizures often accompany strokes. Sudden poststroke changes may occur and include confusion, disorientation, trouble speaking or understanding speech, sudden headache, difficulty walking, poor balance, and numbness or paralysis on one side of the face or the body.	Cognitive changes may occur suddenly after a stroke, or they may have a slower onset. Progression typically follows a "sawtooth" pattern of strokes/ministrokes, followed by decline and stabilization until another vascular event occurs.

Sources: Based on Alzheimer's Association (2020j); Alzheimer's Society UK (2020); American Psychiatric Association (2013); Black and Andreasen (2020); Sadock, Sadock, and Ruiz (2020). Table first appeared in Potter and Moller (2016).

TABLE 23.4 Comparison of Delirium, Dementia, and Depression

	Delirium	Dementia	Depression
Onset	Acute, sudden, rapid	Slow, progressive	Variable
Duration	Hours to days	Months to years	Episodic
Cognitive impairment	Memory, consciousness	Abstract thinking, memory	Memory and concentration
Mood	Rapid mood swings	Depression, apathy	Sadness, anxiety
Delusions/hallucinations	Both; often visual	May present in later stages	Delusions only
Outcome	Recovery possible	Poor	Recovery possible

Source: From Potter and Moller (2020). Pearson Education, Inc., Hoboken, NJ.

Nurses and other healthcare professionals need to recognize that a variety of conditions can mimic dementia, especially in older individuals. Depression and emotional problems may cause cognitive slowing and disorientation. It may also be difficult to distinguish symptoms of delirium from those of dementia. **Table 23.4** » provides a comparison of the manifestations of delirium, dementia, and depression.

Schizophrenia Spectrum and Other Psychotic Disorders

As mentioned previously, psychotic disorders encompass a broad range of cognitive alterations that result in altered perceptions of reality and abnormal thinking in the absence of an underlying condition. Schizophrenia represents one type of psychotic disorder identified in the DSM-5 and is discussed in detail as an exemplar for cognition. Approximately 1–4% of the population experiences some type of psychotic disorder, and up to 1% of the worldwide population meets the criteria for schizophrenia (National Alliance on Mental Illness, 2020). The DSM-5 identifies a number of psychotic disorders in addition to schizophrenia spectrum disorder. Because psychosis can result from an underlying medical condition or ingestion of one or more substances, diagnostic tests should be run to rule out any underlying illness or causative agent.

Risk Factors for Altered Cognitive Function

Although risk factors for impaired cognition vary according to the conditions described in this section, a few general principles apply. Most developmental and acquired cognitive disorders have a nonmodifiable familial/genetic component that predisposes individuals to the development of a specific disorder, such as dementia or schizophrenia. Other categories of risk factors include population-specific factors, lifestyle behaviors, environmental exposures, and certain health conditions. Most cognitive disorders are believed to be multifactorial or the consequence of genetic factors and age, sex, lifestyle behaviors, environmental exposures, or other health conditions.

Case Study » Part 1

Victor Wallace is a 74-year-old man who was diagnosed with mild NCD due to Alzheimer disease 2 years ago. He lives with his 50-year-old daughter, Anne Marie, who is his primary caregiver. His wife of 52 years died of pancreatic cancer 18 months ago.

Mr. Wallace presents at his gerontologist's office at 9:30 on Thursday morning. Ms. Wallace requested the appointment because she is concerned about the changes she has seen in her father over the past month. As the nurse working with Mr. Wallace's gerontologist, you conduct an initial assessment and interview with him and his daughter. Ms. Wallace reports that Mr. Wallace has exhibited increased confusion and anxiety at home and at the adult daycare center he attends each day while she is at work. In the past, he had these problems only in unfamiliar settings. He is also experiencing a decline in language, increasingly using the wrong words to describe common objects and relying on scanning speech to find words. However, Ms. Wallace's main concern is her father's refusal to carry out the basic ADLs he is still capable of performing. When you ask Mr. Wallace about the ADLs, he says, "There's no point in trying because I won't be able to do them much longer."

As you observe Mr. Wallace, you note that he seems agitated. He is sitting on the edge of his chair, tapping his foot and rapping his hands on his knees. When you ask him basic questions, he has a hard time coming up with answers. When he can't find the words he wants, he just repeats the phrase, "That's how it is."

Mr. Wallace's vital signs and weight are normal, and his physical condition is good for a man his age. You administer the Cornell Scale for Depression in Dementia and his score is 17, indicating high probability of depression. His Mini-Mental State Examination score is 14—down 2 points from his last assessment nearly 6 months ago. The gerontologist increases Mr. Wallace's dose of memantine (Namenda) from 21 mg to 28 mg per day to try to slow the progression of his Alzheimer symptoms. She then adds sertraline (Zoloft), a selective serotonin reuptake inhibitor (SSRI), to treat his depression symptoms. Mr. Wallace is to start out taking 50 mg of sertraline per day, gradually working up to 150 mg per day over a 6-week period.

Clinical Reasoning Questions Level I

1. How do your observations of Mr. Wallace correlate with the changes Ms. Wallace reports?
2. What aspects of Mr. Wallace's presentation prompt you to test him for depression?
3. Why might Mr. Wallace's increased confusion in familiar settings be a concern for Ms. Wallace?

Clinical Reasoning Questions Level II

4. Why is it important to distinguish between Mr. Wallace's refusal to perform ADLs and an inability to do so?
5. Would speech therapy be an appropriate intervention for Mr. Wallace? Why or why not?
6. *Refer to the exemplar on Alzheimer disease in this module:* How would a change in Mr. Wallace's Alzheimer medication from an *N*-methyl-D-aspartate (NMDA) receptor antagonist, like memantine, to a cholinesterase inhibitor, like donepezil, affect the doctor's choice of SSRI for depression?

Concepts Related to Cognition

Cognitive function and other systems tend to be interdependent, so determining the extent to which other concepts or systems are involved can be difficult. For example, cerebral perfusion is necessary for normal cognitive functioning but depends on the adequate intake of oxygen and osmotic pressure needed to maintain adequate blood flow. Even subtle variations in perfusion can result in acute alterations in cognitive function, such as delirium, with older adults being more sensitive to these changes because of diminished functional reserves (Wolters et al., 2017).

Cerebral perfusion and cognitive integrity depend on normal gas exchange. Chronic and subtle mechanisms involved in decreased oxygen supply to the brain (as seen in chronic obstructive pulmonary disease [COPD] and anemia) can negatively impact the neurochemical signaling and synaptic plasticity necessary for normal cognitive development and function (Lawley, Macdonald, Oliver, & Mullins, 2017).

Genetic factors and early environmental insults can influence development in utero or in the child's first years, affecting learning, cognition, and speech and language development. Exposure to alcohol or other toxins during pregnancy can have long-term implications for child health and cognition.

Inflammation appears to play a key role in altered cognitive function. Stress, infection, surgery, and cancer all result in an inflammatory response and the release of cytokines. Inflammation can occur in the brain and CNS as a direct result of trauma, cerebral infarction, or infection. Peripheral inflammation (outside of the CNS) causes a cascade of physiologic events with implications for an array of affective, cognitive, and behavioral responses (Gil Montoya et al., 2017; Hayden et al., 2017; Rincon, Serruya, & Jallo, 2020; Yarlott, Heald, & Forton, 2017). Initially, these changes are adaptive, enabling individuals to conserve energy necessary for healing. However, chronic or persistent inflammation can lead to irreversible neuronal changes.

Substances such as alcohol, illicit drugs, and some pharmaceuticals can impact cognitive function. Immediate and long-term consequences of substance intoxication and abuse are discussed in Module 22.

Alterations in cognitive function have the potential to impact an individual's competency to make healthcare decisions and consent to certain treatments and procedures. Patients with mental health disorders, intellectual disabilities, and other cognitive conditions are often unable to advocate for themselves and are considered vulnerable populations. Establishing advance directives during mild stages of cognitive dysfunction or relapse is essential.

The following feature links some, but not all, of the concepts related to cognition. They are presented in alphabetical order.

Health Promotion

A health-promotion model for cognition views cognitive function on a continuum from optimal to impaired function, with the goal being to support independence and quality of life for all individuals at risk for or experiencing an alteration in cognitive function. The CDC (2019a), through its Healthy Brain Initiative, stresses the importance of prevention and early screening to address the public epidemic of cognitive disorders. When individuals are diagnosed with a cognitive disorder, the goal is to provide care that enables them to achieve their fullest potential, maintain their orientation to their families and communities, and live in environments that promote their inherent worth and self-efficacy.

Prevention

Prevention of cognitive disorders includes measures to reduce modifiable risk factors and enhance protective factors. *Universal prevention* of cognitive disorders targets the general population and includes interventions such as public health campaigns regarding the use of seat belts and other safety devices. *Selective prevention* targets subgroups of the population whose risk of developing a cognitive disorder is higher than that of the general population based on an analysis of biological, psychologic, or socioeconomic factors. Examples include early intervention programs for children from disadvantaged backgrounds and counseling following exposure to trauma. *Indicated prevention* is aimed at individuals who have minimal but detectable manifestations of cognitive disorder. An example would be initiating treatment for an individual who demonstrates prodromal symptoms of schizophrenia or has biomarkers for dementia.

Screening and Early Detection

The progression and or impact of many of the cognitive disorders described in this module can be positively impacted through early detection and intervention. A variety of

Concepts Related to
Cognition

CONCEPT	RELATIONSHIP TO COGNITION	NURSING IMPLICATIONS
Addiction	Drugs and alcohol alter normal neuronal functioning, ↓ blood flow and/or waste removal → cognitive impairment.	■ Promote prevention of addiction behaviors; address risk factors. ■ Monitor vital signs. ■ Provide for patient safety. ■ Watch for symptoms of withdrawal and provide supportive care as necessary. ■ Pharmacotherapy to reduce withdrawal symptoms, substance abuse counseling, patient education.
Development	Genetic factors, heredity, and environmental insults → cognitive dysfunction.	■ Refer for genetic counseling. ■ Screen for conditions that may impact cognitive development (e.g., metabolic disorders). ■ Assess for alterations in development, such as cognitive or speech delays. ■ Refer for evaluation. ■ Provide patient/family education and support; collaborate with special education services, psychologists, speech pathologists, occupational therapists, and others.
Inflammation	Inflammation → release of pro-inflammatory proteins that alter neurotransmitter function. Chronic and frequent inflammation → permanent cognitive decline.	■ Promote lifestyle behaviors that decrease inflammation (diet, exercise, prevention of infection, immunizations, injury prevention, use of helmets). ■ Assess for infection or injury that may be causing inflammation. ■ Implement measures to address inflammation/infection (anti-inflammatory agents, antibiotics).
Legal Issues	Recurring or chronic cognitive issues ↓ decision-making capacity and competency. Lack of appropriate services ↑ risk for involvement with the legal system.	■ Advocate for community resources that can enable individuals with cognitive dysfunction to manage the symptoms of their disease and avoid encounters with the criminal justice system. ■ Monitor for signs of abuse and caregiver role strain. ■ Ask whether patient has established an advance directive or is interested in doing so. ■ Document the advance directives and all conversations about it in the patient's chart. ■ Advocate on the patient's behalf by ensuring that the advance directive is followed. ■ If necessary, help vulnerable patients with cognitive deficits to obtain a court-appointed guardian to direct care. ■ *Anticipate:* Patient, family community education, referral to counseling resources, case management services.
Oxygenation	Decreased O_2 reaching the brain → cognitive impairment, coma, and death.	■ Promote prevention of conditions that lead to impaired oxygenation; address modifiable risk factors. ■ Monitor vital signs, arterial blood gases (ABGs), airway clearance, and for signs of impaired perfusion. ■ Administer oxygen and carry out other interventions to support oxygenation.
Perfusion	Inadequate perfusion of brain tissue ↓ O_2 levels and → acute changes in cognitive function. Chronic impairments in perfusion and oxygenation ↑ risk for neurodegeneration.	■ Promote healthy lifestyle; address modifiable risk factors for alterations in perfusion. ■ Monitor vital signs, ABGs, and cardiac sounds. ■ Assess perfusion, including pulses, nail beds, and skin color. ■ *Anticipate:* Pharmacotherapy to maintain blood pressure and cardiac output, intravenous (IV) fluids, stress/exercise tests, echocardiogram, possible cardiac catheterization and/or surgery.

screening tools are identified in the sections on assessment later in this module. Screening and detection of cognitive disorders occur in a number of settings, including but not limited to primary care settings, community health settings, and schools.

Nursing Assessment

A general assessment of cognitive status is an essential component of the nursing assessment of all patients. When a patient presents with the onset of any cognitive changes, the priority assessment focuses on addressing potentially life-threatening factors that may be contributing to the problem through physical assessment, history, and diagnostic procedures, such as laboratory values.

SAFETY ALERT! Any changes in cognition require immediate attention. Cognitive disturbances put patients at increased risk of injury, so rapid initiation of safety measures is critical. Also, prompt assessment of a patient's cognitive impairment may allow the healthcare team to more quickly identify and treat the underlying cause.

Cognitive assessment is performed both for the purposes of initial screening for the presence or absence of cognitive problems and for monitoring changes in cognition over time. An assessment of cognitive status should be performed during an initial provider or home care visit, following any changes in medical treatment and pharmacotherapy, during any transitions in care, and prior to obtaining consent for procedures. Certain individuals are at increased risk for cognitive problems and warrant more frequent assessment of cognitive status. For example, clinical guidelines published by Ellis et al. (2017) suggest that on admission older adults who are hospitalized should receive a comprehensive geriatric assessment (CGA). The CGA is a multidimensional, multidisciplinary assessment of the medical, mental, and functional problems of older people with frailty. Use of the CGA promotes collaborative, integrated care.

Observation and Patient Interview

Initial observation of the patient focuses on appearance and behavioral manifestations that may be indicative of cognitive function. Appearance and dress can provide cues to the patient's mental state and ability to maintain self-care. The nurse may also make general observations related to social skills, motor function, activity level, ability to attend and focus on the assessment, and ability to provide logical and coherent responses to questions. The best source of information comes directly from the patient. However, when assessing pediatric patients or patients with moderate to severe cognitive impairment, a family member or caregiver may be asked to provide information.

During the patient interview, ask direct questions to elicit information related to biophysical and psychosocial history, development, family history, and environmental factors. Use judgment in direct questioning of individuals with established cognitive and perceptual problems, as some may not have the capacity to respond logically. In addition, cognitive problems such as perceptual problems and delusional thinking are likely to increase the patient's anxiety and may result in an escalation of inappropriate behaviors during the patient interview and examination.

Biophysical and Psychosocial History

The medical history includes gathering information about both the presenting problem and the presence or development of altered health patterns across the lifespan.

History of the Current Problem

Initial questions focus on the patient's perception of the problem and what brings the patient to the healthcare setting currently. Initial questions may proceed from broad questions about a typical day, including ADLs, self-care activities, and perceived level of health and wellness. When patients or family members report changes in cognitive function, ask nonthreatening questions such as:

- Can you describe the changes?
- What do you think may be contributing to the changes?
- When did you begin experiencing these changes?
- Are these changes constant and, if not, how frequently do they occur?
- Have you previously sought medical advice or care related to these changes?

More focused questions include the following:

- Are you experiencing any changes in your ability to pay attention or remember things?
- Do you have difficulty planning and organizing things?
- Do you ever hear, see, or smell things that are not apparent to others?
- Have you been experiencing any problems that are making it difficult to learn or function in school (or work)?
- Have you been experiencing any problems expressing yourself or understanding others?

Depending on the patient's responses, seek additional detail about the impact on daily functioning, frequency and duration of symptoms, suspected causes or contributing factors (such as a preexisting medical or psychiatric diagnosis), and how the patient has been treating or managing the symptoms. Be sure to obtain a list of all current medications with the dose, route, and frequency and to inquire about the use of any complementary health approaches.

History of Prior Biophysical and Psychosocial Alterations

A thorough history of patient development, illness and injury, and health behaviors (including substance use) is necessary when working with patients with alterations in cognition. For children, it is necessary to assess for achievement of expected milestones and to note any factors that may impede normal growth and development (such as chronic illness or exposure to trauma).

Ask if any family members had disorders such as dementia, schizophrenia, and/or developmental or learning problems. Because many patients may not have knowledge of the specific diagnoses in family members, use lay terms when inquiring about unusual symptoms and behaviors, such as confusion or memory loss, and treatment history.

Assess for environmental factors that may be contributing to the patient's cognitive status, including nutrition and lifestyle considerations, use of any type of medication or herbal supplement, and any accommodations or services in place to support independent function.

When assessing cognition in children, consider parenting techniques and capabilities, as well as access to activities and stimulation that promote cognitive development, such as age-appropriate activities and toys. Determine the possibility of any current or past exposures to toxic substances at home or at work.

Physical and Mental Status Examination

Once the interview is completed and the patient's history has been obtained, the nurse progresses to a physical assessment of the patient and a mental status examination. The physical examination incorporates an organized pattern of assessment to identify alterations that may be contributing to cognitive dysfunction. The mental status exam includes a series of procedures and tools used to detect alterations in perception and thinking.

Physical Examination

Because changes in cognitive function are often an early sign of decreased oxygenation or perfusion or an alteration in another biophysical process, begin by obtaining a complete set of vital signs and assessing the patient's level of pain. Auscultation of the heart and lungs may reveal an underlying problem with gas exchange or perfusion. For example, murmurs in infants and young children may indicate congenital heart defects associated with other neurodevelopmental problems. An assessment of peripheral perfusion may indicate vascular problems that are compromising cerebral perfusion. An assessment of neurologic signs is an essential component of cognitive evaluation (detailed information can be found in Module 11, Intracranial Regulation). An evaluation of hearing, vision, touch, taste, and smell can help rule out perceptual problems related to impaired sensory function.

» **Skills:** See Skill 1.22, Neurologic Status: Assessing, in Volume 3.

Physical development and height, weight, and fat distribution should be within normal limits for the patient's age. Observable physical alterations may be associated with many cognitive syndromes, including intellectual disabilities and schizophrenia (Bélanger & Caron, 2018; Vancampfort et al., 2017; Vasudevan & Suri, 2017). Examples include small head circumference, wide- or close-set eyes, prominent forehead, folds on the inner corners of the eyes (epicanthic eye folds), asymmetry or malformation of facial features and ears, tongue protrusion, palate and mouth abnormalities, flattened face or nose, limb abnormalities, small stature, poor muscle tone, some birthmarks, palmar folds, and altered posture. Suspicions of genetic and metabolic/biochemical disorders accompanying developmental delay can be investigated through genetic testing and serum and urine tests (Mithyantha, Kneen, McCann, & Gladstone, 2017).

An important component of the physical examination includes an assessment of motor function. Movements should be consistent with age and development. Any changes in gait or other evidence of movement disorders should be noted (Vitrikas, Savard, & Bucaj, 2017).

Mental Status Examination

The mental status exam is a broad screening tool that is used to assess current cognitive functioning of the individual. Many tools are available, and most serve to capture data related to orientation, perception and thought content (including judgment and insight), attention and concentration, memory, speech/language/communication, mood and affect, and psychomotor activity. Other assessments may be used to rule out related conditions such as depression or other mood disorders or to gather information on developmental status or level of functional impairment. **Table 23.5** » lists a variety of common assessment and screening tools that may be used by healthcare professionals to detect alterations in cognitive function. The Mental Status Assessment feature presents an example of an organized formal mental status examination with a description of normal and abnormal findings and patient-centered considerations. Formal assessment often serves to validate findings gathered through observation.

TABLE 23.5 Common Tools Used to Assess Cognition and Mental Status

Assessment Name	Description
Ages & Stages Questionnaires (ASQ),	Set of questionnaires tailored to detect alterations in development in young children.
American Academy of Pediatrics—Bright Futures	Kit for health promotion and prevention published by the American Academy of Pediatrics that includes schedules for screening and care and a variety of questionnaires used to detect health problems, including developmental alterations.
Confusion Assessment Method (CAM)	Five-minute interview-style exam that screens specifically for signs of delirium. Pediatric versions are available for children 5 years and older (pCAM/psCAM-ICU for critically ill infants and children).
Cornell Assessment of Pediatric Delirium	Validated, rapid observational tool for screening children in intensive care for delirium.
Cornell Scale for Depression in Dementia	Nineteen-question tool that involves interviews with both patients and their caregivers; assesses for signs of depression in individuals known to have dementia.
Edinburgh Depression Scale	Validated 10-item questionnaire used to screen for the presence and severity of symptoms of postnatal depression.
Geriatric Depression Scale (GDS)	Brief questionnaire (15 or 30 items) that asks patients how they've felt over the past 7 days; assesses for depression in older adults.
Hamilton Rating Scale for Depression (HRSD)	Twenty-minute, 17-question examination that assesses severity of depression in adult patients. The Weinberg Depression Scale for Children and Adolescents (WDSCA) and the Children's Depression Rating Scale (CDRS-R) are modeled on the HRSD and adapted for children over age 5.

TABLE 23.5 *(continued)*

Assessment Name	Description
Mini-Mental State Examination (MMSE)	Thirty-question interview-style exam that assesses a patient's memory, language skills, attention level, and ability to engage in mental tasks; also known as the Folstein Mini-Mental State Examination. It may be modified for use in children over the age of 4.
Montreal Cognitive Assessment	One-page test that briefly assesses a patient's ability in a variety of cognitive domains, including problem solving and sequencing (traits, similarities), attention (digit span, letter vigilance), memory (word list, orientation), visuospatial construction and reasoning (cube, clock), and language (naming, repetition, word generation).
Nonverbal Learning Disabilities (NVLD) Scale	Assesses deficits in the areas of motor skills, visuospatial skills, and interpersonal skills.
Patient Health Questionnaire (PHQ)	Full-length 11-item tool that screens for depression and anxiety, somatic symptoms, and related disorders; abbreviated forms (PDQ-9 and PDQ-2) are used to more selectively screen for depression.
Positive and Negative Symptoms Scale (PANSS)	Registered nurses and other licensed healthcare providers (HCPs) can administer to detect positive, negative, and other manifestations of psychotic disorders and schizophrenia. May be useful in screening for peripartum psychosis.
Postpartum Depression Predictors Inventory (PDPI)	Validated short inventory that can be integrated into all phases of perinatal care to predict the risk of maternal depression.

Diagnostic Tests

Nurses collaborate with other disciplines to support diagnostic assessment of individuals for cognitive disorders. When individuals present with alterations in cognition, nurses can anticipate that a number of laboratory values and diagnostic tests will be ordered to rule out an underlying medical condition. Priority diagnostic assessment focuses on life-threatening conditions that may manifest in cognitive alterations. Analysis of blood and cerebrospinal fluid (CSF) can identify biomarkers associated with Alzheimer disease and schizophrenia, although this is not typically used for diagnosis. Relevant laboratory tests include the following:

- ***Toxicology screens*** to rule out alcohol or substances as a causative factor for changes in mental status
- ***Drug levels*** to rule out mental status changes related to toxic levels of therapeutic agents
- ***Liver function tests (LFTs), complete blood count (CBC), thyroid function,*** B_1 ***(thiamine), sedimentation rate, urinalysis, HIV titer, and fluorescent treponemal antibody absorption (FTA-abs)*** to rule out metabolic, inflammatory, and infectious conditions that may contribute to alterations in mental status
- ***Blood*** tests to identify biomarkers for schizophrenia
- ***CSF*** and ***blood markers*** to identify biomarkers for certain conditions
- ***Genetic testing*** to identify risk factors or underlying causes of a variety of cognitive disorders
- ***Metabolic screening***, which are newborn screens for 26 to 40 metabolic disorders that can cause learning and intellectual disabilities
- ***Diagnostic imaging*** to detect conditions requiring emergency management, such as cerebral edema, cerebral vascular accidents, tumors, and traumatic injuries
- ***MRIs and CT*** to detect abnormalities that are suggestive of some neurocognitive, neurodevelopmental, and psychotic disorders.

Psychometric tests include a variety of standardized tests that are usually administered by a psychologist or neuropsychologist to measure cognitive function in a variety of areas.

Mental Status Assessment

ASSESSMENT/ METHOD	NORMAL FINDINGS	ABNORMAL FINDINGS	PATIENT-CENTERED CONSIDERATIONS
Step 1: Prepare the Patient			
Tell the patient you will be performing a series of tests. Describe what equipment you'll use. Explain that the exam should be comfortable and ask the patient to inform you should difficulties arise. Provide an overview of the assessment activities and the order in which they will occur.	▪ Patient pays attention and asks questions as appropriate. ▪ Patient may be nervous, but this should not interfere with the assessment process.	▪ Patient displays high levels of confusion, anxiety, or agitation. ▪ Patient shows signs of delusions or hallucinations. ▪ Patient pays no attention to the information you provide. ▪ Patient is partially or fully uncommunicative.	▪ A number of assessment tools are available, with some tailored to specific conditions and/or populations. ▪ Direct questioning may not be appropriate for patients who are experiencing hallucinations, delusions, or extreme anxiety. ▪ Questions for children or individuals with intellectual disabilities should be modified.

(continued on next page)

Mental Status Assessment *(continued)*

ASSESSMENT/ METHOD	NORMAL FINDINGS	ABNORMAL FINDINGS	PATIENT-CENTERED CONSIDERATIONS
Step 2: Observe the Patient			
Take note of the patient's general appearance, including hygiene, posture, body language, and expression. Observe the patient's ability to follow your instructions.	▪ Patient follows directions. ▪ Patient's hygiene and overall appearance are acceptable. ▪ Patient's expressions and body language are appropriate to the situation.	▪ Poor hygiene and/or inappropriate expressions and body language might be reflective of depression, schizophrenia, dementia, or another cognitive disorder.	▪ Poor hygiene may be related to economic circumstances. Patient expressions and body language may be congruent with cultural norms that are different from the provider's.
Step 3: Assess the Patient's Language Abilities			
Note the tone, rate, pronunciation, and volume of the patient's speech throughout the course of the exam. Consider the patient's vocabulary and whether what you are saying is understood.	▪ Patient's tone, rate, pronunciation, and volume are appropriate. ▪ Patient speaks easily and naturally, without searching for words. ▪ Patient understands what you are saying and indicates this through verbal and physical reactions. ▪ Social and language milestones have been met.	▪ Problems with language could be a result of anxiety, dementia, depression, or an expressive or receptive language disorder related to brain injury/illness.	▪ Consider whether the patient's hearing may be impaired, especially when working with older adults. ▪ Don't assume all patients are native English speakers. Some patients may communicate more effectively in another language and require assistance from an interpreter. ▪ Consider the child's stage of development.
Step 4: Assess the Patient's Level of Orientation			
Assess orientation to person, place, time, and situation.	▪ Patient is fully conscious and alert, oriented to self, location, time, and situation.	▪ Reduced or varying consciousness may be due to hypoglycemia, stroke, seizure, delirium, or organic brain disease.	▪ Noticeable decreases in consciousness during the exam may necessitate immediate medical attention. ▪ Modify questions for children according to developmental level.
Step 5: Assess the Patient's Memory			
See whether the patient knows name, birth date, and address. Ask the patient for a brief summary of places lived and jobs held. Attempt to verify all responses.	▪ Patient can recall basic personal information and provide an accurate biography appropriate to age and developmental level.	▪ Inability to recall events from one's past may be suggestive of dementia, especially Alzheimer disease.	▪ In Alzheimer disease, loss of short-term memory typically precedes loss of long-term memory. ▪ Alterations in memory in children may suggest a problem with learning or intellectual function.
Step 6: Assess the Patient's Computational Ability			
Have the patient answer several arithmetic problems. Start with basic facts and work toward more complicated questions. The age and the developmental status of the patient should be considered.	▪ Patient can compute the correct values. Depending on age and cognitive stage, patient may be able to identify numeric symbols and count.	▪ Inability to perform simple calculations may be suggestive of brain disease or learning problems.	▪ Patient's responses may be negatively affected by language barriers, cognitive development, anxiety, and/or limited experience or education in mathematics.

Mental Status Assessment *(continued)*

ASSESSMENT/ METHOD	NORMAL FINDINGS	ABNORMAL FINDINGS	PATIENT-CENTERED CONSIDERATIONS
Step 7: Assess the Patient's Emotions and Mood			
Note the patient's affect. Ask how the patient is feeling and whether this is typical. If not, ask about events that may have prompted the change. Modify questions for children. Children may be asked to draw pictures of how they are feeling or to select from a visual scale.	■ Patient's affect corresponds with the tone and content of speech. ■ Patient's emotions and mood are appropriate given past events and current situation and developmental status.	■ Mismatch between the patient's affect and speech may reflect neurologic or psychologic problems. ■ Absent, excessively subdued, or excessively animated expressions and responses may be indicative of psychologic disorders.	■ Culture, temperament, and development impact emotional expression. Certain developmental stages are associated with increased lability.
Step 8: Assess the Patient's Perceptions and Thinking Abilities			
Note whether the patient's statements are complete, rational, and pertinent, and whether the patient seems aware of reality. Ask the patient to compare two different things or explain the meaning of a common phrase. Ask if the patient can see, hear, smell, or feel things that are not apparent to others.	■ Patient is aware of reality. ■ Patient's statements are logical and complete. ■ Patient correctly compares two objects and/or explains the meaning of a phrase. ■ Patient denies hallucinations of any kind, or perceptual differences may be explained by level of cognitive development or sociocultural factors.	■ Patients who are unaware of reality may be experiencing neurologic disturbances or a mental disorder. ■ Illogical, incomplete statements suggest problems with concrete thought and may be indicative of a mental disorder. ■ Absent or strange comparisons and explanations are frequent symptoms of psychologic disorders.	■ Patient's responses may be negatively affected by language barriers, education level, and/or intellectual disability or level of cognitive development. ■ Perceptual differences in young children may be related to magical thinking and animism. Children may have difficulty distinguishing between what is imagined and what is real.
Step 9: Assess the Patient's Decision-Making Ability			
Ask the patient about a personal situation that requires good judgment. Determine whether the patient's responses reflect consideration of viable options and logical decision making.	■ Patient considers possible, probable, and appropriate options. ■ Patient's thinking and decision-making capabilities are appropriate for age and stage of development.	■ Patient considers impossible, improbable, or inappropriate options. ■ Patient's decision reflects absent or inadequate consideration of available options.	■ Consider whether the patient's options and decisions make sense—not whether they reflect the choice you would make. ■ Decision-making capacity depends on the stage of cognitive development; refer to normal characteristics of thinking associated with each stage.

Comprehensive neuropsychologic testing may include the use of a number of tests administered over a period of several days. Nurses, teachers, parents, and patients may be asked to complete one or more rating scales to contribute to an overall understanding of the presentation of the problem across a variety of domains.

Case Study » Part 2

In the winter after his visit to the gerontologist, Mr. Wallace begins experiencing increased agitation and he wanders in the afternoons and evenings. One afternoon at the adult daycare center, he slips out the door undetected. By the time the daycare providers realize Mr. Wallace is gone, he has left the grounds and is wandering the neighborhood. The daycare providers call Ms. Wallace, his daughter, and 911, and a search for him begins. Ms. Wallace and two police officers find Mr. Wallace 2 miles from the daycare center. He has no idea where he is or how he got there. He has taken a fall, and his face and hands are covered in scrapes.

The officers radio for an ambulance as Ms. Wallace attempts to talk to her father. Mr. Wallace panics because he does not recognize his daughter, and he pushes her to the ground. He then throws punches at the officers when they prevent him from running away. The paramedics arrive and restrain Mr. Wallace. Once he is restrained, Ms. Wallace is able to calm him down. He is then transported to the emergency department (ED), where you are the admitting nurse.

Mr. Wallace is calm on arrival to the hospital, and you are able to treat his injuries without incident. You attempt to speak with him, but he indicates he is tired and promptly falls asleep. You use this opportunity to interview Ms. Wallace. She states that aggression has become fairly common during her father's increasingly frequent periods of confusion. Sometimes Mr. Wallace doesn't recognize her; other times, he mistakes her for his sister. He is also increasingly unable to use basic objects—such as pencils, toothbrushes, and combs—and relies on Ms. Wallace for many basic ADLs. In addition, he occasionally experiences urinary and fecal incontinence. Ms. Wallace is shaken by the day's events and the situation in general, and she begins to cry.

Case Study » Part 2 (*continued*)

When Mr. Wallace's gerontologist arrives in the ED, you inform Ms. Wallace of these developments. She adds 7.5 mg of buspirone two times daily to his treatment regimen to lessen his agitation and aggression. The doctor also tells Ms. Wallace that Mr. Wallace is starting to transition from moderate to severe Alzheimer disease, and she recommends that she consider looking for a nursing home that specializes in the care of individuals with this condition.

Clinical Reasoning Questions Level I

1. What are the priorities for Mr. Wallace's care to decrease his risk of wandering and injury during his remaining time at home?
2. What independent interventions can you perform to address the caregiver role strain felt by Ms. Wallace?
3. What additional information or education do you anticipate Ms. Wallace will need in light of the doctor's recommendation?

Clinical Reasoning Questions Level II

Referring to the exemplar on Alzheimer disease in this module:

4. What cues suggest that Mr. Wallace is transitioning from moderate to severe AD?
5. What steps can Ms. Wallace take at home to lessen the incidence and severity of Mr. Wallace's sundowning episodes?
6. Why might it be necessary for Ms. Wallace to find an institutional care situation for her father now rather than waiting for further progression of symptoms?

Independent Interventions

Given the importance of health promotion with respect to cognitive disorders, nurses should be prepared to carry out a variety of interventions across settings. Nursing interventions include teaching prevention, coordinating care and making appropriate referrals, implementing measures to promote individual/family safety and well-being, and advocating for the needs of individuals impacted by alterations in cognition.

Prevention and Coordination of Care

Nurses in community health and primary care settings play a critical role in addressing health-related behaviors and suggesting protective measures that can reduce the risk of developing cognitive disorders. They also independently carry out routine assessments for cognitive problems and refer patients for further diagnosis and treatment. Examples of independent interventions in this category include:

- Teaching about healthy diet and lifestyle and the importance of preventive healthcare
- Ensuring that patients use protective headgear during sports and activities such as bike riding
- Stressing the importance of developmentally appropriate activities
- Administering routine developmental and cognitive screenings
- Making referrals to other members of the interprofessional team.

Promoting Safety and Well-Being

Nurses in all settings often plan care for individuals that promotes safety and adaptive functioning. For example, the home health nurse may work with individuals with schizophrenia or Alzheimer disease, monitoring adherence (compliance) to treatment, providing emotional support to the patient and family, and assessing comorbid health conditions.

When patients do require hospitalization for acute changes in cognition, the priority is to identify and manage underlying conditions that may be contributing to the problem. Priority interventions address immediate safety. Secondary interventions include teaching patients and families about the illness and prescribed treatments, providing emotional support, and preparing for discharge to settings where they can receive the support necessary to achieve optimal functioning and prevent future hospitalization. Examples of interventions across settings include:

- Evaluating risk of injury or suicide
- Implementing environmental modifications to support patient safety
- Educating patients and families about diseases, medications, and other therapeutic interventions
- Identifying patient and family strengths
- Encouraging the use of adaptive coping skills
- Supporting cultural and spiritual needs
- Providing ongoing emotional support to both patients and families
- Ensuring healthcare needs are met
- Monitoring the effectiveness of care.

Advocating for Patients

Because cognitive disorders have the potential to reduce decision-making capacity, nurses have a role in ensuring that patients are not abused or exploited and are able to partner in healthcare decisions to the greatest degree possible. This includes encouraging patients in remission or in the early stages of neurocognitive dysfunction to establish advance directives and providing teaching about legal protections that may apply to them (see the Patient Teaching feature). Other interventions related to advocacy include providing teaching

Patient Teaching

Legal Protections for Patients with Cognitive Dysfunction

Nurses should teach individuals with cognitive alterations and their families about several key laws that may affect them. For example:

- The Americans with Disabilities Act of 1990 ensures that individuals with disabilities have equal access to government services, employment, and public accommodations.
- The Education for All Handicapped Children Act of 1975 requires that children with any type of disability have access to free public education. An amendment to this act in 1986 provides federal funding to states that offer early intervention services.
- The Developmental Disabilities and Bill of Rights Act of 2000 provides federal funding to state, public, and nonprofit agencies that provide community-based training activities and education to individuals with developmental disabilities. The law also created the U.S. Administration on Developmental Disabilities to oversee these efforts.

related to legal rights and assisting caregivers and community members to understand cognitive disorders. Nurses working in the newborn nursery and in pediatric settings should be familiar with the processes of referring families to area agencies that provide early childhood intervention services.

Collaborative Therapies

When working with individuals at risk for or experiencing alterations in cognitive function, nurses should anticipate collaborating with the patient, family, other members of the healthcare team, and potentially professionals from other disciplines, such as education and law. Table 37.1 in Module 37, Collaboration, provides an overview of select members of the interprofessional team and their roles. Other professionals sometimes involved with assessment, diagnosis, and treatment planning of individuals with cognitive impairments or intellectual disabilities include developmental pediatricians and developmental psychologists, neuropsychologists, and neurologists. Additional resources may be available through local chapters of organizations such as the Alzheimer's Association, the American Psychiatric Association, the American Association of Intellectual and Developmental Disabilities, and the National Alliance on Mental Illness.

Pharmacologic Therapy

Nurses play a key role in medication administration, education, and adherence, and they must be familiar with the different classes of drugs prescribed to individuals with cognitive alterations. Drugs for treating neurocognitive disorders are primarily aimed at slowing further brain changes and deterioration in functioning. Medications used to treat psychosis target the presenting symptoms, in an attempt to balance brain chemistry and help the patient normalize behaviors and restore life functions. Key factors in medication monitoring and education for patients are provided in Exemplar 51.D, Medication Safety, Module 51.

Experienced nurses will check their facility's intranet, use an online database or a current drug reference, and consult with the pharmacist or physician if they have medication questions. Finally, nurses are responsible for educating family and caregivers about administering medications and their side effects, particularly noting adverse drug reactions that require immediate attention. More specific information on medications used in the treatment of patients with cognitive disorders can be found in the exemplars on Alzheimer disease and schizophrenia.

SAFETY ALERT! Nurses must assess patients with cognitive alterations to determine their ability to self-administer medication. Many patients will require caregiver administration of medications. Missed doses may result in a return or exacerbation of symptoms and increase the patient's risk for deterioration or injury. Long-acting drug formulations (e.g., extended-release tablets, transdermal drug patches) may enhance adherence. Assess for factors that affect adherence at each healthcare interaction.

Lifespan Considerations

Cognitive function is mediated by the interaction of genes and experience, both of which provide the foundation for cognitive changes that occur across the lifespan. Nurses use knowledge of these changes to modify assessment and interventions with individuals who are at risk for or are experiencing alterations in cognitive function. A major consideration is the impact of normal growth and development. **Figure 23.5 »** provides a timeline for normal brain development.

Lev Vygotsky (1896–1934), a Russian psychologist, emphasized the importance of social interaction in the development of cognition: When children interact with others, they learn (Myburgh & Tammaro, 2013). Furthermore, he argued that social interactions assist in helping individuals find meaning and form memories and that these interactions can be culturally influenced. Vygotsky's work provided the theoretical underpinnings for collaborative education and online learning.

While Vygotsky viewed learning as a social process, Swiss psychologist Jean Piaget (1896–1980) believed cognitive development is constructed by the individual. Piaget claimed that cognitive development is an orderly, sequential process in which children form adaptive cognitive structures—called *schemes*—in response to environmental stimuli. According to Piaget, as children learn more about the world by physically interacting with it, they actively revise their schemes to better fit with the reality they observe. Over time, as their brains mature and they are exposed to additional stimuli, children become capable of building more complex schemes—and as they do so, they move from one stage of development to the next. In fact, Piaget proposed that all children pass through

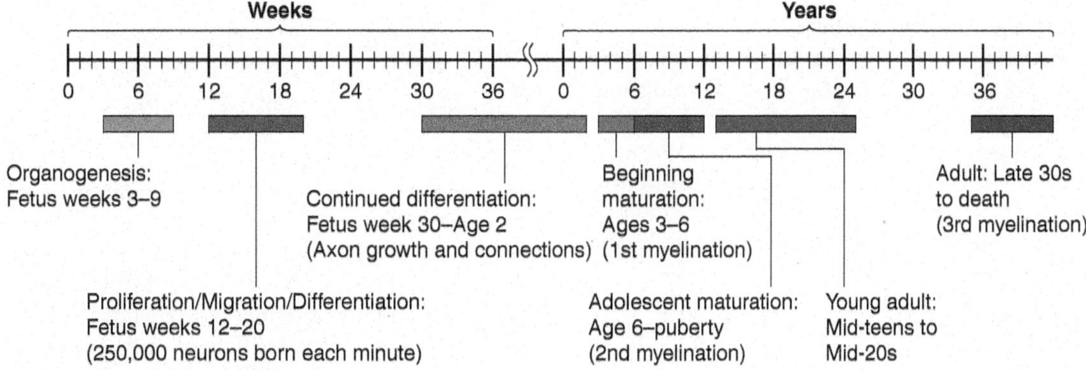

Figure 23.5 » Timeline of brain development.

Source: From Potter and Moller (2020). Pearson Education, Inc., Hoboken, NJ.

TABLE 23.6 Piaget's Stages of Cognitive Development

Stage and Age Range	Description	Developments
Sensorimotor Birth to 2 years	Infants use motor and sensory capabilities to explore the physical environment. Learning is largely trial and error.	Children develop a sense of "self" and "other" and come to understand object permanence. Behavioral schemes begin to produce images or mental schemes.
Preoperational 2–7 years	Young children use symbols (images and language) to explore their environment. Thought is egocentric, and children cannot adopt the perspectives of others.	Children participate in imaginative play and begin to recognize that others don't see the world the same way they do.
Concrete operational 7–11 years	Older children acquire cognitive operations or mental activities that are an important part of rational thought. Logical reasoning is possible but limited to concrete (observable) problems.	Children are no longer fooled by appearances. They understand the basic properties of and relations among objects and events, and they are proficient at inferring motives.
Formal operational 11 years and beyond	Adolescents' cognitive operations are organized in a way that permits them to think about thinking. Thought is now systematic and abstract.	Logical thinking is no longer limited to the concrete or observable. Children engage in systematic, deductive reasoning and ponder hypothetical issues.

four universal stages of cognitive development, as described in **Table 23.6** »: sensorimotor, preoperational, concrete operational, and formal operational (Piaget, 1966; Piaget & Inhelder, 2000).

Cognition from Conception to Adolescence

Simple neuronal connections that shape cognition first occur shortly after the period of conception. These simple connections are then followed by increasingly complex circuits. Any insults during the period of embryonic development—including exposure to toxic substances, maternal stress, nutritional deficits, and illness—can have a devastating impact on cognition (Harvard University Center on the Developing Child, 2020).

Rapid development of neuronal connections occurs during the first few years of life and corresponds with the process through which children assimilate new information, revise cognitive constructs through a process called *accommodation*, and form new thinking structures or schemes to facilitate adaptation. One aspect of normal development is called *pruning*, a process by which unused connections are remodeled or eliminated in order to strengthen cognitive efficiency. Remodeling occurs during sensitive periods of time in brain development. During infancy and early childhood, for example, brains are primed for stimulation of visual pathways and language. If these pathways are not activated, the neuronal pathways required for them will be eliminated, impacting overall cognitive capabilities.

Medical illness and adverse childhood experiences predispose children to alterations in cognitive development and mental function. Nurses recognize that young children have some limitations in the functional reserves required to compensate for certain conditions, such as dehydration or infection. As a result, young children may be more likely to manifest cognitive changes such as confusion or hallucinations when any of these are present.

Cognition from Adolescence to Adulthood

Significant changes in brain structure continue to occur during adolescence, with another period of rapid generation of neuronal pathways and remodeling. Changes in activity in the limbic system are believed to account for increased sensation seeking and need for arousal; at the same time, the underdeveloped prefrontal cortex is unable to mediate impulse control (Mallya, Wang, Lee, & Deutch, 2019; Vijayakumar, Op de Macks, Shirtcliff, & Pfeifer, 2018). Deficits in decision making can place adolescents at increased risk for injuries. These deficits may also make adolescents more prone to use alcohol and other substances. Recent evidence, however, suggests that changes in dopamine systems shift adolescent orientation toward reward-seeking behavior and that self-regulation may be enhanced through the provision of positive reinforcement (Hook & Devereux, 2018).

New-onset cognitive dysfunction in adolescence may signal underlying illness, recent trauma, or a developing mental illness. Adolescents experiencing cognitive dysfunction are at increased risk for a number of problems, including depression, suicide, substance abuse, and antisocial behavior.

For adolescents, the social implications of cognitive disorders can have a devastating impact on self-esteem and peer relationships. Adherence to treatment may be negatively impacted by concerns about being different. Normal changes of adolescence, including the achievement of increased independence, hormonal shifts, and sexual development and a greater need for interaction with peers, may present increased challenges for adolescents with cognitive alterations as well as their parents. Teaching focuses on providing developmentally and cognitively appropriate information on issues such as safety, sexuality, adaptive coping, and management of the cognitive condition.

Cognition from Adulthood through Middle Age

Research indicates that brain maturation, especially areas responsible for executive function, are not fully mature until the mid- to late 20s and that full maturation for men may not occur until the early 30s (Nostro, Müller, Reid, & Eickhoff, 2016; Tang, Shafer, & Ofen, 2017). Middle-aged adults demonstrate an enhanced ability to read other people's emotional states (Oh, Chopik, Konrath, & Grimm, 2020). Vocabulary and other elements of accumulated facts and knowledge have been found to peak even later in life. Nurses can apply this information to dispel myths that surround the belief that cognitive decline is an inevitable aspect of aging, while focusing on the cognitive strengths of patients across the lifespan.

Nursing care of adults with cognitive problems, such as intellectual disabilities or schizophrenia, should consider the patient's need to establish intimate relationships and pursue vocational goals. Teaching about family planning and sexually responsible behaviors should be incorporated into care.

Research is mixed related to the impact of pregnancy and childbirth on maternal cognition, with some studies indicating reduced function in the areas of processing speed, verbal recall, and attention (Davies, Lum, Skouteris, Byrne, & Hayden, 2018; Prado et al., 2018). Hormonal shifts probably account for these changes and are largely adaptive, enabling the mother to be more in tune with the needs of the newborn. Fatigue and sleep deprivation may also contribute to cognitive alterations and may have a role in triggering other mental health issues.

Cognition in Older Adults

As the brain ages, typical changes account for subtle differences in cognitive processing. These may be caused by modest shrinkage of brain tissue and decreased blood flow to the areas of the brain responsible for memory, executive function, and cognitive flexibility. Older adults typically have more difficulty with cognitive functions, such as word retrieval and episodic memory; however, the impact on overall cognitive function should be minimal. The ability to perform visuospatial tasks like drawing may diminish slightly. Nurses should recognize that moderate to severe cognitive decline is not a normal function of aging and that changes may signify an underlying medical or mental health issue (Harrison, Maass, Baker, & Jagust, 2018; Malinowski, Moore, Mead, & Gruber, 2017).

Psychologic problems such as anxiety and depression in older adults may also result in clinical manifestations that may be mistaken for dementia. Screening tools for depression and other mental health issues are used as part of a comprehensive assessment of cognition in older adults.

Case Study » Part 3

After his wandering episode, Mr. Wallace's condition rapidly declines. His communication skills are almost completely gone; he speaks infrequently and uses only two- or three-word sentences. He no longer recognizes Ms. Wallace, cannot perform ADLs, and is indifferent to food. Mr. Wallace's tendency toward wandering and aggression has disappeared. In fact, he rarely leaves his room. For his safety and to allow for provision of the care he needs, Mr. Wallace is admitted to an extended care facility that specializes in treating patients with Alzheimer disease.

You are the nurse assigned to care for Mr. Wallace. As part of his daily assessment, you obtain his vital signs, which include temperature 99.8°F oral, pulse 92 bpm, respirations 32/min, and blood pressure 108/74 mmHg. Auscultation of Mr. Wallace's lungs reveals faint bibasilar crackles. On reviewing his chart, you note that he has experienced a 5% weight loss since the previous month. You notify the attending physician about Mr. Wallace's vital signs, breath sounds, and weight loss. The physician orders a chest x-ray and CBC.

Clinical Reasoning Questions Level I

1. What is the significance of Mr. Wallace's vital signs and breath sounds?
2. What effect might the patient's weight loss have on his cognitive condition?
3. What important cues might be gleaned from tracking Mr. Wallace's food intake and weight?

Clinical Reasoning Questions Level II

4. What is the priority care concern for Mr. Wallace at this time?
5. What independent interventions can you perform to optimize this patient's respiratory status? What positive effects might these have on other aspects of his health?
6. *Refer to the exemplar on Alzheimer disease in this module:* Would Mr. Wallace's condition improve with the addition of a cholinesterase inhibitor to his treatment regimen? Why or why not?

REVIEW The Concept of Cognition

RELATE Link the Concepts

Linking the concept of cognition with the concept of perfusion:

1. Describe how alterations in perfusion can affect a patient's risk for specific types of dementia.
2. What measures might you implement when caring for a patient with impaired perfusion to limit the risk of dementia?

Linking the concept of cognition with the concept of development:

3. What considerations should a nurse apply when designing developmentally appropriate activities for an 8-year-old with Down syndrome?
4. What treatment measures used for patients with ADHD might also be useful for patients with fragile X syndrome? Why?

Linking the concept of cognition with the concept of family:

5. How might a family's normal processes and interactions be affected when one member is diagnosed with a cognitive disorder?
6. What actions can nurses take to support family members of patients with cognitive alterations?

READY Go to Volume 3: Companion Skills Manual

REFER Go to Pearson MyLab Nursing and eText

REFLECT Apply Your Knowledge

Hannah Lister is a 6-year-old first-grade student who frequently presents to the school nurse's office with somatic complaints. Her teacher is increasingly concerned that she is missing valuable class time. The nurse learns that Hannah has a history of learning and behavior problems and was recently diagnosed with nonverbal learning disability. The nurse and classroom teacher meet to discuss the issue with Hannah's parents. Her mother is tearful as she talks about how anxious Hannah is. She states Hannah complains about having to go to school and that other students and teachers are "mean" to her. Hannah's mother says that her oldest child never had any of these problems, and she is at a loss as to how to help Hannah. Her teacher believes that since Hannah is so articulate and has good reading skills, she is capable of doing much better in school. The teacher explains that she has worked with many children with learning disabilities who are not as bright as Hannah. She believes that Hannah should be held accountable for some of her rude and socially inappropriate behaviors and should receive consequences for missing class.

1. What might explain the teacher's misperceptions of Hannah's skills/capabilities?
2. What may make Hannah's learning problems different from those of students with language-based learning disabilities?
3. As the nurse, what kind of teaching could you provide to help teachers and parents understand some of the emotional and behavioral needs of children like Hannah?
4. When providing health teaching to this patient, what kind of approach is most likely to be effective?
5. What types of independent and collaborative interventions may be appropriate to address Hannah's social and emotional needs?

» Exemplar 23.A Alzheimer Disease

Exemplar Learning Objectives

23.A Analyze Alzheimer disease as it relates to cognition.

- Describe the pathophysiology of Alzheimer disease.
- Describe the etiology of Alzheimer disease.
- Compare the risk factors and prevention of Alzheimer disease.
- Identify the clinical manifestations of Alzheimer disease.
- Summarize diagnostic tests and therapies used by interprofessional teams in the collaborative care of an individual with Alzheimer disease.
- Differentiate care of patients with Alzheimer disease across the lifespan.
- Apply the nursing process in providing culturally competent care to an individual with Alzheimer disease.

Exemplar Key Terms

Alzheimer disease (AD), *1772*
Amyloid plaques, *1772*
Caregiver burden, *1772*
Neurofibrillary tangles, *1772*
Relocation syndrome (transfer trauma), *1780*
Sundowning, *1774*

Overview

Alzheimer disease (AD) accounts for approximately 60–80% of all dementia cases in individuals age 65 and older. More than 5 million Americans suffer from AD, and this number is predicted to reach 7 million by 2025 and 14 million by 2050. AD is currently the sixth leading cause of death in the United States (Alzheimer's Association, 2020e).

Although AD usually manifests after age 65, some individuals experience symptoms as early as their 30s. Most individuals with AD survive between 4 and 8 years after diagnosis; those who are diagnosed at younger ages may live up to two decades. Patients typically spend more time in the moderate stage of AD than in any other stage. Eventually, they die from complications of the disease.

One important aspect of AD disease is **caregiver burden**. Caregiver burden refers to the psychologic, physical, and financial cost of caring for an individual with AD (Alzheimer's Association, 2020a; Elif, Taşkapilioğlu, & Bakar, 2017). Alzheimer disease is associated with higher levels of stress and caregiver burden than most other chronic illnesses. Nurses must consider both patient and caregiver needs when working with individuals with AD.

Pathophysiology

There are several types of AD. *Younger* or *early-onset AD* before age 65 can be a familial, or inherited disease, or it can be sporadic, for which there is no known etiology. *Familial AD* (in which AD occurs in multiple generations of a family) has occurred in only a few hundred families worldwide. Scientists have pinpointed several rare genes that are specifically linked to early onset of familial AD (Alzheimer's Association, 2020k). Individuals who inherit these rare genes tend to develop symptoms in their 30s to 50s (Alzheimer's Association, 2020k). The majority of people with younger-onset AD have *sporadic Alzheimer's disease*, which is the most common form and is not attributed to genetics.

Late-onset AD occurs at age 65 or later and accounts for more than 90% of AD cases. Late-onset AD is usually sporadic, affecting people without a family history of the disease (Dutchen, 2018). It shows no clear pattern of inheritance, although genetic factors may increase risk (Condello et al., 2018).

Individuals with AD show a pattern of degenerative changes related to neuronal death throughout the brain. At first, AD typically destroys neurons and their connections in parts of the brain involved in memory, including the entorhinal cortex and hippocampus. It later affects areas in the cerebral cortex responsible for language, reasoning, and social behavior (National Institute on Aging, 2017). Eventually, many other areas of the brain are damaged. Over time, a person with AD gradually loses the ability to live and function independently. Ultimately, the disease is fatal (National Institute on Aging, 2017).

The accompanying figures show the characteristic order of cell death, beginning with neurons in the limbic system, including the hippocampus. Damage to this region results in emotional problems and loss of recent memory. From there, the destruction spreads up and out toward the cerebral surface (see **Figure 23.6** »). Eventually, neuronal death in the cerebral lobes produces a range of symptoms, including loss of remote memory, as outlined in **Table 23.7** ».

As AD progresses and more neurons die, two characteristic abnormalities develop in the brains of affected individuals. The first is thick protein clots called **neurofibrillary tangles**, and the second is insoluble deposits known as **amyloid plaques**. Researchers continue to investigate whether these abnormalities are a cause or a result of AD, as described in the section on etiology.

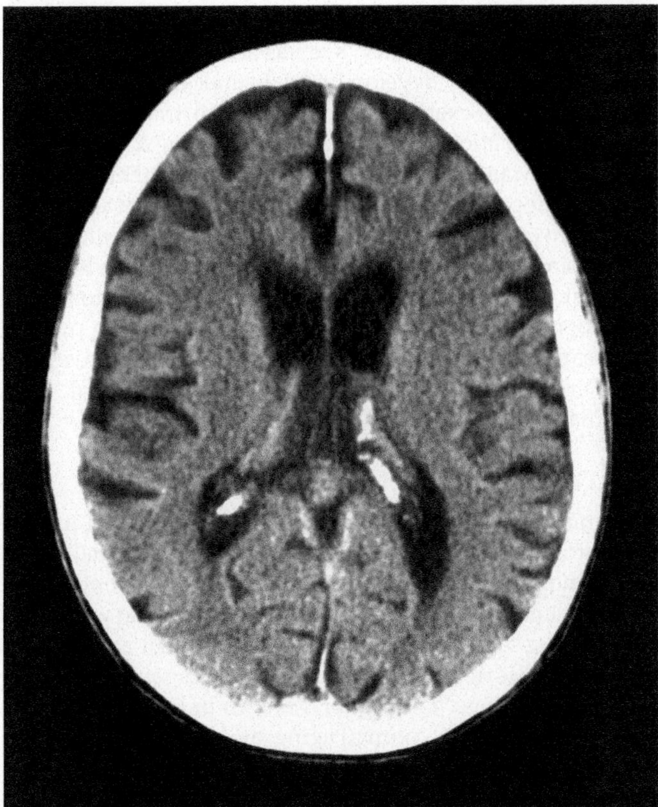

Figure 23.6 » CT scan of 84-year-old man with Alzheimer disease. Note atrophy of the brain.

Source: Scott Camazine/Alamy Stock Photo.

TABLE 23.7 Cerebral Effects of AD

Region	Symptoms of Damage
Limbic system (including hippocampus)	Loss of memory (recent before remote); fluctuating emotions; depression; difficulty learning new information
Frontal lobe	Problems with intentional movement; difficulty planning; emotional lability; loss of walking, talking, and swallowing ability
Occipital lobe	Loss of reading comprehension; hallucinations
Parietal lobe	Difficulty recognizing places, people, and objects; hallucinations; seizures; unsteady movement; expressive aphasia; agraphia; agnosia
Temporal lobe	Impaired memory; difficulty learning new things; receptive aphasia

Etiology

Researchers are not sure why most cases of AD arise, although a variety of genetic, environmental, and lifestyle factors appear to be involved. Moreover, the exact biochemical origins of AD remain unknown, even in patients who clearly have an inherited form of the disease. Researchers have therefore proposed several theories that seek to explain the disease process, including the cholinergic, amyloid, and tau hypotheses.

Cholinergic Hypothesis

The cholinergic hypothesis emerged in the early 1980s after nearly 20 years of investigation into the role of neurotransmitters. Researchers noted that low levels of acetylcholine (a cholinergic neurotransmitter) appeared to produce memory deficits. Autopsies also revealed that brains of individuals with AD had markers characteristic of decreased acetylcholine function. These findings suggested that AD was caused by below-normal production of acetylcholine in the brain, and this led to the development of acetylcholinesterase inhibitor drugs that could inhibit the action of acetylcholinesterase, the enzyme that breaks down acetylcholine. Recent consensus on this theory indicates that cholinergic therapy may slow brain atrophy, but the cholinergic system is only one of several interacting systems failures that contribute to AD pathogenesis (Hampel et al., 2019).

Amyloid and Tau Hypotheses

The amyloid and tau hypotheses have been the mainstream concepts underlying AD research for over 20 years. The original amyloid hypothesis stated that AD arises when the brain cannot properly process a substance called *amyloid precursor-protein (APP)*. Incorrect processing leads to the presence of short, sticky fragments of APP known as *beta-amyloid*. Eventually, the fragments clump together, forming amyloid plaques. These plaques damage the surrounding neurons, eventually killing them and provoking an inflammatory response that may result in further brain damage. However, research of familial AD now indicates that the trigger of AD is closely linked to impairments of APP metabolism and accumulation of APP C-terminal fragments, rather than production and formation of amyloid plaque (Kametani & Hasegawa, 2018). Furthermore, all attempts to develop plaque-targeting drugs to treat AD have ended in failure (Kametani & Hasegawa, 2018).

The tau hypothesis similarly focused on a protein known as tau. Normally, tau holds together the microtubules responsible for intracellular transport within the axons of neurons. With AD, however, individuals have abnormal tau proteins that join and twist, forming neurofibrillary tangles instead of the microtubule network necessary for cellular survival. Recent findings have indicated that the main factor underlying the development and progression of AD is the tau protein, *not* the amyloid protein. Therefore, AD seems to be a disorder that is triggered by impairment of APP metabolism and progresses through tau pathology, not beta-amyloid (Kametani & Hasegawa, 2018).

Recent Research

There have been many other efforts in researching Alzheimer disease in recent years, in particular research around protein misfolding and aggregation, which are known underlying mechanisms of a number of neurodegenerative diseases. For example, Kong et al. (2019) discovered that cellular prion protein plays a role in AD pathogenesis, while University of California San Francisco researchers found proteins central to the pathology of AD disease that act as prions, misshapen proteins that spread through tissue like an infection by forcing normal proteins to adopt the same misfolded shape (Weiler, 2019).

Risk Factors

Nonmodifiable risk factors for AD include age, sex, family history, and genetic factors (Alzheimer's Association, 2020b). Alzheimer disease disproportionately affects Hispanic and African American individuals, although it is not clear whether this relates to underlying biophysical characteristics or socioeconomic or cultural factors that increase modifiable risk factors (CDC, 2019b). AD is almost two times more common in women than in men, primarily because women live longer (CDC, 2019b).

Although developing AD is not a normal or expected consequence of aging, the most prominent risk factor for Alzheimer disease is advancing age. Once an individual reaches the age of 65, the risk of developing the disease doubles every 5 years. After the age of 85, individuals have a 50% chance of developing the disease.

Research has identified cardiovascular risk factors that include diabetes, midlife obesity, midlife hypertension, and hyperlipidemia. Evidence suggests that diabetes increases AD risk through both vascular and metabolic pathways (Mayo Clinic, 2020a). Midlife obesity is correlated with vascular, metabolic, and inflammatory changes that appear to increase the risk of AD (CDC, 2020). Lifestyle risk factors—including cigarette smoking and sedentary lifestyle—also appear to increase risk (Choi, Krishnan, & Ruckmani, 2017; Mosconi et al., 2018).

Several strong and reliable studies have linked the incidence of traumatic brain injury to AD, with individuals exposed to repeated trauma being at the greatest risk (Ramos-Cejudo et al., 2018; Tolppanen, Taipale, & Hartikainen, 2017; Weiner et al., 2017). See Module 11, Intracranial Regulation, for information about traumatic brain injury.

Depression is considered to be both a symptom of and risk factor for Alzheimer disease, with overlapping neurobiological mechanisms responsible for both diseases (Jacus, 2017). There is some research to suggest that the early management of depression with antidepressants may prevent cognitive decline associated with dementia. However, a recent systematic review found that there had been little high-quality research on efficacy of antidepressants, limiting conclusions about their potential role (Orgeta, Tabet, Nilforooshan, & Howard, 2017). Elsworthy and Aldred (2019) suggest that SSRIs may be useful in the early stages of AD because SSRIs appear to slow the conversion from mild cognitive impairment to later stages of AD.

SAFETY ALERT! Research implicates four benzodiazepines—estazolam, quazepam (Doral), temazepam (Restoril), and triazolam (Halcion)—in the development of cognitive deterioration. Certain antihistamines that are also anticholinergics—chlorpheniramine (Chlor-Trimeton), diphenhydramine (Benadryl), doxylamine (Unisom), dimenhydrinate (Dramamine), and meclizine (Bonine)—may actually accelerate cognitive deterioration (Hafdi et al., 2020; Jenraumjit et al., 2020; Moriarty et al., 2020).

Prevention

Evidence-based teaching for the general public with regard to increasing protective factors for AD includes reducing the incidence of cardiovascular disorders and other health problems by adopting a healthy lifestyle. For example, quitting smoking and using safety measures (such as seat belts while driving) can reduce risk for developing Alzheimer disease, and even modest levels of exercise have been demonstrated to improve cognitive function (Cass, 2017; Choi, Choi, & Park, 2018; Kivipelto, Mangialasche, & Ngandu, 2018). Other strategies include adopting a heart-healthy diet, staying socially active and connected with others, seeking appropriate treatment for depression and alterations in sleep, and engaging in activities that exercise cognitive function. Evidence demonstrates that cognitive activities such as reading, completing puzzles, and learning new information or tasks build cognitive resilience and protect against cognitive decline (Hersi et al., 2017; Sardina, Fitzsimmons, Hoyt, & Buettner, 2019).

Clinical Manifestations

The initial symptoms of AD emerge gradually and may be almost unnoticeable. The first manifestation is usually subtle memory loss that becomes increasingly apparent as time passes. Other early signs include difficulty finding words and performing familiar tasks; impaired judgment and abstract thinking; disorientation to time and place; and frequently misplacing things. These alterations go beyond the changes sometimes seen with normal aging, as described in the introduction to this module. Diurnal changes in cognitive function are typical, with patterns of diminished capacity in the evening (also known as **sundowning**). Changes in mood or personality are also common. Early in the course of AD, many individuals exhibit decreased initiative, odd behavior, and signs of depression. As the disease progresses, the continued deterioration in patients' cognition is accompanied by physical decline. At some point, affected individuals lose the ability to perform everyday tasks and must rely entirely on their caregivers.

Alzheimer disease is often described in terms of three general stages: stage 1 (early), stage 2 (moderate), and stage 3 (severe). The Clinical Manifestations and Therapies feature outlines the clinical manifestations associated with each stage along with interventions. Individuals' rate of progression is affected by a variety of factors, including their overall health and the type of care they receive following diagnosis.

Collaboration

The care of patients with AD depends on collaboration among nurses and nurse practitioners; physicians; physical, occupational, and speech therapists; psychologists; family members; volunteers; personal care assistants; social workers; and case managers. In the early to moderate stages of the disease, care is generally community based and involves outpatient visits to primary care providers and a variety of services, including counseling, support groups, in-home care, daycare programs, and assisted living. When individuals are no longer able to be managed in the community setting, they may need to transition to a skilled nursing facility. In this section, diagnostic tests and therapies employed by members of the interprofessional team across settings are summarized.

Diagnostic Tests

There is no definitive way to diagnose AD other than performing a brain autopsy. Instead, practitioners rely on differential

Clinical Manifestations and Therapies

Alzheimer Disease

STAGES	CLINICAL MANIFESTATIONS	CLINICAL THERAPIES
Stage I Mild cognitive impairment	▪ Reduced concentration and memory lapses noticeable by others ▪ Difficulty learning new information ▪ Problems functioning in work or social settings ▪ Frequently losing or misplacing important objects ▪ Difficulties with planning and organization ▪ Forgetting familiar words or the locations of various objects	▪ Patient/caregiver education and training ▪ Environmental modifications to promote safety ▪ Encourage planning for advanced stages of the disease while patients are still able to participate in decision making ▪ Use of cuing devices such as to-do lists, calendars, written schedules, and verbal reminders ▪ Cognitive activity kits ▪ Deliberate establishment of and adherence to daily routines ▪ Referral to community resources, support groups, and/or counseling services ▪ Nonpharmacologic therapies such as validation therapy, reality orientation, and reminiscence therapy ▪ Counseling regarding possible retirement or withdrawal from the more challenging aspects of one's job
Stage II Moderate AD	▪ Inability to carry out ADLs, such as preparing meals for oneself and choosing appropriate clothing ▪ Loss of ability to live independently ▪ Difficulty recalling one's address or phone number ▪ Increased problems finding words and communicating clearly ▪ Inability to recall information from recent memory ▪ Increasing difficulty remembering details from remote memory ▪ Disorientation to time and place ▪ Increased tendency to become lost ▪ Changes in ability to control bladder/ bowels ▪ Changes in sleep patterns ▪ Withdrawal from social situations and challenging mental activity ▪ Increased moodiness, flat affect, or signs of depression and/or anxiety, paranoia	▪ Behavioral interventions such as distraction, provision of meaningful activities ▪ Continued use of cuing devices and established routines ▪ Assistance with ADLs ▪ Administration of anti-AD acetylcholinesterase inhibitors, including rivastigmine (Exelon), galantamine (Razadyne), and donepezil (Aricept); an NMDA inhibitor may be added, including memantine (Namenda) ▪ Administration of SSRIs and/or anxiolytics to address mood-related symptoms of depression and anxiety ▪ Occupational, physical, and speech therapy ▪ Nonpharmacologic therapies such as validation therapy and reminiscence therapy ▪ Consultation with a dietitian or nutritionist ▪ Respite care for family members and other caregivers ▪ May require around-the-clock care or transition to a skilled nursing facility
Stage III Severe AD	▪ Gradual inability to perform any ADLs, including bathing and toileting ▪ Eventual urinary and fecal incontinence ▪ Inability to identify family members and caregivers ▪ Extreme confusion and lack of awareness of one's surroundings ▪ Gradual loss of remote memory and ability to speak ▪ Inability to perform simple mental calculations ▪ Dramatic personality changes, including extreme suspiciousness and fearfulness ▪ Sundowning, delusions, compulsions, agitation, and violent outbursts ▪ Gradual loss of ability to walk, sit unaided, and hold one's head up ▪ Development of abnormal reflexes ▪ Physical rigidity ▪ Loss of swallowing ability	▪ Assistance with all ADLs ▪ Continuation of earlier behavioral and pharmacologic therapies ▪ Round-the-clock care and/or admittance to a skilled nursing facility ▪ Frequent repositioning ▪ Hand feeding and/or liquid nutrition as appropriate ▪ Respite care for family members and other caregivers ▪ End-of-life care

Source: Alzheimer's Association (2020i); Frisoni et al. (2017); L. Y. Wang et al. (2020); Weller and Budson (2018).

diagnosis, ruling out potential causes of a patient's symptoms until AD remains the most likely explanation. When individuals present with signs and symptoms of AD, the nurse can anticipate standard laboratory tests being ordered, including thyroid-stimulating hormone, complete blood count (CBC), serum B_{12}, folate, complete metabolic panel, and testing for sexually transmitted infections. Screening tools and tests that aid in the diagnosis of AD are discussed in detail in the sections on assessment and diagnosis of cognitive disorders. Genetic testing may be conducted under certain clinical guidelines. Researchers have found several genes that increase the risk of AD. *APOE-e4* is the first risk gene identified and remains the gene with strongest impact on risk. Researchers estimate that between 40 and 65% of people diagnosed with AD have the *APOE-e4* gene (Alzheimer's Association, 2020g).

Emerging approaches to diagnosis of AD include the analysis of biomarkers, such as analysis of CSF, brain imaging/neuroimaging, and blood and urine tests. Biomarkers are physiologic, chemical, or anatomic measures that can accurately and reliably indicate the presence of disease. As yet, there are no validated biomarkers for Alzheimer disease (Alzheimer's Association, 2020d).

Researchers are also looking for consistent, measurable changes in urine or blood levels of tau, beta-amyloid, or other biomarkers before AD symptoms appear (Alzheimer's Association, 2020d; Nakamura et al., 2018). Findings from biomarker studies may lead to identifying individuals at risk for developing AD and facilitate early intervention and planning. Other research is investigating whether early AD causes detectable changes in other tissues and structures of the body, such as the lens of the eye.

Imaging research is also taking place. For example, structural imaging provides information about the shape, position, or volume of brain tissue. Structural techniques include magnetic resonance imaging (MRI) and computed tomography (CT) (Alzheimer's Association, 2020d).

Pharmacologic Therapy

There is currently no cure for AD. Two classes of medications are used to slow the progression of the disease. In addition, adjunctive agents may be prescribed to treat associated symptoms of depression, anxiety, or psychosis.

Acetylcholinesterase Inhibitors

Acetylcholinesterase (AChE) inhibitors have been standard treatment for over a decade. They work by inhibiting acetylcholinesterase, an enzyme that normally breaks down acetylcholine. Because individuals with Alzheimer disease are gradually losing neurons that communicate by using acetylcholine, the presence of extra acetylcholine increases communication among the remaining neurons. This appears to temporarily stabilize symptoms related to language, memory, and reasoning for an average of 6 to 12 months.

Commonly prescribed acetylcholinesterase inhibitors include donepezil (Aricept), rivastigmine (Exelon), and galantamine (Razadyne). Galantamine is approved for early to moderate stages of AD, while donepezil and rivastigmine are approved for all stages. Although these drugs all act similarly, not all individuals respond to them in the same way. In fact, about half of individuals who take these drugs experience no delay in symptom progression. AChE inhibitors generally produce mild side effects such as decreased appetite, nausea, diarrhea, headaches, and dizziness. Adverse effects include gastrointestinal (GI) bleeding and bradycardia. Patient and caregiver teaching should include avoiding other medications that may increase the risk of GI bleeding and monitoring pulse rate. The patient's nutritional status and fluid balance should also be monitored. The drug dosage is slowly increased to minimize side effects. Patients and family members should be cautioned not to abruptly stop the medication, as this may cause a sudden worsening of symptoms (Adams, Holland, & & Urban, 2020).

NMDA Receptor Antagonists

NMDA receptor antagonists are believed to block the effects of glutamate, an excitatory neurotransmitter that is present with neuronal damage and appears to be involved in cognitive decline. NMDA receptor antagonists do not reverse existing damage, but they do slow the rate at which new damage occurs. Unlike acetylcholinesterase inhibitors, NMDA receptor antagonists are generally not prescribed until an individual is in the moderate-to-severe stages of AD.

Currently, memantine (Namenda) is the only NMDA receptor antagonist approved by the U.S. Food and Drug Administration (FDA). Namzaric, the trade name, a combination of memantine and donepezil, is approved for use in individuals with moderate to severe AD. Side effects of NMDA inhibitors are less common and usually milder than those associated with donepezil, rivastigmine, and galantamine. They include dizziness, constipation, confusion, headache, fatigue, and increased blood pressure. Patients and family members should be cautioned about performing activities requiring mental alertness or coordination until tolerance is established. The medication should be taken with food if stomach upset occurs (Adams et al., 2020; Alzheimer's Association, 2020h). See **Medications 23.1**, Drugs Used to Treat Alzheimer Disease, for additional information on medications used in the treatment of AD and other dementias.

Other Medications Used to Treat AD Symptoms

Drug classes used to manage the symptoms of AD include antipsychotics (to treat delusions or hallucinations), anxiolytics (to treat anxiety), and SSRI antidepressants (to treat depression). Because there is some evidence that these agents may actually increase the risk of cognitive decline, patients and their families should be encouraged to discuss the risks versus benefits with their providers. For more details on these drugs, please refer to Module 31, Stress and Coping, and Module 28, Mood and Affect.

Nonpharmacologic Therapy

Nonpharmacologic interventions that have been demonstrated to be effective in treating AD include exercise, reality orientation therapy, validation therapy, and reminiscence therapy.

Reality Orientation Therapy

Reality orientation is a structured approach to orienting individuals to person, time, place, and situations at regular intervals and as needed through verbal communication and the use of visual cues (pictures, clocks, calendars, orientation boards).

Medications 23.1
Drugs Used to Treat Alzheimer Disease

CLASSIFICATION AND DRUG EXAMPLES	MECHANISMS OF ACTION	NURSING IMPLICATIONS
Acetylcholinesterase Inhibitors ***Drug examples:*** donepezil (Aricept) galantamine (Razadyne) rivastigmine (Exelon) ***N*-Methyl-D-aspartate (NMDA) Receptor Antagonists** ***Drug examples:*** memantine (Namenda) Namzaric (combination NMDA receptor antagonist memantine and acetylcholinesterase inhibitor donepezil)	Acetylcholinesterase inhibitors reduce acetylcholine breakdown, whereas NMDA receptor antagonists limit the effects of glutamate. Both drug classes have a modest effect in slowing an individual's rate of cognitive decline in AD. ***May also be used for:*** ■ Vascular dementia ■ Parkinson-related dementia Combination drug donepezil and memantine (Namzaric) used only after patients have been stabilized on memantine and donepezil	■ Explain the importance of taking medication as directed; teach about discontinuation and resulting decline in function. ■ Provide patient and caregiver education regarding side effects of dizziness, headache, GI upset, and fatigue. ■ Promote adequate fluid intake. ■ Monitor patient's pulse rate. ■ Use with caution in patients with respiratory conditions (e.g., asthma, COPD). ■ Avoid the use of antipsychotics, beta adrenergic blockers, corticosteroids, and anticholinergic drugs because of their antagonistic or synergistic effects.

Source: Based on Adams et al. (2020).

Reality orientation therapy is a collaborative intervention that is carried out by all members of the healthcare team and should be part of routine care (Chiu, Chen, Chen, & Huang, 2018). However, reorientation to certain situations or information may be upsetting in some cases and should be used judiciously.

Validation Therapy

Validation therapy involves searching for emotion or intended meaning in verbal expressions and behaviors. The basic premise is that seemingly purposeless behaviors and incoherent speech have significance to the patient and can be related to current needs (Berg-Weger & Stewart, 2017). For example, if an individual is wandering and crying out for her mother, instead of reminding the patient that her mother is not available, the nurse may say something like, "You are looking for Mother. Is there something you need from her?" The goal is to elicit a response that identifies an unmet need, such as, "Yes, I need her to give me my dinner." The nurse can then address the wandering and associated anxiety by offering the patient something to eat or reassuring her that dinner will be available soon. Unlike reality orientation, validation therapy does not unnecessarily challenge the patient's perception of reality.

Reminiscence Therapy

Reminiscence therapy uses the process of purposely reflecting on past events. The nurse or other HCP may encourage the patient to talk about events that occurred in the past, often facilitated by using scrapbooks, photo albums, music, or other items (Lök, Bademli, & Selçuk-Tosun, 2019). In addition to helping patients to retain long-term memory, reminiscence therapy may be comforting; provides a source of self-esteem, identity, and purpose; and can help to prevent isolation and withdrawal (Potter & Moller, 2020; Woods, O'Philbin, Farrell, Spector, & Orrell, 2018).

Complementary Health Approaches

Currently, there is no strong evidence that any complementary health approach or diet can prevent cognitive impairment (National Center for Complementary and Integrative Health [NCCIH], 2020). Studies on the use of dietary supplements such as ginkgo biloba, fish oil/omega-3 fatty acids, B vitamins, curcumin, and melatonin have not proven of use in preventing or delaying cognitive decline. Patients taking supplements should be educated about risks, such as interaction with other drugs and toxicity.

There is some research indicating that complementary and alternative measures such as music and art therapy can relieve some of the distressing symptoms associated with cognitive decline, such as pain and agitation (Anderson, Deng, Anthony, Atalla, & Monroe, 2017) and hypertension (Chen et al., 2017). For caregivers, one study showed that taking a mindfulness meditation class or a caregiver education class reduced stress more than just getting time off from providing care (NCCIH, 2020).

NURSING PROCESS

The primary goal of nursing care is to provide a safe, supportive environment that meets patients' changing abilities and needs. The nurse must also take steps to support patients' family members as they cope with the emotional and physical demands of caring for a loved one with AD. Various tools and techniques for providing nursing care for patients and families with AD can be accessed from reliable sources such as The Hartford Institute for Geriatric Nursing, the Alzheimer's Association, and the Agency for Healthcare Research and Quality. Highlights of standards of current practice are provided in this section.

Assessment

Current clinical guidelines for the nursing assessment of individuals with AD include completion of a health history and assessment of physical status, cognitive function, functional status, behavioral presentation, and caregiver/environment (NYU Hartford Institute of Geriatric Nursing, 2020a). Serial assessments allow the nurse to monitor changes indicative of disease progression and the ability of the patient to manage safely in the current living environment.

Observation and Patient Interview

Start the assessment by observing the patient and caregivers. Patients with mild dementia may not present any signs or symptoms notable on appearance. At this stage, family members' reports of noticeable changes in memory or cognitive abilities in certain areas may be the first clue that there is a problem. As dementia progresses, patients exhibit signs of difficulty maintaining self-care, such as dressing inappropriately for the weather or an unkempt appearance; difficulty focusing on simple tasks or paying attention during the patient interview; and changes in gait. The patient interview should address family history of AD and other dementias; medical history; current medications and use of any supplements; changes in cognition, communication, memory, and behavior; alterations in mood, sleep patterns, and ability to perform ADLs; drug and alcohol use; and risk for or history of exposure to environmental toxins.

Mental Status Examination

For patients with AD, a thorough mental status examination is critical. Nurses can choose from a variety of assessment instruments, as described in the Assessment section. The MMSE is the test most commonly used to assess cognitive status.

Physical Examination

During the physical assessment, evaluate the patient's height, weight, vital signs, and overall physical condition. Throughout the exam, remain alert for possible signs of abuse, neglect, depression, malnutrition, elimination difficulties, and alterations in skin integrity, as AD increases the risk for all of these.

A number of other conditions can mimic the symptoms of dementia and AD. A useful mnemonic for remembering to assess for these conditions is DEMENTIA:

Drugs and alcohol
Eyes and ears
Metabolic and endocrine disorders
Emotional disorders
Neurologic disorders
Trauma or tumors
Infection
Arteriovascular disease.

Functional Status

An assessment of functional status addresses any changes in ability to manage day-to-day ADLs, such as eating or dressing, and instrumental activities of daily living (IADLs). This can be addressed through direct questioning of patients or family members (e.g., "Over the past 7 days, have you noticed any changes in your family member's ability to complete getting dressed?"). Screening tools such as the Functional Activities Questionnaire (FAQ) may also be used (NYU Hartford Institute of Geriatric Nursing, 2020b).

Functional decline is the result of progressive deficits in cognitive, emotional, and physical function that lead to loss of independence (Callahan et al., 2017). Individuals with AD typically lose function over time managing the following activities: telephone use, meal preparation, handling medications, managing finances, housekeeping, shopping, traveling within the community, bathing, dressing, eating, toileting, walking across a small room, and transferring from bed to chair (Wang et al., 2018). Functional performance declines with aging regardless of AD status, but individuals with AD experience a more rapid decline (Wang et al., 2018).

Behavior Assessment

The behavioral assessment consists of direct observation of the patient and direct questioning of the patient and caregivers as well as the use of valid assessment tools. Assess for behavior changes associated with AD, including behaviors indicative of depression, anxiety, irritability, impulsivity, poor judgment, paranoia, delusions, and hallucinations. Inquire about events that precipitate any behavior changes (such as a poor night's sleep) so that potential triggers can be identified and eliminated. The Geriatric Depression Scale (GDS) may be used to detect changes in mood. The BEHAVE-AD is a 25-item assessment tool that nurses can use to elicit caregiver reports about a variety of behaviors. These are then scored to determine the magnitude of the disturbance in terms of patient and caregiver safety (Reisberg et al., 2014).

Caregiver/Living Environment

The final area of assessment addresses the needs of the caregiver and the adequacy of the living environment. Ask the caregiver(s) to share perspectives on the patient's ability to function in light of current support. It is also important to determine the impact that patient behaviors have on the caregiver and to gather data about the quality of the caregiving relationship. Two practical tools for assessing caregiver burden include the Zarit Burden Interview (ZBI) and the Caregiver Role Strain Index (CRI). Also assess current knowledge of effective caregiving interventions and the capacity to employ these interventions in the current living environment. Remember to assess for cultural values, beliefs, and practices and even barriers that may affect provision of care or the patient–family relationship (see Focus on Diversity and Culture: Addressing Cultural Factors That Increase Stigma and Caregiver Burden).

Diagnosis

Care priorities for patients with AD vary by stage of the disease and patient and family preferences and needs. Although physiologic and safety needs remain the priority, common problems faced by patients with AD include:

- Cognitive impairment
- Risk of injury
- Inadequate health maintenance
- Inability to perform self-care
- Undernutrition

Focus on Diversity and Culture

Addressing Cultural Factors That Increase Stigma and Caregiver Burden

The stigma associated with having a family member with Alzheimer disease is influenced by a variety of cultural factors, and it has been demonstrated to increase caregiver burden by reinforcing negative emotional responses and limiting external sources of support, especially demonstrated by employment and health insurance discrimination (Stites, Rubright, & Karlawish, 2018). Lack of awareness about dementia and AD is common to many cultures, and there are varying beliefs regarding the cause of the disease and appropriate management of care. Family values may reinforce the caregiver's sense that they have primary responsibility for caring for parents or other family members. Nurses play a key role in assessing family/caregiver beliefs about AD. Family members may be asked open-ended questions such as "What do you or your family members believe caused this disease?" and "Who do you or your family members believe is responsible for caring for your parent/family member?" Once cultural barriers to care are identified, nurses can initiate teaching to address misperceptions and collaborate with other healthcare professionals to address barriers to care, such as lack of social support (Spector, 2017).

- Impaired memory
- Impaired communication
- Fear
- Caregiver burden
- Compromised swallowing
- Compromised physical mobility
- Wandering
- Compromised functional status
- Powerlessness
- Grieving.

Planning

The planning portion of the nursing process involves identifying desired patient outcomes and formulating steps for achieving them. Appropriate goals and actions will vary depending on a patient's physical and mental status and current living situation, and they may include the following:

- Patient will remain free from injury.
- Patient will utilize lists, calendars, and other memory aids as needed.
- Patient will perform IADLs with caregiver assistance.
- Patient will exhibit reduced anxiety, agitation, and restlessness.
- Patient will take all medications as prescribed.

The nurse should also consider caregiver and family needs during the planning process. Some suggested outcomes are as follows:

- Caregiver will utilize respite care resources as necessary.
- Caregiver will learn effective strategies for coping with the stresses of supporting a loved one with AD.
- Caregiver will obtain the sleep and nutrition necessary to preserve personal health.
- Caregiver will engage palliative care and hospice services for end-of-life care of the patient.

Communicating with Patients

Working Phase

Older adults with Alzheimer disease lose language skills over time. In the early stages, the person is still able to participate in conversation and engage in social activities. However, he may repeat himself, have difficulty word finding, and be overwhelmed by excessive stimulation. Knowing this, the nurse should modify the assessment to accommodate the patient at this stage.

- Mr. Jones, tell me about your back pain.

Give the patient adequate time to respond. If a prompt is needed, you can say something like:

- That's okay. We have time to talk.

If the patient is unable to respond or exhibits distress at trying to respond after being given an appropriate amount of time, ask the patient's permission to ask questions of the caregiver:

- Mr. Jones, I see that it is hard for you to answer these questions about your medications. Is it okay for me to talk with your wife about this?

Implementation

Implementation of nursing interventions depends on patient and family needs and integrates an understanding of principles of health promotion in relation to the stages of the illness. The Progressively Lowered Stress Threshold (PLST) intervention model is supported by current clinical guidelines and is an approach that should guide nursing care during all stages of the illness (Robinson, Crawford, Buckwalter, & Casey, 2018). This model proposes that individuals with dementia and Alzheimer disease require a combination of environmental modifications in order to cope with progressive cognitive decline. An escalation in anxiety, depression, or behaviors such as wandering is likely to indicate inappropriate or inadequate environmental modifications.

Promote Safety and Physiologic Integrity

The safety and physiologic integrity of patients and family members, especially those providing care, is priority, even when significant changes in functional capacity have not yet occurred. The nurse should ensure that patients and families understand the role of health behaviors such as exercise and diet in slowing the progression of the disease. Emphasize the importance of adequate sleep, rest, nutrition, elimination, and pain control. Provide information on minimizing exposure to illness and the timely management of comorbid conditions that impact quality of life or that may hasten the rate of cognitive decline.

Injury prevention requires a comprehensive approach that incorporates collaboration with other members of the healthcare team. Principles of environmental safety are discussed in detail in the modules on Safety and Mobility and include but are not limited to fall precautions, skin integrity, and medication adherence. The risks and benefits of devices such as medic alert systems and patient tracking or alert systems should be discussed with patients and families. The use of physical and pharmacologic restraints should be avoided.

>> **Stay Current:** For more information on strategies that can be employed to avoid the use of restraints, see Avoiding Restraints in Patients with Dementia at the Hartford Institute for Geriatric Nursing at https://hign.org/consultgeri/try-this-series/avoiding-restraints-patients-dementia.

Nurses should also address the patient's ability to continue occupational, recreational, and practical activities, such as driving, that may be negatively impacted by impaired cognition. Research shows that the rate of accidents in individuals following the diagnosis of AD dramatically increases (Alzheimer's Association, 2020f). Loss of driving ability can be a point of contention for both patients and family members. Signs that indicate that driving is no longer safe include minor fender benders, getting lost, or ignoring stop signs or other traffic signals. Driver rehabilitation specialists have expertise in evaluating driving abilities and making recommendations for terminating driving privileges.

>> **Stay Current:** For more information on assessment and intervention of driving in older adults with dementia and related disorders, visit https://seniordriving.aaa.com.

SAFETY ALERT! The use of physical and pharmacologic restraints in individuals with AD and dementia significantly increases the risk of injury and death and is never considered therapeutic. Although safety is frequently cited as the rationale for using restraints, the risks of use clearly outweigh the benefits. The use of restraints and other measures to restrict movement can be avoided entirely through behavioral strategies such as distraction, consistent caregiving, provision of meaningful activities, and human monitoring.

Promote Adaptive Functioning and Coping

In the early stages of the disease, the nurse supports adaptive functioning by providing patient and family education and training, facilitating advanced planning, and supporting the emotional needs of both the family and the individual as they come to terms with the diagnosis.

Communication strategies for individuals with AD include the following:

- Establish eye contact.
- Begin every interaction by introducing yourself and stating the patient's name.
- Talk in a calm, reassuring tone.
- Use simple vocabulary and brief, straightforward sentences.
- Ask only one question at a time. Use questions that require yes or no answers and provide sufficient response time.
- Repeat questions, explanations, and instructions as required.
- Be careful about challenging the patient's interpretation of reality, as this may lead to agitation and noncompliance.

As the disease progresses, the emphasis of nursing care focuses on addressing behavioral manifestations of the disease, including neuropsychiatric symptoms such as agitation, depression, and anxiety. Caregivers may need guidance in recognizing the unmet needs that behaviors such as wandering and restlessness represent. Prevention of fatigue, consistency in caregiving, using simple and direct communication, providing comforting and meaningful activities (art, music, reminiscence), scheduling quiet time, and reducing stimulation are effective behavioral strategies.

Nurses are often in a key position to counsel family members as they struggle with ambivalence and guilt related to the decision to transition the patient to a skilled nursing facility. It is important for the nurse to address cultural beliefs that may compound the difficulty associated with making such a decision. Nurses can guide caregivers to select services and placements that best meet the unique needs of the patient and the family and that optimize the family's ability to continue to participate in caregiving. Nurses should be cognizant of the phenomenon of **transfer trauma** or **relocation syndrome**—a worsening of symptoms associated with the stress of moving to a new environment. Strategies to address the transition include retaining as many aspects of the home environment and previous routine as possible.

Provide End-of-Life Care

Nursing care for patients in the final stage of AD focuses on promoting quality of life and minimizing discomfort associated with physiologic decline and profound deficits in cognitive function. Principles of palliative care are discussed in detail in Modules 3, Comfort, and Module 27, Grief and Loss, and encompass a holistic approach to care. Palliative care with individuals with AD is challenged by the patient's inability to communicate needs. Family members and caregivers who have not resolved relationship issues during earlier stages of the illness may have more difficulty with treatment decisions and are at increased risk for complicated grieving. See Exemplar 3.B, End-of-Life Care, for more information.

Evaluation

Evaluation of patient outcomes is based on an understanding that patients may only be able to achieve a series of short-term outcomes based on the stage of disease progression. The focus is on ensuring that the patient and family achieve the optimal level of wellness for the particular stage of the disease. Evaluation also focuses on the caregivers' ability to manage the progression of the disease while meeting their own health and emotional needs. The following are examples of anticipated outcomes of care.

- The patient utilizes strategies to maintain independent functioning.
- The safety of the patient and others is maintained.
- The patient and/or family adheres to the prescribed treatment.
- Caregivers verbalize that self-care needs are met.
- Caregivers verbalize understanding of palliative and end-of-life care.

The unmet outcomes may indicate that the level of support being provided to the patient and family is no longer sufficient. In addition, it is possible that goals or certain interventions are no longer appropriate for the stage of the disease. In both cases the nurse would modify the plan of care.

Nursing Care Plan

A Patient with Alzheimer Disease

Sixty-one-year-old Loretta Gordon arrives at her general practitioner's office complaining of memory problems and depression that began about a month ago. Ms. Gordon is currently taking sertraline for her depression. She is afraid her medication is causing her current complaints, so she came to see the doctor.

ASSESSMENT	DIAGNOSES	PLANNING
Gretchen Burchett, RN, obtains a patient history and conducts a physical examination of Ms. Gordon. Nurse Burchett notes that Ms. Gordon retired 2 years ago after 35 years as an elementary school music teacher. Shortly after retirement, Ms. Gordon began to experience depression and was prescribed sertraline; until recently, her symptoms were well controlled by the medication. Ms. Gordon receives a "comfortable pension" from the school and lives alone in a small house. She has never been married and has no children, but she maintains a close relationship with her brother, who is 15 years younger. Her primary social outlet is a group of women friends she's known since college, although she says she hasn't been attending their weekly get-togethers because she "has a hard time following the conversation." Ms. Gordon is an avid piano player but admits to recent frustration over her inability to follow sheet music. Ms. Gordon is clean and well groomed, and her weight is healthy for someone her age and height. She struggles to find the right words when answering Nurse Burchett's questions. The nurse also notes a family history of AD and that Ms. Gordon sustained a serious head injury in a car accident 8 years ago. Ms. Gordon's vital signs include T 99.0°F oral; P 67 bpm; R 18/min; and BP 116/72 mmHg. Suspecting mild or early-stage AD, Nurse Burchett administers the MMSE. Ms. Gordon scores 23, indicating mild cognitive impairment. The physician orders blood tests to check for metabolic and endocrine problems and an MRI to assess for impaired blood flow and fluid accumulation in the brain. All of Ms. Gordon's test results are negative, and a diagnosis of probable mild or early-stage AD is made. The physician prescribes donepezil, 5 mg orally, increasing to 10 mg after 6 weeks. He also increases her sertraline from 150 mg orally to 175 mg and instructs her to return in 6 months.	■ Risk of injury related to impaired cognitive function ■ Memory impairment related to diminished neurologic function ■ Confusion related to deterioration of cognitive function ■ Impaired communication related to intellectual changes ■ Anxiety related to awareness of physiologic and cognitive changes	Goals for Ms. Gordon's care include: ■ The patient will remain free from injury. ■ The patient will verbalize an understanding of her disease and its stages. ■ The patient will utilize lists, calendars, and other memory aids as needed. ■ The patient will participate in speech and language therapy. ■ The patient will exhibit decreased signs and symptoms of anxiety and depression. ■ The patient will take all medications as prescribed. ■ The patient will remain in the home environment as long as possible.

IMPLEMENTATION

- Teach about AD and provide informational materials and recommendations for community resources.
- Collaborate with other members of the healthcare team to ensure advance planning and decision making, including advance directives, financial planning, and legal concerns related to guardianship and estate planning.
- Collaborate with the primary care provider and other members of the healthcare team about home visits to regularly assess the patient's functional capabilities and identify any safety concerns.
- Emphasize the use of calendars and electronic devices to record appointments and alert to important activities, such as medication administration.
- Instruct about the prescribed medications, potential side effects, and dietary changes that can minimize negative side effects.
- Refer to speech and occupational therapy.
- Teach about strategies to address behavioral changes and anxiety associated with AD, including decreasing environmental stress, regular sleep and meal schedules, redirection and distraction, minimizing unexpected changes, and counseling, relaxation, and music therapy for both patients and families.
- Promote therapeutic environments and activities that encourage physical, social, emotional, and cognitive well-being, including physical activity, diet, prevention and management of health problems, cognitive exercises, games, puzzles, and social engagement.

EVALUATION

Nurse Burchett refers Ms. Gordon to a speech therapist, and therapy sessions are scheduled for twice weekly. During therapy, she engages in a series of exercises designed to slow her decline in communication skills. Ms. Gordon has also mastered the electronic calendar and alarm on her cell phone, programming reminders for even basic daily functions. She enjoys an hour of music in the evenings, although she listens to recordings rather than playing her piano. After 6 months of pharmacologic treatment and speech therapy, Ms. Gordon's cognitive condition is stable and she once again scores 23 on her MMSE.

Ms. Gordon continues to display symptoms of depression, primarily stemming from the realization that there is no cure for her condition. She attends a local AD support group, which helps her verbalize and cope with her anxiety. With the help of her brother, who has invited Ms. Gordon to move into his home, she has created a long-term care plan.

(continued on next page)

Nursing Care Plan *(continued)*

CRITICAL THINKING

1. Ms. Gordon is fortunate that her brother is willing to be involved in her care. How would you adapt the care plan if Ms. Gordon had no family or her family was unwilling to be involved?
2. Ms. Gordon finds comfort in a support group for AD patients. Identify resources in your area that provide these kinds of services to AD patients and caregivers.
3. Develop a care plan to promote Ms. Gordon's ability to perform self-care.

REVIEW Alzheimer Disease

RELATE Link the Concepts and Exemplars

Linking the exemplar of Alzheimer disease with the concept of tissue integrity:

1. Why might patients with AD be at a heightened risk for impaired skin integrity? What types of impairments would you most expect to see, and during which stages of AD would they most likely occur?
2. When caring for the patient with AD, what nursing interventions are appropriate when seeking to limit the risk of impaired skin integrity?

Linking the exemplar of Alzheimer disease with the concept of spirituality:

3. How might a patient's spirituality be affected by a diagnosis of AD? How might a patient's diagnosis of AD affect her family and loved ones?
4. What nursing interventions might be appropriate for patients and families who are experiencing a spiritual crisis related to the cognitive and physical alterations associated with AD?

Linking the exemplar of Alzheimer disease with the concept of legal issues:

5. Why are issues of informed consent often problematic for individuals with AD?
6. What actions might nurses recommend to prevent such issues from arising?

READY Go to Volume 3: Clinical Nursing Skills

REFER Go to Pearson MyLab Nursing and eText

REFLECT Apply Your Knowledge

Robert Moser, a 75-year-old man, is brought to the emergency department by State Trooper Kelly just before midnight. Law enforcement had received reports of a car driving erratically along the highway and pulled Mr. Moser over. Trooper Kelly tells you that when he stopped Mr. Moser, Mr. Moser was able to get out his wallet but unable to tell Trooper Kelly his name. Mr. Moser stated he was trying to find the hospital where his wife is located, but he could not name the hospital or say where it is. Trooper Kelly pulled up the list of contacts in Mr. Moser's cell phone. When Mr. Moser confirmed one of the contacts was his son, Trooper Kelly contacted the son and asked him to meet them at the hospital. The son, who informs Trooper Kelly that his father was recently diagnosed with Alzheimer disease, lives out of town and will arrive in about an hour. Mr. Moser is polite and compliant, but he keeps asking "Is this a hospital?" over and over again. As you begin your assessment, Mr. Moser has difficulty finding the words he needs to respond.

1. What additional assessment information do you need?
2. Identify three other conditions that may produce symptoms that mimic dementia.
3. How will you go about the assessment given that Mr. Moser is unable to participate fully?
4. What are Mr. Moser's priorities for care *at this time*?
5. What stage of Alzheimer disease is this patient likely experiencing?

Exemplar 23.B Delirium

Exemplar Learning Objectives

23.B Analyze delirium as it relates to cognition.

- Describe the pathophysiology of delirium.
- Describe the etiology of delirium.
- Compare the risk factors and prevention of delirium.
- Identify the clinical manifestations of delirium.
- Summarize diagnostic tests and therapies used by interprofessional teams in the collaborative care of an individual with delirium.
- Differentiate care of patients with delirium across the lifespan.
- Apply the nursing process in providing culturally competent care to an individual with delirium.

Exemplar Key Terms

Confusion, *1783*
Confusion Assessment Method (CAM), *1786*
Delirium, *1783*
Sundowning, *1784*

Overview

Delirium is an abrupt, generally transient, and often fluctuating change in mental state and consciousness characterized by disorganized thinking, disorientation, perceptual disturbances, restlessness, agitation, and lability. **Confusion** is a closely related term, broadly used to describe increased difficulty in thinking clearly, making judgments, focusing attention, and maintaining orientation. The terms *acute confusion* and *delirium* have been used interchangeably; however, delirium is recognized as a distinct disorder.

Delirium generally signals the presence of a reversible but potentially life-threatening condition. Delirium is associated with a number of adverse outcomes, including increased mortality, institutionalization, and dementia. The best patient outcomes are associated with the prevention of delirium; however, early detection and management may mitigate the consequences of the condition. It is believed that at least one out of 10 hospitalized patients will experience delirium in the hospital setting, but the likelihood increases significantly according to age and variables such as diagnosis and treatment. Older adults experience delirium at rates up to six times that of the general hospital population, with occurrence rates ranging from 29 to 64% depending on patient population (Hospital Elder Life Program, 2020). Delirium affects more than 2.6 million older adults per year in the United States, accounting for more than $164 billion annually in excess Medicare expenditures (American Geriatric Society, 2019).

The incidence of delirium in community health settings is difficult to estimate and may be underdiagnosed at hospital admission because of underlying cognitive and neurological conditions (Magny et al., 2018). Unfortunately, regardless of care setting, delirium often goes undetected. Some research has shown that delirium is only recognized by one-third of physicians and nurses (Hospital Elder Life Program, 2020).

Pathophysiology

The exact pathophysiology of delirium is unknown. It is theorized that the conditions that lead to delirium increase cerebral oxidative stress and impair neurotransmitter action through a variety of structural, inflammatory, metabolic, and neurochemical pathways. For example, psychologic and physiologic stress both activate the sympathetic nervous system, impairing cholinergic transmission. The net result of these changes is diminished cerebral function and alterations in arousal mechanisms of the RAS and thalamus (Soysal & Isik, 2018).

Etiology

A wide variety of conditions can result in delirium, including infections, metabolic imbalances, trauma, nutritional deficiencies, CNS disease, hypoxia, hypothermia, hyperthermia, circulatory problems, low blood glucose, toxin exposure, sleep deprivation, and drug and alcohol use and withdrawal (Schroeder, 2019).

Iatrogenic (treatment-related) factors also may precipitate delirium and are addressed by interventions such as medication, surgery, and anesthesia and, in special cases, electroconvulsive therapy. Hospitalized patients are much more likely to experience delirium because of the presence of predisposing illnesses, exposure to multiple medical interventions that may contribute to cognitive changes, and being in an environment that is unfamiliar, stimulating, and not conducive to maintaining normal diurnal rhythms. Transfer trauma or relocation syndrome is a major cause of stress in individuals of all ages and a contributing factor to the high incidence of delirium in hospitalized patients. Delirium occurs in up to 61% of the general hospital population, 51% of postoperative patients, and 82% of patients in the intensive care unit (Hospital Elder Life Program, 2020). Among hospitalized individuals over age 65, dementia with superimposed delirium is common (Reynish et al., 2017).

Risk Factors

Although anyone can develop delirium, certain factors increase individual risk. Age is a major risk factor. Older adults are at higher risk due to normal age-related cognitive decline. Age-related vision and hearing loss can contribute to delirium by impairing individuals' ability to accurately and effectively interpret their surroundings. Older patients are also more likely to experience many of the underlying physical causes of delirium, such as CNS and circulatory disease. Children are more prone to delirium than are adolescents and younger adults. Again, physiology is a primary factor, as children's bodies are less equipped to cope with insults such as fever, infection, and toxin exposure.

Other factors that can contribute to delirium include the presence of a chronic illness, onset of a new illness, or exacerbation of a current condition. The use of drugs, alcohol, or prescription medications such as hypnotics/sedatives, anxiolytics, antidepressants, antipsychotics, anti-Parkinson drugs, anticonvulsants, or antispasmodics also increase the risk of delirium (Kassie, Nguyen, Ellett, Pratt, & Roughead, 2017).The strain of illness or environmental change, such as hospitalization, may increase risk of delirium in patients with a preexisting anxiety, cognitive, or mood disorder.

Nonpharmacologic approaches that focus on risk factors such as immobility, functional decline, visual or hearing impairment, dehydration, and sleep deprivation are effective to prevent delirium and also are recommended for delirium treatment (Oh, Fong, Hshieh, & Inouye, 2017).

Prevention

Prevention focuses on reducing the incidence or presence of physiologic and psychosocial factors that lead to delirium, early detection of delirium, and a holistic approach to managing delirium in affected individuals. For individuals with predisposing conditions, proper medical management can reduce the likelihood of delirium. Standardized protocols should be implemented in healthcare settings to address the prevention, detection, and management of delirium (American Geriatric Society, 2019; Mudge et al., 2017; Y.-Y. Wang et al., 2020).

Clinical Manifestations

Typical manifestations of delirium include reduced awareness, impaired thinking skills, and/or changes in activity level and behavior. The Clinical Manifestations and

Therapies table provides an overview of common signs and symptoms from each of these categories. The intensity of manifestations varies, with some patients having only subtle symptoms and others experiencing acute loss of most or all cognitive function. Note that diagnostic markers of delirium may vary somewhat depending on the patient's cultural background.

Delirium is marked by vacillating symptoms. An individual may be largely unresponsive at one point in the day but hypervigilant just a few hours later, with a period of normal behavior in between. In addition, the individual's psychomotor activity may be hyperactive, hypoactive, or a mixture of both at various times throughout the day. Confusion that intensifies in the evening or at bedtime is referred to as **sundowning**. Sundowning is not a disorder in and of itself; rather, it is a feature of delirium and dementia that affects some individuals.

Collaboration

Nurses must be familiar with a range of collaborative interventions related to delirium. These include diagnostic tests, medications, and nonpharmacologic therapies. Psychosocial considerations are directed toward both patients and their family members.

Diagnostic Tests

Medical professionals use any number of diagnostic procedures to determine the underlying source of a patient's delirium. The first steps usually include conducting a physical exam and obtaining a detailed medical history. Cognitive testing, such as the CAM test (described later in this exemplar), can also be useful for determining whether a patient is experiencing reversible confusion or another form of impairment. Advances in diagnosis have also included the development of brief screening tools, such as the 3-Minute Diagnostic Assessment; 4 A's Test; and proxy-based measures such as the Family Confusion Assessment Method. Measures of severity, such as the Confusion Assessment Method–Severity Score, can aid in monitoring response to treatment, risk stratification, and assessing prognosis (Oh et al., 2017).

Based on assessment data, the primary care provider will choose appropriate diagnostic procedures. Examples of tests that may be appropriate for identifying underlying causes of confusion include a detailed neurologic examination; drug and alcohol screening; laboratory tests for signs of infection and metabolic, nutritional, and other imbalances; and screening for depression and other psychiatric conditions.

Pharmacologic Therapy

No one drug or class of drugs is appropriate for all patients with delirium, but some medications may effectively treat the causative condition. For example, antipsychotics may be appropriate for patients with delirium related to an underlying psychotic disorder with symptoms of hallucinations, delusions, aggressiveness, or disorganized thoughts. Lithium and mood stabilizers may be prescribed for mania, hyperactivity,

Clinical Manifestations and Therapies

Delirium*

<table>
<tr><th>CUES</th><th>CLINICAL MANIFESTATIONS</th><th>CLINICAL THERAPIES</th></tr>
<tr><td>Reduced awareness</td><td>▪ Limited attention span
▪ Difficulty focusing or logically shifting from one topic to another
▪ Inability to answer questions or engage in conversation
▪ Limited response to the environment</td><td rowspan="3">▪ Physical interventions aimed at correcting biological causes of delirium:
• Supplemental oxygen
• IV fluids and/or electrolytes
• Supplemental nutrition
▪ Environmental interventions:
• Preventing under- or overstimulation
• Instituting safety measures
• Promoting consistency
▪ Cognitive interventions:
• Orienting patient to place, time, date, and/or person
• Providing reassurance that delirium is temporary
▪ Pharmacologic therapies aimed at the underlying cause of delirium (as appropriate)
▪ Surgical treatment of the underlying cause of delirium (as appropriate)</td></tr>
<tr><td>Impaired thinking</td><td>▪ Impaired memory (especially recent memory)
▪ Disorganized thought
▪ Disorientation to place, time, date, and/or person
▪ Impaired speaking, reading, and comprehension ability
▪ Rambling incoherent or illogical speech
▪ Hallucinations or delusions</td></tr>
<tr><td>Behavioral changes</td><td>▪ Hyperactivity, hypoactivity, or a combination thereof
▪ Hallucinations
▪ Agitation and/or restlessness
▪ Fear, anxiety, and/or depression
▪ Altered sleep patterns
▪ Mood swings
▪ Withdrawal</td></tr>
</table>

*Characterized by acute, sudden onset, and fluctuation of symptoms.

and mood swings. In other cases, discontinuation of medications may be the best course of action, especially for individuals who are experiencing drug-related delirium.

Nonpharmacologic Therapy

Numerous nonpharmacologic interventions may benefit individuals with delirium, depending on their pathology. These interventions fall into three categories: physical, environmental, and cognitive.

- *Physical interventions* target anatomic or biological factors that may be contributing to delirium. Common physical interventions that promote enhanced cognition include oxygen administration, IV delivery of fluids and/or electrolytes, and provision of appropriate nutrition.
- *Environmental interventions* involve enhancing patients' level of comfort within their surroundings, as this helps minimize the likelihood of confusion. Often, these interventions focus on preventing under- or overstimulation, maintaining safety, and promoting consistency. (See the Nursing Process section.)
- *Cognitive interventions* involve orienting patients to person, place, and time, as well as providing reassurance that they are safe and that their delirium will be resolved. Validation therapy may also be an effective way of meeting patient needs (see Exemplar 23.A, Alzheimer Disease, and the Nursing Process section below.)

SAFETY ALERT! Older adults and individuals with dementia or other cognitive disorders and mental illnesses are at increased risk for a misdiagnosis related to the perception that changes in mental status are related to age or a psychiatric condition. In addition, it is easy to confuse diurnal changes in cognition (such as sundowning) with delirium caused by an underlying medical condition. Nurses should never assume that cognitive changes are related to age, mental health issues, or the time of day. A thorough assessment is essential to rule out underlying medical causes of any changes in mental status.

Lifespan Considerations

Although individuals of all ages are susceptible to delirium under certain conditions, risk factors and common etiologies of the condition are associated with different stages of the lifespan. Manifestations of delirium may also vary with different age groups.

Delirium in Children

Like older adults, children lack the functional reserves necessary to cope with both environmental and physiologic stressors and are at increased risk for delirium. In general, children with intellectual and developmental disabilities are at increased risk for delirium. The prevalence of delirium in hospitalized children ranges from 10 to 44% and is more common in younger and critically ill children or those emerging from anesthesia. Any febrile illness may cause symptoms of delirium in the hospital or home settings. Manifestations of delirium may be confused with willful or oppositional behavior or be extremely frightening for parents. The Cornell Assessment of Pediatric Delirium and the Pediatric and Preschool Confusion Assessment Method–Intensive Care Unit (pCAM-ICU) are two instruments that can be used to detect delirium in children. Besides the prevention and management of the underlying medical condition, the presence of parents and family members has been found to reduce the incidence of delirium. Overall, the prognosis for children with delirium is better than that for older individuals (Bettencourt & Mullen, 2017; Meyburg, Dill, Traube, Silver, & von Haken, 2017).

Delirium in Adolescents

By adolescence, the ability to compensate for physiologic alterations that may precipitate delirium has improved; however, some of the common causes of delirium in adolescents are different. Adolescents may be at increased risk for head trauma as a result of participation in contact sports or a tendency toward impulsive, risk-taking behaviors. Drug and substance abuse and withdrawal are another common cause of delirium in this age group (Gerson, Malas, & Mroczkowski, 2018).

Delirium in Pregnant and Postpartum Women

Delirium during pregnancy or in the postpartum period is a serious sign and may indicate the presence of a life-threatening condition such as preeclampsia and HELLP (hemolysis, elevated liver enzymes, low platelet count) syndrome, sepsis, hypo- or hyperglycemia, or fluid and electrolyte imbalance (possibly as a result of hyperemesis gravidarum). Delirium may also be associated with the stress of labor or the use of anesthetic agents. Symptoms of delirium may be difficult to distinguish from postpartum psychosis. Priority care focuses on the patient and determining the underlying cause. This includes monitoring fetal well-being as well as ensuring the safety of the newborn (Davies, 2017; Wisner et al., 2018).

Delirium in Older Adults

In older patients, delirium may be confused with normal forgetfulness or dementia, especially when presenting in healthcare settings where staff are unfamiliar with the patient's history and prior cognitive status. Individuals with dementia are at increased risk of acute mental status changes associated with delirium, and therefore any change from baseline should be considered significant (Hospital Elder Life Program, 2020). Delirium is often the most prominent manifestation of conditions such as dehydration, respiratory infections, urinary tract infections, and urinary retention, and adverse drug events may occur in the absence of symptoms such as fever or discomfort. The possibility of intracranial events (stroke, bleeding) and acute pulmonary and myocardial events should also be considered. Prompt recognition and management of delirium is essential because the risk of long-term disability and death also increases exponentially in older adults (American Geriatric Society, 2019; Oh et al., 2017).

NURSING PROCESS

One of the nurse's primary duties in caring for a patient with delirium is to promote resolution of whatever condition is causing the patient's cognitive impairment. The nurse must also take steps to keep the patient safe, support cognitive functioning and comfort, and minimize the likelihood of further episodes of confusion. When assessing an individual's cognitive skills and orientation, the nurse accounts for variables such as age and development, level of education, and culture.

Assessment

Nursing assessment for the patient with delirium typically involves three main elements: a health history, a physical examination, and a mental status examination.

Observation and Patient Interview

Observe the patient for behavioral manifestations of delirium, including extreme distractibility, disorganized thinking, rambling, irrelevant and incoherent speech, and purposeless motor activity. Fluctuations in psychomotor activity may also be observed with periods of restlessness and agitation to stupor, catatonia, and somnolence. Mood instability may be manifested by episodes of alternating distress or euphoria. The patient may also appear flushed and diaphoretic.

The history is critical to identifying potential causes of the patient's confusion and highlighting areas that require further assessment. Because the patient may not be able to provide a reliable history, a family member or caregiver may need to be interviewed. For the patient with delirium, basic components of the health history include the following:

- Age
- History of other disease processes
- Recent history of infection or fever
- Vision or hearing loss
- Alcohol and drug use (including medications)
- Possible toxin exposure (e.g., in the workplace)
- Dietary patterns and fluid intake
- Untreated or undertreated pain
- History of depression or other mood disorders
- Recent life changes that may be contributing to cognitive and/or emotional upset.

The **Confusion Assessment Method (CAM)** is helpful in differentiating delirium from dementia. The nurse should also screen the patient for depression, as it is often linked to confusion in older adults. For discussion of testing instruments designed for this purpose, refer to the Nursing Assessment section in this module.

Because delirium has a fluctuating course, ongoing assessment is important. The nurse should reassess patients with delirium frequently. Some patients may require one-on-one monitoring.

>> **Stay Current:** A current version of the CAM can be accessed online at https://hign.org/consultgeri/try-this-series/confusion-assessment-method-cam.

Physical Examination

During the physical examination, evaluate the patient's height, weight, vital signs, and overall condition. In addition to a focused assessment of perfusion, oxygenation, intracranial regulation, infection, and inflammation, assess for physical findings associated with any cues brought up during the health history. For example, for a patient who reports a hearing deficit, attempt to determine the degree of impairment and explore the possibility that this impairment may be contributing to the patient's confusion.

Diagnosis

Care priorities diagnoses for patients with delirium vary depending on the cause and severity of their condition. Still, some problems are likely to apply to many, if not most, patients with acute confusion. These include:

- Risk of injury
- Lack of knowledge about delirium
- Inability to perform self-care
- Sleep disturbance
- Confusion
- Impaired communication.

Planning

The planning portion of the nursing process involves identifying desired outcomes and choosing evidence-based interventions that facilitate their achievement. Again, goals and interventions will vary depending on the cause and severity of a patient's delirium. Appropriate outcomes may include the following:

- Patient will remain free from injury.
- Patient will be oriented to time, place, date, and person.
- Patient will return to baseline cognitive status (i.e., status prior to onset of confusion).
- Patient will demonstrate the ability to communicate in a clear and logical manner.
- Patient will obtain adequate sleep and rest.
- Patient will exhibit reduced anxiety, agitation, and restlessness.
- Patient will be able to perform ADLs.

Implementation

Provide a Safe Environment for the Hospitalized Patient

Typically, nursing interventions for the patient with confusion revolve around providing a safe, therapeutic environment that prevents further cognitive impairment and promotes resolution of the condition causing the patient's delirium. The following measures may be useful for most patients:

- Maintaining appropriate levels of noise and lighting in an attempt to prevent under- or overstimulation
- Preventing access to potential hazards (such as lighters, knives, or chemicals)
- Using behavioral interventions and monitoring systems to address wandering
- Promoting consistency by assigning the same caregivers and scheduling activities at the same time each day
- Providing an environment that supports normal sleep–wake cycles

- Ensuring access to assistive devices, including glasses and hearing aids
- Providing adequate pain management
- Keeping familiar items in the patient's environment without allowing the environment to become disorganized or cluttered
- Using calendars, clocks, and signs to help orient the patient to time, date, and place
- Encouraging loved ones to visit the patient.

The nurse can also employ various communication strategies to limit confusion. The nurse should always wear a name tag and make an introduction during patient interactions. The nurse should then verbally orient the patient to date, time, and place. When talking with the patient, the nurse should speak clearly and allow time for a response. All explanations of treatments or procedures should be brief and as easy to understand as possible. The nurse should reinforce reality by helping patients interpret confusing or unfamiliar stimuli. Any misconceptions of events or situations should be gently corrected. The nurse should also reassure patients that their delirium is temporary.

Communicating with Patients

Working Phase

Older adults with delirium can be confused, restless, irritable, paranoid, hyperalert, and somnolent, among other symptoms. Many times, they have hallucinations, mix up their days and nights, and make no sense when they talk.

How can the nurse best communicate with the patient without increasing agitation? Speaking clearly, using short sentences, and easing fears are three helpful strategies. Here are some examples:

- Hello, Mrs. Palchek. I am Nurse Rivera. I will be your nurse tonight.
- I know you are frightened. I will stay with you. You are safe here.
- Mrs. Palchek, here are your glasses. . . let me help you put them on.

» **Stay Current:** The Hospital Elder Life Program (HELP) is a comprehensive, evidence-based patient-care program that provides optimal care for older persons in the hospital and has extensive resources for healthcare professionals on the prevention, identification, and management of delirium in hospitalized patients. For more information, visit http://www.hospitalelderlifeprogram.org/for-clinicians/about-delirium/.

Promote Safe Patient Care in the Home

Teaching is especially important when patients have an ongoing health issue that predisposes them to delirium. For example, if patients are taking medications that increase their risk of cognitive changes, they and their loved ones should be informed of common symptoms of delirium and what to do when these symptoms arise. Similarly, patients with diabetes should be taught about signs of confusion related to abnormal blood glucose. In addition, family members and caregivers should be assisted with developing an action plan for assisting the patient during hyperglycemic or hypoglycemic episodes.

Evaluation

Ongoing evaluation is critical for all patients with delirium, as it allows nurses adjust the nursing plan of care as needed. Some examples of potential achieved outcomes include the following:

- Patient sustains no injuries.
- Patient is oriented to time, place, date, and person or has returned to previous baseline
- Patient demonstrates an absence of manifestations of delirium related to hospitalization.
- Patient demonstrates an absence of manifestations of delirium related to poorly managed chronic health conditions.
- Patient communicates clearly and transitions logically between topics or returns to baseline.
- Patient is able to perform ADLs or returns to baseline level of functioning.

Individuals with delirium may demonstrate permanent changes in neurocognitive function, especially when conditions such as dementia were already present. Family members and caregivers may be more aware of subtle differences indicating that the patient has not returned to previous levels of function. Even when cognitive status has improved, the nurse recognizes that individuals who have experienced delirium are at increased risk for future episodes. The resolution of delirium may allow the nurse to modify the plan of care and provide teaching that emphasizes the prevention, detection, and treatment of precipitating health issues.

REVIEW Delirium

RELATE Link the Concepts and Exemplars

Linking the exemplar of confusion with the concept of infection:

1. How might delirium increase the patient's risk of infection?
2. Why are patients with infection at a heightened risk for delirium? What types of infections do you think would most increase a patient's likelihood of delirium?

Linking the exemplar of confusion with the concept of stress and coping:

3. Why are patients more likely to experience delirium during periods of increased stress? What sorts of events are likely to be most stressful and thus result in confusion?
4. For the patient experiencing delirium, what nursing interventions could be implemented to help reduce stress and promote effective coping?

Linking the exemplar of delirium with the concept of safety:

5. How might caring for patients with delirium put nurses' safety in jeopardy?
6. What interventions could nurses implement to protect their own safety when caring for a patient with delirium? What legal or ethical issues are associated with these measures?

READY Go to Volume 3: Clinical Nursing Skills

REFER Go to Pearson MyLab Nursing and eText

REFLECT Apply Your Knowledge

Mike Finimore is a 64-year-old man who has been married to his wife, Elise, for 40 years. Their only child, 24-year-old Sasha, has Down syndrome and lives with them. Mr. Finimore is a middle manager for a manufacturing company where he has worked for the past 20 years.

Overall, Mr. Finimore is in good health, although he has recently been undergoing conservative treatment for benign prostatic hyperplasia. He has a history of depression, including a brief episode during college for which he did not seek treatment. Mr. Finimore had another episode shortly after his daughter was born and, at the encouragement of his wife, he sought treatment, which consisted of counseling and antidepressant medications. He quit taking the medications after 6 months and decided he would just learn to deal with the depression on his own. Although he has had several mild episodes of depression since that time, Mr. Finimore has been unwilling to seek treatment because he fears the social stigma of being labeled medically depressed and is concerned that his employer will discover it through use of his medical benefits. It is Mr. Finimore's opinion that his employer would perceive depression as a sign of weakness. Overall, he has done well without the medications.

Mr. Finimore has been thinking about retiring in the next few years. He and his wife have always planned to do some traveling, but mostly he looks forward to escaping his busy, stressful work environment. Mr. Finimore and his daughter are involved in church activities; they also enjoy a walk each evening after supper. He belongs to a bowling league and is at the bowling alley a couple of evenings a week.

Mr. Finimore is admitted to the acute care hospital for a transurethral resection of the prostate (TURP). He has been very anxious about the procedure because of the risk of impotence. The surgery goes smoothly, and he experiences no complications. In the immediate postoperative period, Mr. Finimore has a three-way indwelling urinary catheter inserted, with continuous bladder irrigation. He experiences pain and occasional bladder spasms because of blood clots. The day after surgery, the nurse enters Mr. Finimore's room, and he asks why the hospital bed was brought to his room and calls the nurse by his wife's name. He appears restless and agitated. The nurse assesses Mr. Finimore and determines that he is experiencing delirium.

1. What factors may increase the risk of delirium in this patient?
2. What interventions would the nurse initiate for Mr. Finimore?
3. What is the priority problem for this patient? Why?
4. What assessment tools would the nurse use to assess Mr. Finimore?

Exemplar 23.C Schizophrenia

Exemplar Learning Objectives

23.C Analyze schizophrenia as it relates to cognition.

- Describe the pathophysiology of schizophrenia.
- Describe the etiology of schizophrenia.
- Compare the risk factors and prevention of schizophrenia.
- Identify the clinical manifestations of schizophrenia.
- Summarize diagnostic tests and therapies used by interprofessional teams in the collaborative care of an individual with schizophrenia.
- Differentiate care of patients with schizophrenia across the lifespan.
- Apply the nursing process in providing culturally competent care to an individual with schizophrenia.

Exemplar Key Terms

Akathisia, *1796*
Alogia, *1792*
Anhedonia, *1792*
Assertive community treatment (ACT), *1798*
Avolition, *1792*
Catatonia, *1791*
Cognitive symptoms, *1792*
Concrete thinking, *1792*
Delusions, *1791*
Disorganized thinking, *1791*
Dystonia, *1796*
Electroconvulsive therapy (ECT), *1798*
Epigenetic, *1789*
Extrapyramidal symptoms (EPS), *1796*
Hallucinations, *1791*
Loose association, *1791*
Negative symptoms, *1792*
Neuroleptic malignant syndrome (NMS), *1796*
Positive symptoms, *1791*
Recovery, *1790*
Rehabilitation, *1790*
Relapse, *1790*
Schizophrenia, *1788*
Tardive dyskinesia (TD), *1796*

Overview

Schizophrenia is a profound neurobiological disorder that is characterized by psychotic symptoms, diminished capacity to relate to others, and behaviors that are appear odd or bizarre. Approximately 1% of persons living in the United States experience schizophrenia (National Institute of Mental Health, 2018). Although many people associate the disorder with perceptual alterations such as hallucinations, the most chronic and disabling aspects of the disease relate to functional deficits caused by alterations in communication, cognition, attention, memory, emotional regulation, initiative, and social interactions. (See the section Clinical Manifestations for more information.) Schizophrenia typically emerges during early adulthood, but it can also occur during childhood and adolescence or first manifest later in life. Schizophrenia is also associated with a 10- to 25-year reduction in life expectancy as a result of comorbid medical conditions and high rates of suicide (Brink et al., 2019; Moradi, Harvey, & Helldin, 2018). Stigma associated with the disorder is perhaps one of the greatest challenges for individuals impacted by the disease (Thibodeau, Shanks, & Smith, 2018).

Even though schizophrenia is a single diagnosis, it is one of several disorders included in the DSM-5 within the category of "schizophrenia spectrum and other psychotic disorders" (APA, 2013). Manifestations of schizophrenia range in severity, with symptoms and etiologies that overlap with other psychotic disorders.

Pathophysiology

Currently the known pathologic mechanisms associated with schizophrenia include anatomic alterations, neurotransmitter abnormalities, and impairments in immune function. The relationship between these mechanisms is complex, and it is not always clear which alterations are a cause of or a consequence of the disease.

Structural Anatomic Alterations

Brain imaging studies of individuals with schizophrenia consistently reveal a pattern of structural abnormalities that include decreased volumes of gray matter in the prefrontal cortex, temporal lobes, hippocampus, and thalamus; enlarged ventricles and sulci; and decreased blood flow to the frontal lobe, thalamus, and temporal lobes. Positron emission tomography (PET) scans of individuals with schizophrenia reveal alterations in cerebral blood flow and glucose metabolism (Mitelman et al., 2018; Zhu et al., 2017). Although brain abnormalities are present prior to the onset of symptoms, they are difficult to detect and become more pronounced with the first and subsequent episodes of psychotic symptoms.

Neurotransmitter Abnormalities

Abnormalities in neurotransmitter function contribute to the manifestations of schizophrenia. Alterations in the dopaminergic system have been implicated, in part because antipsychotic medications block D_2 (dopamine) receptors, as well as norepinephrine receptors and serotonin (5-HT) receptors. Alterations in the GABA and acetylcholine neurotransmitter systems are also believed to be involved. Nicotinic acetylcholine receptors (nAChR) appear to be diminished in the hippocampus of individuals with schizophrenia, resulting in disturbances in inhibitory gateways. It has been proposed that nicotine stimulates these receptors, providing temporary relief of symptoms of schizophrenia (Koukouli et al., 2017). Research also implicates dysregulation in the NMDA subclass of glutamate receptors in the disease (Nakazawa, Jeevakumar, & Nakao, 2017; Nakazawa & Sapkota, 2020; Snyder & Gao, 2020). Glutamate is required for the degradation of dopamine and several other neurotransmitters that influence prefrontal information processing. Glutamate receptors also play an important role in migration of neurons during brain development. Individuals with schizophrenia have been shown to have abnormally low levels of glutamate in the CSF.

Immunologic and Inflammatory Pathways

Multiple studies support the involvement of inflammatory/immune pathways with an association with chronic oxidative stress (Müller, 2018; Tanaka et al., 2017). Microglia normally serve as a first line of defense against pathogenic invasion in the CNS. They are also involved in other essential brain functions, including the pruning and maintenance of synapses and the consumption of fragments of damaged cells. When activated, microglia produce inflammatory cytokines, resulting in a cascade of events that alter brain function. One consequence appears to be an interruption of metabolic processes responsible for NMDA receptor activity and dopamine regulation (Errico, Nuzzo, Carella, Bertolino, & Usiello, 2018; Weinstein et al., 2017). It is known that individuals with schizophrenia have increased levels of cytokines, especially during periods of acute psychosis or relapse (Misiak et al., 2018). It is believed that additional insults such as illness and stress overwhelm an already compromised neuroimmune system, resulting in an exacerbation of cognitive dysfunction (Altmann, 2018; Jeffries et al., 2018; Pruessner, Cullen, Aas, & Walker, 2017).

Etiology

The exact causes of schizophrenia are not understood. The preponderance of evidence seems to suggest that some individuals have a polygenic predisposition and that a combination of factors, such as prenatal health issues and environmental factors, lead to manifestations of the disorder (Skene et al., 2018). Although no single environmental factor is implicated in the development of schizophrenia, it is clear that genetics plays a role: An individual with a biological parent who has schizophrenia has a 30% higher risk of developing it than the general population and that risk increases substantially if both parents have schizophrenia (Rasic, Hajec, Alda, & Uher, 2014).

The risk of schizophrenia increases incrementally with advancing paternal age as a result of cumulative mutations in sperm. Children born to fathers age 60 and older have an almost twofold risk of developing the disorder (Fond et al., 2017; Janecka et al., 2017). Some evidence also indicates that advanced maternal age is a risk factor for schizophrenia (Fountoulakis et al., 2018; Kollias, Dimitrakopoulos, Xenaki, Stefanis, & Papageorgiou, 2019). Research also highlights an overlap in the genetic influences of schizophrenia and other neurodevelopmental disorders such as autism (Gudmundsson et al., 2019; Owen & O'Donovan, 2017).

Most researchers now agree that external modifications to genes (**epigenetic** factors) must occur for schizophrenia to manifest. Many studies have focused on the impact of external events such as birth complications, in utero viral exposure, poor prenatal care, and marijuana use on gene expression in schizophrenia (Cromby, Chung, Papadopoulos, & Talbot, 2019; Föcking et al., 2019; Swathy & Banerjee, 2017). Research has implicated *Toxoplasma gondii* infection (toxoplasmosis) during pregnancy and early childhood in the development of the disease. *T. gondii* is spread via contact with cat feces, and therefore it is recommended that pregnant women and children do not handle cat litter and that litter boxes be changed daily (Chorlton, 2017; Xiao et al., 2018).

SAFETY ALERT! An estimated 20–40% of individuals diagnosed with schizophrenia attempt suicide. Risk factors include (but are not limited to) greater awareness of the illness, younger age, recent loss, limited support, recent discharge, and treatment failure. Regardless of the treatment phase or the presence of additional risk factors, all individuals with schizophrenia should be closely monitored for suicide.

Risk Factors

One of the challenges of schizophrenia is that many of the associated risk factors lack the specificity or strength to guide preventative health measures. Certain psychosocial and development factors appear to play a role.

Early life adversity (including exposure to chronic and acute stressors such as poverty, violence, and trauma) has been implicated in schizophrenia. Psychosocial risk factors are increased in instances where disparities in healthcare exist, such as with recent immigrant populations. Biochemical mechanisms involved in the stress response may have an epigenetic influence or exacerbate preexisting neuronal pathology (Howes, McCutcheon, Owen, & Murray, 2017).

There is evidence to suggest that children and adolescents who display certain alterations in emotional, cognitive, language, and motor development are at an increased risk for developing schizophrenia. These findings may relate to manifestations of neurodevelopmental problems that precede the prodromal and active phases of the illness (Birnbaum & Weinberger, 2017; Riglin et al., 2017). Stress that occurs during certain developmental periods such as early childhood or adolescence may confer a greater risk of developing the disorder.

Prevention

Research demonstrates that early screening and detection of cognitive, developmental, and behavioral alterations associated with schizophrenia and other mental illnesses may result in better outcomes for individuals, especially when accompanied by coordinated specialty care and nonpharmacologic interventions such as cognitive-behavioral therapy (CBT; Dixon, 2017; Ganguly, Soliman, & Moustafa, 2018; Maziade, 2017). Some aspects of secondary prevention of schizophrenia present ethical challenges, such as the practice of initiating antipsychotic treatment when prodromal symptoms are apparent. The risks associated with labeling and treating individuals who may or may not go on to develop the disorder need to be considered (Hasan & Musleh, 2018).

An important component of health promotion for patients with schizophrenia is to emphasize the possibility of **recovery** and **rehabilitation**. In the *recovery* phase, the symptoms of the disorder are present but under control. The emphasis for healthcare is on learning strategies to maintain health, such as adhering to treatment, reducing stress, and using effective coping strategies. The goal is the prevention of **relapse** (or a return to the acute phase of the illness). *Rehabilitation* refers to a level of wellness in which symptoms of the condition are under control to the extent that the affected individual can engage in goal-directed activities, such as maintaining a job and carrying out self-care (Potter & Moller, 2020).

Clinical Manifestations

The clinical manifestations of schizophrenia may be classified according to the stage of illness as well as the types of symptoms that are observed. Presenting symptoms may vary from person to person, with periods of exacerbation and remission. The trajectory of the illness must be recognized and understood in order to address the unique needs of individuals with the disorder. Many, but not all, individuals with schizophrenia experience sufficiently severe clinical manifestations that they have difficulty engaging in ADLs and IADLs and functioning independently (see the Clinical Manifestations and Therapies table). These patients may benefit from in-home services, day treatment programs, group homes or residential care, or psychiatric rehabilitation through community services.

Clinical Manifestations and Therapies

Schizophrenia

SYMPTOM CATEGORY	CLINICAL MANIFESTATIONS	CLINICAL THERAPIES
Positive symptoms of psychosis	▪ Hallucinations ▪ Delusions ▪ Thought disorders ▪ Disorganized behavior ▪ Movement disorders	▪ Administration of conventional antipsychotics, atypical antipsychotics, and/or dopamine system stabilizers ▪ CBT ▪ Electroconvulsive therapy ▪ Transcranial magnetic stimulation
Negative symptoms of psychosis	▪ Anhedonia ▪ Impaired memory ▪ Flat affect ▪ Avolition ▪ Poverty of speech ▪ Poor personal hygiene	▪ Administration of atypical antipsychotics and/or dopamine system stabilizers ▪ Psychiatric/psychosocial rehabilitation, including education about symptom management and signs of relapse and community service interventions such as assertive community treatment (ACT) ▪ CBT; group, individual, and family therapy
Cognitive symptoms of schizophrenia	▪ Concrete thinking ▪ Impaired memory (problems with word finding and facial recognition) ▪ Inattention and difficulty filtering out information ▪ Poor planning, organization, and problem-solving skills	▪ Cognitive remediation, CBT, social skills training ▪ Modify the environment to reduce stimuli; break tasks down into small parts ▪ Use lists and organizational aids ▪ Psychosocial rehabilitation through community service models

Clinical Manifestations and Therapies *(continued)*

SYMPTOM CATEGORY	CLINICAL MANIFESTATIONS	CLINICAL THERAPIES
Impaired social functioning	▪ Withdrawal ▪ Isolation ▪ Difficulty maintaining relationships	▪ Social skills training and guided practice in social situations ▪ Psychosocial rehabilitation through community service models
Impaired occupational functioning	▪ Unemployment, difficulty maintaining a job	▪ Occupational therapy ▪ Job training and placement

Symptom Types

The symptoms of schizophrenia are generally divided into positive, negative, and cognitive types, as depicted in **Figure 23.7 ››**. There is some overlap in the classification of symptoms, and the presence of these manifestations does not necessarily indicate that an individual has schizophrenia. Affective symptoms are normally not included in these classifications but are common in schizophrenia and are also discussed in this section. The manifestation of symptoms varies according to the phase of the illness.

Positive Symptoms

Positive symptoms are characterized by the psychotic features of the disorder that generally do not occur in healthy people and are outside of the range of normal experiences. Hallucinations, delusions, abnormal movements, and problems with speech or disordered thinking are all classified as positive symptoms.

Hallucinations are abnormal perceptual experiences that usually occur in the absence of external stimuli. Types of hallucinations are discussed in more detail in the Alterations section of this module. In individuals with schizophrenia, auditory hallucinations are generally most prevalent and often have threatening or accusatory content (Galletti, Paolini, Tortorella, & Compton, 2017; Rathee, Luhrmann, Bhatia, & Deshpande, 2018).

Delusions are false beliefs that are based on faulty perceptions and inferences. The most common delusions seen in patients with schizophrenia are those of *reference*, which incorporate the belief that certain events occur for the benefit of the individual. Nihilistic delusions encompass beliefs that the individual is nonexistent or dead. Religious delusions involve the belief that the individual is a religious figure. Grandiose delusions involve beliefs that the individual has special power or significance. Persecutory delusions involve the belief that others wish to harm the individual. Delusions may take on bizarre or implausible features such as thought broadcasting (belief that others can hear thoughts), withdrawal (belief that others can remove thoughts), control (belief that others can control thoughts), and insertion (belief that others can insert thoughts into the person's mind).

Motor symptoms are common in individuals with schizophrenia and range from motor retardation or slowing to posturing and catatonic states. **Catatonia** is a state of unresponsiveness in an individual who is conscious. It may incorporate features such as *mutism* (lack of speech), *echopraxia* (repeating the movements of others), *echolalia* (repeating the words of others), *waxy flexibility* (maintaining whatever position the individual is placed in), and *automatic obedience* (automatic, robotic cooperation with requests). Catatonia can also manifest as an excited state that includes combativeness and impulsivity. Other psychomotor symptoms may be the result of associated neurologic abnormalities and include oculomotor abnormalities, grimacing, and problems with motor sequencing and coordination (Dean et al., 2020; Maes, Sirivichayakul, Kanchanatawan, & Carvalho, 2020; Ungvari, Gerevich, Takács, & Gazdag, 2018).

Disorganized thinking, also referred to as a *formal thought disorder (FTD)*, is generally manifested in disruption of the form and organization of speech. Individuals with FTD lack appropriate, goal-directed thought processes and demonstrate a pattern of abnormal speech, including **loose associations**, tangentiality, incoherence, circumstantiality, and pressured speech. Table 23.1 provides definitions for these indicators of disorganized thinking.

Positive Symptoms	Negative Symptoms	Cognitive Symptoms
Additions to normal experiences: • Delusions • Hallucinations • Abnormal movements • Formal thought disorder	Diminished affects and behaviors: • Flat or blunted affect • Thought blocking • Avolition • Poverty of speech • Social withdrawal	Cognitive issues may include: • Memory deficits • Attention deficits • Language difficulties • Loss of executive function

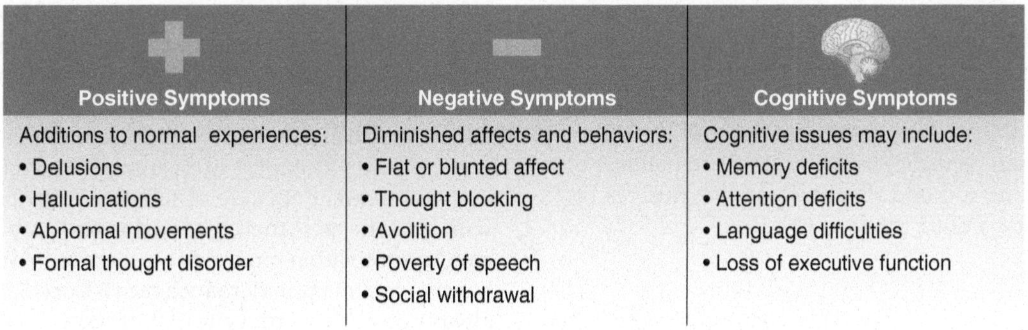

Figure 23.7 ›› The symptoms of schizophrenia have been categorized as positive, negative, and cognitive.
Source: From Potter and Moller (2020). Pearson Education, Inc., Hoboken, NJ.

Negative Symptoms

Negative symptoms refer to affects and behaviors that are diminished or absent in individuals with schizophrenia. These include having a flat or blunted affect, thought blocking (a sudden interruption in speech without explanation), **alogia** (poverty of thought and speech), **anhedonia** (inability to experience pleasure), **avolition** (lack of motivation or initiative), and social withdrawal. Negative symptoms tend to persist during all phases of the illness, are difficult to treat, and account for the some of the most disabling manifestations of the illness.

Cognitive Symptoms

Cognitive symptoms of schizophrenia include deficits in memory, attention, language, visuospatial awareness, social and emotional perception, and intellectual and executive function. Memory deficits impact verbal processing, and individuals with schizophrenia may have difficulty with verbal fluency, pragmatics, and other aspects of spontaneous language. Visual memory deficits and impaired spatial processing also contribute to impaired social interactions. Individuals with schizophrenia often demonstrate poor facial recognition (facial agnosia) and may have difficulty with proxemics and nonverbal processing (e.g., modulating how close to stand to someone or interpreting nonverbal gestures). Individuals with schizophrenia demonstrate difficulty with attention and vigilance and may have difficulty concentrating on tasks that require a sustained focus. They are prone to sensory overload due to difficulty filtering out extraneous information. Studies have demonstrated an association between diminished global intellectual functioning and schizophrenia, with many affected individuals having difficulty with measures of both verbal and perceptual reasoning. Patients with schizophrenia frequently demonstrate **concrete thinking**, focusing on literal aspects of facts and details, and exhibit limited insight (Bora, 2017). Problems with executive functioning may manifest as difficulty with planning and organization, problem solving, and modulating impulses. Studies have shown that higher levels of cognitive impairment in individuals with schizophrenia are associated with poorer overall outcomes (Strassnig et al., 2018).

Affective Symptoms

In addition to positive, negative, and cognitive symptoms, patients with schizophrenia may also exhibit a number of affective symptoms, especially depression. Affective symptoms such as depression and mania significantly increase the risk of suicide in patients with schizophrenia, especially in combination with other variables such as younger or older age, high IQ, higher levels of premorbid function, proximity to onset, male sex, and recent discharge from the hospital (Beckmann, Schnitzer, & Freudenreich, 2020; Gooding, Littlewood, Owen, Johnson, & Tarrier, 2019). In patients with schizophrenia and a mood disorder, the diagnosis is often modified to *schizoaffective disorder*.

Phases of the Illness

The classic course of schizophrenia consists of premorbid, prodromal, acute, and residual phases. Research demonstrates that acute symptoms of the disorder appear to diminish as individuals grow older, with negative and cognitive symptoms becoming more pronounced and disabling. Some individuals may actually achieve complete remission of psychotic symptoms (Lally et al., 2017). Possible explanations for this include age-related dopaminergic activity changes.

Premorbid

Although 75% of patients with schizophrenia are diagnosed during adolescence or early adulthood, a number of alterations may be evident during childhood and the period immediately preceding the onset of the illness. *Premorbid* manifestations occurring in childhood include a number of nonspecific emotional, cognitive, and motor delays that have been identified in individuals who went on to develop schizophrenia (Noguera et al., 2018).

Prodromal Phase

The *prodromal phase* is a symptomatic period that signals a definite shift from premorbid functioning and continues until psychotic symptoms emerge. Manifestations include sleep disturbance, poor concentration, social withdrawal, perceptual abnormalities, and other attenuated or weakened symptoms of psychosis. A dramatic drop in functional or adaptive capabilities may occur with academic and vocational failure. The length of the prodromal period varies considerably, but for most individuals it lasts for 2 to 5 years (McCutcheon, Reis Marques, & Howes, 2020; Powers et al., 2020).

Acute Phase

The *acute phase* of the illness is marked by the onset of florid psychotic/positive symptoms. It generally follows the prodromal period but, in some instances, appears suddenly. This period causes significant distress for the individual and is often the first time that help is sought. If the behavior represents a danger to the individual or others, short-term hospitalization may be required. The number of acute phases experienced by individuals is highly variable and depends, in part, on the ability to access high-quality treatment. In general, longer durations of untreated acute psychosis are associated with poorer long- and short-term patient outcomes (Sarpal et al., 2017).

Residual Phase

The *residual phase* of schizophrenia can be further broken down into the stabilization phase (6 to 18 months after the resolution of the acute phase) and the maintenance phase, during which patients are able to resume full functioning, although perhaps not at preillness levels. The stabilization phase involves the movement to immediate recovery (mentioned earlier) and then toward rehabilitation and fuller functioning. It is important to remember that disabling cognitive and negative symptoms may persist during the residual phase. In addition, the patient may continue to demonstrate odd patterns of thinking and behavior. The level of dysfunction often increases with each subsequent episode of relapse. Patients often struggle with side effects of their medication and may lack the insight and/or motivation required to adhere to treatment. Comprehensive treatment may reduce the risk of relapse, but it is not always possible to prevent it altogether. Careful monitoring of symptoms can often detect a shift toward the active state of the illness (Lecomte et al., 2019).

Comorbid Disorders

Schizophrenia is associated with a number of psychiatric and medical comorbidities, which are described in this section. The presence of these conditions adds to the overall burden of the illness and accounts for the significant reduction in lifespan for affected individuals. Contributing factors to comorbid illness include self-care deficits, sedentary lifestyles, social isolation, lack of access to quality healthcare, and poor dietary habits.

Individuals with schizophrenia are at increased risk for cardiovascular disease, diabetes, COPD, and many infectious diseases. Approximately 50–60% of individuals with schizophrenia smoke cigarettes, possibly because of the short-term relief of symptoms associated with nicotine and its effect on nicotinic receptors (Šagud et al., 2018). Some studies suggest that cardiovascular problems in patients with schizophrenia are frequently undertreated by HCPs (Attar et al., 2018; Correll et al., 2017). Treatment with antipsychotic medications contributes to the overall risk of both cardiovascular disease and diabetes, as common effects include sedation, increased food intake, hyperlipidemia, and alterations in glucose regulation (Jeon & Kim, 2017; MacKenzie et al., 2018).

Comorbid substance abuse is found in almost 50% of all individuals with schizophrenia (Hunt, Large, Cleary, Lai, & Saunders, 2018). Apart from caffeine and nicotine, the main substances of abuse used by individuals with schizophrenia are alcohol, cannabis, and opioids (Center for Behavioral Health Statistics and Quality, 2019). Comorbid depression occurs in an estimated 40–60% of individuals with schizophrenia (Upthegrove, Marwaha, & Birchwood, 2017). Interestingly, multiple studies indicate that individuals with higher levels of premorbid function and greater awareness of the implications of their disorder are more likely to experience depression. Anxiety disorders also occur with greater frequency in schizophrenia, with a rate of about 30% (Bulbena-Cabre & Bulbena, 2018). Posttraumatic stress disorder may be seen in 15% of all patients, roughly double the rate of the general population (Okkels, Trabjerg, Arendt, & Pedersen, 2017).

Collaboration

The management of schizophrenia is challenging for both patient and HCPs. A number of factors complicate treatment. These include characteristic clinical manifestations such as avolition and disordered thought processes and insufficient availability of and access to quality mental health care. Although schizophrenia is a biological illness, many insurance policies continue to place restrictions on the types of services that can be accessed. Another factor complicating the diagnosis and treatment of schizophrenia relates to cultural biases and influences. See Focus on Diversity and Culture: Schizophrenia.

Because of these many factors, the time from diagnosis to recovery is lengthy—often taking as long as four years for patients to be able to adhere to treatment independently and begin working toward goals they had before the onset of psychosis (Potter & Moller, 2020).

Focus on Diversity and Culture

Schizophrenia

Another factor that affects diagnosis and treatment of schizophrenia is provider bias. Numerous studies have demonstrated that people of African and Hispanic heritage are up to three times more likely to be diagnosed with schizophrenia than are Caucasian people (Olbert, Nagendra, & Buck, 2018). Researchers have concluded that this phenomenon occurs even in the absence of a genetic predisposition to the disorder within these populations, suggesting that provider bias plays a significant role (Olbert et al., 2018; Schwartz, Docherty, Najolia, & Cohen, 2019). Psychiatric diagnoses rely, in part, on provider judgment as to whether or not certain behaviors deviate from the norm. In many instances, providers do not account for cultural variances or the context in which behaviors occur (Andrews, Boyle, & Collins, 2020). As a result, it is possible that individuals from communities of color may be more reluctant to report affective symptoms that suggest other disorders. Nurses and other HCPs need to assess individual variables that may lead to misdiagnosis. Nursing care should not depend on diagnostic labels that may not consider patient-centered needs.

Diagnostic Tests

Qualified mental health providers diagnose schizophrenia on the basis of findings obtained during a psychiatric evaluation of the patient. The evaluation generally includes a history and examination and may incorporate the use of screening tools and psychometric tests. Medical tests such as laboratory values and imaging studies are used to rule out other conditions. The patient must meet the criteria identified in the DSM-5, as exemplified by clinical manifestations described earlier. Diagnostic criteria specify that the individual must have experienced significant impairment of functioning for 6 or more months in one or more areas, such as home, work, and self-care. Other mental disorders, such as bipolar disorder, and substance use also must be ruled out for a diagnosis of schizophrenia to be made (APA, 2013; Dollfus & Lyne, 2017; Parnas & Zandersen, 2018).

Like other neurocognitive disorders discussed in this module, a number of biomarkers have been identified for schizophrenia, including the brain-imaging findings depicted in **Figure 23.8** ⟫. Presently, biomarker analysis and diagnostic imaging are in the research stage, but there have been studies on metabolite biomarkers, such as reduced levels of essential polyunsaturated fatty acids, vitamin E, and creatinine; elevated levels of lipid peroxidation metabolites and glutamate (Davison, O'Gorman, Brennan, & Cotter, 2018); analysis of gut microbiota diversity (Shen et al., 2018); peripheral blood micro RNA (He, Guo, He, & Shi, 2017); and abnormal visual saccades (eye movements) (Caldani et al., 2017). In the future, biomarkers and imaging may be used to confirm preclinical findings or to validate a diagnosis of schizophrenia.

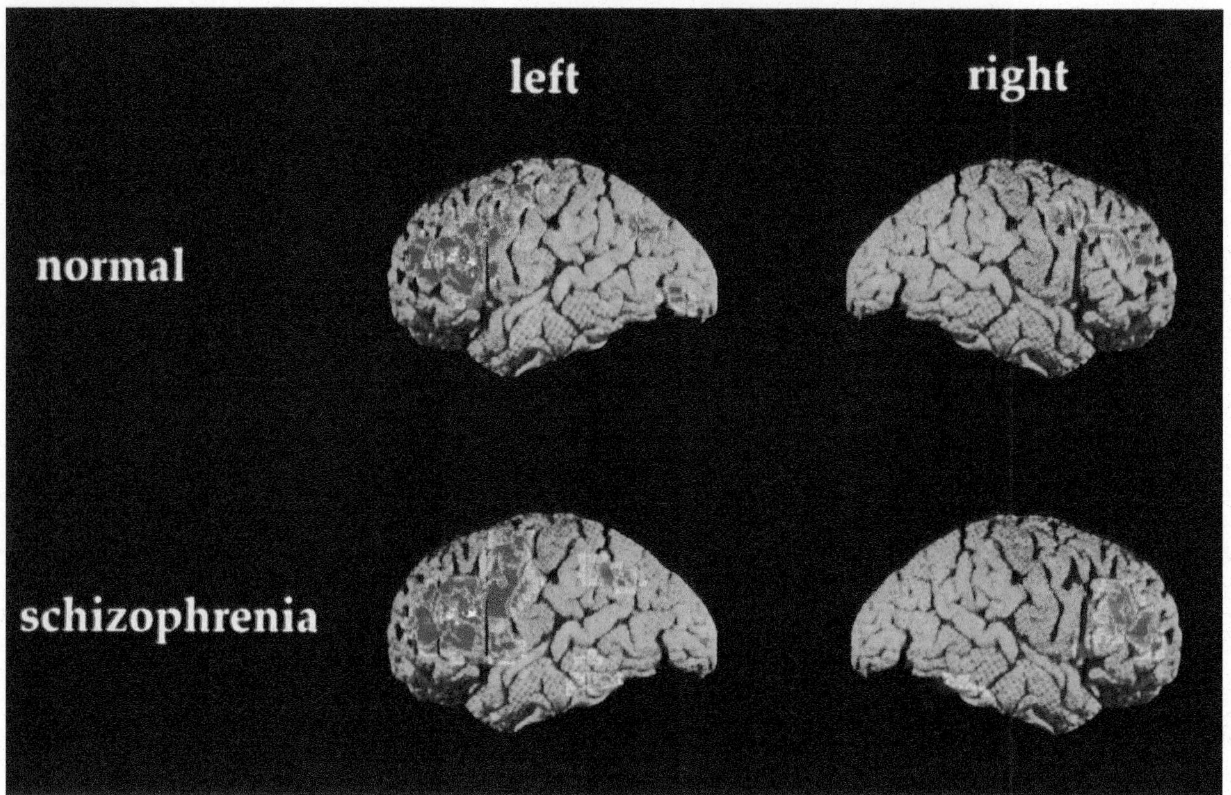

Figure 23.8 ›› These PET scans show the difference between the brains of a normal patient and a patient with schizophrenia during a verbal fluency task—that is, the patients were asked to speak words. The red and yellow areas were activated when the subjects spoke the words. In the normal subject (*top row*), the brain shows much activity in the prefrontal and motor areas and less activity in the parietal area on the left side. In the subject with schizophrenia (*bottom row*), there is also activity in the middle temporal gyrus (lower center of brain), which is not seen in the normal subject.

Source: Wellcome Department of Cognitive Neurology/Science Source.

Pharmacologic Therapy

The first line of intervention for schizophrenia is pharmacologic treatment with antipsychotic medications. The primary goal of pharmacotherapy is to decrease the positive symptoms (such as hallucinations and delusions) of the disorder to a level that enables the individual to maintain social relationships and complete ADLs with minimal assistance. Antipsychotics do not cure schizophrenia, and they elicit a therapeutic response in only about 50% of patients (Leucht et al., 2017; Zhang et al., 2019). In patients who benefit from antipsychotic medication, those positive symptoms improve more than negative symptoms (such as depression and a lack of emotional expression, social interaction, and motivation) (Leucht et al., 2017). The relapse rate for individuals who discontinue medication therapy is approximately 50-80%; patients who take breaks in medication have five times the chance of relapse than patients who adhere to their medication regimen (Adams et al., 2020; Winton-Brown et al., 2017). Adherence to pharmacologic treatment is challenged by factors such as denial or poor insight into the illness, self-care deficits, and the incidence of common and serious adverse effects.

Life-threatening issues that should be considered with the use of antipsychotics include an increased risk of suicide. Early research showed that antipsychotics protected against suicide, but more current research has shown that the medications may actually increase the rate of suicide, likely because of unpleasant side effects (Adams et al., 2020). One 4-year study showed that there was a high prevalence, in up to 48% of the study population, of antipsychotics detected in toxicology screenings in 477 people who committed suicide (Methling, Krumbiegel, Hartwig, Parr, & Tsokos, 2019).

SAFETY ALERT! Antipsychotics, which are sedating, have been used to treat behavioral and psychological symptoms of dementia. However, they have been linked with increased risk for older adults of hospitalization, cardiovascular events, hip fractures, and mortality, among other adverse health events (Cioltan et al., 2017). The atypical (second-generation antipsychotics) carry a black box warning that they are not to be used for patients with dementia-related psychosis due to an increased risk of death (Adams et al., 2020).

Antipsychotic medications include older, conventional agents called typical antipsychotics (first generation), atypical antipsychotics (second generation), and dopamine system stabilizers (third generation), as outlined in **Medications 23.2**, Drugs Used to Treat Schizophrenia. The efficacy of all classes of antipsychotics in treating the acute symptoms of the disease is about the same. However, within each drug class, different drugs have properties that may make them more or less suitable for treating certain target symptoms within the scope of antipsychotic symptoms. In addition, the profile of each drug's side effects and adverse effects may differ. When selecting a drug to treat psychotic symptoms, clinicians consider factors such as the severity of symptoms, prior degree of symptom response, adherence factors (such as dosing convenience or cost), side effect profile, and patient needs (Citrome, 2017; Miyamoto & Fleischhacker, 2017). Long-acting injectable formulations may increase adherence. An adequate treatment trial that demonstrates a full response to the medication may take anywhere from 3 to 10 weeks and is necessary to evaluate efficacy, although symptoms such as hallucinations and delusions may diminish within days.

Typical or conventional antipsychotics include the phenothiazine type (such as chlorpromazine) and nonphenothiazine type (such as haloperidol). This was the "first generation" of drugs introduced to treat schizophrenia. The mechanism of action for both phenothiazine and nonphenothiazine

Medications 23.2

Drugs Used to Treat Schizophrenia

CLASSIFICATION AND DRUG EXAMPLES	MECHANISMS OF ACTION	NURSING IMPLICATIONS
First-Generation (Typical or Conventional) Antipsychotics **Phenothiazines** ***Drug examples:*** chlorpromazine fluphenazine perphenazine thioridazine trifluoperazine **Nonphenothiazines** ***Drug examples:*** haloperidol (Haldol) loxapine (Adasuve)* molindone pimozide (Orap) thiothixene	Both phenothiazines and nonphenothiazines block D_2 dopamine receptors in the brain, increasing synaptic levels of dopamine and leading to a decrease in positive symptoms of psychosis (including delusions and hallucinations). ***May also be used for:*** ■ Other psychotic disorders, bipolar disorder, severe combativeness, nonpsychotic anxiety ■ Tourette syndrome	■ First-generation antipsychotic drugs are given orally or by intramuscular or intravenous injection. Loxapine (Adasuve) is a powder that is inhaled. ■ Monitor for anticholinergic symptoms, such as dry mouth, orthostatic hypotension, constipation, urinary retention, sedation, and sexual dysfunction. ■ Teach patient strategies to address anticholinergic effects (e.g., rising slowly, increasing fluid intake, and increasing fiber intake). ■ Monitor for EPS, such as acute dystonia, akathisia, parkinsonism, and TD. ■ Monitor for signs of hyperprolactemia (menstrual irregularities, decreased libido, gynecomastia, and osteoporosis). Adjunctive therapies, counseling, or changing to a different agent may improve some aspects of sexual dysfunction. ■ Monitor for autonomic instability associated with neuroleptic malignant syndrome and teach patients to seek emergency help if NMS presents. ■ Teach patients importance of adhering to medication regimen and not to abruptly discontinue medication. ■ Monitor for increased risk of suicide. ■ Teach patients importance of wearing sunscreen.
Second-Generation (Atypical) Antipsychotics ***Drug examples:*** asenapine (Saphris, Secuado) clozapine (Clozaril) iloperidone (Fanapt) lurasidone (Latuda) olanzapine (Zyprexa, Zyprexa Relprevv) paliperidone (Invega, Invega Sustenna, Invega Trinza) pimavanserin (Nuplazid) quetiapine (Seroquel) risperidone (Perseris, Risperdal) ziprasidone (Geodon)	Block D_2 dopamine and 5-HT serotonin receptors; treat both positive and negative symptoms of schizophrenia and psychotic disorders and exert mood-stabilizing effect. ***May also be used for:*** ■ Other psychotic disorders ■ Bipolar disorder	■ Second-generation antipsychotic drugs are all given orally. Olanzapine, risperidone, and ziprasidone can also be given by the intramuscular route. Paliperidone can also be given IM every month (Invega Sustena) or every 3 months (Invega Trinza). Asenapine is the first FDA-approved antipsychotic drug available as a transdermal patch (Secuado). ■ Monitor for adverse effects, such as alterations in glucose metabolism, hyperlipidemia, cardiovascular and cerebrovascular alterations, and blood abnormalities. ■ Teach importance of healthy diet and exercise. ■ Monitor for EPS and neuroleptic malignant syndrome. ■ Monitor patients on clozapine (Clozaril) for agranulocytosis and severe granulocytopenia. ■ Monitor for increased risk of suicide. ■ *FDA Black Box Warning:* Do not use in patients with dementia; increased risk of death due to pneumonia.

(continued on next page)

Medications 23.2 *(continued)*

CLASSIFICATION AND DRUG EXAMPLES	MECHANISMS OF ACTION	NURSING IMPLICATIONS
Dopamine system stabilizers (DSS) ***Drug examples:*** aripiprazole (Abilify,* Abilify Maintena) brexpiprazole (Rexulti) cariprazine (Vraylar) *See the Stay Current feature.	Partial agonists of D_2 receptors, also block serotonin receptors. Treat both positive and negative symptoms of schizophrenia and psychotic disorders, exert mood-stabilizing effect. Block 5-HT receptors. Only partially block D_2 receptors and also partially activate D_2 receptors. This provides a stabilizing effect, in that the excessive dopamine that causes schizophrenia is decreased but a total lack of dopamine that causes anticholinergic side effects is avoided.	■ Although generally well tolerated, patients should still be monitored for EPS, NMS, and medical effects associated with atypical antipsychotics. ■ Akathisia and restlessness may be more pronounced with these medications. ■ Teaching should address healthy diet and exercise, importance of adherence, and recognizing and reporting adverse effects. ■ Monitor for increased risk of suicide

Source: Based on Adams et al. (2020).

antipsychotics is believed to be the blocking of postsynaptic D_2 receptors. First-generation antipsychotics mainly treat the positive symptoms of schizophrenia. Unfortunately, there are numerous adverse effects associated with typical antipsychotics that range from uncomfortable to disabling and life-threatening.

Anticholinergic effects occur, such as dry mouth, sedation, constipation, postural hypotension, and urinary retention. These effects are uncomfortable and place patients at increased risk of injury and infection. Sexual side effects such as ejaculation disorders and delay in achieving orgasm may be troubling for patients. Endocrine effects such as hyperprolactinemia can lead to osteoporosis, menstrual irregularities, decreased libido, gynecomastia, lactation, and erectile dysfunction.

Extrapyramidal symptoms (EPS) frequently occur with first-generation antipsychotics and include *akathisia, dystonia,* secondary *parkinsonism,* and *tardive dyskinesia.* The most common EPS is **akathisia**, a feeling of uncomfortable restlessness that is often not recognized and managed appropriately. **Dystonia** often results in sudden and severe muscle spasms in the face, neck, and torso that can be frightening and painful for patients and have the potential to lead to airway obstruction if not identified and reversed. Secondary parkinsonism has some of the symptoms of Parkinson disease, as manifested by tremors, muscle rigidity, masked facies (lack of facial expression), stooped posture, and shuffling gait. **Tardive dyskinesia (TD)** is an often-irreversible condition characterized by unusual facial movements, lip smacking, and wormlike movements of the tongue. **Neuroleptic malignant syndrome (NMS)** is a potentially fatal condition characterized by severe autonomic instability. Manifestations include high fever, confusion, changes in level of consciousness, muscle rigidity, and hyperthermia.

Management of adverse effects such as anticholinergic symptoms and EPS often includes the concurrent use of antiparkinsonian anticholinergic medications, such as benztropine (Cogentin) and trihexyphenidyl normalize the level of dopamine to help decrease stiffness and rigidity. Parenteral benztropine and diphenhydramine (Benadryl) can quickly reverse dystonia and extrapyramidal symptoms. TD is usually managed with a reduction in dose or a switch to another agent. If NMS is suspected, antipsychotic agents are immediately discontinued and the patient is admitted to the intensive care unit for supportive care.

Atypical antipsychotics (also called second-generation antipsychotics) are believed to also block D_2 receptors, although they have a weaker affinity that may account for the lower profile of certain side effects. In addition, atypical antipsychotics also block serotonin and alpha-adrenergic receptors. Atypical antipsychotics treat both positive and negative symptoms of the illness, although definitive proof and high-quality research on efficacy for treating negative symptoms is lacking (Veerman, Schulte, & de Haan, 2017). Examples of atypical antipsychotics include risperidone (Risperdal), lurasidone (Latuda), and olanzapine (Zyprexa). One advantage of atypical antipsychotics seems to be a lower incidence of EPS and TD at therapeutic doses. However, adverse effects can still be quite severe, with an increased risk of medical problems such as metabolic syndrome, cardiovascular and cerebrovascular events, type 2 diabetes mellitus, blood dyscrasias, seizures, and sudden death, especially for older adults with dementia. Anticholinergic effects, endocrine effects, TD, and NMS can also occur with these atypical antipsychotic medications.

Dopamine-serotonin system stabilizers (DSSs)—also called dopamine partial agonists or third-generation antipsychotics—have therapeutic benefits similar to those of atypical antipsychotics, but with an even lower profile of adverse effects. These drugs are generally well tolerated, with very few anticholinergic side effects and a lower incidence of weight gain. They also seem to target affective symptoms, such as anxiety and depression. DSSs are rarely used as a first-line treatment, but they are often useful as an adjunct therapy.

In addition to antipsychotics, individuals may be treated with adjunctive medications such as antianxiety agents, antidepressants, and mood stabilizers. These medications are discussed in Module 31, Stress and Coping, and in Module 28, Mood and Affect.

>> **Stay Current:** The dopamine system stabilizer aripiprazole (Abilify) is available as an oral tablet (called Abilify MyCite) that contains an ingestible event marker (IEM). The tablet comes with a sensor that is worn on the skin above the lower edge of the left rib cage. When the tablet is ingested, the IEM transmits data to an app on a smartphone. This helps with patient adherence (compliance) with the antipsychotic drug. The app also messages the smartphone when it is time to change the patch (weekly).

Nonpharmacologic Therapy

As mentioned previously, the recovery and rehabilitation model is the overarching approach to caring for individuals with schizophrenia outside of hospital and institutional settings. This model does not represent any single distinct pathway to care, but instead recognizes that individuals maintain their own life goals and should be provided with a variety of resources that will empower them to make informed decisions and build on their own strengths in order to regain control of their lives. Pharmacologic interventions alone are insufficient to address the complex needs of individuals with schizophrenia. Nurses providing care to patients with schizophrenia across all settings can anticipate interfacing with a variety of team members, including psychiatrists, social workers, occupational therapists, psychologists, psychiatric rehabilitation specialists, and mental health workers.

Family Intervention and Psychoeducation

Research demonstrates that the provision of family interventions, such as psychoeducation and counseling, can reduce the relapse rate for schizophrenia from 20 to 40% (Camacho-Gomez & Castellvi, 2019). Studies indicate that the best results are achieved when family interventions continue over several months and are combined with pharmacologic interventions and other treatment modalities. Some studies indicate that family psychoeducation in particular reduces the subjective burden of schizophrenia and leads to a more positive family atmosphere (Soliman, Mahdy, & Fouad, 2018).

Social Skills Training

Schizophrenia is characterized by deficits in social cognition that have a profound effect on the individual's ability to accurately read social cues and respond appropriately. Social skills training employs a systematic approach to teaching individuals with schizophrenia how to interact with others. One particularly effective approach is *social cognition and interaction training (SCIT)*. SCIT is a group intervention delivered over a 6-month period. Participants work with trained therapists on three phases that consist of learning about emotions, figuring out situations, and practicing what was learned. Computerized exercises, videos, and other tools may be used to enhance learning. The overall effectiveness of such programs is still under investigation; however, some studies suggest that that the best results are achieved when SCIT is combined with cognitive remediation (Darmedru, Demily, & Franck, 2017; Gordon et al., 2018; Grant, Lawrence, Preti, Wykes, & Cella, 2017; Horan & Green, 2019).

Cognitive-Behavioral Therapy

CBT is a psychosocial treatment that may be helpful in assisting patients with schizophrenia to cope with their symptoms by using distraction, positive self-talk, or behavioral processes such as exercising and deep breathing. In CBT, patients are encouraged to reframe symptoms of psychosis as attempts to cope. Problem-solving techniques are used to identify and make use of new coping strategies. Although earlier studies supported the efficacy of CBT for schizophrenia, during the past decade, research has questioned the benefit of CBT, claiming that it results in only modest therapeutic effects (Jauhar, Laws, & McKenna, 2019; Laws, Darlington, Kondel, McKenna, & Jauhar, 2018). Some researchers argue that these findings fail to consider benefits outside improvement in positive and negative symptoms (such as improvements in coping mechanisms) (Jones et al., 2018). Since the evidence available is not robust, high-quality research is needed about the efficacy of CBT (Bighelli et al., 2018).

Cognitive Remediation

Cognitive remediation or rehabilitation includes strategies aimed to address cognitive deficits associated with schizophrenia. Techniques are similar to educational interventions employed in special education and focus on compensatory strategies as well as drill-and-practice techniques aimed at strengthening specific cognitive functions, such as working memory. Compensatory techniques include organizing and modifying the home environment to support adaptive function (labeling items, making lists, posting emergency numbers) and assisting patients to break down new skills into smaller steps that are then overlearned. Rehabilitation techniques include the use of computer programs that "exercise" certain cognitive functions through engaging games and activities. Because many models are used, the efficacy of these programs is difficult to measure; however, studies suggest that the programs are beneficial and incorporate opportunities for real-world practice (Bryce et al., 2018; Tripathi, Kar, & Shukla, 2018).

Vocational Training

Vocational rehabilitation or training encompasses a variety of services aimed at increasing functional capacity and reducing unemployment for individuals with schizophrenia. Vocational programs aim to increase employability by providing skills training. Supported employment programs assist patients to find and maintain employment. Vocational training may be incorporated into one of the community service models discussed in this section.

Community Service Models

A variety of community service models are available to address the needs of individuals with schizophrenia. Some of the most common models include crisis intervention teams, case management, and ACT.

Crisis intervention refers to short-term, intensive measures to address symptoms or behaviors that impact the safety and equilibrium of the patient and others. The portal of entry into crisis intervention may be the emergency department or through a mobile crisis intervention or outreach team. After an assessment is made, interventions such as medication adjustment, 24-hour monitoring, ECT, or a change in services are implemented in the least restrictive environment possible. For some patients, this may mean a short inpatient stay; for others, services may be provided in the community in the patient's home, in a residential treatment center, or through a combination of partial day treatment and home care. *Mobile crisis outreach teams* consist of interprofessional team members who are deployed to the site of the crisis for assessment and intervention. They have special training that may be used to effectively deescalate the situation and usually work in collaboration with law enforcement.

>> **Stay Current:** For more information on mobile outreach teams and other crisis intervention services, visit the National Alliance for the Mentally Ill "Getting Treatment During a Crisis" at https://www.nami.org/Learn-More/Treatment/Getting-Treatment-During-a-Crisis.

Case management is a method of coordinating care by assigning each individual to a case manager or a qualified person who completes an assessment of patient needs, develops a plan, coordinates appropriate services, monitors the quality of care being provided, and maintains a collaborative relationship with the affected individual (see Module 39, Managing Care). Most clinicians agree that competent case management is essential for community-dwelling patients (Díaz-Fernández, Frías-Ortiz, & Fernández-Miranda, 2019).

Assertive community treatment (ACT) aims to meet many of the same goals as case management, but ACT is a service delivery model in which interprofessional team members share accountability for meeting patient needs in a collaborative and often intensive manner. Most individuals involved in ACT can expect to meet with more than one team member on a weekly basis. Services are available 24 hours a day and 7 days a week. ACT models follow a specific high-fidelity framework for meeting patient needs (such as medical care, housing, social support, and employment) by limiting team-member caseloads and by providing services directly rather than relying on referrals to agencies. The usefulness of ACT has been validated by research, which shows that ACT decreases patient hospitalization time and severity of symptoms while improving stability and quality of life (Schmidt et al., 2018; Schöttle et al., 2018).

Electroconvulsive Therapy

Electroconvulsive therapy (ECT) is a procedure that delivers small electric currents through the brain under general anesthesia, usually without intubation. ECT is not typically used to treat schizophrenia but appears to demonstrate some efficacy for emergency situations or treatment-resistant schizophrenia with certain symptoms, such as depression, paranoia, catatonia, and suicidal ideation (Sanghani, Petrides, & Kellner, 2018; Sinclair et al., 2019). ECT is most effective when used in conjunction with medication. For more information on this procedure, refer to Module 28, Mood and Affect.

Repetitive Transcranial Magnetic Stimulation

Repetitive transcranial magnetic stimulation (rTMS) is a type of therapy that uses an electromagnet placed on the scalp to deliver pulses roughly equivalent to the strength of an MRI. The FDA has approved rTMS for the treatment of depression. The efficacy of rTMS in treating auditory hallucinations and other symptoms of schizophrenia has been the subject of research for several years. Recent research suggests that rTMS may help reduce auditory hallucinations (He et al., 2017). However, there is currently insufficient robust evidence to conclude that rTMS is an effective standardized treatment for schizophrenia (Iimori et al., 2019; Marzouk, Winkelbeiner, Azizi, Malhotra, & Homan, 2019).

Complementary Health Approaches

Integrative and complementary treatments for schizophrenia include the use of nutritional interventions and supplements and the use of mind–body practices. There is no evidence to suggest that any of these treatments are effective alternatives to the collaborative interventions just discussed.

Research on nutritional interventions has focused on potential risks and benefits of supplementation with B vitamins, vitamin D, and omega-3 fatty acids. Currently the most positive and conclusive findings support the use of omega-3 fatty acids in the prodromal and residual phases of the disease (Markulev et al., 2017; Satogami, Takahashi, Yamada, Ukai, & Shinosaki, 2017). However, some research suggests that the use of omega-3 fatty acids has no impact on schizophrenia symptoms (Qiao et al., 2020). Safety and practical considerations should guide the use of nutritional interventions. The use of supplements should be discussed with HCPs so that an individual assessment of the risks versus potential benefits can be made.

Lifespan Considerations

As previously stated, the majority of individuals with schizophrenia experience an emergence of symptoms in early adulthood with a classic course preceded by prodromal symptoms and a lessening of positive symptoms with aging. The remainder of individuals with schizophrenia may be grouped into those with *early-onset schizophrenia (EOS)* (before the age of 18) or a pattern of later onset (after the age of 40), sometimes referred to as *late-onset schizophrenia (LOS)*.

Early-Onset Schizophrenia

EOS generally refers to the emergence of symptoms of schizophrenia before 17 to 18 years of age. Onset prior to puberty is extremely rare, occurring in less than one case per 10,000 population, and is further classified as *childhood-onset schizophrenia (COS)*. In general, childhood schizophrenia may be more difficult to diagnose. Hallucinations are less complex and may focus on childhood themes such as monsters and toys, making them difficult to distinguish from fantasy play (Mayo Clinic, 2020b). Symptoms such as obsessive–compulsive disorder, disordered speech, motor deficits, cognitive deficits, and social withdrawal may overlap with manifestations of developmental disorders such as autism spectrum disorders (Baytunca et al., 2017; Martinez et al., 2019).

Adolescents who experience EOS demonstrate symptoms similar to the adult variants of the disorder. Onset in adolescence seems to be at least slightly more prevalent in boys and is associated with an increased risk of suicide, especially in those with a history of abuse or trauma (Mayo Clinic, 2020b; Mohammadzadeh, Azadi, King, Khosravani, & Sharifi Bastan, 2019). The overall prognosis for both children and adolescents with EOS is poor and is associated with greater symptom burden and higher levels of disability (Grover, Sahoo, & Nehra, 2019; Knorr, 2017). Management of EOS includes many of the same treatments and therapies that are used with adults with appropriate developmental modifications. Significant side effects include weight gain, metabolic side effects, extrapyramidal symptoms, sedation, somnolence, and unexpected death (Ayub, Ramtekkar, & Reiersen, 2018; Pillay et al., 2018; Ray et al., 2019). Children are at increased risk of adverse effects from psychotropic medications, and many agents do not demonstrate the same efficacy as is observed in adults.

Late-Onset Schizophrenia

About 20–30% of all patients do not experience symptoms of schizophrenia until after age 40. The incidence of LOS seems to be greater in women, but other risk factors for the disease are comparable to those associated with an earlier onset. Typically, positive symptoms of the disease are more predominant, with paranoia, elaborate delusions, and hallucinations (Van Assche et al., 2018). Both cognitive and negative manifestations of the disease are higher than in the general population but lower than what is commonly observed in adult-onset schizophrenia. Patients with LOS often respond to lower doses of antipsychotic medication. These findings have led some scientists to suggest that late-onset schizophrenia may even represent a distinct disorder (Belbeze & Gallarda, 2020).

When symptoms of schizophrenia do not emerge until after age 60, the condition is often referred to as *very-late-onset schizophrenia (VLOS)*. VLOS can be distinguished from other variants by a lower genetic load and a higher level of premorbid function. The etiology of VLOS is believed to be neurodegenerative and organic factors. The incidence is higher in immigrant populations, suggesting that sociocultural factors also play a role (Häfner, 2019). Management may include lower-dose antipsychotics and psychosocial interventions.

NURSING PROCESS

The application of the nursing process depends on many factors, including the phase of the illness the patient is experiencing. Primarily, nursing goals for patients with schizophrenia include promoting symptom control and facilitating effective coping to help the patient achieve optimal mental, physical, and social functioning. Ideally, the patient will avoid further episodes of psychosis and be able to function successfully in the community to the greatest degree possible.

Assessment

Nursing assessment of a patient with schizophrenia typically involves three main elements: a patient interview, a physical examination, and a mental status examination.

Observation and Patient Interview

Nurses and others may notice a number of symptoms in patients with schizophrenia: deteriorating personal appearance and neglect of personal hygiene; weight loss; unusual gestures; pacing; or incoherence characterized by making up words or speaking in sentences that make no sense (word salad). Many individuals with schizophrenia smoke, so a noticeable odor of smoke or tobacco may be present. A lack of insight is characteristic of schizophrenia, so patients may be unaware of these changes or actions.

For the patient with known or suspected schizophrenia, elements of the health history should include age; family history and paternal age; history of perinatal health problems or exposures, developmental delays, or exposure to trauma or adversity; history of behaviors such as substance abuse; history of positive, negative, cognitive, and affective manifestations; family coping; history of commonly comorbid mental illness (such as substance use or mood disorders); and presence or emergence of major life stressors.

For the patient diagnosed with schizophrenia, ask about possible risk factors for exacerbations or signs of relapse, such as:

- Poor adherence to the prescribed treatment regimen (especially pharmacologic therapy)
- Possible development of resistance to antipsychotic medications
- Presence of mild to full-blown symptoms of psychosis
- Recent life events that may increase the likelihood of relapse.

Physical Examination

Next, during the physical examination, evaluate the patient's overall physical condition. Throughout the physical exam, remain alert for possible signs of metabolic problems, cardiovascular problems, drug/alcohol abuse, and poor self-care, as schizophrenia increases the risk for all of these. Note any evidence of side effects from medications, such as movement problems, weight gain, or changes in vital signs.

Mental Status Examination

Finally, individuals with known or suspected schizophrenia should receive a thorough mental status examination. Nurses can choose from a variety of assessment instruments, as described in the Mental Assessment feature. Regardless of which tool is used, closely monitor for possible manifestations of schizophrenia throughout the mental status exam. Also keep in mind the patient's cultural and religious background, as this can affect an individual's description and interpretation of symptoms such as auditory and visual hallucinations.

Following the health history, physical exam, and mental status examination, several steps may be appropriate. For an individual suspected of having (but not yet diagnosed with) schizophrenia, referral to a psychologist or to a psychiatrist or other physician may be warranted. Laboratory testing and imaging studies may also be necessary to rule out other potential health problems. When working with a patient who has already been diagnosed with schizophrenia, note any significant changes in the patient's signs, symptoms, and behaviors since the last assessment. In addition, investigate the patient's living situation and adherence to the prescribed treatment regimen.

Diagnosis

Appropriate care priorities for patients with schizophrenia vary depending on symptoms and level of functioning. Still, some patients are likely to have similar needs related to the severity of the illness. Examples of these include:

- Risk of suicide
- Risk of injury
- Lack of knowledge about schizophrenia
- Inability to perform self-care
- Self-neglect
- Impaired verbal communication
- Inadequate social skills
- Inadequate coping skills
- Nonadherence
- Altered cognition
- Disturbed thought processes.

Planning

The planning portion of the nursing process involves identifying desired patient outcomes and formulating steps for achieving those outcomes. For patients with schizophrenia, appropriate nursing outcomes typically fall into one of three broad categories: symptom reduction, improved quality of life, and helping patients achieve life goals. Planning and interventions to help patients achieve life goals will come later in the recovery process. Immediate symptom reduction is needed to ensure patient safety and improve quality of life.

Outcomes Related to Symptom Reduction

- Patient will experience a reduction in hallucinations and delusions.
- Patient will experience a reduction in disordered thoughts.
- Patient will demonstrate appropriate affect.
- Patient will experience fewer negative symptoms of schizophrenia.
- Patient will take all medications as prescribed.

Outcomes Related to Quality of Life

- Patient will demonstrate appropriate self-care and personal hygiene.
- Patient will obtain adequate sleep.
- Patient will avoid injury and risky behaviors.
- Patient will refrain from use of alcohol and/or illicit drugs.
- Patient will demonstrate improved coping skills.
- Patient will make a concerted effort to interact with others and avoid social isolation.
- Patient and caregivers will voice understanding of the disease process and make plans for emergency care.

Communicating with Patients

Working Phase

Patients experiencing acute symptoms may exhibit hallucinations, delusions, or disordered thinking. The nurse needs to modify conversations with these patients to accommodate their presenting symptoms. When working with patients whose thinking is far removed from reality, stand at least an arm's length away and tell the patient what you are going to do before you do it.

- Mr. Moore, I am going to stand here in the doorway while I ask you some questions.
- So, the voices in your head started coming back when we changed your medicine?
- You say your medication makes your bones feel strange. Tell me what happens?

Implementation

Implementation involves evidence-based nursing interventions that facilitate the patient's achievement of identified goals of care. Although appropriate interventions will vary, the following principles apply to most patients diagnosed with schizophrenia. Patients who are actively suicidal or are experiencing hallucinations or delusions will not be able to engage in safety planning and will require interventions and monitoring per agency policy.

Prevent Injury

The nurse's first priority of care should be to provide a safe environment for patients with schizophrenia and prevent them from engaging in violence toward self or others. When hallucinating or interpreting others' actions and statements from the standpoint of delusions, the patient may believe to be in danger, regardless of whether there is a factual basis for the fear. Nursing interventions directed toward promoting safety and preventing injury may include administering antipsychotic medications as ordered, ensuring that the patient's surroundings are free of potentially harmful objects, minimizing environmental stimuli, and monitoring for suicidal behavior. Nursing care for patients who are suicidal can be found in Module 28, Mood and Affect. **Box 23.1** » outlines interventions for patients who are experiencing hallucinations or delusions.

Provide Symptomatic Treatment

The nurse's second priority should be promoting control of patients' current symptoms and minimizing the likelihood that additional symptoms will arise. Applicable nursing interventions may include orienting patients to person and place; avoiding overwhelming or overstimulating patients; remaining calm and consistent when speaking with patients; and always informing patients before touching them. Assess the patients' ability to understand and follow the treatment regimen. Many times, patients will require referral to various community agencies that can assist them with activities such as finding support groups, remembering to take their medications, and obtaining transportation to and from doctors' appointments and therapy sessions.

Educate Patients and Significant Others

Teaching and encouragement are another vital area of intervention for both patients with schizophrenia and their families. Inform patients and their loved ones about the symptoms and course of the disease, available therapeutic options and how they work, possible medication side effects, and potential signs of relapse. The nurse should also

Box 23.1

Selected Nursing Interventions for Patients Experiencing Acute Hallucinations or Delusions

For both hallucinations and delusions, the nurse and healthcare team should rule out any underlying cause, such as a metabolic disorder or hospitalization. The nurse should try to identify any event or situation that may have triggered the symptoms, such as excess noise on the unit or onset of acute illness. Do not confront the patient about hallucinations or delusions, but let the patient know that although you are not experiencing them, you understand that they are real for the patient.

Hallucinations

- Remain calm and ask the patient to describe the hallucination.
- Assess for an event or situation that may have triggered the hallucination.
- Reinforce that the patient is safe.
- Use interventions to reduce patient anxiety.
- Administer PRN medications, if ordered.

Delusions

- Gently question the information the patient provides. Let the patient know you are trying to help process the situation without validating incorrect information.
- Help patient identify fears or anxieties.
- Attempt interventions to help reduce the patient's anxiety level.

Sources: Adapted from Potter and Moller (2020); Price (2016).

explore patients' and families' current communication and coping skills and encourage the development of new and potentially more effective strategies (see Patient Teaching: Communication Techniques for Families with a Member with Schizophrenia). Encourage patients to adopt healthier behaviors, such as discontinuing use of nicotine and alcohol, obtaining adequate sleep, and eating a balanced diet. Referrals for social skills and occupational training are often appropriate, as is encouraging patients to participate in activities that minimize their likelihood of social isolation and withdrawal. To keep patients on the path toward fuller functioning and possibly even independent living, the nurse should be sure to provide frequent positive reinforcement for desired actions and behaviors.

Advocate for Patients

The nurse must take steps to advocate on behalf of patients with schizophrenia. For example, the nurse should ensure that all interventions and therapies are actually in a patient's best interests and not merely intended to ease the burden on the patient's family and caregivers. The nurse should also make sure patients understand their legal rights to the greatest degree possible. Because individuals with schizophrenia are often unable to understand or independently exercise these rights during periods of acute psychosis, they should be encouraged to develop advance directives and similar documents explaining their wishes for times when the disorder is not controlled. During periods when psychosis is not present, patients may decide to execute a psychiatric or mental health advance directive (PAD), a legal tool that allows a person with mental illness to state their preferences for treatment in advance of a crisis or that certain family members cannot receive confidential patient information. PADs serve to protect a person's autonomy and ability to self-direct care.

Evaluation

Ongoing evaluation is critical for patients with schizophrenia, as it allows nurses to monitor their condition and adjust any patient-specific diagnoses, goals, and interventions as necessary. Some general examples of potential achieved outcomes for patients with schizophrenia include the following:

- The patient experiences a reduction in symptoms.
- The patient demonstrates appropriate affect.
- The patient adheres to the medication regimen.
- The patient demonstrates appropriate self-care.
- The patient reports improvement in sleep quality and quantity.
- The patient remains safe and free of injury.
- The patient refrains from use of nicotine, alcohol, and illicit drugs.
- The patient demonstrates improved coping skills.
- The patient reports increased social interactions with others.
- The patient has an emergency plan in place.

Patient Teaching

Communication Techniques for Families with a Member with Schizophrenia

Families are often overwhelmed by the stress associated with having a member affected by schizophrenia. Without specific tools to cope, ineffective communication patterns can arise and have the potential to contribute to poor patient outcomes. Nurses can teach family members strategies to improve communication. For example, if a family is concerned about a patient's behavior, the nurse can guide them through the use of some of the following techniques:

- Using "I" language to express positive feelings (e.g., "I am happy when you decide to sit down for dinner with us")
- Engaging in active listening (by asking questions and nodding in agreement when another person speaks)
- Making positive, specific requests for change that are linked to emotions (e.g., "I would really like it if you could play a game with us tonight")
- Expressing negative feelings with "I" rather than "you" language (for example, saying "I'm worried that you may not be getting enough sleep" instead of "You never get enough sleep at night").

After teaching these skills, the nurse should have family members schedule a time for practice. It is also important for the nurse to emphasize that the more often family members use these skills, the more natural they will become.

Nursing Care Plan

A Patient with Schizophrenia

Lauren Hildebrand, age 22, is brought to a private mental health center by her father, Peter, who is concerned about recent changes in her behavior. He reports that she is demonstrating increasing difficulty expressing her thoughts and that she often stops talking midsentence, as though she's forgotten what she was saying. He also states that Ms. Hildebrand dropped out of her graduate program in engineering 4 months ago because she suddenly was unable to maintain her grades. Mr. Hildebrand believes these problems are tied to cocaine use.

ASSESSMENT

Angel Sanchez, the RN at the health center, obtains a patient history and physical examination of Ms. Hildebrand. Mr. Sanchez notes that she was adopted as an infant and little is known about her birth mother beyond the fact that she was homeless at the time Ms. Hildebrand was born. Until 10 months ago, Ms. Hildebrand was an A student at the local university and was awarded a position as a graduate assistant in the engineering department. Shortly after beginning her assistantship, she began having problems expressing herself. At first, she simply seemed distracted, rapidly switching from one topic to another in conversation; this eventually segued into problems logically connecting thoughts and completing sentences. Within 6 months, Ms. Hildebrand was no longer able to maintain her grades and job responsibilities and was forced to drop out of the graduate program. Around this time, her friends became aware of her drug problem. Out of concern, they contacted her parents.

Ms. Hildebrand's clothes are relatively new and fashionable, but they are rumpled and smell strongly of body odor. It appears that Ms. Hildebrand hasn't bathed or combed her hair in several days. Her affect is flat. Mr. Sanchez detects redness in and around Ms. Hildebrand's nostrils and notices that she frequently rubs her nose, both of which suggest insufflation of cocaine. Ms. Hildebrand admits that she uses cocaine but states that she hasn't used it in 3 days. She has difficulty answering Mr. Sanchez's other questions; her speech is garbled and relies heavily on rhyming words that do not make sense when strung together. Ms. Hildebrand is very thin, and the shape of her arm, hand, and clavicle bones stands out clearly under her skin. Her vital signs include T 100.1°F oral; P 95 bpm; R 22/min; and BP 131/88 mmHg.

Based on his mental status assessment of Ms. Hildebrand, Mr. Sanchez suspects schizophrenia. The psychiatrist orders an MRI to rule out abnormalities such as brain tumors. Aside from slightly enlarged ventricles, Ms. Hildebrand's MRI does not reveal any unusual findings. After speaking with Ms. Hildebrand's father, the psychiatrist interviews her, after which he diagnoses her with probable acute schizophrenia. Based on her mental state and substance abuse, the psychiatrist recommends Ms. Hildebrand be admitted as an inpatient at the mental health center, where she will receive treatment for her psychiatric condition and substance abuse. He also prescribes olanzapine, 5 mg/day for 1 week, to be followed by 2.5 mg/day increases each week until Ms. Hildebrand exhibits improvement, not to exceed 20 mg/day.

DIAGNOSES

- Risk of injury related to disorganized thinking patterns and substance abuse
- Inadequate social skills related to altered cognitive function
- Impaired communication related to perceptual and cognitive impairment
- Inability to perform self-care related to perceptual and cognitive impairment and substance abuse
- Undernutrition related to cognitive impairment and substance abuse

PLANNING

Goals for Ms. Hildebrand's care include:

- The patient will remain free from injury.
- The patient will demonstrate clear communication patterns.
- The patient will verbalize logical thought processes.
- The patient will exercise appropriate self-care and hygiene measures, including bathing or showering daily and completing oral hygiene care twice daily.
- The patient will discontinue cocaine use.
- The patient will gain 1 to 2 lb per week.
- The patient will engage in appropriate rehabilitation and group therapy activities while hospitalized and after release.

IMPLEMENTATION

- Monitor the patient for indicators that suggest the potential for injury to self or others.
- Ensure the patient receives care that promotes physical and psychologic safety.
- Administer all medications as ordered.
- Monitor for signs and symptoms of cocaine withdrawal and address the need for substance abuse treatment.
- Assist the patient with establishing a pattern of self-care that includes adequate nutritional intake and hygiene.
- Teach patient and family members how to cope with schizophrenia and how to respond to signs of relapse.
- Encourage the patient to attend and engage in group therapy sessions.
- Ensure appropriate postdischarge services such as ACT.

Nursing Care Plan *(continued)*

EVALUATION

Mr. Sanchez works closely with Ms. Hildebrand during her stay at the mental health center. While at the center, she receives education about her disorder, its causes and symptoms, and complications commonly associated with it. She also receives substance abuse counseling, CBT, and a referral to vocational counseling to prepare her to find a job after she is released. Her medication is gradually increased over the course of her stay until she reaches an effective dose of 12.5 mg/day. By the end of her inpatient stay, Ms. Hildebrand is able to demonstrate appropriate self-care skills related to hygiene, nutrition, and medication administration. She can also clearly and logically describe the symptoms of her condition and verbalize strategies for coping with them. She is scheduled to return to the center twice each week for group therapy and has an appointment to meet with an ACT provider.

CRITICAL THINKING

1. Based on the little we know of Ms. Hildebrand's birth mother, can we draw any conclusions about either Ms. Hildebrand's genetic predisposition to schizophrenia or environmental factors prior to her birth that may have predisposed her to this disorder? Why is it reasonable to draw these conclusions?
2. Research community services for individuals with schizophrenia in your geographical area. What types of services are offered, and which of these services would you recommend to Ms. Hildebrand if she were your patient? Why would you recommend them?
3. Develop a care plan to reduce the risk of self-directed violence related to disruptions in cognitive processes.

REVIEW Schizophrenia

RELATE Link the Concepts and Exemplars

Linking the exemplar of schizophrenia with the concept of immunity:

1. Why might patients with schizophrenia be at a heightened risk of HIV infection and AIDS?
2. What measures might you implement when caring for a patient with schizophrenia to limit the risk of HIV exposure?

Linking the exemplar of schizophrenia with the concept of addiction:

3. Why are patients with schizophrenia more likely to abuse nicotine, alcohol, and illicit drugs? Be sure to explore physical, social, and psychologic factors in your response.
4. What special challenges might arise when addressing addiction behaviors in patients with schizophrenia (as opposed to other patients)? Why? How might the nurse attempt to overcome these challenges?

Linking the exemplar of schizophrenia with the concept of managing care:

5. Why are care coordination and case management especially important for patients with schizophrenia?
6. What sort of professionals might be involved in the overall plan of care for a patient with schizophrenia? How could the nurse promote better collaboration and communication among these providers?

READY Go to Volume 3: Clinical Nursing Skills

REFER Go to Pearson MyLab Nursing and eText

REFLECT Apply Your Knowledge

Dwight Gibson, a 46-year-old man, is brought to the emergency department by his landlord, Ms. Alder. Ms. Alder is concerned about Mr. Gibson's current mental state. She reports that his behavior has always been eccentric for the 5 years she's known him. For example, he perpetually seems worried that someone is "out to get him" and has installed extra locks on his doors and windows.

Lately, however, Ms. Alder has felt that Mr. Gibson's behavior is progressing from merely unusual to severely disturbed. Ms. Alder explains that she lives in the apartment below Mr. Gibson's, and several times over the past month, she's heard him yelling. When she goes to check on him, he tells her he's arguing with the "voices," yet there's never anyone else in the apartment with him. Ms. Alder also mentions that Mr. Gibson seems to be letting garbage accumulate in his apartment, as it smells quite bad. Upon observation, Mr. Gibson's hair is dirty and his clothes are stained and torn. As the nurse conducting his initial assessment, you introduce yourself to him and ask how he is feeling. He replies that he is feeling fine. Next, you ask Mr. Gibson if you may check his blood pressure. He appears agitated and states, "They told you to do that, didn't they? They're trying to steal my spirit. They're afraid my spirit will tell me the truth. I will not let you do that."

1. What additional assessment information do you need?
2. How should you respond to Mr. Gibson's refusal to allow you to assess his blood pressure?
3. What are this patient's priorities of care at this time?
4. Should Mr. Gibson be determined to be experiencing schizophrenia, what nursing care priorities would be appropriate for inclusion in his plan of care?

References

Adams, M. P., Holland, L. N., & & Urban, C. (2020). *Pharmacology for nurses: A pathophysiologic approach* (6th ed.). Pearson Education.

Altmann, D. M. (2018). Neuroimmunology and neuroinflammation in autoimmune, neurodegenerative and psychiatric disease. *Immunology, 154*(2), 167–168. https://doi.org/10.1111/imm.12943

Alzheimer's Association. (2020a). *Caregiver stress.* https://www.alz.org/help-support/caregiving/caregiver-health/caregiver-stress

Alzheimer's Association. (2020b). *Causes and risk factors for Alzheimer's disease.* https://www.alz.org/alzheimers-dementia/what-is-alzheimers/causes-and-risk-factors

Alzheimer's Association. (2020d). *Earlier diagnosis.* https://www.alz.org/alzheimers-dementia/research_progress/earlier-diagnosis

Alzheimer's Association. (2020e). *Facts and figures.* https://www.alz.org/alzheimers-dementia/facts-figures

Alzheimer's Association. (2020f). *Home safety.* https://www.alz.org/help-support/caregiving/safety/home-safety

Alzheimer's Association. (2020g). *Is Alzheimer's genetic?* https://www.alz.org/alzheimers-dementia/what-is-alzheimers/causes-and-risk-factors/genetics

Alzheimer's Association. (2020h). *Medications for memory.* https://www.alz.org/alzheimers-dementia/treatments/medications-for-memory

Alzheimer's Association. (2020i). *Stages of Alzheimer's.* https://www.alz.org/alzheimers-dementia/stages

Alzheimer's Association. (2020j). *Vascular dementia.* https://www.alz.org/alzheimers-dementia/what-is-dementia/types-of-dementia/vascular-dementia

Alzheimer's Association. (2020k). *Younger/early-onset Alzheimer's.* https://www.alz.org/alzheimers-dementia/what-is-alzheimers/younger-early-onset

Alzheimer's Society UK. (2020). *Huntington's disease.* https://www.alzheimers.org.uk/about-dementia/types-dementia/huntingtons-disease#content-start

American Association of Intellectual and Developmental Disabilities. (2020). *Definition of intellectual disability.* https://www.aaidd.org/intellectual-disability/definition

American Geriatric Society. (2019). *With AGS CoCare: Help, AGS seeks to expand the reach of a seminal program that puts delirium prevention on the map.* https://www.americangeriatrics.org/media-center/news/ags-cocare-helptm-ags-seeks-expand-reach-seminal-program-put-delirium-prevention

American Psychiatric Association (APA). (2013). *Diagnostic and statistical manual of mental disorders* (5th ed.). Author.

American Speech Language and Hearing Association. (2020). *Social communication.* https://www.asha.org/public/speech/development/social-communication/

American Stroke Association. (2020). *Controlling post-stroke seizures.* Retrieved from https://www.stroke.org/en/about-stroke/effects-of-stroke/physical-effects-of-stroke/physical-impact/controlling-post-stroke-seizures

Anderson, A. R., Deng, J., Anthony, R. S., Atalla, S. A., & Monroe, T. B. (2017). Using complementary and alternative medicine to treat pain and agitation in dementia: A review of randomized controlled trials from long-term care with potential use in critical care. *Critical Care Nursing Clinics, 29*(4), 519–537. https://doi.org/https://doi.org/10.1016/j.cnc.2017.08.010

Andrews, M. M., Boyle, J. S., & Collins, J. W. (2020). *Transcultural concepts in nursing care* (8th ed.). Wolters Kluwer.

Attar, R., Valentin, J. B., Freeman, P., Andell, P., Aagaard, J., & Jensen, S. E. (2018). The effect of schizophrenia on major adverse cardiac events, length of hospital stay, and prevalence of somatic comorbidities following acute coronary syndrome. *European Heart Journal: Quality of Care and Clinical Outcomes, 5*(2), 121–126. https://doi.org/10.1093/ehjqcco/qcy055

Ayub, S., Ramtekkar, U. P., & Reiersen, A. M. (2018). Use of antipsychotic drugs for psychotic disorders in children. *Current treatment options in psychiatry, 5*(1), 30–55. https://doi.org/10.1007/s40501-018-0137-1

Barkmeier-Kraemer, J. M., Louis, E. D., & Smith, M. E. (2020). Essential tremor. In P. A. Weissbrod & D. O. Francis (Eds.), *Neurologic and neurodegenerative diseases of the larynx* (pp. 205–214). Springer.

Baytunca, B., Kalyoncu, T., Ozel, I., Erermis, S., Kayahan, B., & Öngur, D. (2017). Early onset schizophrenia associated with obsessive-compulsive disorder: Clinical features and correlates. *Clinical Neuropharmacology, 40*(6), 243–245. https://doi.org/10.1097/WNF.0000000000000248

Beckmann, D., Schnitzer, K., & Freudenreich, O. (2020). Approach to the diagnosis of schizoaffective disorder. *Psychiatric Annals, 50*(5), 195–199. https://doi.org/10.3928/00485713-20200408-01

Bélanger, S. A., & Caron, J. (2018). Evaluation of the child with global developmental delay and intellectual disability. *Paediatrics & Child Health, 23*(6), 403–410. https://doi.org/10.1093/pch/pxy093

Belbeze, J., & Gallarda, T. (2020). Very late onset psychotic symptoms: Psychosis or dementia? A phenomenological approach. A systematic review. *Geriatrie et Psychologie Neuropsychiatrie du Vieillissement, 18*(1), 77–87. https://doi.org/10.1684/pnv.2019.0828

Berg-Weger, M., & Stewart, D. B. (2017). Non-pharmacologic interventions for persons with dementia. *Missouri Medicine, 114*(2), 116–119. Retrieved from https://www.ncbi.nlm.nih.gov/pmc/articles/PMC6140014/

Berti, V., Walters, M., Sterling, J., Quinn, C. G., Logue, M., Andrews, R., et al. (2018). Mediterranean diet and 3-year Alzheimer brain biomarker changes in middle-aged adults. *Neurology, 90*(20), e1789. https://doi.org/10.1212/WNL.0000000000005527

Bettencourt, A., & Mullen, J. E. (2017). Delirium in children: Identification, prevention, and management. *Critical Care Nurse, 37*(3), e9–e18. https://doi.org/10.4037/ccn2017692

Bighelli, I., Salanti, G., Reitmeir, C., Wallis, S., Barbui, C., Furukawa, T. A., & Leucht, S. (2018). Psychological interventions for positive symptoms in schizophrenia: Protocol for a network meta-analysis of randomised controlled trials. *BMJ Open, 8*(3), e019280. https://doi.org/10.1136/bmjopen-2017-019280

Birnbaum, R., & Weinberger, D. R. (2017). Genetic insights into the neurodevelopmental origins of schizophrenia. *Nature Reviews Neuroscience, 18*(12), 727–740. https://doi.org/10.1038/nrn.2017.125

Black, D. W., & Andreasen, N. C. (2020). *Introductory textbook of psychiatry* (7th ed.). American Psychiatric Association Publishing.

Bora, E. (2017). Relationship between insight and theory of mind in schizophrenia: A meta-analysis. *Schizophrenia Research, 190*, 11–17. https://doi.org/10.1016/j.schres.2017.03.029

Briley, D. A., & Tucker-Drob, E. M. (2017). Comparing the developmental genetics of cognition and personality over the life span. *Journal of Personality, 85*(1), 51–64. https://doi.org/10.1111/jopy.12186

Brink, M., Green, A., Bojesen, A. B., Lamberti, J. S., Conwell, Y., & Andersen, K. (2019). Excess medical comorbidity and mortality across the lifespan in schizophrenia: A nationwide Danish register study. *Schizophrenia Research, 206*, 347–354. https://doi.org/10.1016/j.schres.2018.10.020

Bryce, S. D., Rossell, S. L., Lee, S. J., Lawrence, R. J., Tan, E. J., Carruthers, S. P., & Ponsford, J. L. (2018). Neurocognitive and self-efficacy benefits of cognitive remediation in schizophrenia: A randomized controlled trial. *Journal of the International Neuropsychological Society, 24*(6), 549–562. https://doi.org/10.1017/S1355617717001369

Bulbena-Cabre, A., & Bulbena, A. (2018). Schizophrenia and anxiety: Yes, they are relatives not just neighbours. *British Journal of Psychiatry, 213*(2), 498–498. https://doi.org/10.1192/bjp.2018.126

Caldani, S., Bucci, M. P., Lamy, J.-C., Seassau, M., Bendjemaa, N., Gadel, R., et al. (2017). Saccadic eye movements as markers of schizophrenia spectrum: Exploration in at-risk mental states. *Schizophrenia Research, 181*, 30–37. https://doi.org/10.1016/j.schres.2016.09.003

Callahan, C. M., Boustani, M. A., Schmid, A. A., LaMantia, M. A., Austrom, M. G., Miller, D. K., et al. (2017). Targeting functional decline in Alzheimer disease: A randomized trial. *Annals of Internal Medicine, 166*(3), 164–171. https://doi.org/10.7326/M16-0830

Cacioppo, J. T., & Cacioppo, S. (2014). Social relationships and health. The toxic effects of perceived social isolation. *Social and Personality Psychology Compass, 8*(2), 58–72.

Camacho-Gomez, M., & Castellvi, P. (2019). Effectiveness of family intervention for preventing relapse in first-episode psychosis until 24 months of follow-up: A systematic review with meta-analysis of randomized controlled trials. *Schizophrenia Bulletin, 46*(1), 98–109. https://doi.org/10.1093/schbul/sbz038

Cass, S. P. (2017). Alzheimer's disease and exercise: A literature review. *Current Sports Medicine Reports, 16*(1), 19–22. https://doi.org/10.1249/JSR.0000000000000332

Center for Behavioral Health Statistics and Quality. (2019). *Key substance use and mental health indicators in the United States: Results from the 2018 National Survey on Drug Use and Health* (HHS Publication No. PEP19-5068, NSDUH Series H-54). Substance Abuse and Mental Health Services Administration. https://www.samhsa.gov/data/sites/default/files/cbhsq-reports/NSDUHNationalFindingsReport2018/NSDUHNationalFindingsReport2018.pdf

Centers for Disease Control and Prevention (CDC). (2019a). *Healthy Brain Initiative.* https://www.cdc.gov/aging/healthy-brain/index.htm

Centers for Disease Control and Prevention (CDC). (2019b). *Minorities and women are at greater risk for Alzheimer's disease.* https://www.cdc.gov/aging/publications/features/Alz-Greater-Risk.html

Centers for Disease Control and Prevention (CDC). (2019c). *What is Down syndrome?* https://www.cdc.gov/ncbddd/birthdefects/downsyndrome.html

Centers for Disease Control and Prevention (CDC). (2020). *Alzheimer's disease.* https://www.cdc.gov/aging/aginginfo/alzheimers.htm

Chen, K.-H., Yeh, M.-H., Livneh, H., Chen, B.-C., Lin, I. H., Lu, M.-C., et al. (2017). Association of traditional Chinese medicine therapy and the risk of dementia in patients with hypertension: A nationwide population-based cohort study. *BMC Complementary and Alternative Medicine, 17*(1), 178. https://doi.org/10.1186/s12906-017-1677-4

Chiu, H.-Y., Chen, P.-Y., Chen, Y.-T., & Huang, H.-C. (2018). Reality orientation therapy benefits cognition in older people with dementia: A meta-analysis. *International Journal of Nursing Studies, 86*, 20–28. https://doi.org/10.1016/j.ijnurstu.2018.06.008

Choi, D., Choi, S., & Park, S. M. (2018). Effect of smoking cessation on the risk of dementia: A longitudinal study. *Annals of Clinical and Translational Neurology, 5*(10), 1192–1199. https://doi.org/10.1002/acn3.633

Choi, S., Krishnan, J., & Ruckmani, K. (2017). Cigarette smoke and related risk factors in neurological disorders: An update. *Biomedicine & Pharmacotherapy, 85*, 79–86. https://doi.org/10.1016/j.biopha.2016.11.118

Chorlton, S. D. (2017). Toxoplasma gondii and schizophrenia: A review of published RCTs. *Parasitology Research, 116*(7), 1793–1799. https://doi.org/10.1007/s00436-017-5478-y

Cioltan, H., Alshehri, S., Howe, C., Lee, J., Fain, M., Eng, H., et al. (2017). Variation in use of antipsychotic medications in nursing homes in the United States: A systematic review. *BMC Geriatrics, 17*(1), 32. https://doi.org/10.1186/s12877-017-0428-1

Citrome, L. (2017). Activating and sedating adverse effects of second-generation antipsychotics in the treatment of schizophrenia and major depressive disorder: Absolute risk increase and number needed to harm. *Journal of Clinical Psychopharmacology, 37*(2). https://doi.org/10.1097/JCP.0000000000000665

Condello, C., Lemmin, T., Stöhr, J., Nick, M., Wu, Y., Maxwell, A. M., et al. (2018). Structural heterogeneity and intersubject variability of Aβ in familial and sporadic Alzheimer's disease. *Proceedings of the National Academy of Sciences, 115*(4), E782–E791. https://doi.org/10.1073/pnas.1714966115

Correll, C. U., Ng-Mak, D. S., Stafkey-Mailey, D., Farrelly, E., Rajagopalan, K., & Loebel, A. (2017). Cardiometabolic comorbidities, readmission, and costs in schizophrenia and bipolar disorder: A real-world analysis. *Annals of General Psychiatry, 16*(1), 9. https://doi.org/10.1186/s12991-017-0133-7

Cowan, N. (2017). The many faces of working memory and short-term storage. *Psychonomic Bulletin & Review, 24*(4), 1158–1170. https://doi.org/10.3758/s13423-016-1191-6

Crawford, P., & Zimmerman, E. E. (2018). Tremor: Sorting through the differential diagnosis. *American Family Physician, 97*(3), 180–186.

Cromby, J., Chung, E., Papadopoulos, D., & Talbot, C. (2019). Reviewing the epigenetics of schizophrenia. *Journal of Mental Health, 28*(1), 71–79. https://doi.org/10.1080/09638237.2016.1207229

Darmedru, C., Demily, C., & Franck, N. (2017). Cognitive remediation and social cognitive training for violence in schizophrenia: A systematic review. *Psychiatry Research, 251*, 266–274. https://doi.org/10.1016/j.psychres.2016.12.062

Davies, S. J., Lum, J. A. G., Skouteris, H., Byrne, L. K., & Hayden, M. J. (2018). Cognitive impairment during pregnancy: A meta analysis. *Medical Journal of Australia, 208*(1), 35–40. https://doi.org/10.5694/mja17.00131

Davies, W. (2017). Understanding the pathophysiology of postpartum psychosis: Challenges and new approaches. *World Journal of Psychiatry, 7*(2), 77–88. https://dx.doi.org/10.5498%2Fwjp.v7.i2.77

Davison, J., O'Gorman, A., Brennan, L., & Cotter, D. R. (2018). A systematic review of metabolite biomarkers of schizophrenia. *Schizophrenia Research, 195*, 32–50. https://doi.org/10.1016/j.schres.2017.09.021

Dean, D. J., Woodward, N., Walther, S., McHugo, M., Armstrong, K., & Heckers, S. (2020). Cognitive motor impairments and brain structure in schizophrenia spectrum disorder patients with a history of catatonia. *Schizophrenia Research.* https://doi.org/10.1016/j.schres.2020.05.012

Denny, L., Coles, S., & Blitz, R. (2017). Fetal alcohol syndrome and fetal alcohol spectrum disorders. *American Family Physician, 96*(8), 515–522.

Díaz-Fernández, S., Frías-Ortiz, D. F., & Fernández-Miranda, J. J. (2019). Mirror image study (10 years of follow-up and 10 of standard pre-treatment) of psychiatric hospitalizations of patients with severe schizophrenia treated in a community-based, case-managed programme. *Revista de Psiquiatria y Salud Mental.* https://doi.org/10.1016/j.rpsm.2019.04.004.

Dixon, L. (2017). What it will take to make coordinated specialty care available to anyone experiencing early schizophrenia: Getting over the hump. *JAMA Psychiatry, 74*(1), 7–8. https://doi.org/10.1001/jamapsychiatry.2016.2665

Dollfus, S., & Lyne, J. (2017). Negative symptoms: History of the concept and their position in diagnosis of schizophrenia. *Schizophrenia Research, 186*, 3–7. https://doi.org/10.1016/j.schres.2016.06.024

Dutchen, S. (2018). *Sporadic Alzheimer's in a dish: New cell model of most common form of Alzheimer's points to molecular causes, drug target.* Harvard Medical School. https://hms.harvard.edu/news/sporadic-alzheimers-dish

Elif, K., Taşkapilioğlu, Ö., & Bakar, M. (2017). Caregiver burden in different stages of Alzheimer's disease. *Archives of Neuropsychiatry, 54*(1), 82. https://dx.doi.org/10.5152%2Fnpa.2017.11304

Ellis, G., Gardner, M., Tsiachristas, A., Langhorne, P., Burke, O., Harwood, R. H., et al. (2017). Comprehensive geriatric assessment for older adults admitted to hospital. *Cochrane Database of Systematic Reviews*, Issue 9, Article No. CD006211. https://doi.org/10.1002/14651858.CD006211.pub3

Elsworthy, R. J., & Aldred, S. (2019). Depression in Alzheimer's disease: An alternative role for selective serotonin reuptake inhibitors? *Journal of Alzheimer's Disease, 69*, 651–661. https://doi.org/10.3233/JAD-180780

Eramudugolla, R., Mortby, M. E., Sachdev, P., Meslin, C., Kumar, R., & Anstey, K. J. (2017). Evaluation of a research diagnostic algorithm for DSM-5 neurocognitive disorders in a population-based cohort of older adults. *Alzheimer's Research & Therapy, 9*(1), 15. https://doi.org/10.1186/s13195-017-0246-x

Errico, F., Nuzzo, T., Carella, M., Bertolino, A., & Usiello, A. (2018). The emerging role of altered d-aspartate metabolism in schizophrenia: New insights from preclinical models and human studies. *Frontiers in Psychiatry, 9*(559). https://doi.org/10.3389/fpsyt.2018.00559

Föcking, M., Doyle, B., Munawar, N., Dillon, E. T., Cotter, D., & Cagney, G. (2019). Epigenetic factors in schizophrenia: Mechanisms and experimental approaches. *Molecular Neuropsychiatry, 5*(1), 6–12. https://doi.org/10.1159/000495063

Fond, G., Godin, O., Boyer, L., Llorca, P.-M., Andrianarisoa, M., Brunel, L., et al. (2017). Advanced paternal age is associated with earlier schizophrenia onset in offspring: Results from the national multicentric FACE-SZ cohort. *Psychiatry Research, 254*, 218–223. https://doi.org/10.1016/j.psychres.2017.04.002

Foti, D., Perlman, G., Bromet, E. J., Harvey, P. D., Hajcak, G., Mathalon, D. H., & Kotov, R. (2020). Pathways from performance monitoring to negative symptoms and functional outcomes in psychotic disorders. *Psychological Medicine.* https://doi.org/10.1017/S0033291720000768

Fountoulakis, K. N., Gonda, X., Siamouli, M., Panagiotidis, P., Moutou, K., Nimatoudis, I., & Kasper, S. (2018). Paternal and maternal age as risk factors for schizophrenia: A case-control study. *International Journal of Psychiatry in Clinical Practice, 22*(3), 170–176. https://doi.org/10.1080/13651501.2017.1391292

Frisoni, G. B., Boccardi, M., Barkhof, F., Blennow, K., Cappa, S., Chiotis, K., et al. (2017). Strategic roadmap for an early diagnosis of Alzheimer's disease based on biomarkers. *The Lancet Neurology, 16*(8), 661–676. https://doi.org/10.1016/S1474-4422(17)30159-X

Galletti, C., Paolini, E., Tortorella, A., & Compton, M. T. (2017). Auditory and non-auditory hallucinations in first-episode psychosis: Differential associations with diverse clinical features. *Psychiatry Research, 254*, 268–274. https://doi.org/10.1016/j.psychres.2017.04.056

Ganguly, P., Soliman, A., & Moustafa, A. A. (2018). Holistic management of schizophrenia symptoms using pharmacological and non-pharmacological treatment. *Frontiers in Public Health, 6*(166). https://doi.org/10.3389/fpubh.2018.00166

Ganos, C., Rothwell, J., & Haggard, P. (2018). Voluntary inhibitory motor control over involuntary tic movements. *Movement Disorders, 33*(6), 937–946. https://doi.org/10.1002/mds.27346

Gerson, R., Malas, N., & Mroczkowski, M. M. (2018). Crisis in the emergency department: The evaluation and management of acute agitation in children and adolescents. *Child and Adolescent Psychiatric Clinics, 27*(3), 367–386. https://doi.org/10.1016/j.chc.2018.02.002

Gil Montoya, J. A., Barrios, R., Santana, S., Sanchez Lara, I., Pardo, C. C., Fornieles Rubio, F., et al. (2017). Association between periodontitis and amyloid β peptide in elderly people with and without cognitive impairment. *Journal of Periodontology, 88*(10), 1051–1058. https://doi.org/10.1902/jop.2017.170071

Gooding, P. A., Littlewood, D., Owen, R., Johnson, J., & Tarrier, N. (2019). Psychological resilience in people experiencing schizophrenia and suicidal thoughts and behaviours. *Journal of Mental Health, 28*(6), 597–603. https://doi.org/10.1080/09638237.2017.1294742

Gordon, A., Davis, P. J., Patterson, S., Pepping, C. A., Scott, J. G., Salter, K., & Connell, M. (2018). A randomized waitlist control community study of Social Cognition and Interaction Training for people with schizophrenia. *British Journal of Clinical Psychology, 57*(1), 116–130. https://doi.org/10.1111/bjc.12161

Grant, N., Lawrence, M., Preti, A., Wykes, T., & Cella, M. (2017). Social cognition interventions for people with schizophrenia: A systematic review focusing on methodological quality and intervention modality. *Clinical Psychology Review, 56*, 55–64. https://doi.org/10.1016/j.cpr.2017.06.001

Grimm, O., Kranz, T. M., & Reif, A. (2020). Genetics of ADHD: What should the clinician know? *Current Psychiatry Reports, 22*(4), 1–8.

Grover, S., Sahoo, S., & Nehra, R. (2019). A comparative study of childhood/adolescent and adult onset schizophrenia: Does the neurocognitive and psychosocial outcome differ? *Asian Journal of Psychiatry, 43*, 160–169. https://doi.org/10.1016/j.ajp.2019.05.031

Gudmundsson, O. O., Walters, G. B., Ingason, A., Johansson, S., Zayats, T., Athanasiu, L., et al. (2019). Attention-deficit hyperactivity disorder shares copy number variant risk with schizophrenia and autism spectrum disorder. *Translational Psychiatry, 9*(1), 258. https://doi.org/10.1038/s41398-019-0599-y

Haertel, E. H. (2018). Tests, test scores, and constructs. *Educational Psychologist, 53*(3), 203–216. https://doi.org/10.1080/00461520.2018.1476868

Hafdi, M., Hoevenaar-Blom, M. P., Beishuizen, C. R. L., Moll van Charante, E. P., Richard, E., & van Gool, W. A. (2020). Association of benzodiazepine and anticholinergic drug usage with incident dementia: A prospective cohort study of community-dwelling older adults. *Journal of the American Medical Directors Association, 21*(2), 188–193. https://doi.org/10.1016/j.jamda.2019.05.010

Häfner, H. (2019). From onset and prodromal stage to a life-long course of schizophrenia and its symptom dimensions: How sex, age, and other risk factors influence incidence and course of illness. *Psychiatry Journal, 2019*, 9804836. https://doi.org/10.1155/2019/9804836

Hagerman, R. J., Berry-Kravis, E., Hazlett, H. C., Bailey, D. B., Moine, H., Kooy, R. F., et al. (2017). Fragile X syndrome. *Nature Reviews Disease Primers, 3*(1), 1–19. https://doi.org/10.1038/nrdp.2017.65

Hampel, H., Mesulam, M. M., Cuello, A. C., Khachaturian, A. S., Vergallo, A., Farlow, M. R., et al. (2019). Revisiting the cholinergic hypothesis in Alzheimer's disease: Emerging evidence from translational and clinical research. *Journal of Prevention of Alzheimer's Disease, 6*(1), 2–15. https://doi.org/10.14283/jpad.2018.43

Han, Y. M. Y., & Chan, A. S. (2017). Disordered cortical connectivity underlies the executive function deficits in children with autism spectrum disorders. *Research in Developmental Disabilities, 61*, 19–31. https://doi.org/10.1016/j.ridd.2016.12.010

Harrison, T. M., Maass, A., Baker, S. L., & Jagust, W. J. (2018). Brain morphology, cognition, and β-amyloid in older adults with superior memory performance. *Neurobiology of Aging, 67*, 162–170. https://doi.org/10.1016/j.neurobiolaging.2018.03.024

Harvard University Center on the Developing Child. (2020). *In brief: Connecting the brain to the rest of the body.* https://developingchild.harvard.edu/resources/inbrief-connecting-the-brain-to-the-rest-of-the-body/

Hasan, A. A.-H., & Musleh, M. (2018). Self-stigma by people diagnosed with schizophrenia, depression and anxiety: Cross-sectional survey design. *Perspectives in Psychiatric Care, 54*(2), 142–148. https://doi.org/10.1111/ppc.12213

Hayden, K. M., Beavers, D. P., Steck, S. E., Hebert, J. R., Tabung, F. K., Shivappa, N., et al. (2017). The association between an inflammatory diet and global cognitive function and incident dementia in older women: The Women's Health Initiative Memory Study. *Alzheimer's & Dementia, 13*(11), 1187–1196. https://doi.org/10.1016/j.jalz.2017.04.004

He, H., Lu, J., Yang, L., Zheng, J., Gao, F., Zhai, Y., et al. (2017). Repetitive transcranial magnetic stimulation for treating the symptoms of schizophrenia: A PRISMA compliant meta-analysis. *Clinical Neurophysiology, 128*(5), 716–724.

He, K., Guo, C., He, L., & Shi, Y. (2017). MiRNAs of peripheral blood as the biomarker of schizophrenia. *Hereditas, 155*(1), 9. https://doi.org/10.1186/s41065-017-0044-2

Hersi, M., Irvine, B., Gupta, P., Gomes, J., Birkett, N., & Krewski, D. (2017). Risk factors associated with the onset and progression of Alzheimer's disease: A systematic review of the evidence. *NeuroToxicology, 61*, 143–187. https://doi.org/10.1016/j.neuro.2017.03.006

Heyselaar, E., Segaert, K., Walvoort, S. J. W., Kessels, R. P. C., & Hagoort, P. (2017). The role of nondeclarative memory in the skill for language: Evidence from syntactic priming in patients with amnesia. *Neuropsychologia, 101*, 97–105. https://doi.org/10.1016/j.neuropsychologia.2017.04.033

Hook, J., & Devereux, D. (2018). Boundary violations in therapy: The patient's experience of harm. *Trends in Neurosciences, 24*(6), 366–373. https://doi.org/10.1192/bja.2018.26

Horan, W. P., & Green, M. F. (2019). Treatment of social cognition in schizophrenia: Current status and future directions. *Schizophrenia Research, 203*, 3–11. https://doi.org/10.1016/j.schres.2017.07.013

Hospital Elder Life Program. (2020). *Why delirium is important.* https://www.hospitalelderlifeprogram.org/for-clinicians/why-delirium-is-important/

Howes, O. D., McCutcheon, R., Owen, M. J., & Murray, R. M. (2017). The role of genes, stress, and dopamine in the development of schizophrenia. *Biological Psychiatry, 81*(1), 9–20. https://doi.org/10.1016/j.biopsych.2016.07.014

Hunt, G. E., Large, M. M., Cleary, M., Lai, H. M. X., & Saunders, J. B. (2018). Prevalence of comorbid substance use in schizophrenia spectrum disorders in community and clinical settings, 1990–2017: Systematic review and meta-analysis. *Drug and Alcohol Dependence, 191*, 234–258. https://doi.org/10.1016/j.drugalcdep.2018.07.011

Iimori, T., Nakajima, S., Miyazaki, T., Tarumi, R., Ogyu, K., Wada, M., et al. (2019). Effectiveness of the prefrontal repetitive transcranial magnetic stimulation on cognitive profiles in depression, schizophrenia, and Alzheimer's disease: A systematic review. *Progress in Neuro-Psychopharmacology and Biological Psychiatry, 88*, 31–40. https://doi.org/10.1016/j.pnpbp.2018.06.014

Jacus, J.-P. (2017). Awareness, apathy, and depression in Alzheimer's disease and mild cognitive impairment. *Brain and Behavior, 7*(4), e00661. https://doi.org/10.1002/brb3.661

Janecka, M., Mill, J., Basson, M. A., Goriely, A., Spiers, H., Reichenberg, A., et al. (2017). Advanced paternal age effects in neurodevelopmental disorders—Review of potential underlying mechanisms. *Translational Psychiatry, 7*(1), e1019–e1019. https://doi.org/10.1038/tp.2016.294

Jauhar, S., Laws, K. R., & McKenna, P. J. (2019). CBT for schizophrenia: A critical viewpoint. *Psychological Medicine, 49*(8), 1233–1236. https://doi.org/10.1017/S0033291718004166

Jeffries, C. D., Perkins, D. O., Fournier, M., Do, K. Q., Cuenod, M., Khadimallah, I., et al. (2018). Networks of blood proteins in the neuroimmunology of schizophrenia. *Translational Psychiatry, 8*(1), 112. https://doi.org/10.1038/s41398-018-0158-y

Jenraumjit, R., Chinwong, S., Chinwong, D., Kanjanarach, T., Kshetradat, T., Wongpakaran, T., & Wongpakaran, N. (2020). Anticholinergics and benzodiazepines on cognitive impairment among elderly with Alzheimer's disease: A 1 year follow-up study. *BMC Research Notes, 13*(1), 4. https://doi.org/10.1186/s13104-019-4874-z

Jeon, S. W., & Kim, Y.-K. (2017). Unresolved issues for utilization of atypical antipsychotics in schizophrenia: Antipsychotic polypharmacy and metabolic syndrome. *International Journal of Molecular Sciences, 18*(10), 2174. https://doi.org/10.3390/ijms18102174

Jones, C., Hacker, D., Meaden, A., Cormac, I., Irving, C. B., Xia, J., et al. (2018). Cognitive behavioural therapy plus standard care versus standard care plus other psychosocial treatments for people with schizophrenia. *Cochrane Database of Systematic Reviews*, Issue 11, Article No. CD008712. https://doi.org/10.1002/14651858.CD008712.pub3

Kametani, F., & Hasegawa, M. (2018). Reconsideration of amyloid hypothesis and tau hypothesis in Alzheimer's disease. *Frontiers in Neuroscience, 12*(25). https://doi.org/10.3389/fnins.2018.00025

Kassie, G. M., Nguyen, T. A., Ellett, L. M. K., Pratt, N. L., & Roughead, E. E. (2017). Preoperative medication use and postoperative delirium: A systematic review. *BMC Geriatrics, 17*(1), 298. https://doi.org/10.1186/s12877-017-0695-x

Kivipelto, M., Mangialasche, F., & Ngandu, T. (2018). Lifestyle interventions to prevent cognitive impairment, dementia and Alzheimer disease. *Nature Reviews Neurology, 14*(11), 653–666.

Knorr, J. (2017). Childhood-onset schizophrenia spectrum disorders. In S. Goldstein & M. DeVries (Eds.), *Handbook of DSM-5 disorders in children and adolescents* (pp. 107–122). Springer.

Kollias, C., Dimitrakopoulos, S., Xenaki, L. A., Stefanis, N., & Papageorgiou, C. (2019). Evidence of advanced parental age linked to sporadic schizophrenia. *Psychiatrike, 30*(1), 24–31. https://doi.org/10.22365/jpsych.2019.301.24

Kong, C., Xie, H., Gao, Z., Shao, M., Li, H., Shi, R., et al. (2019). Binding between prion protein and Aβ oligomers contributes to the pathogenesis of Alzheimer's disease. *Virologica Sinica, 34*(5), 475–488. https://doi.org/10.1007/s12250-019-00124-1

Koukouli, F., Rooy, M., Tziotis, D., Sailor, K. A., O'Neill, H. C., Levenga, J., et al. (2017). Nicotine reverses hypofrontality in animal models of addiction and schizophrenia. *Nature Medicine, 23*(3), 347–354. https://doi.org/10.1038/nm.4274

Lally, J., Ajnakina, O., Stubbs, B., Cullinane, M., Murphy, K. C., Gaughran, F., & Murray, R. M. (2017). Remission and recovery from first-episode psychosis in adults: Systematic review and meta-analysis of long-term outcome studies. *British Journal of Psychiatry, 211*(6), 350–358. https://doi.org/10.1192/bjp.bp.117.201475

Lawley, J. S., Macdonald, J. H., Oliver, S. J., & Mullins, P. G. (2017). Unexpected reductions in regional cerebral perfusion during prolonged hypoxia. *Journal of Physiology, 595*(3), 935–947. https://doi.org/10.1113/jp272557

Laws, K. R., Darlington, N., Kondel, T. K., McKenna, P. J., & Jauhar, S. (2018). Cognitive behavioural therapy for schizophrenia—Outcomes for functioning, distress and quality of life: A meta-analysis. *BMC Psychology, 6*(1), 32. https://doi.org/10.1186/s40359-018-0243-2

Learning Disabilities Association of America. (2020). *Types of learning disabilities*. https://ldaamerica.org/types-of-learning-disabilities/

Lecomte, T., Potvin, S., Samson, C., Francoeur, A., Hache-Labelle, C., Gagné, S., et al. (2019). Predicting and preventing symptom onset and relapse in schizophrenia—A metareview of current empirical evidence. *Journal of Abnormal Psychology, 128*(8), 840–854. https://doi.org/10.1037/abn0000447

Leucht, S., Leucht, C., Huhn, M., Chaimani, A., Mavridis, D., Helfer, B., et al. (2017). Sixty years of placebo-controlled antipsychotic drug trials in acute schizophrenia: Systematic review, Bayesian meta-analysis, and meta-regression of efficacy predictors. *American Journal of Psychiatry, 174*(10), 927–942. https://doi.org/10.1176/appi.ajp.2017.16121358

Lök, N., Bademli, K., & Selçuk-Tosun, A. (2019). The effect of reminiscence therapy on cognitive functions, depression, and quality of life in Alzheimer patients: Randomized controlled trial. *International Journal of Geriatric Psychiatry, 34*(1), 47–53. https://doi.org/10.1002/gps.4980

MacKenzie, N. E., Kowalchuk, C., Agarwal, S. M., Costa-Dookhan, K. A., Caravaggio, F., Gerretsen, P., et al. (2018). Antipsychotics, metabolic adverse effects, and cognitive function in schizophrenia. *Frontiers in Psychiatry, 9*(622). https://doi.org/10.3389/fpsyt.2018.00622

Maes, M., Sirivichayakul, S., Kanchanatawan, B., & Carvalho, A. F. (2020). In schizophrenia, psychomotor retardation is associated with executive and memory impairments, negative and psychotic symptoms, neurotoxic immune products and lower natural IgM to malondialdehyde. *World Journal of Biological Psychiatry*. https://doi.org/10.1080/15622975.2019.1701203

Magny, E., Le Petitcorps, H., Pociumban, M., Bouksani-Kacher, Z., Pautas, É., Belmin, J., et al. (2018). Predisposing and precipitating factors for delirium in community-dwelling older adults admitted to hospital with this condition: A prospective case series. *PLoS One, 13*(2), e0193034. https://doi.org/10.1371/journal.pone.0193034

Malinowski, P., Moore, A. W., Mead, B. R., & Gruber, T. (2017). Mindful aging: The effects of regular brief mindfulness practice on electrophysiological markers of cognitive and affective processing in older adults. *Mindfulness, 8*(1), 78–94. https://doi.org/10.1007/s12671-015-0482-8

Mallya, A. P., Wang, H.-D., Lee, H. N. R., & Deutch, A. Y. (2019). Microglial pruning of synapses in the prefrontal cortex during adolescence. *Cerebral Cortex, 29*(4), 1634–1643. https://doi.org/10.1093/cercor/bhy061

Markulev, C., McGorry, P. D., Nelson, B., Yuen, H. P., Schaefer, M., Yung, A. R., et al. (2017). NEURAPRO-E study protocol: A multicentre randomized controlled trial of omega-3 fatty acids and cognitive-behavioural case management for patients at ultra high risk of schizophrenia and other psychotic disorders. *Early Intervention in Psychiatry, 11*(5), 418–428. https://doi.org/10.1111/eip.12260

Marsman, A., Mandl, R. C. W., Klomp, D. W. J., Cahn, W., Kahn, R. S., Luijten, P. R., & Hulshoff Pol, H. E. (2017). Intelligence and brain efficiency: Investigating the association between working memory performance, glutamate, and GABA. *Frontiers in Psychiatry, 8*, 154. https://doi.org/10.3389/fpsyt.2017.00154

Martinez, G., Mosconi, E., Daban-Huard, C., Parellada, M., Fananas, L., Gaillard, R., et al. (2019). "A circle and a triangle dancing together": Alteration of social cognition in schizophrenia compared to autism spectrum disorders. *Schizophrenia Research, 210*, 94–100. https://doi.org/10.1016/j.schres.2019.05.043

Martino, D., & Hedderly, T. (2019). Tics and stereotypies: A comparative clinical review. *Parkinsonism & Related Disorders, 59*, 117–124. https://doi.org/10.1016/j.parkreldis.2019.02.005

Marzouk, T., Winkelbeiner, S., Azizi, H., Malhotra, A. K., & Homan, P. (2019). Transcranial magnetic stimulation for positive symptoms in schizophrenia: A systematic review. *Neuropsychobiology*. https://doi.org/10.1159/000502148

Mayo Clinic. (2020a). *Alzheimer's treatments: What's on the horizon?* https://www.mayoclinic.org/diseases-conditions/alzheimers-disease/in-depth/alzheimers-treatments/art-20047780

Mayo Clinic. (2020b). *Childhood schizophrenia*. https://www.mayoclinic.org/diseases-conditions/childhood-schizophrenia/symptoms-causes/syc-20354483

Mayo Clinic. (2020c). *Vascular dementia*. https://www.mayoclinic.org/diseases-conditions/vascular-dementia/symptoms-causes/syc-20378793

Maziade, M. (2017). At risk for serious mental illness—Screening children of patients with mood disorders or schizophrenia. *New England Journal of Medicine, 376*(10), 910–912.

McCutcheon, R. A., Reis Marques, T., & Howes, O. D. (2020). Schizophrenia—An overview. *JAMA Psychiatry, 77*(2), 201–210. https://doi.org/10.1001/jamapsychiatry.2019.3360

Methling, M., Krumbiegel, F., Hartwig, S., Parr, M. K., & Tsokos, M. (2019). Toxicological findings in suicides—Frequency of antidepressant and antipsychotic substances. *Forensic Science, Medicine and Pathology, 15*(1), 23–30. https://doi.org/10.1007/s12024-018-0041-4

Meyburg, J., Dill, M.-L., Traube, C., Silver, G., & von Haken, R. (2017). Patterns of postoperative delirium in children. *Pediatric Critical Care Medicine, 18*(2), 128–133. https://doi.org/10.1097/PCC.0000000000000993

Misiak, B., Stanczykiewicz, B., Kotowicz, K., Rybakowski, J. K., Samochowiec, J., & Frydecka, D. (2018). Cytokines and C-reactive protein alterations with respect to cognitive impairment in schizophrenia and bipolar disorder: A systematic review. *Schizophrenia Research, 192*, 16–29. https://doi.org/10.1016/j.schres.2017.04.015

Mitelman, S. A., Bralet, M.-C., Mehmet Haznedar, M., Hollander, E., Shihabuddin, L., Hazlett, E. A., & Buchsbaum, M. S. (2018). Positron emission tomography assessment of cerebral glucose metabolic rates in autism spectrum disorder and schizophrenia. *Brain Imaging and Behavior, 12*(2), 532–546. https://doi.org/10.1007/s11682-017-9721-z

Mithyantha, R., Kneen, R., McCann, E., & Gladstone, M. (2017). Current evidence-based recommendations on investigating children with global developmental delay. *Archives of Disease in Childhood, 102*(11), 1071. https://doi.org/10.1136/archdischild-2016-311271

Miyamoto, S., & Fleischhacker, W. W. (2017). The use of long-acting injectable antipsychotics in schizophrenia. *Current Treatment Options in Psychiatry, 4*(2), 117–126. https://doi.org/10.1007/s40501-017-0115-z

Mohammadzadeh, A., Azadi, S., King, S., Khosravani, V., & Sharifi Bastan, F. (2019). Childhood trauma and the likelihood of increased suicidal risk in schizophrenia. *Psychiatry Research, 275*, 100–107. https://doi.org/https://doi.org/10.1016/j.psychres.2019.03.023

Moradi, H., Harvey, P. D., & Helldin, L. (2018). Correlates of risk factors for reduced life expectancy in schizophrenia: Is it possible to develop a predictor profile? *Schizophrenia Research, 201*, 388–392. https://doi.org/10.1016/j.schres.2018.05.035

Moriarty, F., Savva, G. M., Grossi, C. M., Bennett, K., Fox, C., Maidment, I., et al. (2020). Cognitive decline associated with anticholinergics, benzodiazepines, and Z-drugs: Findings from The Irish Longitudinal Study on Ageing (TILDA). *medRxiv*. https://doi.org/10.1101/2020.05.09.20095661

Mosconi, L., Walters, M., Sterling, J., Quinn, C., McHugh, P., Andrews, R. E., et al. (2018). Lifestyle and vascular risk effects on MRI-based biomarkers of Alzheimer's disease: A cross-sectional study of middle-aged adults from the broader New York City area. *BMJ Open, 8*(3), e019362. https://doi.org/10.1136/bmjopen-2017-019362

Mudge, A. M., Banks, M. D., Barnett, A. G., Blackberry, I., Graves, N., Green, T., et al. (2017). CHERISH (Collaboration for Hospitalised Elders Reducing the Impact of Stays in Hospital): Protocol for a multi-site improvement program to reduce geriatric syndromes in older inpatients. *BMC Geriatrics, 17*(1), 11. https://doi.org/10.1186/s12877-016-0399-7

Mukherjee, R. A. S., Cook, P. A., Norgate, S. H., & Price, A. D. (2019). Neurodevelopmental outcomes in individuals with fetal alcohol spectrum disorder (FASD) with and without exposure to neglect: Clinical cohort data from a national FASD diagnostic clinic. *Alcohol, 76*, 23–28. https://doi.org/10.1016/j.alcohol.2018.06.002

Müller-Vahl, K. R., Sambrani, T., & Jakubovski, E. (2019). Tic disorders revisited: Introduction of the term "tic spectrum disorders." *European Child and Adolescent Psychiatry, 28*(8), 1129–1135.

Müller, N. (2018). Inflammation in schizophrenia: Pathogenetic aspects and therapeutic considerations. *Schizophrenia Bulletin, 44*(5), 973–982. https://doi.org/10.1093/schbul/sby024

Myburgh, S., & Tammaro, S. M. (2013). *Vgotsky's theory*. Science Direct. https://www.sciencedirect.com/topics/psychology/vygotskys-theory

Myers, K. A., van't Hof, F. N. G., Sadleir, L. G., Legault, G., Simard-Tremblay, E., Amor, D. J., & Scheffer, I. E. (2019). Fragile females: Case series of epilepsy in girls with FMR1 disruption. *Pediatrics, 144*(3), e20190599. https://doi.org/10.1542/peds.2019-0599

Nakamura, A., Kaneko, N., Villemagne, V. L., Kato, T., Doecke, J., Doré, V., et al. (2018). High performance plasma amyloid-β biomarkers for Alzheimer's disease. *Nature, 554*(7691), 249–254. https://doi.org/10.1038/nature25456

Nakazawa, K., Jeevakumar, V., & Nakao, K. (2017). Spatial and temporal boundaries of NMDA receptor hypofunction leading to schizophrenia. *NPJ Schizophrenia, 3*(1), 7. https://doi.org/10.1038/s41537-016-0003-3

Nakazawa, K., & Sapkota, K. (2020). The origin of NMDA receptor hypofunction in schizophrenia. *Pharmacology & Therapeutics, 205*, 107426. https://doi.org/10.1016/j.pharmthera.2019.107426

National Alliance on Mental Illness. (2020). *Schizophrenia*. https://www.nami.org/About-Mental-Illness/Mental-Health-Conditions/Schizophrenia

National Center for Complementary and Integrative Health. (2020). *Alzheimer's disease at a glance*. https://www.nccih.nih.gov/health/alzheimers-disease-at-a-glance

National Down Syndrome Society. (2020). *What is Down syndrome?* https://www.ndss.org/about-down-syndrome/down-syndrome/

National Fragile X Foundation. (2020). *Fragile X syndrome (FSX)*. https://fragilex.org/understanding-fragile-x/fragile-x-syndrome/

National Institute on Aging. (2017). *What happens to the brain in Alzheimer's disease?* Retrieved from https://www.nia.nih.gov/health/what-happens-brain-alzheimers-disease

National Institute of Mental Health. (2018). *Statistics: Schizophrenia*. https://www.nimh.nih.gov/health/statistics/schizophrenia.shtml

National Institute of Mental Health. (2020). *Schizophrenia: Risk factors*. https://www.nimh.nih.gov/health/topics/schizophrenia/index.shtml#part_145429

National Institute of Neurological Disorders and Stroke. (2019). *Dementia*. https://www.ninds.nih.gov/Disorders/All-Disorders/Dementia-Information-Page

National Organization on Fetal Alcohol Syndrome. (2020). *Recognizing FASD*. https://www.nofas.org/recognizing-fasd/

Nguyen, T. T., Kovacevic, S., Dev, S. I., Lu, K., Liu, T. T., & Eyler, L. T. (2017). Dynamic functional connectivity in bipolar disorder is associated with executive function and processing speed: A preliminary study. *Neuropsychology, 31*(1), 73. https://doi.org/10.1037/neu0000317

Nitza, G., Winer, A., & Zaks, B. (2017). Challenging the six-minute myth of online video lectures: Can interactivity expand the attention span of learners? *Online Journal of Applied Knowledge Management, 5*(1), 101–111.

Noguera, A., Castro-Fornieles, J., Romero, S., de la Serna, E., Sugranyes, G., Sánchez-Gistau, V., et al. (2018). Attenuated psychotic symptoms in children and adolescent offspring of patients with schizophrenia. *Schizophrenia Research, 193*, 354–358. https://doi.org/10.1016/j.schres.2017.07.050

Nostro, A. D., Müller, V. I., Reid, A. T., & Eickhoff, S. B. (2016). Correlations between personality and brain structure: A crucial role of gender. *Cerebral Cortex, 27*(7), 3698–3712. https://doi.org/10.1093/cercor/bhw191

NYU Hartford Institute of Geriatric Nursing. (2020a). *The AD8: The Washington University Dementia Screening Test.* https://hign.org/consultgeri/try-this-series/ad8-washington-university-dementia-screening-test

NYU Hartford Institute of Geriatric Nursing. (2020b). *Use of the Functional Activities Questionnaire in older adults with dementia.* https://hign.org/consultgeri/try-this-series/use-functional-activities-questionnaire-older-adults-dementia

Oberer, N., Gashaj, V., & Roebers, C. M. (2018). Executive functions, visual-motor coordination, physical fitness and academic achievement: Longitudinal relations in typically developing children. *Human Movement Science, 58*, 69–79. https://doi.org/10.1016/j.humov.2018.01.003

Oh, E. S., Fong, T. G., Hshieh, T. T., & Inouye, S. K. (2017). Delirium in older persons: Advances in diagnosis and treatment. *Journal of the American Medical Association, 318*(12), 1161–1174. https://doi.org/10.1001/jama.2017.12067

Oh, J., Chopik, W. J., Konrath, S., & Grimm, K. J. (2020). Longitudinal changes in empathy across the life span in six samples of human development. *Social Psychological and Personality Science, 11*(2), 244–253. https://doi.org/10.1177%2F1948550619849429

Okkels, N., Trabjerg, B., Arendt, M., & Pedersen, C. B. (2017). Traumatic stress disorders and risk of subsequent schizophrenia spectrum disorder or bipolar disorder: A nationwide cohort study. *Schizophrenia Bulletin, 43*(1), 180–186. https://doi.org/10.1093/schbul/sbw082

Olbert, C. M., Nagendra, A., & Buck, B. (2018). Meta-analysis of Black vs. White racial disparity in schizophrenia diagnosis in the United States: Do structured assessments attenuate racial disparities? *Journal of Abnormal Psychology, 127*(1), 104–115. https://doi.org/10.1037/abn0000309

Orgeta, V., Tabet, N., Nilforooshan, R., & Howard, R. (2017). Efficacy of antidepressants for depression in Alzheimer's disease: Systematic review and meta-analysis. *Journal of Alzheimer's Disease, 58*, 725–733. https://doi.org/10.3233/JAD-161247

Owen, M. J., & O'Donovan, M. C. (2017). Schizophrenia and the neurodevelopmental continuum: Evidence from genomics. *World Psychiatry, 16*(3), 227–235. https://doi.org/10.1002/wps.20440

Parnas, J., & Zandersen, M. (2018). Self and schizophrenia: Current status and diagnostic implications. *World Psychiatry, 17*(2), 220–221. https://doi.org/10.1002/wps.20528

Piaget, J. (1966). *Time perception in children.* Norton.

Piaget, J., & Inhelder, B. (2000). *The psychology of the child* (2nd ed.). Basic Books.

Pillay, J., Boylan, K., Newton, A., Hartling, L., Vandermeer, B., Nuspl, M., et al. (2018). Harms of antipsychotics in children and young adults: A systematic review update. *Canadian Journal of Psychiatry, 63*(10), 661–678. https://doi.org/10.1177/0706743718779950

Potter, M. L., & Moller, M. D. (Eds.). (2020). *Psychiatric-mental health nursing: From suffering to hope* (2nd ed.). Pearson Education.

Powers, A. R., Addington, J., Perkins, D. O., Bearden, C. E., Cadenhead, K. S., Cannon, T. D., et al. (2020). Duration of the psychosis prodrome. *Schizophrenia Research, 216*, 443–449. https://doi.org/10.1016/j.schres.2019.10.051

Prado, E. L., Ashorn, U., Phuka, J., Maleta, K., Sadalaki, J., Oaks, B. M., et al. (2018). Associations of maternal nutrition during pregnancy and post partum with maternal cognition and caregiving. *Maternal & Child Nutrition, 14*(2), e12546. https://doi.org/10.1111/mcn.12546

Price, B. (2016). Continuing professional development: Hallucinations: Insights and supportive first care. *Nursing Standard, 30*(21), 49–60. https://doi.org/10.7748/ns.30.21.49.s45

Pruessner, M., Cullen, A. E., Aas, M., & Walker, E. F. (2017). The neural diathesis-stress model of schizophrenia revisited: An update on recent findings considering illness stage and neurobiological and methodological complexities. *Neuroscience & Biobehavioral Reviews, 73*, 191–218. https://doi.org/10.1016/j.neubiorev.2016.12.013

Qiao, Y., Liu, C. P., Han, H. Q., Liu, F. J., Shao, Y., & Xie, B. (2020). No impact of omega-3 fatty acid supplementation on symptoms or hostility among patients with schizophrenia. *Frontiers in Psychiatry, 11*(312). https://doi.org/10.3389/fpsyt.2020.00312

Ramos-Cejudo, J., Wisniewski, T., Marmar, C., Zetterberg, H., Blennow, K., de Leon, M. J., & Fossati, S. (2018). Traumatic brain injury and Alzheimer's disease: The cerebrovascular link. *EBioMedicine, 28*, 21–30. https://doi.org/10.1016/j.ebiom.2018.01.021

Rasic, D., Hajek, T., Alda, M., & Uher, R. (2014). Risk of mental illness in offspring of parents with schizophrenia, bipolar disorder, and major depressive disorder: A meta-analysis of family high-risk studies. *Schizophrenia Bulletin, 40*(1), 28–38.

Rathee, R., Luhrmann, T. M., Bhatia, T., & Deshpande, S. N. (2018). Cognitive insight and objective quality of life in people with schizophrenia and auditory hallucinations. *Psychiatry Research, 259*, 223–228. https://doi.org/10.1016/j.psychres.2017.09.032

Ray, W. A., Stein, C. M., Murray, K. T., Fuchs, D. C., Patrick, S. W., Daugherty, J., et al. (2019). Association of antipsychotic treatment with risk of unexpected death among children and youths. *JAMA Psychiatry, 76*(2), 162–171. https://doi.org/10.1001/jamapsychiatry.2018.3421

Reisberg, B., Monteiro, I., Torossian, C., Auer, S., Shulman, M. B., Ghimire, S., et al. (2014). The BEHAVE-AD assessment system: A perspective, a commentary on new findings, and a historical review. *Dementia and Geriatric Cognitive Disorders, 38*(1–2), 89–146. https://doi.org/10.1159/000357839

Reynish, E. L., Hapca, S. M., De Souza, N., Cvoro, V., Donnan, P. T., & Guthrie, B. (2017). Epidemiology and outcomes of people with dementia, delirium, and unspecified cognitive impairment in the general hospital: Prospective cohort study of 10,014 admissions. *BMC Medicine, 15*(1), 140–140. https://doi.org/10.1186/s12916-017-0899-0

Riglin, L., Collishaw, S., Richards, A., Thapar, A. K., Maughan, B., O'Donovan, M. C., & Thapar, A. (2017). Schizophrenia risk alleles and neurodevelopmental outcomes in childhood: A population-based cohort study. *The Lancet Psychiatry, 4*(1), 57–62. https://doi.org/10.1016/S2215-0366(16)30406-0

Rincon, F., Serruya, M., & Jallo, J. (2020). Arterial hyperoxia is associated with poor functional outcome and cognitive impairment after TBI: A retrospective multi-center cohort study. *Neurology, 94*, 1272–1279.

Robinson, K. M., Crawford, T. N., Buckwalter, K. C., & Casey, D. A. (2018). Outcomes of a two-component intervention on behavioral symptoms in persons with dementia and symptom response in their caregivers. *Journal of Applied Gerontology, 37*(5), 570–594. https://doi.org/10.1177/0733464816677549

Rutter, L. A., Dodell-Feder, D., Vahia, I. V., Forester, B. P., Ressler, K. J., Wilmer, J. B., & Germine, L. (2019). Emotion sensitivity across the lifespan: Mapping clinical risk periods to sensitivity to facial emotion intensity. *Journal of Experimental Psychology: General, 148*(11), 1993–2005. https://doi.org/10.1037/xge0000559

Sadock, B., Sadock, V. A., & Ruiz, P. (2020). *Kaplan & Sadock's synopsis of psychiatry: Behavioral sciences/Clinical psychiatry* (11th ed.). Wolters Klower.

Šagud, M., Vuksan-Cusa, B., Jakšic, N., Mihaljevic-Peleš, A., Rojnic Kuzman, M., & Pivac, N. (2018). Smoking in schizophrenia: An updated review. *Psychiatria Danubina, 30*(4), 216–223.

Sanghani, S. N., Petrides, G., & Kellner, C. H. (2018). Electroconvulsive therapy (ECT) in schizophrenia: A review of recent literature. *Current Opinion in Psychiatry, 31*(3), 213–222. https://doi.org/10.1097/YCO.0000000000000418

Sardina, A. L., Fitzsimmons, S., Hoyt, C. M., & Buettner, L. L. (2019). A mentally stimulating activities program for the treatment of neuropsychiatric symptoms in Alzheimer's disease. *American Journal of Recreation Therapy, 18*(4), 27–37. https://doi.org/10.5055/ajrt.2019.0200

Sarpal, D. K., Robinson, D. G., Fales, C., Lencz, T., Argyelan, M., Karlsgodt, K. H., et al. (2017). Relationship between duration of untreated psychosis and intrinsic corticostriatal connectivity in patients with early phase schizophrenia. *Neuropsychopharmacology, 42*(11), 2214–2221. https://doi.org/10.1038/npp.2017.55

Satogami, K., Takahashi, S., Yamada, S., Ukai, S., & Shinosaki, K. (2017). Omega-3 fatty acids related to cognitive impairment in patients with schizophrenia. *Schizophrenia Research: Cognition, 9*, 8–12. https://doi.org/10.1016/j.scog.2017.05.001

Schmidt, S. J., Lange, M., Schöttle, D., Karow, A., Schimmelmann, B. G., & Lambert, M. (2018). Negative symptoms, anxiety, and depression as mechanisms of change of a 12-month trial of assertive community treatment as part of integrated care in patients with first- and multi-episode schizophrenia spectrum disorders (ACCESS I trial). *European Archives of Psychiatry and Clinical Neuroscience, 268*(6), 593–602. https://doi.org/10.1007/s00406-017-0810-1

Schöttle, D., Schimmelmann, B. G., Ruppelt, F., Bussopulos, A., Frieling, M., Nika, E., et al. (2018). Effectiveness of integrated care including therapeutic assertive community treatment in severe schizophrenia-spectrum and bipolar I disorders: Four-year follow-up of the ACCESS II study. *PLoS One, 13*(2), e0192929. https://doi.org/10.1371/journal.pone.0192929

Schroeder, M. E. (2019). Delirium in the elderly. In A. Abd-Elsayed (Ed.), *Pain* (pp. 1117–1120). Springer.

Schwartz, E. K., Docherty, N. M., Najolia, G. M., & Cohen, A. S. (2019). Exploring the racial diagnostic bias of schizophrenia using behavioral and clinical-based measures. *Journal of Abnormal Psychology, 128*(3), 263. https://psycnet.apa.org/doi/10.1037/abn0000409

Shen, Y., Xu, J., Li, Z., Huang, Y., Yuan, Y., Wang, J., et al. (2018). Analysis of gut microbiota diversity and auxiliary diagnosis as a biomarker in patients with schizophrenia: A cross-sectional study. *Schizophrenia Research, 197*, 470–477. https://doi.org/10.1016/j.schres.2018.01.002

Sinclair, D. J. M., Zhao, S., Qi, F., Nyakyoma, K., Kwong, J. S. W., & Adams, C. E. (2019). Electroconvulsive therapy for treatment resistant schizophrenia. *Cochrane Database of Systematic Reviews*, Issue 3, Article No. CD011847. https://doi.org/10.1002/14651858.CD011847.pub2

Skene, N. G., Bryois, J., Bakken, T. E., Breen, G., Crowley, J. J., Gaspar, H. A., et al. (2018). Genetic identification of brain cell types underlying schizophrenia. *Nature Genetics, 50*(6), 825–833. https://doi.org/10.1038/s41588-018-0129-5

Snyder, M. A., & Gao, W.-J. (2020). NMDA receptor hypofunction for schizophrenia revisited: Perspectives from epigenetic mechanisms. *Schizophrenia Research, 217*, 60–70. https://doi.org/10.1016/j.schres.2019.03.010

Soliman, E. S., Mahdy, R. S., & Fouad, H. A. (2018). Impact of psychoeducation program on quality of life of schizophrenic patients and their caregivers. *Egyptian Journal of Psychiatry, 39*(1), 35. https://doi.org/10.4103/ejpsy.ejpsy_34_17

Soysal, P., & Isik, A. T. (2018). Pathogenesis of delirium. In A. T. Isak & G. T. Grossberg (Eds.), *Delirium in elderly patients* (pp. 7–18). Springer.

Spector, S. E. (2017). *Cultural diversity in health and illness* (9th ed.). Pearson.

Steingartner, W., Novitzká, V., Bačíková, M., & Korečko, _. (2018). New approach to categorical semantics for procedural languages. *Computing and Informatics, 36*(6), 1385–1414.

Stites, S. D., Rubright, J. D., & Karlawish, J. (2018). What features of stigma do the public most commonly attribute to Alzheimer's disease dementia?: Results of a survey of the US general public. *Alzheimer's & Dementia, 14*(7), 925–932. https://doi.org/10.1016/j.jalz.2018.01.006

Strassnig, M., Bowie, C., Pinkham, A. E., Penn, D., Twamley, E. W., Patterson, T. L., & Harvey, P. D. (2018). Which levels of cognitive impairments and negative symptoms are related to functional deficits in schizophrenia? *Journal of Psychiatric Research, 104*, 124–129. https://doi.org/10.1016/j.jpsychires.2018.06.018

Swathy, B., & Banerjee, M. (2017). Understanding epigenetics of schizophrenia in the backdrop of its antipsychotic drug therapy. *Epigenomics, 9*(5), 721–736. https://doi.org/10.2217/epi-2016-0106

Tanaka, T., Matsuda, T., Hayes, L. N., Yang, S., Rodriguez, K., Severance, E. G., et al. W. (2017). Infection and inflammation in schizophrenia and bipolar disorder. *Neuroscience Research, 115*, 59–63. https://doi.org/10.1016/j.neures.2016.11.002

Tang, L., Shafer, A. T., & Ofen, N. (2017). Prefrontal cortex contributions to the development of memory formation. *Cerebral Cortex, 28*(9), 3295–3308. https://doi.org/10.1093/cercor/bhx200

Thibodeau, R., Shanks, L. N., & Smith, B. P. (2018). Do continuum beliefs reduce schizophrenia stigma?: Effects of a laboratory intervention on behavioral and self-reported stigma. *Journal of Behavior Therapy and Experimental Psychiatry, 58*, 29–35. https://doi.org/10.1016/j.jbtep.2017.08.002

Tolppanen, A.-M., Taipale, H., & Hartikainen, S. (2017). Head or brain injuries and Alzheimer's disease: A nested case-control register study. *Alzheimer's & Dementia, 13*(12), 1371–1379. https://doi.org/10.1016/j.jalz.2017.04.010

Tripathi, A., Kar, S. K., & Shukla, R. (2018). Cognitive deficits in schizophrenia: Understanding the biological correlates and remediation strategies. *Clinical Psychopharmacology and Neuroscience, 16*(1), 7–17. https://doi.org/10.9758/cpn.2018.16.1.7

U.S. National Library of Medicine. (2020). *Fragile-X-syndrome.* https://ghr.nlm.nih.gov/condition/fragile-x-syndrome

Ungvari, G. S., Gerevich, J., Takács, R., & Gazdag, G. (2018). Schizophrenia with prominent catatonic features: A selective review. *Schizophrenia Research, 200,* 77–84. https://doi.org/10.1016/j.schres.2017.08.008

Upthegrove, R., Marwaha, S., & Birchwood, M. (2017). Depression and schizophrenia: Cause, consequence, or transdiagnostic issue? *Schizophrenia Bulletin, 43*(2), 240–244. https://doi.org/10.1093/schbul/sbw097

Van Assche, L., Van Aubel, E., Van de Ven, L., Bouckaert, F., Luyten, P., & Vandenbulcke, M. (2018). The neuropsychological profile and phenomenology of late onset psychosis: A cross-sectional study on the differential diagnosis of very-late-onset schizophrenia-like psychosis, dementia with Lewy bodies and Alzheimer's type dementia with psychosis. *Archives of Clinical Neuropsychology, 34*(2), 183–199. https://doi.org/10.1093/arclin/acy034

Vancampfort, D., Firth, J., Schuch, F. B., Rosenbaum, S., Mugisha, J., Hallgren, M., et al. (2017). Sedentary behavior and physical activity levels in people with schizophrenia, bipolar disorder and major depressive disorder: A global systematic review and meta-analysis. *World Psychiatry, 16*(3), 308–315. https://doi.org/10.1002/wps.20458

Vasudevan, P., & Suri, M. (2017). A clinical approach to developmental delay and intellectual disability. *Clinical Medicine, 17*(6), 558–561. https://doi.org/10.7861/clinmedicine.17-6-558

Veerman, S. R. T., Schulte, P. F. J., & de Haan, L. (2017). Treatment for negative symptoms in schizophrenia: A comprehensive review. *Drugs, 77*(13), 1423–1459. https://doi.org/10.1007/s40265-017-0789-y

Vijayakumar, N., Op de Macks, Z., Shirtcliff, E. A., & Pfeifer, J. H. (2018). Puberty and the human brain: Insights into adolescent development. *Neuroscience & Biobehavioral Reviews, 92,* 417–436. https://doi.org/10.1016/j.neubiorev.2018.06.004

Vitrikas, K. R., Savard, D., & Bucaj, M. (2017). Developmental delay: When and how to screen. *American Family Physician, 96*(1), 36–43.

Wang, D., Schultz, T., Novak, G. P., Baker, S., Bennett, D. A., & Narayan, V. A. (2018). Longitudinal modeling of functional decline associated with pathologic Alzheimer's disease in older persons without cognitive impairment. *Journal of Alzheimer's Disease 62*(2), 855–865. https://doi.org/10.3233/JAD-170903

Wang, L. Y., LaBardi, B. A., Raskind, M. A., & Peskind, E. R. (2020). Alzheimer's disease and other neurocognitive disorders. In N. Hantke, A. Etkin, & R. O'Hara (Eds.), *Handbook of mental health and aging* (pp. 161–183). Elsevier.

Wang, Y.-Y., Yue, J.-R., Xie, D.-M., Carter, P., Li, Q.-L., Gartaganis, S. L., et al. (2020). Effect of the tailored, family-involved Hospital Elder Life Program on postoperative delirium and function in older adults: A randomized clinical trial. *JAMA Internal Medicine, 180*(1), 17–25. https://doi.org/10.1001/jamainternmed.2019.4446

Weiler, N. (2019). *Alzheimer's disease is a "double-prion disorder," study shows: Self-propagating amyloid and tau prions found in post-mortem brain samples, with highest levels in patients who died young.* University of California San Francisco. https://www.ucsf.edu/news/2019/05/414326/alzheimers-disease-double-prion-disorder-study-shows

Weiner, M. W., Harvey, D., Hayes, J., Landau, S. M., Aisen, P. S., Petersen, R. C., et al. (2017). Effects of traumatic brain injury and posttraumatic stress disorder on development of Alzheimer's disease in Vietnam Veterans using the Alzheimer's Disease Neuroimaging Initiative: Preliminary report. *Alzheimer's & Dementia: Translational Research & Clinical Interventions, 3*(2), 177–188. https://doi.org/10.1016/j.trci.2017.02.005

Weinstein, J. J., Chohan, M. O., Slifstein, M., Kegeles, L. S., Moore, H., & Abi-Dargham, A. (2017). Pathway-specific dopamine abnormalities in schizophrenia. *Biological Psychiatry, 81*(1), 31–42. https://doi.org/10.1016/j.biopsych.2016.03.2104

Weller, J., & Budson, A. (2018). Current understanding of Alzheimer's disease diagnosis and treatment. *F1000Research, 7.* doi:10.12688/f1000research.14506.1

Wideman, C. E., Jardine, K. H., & Winters, B. D. (2018). Involvement of classical neurotransmitter systems in memory reconsolidation: Focus on destabilization. *Neurobiology of Learning and Memory, 156,* 68–79. https://doi.org/10.1016/j.nlm.2018.11.001

Winton-Brown, T. T., Elanjithara, T., Power, P., Coentre, R., Blanco-Polaina, P., & McGuire, P. (2017). Five-fold increased risk of relapse following breaks in antipsychotic treatment of first episode psychosis. *Schizophrenia Research, 179,* 50–56. https://doi.org/10.1016/j.schres.2016.09.029

Wisner, K. L., Sit, D. K. Y., Bogen, D. L., Altemus, M., Pearlstein, T. B., Svikis, D. S., et al. (2018). Mental health and behavioral disorders in pregnancy. In M. B. Landon, et al. (Eds.), *Gabbe's obstetrics essentials: Normal and problem pregnancies e-book* (pp. 408–410). Elsevier.

Wolters, F. J., Zonneveld, H. I., Hofman, A., van de Lugt, A., Koudstaal, P. J., Vernooij, M. W., & Ikram, M. A. (2017). Cerebral perfusion and the risk of dementia. *Circulation, 136*(8), 719–728. https://doi.org/10.1161/CIRCULATIONAHA.117.027448

Woods, B., O'Philbin, L., Farrell, E. M., Spector, A. E., & Orrell, M. (2018). Reminiscence therapy for dementia. *Cochrane Database of Systematic Reviews,* Issue 3, Article No. CD001120. https://doi.org/10.1002/14651858.CD001120.pub3

Xiao, J., Prandovszky, E., Kannan, G., Pletnikov, M. V., Dickerson, F., Severance, E. G., & Yolken, R. H. (2018). Toxoplasma gondii: Biological parameters of the connection to schizophrenia. *Schizophrenia Bulletin, 44*(5), 983–992. https://doi.org/10.1093/schbul/sby082

Yarlott, L., Heald, E., & Forton, D. (2017). Hepatitis C virus infection, and neurological and psychiatric disorders: A review. *Journal of Advanced Research, 8*(2), 139–148. https://doi.org/10.1016/j.jare.2016.09.005

Zhang, J. P., Robinson, D., Yu, J., Gallego, J., Fleischhacker, W. W., Kahn, R. S., et al. (2019). Schizophrenia polygenic risk score as a predictor of antipsychotic efficacy in first-episode psychosis. *American Journal of Psychiatry, 176*(1), 21–28. https://doi.org/10.1176/appi.ajp.2018.17121363

Zhu, J., Zhuo, C., Xu, L., Liu, F., Qin, W., & Yu, C. (2017). Altered coupling between resting-state cerebral blood flow and functional connectivity in schizophrenia. *Schizophrenia Bulletin, 43*(6), 1363–1374. https://doi.org/10.1093/schbul/sbx051

Module 24

Culture and Diversity

Module Outline and Learning Outcomes

The Concept of Culture and Diversity

Cultural Diversity

24.1 Describe the language used to describe cultural diversity.

Values and Beliefs

24.2 Analyze how values and beliefs are components of cultural diversity.

Disparities and Differences

24.3 Describe how cultural disparities and differences affect healthcare.

Concepts Related to Culture and Diversity

24.4 Outline the relationship between culture and diversity and other concepts.

Developing Cultural Competence

24.5 Analyze the need for developing cultural competence.

Nursing Process

24.6 Summarize the nursing process in the context of cultural competence.

» The Concept of Culture and Diversity

Concept Key Terms

Acculturation, **1812**
Ageism, **1815**
Alternative therapies, **1823**
Assimilation, **1812**
Bias, **1813**
Classism, **1814**
Complementary therapies, **1823**
Cultural competence, **1820**
Cultural groups, **1809**
Cultural humility, **1810**
Cultural values, **1810**
Culture, **1809**
Discrimination, **1812**
Diversity, **1809**
Enculturation, **1812**
Ethnic groups, **1810**
Health disparity, **1816**
Heterosexism, **1815**
Homophobia, **1815**
Minority, **1813**
Multiculturalism, **1809**
Poverty, **1814**
Prejudice, **1821**
Race, **1813**
Racism, **1813**
Sexism, **1813**
Sexual orientation, **1815**
Social justice, **1812**
Stereotyping, **1813**
Subculture, **1809**
Transgender, **1813**
Vulnerable populations, **1816**
Worldview, **1811**

Culture refers to the patterns of behavior and thinking that people living in social groups learn, develop, and share. The term **diversity** refers to the array of differences among individuals, groups, and communities. Today's nurses must be able to work with diverse populations of patients—patients of varying socioeconomic, cultural, and spiritual backgrounds and patients with varying values and belief systems. To be able to provide culturally aware nursing, nurses must examine their own cultural values and beliefs.

Cultural Diversity

Cultural groups can be categorized around racial, ethnic, religious, or socially common practice patterns. Race, however, does not equate with culture. Cultural groups often share common characteristics such as history of origin; general worldview, language, customs, beliefs, and values; experiences of power, stigma, and discrimination; religious beliefs and practices; food practices and eating patterns; health and illness beliefs and behaviors; and concept of time, self, and personal space (Purnell & Fenkl, 2019; Spector, 2017). **Subculture** is a term that refers to a group of people within a culture whose practices or beliefs are distinct or separate from the dominant or parent culture. Subculture is a term often defined more broadly and has been used to describe certain religious sects, ethnic groups, and even devotees of some genres of music or philosophy.

Multiculturalism is defined as many cultures and subcultures coexisting within a given society in which no one culture dominates. In a multicultural society, human differences are accepted and respected. Classrooms in an academic setting may be considered multicultural when all students are socialized to succeed and all learning styles are valued and understood.

In the United States, one driver of multiculturalism has been immigration. People from every country in the world have come to the United States. Each year, more than one million individuals obtain legal permanent resident status in the United States.

The majority of those who immigrate to the United States are from Mexico, followed by China and the Philippine Islands (U.S. Department of Homeland Security, 2020).

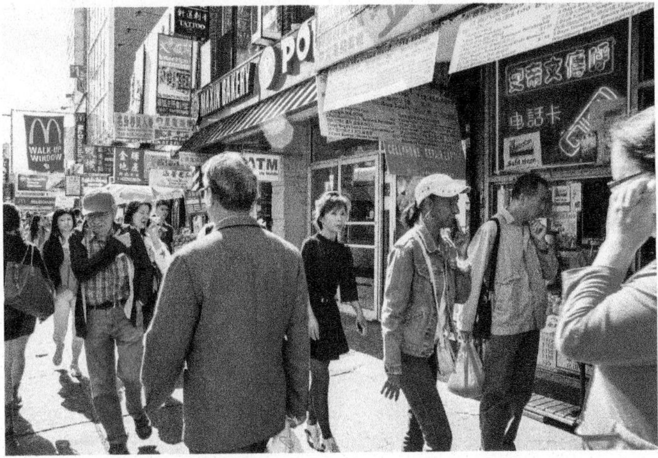

Figure 24.1 » A crowded street in the Chinatown area of Flushing, Queens, New York. More than half a million Chinese Americans live in New York City.

Source: sx70/iStock Editorial/Getty Images.

The reasons for immigration vary: some immigrants are fleeing an oppressive government, civil unrest, or war; some come seeking religious and/or political freedom; still others come to the United States to join familly or to pursue advanced education (**Figure 24.1 »**). In 2018, more than 1 million people came into the United States under legal status, some 53,000 claiming either refugee status or asylum from political oppression (U.S. Department of Homeland Security, 2020). Many immigrants coming to the United States have fled horrific experiences such as gang violence, rape, torture, and starvation.

Each family or group of immigrants brings its own culture, adding to what has been described as the "melting pot" that is the United States. The image of a melting pot implies the assimilation of multiple ethnic groups and their cultural practices into a single national identity. However, as these groups become established in the American culture, part or all of their ethnic identity remains. Instead of a melting pot, the United States should be considered a mosaic of the unique qualities of the cultural groups, coming together to make one America.

Members of each of these **ethnic groups** have common characteristics, including nationality, language, values, and customs, and they share a cultural heritage. Examples of ethnic groups are Cuban Americans, Appalachians, Samoan Americans, and American Creole.

In addition to different cultural and ethnic groups, individuals in the United States belong to one or more races. The U.S. Census Bureau (2020) identifies the following races:

- White
- Black or African American
- American Indian or Alaska Native
- Asian
- Native Hawaiian or Other Pacific Islander.

Individuals of Hispanic, Latino, or Spanish origin may identify as members of any race.

Cultural, ethnic, racial, and other differences make nursing care both a privilege and a challenge. Nurses who do develop cultural competence and practice evidence-based care that is relevant to all of their patients will gain confidence in their abilities and greater personal benefit from their work. A culturally competent practice begins with gaining a greater understanding of the differing values and beliefs of others (**Box 24.1 »**) and recognizing how these differing values and beliefs affect patients in all aspects of providing care.

Box 24.1

Nurses' Self-Awareness and Cultural Humility

Professional nurses must possess self-awareness. Self-awareness is critical to developing sensitivity to differences while supporting a sense of cultural humility rather than superiority over others. **Cultural humility** has been described as "a lifelong commitment to self-evaluation and critique, to redressing power imbalances . . . and to developing mutually beneficial and non-paternalistic partnerships with communities on behalf of individuals and defined populations" (Tervalon & Murray-Garcia, 1998, p. 123).

As a nursing student, you may find your personal values conflict with professional values. For example, you may find yourself uncomfortable with a certain ethnic group or religious faith. Yet a nurse, or any healthcare provider (HCP), cannot refuse to care for a person based on cultural identity. Instead, your profession calls you to practice cultural humility, realizing that the person needs care, not judgment.

Following the June 2016 Orlando club shooting in which 49 people died and 53 others were wounded, a surgeon who took care of many of the victims posted a picture on Facebook of his bloodied shoes and wrote: "I don't know which [of the patients] were straight, which were gay, which were black or which were Hispanic. . . . And somehow, in that chaos, doctors, nurses, technicians, police, paramedics, and others performed super-human feats of compassion and care" (Itkowitz, 2016, para 6, 7). This example illustrates the essence of cultural humility.

Values and Beliefs

Culture includes a society's values, beliefs, assumptions, principles, myths, legends, and norms. People living within a culture typically share many of the prevailing society's values and beliefs. People use these values and beliefs to help them define meaning, identify acceptable behaviors, choose emotional reactions, and determine appropriate actions in given situations. Values and belief systems are part of a culture, as are family relationships and roles. To understand patient behaviors in more depth, a nurse must identify which cultures are prevalent demographically in a given area, learn more about those cultures, and apply that knowledge and experience when providing patient care.

Values reflect an underlying system of beliefs. **Cultural values** describe preferred ways of behaving or thinking that are sustained over time and used to govern or guide a cultural group's actions and decisions. When people live together in a society, cultural values often determine the rules people live by each day. These rules may be variously stated, but they basically address similar values. Curry, Mullins, and Whitehouse (2019) identified seven universal values that are used to build cooperation and morality within a culture: family values, group loyalty, reciprocity, bravery, respect, fairness, and property rights.

Cultural characteristics include observable behaviors as well as the unseen values that influence those behaviors. Cultural practices have meanings that give the group its worldview and that reflects the social organization of the culture. The organization of a culture or society includes the following elements:

- ***A physical element.*** The geographic area in which a society is located
- ***An infrastructure element.*** The framework of the systems and processes that keep a society functioning
- ***A behavioral element.*** The way people in a society act and react to each other
- ***A cultural element.*** All the values, beliefs, assumptions, and norms that make up a code of conduct for acceptable behaviors within a society.

Each culture has its own worldview or understanding of the world. **Worldview** refers to how the people in a culture perceive ideas and attitudes about the world, other people, and life in general. A culture's worldview supports its overall *belief system*, which is developed to explain the mysteries of the universe and of life that each society tries to understand, including:

- What is the meaning and purpose of life?
- Is there a God or higher power?
- What happens after death?

A cultural belief system influences an individual's decisions and actions in society regarding everything from preparing food and caring for the sick to rituals of death and burial. Scientific and medical advancements may or may not impact a culture's belief systems. The beliefs of a society are passed from generation to generation by word of mouth and by rituals, such as reading, telling certain stories, and observing holidays (**Figure 24.2** »). In many cases, cultural practices are rooted in the individual's religious faith or practices (see Module 30, Spirituality). Children observe and learn the belief system of their culture from parents, family members, and other caregivers who teach them any number of values and beliefs. Differing opinions may originate from religious beliefs or social conditions. People make decisions about "right or wrong," and as things change, people adapt, and the culture evolves.

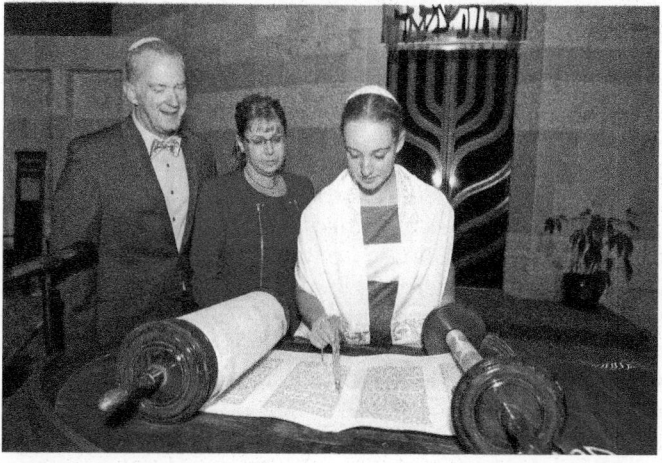

Figure 24.2 » Cultures try to understand and give meaning to life through spiritual beliefs, social values, and acceptable behaviors. In this picture, a 12-year-old girl is seen reading the Torah with her parents as she is acknowledged as a Bat Mitzvah, a Jewish adult.

Source: Donna Ellen Coleman/Shutterstock.

Belief systems are based on people's experiences and exposures to differences found in our world. As people's knowledge and understanding grow, their belief systems expand. Knowing why we believe what we do builds self-awareness and understanding of differences in our own beliefs compared with the beliefs of others.

Culturally based beliefs and traditions can affect the course and outcome of disease and illness. Healthcare providers and patients bring their respective cultural backgrounds and expectations to each interaction. These differences can impact both the expectations and practices of the patient and the provision of services by nurses and other healthcare professionals. Some differences in core beliefs have been described as *Western* (a term that generally refers to healthcare favored in North America and western Europe) and *Eastern*, referring to South America and the Asian and some African countries. Some of these are listed in **Table 24.1** ».

Cultural differences can present barriers to necessary care. Some areas in which barriers can arise include the following (Purnell & Fenkle, 2019; Spector, 2017):

- The importance, or lack of importance, of family members' involvement in managing illness and disease
- Lack of trust in the healthcare system and HCPs
- Lack of certified, dialect-specific interpreters
- Insufficient support for cultural competency at the institutional level
- Belief that illnesses are not linked to scientific pathophysiology
- Refusal of modern HCPs to believe the mind–body connection

TABLE 24.1 Examples of Differences in Core Beliefs

North American and "Western" Cultures	South American and "Eastern" Cultures
Health is viewed by many as the absence of disease.	Health is a state of harmony that encompasses the mind, body, and spirit.
Use of specialty practitioners (e.g., pediatricians, obstetricians)	Preference for respected healers from the culture of origin (e.g., herbalists, midwives, curanderos)
Recognition that food affects biophysical processes and functions	Belief that food can restore imbalances
Independence, individualism, and freedom are valued	Interdependence with family, community, and group acceptance are valued
Emphasis on use of modern healthcare practices to maintain or treat health issues	Emphasis on traditional methods of maintaining, protecting, and restoring health (such as through the use of traditional Chinese medicine [TCM])

Source: Based on Spector (2017).

- Fear or denial of death or life after death
- Cultural assumptions about disease and illness that may influence the presentation of symptoms or the response to treatments.

Although cultural beliefs and behaviors change over the years as a cultural group adapts to new ideas and conditions, some individuals may retain traditional behaviors and thinking. For instance, some cultures see health providers as authority figures and, as a result, patients may not communicate their discomforts, leading to the provision of unintentional substandard care (Li, Abdulkerim, Jordan, & Ga Eun Son, 2017). Tension can arise when different health belief systems conflict with each other. The result may be anxiety, anger, or fear. Nurses and other HCPs may reduce a patient's discomfort and promote trust by showing a nonjudgmental attitude of respect. Nurses must also recognize the common defense mechanisms such as anger, avoidance, denial, intellectualization, or projection that may be used when an individual feels threatened. (See Module 31, Stress and Coping, for information about defense mechanisms.)

Professional nurses work with and care for people who have differing values and beliefs. It is important for nurses to understand how their own cultural beliefs and practices inform who they are as nurses, in part to strengthen their own value systems but also to ensure they are sufficiently self-aware to keep from projecting their own beliefs and values onto their patients.

Cultural Transmission

A society is a group of people who share a common culture, rules of behavior, and basic social organization. Culture is transmitted, or learned and shared, by people living together in a society. Cultural characteristics—such as customs, beliefs, values, language, and socialization patterns—are passed from generation to generation.

Culture is transmitted from one generation to the next through language, material objects, rituals, customs, institutions, and art. Using a common language, people learn how to live by the rules governing the society and how to earn money or trade goods or services to meet basic needs, such as food and shelter. Culture can influence everything the members of a society think and do.

Enculturation, or cultural transmission, is exemplified by how children learn cultural characteristics from adults. These characteristics are often normalized as acceptable rules and procedures of behaviors. People biologically inherit physical traits and behavioral instincts, but they socially inherit cultural characteristics. Enculturation occurs in families until the children are ready to leave and establish their own values, beliefs, and practices through exposure to other cultural or societal practices through work, marriage, or higher education. However, enculturation may continue among family members who live close to each other, celebrate religious holidays together, or otherwise work to maintain the culture within their family and limit their exposure to other cultures.

People in a society have cultural characteristics that are embedded in art, music, food, religion, and traditions. Because culture is adaptive, these characteristics may be modified over the years as people use culture to adjust to changes in the world around them. Cultural behaviors are learned by:

- Observing others' actions
- Hearing instructions on what behaviors are right or wrong
- Imitating others doing a behavior
- Getting reinforcement (either positive or negative) for enacting a behavior
- Internalizing behaviors
- Spontaneously doing the behaviors without thinking about it.

Different societies can come together and share or exchange cultures as well. People may evolve from one cultural group to another. **Assimilation** is the process of adapting to and integrating characteristics of the dominant culture as one's own. People typically benefit by exchanging ideas, natural resources, and goods. **Acculturation** is the process of not only adapting to another culture but also accepting the majority group's culture as one's own. Because culture is complex, members of a cultural group may engage in many behaviors and habits unconsciously, making them difficult to explain to others. Sometimes assimilation and acculturation are implicit and covert, whereas other times assimilation can be overt and coercive.

As individuals go through the process of acculturation, they may choose to discard some practices from their culture of origin in exchange for practices of the dominant culture. Therefore, nurses need to ask appropriate questions to assess individual cultural practices rather than make assumptions. For example, some patients of Chinese background may be practicing Buddhists; others may prefer traditional Chinese practices such as herbs and acupuncture; others may be Christian and completely embrace Western medicine; while still others may blend practices in ways that make sense to them. Careful assessment of the individual patient is necessary to avoid making assumptions and stereotyping.

Diversity

Cultural differences are not the only hallmarks of diversity. Gender, race, class, sexual orientation, and age are just a few of the differences among individuals living in the United States. In many instances, these factors carry important implications for nursing. For example, African American men are at greater risk for stroke than any other single population (Centers for Disease Control and Prevention [CDC], 2019) and transgender people may delay seeking care due to previous negative encounters with healthcare professionals. Nurses must be prepared to work with everyone who walks in the door, regardless of that individual's personal background.

The concept of **social justice** recognizes that in society, not all groups are treated equally. **Discrimination**, or the restriction of justice, rights, and privileges of individuals or minority groups, may occur when dominant groups reinforce their rules and regulations in a way that limits opportunities for others. A dominant group may be one that is dominant by reason of its numbers or having influence, power, money, and position to remain dominant while reinforcing rules and norms that benefit its own interests. The term **minority** usually refers to an individual or group of individuals who are outside the dominant group. Although demographics can vary from one area to another, in the United States, African Americans, Hispanics, Asian Americans, and American Indians/Alaska Natives are among those generally referred to as minority groups, even in situations when they are not in the numerical minority. **Stereotyping** is an overgeneralization of group characteristics that reinforces societal biases and distorts individual characteristics.

Culturally competent nurses should respect and advocate for human dignity. Stereotyping, prejudice, and discrimination can threaten the delivery of healthcare services and adversely affect patient outcomes. Nurses need to understand and recognize these attitudes in themselves and others to reduce their effects on the patients they serve. To overcome barriers to multiculturalism, nurses must have a deep understanding of vulnerable patients who are impacted by racism, sexism, classism, and heterosexism.

Gender and Sex

Traditionally gender has been dichotomized into two groups: men and women. However, it is now known that some people do not fit neatly into these categories of gender. The term **transgender** refers to individuals whose gender is not the same as their assigned sex. Gender identity is explored in more detail in the Concept of Sexuality.

Differences between men and women go beyond anatomy and physiology and cultural or social definitions. Evidence indicates that men and women have definite gender differences in personality, language skills, and visuospatial skills. Men tend to have greater visuospatial skills and less verbal skills than women; women tend to be more nurturing and have greater emotional memory (Goldman, 2017). Even within genders, individual diversity is expected. For example, male nurses often are stereotyped to lack the ability to nurture and communicate with care, which is not necessarily true (Christensen, Welch, & Barr, 2018). No conclusion about an individual can ever be drawn based on a simple term such as *woman* or *man*.

Differences also exist in access to and control over resources and decision-making power in the family and community. The extent of these differences is often informed by social and cultural contexts. Gender roles, often in interaction with socioeconomic circumstances, influence exposure to health risks, access to health information and services, health outcomes, and the social and economic consequences of ill health. Therefore, nurses must recognize the root causes of gender inequities when designing a nursing plan of care. To obtain positive outcomes, health promotion and disease prevention and treatment need to address gender differences. For example, millions of women are injured as the result of spousal or significant other abuse, but the magnitude and health consequences of interpersonal violence against women have often been neglected in both research and policy.

In addition to the way in which men and women respond to health promotion, they also display different needs regarding their response to the same diagnosis. For example, the traditional symptom of crushing chest pain as a primary indicator of myocardial infarction has been found to be primarily a male response. Women with myocardial infarction are more likely to experience extreme fatigue that extends to pain in the jaw, back, or shoulder if not treated early. Biological differences such as genetics, hormones, and metabolic influences combine to play a part in shaping different symptoms as well as morbidity and mortality rates (National Heart, Lung, and Blood Institute, 2019; Schuiling & Likis, 2017).

By improving their understanding of how gender differences impact patient health, nurses can develop a plan of care that meets the specific and unique healthcare needs of each patient. It is important that nurses not allow their own gender bias or preconceived beliefs to affect their ability to assess and plan appropriate care for the individual patient. Nurses should promote an environment in which patients can access essential services that address the differences between men and women in an equitable manner. When planning care, nurses who consider the biological differences and social vulnerability of men and women are more likely to see positive outcomes for their patients.

Bias can be defined as favoring a group or individual over another. Gender bias results in **sexism** and occurs when the values, activities, or needs of one gender are preferred over the other. Sexism may be overt or covert. Institutional bias related to gender results in sexist practices within an organization. Nurses need an awareness of cultural variations of gender, as they will be caring for diverse patient needs. What might be considered sexism by one culture may not be in another. The wearing of a *hijab*, or head scarf, is an example. In some regions of the world, women are required by Islamic tradition to cover; however, in other areas of the world women have a choice to cover their heads. Some Muslim women find wearing the hijab empowering, believing that because their bodies are covered, they cannot be sexualized (Yusef, 2015). Because many women view wearing a hijab as an expression of faith, doing so should not necessarily be seen as a sign of sexism.

Race

The concept of race is complex. Historically, **race** has often been defined by physical attributes linked to continents of origin: Asia, Europe, Africa, and the Americas. Variations of skin color and hair texture have traditionally been used as markers of race. As the U.S. population becomes more multiracial, more individuals identify as two or more races. The 2000 U.S. Census was the first to allow individuals to choose more than one race. The 2020 U.S. Census asks individuals for more information regarding their origins with specifics country of origin (i.e., England, Nigeria) for those who are White and Black (Brown, 2020).

» **Stay Current:** To learn more about the U.S. census racial categories, search the U.S. Census Bureau's website at https://www.census.gov/topics/population/race.html.

The discrimination, oppression, and/or prejudice of a group of people based on perceived race or ethnic group is known as **racism**. Often racism is directed toward minority groups. Although racism is often perceived as overt acts of hostility, racism can also be insidious policies, procedures, systems, traditions, or rules that benefit one group of people over another.

Racism is a social determinant of health (Paradies et al., 2015). Health inequities are a result of socioeconomic conditions, including racism (World Health Organization [WHO], 2008). Racism has been linked to poorer mental health and physical health, especially among children. Racial residential segregation (such as Indian reservations and low-income housing zones) makes it difficult for many Native Americans and other people of color to access equitable healthcare systems, affordable fresh food, and other resources (Capatides, 2020; Williams, Lawrence, & Davis, 2019).

Class

Socioeconomic variations contribute to a society stratification based on money and access to resources. **Classism** is the oppression of groups of people based on their socioeconomic status. The lack of access to resources is apparent in some of the people at the lowest economic level such as the homeless, those living in poverty, and undocumented immigrants.

Homelessness

Among the most vulnerable patients are those who are homeless. According to the U.S. Department of Housing and Urban Development (2019), more than 500,000 individuals report being homeless each year.

Homeless patients present unique and complex challenges because they often live in dangerous, unsanitary conditions; have diets that are severely lacking in nutrients; and have very few resources for coping with illness. They must find shelter and food every day and cannot predict what the next day will bring. People who are homeless have difficulty obtaining, keeping, and storing medications and have difficulty maintaining self-care regimens. Women without adequate support systems, often with children, find themselves homeless when faced with long-term job loss or when fleeing domestic/intimate partner violence. The COVID-19 pandemic that emerged in 2020 created even more challenges for those who were homeless because they could not "stay and shelter" and put more people at risk of homelessness or inadequate housing due to extensive job losses.

An important nursing intervention in addition to providing care to those who are homeless is to identify resources to help them.

» **Stay Current:** The National Alliance to End Homelessness is a nonprofit organization that advocates for the homeless through the use of data and evidence to find solutions to homelessness: https://endhomelessness.org.

Poverty

Although people who are homeless can be considered impoverished, many families with adequate shelter live in poverty. **Poverty** is defined as a lack of income to meet basic needs that include food and nutrition, education and other basic services, productive resources for income, and healthcare (United Nations, n.d.). In the United States, poverty level is determined by the number of people in a household and the income of the household (U.S. Census, 2019a). For example, poverty-level income for two adults living in a household with one child was $17,622 in 2019 (U.S. Census, 2019b).

Children and those living in households headed by women are at greatest risk of living in poverty (U.S. Census Bureau, 2019c). According to the U.S. Census Bureau (2019c):

- The overall poverty rate in the United States is 12.8% with 41.4 million living in poverty.
- 13.7% of children live in poverty, roughly 10 million children.
- The poverty rate for people age 65 and over increased from 8.8% to 13.6% between 2015 and 2019.
- More individuals living in poverty are uninsured than in previous years, with 24.4%% reporting they are uninsured.

The U.S. Census Bureau (2020) does not identify American Indians and Alaska Natives, Native Hawaiians and other Pacific Islanders, or those who identify as two or more races in their poverty statistics. However, according to the Kaiser Family Foundation (2018), 24% of American Indians/Alaska Natives live in poverty in the United States, the greatest percentage of all races. Over 51% of American Indians/Alaska Natives in South Dakota live in poverty (Kaiser Family Foundation, 2020).

Undocumented Immigrants

Undocumented immigrants often do not seek healthcare until their condition becomes critical. This behavior results from a complex combination of factors, including the threat of arrest and deportation. Most are uninsured, do not speak English, and have not yet learned the culture of their new homeland. For some, the differences between the U.S. healthcare system and the medical practices and beliefs of their culture of origin create an additional barrier. These factors combine to create fear in the undocumented immigrant patient who needs medical attention, often resulting in delay or refusal to seek diagnosis and care. In addition, many undocumented immigrants live in community with others in small spaces, increasing their risk for viral infections, such as COVID-19 (Chishti & Pierce, 2020).

Special healthcare concerns related to this population include lack of preventive care for chronic diseases such as obesity and diabetes, inadequate immunization status, exposure to untreated or undertreated infectious diseases such as tuberculosis, mental health concerns due to trauma exposure, and lack of past medical records (Rosales, 2017). Barriers to access to timely and appropriate medical care include lack of medical insurance, lack of culturally competent medical services, and a preference for maintaining health practices from the country of origin (Andrews, Boyle, & Collins, 2020).

States and regional politics vary across the country as to whether government or healthcare facilities are required to ask for proof of citizenship when providing care. Furthermore, some states require reporting undocumented people, which also impedes their willingness to seek care. Nurses need to be familiar with the laws of the state in which they practice. When providing care to patients who may be or are known to be undocumented immigrants, the nurse has the ethical and moral imperative to deliver the same high-quality care delivered to any patient. Use of an interpreter or interpreter system will improve the quality of communication if the patient does not speak English or does not speak English well enough to understand the information presented. Thorough screening, nursing history, and assessment contribute to determining both current condition as well as risks, preventive care needs, and understanding of self-care upon discharge. Respectful, appropriate, culturally congruent care by the nurse and the healthcare team promotes trust in the healthcare system and increases the likelihood of patient adherence to treatment. Because access to healthcare for this population is unpredictable, nurses should maximize each opportunity to care for and teach self-care to these patients.

Sexual Orientation

Sexual orientation is a continuum ranging from those who have a strong preference for a partner of the same sex to those who strongly prefer someone of the opposite sex. *Homosexual* individuals prefer a partner of the same sex, with the term *lesbian* often used to describe women who prefer to develop intimate relationships with other women. The term *gay* may refer to homosexual women or men. *Heterosexual* individuals prefer to develop an intimate relationship with a partner of the opposite sex. *Bisexual* individuals are physically attracted to both males and females. The most common biases related to sexual orientation are **homophobia** (fear, hatred, or mistrust of gays and lesbians often expressed in overt displays of discrimination) and **heterosexism** (view of heterosexuality as the only correct sexual orientation).

Historically, homosexuality was not acceptable in many cultures and societies. In some countries, being a homosexual was punishable by death. However, over the past 20 years, homosexuality continues to gain acceptance and legal status globally (Kenny & Patel, 2017). Yet, LGBTQ (lesbian, gay, bisexual, transgender, and queer/questioning) individuals continue to report discrimination and harassment, despite changing attitudes in society, even in the healthcare setting. Members of the LGBTQ community are also at greater risk for healthcare disparities and health issues. According to the Health Resources and Services Administration (n.d.), LGBTQ individuals are at higher risk for such health problems as obesity, mental health issues, substance abuse, and violence. Transgender individuals face greater discrimination in healthcare than lesbians and gays.

Transgender individuals often delay seeking healthcare for fear of discrimination (Seelman, Colón-Diaz, LeCroix, Xavier-Brier, & Kattari, 2017). Transgender persons are more likely to have mental health issues, including depression and anxiety, as well as abuse drugs and alcohol in order to cope with the difficulties involved in being transgender. According to a study by Seelman et al. (2017), transgender individuals are approximately three times more likely to experience depression and suicidal ideation than nontransgender individuals, and they are nearly four times more likely to attempt suicide.

The nurse should recognize that the LGBTQ individual will have specific and distinct healthcare needs, including risk for some infectious diseases, suicide attempt, substance abuse, and violence (SAMHSA, 2012). Additionally, the nurse will need to consider ways to overcome the health disparities that the LGBTQ population faces.

Disability Status

Many patients have physical or cognitive disabilities. Patients with an intellectual disability and their families experience poorer healthcare compared with the general population. Living with an intellectual disability is often challenged by coexisting complex and chronic conditions and can lead to economic hardship and family conflict. Both intellectual and physical disability can impair the individual patient's ability to participate in health promotion and to provide self-care.

Nurses working with patients with disabilities must develop trusting relationships so they can successfully assist those patients and their families and caregivers and enable them to find resources.

Age

Children and older adults are considered vulnerable populations. Both older adults and children often depend on others for nutrition, healthcare, transportation, and personal safety. Children's vulnerability is based in their immature immune status (especially for infants and young children), their reliance on others to meet their basic needs, and the fact that they lack autonomy and judgment to make critical decisions independently

Many older adults live on limited incomes, and more than 7.1 million (13.6%) live in poverty (U.S. Census Bureau, 2019a). In 2016, there was a great disparity between men's and women's income for those over age 65: the average income for a man was $31,168; for women, it was $18,380 (Administration for Community Living, 2018). Due to changes in Medicare and supplemental insurance, older adults are paying more for medical expenses, including prescription drugs (Administration for Community Living, 2018).

Ageism is defined as discrimination against older adults. U.S. culture places an emphasis on youth, beauty, and productivity, which minimizes respect and access to opportunities for older adults. The increasing use of the internet and technology as a primary means of sharing and retrieving information also has implications. More and more older adults are embracing technology and the internet, particularly in those with higher education and/or spouses (Vroman, Arthanat, & Lysack, 2015). However, those who have less education or do not have access to technology resources are left behind. The nurse should consider access to technology when recommending online educational resources or sending results to online personal charts.

Disparities and Differences

In many ways the United States is a nation that celebrates culture and diversity. From Greek festivals to soul food to Tex-Mex, from gay pride parades to Tibetan New Year to Octoberfest, there is plenty of diverse heritage and society to celebrate. Unfortunately, these differences also give rise to disparities of opportunity, and these include disparities that relate to healthcare. In 2002, the Institute of Medicine released a report on disparities in the United States regarding the types and quality of health services that racial and ethnic groups receive. This historic report explored factors that may contribute to inequities in care and recommended policies and practices to eliminate these inequities. Years later, despite much progress, inequities still exist, and researchers are attempting to identify and prevent the causes of disparities (**Figure 24.3** »).

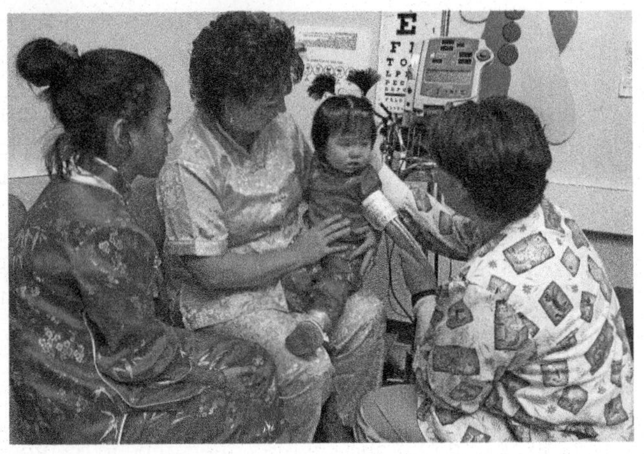

Figure 24.3 ›› Although much has been done to improve the quality of health services received by American cultural and ethnic minorities, these services are still in need of continued reform.

Source: Pearson Education, Inc.

Nurses should be alert to practices in their work environment that impact the quality of care offered to individuals of any ethnic or cultural group. Healthcare practices should be accessible and culturally relevant, and patient preferences should be at the core of decision making. Nurses should work collaboratively to ensure quality care and provision of best-practice methods to all patients.

Recommendations for reducing these disparities in healthcare include increasing awareness of them among the public, HCPs, insurance companies, and policymakers. See Module 47, Health Policy, for more information.

›› **Stay Current:** The U.S. Department of Health and Human Services offers a free online course to educate nurses and other healthcare workers on culturally competent care to help educate nurses and narrow the healthcare disparities gap and improve overall health in different populations: https://www.thinkculturalhealth.hhs.gov/education/nurses.

Vulnerable Populations

The term **vulnerable population** refers to groups in a society who are at greater risk for diseases and reduced lifespan due to lack of resources and exposure to more risk factors. Poverty is a major culprit in vulnerable populations (United Nations, n.d.; World Health Organization, 2016). Persons in poverty are at risk for malnutrition, poor housing, violence, and limited or no access to healthcare. Other conditions associated with vulnerability include age, disability, health/disease state, education status, language spoken, and socioeconomic situation. For example, older adults with frailty are at increased risk for malnutrition if they do not have assistance with obtaining healthy foods.

Oppression, or the systematic limitation of access to resources, may be covert or subtle and is typically linked to laws, education, or even healthcare norms and regional access to services and transportation. All vulnerable populations are less able than others to safeguard their needs and interests adequately. In conceptual terms, the most vulnerable are those households with the fewest choices and the greatest number of disabling factors.

Patients from vulnerable populations are more likely to develop health problems because they have the greatest number of risk factors and the fewest options for managing those risks. These individuals often have limited access to healthcare and are more dependent on others for helping them meet their healthcare needs. Those from vulnerable populations are likely to be living in poverty, homeless, in abusive relationships, mentally ill, or chronically ill. Vulnerability is greater among children and older adults.

It is not uncommon for vulnerable individuals to belong to more than one of these groups (see the Reflect case study at the end of this module). They face multiple challenges, statistically poorer outcomes and shorter lifespans, and higher mortality and morbidity rates due to cumulative or combinations of risk factors. They may be from any culture, ethnicity, age, or gender, although they are more likely to be women than men.

Nurses face many challenges when caring for individuals who are vulnerable. Their physical, social, and emotional needs are complex, and many have multiple chronic conditions that can complicate care still further. Other barriers to health and healthcare include accessibility and transportation. For example, children who live in impoverished rural communities may not have access to fluoridated water and may be an hour or more from the nearest dentist who accepts Medicaid. Assessing the patient from a vulnerable population requires the nurse to investigate all systems, determine stressors and coping mechanisms, and help the patient identify potential resources.

A primary focus of healthcare at federal and local levels is to reduce the disparity of access to healthcare among groups. **Health disparity** has been defined as a preventable difference in the effects or experiences of illness, injury, violence, or opportunities experienced by medically underserved and socioeconomically disadvantaged populations (CDC, 2008). Some examples of vulnerable group affiliations are highlighted in this module.

Birth Equity

Birth equity describes optimal maternal and child outcomes for pregnant and postpartum women and their babies. The United States has the highest maternal mortality (deaths among pregnant and laboring mothers) of all developed countries (United Health Foundation, 2020). Pregnancy-related deaths have been steadily climbing over the past three decades. In 1987, the pregnancy-related mortality was 7.2 deaths per 100,000 live births compared to 16.9 deaths per 100,000 live births in 2016 (National Center for Chronic Disease Prevention and Health Promotion, 2020). Rates of maternal death are highest among Black women and women of American Indian heritage.

The California Maternal Quality Care Collaborative (CMQCC) has identified a number of factors that contribute to the high rates of maternal morbidity and mortality among Black mothers in the United States. These include social determinants of health (such as poverty and access to affordable fresh food), health disparities (including lack of health insurance and difficulty accessing adequate prenatal care), and racism, including racial bias of HCPs. Many of these disparities also drive high maternal death rates among women from other groups. However, when controlling for all other factors, Black mothers continue to die at higher rates than mothers from any other racial group (42.4 deaths per 100,000 live births compared to 11.3 deaths per 100,000 White women; Peterson et al., 2019).

Nurses and other HCPs can use several strategies to try to reduce or mitigate factors that lead to maternal morbidity, including by (CMQCC, 2020; Minority Nurse, 2018):

- Ensuring all mothers receive timely and thorough antepartum assessments
- Ensuring all mothers receive best practice care at each interaction with the healthcare system
- Listening to mothers' concerns and responding quickly to maternal expressions of distress
- Participating in and advocating for racial equity training and quality improvement initiatives
- Working with their institutions to develop quality standards for maternal care
- Increasing their own awareness of maternal care issues
- Advocating for expanded Medicaid coverage to cover the full postpartum period.

Social Differences

People learn the social behaviors practiced in their cultures and communities. These behaviors differ from culture to culture and from community to community. They may also be practiced by members of subcultures who decide to maintain traditional cultural practices, whereas others from the same culture living nearby may choose to adapt to the dominant culture (**Figure 24.4** »). The terms *subculture* and *minority* are sometimes used to label groups characterized by specific norms, beliefs, and values that coexist or even oppose those of the dominant culture. Some common social behavioral variations among people of different cultures involve communication, environmental control, hygiene, space, time, and social organization. These ethnic differences exist within smaller cultural groups within a larger society. Within the United States, social differences are evolving as individuals from different cultural groups relocate for college or work and interact with people from other cultures, and as the numbers of individuals of different cultural groups change over time. For example, Hmong culture has traditionally been a patriarchal society where a man's identity is that of an income earner and a woman's identity is that of a daughter, wife, and mother (Xiong, 2018). However, many Hmong women born in the United States have pursued higher education and professions. Consequently, there has been a change in gender norms within the culture as women have begun earning money (Lo, 2017; Xiong, 2018). Religious differences can also create some social differences and play different roles in different communities. For example, some religions specify what foods may be eaten and how they should be prepared. See Module 30, Spirituality, for more information.

Communication

Cultural groups and subcultures may speak a unique language or a variation of another language. (**Figure 24.5** »). The meaning of words can differ among various groups of people, and misunderstandings may result from lack of common communication. Languages vary in terms of references to time, gender, roles, or common concepts and definitions. Translation of concepts from one language to another may miss contextual embedded meanings and lead to misunderstandings. Misinterpretation of nonverbal communication also may lead to problems. Direct eye contact may show disrespect in some cultures and be a sign of interest and active listening in others. In some cultures, nodding does not reflect agreement, but instead is an attempt to acknowledge respect for authority.

Environmental Control

Relationship to the environment varies among cultures. Different health practices, values, and experiences with illness can be associated with an external or internal locus of control. Rotter (1966) theorized that individuals believe either that they can control certain aspects of their lives (internal locus of control) or that outside sources control their lives (external locus of control).

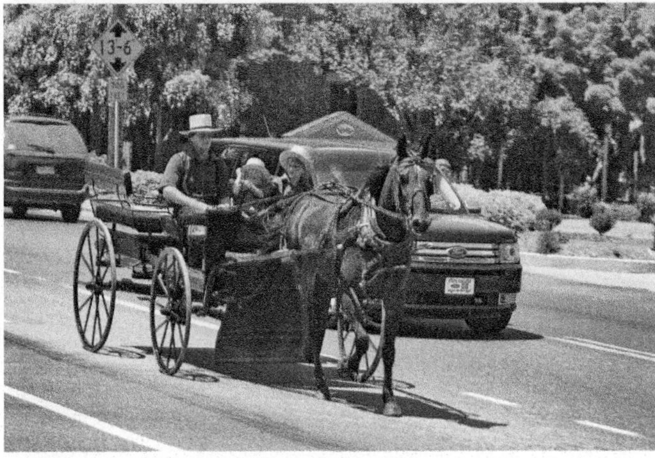

Figure 24.4 » Subcultures can maintain heritage and identity through dress, foods eaten, and cultural festivities. This Amish family in Bird-in-Hand, Pennsylvania, wears traditional plain clothing and drives a horse-drawn buggy while sharing the road with the larger community of non-Amish Pennsylvanians who drive cars.

Source: George Sheldon/Shutterstock.

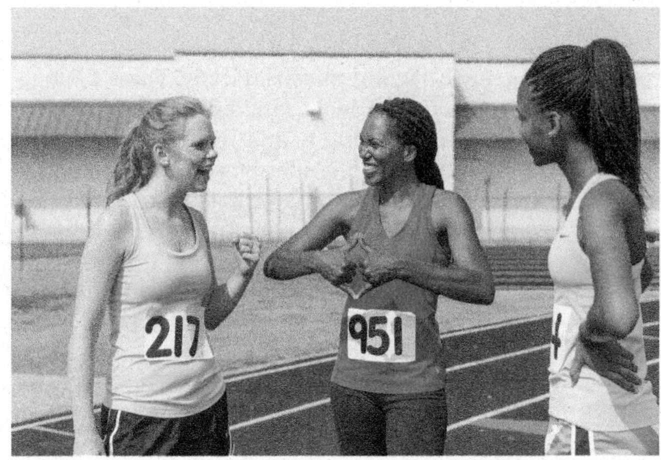

Figure 24.5 » American Sign Language (a method of communicating through the use of hand gestures and facial expressions) is considered an essential part of culture and identity among many people who are born deaf or nearly deaf.

Source: Lokibaho/iStock/Getty Images.

Those who believe in an internal locus of control over their health will be motivated to eat healthy, exercise, and make use of other wellness measures. Those who follow an internal locus of control tend to respond well to preventive medicine. Those with an external locus of control will feel that outside influences will care for their health.

Personal Space

Culture defines an individual's perception of personal space. Comfort may result from honoring the boundaries of personal space, whereas anxiety can result when these boundaries are not followed. Practices regarding proximity to others, body movements, and touch differ among groups. Variations of intimate zones and social public distance occur among cultural groups, and HCPs need to be aware that what they perceive as normal or appropriate may be produce anxiety for others (Dayer-Berenson, 2013). For example, in many Asian cultures, it is considered rude or inappropriate to touch someone on the head (Giger & Haddad, 2021).

Time

The concepts of time, duration of time, and points in time vary among cultures. Past-oriented cultures, for example, value tradition. Individuals from cultures that closely follow tradition may not be receptive to new procedures or treatments. Present-oriented cultures focus on the here and now, and individuals from these cultures may not be receptive to preventive healthcare measures. Different cultures value time differently, which can have implications for healthcare in a system that is very regulated by clock hours (Andrews et al., 2020). For example, many people from the United States and northern Europe are considered *monochronic* because of the way they view time as a commodity, something that can be "lost" or "wasted." Many people from these countries consider it rude for someone to be late to an appointment. But people from other areas, including the Middle East and Latin America, are *polychronic* and believe that time is flexible. They may not leave one event for the next until the first event has concluded, even if that means being late for the next appointment (Giger & Haddad, 2021).

Biological Variations

People differ genetically and physiologically. These biological variations among individuals, families, and groups produce differences in susceptibility and response to various diseases. The field of ethnopharmacology addresses variations in pharmacodynamics and pharmacokinetics among cultural groups. Nurses are responsible for monitoring patients' responses to the drugs they give and thus must be aware of these differences. ACE inhibitors are well known to cause angioedema in African Americans, particularly African American women (Guyer & Banerji, 2020). In addition, some enzyme deficiencies occur more commonly in some cultural groups. For example, lactose deficiency (the inability to absorb milk by-products) is often present in Asian and African cultural groups.

Susceptibility to Disease

Certain ethnic groups or races may tend toward developing specific diseases. African Americans, for example, have a higher incidence of hypertension and sickle cell disease. Cystic fibrosis occurs almost exclusively in white populations. Native Americans have a higher incidence of death due to diabetes than any other group (Heron, 2019). Sometimes, however, an individual's susceptibility to disease is not so obvious but may be discerned as a nurse takes a health history, including the health of any parents, grandparents, and siblings.

Skin Color

Historically, skin color has been associated with racial definitions. However, labeling of people based on their skin color should be avoided. Healthcare providers need to explore ethnic variations and not make assumptions based on skin color. As a nurse, when doing skin assessment, it is important to know that darker skin tones require closer inspection and enhanced lighting to observe changes (e.g., when assessing for changes in oxygenation). Skin color changes such as erythema and cyanosis are subtle, and palpation and lighting will need to be used for skin assessment. In addition, skin color does impact some prevalence statistics: African Americans and American Indians have lower incidences of skin cancer due to higher levels of melanin.

Additional cultural and social differences are outlined in **Table 24.2** ».

TABLE 24.2 Additional Cultural and Social Differences

Category	Implications
Hygiene	Cleanliness practices can vary among cultural groups. Whether or not body odor is disguised, ignored, or enhanced can vary by culture, as can hairstyles and grooming practices.
Nutrition	Food preferences can be an indicator of or a cause of disease. Cooking techniques vary and may increase risk for disease in susceptible populations. Social patterns around eating and food choices also have implications for health promotion and direct nursing care.
Skeletal and growth and development differences	Skeletal variations occur across racial and cultural lines. For example, small-framed American women of European descent are at greater risk for osteoporosis. Pubertal developmental changes occur at different times.
Social organization	Across cultures and communities, the roles of older adults and the respect given them vary. Differences among who is the recognized head of household and gender roles also exist. Work and recreational patterns and norms vary. The role of adult children and caretaking expectations also vary among groups.

Clinical Example A

Naomi Moore is a 16-year-old girl who comes with her mother to a local family practice clinic for a first-time appointment. She is complaining of abdominal pain that is later revealed to be painful, irregular, and heavy menstrual periods. Naomi's assessment is notable for her lack of participation in regular medical care. Her parents homeschool Naomi and her sisters, and her mother tells you that they hardly ever see a physician unless "absolutely necessary." Following a thorough nursing assessment and physical examination, the family nurse practitioner diagnoses Naomi with endometriosis and recommends hormonal contraceptives. Naomi's mother is adamant that Naomi will not take any medication, saying they believe in using only "natural" therapies and do not use prescription drugs. Naomi begins to cry, complaining of how much pain she is in constantly, and she pleads with her mother to let her try the medication.

Critical Thinking Questions

1. What are the priorities for care for Naomi based on the information presented here?
2. How can you show cultural sensitivity to Naomi and her mother and promote evidence-based care?
3. Using therapeutic communication, what could you say or do to affect Naomi's mother's decision regarding her daughter's treatment?

Concepts Related to Culture and Diversity

Differences among patients that are attributable to culture, ethnicity, race, gender, sexuality, and vulnerability impact the nursing care of patients in a variety of ways.

Two meta-analyses (Kim et al., 2017; Rahim-Williams, Riley, Williams, & Fillingim, 2012) found that African Americans and other people of color report lower tolerance for pain and higher pain ratings than White Americans. Yet a number of studies have documented racial disparities in the use of pain medication in emergency departments, including disparities in the treatment of pain in Black children (Cheng, Goodman, & Committee on Pediatric Research, 2015; Goyal, Kuppermann, Cleary, Teach, & Chamberlain, 2016). Factors implicated in undertreatment of pain in people of color include provider bias, leading to inadequate assessment and treatment, and distrust of the system on the part of patients, leading some patients to withhold information (Andrews et al., 2020).

Within the concept of communication, it is important to understand that patients use language differently, speak different languages, and recognize nonverbal cues differently. Therapeutic communication, interpreters, shared languages, and awareness of nonverbal cues can help nurses communicate more effectively with patients from diverse backgrounds.

Patients' relationship to healthcare resources and systems vary according to their own resources, including access to transportation and understanding of health information. Nurses should consider these issues as well as financial implications of the resources and limits in health insurance/no insurance. Referring a post–knee surgery patient to aqua therapy is not realistic to a patient who lives in a rural area with no indoor pools. Likewise, referring Medicaid patients to specialists who do not take Medicaid can create financial hardships or no follow-up. Patients who live in poverty or who are homeless may need referrals to additional resources. Nurses must advocate for services, such as interpreters or mental health resources, for their patients who do not have the awareness or influence to ask on their own.

The professional behavior of nurses must be built on a moral and ethical code. Nursing as a discipline has a culture of its own. Nurses must understand collegial and regional differences to effectively work collaboratively with diverse interprofessional teams. Self-awareness, emotional intelligence, and lifelong learning should be characteristics of a nurse's professional behavior.

Another concept related to culture and diversity is sexuality. Gender roles and the timing and type of sexual relationships vary among groups of people. Heterosexual and homosexual variations may also be culturally embedded.

For many people, their spirituality is closely tied to their culture of origin. Although spirituality may be defined more broadly than religion, cultural variations exist among different religious communities and faiths. Religious practices commonly influence eating or fasting patterns, types of worship, and family roles and responsibilities. The Concepts Related to Culture and Diversity feature lists some, but not all, of the concepts integral to providing culturally aware nursing.

Concepts Related to **Culture and Diversity**

CONCEPT	RELATIONSHIP TO CULTURE AND DIVERSITY	NURSING IMPLICATIONS
Comfort	Individual tolerance for pain and expressions of pain vary; however, evidence indicates that people of color have lower pain tolerance than White populations and often receive inadequate treatment for pain.	■ Use therapeutic communication skills. ■ Conduct a holistic nursing assessment that includes a thorough assessment of pain of all patients who present with pain or with a condition for which pain is normally a key symptom. ■ Use language that the patient understands. ■ Before discharge, make sure patient knows what to do if pain becomes worse or returns.
Communication	Listening, clarification, reflection, and all therapeutic communication techniques are important when communicating with people different from you.	■ Use therapeutic communication skills. ■ Identify translation and interpreter resources in your organization. ■ Use language that the patient understands.

(continued on next page)

Concepts Related to *(continued)*

CONCEPT	RELATIONSHIP TO CULTURE AND DIVERSITY	NURSING IMPLICATIONS
Healthcare Systems	Availability of healthcare services for vulnerable populations may be low. Availability of resources varies by community.	▪ Recognize and address unequal distribution of facilities and resources. ▪ Recognize cultural and group differences among HCPs. Seek to advocate for vulnerable populations. ▪ Refer patients in need of additional resources to social services and nonprofit service agencies.
Professional Behaviors	Recognize personal values and professional values.	▪ Providing culturally competent care improves patient outcomes and promotes patient trust in the healthcare system.
Sexuality	Sexual orientation, homophobia, heterosexism.	▪ Assist in advocating for LGBTQ healthcare needs and access. ▪ Recognize same-sex partners as family and patient support. ▪ Refer to transgender patients by preferred name (rather than legal name). ▪ Ask for patients' preferred use of pronoun (*he/she/they*)
Spirituality	Recognize religious beliefs related to dietary regimen or times of fasting.	▪ Show respect for religious differences, leaders, and practice. ▪ Recognize that your personal spiritual and religious beliefs will not be universally shared with your patients. ▪ Be nonjudgmental of differences. ▪ Support patient religious practices.

Developing Cultural Competence

Cultural competence is the ability to apply the knowledge and skills needed to provide high-quality, evidence-based care to patients of diverse backgrounds and beliefs to overcome barriers and access resources promoting health and wellness. Cultural competence has some basic characteristics:

1. Valuing diversity
2. Capacity for cultural self-assessment
3. Awareness of the different dynamics present when cultures interact
4. Knowledge about different cultures
5. Adaptability in providing nursing care that reflects an understanding of cultural diversity.

Cultural competence can be considered a process as well as an outcome, although no one person can be competent in dealing with all types of cultural variations. The American Association of Colleges of Nursing (2008) has identified five competencies considered essential for baccalaureate nursing graduates to provide culturally competent care in partnership with the interprofessional team:

- ***Competency 1.*** Apply knowledge of social and cultural factors that affect nursing and healthcare across multiple contexts.
- ***Competency 2.*** Use relevant data sources and best evidence in providing culturally competent care.
- ***Competency 3.*** Promote achievement of safe and quality outcomes of care for diverse populations.
- ***Competency 4.*** Advocate for social justice, including commitment to the health of vulnerable populations and the elimination of health disparities.
- ***Competency 5.*** Participate in continuous cultural competence development.

Because the concept of culture is very complex, scholars have identified models of cultural competence to facilitate the continuous process of cultural competence. The purpose of using a model is to help communicate and enhance the understanding of a complex concept. A theoretical model may provide a nurse or student with a deeper understanding of how concepts are related. Many models have been published. One of the oldest, yet still relevant, nursing theories regarding culture is Madeleine Leininger's (2002) Culture Care Diversity and Universality theory. Leininger developed this theory with a unique emphasis on cultural care and the nurse. See Module 35, Caring Interventions, for more information regarding Leininger's Theory of Culture Care Diversity and Universality.

Nurses' journey toward cultural competency begin with self-awareness, with identifying areas in which nurses can improve how they relate to and communicate with individuals with values and beliefs different from their own. See the Focus on Diversity and Culture feature for a values clarification checklist to help you begin to cultivate self-awareness.

The LEARN model (Association of American Medical Colleges, 2005; Berlin & Fowkes, 1983) can be used as a tool for developing cultural competency. Below is a modification of the **LEARN** model that can help nurses include cultural behaviors in a patient's care:

Listen to the patient's perception of the problem.

Explain your perception of the problem and of the treatments ordered by the provider.

Acknowledge and discuss the differences and similarities between these two perceptions.

Review the ordered treatments while remembering the patient's cultural parameters.

Negotiate agreement. Assist the patient in understanding the medical treatments ordered by the provider and have the patient help to make decisions about those treatments as appropriate (such as choosing culturally acceptable foods that are permitted on an ordered diet).

In addition to the LEARN model, nursing scholars have identified models that illuminate a variety of areas for nurses to explore to deepen their understanding of cultural competence.

Purnell's (Purnell & Fenkl, 2019) model of cultural competence identifies how individuals, families, communities, and the global society all possess 12 domains of culture:

1. Overview, inhabited localities, and topography
2. Communication
3. Family roles and organization
4. Workforce issues
5. Biocultural ecology
6. High-risk behaviors
7. Nutrition
8. Pregnancy and childbearing practices
9. Death rituals
10. Spirituality
11. Healthcare practices
12. Healthcare practitioners.

No one becomes culturally aware or culturally competent overnight. As HCPs, it is imperative that nurses recognize common prejudices. **Prejudices** are prejudgments about cultural groups or vulnerable populations that are unfavorable or false because they have been formed without the background knowledge and context on which to base an accurate opinion. There is a process by which nursing students (and other individuals) learn cultural confidence, with learning taking place in a fairly predictable sequence:

1. Students begin by developing cultural awareness of how culture shapes beliefs, values, and norms.
2. Students develop cultural knowledge about the differences, similarities, and inequalities in experience and practice among various societies.
3. Students develop cultural understanding of problems and issues facing societies and cultures when values, beliefs, and behaviors are compromised by another culture.
4. Students develop cultural sensitivity to the cultural beliefs, values, and behaviors of their patients. This reflects an awareness of their own cultural beliefs, values, and behaviors that may influence their nursing practice.
5. Students and nurses develop cultural competence and provide care that respects the cultural values, beliefs, and behaviors of their patients.
6. Nurses practice lifelong learning through ongoing education and exposure to cultural groups.

Focus on Diversity and Culture

How Culturally Competent Are You?

To help you identify areas where you can improve when providing nursing care to culturally different people, answer the following questions by checking "Yes" or "No":

_____ Yes _____ No I accept values of others even when different from my own.

_____ Yes _____ No I accept beliefs of others even when different from my own.

_____ Yes _____ No I accept that feminine and masculine roles may vary among different cultures.

_____ Yes _____ No I accept that religious practices may influence how a patient responds to illness, health problems, and death.

_____ Yes _____ No I accept that alternative medicine practices may influence a patient's response to illness and health problems.

_____ Yes _____ No I accept cultural diversity in my patients.

_____ Yes _____ No I attend educational programs to enhance my knowledge and skills in providing care to diverse cultural groups.

_____ Yes _____ No I understand that patients who are unable to speak English are fluent in their own languages.

_____ Yes _____ No I try to have written materials in the patient's language available when possible.

_____ Yes _____ No I use interpreters when available to improve communication.

If you have more No responses than Yes responses, you may not be as culturally competent as you could be. The purpose of this self-assessment is to increase your awareness of areas where you can improve your cultural competence.

Clinical Example B

Mr. and Mrs. Ali come to a local clinic because Mrs. Ali, who is 6 months pregnant, is not feeling well. Mr. Ali speaks English fluently, but his wife's proficiency in English is more limited. Both are dressed in American-style clothes. During the assessment, the registered nurse determines that the couple has a 9-month-old and a 2-year-old at home. Ms. Smith also learns that Mr. Ali is the head of the household, making most of the major decisions for the family, and that Mrs. Ali has sole responsibility for the family's care and daily living needs. Mrs. Ali presents with exhaustion and elevated blood pressure. After obtaining a urine specimen, the provider diagnoses toxemia and orders Mrs. Ali to be on strict bedrest and to return in 2 weeks. While Mr. Ali conveys concern for his wife's health, he is reluctant to have her treatment disrupt the household routine.

Critical Thinking Questions

1. What are the priorities of care for Mrs. Ali?
2. What additional information would you like to collect about this family?
3. Using the LEARN model, describe how the nurse working with this family could understand and address this situation and the physician's recommendations with both the husband and wife.

Standards of Competence

Maintaining cultural competence is an ongoing process. Nurses continually assess, modify, and evaluate the care provided to culturally diverse patients. The American Nurses Association has identified culturally congruent practice as one of its standards of nursing practices. Competencies associated with culturally congruent practice include (Marion et al., 2017):

- Demonstrating respect for all individuals, regardless of cultural background or heritage
- Participating in lifelong continuing education related to cultural awareness and competency
- Considering the effect of discrimination on vulnerable individuals and groups
- Communicating with appropriate language and behaviors, using interpreters and translators as appropriate and with permission from the patient.

Institutions such as hospitals also need to develop and implement cultural competence to address the cultural and language needs of an increasingly multicultural patient population.

Using an Interpreter

Many patients do not speak English, and many who do speak some English are of limited proficiency. Any facility receiving federal funding from the U.S. Department of Health and Human Services is required to communicate effectively with patients or risk the loss of that funding.

Having bilingual nurses available is one strategy to address the language barrier. Another strategy is providing access to interpreters through telephone or telehealth systems. However, the nurse should be aware that some cultures find it offensive to discuss medical issues with a member of the opposite gender. The nurse should collaborate with the patient and family regarding specifics for an interpreter. Most organizations discourage use of family members for interpretation for a variety of reasons, including the possibility that information may be mistranslated or withheld from the patient. Children should not be used for interpreting medical information as they may lack the maturity to understand what is being said. There is a host of other potential problems with having children interpret for parents, such as being included in discussions about interpersonal violence, pregnancy, and "bad news" (Finlay, Dunne, & Guiton, 2017).

Guidelines for using an interpreter include the following:

- When possible, use a certified medical interpreter to translate and provide meaning behind the words.
- If requested, provide an interpreter of the same gender as the patient.
- Address your questions to the patient, not the interpreter, but maintain eye contact with both the patient and the interpreter.
- Avoid using metaphors, medical jargon, similes, and idiomatic phrases.
- Observe the patient's nonverbal communication.
- Plan what to say and avoid rephrasing or hesitating.
- Use short questions and comments. Ask one question at a time.
- Speak slowly and distinctly, but not loudly.
- Provide written materials in the patient's language as available.

Clinical Example C

Henry Lee is approximately 55 years old. Born in South Korea, he has been living in the United States for the past 10 years, working as a professor at a local university. Following surgery for a broken arm, he refuses pain medication, explaining that his discomfort is bearable and he can survive without medication.

When you next check on Mr. Lee, you find him restless and uncomfortable. You have a standing order to administer medication as needed and again offer to administer medication. Mr. Lee again refuses, saying that your other responsibilities are more important than his discomfort and he does not want to impose.

Critical Thinking Questions

1. What do you think is behind Mr. Lee's refusal to accept medication?
2. What can you do or say to change Mr. Lee's perception of the situation?
3. What additional information might influence your nursing care?

NURSING PROCESS

The nursing process is interwoven in providing culturally competent care. In each step, the nurse should be considerate of the patient's cultural background and practices. This holistic approach will help both the patient and the nurse create a therapeutic plan of care.

Assessment

The provision of culturally competent care begins with incorporating culture into the initial nursing assessment. Areas for assessment include the use of traditional healing practices such as herbal supplements or mind–body practices (e.g., cupping, acupuncture); cultural practices related to food preparation and preferences; religious or cultural practices at specific times of day or during the week; health beliefs; and preferences for care, such as whether or not women prefer to be examined by a female nurse.

Minimal cultural assessment information from patients can be obtained with the following questions:

- What languages do you speak?
- How long have you lived here?
- Where else have you lived?
- Describe the illness or problem that brings you here today.
- What do you think caused your problem?
- When did it start?
- Why do you think it started when it did?
- What does your sickness do to you?
- How severe is your sickness?
- What helps make it better? Worse?
- What kind of treatment do you think you need?
- Are there any religious practices we need to know about?
- Who is your family?
- Who makes decisions most of the time?
- Who can you go to for help when you need it?

Assessment of cultural influences and practices is imperative because differences in cultural behaviors, beliefs, and values may result in barriers to patients achieving positive outcomes. Cultural misunderstandings or miscommunications also may result from different perceptions of health and of the illness diagnosed.

Nursing assessment of the patient's values and beliefs includes assessing for the use of complementary and alternative therapies. The term **complementary therapies** (also called *complementary health approaches*) refers to any of a diverse array of practices, therapies, and supplements that are not considered part of conventional or Western medicine and that are used *in addition to* conventional treatments. **Alternative therapies** is a term used to describe use of these diverse therapies *instead of* conventional therapies (see the Focus on Integrative Health feature). Assessing the patient for use of these therapies is important to determine patient preferences for care and if there are any therapies the patient is currently using that are contraindicated.

Diagnosis

Once the assessment is complete, nurses can begin to identify priorities for care appropriate to the individual or family seeking care. Examples of patient needs and/or nursing priorities may include:

- Powerlessness
- Interrupted religious practice
- Fear
- Lack of knowledge about healthcare options or healthcare system
- Anxiety
- Hopelessness
- Inadequate family coping skills or resources
- Potential for compromised human dignity.

Focus on Integrative Health

Overview of Complementary Health Approaches

The National Center for Complementary and Integrative Health (NCCIH; 2018) reports the use of complementary health approaches is on the rise among both children and adults, including use of yoga, meditation, and chiropractors (see also Clarke et al., 2018). Types and examples of these approaches include:

- ***Natural products.*** Dietary supplements, including fish oil and herbal supplements such as turmeric
- ***Mind and body practices.*** Meditation, yoga, acupuncture, chiropractic medicine, massage therapy

» **Stay Current:** For more information on complementary and alternative therapies, go to the NCCIH website at https://nccih.nih.gov.

Planning

Planning care in collaboration with the patient increases the likelihood that the patient will follow the care plan, particularly if the plan is culturally sensitive. At times it can be challenging to incorporate a patient's cultural preferences and practices into the care plan, especially in the hospital setting. For example, the culture of India tends to encourage strong multigenerational family ties. When a person becomes ill, several family members may come to the hospital and gather in the room, causing crowding. Typically, the mother will provide care for the patient, no matter the age of the patient. This can cause conflict, as many from India believe in self-medication and herbal medicines and may be trying to complement the hospital care. The nurse, therefore, should collaborate with the patient and family to provide safe, effective care.

Appropriate goals for patients will include the following:

- The patient will remain safe through the use of interpreters, educational materials written in the patient's primary language, and other cultural bridges of communication between the healthcare team and the patient.
- The patient will meet nutritional needs during hospitalization through meal accommodation, nutritional counseling, and incorporation of preferred foods in the meal plan.
- The patient will perform ADLs and increase mobility when appropriate.
- Both patient and family members will verbalize understanding of necessity of early mobility and independence with ADLs.

Implementation

Implementation should involve a care plan that incorporates the patient's cultural beliefs and practices.

Promote Safety

There is great potential for harm due to cultural and language issues. Patients who do not understand the language of the nurse may not adhere to safety instructions, including using a call light before getting out of bed. Family members may bring comfort foods from home that might interfere with fluid or diet restrictions. Some might want to complement the patient's care with traditional healing remedies that may interact with medications. The nurse must create an open channel of communication with family members and the patient to provide safe and culturally sensitive care. Additional assessment and patient teaching regarding safety procedures, medication side effects and interactions, and other areas of care may be necessary.

Provide Adequate Nutrition

In the hospital setting, international foods are often not available. Many cultures see food as a way to provide healing and comfort. Some patients may not eat hospital food because it is foreign or taboo. For instance, some people of Jewish heritage may not eat the food provided in a hospital if it is not prepared and served correctly in a kosher manner. Vietnamese patients who follow traditional cultural practices regarding eating certain foods during illness may ignore Western food or diet recommendations. Regardless of the patient's background, carefully assess patient and family expectations and practices regarding foods and beverages and incorporate these into the plan of care when it is safe to do so.

Communicating with Patients

Introductory Phase

Patients who are experiencing their first admission to a hospital can be particularly nervous about the experience. You can help alleviate their anxiety by taking the time to find out what makes them comfortable and what their concerns are.

- You said this is your first time being admitted to the hospital. What could I do to make you more comfortable?
- Are there any particular comfort foods you like to eat when you're sick? I could check with the nutrition team and see what is available that you might enjoy.
- Are there any cultural or religious practices that you would like to maintain while you're here in the hospital?
- What concerns do you have about your hospital stay?

Promote Physical Mobility

Many cultures believe that the sick must remain in bed with little physical activity until deemed well. The belief is that the sick person must gain strength. The cultural belief of restricted activity may cause conflict with nurses who wish to promote activity to prevent skin integrity breakdown, clots, and other complications with immobility. The nurse can take this opportunity to educate as well as collaborate. The nurse should collaborate with the family to implement a plan that does include mobility, but also appreciates the cultural need for rest.

Evaluation

The evaluation of the nurse's plan of care will involve the underlying goals that include a culture component. Goals may include:

- The patient expresses that cultural needs were met.
- The patient is able to verbalize understanding of medical diagnosis and treatment plan.
- The patient is able to collaborate with the care team when using complementary therapies.
- The patient is able to meet nutritional needs.

Evaluating how successfully the patient is able to follow the treatment regimen while observing cultural practices and rituals is essential to determining patient outcomes but also provides a way for nurses to evaluate whether or not they provided culturally competent care that promoted improved patient outcomes.

REVIEW The Concept of Culture and Diversity

RELATE Link the Concepts

Linking the concept of culture and diversity with the concept of development:

1. How might a pediatric patient's development be impacted if their parent is homeless?
2. How might an adolescent's development be impacted by the realization that they are transgender?

You are a nurse working in a children's rehabilitation center in the United States. A 6-year-old girl who is recovering from a motor-vehicle accident comes to your center for an extended stay. The family speaks French as their primary language, and the father speaks limited English. The mother cares for their two children at home, homeschooling them through an international homeschool organization. The father, who has a driver's license, works long hours at two jobs. The mother has not yet qualified for a driver's license. The bus service from their home to the facility requires a half-mile walk from their home to the nearest bus station, and then two transfers to get to the facility.

Linking the concept of culture and diversity with the concept of communication:

3. How might the nurse assess this family's values and beliefs in light of the language barrier?
4. How might involvement of an interpreter to facilitate communication impact the patient and her family's values and beliefs? How can you overcome this problem?

Linking the concept of culture and diversity with the concept of advocacy:

5. How can you advocate for this patient's values and beliefs while she is in the rehabilitation center?
6. The patient's family wishes to pray at the child's bedside using candles, which are not allowed because of the risk for fire related to oxygen use. How can you advocate for this family while maintaining safety?
7. How can you advocate for the mother with regard to transportation if the father is working and unable to bring the mother to the facility?

REFER Go to Pearson MyLab Nursing and eText

REFLECT Apply Your Knowledge

Elam Avromovitch, a 76-year-old man, is visiting his son's family in the United States when he develops chest pain. A native of Israel and a follower of ultra-Orthodox Judaism, he speaks Yiddish as his first language. Tests reveal he is having an acute myocardial infarction and needs intervention in a cardiac catheterization lab. The nurses on the cardiac floor are attempting to prepare Mr. Avromovitch for the procedure while his son translates. The nurse attempts to call for a translator for the consent, but the son declines a translator, stating that he will serve instead. When attempting to undress Mr. Avromovitch for a required admission skin assessment before the procedure, the patient starts to "shoo" away the female nurses and tries to cover up.

The son explains that women are not permitted to see him undressed, particularly women who are not of his faith.

1. Is the use of the son for interpretation valid for a legal consent for treatment?
2. How can the nurse respect Mr. Avromovitch's diversity requirements while maintaining facility policy and meeting the patient's healthcare needs?
3. What nursing diagnoses and interventions would be appropriate for Mr. Avromovitch's plan of care?

References

Administration for Community Living. (2018). *A profile of older Americans: 2017.* U.S. Administration on Aging, Department of Health and Human Services. https://acl.gov/sites/default/files/Aging%20and%20Disability%20in%20America/2017OlderAmericansProfile.pdf

American Association of Colleges of Nursing. (2008). *Cultural competency in baccalaureate nursing education.* http://www.aacn.nche.edu/leading-initiatives/education-nbvcfg/-competency.pdf

Andrews, M. A., Boyle, J. S., & Collins, J. (2020) *Transcultural concepts in nursing care* (8th ed.). Wolters Kluwer.

Association of American Medical Colleges. (2005). *Cultural competence education.* https://www.aamc.org/download/54338/dataf

Berlin, E. A., & Fowkes, W. C. (1983). A teaching framework for cross-cultural health care. *Western Journal of Medicine, 139,* 934–938.

Brown, A. (2020, February 25). *The changing categories the U.S. census has used to measure race.* Pew Research Center. https://www.pewresearch.org/fact-tank/2020/02/25/the-changing-categories-the-u-s-has-used-to-measure-race/

California Maternal Quality Care Collaborative (CMQCC). (2020). *California Birth Equity Collaborative: Improving care, experiences, and outcomes for Black mothers.* https://www.cmqcc.org/qi-initiatives/birth-equity

Capatides, C. (2020). *Doctors Without Borders dispatches team to the Navajo Nation.* CBS News. https://www.cbsnews.com/news/doctors-without-borders-navajo-nation-coronavirus/

Centers for Disease Control and Prevention (CDC). (2008). *Health disparities among racial/ethnic populations.* U.S. Department of Health and Human Services.

Centers for Disease Control and Prevention (CDC). (2019). *Men and stroke.* https://www.cdc.gov/stroke/men.htm

Cheng, T. L., Goodman, E., & Committee on Pediatric Research. (2015). Race, ethnicity, and socioeconomic status in research on child health. *Pediatrics, 135*(1), e225–e237.

Chishti, M., & Pierce, S. (2020, March 26). *Crisis within a crisis: Immigration in the United States in a time of COVID-19.* Migration Policy Institute. https://www.migrationpolicy.org/article/crisis-within-crisis-immigration-time-covid-19

Christensen, M., Welch, A. Y., & Barr, J. (2018). Men are from Mars: The challenges of communicating as a male nursing student. *Nurse Education in Practice, 33,* 102–106. https://doi.org/10.1016/j.nepr.2018.04.014

Clarke, T.C., Barnes, P. M., Black, L. I., Stussman, B. J., & Nahin, R. L. (2018). *Use of yoga, meditation, and chiropractors among U.S. adults aged 18 and over* (NCHS Data Brief No. 325). National Center for Health Statistics.

Curry, O. S., Mullins, D. A., & Whitehouse, H. (2019). Is it good to cooperate?: Testing the theory of morality-as-cooperation in 60 societies. *Current Anthopology, 60*(1), 47–49. https://doi.org/10.1086/701478

Dayer-Berenson, L. (2013). *Cultural competencies for nurses: Impact on health and illness* (2nd ed.). Jones & Bartlett.

Finlay, F. Dunne, J., & Guiton, G. (2017). G54(P) Children acting as interpreters. *Archives of Disease in Childhood, 102*(A23). http://dx.doi.org/10.1136/archdischild-2017-313087.53

Giger, J. N., & Haddad, L. G. (2021). *Transcultural nursing: Assessment and intervention* (8th ed.). Elsevier.

Goldman, B. (2017, Spring). *Two minds: The cognitive differences between men and women.* Stanford Medicine. https://stanmed.stanford.edu/2017spring/how-mens-and-womens-brains-are-different.html#

Goyal, M. K., Kuppermann, N., Cleary, S. D., Teach, S. J., & Chamberlain, J. M. (2016). Racial disparities in pain management of children with appendicitis in emergency departments. *JAMA Pediatrics, 169*(11), 996–1002.

Guyer, A. C., & Banerji, A. (2020). *ACE inhibitor-induced angioedema.* UpToDate. https://www.uptodate.com/contents/ace-inhibitor-induced-angioedema

Health Resources and Services Administration. (n.d.). *LGBT health.* http://www.hrsa.gov/lgbt/

Heron, M. (2019, June). Deaths: Leading causes for 2017. *National Vital Statistics Reports, 68*(6). https://www.cdc.gov/nchs/data/nvsr/nvsr68/nvsr68_06-508.pdf?fbclid=IwAR0ShnhUypiDEhFAJvjgxEjArda8ujdLSJj97y3cORXzUHID_cLPdmzdSdY

Intersex Society of North America. (n.d.). *What is intersex?* http://www.isna.org/faq/what_is_intersex.

Itkowitz, C. (2016, June 21). An Orlando doctor's bloodied shoes—the story behind the viral story. *Washington Post.* https://www.washingtonpost.com/news/inspired-life/wp/2016/06/21/im-carrying-them-on-me-all-the-time-the-orlando-doctor-whose-bloody-shoes-went-viral/

Kaiser Family Foundation. (2020) *Poverty rate by race/ethnicity 2018.* Retrieved from https://www.kff.org/other/state-indicator/poverty-rate-by-raceethnicity/?currentTimeframe=0&sortModel=%7B%22colId%22:%22Location%22,%22sort%22:%22asc%22%7D

Kenny, C., & Patel, D. (2017). *Norms and reform: Legalizing homosexuality improves attitudes* (Working Paper No. 465). Center for Global Development. https://www.cgdev.org/publication/norms-and-reform-legalizing-homosexuality-improves-attitudes

Kim, H. J., Yang, G. S., Greenspan, J. D., Downton, K. D., Griffith, K. A., Renn, C. L., et al. (2017). Racial and ethic differences in experimental pain sensitivity: Systematic review and meta-analysis. *Pain, 158*(2), 194–211.

Leininger, M. (2002). Culture care theory: A major contribution to advance transcultural nursing knowledge and practices. *Journal of Transcultural Nursing, 13,* 189–192. https://doi.org/10.1177/10459602013003005

Li, C., Abdulkerim, N., Jordan, C. A., & Ga Eun Son, C. (2017). Overcoming communication barriers to healthcare for culturally and linguistically diverse patients. *North American Journal of Medicine and Science, 10*(3), 103–109. https://doi.org/10.7156/najms.2017.1003103]

Lo, B. (2017). Gender, culture, and the educational choices of second generation Hmong American girls. *Journal of Southeast Asian American Education and Advancement, 12*(1), Article No. 4. https://doi.org/10.7771/2153-8999.1149

Marion, L., Douglas, M., Lavin, M. A., Barr, N., Gazaway, S., Thomas, E., & Bickford, C. (2017). Implementing the New ANA standard 8: Culturally congruent practice. *Online Journal of Issues in Nursing, 22*(1). https://ojin.nursingworld.org/MainMenuCategories/ANAMarketplace/ANAPeriodicals/OJIN/TableofContents/Vol-22-2017/No1-Jan-2017/Articles-Previous-Topics/Implementing-the-New-ANA-Standard-8.html

Minority Nurse. (2018). *Reversing the rise in maternal deaths: Implications for nursing awareness and advocacy.* https://minoritynurse.com/reversing-the-rise-in-maternal-death-rates-implications-for-nursing-awareness-and-advocacy/

National Center for Chronic Disease Prevention and Health Promotion. (2020). *Pregnancy mortality surveillance system.* Centers for Disease Control and Prevention. https://www.cdc.gov/reproductivehealth/maternal-mortality/pregnancy-mortality-surveillance-system.htm

National Heart, Lung, and Blood Institute. (2019, May). *Coronary heart disease: Women and heart disease.* https://www.nhlbi.nih.gov/health-topics/coronary-heart-disease

Paradies, Y., Ben, J., Denson, N., Elias, A., Priest, N., Pieterse, A., et al. (2015). Racism as a determinant of health: A systematic review and meta-analysis. *PLoS One, 10*(9), e0138511. https://doi.org/10.1371/journal.pone.0138511

Peterson, E. E., Davis, N. L., Goodman, D., Cox, S., Mayes, N., Johnston, E., . . . , & Barfield, W. Vital signs: Pregnancy-related deaths, United States, 2011–2015, and strategies for prevention, 13 states, 2013–2017. *MMWR Morbidity and Mortality Weekly Report, 68*(18), 423–429.

Purnell, L. D., & Fenkl, E. A. (2019). *Handbook for culturally competent care.* Springer.

Rahim-Williams, B., Riley, J., Williams, A. K., & Fillingim, R. B. (2012). A quantitative review of ethnic group differences in experimental pain response: Do biology, psychology, and culture matter? *Pain Medicine, 13*(4), 522–540.

Rosales, C. B. (2017). *Emergent public health issues in the US–Mexico border region.* Frontiers Media.

Rotter, J. B. (1966). Generalized expectancies for internal versus external control of reinforcement. *Psychological Monographs: General and Applied, 80*(1), 1–28. http://dx.doi.org/10.1037/h0092976

Seelman, K. L., Colón-Diaz, M. J. P., LeCroix, R. H., Xavier-brier, M., & Kattari, L. (2017). General health and mental health among transgender adults. *Transgender Health, 2*(1). https://doi.org/10.1089/trgh.2016.0024

Schuiling, K. D., & Likis, F. E. (2017). *Women's gynecologic health* (2nd ed.). Jones & Bartlett.

Spector, R. E. (2017). *Cultural diversity in health and -illness* (9th ed.). Pearson.

Substance Abuse and Mental Health Services Administration. (2012). *Top health issues for LGBT populations information & resource kit.* https://store.samhsa.gov/sites/default/files/d7/priv/sma12-4684.pdf

Tervalon, M., & Murray-Garcia, J. (1998). Cultural humility versus cultural competence: A critical distinction in defining physician training outcomes in multicultural education. *Journal of Health Care for the Poor and Underserved,* 9, 117–125.

Vanderbilt University. (2017). *Lesbian, gay, bisexual, transgender, queer, and intersex life: Definitions.* https://www.vanderbilt.edu/lgbtqi/resources/definitions

United Health Foundation. (2020). Maternal mortality. https://www.americashealthrankings.org/explore/health-of-women-and-children/measure/maternal_mortality_a

United Nations. (n.d.) *Ending poverty.* https://www.un.org/en/sections/issues-depth/poverty/

U.S. Census Bureau. (2020). *Race: About.* http://www.census.gov/topics/population/race/about.html

U.S. Census Bureau. (2019a). *How the Census Bureau measures poverty.* https://www.census.gov/topics/income-poverty/poverty/guidance/poverty-measures.html

U.S. Census Bureau. (2019b). *Poverty thresholds.* https://www.census.gov/data/tables/time-series/demo/income-poverty/historical-poverty-thresholds.html

U.S. Census Bureau. (2019c, October 7). *The supplemental poverty measure: 2018.* https://www.census.gov/library/publications/2019/demo/p60-268.html

U.S. Department of Homeland Security. (2020, January 6). *Yearbook of immigration statistics: 2018.* https://www.dhs.gov/immigration-statistics/yearbook/2018

U.S. Department of Housing and Urban Development. (2019). *Homeless populations and sub-populations.* https://www.hudexchange.info/programs/coc/coc-homeless-populations-and-subpopulations-reports/

Vanderbilt University. (2017). *Lesbian, gay, bisexual, transgender, queer, and intersex life: Definitions.* https://www.vanderbilt.edu/lgbtqi/resources/definitions

Vroman, K. G., Arthanat, S., & Lysack, C. (2015). "Who over 65 is online?" Older adults' - dispositions toward information communication technology. *Computers in Human Behavior, 43,* 156–166. http://dx.doi.org/10.1016/j.chb.2014.10.018

Williams, D. R., Lawrence, J. A., & Davis, B. A. (2019). Racism and health: Evidence and needed research. *Annual Review of Public Health, 40,* 105–125. https://doi.org/10.1146/annurev-publhealth-040218-043750

World Health Organization (WHO). (2008). *Social determinants of health.* https://www.who.int/social_determinants/thecommission/finalreport/key_concepts/en/

World Health Organization (WHO). (2016). *Vulnerable groups.* http://www.who.int/environmental_health_emergencies/vulnerable_groups/en/

Xiong, L. (2018). *Negotiating two cultural worlds: The development of career aspirations* Unpublished doctoral dissertation, California State University, Stanislaus. http://scholarworks.csustan.edu/handle/011235813/1219

Yusef, H. (2015, June 24). My hijab has nothing to do with oppression: It's a feminist statement. *The Guardian.* https://www.theguardian.com/commentisfree/video/2015/jun/24/hijab-not-oppression-feminist-statement-video

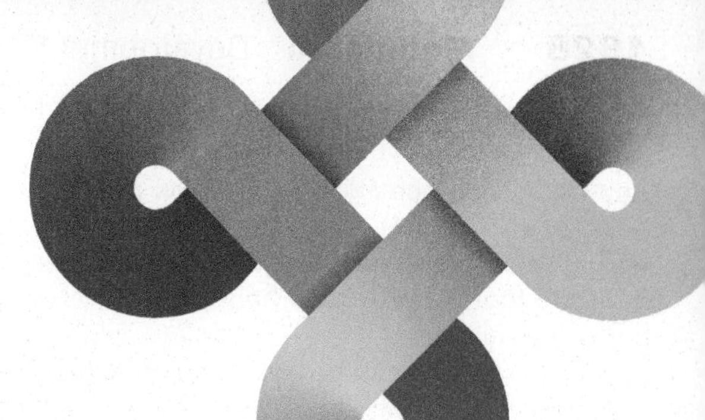

Module 25

Development

Module Outline and Learning Outcomes

The Concept of Development

Normal Development

25.1 Describe the course of normal development.

Theories of Growth and Development

25.2 Analyze theories of growth and development

Growth and Development Through the Lifespan

25.3 Summarize the developmental milestones of individuals across the lifespan.

Alterations to Development

25.4 Differentiate alterations in development.

Concepts Related to Development

25.5 Outline the relationship between development and other concepts.

Health Promotion

25.6 Explain the promotion of healthy development.

Nursing Assessment

25.7 Differentiate common assessment procedures and tests used to examine development.

Independent Interventions

25.8 Analyze independent interventions nurses can implement for patients with alterations in development.

Collaborative Therapies

25.9 Summarize collaborative therapies used by interprofessional teams for patients with alterations in development.

Lifespan Considerations

25.10 Differentiate considerations related to the assessment and care of patients with alterations in development throughout the lifespan.

Development Exemplars

Exemplar 25.A Attention-Deficit/Hyperactivity Disorder

25.A Analyze ADHD as it relates to development.

Exemplar 25.B Autism Spectrum Disorder

25.B Analyze ASD as it relates to development.

Exemplar 25.C Cerebral Palsy

25.C Analyze CP as it relates to development.

Exemplar 25.D Failure to Thrive

25.D Analyze failure to thrive as it relates to development.

The Concept of Development

Concept Key Terms

Accommodation, 1832
Adaptation, 1832
Adaptation phase, 1833
Adjustment phase, 1833
Assimilation, 1832
Associative play, 1840
Centration, 1840
Cephalocaudal, 1829
Cognitive development, 1831
Conservation, 1840
Cooperative play, 1843
Development, 1828
Developmental milestones, 1835
Developmental stage, 1828
Developmental task, 1830
Dramatic play, 1841
Ecologic theory, 1833
Egocentrism, 1840
Expressive jargon, 1839
Expressive speech, 1838
Growth, 1828
Individualized education plan, 1857
Individualized family service plan, 1857
Magical thinking, 1840
Moral behavior, 1834
Moral development, 1834
Morality, 1834
Morals, 1834
Nature, 1833
Nurture, 1833
Object permanence, 1835
Parallel play, 1838
Personality, 1829
Protective factors, 1833
Proximodistal, 1829
Puberty, 1844
Receptive speech, 1838
Resilience, 1833
Risk factors, 1833
Self-efficacy, 1832
Solitary play, 1836
Temperament, 1833
Transductive reasoning, 1840

Jean Piaget (1970) wrote: "It is with children that we have the best chance of studying the development of logical knowledge, mathematical knowledge, physical knowledge, and so forth" (p. 14). Understanding lifespan development and applying that knowledge can provide the nurse with valuable tools to provide a holistic approach to caring for patients of all ages.

Human growth and development are dynamic processes that occur throughout the lifespan in humans, from conception through young adulthood to old age. **Growth** is measurable and refers to a physical increase in size and mass, such as height and weight. The rate of growth changes, from conception through adulthood, with a faster rate of growth occurring through adolescence, slowing down into young adulthood, and only nominal growth occurring beyond young adulthood. While growth progresses in a similar pattern in all individuals, it is affected by factors such as nutrition, genetics, and health.

Development is a change in function, complexity, and skill level that progresses gradually throughout the lifespan. Development is characterized by behavioral changes and moves from simple, to more integrated, to complex skills.

Normal Development

Children proceed through predictable stages of growth and development (**Table 25.1** »). Each child, however, moves through these stages in an individualized manner. Normal growth and development follow certain patterns:

- Growth and development proceed in an organized manner that is affected by an interplay of genetic and environmental influences.
- Maturation affects growth and development. Maturation of the brain and nervous system must occur to allow a child to progress and acquire new skills, such as communication. As the brain and nervous system mature, the child can move from communicating discomfort by crying to communicating needs with words.
- Growth and development proceed in a predictable manner in all children, yet each child is unique in timing, duration, and impact of the stage.
- Each **developmental stage** (a level with defined accomplishments) is unique and builds on the achievements gained at previous stages. For example, Erikson (1963, 1968)

TABLE 25.1 Stages of Growth and Development

Stage	Age	Significant Characteristics	Nursing Implications
Neonatal	Birth–28 days	Behavior is largely reflexive and develops to more purposeful behavior.	Assist parents to identify and meet unmet needs.
Infancy	1 month–1 year	Physical growth is rapid.	Control the infant's environment so that physical and psychologic needs are met.
Toddlerhood	1–3 years	Motor development permits increased physical autonomy. Psychosocial skills increase.	Safety and risk-taking strategies must be balanced to permit growth.
Preschool	3–6 years	The preschooler's world is expanding. New experiences and the preschooler's social role are tried during play. Physical growth is slower.	Provide opportunities for play and social activity.
School age	6–12 years	This stage includes the preadolescent period (10–12 years). Peer group increasingly influences behavior. Physical growth is slower.	Allow time and energy for the school-age child to pursue hobbies and school activities. Recognize and support child's achievement.
Adolescence	12–18 years	Self-concept changes with biological development. Values are tested. Physical growth accelerates. Stress increases.	Assist adolescents to develop coping behaviors. Help adolescents develop strategies for resolving conflicts.
Young adulthood	18–40 years	A personal lifestyle develops. Individuals may establish commitments to others and to services or organizations; many become parents. Physical growth slows and then stops (except for weight gain). Metabolism begins to slow down.	Accept adult's chosen lifestyle and assist with necessary adjustments relating to health. Recognize the individual's commitments. Support change as necessary for health.
Middle adulthood	40–65 years	Lifestyle changes because of other changes; for example, children leave home, occupational goals change. Physical changes may include weight gain, diminished vision and hearing, onset of wrinkles, hair loss in men. Risk for onset of chronic illness greatest during this time.	Assist patients to plan for anticipated changes in life, to recognize the risk factors related to health, and to focus on strengths rather than weaknesses.
Older adulthood			
Young-old	65–74 years	Adaptation to retirement and changing physical abilities is often necessary. Chronic illness may develop/continue.	Assist patients to stay mentally, physically, and socially active and to maintain peer group interactions.
Middle-old	75–84 years	Adaptation to decline in speed of movement, reaction time, and balance issues. Increasing dependence on others may be necessary.	Assist patients to cope with loss (e.g., hearing, sensory abilities, eyesight, death of loved one). Provide necessary safety measures.
Old-old	85 years and older	Increasing physical problems may develop. Many need help with self-care.	Assist patients with self-care as required and with maintaining as much independence as possible.

Source: Berman, Snyder, and Frandsen (2021). Pearson Education, Inc., Hoboken, NJ.

explained how infants must move through the stage of trust versus mistrust and achieve a level of basic trust before moving on to the next stage of autonomy versus shame and doubt.

- Growth and development proceed in a head to toe or **cephalocaudal** direction. For example, a child first gains control of the head, then develops coordination of the arms, followed by the legs. At birth, the head is much larger than the rest of the body (**Figure 25.1** »).
- Growth and development also proceed in a **proximodistal** manner, from the center of the body to the periphery. Following this principle, a child develops control of the arms before the fingers. For example, a child waves the arms before being able to grasp an object.
- Development progresses from general to specific, from simple to complex actions. To be able to accomplish the act of eating finger foods, the infant needs to progress through certain stages: First, the infant learns to reach out with the arms before being able to grasp an object; then the infant begins to move the object to the mouth. At the same time, the infant develops the integrated actions of the mouth needed to eat and swallow.
- Development follows the principle of differentiation. Through differentiation, the child develops a progressive ability to act and respond. At first, the infant smiles at everyone, then later learns to differentiate and recognize family members.
- The rate of growth and development is marked by periods of slow growth and spurts. During the early years of life, growth and development are rapid. For example, during infancy the head grows at a rapid rate and continues to grow at a slower rate in the following years. In puberty, growth spurts and sexual maturation occur before slowing down in young adulthood.

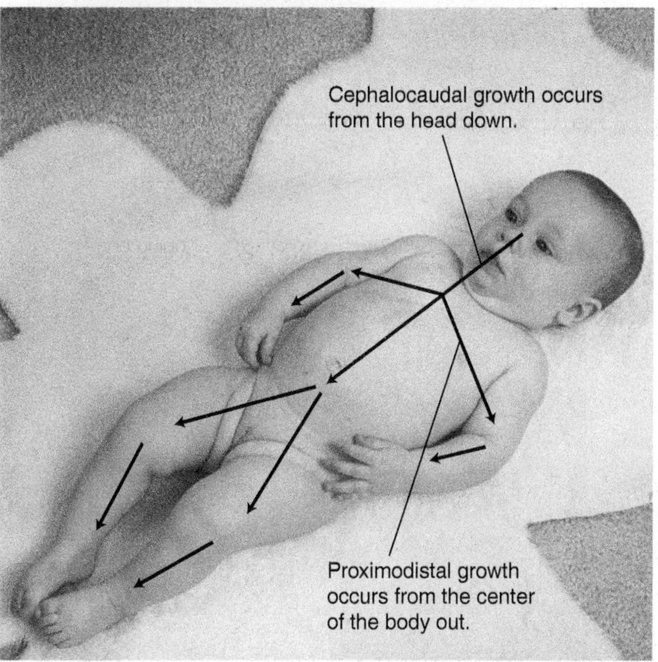

Figure 25.1 » In normal cephalocaudal growth, the child gains control of the head and neck before the trunk and limbs. In normal proximodistal growth, the child controls arm movements before hand movements. For example, the child reaches for objects before being able to grasp them. Children gain control of their hands before their fingers; that is, they can hold things with the entire hand before they can pick something up with just their fingers.

Source: Pearson Education, Inc.

Theories of Growth and Development

Theories of growth and development explain how individuals change over the lifespan. Theories tend to focus on one developmental perspective, such as psychosocial, cognitive, or moral growth. Depending on the background of the theorist, a theory may explain changes that occur over the lifespan or may focus on a specific developmental stage from birth through older adulthood. Developmental stages may include infancy, early childhood, school age, adolescence, and adulthood, from young adults to older adults.

Theories attempt to explain and predict changes in growth and development that occur in an individual and provide guidance on developmental norms. These norms allow anticipatory guidance and serve as guides to indicate whether or not an individual is meeting expected milestones for that stage of development. However, theories also have limitations. Typically, theories only describe one particular aspect of growth and development during a specific time frame, segmenting an individual's life rather than examining the person as a whole. Observing an individual through the lens of several theories of growth and development may provide a broader and more holistic understanding of the individual.

According to certain theories, developmental tasks occur within a specified age range. Most children meet these developmental norms within the identified age range of the theory whereas others may achieve a developmental task earlier or later than expected. These variations from the specified milestones of the theory can be within normal ranges or may be a red flag for a developmental problem.

Theories of growth and development can be categorized by their domain. Common domains include the psychosocial, cognitive, moral, spiritual, and physical theories. Other domains that theorists have used to describe growth and development include behavioral, social learning, temperament, resiliency, and ecologic theories. These theories delineate developmental stages within their domain and the ages that children typically reach these milestones.

Psychosocial Theories

Psychosocial theories emphasize personality development and the social nature of humans. An individual's **personality** consists of beliefs, attitudes, and social interactions. Personality is the distinct, visible display of an individual's thoughts, feelings, and behaviors (Costa, McCrae, & Löckenhoff, 2019). An individual's personality tends to be stable across life stages, but is influenced by factors such as environment, life events, and education.

Sigmund Freud (1856–1939) presented one of the first theories on personality development. He proposed that personality developed through five psychosexual stages. When ego defense mechanisms are stressed with healthcare crises, individuals may develop anxiety and phobias that affect their recovery. This topic is discussed in Module 31, Stress and Coping module.

TABLE 25.2 Erikson's Eight Stages of Development

Stage	Age	Primary Task	Outcomes of Successful Task Accomplishment	Outcomes of Failed Task Accomplishment
Infancy	Birth–18 months	Trust versus mistrust	Development of basic trust and sense of security	Lack of trust, sense of fear
Early childhood	18 months–3 years	Autonomy versus shame and doubt	Basic awareness of independence; sense of autonomy and self-control	Self-doubt, sense of helplessness, heightened dependence on caregivers
Late childhood	3–5 years	Initiative versus guilt	Emergence of basic sense of self-guidance and self-discipline	Impaired self-initiative, insecurity regarding leadership ability
School age	6–12 years	Industry versus inferiority	Confidence in ability to attain goals, initial formation of identity apart from nuclear family, successful peer group integration	Sense of incompetence, low self-esteem, difficulty integrating into peer groups
Adolescence	12–20 years	Identity versus role confusion	Formation of strong sense of identity as an individual and as a member of society, identification of personal and occupational goals	Role confusion, social alienation, potential substance misuse or abuse, potential development of antisocial personality disorder
Young adulthood	18–25 years	Intimacy versus isolation	Development of healthy romantic relationships without compromising personal identity	Avoidance of intimacy, fear of commitment, isolation
Adulthood	25–65 years	Generativity versus stagnation	Productivity and creativity, desire to care for and guide offspring (or, if child-free, to guide the next generation)	Self-preoccupation, primary attainment of pleasure through self-indulgence, stagnation
Maturity	65 years–death	Integrity versus despair	Sense of peace concerning life experiences, life choices framed within a meaningful context, development of wisdom	Life experiences framed by bitterness and/or regret; may progress to hopelessness and depression

Sources: Based on Berk (2018); Erikson (1963); Weber and Kelley (2018).

Erikson (1902–1994)

Erik H. Erikson's (1963, 1968) theory of psychosocial development consists of eight stages that span infancy through adulthood. According to Erikson, individuals are continually developing throughout their lives (**Table 25.2** »).

Erikson believed that individuals move through a series of eight predetermined stages of development. During each stage, an individual faces a **developmental task** (a skill or behavior that is accomplished during a specific stage of development) that must be resolved or met to develop a healthy personality and engage confidently in society. Successfully mastering the stage or resolving the conflict helps the individual develop into a confident adult. Unsuccessful resolution of the conflict leads to feelings of inadequacy. During Erikson's first stage of development, trust versus mistrust, for example, the infant learns trust as adults act to meet the infant's basic needs. The infant learns to feel safe and that the environment is predictable. The infant whose needs are not successfully met does not develop trust and learns that the world is unpredictable. See **Figure 25.2** » and **Figure 25.3** ».

When developing a plan of care, the nurse should consider the individual's stage of development and the developmental task that needs to be achieved. The care plan should include interventions to help the patient successfully meet the stressors occurring at the specific developmental stage. The nurse caring for a 13-year-old, during the stage of identity versus role confusion, can encourage the hospitalized adolescent to maintain contact with friends through social media. During this stage of development, a teenager wants to feel a sense of independence from the parents and be part of a peer group.

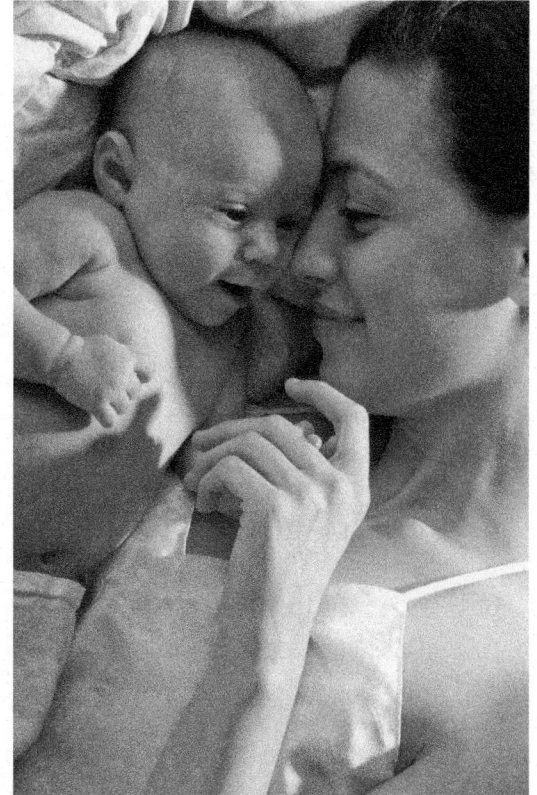

Figure 25.2 » This infant is clearly on his way to accomplishing a sense of basic trust in and security with his mother.
Source: Purestock/Getty Images.

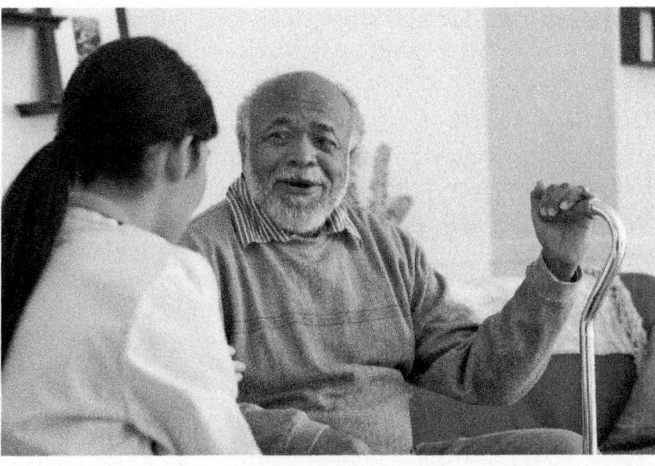

Figure 25.3 » Regular visits from a home health nurse can help older adults maintain their health and independence, contributing to the achievement of integrity versus despair.
Source: Jupiter Images/Stockbyte/Getty Images.

In contrast, the care plan for an older adult, in the stage of integrity versus despair, for example, should include interventions that promote a sense of satisfaction with life. Reminiscence allows older adults to reflect on whether they have lived a meaningful life. The nurse can help the older adult make social connections and remain connected to others to avoid loneliness and despair.

Erikson noted that development may be affected by environment. For example, a crisis, such as illness and hospitalization, may interfere with an individual's mastery of a stage and cause that person to revert to a previous stage or remain stuck in the present stage. A sick toddler, in the stage of autonomy versus shame and doubt, who was previously toilet-trained may revert back to needing a diaper and need time to return to independent toileting once the illness has resolved.

Gould (1935–)

Roger Gould also studied the transitions that occur in adulthood. He believes that adults move through development stages as they progress from young adulthood to older adulthood and that at each stage, they view life differently. At each sequential stage, Gould (1972) maintained that specific assumptions from childhood needed to be resolved:

- **Ages 16 to 18.** Individuals believe they will always be a part of a family, but they begin to separate from family and build an identity as an adult. They perceive a vague future view of themselves.
- **Ages 18 to 22.** Individuals are still working on autonomy from parents and the family unit and fear being drawn back into the family. They feel only partially in the adult world. Real life is imminent.
- **Ages 22 to 28.** Individuals feel autonomous and distinct from the family and work on being an adult. Energy is focused on building an adult life and proving to parents that they are adults. Their work is on being who they believe they should be. There may be a commitment to a spouse.
- **Ages 28 to 34.** Individuals have established careers, married, and may have young children. Individuals no longer feel the need to prove themselves and want acceptance as they are. They question what life is about and if their path is their only choice. They are tired of being who they are supposed to be.
- **Ages 34 to 43.** Individuals look inward and question their values, life, and self. There is a realization that their children are growing up and that their time to influence them is limited. They want to spend time being who they are and become increasingly aware of the passage of time.
- **Ages 43 to 50.** Individuals see there is still time to follow dreams. They believe their personalities are established. They desire social activities and friends, but more superficially than previous stages. They are watching their children become adults and separate from them.
- **Ages 50 to 60.** There is a decrease in the negativity of the 40s. Individuals are more positive in relationship to themselves, their parents, and their grown children. Mortality is a reality and individuals question the meaning of life.

Peck (1919–2002)

As individuals are living longer and healthier lives, theorists have started looking at stages of development in the older adult. While Erikson viewed the last stage of personality development as occupied by one developmental task, that of integrity versus despair, Robert Peck (1968) suggested that the older adulthood moved through three distinct stages of development:

1. ***Ego differentiation versus work-role preoccupation***. Older adults whose role has been defined by work must now redefine their role in a way that does not relate to their occupational role. They must learn to find self-worth and self-esteem and other rewarding roles.
2. ***Body transcendence versus body preoccupation***. Due to physical limitations, the task of older adults in this stage is to maintain well-being in other ways, such as through cognitive or social tasks.
3. ***Ego transcendence versus ego preoccupation***. The task at this stage is to accept the reality of death without fear. During this stage, the individual takes meaningful actions that will extend beyond one's life and positively affect future generations.

Cognitive Theory

Cognitive development describes the process of intellectual development from infancy through adulthood. This process includes the development of thought, judgment, and knowledge. During cognitive development, an individual's intellectual abilities progress from concrete thinking to abstract ideas. As cognitive abilities develop, children advance from illogical to logical thinking. This advancement allows them to move from uncomplicated problem-solving to multifaceted problem solving. Jean Piaget (1896–1980) developed a well-known and influential theory of cognitive development based on his observations of children at different ages.

Piaget proposed that children's cognitive development progressed through four stages that occurred in a preset order. The first stage is the sensorimotor stage, followed by the preoperational reasoning stage, concrete operational reasoning stage, and the formal operational reasoning stage. Module 23, Cognition, presents these stages in detail along with a discussion on how the nurse can utilize these stages when developing plans of care for clients.

Piaget believed that individuals moved through these stages in order and that each cognitive stage had distinct characteristics built on the previous stage (**Table 25.3** »). In Piaget's theory, schemas are the foundation or building blocks of cognition. During each phase, the individual uses assimilation, accommodation, and adaptation to engage in cognitive development. In **assimilation**, an individual uses preexisting schema to understand new situations. **Accommodation** occurs when a schema is changed or a new one is created to match new information and situations. To accommodate, an individual must assimilate new knowledge. **Adaptation** is the process of adjusting to new information and demands through assimilation and accommodation.

Nurses need to provide developmentally appropriate care to individuals throughout the lifespan. For example, the nurse can use Piaget's theory of cognitive development when forming the plan of care. The plan of care for an 18-month-old should take into account that rituals are important in this stage of development. Nursing interventions focus on maintaining consistency, such as keeping the schedule of care the same each day. Because 11-year-olds are beginning to use rational thinking, the nurse should explain the reason for blood glucose monitoring to the preteen with diabetes as well as the consequences of not monitoring blood glucose levels. The 11-year-old can then begin to participate in and understand care decisions. Since individuals move through cognitive stages at their own pace, the nurse must assess each patient to determine the developmental stage. Cognitive stages for adults span a wide age range; therefore, the nurse should determine how each adult prefers to learn.

Behaviorism

According to behaviorist theory, learning occurs when an individual interacts with the environment. The individual's behavior is shaped through positive or negative reinforcement. Reinforcement that is positive, consistent, and delivered quickly increases the likelihood a behavior will be learned.

According to B. F. Skinner (1904–1990), organisms learn through the process of "operating on" or reacting to their environment. In this process, called *operant conditioning*, a behavior elicits a consequence. If the behavior is reinforced or rewarded, it will continue. Behavior that is punished weakens or decreases the behavior.

Social Learning Theory

Albert Bandura's (1925–) social learning theory asserts that children observe and model the behaviors, attitudes, and emotions of their peers, family members, and other adults. Children model the external behaviors they have observed and use these behaviors as a guide on how to act. They are more likely to model a behavior if the outcome is important to them and the consequences are rewarding. Bandura also believes that an individual's mental state and motivation can affect learning. A child might, for example, be motivated to act due to an internal reward, such as a feeling of accomplishment or pride. Learning, therefore, involves both the internal and external environments (Bandura, 1986, 1997a).

According to Bandura, individuals have **self-efficacy**, the belief that their actions can produce a specific result. A school-age child who believes that studying equates with academic success is more likely to study. A teen with diabetes who has confidence in the ability to control blood glucose levels has a greater chance of following healthy eating guidelines.

TABLE 25.3 Piaget's Phases of Cognitive Development

Phases and Stages	Age	Significant Behavior
Sensorimotor phase	Birth–2 years	
Stage 1: Use of reflexes	Birth–1 month	Uses reflexes: sucking, rooting, grasping.
Stage 2: Primary circular reaction	1–4 months	Infant responds reflexively. Objects are extension of self.
Stage 3: Secondary circular reaction	4–8 months	Awareness of environment grows. Changes in the environment are actively made as infant recognizes cause and effect.
Stage 4: Coordination of secondary schemata	8–12 months	Intentional behavior occurs. Object permanence begins.
Stage 5: Tertiary circular reaction	12–18 months	Toddlers discover new goals and ways to attain goals. Rituals are important.
Stage 6: Mental combinations	18–24 months	Language gives toddlers a new tool to use.
Preoperational phase	2–7 years	Young children think by using words as symbols. Everything is significant and relates to "me." They explore the environment. Language development is rapid. Words are associated with objects. As children get older, egocentric thinking diminishes. They think of one idea at a time. Words express thoughts.
Concrete operational phase	7–11 years	Children solve concrete problems, begin to understand relationships such as size, understand right and left, and recognize various viewpoints.
Formal operational phase	11 years and up	Children use rational thinking. Reasoning is deductive and futuristic.

Source: Data from Piaget (1966). Copyright © 1966 International Universities Press, Inc.

Adults who have confidence in their parenting skills have a better probability of becoming successful parents (Bandura, 1997b).

Temperament Theory

In contrast to personality, **temperament** refers to innate characteristics, such as nervousness or sensitivity, that do not change over time. Chess and Thomas (1995, 1996) recognize the innate qualities of personality that each individual brings to the events of daily life. They view the child as an individual who both influences and is influenced by the environment. However, Chess and Thomas focus on one specific aspect of development: the wide spectrum of behaviors possible in children and how they respond to daily events. Infants generally display clusters of responses, which Chess and Thomas have classified into three major personality types (**Box 25.1** »). Although most children do not demonstrate all behaviors described for a particular type, they usually show a grouping indicative of one personality type (Chess & Thomas, 1995, 1996).

Longitudinal research has demonstrated that personality characteristics displayed during infancy are often consistent with those seen later in life. The ability to predict future characteristics is not possible, however, because of the complex and dynamic interaction of personality traits and environmental reactions.

Resiliency Theory

The concept of resilience first appeared in the literature in the early 1970s. Werner, Bierman, and French (1971) studied a cohort of children from Kauai, Hawaii, in efforts to understand why some children who grow up in poverty and other challenging situations did not follow in the footsteps of their parents, many of whom were alcoholics and/or had mental illness. The researchers felt those children grew up "resilient" to challenging situations (Werner et al., 1971). Resiliency theory examines the individual's characteristics as well as the interaction of those characteristics with the environment. **Resilience** is the ability to function with healthy responses, even when experiencing significant stress and adversity (Masten, 2018). In this model, the individual or family members experience a crisis that provides a source of stress, and the family interprets or deals with the crisis based on resources available. Families and individuals have **protective factors** that provide strength and assistance in dealing with crises and **risk factors** that promote or contribute to their challenges (Masten, 2018). Protective factors and risk factors can be identified in children, their families, and their communities. A typical crisis for a young child might be a transfer to a new child care provider. Protective factors for a child transferring to a new provider could involve past positive experiences with new people and an "easy" temperament. An additional protective factor might be the level of understanding the new childcare provider has about the adaptation needs of young children to new experiences. Risk factors for a child experiencing this type of transition might include repeated moves to new care providers, limited close relationships with adults, and a "slow-to-warm-up" temperament. See the Evidence-Based Practice feature for a discussion of resiliency in nursing.

Once confronted by a crisis, the child and family first experience the **adjustment phase**. During this phase the family works to achieve a state of homeostasis following the crisis (Faccio, Renzi, Giudice, Pravettoni, 2018). In the **adaptation phase**, the child and family meet the challenge and use resources to deal with the crisis. Adaptation may lead to increasing resilience as the child and family learn about new resources and inner strengths and develop the ability to deal more effectively with future crises.

Box 25.1

Patterns of Temperament—Chess and Thomas

- ***"Easy" child.*** The "easy" child is moderately active; shows regularity in patterns of eating, sleeping, and elimination; and is usually positive in mood and when subjected to new stimuli. The easy child adapts to new situations, accepts rules, and works well with others. About 40% of children in the New York Longitudinal Study displayed this personality type.
- ***"Difficult" child.*** The "difficult" child displays irregular schedules for eating, sleeping, and elimination; adapts slowly to new situations and persons; and displays a predominantly negative mood. Intense reactions to the environment are common. The New York Longitudinal Study found that approximately 10% of children display this personality type.
- ***"Slow-to-warm-up" child.*** The "slow-to-warm-up" child has reactions of mild intensity and is slow to adapt to new situations. The child displays initial withdrawal followed by gradual, quiet, and slow interactions with the environment. About 15% of children in the New York Longitudinal Study displayed this personality type.

The remaining 35% of children studied showed some characteristics of each personality type.

Source: Data from Chess and Thomas (1996).

Ecologic Theory

The relative importance in human development of heredity versus environment—or nature versus nurture—is controversial among theorists. **Nature** refers to the genetic or hereditary capability of an individual. **Nurture** refers to the effects of the environment on a person's performance. Contemporary developmental theories increasingly recognize the interaction of nature and nurture in determining the individual's development.

The ecologic theory of development was formulated by Urie Bronfenbrenner (1917–2005) to explain the individual's unique relationship in all of life's settings, from influences close to the child to more widespread forces (Bronfenbrenner, 1986, 2005; Bronfenbrenner, McClelland, Ceci, Moen, & Wethington, 1996). **Ecologic theory** emphasizes the presence of mutual interactions between the individual and these various settings. Neither nature nor nurture is considered more important. Bronfenbrenner believed that each individual brings a unique set of genes—and specific attributes such as age, sex, health, and other characteristics—to their interactions with the environment.

Evidence-Based Practice

Nurse Resiliency

Problem

Nurses today face high levels of stress and burnout. Nurses encounter constant stress from many different sources, including but not limited to patient acuity, infection exposure, short staffing, family dynamics, poor support systems, bullying, and ethical challenges. Nurses who are resilient are able to use effective coping strategies to overcome stress (Brown, Whichello, & Price, 2018).

Evidence

In an integrative review of the literature on the impact of nurse resiliency on burnout, Brown and colleagues (2018) identified that the harmful effects of burnout affected nurses, patients, and the interprofessional team. Nurses reported anxiety, depression, impaired sleep, health-related complaints, compassion fatigue, increased job turnover, leaving the profession, and depersonalization. The impact of burnout on patients and families included reduced satisfaction with care and poorer outcomes. As interpersonal relationships and patient care were affected, the interprofessional team also suffered.

Factors that promoted a high level of resiliency in nurses included hope, flexibility, optimism, self-efficacy, creative thinking, and problem solving (Brown et al., 2018). Brown and colleagues (2018) found that mindfulness training, conflict instruction, emotional distancing, and event trigger education improved resiliency. Other techniques that positively affected resiliency were writing, relaxation training, and exercise.

Implications

Providing education and training to improve resiliency is a worthy investment for nurse managers and healthcare facilities to make, as the outcomes of improved mental health and coping skills are likely to lower burnout and error rates and improve retention rates. Likewise, nurses should be aware of the benefits of developing resiliency. Nurses can nurture their own personal resilience through self-care, exercise, relaxation techniques, and other positive coping skills. Nurses can apply this concept of resilience in several different ways.

Critical Thinking Application

1. You are working as the staff educator on an oncology unit. In what ways is this evidence-based resilience training applicable to your unit? Give a rationale for your answer.
2. You are working as a nurse manager of a 28-bed ICU. You want to incorporate resilience training for your staff. Should the training be part of the new hire orientation? Should the training be delayed until the new staff member is off probation and has been working on the unit for 6 or more months? Should resilience training be part of the yearly staff education? Give rationales for your answers.

The individual then interacts in many settings at different levels or systems, such as family, school or work, and sports team or interest club. The systems the individual encounters affect both the individual and the other systems. For example, communication between the parent, the pediatrician's office, and the school may help ensure that a child has an asthma action plan in time for the school nurse to review it with the child's teachers and bus drivers.

Moral Theories

Moral development is a complicated and progressive process in which a child learns what an individual should and should not do in society. Moral development emerges progressively, as the child develops. **Morals** are a code of acceptable behavior, a sense of right and wrong, what a person ought to do. **Morality** denotes the standards of behavior for people to live by in a particular society. **Moral behavior** is how an individual follows the standards of behaviors. **Moral development** is the manner in which children progressively develop moral behaviors as they age.

Kohlberg (1927–1987)

Lawrence Kohlberg's theory focuses on changes in moral development from childhood through adulthood and is based on Piaget's cognitive development. He believed that morals are actively learned and follow a progression of six stages through three levels. At the earliest preconventional level in young children, moral reasoning is externally controlled, with actions based on consequences. At the level of conventional morality, individuals accept the laws and rules of society because it is for the good of all. The level of postconventional morality, which not everyone will reach, is marked by abstract principles and values. An individual might, perhaps, question whether some laws are unjust. Kohlberg's theory has been criticized as being biased, with women attaining stage 3 while men attained stage 4 morality. Gilligan (1982) argued that Kohlberg's model was based on research involving only white upper-class males and that females reason differently than males. Males, she claimed, valued principles of justice while females valued caring.

Gilligan (1936–)

While Carol Gilligan worked as a research assistant to Kohlberg, she began concentrating on moral development in girls. She believed that women focused on caring and relationships in their moral development and proposed a model based on three stages of moral development (Gilligan, 1982). In the preconventional stage, morality focuses on the self and self-interest. The conventional stage of moral development is characterized by selflessness and responsibility for others. In the final postconventional stage, women focus on responsibility for consequences of their actions. This moral theory is based on caring and relationships in which decisions do not cause harm to others (Copraro & Sippel, 2017).

In contrast to Kohlberg, Gilligan proposed that men and women view morality differently. Men view morality from a rules and justice point of view while women perceive it from a relationship and caring standpoint. Gilligan emphasized that neither way of viewing morality was better; rather, they were different ways of perceiving it (Kakkori & Huttunen, 2017).

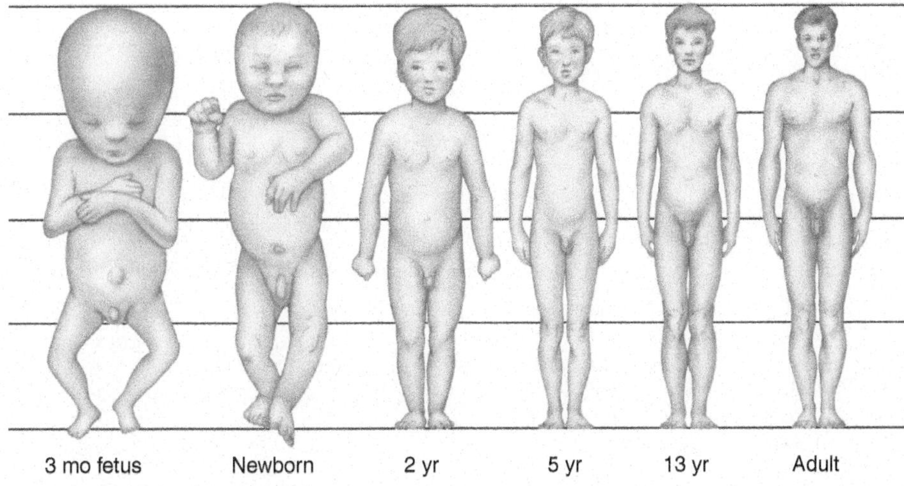

Figure 25.4 ⟫ Body proportions at various ages.

Growth and Development Through the Lifespan

Individuals constantly change and evolve throughout their lives. While some changes are subtle and highly individualized, others are apparent and represent **developmental milestones** common to all human beings at or near a specific phase of growth and development. The stages of sexual development are covered in Module 19, Sexuality.

Infants (Birth to 1 Year)

Immense changes occur during a child's first year of life. The child emerges totally dependent on others, with actions primarily reflexive in nature. By the end of the first year, the infant can walk and communicate. Never again in life is development so swift.

Physical Growth and Motor Development

The infant's birth weight usually doubles by about 5 months and triples by the end of the first year. Height increases by approximately 1 foot during this year. Teeth begin to erupt at about 6 months, and by the end of the first year, the infant has six to eight deciduous teeth. Physical growth is closely associated with type and quality of feeding.

Body organs and systems, although not fully mature at 1 year of age, function differently than they did at birth. Kidney and liver maturation help the 1-year-old excrete drugs or other toxic substances more readily than in the first weeks of life. The changing body proportions mirror changes in developing internal organs (**Figure 25.4** ⟫). Maturation of the nervous system is demonstrated by increased control over body movements, enabling the infant to sit, stand, and walk. Sensory function also increases as the infant begins to discriminate visual images, sounds, and tastes (**Table 25.4** ⟫).

Cognitive Development

The brain continues to increase in complexity during the first year of life. Most of the growth involves maturation of cells, with only a small increase in cell number. This growth of the brain is accompanied by development of its functions, something easily understood when one compares the behavior of the newborn to that of the 1-year-old. The newborn's eyes widen in response to sound; the 1-year-old turns to the sound and recognizes its significance. The 2-month-old cries and coos; the 1-year-old says a few words and understands many more. The 6-week-old grasps a rattle for the first time; the 1-year-old reaches for toys and begins to feed self. At 8 to 12 months of age, **object permanence** (ability to understand that when something is out of sight it still exists) is evolving. Before development of object permanence, babies will not look for toys or other objects out of sight; as the concept is developing, they are concerned when a parent or primary caregiver leaves because they are not certain that person will return.

The infant's behaviors provide clues about thought processes. Piaget's work outlines the infant's actions in a set of rapidly progressing changes in the first year of life. The infant receives stimulation through sight, sound, and feeling, which the maturing brain interprets. This input from the environment interacts with internal cognitive abilities to enhance cognitive functioning.

Psychosocial Development

The infant relies on interactions with primary care providers to meet needs and then begins to establish a sense of trust in other adults and in children. As trust develops, the infant becomes comfortable in interactions with a widening array of people.

Play

The play of infants begins in a reflexive manner. When infants move extremities or grasp objects, they experience the foundations of play. They gain pleasure from the feel and sound of these activities, and gradually perform them purposefully. For example, when a parent places a rattle in the hand of a 6-week-old infant, the infant grasps it reflexively. As the hands move randomly, the rattle makes an enjoyable sound. The infant learns to move the rattle to create the sound and then finally to grasp the toy at will to play with it.

TABLE 25.4 Growth and Development Milestones During Infancy

Age	Physical Growth	Fine Motor Ability	Gross Motor Ability	Sensory Ability
Birth–1 month	Gains 140–200 g (5–7 oz)/week. Grows 1.5 cm (1/2 in.) in first month. Head circumference increases 1.5 cm (1/2 in.)/ month.	Forms hand into a fist. Draws arms and legs to body when crying.	Inborn reflexes such as startle and rooting are predominant activity. May lift head briefly if prone. Alerts to high-pitched voices. Comforts with touch.	Prefers to look at faces and black-and-white geometric designs. Follows objects in line of vision.
2–4 months	Gains 140–200 g (5–7 oz)/week. Grows 1.5 cm (1/2 in.)/month. Head circumference increases 1.5 cm (1/2 in.)/month. Posterior fontanel closes. Eats 120 mL/kg/ 24 hr (2 oz/lb/24 hr).	Holds rattle when placed in hand. Looks at and plays with own fingers. Brings hands to midline.	Moro reflex fading in strength. Can turn from side to back and then return. Head lag when pulled to sitting position decreases; sits with head held in midline with some bobbing. When prone, holds head and supports weight on forearms.	Follows objects 180 degrees. Turns head to look for voices and sounds.
4–6 months	Gains 140–200 g (5–7 oz)/week. Doubles birth weight in 5–6 months. Grows 1.5 cm (1/2 in.)/month. Head circumference increases 1.5 cm (1/2 in.)/month. Teeth may begin erupting by 6 months. Eats 100 mL/kg/24 hr (1 1/2 oz/lb/24 hr).	Grasps rattles and other objects at will; drops them to pick up another offered object. Mouths objects. Holds feet and pulls to mouth. Holds bottle. Grasps with whole hand (palmar grasp). Manipulates objects.	Holds head steady when sitting. Has no head lag when pulled to sitting. Turns from abdomen to back by 4 months and then back to abdomen by 6 months. When held standing, supports much of own weight.	Examines complex visual images. Watches the course of a falling object. Responds readily to sounds.
6–8 months	Gains 85–140 g (3–5 oz)/week. Grows 1 cm (3/8 in.)/month. Growth rate slower than first 6 months.	Bangs objects held in hands. Transfers objects from one hand to the other. Pincer grasp begins at times.	Most inborn reflexes extinguished. Sits alone steadily without support by 8 months. Likes to bounce on legs when held in standing position.	Recognizes own name and responds by looking and smiling. Enjoys playing with small and complex objects.
8–10 months	Gains 85–140 g (3–5 oz)/week. Grows 1 cm (3/8 in.)/month.	Picks up small objects. Uses pincer grasp well.	Crawls or pulls whole body along floor by arms. Creeps by using hands and knees to keep trunk off floor. Pulls self to standing and sitting by 10 months. Recovers balance when sitting.	Understands words such as "no" and "cracker." May say one word in addition to "mama" and "dada." Recognizes sound without difficulty.
10–12 months	Gains 85–140 g (3–5 oz)/week. Grows 1 cm (3/8 in.)/month. Head circumference equals chest circumference. Triples birth weight by 1 year.	May hold crayon or pencil and make mark on paper. Places objects into containers through holes.	Stands alone. Walks holding onto furniture. Sits down from standing.	Plays peek-a-boo and patty cake.

Source: Ball, Bindler, and Cowen (2022). Pearson Education., Inc. Hoboken, NJ.

The next phase of infant play focuses on manipulative behavior. The infant examines toys closely, looking at them, touching them, and placing them in the mouth. The infant learns a great deal about texture, qualities of objects, and all aspects of the surroundings. At the same time, interaction with others becomes an important part of play. The social nature of play is obvious as the infant plays with other children and adults. For example, when a parent walks by, the infant laughs and waves hands and feet wildly (**Figure 25.5** »). The infant plays primarily alone with toys (**solitary play**) but enjoys the presence of adults or other children. Physical capabilities enable the infant to move toward and reach for objects of interest.

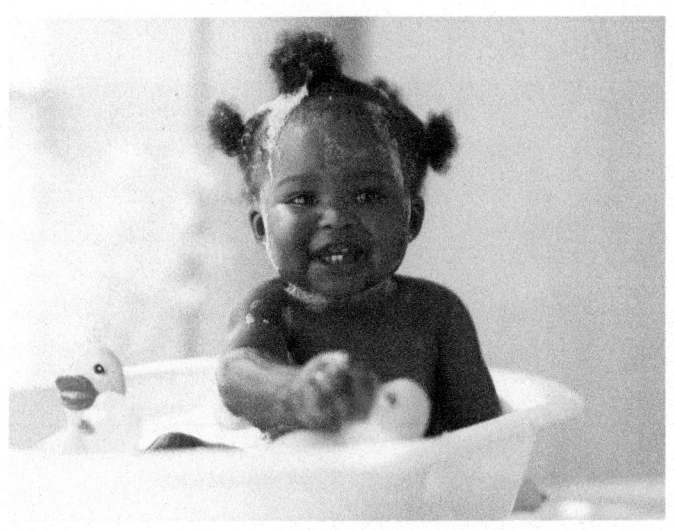

Figure 25.5 » This infant girl demonstrates physical, cognitive, and social capabilities while playing in the tub.
Source: LWA/Dann Tardif/Getty Images.

Cognitive ability is reflected in manipulation of blocks to create different sounds. Social interaction enhances play. The presence of a parent or other individual increases interest in surroundings and teaches the infant different ways to play.

Toward the end of the first year, the infant's ability to move in space enlarges the sphere of play. Once infants crawl or walk, they can get to new places, find new toys, discover forgotten objects, or seek out other people for interaction. Play is a reflection of every aspect of development, as well as a method for enhancing learning and maturation (**Table 25.5** »).

Personality and Temperament

Personality and temperament vary widely among infants. For example, one infant will awaken frequently in the night, whereas another will sleep soundly for 8 to 10 hours. One infant may smile and react positively to interactions, whereas another withdraws around unfamiliar people and frequently frowns and cries. Such differences in responses to the environment are believed to be inborn characteristics of temperament. Infants are born with a tendency to react in certain ways to noise and to interact differently with people. They may display varying degrees of regularity in activities of eating and sleeping and manifest a capacity for concentrating on tasks for different amounts of time. Although an infant's temperament cannot be changed, parents can modify the environment to promote adaptation. Strategies include using only one or two consistent babysitters or caregivers, rather than engaging new or changing caregivers frequently, and feeding the infant in a quiet setting to encourage a focus on eating.

Focus on Diversity and Culture

Reaching Developmental Milestones

In some cultures, children are allowed to unfold and develop naturally at their own pace. Children wean and toilet-train themselves with little interference or pressure from parents. The nurse should be sensitive to the childrearing practices of the family and support them in these culturally accepted practices.

For example, the developmental milestone for sleeping through the night is typically reached at age 4 to 5 months (Andrews, Boyle, & Collins, 2019). However, in many cultures, including American Indian, Alaskan Native, and First Nation tribes, infants sleep with their mothers. Infants will wake and nurse typically every 4 hours through the night. The mothers are usually not disturbed by this on-demand feeding practice, so there is less motivation for the mother to have the child sleep through the night. Therefore, these infants do not reach the milestone of sleeping 8 hours a night until later in their development than infants who do not sleep with their mothers.

TABLE 25.5 Psychosocial Development During Infancy

Age	Play and Toys	Communication
Birth–3 months	■ Prefers visual stimuli of mobiles, black-and-white patterns, mirrors. ■ Responds to auditory stimuli such as music boxes, video/audio sounds, soft voices. ■ Responds to rocking and cuddling. ■ Moves legs and arms while adult sings and talks. ■ Likes varying stimuli—different rooms, sounds, visual images.	■ Coos. ■ Babbles. ■ Cries.
3–6 months	■ Prefers noise-making objects that are easily grasped, like rattles. ■ Enjoys stuffed animals and soft toys with contrasting colors.	■ Vocalizes during play and with familiar people. ■ Laughs. ■ Cries less. ■ Squeals and makes pleasure sounds. ■ Babbles multisyllabically ("mamamamama").
6–9 months	■ Likes teething toys. ■ Increasingly desires social interaction with adults and other children. ■ Favors soft toys that can be manipulated and mouthed.	■ Increases vowel and consonant sounds. ■ Links syllables together. ■ Uses speechlike rhythm when vocalizing with others.
9–12 months	■ Enjoys large blocks, toys that pop apart and go back together, nesting cups and other objects. ■ Laughs at surprise toys like a jack-in-the-box. ■ Plays interactive games like peek-a-boo. ■ Uses push-and-pull toys.	■ Understands "no" and other simple commands. ■ Says "dada" and "mama" to identify parents. ■ Learns one or two other words. ■ Receptive speech surpasses expressive speech.

Source: Ball et al. (2022). Pearson Education., Inc. Hoboken, NJ.

TABLE 25.6 Growth and Development Milestones During Toddlerhood

Age	Physical Growth	Fine Motor Ability	Gross Motor Ability	Sensory Ability
1–2 years	▪ Gains 227 g (8 oz) or more per month. ▪ Grows 9–12 cm (3.5–5 in.) during this year. ▪ Anterior fontanel closes.	▪ By end of second year, builds a tower of four blocks. ▪ Scribbles on paper. ▪ Can undress self. ▪ Throws a ball.	▪ Runs. ▪ Walks up and down stairs. ▪ Likes push-and-pull toys.	Visual acuity 20/50
2–3 years	▪ Gains 1.4–2.3 kg (3–5 lb)/year. ▪ Grows 5–6.5 cm (2–2.5 in.)/year.	▪ Draws a circle and other rudimentary forms. ▪ Learns to pour. ▪ Is learning to dress self.	▪ Jumps. ▪ Kicks ball. ▪ Throws ball overhand.	

Source: Ball et al. (2022). Pearson Education., Inc. Hoboken, NJ.

Communication

Communication skills are evident even at a few weeks of age. Infants communicate and engage in two-way interaction; they express comfort by soft sounds, cuddling, and eye contact. The infant displays discomfort by thrashing the extremities, arching the back, and crying vigorously. From these rudimentary skills, communication ability continues to develop until the infant speaks several words at the end of the first year of life (see Table 25.5). Nonverbal methods continue to be a primary method of communication between parent and child.

Nurses assess communication to identify possible abnormalities or developmental delays. Language ability may be assessed with a specialized language screening tool. Normally developing infants and toddlers understand (**receptive speech**) more words than they can speak (**expressive speech**). Abnormalities may be caused by a hearing deficit, developmental delay, or lack of verbal stimulation from caregivers. Further assessment may be required to pinpoint the cause of the abnormality.

Nursing interventions focus on providing a stimulating and comforting environment and encouraging parents to speak to infants and teach words. Nurses should include the infant's known words when providing care and offer nonverbal support by hugging and holding. Nurses planning interventions should consider the family's cultural patterns for communications and development.

Toddlers (1 to 3 Years)

Toddlerhood is sometimes called the first adolescence. The child from 1 to 3 years of age, who months before was merely an infant, is now displaying independence and negativism. Pride in newfound accomplishments emerges during this time.

Physical Growth and Motor Development

The rate of growth slows during the second year of life. The child requires limited food intake during this time, a change that may cause concern to the parent. The nurse reassures parents that reduced nutritional intake is a normal occurrence in their child's development. By age 2 years, the birth weight has usually quadrupled and the child is about one-half of the adult height. Body proportions begin to change, with longer legs and a smaller head in proportion to body size than during infancy. The toddler has a pot-bellied appearance and stands with feet apart to provide a wide base of support. By approximately 33 months, eruption of the 20 deciduous teeth is complete.

Gross motor activity develops rapidly (**Table 25.6** »)) as the toddler progresses from walking to running, kicking, and riding a tricycle. As physical maturation occurs, the toddler develops the ability to control elimination patterns.

Cognitive Development

During the toddler years, the child moves from the sensorimotor to the preoperational stage of development. The early use of language awakens in the 1-year-old the ability to think about objects or people when they are absent. Object permanence is well developed.

At about 2 years of age, the increasing use of words as symbols enables the toddler to use preoperational thought. Rudimentary problem solving, creative thought, and an understanding of cause-and-effect relationships are now possible.

Psychosocial Development

The toddler is soundly rooted in a trusting relationship and feels more comfortable asserting autonomy and separating from primary care providers. It is important for toddlers to begin asserting their autonomy within the context of safe places and relationships that promote their interaction with both adults and other children.

Play

Patterns of play emerge and change between infancy and toddlerhood. The toddler's motor skills enable banging pegs into a pounding board with a hammer. The social nature of toddler play is also visible. Toddlers find the company of other children pleasurable, even though socially interactive play may not occur. Toddlers tend to play with similar objects side by side, occasionally trading toys and words (**Figure 25.6** »)). This is called **parallel play**. Playing with other children assists toddlers to develop social skills. Toddlers engage in play activities they have seen at home, such as pounding with a hammer and talking on the phone. This imitative behavior helps them to learn new actions and skills.

Physical skills are manifested in play as toddlers push and pull objects, climb in and out and up and down, run, ride a Big Wheel, turn the pages of books, and scribble with a pen. Both gross motor and fine motor abilities are enhanced during this age period.

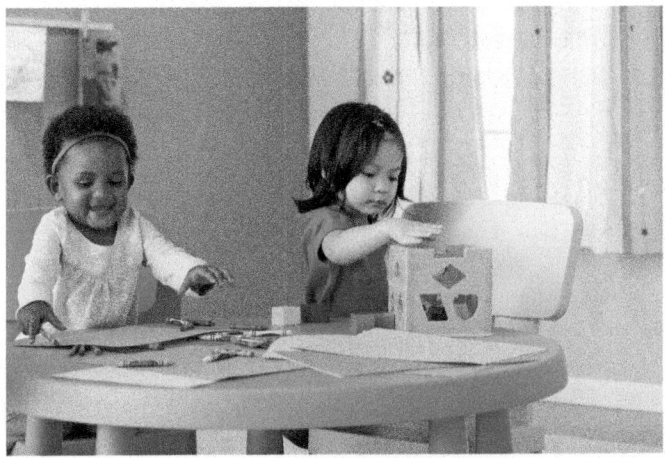

Figure 25.6 ›› These toddlers display typical parallel play at daycare, playing next to but not with each other.
Source: Jupiter Images/Stockbyte/Getty Images.

Cognitive understanding enables the toddler to manipulate objects and learn about their qualities. Stacking blocks and placing rings on a building tower teach spatial relationships and other lessons that provide a foundation for future learning. Various kinds of play objects should be provided for the toddler to meet play needs. These play needs can easily be met whether the child is hospitalized or at home (**Table 25.7** ››).

Personality and Temperament

The toddler retains most of the temperamental characteristics identified during infancy but may demonstrate some changes. The normal developmental progression of toddlerhood plays a part in responses. For example, the infant who previously responded positively to stimuli, such as a new babysitter, may appear more negative in toddlerhood. The increasing independence characteristic of this age is shown by the toddler's use of the word *no*. The parent and child constantly adapt their responses to each other and learn anew how to communicate with each other.

Communication

Because the child's capacity for development of language skills is greatest during the toddler period, adults should communicate frequently with children in this age group. This communication is critical not only to the toddler's ability to communicate simple wants and needs, but also to cognitive and language development, which affects the toddler's future literacy. Toddlers also begin to learn the social interactions and nonverbal gestures that they observe.

At the beginning of toddlerhood, the child may use four to six words in addition to "mama" and "dada." Receptive speech (the ability to understand words) far outpaces expressive speech. By the end of toddlerhood, however, the 3-year-old has a vocabulary of almost 1000 words and uses short sentences. Toddler communication includes pointing, pulling an adult over to a room or object, and speaking in **expressive jargon** (using unintelligible words with normal speech intonations as if truly communicating in words). Communication methods may also include crying, pounding or stamping feet, displaying a temper tantrum, or other means that illustrate dismay. These powerful communication methods can upset parents, who often need suggestions for handling them. Adults can best assist the toddler by verbalizing the feelings shown by the toddler, by saying things like "You must be very upset that you cannot have that candy. When you stop crying you can come out of your room." Verbalizing the child's feeling and then ignoring further negative behavior ensures that the parent is not unintentionally reinforcing the inappropriate behavior. While the toddler's search for autonomy and independence creates a need for such behavior, an upset toddler may respond well to holding, rocking, and stroking.

Parents and nurses can promote a toddler's communication by speaking frequently, naming objects, giving single-step directions, explaining procedures in simple terms, expressing feelings that the toddler seems to be displaying, and encouraging speech. The toddler is at an optimal age to learn two languages. For example, if the parents wish for their child to learn two languages, the toddler will benefit from a child care experience that includes exposure to a second language in addition to the language her family speaks at home.

The nurse who understands the communication skills of toddlers is able to assess expressive and receptive language and communicate effectively, thereby promoting positive healthcare experiences for these children. Parents often need suggestions for ways to communicate with the young child.

Preschool Children (3 to 6 Years)

The preschool years are a time of new initiative and independence. Most children are in a childcare center or school for part of the day, and they learn a great deal from this social contact. Language skills are well developed, and the child is able to understand and speak clearly. Endless projects

TABLE 25.7 Psychosocial Development During Toddlerhood

Age	Play and Toys	Communication
1–3 years	■ Refines fine motor skills by use of cloth books, large pencil and paper, wooden puzzles. ■ Facilitates imitative behavior by playing kitchen, grocery shopping, toy telephone. ■ Learns gross motor activities by riding Big Wheel tricycle, playing with a soft ball and bat, molding water and sand, tossing ball or beanbag. ■ Develops cognitive skills through exposure to educational television shows, music, stories, and books.	■ Increasingly enjoys talking. ■ Vocabulary grows exponentially, especially when spoken and read to. ■ Needs to release stress by pounding board, frequent gross motor activities, and occasional temper tantrums. ■ Likes contact with other children and learns interpersonal skills.

Source: Ball et al. (2022). Pearson Education., Inc. Hoboken, NJ.

TABLE 25.8 Growth and Development Milestones During the Preschool Years

Physical Growth	Fine Motor Ability	Gross Motor Ability	Sensory Ability
Gains 1.5–2.5 kg (3–5 lb)/year. Grows 4–6 cm (1½–2½ in.)/year.	Uses scissors. Draws circle, square, cross. Draws at least a six-part person. Enjoys art projects such as pasting, stringing beads, using clay. Learns to tie shoes at end of preschool years. Buttons clothes. Brushes teeth. Eats three meals, with snacks. Uses spoon, fork, and knife.	Throws a ball overhand. Climbs well. Rides tricycle.	Visual acuity continues to improve. Can focus on and learn letters and numbers.

Source: Ball et al. (2022). Pearson Education., Inc. Hoboken, NJ.

characterize the world of busy preschoolers. They may work with play dough to form animals, then cut out and paste paper, then draw and color.

Physical Growth and Motor Development

Preschoolers grow slowly and steadily, with most growth taking place in long bones of the arms and legs. The short, chubby toddler gradually gives way to a slender, long-legged preschooler (**Table 25.8** »).

Physical skills continue to develop. The preschooler runs with ease, holds a bat, and throws balls of various types. Writing ability increases, and the preschooler enjoys drawing and learning.

The preschool period is a good time to encourage healthy dental habits. Children can begin to brush their own teeth with parental supervision and help in reaching all tooth surfaces. Parents should floss children's teeth, give fluoride as prescribed if the water supply is not fluoridated, and schedule the first dental visit so the child can become accustomed to the routine of periodic dental care.

Cognitive Development

The preschooler exhibits characteristics of preoperational thought. Symbols or words are used to represent objects and people, enabling the young child to think about them. This is a milestone in intellectual development; however, the preschooler still has some limitations in thought (**Table 25.9** »). It is important to understand the preschooler's thought processes in order to plan appropriate teaching for healthcare and development of health habits.

Psychosocial Development

The preschooler is more independent in establishing relationships with others. The child interacts closely with children and adults and is able to plan and carry out activities.

Play

Play for preschoolers takes on a new dimension as they begin to interact with others. One child cuts out colored paper while a friend glues it on paper in a design. This new type of interaction is called **associative play**.

TABLE 25.9 Characteristics of Thought Identified by Piaget

Characteristic	Definition	Development Stage	Nursing Implications
Egocentrism	Ability to see things only from one's own point of view	Preoperational thought	Peers or others who have gone through an experience will not impress the preschooler; teaching should focus on what an experience will be like for the child.
Transductive reasoning	Connecting two events in a cause-and-effect relationship simply because they occur together in time	Preoperational thought	Ask what the child thinks caused an occurrence; ask how the two events are connected; correct misconceptions to lessen child's guilt.
Centration	Focusing only on one particular aspect of a situation	Preoperational thought	Listen to the child's comments and deal with concerns in order to be able to present new concepts to the child.
Magical thinking	Believing that events occur because of one's thoughts or actions	Preoperational thought	Ask how the young child became ill or what caused a parent's or sibling's illness. Correct misconceptions when the child blames self for causing problems by wishing someone ill or having bad behavior.
Conservation	Knowing that matter is not changed when its form is altered	Concrete operational thought	Before conservation of thought is reached, the child may think that gender can be changed when hair is cut or that a broken leg under a cast is broken into separate pieces. Ask about perceptions and clarify misconceptions.

Source: Ball et al. (2022). Pearson Education., Inc. Hoboken, NJ.

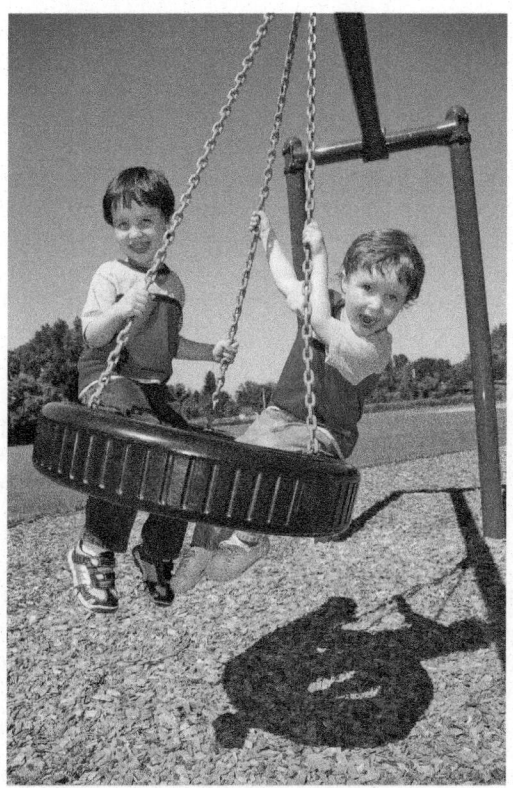

Figure 25.7 ›› Preschoolers have well-developed large motor skills and enjoy activities such as swinging.
Source: Rossario/Shutterstock.

In addition to this social dimension, other aspects of play also differ. The preschooler enjoys large motor activities such as swinging, riding a tricycle, and throwing a ball (**Figure 25.7** ››). Preschoolers demonstrate increasing manual dexterity as they create more complex drawings and manipulations of blocks and modeling. Because fantasy life is so powerful at this age, the preschooler readily uses props to engage in **dramatic play** (the living-out of the drama of human life).

The nurse can use playtime to assess the preschooler's developmental level, knowledge about healthcare, and emotions related to healthcare experiences. Observations about objects chosen for play, content of dramatic play, and pictures drawn can provide important assessment data. The nurse can also use play periods to teach the child about healthcare procedures and offer an outlet for expressing emotions (**Table 25.10** ››).

The use of media such as smartphones, tablets, and computers is becoming more of the preschooler's life than ever before. An estimated 46% of children under the age of 2 have used media on a mobile device, and they spend 42 minutes per day using screen media (Common Sense, 2017). The nurse might find that hospitalized children can be soothed and distracted by portable media devices such as tablets. However, the nurse should be aware that the research is very limited on what can be considered too much screen time. The American Academy of Pediatrics (AAP) recommends that parents and other caregivers discourage the use of screen time for children under 18 months unless it is for video chatting with a loved one. For older toddlers and preschoolers, the AAP recommends limiting screen time to an hour a day and then only for educational programming or video chatting. Young children should not engage in screen time during meals and for at least an hour before bedtime (AAP, 2016).

As with television, ask how parents decide which technology and content is best for their children and how they monitor and set rules for use. Violence on mobile media should be avoided and, when encountered, parents and caregivers should help their children understand it. Providers can recommend age-appropriate, educational content and suggest the use of resources such as PBS Kids (www.pbskids.org), Sesame Workshop (www.sesameworkshop.org), or Common Sense Media (www.commonsensemedia.org) to guide media choices.

Personality and Temperament

Characteristics of personality observed in infancy tend to persist over time. The preschooler may need assistance as these characteristics are expressed in the new situations of preschool or nursery school. An excessively active child, for example, will need gentle, consistent handling to adjust to the structure of a classroom. Encourage parents to visit preschool programs to choose the one that would best foster growth in their child. Some preschoolers enjoy the structured learning of a program that focuses on cognitive skills, while others are happier and more open to learning in a small group that provides much time for free play. Nurses can help parents identify their child's personality or temperament characteristics and to find the best environment for growth.

Communication

Language skills blossom during the preschool years. The vocabulary grows to over 2000 words, and children speak in complete sentences of several words and use all parts of speech.

TABLE 25.10 Psychosocial Development During the Preschool Years

Age	Play and Toys	Communication
3–6 years	Associative play is facilitated by simple games, puzzles, nursery rhymes, songs. Dramatic play is fostered by dolls and doll clothes, playhouses and hospitals, dress-up clothes, puppets. Stress is relieved by pens, paper, glue, scissors. Cognitive growth is fostered by educational television shows, music, stories, books.	Develops and uses all parts of speech, occasionally incorrectly. Communicates with a widening array of people. Play with other children is a favorite activity. Health professionals can: ▪ Verbalize and explain procedures to children. ▪ Use drawings and stories to explain care. ▪ Use accurate names for bodily functions. ▪ Allow the child to talk, ask questions, and make choices.

Source: Ball et al. (2022). Pearson Education., Inc. Hoboken, NJ.

They practice these newfound language skills by endlessly talking and asking questions.

The sophisticated speech of preschoolers mirrors the development occurring in their minds and helps them to learn about the world around them. However, this speech can be quite deceptive. Although preschoolers use many words, their grasp of meaning is usually literal and may not match that of adults. These literal interpretations have important implications for healthcare providers (HCPs). For example, the preschooler who is told they will be "put to sleep" for surgery may think of a pet recently euthanized; the child who is told that a dye will be injected for a diagnostic test may think they are going to die; mention of "a little stick" in the arm can cause images of tree branches rather than of a simple immunization.

Concrete visual aids such as pictures of a child undergoing the same procedure or a book to read together enhance teaching by meeting the child's developmental needs. Handling medical equipment such as intravenous bags and stethoscopes increases interest and helps the child to focus. Teaching may have to be done in several short sessions rather than one long session.

Some general approaches include the following:

- Allow time for the child to integrate explanations.
- Verbalize frequently to the child.
- Use drawings and stories to explain care.
- Use accurate names for bodily functions.
- Allow choices.

The preschooler's social growth and increased communication skills make these years the perfect time to introduce concepts related to problem solving and conflict resolution. Puzzles and manipulative toys help foster early problem-solving skills. Children in this age group can learn to calm themselves by teaching them how to take deep breaths and count to three or five when they are upset. Many preschool programs employ special curricula that help teachers and parents assist children in developing essential conflict-resolution skills. Using language to resolve conflict is a protective factor that decreases the likelihood of children choosing inappropriate or violent behavior to try to get what they want or bring a distressing interaction to a close.

School-Age Children (6 to 12 Years)

School-age children demonstrate common characteristics of their age group. They are in a stage of industry in which it is important to the child to perform useful work. Meaningful activities take on great importance and are usually carried out in the company of peers. A sense of achievement in these activities is important for developing self-esteem and preventing a sense of inferiority or poor self-worth.

Physical Growth and Motor Development

School age is the last period in which girls and boys are close in size and body proportions. As the long bones continue to grow, leg length increases (see Figure 25.4). Fat gives way to muscle, and the child appears leaner. Jaw proportions change as the first deciduous tooth is lost at 6 years and permanent teeth begin to erupt. Body organs and the immune system mature, resulting in fewer illnesses among school-age children. Medications are less likely to cause serious side effects because they can be metabolized more easily. The urinary system can adjust to changes in fluid status. Physical skills are also refined as children begin to play sports, and fine motor skills are well developed through school activities.

Although it is commonly believed that the start of adolescence (age 12 years) heralds a growth spurt, the rapid increases in size commonly occur during school age. Girls may begin a growth spurt as early as 9 or 10 years of age and boys a year or so later (**Figure 25.8** »). Nutritional needs increase dramatically with this spurt.

The loss of the first deciduous teeth and the eruption of permanent teeth usually occur at about age 6 years, or at the beginning of the school-age period. Of the 32 permanent teeth, 22 to 26 erupt by age 12 years and the remaining molars follow during the teenage years. See Module 7, Health, Wellness, Illness, and Injury, for a discussion of oral care for school-age children.

Cognitive Development

The child enters the stage of concrete operational thought at about age 7 years. This stage enables school-age children to consider alternative solutions and solve problems. However, school-age children continue to rely on concrete experiences and materials to form their thought content.

During the school-age years, the child learns the concept of conservation (that matter is not changed when its form is altered). At earlier ages, a child believes that when water is poured from a short, wide glass into a tall, thin glass, there is more water in the taller glass. The school-age child recognizes that, although it may look like the taller glass holds more water, the quantity is the same. The concept of conservation is helpful when the nurse explains medical treatments. The school-age child understands that an incision will heal, that a cast will be removed, and that an arm will look the same as before once the intravenous infusion needle is removed. The child learns to read during this period and can concentrate for longer periods.

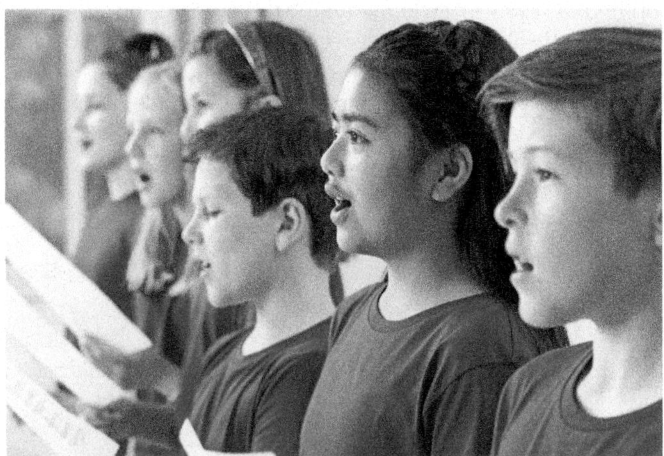

Figure 25.8 » Because girls have a growth spurt earlier than boys, girls often are taller than boys of the same age, as shown in this group of middle schoolers in a dress rehearsal for a choral performance.

Source: Highwaystarz-Photography/iStock/Getty Images.

Psychosocial Development

The school-age child has many friends and cooperatively interacts with others to accomplish tasks. The child develops a sense of accomplishment from activities and relationships.

Play

Play for the school-age child is enhanced by increasing fine and gross motor skills. By 6 years of age, children have acquired the physical ability to hold a bat properly and may occasionally hit the ball. School-age children also understand that everyone has a role—the pitcher, the catcher, the batter, the outfielders. They cooperate with one another to form a team, are eager to learn the rules of the game, and want to ensure that these rules are followed exactly (**Table 25.11** »).

The characteristics of play exhibited by the school-age child include cooperation with others and the ability to play a part in order to contribute to a unified whole. This type of play is called **cooperative play**. The concrete nature of cognitive thought leads to a reliance on rules to provide structure and security. Children have an increasing desire to spend much of their playtime with friends, which demonstrates the social component of play. Play is an extremely important method of learning and living for the school-age child. Active physical play has decreased in recent years as television viewing and video-game playing have increased, leading to poor nutritional status and high rates of overweight among children.

When a child is hospitalized, the separation from playmates can lead to feelings of sadness and purposelessness. Normal, rewarding parts of play should be integrated into care. Friends should be encouraged to visit or call a hospitalized child. Discharge planning for the child who has had a cast or brace applied should address the activities in which the child can participate and those the child must avoid. Nurses should reinforce the importance of playing games with friends to both parents and children.

Personality and Temperament

Characteristics seen in earlier years tend to endure in the school years. The child classified as "difficult" at an earlier age may now have trouble in the classroom. Nurses may advise parents to provide a quiet setting for homework and to reward the child for concentration. For example, after completing homework, the child may be allowed to have "screen time" (play a video game, watch television, or play on the computer or tablet). Creative efforts and alternative methods of learning should be valued. Encourage parents to see their children as individuals who may not all learn in the same way. The "slow-to-warm-up" child may need encouragement to try new activities and to share experiences with others, whereas the "easy" child will readily adapt to new schools, people, and experiences.

Communication

During the school-age years, children should learn how to use language correctly, including correcting any lingering pronunciation or grammatical errors, and learning the pragmatic (social) uses of language. Vocabulary increases, and the child learns about parts of speech in school. Children also are becoming more technologically savvy with their communication. According to the Pew Research Center, 95% of children 13 to 17 years of age own or have access to a smartphone (Anderson & Jiang, 2018).

School-age children enjoy writing and, while in the hospital, can be encouraged to keep a journal of their experiences as a method of dealing with anxiety. The literal translation of words characteristic of preschoolers is uncommon among school-age children.

Some communication strategies helpful with the school-age child include:

- Provide concrete examples of pictures or materials to accompany verbal descriptions.
- Assess knowledge before planning the instruction.
- Allow child to select rewards following procedures.
- Teach techniques such as counting or visualization to manage difficult situations.
- Include child in discussions and history taking with the parent.

Sexuality

Awareness of gender differences and sexuality becomes more pronounced during the school years. Although children become aware of sexual differences during preschool years, they deal much more consciously with sexuality during the school-age years. As children mature physically, they need information about their bodily changes so that they can develop a healthy self-image and an understanding of the relationships between their bodies and sexuality. Children become interested in sexual issues and are often exposed to erroneous information on television shows, in magazines, from internet sources, or from friends and siblings. Schools and families need to use opportunities to teach school-age

TABLE 25.11 Psychosocial Development During the School-Age Years

Age	Activities	Communication
6–12 years	Gross motor development is fostered by ball sports, skating, dance lessons, water and snow skiing/boarding, biking. A sense of industry is fostered by playing a musical instrument, gathering collections, starting hobbies, playing board and video games. Cognitive growth is facilitated by reading, crafts, word puzzles, schoolwork.	Use of language is mature. Is able to converse and discuss topics for increasing lengths of time. Spends many hours at school and with friends in sports or other activities. Health professionals can: ■ Assess child's knowledge before teaching. ■ Allow the child to select rewards following procedures. ■ Teach techniques such as counting or visualization to manage difficult situations. ■ Include both parent and child in healthcare decisions.

Source: Ball et al. (2022). Pearson Education., Inc. Hoboken, NJ.

children factual information about sex and to foster healthy concepts of self and others. It is advisable to ask occasional questions about sexual issues to learn how much the child knows and to provide correct information when answers demonstrate confusion.

Both friends and the media are common sources of erroneous ideas. Appropriate and inappropriate touch should be discussed, with lists of trusted people who can be approached (teachers, clergy, school counselors, family members, neighbors) to discuss any episodes with which the child feels uncomfortable. Because even these trusted people can be implicated in inappropriate episodes, the nurse should encourage the child to go to more than one person, an important approach if the child is uncomfortable about a relationship with any individual.

Adolescents (12 to 18 Years)

Adolescence is a time of passage signaling the end of childhood and the beginning of adulthood. Although adolescents differ in behaviors and accomplishments, they are all in a period of identity formation. If a healthy identity and sense of self-worth are not developed during this period, role confusion and purposeless struggling will ensue. The adolescents in the healthcare setting will represent various degrees of identity formation, and each will offer unique challenges.

Physical Growth and Motor Development

The physical changes ending in **puberty**, or sexual maturity, begin near the end of the school-age period. The prepubescent period is marked by a growth spurt at an average age of 10 years for girls and 13 years for boys, although there is considerable variation among children. The increase in height and weight is generally remarkable and is completed in 2 to 3 years. The growth spurt in girls is accompanied by an increase in breast size and growth of pubic hair. Menstruation occurs last and signals achievement of puberty. In boys, the growth spurt is accompanied by growth in size of the penis and testes and by growth of pubic hair. Deepening of the voice and growth of facial hair occur later, at the time of puberty. For both boys and girls, some lack of coordination is common during growth spurts.

During adolescence, children grow stronger and more muscular and establish characteristic male and female patterns of fat distribution. The apocrine and eccrine glands mature, leading to increased sweating and a distinct odor to perspiration. All body organs are now fully mature, enabling the adolescent to take adult doses of medications.

The adolescent must adapt to a rapidly changing body for several years. These physical changes and hormonal variations offer challenges to identity formation. See the Focus on Integrative Health.

Cognitive Development

Adolescence marks the beginning of Piaget's last stage of cognitive development, the stage of formal operational thought. The adolescent no longer depends on concrete experiences as the basis of thought but develops the ability to reason abstractly. The adolescent can understand concepts such as justice, truth, beauty, and power. The adolescent revels in this newfound ability and spends a great deal of time thinking, reading, and talking about abstract concepts.

Focus on Integrative Health

Weight Loss Supplements

Many adolescents are consumers of complementary and alternative medicine products, including dietary supplements and herbal therapies. The primary reasons adolescents use dietary supplements include weight loss, muscle building, and energy. Unfortunately, many "holistic" products are unregulated and may be poisonous when not taken as directed or when taken in combination with other substances. These characteristics may escape the attention of the adolescent (Or, Kim, Simms, & Austin, 2019). Dietary supplements, particularly those for weight loss and energy, can cause cardiac symptoms, including chest pain, tachycardia, and heart palpitations. Supplements used for muscle building can lead to testicular cancer. Adolescents most likely are not aware of the dangerous effects of these supplements. The nurse should encourage both parents and adolescents to report any use of supplements, herbal remedies, or other complementary medicines.

Adolescents seek to establish their own identity and values. They may rebel against parental authority as they try out new activities and behaviors. Although this is normal for adolescents, it can create a number of difficulties at home and school as adolescents try to balance their need to express themselves against the expectations of parents, teachers, and other authority figures.

Psychosocial Development

The adolescent is mature in relationships with others. The key aspect that teens work on during relationships and activities is establishing a meaningful identity.

Activities

Increasing desire for both peer contact and independence leads to a focus on activities for the adolescent. Some activities are maturational, as adolescents arrange for their own transportation to events and begin to drive independently. Sports, the arts, and other extracurricular activities provide opportunities for exercise, self-impression, and more directed ways of interacting with peers. Other activities include attending movies, concerts, or sporting events with friends. Healthy peer relationships can promote establishment of identity and provide meaning. Interest in romantic relationships begins, although most adolescents continue to maintain focus on their core friendships. Adolescents begin to participate in activities such as school dances that promote social interactions. Adolescence also marks the beginning of development of abstract thought and analysis.

Adolescents may socialize through social media, texting, and other technologies. Adolescents "hang out" not only in coffee shops and malls, but also in chat rooms, online games, and via group texts. According to a Pew survey (Anderson & Jiang, 2018), 31% of teens believed that social media has a positive effect on their lives, about 24% felt it had a negative effect, and 45% were neutral about the impact of social media on their lives.

Personality and Temperament

Characteristics of temperament manifested during childhood usually remain stable in the teenage years. For instance, the adolescent who was a calm, scheduled infant and child often demonstrates initiative to regulate study times and other routines. Similarly, the adolescent who was an easily stimulated infant may now have a messy room, a harried schedule with assignments always completed late, and an interest in many activities. It is also common for an adolescent who was an easy child to become more difficult because of the psychologic changes of adolescence and the need to assert independence.

As during the child's earlier ages, the nurse's role may be to inform parents of different personality types and to help them support the teen's uniqueness while providing necessary structure and feedback. Nurses can help parents understand their teen's personality type and work with the adolescent to meet expectations of teachers and others in authority.

Communication

Adolescents understand and use all parts of speech. They commonly use colloquialisms and slang when speaking—or texting—with their peers.

The adolescent increasingly leaves the home base and establishes close ties with peers. These relationships become the basis for identity formation. A period of stress or crisis generally occurs before a strong identity can emerge. The adolescent may try out new roles by learning a different sport or other skills, experimenting with drugs or alcohol, wearing different styles of clothing, or other activities. It is important to provide positive role models and a variety of experiences to help the adolescent make wise choices.

The adolescent also has a need to leave the past, to be different, and to change from former patterns to establish a self-identity. Rules that are repeated constantly and dogmatically will probably be broken in the adolescent's quest for self-awareness. This poses difficulties when the adolescent has a health problem that requires ongoing care, such as diabetes or cardiac illness. Introducing the adolescent to other teens who manage the same problem appropriately is usually more successful in getting the adolescent to comply with a care plan than telling the adolescent what to do.

Teens need privacy during patient interviews or interventions. Even if a parent is present for part of a health history or examination, the adolescent should be given the opportunity to relay information to or ask questions of the HCP alone. The adolescent should be given a choice of whether to have a parent present during an examination or while care is provided. Most information shared by an adolescent is confidential. Some states mandate disclosure of certain information to parents such as an adolescent's desire for an abortion. In these cases, the adolescent should be informed of what information will be disclosed to the parent.

In the hospital setting, nurses should allow adolescents the freedom of choice whenever possible, including preferences for evening or morning bathing, the type of clothes to wear while hospitalized, timing of treatments, and visitation guidelines. Use of contracts with adolescents may increase adherence with healthcare recommendations. Firmness, gentleness, choices, and respect must be balanced during care of adolescent patients.

Some specific communication strategies that help with the adolescent:

- Provide written and verbal explanations.
- Direct history and explanations to teen alone, then include parent.
- Allow for safe exploration of topics by suggesting that the teen is similar to other teens ("Many teens with diabetes have questions about. . . . How about you?").
- Arrange meetings for discussions with other teens.

Sexuality

Sexuality is influenced by physical maturation and increased hormonal secretion, which are integral to the adolescent's development of physiologic sexual maturity. Adolescents begin to engage in social interactions with those to whom they are sexually attracted, a complex process of both casual interactions on a day-to-day basis and more formal interactions at events such as dances and other social events. Some adolescents begin to engage in sexual activities and may have regular sexual interactions.

Adolescents begin exploring feelings of sexuality, learning if they are attracted to members of the same or opposite sex. Some may begin to identify as bisexual (attracted to both girls and boys). Most adolescents who feel supported and safe will have a positive adolescence (Centers for Disease Control and Prevention [CDC], 2017a). Unfortunately, LGBTQ (lesbian, gay, bisexual, transgender, queer/questioning) youth experience high rates of bullying, violence, and harassment (CDC, 2017a). Partially because of negative interactions with peers and society, LGBTQ youth are more likely to abuse substances or report mental health problems such as anxiety and depression and are more likely to attempt suicide than their peers (CDC, 2017a). Nurses can support LBGTQ youth by providing accurate information, promoting inclusion of LGBTQ contact in sexual education teaching, promoting safety by identifying and addressing bullying early, and providing referrals for healthcare and social support as needed. School nurses can play a particularly positive role in the safety and security of LGBTQ youth. School nurses can provide confidential healthcare and education to the LGBTQ student, collaborate with faculty and staff at school, and provide support, education, and resources for parents and community members (National Association of School Nurses, 2016).

Trends indicate that adolescents are not as sexually active as in the past. According to the CDC (2020i), 40% of high school students have had sexual intercourse. Thirty percent of high school students reported having sex in the past 3 months (CDC, 2020i). High school students who are sexually active may be engaged in risky behaviors. For example, 46% reported not using a condom during their last sexual encounter, 14% reported not using any form of birth control, and less than 10% have had HIV testing (CDC, 2020i). Many schools now provide some education on sex, HIV, and sexually transmitted infections. Some high schools even provide onsite health clinics offering primary care, mental health, and prevention services.

Adolescents benefit from clear information about sexuality, an opportunity to develop relationships with adolescents in various settings, an open atmosphere at home and school where problems and issues can be discussed, and previous experience in problem solving and decision making. Alternatives and support for their decisions should be available.

In addition, the nurse who encounters a sexually active teenager may be the very first HCP with whom the teenager discusses sexuality. The nurse who refrains from asserting personal beliefs and who emphasizes open communication and active listening will strengthen the teen's confidence in the healthcare system and increase the likelihood that the teen will seek help from a healthcare professional in the future.

Adults

The transition from adolescence to adulthood is complex. Unlike when individuals were infants and children with very clear milestones, adulthood does not have such defined markers. Yet, the adult continues to pass through stages or complete tasks that encompass the individual's physical, emotional, social, spiritual, and economic self.

Young Adults

Many societies, such as those in the United States, consider adulthood to start at the age of 18 years. At this age, many adolescents begin to enjoy adult privileges, such as voting and opening a bank account. At the age of 18, individuals can seek medical care without parental consent and can make medical decisions independently. With new laws regarding medical insurance in place, many young adults stay on their parents' insurance plans. The individual is still depending on the parents' insurance but is able to make medical decisions.

Economic status is no longer a sign of adulthood. In addition to staying on their parents' health insurance plans, many young adults are living with their parents into their mid-20s or later. Many are delaying marriage and childrearing until later in adulthood. The average age for first birth is 26.3, with a growing number of women having their first child between ages 30 and 35 (National Center for Health Statistics, 2016). Prominent life changes and stressors for young adults include going to (and paying for) college, choosing and establishing a career, and finding a significant other or spouse.

In terms of physical development, most individuals are still growing. In particular, men may not reach their full height until around age 20. Studies continue to show that the human brain is not fully mature until around the age of 25 (Hochberg & Konner, 2020). In the early to mid-20s, most individuals are at their peak physical condition. Causes of mortality and morbidity are mainly attributed to unintentional injury (i.e., motor-vehicle crashes) and intentional trauma (homicide and suicide) (Heron, 2019).

The health assessment of the young adult should include vital signs, height, and weight (**Table 25.12** »). Vision and hearing screenings should also be considered, particularly since many young people are of the "earbud generation." Assessment questions should address stressors, diet recall, activity level and exercise, family history, smoking history, and alcohol/substance use. Additional data necessary to appropriately assess young adults include sexual history and activity, menstrual concerns and patterns, and use of birth control, including condom use. As with the adolescent patient, the nurse should be open to questions and ready to educate the patient on sexual concerns. Health screenings should include STIs.

TABLE 25.12 Physical Status and Changes in the Young Adult Years

Assessment	Status During the 20s	Status During the 30s
Skin	Smooth, even temperature	Beginning of wrinkles
Hair	Slightly oily, shiny Beginning of balding	Beginning of graying Balding
Vision	Snellen 20/20	Some loss of visual acuity and accommodation
Musculoskeletal	Strong, coordinated	Some loss of strength and muscle mass
Cardiovascular	Maximum cardiac output 60–90 beats/min Mean BP: 120/80	Slight decline in cardiac output 60–90 beats/min Mean BP: 120/80
Respiratory	Rate: 12–20 Full vital capacity	Rate: 12–20 Decline in vital capacity

Source: Bauldoff, Gubrud, and Carno (2020). Pearson Education, Inc., Hoboken, NJ.

Middle Adults

The "middle" years of adulthood are typically considered to be between the ages of 40 and 65 years. Often called the "sandwich" generation, those who are in this stage of life often find themselves taking care of both their children (and sometimes, grandchildren) and their own aging parents. This creates a new set of stressors. In some cases, the individual must also cope with divorce or loss of a significant other.

In this stage of life, the body begins to experience changes related to aging (**Table 25.13** »). Risk factors for

TABLE 25.13 Physical Changes in the Middle Adult Years

Assessment	Changes
Skin	■ Decreased turgor, moisture, and subcutaneous fat result in wrinkles. ■ Fat is deposited in the abdominal and hip areas.
Hair	■ Loss of melanin in hair shaft causes graying. ■ Hairline recedes in men.
Sensory	■ Visual acuity for near vision decreases (presbyopia) during the 40s. ■ Auditory acuity for high-frequency sounds decreases (presbycusis); more common in men. ■ Sense of taste diminishes.
Musculoskeletal	■ Skeletal muscle mass decreases by about age 60. ■ Thinning of intervertebral discs results in loss of height (about 2.5 cm [1 in.]). ■ Postmenopausal women may have loss of calcium and develop osteoporosis.
Cardiovascular	■ Blood vessels lose elasticity. ■ Systolic blood pressure may increase.
Respiratory	■ Loss of vital capacity (about 1 L from age 20 to 60) occurs.
Gastrointestinal	■ Large intestine gradually loses muscle tone; constipation may result. ■ Gastric secretions are decreased.
Genitourinary	■ Hormonal changes occur; menopause, women (↓ estrogen), andropause, men (↓ testosterone).
Endocrine	■ Gradual decrease in glucose tolerance occurs.

Source: Bauldoff, Gubrud, and Carno (2020). Pearson Education, Inc., Hoboken, NJ.

Multisystem Effects of Aging

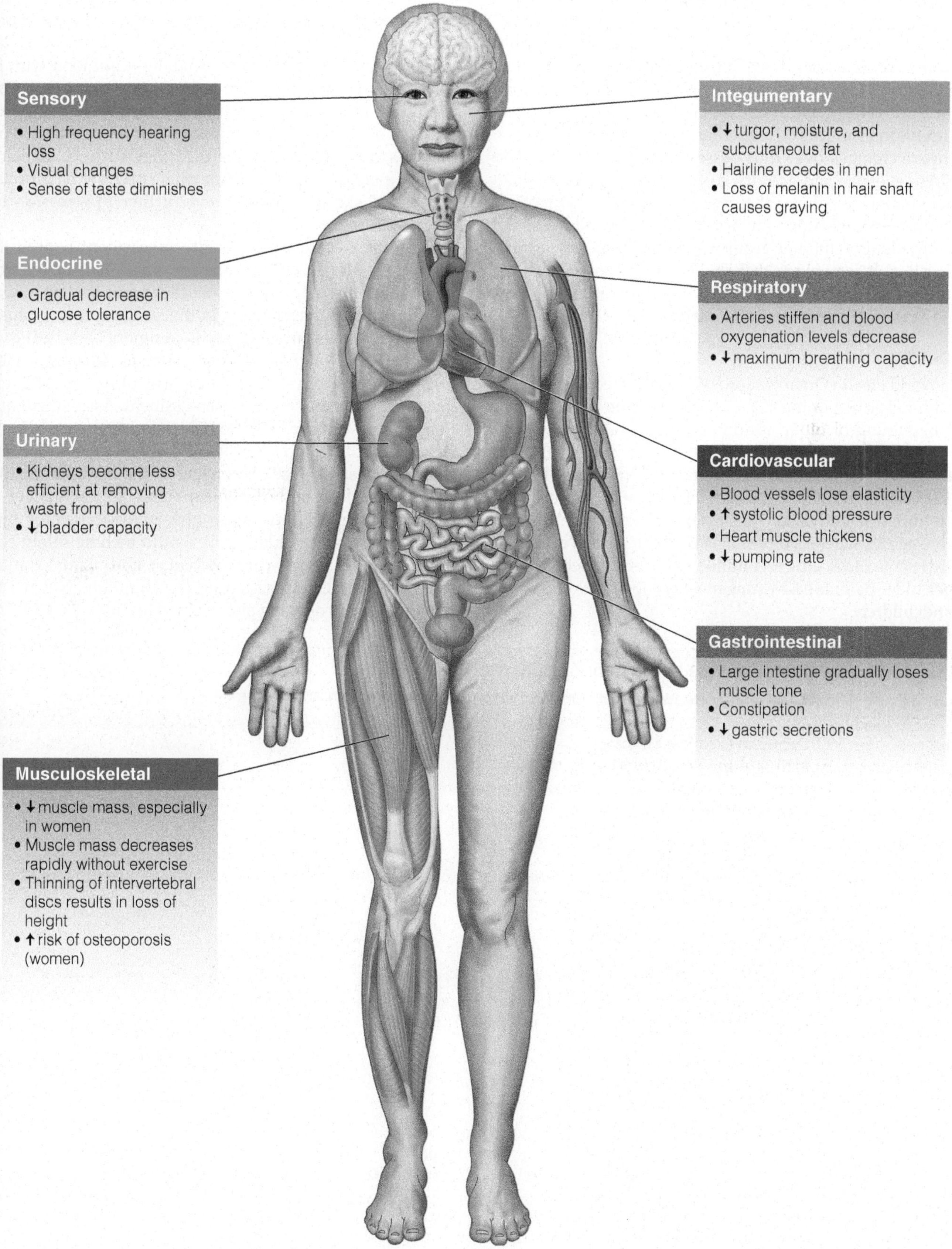

Sensory
- High frequency hearing loss
- Visual changes
- Sense of taste diminishes

Endocrine
- Gradual decrease in glucose tolerance

Urinary
- Kidneys become less efficient at removing waste from blood
- ↓ bladder capacity

Musculoskeletal
- ↓ muscle mass, especially in women
- Muscle mass decreases rapidly without exercise
- Thinning of intervertebral discs results in loss of height
- ↑ risk of osteoporosis (women)

Integumentary
- ↓ turgor, moisture, and subcutaneous fat
- Hairline recedes in men
- Loss of melanin in hair shaft causes graying

Respiratory
- Arteries stiffen and blood oxygenation levels decrease
- ↓ maximum breathing capacity

Cardiovascular
- Blood vessels lose elasticity
- ↑ systolic blood pressure
- Heart muscle thickens
- ↓ pumping rate

Gastrointestinal
- Large intestine gradually loses muscle tone
- Constipation
- ↓ gastric secretions

heart disease, such as hypertension and elevated lipids, and related vascular problems start during this life period. Arthritis and back problems often arise during middle adulthood. Difficulty in mobility, most commonly due to spinal/back issues and arthritis, may cause disability in individuals in this age group.

The health assessment of the middle-aged adult should include vision and hearing screenings and vital signs, as well as height, weight, and body mass index (BMI). Along with a complete physical assessment, these indicators can all be useful in establishing a baseline against which HCPs can compare changes over time. Assessment questions should address exercise and activity levels, diet and food choices, family history, alcohol/substance use, smoking history, and stressors. Sexual history and activity should be addressed in all individuals in this age group, even those who are married. Other health screenings that should be discussed with the adult patient include Pap smears, mammography, colonoscopy, fasting glucose, and lipid panels.

Older Adults

The World Health Organization (WHO; 2016) recognizes older adulthood as beginning at the age of 60. In the United States, the beginning of older adulthood is generally recognized as age 65, in part because at this age Americans qualify for Medicare benefits (Administration for Community Living, 2018). The experiences of older adulthood vary considerably from one individual to the next. Some may retire at or before age 65, whereas others may work for many years afterward. Some older adults continue to be "sandwiched" with much older parents and younger generations of children and grandchildren.

Older adulthood is often thought of as a stage of loss and mourning. Many older adults experience loss of friends, relatives, and spouses. Some mourn physical loss, such as mobility due to arthritis. Yet, many older adults continue to live healthy, active, happy lives. Older adults also continue to be sexually active well into their 80s and 90s. Because of advancements in preventive medicine and healthcare, many individuals are transitioning into older adulthood with few chronic conditions. However, as the body matures, chronic conditions can be complicated by the normal stages of aging. Risk for developing cardiovascular disease, cancer, type 2 diabetes, and neurocognitive disorders such as Alzheimer disease increases. Therefore, the nurse needs to be especially concerned about screening and further progression of a chronic disease.

As with all adults, the health assessment begins with vital signs. Height and weight are especially important, as it is during this stage in life that older adults start to experience degenerative changes in the spinal column, causing shrinking. Loss of muscle mass is common. Older adults are at greater risk for sensory losses, such as hearing or vision loss. A complete physical assessment of all systems should be included in the nurse's health assessment. Assessment questions should include exercise habits and tolerance, diet and appetite, ability to do activities of daily living, and tobacco/alcohol/substance use. According to the National Institute on Alcohol Abuse and Alcoholism (n.d.), approximately 40% of older adults drink alcohol, which increases risk for injury. Assessments of the older adult should include safety, functional status (e.g., self-care, mobility), and mental status to establish a baseline (see Module 23, Cognition). Normal age-related changes of aging are outlined in **Table 25.14** ».

TABLE 25.14 Physical Changes in the Older Adult Years

Assessment	Changes
Skin	■ Decreased turgor and sebaceous gland activity result in dry, wrinkled skin. ■ Melanocytes cluster, causing "age spots" or "liver spots."
Hair and nails	■ Scalp, axillary, and pubic hair thins; nose and ear hair thicken. Women may develop facial hair. ■ Nails grow more slowly; may become thick and brittle.
Sensory	■ Visual field narrows, and depth perception is distorted. ■ Pupils are smaller, reducing night vision. ■ Lenses yellow and become opaque, resulting in distortion of green, blue, and violet tones and increased sensitivity to glare. ■ Production of tears decreases. ■ Sense of smell decreases. ■ Age-related hearing loss progresses, involving middle- and low-frequency sounds. ■ Threshold for pain and touch increases. ■ Alterations in proprioception (sense of physical position) may occur.
Musculoskeletal	■ Loss of overall mass, strength, and movement of muscles occurs; tremors may occur. ■ Loss of bone structure and deterioration of cartilage in joints result in increased risk of fractures and limitation of range of motion.
Cardiovascular	■ Systolic blood pressure rises. ■ Cardiac output decreases. ■ Peripheral resistance increases, and capillary walls thicken.
Respiratory	■ Loss of vital capacity continues as the lungs become less elastic and more rigid. ■ Anteroposterior chest diameter increases; kyphosis occurs. ■ Although blood carbon dioxide levels remain relatively constant, blood oxygen levels decrease by 10–15%.
Gastrointestinal	■ Production of saliva decreases, and declining number of taste buds reduces the number of accurate receptors for salt and sweet. ■ Gag reflex is decreased, and stomach motility and emptying are reduced. ■ Both large and small intestines undergo some atrophy, with decreased peristalsis. ■ The liver decreases in weight and storage capacity; incidence of gallstones increases; pancreatic enzymes decrease.

TABLE 25.14 Physical Changes in the Older Adult Years (*continued*)

Assessment	Changes
Genitourinary	■ Kidneys lose mass, and the glomerular filtration rate is reduced (by nearly 50% from young adulthood to old age). ■ Bladder capacity decreases, and the micturition reflex is delayed. Urinary retention is more common. ■ Women may have stress incontinence; men may have an enlarged prostate gland. ■ Reproductive changes in men include decreases in sperm count and testosterone; the testes becoming smaller; and an increase in the length of time to achieve an erection. ■ Reproductive changes in women include a decrease in estrogen levels, breast tissue, and vaginal lubrication; alkalinization of vaginal secretions; and atrophy of the vagina, uterus, ovaries, and urethra.
Endocrine	■ Pituitary gland loses weight and vascularity. ■ Thyroid gland becomes more fibrous, and plasma T3 decreases. ■ Pancreas releases insulin more slowly; increased blood glucose levels are common. ■ Adrenal glands produce less cortisol.

Alterations to Development

Developmental disabilities are a cluster of conditions that occur as the result of impairment in motor function, speech and language development, behavioral patterns, or learning ability. To recognize delays or deviations from normal patterns of development, the nurse must be knowledgeable about normal developmental milestones. Although this module focuses on impairments that affect pediatric development, it is important to remember that development continues throughout the lifespan and alterations may occur at any point. Any noted alteration should be investigated further. Management of developmental delays varies and may require use of an interprofessional team, depending on the nature of the alterations and the individual's needs. In addition, nurses assess each patient's individual developmental level and incorporate that into the plan of care. This is especially important when considering patient teaching and planning for the patient's care needs following discharge.

Alterations and Manifestations

Alterations in development may occur in a single area or multiple areas. Alterations may be referred to as a delay, a deficit, or a disorder. While developmental delays are primarily thought of as childhood disorders and improve or disappear with intervention and use and practice of skills, some (such as attention-deficit/hyperactivity disorder and autism spectrum disorder) will challenge the individual for the length of the lifespan. In addition, deficits in any area may occur in adulthood as the result of injury, stroke, or other trauma.

Communication

The term *communication disorder* refers to any delay or deficit in one of the following areas: speech, language, voice, or swallowing. A child with a speech delay has difficulty making the sounds of language—that is, not being able to articulate specific sounds or speaking with a stutter. A child with a language delay may have difficulty accessing receptive language or may have difficulty expressing language. Language delays also encompass the acquisition of vocabulary. A child with a pragmatic language delay has difficulty using language in social contexts (American Speech-Language-Hearing Association, 2017).

Although hearing children may not necessarily benefit from learning sign language, research has shown that children with developmental delays and cognitive differences do benefit from learning sign language. Sign language has been particularly beneficial to those born with Down syndrome as a nonverbal means of communication (Barbosa et al., 2018).

Motor Function

Motor delays are often more easily identified as a child fails to achieve certain milestones or experiences losses of previous gains. Motor delays may be seen in fine motor skills, gross motor skills, or both. Some 5–6% of children will experience developmental coordination disorder, which is usually identified when the child enters kindergarten. While some children will achieve all milestones, just at a later age, others, such as those with cerebral palsy, may never meet certain milestones (Blank et al., 2019). Tic disorders, such as Tourette syndrome, are characterized by rapid, recurrent movements or vocalizations and are considered a form of motor disorder. Tics are common in childhood but generally abate as the child matures.

For children having difficulty with fine motor skills, such as grasping and transferring objects, evaluation by an occupational therapist is recommended. Children who have difficulty meeting gross motor milestones will require evaluation by a physical therapist.

Cognition

A child experiencing a cognitive delay has difficulty with thinking and problem solving in relation to developmental milestones. For example, a 3-year-old who is unable to work with everyday objects (e.g., button, zipper), turn a door handle, or put together a three- or four-piece puzzle is showing evidence of not meeting developmental milestones for cognitive ability (CDC, 2020h). Preterm infants are at greater risk for cognitive delays than full-term infants (Anderson, 2017). Cognitive delays are seen in children with a variety of disorders, including autism spectrum disorder, cerebral palsy, and Down syndrome. Children with intellectual disability will exhibit cognitive delays as well as difficulty with adaptive functioning. Children experiencing cognitive delays benefit from evaluation by an interprofessional team that includes a child psychologist, speech-language pathologist, occupational therapist, and physical therapist, as well as a nurse and the child's primary care provider.

Adaptive Functioning

Adaptive functioning encompasses life and social skills. Individuals who have difficulty adapting to different people and environments—at home, work, and school—face many challenges. Adaptive functioning and cognition are closely linked. While a number of studies have found a correlation between executive function and adaptive behavior in children with attention-deficit/hyperactivity disorder (ADHD), researchers are also finding that poor executive functioning is associated with poor adaptive behavior in children with histories of heavy prenatal alcohol exposure (Mattson, Bernes, & Doyle, 2019). These children also benefit from evaluation by an interprofessional team.

Etiology

Certain alterations in development have a single manifestation; however, the alteration may stem from one of many different etiologies. For example, congenital anomalies, infantile glaucoma, and retinopathy of prematurity can all lead to visual impairment in neonates. In other cases, a single defect may manifest in an array of signs and symptoms. Fragile X syndrome is a genetic disorder in which the absence of one protein impairs brain development and may yield multiple effects, including impairments related to language, learning, and social interaction (CDC, 2020k). Other developmental disabilities come about from exposure to fetal toxins, such as alcohol. Fetal alcohol spectrum disorders (FASDs) occur when pregnant mothers consume alcohol. Those born with FASDs have a host of challenges, including intellectual and neurologic, visual and hearing, as well as behavioral and mental health (CDC, 2020e). Infectious agents, such as viruses and bacteria, can cause fetal harm. Zika, a virus transmitted by certain breeds of mosquitoes, has been linked to miscarriage, impaired growth, microcephaly, neurologic deficits, eye damage, and hearing loss (CDC, 2019a).

Other developmental disabilities include ADHD, intellectual disability (ID), Down syndrome (or trisomy 21), muscular dystrophy, and Tourette syndrome. The exemplars in this module explore three developmental impairments commonly diagnosed initially in pediatric patients—ADHD, autism spectrum disorder (ASD), and cerebral palsy (CP)—and one seen in infants and older adults—failure to thrive.

>> **Stay Current:** For discussion of additional pediatric developmental disorders, visit the CDC's information center at http://www.cdc.gov/ncbddd/developmentaldisabilities/index.html.

Prevalence

Approximately 1 in 6 children in the United States is impaired by one or more developmental disabilities or by other forms of developmental delays (CDC, 2019f). Trends show an increase in developmental disabilities from 2009–2011 and 2015–2017 in children age 3 to 17 (CDC, 2019f). In particular, increases were seen in the numbers of children diagnosed with ADHD, ASD, and intellectual disabilities. There are many different theories as to the cause of the rise in ASD diagnoses, including greater awareness of autism, better diagnostic tools, and change in the language used to survey parents. Other disabilities tracked by the CDC include ID, CP, vision loss, and hearing loss. Currently, the CDC's Metropolitan Atlanta Developmental Disabilities Surveillance Program (MADDSP) is the hallmark tracking site for trends in childhood disabilities (CDC, 2017b).

Genetic Considerations and Nonmodifiable Risk Factors

In some cases, developmental delays are inevitable because of genetic abnormalities. Because chromosomes and genes carry messages that encode for certain characteristics, they also can carry diseases. Although some genetic mutations are incompatible with life and result in fetal death, live births can occur with others.

Chromosomal disorders may be caused by an array of factors, such as radiation exposure, parental age, exposure to infectious agents, or parental disease states; however, sometimes their causes cannot be determined. Some children inherit genes that lead to diseases such as cystic fibrosis; others may have a mutation that manifests in the disease. A family history of these diseases is usually present, but because genes sometimes mutate, an initial incidence of a genetic disorder may appear with no identifiable history.

Premature birth, multiple gestation, and low birth weight are also linked to an increased risk for several types of developmental disorders (CDC, 2019h). In all cases, early identification and referral to appropriate resources can help a patient to achieve the highest level of developmental functioning possible based on the abnormality.

Case Study >> Part 1

Farah Mohamed, 24 years old, is a Somali refugee who immigrated to the United States at the age of 10. She is married and has a 2-year-old son, Amiir Yusef. She brings Amiir to the family practice clinic for his well-child visit. As his mother carries him from the lobby, you notice Amiir squirming the entire time. When you reach the examination room, Amiir screams in a high pitch and pulls away from his mother. During the assessment, you notice that Amiir is rocking back and forth on the floor as he sits with a toy vacuum making R-noises. The mother remarks, "He loves vacuums. Sometimes, he screams and screams at the closet until I bring him the vacuum. I have to turn it on, and then he is happy. That toy vacuum is his favorite toy. He shows more love to the vacuum than he does to me."

When discussing Amiir's development, Ms. Mohamed tells you that he was born early, at 36 weeks, after she had been on bed-rest for early cervical effacement. She shares that her pregnancy was difficult because she had hyperemesis gravidarum (intractable vomiting) through much of her pregnancy. She tells you that he was a quiet baby, and he did not like to be touched. She reports he still does not like to be held. She tells you, "I think he was angry I did not take better care of him when I was pregnant. He still is angry with me."

As your conversation and assessment progresses, you learn:

- Amiir was sitting by himself at 6 months.
- He did not crawl but was able to pull himself up at 10 months.
- He walked independently at 13 months.
- He has difficulty holding a spoon and fork; instead, he likes to eat with his hands.
- His vocabulary is very limited.

Ms. Mohamed tells you she is worried about her son because he doesn't seem like other children. She shares, "My husband just graduated from college and is starting a new job. I am now going to college, and so I am not home much with Amiir. He spends most of his time with my mother. She does not speak English, and she puts Amiir in front of the television so that he will learn English. Is this why he doesn't really speak? Is it because he is confused about which language he should learn?"

Clinical Reasoning Questions Level I

1. Identify two or more developmental milestones that Amiir has met and two that he has not met. At what age should he have met the milestones that he has not met?
2. Using Erikson's theory of developmental stages, what is Amiir's current developmental task? What is Ms. Mohamed's developmental task?
3. Ms. Mohamed blames Amiir's vocabulary on the fact that he is growing up in a bilingual family. Could this indeed be the cause of Amiir's limited vocabulary? Why or why not?

Clinical Reasoning Questions Level II

4. Identify two nursing priorities for this case study that could be used in the plan of care of Amiir and/or Ms. Mohamed.
5. Ms. Mohamed blames herself for Amiir's behavior. How would the nurse respond to Ms. Mohamed's comments regarding blame for her difficult pregnancy?
6. After you complete your assessment, you are concerned that Amiir may have autism. What data collected during the assessment support or refute your suspicion? What additional data should be collected?

Concepts Related to Development

Most people with mild alterations in development, whether they occur in childhood or as the result of injury or trauma in adulthood, will be able to cope with them with appropriate interventions. For those with more significant delays or alterations, however, the implications for health, wellness, illness, injury, and functioning in all areas of life are great. The presence of a developmental disability increases the individual's risk for injury, abuse, and exploitation and increases difficulty with self-care, activities of daily living, and responding to and participating in treatment for acute or chronic illness.

Selected concepts integral to development are presented in the Concepts Related to Development feature. They are presented in alphabetical order.

Concepts Related to **Development**

CONCEPT	RELATIONSHIP TO DEVELOPMENT	NURSING IMPLICATIONS
Assessment	Language, motor, cognitive, and adaptive functioning delays or deficits can make assessment a challenge.	■ Adapt the assessment to the individual's developmental level. ■ Include family and caregivers in the assessment as appropriate but take care to promote autonomy and maintain confidentiality on the part of the patient.
Family	Moderate to severe alterations in development may disrupt family processes as family members struggle to integrate the individual who is delayed or disabled into family activities and communication patterns. Families also must integrate therapies and interventions into their daily schedules.	■ Assess family functioning. ■ Assess family supports. ■ Provide referrals to area resources as needed.
Health, Wellness, Illness, and Injury	Individuals with developmental deficits or disorders benefit from appropriate nutrition, rest, and physical exercise. By reducing risk factors related to these areas, patients will be more likely to achieve better outcomes and integrate more successfully at home, work, and school. Illness can interfere with normal developmental processes. For example, toddlers who previously were toileting independently may regress during periods of hospitalization. In older adults, hospitalization can cause cognitive disturbances and impair functioning in other areas.	■ Assess sleep and rest patterns. ■ Assess meal patterns and dietary intake. ■ Assess level, amount, and type of exercise. ■ Encourage patients and families to participate in healthy behaviors related to sleep hygiene, eating habits, and exercise. ■ Provide referrals as needed for evaluation or support in these areas. ■ Assess functioning before hospitalization to establish baseline. ■ Communicate developmental level to providers who will be working with the patient. ■ Plan interventions and communications according to developmental level. ■ Assess for regression or deterioration at regular intervals. ■ Provide interventions necessary to promote return to functioning.

(continued on next page)

Concepts Related to *(continued)*

CONCEPT	RELATIONSHIP TO DEVELOPMENT	NURSING IMPLICATIONS
Safety	Deficits or delays may increase an individual's risk for injury or illness. For example, an individual with cognitive and adaptive functioning deficits may not recognize illness or injury requiring attention from a HCP. Similarly, an individual with cognitive or adaptive functioning deficits may have difficulty following a treatment regimen without adequate supervision.	■ Assess personal, home, and environmental safety factors. ■ Link patients and families with resources that can promote skills that increase safety. ■ Simplify treatment instructions and regimen whenever possible.
Stress and Coping	Developmental delays or deficits can cause distress to the individual, caregivers/family, and those with whom the individual interacts at school and work.	■ Assess individual and family coping mechanisms. ■ Provide developmentally appropriate suggestions for improving coping skills.
Trauma	Individuals with developmental delays and disabilities are at increased risk for abuse from family members and strangers and at increased risk for sexual exploitation. Families and providers can be reluctant to discuss personal safety with these patients, putting them at even greater risk.	■ Assess patient and family understanding of the risks for abuse. ■ Provide patient and family education related to risks and personal safety practices.

Health Promotion

Health promotion to reduce risk for developmental disabilities in children focuses on maternal well-being. Preterm birth is the number one cause of long-term neurologic disabilities in children (CDC, 2019h). Several maternal factors have been linked with early deliveries, including age, race, socioeconomic status, health status, pregnancy abnormalities, and behavioral issues (CDC, 2019h). Behavioral factors include substance use, inadequate prenatal care, and psychologic influences (CDC, 2019h). Infants who are premature have immature body systems, requiring medical support in the newborn period.

Some developmental delays can be prevented by educating the pregnant patient in the care of her baby in utero. Education regarding proper prenatal care should start with the first prenatal visit. The nurse has the opportunity to begin the educational process of lifelong health promotion by starting with prenatal education. After birth, the focus shifts to helping parents raise a healthy child in a safe environment, giving that child the optimal ability to develop and thrive.

Prenatal Considerations

The mother's nutrition and general state of health play a part in pregnancy outcome. Even before the woman considers becoming pregnant, it is recommended she take a prenatal vitamin with at least 400 mcg of folic acid for at least 1 month before conceiving to prevent such birth defects as anencephaly and spinal bifida (CDC, 2020d, 2020f). The use of prenatal vitamins should continue throughout the pregnancy and postpartum stages to prevent anemia in the mother and baby, as well as other vitamin and mineral deficiencies.

Prescription medications, over-the-counter medications, and herbal supplements are not necessarily safe for the fetus. Various substances can cause *teratogenesis* (abnormal development of the fetus) or *mutagenesis* (permanent changes in the fetus's genetic material). Effects can be long term and range from hearing loss to severe congenital abnormalities. In 2014, the U.S. Food and Drug Administration (FDA; 2020) published the Pregnancy and Lactation Labeling Rule, which requires that drug labels be formatted to assist HCPs in assessing risk versus benefit for pregnant women and nursing mothers who need to take medication.

>> **Stay Current:** See samples of drug labels at http://www.fda.gov/Drugs/DevelopmentApprovalProcess/DevelopmentResources/Labeling/ucm093307.htm.

Although some medications are safe during certain stages of the pregnancy, there is the potential for those same medications to be dangerous in other stages, depending on fetal development and approaching delivery. For example, ibuprofen, a nonsteroidal anti-inflammatory drug, has been found in a few studies to interfere with conception and cause miscarriages. In the later portion of the first trimester and second semester, there are no reported problems. However, after 30 weeks of pregnancy, the mother is advised not to take ibuprofen because of its potential to decrease amniotic fluid and increase the risk of heart defects in the fetus (Organization of Teratology Information Specialists, 2019). To help HCPs and pharmacists to provide evidence-based information regarding safe medication use by pregnant women and breastfeeding mothers, the CDC has paired with the Organization of Teratology Information Specialists (OTIS) to create a clearinghouse for information at www.mothertobaby.org.

Some maternal illnesses are harmful to the developing fetus. Cytomegalovirus (CMV) infection is quite common in adults, children, and newborn babies. The CDC (2020c) estimates that 1 in 200 babies are born each year with this virus. Although many babies are infected via their mothers, few will have lasting effects. However, some infected babies may be born with microcephaly, hearing loss, vision loss, intellectual disabilities, and major organ issues (CDC, 2020b). A fetus can also acquire chronic infections, such as HIV/AIDS or hepatitis B, from the mother.

Chronic maternal distress, anxiety, and depression can affect the fetus. Excess stress hormones, such as cortisol, pass through the placenta and can result in lower birth weight and size. Moreover, maternal stress can affect behavioral and emotional child development (Lima et al., 2018). Maternal psychological distress and anxiety have even been linked to increased BMI and likelihood of childhood obesity (Vehmeijer et al., 2019).

In addition to abstaining from use of drugs, alcohol, and tobacco products, healthy eating, regular exercise, early prenatal care, and infection prevention are the best ways to promote safe delivery of a healthy newborn.

Environmental Factors

Appropriate prenatal and early nutrition are essential to promoting healthy growth and development. For example, children who do not receive adequate nutrition are at greater risk of infection than children who are well nourished. Infection, then, can cause further malnutrition as the individual may not want to eat or, because of such compensatory reactions as diarrhea, may not be able to absorb nutrition. Inadequate nutrition in pregnancy and in the first years of life may result in growth restriction or impact brain development. See Module 14, Nutrition, for more information.

Other environmental factors that can influence growth and development are the living conditions of the child, socioeconomic status, climate, and community. Illness or injury can affect growth and development. Being hospitalized is stressful for a child and can affect the child's coping mechanisms. Prolonged or chronic illness may affect normal developmental processes, including psychosocial development. See Exemplar 43.A, Environmental Quality, in Module 43, Advocacy, for more information.

SAFETY ALERT Environmental lead exposure can have devastating effects on infant and child development. Potential consequences of pediatric lead exposure include slower growth and development, learning disabilities, hearing and speech deficits, and behavior problems (CDC, 2020g; Ruckart et al., 2019).

Screenings

Well-child visits are perhaps the most effective initial method of screening for developmental disorders. Through regularly assessing the child at set intervals, the HCP can identify the child's degree of achievement of milestones related to growth and development. Developmental assessments are performed in the clinical setting, as well as in home, school, and community settings. Numerous screening instruments are available for use by HCPs and school systems (New York City Health Department, 2015; Ringwalt, 2008). Two commonly used screening tools are the Ages and Stages Questionnaire (ASQ) and the Battelle Developmental Inventory Screening Test (BDIST). The ASQ is appropriate for infants and young children and relies on the parent's report of the child's communication and motor skills, social skills, and problem-solving ability. The BDIST is appropriate for children birth to 7 years 11 months old and uses both parent report and direct observation of the child to assess skills in a variety of areas. Screening instruments used to screen for ASD and ADHD are outlined in those exemplars.

>> Stay Current: For more information on specific developmental screenings, visit the CDC's child development and screening information center at https://www.cdc.gov/ncbddd/childdevelopment/screening.html.

Anticipatory Guidance

Anticipatory guidance related to developmental and age-related risks for injury is discussed in Module 51, Safety.

Nursing Assessment

When performing a nursing assessment, the nurse can utilize developmental theories and stages of development to guide the assessment. Developmental theory can help the nurse individualize the assessment to match the child's stage of development and to anticipate the response of the child to the assessment. For example, the nurse understands that the modesty of an adolescent should be preserved during a physical examination. Knowledge of developmental theory also allows the nurse to notice any deviations of milestones that have been missed or delayed.

Knowledge of adult theories of development can help the nurse provide care appropriate to the adult's stage of development. The nurse needs to be aware of the physical changes that are part of the aging process as well as the cognitive and psychological changes that occur with aging as well. With this knowledge, the nurse understands that an individual in middle adulthood may have increased stress caring for both children as well as older parents.

Assessment of those with developmental differences requires that the nurse have not only a firm foundation in developmental theories and concepts, but also an understanding of the impact of those differences. For example, many cognitive tests require the individual to read or respond to pictures, actions that may not be possible for an individual with limited vision.

Pain is a subjective experience that is perceived differently across the lifespan. HCPs often do not take into account Piaget's stages of cognitive development; yet, by doing so, the nurse can have a better understanding of the patient's perspective of pain and treat accordingly (Freund & Bolick, 2019). For example, toddlers and young children in the preoperative phase are not able to connect illness with pain, and therefore will blame others for their pain. The toddler having a surgical procedure will likely associate postoperative pain with the nurse who provides treatments.

Older adults see pain as a natural progression of aging. There is the misconception held by both patients and providers that pain is a normal of function of aging. Many elderly patients may downplay the extent of their pain for a variety of reasons, which leads to undertreatment of pain. The nurse should be aware that when assessing for pain, older adults might not rate their pain realistically.

Children with developmental delays or sensory deficits, such as those seen in ASD, often do not sense pain as others do. One child may giggle or laugh with shots, saying they "tickle," whereas another child will not tolerate the feel of mittens on the hands. Even though these children may not perceive pain as others might, they do experience pain. Unfortunately, many children with developmental delays and sensory deficits are not able to communicate their discomforts (Hauer, Houtrow, & Council on Children with Disabilities, 2017). Allowing parents and caregivers to have an active role in the child's pain management is crucial in providing relief to children with developmental and sensory deficits, especially those who are nonverbal (Hauer et al., 2017).

Observation and Patient/Family Interview

Parents and caregivers of children are reliable resources of information about their child's behaviors and milestones. The assessment should be conducted in a well-lit, quiet room with space for the family, patient, and nurse. Small spaces may make it difficult to observe the pediatric patient at play; dim rooms may make it difficult for the older patient to see. The nurse should plan for plenty of time for the interview and should not rush the observation/interview process.

During the assessment interview, the nurse can observe the child for certain behaviors and physical traits. For example, the nurse would observe if an infant at the 6-month well-baby check can hold the head upright. With toddlers and older children, the nurse can provide age-appropriate

Development Assessment

GENERAL HEALTH	GROWTH AND DEVELOPMENT	PSYCHOSOCIAL HEALTH	NURSING CONSIDERATIONS
Newborns and Infants			
■ Feeding patterns and practices ■ Sleeping patterns and practices ■ Metabolic screening ■ Vision, hearing screenings ■ Immunizations ■ Tobacco/drug exposure ■ Risk for sudden infant death syndrome (SIDS) ■ Hand hygiene and infection prevention	■ Length, height, head circumference ■ Meets developmental milestones (Table 25.4 and Table 25.5)	■ Family attachment ■ Cultural practices ■ Self-soothing/self-regulation ■ Separation, stranger anxiety normal at this age	■ Be alert for significant changes from one well visit to the next (e.g., significant decrease or increase in percentile for length and weight requires evaluation) ■ Lethargy or failure to meet milestones requires evaluation; may indicate poor nutritional intake.
Toddlers and Preschoolers			
■ Eating habits and meal patterns ■ Sleep and rest patterns ■ Immunizations ■ Oral health ■ Physical activity ■ Screen and TV time	■ Height and weight ■ Head circumference until 1 to 2 years old ■ Toilet training ■ Meets developmental milestones (Tables 25.6, 25.7, 25.8, and 25.10)	■ Signs of independence versus reliance ■ Parent and child interactions ■ Self-regulation ■ Beginning awareness of sex and gender ■ Self-regulation	■ < 5th percentile weight or BMI or > 85th percentile requires further evaluation ■ Provide anticipatory guidance related to changing risks for injury as child develops ■ Provide patient education regarding promoting healthy self-concept (e.g., praise, appreciation, limit-setting)
School-Age Children			
■ Eating habits and meal patterns ■ Sleep and rest patterns ■ Immunizations ■ Oral health ■ Physical activity ■ Screen and TV time, internet access and safety	■ Height, weight, BMI ■ Slow, steady growth normal until puberty ■ Assess risk and protective factors for obesity ■ Meets developmental milestones (Table 25.11)	■ Assess self-esteem, self-concept, including body image ■ Child should be exhibiting increasing independence, responsibility for self ■ Inquire about family relationships and stressors ■ Assess family supports and resources	■ Provide patient education regarding physical activity, making good food choices, and the need for parents to model healthy behaviors ■ Teaching for children at this age is most effective when children are actively engaged in learning. ■ Unusual complaints may require follow-up ■ Provide anticipatory guidance related to changing risks for injury as child develops

Development Assessment *(continued)*

GENERAL HEALTH	GROWTH AND DEVELOPMENT	PSYCHOSOCIAL HEALTH	NURSING CONSIDERATIONS
Adolescents			
▪ Eating habits and meal patterns ▪ Sleep and rest patterns ▪ Immunizations ▪ Oral health ▪ Physical activity ▪ Screen and TV time, internet access and safety ▪ Extracurricular activities	▪ Height, weight, BMI ▪ Scoliosis screening ▪ Sexual maturity rating (Tanner stages) ▪ Breast/testicular exam ▪ Sexually transmitted infection screenings, pelvic exam, Pap smear for those who are sexually active ▪ Meets developmental milestones	▪ Assess self-esteem, self-concept, including body image ▪ Child should be exhibiting increasing independence, responsibility for self ▪ Inquire about family relationships and stressors ▪ Assess family supports and resources ▪ Assess risks for injury related to extracurricular activities	▪ Develop a partnership with the adolescent ▪ Provide patient teaching relating to nutrition, physical activity, sleep hygiene ▪ Provide anticipatory guidance related to changing risks for injury
Adults			
▪ Eating habits and meal patterns ▪ Sleep and rest patterns ▪ Immunizations ▪ Oral health ▪ Physical activity ▪ Risk and protective factors for health and mental health	▪ Height, weight, BMI ▪ Sexual activity/risks ▪ Breast and pelvic or testicular exams ▪ Use of tobacco, alcohol, drugs ▪ Changes in health status are appropriate for age (Table 25.12 and Table 25.13)	▪ Assess self-esteem, self-concept, including body image ▪ Inquire about family relationships and stressors ▪ Assess family supports and resources	▪ Develop a therapeutic alliance with the patient ▪ Provide anticipatory guidance and health teaching based on assessment and individual risk factors
Older Adults			
▪ Eating habits and meal patterns ▪ Sleep and rest patterns ▪ Immunizations ▪ Oral health ▪ Physical activity ▪ Risk and protective factors for health and mental health ▪ Presence of chronic illness ▪ Polypharmacy	▪ Height, weight, BMI ▪ Sexual activity/risks ▪ Breast and pelvic or testicular exams ▪ Use of tobacco, alcohol, drugs ▪ Changes in health status are appropriate for age (Table 25.14)	▪ Assess self-esteem, self-concept, including ability to engage in meaningful activity ▪ Inquire about family relationships and stressors ▪ Assess family supports and resources	▪ Develop a therapeutic alliance ▪ Assess for malnutrition, elder abuse ▪ Assess ability to perform ADLs, access to resources

toys, puzzles, and crayons, pencils, and paper. The nurse can observe for eye contact, overall appearance, interaction with family members and the nurse, and other visuals, such as body language, that can help the nurse gather the data to make an appropriate nursing plan.

The nursing interview is family-centered, culturally competent, and specific to the patient's age and developmental stage. Use open-ended questions and allow plenty of time for the patient and family members to answer questions and interject.

As necessary, provide an interpreter for patients whose primary language is not that of the nurse interviewer. Be aware of any cultural considerations during the interview. In some cultures, the patient does not answer direct questions; rather, a spokesperson answers for the patient. In other cultures, the parents might find it disrespectful for the child to play while the nurse is doing the interview. The nurse can explain the importance of watching the child for certain developmental behaviors.

As with any nursing assessment, the interview should include a complete health history. Interviews involving pediatric patients typically include prenatal and birth history, as well as any complications. Biographical data and health history, including immunizations, current medications, and family history, should be included in this assessment, as well as a review of systems. See Module 34, Assessment, for more information.

Nurses use information about developmental milestones to assess children and determine if any additional screening or assessment for developmental delays is necessary. Information from the initial assessment and health history may signal risk factors that suggest a need for more frequent assessment or follow-up. As appropriate, nurses may make referrals for further evaluation and use the results to plan appropriate nursing interventions.

Cultural Considerations

Culture influences development in numerous ways. For example, nutritional habits of different ethnic groups may affect growth rate in infants. In some cultures, children are carried next to the parent or caregiver rather than carried in a car seat or pushed in a stroller. Ensuring cultural competency in developmental screening is difficult when tests are not culturally sensitive and can inaccurately predict a child's pattern of development. Cultural norms among some groups may result in differences in parents' views of "normal" behaviors or milestones. Language barriers may render parent self-report assessments unhelpful or unreliable. In some situations, this may result in a delay in diagnosis of a developmental delay.

All cultural groups have patterns of language acquisition and social interactions. Young children in homes that speak multiple languages or engage children in talking early may be at an advantage in developing language skills over children who grow up in homes where language is used less frequently. Attitudes toward touching, play, movement, and other developmental skills vary among cultures. Genetic traits of families and their cultures of origin may influence physical growth and characteristics.

Physical Examination

The physical examination includes a review of systems as well as height, weight, and, for children older than 2 years of age, a BMI assessment. In young children especially, any physical distress or change in weight/BMI or motor function may be an early indicator of nutritional or developmental issues. The feature on Development Assessment lists broad categories of areas to assess for individuals at various ages.

Diagnostic Tests

Laboratory diagnostic tests are generally not used to determine developmental status. Medical evaluations typically rule out organic reasons for developmental delays, such as lead poisoning, but from there, most developmental delays are diagnosed through other means. Observational tools, questionnaires, and screening tests are some of the tools that are most helpful in determining developmental status.

Case Study » Part 2

After you complete your assessment of Amiir Yusef, you share your findings with the nurse practitioner. The nurse practitioner also is concerned after her assessment. As you did, she found that Amiir would not make eye contact, showed affection toward an inanimate object, had limited vocabulary, skipped a milestone (crawling), and seems to not like tactile stimuli. She arranges for Amiir to have comprehensive testing by a child neuropsychologist.

As you are reviewing the discharge instructions with Ms. Mohamed, she begins to cry. She tells you, "I don't understand what this means. I have heard of this autism, but what is it? Is this from his vaccinations? I have heard in my community that I should not do vaccinations. What have I done? It is Allah's will."

Clinical Reasoning Questions Level I

1. Ms. Mohamed is visibly upset by the potential diagnosis of her son having autism. Reflect on therapeutic communication techniques to use when talking with Ms. Mohamed. What actions would you take and how would you respond to Ms. Mohamed?
2. Ms. Mohamed, who is Muslim, made the comment, "It is Allah's will." What does that mean in terms of Ms. Mohamed's spiritual self?

Clinical Reasoning Questions Level II

3. *Refer to Exemplar 25.B, Autism Spectrum Disorder*. How would you explain the definition of autism to Ms. Mohamed?
4. What are possible causes of autism? How would you respond to Ms. Mohamed's question regarding vaccinations causing autism?
5. Ms. Mohamed requests information regarding diagnostic testing for autism. What information would you give Ms. Mohamed regarding how autism is diagnosed?

Independent Interventions

Often, patients with impaired development will demonstrate alterations in more than one area of function. For that reason, the treatment approach is varied.

As with all patient care, safety is the highest priority. All children with impaired mobility are at an exceptionally high risk for injury. For ambulatory children with mobility impairments, the nurse should ensure that the child is assisted with activities as needed and that properly fitted orthotic devices are being effectively used. In addition, range-of-motion (ROM) exercises should be implemented in order to promote flexibility and reduce contracture formation. Families and caregivers should be instructed about injury prevention within the home, including keeping walkways free from loose rugs, electrical cords, or any other obstacles.

Patients affected by developmental impairment, as well as their caregivers and family members, face challenges that extend into the physical and psychosocial realm. For those individuals who require lifelong treatment of a severe condition, financial stress and caregiver burden are serious concerns. The nurse caring for these individuals and their families should offer to facilitate connections with support groups and community resources, including agencies that offer assistance through financial aid or services.

Teaching patient safety will be based on the individual's needs, family situation, and home environment. General needs include the following:

- ***Health needs:*** Provide demonstrations of interventions to be done at home (e.g., trach care or tube feedings) and ask for return demonstrations.
- ***Physical environment:*** Provide safety instructions about smoke detectors, use of strobe lights as signals for the hearing impaired, and other safety devices. Provide patient and family education related to potential hazards in the home.
- ***Communication needs:*** Develop a safety plan for emergencies that the patient and family can communicate and practice often. If the patient is nonverbal, collaborate with the family to create a visual or symbol safety plan for the patient.

- Instruct the family to contact the local emergency dispatch and have the house "flagged" that a patient with communication and/or other special needs lives at that number. Those with limited communication or cognitive delays can be taught to call 911 and know that help will arrive.
- Watch the patient demonstrate how to call 911. If possible, have the patient demonstrate how to call other important numbers.

- ***Cognitive needs:*** Encourage parents to let their child explore and experience their surroundings. Humans on all cognitive levels experience and learn via sensory input. Consult with school providers and other healthcare team members to find adaptive equipment that the child can use to participate in different activities safely.

Collaborative Therapies

Collaborative interventions for individuals with developmental delays and disabilities are highly individualized and yet are partially determined by the services available in the community. For individuals of all ages, the goal is to help the patient achieve the greatest level of independence in the least restrictive environment possible.

Early Intervention Services

In the United States, growth and development surveillance begins at birth. Nurses and other providers conduct routine and specific assessments following labor and delivery, prior to discharge, and in the neonatal intensive care unit. Early intervention services may begin that soon for children who are identified with a growth or development issue in the hospital. Early intervention services are designed to enhance both the health and development of infants and young children with or at risk for disabilities.

Developmental screenings continue at well-child visits and follow the recommendations of the AAP (Lipkin, Macias, & Council on Children with Disabilities, 2020). For children whose screenings suggest the need for further evaluation, the family is typically referred to the agency that oversees early intervention services in their community. Funding for early childhood intervention services is usually a combination of federal and state sources and is authorized under Part C of the Individuals with Disabilities in Education Act. Early intervention agencies employ nurses, pediatricians, child psychologists or other mental health professionals, speech-language pathologists (SLPs), occupational therapists (OTs), physical therapists (PTs), and other professionals as necessary to diagnose and meet the needs of children in their communities. Early childhood intervention agencies serve children ages 0 to 3. Together with the parent, the interprofessional team will develop an **individualized family service plan** that identifies the child and family's strengths and weaknesses and designs activities and goals to help the child meet developmental milestones. The family is included to ensure that parents receive appropriate education and to help them learn how to support their child's development.

Nurses working in early childhood intervention may assist with both physical and health screenings and assessments. In addition, they may provide direct follow-up services for children who are medically fragile or have a medical need with or without a co-occurring developmental issue. For example, a nurse from the local health department or the early childhood intervention agency may assist a child in daycare with parenteral feedings or administer growth hormone shots to a child who has been found to have a deficiency in growth hormone.

Early identification of children in need of these services is critical to ensure the best possible outcomes. In a systematic review of best evidence for early intervention in infants with CP, the reviewers noted the importance of early intervention to improve infant motor function and cognitive plasticity. Infants with CP who received early, specific, and intensive intervention at home demonstrated better motor and cognitive function at age 1 than infants with CP who did not receive this intervention (Novak et al., 2017).

School-Based Interventions

Once a child turns 3, responsibility for oversight of developmental delay interventions passes to the child's public school system. Public schools employ early childhood specialists, SLPs, OTs, PTs, and child mental health professionals to assist in diagnosis and planning for children with special needs. Children with special health needs may benefit from a 504 plan that the interprofessional team and parent develop. These plans may include accommodations (such as sitting at the front of the class) or ensure the provision of health-related interventions. For children who need educational support to address their developmental needs, the parent and the interprofessional team will develop an **individualized education plan** (IEP). As with early intervention services, most funding for IEP services is made possible by a combination of federal funding through the Individuals with Disabilities Act and state funds.

Illness, Injury, and Trauma

At any stage of life, the onset of acute or chronic illness, injury, or trauma can impair development or function. For all patients, nurses working in acute and long-term/rehabilitation settings conduct functional assessments and work to ensure that patients do not regress or lose ability to function. Individuals who have lost or have impaired functioning of a limb or body part require evaluation by an OT and/or PT. Those who have lost any speech, language, or communication function due to stroke, injury, or other trauma should be evaluated by an SLP.

Lifespan Considerations

As stated earlier, many developmental delays may be overcome with timely and appropriate interventions. Some children, however, face long-term challenges and even disability. Individuals with developmental disability face greater risks for abuse and neglect, inappropriate treatment, and placement in more restrictive environments. At all ages and stages, the nurse acts as an advocate for the patient, seeking solutions that will help the patient live the fullest, best life in the least restrictive environment possible.

Adolescents and Younger Adults

The transition from childhood to adolescence and early adulthood is a challenging time for the individual and a stressful one for parents and family members. Just like their peers, teens with developmental differences typically seek greater independence from their parents, and parents and their growing children experience new stressors as the child matures toward adulthood. Gaining independence is key for both parents and children alike. Some children with developmental impairments may have difficulty attaining independence and need greater support or encouragement than others.

Children "age out" of the school system at 18 or on graduation from high school, and many of the supports once available to adolescents and their parents are no longer available. Challenges associated with this stage of development include transitioning to work or, for some, college; augmenting strained financial resources; and navigating disability program requirements and restrictions. Children with significant cognitive or adaptive impairments may leave home later in life; some may never leave home and will always require some level of supervision. Aging parents worry about how to plan for their adult child's safety after their deaths.

Risks for abuse and exploitation continue as the adolescent and young adult begin to take public transportation, go to work, or engage in new situations such as moving into a group home or various levels of assisted living situations. These housing alternatives can provide helpful, safe environments where adults with disabilities can thrive and gain independence.

Nurses working with adolescents and young adults with disabilities can provide support and encouragement to these patients and their families. Specific interventions may include assessing and providing information regarding personal and environmental safety; referring patients and families to peer support and vocational education programs; establishing case management services; and encouraging parents and families to make legal and financial arrangements for the patient.

Pregnant Women

Evidence suggests that women with intellectual and developmental disabilities (IDD) are at risk for maternal and neonatal complications. When compared to women in the general population, pregnant women with IDD more likely to experience preterm birth, stillbirth, and babies with low birth weight (Akobirshoev, Parish, Mitra, & Rosenthal, 2017). In addition, pregnant women with IDD experience poor prenatal care and are more likely to have gestational diabetes and preeclampsia than women without IDD (Mueller, Crane, Doody, Stuart, & Schiff, 2019). Implications for nursing are clear: Pregnant women with IDD require careful interprofessional care during and following pregnancy. Nurses caring for these women must familiarize themselves with area resources in order to provide timely and helpful referrals.

Older Adults

Many older adults with developmental disabilities live independently or with a spouse, with the majority living with a family member of some kind. Still others live in group homes, assisted living facilities, or in skilled nursing units. Preexisting disability in the older adult increases the individual's risk for type 2 diabetes due to a number of factors, including sedentary lifestyle, higher rate of obesity, and reduced participation in health screenings (Taggart, Truesdale, Dunkley, House, & Russell, 2018). For older adults with intellectual or developmental disabilities who present with symptoms of an emerging neurocognitive disorder, a thorough assessment is necessary to determine whether the adverse effects of a medication or environmental changes may be causing the alterations in cognition. Communication deficits can result in challenging behaviors in the older adult with a developmental disability. This, combined with the increased cost for care and often fragmented resources, creates an increased risk for patient frustration and caregiver burnout (Bishop & Lucchino, n.d.). Older adults with developmental disabilities also experience long wait lists for services (Cross Network Collaboration for Florida, n.d.). Nurses working with this population serve as advocates to help these patients navigate the services in their communities; assess patients' physical and mental health as well as adaptive and social functioning; and assess both patient and family needs.

Case Study » Part 3

Ms. Mohamed returns to the clinic for a follow-up appointment with her mother, Fartuun Eyl, and husband, Yuusef Yusef. Amiir has been diagnosed with autism by a pediatric neuropsychologist. During your initial interview, Mr. Yusef shares he does not trust the diagnosis of the neuropsychologist. He tells you, "This doctor, he did not know my son. How can he tell if my son has autism? I do not believe him."

While Mr. Yusef is talking to you, his wife starts to cry. Amiir's grandmother starts speaking in Somali, and the family has a discussion in their primary language. During this time, Amiir is sitting on the ground, hugging his toy vacuum. The volume of the family discussion becomes louder. Amiir starts to scream in a high pitch. The family stops talking, and Ms. Mohamed attempts to comfort Amiir, but he pulls away. Mr. Yusef apologizes, telling you, "This is very hard for my wife and me. We love our son very much. We want only the best for him."

After meeting with the nurse practitioner regarding the results of the testing, the family meets with you for further education. Both Mr. Yusef and Ms. Mohamed express concern for Amiir's future. They tell you that in Somalia, children do not have autism, so the concept of autism is very new for them. The grandmother, who does not speak English, also asks questions through the daughter who interprets for her. The family is referred to a specialty center for different therapies.

Clinical Reasoning Questions Level I

1. *Refer to Exemplar 25.B, Autism Spectrum Disorder, and other resources.* Explain why Amiir began to scream when the family's discussion became louder. How can the family avoid such events in the future?
2. The family makes the statement that autism does not exist in Somalia. How does the nurse explain this discrepancy?
3. What resources are available in your own community to support children ages 2 through 5 who are determined to have autism? Which of these might be appropriate for or helpful to Amiir and his family? Why?

Clinical Reasoning Questions Level II

4. *Refer to Module 27, Grief and Loss.* Is there a possibility that Amiir's caregivers are grieving his diagnosis? Why or why not? If the family is grieving, using a theory of grieving, categorize the family in a stage or phase of grieving. How can the nurse help the family cope with this diagnosis?
5. You notice that Ms. Mohamed and Mr. Yusef are translating for Ms. Eyl. She appears to have many questions. How should you respond to Ms. Eyl's language barrier?

REVIEW The Concept of Development

RELATE Link the Concepts

Linking the concept of development with the concept of infection:

1. Explain the impact of infection on prenatal development.
2. When caring for pregnant patients, how might the nurse promote infection prevention for both mother and fetus?

Linking the concept of development with the concept of family:

4. Explain the interrelationship between an individual's successful achievement of developmental milestones and the developmental health of the individual's family unit.
5. Describe specific aspects of family function that may be impacted when one family member is diagnosed with a developmental disorder.

Linking the concept of development with the concept of ethics:

6. You are caring for an 8-month-old infant who appears to be undernourished. Along the infant's arms and back, you note what appear to be bruises. The child's mother reports that she recently lost her job and can barely afford to pay her rent or other bills. As a nurse, what is the primary issue and what actions are required of you?
7. Identify potential ethical concerns that may arise as a result of using prenatal testing (e.g., amniocentesis and chorionic villus sampling) to diagnose developmental disorders in utero.

READY Go to Volume 3: Clinical Nursing Skills

REFER Go to Pearson MyLab Nursing and eText

REFLECT Apply Your Knowledge

Abby is a 15-year-old girl who has recently entered high school. She has a diagnosis of Down syndrome and is considered moderate-to-high functioning. The school nurse is attending her IEP meeting with the rest of the school team. When Abby's mother is asked how she feels about the transition from the small middle school to the larger high school, the mother relates, "I am worried about Abby. She has become involved in so many things. She talks about new friends and wants to go to so many activities. She even has started dating! This boy has asked Abby to go to Homecoming, but I am nervous! Should I let her go?"

1. Why is the school nurse part of an IEP team?
2. How should the school nurse answer the mother's question?
3. What role can the school nurse have in Abby's development and safety? What education can the school nurse provide the mother? Provide Abby?

Exemplar 25.A Attention-Deficit/Hyperactivity Disorder

Exemplar Learning Outcomes

25.A Analyze ADHD as it relates to development.

- Describe the pathophysiology of ADHD.
- Describe the etiology of ADHD.
- Compare the risk factors and prevention of ADHD.
- Identify the clinical manifestations of ADHD.
- Summarize diagnostic tests and therapies used by interprofessional teams in the collaborative care of an individual with ADHD.
- Differentiate care of patients with ADHD across the lifespan.
- Apply the nursing process in providing culturally competent care to an individual with ADHD.

Exemplar Key Terms

Attention-deficit disorder (ADD), *1860*
Attention-deficit/hyperactivity disorder (ADHD), *1859*

Overview

At one time, **attention-deficit/hyperactivity disorder (ADHD)** was considered a childhood condition, outgrown in adolescence and of little consequence for adults. Research indicates, however, that the disorder persists into adulthood in 60% of individuals (Sibley et al., 2017). Classic characteristics of ADHD include difficulty completing tasks that require focused concentration, hyperactivity, and impulsivity (American Psychiatric Association, 2017). Hyperactivity and impulsivity may improve as the child nears adulthood, with inattentiveness appearing as the most persistent characteristic (Cabral, Liu, & Soares, 2020).

ADHD is often a missed diagnosis in the adolescent and adult. The adolescent's diagnosis is often complicated by other co-occurring behaviors and mental health diagnoses during this developmental stage (CDC, 2019g). The adolescent may have difficulty due to the increasing cognitive demands of school and socialization. As a result, what parents, educators, and other adults see as "just being a teen" or as defiant behavior might be ADHD. Among adults, ADHD is a known risk factor for antisocial behavior, substance abuse, involvement in serious accidents, academic underachievement, and low occupational success. In adults, inattention is more persistent than hyperactivity or impulsivity (Hackett et al., 2020).

Roughly one-third of adults with ADHD are not diagnosed until after 18 years of age. Approximately 33% of men diagnosed with ADHD as children go on to have a child with the disorder, suggesting a genetic component to the disease (American Academy of Child and Adolescent Psychiatry, n.d.). More boys (12.9%) are diagnosed with ADHD than girls (5.6%) (CDC, 2019d), possibly because girls tend to present with inattention manifestations as well as anxiety and depression, which are not as disruptive and obvious as hyperactivity (Wolraich et al., 2019a). Adult women, in particular, are often misdiagnosed before a diagnosis of ADHD is reached (Children and Adults with Attention-Deficit/Hyperactivity Disorder [CHADD], 2019).

The term **attention-deficit disorder (ADD)** is sometimes used to describe individuals who experience the inattentiveness and difficulty concentrating related to ADHD, but who are without the associated hyperactivity that accompanies it. However, in the fifth edition of the *Diagnostic and Statistical Manual of Mental Disorders* (DSM-5), the American Psychiatric Association (2013) officially recognizes only ADHD, the manifestations of which are described using specifiers.

Pathophysiology

The pathophysiology of ADHD is unclear, although dopamine (involved in reward, impulsivity, and mood) and norepinephrine (which modulates attention and arousal) are implicated. More recent research has implicated neuroanatomical alterations in the prefrontal and frontal cortex areas (Soref, 2019). Inability to regulate both input from and responses to stimuli combined with decreased self-regulation leads to the hallmark symptoms of ADHD. Children may experience ADHD alone or with additional manifestations such as learning disabilities, aggressive behaviors, or motor dysfunction.

Etiology

Although a variety of physical and neurologic disorders are associated with ADHD, children with identifiable causes represent a small proportion of this population. ADHD may result from several different mechanisms involving interaction of genetic, biological, and environmental risk factors. Although ADHD occurs more commonly within families (25% have a first-degree relative with the disorder), a single gene has not been located and a specific mechanism of genetic transmission is not known. It is believed that a genetic predisposition interacts with the child's environment, so that both factors contribute to the appearance of the condition. Family stress, poverty, and poor nutrition may be contributing factors in some cases.

Prevalence rates for ADHD vary somewhat based on race and ethnicity, family poverty level, and parental education. Among children age 3 to 17, non-Hispanic Black children are more likely to be diagnosed with ADHD or a learning disability (16.9%) compared to non-Hispanic white children (14.7%) and Hispanic children (11.9%). Overall, children from families below federal poverty level are more likely to be diagnosed (18.7%) with ADHD or a learning disability than those living at or above poverty level (12.7%). Similarly, children of parents with a high school education or less are more likely to be diagnosed with ADHD or a learning disability than children whose parents attended some level of college or educational program after high school (Zablotsky & Alford, 2020).

Risk Factors

Multiple risk factors for ADHD have been identified. Maternal factors, such as smoking cigarettes and drinking alcohol during pregnancy, increase the risk of ADHD in offspring (Cabral et al., 2020). Other prenatal factors associated with a higher incidence of ADHD include preterm labor, impaired placental functioning, and impaired oxygenation. Sleep disorders, seizures, and other neurologic disorders are additional potential associations (Wesemann & Van Cleve, 2018). ADHD has also been linked to exposure to heavy metals, such as lead and mercury, and to chemicals, such as organophosphate pesticides (Cabral et al., 2020).

Prevention

At this time, there is no known way to prevent the development of ADHD. Women should avoid smoking, drugs, and alcohol during pregnancy to reduce the risk of ADHD and other disorders in their children. Likewise, women should seek prenatal care to avoid preterm birth and monitor for low fetal growth. Exposure to environmental toxins, such as lead and mercury, should be limited during pregnancy and early childhood.

Clinical Manifestations

Children with ADHD have problems related to decreased attention span, impulsiveness, and/or increased motor activity (**Figure 25.9** »). ADHD in school-age children and adolescents is marked by a persistent pattern of six or more symptoms in the inattentive category and at least six or more symptoms in the hyperactive/impulsive category that occur

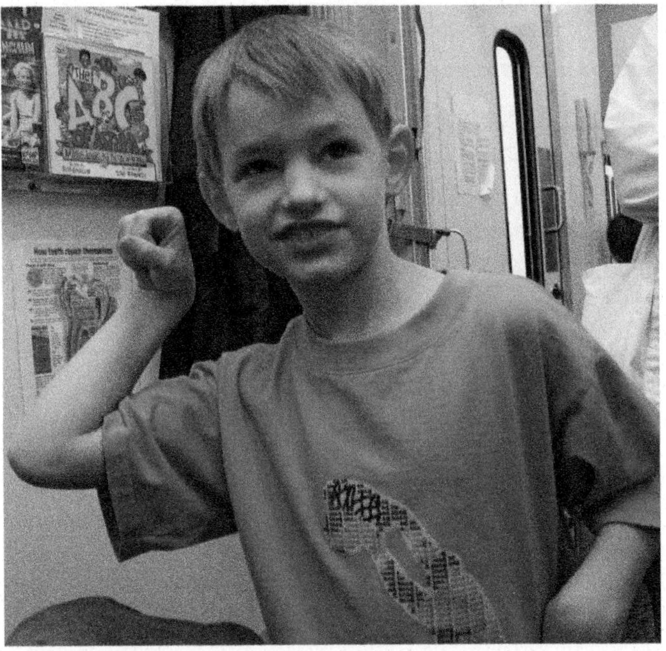

Figure 25.9 » This child with ADHD was challenged by a visit to a healthcare facility for dental care. He found it difficult to remain in the chair for the examination, and once it was over, he rapidly ran from one piece of equipment to another in the facility. He asked what things were for but did not wait for answers. His engaging personality emerged as he posed briefly for a picture. Such behaviors can be exhausting for parents to manage and may create safety hazards in the healthcare setting.

Source: George Dodson/Pearson Education, Inc.

in multiple areas (e.g., home, school, or job) of daily life. Symptoms must occur over a period of 6 months or more for a diagnosis of ADHD to be considered. Some symptoms must have been present prior to age 7 (Wolraich et al., 2019b).

Symptoms of ADHD can range from mild to severe. The child has difficulty completing tasks, fidgets constantly, is frequently loud, and interrupts others. Sleep disturbances are common. Because of these behaviors, the child often has difficulty developing and maintaining social relationships and may be shunned or teased by other children. While children with ADHD are at higher risk of being bullied than children without ADHD, those with hyperactive and impulsive behaviors were more likely to be the victims of bullying (Winters, Blake, & Chen, 2018). Typically, girls with ADHD show less aggression and impulsiveness than boys, but far more anxiety, mood swings, social withdrawal, rejection, and cognitive and language problems (Wolraich et al., 2019a). Girls tend to be older at the time of diagnosis.

Children with ADHD tend to have social impairments, such as difficulty making and keeping friends, that tend to persist into adulthood. Friendships are often fraught with conflict and a lack of intimacy. Other psychosocial problems include delinquent behaviors, aggression, unsportsman-like behaviors, substance abuse, and lack of attention to social cues (Mikami, Smit, & Khalis, 2017).

Collaboration

The successful diagnosis and treatment of the child or adult with ADHD requires a collaborative effort that may involve any combination of the following: parents, nurses, and physicians; teachers, school nurses, and school psychologists or other mental health specialists; and speech-language pathologists.

Diagnostic Tests

Diagnosis begins with a careful history of the child, including family history, birth history, growth and developmental milestones, behaviors such as sleep and eating patterns, progression and patterns in school, social and environmental conditions, and reports from parents and teachers. A physical examination should be performed to rule out neurologic diseases and other health problems.

The mental health specialist then tests the child and administers questionnaires to parents and teachers. Behaviors at home and school or at daycare must be evaluated because abnormal patterns in two settings are needed for diagnosis. A variety of tests are available to use in establishing the diagnosis (**Table 25.15** »). It is also important to identify other conditions that may mimic ADHD or exist in conjunction with the disorders. These conditions may include depression, anxiety, learning disorder, conduct disorder, oppositional defiant disorder, or sleep disturbances (CHADD, 2020a).

» **Stay Current:** Visit NICHQ Vanderbilt Assessment Scales at https://www.nichq.org/sites/default/files/resource-file/NICHQ_Vanderbilt_Assessment_Scales.pdf to learn more about a screening for parents and teachers to use to identify ADHD behaviors for diagnosis and to follow the disorder over time.

Based on the assessment findings, desired outcomes are established for the child's performance and management of

Clinical Manifestations and Therapies

ADHD

CUES	CLINICAL MANIFESTATIONS	CLINICAL THERAPIES
Hyperactivity	▪ Fidgets, squirms ▪ Talks excessively ▪ Leaves seated position when supposed to be seated ▪ Difficult to engage in tasks or activities quietly ▪ Restless ▪ Always moving	▪ Make environmental modifications. ▪ Reduce environmental stimuli. ▪ Encourage planned seating in classrooms, group settings. ▪ Promote consistent limit setting. ▪ *Behavioral therapy:* • Reward appropriate behavior. • Apply timely, appropriate consequences for inappropriate behavior. • Teach strategies to improve focus and coping. • Teach social and peer skills. • Apply behavioral management in the classroom. • Carry out individualized education plan and/or 504 plan. • Teach parent training in behavioral management. ▪ *Medications:* See Medications 25.1.
Impulsive behavior	▪ Blurts out answers ▪ Can't take turns ▪ Interrupts others	
Inability to pay attention	▪ Makes careless mistakes ▪ Problems maintaining attention on tasks or play activities ▪ Loses things needed to accomplish tasks ▪ Does not seem to listen when spoken to ▪ Forgets to do things ▪ Does not finish tasks ▪ Distracts easily ▪ Has trouble with organization ▪ Avoids activities requiring attention	

TABLE 25.15 Screening Tests for ADHD

Test	Description
Vanderbilt Parent and Teacher Scales	Completed by parents and teachers to diagnose and follow up on ADHD in children age 6–12
Conners' Parent and Teacher Rating Scales	Completed by parents and teachers to diagnose children for ADHD; can identify comorbidities such as oppositional defiant disorder
Swanson, Nolan, and Pelham Questionnaire IV Teacher and Parent Rating Scale (SNAP-IV)	Completed by parents and teachers in the diagnosis of children with ADHD
Disruptive Behavior Disorder Scale	Completed by parents and teachers in the diagnosis of children with ADHD, oppositional defiant disorder, and conduct disorder in children and adolescents
ADHD Rating Scale IV	Completed by parents to determine frequency of behaviors of ADHD to diagnose ADHD and monitor therapy
Revised Behavior Problem Checklist	Used to rate problem behaviors (conduct disorder, socialized aggression, attention, anxiety/withdrawal, psychotic, motor) in children and adolescents
Adult Self-Report Scale for ADHD	Used for self-assessment of ADHD symptoms in patients age 18 years or older

the disorder. Treatment is established to meet the desired behavioral outcomes and includes a combination of approaches, such as environmental changes, behavior therapy, skills training, and pharmacotherapy.

Children are usually brought for evaluation when behaviors escalate to the point of interfering with the daily functioning of teachers or parents. When children have learning disabilities or anxiety disorders, the problem is commonly misdiagnosed as ADHD without further evaluation of the child's symptoms. ADHD can be diagnosed by a mental health professional or a medical provider. Careful management of ADHD in childhood may lead to better social functioning later in life, as well as better relationships with family and peers. Nonpharmacologic therapies are typically tried first, with medication added later if other interventions do not provide enough support.

Pharmacologic Therapy

Children with moderate to severe ADHD are treated with pharmacotherapy (see **Medications 25.1**). Stimulants are primarily prescribed; however, there are three nonstimulant medications approved by the FDA for children: Strattera (atomoxetine), Intuniv (guanfacine), and Kapvay (clonidine) (Wolraich et al., 2019a). Paradoxically, in patients with ADHD, psychostimulants help improve focus and attention, as opposed to yielding increased hyperactivity. Usually, a favorable response (a decrease in impulsive behaviors and an increase in the ability to sit still and attend to an activity for at least 15 minutes) is seen in the first 10 days of treatment and frequently with the first few doses. Stimulants are started at a low dose and slowly increased to behavioral goals with less adverse effects (Wesemann & Van Cleve, 2018). All psychostimulants are Schedule II drugs, which means that a monthly prescription must be obtained from a HCP. The child's growth pattern should be carefully monitored while taking these medications. A "drug holiday," during which the child does not take the medication during weekends or over school breaks, can be considered and discussed with the prescribing provider.

SAFETY ALERT Many medications used to treat ADHD are central nervous system (CNS) stimulants. As such, they have a potential for abuse, especially among teens and young adults who take them as an appetite suppressant or in order to stay awake (Wolraich et al., 2019a). In the adult population, the nurse should be aware of the increased risk of potentially fatal cardiovascular effects of stimulant medication (FDA, 2018).

Nonpharmacologic Therapy

Environmental modifications, behavioral therapy, and skills training are important components of the treatment plan for individuals with ADHD to improve outcomes and enhance quality of life. These treatments can be used alone or in conjunction with ADHD medications. In a hallmark study conducted by the National Institute of Mental Health (NIMH), behavioral therapy in combination with medication has shown to be the best practice for treatment of ADHD (Molina et al., 2009). Preschool-age children should first be treated with behavioral therapy and later treated with medications if symptoms continue to be troublesome (Wolraich et al., 2019b).

Environmental Modification

Reducing environmental stimuli and distractions, such as by turning off the television and keeping the study area free of clutter and toys, can help improve children's focus. Placing the child with ADHD in a smaller class with a structured routine or having the child sit at the front of the classroom are examples of environmental modifications that can be implemented at school. Routines and signaled transitions help the child to feel organized. Children with ADHD also benefit from consistent limits and expectations at school and at home.

Behavioral Therapy

Behavioral therapy is implemented to reduce the manifestations of ADHD and includes behavioral management in the classroom and parent training in behavior management (PTBM).

Medications 25.1

Drugs Used to Treat ADHD

CLASSIFICATION AND DRUG EXAMPLES	MECHANISMS OF ACTION	NURSING CONSIDERATIONS
CNS Stimulants ***Drug examples:*** amphetamine-dextroamphetamine (Adderall) dexmethylphenidate (Focalin) dextroamphetamine (Dexedrine) lisdexamfetamine (Vyvanse) methamphetamine (Desoxyn) methylphenidate (Concerta, Ritalin)	The mechanisms of action for stimulants in the treatment of ADHD is poorly understood. It is thought to block the reuptake of dopamine and norepinephrine. *May also be used for:* Narcolepsy	■ Teach patients and parents about side effects such as headaches, insomnia, and anorexia. ■ Monitor patient's growth while on this medication. ■ Check heart rate and blood pressure, which can increase in some children. ■ Ask about a "drug holiday" on weekends and school breaks. ■ *Potential for abuse:* Some children may sell the drug at school.
Nonstimulants ***Drug examples:*** atomoxetine (Strattera) clonidine (Kapvay) guanfacine (Intuniv)	The mechanism of action of nonstimulants in the treatment of ADHD is poorly understood. Atomoxetine is a selective norepinephrine reuptake inhibitor. Both clonidine and guanfacine are antihypertensives that are also used for ADHD. They are best used conjunctively with a stimulant.	■ Has less abuse potential since nonstimulant. ■ Teach parents to be alert for serious side effects, including psychosis and suicidal tendencies, particularly with atomoxetine. ■ Monitor hepatic function while on atomoxetine. ■ Monitor blood pressure while on clonidine or guanfacine. ■ Use with caution in patients with heart disease. ■ Taper guanfacine and clonidine when discontinuing to avoid rebound hypertension. ■ Assess for sleepiness, dry mouth, dizziness, irritability, headache, bradycardia, hypotension, and abdominal pain with extended-release guanfacine and clonidine
Psychostimulant Skin Patch ***Drug example:*** methylphenidate (Daytrana)	The mechanism of action for stimulants in the treatment of ADHD is poorly understood. It is thought to block the reuptake of dopamine and norepinephrine.	■ Teach patients to alternate patch placement between left and right hips. ■ Watch for skin irritation. ■ Has been known to cause permanent leukoderma in some children. ■ Teach patient to remove patch after 9 hours. ■ Same side effect profile as oral medications.

Source: Data from Adams, Holland, and Urban (2020).

In behavioral therapy, the child is rewarded for desired behaviors and consequences are applied for undesirable behaviors. Children may be rewarded by praise or earn points toward a movie or another desired outing for staying seated during meals or quietly listening in a classroom. Cues are established so that a child can subtly be reminded when impulsive or hyperactive behaviors are escalating. Behavioral therapy is most effective when all adults who are in close contact with the child, such as parents and teachers, are involved in and supportive of the program. The desired behaviors produced by behavioral therapy are more persistent than those produced by medication, which stop when the medication is discontinued (Wolraich et al., 2019b).

Using a daily report card, the teacher marks progress toward behavioral goals. This report card is shared daily with parents and when certain criteria are met, the child receives a reward. The teacher also works with the child on time management, planning, and organizational skills (CHADD, 2018). Due to laws about providing services to children with conditions such as ADHD, the child may have an individualized education plan (to provide for the unique needs of the child) or a 504 plan (to provide accommodations to meet the child's educational needs) (CDC, 2020a).

>> **Stay Current:** Visit the Children and Adults with Attention-Deficit/Hyperactivity Disorder website at https://chadd.org/for-educators/overview/ to learn more about how teachers can help the child with ADHD in the classroom.

PTBM can be applied to any child with ADHD and is the first-line treatment for children who are 4 years of age until the 6th birthday. Interventions in PTBM teach parents appropriate developmental expectations for the child's age, behaviors that promote a strong relationship between parents and child, and skills to manage the child's behaviors. A benefit of PTBM is that it can be started before a diagnosis of ADHD is made (Wolraich et al., 2019b).

Skills Training

Individuals with ADHD can be aggressive, have intense emotions, and miss social cues, making it difficult to make and keep friends. Skills training can help these individuals improve social and peer interactions. Although studies of these interventions show limited effectiveness, providing direction and reinforcement during actual peer interactions rather than in a treatment program has been shown to be more successful (Mikami et al., 2017). These interventions involve teachers and parents coaching and rewarding positive social skill behaviors.

Complementary Health Approaches

According to the National Center for Complementary and Integrative Health (NCCIH; 2019b), there is no scientific evidence supporting the use of complementary health approaches in the treatment of ADHD. Several areas of complementary medicine have been studied, including diet regimens, dietary supplements, and neurofeedback (NCCIH, 2019b). Although it does not help reduce hyperactivity and other symptoms of ADHD, melatonin may help some patients who have difficulty with sleep. Yoga may improve symptoms of attention, hyperactivity, and impulsivity (NCCIH, 2019a) and may help with sleep.

Lifespan Considerations

Although ADHD was once thought of as a childhood disorder, it is now being diagnosed in younger children and in adults. ADHD manifests in different ways across the lifespan. Nurses should be alert for the following signs of ADHD in patients of all ages.

ADHD in Toddlers and Preschoolers

Diagnosing ADHD in toddlers is difficult. Many of the normal behaviors of toddlers and preschoolers are similar to those seen in ADHD, such as trouble concentrating or taking turns. However, children as young as 3 years of age can be diagnosed with ADHD (NIMH, 2019). Young children with ADHD tend to be more disruptive than those without. Some children are so disruptive they are expelled from preschool. Often, children with ADHD tend to get special education placement. Young children with ADHD tend to have more injuries and take greater risks than their peers. Behavioral classroom interventions and PTBM are the preferred treatments for preschoolers (Wolraich et al., 2019b).

ADHD in School-Age Children and Adolescents

ADHD is typically diagnosed once the child reaches school age and the hyperactivity and impulsivity prevalent with this disorder manifest in the classroom setting. Children with ADHD often have academic difficulties regardless of their cognitive abilities. Creating peer relationships is an important part of development, but because of the behaviors of ADHD, children sometimes struggle with making and maintaining friends. Children with ADHD also are more prone to accidents and injuries due to risk-taking behaviors and lack of forethought.

As a child with ADHD progresses into adolescence, there is less hyperactivity, but fidgeting and restlessness are still present. Impulsive behaviors and inattentiveness persist and can continue into adulthood. Many of the behaviors of ADHD in adolescence could be considered antisocial, which in turn makes it difficult for the teen with ADHD to make and keep friends. School typically continues to be a challenge because of inability to focus and stay organized.

SAFETY ALERT Diversion of stimulant medications is of concern in adolescents and young adults with ADHD. Stimulants may be misused to stay awake or suppress appetite and the adolescent or young adult with ADHD may face pressure to share or sell these medications. Teach adolescents and young adults about the legal and health risks of sharing and talk with them about how to say no when asked (Maitland, 2020).

ADHD in Adults

The diagnosis of ADHD in the adult may be accompanied by a sense of relief. As children, these adults often exhibit mild symptoms and therefore were not diagnosed. As they moved into adulthood, they continued to struggle with personal and social relationships, workplace responsibilities, and time management. Both young and older adults with ADHD may exhibit antisocial behavior, have difficulties maintaining jobs, and participate in risky behaviors. Chemical dependency, assault, and trauma are commonly seen in adults with ADHD, particularly those who have gone undiagnosed and untreated. Compared to women without ADHD, adult women with ADHD are more likely to experience depression, stress, anxiety, and lower self-esteem (CHADD, 2020c).

NURSING PROCESS

Care of the patient with ADHD requires a coordinated approach by the healthcare team, including teachers, parents, and caregivers. When caring for pediatric patients, parents and caregivers are integral to each phase of the nursing process. Because collection of assessment data depends largely on interviews, the nurse should establish effective communication patterns with the patients, parents, and caregivers. Coordination between parents and teachers is key to providing consistent interventions to the child with ADHD.

Assessment

Families often present to the pediatric provider's office with concern about a child's behavior prior to a diagnosis being made. Assessment of a patient with ADHD can sometimes be difficult, as it is a complex neurodevelopmental disorder that is not always obvious. Moreover, the time a nurse spends with a patient is usually short, and the diagnosis of ADHD typically requires many interactions.

- ***Observation and patient interview***. Because ADHD has three clusters of symptoms, (inattentive, hyperactive, and impulsive), the nurse should look for signs of these behaviors. Watch to see if the patient appears to be listening and paying attention to the nurse during discussions. Observe for signs of hyperactivity, such as fidgeting and inability to sit in one place. Listen for rapid, excessive speech patterns. Usually within a few minutes in an unstructured setting or waiting area, the child with ADHD becomes restless and searches for distraction. Gather information about the child's activity level and impulsiveness. Find out how the family manages at home and what treatments are being applied.

For all patients, ask about family and birth history. For children, ask parents to describe behaviors they or others have observed. Ask about any problems in school and social settings. The nurse may perform developmental screenings, if appropriate, but may be more likely to facilitate screening with the pediatric provider and then a referral to early childhood intervention services or a mental health specialist (see Focus on Diversity and Culture: Racial and Ethnic Differences in ADHD Diagnosis).

Adults can be diagnosed by either a mental health provider or a primary care provider, preferably someone with whom the patient has a long-term relationship. For the adult, data collection and assessment for ADHD is more complicated. Like the pediatric patient, the adult patient may become inattentive, restless, or fidgety. A rating scale such as the Adult ADHD Self-Report Scale may be used for assessing symptoms in individuals over age 18 (Hackett et al., 2020).

- ***Physical examination***. The physical exam of the patient with ADHD across the lifespan will not show any physical abnormalities unless the patient is being seen for injuries related to hyperactive and impulsive behaviors.

Diagnosis

Examples of patient problems or care priorities that may be appropriate for a patient of any age who has ADHD include the following:

- Risk of injury
- Undernutrition
- Inadequate social skills
- Poor impulse control
- Chronic low self-esteem
- Caregiver burden
- Sleep disturbances.

Planning

Planning for the patient with ADHD may include the following goals:

- The patient will adhere to the treatment regimen.
- The patient will demonstrate appropriate behaviors at home and at school or work.
- The patient will demonstrate more successful interactions with peers.
- The adult patient will have a plan to meet workplace expectations and responsibilities.
- The patient will remain safe from self-harm and physical injury.
- The patient will consume adequate calories based on age and activity.
- The patient will develop normal sleep patterns.
- The patient will develop individual coping skills.
- The patient will demonstrate improved self-esteem.
- The parents of the pediatric patient will verbalize satisfaction with parenting skills.

Implementation

Parents and teachers of children with ADHD often feel overwhelmed and require significant support and education from the nurse. A key role of the nurse is providing education and may include information about medications and their side effects; decreasing environmental stimuli and minimizing distractions; and following a consistent behavior plan. In many cases, multiple trials may be necessary before finding the combination of medication and behavior strategies that work best for the individual child.

Implementation of the nursing plan with the adult patient is a challenge because much of the responsibility of follow-through rests with the individual. The adult patient may not have the support system a child has and may benefit from case management to assist with medication adherence, support systems, and community resources.

Administer Pharmacologic Treatments

Stimulant and nonstimulant medications increase the patient's attention span and decrease distractibility. Interventions related to pharmacologic treatment include the following:

- Teach patient and parents or family members to be alert for the common side effects of these medications, including anorexia (loss of appetite), insomnia, and tachycardia.
- Administer medication early in the day to help alleviate insomnia. Anorexia can be managed by giving medication at mealtimes.
- Perform periodic monitoring of weight, height, and blood pressure.
- Instruct families about the abuse potential of stimulant drugs; these drugs should be locked up and administered only as directed.

Focus on Diversity and Culture

Racial and Ethnic Differences in ADHD Diagnosis

Current trends of ADHD and ethnicity and race show a greater percentage of non-Hispanic Black and white children diagnosed with ADHD or a learning disability than Hispanic children (Zablotsky & Alford, 2020). Culture might play a significant factor in diagnosis. For example, in some cultures, energetic behaviors and fidgeting are not viewed as undesirable in children. As a result, parents might not seek out a diagnosis. Parenting style, which is influenced by culture, may also play a part in differential diagnosis (Gómez-Benito, Van de Vijver, Balluerka, & Caterino, 2019). Practitioners of one culture might not appreciate the behaviors of a child of another culture. Other factors involved in diagnostic disparities may include financial means, lack of access to specialty providers, mistrust of providers from the dominant culture, and stigma.

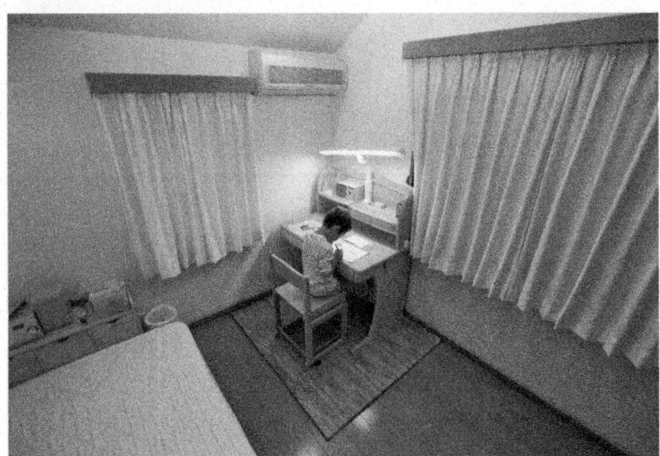

Figure 25.10 ›› Managing the environment to provide quiet places with minimal distractions is often necessary for the child with ADHD. This boy reads and does homework in a room with no pictures, no music, and only his homework on his desk. He also is assisted by structure, such as a scheduled time for homework, with short breaks to walk around every 10 to 15 minutes.

Source: MIXA next/Getty Images.

Minimize Environmental Distractions

Patients with ADHD benefit from fewer environmental distractions. For children:

- Keep potentially harmful equipment out of reach.
- Limit and monitor screen time.
- Provide a quiet, clutter-free area for study time.
- Use shades to darken the room during naps or at bedtime and minimize noise.
- Teach parents to minimize distractions at home during periods when the child needs to concentrate (e.g., when doing schoolwork) (**Figure 25.10** ››).
- When the child is hospitalized, minimizing environmental distractions may mean placement in a private room.

Adults may benefit from similar environmental modifications, including maintaining a quiet, clutter-free area for work and limiting screen time, especially when completing tasks and for an hour or more before bedtime.

Implement Behavioral Management Plans

Behavior modification programs can help reduce specific impulsive behaviors. An example is setting up a reward program for the child who has taken medication as ordered or completed a homework assignment. Depending on the child's age, the rewards may be daily as well as weekly or monthly. For example, one completed homework assignment might be rewarded with 30 minutes of basketball or a bike ride, and assignments completed for a week might be rewarded with participation in an activity of the child's choice on the weekend.

Communicating with Patients

Working Phase

Because children with ADHD are easily distracted, avoid overwhelming the child by giving directions one at a time in a positive tone. For example, if the parent needs the child to get ready for school, the following directions can help to break down the tasks:

- Here are your clothes. I need you to put them on.
- Great job with your clothes. Please go brush your teeth.
- You are almost done. Find your shoes and I will help you tie them.

Provide Emotional Support

Family support is essential. Educate family members and patients about the importance of appropriate expectations and consequences of behaviors. Teach skills such as making lists of tasks to accomplish; following routines for eating, sleeping, recreation, and, for children, schoolwork; and minimizing stimuli in the environment when completing work.

Patients who are diagnosed with ADHD as adults may also need emotional support. While some are relieved to understand the cause of some of the hardships in their lives, others are dismayed by the diagnosis. Refer adult patients to mental health counselors as appropriate. Evidence has shown that cognitive-behavioral therapy combined with medications improves outcomes for adults with ADHD (Scrandis, 2018).

Promote Self-Esteem

Patients with ADHD are easily frustrated, in part by their own behaviors and in part by the reactions of others. This frustration easily leads to loss of self-esteem. Nurses can help patients with ADHD understand the disorder at a developmentally appropriate level and also facilitate a trusting relationship with HCPs. Patients of all ages with ADHD who build healthy relationships with HCPs are more likely to seek help. Interventions to promote self-esteem may include:

- Emphasize the positive aspects of behavior and treat instances of negative behavior as learning opportunities.
- Encourage skills at which the patient excels and consider the use of support groups in school or in the community.
- Offer praise for successfully following tasks or meeting goals. For example, praise the adult patient whose spouse reports improved communication with children and other family members or the hospitalized child who helps carry toys around to other children.

Educate Families

Parents of children with ADHD need support to understand the diagnosis and to learn how to manage the child. Explain the diagnosis and what is known about attention-deficit disorders. Provide written materials, credible internet sites, and an opportunity to ask questions.

Emphasize the importance of a stable environment at home as well as at school. At home, the child may have difficulty staying on task. Parents need to consider the child's age and developmental appropriateness of tasks, give clear and simple instructions, and provide frequent reminders to ensure completion. Routines in the evening can promote good sleep patterns.

The nurse can serve as a liaison to teachers and school personnel or as the case manager for the child. See the Patient Teaching box for suggestions on how parents and teachers

Patient Teaching

Optimizing the Educational Experience for the Child with ADHD

Schools are now changing their perspective on children with ADHD. Prior to the DSM-5, ADHD was seen as a disruptive behavior disorder that highly impacted the school setting. Now that ADHD is seen as a neurodevelopmental disorder, schools are approaching the behaviors of ADHD students differently. The key to supporting the child with ADHD in school is a strong parent–teacher relationship. Parents can work with teachers to provide a school environment that fosters attention and learning. Some ideas that may be helpful include the following:

- Have the child sit near the front of the class, preferably away from doors or windows.
- Plan a reminder (for the child) that is apparent to the teacher and the child but not to other students when the child needs to concentrate on attention. This might be an object placed on the student's desk or a light hand placed on the shoulder or arm.
- Go over assignments and tests with the child to explain areas that are understood and those that need attention. Give instructions verbally and in written form and repeat them more than once.
- Provide opportunities to take notes and make lists of assignments and mark off when accomplished. Have a planned time to go through the child's backpack daily to find notices and to ensure that homework is completed and in a uniform location.
- Use computers, note-taking partners, or recording devices for making lists and taking notes.
- Integrate motor movement into learning situations whenever possible. Allow the child to run occasional errands to provide additional opportunities for movement.
- Provide quiet places with minimal distraction for examinations. Offer additional time.
- Allow time for organizing clothing, desk, and other areas.
- Find the child's areas of excellence and allow for performance in these ways. Some children are talented in dance, others in art or extemporaneous speech.
- Never call the child names, make fun of behavior or performance, or call the child "hyperactive" in front of other children, teachers, or parents.
- Incorporate behavioral skills into the child's learning plan.
- Reinforce social skills as the child interacts with other children.

Sources: Centers for Disease Control and Prevention (2020a); Children and Adults with Attention-Deficit/-Hyperactivity Disorder (2020b); National Alliance on Mental Illness (n.d.).

can work together to optimize the child's educational experience. An IEP may be needed, with clear expected outcomes stated for the child's behaviors. IEPs or periods of instruction free from the distractions of the entire class may enable the child to improve school performance. Parents may have difficulty understanding the need for these approaches because the child often tests at above-average intelligence.

As the child grows older, provide explanations about the disorder and information about techniques that will assist in dealing with problems. Emphasize the importance of doing homework or other tasks requiring concentration in a quiet environment without background noise from a television or radio. Encourage children with ADHD to keep assignment notebooks and use checklists to help them accomplish specific tasks.

Evaluation

Expected outcomes of nursing care for the child with ADHD include the following:

- The family accurately and safely manages medication administration.
- The child maintains a weight that is within normal limits.
- The child demonstrates an increase in attentiveness and a decrease in hyperactivity and impulsivity.
- The child receives adequate rest each night and wakes up well rested.
- The child displays formation of a positive self-image.
- The child manifests formation of healthy social interactions with peers and family.
- The parents verbalize satisfaction with parenting skills.

Expected outcomes for an adult with ADHD are similar to that of a child and may also include:

- The patient remains safe and free from self-harm.
- The patient adheres to the treatment regimen.
- The patient verbalizes workplace responsibilities are being met.

Nursing Care Plan

A Patient with ADHD

Melanie Taylor, age 8, visits her pediatrician's office for a routine checkup. Her mother, Mrs. Taylor, reports that Melanie is not doing well in school and that she is a difficult child to raise. Upon further questioning, Mrs. Taylor reports that her daughter is forgetful, has trouble focusing, and often does not respond to her name being called. She repeatedly asks Melanie to perform her chores, get ready for bed, or do her homework. Melanie does not sleep well at night, and most nights she crawls into her parents' bed. One night, Mrs. Taylor awoke to find Melanie watching TV at 2:00 a.m. in the family room. Melanie's teacher has suggested she be evaluated for possible ADHD.

(continued on next page)

Nursing Care Plan *(continued)*

ASSESSMENT

The nurse interviews Melanie, who says she doesn't like school because "it's too hard" and the teacher "always tells me to sit still."

Upon reviewing Melanie's medical history, the nurse finds the patient's growth and development have been normal to date. Mrs. Taylor's pregnancy and delivery were unremarkable.

The physical examination is normal, although the nurse notes that Melanie often requires repetition of instructions such as "Touch your finger to your nose" before she complies. Both Melanie and her mother appear tired and yawn several times during the nurse's time with them.

The practitioner speaks with Melanie and Mrs. Taylor, suggesting that the signs and symptoms are suggestive of ADHD, and provides a referral for the family to meet with a psychologist specializing in the care of patients with this disorder.

The nurse provides Mrs. Taylor with a Conners' Parent Rating Scale to complete and gives her a copy of the Teacher Rating Scale to give to Melanie's teacher for completion before seeing the counselor, who will evaluate the results.

DIAGNOSES

- Chronic low self-esteem
- Sleep disturbance
- Caregiver burden
- Fatigue

PLANNING

- The patient (Melanie) will sleep through the night, remaining in her own bed.
- The patient will participate in a therapeutic regimen as recommended by the HCP.
- The patient's parents and teachers will participate in the therapeutic regimen.
- The patient will increase her ability to remain on task by 5-minute intervals over a period of 6–8 weeks, until she can remain on task for a minimum of 20 minutes at a time.
- The patient will keep track of her belongings.
- The patient will respond when spoken to the first time.

IMPLEMENTATION

- Explain the diagnosis in terms Melanie can understand and help her understand that she is not "abnormal" but "unique" in how her brain works.
- Help Mrs. Taylor set rules related to sleep that will promote Melanie's sleep hygiene.
- Assist patient to understand how her potential diagnosis of ADHD impacts her thinking as well as how treatment can help her perform better in school.
- Determine if Melanie or Mrs. Taylor have questions related to ADHD.
- Suggest strategies for helping Melanie improve her concentration and memory.
- Teach positive behavioral skills through role play, role modeling, and discussion.
- Convey confidence in patient's and mother's ability to handle situation.
- Encourage increased responsibility for self, as appropriate.
- Encourage Melanie to accept new challenges.
- Monitor Melanie's statements of self-worth and frequency of self-negating verbalizations.

EVALUATION

Mrs. Taylor and Melanie return at the end of 3 months. Mrs. Taylor reports that Melanie is doing better at paying attention both at home and at school and that she is able to maintain attention for 20 minutes "most of the time." Both of them are sleeping better. Melanie is able to answer the nurse's questions readily and describes things that she does to keep track of her belongings and try to stay on task. Melanie voices pride in her improvement at school.

CRITICAL THINKING

1. Mrs. Taylor asks the nurse, privately out of range of Melanie's hearing, if the diagnosis resulted from something she did as a parent or while pregnant. How would you respond?
2. Melanie tells the nurse, "I'm so stupid compared to the other kids in my class. I guess ADHD means I'm brain-damaged." How would you respond?
3. Is it possible to adequately treat ADHD without the use of medications? Explain your answer.

REVIEW Attention-Deficit/Hyperactivity Disorder

RELATE Link the Concepts and Exemplars

Linking the exemplar of attention-deficit/hyperactivity disorder with the concept of family:

1. How can the nurse support the family of a child with ADHD?

2. What if the family is a single parent? A grandparent?

Linking the exemplar of attention-deficit/hyperactivity disorder with the concept of safety:

3. What interventions are important for the nurse to initiate to maintain the safety of a patient with ADHD?

4. When caring for an adolescent with ADHD, how would you teach automobile safety?

READY Go to Volume 3: Clinical Nursing Skills

REFER Go to Pearson MyLab Nursing and eText

REFLECT Apply Your Knowledge

Jason is an active, healthy 11-year-old boy. He is in fifth grade at the public elementary school near his home. He lives with his mother Evelyn and his 14-year-old sister Jenna. He has not had much contact with his father. Jason's home life has been somewhat stressful the past year or so because of ongoing fights between his mother and oldest sister Jessica; the conflict resulted in Jessica moving out of the house. Jason gets along well with his mother, but he has typical sibling conflicts with Jenna.

Jason has been having trouble in school for some time. Teachers report that he has difficulty staying on task and won't follow directions. Although he made some progress last year with his fourth-grade teacher, his grades have been consistently poor. His mother tries to help him with homework after school or in the evening; these sessions frequently turn into battlegrounds. It takes Jason hours to complete fairly simple assignments, resulting in frustration for both Jason and his mother. The fact that he frequently comes home from school with headaches further aggravates the situation.

In addition to problems with academics, Jason has problems with social interactions. His teachers find him to be disruptive in the classroom. During the past year, he has often been sent to the principal's office for misbehaving. He has few friends and is a frequent target of bullying at school. Most of his time at home is spent playing video and computer games and watching TV.

1. What are the priorities of nursing care for Jason?
2. What outcomes would be appropriate for this patient?
3. What independent nursing interventions would you initiate for this patient?

Exemplar 25.B Autism Spectrum Disorder

Exemplar Learning Outcomes

25.B Analyze ASD as it relates to development.

- Describe the pathophysiology of ASD.
- Describe the etiology of ASD.
- Compare the risk factors and prevention of ASD.
- Identify the clinical manifestations of ASD.
- Summarize diagnostic tests and therapies used by interprofessional teams in the collaborative care of an individual with ASD.
- Differentiate care of patients with ASD across the lifespan.
- Apply the nursing process in providing culturally competent care to an individual with ASD.

Exemplar Key Terms

Autism spectrum disorder (ASD), *1869*
Echolalia, *1870*
Stereotypy, *1870*

Overview

The patient with **autism spectrum disorder (ASD)** characteristically demonstrates impaired communication and social interaction patterns and the presence of repetitive, restrictive behaviors. Manifestations of ASD range across a spectrum from mild to severe. Children and adults with ASD often experience impairments of language, behaviors, and social skills that make them seem different from others. The prevalence of ASD is approximately 1 in 54 children in the United States. It is four times more common in males than in females (CDC, 2020d). Other conditions that have a high co-occurrence with autism include intellectual differences, mood or other mental health disorders, seizures, eating issues, and gastrointestinal (GI) problems. Managing ASD can be stressful for both patients and family members. Nurses play an essential role in providing information and emotional support related to managing the diagnosis and promoting health and wellness for both the patient with autism and family members and caregivers.

>> **Stay Current:** Keep abreast of statistics, research, and treatment at www.autismspeaks.org.

Pathophysiology

The pathophysiology of autism is not well understood. What is known is that those with autism have defects in the genes and gene expression in the areas of cell-cycle expression. The construction of the brain is atypical in comparison to those without autism. MRIs and other imaging have shown there are abnormalities of neurons of the cerebral cortex. The frontal and temporal lobes are particularly susceptible to these abnormal neuron patches. The frontal lobe is responsible for social behaviors, motor function, problem solving, and other higher functions. The temporal lobe is responsible for language and sensory input. These neuron irregularities are thought to be responsible for the dysfunction and behaviors associated with autism. These abnormalities are created during fetal development. Because the infant brain continues to develop, with early intervention the brain can develop neuron networking around the defective neuron abnormalities and/or use pathways from nearby areas of the brain (Brasic, 2020).

Etiology

Although the etiology of ASD remains unknown, it is believed to be associated with a complex interplay between genetic, epigenetic, immunologic, and environmental factors. More than 800 ASD predisposition genes have been implicated in the development of ASD (Yin & Schaaf, 2017). Children with genetic abnormalities such as tuberous sclerosis, fragile X syndrome, Down syndrome, and neurofibromatosis have an increased occurrence of autism. Children who have family members with autism are more likely to have it. Boys have a higher rate of ASD than girls.

Risk Factors

There are a number of factors that increase the risk of a child having ASD. Prenatal factors that increase the risk include pregnancies occurring close together, multiple pregnancies, maternal obesity, gestational bleeding, diabetes, advanced maternal and paternal age, maternal use of valproate or thalidomide during pregnancy, and maternal infections (such as rubella and cytomegalovirus). Perinatal risks associated with the fetus that are associated with increased risk for ASD include prematurity, low birth weight, small for gestational age, hypoxia, and encephalopathy (Hyman, Levy, Myers, & Council on Children with Disabilities, 2020).

Prevention

As with the prevention of any developmental condition, prenatal care is essential to helping prevent autism. If the mother is on medication, including antiepileptics, she should discuss the benefits and risks of taking medication through pregnancy with her HCP. The woman should also discuss genetic counseling with her provider if there are family members with autism.

It is important to emphasize that multiple studies have found no link between immunizations and autism (Hyman et al., 2020; Taylor, Swerdfeger, & Eslick, 2014). During pregnancy, the mother should avoid alcohol, tobacco, infection, toxic substances, and other known causes of birth defects. While these measures might not necessarily prevent autism, they will help improve the chances of giving birth to a healthy baby.

Clinical Manifestations

The core characteristics of autism fall into two developmental areas and usually manifest by the time the child is 3 years old: (1) social interaction and communication and (2) restrictive and repetitive behaviors. **Table 25.16** » outlines common deficits and examples of how they manifest.

Signs of ASD can be detected in children as young as 18 months (CDC, 2020d). Clues for ASD can be detected in some children as early as the first few months of life. Other children may show typical development until 18 to 24 months old, when skill acquisition stops or skills begin to deteriorate. Up to half of parents of children with ASD suspected a problem in the child by age 1, and 89–90% noted problems by age 2 (CDC, 2019i).

Children with ASD have difficulties with social interactions, communication, and restrictive, repetitive behaviors. Social interactions are always complex and involve perceptions of the other individual as well as social behaviors. The patient with ASD does not learn the common characteristics of these social interchanges. As a result, the patient may be unable to converse normally, may fail to initiate conversations, and/or may fail to understand or observe nonverbal behavior.

Communication difficulties or delays in speech and language are common and are often the first symptoms that lead to diagnosis. Absence of babbling and other communication by 1 year of age, absence of two-word phrases by 2 years, and deterioration of previous language skills are characteristic of autism. Language acquisition, including verbal and nonverbal communication patterns, such as eye contact, will vary based on the severity of the disorder. Some children and adults with ASD can participate fully in conversations, but they may show characteristic behaviors such as marked lack of eye contact and lack of emotional reciprocity. They may or may not understand humor and other subtleties of language.

For children with ASD, speech patterns are likely to show certain abnormalities, such as the following:

- Using *you* in place of *I*
- Engaging in **echolalia** (a compulsive parroting of a word or phrase just spoken by another)
- Repeating questions rather than answering them
- Being fascinated with rhythmic, repetitive songs and verses.

In addition to social and communication problems, **stereotypy**, or rigid and obsessive behavior, may be observed. Characteristically, these repetitive behaviors in affected children include head banging, twirling in circles, biting themselves, and flapping their hands or arms. The child's behavior may be self-stimulating or self-destructive. Responses to sensory stimuli are frequently abnormal and include an extreme aversion to touch, loud noises, and bright lights (**Figure 25.11** »). Emotional lability (rapid, significant mood changes) is common.

TABLE 25.16 Characteristics of Autism

Social Interaction and Communication	
Impaired social and emotional interactions Impaired nonverbal interactions Lack of understanding of relationships	▪ Restricted affect ▪ Inability to initiate and participate in social interactions (i.e., communication, cooperative or collaborative play) ▪ Abnormal, incongruent, or lacking verbal and nonverbal communication ▪ Apparent disinterest in relationships, peers
Restrictive and Repetitive Behaviors	
Stereotypes or repetitive movements, use of objects, or speech Extremely intense fixations on interests	▪ Immature motor control affecting speech patterns (e.g., echolalia) ▪ Repetitive behaviors such as twirling, biting (of self), arm flapping ▪ Restricted, repetitious play (often with a single object of preoccupation, such as toy trains)
Insistence on consistency, inflexibility of routines and rituals	▪ Difficulty or inability to adjust behavior to context ▪ Significant distress at changes in routine or environment ▪ Rigid routines and rituals (such as the order of tasks, need to eat the same food every day)
Hyper- or hyposensitivity to aspects of the environment	▪ Indifference or excessive response to temperature, sound, pain, light, textures, or other aspects of the environment

Source: Adapted from American Psychiatric Association (2013); Hyman et al. (2020).

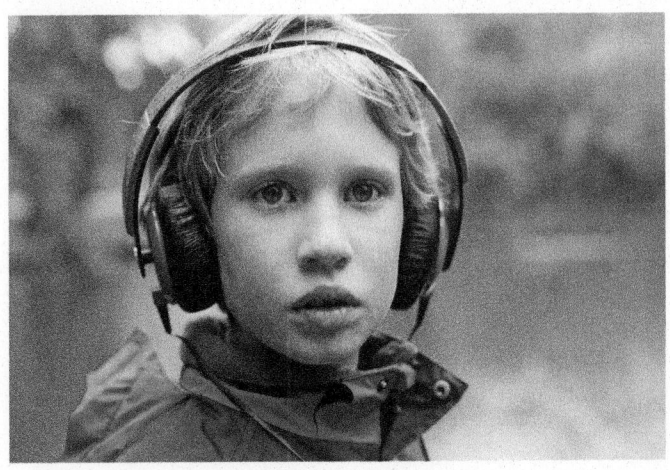

Figure 25.11 ›› This child with autism chooses to wear headphones whenever he leaves the house because loud noises hurt his ears and frighten him. The headphones give him a sense of security, making it easier for him to go out and interact with others.
Source: Maria Dubova/iStock/Getty Images.

Children with ASD may have a great difficulty dealing with new situations and typically show agitation and withdrawal when routines are changed. Children with ASD do not commonly explore objects but have stereotyped behaviors. They may line up objects, play with the same objects over and over, and have certain rituals that must be performed. They often become upset if these normal routines are disrupted. Rituals may involve eating only certain types or colors of foods or eating in specific patterns.

Pediatric patients may be cognitively impaired, but they can demonstrate a wide range of intellectual ability and functioning. Cognitive impairment may be manifested early in life by slow developmental progression, particularly in social skills. Some children with ASD are of at least average intelligence, and some are highly gifted. Some children with ASD are impaired in particular areas of development, whereas others are above normal.

Most children with autism do not present with physical signs. Unfortunately, this can create problems for the higher-functioning child, who might be perceived as "odd" or socially aloof. These individuals are often bullied and ostracized as a result. A minority of those with autism have macrocephaly, or brain overgrowth. Approximately 16% of young children with autism will develop a head circumference measuring above the 97th percentile (Hyman et al., 2020).

The clinical manifestations and therapies for ASD are outlined in the following feature.

Clinical Manifestations and Therapies

Autism Spectrum Disorder

SEVERITY	CLINICAL MANIFESTATIONS	CLINICAL THERAPIES*
Communication Deficits		
Mild	■ Difficulty initiating and maintaining social interactions ■ Reduced or unusual responses to overtures or communication from others	■ Visual cues and reminders; visual schedules ■ Speech-language therapy ■ Occupational therapy ■ Applied behavior analysis ■ Focused interventions ■ Environmental interventions
Moderate–Severe	■ Moderate to severe deficits in multiple areas of language/communication ■ Unable to initiate or sustain social interactions ■ Minimal or inappropriate responses to social overtures from others	All of the above, plus: ■ Sign language ■ Assistive communication devices
Repetitive/Restrictive Behaviors		
Mild	■ Inflexible behaviors that affect functioning at home and/or school ■ Problems with organization and planning ■ Some distress at switching activities, changes in routines ■ Mildly distressing repetitive behaviors, such as arm flapping	■ Behavior therapy or reinforcements ■ Environmental interventions
Moderate–Severe	■ Inflexible or restricted behaviors that severely impact functioning ■ Moderate to severe difficulty coping with change that severely impacts functioning ■ Moderate to severe distress at switching activities, changes in routines ■ Alarming and potentially dangerous repetitive behaviors such as biting self, head banging	

*Strengths-based approaches use a variety of evidence-based strategies to help children build skills and competencies. Selected therapy categories are mentioned here. Early diagnosis and intervention are essential to help children become more functional and independent.

Collaboration

Nurses frequently serve on interprofessional teams to ensure that medical and mental health needs of children with ASD are included in supportive plans. Team members may include parents, nurses, physicians, teachers, mental health professionals, speech-language pathologists, occupational therapists, and physical therapists. It is the role of the team to support and educate the family so they can make informed decisions regarding care, participate in the treatment process, and begin early interventions (Hyman et al., 2020).

A number of agencies and resources are available to support the child with ASD. Many communities have an interprofessional committee or team that meets regularly to review services available in their area for children with special needs, including ASD. By law, public schools are charged with the responsibility of facilitating and providing services for children age 3 and up with ASD and other disabilities. For preschool-age children, services may be provided directly by the school system or in collaboration with a preschool developmental day center. Some private schools do accept and provide accommodations for children with autism, and some private schools are created exclusively for students with learning challenges. However, private schools are not required by law to provide accommodations for children with disabilities.

Comorbid conditions that may occur in children with ASD include sleep disorders, seizures, GI symptoms, feeding problems, pica, obesity, and wandering. Depending on the individual needs of each child, other specialists may be part of the patient's care team. Behavioral diagnoses and disorders that may occur with ASD include ADHD, anxiety, mood disorders, food refusal, self-injurious behavior, and aggression. About one-third of children with ASD will also be affected by intellectual disability.

The overall prognosis for children with ASD to become functioning members of society is guarded. The extent to which adequate adjustment is achieved varies greatly. Successful adjustment is more likely for children with higher IQs, adequate speech, and access to specialized programs.

Diagnostic Tests

Diagnosis of autism is based on the presence of specific criteria, as described in the DSM-5 (Hyman et al., 2020). Symptoms must be persistent and cause impairments in everyday functioning. An early childhood intervention specialist, who may be a pediatrician or other licensed HCP, may conduct an initial screening as well as testing to rule out a medical cause of the child's behavior. Depending on the needs of the child, tests may include neuroimaging (CT scan or MRI), lead screening, DNA analysis, and electroencephalography.

Developmental screenings for language, cognition, and motor function should occur at 9, 18, and 30 months of age during well-child visits to allow for early identification of any deviations from normal developmental milestones. Children should be screened for ASD using a standardized tool at 18 and 24 months of age (Hyman et al., 2020). These early screenings allow for detection of at-risk children at a young age when interventions can improve outcomes. These screenings include asking parents about specific milestones and behaviors and through use of screening tools.

Focus on Diversity and Culture

Disparities in Diagnosis Narrowing

Data from the Autism and Developmental Disabilities Monitoring Network (2020) show that the prevalence of ASD in the United States is now approximately equal for white, Black, and Asian/Pacific Islander children and lower for Hispanic children. These data indicate that the racial and ethnic disparities that were formerly identified in the diagnosis of children with ASD may be narrowing. Discrepancies still exist, however, in the age at which a child is diagnosed with ASD. White children are more likely to be evaluated at an earlier age than Black and Hispanic children. This impairs the ability to provide early intervention in these children to improve their outcomes. To reduce disparities in identifying children with ASD at earlier ages in Black and Hispanic children, the CDC recommends that children be evaluated for ASD at the time parents, teachers, or others note any developmental issues. Community programs in targeted areas can further help to reduce this gap.

The Modified Checklist for Autism in Toddlers (M-CHAT) is commonly used for screening for ASD in toddlers. Based on the screening results, children are referred for further diagnostic testing, and early intervention is recommended. While ASD can be diagnosed in children as young as 18 months of age, children who have mild symptoms or whose intelligence is at or above average may not be diagnosed until they are older. As a result, screenings should be ongoing. Since girls tend to have less intense symptoms and external behaviors, ASD may not be diagnosed in girls as readily (Hyman et al., 2020). A diagnostic workup should also include language, cognitive, adaptive ability, and sensory assessments.

Pharmacologic Therapy

It is important for the nurse to teach families and patients that there is no medication that will "cure" autism. The FDA (2019) warns consumers about false advertising and cures for autism, including chelation therapy and mineral solutions. These "treatments" have been known to cause adverse effects, including nausea, vomiting, and electrolyte imbalances.

Medications are generally not used in the treatment of ASD. They may, however, be used to treat co-occurring conditions, such as sleep disorders, seizures, ADHD or other mental health condition, and GI problems (Hyman et al., 2020). GI problems may be related to sensory issues, restrictive eating patterns, delayed oral motor development, or a combination of these. Clinical guidelines recommend considering medication only after careful evaluation of behaviors, triggers, and functional assessment, as some conditions may be managed through behavioral or other nonpharmacologic interventions (Hyman et al., 2020).

SAFETY ALERT Many medications, in particular psychotropics, lack sufficient evidence related to safe use in children and adolescents (Solmi et al., 2020). A common-sense strategy is to start at the lowest dose and monitor children closely when initiating or changing doses. Nurses can encourage parents considering medications to ask such questions as (Jung Kim, 2020):

- How will this medication help my child?
- Is this the only option available?
- What are the potential side effects?
- What monitoring is recommended?
- Is it safe to stop taking it suddenly?

Nonpharmacologic Therapy

The goals of therapy for the child with ASD are to reduce deficits in social communication and interaction and minimize restrictive, repetitive behaviors; teach adaptive skills to improve functional independence; and reduce rigidity or stereotypy (repetitive, obsessive, machine-like movements) and other inappropriate behaviors. An individualized treatment plan is developed for each child, based on factors such as the intensity of symptoms, developmental level, and degree of cognitive impairment (Hyman et al., 2020). The best outcomes are achieved when intensive interventions are started early and include the family.

The infant brain is still developing and creating pathways and neurons. Research has shown a strong link between brain development and autism. As a result, early intervention to help facilitate healthy brain development may decrease the severity of symptoms and behaviors in the young child with ASD. In addition, those children who receive intense therapies in early childhood have better long-term outcomes and maintain higher functionality (Hyman et al., 2020).

Treatment focuses on behavior management to reward appropriate behaviors, foster positive or adaptive coping skills, and facilitate effective communication. Applied behavior analysis (ABA) is a commonly used treatment approach for autism. Based on the principles of B. F. Skinner's model that behaviors are reinforced with either positive or negative consequences, children with autism are taught behaviors with positive reinforcement or rewards. For example, a toddler who does not make eye contact may be taught to do so by being rewarded with a piece of cereal, or a 5-year-old might get a sticker on his shirt every time they complete a sentence.

Applied behavior analysis is very structured, intense, and lengthy, typically 6 to 8 hours a day for a minimum of 25 hours a week with a certified therapist. Parents continue the therapy when the therapist is not in the home (CDC, 2019b). However, ABA is only one of several evidence-based approaches, and individually based ABA therapy is not easily applied in a classroom setting, as most schools employ their own therapists and do not permit independent therapists to practice on site.

Focused interventions based on a functional analysis of behaviors as well as evaluations by a speech-language pathologist may also be included in the treatment plan to deal with specific skills, for example, developing social communication skills (Fuentes, Hervas, Howlin, & ESCAP ESD Working Party, 2020; Hyman et al., 2020). A variety of strategies have some evidence for usefulness and may be applied across settings and regardless of approach. These include incorporating interventions into daily routines, making environmental adaptations, providing positive reinforcement that has meaning to the child, and parent teaching (Bottema-Beutel & Crowley, 2020).

Complementary Health Approaches

When faced with the diagnosis of autism in a child, many parents seek complementary and alternative therapies, despite the fact that research continues to show that most complementary and alternative therapies are not effective in the treatment of autism (Hyman et al., 2020).

A popular option with parents of children with ASD is implementation of a gluten-free, casein-free (GFCF) diet. This has gained popularity and there are websites and programs devoted to this diet. Essentially, the GFCF diet eliminates the proteins gluten and casein; however, evidence to support this diet is lacking (Hyman et al., 2020). Nurses working with parents considering the GFCF diet should encourage them to consult with a nutritionist or registered dietitian who can help them make sure that they plan GFCF meals that will meet their child's nutritional needs.

Nurses can help parents evaluate studies on complementary care and encourage parents to initiate only one treatment at a time; the effectiveness of any one treatment cannot be measured properly if it is initiated in conjunction with other therapies. At each healthcare interaction, the nurse working with a patient with ASD should ask about therapies being used and discuss safeguards to avoid any undesired side effects.

Lifespan Considerations

Childhood ASD persists into adulthood. Children who receive timely intervention and whose parents and treatment teams collaborate to find the best treatment for them as individuals have the greatest chance of becoming successfully functioning adults. Even high-functioning adults with ASD continue to struggle with communication skills, especially understanding nonverbal communication and socialization. Adults with ASD are most successful when they seek employment opportunities and activities that play to their strengths.

Many communities provide job training and supervised work programs for adults with ASD. Adults with less severe ASD may be active community members, becoming fully employed and living independently. Others need more support and may choose to continue to live with their parents or to reside in a group living environment that provides additional support. A number of government programs assist these individuals with financial support. Information on these programs is available from the Social Security Administration as well as local, state, and county social services. In addition, such nonprofit organizations as Easter Seals and Goodwill offer employment opportunities and resources. Finally, several internet resources, such as AutismSpeaks.org, are available for adults with autism to navigate different systems.

Few clinics exist that specifically treat adults with ASD, making it challenging for adults to get the best level of care. Many adults with ASD who cannot function independently or whose families can no longer provide care for them end up being financially subsidized by the state. With the steady rise in the number of children diagnosed with this disorder comes a resulting increase in the number of adults with the disorder. The financial impact on state governments is significant and is likely to increase steadily for many years. This is another reason why children with ASD need to be identified early, so that they may have access to treatments and therapies that give them the best chance to become fully functioning adults.

As the person with autism matures, the likelihood of developing a mental health condition, such as anxiety or depression, also increases. The person with autism may not recognize the signs of mental illness; likewise, practitioners might not recognize signs of mental illness in the adult autistic patient (Huang, Arnold, Foley, & Trollor, 2020). In turn, the individual with ASD may show decreased functioning that is not related to autism but, rather, to undiagnosed mental illness. This adds to the burden of care.

Autism is a lifelong condition, but the greater concentration of research, resources, funding, and support is focused on children and young adults. Research on adults with ASD remains lacking, especially for the geriatric population, and diagnosis in this population is rarely done.

NURSING PROCESS

Throughout the nursing process, the patient's parents and family will be integral team members. Because much of the assessment data are collected by way of interview, the nurse should establish effective, open communication patterns with the parents. Developing good communication with parents will help to develop a trusting relationship in the care of the child with ASD.

Assessment

Initial concerns about a child with ASD may arise related to a possible hearing, speech, or developmental delay. Even though all children develop at their own pace, standardized ASD screening at 18 and 24 months along with early screening for developmental milestones will help identify potential problems at a younger age. This is essential since the earlier intervention is offered, the more likely the child is to achieve positive, long-term outcomes (Hyman et al., 2020).

- ***Observation and patient/family interview***. Parents may report that their child has abnormal interaction such as lack of eye contact, disinterest in cuddling, minimal facial responsiveness, and failure to talk. Be alert to observations by the parents that the baby or young child does not look at them or provide other developmental or behavioral cues. Initial assessment focuses on language development, response to others, and hearing acuity. Become familiar with the following "red flags" that require immediate evaluation (CDC, 2019i), such as:

  - No reaction to name by 12 months
  - No pointing to objects of interest by 14 months
  - No pretend play by 18 months
  - No eye contact
  - Delayed speech and language abilities.

  Note both maternal and parental ages at the time the child was born. Consider genetic history of autism or like behaviors in the patient's families. Ask about prenatal history, including possible neonatal exposure to toxins or medications such as antiepileptics. Carefully evaluate the child for history of developmental milestones. Participate in developmental screening, including motor activity, social skills, and language, or refer the family to a professional or community resource that provides such screenings. Recall that the child may have normal performance in one area such as motor skills but delayed development in another area such as language skills. Likewise, language may be normal for age, but social interactions are delayed. Include questions about adaptive skills such as toilet training and feeding patterns. Inquire about school performance because some areas may be normal while others are delayed. Observe the child in play situations and evaluate the use of creative and exploratory play versus more repetitive patterns.

  When a child with a diagnosis of ASD is hospitalized for a concurrent problem, obtain a history from the parents regarding the child's routines, rituals, and likes and dislikes, as well as ways to promote interaction and cooperation. Children with ASD may carry a special toy or object that they play with during times of stress. Ask parents about these objects and their use. Ask about the child's behaviors and observe them on admission. Obtain a history of acute and chronic illnesses and injuries. Ask about eating patterns and food restrictions. Inquire about complementary health approaches in a nonjudgmental and supportive manner.

  For the adult patient with ASD, the nurse should remember that behaviors of other mental health conditions are similar and may overlap autism behaviors. These conditions include schizophrenia, ADHD, and obsessive–compulsive disorder (NIMH, 2018). Similar behaviors regarding ability to socialize, eye contact, sensory disorders, and repetitive behaviors will be present in the adult with ASD. Adults who are diagnosed later in life are typically higher functioning and may have careers and families. Many adults initiate the diagnosis with their provider and may express relief after their diagnosis, as their behaviors have an etiology. Yet others may express sadness because there is no "cure" for ASD.

  Just as with the evaluation of a child who potentially has autism, the nurse will question the adult patient regarding family history, neonatal exposures, birth history, and developmental history. Family members and others close to the patient are helpful in filling in any details the patient is unable to provide.

- ***Physical examination***. The physical exam for autism often will reveal no abnormalities because of the neurodevelopmental nature of this disorder. However, the nurse may face challenges in the physical assessment because of behavioral issues. The nurse will have to adapt the physical exam according to the patient's temperament, cognitive level, sensory perceptions, and developmental stage.

  Patients with ASD who have sensory deficits or behaviors often do not like being touched. The patient might complain that a light touch hurts, yet giggle with immunizations. If asked to change into a gown, the patient may not like the material of the gown against the skin, becoming irritable or focused on the gown rather than the exam.

  The patient may not sit still for the exam or may display flapping, rocking, or head-banging to self-soothe during the exam. If the patient becomes overwhelmed, the patient might have what is perceived as a temper tantrum, otherwise known colloquially as an "autistic meltdown." The nurse should stop the examination, reduce sensory stimuli, and ensure the patient's safety during this time.

Many individuals with ASD do not like quick transitions. Just as with neurotypical children, the nurse should tell the patient before doing certain assessments. For example, before assessing a patient's eyes with a penlight, the nurse should tell the patient first before shining a bright beam.

If the patient is nonverbal, the nurse should not assume the patient does not understand language. The nurse should continue to talk and explain each step during the assessment. The nurse should also consider alternative communication tools to ask the patient questions. Some patients use pictures, sign language, and technology (e.g., smartphone apps that convert pictures into spoken words) to communicate.

Encourage the patient or parents to bring an item that offers comfort, such as a blanket or favorite object. Perform the exam in small, short steps and consider giving the patient a reward with each step (as typically done in ABA treatments). The nurse should never restrain a patient, particularly an older child or adult, to complete an exam. Examination of the adult patient will be very similar but is likely to be less challenging than examining a child. However, many adults with ASD do have sensory perception issues and others have difficulty with communication. The communication challenges may manifest as social awkwardness during the exam. The patient might pull away from certain aspects of the physical exam. The nurse should advise the patient of each step of the exam, paying careful attention to transitions and actions.

Diagnosis

Priorities for care vary depending on the needs of the individual patient and family. Common issues that may be appropriate for inclusion in the plan of care for the patient as well as the family include:

- Risk of injury
- Potential for developmental delay
- Lack of knowledge about condition, needs, or appropriate care
- Impaired verbal communication
- Inadequate social skills
- Caregiver burden
- Inadequate family coping skills or resources.

Planning

Nursing care of children with ASD focuses on preventing injury, stabilizing environmental stimuli, providing supportive care, enhancing communication, giving the parents anticipatory guidance, and providing emotional support. Appropriate outcomes for a child with ASD and the family may include the following:

- The child will remain free of injury.
- The child will acquire strategies that enable communication with others.
- The child will be able to perform self-care to maximum potential.
- The child will demonstrate consistent developmental progress.
- The child will participate in small-group activities with family members or peers.
- The child's symptoms will be managed successfully.
- The parents will verbalize confidence in caregiver skills.

Nursing care of adults with a new diagnosis of ASD focuses on education and coping. Care of the adult with a current diagnosis of ASD focuses on assessing and promoting social interactions, continued education regarding diagnosis, and establishing and maintaining individual functions. Planning may include the following goals:

- The patient will remain free from injury.
- The patient will verbalize understanding of diagnosis.
- The patient will demonstrate positive coping skills.
- The patient will participate in social activities with peers, coworkers, and family members.
- The patient will maintain independence to the full potential of the individual.

Implementation

Working with families, particularly with children and their parents, is critical to caring for children with ASD. Patience and understanding are essential when providing care to families with loved ones with ASD. Parental responses may range from aggressive attempts to gain information and resources to exhaustion from caring for a child with communication deficits and challenging behaviors that require constant monitoring. The nurse may be the most accessible, most caring professional available to them.

Adults with ASD will want to have structure and a predictable course of action. Adults with ASD often are very punctual and time-conscious. Nurses should be aware that any delay in treatments may cause anxiety in the adult with ASD. Nurses should provide education for the adult patient, as well as any family members involved. Emotional support may be needed, particularly for the adult patient who will not benefit from ABA and other early interventions. Support services and groups may not be readily available for the adult patient. However, there are internet support groups through such websites as Autism Speaks and the National Autism Network. Case management services may help the adult with ASD navigate through the healthcare system.

Prevent Injury

Monitor children with ASD at all times, including bath time and during play time. Close supervision ensures that the child does not obtain any harmful objects or engage in dangerous behaviors. For the child who engages in head banging or other harmful behaviors, bicycle helmets and hand mitts can be the least restrictive method for providing safety. These items enable the child to participate in activities and engage in a social environment to the degree possible.

Provide Anticipatory Guidance

Many children with ASD will require lifelong supervision and support, especially if the disorder is accompanied by intellectual disability. Some children may grow up to lead independent lives, although they may have social limitations with impaired interpersonal relationships. Encourage parents to promote the child's development through behavior modification and specialized educational programs. The overall goal is to provide the child with the guidance, education, and support necessary for optimal functioning.

Address Environmental Issues

Patients with ASD interpret and respond to the environment differently than other individuals. Sounds that are not distressing to other individuals may be interpreted as loud, frightening, and overwhelming to children with ASD. They may respond to different sounds or environments by withdrawing, crying, or using ritualistic behaviors such as arm flapping, which may or may not be self-injurious.

The patient with ASD needs to be oriented to new settings such as a hospital room and should be encouraged to bring familiar items from home. To avoid distressing the patient, minimize relocation of objects within the environment.

Provide Supportive Care

Developing a trusting relationship with the patient who has ASD is often difficult. Adjust communication techniques and teach to the patient's developmental level. Ask about the patient's usual home routines and maintain these routines as much as possible when the patient is out of the home.

Because self-care abilities are often limited, the child or adult with ASD may need assistance to meet basic needs. When possible, schedule daily care and routine procedures at consistent times to maintain predictability. Identify rituals for naptime and bedtime and maintain them to promote rest and sleep. Integrate patterns that facilitate intake of nutritious foods at mealtimes. If the child is hospitalized, encourage parents to remain with the child and to participate in daily care planning.

All patients with ASD need emotional support. Children who are developing successfully may face new challenges with the onset of the emotional and hormonal changes of adolescence. As social circles develop in middle and high school, the adolescent with autism may become more aware of being different from peers. The nurse may see this when a parent brings in a child after a scuffle at school or for help with increasingly self-destructive behaviors as the child struggles to deal with the many changes inherent in adolescence. The nurse can provide crucial information about the physical changes adolescents experience and help the parent modify the plan of care to include opportunities for building new skills the child needs to navigate this difficult time.

Enhance Communication

Because patients with autism have impaired communication skills, nursing care focuses on improving communication with the patient. When speaking, use short, direct sentences and keep distractions to a minimum (Zanotti, 2018). If the patient responds well to visual cues, then pictures, computers, and other visual aids may form an important part of interaction. Some patients with limited verbal skills learn and communicate through sign language, pictures, talking boxes, and smartphone apps.

Children with ASD benefit from speech and language therapy. Encourage parents to maintain close contact with speech therapists. Use of consistent communication techniques at home and at school provides further stability for the child and increases opportunities for successful communication.

Communicating with Patients

Working Phase

When communicating with a child with ASD, take a deep breath and slow down. Reduce sensory stimulation, such as by closing the door to shut out noise and dimming the lights. Use short sentences and concrete words. Avoid abstract words and metaphors. For example, if the nurse needs to obtain a child's weight at an office visit, rather than saying "Let's get a weight and see how much you've grown. . . . Oh my, you are growing like a wildflower," the nurse might say the following:

- I need you to take off your shoes.
- Good work. Now, step up on the scale.
- You weigh 53 pounds, that's 3 more pounds than you weighed last visit.

Facilitate Community-Based Care

Families need strong support to cope with the challenges of caring for the child or adult family member with ASD. Many communities offer training programs for parents, in addition to support groups. Help parents identify resources for childcare, such as special toddler programs and preschools. Provide resources for case management, respite care, and governmental services, including Social Security benefits to help with the added cost of ASD treatments.

Nurses working in these community training programs and support services can help parents cope with the stresses of having a child with ASD. Nurses can provide guidance in stress-reduction techniques, stress management, self-care, and mind–body therapies.

The patient may need specialized transportation services and other social supports. The school-age child will need an IEP. School programs and IEPs can help the child learn self-care skills. Parents are integral parts of the treatment team when the child's learning goals are established in early intervention or school programs.

The parent or primary caregiver may have difficulty obtaining respite care and may need assistance to find suitable resources. Siblings of children with autism may need help explaining the disorder to their friends or teachers. The nurse can be instrumental in assisting these siblings in understanding and explaining autism.

Local support groups for parents of autistic children are available in most areas. Families can also be referred to local chapters of national autism programs. There are support groups for teens and adults with ASD as well. Many connect via social media networks and internet resources. Social media is becoming a more popular way for those with ASD to socialize and plan get-togethers. Social media may be used to find friends, which might be difficult in other social settings.

» **Stay Current:** Patients of all ages with ASD and their families can find support online and in their communities. Autism Speaks, https://www.autismspeaks.org; Autism Society of America, http://www.autism-society.org; and the National Autism Association, https://nationalautismassociation.org are websites that are current on best practices for autism in several areas, including research, education, therapies, and other things related to autism.

Evaluation

At each healthcare interaction, the nurse discusses the child's progress with the parents, including any injuries that have occurred since the previous visit and the steps being taken to prevent recurrence. The nurse asks parents what type of environments the child is in during the day, paying particular attention to the frequency of transitions and changes in caregivers. For example, a child with ASD who attends school or an early intervention program at a preschool will do well having the same caregiver drop off the child in the morning and pick up the child at the end of the school day.

Children who are enrolled in early intervention programs or who have IEPs at school may benefit from having the nurse participate as part of the treatment team. If this is not possible, the nurse should ask the parent how the child's treatment is progressing and continue to encourage open communication between the parents and the treatment team. For children who are taking medication to treat a comorbid disorder, such as depression or ADHD, the nurse should, with parent permission, provide the necessary information to the treatment team so that the team is aware of potential side effects.

For adult patients with ASD, the nurse should inquire about coping strategies, workplace relationships, family relationships, anxieties, and social connections. Nurses may also ask about the usefulness of resources and support services. If the adult is taking medications, the nurse can evaluate for the desired effects and side effects of the medication.

REVIEW Autism Spectrum Disorder

RELATE Link the Concepts and Exemplars

Linking the exemplar of autism spectrum disorder with the concept of family:

1. How can the nurse support the family of a child with ASD?
2. How might other children in the family be impacted by a sibling with ASD?

Linking the exemplar of autism spectrum disorder with the concept of safety:

3. What interventions are important for the nurse to initiate to maintain the safety of a patient with autism?
4. What safety interventions would be important at school?

READY Go to Volume 3: Clinical Nursing Skills

REFER Go to Pearson MyLab Nursing and eText

REFLECT Apply Your Knowledge

Four-year-old Finn was recently diagnosed with ASD. Finn's parents are struggling with the diagnosis, wondering if the treatment team has misdiagnosed their child. They have told the treatment team that Finn is just a little slow and will catch up. At the same time, they are trying to cope with his challenging behaviors, which include banging his head against the wall and wearing a pull-up diaper at all times for urinary incontinence.

1. Based on the case study, what are the priorities of nursing care for Finn?
2. Based on the statement made by Finn's parents, what are his parents experiencing?
3. How might the nurse locate resources to help Finn's parents learn more about having a child with autism? What resources might the nurse find?

» Exemplar 25.C Cerebral Palsy

Exemplar Learning Outcomes

25.C Analyze CP as it relates to development.

- Describe the pathophysiology of CP.
- Describe the etiology of CP.
- Compare the risk factors and prevention of CP.
- Identify the clinical manifestations of CP.
- Summarize diagnostic tests and therapies used by interprofessional teams in the collaborative care of an individual with CP.
- Differentiate care of patients with CP across the lifespan.
- Apply the nursing process in providing culturally competent care to an individual with CP.

Exemplar Key Term

Cerebral palsy (CP), *1877*

Overview

Cerebral palsy (CP) is a group of chronic conditions affecting body movement, coordination, and posture that results from a nonprogressive abnormality of the immature brain. CP often is the result of some type of insult to the developing brain of the fetus, neonate, or infant that occurs in the later stages of pregnancy, during birth, or within the first 2 years after birth. The impact of the disease can range from mild to profound mobility issues (**Figure 25.12** »). CP may or may not include intellectual disability.

Cerebral palsy occurs in an estimated 1 in 323 children (CDC, 2019h). Four types of motor dysfunction are seen with CP—spastic, dyskinetic, ataxic, and mixed—and are related

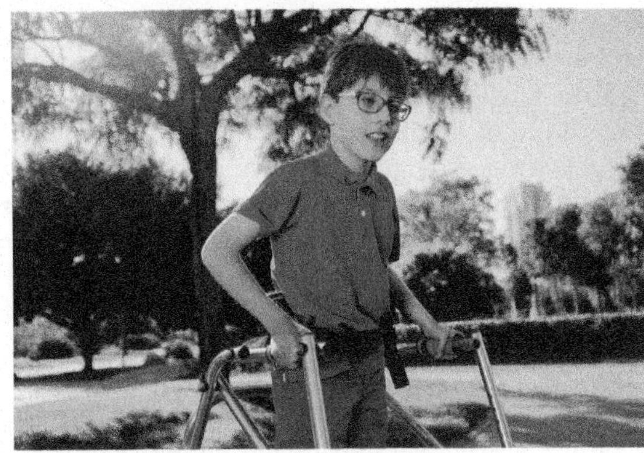

A

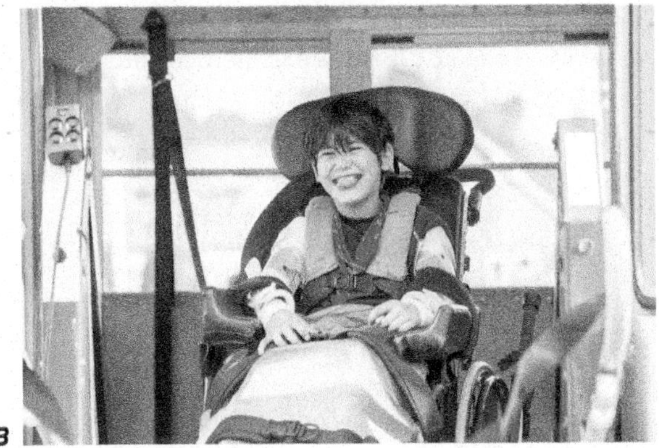

B

Figure 25.12 ›› Individuals with CP can have mild to profound mobility issues and may be able to walk unaided, need an assistive device ***A***, or use a wheelchair ***B***.

Sources: ***A***, Sweetmonster/iStock/Getty Images; ***B***, Jaren Wicklund/iStock/Getty Images.

to the location of brain insult. Spastic CP, the most common type, affects approximately 80% of those diagnosed with CP (CDC, 2020j).

Pathophysiology

Cerebral palsy involves abnormal development or damage to the immature brain that affects motor function and muscles (CDC, 2019e). There are two main categories: congenital and acquired. Congenital CP occurs during fetal development, birth, and the neonatal period. Acquired CP happens after the first 28 days of life. The specific insult leading to CP may not be identifiable if it occurs during the prenatal period. Moreover, since brain formation begins during the early embryonic period, timing of the insult is important. After the neonatal period, it may be easier to detect the reason for CP in a child, for example, an environmental or genetic cause. CP may result in changes in muscle tone, muscle reflexes, postural reactions, and primitive reflexes; it may also result in seizures, intellectual or learning disabilities, and hearing problems. The outcome depends on the area of the brain affected, the severity of the event, the duration of the insult, and the child's age at the time of the event.

Pathogenesis of CP is multifactorial and depends on the cause of the insult to the brain. Brain damage associated with cerebral palsy occurs in the motor areas of the brain, impairing the body's ability to control movement and adjust posture appropriately. CP cannot be cured, but the associated symptoms can be managed.

CP often is identified when children fail to meet expected developmental milestones and diagnostic testing is ordered to pinpoint the reason for the delay. Symptoms and manifestations vary from person to person depending on the exact neurologic impact of the event.

Etiology

Approximately 85–90% of children with CP are diagnosed with congenital CP (CDC, 2019c). At one time, hypoxia was considered the primary culprit for congenital CP; however, research now indicates that it is only responsible for a small number of cases. Instead, pathogens, toxins, trauma, and genetic mutations that affect the development of the brain are now suspected causes of CP.

The pathology of the brain injury depends on the etiology. For instance, pathogens that directly attack the brain—such as *Streptococcus pneumoniae* (pneumococcus), which is responsible for the majority of meningitis in infants—cause cellular damage through the consumption of the brain's tissue and production of the by-product lactic acid. Trauma stretches and shears neural pathways and brain tissue. Neurotoxins, such as bilirubin, accumulate in the bloodstream and eventually injure the nerve cells in the brain.

Risk Factors

Risk factors for cerebral palsy include events and exposures that may cause damage to the developing brain. Risk factors do not necessarily mean, however, that the infant has or will develop cerebral palsy. For instance, children conceived via assisted reproductive technology (ART) have a greater incidence of cerebral palsy; however, many conceived via ART do not develop CP.

Risk factors associated with congenital CP occurring in utero include infections such as pelvic inflammatory disease, rubella, chickenpox, CMV, and bacterial infections. Fevers in the mother prior to birth also may contribute to the development of CP. Cytokines, which are produced with fevers and certain infections, are thought to cause inflammation and damage to neurons in the developing fetus's brain (CDC, 2019c). Blood type incompatibility between the fetus and mother may cause CP. If the mother is exposed to toxins, such as mercury, there is a greater chance of CP (Abdel-Hamid, 2018). Likewise, if the mother has such conditions as seizures, thyroid disease, or proteinuria, there is a slightly greater chance of CP.

Birth and the health of the neonate are significant factors that contribute to the risk of developing CP. Risk factors associated with delivery include breech delivery, tight and nuchal cords, shoulder dystocia, uterine rupture, placenta previa, and fetal stress and hypoxia (Abdel-Hamid, 2018; CDC, 2019c; Mayo Clinic, 2019).

Preterm birth is also a risk factor for CP. Studies have found that the earlier in gestational age the infant is born, the greater the likelihood the infant will have CP (Mayo Clinic, 2019). Multiple fetuses are also at risk, partially due to the greater chance of preterm birth. Low birth weight, also associated with preterm birth and/or multiples, is also considered a risk factor. Neonates delivered with low Apgar scores have a greater risk of CP (Persson, Razaz, Tedroff, Joseph, & Cnattingius, 2018).

During the neonatal period, infants who have severe jaundice are at risk for developing CP due to hyperbilirubinemia. Bilirubin is considered a neurotoxin and can damage the fragile neonatal brain on the cellular level. Because the neonatal immune system is immature, the infant is particularly susceptible to meningitis and encephalitis, two conditions also associated with CP.

Brain trauma is also a risk factor for CP (CDC, 2019c). Neonates may experience trauma during birth from precipitous delivery, prolonged delivery, and other causes. After delivery, infants may experience trauma from shaken baby syndrome, being dropped, or improper placement in a car seat, as well as other means. The damage from these traumas puts the infant at risk for CP.

Prevention

A major factor in reducing the risk for CP is preventing premature and low-birth-weight births (Patel, Neelakantan, Pandher, & Merrick, 2020). Nurses should educate mothers-to-be on the prevention of preterm labor, including encouraging good prenatal care and visits with a provider. Nurses should also educate the pregnant patient on the signs and symptoms of preterm labor. Mothers with multiple fetuses require close monitoring. If the mother is placed on bedrest, the nurse should encourage the mother to comply with treatment in order to deliver a healthy baby.

Because maternal infection is associated with the development of CP, infection prevention, including maintaining good hand hygiene, is a primary goal (CDC, 2019c). Keeping current with vaccinations can also help the pregnant patient reduce the risk for having a baby born with CP. After birth, parents should avoid exposure of their infant to infection, including using good hand hygiene when caring for the infant. Vaccinations are essential in preventing certain infections that may cause CP, including the *Haemophilus influenzae* vaccination that helps prevent the most common form of bacterial meningitis.

Injury prevention, including properly securing infants during motor-vehicle travel and taking measures to prevent falls, serves to protect the child from brain trauma. Nurses should also educate parents on stress reduction and prevention of shaken baby syndrome.

>> **Stay Current:** Shaken baby syndrome, also referred to as abusive head trauma or shaken infant syndrome, occurs when a parent or caregiver severely shakes a baby. For more information, go to the National Center on Shaken Baby Syndrome, www.dontshake.org.

Clinical Manifestations

Abnormal muscle tone and lack of coordination, usually (but not always) accompanied by spasticity, are characteristic of CP. Symptoms vary by age, area of the brain involved, and degree of the insult to the brain. **Table 25.17** >> outlines typical symptoms of CP. The Clinical Manifestations and Therapies feature links clinical characteristics to the area of the brain involved.

Children with CP are usually delayed in meeting developmental milestones. For example, at 6 months of age, they may have persistent back arching, show little spontaneous movement, and be unable to sit up. They frequently have other problems, including visual defects such as strabismus (abnormal alignment of the eyes or "crossed eyes"), nystagmus (involuntary rapid eye movement), or refractory errors; hearing loss; language delay; speech impediment; or seizures. Feeding may be difficult because of oral motor involvement.

TABLE 25.17 Clinical Characteristics of Cerebral Palsy

Clinical Characteristics	Definitions
Hypotonia	Floppiness, increased range of motion of joints, diminished reflex response
Hypertonia, rigidity, spasticity	Tense, tight muscles Uncoordinated, awkward, stiff movements; scissoring or crossing of the legs; exaggerated reflex reactions
Athetosis	Constant involuntary writhing motions that are more severe distally
Ataxia	Poor muscle control during voluntary movement, poor balance
Hemiplegia	Involvement of one side of the body, with the upper extremities being more dysfunctional than the lower extremities
Diplegia	Involvement of all extremities, but the lower extremities are more affected than the upper, usually spastic
Quadriplegia	Involvement of all extremities with the arms in flexion and legs in extension

Source: Adapted from Ball et al. (2022).

Intellectual impairment is seen in approximately 49% of individuals with CP (Novak et al., 2017). Intellectual challenges are more commonly seen in those with spastic quadriplegia, whereas those with CP and a seizure disorder are most likely to have an intellectual disability (Sadowska, Sarecka-Hujar, & Koptya, 2020).

Collaboration

Care of the patient with CP requires an interprofessional team of nurses, physicians, physical therapists, occupational therapists, speech-language pathologists, dietitians, and social workers or case managers. Cerebral palsy is a lifelong condition that requires special consideration, particularly in the growing child who quickly outgrows assistive devices and must meet changing developmental needs.

>> **Stay Current:** For more information on CP, visit the National Institutes of Health at www.nlm.nih.gov/medlineplus/cerebralpalsy.html.

Diagnostic Tests

Diagnosis is usually based on clinical findings, including a history, standardized motor and neurological assessments, and brain imaging (Novak et al., 2017). The history should include signs and symptoms of CP, developmental milestones, and information about the pregnancy and perinatal and postnatal periods. Assessment tools to evaluate motor and neurological function, depending on the infant's age, include the Prechtl Qualitative Assessment of General Movements, Hammersmith Infant Neurological Examination, and Developmental

Clinical Manifestations and Therapies

Cerebral Palsy

ETIOLOGY	CLINICAL MANIFESTATIONS	CLINICAL THERAPIES*
Spastic *Cerebral cortex or pyramidal tract injury; most common form of CP, comprising 80% of cases (CDC, 2020j)*	▪ Persistent hypertonia, rigidity ▪ Exaggerated deep tendon reflexes ▪ Persistent primitive reflexes ▪ Leads to contractures and abnormal curvature of the spine	▪ Physical therapy ▪ Occupational therapy ▪ Speech therapy ▪ Canes, crutches, walkers, braces, splints, and other orthotics to promote mobility ▪ Special education ▪ Muscle relaxants ▪ Surgery to loosen contractures or to repair curvature of the spine
Dyskinetic—Athetosis *Extrapyramidal, basal ganglia injury*	▪ Abnormal muscle tone affecting all areas of body ▪ Difficulty with fine and purposeful motor movements ▪ Bizarre twisting movements	
Dyskinetic—Dystonia *Extrapyramidal injury, basal ganglia*	▪ Impairment of voluntary muscle control accompanied by appearance of involuntary movements (e.g., tics, chorea) ▪ Rigid muscle tone when awake and normal or decreased muscle tone when asleep ▪ Tremors ▪ Exaggerated posturing ▪ Inconsistent muscle tone that may change hour to hour or day to day	
Ataxic *Cerebellar (extrapyramidal) injury*	▪ Abnormalities of voluntary movement involving balance and position of the trunk and limbs ▪ Difficulty holding posture ▪ Muscle instability and wide-based, unsteady gait ▪ Difficulty controlling hand and arm movements when reaching ▪ Increased or decreased muscle tone ▪ Hypotonia in infancy	
Mixed *Injuries to multiple areas*	▪ No dominant motor pattern ▪ Unique compensatory movements and posture to maintain control over specific neuromotor deficits ▪ Combination of characteristics from other types	

*Therapies are based on clinical presentation of the individual and not by "type."

Source: Adapted from Ball et al. (2022).

Assessment of Young Children. Imaging tests that may be performed to detect brain abnormalities associated with CP include ultrasonography and MRI (Novak et al., 2017).

Cerebral palsy is more difficult to diagnose in the early months of life because it must be distinguished from other neurologic conditions and signs may be subtle. Cerebral palsy is usually diagnosed between 12 and 24 months of age (Novak et al., 2017). However, earlier diagnosis is recommended, particularly in those children with high risk factors, so that interventions can be initiated to improve neuromotor function.

Suspicious findings include an infant who is small for age or has a history of prematurity; low birth weight; low Apgar score (0 to 3 at 5 minutes); or the occurrence of an inflammatory, traumatic, or anoxic event (Persson et al., 2018). However, the majority of children who develop CP have normal Apgar scores at birth.

Surgery

Surgical interventions may be required to improve function by balancing muscle power and stabilizing uncontrollable joints. The Achilles tendon may be lengthened to increase range of motion in the ankle, which allows the heel to touch the floor and thus improves ambulation. The hamstrings may be released to correct knee flexion contractures. Other procedures may be performed to improve hip adduction or correct the foot's natural position.

Selective dorsal rhizotomy is a surgical procedure that disconnects afferent nerves in order to reduce spasticity and improve the ability to sit, stand, and walk. This is most commonly done in the spastic diplegia subtype of CP. Although this surgery helps reduce spastic muscles and has been shown to increase functionality, it can have troubling aftereffects, including muscle weakness (Wang, Munger, Chen, & Novacheck, 2018).

Pharmacologic Therapy

Medications are given to control seizures, reduce spasms (skeletal muscle relaxants, baclofen, and benzodiazepines), and minimize GI side effects (cimetidine or ranitidine). Baclofen is administered by intrathecal pump to decrease muscle tone and vasospasms when oral administration is ineffective or causes side effects (Adams et al., 2020).

Botulinum toxin (BT-A) injections are used to decrease focal spasticity and are considered standard practice. BT-A helps relax the contracted muscle (see **Medications 25.2**, Drugs Used to Treat Cerebral Palsy). Used in conjunction with a stretching program, those who undergo this treatment report good results (Sadowska et al., 2020). For an overview of seizure medications, see Exemplar 11.B, Seizure Disorders, in Module 11, Intracranial Regulation.

Medications 25.2

Drugs Used to Treat Cerebral Palsy*

CLASSIFICATIONS AND DRUG EXAMPLES	MECHANISMS OF ACTION	NURSING CONSIDERATIONS
Alpha$_2$-Adrenergic Antagonists ***Drug example:*** tizanidine (Zanaflex)	Increase presynaptic inhibition of motor neurons at the spinal cord level, reducing skeletal muscle spasms.	Monitor for effectiveness (decreased muscle tone). Contraindicated with ciprofloxacin and fluvoxamine. Monitor for and report orthostatic hypotension or bradycardia. Teach patients to monitor for sedation and to report hallucinations or delusions.
Benzodiazepines ***Drug example:*** diazepam (Valium)	Depending on dosage, diazepam can affect skeletal muscle relaxation and act as an anticonvulsant due to its action on the CNS. Only the oral and IM routes of administration are indicated for muscle spasticity.	Monitor for therapeutic effectiveness as tolerance may develop. Prolonged use requires periodic complete blood counts and liver function tests (LFTs). Prolonged use should be accompanied by periodic risk–benefit analysis due to risks associated with long-term use of benzodiazepines. Monitor for signs of depression and suicidal ideation in patients with comorbid depression or anxiety.
Muscle Relaxants ***Drug examples:*** baclofen (Gablofen, Lioresel, Ozobax)	Depress afferent reflex activity at the spinal cord, stimulate GABA receptors, decreasing excitatory messages to alpha-motor neurons.	Monitor for: ■ Orthostatic hypotension, ambulation problems ■ CNS side effects: confusion, depression, hallucinations ■ Baseline and periodic blood glucose and LFTs. There is a *black box warning* related to abrupt discontinuation of baclofen. Caution patients not to stop taking baclofen without consultation with HCP.
dantrolene (Dantrium)	Interferes with the release of calcium ions from skeletal muscle cells.	Monitor for: ■ Signs of hepatotoxicity (jaundice, clay-colored stools, dark urine, abdominal discomfort) ■ Weakness, dizziness ■ Vital signs, electrocardiogram, central venous pressure during infusion; serum potassium There is a *black box warning* for dantrolene related to risk of hepatotoxicity. Report: ■ Lack of response within 45 days of treatment Safe use in children younger than 5 years old has not been established.
Neuromuscular Blockers ***Drug example:*** abobotulinumtoxinA (Dysport)	Botulinum toxin type A (a neurotoxin produced by the bacillus *Clostridium botulinum*) inhibits release of acetylcholine, the neurotransmitter involved in voluntary contraction of skeletal muscle.	Monitor for and report: ■ Anaphylaxis ■ Difficulty breathing or swallowing ■ Difficulty speaking ■ Unusual bleeding, bruising, or swelling around injection site

*Antiseizure drugs are covered in Exemplar 11.B, Seizure Disorders, in Module 11, Intracranial Regulation.

Nonpharmacologic Therapy

Clinical therapy focuses on helping the child develop to a maximum level of independence. Early intervention services are key and may include a combination of physical, occupational, and speech therapy, as well as special education. Physical therapy helps to improve motor function, ability, strength, and range of motion and reduce contractures (Patel et al., 2020). Interventions vary depending on the child's needs. Braces and splints, serial casting, and positioning devices (prone wedges, standers, and sidelyers) are used to promote range of motion, skeletal alignment, stability, and control of involuntary movements. Constraint-induced movement therapy (CIMT) has been shown to be helpful for those with hemiplegia. In CIMT, the less or nonaffected arm is restrained to promote use of the more affected arm (Novak et al., 2017). Another therapy, Goals-Activity-Motor Enrichment (GAME) is an intensive family- and home-based program of enriched task-specific interventions managed by physical and occupational therapists to improve motor function (Novak et al., 2017).

Occupational therapy focuses on improving fine motor control and use of adaptive devices to promote as much independence as possible with self-care (Patel et al., 2020). Speech therapy can assess the individual's ability to swallow food and teach both the individual and caregiver safe feeding techniques. Tube feedings may be needed if the child is unable to safely swallow. The speech therapist can also help parents to promote communication and to learn alternative communication measures when the child is unable to communicate orally. Social and psychological support can help to improve quality of life for the child, parents, and family.

Lifespan Considerations

Many children with CP grow up to be independent, functioning adults with careers, families, and social support systems (**Figure 25.13** ››). Having CP does take a toll on the adult body. Many adults with CP have chronic pain due to contractions of the muscles, arthritis due to the wear and tear on the joints, and persistent fatigue due to the extended energy needed to work against the contracted muscles.

Because CP puts the body in a continual stress state, many adults experience signs of premature aging by their early 40s, including atherosclerosis, osteoarthritis, and hypertension (Whitney et al., 2018; Yi, Jung, & Bang, 2019). As individuals with CP age, they are more prone to urinary and bowel incontinence, which can hamper their quality of life. With all these factors affecting the patient with CP, depression is not uncommon. Comorbidities such as seizures and respiratory disorders often shorten the life of the person with CP.

NURSING PROCESS

Nursing care focuses on early intervention, prevention of complications, and support of children and families to help them cope with the diagnosis of CP.

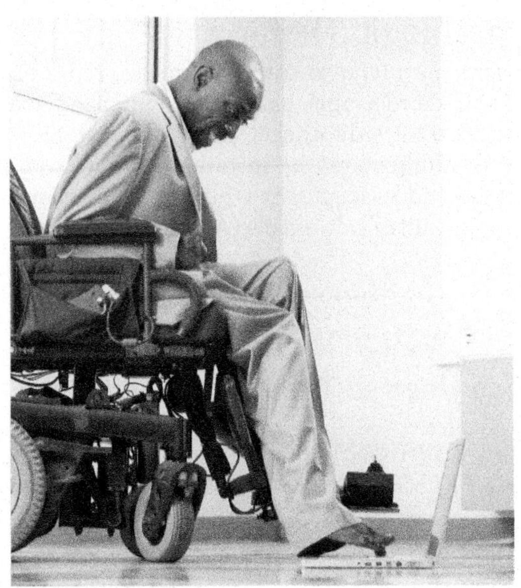

Figure 25.13 ›› This man with CP uses a wheelchair and works on his laptop using his foot.
Source: Huntstock/Getty Images.

Assessment

Be alert for children whose histories indicate an increased risk for CP. It is not uncommon for children who are delayed in meeting developmental milestones or have neuromuscular abnormalities at 1 year of age to show gradual improvement in function. The child with mild symptoms may not be diagnosed as early as a child with a more severe presentation.

Assess all children at each healthcare visit for developmental delays. Note any orthopedic, visual, auditory, or intellectual deficits. Assess for newborn reflexes, which may persist beyond the normal age in a child with CP. Identify infants who appear to have abnormal muscle tone or abnormal posture (child has an arched back, child becomes stiff when moving against gravity, child's neck or extremities have increased or decreased resistance to passive movement). A child with asymmetric or abnormal crawling using two or three extremities indicates a motor problem. Hand dominance before the preschool years is another sign of a motor problem. Record dietary intake as well as height and weight percentiles for children suspected to have or to be diagnosed with the condition.

Evaluate all infants who show symptoms of developmental delays, feeding difficulties caused by poor sucking, or abnormalities of muscle tone. Two simple screening assessments are helpful:

- Place a clean diaper on the 6- to 12-month-old infant's face. The infant without special needs will use two hands to remove it, but the infant with CP will use one hand or will not remove the cloth at all.
- Turn the infant's head to one side. A persistent asymmetric tonic neck reflex (beyond 6 months of age) indicates a pathologic condition. Suspect CP in any infant who has persistent primitive reflexes.

Diagnosis

Patient care needs vary depending on the type of CP, the particular child's symptoms and age, and the family situation. Examples of priorities relevant to caring for the patient with CP may include the following:

- Risk of injury
- Compromised physical mobility
- Potential for undernutrition
- Potential for impaired tissue integrity
- Impaired verbal communication
- Pain
- Caregiver burden.

Planning

Because CP can range from mild to severe and may involve numerous manifestations, care planning must be highly individualized based on the specific needs of each individual. It may include the following goals:

- The patient will remain free from injury.
- The patient will demonstrate appropriate growth and development.
- The patient will maintain an appropriate diet to meet nutritional needs.
- The patient will be able to communicate basic needs.
- The patient will indicate that discomfort is at a tolerable level.
- The patient's skin will remain intact and free of injury.
- The parents utilize effective coping strategies.

Implementation

Interventions are tailored to the needs of each child and family. Many of the child's interventions will be provided through therapists and/or in an educational setting. Nurses provide family-focused care that includes patient teaching related to safety, nutrition, overall growth and development, day-to-day care for the child, and emotional support. Because children with CP are at increased risk for skin conditions, nursing care should include patient and family education about maintaining skin integrity.

Prevent Injury

Patients with CP have varying degrees of mobility. The nurse should ensure that the patient receives the degree of assistance required for safe ambulation and that orthotic and assistive devices are used properly. Maintaining a safe environment includes eliminating all potential obstacles from walkways and providing adequate lighting. Assess caregivers and family members for awareness of safety precautions and provide teaching as needed, especially related to the use of safety belts in strollers and wheelchairs, as well as adaptive safety seats for transportation in vehicles. Physical therapy can help reduce the risk of injury through strength, mobility, posture, and balance training. Children with chronic seizures may need to wear helmets to protect them from head injury.

Communicating with Families

Working Phase

Feeding the child with CP can be stressful, messy, lengthy, and, overall, not an enjoyable experience. Additionally, the caregiver needs to be mindful of the increased caloric needs of the child with CP as well as the risk for aspiration (Scarpato et al., 2017). Here are some helpful openings and responses by the nurse when addressing the issue of feeding with a parent:

- Tell me about mealtime in your house.
- That sounds stressful. Let's talk more about your fear of your child choking.
- I'd like to help you feed your child lunch today. Then we can talk about how it went.

Promote Community-Based Services

Children with CP need continuous support in the community. A case manager is often needed to coordinate care. Parents may need financial assistance to provide for the child's needs and to obtain appliances such as braces, wheelchairs, or adaptive utensils. As they grow, children need new adaptive devices, ongoing developmental assessment and care planning, and sometimes surgery. Although the brain lesion does not change, it manifests differently as the child grows. For example, once the child begins to walk, the extensor tone may cause tightening of the Achilles cord. Braces may decrease deformities, but surgery may be needed eventually. The nurse or HCP is often the one to make referrals to early intervention programs to assist parents in meeting their child's needs. In addition, the nurse makes referrals, as appropriate, to support groups and organizations such as the United Cerebral Palsy Association and Shriners Hospitals.

An individualized transition plan developed during adolescence assists the family and adolescent with CP to develop plans for adult living. Vocational training options can be explored. The young adult (18 to 21 years) may be able to move into a group home or live independently if desired.

Provide Adequate Nutrition

Because children with CP require greater energy for movement and muscle contraction, they need high-calorie meals and snacks and/or supplements to their diets to meet their energy needs. Problems with swallowing, sucking, chewing, and movements in the mouth and jaw also cause nutritional challenges. Children who are able to eat may need soft foods in small amounts and adaptive utensils that are easier for them to use. Individuals with CP may also have dysphagia (difficulty swallowing), which affects nutrition and carries the risk of aspiration (Benfer et al., 2017).

» **Skills:** See Skill 10.3, Eating Assistance: Providing, in Volume 3.

Oral hygiene can sometimes be an issue. Dental caries and gum disease are common in patients with CP because of difficulties with brushing teeth. This can also add to nutritional deficits if pain occurs with eating.

Maintain Skin Integrity

Children with CP are at risk for skin breakdown at bony prominences and with use of splints or braces. Monitor and provide parent teaching related to skin surveillance and care. If skin underneath a brace or splint is red, the device should be removed and not used again until the redness is gone.

Children should maintain proper body alignment. Infants with "floppy" heads will need head and body support. Pillows, bolsters, and towels should be used when the child is in a bed or chair. Spasticity can cause scissored, extended legs. Some children may be difficult to carry or transport, especially if they have athetoid movements.

Promote Physical Mobility

Range-of-motion exercises are essential to maintain joint flexibility and prevent contractures. Consult with the child's physical therapist and help with recommended exercises. Teach parents to position the child to foster flexion rather than extension so that the child can more easily interact with the environment (e.g., by bringing objects closer to the face). Consider the use of therapeutic massage and ROM exercise to help strengthen muscles and promote flexibility.

As the child grows, adaptive and assistive technology may be needed to promote mobility. Assistive technology is any item, equipment, or product customized for use to promote the functional capabilities and independence of an individual with disabilities. Examples include computers, adaptive utensils, and customized wheelchairs. Refer parents to the appropriate resources for help obtaining adaptive devices. Encourage parents to bring in the child's adaptive appliances (braces, positioning devices) for use during hospitalization.

Promote Growth and Development

Many children with CP have physical disabilities but not necessarily intellectual disabilities. Use terminology appropriate for the child's developmental level. Help the child develop a positive self-image to ensure emotional health and social growth. Adaptive devices may be available to help the child with CP to communicate more independently. Children with hearing loss may need a referral to learn American Sign Language or other communication methods. Provide audio and visual activities for the child who is quadriplegic.

Provide Parent Education

Teach parents about the disorder and their child's special needs. Teach administration, desired effects, and side effects of medications prescribed for seizures. Make sure parents are aware of the need for dental care for children, especially those taking anticonvulsants and other medications that can impact oral health. Parents also may need suggestions for promoting the child's autonomy and abilities.

Provide Emotional Support

Parents require emotional support to help them cope with the diagnosis. Listen to the parents' concerns and encourage them to express their feelings and ask questions. Explain what they can expect from future treatment. Refer parents to individual and family counseling and support groups, if appropriate. Work with other healthcare professionals to help families adjust to this chronic disease.

EVALUATION

Patients are evaluated based on their ability to meet goals identified in the plan of care, which may include the following:

- Patient's growth is appropriate for age.
- Patient meets developmental milestones appropriate for age.
- Patient's nutritional status is adequate for age and energy needs.
- Patient is able to communicate needs.
- Patient does not show evidence of skin breakdown.
- Patient verbalizes an adequate comfort level.
- Parents report they are attending a support group.

Nursing Care Plan

A Patient with Cerebral Palsy

Justine McBride is a 2-year-old girl. Her mother was age 37 and her father was age 45 when Justine was born. She is the seventh child in the family. Her mother works as a chemist in a local laboratory and her father is an accountant for a large firm.

ASSESSMENT	DIAGNOSES	PLANNING
Justine's mother became concerned that Justine was not walking when she turned 14 months old; all her other children were walking by 12 months of age. Testing was performed, and Justine was diagnosed with spastic CP. Examination of Justine demonstrates scissoring of the legs when prone, stiff movements of arms and legs, hyperreflexia, and muscular rigidity.	■ Compromised physical mobility related to decreased muscle strength and control ■ Undernutrition related to difficulty in chewing and swallowing and high metabolic needs ■ Inadequate family health maintenance related to excessive demands made on family with child's complex care needs	Goals for Justine's care include the following: ■ Justine will reach maximum physical mobility and developmental milestones. ■ Justine will receive adequate visual sensory/perceptual input to maximize developmental outcome. ■ Justine will exhibit normal growth patterns for height, weight, and other physical parameters. ■ Justine's family will successfully support all of its members. ■ Justine will participate in activities to maximize development.

Nursing Care Plan *(continued)*

IMPLEMENTATION

Recreation Therapy: *Purposeful use of recreation to promote relaxation and enhancement of social skills.*

- Refer the family to an early intervention program. Encourage contact with other children through play groups or early intervention programs.
- Investigate recreational programs for children with disabilities and share information with the parents.

Family Mobilization: *Utilization of family strengths to influence Justine's health in a positive direction.*

- Encourage parents to verbalize the impact of CP on the family. Refer them to other parents and support groups.
- Explore community services for rehabilitation, respite care, child care, and other needs and refer family as appropriate.
- During home and office visits, review Justine's achievements and praise the family for care provided.
- Teach the family skills needed to manage Justine's care (e.g., medication administration, muscle stretching, physical rehabilitation, seizure management).
- Teach case management techniques.
- Assess needs of siblings; involve them in Justine's care as appropriate. Review with parents the needs of all children in the family.

Nutrition Management: *Assistance with or provision of a balanced dietary intake of foods and fluids.*

- Monitor height and weight and plot on a growth grid. Perform hydration status assessment.
- Teach the family techniques to promote caloric and nutrient intake.
- Position Justine upright for feedings.
- Place foods far back in the mouth to overcome tongue thrust.
- Use soft and blended foods.
- Allow extra time for chewing and swallowing.
- Obtain adaptive handles for utensils and encourage self-feeding skills.
- Apply manual jaw control technique if it helps the child to control jaw movement.
- Perform frequent respiratory assessment. Teach the family to avoid aspiration pneumonia.

Exercise Therapy, Joint Mobility: *Use of active and passive body movement to maintain or restore joint flexibility.*

- Perform developmental assessment and record age of achievement of milestones (e.g., reaching for objects, sitting).
- Plan activities to use gross and fine motor skills (e.g., holding a crayon or eating utensils, reaching for toys and rolling over).
- Allow time for the child to complete activities.
- Perform ROM exercises for the child who is unable to move body parts. Position the child to promote tendon stretching (e.g., foot plantar flexion instead of dorsiflexion, legs extended instead of flexed at knees and hips).
- Arrange for and encourage parents to keep appointments with physical or rehabilitation therapist and other members of the collaborative team.

EVALUATION

The patient's progress in meeting the goals of care is based on the following expected outcomes:

- Justine reaches maximum physical mobility and developmental milestones.
- Justine shows normal growth patterns for height, weight, and other physical parameters.
- Justine demonstrates appropriate growth and developmental progress. The family successfully supports all of its members.
- Justine engages in activities to maximize development.

CRITICAL THINKING

1. What support groups or professional organizations exist in your area that could help Justine's family cope with this diagnosis?
2. Why is involvement of the older siblings important?
3. How would you assess Justine's cognitive ability? Is cognition always impacted by CP?

REVIEW Cerebral Palsy

REVIEW Link the Concepts and Exemplars

Linking the exemplar of cerebral palsy with the concept of comfort:

1. How might you promote comfort in a child with CP who is required to wear braces and orthotics to bed at night?
2. If spasticity of muscles causes pain, what nonpharmacologic strategies might you recommend?

Linking the exemplar of cerebral palsy with the concept of cognition:

3. While caring for a child diagnosed with CP who also has mild cognitive impairment, how would you help the child become increasingly autonomous in performing ROM exercises?
4. How might you encourage this child's parents to promote autonomy?

READY Go to Volume 3: Clinical Nursing Skills

REFER Go to Pearson MyLab Nursing and eText

REFLECT Apply Your Knowledge

Frangelica Gonzalez, 12 years old, was born with CP. She began working with physical therapists when she was less than 1 year old and has worn braces on her legs and used crutches to allow her greater mobility for as long as she can remember. Her mother and father have always told her she can overcome any challenge and do anything other children do if she tries hard enough. As a result of her parent's encouragement and support, Frangelica is a member of the school swim team, plays jazz piano, and has a large circle of friends. She has a younger brother who is 9 years old, an older brother who is 15 years old, and an identical twin sister who is healthy and does not have CP.

Lately her parents have noticed that Frangelica is moody, often seeming depressed, and her twin sister told their mother that Frangelica is "tired of being different." Frangelica has been waking in the morning offering various physical complaints as reasons why she can't go to school that day, ranging from a stomachache to a sore foot.

1. What might explain Frangelica's moodiness and trying to find reasons not to go to school?
2. What strategies might you recommend to Frangelica's parents to help her cope with the developmental changes she is experiencing?
3. What strategies might you recommend to Frangelica to explore and cope with her feelings?

Exemplar 25.D Failure to Thrive

Exemplar Learning Outcomes

25.D Analyze failure to thrive as it relates to development.

- Describe the pathophysiology of failure to thrive.
- Describe the etiology of failure to thrive.
- Compare the risk factors and prevention of failure to thrive.
- Identify the clinical manifestations of failure to thrive.
- Summarize diagnostic tests and therapies used by interprofessional teams in the collaborative care of an individual with failure to thrive.
- Differentiate care of patients with failure to thrive across the lifespan.
- Apply the nursing process in providing culturally competent care to an individual with failure to thrive.

Exemplar Key Terms

Failure to thrive (FTT), *1886*
Food insecurity, *1887*
Geriatric failure to thrive (GFTT), *1886*

Overview

Failure to thrive (FTT), also referred to as *faltering growth*, most commonly describes a syndrome in which an infant falls below the 5th percentile for weight and height on a standard growth chart or is falling in percentiles on a growth chart. The most common cause is malnutrition (Homan, 2016; Sirotnak & Chiesa, 2018). Prevalence rates are thought to be between 5 and 10% of children seen in primary care settings (Motil & Duryea, 2020). However, many parents of children with FTT do not or cannot seek proper and regular medical care, so prevalence rates may be higher.

Geriatric failure to thrive (GFTT) is a condition in which older adults experience a multidimensional decline in physical functioning that is characterized by weight loss of more than 5% of baseline body weight, decreased appetite, undernutrition, dehydration, depression, and cognitive and immune impairment. Similar to pediatric failure to thrive, GFTT can lead to death if left untreated (Ali, 2020).

Pathophysiology

FTT and GFTT may stem from inadequate caloric intake, inadequate caloric absorption, or excessive caloric expenditure. In all cases, undernutrition results. In infants, FTT affects weight, followed by body length and head circumference. Immune function and neurocognitive skills are also impaired (Lezo, Baldini, & Asteggiano, 2020). Additionally, the child is at risk for short stature, developmental delays, behavioral problems, and poor academic success (Murray, 2018).

As the adult body ages, weight typically increases until late middle age and declines between age 65 and 70. With this decline, lean body mass is lost resulting in a decrease in resting metabolic rate. Fat mass, however, increases. Age-related changes that impact food intake and digestion include decreased sense of taste, secretion of digestive enzymes, GI motility, and salivation.

While metabolic rate and energy consumption are changing in the older adult, decreased efficiency of body systems makes it increasingly difficult to maintain homeostasis. To compensate for these changes, homeostatic mechanisms require extra energy that may not be available due to dietary changes. Neurologic and psychologic changes can further compound these problems. Although many older adults experience good physical and cognitive health, some experience motor and cognitive decline, making it difficult to purchase food and prepare meals, and sometimes making it difficult to remember mealtimes and whether or not they have eaten.

Etiology

FTT may result from an insufficient intake of calories, reduced absorption of nutrients, or increased metabolic processes (Homan, 2016; Vachani, 2018). Causes of insufficient intake of calories include difficulties with breastfeeding, issues with feeding, inadequate feeding habits, impaired oromotor coordination, neglect, and abuse. FTT due to reduced absorption of nutrients include conditions such as celiac disease, cystic fibrosis, gastroesophageal reflux, and inflammatory bowel disease, among others. Increased metabolic processes that can lead to FTT may be caused by hyperthyroidism, infection, genetic disorders, and heart, lung, and kidney disease. Causes of FTT can also be classified as organic or inorganic. *Organic* causes of FTT are due to medical conditions, whereas *inorganic* causes include environmental, psychosocial, or family concerns, such as neglect and abuse or not preparing formula correctly. Most children, however, have FTT due to inorganic causes (Vachani, 2018).

Chronic diseases can impact the older person's ability to maintain weight and nutritional status. Diabetes can cause malabsorption and end-organ damage. Parkinson disease can cause dysphagia and tremors that make it difficult to get food into the mouth. Other chronic diseases that can affect the body's ability to get and maintain nutrition include cancer, inflammatory diseases, chronic lung diseases, cardiovascular disease, neurological disorders, and chronic renal insufficiency. Mental health disorders, especially depression, put the older adult at risk for developing GFTT.

Anorexia of aging, which can lead to GFTT, is a decrease in appetite and consequential decrease of nutrition intake (Landi, Picca, Calvani, & Marzetti, 2017). Vitamin and nutrient deficiencies are also common and decrease the older patient's ability to recover from injury, illness, and infection. This impaired immunity makes older patients more susceptible to both chronic and acute illnesses; illness, in turn, makes patients more susceptible to GFTT.

Risk Factors

Infants who are deprived of mothering will not learn to form significant relationships or to trust others (Hornor, 2019). Touch, cuddling, and visual and auditory stimulation are all critical for the infant. Through these mechanisms, the baby comes to know self and the environment. Infants who fail to establish a loving, responsive relationship with a caregiver often fail to develop normally.

Infants and children whose parents or caregivers experience depression, substance abuse, or psychosis or who have a history of abuse are at risk for FTT (Vachani, 2018). Their parents may be socially and emotionally isolated or may lack knowledge of infant nutritional and nurturing needs. A multifactorial and reciprocal interaction pattern may exist whereby the parent does not offer enough food or is not responsive to the infant's hunger cues and, as a result, the infant is irritable, not soothed, and does not give clear cues about hunger.

Children living in poverty and rural areas are also at risk for FTT. When food is scarce due to **food insecurity** (without reliable access to sufficient quantities of nutritious food), there is greater potential for undernutrition (Lezo et al., 2020).

Risk factors for the older adult developing GFTT involve conditions that lead to undernutrition. There is a greater chance of anorexia leading to malnutrition if the elderly patient is on more than four medications. Medications, such as anticholinergic drugs, beta blockers, and selective serotonin reuptake inhibitors, can cause anorexia in older adults. Other risks for GFTT include sensory deficits; confusion, delirium, or dementia; and alcohol or substance abuse.

Residents in nursing homes, particularly veterans, show a greater risk of GFTT than those who live in the community (Ali, 2020). As with children in poverty, adults who live in poor conditions and are food insecure are more likely to develop GFTT. Social isolation, widowhood, and abandonment by family/friends are also considered risk factors.

Dentition is also affected by aging, with many older adults experiencing tooth loss, gum disease, and other painful mouth conditions. These changes make eating more difficult and less enjoyable, leading to older adults consuming fewer calories.

Prevention

Educating caregivers regarding an infant's dietary and nutritional needs may help guard against development of FTT in children. Nurses can provide resources for family with food insecurity, including referrals to local food pantries, school meals, and state and federal food assistance. Likewise, home nursing visits have been shown to significantly impact caregivers' delivery of adequate nutrition to children within the home (Homan, 2016). To promote successful outcomes for both children and families, nurses working with parents and other caregivers should encourage their participation in the care plan and not make them feel embarrassed or ashamed.

Prevention of GFTT is complicated. The nurse can review the patient's medications, assessing for medications that may cause decreased appetite. Patients can be taught to eat high-calorie, nutritionally dense foods. Other nutritional strategies can also be discussed with the patient, including eating small, frequent meals.

Nurses can refer patients to social support groups and senior programs to help decrease isolation. Various organizations can be used to help the senior have meals delivered to the home. Case management should be considered for those individuals with several chronic diseases, as well as for those in need of financial and/or transportation assistance to buy food.

Clinical Manifestations

The characteristics of FTT are persistent failure to eat adequately with no weight gain or with weight loss in a child over time (Homan, 2016). Infants with feeding disorders refuse food, may have erratic sleep patterns, are irritable and difficult to soothe, fall well under expected growth patterns, and are often developmentally delayed (**Figure 25.14** »).

Infants with inorganic FTT show delayed development without any physical cause. They are often malnourished and fail to gain weight and grow normally. Behavior may be apathetic and withdrawn, and the child may demonstrate poor eye contact and lack anticipated stranger danger.

Patients with GFTT typically present with unintended weight loss, lack of appetite and energy, and diminished physical activity and strength. Muscle tone is poor; limbs are cachectic, though fat deposits appear around the midsection. Skin is dry and scaly, and wounds heal slowly and poorly. Hair is thin and nails are weak, discolored, and misshapen. Patients may complain of bone or joint pain, and edema may be present. Blood tests reveal anemia, low serum albumin and prealbumin levels, and low serum cholesterol levels.

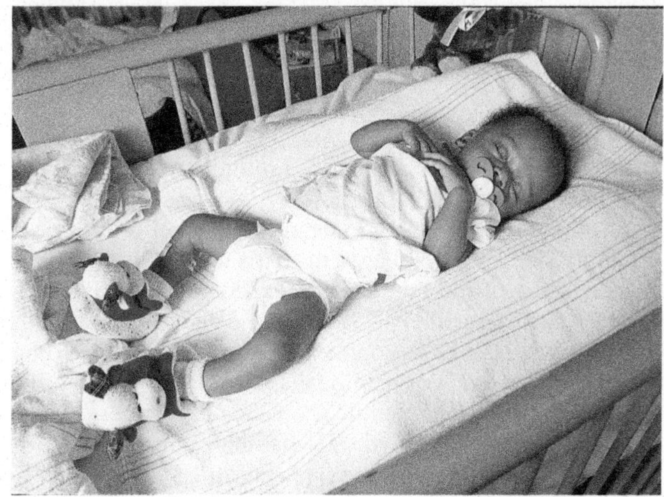

Figure 25.14 » Infants with failure to thrive may not look severely malnourished, but they fall well below the expected weight and height norms for their age and population. This infant, who appears to be about 4 months old, is actually 8 months old. He has been hospitalized for examination of his failure to thrive and treatment of an eating disorder.

Source: Pearson Education, Inc.

GFTT patients are sometimes described as being "wasted" or "frail." Wasting refers to gradual physical deterioration accompanied by a loss of strength and appetite. Frailty refers to cumulative physiologic decline that manifests itself in a wasted appearance, impaired physical abilities, decreased resistance to stressors, and diminished cognitive function. Resistance to stressors and cognitive functioning are important to consider when diagnosing GFTT because active older patients may consume fewer calories than required and experience weight loss but be resilient to stress and have high cognitive functioning. In other words, weight loss alone is not indicative of GFTT.

Collaboration

A thorough history and physical examination are needed to rule out any chronic illness in the child or adult with FTT. The goals of treatment are to provide adequate caloric and nutritional intake. For the child, the nurse promotes normal growth and development and assists parents in developing feeding routines and responding to the infant's cues of physical and psychologic hunger. For the older adult, the nurse collaborates to maximize functional status, treat depression, and manage any chronic illnesses (Ali, 2020).

In addition to the physician and nurse, a registered dietitian and social worker are key members of the interprofessional team caring for a child or older adult with FTT. For the older adult, physical and occupational therapists may be involved to reduce functional impairment. A pharmacist may work with the healthcare team to review medications that may be contributing to GFTT and discuss issues of polypharmacy. A geriatrician, specializing in the care of the older adult, can help the healthcare team when multiple and complex conditions are present.

>> **Stay Current:** For a description of a collaborative healthcare team addressing FTT, visit the website of the Kennedy Krieger Institute's Feeding Disorder Clinic at www.kennedykrieger.org/patient-care/patient-care-programs/outpatient-programs/feeding-disorders-clinic.

Diagnostic Tests

Diagnosis of FTT occurs primarily through assessments made over time (Homan, 2016).

Height and weight should be measured and plotted on a growth chart. The WHO growth charts are utilized for children up to age 2 and the CDC growth charts for individuals from 2 to 20 years old. FTT is identified by weight less than the 5th percentile based on sex and age. FTT may also be diagnosed if weight-for-length falls below the 5th percentile, BMI below the 5th percentile, or if the child experiences a marked decrease in growth rate (falling by more than two percentile markers) over time (Homan, 2016).

In addition to growth parameters, nutritional assessments are useful when evaluating all patients for FTT. Twenty-four-hour recall (by the adult patient or the parent if the patient is a child) is commonly used, although 3- or 7-day food diaries and food frequency questionnaires tend to be more accurate. The Malnutrition Universal Screening Tool (MUST) and Mini Nutrition Assessment (MNA) may be used for identifying adults who are undernourished or at risk of being undernourished.

Body mass index should be assessed, although BMI carries limitations in older patients. Changes in height, posture, and muscle tone impact its overall accuracy as a health measure. Tricipital skinfold measurement, mid-upper-arm circumference, and biometric impedance analysis are other useful anthropometric assessments of lean mass and fat mass.

A psychosocial assessment can also determine if neglect, abuse, or economic factors are contributing to FTT in the child or older adult. Psychosocial assessment should be performed on older adults, especially if they have risk factors for depression, such as the loss of a spouse or a change in living arrangements. See Exemplar 28.A, Depression, in Module 28, Mood and Affect, for information about assessing older adults for depression.

Diagnostic laboratory tests also are appropriate when assessing for GFTT. Serum proteins—including albumin, transferrin, retinol-binding proteins, and thyroxine-binding prealbumin—are typically assessed. Decreases in any of these proteins can be indicative of GFTT. These values should be considered cautiously, however, because they also serve as markers for other problems commonly associated with aging, such as inflammation and infection. Serum cholesterol and vitamin levels are also assessed.

Surgery

Surgical management of the patient with FTT will vary based on the physiologic impairment. For example, possible surgical interventions may include cleft palate repair or alleviation of a bowel obstruction. The type and appropriateness of such surgical interventions depend on the specific condition.

Pharmacologic Therapy

No medications are indicated for primary treatment of FTT. Rather, the approach to treatment includes identifying the cause, resolving any barriers to obtaining and absorbing adequate caloric intake, and providing nutritional supplementation to treat deficiencies. Because the older adult is at risk for polypharmacy, review the current list of medications for those that may be contributing to a lack of appetite or weight loss (Ali, 2020).

Pharmacologic therapies for the treatment of GFTT may involve vitamin regimens. Vitamins D, B_{12}, and folate are commonly prescribed supplements for GFTT patients. Vitamin D and folate deficiencies typically stem from altered dietary intake; B_{12} deficiencies, on the other hand, are most commonly caused by disease states.

Nonpharmacologic Therapy

Developmentally appropriate education for caregivers regarding nutrition and home care visits is believed to reduce the incidence of FTT among children. For parents who choose to breastfeed, the nurse should assess the parent's knowledge and efficacy and provide or facilitate the provision of additional teaching as needed. Families with food insecurity should be referred to social services to identify community resources for food (Homan, 2016).

Nonpharmacologic therapies tend to focus on improving oral intake of foods and fluids. Therapies may include providing smaller, more manageable portions to decrease patient anxiety about wasted food. Portions may be fortified with additional vitamins and nutrients, and they may be softer in texture for patients with dentition problems. Snacks should be offered, and patients should be allowed choice in menu selection whenever possible. Patients with alterations in mobility or illness should receive nursing assistance at mealtimes.

Care of the pediatric or the older adult patient also includes addressing any underlying medical condition that may be contributing to FTT. For a child this may include repairing a cleft lip or palate or treating celiac disease. The older adult may require maximizing treatment for chronic conditions, such as chronic obstructive pulmonary disease or congestive heart failure.

For older adults with GFTT, oral liquid, energy-dense, and high-quality protein supplements may be appropriate (Ali, 2020). For severely undernourished patients or those who cannot take food orally, enteral feeding may be appropriate.

NURSING PROCESS

Nursing care of the child with FTT is directed toward improving the child's nutritional intake and increasing the growth and health of the child. This may be accomplished through parent teaching; observation of child–parent interactions, especially during feeding times; and careful recording of height and weight on growth charts.

Nursing care of the older adult with GFTT involves both the acute care of the GFTT and the chronic care of any underlying disease processes. Assisting the patient to meet nutritional needs is a priority. This may include helping the patient make food choices that are nutritionally dense and easy to eat. Referral to a dietitian may be necessary. The nurse may also engage in therapeutic communication for the older adult who might be depressed, socially isolated, or coping with loss.

Assessment

Assessment of the child is essential for establishing an intervention plan. Take accurate measurement of weight, height, BMI, and percentiles each time a child interacts with a HCP to develop an important record of growth patterns over time. The child's activity level, developmental milestones, and interaction patterns also provide important information.

When feeding the child, observe how the child indicates hunger or satiety, the ability of the child to be soothed, and general interaction patterns such as eye contact, touch, and cuddliness.

Ask parents about stressors in their lives that may prevent or interfere with appropriate interaction with the child. Questions about the pregnancy and delivery can elicit information about early disturbances in the child–parent relationship. Ask whether there are other children in the family and whether they have experienced feeding problems. It is important for the nurse to observe the child's and parents' behaviors when the parents feed the child; cues given by each individual and interactional modes such as rocking, singing, talking, and body postures are important. For the bottle-fed infant, check on preparation of formula (Lezo et al., 2020).

For older adults, assess the patient's opportunity for socializing during meals; intake tends to improve when others are present. For patients living at home, assess the food preparation area to ensure that patients are physically capable of using necessary appliances and navigating the space. If patients in the home environment cannot prepare meals on their own, social services (e.g., Meals on Wheels) should be considered. Review prescribed and over-the-counter drugs and herbal supplements that the patient takes for those that can affect appetite, nutrition, and weight. Assess the older adult for support systems, social activities, loneliness, and depression.

Diagnosis

Care priorities of the young child with FTT may include the following:

- Undernutrition
- Potential for developmental delay
- Inadequate parenting.

Priorities for care of the older adult with GFTT may include:

- Undernutrition
- Fatigue
- Inability to perform self-care.

Planning

The goals of nursing care for the child with FTT may include the following:

- Child will attain adequate growth and normal development.
- The parent–child relationship will demonstrate appropriate behaviors based on child's developmental level.
- Parents will verbalize understanding of the child's nutritional requirements.

Goals for nursing care of older adults with GFTT may include:

- Patient will choose food items that are nutritionally dense for snacks and meals.
- Patient will have adequate mental health support and services.
- Patient will have stable sources of nutritious food and supplements.
- Patient will be able to obtain food and prepare meals.

Implementation

Nursing care of infants and young children with FTT focuses on performing a thorough history and physical assessment, observing parent–child interactions during feeding times, and providing necessary teaching to enable parents to respond appropriately to their child's needs. Accurate weights, nutritional assessments, and developmental evaluation should be done to see if the child begins to grow more normally.

Additional diagnostic tests may be performed to rule out organic causes of the poor growth.

Observations of feeding and continued careful physical assessments are needed. Teach parents to record carefully the child's intake at each meal or feeding. Help them to understand and respond to the child's cues of hunger and satiety. Reinforce the need to hold, rock, and touch the infant during feeding and to establish eye contact with infants and older children.

Upon discharge, refer parents to an early childhood intervention agency that can continue monitoring the home situation. Agency staff can observe feeding during a home visit and evaluate stresses and behavior patterns among family members. Frequent measurement of growth and development must be ensured so that the child is adequately nourished. Parents may need referral to community resources to help them manage stressful situations and to enhance their parenting skills.

For the older adult patient with GFTT, nursing care centers on weight gain and nutritional improvement. This will require the nurse to monitor caloric intake and nutritional choices. Nurses should encourage nutritionally dense snacks and small, frequent meals. Addressing the underlying causes of the GFTT is also important. For example, if the patient is prescribed several medications, the nurse can collaborate with the pharmacist and HCP to evaluate the medication for anorexic side effects and consider alternatives. The nurse should consider case management for the patient. In nursing homes and transitional care units, the nurse should encourage the resident to participate in social activities, including eating with other residents.

Refer families and older adults who have difficulty obtaining healthy food to social services for support and community services.

Communicating with Patients

Introductory Phase

When assessing the nutritional status of older adults, address them in a thoughtful manner to avoid embarrassing them if they are unable to shop, cook for themselves, or afford to buy food. Begin the discussion by asking questions that encourage the older adult to open up. Ask basic questions that will give you an indication of how well the individual is eating, preparing meals, and feeling satiated after eating. Listen carefully and allow the individual to fully answer the question. Basic questions to begin assessing nutritional status include:

- Tell me what you ate for breakfast/lunch/dinner yesterday.
- Who prepared the meals?
- Were you satisfied after your meals?

Evaluation

The child's outcomes are largely evaluated based on the following:

- Growth and development of the child improve.
- The parent–child relationship improves.
- The parent voices a specific action plan to improve and maintain appropriate growth of child.
- The child experiences no long-term complications as a result of FTT.

Outcomes for older adults with GFTT may include:

- The patient achieves improved nutritional status.
- The patient has food security.
- The patient uses social support systems as necessary to promote health and functioning.

REVIEW Failure to Thrive

RELATE Link the Concepts and Exemplars

Linking the exemplar of failure to thrive with the concept of acid–base balance:

1. How might excessive protein metabolism as the result of inadequate sources of energy supply from dietary intake impact the patient's acid–base balance?
2. How might altered glucose metabolism as a result of inadequate caloric intake impact the patient's acid–base balance?

Linking the exemplar of failure to thrive with the concept of elimination:

3. How might inadequate caloric and nutrient intake impact elimination?
4. If caloric and nutrient intake is increased suddenly, how might the patient's elimination habits be impacted?

READY Go to Volume 3: Clinical Nursing Skills

REFER Go to Pearson MyLab Nursing and eText

REFLECT Apply Your Knowledge

Hilary is born 8 weeks prematurely at 32 weeks' gestation to a single adolescent mother. Hilary remains in the neonatal intensive care unit for 10 weeks until she is stable enough to be discharged. Her mother tries to visit at least once a week and is sometimes able to visit more often depending on whether someone can give her a ride to and from the hospital.

Hilary returns in 6 weeks following discharge and is found to have gained only 2 oz, increasing her weight from 2.32 kg (5 lb 2 oz) to 2.38 kg (5 lb 4 oz). The provider schedules a follow-up visit for 2 weeks later, and the nurse explains Hilary's nutritional requirements. When Hilary returns, she has lost 1 oz in weight.

1. Does Hilary qualify as having FTT? Explain your answer.
2. Do you suspect an organic or inorganic cause of her failure to gain weight? What cues led you to your answer?
3. Develop a nursing plan of care for Hilary.

REFLECT Apply Your Knowledge

Tom and Jenny Fordham, both in their 70s, have lived in the same home for more than 20 years. Mr. Fordham is a retired media professional; Mrs. Fordham a retired interior designer. In the past 3 years, both have experienced a decline in health. Mr. Fordham is now in the middle stages of Alzheimer disease. He is no longer able to drive and needs to be reminded to do things like take a shower or take his medicine. Mrs. Fordham developed chronic obstructive pulmonary disease several years ago. She now requires oxygen via cannula 24/7, and she uses her tiotropium bromide (Spiriva) and fluticasone (Flovent) inhalers daily as prescribed. Mrs. Fordham also takes calcium and vitamin D daily and ibandronate sodium (Boniva) once a month for osteoporosis. She continues to drive, although she finds it frustrating and does not like to go out often.

You are the nurse at Mrs. Fordham's primary care provider's office. When Mrs. Fordham comes for a routine checkup, you take her height and weight and find that she has lost 5 lb since she was in 3 months ago with acute bronchitis. She complains that Mr. Fordham is in the waiting room because she is too scared to leave him home alone. She relates that she has very little energy these days, and that taking care of him is "wearing me out."

1. What risk factors does Mr. Fordham have for GFTT? Mrs. Fordham?
2. What are your primary concerns about Mrs. Fordham at this time? Why?
3. What additional assessment data do you need to gather? Why?

References

Abdel-Hamid, H. Z. (2018). *Cerebral palsy*. Medscape. https://emedicine.medscape.com/article/1179555-overview#a5.

Adams, M. P., Holland, L. N., & Urban, C. (2020). *Pharmacology for nurses: A pathophysiologic approach* (6th ed.). Pearson Education.

Administration for Community Living. (2018). *2017 profile of older Americans*. U.S. Department of Health and Human Services. https://acl.gov/sites/default/files/Aging%20and%20Disability%20in%20America/2017OlderAmericansProfile.pdf

Akobirshoev, I., Parish, S. L., Mitra, M., & Rosenthal, E. (2017). Birth outcomes among U.S. women with intellectual and developmental disabilities. *Disability and Health Journal, 10*(3), 406–412.

Ali, N. (2020). *Failure to thrive in elderly adults*. Medscape. https://emedicine.medscape.com/article/2096163-overview

American Academy of Pediatrics (AAP). (2016). *Media and young minds: A policy statement*. http://pediatrics.aappublications.org/content/pediatrics/138/5/e20162591.full.pdf

American Academy of Child and Adolescent Psychiatry. (n.d.). *How common is ADHD?* https://www.aacap.org/AACAP/Families_and_Youth/Resource_Centers/ADHD_Resource_Center/ADHD_A_Guide_for_Families/How_Common_is_ADHD.aspx

American Psychiatric Association (APA). (2013). *Diagnostic and statistical manual of mental disorders* (5th ed.). Author.

American Psychiatric Association (APA). (2017). *What is ADHD?* https://www.psychiatry.org/patients-families/adhd/what-is-adhd

American Speech-Language-Hearing Association. (2017). *Social language use: Pragmatics*. Retrieved from http://www.asha.org/public/speech/-development/Pragmatics/

Anderson, C. (2017). Implications of preterm birth for maternal mental health and infant development. *American Journal of Maternal/Child Nursing, 42*(2), 108–114.

Anderson, M., & Jiang, J. (2018). *Teens, social media, and technology 2018*. Pew Research Center. http://publicservicesalliance.org/wp-content/uploads/2018/06/Teens-Social-Media-Technology-2018-PEW.pdf

Andrews, M. M., Boyle, J. S., & Collins, J.W. (2019). *Transcultural concepts in nursing care* (8th ed.). Wolters Kluwer.

Autism and Developmental Disabilities Monitoring Network. (2020). Autism spectrum disorder (ASD). https://www.cdc.gov/ncbddd/autism/materials/addm-factsheet.html

Ball, J. W., Bindler, R. M., & Cowen, K. J. (2022). *Principles of pediatric nursing: Caring for children* (8th ed.). Pearson.

Bandura, A. (1986). *Social foundations of thought and actions: A social cognitive theory*. Prentice Hall.

Bandura, A. (1997a). *Self-efficacy: The exercise of control*. W.H. Freeman.

Bandura, A. (1997b). *Self-efficacy in changing societies*. Cambridge University Press.

Barbosa, R., de Oliveira, A., de Lima Antão, J., Crocetta, T. B., Guarnieri, R., Antunes, T., et al. (2018). Augmentative and alternative communication in children with Down's syndrome: A systematic review. *BMC Pediatrics*, 18(1), 160.

Bauldoff, G., Gubrud, P., & Carno, M. (2020). *LeMone & Burke's medical-surgical nursing* (7th ed.). Pearson.

Benfer, K. A., Weir, K. A., Bell, K. L., Ware, R. S., Davies, P., & Boyd, R. N. (2017). Oropharyngeal dysphagia and cerebral palsy. *Pediatrics, 140*(6), e20170731.

Berk, L. E. (2018). *Development through the lifespan* (7th ed.). Pearson Education.

Berman, A., Snyder, S., & Frandsen, G. (2021). *Kozier & Erb's fundamentals of nursing: Concepts, process, and practice* (11th ed.). Pearson.

Bishop, K. M., & Lucchino, R. (n.d.). *Aging in individuals with a developmental disability*. Aging and Disabilities Resource Center Training for the Cross Network Collaboration of Florida. http://elderaffairs.state.fl.us/doea/ARC/05c_Module_3_Aging_in_Individuals_with_a_Developmental_Disability.pdf

Blank, R., Barnett, A., Cairney, J., Green, D., Kirby, A., Polatajko, H., et al. (2019). International clinical practice recommendations on the definition, diagnosis, assessment, intervention, and psychosocial aspects of developmental coordination disorder. *Developmental Medicine & Child Neurology, 61*, 242–285.

Bottema-Beutel, K., & Crowley, C. (2020). Beyond monolithic packages: Important strategies across early interventions for children and autism. In G. Vivanti, K. Bottema-Beutel, & L. Turner-Brown (Eds.), *Clinical guide to early interventions for children with autism* (pp. 151–161). Springer.

Brasic, J. B. (2020). *Autism spectrum disorder*. Medscape. https://emedicine.medscape.com/article/912781-overview#a3

Bronfenbrenner, U. (1986). Ecology of the family as a context for human development: Research perspectives. *Developmental Psychology, 22*, 723–742.

Bronfenbrenner, U. (Ed.). (2005). *Making human beings human: Bioecological perspectives on human development*. Sage.

Bronfenbrenner, U., McClelland, P. D., Ceci, S. J., Moen, P., & Wethington, E. (1996). *The state of Americans*. Free Press.

Brown, S., Whichello, R., & Price, S. (2018). The impact of resiliency on nurse burnout: An integrative review. *MEDSURG Nursing, 27*(6), 349–354, 378.

Cabral, M. D. I., Liu, S., & Soares, N. (2020). Attention-deficit/hyperactivity disorder: diagnostic criteria, epidemiology, risk factors and evaluation in youth. *Translational Pediatrics*, 9(Suppl. 1), S104–S113.

Centers for Disease Control and Prevention (CDC). (2017a). *LGBT youth*. https://www.cdc.gov/lgbthealth/youth.htm

Centers for Disease Control and Prevention (CDC). (2017b). *Metropolitan Atlanta Developmental Disabilities Surveillance Program (MADDSP)*. https://www.cdc.gov/ncbddd/developmentaldisabilities/maddsp.html

Centers for Disease Control and Prevention (CDC). (2019a). *About Zika*. https://www.cdc.gov/zika/about/index.html

Centers for Disease Control and Prevention (CDC). (2019b). *Autism spectrum disorder: Treatments*. http://www.cdc.gov/ncbddd/autism/treatment.html#ref

Centers for Disease Control and Prevention (CDC). (2019c). *Causes and risk factors of cerebral palsy*. https://www.cdc.gov/ncbddd/cp/causes.html

Centers for Disease Control and Prevention (CDC). (2019d). *Data and statistics about ADHD*. https://www.cdc.gov/ncbddd/adhd/data.html

Centers for Disease Control and Prevention (CDC). (2019e). *Data and statistics for cerebral palsy*. https://www.cdc.gov/ncbddd/cp/data.html

Centers for Disease Control and Prevention (CDC). (2019f). *Facts about developmental disabilities*. https://www.cdc.gov/ncbddd/developmentaldisabilities/facts.html

Centers for Disease Control and Prevention (CDC). (2019g). *Other concerns and conditions with ADHD*. https://www.cdc.gov/ncbddd/adhd/conditions.html

Centers for Disease Control and Prevention (CDC). (2019h). *Preterm birth*. https://www.cdc.gov/reproductivehealth/MaternalInfantHealth/PretermBirth.htm

Centers for Disease Control and Prevention (CDC). (2019i). *Signs and symptoms of autism spectrum disorders*. https://www.cdc.gov/ncbddd/autism/signs.html

Centers for Disease Control and Prevention (CDC). (2020a). *ADHD in the classroom: Helping children succeed in school*. https://www.cdc.gov/ncbddd/adhd/school-success.html.

Centers for Disease Control and Prevention (CDC). (2020b). *Babies born with congenital cytomegalovirus (CMV)*. https://www.cdc.gov/cmv/congenital-infection.html

Centers for Disease Control and Prevention (CDC). (2020c). *Cytomegalovirus (CMV) and congenital CMV infection*. https://www.cdc.gov/cmv/index.html

Centers for Disease Control and Prevention (CDC). (2020d). *Data & statistics on autism spectrum disorder*. https://www.cdc.gov/ncbddd/autism/data.html

Centers for Disease Control and Prevention (CDC). (2020e). *Fetal alcohol spectrum disorders (FASDS)*. https://www.cdc.gov/ncbddd/fasd/

Centers for Disease Control and Prevention (CDC). (2020f). *Folic acid*. https://www.cdc.gov/ncbddd/folicacid/index.html

Centers for Disease Control and Prevention (CDC). (2020g). *Health effects of lead exposure*. https://www.cdc.gov/nceh/lead/prevention/health-effects.htm

Centers for Disease Control and Prevention (CDC). (2020h). *Important milestones: Your child by three years*. https://www.cdc.gov/ncbddd/actearly/milestones/milestones-3yr.html

Centers for Disease Control and Prevention (CDC). (2020i). *Sexual risk behaviors: HIV, STD, & teen pregnancy prevention*. http://www.cdc.gov/HealthyYouth/sexualbehaviors/

Centers for Disease Control and Prevention (CDC). (2020j). *What is cerebral palsy?* https://www.cdc.gov/ncbddd/cp/facts.html

Centers for Disease Control and Prevention (CDC). (2020k). *What is fragile X syndrome*. https://www.cdc.gov/ncbddd/fxs/facts.html

Chess, S., & Thomas, A. (1995). *Temperament in clinical practice*. Guilford Press.

Chess, S., & Thomas, A. (1996). *Temperament: Theory and practice*. Brunner/Mazel.

Children and Adults with Attention-Deficit/Hyperactivity Disorder (CHADD). (2018). *Life skills program holds promise as school-based behavioral intervention for ADHD*. https://chadd.org/adhd-weekly/life-skills-program-holds-promise-as-school-based-behavioral-intervention-for-adhd/

Children and Adults with Attention-Deficit/Hyperactivity Disorder (CHADD). (2019). *Women often diagnosed with ADHD later in life*. https://chadd.org/adhd-weekly/women-often-diagnosed-with-adhd-later-in-life/

Children and Adults with Attention-Deficit/Hyperactivity Disorder (CHADD). (2020a). *Diagnosing ADHD*. https://chadd.org/about-adhd/diagnosing-adhd/

Children and Adults with Attention-Deficit/Hyperactivity Disorder (2020b). *For educators*. https://chadd.org/for-educators/overview/

Children and Adults with Attention-Deficit/Hyperactivity Disorder (CHADD). (2020c). *Women and girls*. https://chadd.org/for-adults/women-and-girls/

Common Sense. (2017). Fact sheet: The Common Sense census: Media use by kids age zero to eight, 2017. https://www.commonsensemedia.org/sites/default/files/uploads/research/0-8census_undertwo_release.pdf

Copraro, V., & Sippel, J. (2017). Gender differences in moral judgment and the evaluation of gender-specified moral agents. *Cognitive Processing, 18*, 399–405.

Costa, P. T., McCrae, R. R., & Löckenhoff, C. E. (2019). Personality across the life span. *Annual Review of Psychology, 70*, 423–448.

Cross Network Collaboration for Florida. (n.d.). *Meeting the needs of aging persons with developmental disabilities and their families*. http://elderaffairs.state.fl.us/doea/ARC/06_DD_Presenters_Manual.pdf

Erikson, E. (1963). *Childhood and society*. Norton.

Erikson, E. (1968). *Identity: Youth and crisis*. Norton.

Faccio, F., Renzi, C., Giudice, A. V., & Pravettoni, G. (2018). Family resilience in the oncology setting: Development of an integrative framework. *Frontiers in Psychology, 9*, 666.

Freund, D., & Bolick, B.N. (2019). Assessing a child's pain. *American Journal of Nursing, 119*(5), 34–41.

Fuentes, J., Hervas, A., Howlin, P., & ESCAP ESD Working Party. (2020). ESCAP practice guidance for autism: a summary of evidence-based recommendations for diagnosis and treatment. *European Child & Adolescent Psychiatry*. https://doi.org/10.1007/s00787-020-01587-4

Gilligan, C. (1982). *In a different voice: Psychological -theory and women's development*. Harvard University Press.

Gómez-Benito, J., Van de Vijver, F. J. R., Balluerka, N., & Caterino, L. (2019). Cross-cultural and gender differences in ADHD among young adults. *Journal of Attention Disorders, 23*(1), 22–31.

Gould, R. L. (1972). The phases of adult life: A study in developmental psychology. *American Journal of Psychiatry, 129*, 33–43.

Hackett, A., Joseph, R., Robinson, K., Welsh, J., Nicholas, J., & Schmidt, E. (2020). Adult attention deficit/hyperactivity disorder in the ambulatory care setting. *Journal of the American Academy of PAs, 33*(8), 12–16.

Hauer, J., Houtrow, A. J., & Council on Children with Disabilities, Section on Hospice and Palliative Care Medicine. (2017). Pain assessment and treatment in children with significant impairment of the central nervous system. *Pediatrics, 139*(6), e1–e27.

Heron, M. (2019). Deaths: Leading causes for 2017. *National Vital Statistics Reports, 68*(6). https://www.cdc.gov/nchs/data/nvsr/nvsr68/nvsr68_06-508.pdf

Hochberg, Z. E., & Konner, M. (2020). Emerging adulthood, a pre-adult life-history stage. *Frontiers in endocrinology, 10*, 918.

Homan, G. J. (2016). Failure to thrive: a practical guide. *American Family Physician, 94*(4), 295–299.

Hornor, G. (2019). Attachment disorders. *Journal of Pediatric Health Care, 33*(5), 612–622.

Huang, Y., Arnold, S. R. C., Foley, K. R., & Trollor, J. N. (2020). Diagnosis of autism in adulthood: A scoping review. *Autism, 24*(6), 1311–1327.

Hyman, S. L., Levy, S. E., Myers, S. M., & Council on Children with Disabilities, Section on Developmental and Behavioral Pediatrics. (2020). Identification, evaluation, and management of children with autism spectrum disorder. *Pediatrics, 145*(1), e20193447.

Jung Kim, H. (2020). *Children, teens, and the safety of psychotropic medications*. Harvard Health Publishing. https://www.health.harvard.edu/blog/children-teens-and-the-safety-of-psychotropic-medicines-2020080620715

Kakkori, L., & Huttunen, R. (2017). Gilligan-Kohlberg controversy. In M. A. Peters (Ed.), *Encyclopedia of educational philosophy and theory*. Springer.

Landi, F., Picca, A., Calvani, R., & Marzetti, E. (2017). Anorexia of aging: Assessment and management. *Clinics in Geriatric Medicine, 33*(3), 315–323.

Lezo, A., Baldini, L., & Asteggiano, M. (2020). Failure to thrive in the outpatient clinic: A new insight. *Nutrients, 12*, 1–16.

Lima, S. A. M., El Dib, R. P., Rodrigues, M. R. K., Ferraz, G., Molina, A. C., Neto, C., et al. (2018). Is the risk of low birth weight or preterm labor greater when maternal stress is experienced during pregnancy?: A systematic review and meta-analysis of cohort studies. *PloS One, 13*(7), e0200594.

Lipkin, P. H., Macias, M. M., & Council on Children with Disabilities, Section on Developmental and Behavioral Pediatrics. (2020). Promoting optimal development: Identifying infants and young children with developmental disorders through developmental surveillance and screening. *Pediatrics, 145*(1), e20193449. https://doi.org/10.1542/peds.2019-3449

Maitland, T. E. L. (2020). *Teaching teens the dangers of sharing ADHD medication*. ADDitude. https://www.additudemag.com/adhd-medication-diversion-teens-sharing-stimulants/

Masten, A. S. (2018). Resilience theory and research on children and families: Past, present, and promise. *Journal of Family Theory & Review, 10*, 12–31.

Mattson, S. N., Bernes, G. A., & Doyle, L. R. (2019). Fetal alcohol spectrum disorders: A review of neurobehavioral deficits associated with prenatal alcohol exposure. *Alcohol: Clinical and Experimental Research, 43*(6), 1046–1062.

Mayo Clinic. (2019). *Cerebral palsy*. https://www.mayoclinic.org/diseases-conditions/cerebral-palsy/symptoms-causes/syc-20353999

Mikami, A. Y., Smit, S., & Khalis, A. (2017). Social skills training and ADHD–What works? *Current Psychiatry Reports, 19*(12), 93.

Molina, B. S. G., Hinshaw, S. P., Swanson, J. M., Arnold, L. E., Vitiello, B., Jensen, P. S., et al. (2009). The MTA at 8 years: prospective follow-up of children treated for combined type ADHD in a multisite study. *Journal of the American Academy of Child and Adolescent Psychiatry, 48*, 484–500.

Motil, K. J., & Duryea, T. K. (2020). *Poor weight gain in children younger than two years in resource-rich countries: Etiology and evaluation*. UpToDate. https://www.uptodate.com/contents/poor-weight-gain-in-children-younger-than-two-years-in-resource-rich-countries-etiology-and-evaluation

Mueller, B. A., Crane, D., Doody, D. R., Stuart, S. N., & Schiff, M. A. (2019). Pregnancy course, infant outcomes, rehospitalization, and mortality among women with intellectual disability. *Disability and Health Journal, 12*(3), 452–459.

Murray, R. D. (2018). Assessing nutritional risk among infants and toddlers in primary care practice. *Pediatric Annals, 47*(11), e465–469.

National Alliance on Mental Illness (NAMI). (n.d.) *Attention deficit hyperactivity disorder (ADHD)*. https://www.nami.org/About-Mental-Illness/Mental-Health-Conditions/ADHD/Support

National Association of School Nurses. (2016). *LGBTQ students: The role of the school nurse. Position statement*. https://www.nasn.org/nasn/advocacy/professional-practice-documents/position-statements/ps-lgbtq

National Center for Complementary and Integrative Health (NCCIH). (2019a). *ADHD and complementary health approaches: What the science says*. https://www.nccih.nih.gov/health/providers/digest/adhd-and-complementary-health-approaches-science

National Center for Complementary and Integrative Health (NCCIH). (2019b). *Attention-deficit hyperactivity disorder at a glance*. https://www.nccih.nih.gov/health/attention-deficit-hyperactivity-disorder-at-a-glance

National Center for Health Statistics. (2016). *Mean age of mothers is on the rise: United States, 2000–2014*. http://www.cdc.gov/nchs/products/databriefs/db232.htm

National Institute on Alcohol Abuse and Alcoholism. (n.d.). *Older adults*. https://want youwww.niaaa.nih.gov/older-adults

National Institute of Mental Health (NIMH). (2018). *Autism spectrum disorder*. https://www.nimh.nih.gov/health/topics/autism-spectrum-disorders-asd/index.shtml?utm_source=rss_readersutm_medium=rssutm_campaign=rss_full

National Institute of Mental Health (NIMH). (2019). *Attention deficit hyperactivity disorder*. Retrieved from https://www.nimh.nih.gov/health/topics/attention-deficit-hyperactivity-disorder-adhd/index.shtml

New York City Health Department. (2015). *Pediatric bundle initiative*. https://www1.nyc.gov/assets/doh/downloads/pdf/hcp/pediatric-bundle-all.pdf.

Novak, I., Morgan, C., Adde, L., Blackman, J., Boyd, R. N., Brunstrom-Hernandez, J., et al. (2017). Early, accurate diagnosis and early intervention in cerebral palsy: Advances in diagnosis and treatment. *JAMA Pediatrics, 171*(9), 897–907.

Or, F., Kim, Y., Simms, J., & Austin, S. B. (2019). Taking stock of dietary supplements' harmful effects on children, adolescents, and young adults. *Journal of Adolescent Health, 65*, 455–461.

Organization of Teratology Information Specialists. (2019). *MotherToBaby/Fact sheet: Ibuprofen*. https://mothertobaby.org/fact-sheets/ibuprofen-pregnancy/pdf/

Patel, D. R., Neelakantan, M., Pandher, K., & Merrick, J. (2020). Cerebral palsy in children: A clinical overview. *Translational Pediatrics, 9*(Suppl. 1), S125–S135.

Peck, R. (1968). Psychological developments in the second half of life. In B. L. Neugarten (Ed.), *Middle age and aging*. University of Chicago Press.

Persson, M., Razaz, N., Tedroff, K., Joseph, K. S., & Cnattingius, S. (2018). Five and 10 minute Apgar scores and risks of cerebral palsy and epilepsy: Population based cohort study in Sweden. *British Medical Journal, 360*, k207. https://doi.org/10.1136/bmj.k207

Piaget, J. (1966). *Origins of intelligence in children*. International Universities Press.

Piaget, J. (1970). *Genetic epistemology*. Norton.

Ringwalt, S. (2008). *Developmental screening and assessment instruments with an emphasis on social and emotional development for young children ages birth through five*. University of North Carolina, FPG Child Development Institute, National Early Childhood Technical Assistance Center.

Ruckart, P. Z., Ettinger, A. S., Hanna-Attisha, M., Jones, N., Davis, S. I., & Breysse, P. N. (2019). The Flint water crisis: A coordinated public health emergency response and recovery initiative. *Journal of Public Health Management and Practice, 25*(Suppl. 1), S84–S90.

Sadowska, M., Sarecka-Hujar, B., & Koptya, I. (2020). Cerebral palsy: Current opinions on definitions, epidemiology, risk factors, classification and treatment options. *Neuropsychiatric Disease and Treatment, 16*, 1505–1518.

Scarpato, E., Staiano, A., Molteni, M., Terrone, G., Mazzocchi, A., & Agostoni, C. (2017). Nutritional assessment and intervention in children with cerebral palsy: A practical approach. *International Journal of Food Sciences and Nutrition, 68*(6), 763–770.

Scrandis, D.A. (2018). Diagnosing and treating ADHD in adults. *The Nurse Practitioner, 43*(1), 8–10.

Sibley, M. H., Swanson, J. M., Arnold, L. E., Hechtman, L. T., Owens, E. B., Stehli, A., et al. (2017). Defining ADHD symptom persistence in adulthood: optimizing sensitivity and specificity. *Journal of Child Psychology and Psychiatry, 58*(6), 655–662.

Sirotnak, A., & Chiesa, A. (2018). *Failure to thrive*. Medscape. http://emedicine.medscape.com/article/915575-overview

Solmi, M., Fornaro, M., Ostinelli, E. G., Zangani, C., Croatto, G., Monaco, F., et al. (2020). Safety of 80 antidepressants, antipsychotics, anti-attention-deficit/hyperactivity medications and mood stabilizers in children and adolescents with psychiatric disorders: A large scale systematic meta-review of 78 adverse effects. *World Psychiatry, 19*(2), 214–232.

Soref, S. (2019). *Attention deficit hyperactivity disorder (ADHD)*. Medscape. https://emedicine.medscape.com/article/289350-overview#a5.

Taggart, L., Truesdale, M., Dunkley, A., House, A., & Russell, A. M. (2018). Health promotion and wellness initiatives targeting chronic disease prevention and management for adults with intellectual and developmental disabilities: Recent advancements in type 2 diabetes. *Current Developmental Disorders Reports, 5*(3), 132–142.

Taylor, L. E., Swerdfeger, A. L., & Eslick, G. D. (2014). Vaccines are not associated with autism: An evidence-based meta-analysis of case-control and cohort studies. *Vaccine, 32*(29), 3623–3629.

U.S. Food and Drug Administration (FDA). (2018). *FDA drug safety communication: Safety review update of medications used to treat attention-deficit/hyperactivity disorder (ADHD) in adults*. http://www.fda.gov/Drugs/DrugSafety/ucm279858.htm

U.S. Food and Drug Administration (FDA). (2019). *Beware of false or misleading claims for treating autism*. http://www.fda.gov/ForConsumers/ConsumerUpdates/ucm394757.htm

U.S. Food and Drug Administration (FDA). (2020). *Pregnancy and lactation labeling (drugs) final rule*. https://www.fda.gov/drugs/labeling-information-drug-products/pregnancy-and-lactation-labeling-drugs-final-rule

Vachani, J. G. (2018). Failure to thrive: Early intervention mitigates long-term deficits. *Contemporary Pediatrics, 35*(4), 14–20.

Vehmeijer, F., Silva, C., Derks, I., El Marroun, H., Oei, E., Felix, J. F., et al. (2019). Associations of maternal psychological distress during pregnancy with childhood general and organ fat measures. *Childhood Obesity, 15*(5), 313–322.

Wang, K. K., Munger, M. E., Chen, B. P-J., & Novacheck, T. F. (2018). Selective dorsal rhizotomy in ambulant children with cerebral palsy. *Journal of Children's Orthopaedics, 12*, 413–427.

Weber, J. R., & Kelley, J. H. (2018). *Health assessment in nursing* (6th ed.). Lippincott Williams & Wilkins.

Werner, E., Bierman, J., & French, F. (1971). *The children of Kauai: a longitudinal study from the prenatal period to age ten*. University of Hawaii Press.

Wesemann, D., & Van Cleve, S. N. (2018). ADHD: From childhood to young adulthood. *The Nurse Practitioner, 43*(3), 8–15.

Whitney, D. G., Hurvitz, E. A., Ryan, J. M., Devlin, M. J., Caird, M. S., French, Z. P., et al. (2018). Noncommunicable disease and multimorbidity in young adults with cerebral palsy. *Clinical Epidemiology, 10*, 511–519.

Winters, R. R., Blake, J. J., & Chen, S. (2018). Bully victimization among children with attention deficit/hyperactivity disorder: A longitudinal examination of behavioral phenotypes. *Journal of Emotional and Behavioral Disorders, 28*(2), 80–91.

Wolraich, M. L., Hagan, J. F., Allan, C., Chan, E., Davison, D., Earls, M., et al. (2019a). Clinical practice guidelines for the diagnosis, evaluation, and treatment of attention-deficit/hyperactivity disorder in children and adolescents. *Pediatrics, 144*(4), 1–25.

Wolraich, M. L., Hagan, J. F., Allan, C., Chan, E., Davison, D., Earls, M., et al. (2019b). Implementing the key action statements: An algorithm and explanation for process of care for the evaluation, diagnosis, treatment, and monitoring of ADHD in children and adolescents. *Pediatrics, 144*(4), SI1–SI21. https://pediatrics.aappublications.org/content/suppl/2011/10/11/peds.2011-2654.DC1/zpe611117822p.pdf

World Health Organization (WHO). (2016). *Definition of an older or elderly person*. http://www.who.int/healthinfo/survey/ageingdefnolder/en/

Yi, Y. G., Jung, S. H., Bang, M. S. (2019). Emerging issues in cerebral palsy associated with aging: A physiatrist perspective. *Annals of Rehabilitative Medicine, 43*(3), 241–249.

Yin, J., & Schaaf, C. P. (2017). Autism genetics—an overview. *Prenatal Diagnosis, 37*, 14–30. http://dx.doi.org/10.1002/pd.4942

Zablotsky, B., & Alford, J. M. (2020). Racial and ethnic differences in the prevalence of attention-deficit/hyperactivity disorder and learning disabilities among U.S. children aged 3–17 years. *NCHS Data Brief* No. 358. National Center for Health Statistics.

Zanotti, J. M. (2018). Handle with care: Caring for children with autism spectrum disorder in the ED. *Nursing2018, 48*(2), 51–53.

Module 26
Family

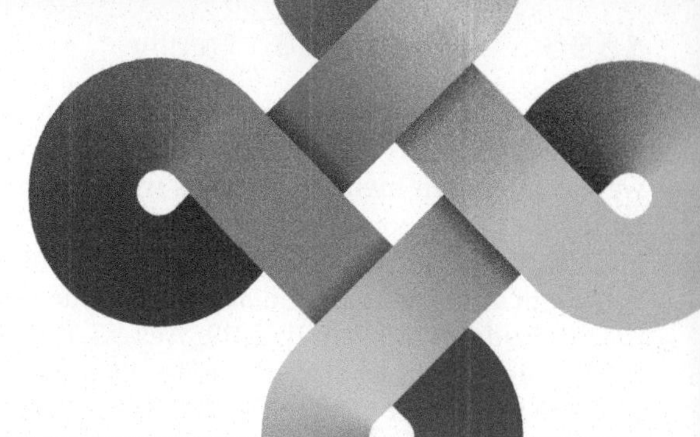

Module Outline and Learning Outcomes

The Concept of Family

Normal Presentation

26.1 Outline the makeup of the family structure.

Factors That Shape Family Development

26.2 Summarize the factors that shape family development.

Selected Influences on the Family System

26.3 Contrast different influences on the family system.

Alterations in Family Function

26.4 Differentiate alterations in family.

Concepts Related to Family

26.5 Outline the relationship between family and other concepts.

Health Promotion

26.6 Explain family health promotion.

Nursing Assessment

26.7 Differentiate common assessment procedures and tests used to examine family.

Independent Interventions

26.8 Analyze independent interventions nurses can implement for patients with alterations in family.

Collaborative Practices

26.9 Summarize collaborative therapies used by interprofessional teams for patients with alterations in family.

Family Exemplar

Exemplar 26.A Family Response to Health Alterations

26.A Analyze family response to health alterations.

›› The Concept of Family

Concept Key Terms

Adolescent family, **1898**
Binuclear family, **1897**
Blended family, **1898**
Childfree family, **1898**
Discipline, **1903**
Ecomap, **1911**
Extended-kin network family, **1897**
Family, **1895**
Family-centered care, **1896**
Family cohesion, **1901**
Family communication, **1900**
Family coping mechanisms, **1901**
Family development, **1899**
Foster family, **1898**
Genogram, **1911**
Intergenerational family, **1898**
Joint custody, **1897**
LGBTQ family, **1898**
Limit setting, **1902**
Nuclear family, **1897**
Punishment, **1903**
Resiliency, **1901**
Single-parent family, **1897**
Two-career family, **1897**

For most individuals, family serves as a primary developmental influence. Numerous family structures exist, from single-parent families to families headed by two mothers or two fathers. Regardless of structural variations, every family is subject to the challenges of life, including economic hardship, illness, and stress. This concept explores the role of the family in terms of development, childrearing, health promotion, and response to alterations in health status. In addition, the nurse's role in caring for the family unit is examined.

Normal Presentation

The *Merriam-Webster Dictionary* (2020) gives no fewer than eight definitions of the word *family*. The basic unit of society, family can be defined as a group of people related to each other, by birth, by marriage, or by choice, who may or may not live together in the same household. The head of a family may be a single individual—for example, a grandfather or elder or a single mother—or a couple who may or may not be married and who may or may not live under the same roof with all members of the family. The U.S. Census Bureau (2019c) defines a **family** as two or more individuals who are joined together by marriage, birth, or adoption and are residing in the same household. This definition is somewhat limiting, however, as there exist legal, social, cultural, and psychologic implications to the term *family* that vary widely depending on the state, region, country, culture, or society in which the family lives. More broadly, families are generally characterized by bonds of emotional closeness, sharing, and support, and one family may define its members very differently from the next.

The Family as a Functional System

As with any unit or organization, the family is more than the sum of its parts or members. Genetic and cultural influences (including beliefs and value systems) and the interactions among its members inform the family's functional ability as well as how each member interacts with others outside the family. In other words, within a family, each individual is interconnected with and interdependent on the other members, both as individuals and as a group (The Bowen Center for the Study of the Family, 2019; Weyers, Zemp, & Alpers, 2019). This is the heart of *family systems theory*. A *system* can be described as a set of parts or elements (or in the case of a family, individuals) that interact purposefully or orderly rather than randomly with each other (von Bertalanffy, 1981). Like any system, the family's purpose or goals are to maintain functioning—a steady state—and to adapt or respond successfully to change. Families that operate with cohesiveness are able to exchange information (for example, by discussing and modeling acceptable behaviors) and resources (such as personal energy necessary to accomplish tasks) to meet problems and find solutions (The Bowen Center for the Study of the Family, 2019). However, families may suffer when stressful situations impact all family members due to the interconnectedness, making it difficult to adapt and overcome.

Precisely because family members are so interconnected and interdependent, when nurses encounter any individual in need of care, they should approach the patient holistically, viewing the patient as part of a whole, as part of the family unit, and not simply as an individual. Consider the following examples:

- Parents/caregivers caring for a toddler with a chronic illness. What hurdles might they face? What thoughts or feelings might they have? How might these impact care of other children? Their relationship as parents?
- A family whose oldest child has a serious mental illness, such as schizophrenia or bipolar disorder.
- A family whose main provider is in a motor-vehicle crash and sustains significant head trauma.
- A woman who comes for a simple procedure (say, a mammogram or DEXA scan) at 3:30 and is still in the waiting room at 4:30 and must pick up her father from eldercare by 5:00 before picking up her teenager from soccer practice by 5:30.

Consider how even small issues can have a large impact and how the nurse and staff may view the issue differently from the patient, as in the last example provided. These and myriad other issues can impact functioning of the entire family system.

A family generally provides an environment for its members to learn group values, norms, and acceptable behaviors. Support and communication provide a way for families to maintain optimal health and functioning. In a healthy, functional family unit, functions have historically included the following:

- Socializing children
- Providing support, both emotional and physical
- Sexual reproduction
- Providing a social identity (Barkan, 2019).

These functions allow for the transmission of beliefs, values, and traditions to be passed on through the socialization of the children as the social identity is formed. Emotional support allows for nurturing and love in a healthy family, while physical support ensures protection and economic support. Healthy family functioning provides a constant system of support to the child members, allowing for health and wellness in physical and psychological aspects.

Within the family unit, members fulfill designated roles to promote day-to-day functioning. These roles are established to support the values and beliefs held by the family, and may be based on religious, cultural, or societal norms. Additional influences may stem from educational levels, and individual life experiences of the adult family members. The parental roles held by adult family members are often learned through socialization during their own childhood. Nurses should respect the family roles and experiences when providing care. Through this respect, the nurse and family can form a partnership that enables **family-centered care** (Institute for Patient- and Family-Centered Care [IPFCC], 2020). Effective decision making regarding the child's health results from a successful partnership.

Recognition of the advantages of involving patient and families across the lifespan directly in their care has resulted in patient- and family-centered care (PFCC), alternatively known as person-centered care. This concept identifies that the healthcare team needs to involve both the patient and the family in making mutually beneficial partnerships for the planning and implementation of healthcare in a variety of settings (IPFCC, 2020; Planetree International, 2018). Nursing care of the patient and family is core to nursing practice, and as such necessitates viewing this as a partnership in a comprehensive, holistic manner.

Providing culturally competent care is imperative to providing family-centered care. Within the United States, the core foundation of the nation's heritage is drawn from families of different cultures. The values and beliefs from a family's culture impact many aspects of daily family functioning, including communication styles, health beliefs and practices, living arrangements, and support and coping methods.

Diversity in Family Structures and Roles

Families may look very different from one another in structure (the individuals within the family) and the roles or responsibilities of those individuals. Data from the U.S. Census Bureau (n.d.) identifies several types of households, including married couples (opposite-sex and same-sex), unmarried couples (opposite-sex or same-sex), multigenerational, single-adult, and nonfamily households. Furthermore, these various household types may be with or without children. The presence of children does not necessarily define a family or household. Family housing units may include houses and apartments located in urban, suburban, or rural areas.

Families provide for physical support in the form of housing, nutrition, and healthcare, and economic resources are essential to support the lifestyle practices within each family. Children are significantly impacted by the physical support for growth and development, as well as the lack of physical support that may stem from a lack of housing, nutrition, or healthcare.

When considering families from the standpoint of the tasks associated with functioning as a unit, many families are similar. However, family units in the United States are diverse in terms of structure and with regard to which family member assumes a given role.

Nuclear Family

A family structure of a mother and father and their offspring is known as the **nuclear family**. In 2018, 65% of children under the age of 18 lived in the same household with two married parents (Federal Interagency Forum on Child and Family Statistics, 2019). This percentage has decreased from nearly 80% in the early 1980s due to evolving family structures (Federal Interagency Forum on Child and Family Statistics, 2019).

When two biological parents divorce but continue to raise their children in partnership with one another, the family may be referred to as **binuclear**. Children in a binuclear family spend significant time with both parents, often going from one house to the other on a mutually agreed-upon schedule. In **joint custody**, both parents have equal legal rights and responsibility regardless of where the children live. The binuclear family model enables both parents to be involved in the children's upbringing and provides additional support and role models in the form of extended family members. Special nursing considerations in this family type involve ensuring that health promotion guidance and education for care of the child with an acute or chronic condition are communicated effectively to both biological parents.

Extended Family

Grandparents, aunts, uncles, cousins, and other relatives are termed *extended family*. Extended family members may live with the family or live away from the family. Regardless of living arrangements, the extended family members may serve as a source of emotional and/or financial support (**Figure 26.1** ›)). An extended family may also share household and childrearing responsibilities with parents, siblings, or other relatives. In 2018, 2.8 million children in the United States lived with a grandparent (The Annie E. Coley Foundation Kids Count Data Center, 2019). Grandparents may raise children when their parents are unable to care for them. Grandparents endure emotional, physical, and financial stresses when taking on the childrearing role for one or more grandchildren.

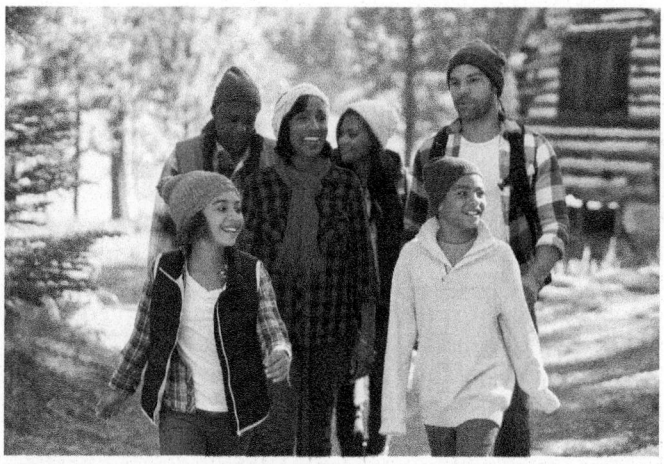

Figure 26.1 ›) Three generations of a family enjoying a walk in the woods.

Source: Shutterstock.

One example of an extended family is the **extended-kin network family**. An extended-kin network family exists when there are two or more nuclear families living in close proximity to one another, allowing for ease of the sharing of responsibilities that can occur with an extended family. The household chores, childrearing, and other daily family responsibilities are shared among the families that account for the extended-kin network. Within certain cultures, this type of arrangement is more common. In the United States, it is most commonly seen among Latino families.

Two-Career Family

In **two-career families** (or *dual-career families*), both partners are employed by choice or by necessity. They may or may not have children. Two-career families have steadily increased since the 1960s because of increased career opportunities for women, a desire to increase the family's standard of living, and economic necessity. The U.S. Bureau of Labor Statistics (2020) reported that the percentage of married dual-career families rose to 64.2% in 2019. Two-career families have to address issues related to child care, household chores, and spending time together, with finding good-quality, affordable child care being one of the greatest stressors. A majority of families opt for center-based child care (54%), while others utilize a home-based option with 18% utilizing a relative and 11% placing children with a home-based nonrelative daycare (Federal Interagency Forum on Child and Family Statistics, 2019). The average cost of daycare for an infant is over $200 per week, which is more than $10,000 annually (Care.com Editorial Staff, 2020). This cost has continued to rise, and it requires a significant portion of income for many families.

Single-Parent Family

In 2018, just over one-quarter (26%) of all children in the United States lived in a **single-parent family**, that is, a family with one parent only (Federal Interagency Forum on Child and Family Statistics, 2019). Single-parent families can result from a variety of situations. Divorce, separation, or the death of a partner lead to single-parent households. Additionally, children may be born to a single woman through planned or unplanned pregnancies. In recent years, adoptions by single men or women have become more common. There are several challenges that may arise when there is only a single parent present in the household, ranging from childcare concerns to economic difficulties. These demands may result in social isolation, role overload, and fatigue. It is essential to the well-being of a single-parent family to identify a support system to help mitigate the difficulties. Single-parent families experience higher rates of poverty, which has important implications for the children. Poverty is highest among single-parent families headed by women, with 40.7% living in poverty, compared to only 8.4% of children in married households that live in poverty (Federal Interagency Forum on Child and Family Statistics, 2019).

Single mothers are at risk for poverty because of lack of child support, unequal pay for work performed, and the high costs of child care. Nurses working with single parents need to assess their strengths and needs related to providing care for their children, fulfilling work commitments, and making healthcare appointments. Availability of afterschool care and backup child care arrangements can affect adherence to treatment regimens and employment status. Nurses also help connect families with available resources such as school breakfast/lunch programs and child care subsidy assistance.

Adolescent Family

The birthrate among teenagers peaked in the early 1990s and has decreased progressively since then to 18.8 births per 1000 women age 15 to 19 in 2017 (U.S. Department of Health and Human Services [DHHS], 2019). While this birth rate shows progress in the Unites States, there are discrepancies among races. Adolescent birth rates are highest among Hispanic and Black females (DHHS, 2019). Furthermore, adolescent birth rates are higher in the United States compared to other developed countries. For example, in 2018, Canada saw 8 births per 1000 women and the United Kingdom 13 births per 1000 women ages 15–19 (World Bank Group, 2020). **Adolescent families** (families in which the parent is an adolescent) will likely face many challenges, including lower educational levels, lower income generation, and more reliance on welfare and other public resources (Gorry, 2019). Adolescent parents are still developing, thus leading to a lack of developmental preparation for childrearing in both physical and emotional arenas. Their children will be impacted by these concerns.

Foster Family

In the United States, more than 260,000 children enter the foster care system each year following a determination that their families are unable to care for them properly (Child Welfare Information Gateway, 2019). A **foster family** makes a legal commitment to provide appropriate care for a child who cannot be cared for by a parent or close family member. Foster parents may accept one or more children into their care after completing a lengthy screening and training process with a local division of child services or other overseeing agency. Ideally, foster children are returned to their birth parent(s) or legally and permanently adopted by another family member or adult. However, many children will grow up and "age out" of foster care without having been placed permanently in a caring home. Of these, approximately 25% become homeless during the first 4 years after leaving foster care (U.S. Department of Housing and Urban Development, 2019).

Childfree Family

Childfree families are a growing trend. In some cases, a family has no children by choice; in other cases, a family has no children because of issues related to infertility or other medical conditions that present risks to the woman or fetus should the woman become pregnant. According to the U.S. Census Bureau (2019a), in 2018, more women in the United States (49.8% of those ages 15 to 44) did not have children than at any other time since the government started tracking childbearing.

Blended Family

A **blended family** consists of two parents with biological children from previous relationships. The parents may be married or may cohabit. This family structure has become increasingly common in the United States because of high rates of divorce and remarriage. In 2018, 8% of children in the United States lived with a stepparent (Federal Interagency Forum on Child and Family Statistics, 2019).

Many benefits arise from blended families, as well as some stressors. Benefits may include improved financial status, as well as increased support in childrearing and role modeling. At times, however, there may be increased stress related to the stepparent and stepchild relationships. Stresses can include discipline issues, adjustment problems, role ambiguity, strain with the other biological parent, and communication issues. When blended families with children form after the divorce or death of a parent, adjustment can be particularly challenged by the normal processes of grief and loss. An important nursing consideration is to direct families to resources that may help reduce the potential conflicts associated with different parenting styles, discipline, and manipulative behaviors of children that can develop within a blended family.

Intergenerational Family

An **intergenerational family** typically includes more than two generations living together, although sometimes a generation may be skipped or missing. Examples include a family with a grandparent, an adult child, and the grandchild living together or a grandparent caring for one or more grandchildren with the parents absent or living elsewhere.

Cohabiting Family

Cohabiting (or communal) families consist of unrelated individuals or families who live under one roof. This may include never-married individuals as well as divorced or widowed persons. In 2018, 8% of children age 0 to 17 in the United States lived with two unmarried, cohabiting parents (Federal Interagency Forum on Child and Family Statistics, 2019). Within the cohabiting family, one or both parents have biological children that are a part of the family and additional children may be born into the family, with all of these scenarios representing a blended cohabitating family.

While there are similar benefits and stresses in the blended cohabiting family compared to the blended (married) family, there is one notable nursing consideration: The nonbiological parent does not have legal authority for the child. The lack of legal authority will impact the ability of the nonbiological parent to seek medical care for the child. However, emergency medical care would be provided without parental consent if there is significant concern regarding loss of life or function. Similar legal considerations may arise with the education system as well.

LGBTQ Families

LGBTQ (lesbian, gay, bisexual, transgender, and queer/questioning) families can have all of the structures outlined previously (e.g., married, single parent, blended, intergenerational, cohabitation) (**Figure 26.2** »). Nearly 200,000 children in the United States live in two-parent same-sex households (Gurrentz & Valerio, 2019). The number of children being raised by a single LGBTQ parent is less clear and much harder to track with current census data.

There are a variety of ways in which children become a part of an LGBTQ household. Some children are born from a previous heterosexual relationship, while others are adopted by one or both members of an LGBTQ couple.

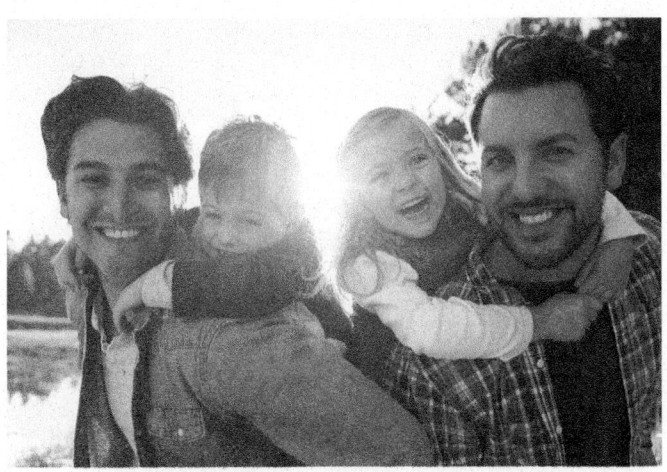

Figure 26.2 » A gay couple and their children.
Source: Shutterstock.

Furthermore, artificial insemination with donor sperm or the use of a surrogate and a donor egg are becoming more common ways to build families. Foster care and adoption are also common methods of family building among LGBTQ families.

Research has identified no differences in the well-being of children raised by an LGBTQ parent, including psychological and developmental well-being (American Psychological Association, 2020). In addition, Farr and Vazquez (2020) report that children of LGBTQ parents report similar levels of parent–child relationship quality when compared to children of heterosexual parents.

SAFETY ALERT When obtaining consent to provide healthcare and medical treatments to children and adolescents, the healthcare provider (HCP) should identify the biological or adoptive parent or confirm a caregiver's possession of legal documentation proving the right to make medical decisions on the child's behalf.

Children in LGBTQ families typically have only one biological or adoptive legal parent even if the parents are legally married. In many states, the other partner is the coparent and has no legal parental status. Various states have now taken legislative action to ensure the security of children whose parents are LGBTQ by guaranteeing access by the second parent to joint adoption rights. Coparent adoption provides for either parent to give consent for healthcare and make other important decisions on behalf of the child. It also has implications for child custody and financial support in the event the parents separate or a death occurs, ensuring the child's right to a continuing relationship with and financial support from both parents. Nursing considerations for individuals in LGBTQ families emphasize respect for the relationship between partners and recognition of the nurturing capacity in these families.

There is a range of legal issues that may arise for LGBTQ families, and these are dynamic and frequently changing. Despite a U.S. Supreme Court decision in 2015 supporting marriage between same-sex partners, many states across the country maintain laws that do not recognize such a union (Cable News Network, 2019). As such, there are many loopholes and discrepancies in laws that contribute to limited access to the same rights and privileges of a heterosexual married couple. Health insurance is available to same-sex married couples, as a result of the 2015 ruling that recognized same-sex marriage across the United States. Prior to that ruling, domestic partner benefits were common for unmarried same-sex partners; however, these benefits have decreased in availability following legalization of same-sex marriage.

» **Stay Current:** The Family Equality Council advocates for family rights of LGBTQ families. For current advocacy initiatives, visit https://www.familyequality.org.

Single Adults Living Alone

Individuals who live by themselves represent a significant portion of today's society. According to the U.S. Census Bureau, in 2019, 28.4% of adults lived alone (U.S. Census Bureau, 2019b). This percentage has increased steadily over the last 50 years. Single adults living alone range in age from young adults who have recently moved out of the family home, to older adults who may be widowed, divorced, or never married.

Stages of Family Development

Family development (the growth or progress of communication patterns, roles, and interactions within a family) occurs over time as a result of childbearing, growth, and other changes that transpire as the family grows together. Many of these changes are unique to each individual family, yet there are theories to support some common stages that are experienced. Duvall (1977) theorized that families go through eight stages in the family life cycle (see **Table 26.1** »). Based on the traditional nuclear family at the time of development of the theory, Duvall noted that the life cycle stages are based on the age of the children in the family, until the children have aged out of the family home. In many families, there is more than one child, so there may be some overlap in staging. While other models exist, many are rooted in this model and were developed to account for other types of families, from LGBTQ, blended, or single parent family types.

TABLE 26.1 Eight-Stage Family Life Cycle

Stage	Characteristics
Stage I	Beginning family, newly married couples*
Stage II	Childbearing family (oldest child is an infant through 30 months of age)
Stage III	Families with preschool children (oldest child is between 2.5 and 6 years of age)
Stage IV	Families with schoolchildren (oldest child is between 6 and 13 years of age)
Stage V	Families with teenagers (oldest child is between 13 and 20 years of age)
Stage VI	Families launching young adults (all children leave home)
Stage VII	Middle-aged parents (empty nest through retirement)
Stage VIII	Family in retirement and old age (retirement to death of both spouses)

* Keep in mind that this was the norm at the time the model was developed, but today families form through many different types of relationships.

Sources: Data from Coehlo (2015); Duvall (1977); Duvall and Miller (1985).

Choosing to become a parent is a major life change for adults. Beginning when they first learn they are expecting a child (whether through pregnancy or adoption), parents experience stresses and challenges along with feelings of pride and excitement. Mothers and fathers adjust their lifestyles to give priority to parenting. Babies and very young children are dependent for total care 24 hours a day, and this often results in sleep deprivation, irritability, less personal time, and less time for the couple's relationship. In addition, the family with a new baby often experiences a change in financial status.

Families progress in their development as children grow and, in many cases, initiate new generations of the family. Parents grow older, seeing their children leave the "nest" and progressing toward retirement. Factors that affect how families adjust to each stage include family communication patterns, resiliency, and parenting styles. These and other factors are outlined later in this module.

As families progress through the developmental stages, adaptation occurs that can either go well or lead to alterations in family development. These alterations may impact the health and wellness of family members and must be considered by the nurse, in addition to the developmental stage of the family.

Factors That Shape Family Development

Changes in the family structure, function, and processes can alter family development. These changes generally occur over time and may be planned or unplanned.

Cultural Practices

Family assessment requires consideration of the ages of all family members, as well as the cultural practices of the family. The age of the child or children will influence the family dynamic; for example, tasks associated with raising a toddler are vastly different from those pertinent to raising a teenager. Family activities and interactions will also vary depending on the age of the child. For example, when raising a toddler, a majority of the parents' focus may be on meeting the child's developmental and social needs, whereas a teenager will generally work to meet these needs on his own, and the parental roles incorporate guiding the teenager in making life choices.

Cultural practices may influence the child's diet, behavior, and even sleep patterns. Some cultural and religious traditions may involve vegetarianism (see **Figure 26.3** »), while others may involve brief periods of fasting. The manner in which a child is expected to behave in public and at home can be impacted by culture, as can the child's degree of respect for older adults. Culture can also affect the behavior of the entire family unit depending on matriarchal or patriarchal views. For example, in a matriarchal structure, the mother may be expected to take responsibility for making family healthcare decisions, to the near exclusion of the father and children. Although it is neither realistic nor necessary for the nurse to be an expert on each culture's beliefs, through open and nonjudgmental communication, the nurse can ascertain a great deal about the family's cultural influences.

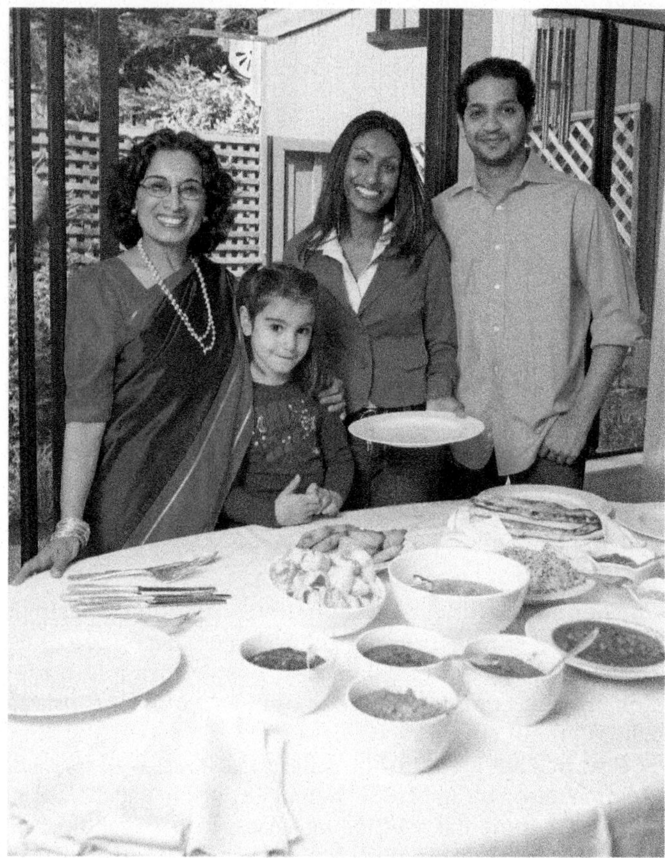

Figure 26.3 » This extended family of Indian Americans are vegetarians in keeping with their Hindu religion's concept of nonviolence against all life forms.
Source: Tanya Constantine/Getty Images.

Emotional Availability

Healthy coping among family members occurs when all members feel safe expressing their feelings—positive and negative—and the emotional environment of the family is one of respect, closeness, and predictability. Predictability refers to the inclusion of family routines on which family members can depend and in which they find comfort. Examples include a reasonably regular schedule of activities (e.g., reading before bed and a consistent bedtime). In a family with healthy coping, members are emotionally available to each other—that is, they have healthy emotional connections (Hajal & Paley, 2020). Emotional availability is correlated to parenting ability (Benton, Coatsworth, & Biringen, 2019). Emotionally available parents are sensitive to their children's needs without being intrusive, provide structure for learning and exploration without exceeding the child's abilities, and are available but not interfering or hostile. These behaviors encourage child responsiveness, respect, and willingness to interact with parents and other family members (Benton et al., 2019).

Family Communication Patterns

Family communication is a key factor in family development. Clear communication, problem solving, and sharing feelings associated with events within the family can help families achieve a high level of functioning and increase self-efficacy among children and other family members (Hemati, Abbasi, Oujian, & Kiani, 2020).

Throughout all family communication, similar to all other types of communication, verbal and nonverbal messages are exchanged. The effectiveness of these various communication styles leads to the family's ability to function in a healthy capacity. Self-efficacy, along with self-esteem, develop from healthy communication patterns in families (Hemati et al., 2020). Family communication contributes to development of values and beliefs, determination of roles within the family, and learning how to function in society.

Family Cohesion

Family cohesion is defined as the emotional bonding between family members. Cohesion among family members can be visualized on a continuum from disengaged (very low cohesion and independence) to enmeshed (very high cohesion and dependence). A family unit may be very cohesive. In addition, there may be very cohesive or very disengaged dyadic or triadic relationships within the family. *Dyadic* refers to the dynamics in a relationship between two people, *triadic* to the dynamics among three people. For example, a dynamic triad may develop between one parent and two children when the other parent is called out of town for work and therefore absent on a regular basis.

Family Coping Mechanisms

Family coping mechanisms reflect the strategies used within a family to manage stress that occurs from internal or external factors. The coping mechanisms may be stable or may change over time as a result of family growth and development. Adult family members will model coping strategies to the children in the family, and children will adopt these strategies (Tiret & Knurek, 2020). Family success may rely on the methods for coping with stress occurring as a result of financial concerns, illness, or many other situations.

Nurses must assess coping mechanisms when working with families and must consider both positive and negative coping strategies in the assessment. Positive coping strategies may include exercise, reading, and relaxation techniques, while negative coping strategies can include drugs and alcohol for stress management (Tiret & Knurek, 2020). Negative coping strategies may lead to additional stress and consequences for the family. In addition to considering positive and negative strategies, the nurse must consider the internal and external resources available to each family. Internal resources may include the communication patterns and family roles that facilitate problem solving, whereas external resources include extended family, friends, and community organizations, including religious or healthcare settings. External resources are not equally available to all families due to factors such as poverty and isolation and are therefore imperative for nurses to assess.

Family Size

Historically speaking, family size referred to the number of children that resulted from a traditional nuclear family union. Given the various family structures that are seen today, it is much more difficult to define family size when taking into consideration blended or single-parent families and other variations in family structure. It is important to consider the difference between family size and household size, as they may be very different. While a child may live with a single parent and one sibling, leading to a household size of three, that same child may be part of an extended-kin network with other family members living nearby who actively participate in the life and support of the child. This would lead to a family size that may be perceived as much different than the household size. Therefore, it is important for nurses to assess family structure and support with not only the family members in the household but any additional close family members that may be actively engaged in the child's life.

Parent–Child Interaction

The interactions between a parent and a child are essential to growth and development and have the ability to impact development in both positive and negative ways. Effective parent–child interactions lead to positive impacts on a child's social behavior and result in positive nurturing interactions (The University of Tennessee Health Science Center, 2020). Stress and coping mechanisms are impacted by these interactions, which can, in turn, impact self-efficacy and self-esteem. Parents express less distress from disruptive child behaviors when the parent–child interaction is effective (The University of Tennessee Health Science Center, 2020). More information on how parenting influences family development can be found later in this module.

Resiliency

Another factor important in shaping a family is **resiliency**—the ability to adapt to change. Having resources and adaptive abilities increases the resilience of a family, thus helping them to overcome adversity, heal from adverse experiences, and progress beyond adversity to fulfillment (Child Welfare Information Gateway, n.d.). Life crises and developmental transitions can stimulate family growth and transformation. Resilient families make it through crises (such as serious injury to a family member) with a renewed sense of confidence and purpose. The U.S. Department of Defense funds a source to promote resiliency in military families, who face singular challenges related to deployment and frequent relocation. Military One Source (2020) has identified several strategies for promoting resiliency in families, including staying smart about stress management, staying connected with family and relationships, and staying positive when challenges arise. In addition, routine and consistent communication among all members of the healthcare team with all family members is an important strategy for enhancing resiliency. Allowing the family to support their family members through providing basic care or through identifying the unique needs of their family member is a supportive action that increases resilience.

Sibling Relationships

Sibling relationships in society today may be impacted by whether or not the siblings reside in the same household. Close sibling relationships may result from gender, age, and residence in the same household, which promotes shared experiences.

Sibling roles vary based on family and environmental experiences. At times a sibling may serve as a confidant, friend, protector, and more, while at the same time both

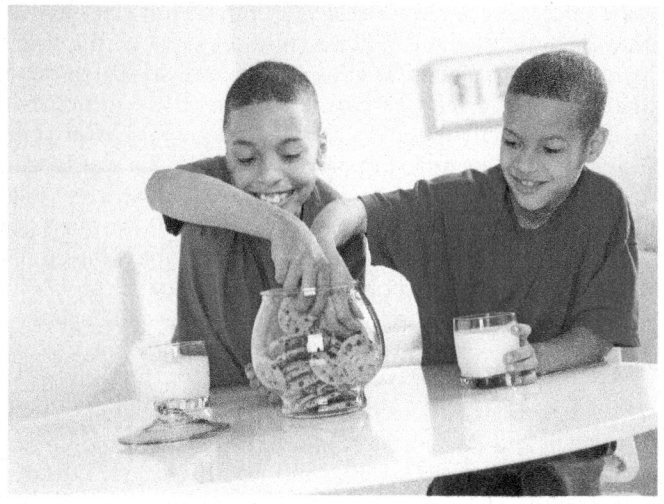

Figure 26.4 » Same-gender siblings who are close in age tend to have close, lifelong relationships.

Source: Andersen Ross Photography Inc/DigitalVision/Getty Images.

sharing and competing with other siblings. Older siblings may reinforce the household rules set by the parents to younger siblings. In many families, siblings learn to work well together to debate household rules (see **Figure 26.4** »). However, sibling rivalry can challenge sibling relationships and may have a long-term impact. Parents should work to encourage positive sibling relationships.

While it is widely thought that birth order has an impact on child temperament and other characteristics, research has not resulted in evidence to support this. Bornstein, Hahn, Putnick, and Pearson (2019) evaluated child temperament through a variety of moderating characteristics, including birth order. The longitudinal study evaluated children at 3, 5, and 6 years of age and noted no significant impact from birth order in relationship to child temperament (activity level, emotionality, shyness, and sociability). In a large study utilizing a within- and between-families design, Boccio and Beaver (2019) similarly noted no differences in the areas of extraversion, neuroticism, agreeableness, conscientiousness, or openness as a result of birth order in adult participants.

Selected Influences on the Family System

Raising a family can be a difficult task. Every day, parents must balance change within the family, their role as parents, and the delicate nature of reward and stress when dealing with their children. Being flexible within the context of parenting is referred to as parenting flexibility. Being able to deal with stressful issues without the need to control psychologic experiences can help the child to learn to cope and can provide the necessary structure for the parent–child relationship and the family unit to thrive.

Parenting Styles

Families will experience frequent changes as they move through the family developmental cycles and the children age. It is imperative for parents to provide stability to children throughout these changes. Nurturing allows for children to feel safe and secure in the family unit, both physically and psychologically. Throughout childhood, children learn values, beliefs, and behaviors from their parents and other family members.

Limit setting is imperative to successful parenting, as it allows children to gain independence as they grow and explore their own boundaries. Exploration and curiosity lead to development of autonomy, which is necessary as children age and progress toward adulthood. Two important factors that impact parenting choices and how successful parents are at setting appropriate limits are parental warmth (affection) and parental control (rule setting). See **Table 26.2** » for selected characteristics of parental warmth and control. In addition to these characteristics, parents' particular parenting styles also impact the success of the parent–child relationship as well as the autonomy and well-being of children later in life.

Brown (2019) noted that four parenting styles originally defined by Diana Baumrind in the 1970s are still applicable today: authoritarian, authoritative, permissive, and neglectful. Families generally tend to use one style, but they may vary their style for certain situations. Although helicopter parenting has not been identified as a specific and separate parenting style, research in this area is increasing. An overview of helicopter parenting can be found in **Box 26.1** ».

TABLE 26.2 Characteristics of Significant Parenting Attributes

Parenting Attribute	Parental Warmth	Parental Control
High level	■ Warm, nurturing ■ Expressing affection and smiling at children frequently ■ Limiting criticism, punishment ■ Expressing approval of child	■ Restrictive control of behavior ■ Surveying and enforcing compliance with rules ■ Encouraging children to fulfill their responsibilities ■ Sometimes limiting freedom of expression
Low level	■ Cool, hostile ■ Quick to criticize or punish ■ Ignoring children ■ Rarely expressing affection or approval ■ Sometimes rejecting children	■ Permissive, minimally controlling ■ Making fewer demands ■ Making fewer restrictions on behavior or expression of emotion ■ Permitting freedom in exploring environment

Source: From Ball, Bindler, and Cowen (2017). Pearson Education., Inc. Hoboken, NJ.

Box 26.1
Helicopter Parenting

Overparenting, often referred to as *helicopter parenting*, refers to the overinvolvement of parents in their children's lives. Behaviors exhibited by helicopter parents may include (Bristow, 2020; Weiland & Kucirka, 2019):

- Low expectations and demands for children to develop independence and self-efficacy, proceed along developmental milestones, or accept consequences for their actions
- Constant monitoring, phoning or messaging, and intrusiveness (micromanaging) in the child's life
- A perception that their child is always right
- Constant instruction regarding behavior, an intense focus on academics, and restriction of experiences with peers.

Although the effects of overparenting are still being studied and may vary from one child to the next, overparenting has been positively associated with increased parental anxiety. Among young adults and adults who experienced overparenting growing up, the overinvolvement of their parents was associated with an increase in ineffective coping skills, which in turn was associated with greater anxiety. The increased anxiety is being seen in increasing numbers on college campuses, as children of helicopter parents try to learn to function independently outside of the home (Weiland & Kucirka, 2019).

Authoritarian Parents

Authoritarian parents are known to be strict and demanding of their children. Parents utilizing this parenting style tend to set strict rules that must be followed or there will be consequences implemented. Children are expected to adhere to the rules without question, and the parents lack responsiveness to the child's feelings or opinions. This style can impact overall child self-esteem and understanding of how his or her own actions can affect others.

Authoritative Parents

Authoritative parents can be described as supportive and fair, yet firm. These parents are highly responsive and open to the child's needs, while maintaining high standards for behavior. Rules are expected to be followed; however, the parents take the time to explain why the rules exist to strengthen the child's development and sense of right and wrong. Flexibility may be granted as appropriate. Authoritative parenting is often considered a very positive parenting approach.

Permissive Parents

Permissive parents are laidback and tolerant of their children. Additionally, these parents are easy to forgive their children, believing they will learn from their own mistakes. Permissive parents may make rules, but they do not often enforce them. Discipline is limited or does not occur at all, which can reinforce bad behavior. This parent style is often considered more of a friend then a parent.

Neglectful Parents

Neglectful parents do not display much interest in their children or in their roles as parents. They are often described as disengaged, distant, and uninvolved. Clear rules are not set for the children, and the child's needs frequently go unnoticed. The effects on children can range from low self-esteem and increased risk for unhealthy behaviors to insufficient access to appropriate food and nutrition and other basic care needs.

Discipline

Discipline is the process for teaching the rules of behavior to a child, including behaviors in a variety of circumstances. **Punishment** describes actions that are taken when the expected behavior is not followed. Both discipline and punishment are determined by the parenting style being followed. Therefore, some children may be disciplined more firmly (authoritarian), whereas others may receive less punishment (authoritative). Children are nurtured by limits on behavior as they feel safe and secure to explore within the boundaries that are set. Punishment for breaking the limits or rules contributes to the development of morals and understanding of the consequences of behavior.

Effects of Stigma on LGBTQ Families

In *Accelerating Acceptance 2018*, GLAAD published the results of surveys conducted among non-LGBTQ Americans on their degree of acceptance of LGBTQ individuals. Thirty percent of Americans reported they would feel either somewhat uncomfortable or very uncomfortable on learning a family member was LGBTQ (GLAAD, 2018). Stigma and discrimination against LGBTQ individuals and families can arise from external influences (community and systemic discrimination) and internal influences (stigma from within the family).

LGBTQ Youth

LGBTQ youth experience disparities in both physical and mental health compared to their heterosexual peers. This has significant implications for both the medical and the larger community. According to The Trevor Project (2019), almost 10.5% (over 2 million) youth ages 13–18 identify as LGBTQ. Of this number, over 45% had considered suicide in the last 12 months (The Trevor Project, 2019). Suicide prevention and mental health care is imperative for this population.

The significance of the role of the family in the health of the LGBTQ child or adolescent cannot be overstated. Failure of the family unit to accept a child or adolescent's identification as LGBTQ can lead to a number of unhealthy outcomes, one of which is homelessness. An estimated 20–40% of the total LGBTQ youth population are homeless, compared to approximately 4–10% of the total youth population in the United States (Homelessness Policy Research Institute, 2019). Additionally, homeless LGBTQ youth are noted to experience more violence, exploitation, and health concerns (both physical and mental) then heterosexual youth who are homeless.

Nurses working with families with an LGBTQ child or adolescent can support both the youth and the family by:

- Providing information on LGBTQ resources in the area
- Encouraging open, respectful communication among all family members
- Encouraging parents to allow their child access to LGBTQ friends and resources
- Helping the family understand that the young person is not to blame for any stigma the family experiences

- Encouraging the parents to talk with their child about identity in an affirming manner
- Advocating in their communities for increased resources and support for LGBTQ children and adolescents.

LGBTQ Parents

In recent years, child well-being has been a focus of research, with specific consideration on the impact of a child being raised in an LGBTQ family. Pollitt, Reczek, and Umberson (2020) note that while children and adults in LGBTQ-led families may experience more psychological distress due to stigma and victimization, these experiences do not lead to disparities in the mental health of children or LGBTQ parents when compared to children of heterosexual parents. As outlined earlier, parenting style and involvement, not the sexual attraction of the parents, seems to be the most important for child outcomes. However, children in LGBTQ families may be at risk because of how they are treated by those in their communities. Nurses should be aware of support groups or other services to assist children in LGBTQ families who are misunderstood in their community.

>> **Stay Current:** LGBTQ acceptance across the country is the focus of GLAAD. For more information on their current work, visit https://www.glaad.org.

Alterations in Family Function

Any number of situations or factors can cause short- or long-term alterations in family function. Trauma, abuse, neglect, addiction, criminal activity, and military deployment are just a few of these situations. Resilient families may overcome alterations or crises with time, patience, and understanding and family and social support. Whenever a family experiences some kind of upheaval or alteration to family functioning, nurses assess for safety, coping mechanisms, and immediate and long-term needs, as well as providing support and making referrals as appropriate.

Alterations and Therapies

Family

ALTERATION	DESCRIPTION	MANIFESTATIONS	INTERVENTIONS AND THERAPIES
Abuse	Physical, emotional, or sexual abuse directed toward another individual	▪ Withdrawn emotions and a decrease in communication and/or socialization with family and friends ▪ Behavioral changes, such as anger, depression, acting out in school or at home, and changes in appetite or sleep patterns ▪ Bruises, broken bones, concussion, and other physical markers ▪ Fear of a specific person or situation (e.g., family events, arguments, school dances)	▪ Follow state laws and agency policies and procedures regarding the reporting of abuse and neglect. ▪ Treat physical injuries (e.g., broken bones, cuts, concussions) and emphasize the importance of follow-up care. ▪ Offer resources for emotional manifestations, for example, counseling or therapy. ▪ Provide proficient, nonjudgmental patient care.
Divorce	The separation of a couple from a marital bond with or without children	▪ Anxiety ▪ Depression ▪ Stress and resulting manifestations such as restlessness, weight loss, headaches, and sleeplessness ▪ Behavioral modifications in children (e.g., acting out in school, withdrawal, anger, confusion, nightmares)	▪ Provide information about counseling, therapy, and support groups. ▪ Advise about healthy coping mechanisms for stress—for example, exercise, new hobbies, and writing. ▪ Educate about the importance of health maintenance and nutrition even during times of high stress and anxiety.
Death of family member	The loss of a spouse, child, parent, or other family member	▪ Grief as evidenced by sadness, anger, denial, and pain associated with the loss ▪ Depression manifested in a lack of enjoyment of normal activities, intense feelings of sadness, and changes in appetite ▪ Sleeplessness ▪ Weight loss or weight gain ▪ Anxiety	▪ Provide information about therapy and support groups. ▪ Teach about healthy coping strategies. ▪ Assess for signs of complicated or traumatic grief. ▪ Facilitate referrals to grief counselors and other professional resources.

Alterations and Therapies *(continued)*

ALTERATION	DESCRIPTION	MANIFESTATIONS	INTERVENTIONS AND THERAPIES
Incarceration	One or both parents are in jail for varying lengths of time	▪ Separation from one or both parents ▪ Possibility of repartnering of parent who is left to raise children ▪ Increase in physical and emotional concerns	▪ Facilitate communication with family counselor. ▪ Recognize changes in child's behavior indicating they are not coping with the situation. ▪ Provide nonjudgmental care and assistance.
Military deployment	Family with one or more members deployed from home (domestic or overseas deployment)	▪ Frequent separations and reunions ▪ Frequent family relocations ▪ Social considerations related to rank ▪ Lack of control over progress in employment, promotion	▪ Encourage and promote open family communication, use of alternative communication methods (e.g., video messaging, email). ▪ Assist family to identify previously helpful coping strategies. ▪ Encourage participation in social and community supports and activities. ▪ Assist family members in mutual goal setting.
Poverty	Individuals and families living near or below the federally designated poverty threshold	▪ Overall poor health ▪ Increased stress ▪ Altered child development ▪ Increased risk for chronic illness	▪ Provide and encourage use of available resources. ▪ Identify support groups. ▪ Monitor child growth and development.

Patient Teaching

Guidelines for Promoting Acceptable Behavior in Children

The nurse can assist parents in handling their child's misbehavior by helping them to:

- Set realistic expectations and directions for behavior based on the child's age and understanding; consistently enforce the expected directions and behaviors.
- Focus on promoting appropriate and desirable behaviors in the child.
- Model or suggest appropriate behavior.
- Review expected behavior for special situations, such as a family party, going to the movies, or other social event.
- Praise or reward the child using appropriate behaviors.
- Tell the child about his or her inappropriate behavior as soon as it begins and offer guidelines for changing behavior or provide a distraction.
- When reprimanding the child, focus on the behavior rather than stating that the child is bad. Explain how the behavior is inappropriate and how it makes you, as the parent, and any other person involved feel. Avoid ridicule or accusation that can take the form of shame or criticism because these actions can affect the child's self-esteem if repeated often enough. Stay calm.
- Remember that loud volume (yelling) is meant to warn of danger. Parents who discipline kindly have more success than those who discipline in anger or frustration.
- Be alert for situations when the child could misbehave, such as when tired or overexcited. Use a distraction to persuade or calm the child.
- Help children gain self-control with friendly reminders (e.g., count to 3, as soon as the clothes are on the doll, as soon as you finish the game) regarding the timing for transition to the next event of the day, such as bedtime, putting the toys away, or washing hands before dinner.

Abuse

Interpersonal (domestic) violence and child abuse and neglect have long-term implications for children and families. In addition to the risks of physical injury and even death, children who grow up with violence or neglect are at greater risk for delinquency, substance abuse, mental illness, and lower school achievement (Federal Interagency Forum on Child and Family Statistics, 2019). More information on the effects of abuse on children and families can be found in Module 32, Trauma.

Death of a Family Member

Death of an immediate family member can interrupt and even permanently alter family functioning and processes in a number of ways. The death of a parent brings both financial and practical concerns to the family as well as profound emotional loss. Loss of income and loss of another adult to assist with transportation to child care, school, doctor's appointments, and extracurricular activities combine to create new burdens for the remaining parent. In divorced families, death of a custodial parent can result in children relocating to new homes and schools. Death of a child has been identified as one of the most stressful events in an adult's life. For adults, death of a parent can result in an array of emotions and may also result in an adult child finding himself caring for the remaining parent, if the parent who died was a caregiver to the other parent.

Divorce

Nearly half of all marriages in the United States end in divorce, leading to many children with divorced parents (Raley & Sweeney, 2020). When the divorce is preceded by long periods of stress and tension between the parents, the family may experience some level of disruption or dysfunction well in advance of the actual divorce. Children may experience guilt in the form of feeling they did something that caused the divorce. If the divorce results in the children seeing significantly less of one parent, one or more of the children may experience feelings of abandonment. Young children especially may fear abandonment by the remaining parent. Divorce can bring disruption to daily schedules and even result in children changing schools or moving to another city or state. Children who lived in a stable household with both parents are disrupted by the changes in household living arrangements. Disruptions that start with divorce and end with persistent family instability can result in child adjustment, academic, or behavior problems (Raley & Sweeney, 2020).

Incarceration

In the United States, approximately 2.7 million children have at least one parent currently incarcerated, while up to 5 million children have a parent incarcerated at some point during their lifetime (Noel & Najowski, 2019). Children of incarcerated parents face many disadvantages that affect their emotional, physical, and mental health. Noel and Najowski (2019) note that children of parents who are in jail or prison are more likely to experience depression, aggression, antisocial behavior, and delinquency. Separation and divorce are not uncommon when one parent is incarcerated and the other is left to care for the children and take on the role responsibilities of both parents (see **Figure 26.5** »). Outcomes may include increased social and economic inequality for these families.

Military Deployment

Throughout history, many families have experienced having a loved one deployed on military service far from home. Of the almost 3 million service members who have been deployed since the terrorist attacks on September 11, 2001, over 45% were parents (Coppola, McCall, Bailey, Mihalec-Adkins, & Wadsworth, 2020). Family members, including children, experience psychological distress as a result of military deployment (see **Figure 26.6** »). Outside of deployment, military families may relocate frequently, leading to challenges in the education of the children in the family (Coppola et al., 2020). Family income may also be affected if the nonmilitary parent has difficulty finding work in the new community or if there is a delay in employment because that parent has to pass state-required certification or testing to begin working.

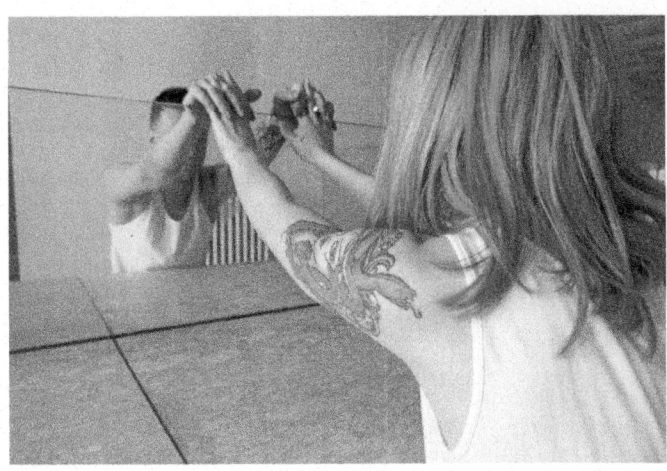

Figure 26.5 » Visiting day in prison is difficult for the incarcerated partner and the one left behind to care for the family.
Source: C_FOR/ iStock/Getty Images.

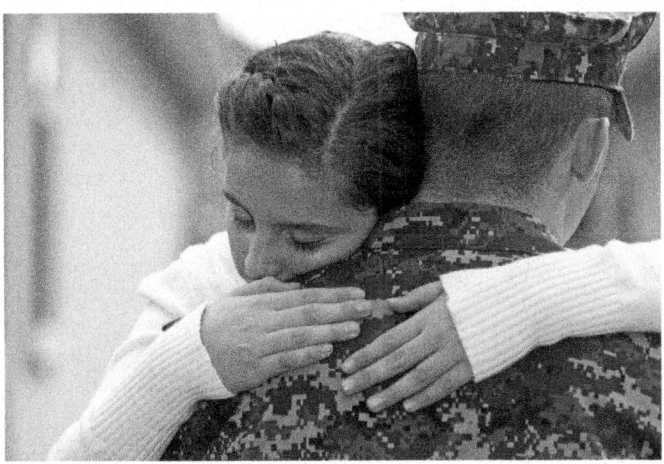

Figure 26.6 » Parental military deployment puts children at increased risk for behavioral and emotional problems.
Source: Kali9/E+/Getty Images.

Poverty

For 2020, the U.S. poverty threshold for a family of four was $26,200 (DHHS, 2020). Nearly 20% of children in the United States live at or near this threshold (Federal Interagency Forum on Child and Family Statistics, 2019). Extreme poverty is defined as below 50% of the poverty threshold (Federal Interagency Forum on Child and Family Statistics, 2019). Approximately 8% of children live in families faced with extreme poverty.

Poverty is associated with poor outcomes for children and families. First, it is linked with substandard housing, homelessness, food insecurity and malnutrition, lack of access to healthcare, unsafe neighborhoods, and inadequate school environments. Consider the issue of access to healthcare. Some may dismiss that as a nonissue because of the existence of Medicaid and Child Health Insurance Programs. But what of the child who lives in a rural area whose parent or parents

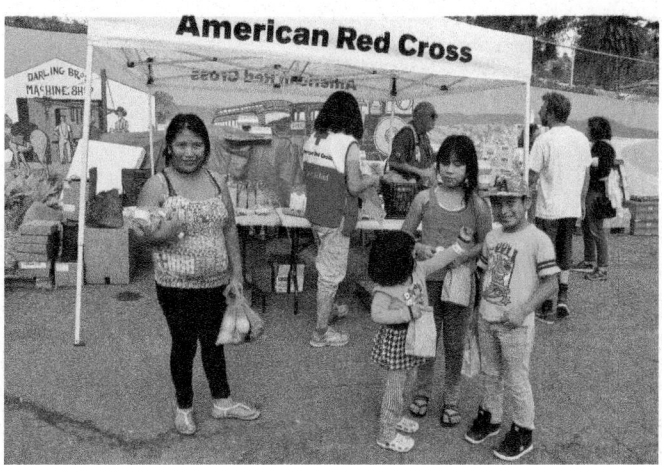

Figure 26.7 ›› This family was forced to evacuate their home during the Kincade Fire in Sonoma County in 2019. Schools across four districts were forced to close for several days. Families displaced from their homes require additional resources to meet basic needs and may experience dysfunction in family coping and communication strategies.

Source: Amy Beth Katz/ZUMA Wire/ZUMA Press, Inc./Alamy Stock Photo.

does not have a car? That family's ability to access healthcare and other resources will be limited.

In children, poverty is associated with an array of short- and long-term consequences. The chronic stress of living in poverty leads to impaired concentration and memory. Poverty leads to decreased access to healthy foods, safe neighborhoods, and stable education. Due to the consequences of poverty, it is considered a social determinant of health, as it can impact health and wellness significantly.

Trauma

When one or more family members experiences a traumatic event, it can upset the rhythms and relationships in the whole household and deplete individual and family coping mechanisms (see **Figure 26.7** ››). Trauma can result from abuse, violence, sexual violence, natural disasters, death, neglect, illness, and more. Children who experience trauma are at risk for trauma-related problems and disorders that disrupt normal family and life functioning (Substance Abuse and Mental Health Services Administration, 2020).

Case Study ›› Part 1

Maria Rodriguez, age 30, and her wife Daniella Marshall, age 32, were recently married and decided to start a family. Following donor insemination, Mrs. Rodriguez became pregnant. The couple arrives at the obstetrician's office for Mrs. Rodriguez's routine health exam. You are familiar with the couple and have provided care to them in the past. Today, you are assigned to care for Mrs. Rodriguez, who is now at 7 months' gestation. After talking to the couple for a few minutes, you notice that Mrs. Rodriguez is more reserved than usual and seems a bit depressed. When you ask how things are coming along with planning for the new arrival, both women are silent. Finally, Mrs. Marshall explains that they are struggling to cope with reactions from other participants of the birthing classes they have been attending, and it is making them both more stressed. Mrs. Rodriguez then tells you that she no longer wishes to attend the birthing classes, even though Mrs. Marshall wishes to complete the course.

Clinical Reasoning Questions Level I

1. What additional information would be useful in assessing the challenges faced by Mrs. Rodriguez and Mrs. Marshall?
2. Which characteristics of communication would best promote open discussion between you and this couple?
3. What are some societal challenges that LGBTQ couples face?

Clinical Reasoning Questions Level II

4. Describe two nursing diagnoses that may be applicable in the care of Mrs. Rodriguez and Mrs. Marshall.
5. What are some of the dangers of stress at this stage in Mrs. Rodriguez's pregnancy?
6. Explain some of the benefits of birthing classes in terms of both safe delivery of the child and family planning.

Concepts Related to Family

Any number of concepts can influence family dynamics. For example, when an individual suffers from addiction to illegal substances or alcohol, his addictive behaviors are likely to affect close family members in a number of ways. Life-threatening health conditions can result in anticipatory grieving, loss of financial security, and caregiver burden, increasing the stresses with which families cope on a daily basis. Alternatively, the birth of a child can result in the strengthening or weakening of bonds and relationships within the family. Family members may be drawn closer through shared interests in the welfare of the child. Conversely, the addition of a new family member can add financial and emotional stressors that strain familial relationships.

Culture and spirituality inform the lifestyles and decision-making process of many families. It is important to note, however, that even within a single family, individual members may engage in different beliefs and practices or experience different degrees of devotion to the culture, religion, or spiritual practices of the family. Culturally competent nursing practice is a critical part of nursing care for children and families. The Concepts Related to Family feature links some, but not all, of the concepts integral to family. They are presented in alphabetical order.

Health Promotion

Health and wellness promotion is an essential aspect of family health and focuses on increasing healthy behaviors and optimizing lifestyle choices. Educating patients and facilitating appropriate referrals (e.g., to nutritionists, educational programs, and community service providers) will not only improve the family's quality of life but also reduce the risk of illness. Depending on the needs of the patient, nurses may collaborate with a variety of healthcare professionals, including physicians, counselors, social workers, and mental health specialists.

Families may be most in need of health promotion and patient teaching during times of transition into new developmental or life stages. From teaching new parents the importance of skin-to-skin contact in the first hours after delivery to helping parents of teenagers identify signs of depression or addiction, nurses are uniquely placed to help parents parent their children successfully and to help families obtain optimal wellness and functioning. Settings in which nurses provide health promotion for patients and

Concepts Related to
Family

CONCEPT	RELATIONSHIP TO FAMILY	NURSING IMPLICATIONS
Addiction	Substance and/or alcohol misuse or abuse can affect individual family members as well as the family unit as a whole. Potential stressors may be psychosocial, physiologic, financial, or spiritual in nature.	■ Be alert to the signs of addiction. ■ Propose interventions appropriate to addiction behavior. ■ Evaluate the individual's potential for being a danger to herself or others. ■ Recommend community resources to family members to help them process and cope with resultant complications.
Culture and Diversity	Cultural beliefs and practices may vary even among generations of the same family. They may impact decision-making processes, how patients and families view procedures, and day-to-day patient and family needs.	■ Explore meaning of culture and diversity as it impacts each family. ■ Identify resources available for families who are diverse or from a different culture.
Grief and Loss	Grief and loss may result in alterations in family dynamics, particularly if the deceased individual was in a position of family leadership or was the primary source of financial support. Grief reactions can also affect how family members relate to one another.	■ Be alert to the signs of intense grief reactions, such as lasting depression, anger, or denial. ■ Consider the nature of the loss and its possible ramifications. ■ Offer appropriate support and referral, such as therapy or grief counseling.
Reproduction	Addition of a family member may strengthen familial bonds through shared interests in the child's welfare or may instead strain relationships in terms of increased physical, emotional, and financial demands.	■ Teach about prenatal care and maternal health. ■ Encourage all family members to engage in educational activities. ■ Assess the involved individuals' responses to the pregnancy and sensitively address potentially harmful issues, such as ineffective communication patterns. ■ Be alert to signs of postpartum depression. ■ Advise parents of potential jealousies and complications with toddlers and new infants.
Stress and Coping	Family stressors are many and may increase risks for physical and mental illness, caregiver burden, and successful family functioning.	■ Encourage open dialog among all family members. ■ Discuss what the issue means to family members. ■ Identify past coping mechanisms used by individual family members. ■ Help family members identify ways to find strength in the change. ■ Allow individuals to grieve. ■ Identify resources available.
Trauma	Trauma may be caused by physical abuse or emotional/verbal abuse or neglect. Trauma may also result from unintentional injuries. See Module 32, Trauma, for more information.	■ Identify and document physical findings associated with physical abuse/neglect. ■ Enlist the aid of counselors/clergy. ■ Provide support to all family members. ■ Encourage open communication.

families include hospitals, physicians' offices and clinics, local health departments, and public schools.

A therapeutic relationship between the nurse and the family stems from effective rapport. Through the development of this relationship, the nurse displays empathy, respect, and attentiveness to the patient and family, leading to a trusting and therapeutic relationship. Within the context of this relationship, the nurse can facilitate progress toward goals established by the family with clear education to facilitate family problem solving.

When working with families, the nurse considers health and wellness not only from an individual perspective but also in terms of the family unit. Family wellness promotion emphasizes addressing each individual family member's contribution to the health and well-being of the family and recognizing that if one member is affected, the entire family is affected. For example, any number of occupational or environmental problems could alter the individual's physical and emotional wellness. A physical ailment—such as a broken leg or lead poisoning—can be treated, but if occupational (e.g., physically demanding and personally unsatisfying hard labor) and environmental (e.g., house with lead-based paint in a dangerous neighborhood) aspects are not addressed, the health of the individual and the family remain at risk.

Family wellness and health promotion strategies involve empowering patients to make beneficial changes in their lives. Some common health promotion strategies include encouraging tobacco cessation, increased exercise, healthy eating habits, and use of stress-reduction techniques. Each individual will have different needs and circumstances, requiring nurses to modify health promotion suggestions. For example, consider a stay-at-home mother of three who is seeking stress relief. For this patient, the nurse might suggest a community activity that promotes exercise (for stress relief) and a chance to connect with others in the community (for social wellness). Patients may decline to follow the nurse's suggestion; however, the nurse's role is to offer health- and wellness-promoting options without judgment and then allow the patient to decide.

Empowering patients requires nurses to help patients set goals for their own personal wellness and the wellness of their families. The choice of goals is dependent on the family's needs, both as individual members and as a unit. One family may set the goal of participating in a family game night once a week to promote emotional, social, and intellectual wellness, whereas another family could set the goal of going hiking or biking every 2 weeks as a family to promote physical and even spiritual wellness. Nurses can help families set goals by working to understand the needs and wants of the family. More information on empowering families and patients can be found in Module 35, Caring Interventions.

Health promotion within the family unit can be challenging. In some cases, family members will respond positively to nursing suggestions and interventions; in other cases, patients may feel they are unable to change their lifestyle because of socioeconomic conditions, stress, or other factors. Individuals also may interpret health promotion as an attempt to control their behaviors. The nurse approaches families on a case-by-case basis, recognizing that each family unit will need different forms of care and different nursing approaches.

Risk and Protective Factors

Risk factors for family dysfunction may not always be evident. At times, risk factors are masked by the absence of obvious problems. Stress, for example, can lead to many problems within a family, as the effects of unmanaged and unresolved stress can impact normal family functioning. Parental coping methods can also determine how children will learn to handle stress because children often model the actions of their parents (Centers for Disease Control and Prevention [CDC], 2020). The response to stressors can be exacerbated by a real or perceived sense of powerlessness over circumstances, such as poverty, unemployment, or abuse. Other risk factors for family dysfunction include family separation, forced migration, and cultural and social isolation.

Protective factors for family health and function include stable living environments, healthy and consistent parenting and supervision, healthy family coping, social and community supports, and financial stability (e.g., adequate shelter, food and nutrition, and access to healthcare).

Recognition and awareness of risk and protective factors and knowledge of community supports can help the nurse identify and plan health and wellness promotion activities for families at risk of alterations in family coping, physical health, and mental health (see **Table 26.3** »).

Care in the Community

Nurses encounter families experiencing stress, trauma, poverty, acute health conditions, and chronic illnesses in all settings. Many times, nurses are called on to assist families in finding resources to alleviate financial burdens or to help them access social supports. Although the names of local resource agencies may vary from one location to another, both public and private resources are available in most communities. Public resources include departments of social services, local health departments, departments of aging, and public schools. Private resources are often available through nonprofit organizations such as literacy centers, homeless and transition shelters, and nonprofits that serve older adults or individuals who are disabled. Nurses should be aware of the resources in their community that support the populations with which they work.

» **Stay Current:** The organization 2-1-1 is a free and confidential service that helps individuals find local resources: www.211.org.

Nursing Assessment

Nursing assessment of a family elicits important information about family functioning and interactions, health status of each family member, family strengths and needs, coping strategies, and parenting and health practices. As the nurse and family become acquainted and the therapeutic relationship progresses, assessment may become more targeted as time goes on and some goals are met and other needs arise.

Observation and Family Interview

An accurate family assessment depends on a trusting relationship between the nurse and the family, preferably performed in a comfortable environment that provides privacy and is free of interruptions. Family assessment may be done in the family home, in a healthcare clinic or office setting, or in the hospital.

Key to any good assessment and health history is observation of how family members interact with and respond to each other, what types of communication patterns they use, the amount of support they provide to one another, and the closeness/distance of each family member as they relate to one another. Interviewing family members individually or as a group, depending on the situation, provides additional valuable information about their knowledge regarding health promotion and illness prevention. The amount of cooperation, identification of norms within the family, and assessing for the potential for the family to engage in positive change are all other important aspects of observation and the interview (Planetree International, 2018). This information should be documented clearly on the electronic health record, whether the nurse is working with the family in the community or an inpatient setting.

The family assessment provides important information about family structure and function, including which

TABLE 26.3 Health and Wellness Promotion for the Family at Risk for Health Alterations

Developmental Stage and Associated Risk Factors	Potential Health Consequences	Health and Wellness Promotion Strategies
Individual, Couple, or Family with Infants and Young Children ■ Lack of knowledge about issues related to sexuality, family planning, and relationship roles ■ Lack of knowledge about prenatal care ■ Nutritional deficiencies, obesity ■ Substance use or abuse ■ Lack of knowledge about child health and safety ■ Poverty, lack of health insurance or access to resources ■ First pregnancy before age 16 or after age 35	■ Unplanned pregnancy ■ Poor health outcomes for newborns (e.g., low birth weight, drug exposure, birth defects) ■ Unintentional injury	■ Promote preconception/prenatal care, if applicable. ■ Obtain detailed history to uncover environmental issues and lifestyle practices that may impact health of individuals and family. ■ Provide education related to contraception and sexually transmitted infection (STI) prevention. ■ Facilitate nutritional assessment and counseling. ■ Offer referrals to appropriate resources for smoking-cessation programs and alcohol/drug abuse counseling. ■ Educate about basic child health and safety protocols. ■ Identify resources for financial assistance and facilitate appropriate referrals. ■ Advocate for safe care of infants and their families.
Family with School-age Children ■ Lack of knowledge about appropriate parenting techniques ■ Working parent(s) with inappropriate or inadequate child care ■ Poverty, lack of health insurance or access to resources ■ Child abuse or neglect ■ Repeated accidents and hospitalizations or sick visits ■ Inadequate nutrition, obesity ■ Lack of knowledge related to maintaining a safe home environment	■ Behavior problems ■ Speech and vision problems ■ Learning disabilities, developmental delays ■ Infectious diseases ■ Abuse/neglect ■ Obesity, underweight	■ Educate about preventive healthcare measures. ■ Provide information about community assistance and healthcare programs. ■ Educate about contraception. ■ Provide information about adequate nutrition. ■ Provide education to children and families regarding risk of certain environmental hazards (i.e., risk of carbon monoxide [CO] poisoning and need for CO monitors in home).
Family with Adolescents and Young Adults ■ Lifestyle choices and behaviors that lead to acute injury (participation in sports) or chronic illness (substance abuse, inadequate diet) ■ Experimental behaviors, lack of problem-solving skills ■ Parent–adolescent conflict	■ Unintentional injury ■ Increased risk for suicide or self-harm ■ Alcohol/drug abuse ■ Unwanted pregnancy ■ STIs ■ Interpersonal or dating violence	■ Promote healthy problem-solving skills. ■ Educate about healthy anger and emotion management techniques. ■ Provide information about healthcare resources. ■ Teach about contraception. ■ Facilitate learning about substance and alcohol abuse prevention.
Family with Middle-Aged Adults ■ Inadequate diet, obesity ■ High blood pressure ■ Tobacco or substance use/abuse ■ Insufficient or inadequate physical activity ■ Poor or inadequate coping mechanisms ■ Environmental exposure (e.g., occupational hazards, sun exposure, water or air pollution) ■ Depression	■ Chronic disease (e.g., cardiovascular disease, type 2 DM) ■ Cancer ■ Unintentional injury ■ Suicide ■ Mental illness	■ Educate about nutrition and exercise and its relationship to cardiovascular disease, diabetes, and certain forms of cancer. ■ Educate regarding changes in relationships, careers, and biologic changes that occur during this time. ■ Provide information about mental health counseling and facilitate referrals. ■ Suggest screening for hypertension, cardiac disease, osteoporosis, colon cancer, breast cancer. ■ Educate regarding occupational safety hazards and risk for exposure to potential carcinogens and risk of accidents, if applicable.
Family with Older Adults ■ Depression ■ Polypharmacy ■ Chronic illness ■ Reduced income ■ Inadequate nutrition and/or exercise ■ Sensory impairments (e.g., vision, hearing) ■ History of environmental exposure and adverse lifestyle choices	■ Unintentional injuries from burns or falls ■ High blood pressure ■ Acute, chronic, or progressive illness ■ Increased risk of infection (influenza, pneumonia, urinary tract infection) ■ Adjustment disorder, grieving, depression ■ Substance use or abuse ■ Relocation syndrome	■ Educate about nutrition and exercise. ■ Provide information about community-based programs for healthcare. ■ Facilitate mental health counseling. ■ Educate about illness prevention and health promotion (i.e., use of prescription medications with herbal remedies). ■ Encourage ways to stay involved and productive (e.g., volunteering, assisting with community projects). ■ Provide referrals regarding wills, advance directive, power of attorney.

individuals are responsible for making healthcare decisions for specific family members. The following data may be useful in informing planning and care:

Family Structure

- Which adults spend the most time with the children? What is the nature of sibling relationships?
- Who has legal custody—that is, who is able to make healthcare decisions for the child?
- For older adults or those living with serious illness, has a family member been legally designated as having a healthcare power of attorney?

Family Roles/Functions/Resources

- Who provides for the child or family financially? Does the child/patient/family have health insurance?
- Who else helps the parent(s) care for the children? What other support systems does the family have in place?

Physical Health

- How is the health of each family member? How do they view their health and healthcare?
- What health promotion and prevention strategies do they use (e.g., immunizations, regular physical examinations for both parents and children, vision and dental care)?

Mental Health Status

- What is the mental health status of each member of the family? How do family members perceive their own health?
- What protective factors are in place? What kind of family or community supports do family members access or participate in?
- What kind of coping mechanisms do individual members use? How does the family cope with stresses together?

Family Interactions and Values

- How do family members communicate with each other?
- What cultural and religious practices does the family observe? How do these affect the health and well-being of both individual family members and that of the family as a whole?
- What type of parenting style is preferred by the parent(s)? Do parents share caregiving responsibilities?
- Are complementary health approaches included in their daily activities? Are they used to promote health and prevent illness?

Communicating with Families

Working Phase

Sudden changes in family structure can create strain on family members. During an office visit, a parent discloses that her partner was recently in a severe accident, and an amputation of the lower leg was required. She is concerned about their daughter. The nurse utilizes empathetic listening and open-ended questions.

- Tell me about how your daughter has responded so far.
- You mentioned that you might consider family counseling to help with the change. How does your partner feel about that option?

Family Assessment Tools

In the context of wellness promotion, nursing assessment includes identifying and optimizing current positive behaviors and lifestyle choices, as well as recognizing the family's needs for disease prevention. In addition to patient interviews and observation of family processes, several tools are available for completing a multifaceted family assessment that takes into consideration a number of factors, including physiologic, psychosocial, spiritual, and environmental components. Presented are some of the more common tools that can be used by nurses to identify strengths and areas where families may need more support, education, or resources in order to strengthen the family unit.

Family Ecomap

A family **ecomap** is a helpful tool to visually represent how a family interacts with various domains, including healthcare, education, family, recreation, and social networks. When families are facing difficulties and are challenged with coping, this visual ecomap assessment tool provides the nurse with information on how the family is organized (see **Figure 26.8** »). The nurse is able to identify patterns among the family and domain interactions on the ecomap, leading to an ability to identify appropriate community resources that may be beneficial. Communication patterns are a key area of the assessment, including verbal and nonverbal communication, listening, and how disagreements are managed.

Family Genogram

Using a genogram assists the nurse to visualize familial relationships and patterns of chronic conditions occurring within the family unit. **Genograms** consist of visual representations of gender showing lines of birth descent through the generations (see **Figure 26.9** »).

Family APGAR

The Family APGAR tool allows for a rapid assessment of family function and/or dysfunction. The tool consists of five items, including adaptation, partnership, growth, affection, and resolve (see **Table 26.4** »). Given its short length, this tool can be administered quickly to family members. Unreliable results may be noted if responses are mostly in the *hardly ever* category or when there is significant variance among family members. When this occurs, coping strategies may need to be investigated.

Home Observation for Measurement of the Environment

Caldwell and Bradley (1984) developed the HOME (Home Observation for Measurement of the Environment) assessment tool to study relationships between aspects of a child's home environment and the child's developmental outcomes.

Each age-specific tool is separated into subscales that include responsivity of the parent, acceptance of child, the physical environment and organization learning materials, variety in experience, and parental involvement. The tool takes up to 90 minutes to complete and the assessment is conducted in the home setting with the child and primary caregiver to observe the overall interactions and relationship. Nursing interventions and suggestions for normal child development may arise following this assessment.

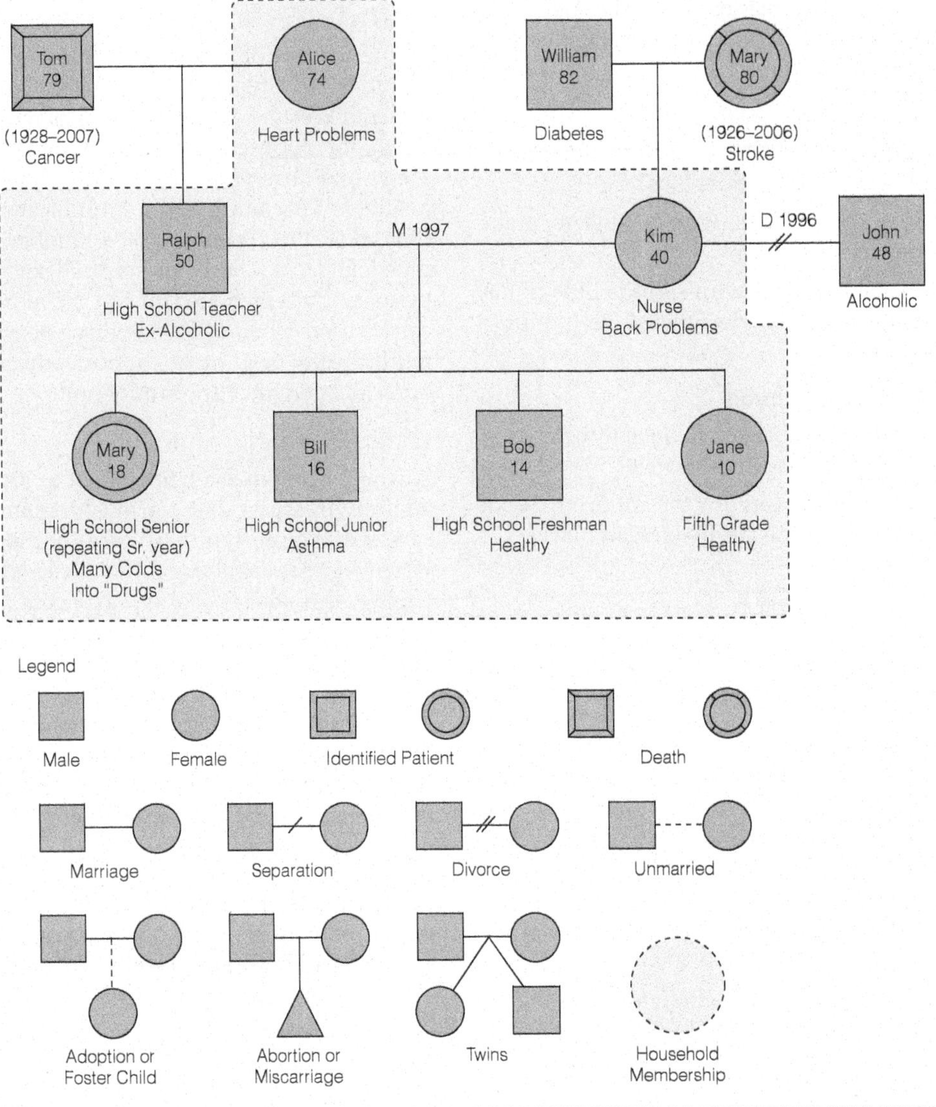

Figure 26.8 ›› Example of a family genogram.

The Friedman Family Assessment Tool

Marilyn Friedman, RN, PhD, developed the Friedman Family Assessment Tool (FFAM) for nurses to utilize in assessing a family to understand family structure, influences, strengths, and weaknesses. The FFAM focuses on environmental influences that can impact the family by assessing the following categories (Friedman, Bowden, & Jones, 2003):

- Identifying data (including name, family composition, cultural background, and religious identification)
- Family structure and developmental stage
- Environmental data (including the family's engagement with community resources and activities)
- Communication patterns and role structures
- Family values
- Socialization and parenting practices
- Healthcare beliefs, values, and behaviors
- Dietary and mealtime practices
- Stressors, strengths, and coping strategies
- Resiliency and adaptation.

Case Study ›› Part 2

After expressing concern for Mrs. Rodriguez and Mrs. Marshall, you begin to explore their birthing class experiences in greater detail. Mrs. Rodriguez explains that many of the other couples in the class are rude to her and her wife and that the woman conducting the class is cold to them. The couple continues to tell you about similarly negative reactions they have experienced while searching for a birthing center. During the discussion, you notice that Mrs. Rodriguez becomes increasingly upset. When Mrs. Marshall asks for a few moments alone with Mrs. Rodriguez, you step out of the room. Upon your return, Mrs. Rodriguez apologizes for "losing control of my emotions." You assure her that she is welcome to express her emotions and that you are committed to providing her with the best possible care, including recommending some potential alternatives to her current birthing classes. You continue your physical assessment of Mrs. Rodriguez. Her vital signs are T 98.8°F oral, P 86 bpm, R 24/min, and BP 168/90 mmHg. Mrs. Rodriguez denies any physical complaints or unusual changes in her condition. You leave the room to talk with the physician. The physician comes in to examine Mrs. Rodriguez and notes that everything appears to be fine but expresses concern about Mrs. Rodriguez's elevated blood pressure.

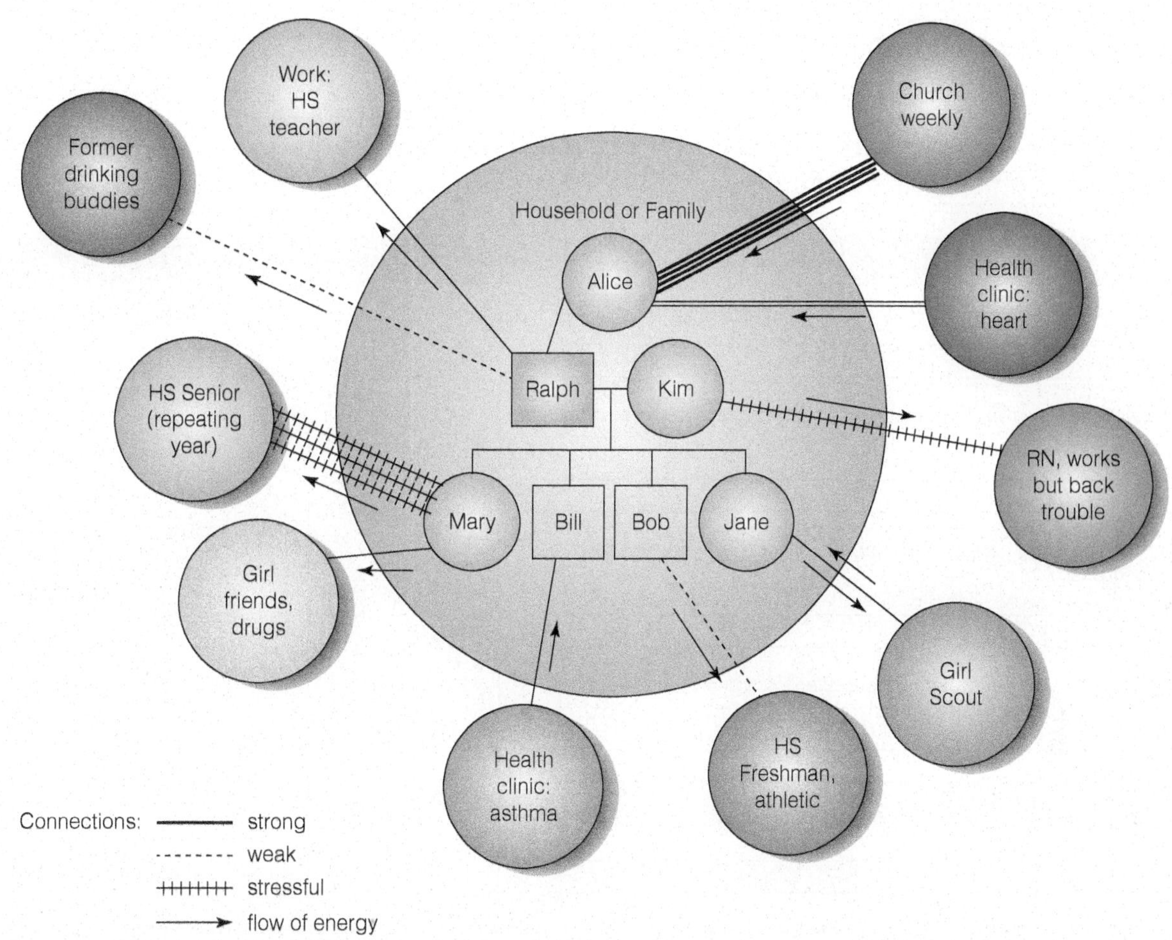

Figure 26.9 ›› Example of a family ecomap. Many more components may be added to the map.

Case Study ›› Part 2 (*continued*)

Clinical Reasoning Questions Level I

1. Presuming that Mrs. Rodriguez has no other health issues and no pregnancy-related complications, why might her blood pressure be elevated?
2. Identify three nursing actions described in this scenario that reflect respect and nonjudgmental care of this couple.

Clinical Reasoning Questions Level II

3. Describe two nursing interventions appropriate for inclusion in the care of this couple.
4. What steps might you take to assist Mrs. Rodriguez with identifying alternative providers of birthing classes?
5. What are some concerns associated with hypertension during the third trimester of pregnancy?

Independent Interventions

Families are shaped by multiple factors, including life experiences, current and past challenges, coping abilities, cultural diversity, individual personalities, and the age of the family members. Nurses can employ numerous interventions to assist families with navigating through challenges or difficult circumstances, as well as to promote the optimal use of each individual's strengths.

Explore Health Beliefs

Families have different and varying beliefs about health, illness, and ways and methods of treating illness. In some cases, these beliefs may be based in cultural or religious practices. As part of the assessment, the nurse asks open-ended questions in a nonjudgmental manner in an attempt to learn about the family's health beliefs, including the use of herbs and supplements and the use of home remedies. By exploring the family's health beliefs, nurses show respect for cultural and religious values and practice and can identify practices that may have a bearing on healthcare and family functioning. For example, consider the Muslim patient who has come in for assessment prior to scheduling a procedure. The nurse recognizes that the holy period of Ramadan is coming up and knows that observances for Ramadan include a month-long period of fasting from sunrise to sunset. One of the medications the patient will have to take during the postoperative period must be taken four times a day with food. Although the Muslim faith respects the need of those who are sick to abstain from fasting, the nurse consults with both the patient and the physician about whether or not the procedure may be scheduled after Ramadan.

Identify Resources

An important nursing role when working with families is to include community resources that will help to meet the

TABLE 26.4 The Family APGAR Questionnaire

Directions: The following questions have been designed to help us better understand you and your family. You should feel free to ask questions about any item in the questionnaire. The space for comments should be used when you wish to give additional information or if you wish to discuss how the question is applied to your family. Please try to answer all questions. Family is defined as the individual(s) with whom you usually live. If you live alone, your "family" consists of persons with whom you now have the strongest emotional ties.*

For each question, check only one box.

	Almost Always 2	Some of the Time 1	Hardly Ever 0
I am satisfied that I can turn to my family for help when something is troubling me. Comments: ________________			
I am satisfied with the way my family talks over things with me and shares problems with me. Comments: ________________			
I am satisfied that my family accepts and supports my wishes to take on new activities or directions. Comments: ________________			
I am satisfied with the way my family expresses affection and responds to my emotions, such as anger, sorrow, and love. Comments: ________________			
I am satisfied with the way my family and I share time together. Comments: ________________			

**Note:* Depending on which member of the family is being interviewed, the interviewer may substitute for the word *family* either *spouse*, *significant other*, *parents*, or *children*. Responses are scored 2, 1, 0 and totaled. The total score ranges from 0 to 10. The higher the score, the greater amount of satisfaction that family member has with family functioning.

Source: Adapted from Smilkstein (1978). Reprinted with permission from Frontline Medical Communications, Inc.

family's needs. A collaborative team approach, including social work, can strengthen the care plan for the family. Appropriate resources may include financial, nutrition, child care, transportation, and housing. The nurse will not only provide information about the resources that are available but will also guide the family through the process of initiating contact with the community agencies that provide the vital resources. Referral to family counseling services may also be considered by the nurse when the family needs extend into areas related to communication and mental health.

Provide Patient and Family Education

When providing education to a patient and family, it is important to consider health literacy. Many people do not have a basic understanding of health and disease. Additionally, the speed at which medicine and healthcare advances makes it difficult for individuals to stay current with health-related information. The growth of available information on the internet has led to health information and misinformation being readily accessible to anyone. It is important for the nurse to ensure that families access reliable information when searching the internet for health-related topics to avoid misinformation being interpreted as accurate.

Collaborative Practices

The interconnectedness and interdependence that are inherent in each family underscore the importance of collaboration as part of family-centered nursing care. Armed with the information from the family assessment, the nurse advocates within the interprofessional care team on behalf of the family and helps family members learn how to advocate for themselves and each other. At all times, the nurse remembers that family members may perceive some needs, issues, and situations differently than the nurse or other members of the healthcare team. **Box 26.2** » illustrates this aspect of family-centered care.

For some families, collaboration may include working with experts who specialize in social work, psychology, or mental healthcare. For families in need of counseling, financial assistance may be available. In some areas, community-funded organizations offer free or discounted services. When making these recommendations, nurses should be aware of stigmas surrounding therapy and counseling and work to assure families of the potential benefits of these modes of care. For new or expectant parents, referral to parenting classes may be valuable. Families facing economic challenges should be made aware of community resources, including wellness

Box 26.2

Family-Centered Collaborative Care

Kayla Harrison is a public health nurse who is part of the early childhood collaborative assessment and referral team in her community. The team also includes a child psychologist, a pediatrician, a speech and language therapist, and an early childhood specialist from the local public school system. The team is meeting with Coretta Simons, the grandmother and foster parent of Alex Simons, a 3-year-old who was referred for evaluation based on an obvious speech deficit and behavior problems reported by his preschool teacher. During the meeting, the team shares the results of Alex's evaluation and listens to Ms. Simon's concerns about her grandson. Ms. Simon is the foster parent for Alex and his two older siblings. She works 40 hours a week driving a van for the local eldercare center, taking older adults to and from the center for the day while their caregivers go to work. Ms. Simon reports that Alex is the youngest, and his behavioral problems are exhausting the entire family. Team members advise her that they would like for Alex to be enrolled in a part-day program offered by the school system. The program specializes in offering services for children based on an individual education plan. The team is also recommending that Alex see a child psychologist to begin to learn some coping skills and for Ms. Simon to participate in therapy as well. Ms. Simon shares she cannot take any more time off from work to attend to Alex's needs, in part because of the number of times she got calls at work from the preschool asking her to come to the center to help intervene with Alex's troublesome behaviors. She also says that she does not think a part-day program is best for Alex. That would mean he would have to be shuttled to and from his current preschool to the public school's part-day program because she works all day. Ms. Simon does not see this as being appropriate for a 3-year-old.

Ms. Harrison, the nurse at the table, hears Ms. Simon's frustrations and recognizes quickly that Ms. Simon understands her needs, Alex's needs, and the needs of their family unit. The early childhood specialist, however, is pushing for Ms. Simon to make the therapy appointments happen, on the argument that this will help her learn to manage Alex's behaviors and help Alex learn some coping mechanisms as well. Ms. Harrison knows that the local preschool developmental day center has some grant funding to provide outreach mental health services to children in other preschool settings. Ms. Harrison suggests that the team begin Alex's treatment plan by starting with speech therapy and by signing Alex up for the outreach services so that a behavioral therapist can work with Alex at school. When possible, Ms. Simon can join in those sessions or observe and work with the therapist to find what works for Alex and perhaps make a home visit to observe the dynamic at home. Ms. Harrison suggests that the team try these options and meet again after a few weeks to see how the plan is working. Ms. Simon replies that this sounds feasible, that she would find it more helpful to meet with a therapist at Alex's preschool instead of having to take him to and from appointments.

clinics and food banks. Additional assistance and collaboration with the school nurse may also help those families whose children require special care during the school day.

Family responsibilities for children do not necessarily end on the child's 18th birthday. This is particularly true for families with children with disabilities and families with children with *serious mental illness (SMI)*. Serious mental illnesses are those that create significant disability in an individual's ability to function and reach life goals. Some community and social supports for individuals with disability or mental illness end when the individual turns 18 or graduates from high school. Parents may find themselves at a loss to cope with an adult child who needs continued support and care. In particular, older adults who have been caring for adult children with disability or SMI may experience increased distress as they plan for the care of their child beyond their own lives (The Arc, n.d.). Nurses may find themselves collaborating with these parents to help them find and access services for adult children.

» **Stay Current:** The Center for Future Planning provides resources to support adults with disablities. Go to https://futureplanning.thearc.org.

Case Study » Part 3

The physician requests that Mrs. Rodriguez remain at the office so that her blood pressure can be reassessed. While Mrs. Rodriguez is relaxing, you check with some of the staff and learn that a newly hired certified nurse midwife (CNM) offers a birthing class once per week. The CNM reports that two of her patients are a lesbian couple and that they are warmly welcomed by the other patients. You also consult with two of the physicians and compile a list of three birthing centers in the area that they prefer.

Upon return to Mrs. Rodriguez's room, you reassess her blood pressure, which is now 122/82 mmHg. You provide the couple with the information you have gathered about the birthing class and the three birthing centers. Both Mrs. Rodriguez and her wife express gratitude for your compassion and efforts to assist them. Mrs. Rodriquez is scheduled to return for a follow-up appointment in 2 weeks. She reports that she has a blood pressure monitor at home and tells you she will check her blood pressure at least once daily. Mrs. Rodriguez agrees to contact the clinic if her blood pressure is elevated or if she has any unusual changes.

Clinical Reasoning Questions Level I

1. Do you think Mrs. Rodriguez and Mrs. Marshall are wellness oriented? Explain your answer.
2. What recommendations would you provide to help Mrs. Rodriguez keep her stress level down during her pregnancy?

Clinical Reasoning Questions Level II

3. What are some of the negative effects of stress on families?
4. According to the laws of your state, when the couple in this case study has their child, who will have parental rights?
5. If Mrs. Rodriguez's blood pressure had not decreased, what interventions could have been proposed?

Nursing Care Plan

A Single-Parent Family with Child Care Issues

ASSESSMENT	DIAGNOSES	PLANNING
Ms. Wilson, a newly divorced single mother, brings her 3-year-old son in for routine immunizations. After he has received his immunizations, while waiting the required 20 minutes before leaving, Ms. Wilson reveals that she recently lost her job because her company was bought by another. She says that she has found a new job, and that the salary is much higher, but the only available shift is from midnight to 7:00 a.m. She asks if there are any certified child care providers who provide services during nighttime hours. Ms. Wilson notes that her parents have offered to keep her son while she is at work, but she is worried about burdening her parents and being viewed as incapable of taking care of her child independently.	■ Ready to learn about resources ■ Ready for education about decision making and child care resources	■ Ms. Wilson will learn of other resources available to help her care for her child in a safe environment. ■ Ms. Wilson will discuss available choices she has without risking her child's safety.

IMPLEMENTATION

- Explore Ms. Wilson's reluctance to accept her parents' offer to assist her.
- Assist with identifying additional sources of support, including support groups and classes geared toward meeting the needs of single parents.
- Reinforce and support Ms. Wilson's concern for her child's well-being, including his physiologic and psychosocial wellness.
- Provide referrals to social services to help meet financial needs.
- Encourage and support patient's desire to be financially self-sufficient.
- Assess patient's knowledge of pediatric vaccination schedules and provide appropriate teaching, including in written form.

EVALUATION

Ms. Wilson agrees to explore the option of accepting her parents' offer to care for her child while she is at work. She also agrees to attend classes designed to educate and assist individuals with overcoming challenges that accompany single parenting.

CRITICAL THINKING

1. Is the nursing diagnosis of ready to learn about resources appropriate? Why or why not?
2. In what ways might Ms. Wilson's recent divorce have affected her family's level of wellness?
3. How might Ms. Wilson's fear of appearing dependent negatively impact her level of personal and family wellness?

REVIEW The Concept of Family

RELATE Link the Concepts

Linking the concept of family with the concept of culture:

1. Explain how culture influences the family unit. What are three values or beliefs that could impact how a family functions?
2. What impact does stereotyping have on family? Describe at least two negative effects stereotyping can have on the family unit.
3. How does the nurse incorporate the family's cultural beliefs into health promotion teaching?
4. How might the family's cultural beliefs impact their health behaviors?

Linking the concept of family with the concept of self:

5. What are two measures that could be implemented for a teenager you suspect is experiencing anorexia nervosa?
6. While you are providing care to a family of four (two parents, two children), the parents ask for advice on helping their daughter, who they believe has become bulimic. What suggestions do you provide the parents? Explain your answers.

Linking the concept of family with the concept of advocacy:

7. How can the nurse advocate for families from vulnerable populations in the community?
8. What responsibilities does the nurse have to advocate for families?

READY Go to Volume 3: Clinical Nursing Skills

REFER Go to Pearson MyLab Nursing and eText

REFLECT Apply Your Knowledge

The home health nurse has been visiting a 90-year-old woman and her younger sister who live together in a large farmhouse. The women have been active in caring for each other and their residence. During one of the home visits, they confide that the farm is too much for them, but they admit that they do not want to tell their families because they are afraid that they will be put into a nursing home.

1. What community resources are available to assist the sisters to live independently?
2. How should the family be involved in the decision making?
3. What signs can alert the nurse that the sisters are unable to care for themselves?
4. Should the nurse contact the family without the sisters' knowledge? Why or why not?

» Exemplar 26.A Family Response to Health Alterations

Exemplar Learning Outcomes

26.A Analyze family response to health alterations.

- Describe the impact of illness on the family system.
- Identify the clinical manifestations of family response to health alterations.
- Outline aspects of collaboration necessary to the care of families experiencing health alterations.
- Apply the nursing process in providing culturally competent care to families with health alterations.

Exemplar Key Terms

Caregiver burden, *1918*
Objective caregiver burden, *1918*
Stigma, *1918*
Subjective caregiver burden, *1918*

Overview

More and more, people identify family based on their personal definitions. Although most people still use the term *family* to describe both close and extended relatives (by birth, marriage, or adoption), many use the term in a larger sense and may have significant relationships with friends that they consider to be familial. The nurse recognizes the importance of the family to the health and well-being of each patient.

The Impact of Illness on the Family System

Illness of a family member disrupts everyday normal family functioning, as family roles are shifted during the illness. Responsibilities normally completed by the individual who has become ill must be distributed to other members of the family to ensure a balance is maintained in the family system. Additionally, new responsibilities result from the care required by the ill family member. These changes in family structure can result in stress and anxiety, which can make it even harder to adjust to the new roles and responsibilities. See **Box 26.3** » for some factors that determine the impact of illness on the family unit.

Successful stress management and coping skills are crucial to the family's response to illness and the changes that result. Clear and consistent communication among all family members is necessary to promote family functioning in the face of updated roles and responsibilities. Timely adjustments to the family plan can occur in response to an evolving situation with the illness. Strong family support is a strength during times of illness in the family, as well as close interactions with the nurse and appropriate referrals. Often, the support that family members provide for each other during an illness lends to growth in the family relationships as they are brought together for a single purpose.

Nurses will interact with both the patient and the family members while navigating the course of the illness. However, the nurse must not share any information with the family members without the permission of the patient. With patient permission, the nurse will work with the patient and family to educate on the illness, disease management, and the plan of care. The nurse will address any changes to family function that may result from the illness. Nurses can also provide helpful suggestions for managing the healthcare system, such as whether the primary caregiver can expect a faster response by telephoning the office or using the patient portal. At the same time, nurses assess family resources to note important variances, such as limited transportation or preferences for voice or email messages instead of text-based communications.

In educating patients on disease management, the nurse must consider the needs of the entire family. For example, the entire family may be impacted when a patient needs to make dietary changes following a cardiac event. The nurse must assess how the changes will impact the family and work with the patient and family to determine feasible solutions for incorporating the new healthcare strategies.

Nurses also support families as they try to find solutions, providing patient education about community resources and the Family and Medical Leave Act (**Box 26.4**) ».

Box 26.3

Factors That Influence the Impact of Illness on the Family

- Severity and duration of the illness
- Family's perception of the significance of the illness related to family coping and burden of care
- Long-term effects, such as reduced functioning or permanent disability
- Effect of the illness on financial resources

Chronic Illness and the Family

The prevalence of chronic illness in the United States has increased dramatically: More than half of the U.S. population experiences a chronic condition, and four out of every 10 Americans have multiple chronic conditions (CDC, 2019). Care for patients with chronic illness usually takes place at home, sometimes with intermittent hospitalizations during times of acute exacerbation. Chronic illness can put an incredible amount of stress on family structure and function.

Factors that affect family responses to chronic illness are varied and relate to financial considerations, other caregiving responsibilities, employment status, the nature and duration of the illness itself, and the age and capacity of the individual family member. In addition, how family members perceive the demands of the illness can affect how individual members respond.

Box 26.4
Family and Medical Leave Act

Parents of both newborns and adopted children may be entitled to 12 weeks of unpaid leave during any 12-month period within the birth or adoption of a child according to the Family and Medical Leave Act (FMLA) of 1993. Many employers allow vacation or sick leave to be used to pay for at least some of the time away from work during this period. FMLA may also be used if a child, spouse, or parent develops a serious illness. There are some additional requirements, including that an employee must have worked for 1250 hours over the previous 12 months prior to taking leave.

» **Stay Current:** More information on the Family and Medical Leave Act can be found at http://www.dol.gov/whd/fmla/employeeguide.htm.

Source: Based on the Family and Medical Leave Act, Public Law 103-3, February 5, 1999. 5 U.S.C. 6381–6387; 5 CFR part 630, subpart L. https://www.govinfo.gov/app/details/CFR-1999-title5-vol1/CFR-1999-title5-vol1-part630

In a recent study, Jehangir, Collier, Shakhatreh, Malik, and Parkman (2019) noted that caregivers are impacted by the severity of the chronic illness and the related increase in the amount of care required. Impacts include missed work due to the need to care for the family member. The responsibilities of the caregivers can lead to increased stress and anxiety that should be addressed by the healthcare team.

Patients with chronic illness, and their families, may be at risk for depression. Caregiver burden, loss of role function, and financial burden are just some of the factors that increase risk for depression in patients with chronic illness and their families. Nursing considerations for a patient with a chronic illness include being alert to symptoms of depression, both in the patient and in his or her close family members.

Serious Mental Illness and the Family

Caring for a family member with a mental illness can result in overwhelming emotional and economic stress on the family system, particularly if caregiver role strain becomes a contributing factor. Symptoms associated with SMI can significantly impair daily functioning, requiring a great deal of time and energy from family members who live with or care for the individual. Thus, it is common for the individual with SMI to become a large focus within the family dynamic, causing other members of the family to feel neglected or even ignored, which contributes to strain on the family. Family members of someone with an SMI may feel stigmatized and choose to keep the illness a secret from others outside of the family as a result (Kallquist & Salzmann-Erikson, 2019).

Caregiver burden generally refers to the stress, tension, and anxiety experienced as a result of caring for someone with a mental (or other chronic) illness (Cao & Yang, 2020). **Objective caregiver burdens** are those that are measurable, such as disruption of family functioning and routines and financial costs of care. **Subjective caregiver burdens** refer to the caregiver's perception of what is burdensome. Significantly higher family burden is associated with a number of variables. For example, well-controlled schizophrenia creates less caregiver burden then treatment-resistant schizophrenia, thus indicating severity of symptoms is a contributing factor (Velligan, Brain, Duvold, & Agid, 2019). Acuity of patient symptoms is highly associated with caregiver burden, with sleep disturbances, lack of motivation, poor hygiene, acting out, and violent behaviors among a number of behaviors that increase family burden. Trapp, Ertl, Gonzalez-Arredondo, Rodriguez-Agudelo, and Arango-Lasprilla (2019) noted that family cohesion could mediate the psychological impacts of caregiver burden on the caregiver. Nurses should therefore support family cohesion within the care plan.

The caregiving process itself can be stressful. Often community resources are not available, not satisfactory, or have long waiting lists. Insufficiency of these resources nationwide has resulted in high rates of homelessness, incarceration, and hospitalization of individuals with mental illness (National Alliance on Mental Illness [NAMI], 2020). Nearly 40% of incarcerated adult individuals have been diagnosed with a mental illness, and 70.4% of youth in the juvenile justice system have a mental health diagnosis (NAMI, 2020). Families of the seriously mentally ill often find themselves negotiating the criminal justice system. Many times, the crimes are misdemeanors; however, research shows that individuals with a mental illness are more likely to be incarcerated for the same crime when compared to someone without a mental illness (Walthall, 2019).

Stigma describes patterns of negative attitudes that lead people, sometimes including healthcare workers, to fear and discriminate against individuals with mental illness and their families. Because mental illness is so widely misunderstood, family members may isolate themselves from others who they feel are unsupportive or critical. Inability of some family members and friends to learn about and accept mental illness may lead to rejection. Furthermore, discrimination resulting from stigma often extends to the family and caregivers (Yin, Li, & Zhou, 2019).

Feelings associated with subjective caregiver burden include frustration, anxiety, hopelessness, and helplessness. Feelings of depression and/or grief and loss may also be present. Chronic sorrow may take hold as family members experience the relapsing nature of the illness.

Families with healthy coping strategies are more likely to experience better outcomes and reduced caregiver burden. Healthy coping strategies for caring for a loved one with SMI include:

- Focusing on the positive aspects of the relationship
- Seeking social and community supports
- Reducing sources of conflict
- Expressing affection.

Moral support, practical support, and motivation to help the loved one improve in functional ability are essential to helping family members with SMI lower their symptom burdens and increase daily functioning (Tamizi et al., 2020). Lower symptom burden and increased functioning lead to decreased caregiver burden. Families that act as stressors increase or create conflict, display stigma and discrimination, or force treatment choices and can impede the recovery of their loved one.

Pediatric Illness and the Family

When providing care for children, collaboration with the family is essential. Parents and other family members who provide care possess helpful information about their child's health and illness, as well as coping strategies and treatments that have helped in the past. Understanding which adult is the primary decision maker as well as what other family members provide care will assist the nurse in developing a family-centered care plan. Elements of a family-centered care plan are outlined in **Table 26.5** ».

Parents often need to assess their strengths in managing their ongoing family and caregiving responsibilities before planning how to add more caregiving responsibilities to their routine. Individuals who become family caregivers are at risk for considerable strain and stress, especially if they are unable to balance their own needs with those of the child. The nurse

TABLE 26.5 Elements of Family-Centered Care and Recommendations for Nursing Practice

Elements	Nursing Practice Recommendations
Family at the Center: ▪ Incorporate into policy and practice the recognition that the family is the constant in a child's life, while the service systems and support personnel within those systems fluctuate, and that the illness or injury of a child affects all members of the family system.	▪ Establish a therapeutic relationship with the family. ▪ Perform a comprehensive family assessment in collaboration with the family, identifying both strengths and needs. ▪ Use the family assessment when working with the family to plan, implement, and evaluate care, considering the impact of the child's illness or injury on the entire family, with special attention to the siblings. ▪ Provide siblings with information about their sibling's illness/injury at an appropriate developmental level and answer questions honestly. ▪ Promote sibling visitation in hospital settings and participation in home care activities. ▪ Identify extended family members who should receive information and be included in the educational process.
Family–Professional Collaboration: ▪ Facilitate family–professional collaboration at all levels of hospital, home, and community care.	▪ Develop provider–family relationships that are guided by the goals and expectations of both the family and the provider. ▪ Ensure that parents are integral and critical collaborators in the decision-making process about their child's care. Involve children and adolescents in the decision-making process as appropriate for their cognitive and emotional development. ▪ Ensure that parents have 24-hour access to their child and facilitate their participation in the child's care. ▪ Provide parents with the option to stay with their child during procedures and tests and provide ways for parents to support the child during the procedure. ▪ Provide comfort and hygiene facilities for families who spend long hours at the facility or travel great distances. ▪ Promote the family's development of expertise in the special care of their child, fostering family independence and empowerment. ▪ Incorporate parents and children into the quality assessment/improvement process. ▪ Integrate family members into institutional and community advisory groups and involve them in policy development.
Family–Professional Communication: ▪ Exchange complete and unbiased information between families and professionals in a supportive manner at all times.	▪ Provide information about the child's problem, prognosis, and needs in a manner that respects the child and family as individuals and promotes two-way dialogue. ▪ Encourage the family to share information about the child and the illness/injury so that care planning and decisions are made in the most informed and collaborative manner.
Cultural Diversity of Families: ▪ Incorporate into policy and practice the recognition and honoring of cultural diversity, strengths, and individuality within and across all families, including ethnic, racial, gender, spiritual, social, economic, educational, and geographic diversity.	▪ Practice family-centered care in a culturally competent manner with respect and sensitivity for the wide range of families with diverse values and beliefs. ▪ Seek to understand the family's beliefs and practices related to race, culture, gender, and ethnicity when developing relationships and collaborating in the child's healthcare. ▪ Seek to understand and respect the family's religious/spiritual beliefs and practices and integrate these into the child's care, as the family desires. ▪ Assist the family to address care issues related to socioeconomic status, insurance status, geography, and access to healthcare. ▪ Integrate training programs on diversity, cultural understanding, and culturally competent care into staff development programs.
Coping Differences and Support: ▪ Recognize and respect different methods of coping. Implement comprehensive policies and programs that provide families with the developmental, educational, emotional, spiritual, environmental, and financial support needed to meet their diverse needs.	▪ Assess the strengths and weaknesses of the family's coping strategies and its resiliency factors and characteristics. Identify maladaptive coping mechanisms and help the family to augment its coping efforts. ▪ Assess and support the family's needs and desires for support and assist the family in accessing and accepting assistance from support networks as needed or desired.

(continued on next page)

TABLE 26.5 Elements of Family-Centered Care and Recommendations for Nursing Practice (*continued*)

Elements	Nursing Practice Recommendations
Family-Centered Peer Support: ■ Encourage and facilitate family-to-family support and networking.	■ Educate parents about parent-to-parent and family support resources and help them to access such resources in the institution and community. ■ Provide access to psychoeducational groups that might be useful to parents, siblings, or ill or injured children.
Specialized Service and Support Systems: ■ Ensure that hospital, home, and community service and support systems for children needing specialized health and developmental care and their families are flexible, accessible, and comprehensive in responding to diverse family-identified needs.	■ Provide collaborative, flexible, accessible, comprehensive, and coordinated services to children and their families. ■ Provide comprehensive case management/care coordination for children and families with ongoing care needs. ■ Along with families, take an active role in advocating for the needs of ill or injured children.
Holistic Perspective of Family-Centered Care: ■ Appreciate families as families and children as children, recognizing that they possess a wider range of strengths, concerns, emotions, and aspirations beyond their need for specialized health and developmental services and support.	■ Encourage attention to the normal developmental needs and developmental tasks of the entire family unit and individual family members. ■ Encourage and facilitate the development of individual and family identities beyond a focus on illness or injury. ■ Facilitate "normalization" as valued and desired by the family.

Source: From National Alliance on Mental Illness (2013). This is a 15-hour in-service training for direct case staff of mental health organizations. The course is taught by a trained team of family members, individuals living with mental illness, and a mental health professional who is also either a family member or living with a mental illness themselves. Copyright © 2013 by NAMI.

and parents should collaborate in developing the plan for the child's care, so as not to conflict with the family's cultural or ethnic illness-related behaviors, experiences, and beliefs. It is important to include children in the care planning process and consider their thoughts and choices throughout the plan. Careful collaboration with the family and child will allow for a smooth transition from the healthcare setting to home with a continued positive relationship between the family and the healthcare system. See **Box 26.5** » for guidelines for effective collaboration.

Family or person-centered care is vital in all healthcare settings. Feedback from patients and families following an interaction with the healthcare system, including inpatient and outpatient experiences, can provide for a better understanding of the family and patient perspective on the care that was provided by the nurses and the other members of the healthcare team. Most healthcare systems regularly send out surveys to patients to collect this data, and to make improvements in the policies and procedures to ensure that the family and patient have the best experience possible.

There are several organizations that healthcare settings can utilize to help develop family-centered care practices, including the Institute for Patient- and Family-Centered Care (IPFCC) and Planetree International. As a nurse advocate, the nurse can emphasize the importance of following these practices when caring for children and their families. Dignity, respect, participation, and collaboration are core concepts of family-centered care (IPFCC, 2020). Additionally, information sharing is considered an important element in the practice of family-centered care, and the nurse should ensure that families have access to appropriate resources to understand the medical diagnosis and care that is needed. These resources

Box 26.5

Guidelines for Effective Parent–Provider Collaboration

Parents have a wealth of information about their child's health, health condition, symptoms and triggers, coping skills, and preferences for everything from foods to stress-reduction strategies. Nurses can encourage parents to share this information and to participate fully in their child's care by suggesting they:

- Use a journal or spreadsheet to track their child's behaviors, eating habits, and illness and symptoms and bring this information with them.
- Keep a copy of all medical records
- Bring a list of questions to the healthcare visit
- Ask all questions and ask for clarification when needed.

Nurse can promote communication with family members and caregivers by:

- Listening to information and concerns shared by parents and family members
- Showing respect for parents' and family members' questions and decisions
- Engaging in problem solving with the family to help identify treatment and care options that meet the family's needs.

Focus on Diversity and Culture

Family-Centered Care

When working to establish a family-centered relationship with families of various cultural or ethnic groups, consider the possibility that an extended family may need to be consulted. For example, some American Indians may consult tribal elders (considered part of the extended family) before agreeing to healthcare for their child. In some Hispanic cultures, major decisions for the child's healthcare are made with input from grandparents and other extended family members. Nurses and other HCPs should work to determine the strengths and coping mechanisms of the family network to facilitate effective and appropriate care planning (Nelson & Jett, 2020).

will facilitate effective informed decisions surrounding the child's health (IPFCC, 2020).

When providing care to children, be aware that the family is central to all healthcare interventions with parents and child as the partners in care. It is important to consider how a healthcare setting's written policies, procedures, and literature for families refer to families and what attitudes these materials convey. Words like *policies, allowed*, and *not permitted* imply that hospital personnel have authority over families in matters concerning their children. Words like *guidelines, working together*, and *welcome* communicate an openness and appreciation for families in the care of their children.

>> **Stay Current:** Planetree International provides certification to healthcare settings in person-centered care. For more information on this certification, visit https://www.planetree.org/certification-resources/top-10-best-practices-in-person-centered-care.

Geriatric Illness and the Family

Adults who care for their own children and one or more of their own parents belong to a group that has come to be known as the "sandwich generation." This group of adults faces an incredible amount of stress trying to meet the diverse needs of young children and adolescents as well as aging parents. One of the chief sources of stress for these families is financial insecurity. A family with limited financial resources may face taking the aging parent into their own home or placing an aging parent who is no longer independent into a senior care facility that is below standard. If a family has very young children, taking an aging parent with dementia into the home can present either real or perceived hazards to the young children, increasing the stress level of the entire family. In addition, a member of the sandwich generation often faces additional stress addressing an older parent's needs while still trying to get children off to school and extracurricular activities and maintaining full-time employment. In-home care and assistance are not always feasible due to financial constraints. Furthermore, end-of-life issues can be a great source of stress and conflict for these families.

The needs of the family caring for an older adult who is ill will vary based on factors already detailed in this module. In some cases, interventions needed are multiple and complex. But that should not stop nurses from helping family members identify needs that can be met in the short term with simple interventions. For example, caregivers may benefit from patient teaching regarding sleep hygiene to improve their own sleep or teaching about deep breathing and other relaxation techniques (see Box 3.1, Guidelines for Sleep Hygiene, in Module 3, Comfort, for strategies that promote sleep). Other nursing interventions may include referrals for respite care, hospice services, or counseling.

>> **Stay Current:** Older adults with neurologic disorders often experience sleep disruption. Research and advocacy organizations such as the Michael J. Fox Foundation for Parkinson's Research and the Alzheimer's Association offer resources to help both professionals and caregivers learn how to help their loved ones. See www.michaeljfox.org for resources for caregivers of individuals with Parkinson disease.

Risk Factors

The physical or mental illness of one family member places the entire family unit at risk for alterations in function. Among families, coping with illness may lead to family disputes, financial difficulties, and caregiver strain, as well as a number of other challenges. Financial challenges associated with illness are multifactorial; however, two common sources include medical bills and a member of the family leaving employment to help take care of another family member. Illness alone adds a considerable amount of stress to each family member's life—financial strains are one element of stress that occurs (Marsack-Topolewski & Church, 2019). High stress levels, especially among family caregivers, have been linked to health problems and an increased risk for premature mortality. Nurses should be aware of any negative coping mechanisms (alcohol or drug use) that may arise among caregivers.

Prevention

Families who are made aware of the challenges associated with illness early in the process may benefit from having additional time to consider and plan for some of the upcoming circumstances. For instance, discussing the wandering behaviors associated with dementia may prompt family members to install alarms on doors or take other measures to prevent wandering before it happens. Talking about the illness as a family can be extremely beneficial, as can family counseling. Nurses can help families by advising them of the challenges they will face and connecting them with the appropriate supportive resources, including counselors and sources of financial assistance as indicated.

Clinical Manifestations

Each family's reaction to a particular illness will vary based on their previous experiences, personal opinions, and cultural influences. Nurses must be alert to manifestations that signal the family is having difficulty coping with managing the illness and be able to respond appropriately to help family members improve their coping skills and access helpful resources (see the Clinical Manifestations and Therapies feature). Primary caregivers may benefit from education about techniques to relieve stress, participation in support groups, and respite care.

Collaboration

Interventions vary based on the identified risks and actual or potential alterations in health. Nurses working with pediatric patients may collaborate with the school nurse, homebound teacher, guidance counselors, and other professionals. Collaboration with parents is key because they often are the experts not only on their child but also on their child's illness, making them an extremely valuable member of the healthcare team. For older adults, nurses and other HCPs should continue to collaborate with the patient as long as the patient is able to participate in care. However, the nurse and the healthcare team may increasingly collaborate with the older adult's primary caregiver in the event of progressive illness or deteriorating condition.

Clinical Manifestations and Therapies

Family Stressors

ETIOLOGY (PRIMARY STRESSOR)	CLINICAL MANIFESTATIONS	CLINICAL THERAPIES
Chronic illness in the family	▪ Increased stress resulting in weight loss or gain, headaches, and anxiety ▪ Lifestyle changes (e.g., job loss and financial difficulties) ▪ Depression as evidenced by fatigue, lack of enjoyment, loss of interest in regular activities ▪ Decreased participation in social activities; withdrawal ▪ Unhealthy coping mechanisms (e.g., smoking, alcohol use, substance use)	▪ Teach about healthy forms of stress management. ▪ Provide resources for family counseling. ▪ Educate about healthy eating habits to reduce risk for further illness and improve nutrition. ▪ Discuss the benefits of exercise for stress relief and health.
Mental illness in the family	▪ Confusion over changes occurring within the family unit ▪ Stress related to helping the family member experiencing mental illness (possibly financial stress) ▪ Anxiety ▪ Depression ▪ Feelings of loss related to changes in family member's behavior ▪ Fear over the changes that are occurring ▪ Changes in social activities, often resulting in decreased socialization	▪ Educate about the benefits of counseling for the family to help with the changes that are occurring. ▪ Advise about healthy stress management techniques. ▪ Provide resources for support groups involving other families in similar circumstances. ▪ Educate about the realities of the mental illness to dispel any misinformation and/or stigmas.
Illness of a child	▪ Fear of death of the child ▪ Anxiety, stress, or depression in accordance with the child's illness and its effect on the parents and family ▪ Decreased job performance, job loss, and financial difficulties resulting from taking the child to doctor appointments or spending time in the hospital ▪ Confusion and anger resulting from a lack of control over the child's illness and health	▪ Promote awareness of available counseling services. ▪ Emphasize the importance of healthy eating habits and exercise. ▪ Advise the primary caregivers to take time for themselves to avoid burnout. ▪ Teach about healthy coping mechanisms and stress management. ▪ Answer any questions the parents may have about their child's illness.
Caring for older parents	▪ Criticism for not caring or not wanting to care for parent ▪ Feeling censured because of reasons for caring for parent ▪ Moral exclusion for not caring for parents	▪ Suggest counseling for adult children of older adult as well as family members. ▪ Provide resources such as respite care/daycare for older adult and adult children.

NURSING PROCESS

Nurses assess both the family and the patient when one family member is experiencing health problems. Families should be assessed for coping abilities, as well as possible complications that can arise from stress as a result of the family member's illness. Data from assessment of the patient and family will determine priorities for care.

Assessment

Assessment of the family facing challenges related to illness leads to the identification of family strengths and weaknesses. When indicated, the nurse also assesses the family's readiness and ability to provide continued care and supervision at home. Key components to consider when performing any family assessment and developing a patient's plan of care include the following:

- Cohesiveness and communication patterns within the family
- Family interactions that support self-care
- Number of friends and relatives available
- Family values and beliefs about health and illness
- Cultural and spiritual beliefs
- Developmental level of the patient and family.

Nursing assessment requires obtaining a complete family history, including genetic influences that may impact health. A family genogram (see Figure 26.9) may be helpful in collecting information, as detailed health histories should incorporate data regarding the patient's parents, siblings, grandparents, and even great-grandparents if information is available. If aunts, uncles, or cousins have had any health concerns, these should be noted as well. When assessing a family's history of mental illness, nurses should be aware that many individuals—especially from older generations—might not have volunteered knowledge about their mental illness. As a result, the patient may not know that a grandparent was diagnosed with a mental illness. Patients who were adopted and have no information about their birth parents will have no genetic health history to report, but information can be gathered about their health and environmental conditions during childhood, such as exposure to secondhand smoke, dietary patterns, or childhood illnesses.

Nurses are in a unique position to focus on care for an individual within the context of the family as partners. Being aware of issues that the family may face when one or more family members becomes ill can be helpful in guiding, teaching, and coordinating care for families. Being mindful of the impact of family function and structure in the particular family being cared for will provide a framework for identifying strengths of families as well as areas/resources needed by the family to recover and establish normal functioning patterns.

Diagnosis

Data gathered during a family assessment may lead to identification of the following family issues:

- Impaired family functioning
- Potential to improve family functioning
- Inadequate family skills or resources
- Inadequate parenting
- Caregiver burden.

Planning

When planning for patient care, the nurse should take into consideration the family network and structure. Determining the family structure will help the nurse to understand who the decision maker is in the family, as this can vary by cultures. In many cultures, the extended family is influential in healthcare decisions. The nurse should consider any cultural practices that should be included in the care plan. The awareness of cultural differences is one way for the nurse to form a trusting and beneficial relationship with the patient and the family.

The care plan should always include SMART (specific, measurable, achievable, realistic, and time-sensitive) goals and outcomes. The nurse should plan for goals that boost family functioning and communication and build on the strengths of the family. In caring for children, anticipatory guidance is crucial to consider, as there are anticipated norms in growth, development, and healthcare that the nurse should acknowledge during the planning phase.

The mutual development of goals between the nurse and the family will facilitate a smooth transition from the hospital to home, as all required resources can be identified and planned for during the hospital stay. Additionally, this careful planning will allow for the family to have a clear understanding of the changes in roles and responsibilities due to the illness and the recovery that is needed by the child.

Implementation

Although teaching is a core nursing intervention, it is important to remember that standardized teaching plans may not be effective for patients with chronic illness and their families. Encourage patients and families to choose appropriate literature and to find self-help or support groups so they can interact with others who have the same illness.

For families who will be providing care in the home setting, extensive teaching may be required. When the plan of care includes medication administration and equipment use, family members and caregivers may feel overwhelmed by the technical aspects of the patient's care. As much as possible, teaching sessions should be organized and divided into segmented presentations to avoid overloading the family and caregivers with information. Teaching sessions may include demonstration of the family's ability to provide care to their family member. In addition, the nurses assist in identifying appropriate community resources.

Communicating with Families

Working Phase

Parents of a child that is newly diagnosed with a chronic illness, such as type 1 diabetes, may experience fear and anxiety. Demonstration of physical presencing will facilitate a therapeutic relationship with the family. Always remember to use open-ended questions:

- Tell me what this diagnosis means to you.
- You mentioned that you are worried about diabetes care during the school day; tell me more about your specific concerns.

Evaluation

In evaluating the efficacy of the family nursing care plan, the nurse identifies the degree to which the family members have achieved the identified outcomes relevant to each nursing diagnosis. During evaluation, the nurse also examines all aspects of the nursing care plan to determine the effectiveness of nursing interventions, as well as to evaluate the continued relevance of original nursing diagnoses. Based on evaluation, the nursing care plan is modified to meet the family's current needs.

While the process of evaluation varies depending on the components of the family-specific nursing care plan, examples of criteria that may reflect successful achievement of identified outcomes include the following:

- Family members demonstrate the ability to identify realistic personal and family goals.
- Family members identify and demonstrate healthy coping strategies.
- Caregiver(s) demonstrate safe and effective implementation of care to their family member.
- Family members demonstrate support of the primary caregiver(s).

REVIEW Family Response to Health Alterations

RELATE Link the Concepts and Exemplars

Mrs. Ann Bell, an 82-year-old widow, was diagnosed with Alzheimer disease several years ago. She lives with her daughter and son-in-law and their two children, ages 16 and 10 years. Mrs. Bell has begun wandering, especially at night, and has started small fires when she attempts to cook and forgets about the pot on the stove. Mrs. Bell's daughter, Laura, accompanies her mother to her physician's appointment today and relates that the stress of caring for her mother, in addition to her other obligations to her husband and children, is becoming increasingly difficult.

Linking the exemplar of family response to health alterations with the concept of grief and loss:

1. How can the nurse help the family members to cope with the loss they feel related to Mrs. Bell's cognitive degeneration?
2. What strategies might help Mrs. Bell's grandchildren identify their feelings of grief and loss and work as a family to deal with these feelings?

Linking the exemplar of family response to health alterations with the concept of stress and coping:

3. What strategies can you suggest that will help this family deal with the stress of Mrs. Bell's cognitive degeneration?
4. What referrals can you make to reduce Mrs. Bell's daughter's caregiver role strain?

REFER Go to Pearson MyLab Nursing and eText

REFLECT Apply Your Knowledge

Coley, a 16-year-old, is recuperating from injuries sustained in a motor-vehicle crash in which he was the passenger. He was not wearing a seat belt and experienced a brain injury after striking the windshield. His cognitive and motor functions are impaired. After a 7-day acute care hospital stay, Coley was moved to an inpatient rehabilitation hospital, where he has been for the past 5 days. He is much more responsive to stimuli and to family members 12 days after his injury. Physical therapy is provided twice a day to promote range of motion and muscle tone and to prevent contractures. Plans are being made to discharge Coley home with outpatient rehabilitation care within the next 5 days. A case manager will be assigned to coordinate his healthcare services.

Coley lives with his mother, two half-brothers (10 and 6 years old), and stepfather. Both his mother and stepfather are employed full time and are trying to determine how to manage care for Coley once he returns home. Coley's father has not been actively involved in his life since his parents divorced 12 years ago. Coley's grandparents reside in the same town and may provide the family some support.

1. What family supports will Coley need as he continues his rehabilitation for the brain injury?
2. What family assessment information is needed to effectively plan nursing care for this adolescent and his family?
3. Identify two strengths and coping strategies that will help Coley's family members adapt to his disability.

Coley's family is coping with his initial survival of a serious brain injury and facing a long rehabilitation process. The family is just now recognizing that life as they have known it is changing. Coley is totally dependent for care, including bathing, toileting, feeding, and mobilizing. While he is expected to regain self-care abilities, the impact of the injury on his cognitive ability and future functioning is unknown.

Coley's extended family has provided support for the family during the past 12 days, but the level of support in the future weeks will decrease because of other family obligations. Coley's mother has already initiated a leave of absence from work so she can care for him when he returns home; however, this will mean the family has reduced income during that time period. Coley's younger brothers have been able to visit him, and they are very anxious because Coley cannot talk with them. They have been trying to avoid bothering their mother and father during this time, but they are wondering when life will be more normal and they can again participate in their usual afterschool activities.

4. What information about the family's strengths, needs, and resilience can be identified from the case study scenario?
5. What additional information would be helpful to know about family strengths and needs prior to developing a nursing care plan?
6. Based on your assessment of the family and challenges facing them, what is the priority nursing diagnosis for Coley and his family at this time? Why do you believe it is the priority?
7. Describe the use of family-centered care principles in planning Coley's nursing care in collaboration with the family.
8. What potential parenting issues could this family anticipate for Coley and his brothers?

References

American Psychological Association. (2020). *Resolution on sexual orientation, gender identity (SOGI), parents and their children*. https://www.apa.org/pi/lgbt/resources/policy/sexual-orientation

The Annie E. Coley Foundation Kids Count Data Center. (2019). *Children in the care of grandparents in the United States*. https://datacenter.kidscount.org/data/tables/108-children-in-the-care-of-grandparents#detailed/1/any/false/37,871,870,573,869,36,868,867,133,38/any/433,434

The Arc. (n.d.). *Center for Future Planning*. https://futureplanning.thearc.org/

Ball, J. W., Bindler, R. M., & Cowen, K. J. (2017). *Principles of pediatric nursing: Caring for children* (7th ed.). Pearson.

Barkan, S. (2019). *Sociology: Understanding and changing the social world*. BCcampus. http://solr.bccampus.ca:8001/bcc/items/78a5958f-17a5-44fa-ac72-53f749f90529/1/

Benton, J., Coatsworth, D., & Biringen, Z. (2019). Examining the association between emotional availability and mindful parenting. *Journal of Child and Family Studies, 28*(6), 1650–1663. https://doi.org/10.1007/s10826-019-01384-x

Boccio, C. M., & Beaver, K. M. (2019). Further examining the potential association between birth order and personality: Null results from a national sample of American siblings. *Personality & Individual Differences, 139*, 125–131. https://doi.org/10.1016/j.paid.2018.11.017

Bornstein, M. H., Hahn, C., Putnick, D. L., & Pearson, R. (2019). Stability of child temperament: Multiple moderations by child and mother characteristics. *British Journal of Developmental Psychology, 37*(1), 51–67. https://doi.org/10.1111/bjdp.12253

The Bowen Center for the Study of the Family. (2019). *Theory*. http://thebowencenter.org/theory/

Bristow, J. (2020). "Helicopter parents", higher education, and ambivalent adulthood. *Revue des politiques sociales et familiales*. https://repository.canterbury.ac.uk/item/8qqw3/-helicopter-parents-higher-education-and-ambivalent-adulthood

Brown, J. (2019). *Parenting styles: Types of effective parenting explained*. Find My Kids. https://findmykids.org/blog/en/parenting-styles

Cable News Network. (2019). *Same-sex marriage fast facts*. https://www.cnn.com/2013/05/28/us/same-sex-marriage-fast-facts/index.html

Caldwell, B. M., & Bradley, R. H. (1984). The HOME Inventory and family demographics. *Developmental Psychology, 20*(2), 315–320.

Cao, Y., & Yang, F. (2020). Objective and subjective dementia caregiving burden: The moderating role of immanent justice reasoning and social support. *International Journal of Environmental Research and Public Health, 17*(2), 455. https://doi.org/10.3390/ijerph17020455

Care.com Editorial Staff. (2020). *Child care costs more in 2020, and the pandemic has parents scrambling for solutions*. https://www.care.com/c/stories/2423/how-much-does-child-care-cost/

Centers for Disease Control and Prevention (CDC). (2019). *About chronic diseases*. https://www.cdc.gov/chronicdisease/about/index.htm

Centers for Disease Control and Prevention (CDC). (2020). *Helping children cope*. https://www.cdc.gov/coronavirus/2019-ncov/daily-life-coping/for-parents.html

Child Welfare Information Gateway. (n.d.). *Parental resilience.* U.S. Department of Health and Human Services. https://www.childwelfare.gov/topics/preventing/promoting/protectfactors/resilience/

Child Welfare Information Gateway. (2019). *Foster care statistics 2017.* https://www.childwelfare.gov/pubPDFs/foster.pdf#page=3&view=Children%20in,%20entering,%20and%20exiting%20care

Coehlo, D. P. (2015). Family child health nursing. In J. R. Kaakinen, D. P. Coehlo, R. Steele, A. Tabacco, & S. M. H. Hanson (Eds.), *Family health care nursing: Theory, practice, and research* (5th ed., pp. 387–432). F. A. Davis.

Coppola, E. C., McCall, C. E., Bailey, K., Mihalec-Adkins, B. P., & Wadsworth, S. M. (2020). *Understanding the challenges and meeting the needs of military and veteran families.* National Council on Family Relations. https://www.ncfr.org/resources/research-and-policy-briefs/understanding-challenges-and-meeting-needs-military-and-veteran-families

Duvall, E. M. (1977). *Marriage and family development* (5th ed.). Lippincott.

Duvall, E. M., & Miller, B. C. (1985). *Marriage and family development* (6th ed.). Harper Row.

Farr, R. H., & Vazquez, C. P. (2020). Stigma experiences, mental health, perceived parenting competence, and parent–child relationships among lesbian, gay, and heterosexual adoptive parents in the United States. *Frontiers in Psychology, 11*(445), 1–16. https://doi.org/10.3389/fpsyg.2020.00445

Federal Interagency Forum on Child and Family Statistics. (2019). *America's children: Key national indicators of well-being, 2019.* https://www.childstats.gov/pdf/ac2019/ac_19.pdf

Friedman, M. M., Bowden, V. R., & Jones, E. G. (2003). *Family nursing: Research, theory, and practice* (5th ed.). Pearson.

GLAAD. (2018). *Accelerating Acceptance 2018.* https://issuu.com/glaad/docs/accelerating_acceptance_2018

Gorry, D. (2019). Heterogeneous consequences of teenage childbearing. *Demography, 56,* 2147–2168. https://doi.org/10.1007/s13524-019-00830-1

Gurrentz, B., & Valerio, T. (2019). *More than 190,000 children living with two same-sex parents in 2019.* U.S. Census Bureau. https://www.census.gov/library/stories/2019/11/first-time-same-sex-couples-in-current-population-survey-tables.html

Hajal, N. J., & Paley, B. (2020). Parental emotion and emotion regulation: A critical target of study for research and intervention to promote child emotion socialization. *Developmental Psychology, 56*(3), 403–417. https://doi.org/10.1037/dev0000864

Hemati, Z., Abbasi, S., Oujian, P., & Kiani, D. (2020). Relationship between parental communication patterns and self-efficacy in adolescents with parental substance abuse. *Iranian Journal of Child Neurology, 14*(1), 49–56.

Homelessness Policy Research Institute. (2019). *LGBTQ youth experiencing homelessness.* https://socialinnovation.usc.edu/wp-content/uploads/2019/08/LGBTQ-Youth-Lit-Review-Final.pdf

Institute for Patient- and Family-Centered Care. (2020). *Patient- and family-centered care.* https://www.ipfcc.org/about/pfcc.html

Jehangir, A., Collier, A., Shakhatreh, M., Malik, Z., & Parkman, H. P. (2019). Caregiver burden in gastroparesis and GERD: Correlation with disease severity, healthcare utilization, and work productivity. *Digestive Diseases and Sciences, 64,* 3451–3462. https://doi.org/10.1007/s10620-019-05723-2

Kallquist, A., & Salzmann-Erikson, M. (2019). Experiences of having a parent with serious mental illness: An interpretive meta-synthesis of qualitative literature. *Journal of Child and Family Studies, 28,* 2056–2068. https://doi.org/10.1007/s10826-019-01438-0

Marsack-Topolewski, C. N., & Church, H. L. (2019). Impact of caregiver burden on quality of live for parents of adult children with autism spectrum disorder. *American Journal on Intellectual and Developmental Disabilities, 124*(2), 145–156. https://doi.org/10.1352/1944-7558-124.2.145

Merriam-Webster Dictionary. (2020). *Family.* https://www.merriam-webster.com/dictionary/family

Military One Source. (2020). *Tips for building family resilience.* https://www.militaryonesource.mil/family-relationships/family-life/keeping-your-family-strong/family-resilience-protective-factors

National Alliance on Mental Illness. (2013). *NAMI Provider Education program.* https://www.nami.org/Support-Education/Mental-Health-Education/NAMI-Provider

National Alliance on Mental Illness. (2020). *Mental health by the numbers.* https://www.nami.org/mhstats

Nelson, L., & Jett, E. (2020). *Identifying family strengths in times of crisis.* Southern New Hampshire University. https://www.snhu.edu/about-us/newsroom/2020/05/identifying-family-strengths-in-times-of-crisis

Noel, M., & Najowski, C. (2019). When parents are incarcerated, their children are punished, too. *Monitor on Psychology, 50*(8). http://www.apa.org/monitor/2019/09/jn

Planetree International. (2018). *Top 10 best practices in person-centered care.* https://www.planetree.org/certification-resources/top-10-best-practices-in-person-centered-care

Pollitt, A. M., Reczek, C., & Umberson, D. (2020). LGBTQ-parent families and health. In A. Goldberg & K. Allen (Eds.) *LGBTQ parent families.* New York, NY: Springer, 105–124.

Raley, R. K., & Sweeney, M. M. (2020). Divorce, repartnering, and stepfamilies: A decade in review. *Journal of Marriage and Family, 82*(1), 81–99. https://doi.org/10.1111/jomf.12651

Smilkstein, G. (1978). The family APGAR: A proposal for a family function test and its use by physicians. *Journal of Family Practice, 6,* 1231–1239.

Substance Abuse and Mental Health Services Administration. (2020). *Understanding child trauma.* https://www.samhsa.gov/child-trauma/understanding-child-trauma

Tamizi, Z., Fallahi-Khoshknab, M., Dalvandi, A., Mohammadi-Shahboulaghi, F., Mohammadi, E., & Bakhshi, E. (2020). Caregiving burden in family caregivers of patients with schizophrenia: A qualitative study. *Journal of Education and Health Promotion, 9*(12), 1–17. https://doi.org/10.4103/jehp.jehp_356_19

Tiret, H., & Knurek, S. (2020). *Strategies to cope with family stress.* Michigan State University. https://www.canr.msu.edu/news/strategies_to_cope_with_family_stress

The Trevor Project. (2019). *National estimate of LGBTQ youth seriously considering suicide.* https://www.thetrevorproject.org/wp-content/uploads/2019/06/Estimating-Number-of-LGBTQ-Youth-Who-Consider-Suicide-In-the-Past-Year-Final.pdf

Trapp, S. K., Ertl, M. M., Gonzalez-Arredondo, S., Rodriguez-Agudelo, Y., & Arango-Lasprilla, J.C. (2019). Family cohesion, burden, and health-related quality of life among Parkinson's disease caregivers in Mexico. *International Psychogeriatrics, 31*(7), 1039–1045. http://dx.doi.org/10.1017/S1041610218001515

The University of Tennessee Health Science Center. (2020). *Parent–child interaction therapy.* https://www.uthsc.edu/cdd/services/parent-child-interaction.php

U.S. Bureau of Labor Statistics. (2020). *Families with own children: Employment status of parents by age of youngest child and family type, 2018–2019 annual averages.* https://www.bls.gov/news.release/famee.t04.htm

U.S. Census Bureau. (n.d.) *Glossary: Household type.* https://www.census.gov/glossary/#term_Householdtype

U.S. Census Bureau. (2019a). *Fertility historical time series visualizations.* https://www.census.gov/library/visualizations/time-series/demo/his-cps.html

U.S. Census Bureau. (2019b). *One-person households on the rise.* https://www.census.gov/library/visualizations/2019/comm/one-person-households.html

U.S. Census Bureau. (2019c). *Subject definitions.* https://www.census.gov/programs-surveys/cps/technical-documentation/subject-definitions.html

U.S. Department of Health and Human Services (DHHS). (2019). *Trends in teen pregnancy and childbearing.* https://www.hhs.gov/ash/oah/adolescent-development/reproductive-health-and-teen-pregnancy/teen-pregnancy-and-childbearing/trends/index.html

U.S. Department of Health and Human Services (DHHS). (2020). *HHS poverty guidelines for 2020.* https://aspe.hhs.gov/poverty-guidelines

U.S. Department of Housing and Urban Development (HUD). (2019). *HUD launches initiative to prevent and end homelessness among young people aging out of foster care.* https://www.hud.gov/press/press_releases_media_advisories/HUD_No_19_111

Velligan, D. I., Brain, C., Duvold, L. B., & Agid, O. (2019). Caregiver burdens associated with treatment-resistant schizophrenia: A quantitative caregiver survey of experiences, attitudes, and perceptions. *Frontiers in Psychiatry, 10,* Article No. 584. https://doi.org/10.3389/fpsyt.2019.00584

von Bertalanffy, L. (1981). *A systems view of man.* Westview Press.

Walthall, J. (2019). *Features and news.* Treatment Advocacy Center. https://www.treatmentadvocacycenter.org/fixing-the-system/features-and-news/4204-research-weekly-serious-mental-illness-and-likelihood-of-incarceration-after-arrest-

Weiland, D. M., & Kucirka, B. G. (2019). Helicopter parenting and the mental health of iGen college students. *Journal of Psychosocial Nursing and Mental Health Services, 58*(5), 16–22. https://doi.org/10.3928/02793695-20191210-01

Weyers, L., Zemp, M., & Alpers, G. W. (2019). Impaired interparental relationships in families of children with attention-deficit/hyperactivity disorder (ADHD): A meta-analysis. *Zeitschrift für Psychologie, 227*(1), 31–41. https://doi.org/10.1027/2151-2604/a000354

World Bank Group. (2020). *Adolescent fertility rate (births per 1,000 women ages 15–19).* https://data.worldbank.org/indicator/SP.ADO.TFRT?name_desc=false

Yin, M., Li, Z., & Zhou, C. (2019) Experience of stigma among family members of people with severe mental illness: A qualitative systematic review. *International Journal of Mental Health Nursing, 29*(2), 141–160. https://doi.org/10.1111/inm.1266

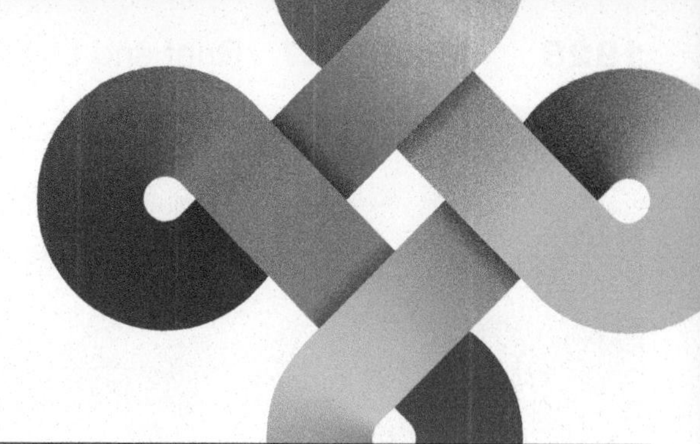

Module 27
Grief and Loss

Module Outline and Learning Outcomes

The Concept of Grief and Loss

The Process of Grieving

27.1 Analyze the process of grieving.

Factors That Affect the Grieving Process

27.2 Analyze factors that affect the grieving process.

Concepts Related to Grief and Loss

27.3 Outline the relationship between grief and loss and other concepts.

Nursing Assessment

27.4 Differentiate common assessment procedures used to examine patients or families who are grieving.

Independent Interventions

27.5 Analyze independent interventions nurses can implement for patients who are grieving.

Collaborative Therapies

27.6 Summarize collaborative therapies used by interprofessional teams for patients experiencing grief and loss.

Children's Grief Responses

27.7 Differentiate considerations related to the assessment and care of children who are dying or experiencing significant loss.

Perinatal Loss

27.8 Differentiate considerations related to the assessment and care of a family who experiences a perinatal loss.

Older Adults' Responses to Loss

27.9 Differentiate considerations related to the assessment and care of older adults experiencing a significant loss.

>> The Concept of Grief and Loss

Concept Key Terms

Actual loss, **1928**
Ageism, **1946**
Anticipatory grief, **1928**
Anticipatory loss, **1928**
Bereavement, **1927**
Childhood traumatic grief, **1940**
Death anxiety, **1938**
Disenfranchised grief, **1928**
Disseminated intravascular coagulation (DIC), **1942**
Fetal demise, **1942**
Grief, **1927**
Hospice, **1937**
Intrauterine fetal death (IUFD), **1942**
Loss, **1927**
Miscarriage, **1942**
Mourning, **1927**
Perceived loss, **1928**
Perinatal loss, **1942**
Placental abruption, **1942**
Prolonged grief disorder, **1928**
Rh disease, **1942**
Spontaneous abortion, **1942**
Stillbirth, **1942**

Loss and grief are inherent in the human experience. Even so, reactions to loss and manifestations of grief vary widely. Each individual's methods of processing and coping with grief are influenced by numerous variables, including personality, age, culture, the nature of the loss, and the availability of a functional support system. **Loss** occurs when something or someone of value is rendered inaccessible or drastically changed. In addition to the loss of a loved one, numerous other sources of loss can also prompt grief reactions. Examples include the loss of a friend or relationship, loss of mobility, loss of independence, loss of a limb, and loss of hair from illness (**Figure 27.1** >>). By understanding the emotional and physical aspects associated with grief, nurses are better prepared to care for patients who have experienced loss, as well as to support these patients during the grieving process.

The Process of Grieving

Grief is the combination of various psychologic, biological, and behavioral responses to a loss. Psychologic responses may include anger, denial, and depression. Biological responses to grief include sleep disturbances, decreased appetite, and weight loss. Behavioral responses include personality changes and decreased socialization. Bereavement and mourning can also accompany grief. **Bereavement** is the response to having lost another through death. **Mourning** involves the processing and resolution of grief, generally through cultural and/or spiritual beliefs and practices. Grief can be triggered by any number of situations or occurrences, such as the loss of a loved one or acquaintance or being diagnosed with a terminal illness. Grief can also result from the end of a significant relationship with a partner or a close

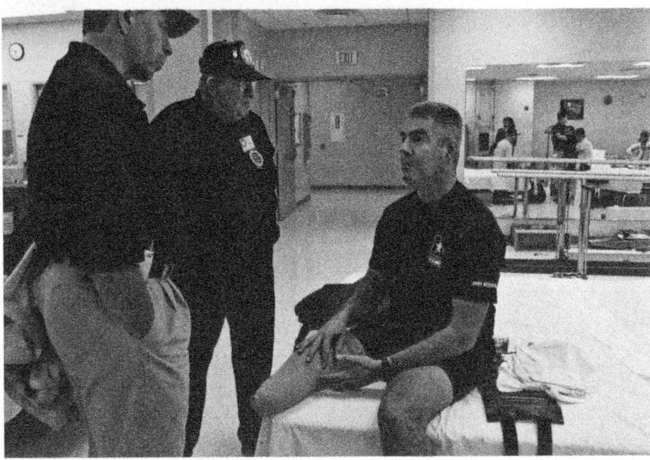

Figure 27.1 » Loss of an aspect of self is common in those serving in the military, as loss of an appendage or a functional ability is one of the hazards of serving in combat.
Source: David S. Holloway/Getty Images.

friend. In most cases, grief is a normal, healthy reaction to loss, as it helps the individual to process the situation. Grief should not be avoided, as avoidance often prolongs and intensifies the experience. For some individuals, the grieving process may also be prolonged by failure to mourn the loss according to an individual's cultural or spiritual practices.

The process of grieving is different for all who experience a loss. There is no correct way to grieve, nor is there a timetable for how long the grieving process should last. Manifestations associated with grief are highly individualized and depend on numerous factors such as the nature of the loss, the circumstances surrounding the loss, the developmental age and personality of the individual who is grieving, and the individual's history of grief and/or depression. Intense feelings of grief over the loss of a loved one are generally believed to lessen over a few months, and to resolve—or at least partly resolve—within 1 to 2 years (Walsh, 2012). This timetable does not apply in every case, and if the grief becomes complicated in any way—for example, when a loss is especially sudden or traumatic—resolution and acceptance take longer. Different types of grief should also be considered, as these often coincide with the type of loss experienced.

Types and Sources of Loss

Everyone experiences various types of loss over the course of a lifetime. The three main types of loss are **actual loss**, loss that is identified and recognized by others, such as the loss of a spouse; **anticipatory loss**, which occurs when an individual knows a loss is coming, such as the impending death of a close friend or family member from a fatal illness; and **perceived loss**, which is felt by an individual but cannot be verified as a loss from outside—for example, loss of control or loss of self-esteem.

The source of the loss may impact the range of an individual's emotional responses. For example, individuals who have lost a limb because of amputation lose an aspect of the self. They may experience disturbance of body image, depression, loss of independence, and frustration as they learn to live without use of the limb. Loss of an aspect of self can be very similar to loss of a loved one, in that the individual must learn to function despite the loss. Loss of independence itself is a serious loss, and it may occur with the loss of mobility due to injury or with debilitating illnesses such as dementia or multiple sclerosis.

The COVID-19 pandemic resulted in enormous losses for individuals and families. Actual losses—deaths, income and employment losses—were often accompanied by more intangible losses, such as the loss of routine as many people were prevented from participating in normal daily activities. Strategies for coping with grief discussed in this module are appropriate for patients who are grieving, regardless of the type of loss. Additional strategies for coping in times of crisis can be found in Exemplar 31.B, Crisis.

Types of Grief

Grief presents itself in many different forms, ranging from anticipatory grief to complicated grief. Similar to anticipatory loss, **anticipatory grief** is grief that is experienced before the event occurs. This can occur in anticipation of the death of a loved one or in response to the diagnosis of an individual's own terminal illness. For example, a man's wife has a terminal illness and is expected to live only another 3 months. He may experience anticipatory grief in advance of his wife's death, grieving for her while she is still alive. Not all individuals experience anticipatory grief. Despite many debates on the subject, no conclusive studies have proven whether anticipatory grief actually lessens the grieving process after a loved one has died.

Disenfranchised grief occurs when individuals cannot acknowledge their loss to others, typically when the loss is not one that is socially recognized (sometimes referred to as an *ambiguous loss*). Disenfranchised grief may result from the loss of a partner in a socially unrecognized relationship, the loss of a child due to abortion, the loss of someone from suicide or a drug overdose, or even the loss of a pet. LGBTQ individuals may experience disenfranchised grief over losses associated with social stigma: for example, when a family member fails to respect their sexuality or a spouse or partner. When a loss is considered socially unacceptable, the individual grieving the loss may experience not only intense grief but also feelings of isolation. Unable to participate in culturally appropriate expressions of mourning, the bereaved may find it very difficult to resolve their feelings and responses to the loss.

Prolonged grief disorder (PGD) may be diagnosed when a person persistently mourns a loss for longer than 6 months. Recently added to the World Health Organization's 11th Revision of the *International Classification of Diseases* (ICD-11), those who suffer PGD are typically those who suffer intimate losses, such as the loss of a romantic partner or a child. Losses resulting in PGD are often sudden or violent, such as suicide or an accident. Those who suffer from PGD often have associated posttraumatic stress disorder (PTSD) or complex PTSD (Killikelly & Maercker, 2018; Weir, 2018; see Exemplar 32.C, Posttraumatic Stress Disorder, in Module 32, Trauma).

Theories of Grieving

Different theories have been proposed to explain the grieving process. Typically, these theories identify different stages of grief. There are several different theories regarding grief.

Alterations and Therapies
Grief

ALTERATION	DESCRIPTION/DEFINITION	MANIFESTATIONS	INTERVENTIONS AND THERAPIES
Disenfranchised grief	The result of being unable to acknowledge a loss to others, generally because the grief is not socially recognized	▪ Hiding grief from others as opposed to allowing support from friends and family ▪ Not seeking support after a loss because of feelings of shame, guilt, or lack of recognition of the loss ▪ Intensified emotions associated with grief as opposed to those found in a normal grief reaction ▪ More pronounced feelings of anger and depression due to resentment over the unacknowledged loss	▪ Refer the patient to support groups that acknowledge the loss and feelings of grief. ▪ Recognize and support the patient's right to grieve the loss. ▪ Facilitate the patient's spiritual and cultural needs.
Prolonged grief disorder	Prolonged grief that impairs the individual's ability to perform daily activities and impairs social interactions.	▪ At least 6 months of longing for the deceased with little to no change in the mourning process ▪ Inability to participate in daily activities ▪ Decreased sense of self and/or loss of identity ▪ Difficulty with social interactions or avoidance of social settings ▪ Avoidance of things/places that remind of the deceased ▪ Feelings of anger, distrust, depression, or meaninglessness or void of all feelings.	

Some propose "stepwise" or "stage" models that a person completes; other theories consider grief "work" and grief "process."

Kübler-Ross and the Five Stages of Grief

One of the first grief theorists, Elisabeth Kübler-Ross (1969), proposed five stages of grief: denial, anger, bargaining, depression, and acceptance. A psychiatrist, Kübler-Ross based her theory on work she did with dying patients, so some criticism holds that these stages cannot, therefore, be ascribed to those mourning the loss of another. Other critics contend that the stages of grief do not always occur sequentially, as Kübler-Ross described them; stages can overlap or occur individually.

Denial, the first stage of grieving, may serve to soften the initial blow of the loss. A small amount of denial early in the grieving process is healthy, as it allows individuals who have undergone a loss to retreat into themselves to eventually accept the loss more fully. Nurses working with patients in denial should not force their patients to accept the loss; neither should they reinforce the denial. Denial generally occurs for only a short time, as most individuals eventually begin to accept the loss in their own way, so nurses should be understanding and supportive.

Anger is one of the most difficult stages for all those involved. During this stage, bereaved individuals direct their anger toward anyone who is around them, sometimes without even the slightest apology. Patients who are angry in their grief over a significant loss may direct their anger at others, including nurses. This behavior should not be taken personally.

The third stage is *bargaining*. Those who are in this phase of grieving try to make a bargain, generally with a higher power (such as God) or others in perceived power, such as a provider, for more time. Kübler-Ross (1969) found through interviews with patients that this stage sometimes results from the individual's guilt over something from the past. A nurse can help during this stage by listening sympathetically to the patient's expression of fear and guilt.

Depression follows the bargaining stage. Depression, a profound sense of deep and penetrating loss felt during the grieving period, is part of the normal work of loss. Nurses support patients during this phase by encouraging and allowing them to express their sadness and sometimes simply by sitting with them silently as they work through these emotions on their own.

After depression, the final stage of the grieving process is *acceptance*. During acceptance, the patient is free from anger and depression; this is not a happy stage, but a stage almost lacking in emotions. Generally, during this time, a terminally ill patient's family needs more support and comfort than the patient, who often experiences a decreased desire for visits from family and loved ones. At this point, the dying individual has fully accepted the loss and gone through the various stages of grieving to arrive at acceptance.

David Kessler, a colleague of Kübler-Ross and a trauma and grief specialist, proposed a sixth stage of grief: *finding meaning*. That after acceptance, people often seek to find new meaning in their lives in response to a loss. For some, it may be creating a memorial event (such as a race to raise funds for a charitable organization) or making new connections with others (Kessler, 2019).

Stroebe and Schut

Margaret Stroebe and Henk Schut (2010) propose that bereavement is actually two related processes: loss-oriented process and restoration process. The loss-oriented process focuses on the loss the individual has experienced, recognizing it, and eventually accepting the loss. With the loss-oriented process, the person will experience depression, anxiety, anger, and other emotions related to the pain of the loss. The restoration-orientated process focuses on the change of identity, role, and life without the loss. The person will create new roles and meanings of life. The two processes "oscillate" between each other during the bereavement period.

Manifestations of Grief

Normal grief reactions are difficult to define, as all individuals grieve differently. In general, it is normal to experience sadness, anxiety, guilt, anger, confusion, sleep disturbances, and loss of appetite, among other reactions. The amount of time these emotions last varies. Typically, however, the intense feelings of grief begin to dissipate over the first 3 to 6 months following the loss, resurfacing on holidays, birthdays, and other important reminders of the loss. When grief becomes complicated, the intense emotions begin to impact the individual's ability to carry out daily activities. Similarly, these forms of grief may begin to affect the individual's health through loss of appetite, extreme depression, and sleeplessness. It is important for nurses to know the signs of different forms of grief reactions. Disenfranchised grief, described earlier, may result in a prolonged grief reaction, in part due to the individual's inability to mourn the loss in a socially acceptable way. Consider, for example, the case of a parent losing a child to a drug overdose. Despite the fact that unintentional drug overdoses are on the rise, social stigma around this type of loss remains. The parent may not feel comfortable mourning the loss openly because the child died doing something illegal and socially unacceptable.

It is critical that nurses provide nonjudgmental physical care and psychosocial support to patients experiencing grief, especially those dealing with disenfranchised grief. Often, the nurse's willingness to listen without offering advice provides a safe, nonjudgmental place for the patient to grieve.

Individuals experiencing PGD have ongoing difficulty in accepting loss, often a loss that is sudden and unexpected. For example, a mother may experience PGD after the death of a child from suicide. Often, PTSD and PGD are intertwined. Growing evidence indicates that 1 in 10 of those in mourning will develop PGD (Lundorff, Holmgren, Zachariae, Farver-Vestergaard, & O'Connor, 2017). In a meta-analysis study, the higher the mean age, the greater the prevalence of PGD. Meaning, the older the person experiencing a sudden loss, the greater the chances of experiencing PGD. Individuals with PGD are more likely to withdraw from society, have difficulty with daily tasks, and be prone to suicidal thoughts and attempts. These individuals are also more likely to have issues with substance abuse, sleep disorders, and depressed immunity and therefore should be referred to a mental health professional. In the meantime, the nurse can provide care by providing a safe environment and supportive care that includes screening for substance abuse and suicide assessment.

Factors That Affect the Grieving Process

When considering the process of grieving, it is important to consider the nature of the individual's loss as well as the support system. The nature of the loss and the individual's current health and financial status affect the amount and type of support needed. A loss that impacts daily functioning, such as the death of an income-earning spouse or of a primary caregiver, results in a variety of consequences. Individuals experiencing this type of loss typically require greater support than those who experience the loss of a distant relative or casual acquaintance. Similarly, individuals who experience ambiguous losses—such as perinatal loss, the death of a pet, or the death of an ex-spouse—require a wholly different form of support. In general, individuals seek support from those who were close to the deceased or from those who have experienced similar losses. Likewise, grieving individuals can find support through social means, including in-person support groups and virtual groups. With emerging technology, more and more virtual support groups have become available. A qualitative study found that online support groups, in conjunction with grief therapy, can be therapeutic for grieving individuals. However, the nurse should be aware that online support groups should not be solely recommended; evidence shows that virtual support groups alone are not as effective as and should be used to complement counseling (Robinson & Pond, 2019).

Cumulative loss is defined as several losses within a short period, one after another after another. The individual who experiences cumulative loss may not recover from the initial loss before the next loss occurs. Each loss has the potential to compound the grief of previous loss to the point where the individual becomes paralyzed with grief (Thompson, 2012). An example of a cumulative loss would be an individual who experiences the death of a friend, then a short time later experiences the death of a spouse, and soon after is diagnosed with a serious illness. The individual may not be able to fully grieve the loss of the friend when having to then cope with the loss of the spouse. The grief then could be compounded with the diagnosis of a serious illness when faced with the individual's own mortality.

Likewise, nurses should be aware of their own cumulative loss in the workplace. Some nurses may experience multiple losses of patients and may not have the ability to cope with several deaths. Cumulative grief may take a toll on the nurse's mental health. Strategies to help reduce or mitigate the stress of cumulative losses in the workplace are discussed later in this module.

Age

Children who experience loss at an early age are at greater risk of an intense grieving period, especially children who lose a parent or primary caregiver. This risk increases further when the remaining parent or caregiver fails to recognize the child's grief and assumes that the child is too young to be affected by the loss. If children do not receive support and explanation after a substantial loss, they may view the loss as a betrayal, giving rise to feelings of guilt and anger. This reaction may result in the development of trust issues later in life (Walsh, 2012). More information about children's responses to loss follows later in this chapter.

Adults' reactions to grief and loss can become abnormal if the loss cannot be, or is not, acknowledged by others, or if extreme grief responses do not lessen after a substantial amount of time. The complicated or disenfranchised grief responses in adults have more to do with personality, circumstance, support systems, and other factors. By middle adulthood, loss and grief begin to be expected and accepted as a normal occurrence. Although losses are certainly not easy, they are typically processed in a healthy manner. Older adults may be at greater risk for PGD because their support system may have become limited as a result of past losses, including the death of close family members and friends and even children and grandchildren. For example, an older adult who has already lost a spouse may be more likely to experience PGD if her child dies, as she finds herself without her partner to help her mourn the loss of their child. As described earlier, these cumulative, substantial losses may result in PDG. Having a history of numerous losses may make the grieving process harder for older adults, as the individual may not have had time to resolve a previous loss.

Symbolic losses are also more prevalent among older adults; for example, older adults are more at risk than other age groups of losing their independence, their memory, and their mobility, as well as other significant assets. Symbolic losses may occur because of the death of a spouse or caregiver. For example, a husband with limited mobility may rely on his wife for transportation, cooking, and assistance with daily living. If she dies, the husband faces numerous losses in addition to his wife's death (**Figure 27.2** »).

Sex

Sex often is a factor in grief when society or culture influences how individuals perceive the grieving process. In some cultures, men cannot show sadness or tears, whereas women are expected to do so. In other cultures, only men can attend funerals, while women must stay at home and grieve privately (Purnell & Fenkl, 2019). Grief reactions in general, though, cannot truly be understood or analyzed based on the individual's sex alone. Factors such as age, personality, culture, family dynamics, and the nature of the loss must also be considered when assessing grief reactions.

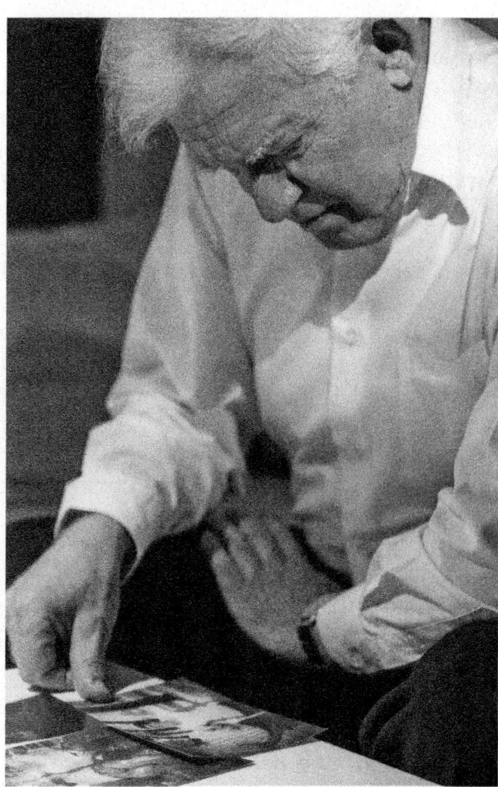

Figure 27.2 » A widower mourns the loss of his wife and needs to learn to cook for himself and clean the house, tasks his wife handled during their 60 years of marriage.

Source: KatarzynaBialasiewicz/iStock/Getty Images.

Substance and Alcohol Abuse

Periods of grief and loss are very vulnerable times. Grief can have devastating effects that, if not acknowledged and dealt with, can result in various forms of self-medicating. Nurses encourage healthy coping mechanisms such as seeking counsel from support systems, seeking comfort from religious practices, going to support groups, and doing therapeutic writing. Unhealthy coping mechanisms can complicate grief, resulting in alcohol or drug use to escape the pain of loss. The use of unhealthy coping mechanisms, including drugs or alcohol, can further prolong the grieving process. In situations where the nurse suspects alcohol or substance abuse, the nurse remains nonjudgmental and uses a therapeutic approach to ask how the patient has been handling the grief and adjusting to the loss. If patients admit to depending on alcohol or substances, the nurse can provide support and referral for the dependency and can also provide patient teaching related to healthy coping responses.

Resilience

Experiencing a loss, or many losses, can be a challenge for individuals to cope and recover. Resilience, in this case, is how quickly individuals can return to their normal state of being. Individual resilience depends on many factors. One impact on resilience is the cause of the loss. Those who experience loss unexpectedly or through trauma or violence may have more difficulty returning to normal than those who anticipate a loss due to illness. For example, a patient who must have an amputation because of a prolonged struggle with a nonhealing wound will be more likely to cope than a patient who loses a limb in a car accident. Similarly, in the case of loss due to death, the relationship between the deceased and the bereaved can also be a factor in the individual's resilience in the situation. Finally, those who experience loss and trauma simultaneously, such as surviving a bombing during a conflict, but lose family members in the process are less likely to have resilience in this situation.

The physical health of the individual at the time of loss can also affect resilience. A study found that bereaved spouses who were in good physical health were less likely to report somatic symptoms and/or depression after the loss of a spouse compared to those who were not in good health at the time of their spouse's death (Utz, Caserta, & Lund, 2012). Other factors that can influence an individual's resilience in the time of loss include mental and cognitive state, support systems, and spiritual strength.

Asking for Help

Depending on an individual's paradigm, as well as the views of society or an individual's culture, grief may carry a stigma. Neglecting to grieve or being unable to seek comfort and strength from support systems can lead to feelings of isolation. Nurses encourage patients to ask for help if they feel that the effects of loss are becoming overwhelming. Nurses also provide information about support systems and services available in the community. A strong support system can positively impact the grieving process.

Case Study » Part 1

Josie Duncan is a 32-year-old woman whose 7-year-old daughter, Tasha, died 3 months ago after fighting leukemia. Mrs. Duncan took a week off from work after her daughter died and then returned to her job. She visits her primary care physician's office complaining of difficulty falling asleep over the past 2 weeks. After checking her vital signs, weight, and temperature, you notice that Mrs. Duncan has lost 15 pounds since her last visit 6 months ago. Her blood pressure and temperature are both normal. You observe that she looks exhausted and has deep circles under her eyes; the clothes she is wearing are at least a size too large. She also seems to be very distracted.

Clinical Reasoning Questions Level I

1. Why might Mrs. Duncan be having trouble sleeping?
2. What are some factors that influence an individual's grief response?
3. What additional questions would you want to ask Mrs. Duncan? Why?

Clinical Reasoning Questions Level II

4. Is Mrs. Duncan at risk for a prolonged grief disorder? Explain your answer.
5. Do you think the doctor will prescribe medication for Mrs. Duncan's sleeplessness? What other interventions could be performed?

Concepts Related to Grief and Loss

Grief is an important consideration when working with end-of-life patients. Not only are these patients learning how to come to terms with the loss of their own lives, but also their families experience a variety of hardships during this time, from the financial burden of caring for the dying to anticipatory grieving. Nurses need to understand the grieving process to help end-of-life patients and their families work through grief. When working with grieving patients, it is equally important to obtain a full history to determine if those patients have a history of anxiety or depression, as these conditions can complicate or elongate the grieving process. Patients who have experienced a traumatic loss, such as a perinatal loss or a death due to violence, or who have witnessed a death are at risk for developing PTSD and should be made aware of the signs. Similarly, patients who have a history of PTSD have a higher risk of developing PGD later in life. When grief becomes overwhelming, some individuals turn to alcohol or other substances to numb their emotions.

The Concepts Related to Grief and Loss feature links some, but not all, of the concepts integral to grief and loss. They are presented in alphabetical order.

Concepts Related to
Grief and Loss

CONCEPT	RELATIONSHIP TO GRIEF AND LOSS	NURSING IMPLICATIONS
Addiction	Alcohol and substance abuse can mask the emotions associated with grief and cause a longer and sometimes more intensified grief reaction.	■ Look for signs of alcohol or substance use as an unhealthy coping mechanism for grief. ■ Teach the patient about healthy coping mechanisms. ■ Maintain a nonjudgmental attitude. ■ Refer to a specialist.
Comfort	Palliative care can help further the grieving process for both patients and their families, providing both physical and psychologic comfort.	■ Help dying patients to grieve for their own loss of life. ■ Assist family members in understanding the signs of grief and acceptance of death. ■ Provide referral to such assistance as hospice, support groups, and spiritual resources.
Culture and Diversity	Response to loss and the display of grief will be different from culture to culture. Culture also dictates how different family members, including males and females, are to respond to loss.	■ Be aware that grief and loss response is culturally influenced. ■ Ask the patient how cultural needs can be met during the time of loss and grief.

Concepts Related to *(continued)*

CONCEPT	RELATIONSHIP TO GRIEF AND LOSS	NURSING IMPLICATIONS
Legal Issues	Death of a spouse or parent may result in additional financial hardships due to medical bills. If the death was unexpected, an autopsy may be required. If a crime was involved with the death, the survivor may have to endure the judiciary process.	■ Refer the surviving family to a social worker or elder law attorney for resources regarding financial obligations after death. ■ Educate the family on the local coroner's office procedures and policies, such as release of the body. ■ Refer the family to advocacy groups or the local district attorney's office regarding court procedures.
Mood and Affect	Situational depression is common in those who experience loss. Those effects may include feelings of extreme sadness, guilt, worthlessness, and other such emotions. Physically, the individual may complain of fatigue, lack of appetite, and sleep pattern disruption.	■ Assess for suicidal ideation. ■ Engage the patient in therapeutic communication. ■ Provide resources for support groups. ■ Refer the patient to a healthcare provider for evaluation and potential medications.
Nutrition	Those who are grieving may not eat as they did previously. They are more likely to eat alone and eat less. Along with decreased caloric intake, bereaved people tend to have nutritional deficits as well.	■ Assess the patient for signs of malnutrition. ■ Monitor the patient's weight. ■ Obtain a 24-hour food diary and make recommendations based on the findings. ■ Provide and teach a nutrition plan based on the patient's needs. ■ Suggest nutritionally dense, small meals to help promote weight stability and to meet nutritional needs.
Spirituality	Grief and loss can have either a positive or negative impact on the patient's spiritual foundation.	■ Assess the patient's attitude and current state of spirituality. ■ Refer the patient to a rabbi, priest, pastor, imam, chaplain, or other spiritual counselor.
Stress and Coping	Existing anxiety/stress disorders and PTSD can prolong or intensify the effects of grief.	■ Assess patient's anxiety level and trauma history and any co-occurring stressors (such as loss of income). ■ Assess history of losses and level of current functioning. ■ Encourage patients who are already in treatment to continue their treatment plan and to communicate their loss to their provider.

Nursing Assessment

Assessment related to grief and loss should include exploration of the patient's current grief, as well as interviewing the patient regarding any past significant losses. Obtaining a complete history of any medical conditions is also necessary. A mental health assessment and information about current coping abilities should also be obtained. A complete nursing assessment also includes identifying the patient's cultural and spiritual needs.

Observation and Patient Interview

Assessment of the patient who has experienced a loss includes assessing the many factors that contribute to an individual's grief reaction, such as the patient's age, coping mechanisms, support system, history of previous losses, history of depression, culture, cause of the loss, and personality. When conducting an assessment, be attentive to the patient's needs and maintain a nonjudgmental attitude. If the patient has an extensive history of loss, ascertain how the patient dealt with those losses and whether the patient has achieved resolution or acceptance of them. A sensitive and thorough assessment promotes openness and creates an environment in which the patient can feel safe in discussing emotions. The following questions may be included in the patient interview.

Current Loss

- When did the loss occur?
- What was the nature of the loss?
- Are you having trouble carrying on with your normal activities?
- Have you experienced any trouble sleeping or eating?
- Have you talked to anyone about the loss (e.g., spouse, friends, family, or counselor)?
- Are you taking any medications and/or antidepressants?

History of Loss and Grief Reactions

- Have you experienced similar losses in the past?
- Did your grief manifest in ways similar to those for your grief for this loss?
- Are you experiencing any unresolved grief?

Grief and Loss Assessment

ASSESSMENT/ METHOD	NORMAL FINDINGS	ABNORMAL FINDINGS	LIFESPAN OR DEVELOPMENTAL CONSIDERATIONS
Loss Assessment			
Ask about previous losses. Discover the different types of losses, as well as their frequency.	Experiencing several losses is normal at almost any age. In the first few months after the loss, sadness, sleep disturbance, loneliness, and intermittent periods of decreased motivation or activity are to be expected.	▪ Inability or unwillingness to process the loss ▪ Denial of the loss for a prolonged time ▪ Inability or unwillingness to discuss the loss ▪ Accumulation of losses with little to no resolution ▪ Grief that interferes with daily functioning and lasts 6 months or longer should trigger additional assessment	▪ Children and adolescents are likely to process losses differently from adults; it should not be assumed that they do not understand loss because of their age. ▪ Older adults are likely to have numerous losses over their lifetime, and these can begin to have a cumulative effect.
Grief Assessment			
Assess patient's current and past grief reaction. Determine the nature of the loss causing the grief.	Grief is intense over the first 2–6 months after the loss and then begins to lessen. Resolution/acceptance generally occurs within 1–2 years after the loss.	▪ Inability to return to usual activities (such as work or school) ▪ Inability to maintain activities of daily living, self-care	▪ Children who do not receive appropriate support or who experience a traumatic death may be at risk for developing a prolonged or complicated grief reaction. ▪ Older adults are at high risk for depression. Loss of a spouse or caregiver may impact independence and requires additional assessment and referral.

Lifestyle

- Do you have an active support system?
- Do you drink alcohol and/or use substances on a regular basis?
- What types of coping mechanisms have you employed to work through your grief?

Physical Examination

Physical examination of the grieving patient should include a complete physical assessment. Patients may have somatic complaints, such as abdominal pain or headaches, that will need focused assessments. Other focused assessments include looking for signs of self-harm, self-neglect, and nutritional status. Evaluate the patient's hair, skin, and nails for signs of malnutrition and wounds. Evaluate energy level, functional status, and mental status.

Assessing Family Functioning

Family bonds are often challenged when coping with loss. Some families are able to come together and grow stronger; other families become distant and detached. Assessment of the family unit is primarily an interview process. Questions to ask of family members include:

- What impact is the loss having on the family?
- What are the strengths of the family?
- What are the support systems of the family?
- What needs does the family have?
- How does the family perceive how they are coping?
- How are family members expressing their feelings?
- How is each family member's current health status?

See Module 26, Family, for more information regarding assessment of the family.

Spiritual and Cultural Considerations

Accurate assessment of the grieving process requires awareness of an individual's cultural influences. While it would be unreasonable to expect nurses and other medical professionals to know the practices and beliefs of every culture, in many cases valuable information can be gleaned during a simple patient interview. Understanding the patient's culture may also give meaning to unusual or unexpected reactions toward professionals who offer assistance, particularly as certain cultural or religious practices view seeking help as a sign of weakness. Nurses should avoid the tendency to view individual behaviors and cultural practices through personal worldviews. In most settings, patient populations offer a diversity of cultural backgrounds. Respect for the practices of others is essential to building trust, establishing a relationship, and, ultimately, providing effective patient care.

Awareness of the patient's cultural beliefs and values can prevent miscommunication and conflict. For example, some cultures see death as a beginning rather than an end and choose to celebrate the individual's life on Earth and the movement to the next life. Misinterpretation of cultural belief may lead nurses to try to promote coping mechanisms that may not be effective. It is important to understand that patients view death and grief from their own perspective.

Mourning practices vary widely among cultures and religions. Some mourn openly and in public, whereas others mourn at home for a set period before moving back into society. In the Jewish faith, for example, followers practice the tradition of *shivah* (or *shiv'a*), a 7-day mourning period during which the closest family members—such as parents, siblings, and spouse—stay together to mourn their loss and receive visitors. Other cultures may emphasize the need to continue with normal activities, such as school or work, during the mourning period, in place of taking time away to mourn privately.

Similarly, cultural and religious practices are important to a patient who is dying. If a patient has specific spiritual or religious requests, such as seeing a priest or a rabbi or having ceremonial traditions performed by an elder of the religion, nurses and other staff should facilitate these requests whenever possible. Those who practice Catholicism, for example, believe the dying person should receive the Sacrament of the Sick (sometimes referred to as Last Rites) to receive God's grace before death. Some requests have greater impact on nursing and clinical staff than others. As part of Jewish practice, if the person dies on the Sabbath, the body cannot be removed from the place of death. This means the body cannot be removed from a hospital room until the Sabbath is over. Some cultures and religions have ritualistic cleaning of the deceased by same-gender attendants. In those cases, opposite-gender nurses should not prepare a body for the morgue. Even more so, some faiths do not want those who are not of the faith to touch the deceased. When a Muslim person dies, the body is typically prepared for burial by Muslims of the same gender (Purnell & Fenkl, 2019), and nurses should limit the amount of contact with the deceased. Even within cultures some patients may have individual preferences. Respectful assessment is necessary to identify and promote patient preferences.

Case Study » Part 2

Mrs. Duncan tells you that she has been working a lot since her daughter died because she needs something to occupy her mind. For the last year of Tasha's life, Mrs. Duncan spent a great amount of time taking her to doctor appointments and treatments; now that Tasha is gone, Mrs. Duncan does not know what to do with her spare time. She reports that her appetite decreased before her daughter died, and she has not really had any desire to eat since then. Lately she has not wanted to see any of her friends because they act differently around her. Mrs. Duncan admits she does not want to be around children right now. She reports her sleeplessness started 2 weeks ago, shortly after the Christmas holiday. She and her husband tried to celebrate, but they felt it was not the same without their daughter. Mrs. Duncan admits that she does not think her husband understands how upset she is over their loss.

Clinical Reasoning Questions Level I

1. Why was Mrs. Duncan's appetite poor before her daughter died?
2. What are two nursing diagnoses that apply to Mrs. Duncan?

Clinical Reasoning Questions Level II

3. Based on what you know about grief and loss, why do you think Mrs. Duncan began to experience sleep disturbances after Christmas?
4. How would you characterize this patient's support system? Is it strong, moderate, or weak? Explain your answer.
5. Do you think Mrs. Duncan is working through the grieving process, avoiding grief, or both? Justify your answer using data from the case study.

Independent Interventions

When an individual is grieving, it is sometimes hard to know what to say or do, and nurses may find themselves reluctant to pose questions. It is important to know that there are many ways to offer a patient support and a forum to discuss any difficulties (**Figure 27.3** »). Open-ended questions, such as asking how the patient has been doing since the loss or what challenges the patient is facing, may be effective for engaging the patient in discussion. Once the patient begins to speak, the nurse should use active listening techniques to show full engagement in the interaction. Body language also conveys the nurse's engagement in the conversation. A nurse's body language should be open and attentive and, when possible, both individuals should be positioned so they are at eye level with one another. (See Exemplar 38.B, Therapeutic Communication, in Module 38, Communication, for a discussion of active listening techniques.)

Implementation of the patient's care depends on different factors, including the nature of the loss, the patient's health, the patient's use of coping mechanisms, and the patient's personality. Interventions helpful in working with adults and older adults who are grieving include:

- Teach the patient about the grieving process and its general progression.
- Discuss the benefits of different forms of therapy, as well as the differences between modes of therapy such as group therapy, psychotherapy, and one-on-one therapy.

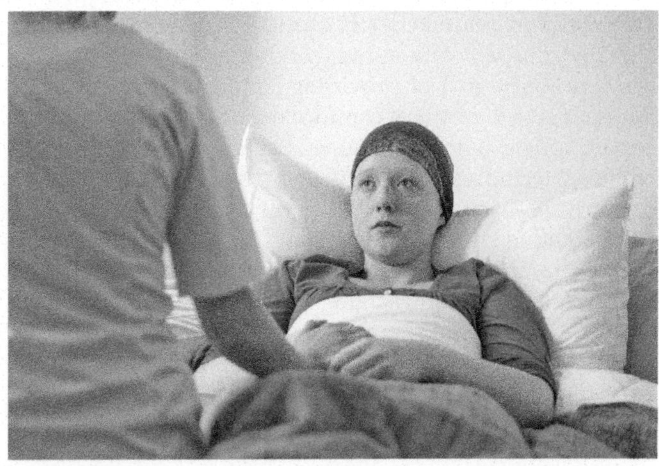

Figure 27.3 » Finding the time to talk with patients and actively listening to their concerns is an important component of nursing.
Source: KatarzynaBialasiewicz/iStock/Getty Images.

- Inform the patient about the warning signs of intense depression and/or suicidal thoughts.
- Teach the patient about healthy coping mechanisms.
- Provide a judgment-free area for the patient to discuss experiences and fears about grief.
- Encourage the patient to share emotions and fears with close family members or friends.
- Provide referral to resources that can assist the patient to maintain as much independence as possible.

Supporting Anticipatory Grief

With anticipatory grief, the individual begins to grieve before the actual loss occurs. For example, a family member may begin the mourning process when given the news that another family member has a terminal condition. Sometimes, individuals complete the grieving process before the loss occurs and, as a result, become detached. As in the previous example, the family member of the individual who is diagnosed with the terminal illness may complete mourning for the loved one before death actually occurs. The family member may seem distant to the dying individual, causing isolation and loneliness for the terminally ill individual. The nurse can help both the family member and the dying individual by encouraging them to share feelings about the impending death. The nurse should also encourage family members to create positive moments that may include storytelling and memory sharing. Educating the family and individual on a typical course of care and the dying process can reduce anxiety about both processes. Many hospice programs use written materials to educate on death and dying. See Exemplar 3.B, End-of-Life Care, in Module 3, Comfort.

Helping the Patient to Cope with Death

The dying patient also experiences stages of grief. The nurse can apply techniques and strategies for those experiencing the loss of their life just as others will be experiencing the loss of a loved one.

Preparing for death is a process that is unique to each individual. Some patients will embrace death as relief from their pain and find peace in death; others will be fearful of death and find despair. The nurse working with dying patients has a primary goal of providing comfort. This comfort is not exclusive to physical comfort: the nurse should help the patient cope in a holistic manner. Patients may feel a variety of things, including social distress, psychologic distress, and/or spiritual distress, along with physical distress (Hospice and Palliative Nurses Association, n.d.).

Some might find talking with a dying person awkward or uncomfortable. Acknowledging these feelings is important for the nurse to address. From there, the nurse should let the dying patient lead the conversation (Canadian Virtual Hospice, 2015). The nurse can offer support and provide care that the patient directs. If the patient expresses spiritual distress, the nurse can collaborate with a spiritual counselor; if the patient requests relief from pain, the nurse can provide comfort measures. During these conversations with the dying patient, the nurse should always be honest regarding the patient's health status unless this is not culturally acceptable (some cultures do not believe in telling individuals they are dying).

Coping with the Loss of a Patient

All nurses will encounter death of a patient at some point in their practice, although nurses in care settings such as oncology, hospice, emergency departments, and intensive care units will experience patient deaths with some frequency. Nurses are particularly vulnerable to *compassion fatigue*, a symptom of persistent loss that causes nurses to lose interest in caring for patients (Perregrini, 2019). All nurses should assess their own needs to grieve and process a loss. Nurses who are experiencing compassion fatigue should practice excellent self-care and employ strategies such as connecting with colleagues, maintaining helpful self-talk, and fostering a spirit of helpfulness and teamwork (U.S. Department of Veterans Affairs, 2020). Excellent self-care includes health promotion activities such as getting regular exercise and maintaining a healthy diet, as well as taking regular breaks at work for refreshment and stress reduction activities (e.g., deep breathing).

Nurses not accustomed to working with dying patients should also assess their own feelings regarding death. Peters et al. (2013) found that nurses who have strong anxiety regarding death tend to be more uncomfortable with caring for the dying patient. Nurses who are not comfortable with the topic of dying may not be prepared when confronted by a patient who is dying and in need of support. When this happens, nurses may cope by encouraging the patient or family member to talk about something else. While this may seem more conducive to the patient's happiness, it can be detrimental to the patient's overall well-being. Similarly, the nurse who is uncomfortable with the topic of death may try to avoid the topic by providing the patient with false hope, saying such things as "You are going to be fine; don't worry." This type of false reassurance is not beneficial to either the patient or the family (Potter & Moller, 2020). Nurses need to honestly assess their own feelings about death and dying, otherwise, patient care may be affected. For example, a nurse who is obviously anxious about and fearful of death can make a patient more fearful of death.

When working with a patient who is dying, it is easy for a nurse to bond with the patient. These bonds can result not only in normal feelings of grief, such as sorrow, but also in feelings of guilt, perhaps because the nurse cannot save the patient. In such cases, it is important that nurses acknowledge and process their feelings of guilt rather than ignore them. Similarly, nurses should seek support for any grief they may feel at the loss of a patient (**Figure 27.4** »). Resources for support may include coworkers, professional therapists or social workers, and grief counseling resources offered through employers. It is important that nurses make time to seek and find the support they need to process their own grief in a healthy manner. In acknowledging and processing their grief over a patient's death, nurses will be better able to help future patients and their families through the processes of death and grief.

Collaborative Therapies

Collaboration may include facilitating meetings between a spiritual care provider and the patient and/or the family. A referral to a social worker can provide expert guidance about coping with loss and assist with linking patients with

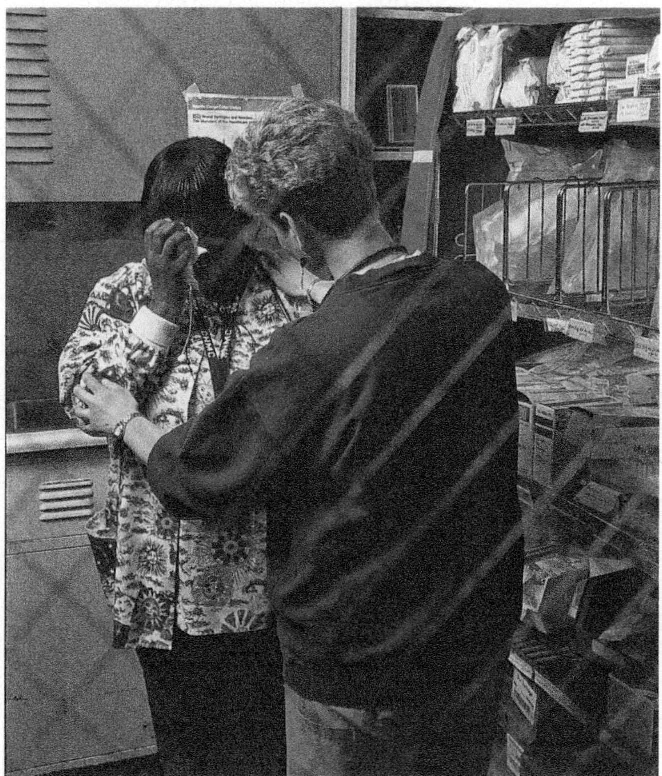

Figure 27.4 » Nurses need to express their own grief in a supportive environment after a child's death. Sharing with colleagues the sadness and grief or futility of resuscitation efforts often helps nurses provide supportive care to the next family who needs it.
Source: Pearson Education, Inc.

additional resources. Group therapy, bereavement groups, and grief therapists can all be resources for patients who have experienced a loss. **Hospice** is an organization that provides end-of-life care for patients either in their homes or in a hospital setting. Area hospice programs also provide an array of other services, depending on the community resources available.

Treatment of PGD is often in the form of psychotherapy, targeting specific symptoms related to the disorder. Katherine Shear and colleagues (2005) developed *complicated grief treatment (CGT)*, a form of psychotherapy administered over 16 sessions in accordance with a published manual that describes this treatment. The use of CGT has proven to be effective in the treatment of PGD. Greater success has been found with the use of antidepressants, such as citalopram, along with CGT (Shear et al., 2016).

Pharmacologic Therapy

Because grief on its own is not a disease, psychotherapy is favored over pharmacologic therapy. Antidepressants are usually reserved for PGD cases but may be prescribed in certain cases. Psychotherapy is preferred over prescribing medications for sleep, and CGT has been reported as helpful in improving sleep patterns (Szuhany et al., 2020). Sleep aids are rarely prescribed as their benefits are outweighed by their detriments.

Nonpharmacologic Therapy

Finding support sources is one of the primary ways that the nurse can provide nonpharmacologic therapy for the person experiencing loss. Support can come in many forms, including support groups, family support, community support, faith community support, and individual counseling. The nurse can also provide support to the individual.

Complementary health approaches, including stress management techniques, may be helpful. Those grieving might find comfort in gentle exercise, such as yoga and t'ai chi. Others might find massage and healing touch helpful. Aromatherapy might also be a useful tool to use for coping.

Case Study » Part 3

Before the healthcare provider talks with Mrs. Duncan, you discuss her complaints of sleeplessness and weight loss with him. You also inform him of Mrs. Duncan's difficulties since her daughter died. After the HCP talks to Mrs. Duncan, he recommends that she consider talking with a grief counselor about the loss of her daughter. He also recommends that she try to eat more and that she begin exercising at least three times a week—even if she only goes for a 10-minute walk. Mrs. Duncan and the HCP agree that she should try a combination of counseling, a healthy diet, and exercise before they consider the possibility of pharmacotherapy. Mrs. Duncan schedules a follow-up appointment for next month.

Clinical Reasoning Questions Level I

1. Why do you think the HCP recommended exercise?
2. What are some of the benefits of grief counseling?

Clinical Reasoning Questions Level II

3. Do you think Mrs. Duncan's grief reaction is normal after the loss of a child? Explain your answer.
4. Why did the doctor not prescribe pharmaceutical sleep aids immediately? What are some risk factors associated with taking controlled substances while grieving?
5. Do you think Mrs. Duncan has demonstrated healthy coping mechanisms for dealing with her grief?

Children's Grief Responses

Children and adults experience grief differently, and manifestations of grief vary across the lifespan (**Figure 27.5 »**). Children do not generally show or express their emotions regarding loss as openly as adults. Because young children may not express their grief in a way that is expected by an adult, they are sometimes believed to be too young to fully recognize the loss. However, this is not always the case. Children may be grieving in their own way and sometimes express this grief after loss through art, imaginary games, playing, or behavioral changes. Behavioral changes, such as decreased socialization, irritability, and confusion, may occur more frequently in adolescents than in very young children (Walsh, 2012). Losses experienced by children that may result in grieving include any of the following: loss of parent or primary caregiver, grandparent, or sibling; loss of a pet; loss of a relationship with a parent due to divorce; loss of a childhood friend or mentor; and loss of support systems if the family relocates to another city or country.

Children's grief responses vary depending on a variety of factors, most notably the child's developmental stage and the significance of the loss. When caring for a grieving child, it is important to remember that cognitive development greatly influences grief response. While young children have the capacity to understand loss to some degree, their grief

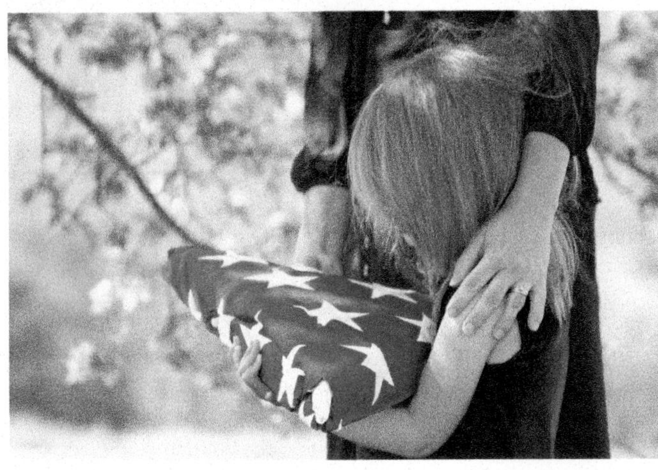

Figure 27.5 ›› Children who experience the death of a parent may be concerned about losing their other parent as well. Nurses can help by inviting children to talk about their grief and answering questions they may have.

Source: Stephanie Frey/iStock/Getty Images.

is displayed in ways that differ from grief reactions seen in other age groups. Children also experience **death anxiety**, which manifests as feelings of fear and/or apprehension connected with death.

Developmental Stage

Children grieve differently at different stages of development. Quite a few similarities exist as well. Grief responses in children across the developmental stages are often behavioral: The child acts out emotionally or physically in one way or another.

Worden and Silverman (1996) proposed four tasks that help children adapt to loss:

1. Accept the loss and its permanence.
2. Experience the emotions associated with grief, such as anger, fear, sadness, guilt, and loneliness.
3. Adjust to daily life without the individual who has been lost.
4. Come to see the relationship with the deceased as one based on memories in place of continuing experience.

During the first task, the child must come to understand the loss. In the case of a death, the child must understand that the one who has been lost will not return. Many childhood movies, television shows, and books involve storylines in which an important character dies but is then magically brought back to life. Although a child may intellectually understand that this is not possible, the desire for the return of the individual who has been lost may be so great that it is easier for the child to believe that the individual will come back in some way. Although the child should not be forced to accept the death, nurses and other caregivers can explain and reinforce the reality that the beloved individual is not returning. During the second task, children experience emotions similarly to those of adults as they grieve loss. Nurses support children in this task by encouraging emotional expression and by helping parents to understand that these expressions are normal and appropriate. It also is helpful for adults to recognize that emotions can be triggered long after the loss by holidays, birthdays, or other special events. The third and fourth tasks of this model take time to process and accept. Adults can help children in these tasks by listening, by helping children adjust to changes in routines, and by encouraging activities that promote new memories.

Ages 2–4

Children ages 2–4 cannot yet fully comprehend or express the ideas associated with loss. At this stage, they also see death as temporary or even reversible, believing that the individual or pet who has been lost will come home again. Reaction to grief at this age can also result in changes to sleeping and eating habits, as well as regression with toilet training. Other habits also may change in reaction to loss; for example, the child may lose interest in normal activities or may crave more attention and affection. This type of behavior often manifests as the child becoming clingy or screaming when not being held. When dealing with loss at this age, it is best for caregivers to respond to the child's changes from grief by trying to maintain as normal a routine as possible. Similarly, providing extra reassurance and attention can also be helpful. It is easy to believe that children at such a young age do not understand the concept of loss or death, but they most certainly do notice and understand when change occurs. Therefore, it is important for parents to provide honest answers to questions about grief when they are asked.

Ages 5–7

At this stage, children still view death as reversible. It is common during this age span for children to think of death as another place; according to this thinking, the loved one is still alive but has moved to a place the child cannot reach. Other common thought processes at this age revolve around feelings of guilt or blame. In the case of the death of a loved one, a child may fear having caused the death, especially because of negative thoughts about the individual or engaging in some type of misbehavior just before the death. Feelings of responsibility such as these are referred to as *magical thinking* and are quite normal in this stage of development. Children at this age may or may not verbalize these feelings, so parents or caregivers are advised to discuss the loss honestly and help the child realize the loss is not the child's fault. A child experiencing grief at this age may also act as though nothing has changed—this is a common reaction for children at this stage and is not by itself cause for alarm.

Grief responses for children ages 5 to 7 may include changes in eating and sleeping patterns, as well as an increase in nightmares. It is also quite normal for the child to be concerned that other important individuals may die as well. Some children express these fears verbally, whereas others express them through artwork or even writing. Parents and caregivers can help children with reassurances about their safety and well-being and also by inviting children to talk about their grief or ask any questions. It is best for adults to answer questions simply and honestly, providing the child with further explanations when needed.

Ages 8–11

From around ages 8 to 11, children begin to understand that death means the individual is gone and will not be coming back. During this developmental stage, children become more curious about death and what happens after people (or pets) die. As in the previous developmental stage, children in this age group also tend to believe their thoughts or misbehaviors could be the cause of a loved one's death. It is common for a child to feel that the death of a loved one is a form of punishment for some misbehavior. Grief responses at this stage are typically behavioral and may involve becoming more aggressive, acting out in school, or misbehaving at home, or the child may respond by becoming more withdrawn and engaging in solitary activities.

Ages 12–18

By the time children reach adolescence, they are more capable of understanding the abstract idea of death. During this time, children stop believing that their thoughts or behaviors can result in the death of others. Adolescent grief responses are very similar to those of most adults, and adolescents may display a wide range of emotions, including depression, denial, and anger. It is very common for individuals in this age group to direct grief-related anger toward their parents. Adolescents should be encouraged, but not forced, to voice their feelings about the loss. Sometimes individuals in this age group feel more comfortable talking to peers or those outside the family (**Figure 27.6 ›››**).

Significance of the Loss

The significance of a loss impacts the child's grief experience. For many children, their first encounter with loss is the death of a pet; regardless of the type of pet (fish or dog, cat or hamster), the loss carries meaning for the child. With the death of a pet, the child may react with an abbreviated grief response and, depending on age, ask several questions. For more significant losses, though, such as the death of a parent, grandparent, sibling, or friend, a child's grief response is likely to be much more developed.

Death of a Parent

In many ways, the death of a parent, especially for a young child, is one of the most devastating losses the child will experience. The death of a parent is not only the loss of an important person—for many children, the death results in the loss of an entire way of life. Children depend on their parents or caregivers for almost everything, from their home, meals, and security to their sense of love and belonging. Fathers die more frequently than mothers. Children of color and children from households living in poverty are more likely to lose a parent to death (Scherer, 2019).

Depending on the developmental stage of the child, the death of one parent could also introduce profound fear that the other parent will die soon as well. This sense of impending loss can stimulate a great deal of anxiety for the child. How the surviving parent or guardian handles the adjustment period after the death has a large impact on how the child copes with the loss. Many children are said to adjust to a parent's death after about a year, but a large percentage still experience changes in behavior, such as social withdrawal and problems with schoolwork, well beyond the first year.

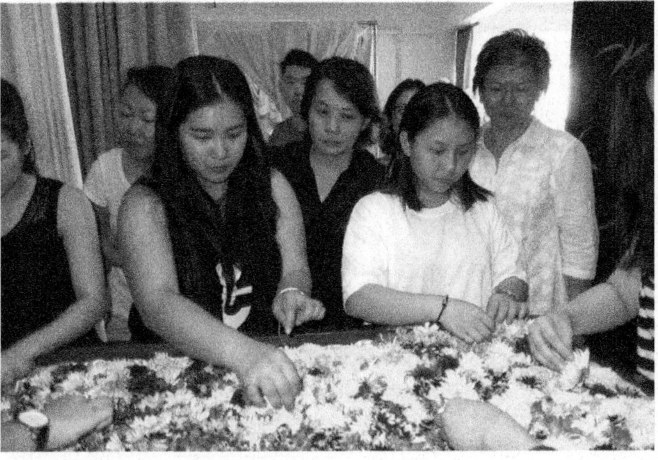

Figure 27.6 ››› Teenagers lay flowers on the casket of the victim of a drive-by shooting.

Source: Chua Wee Boo/agefotostock/Alamy Stock Photo.

Death of a Grandparent

The death of a grandparent generally is one of the first significant losses children experience. How a child handles the death depends on the child's relationship with that grandparent. For example, if the child has met their grandfather only once because he lives in another state and does not visit often, the impact of the loss will be far less than if the grandparent has lived with and helped raise the child. In this case, the impact of the grandparent's death is similar to that of a parent dying. Children who realize the significance of the grandparent's relationship to their own parent may become concerned about the possibility of losing their parents.

Death of a Sibling

In many ways, the loss of a sibling can be as traumatic as losing a parent or primary caregiver. Siblings often spend much of their childhood together, and they share experiences and relationships with loved ones. For siblings who share a bedroom, the connection is intensified. At a minimum, the death of a sibling generates questions about mortality; related concerns may lead to fear and worry. If unaddressed, fear and worry may cause behavioral problems, developmental regression, and a heightened fear of anything the child believes may be harmful. Depending on the developmental stage of the child, feelings of guilt and confusion may also be associated with the death of a sibling. For example, a brother who fights with a sister who later dies in an accident may feel he is responsible for her death.

Death of a Friend

Similar to the death of a sibling, the loss of a friend causes difficulties for children because it is the death of someone their own age. When a parent or grandparent dies, children often fear for the surviving adults; however, when another child dies, children fear for themselves and their friends. This fear can affect the child's sense of security in the world. If a child is friends with a schoolmate who is terminally ill, parents can work to prepare the child for the loss. If the death occurs suddenly, however, there is no time to prepare, and parents and caregivers should work to assure children of their safety.

Other Losses

Like adults, children experience losses other than death that can trigger a grief response. Parental divorce alone can be a significant loss, but it is further complicated if the divorce results in the child's separation from the noncustodial parent by a great distance. Similarly, deployment of a parent serving in the military or other parental absence creates a loss for the child and other family members. Moving can result in loss of school friends, teachers, and other support systems. Long-term or severe acute or chronic illness or injury may result in lifestyle modifications, loss of a limb or body part, or loss of independence. Children experiencing these losses need as much support as, and sometimes more support than, children who experience the death of a loved one.

Complications

Children can experience complications in the grief process as the result of circumstances surrounding the loss, or the significance of the loss. When children experience a significant or traumatic loss, they need a very strong support system to help them work through their feelings of grief, which are most likely difficult for them to understand. Children who do not receive the support they need are at an increased risk for developing a grief reaction that has been complicated in some way.

Complicated Grief Reactions

Children who lose a parent suddenly are more likely to develop mental health disorders such as depression and posttraumatic stress disorder (Pham et al., 2018). These children are also more likely to suffer from PGD, often for more than 2 years.

If a child is abused, the loss of an abuser can create complicated feelings. Feelings of grief are mixed with a sense of relief that the abuse has ended. Regardless of age, coping with mixed emotions related to the death of an abuser presents serious challenges. For children who lack the cognitive ability to fully understand death, the impact is even more complex. Furthermore, if the abuse was hidden, the child's experience can be even more confusing. The child who is grappling with mixed emotions observes the others involved in mourning the loss. With no confidantes, the child has no one with whom to discuss the conflicted feelings. This is an example of disenfranchised grief that can lead to PGD.

Childhood Traumatic Grief

Childhood traumatic grief is a grief reaction to the traumatic death of an individual who is important in a child's life or to witnessing a traumatic event. The child may associate thoughts of the beloved with the circumstances of the death and be unable to separate the beloved from the event.

Several factors influence how a child develops and recovers from a loss, particularly a traumatic loss. These include the available social support system and the child's own coping style (Brooks, Graham-Kevan, Robinson, & Lowe, 2019). The prognosis for grief recovery is less optimistic when a child practices avoidant coping by attempting to avoid the grief and associated memories, places, and things associated with the deceased. For example, if a child's friend died on a playground, the child may refuse to go to playgrounds or even play outside. Children who are unable to overcome loss often experience learning difficulties, behavioral issues, and mental health problems (Child Traumatic Stress Network, n.d.). Both children and adults fare better with grief work when there is strong social support available, along with healthy coping strategies.

Not all children who witness trauma or violence, or lose a loved one to accidental death, develop traumatic grief. In fact, the majority of children recuperate from the loss with no lasting effects if there are strong support systems in place, including parental/family support.

Clinical Manifestations

When children encounter death, they often do not grasp the idea entirely. As a result, their minds often work to protect them from the overwhelming feelings caused by grief. In some cases, children may not even react to loss outwardly. There is nothing wrong with this reaction: Their minds may act to protect them from experiencing emotions for which they have no point of reference. When children do react, though, their reactions often revolve around behavioral changes, which may include emotional and behavioral regression.

Behavioral Responses to Grief

Behavioral responses to grief vary depending on developmental age, temperament, and other factors already mentioned. Behavioral changes following loss may be immediate or may occur over time. A child's behavior change often presents in one of two ways: withdrawal or acting out. Some children are more withdrawn at home but act out more frequently at school. The responses depend on the child. Some who withdraw will be quieter than usual and seem shy around others. Their primary method of play may be in activities they can do alone, such as drawing, reading, or simply engaging in solitary play. In rare cases, a school-age child may revert to total silence, refusing to speak to anyone. If this behavior goes on for an extended period, a mental health professional should be consulted.

Some children may respond to grief with anger and aggression. Anger is typically directed toward the individual who has died, or at the loss itself, but often is taken out on family, friends, or teachers. Other responses may involve trouble eating and sleeping or an overall feeling of anxiety. Adolescents who are grieving may turn to alcohol, tobacco, or drugs as a method of coping with the loss.

Watching a child's behavior change drastically after an individual has died can be terrifying for a parent or guardian. Nurses work to assure parents that the changes they are seeing in their children are a normal response to the loss and that each individual grieves differently. Nurses and other clinicians encourage parents to allow children to express their grief, either verbally or artistically, and provide parents with information about warning signs of unhealthy coping. For example, preoccupation with thoughts of death, engaging in dangerous activities, and drug or alcohol use are considered unhealthy coping mechanisms.

Cultural Considerations

How children handle their grief at the loss of a loved one is greatly influenced by the cultural or spiritual practices of the child's immediate family. For example, children may be raised to believe that someone who dies goes on to an afterlife. Other cultural traditions believe that an individual's soul is reincarnated in a new body after death. Some practices teach that no existence of any sort continues after death, and that death is simply the end of life (Spector, 2017). Nurses take the cultural and spiritual traditions of patients into consideration, especially when speaking to children about grief. For example, if a child's father has told her that the individual who has died will now be reincarnated in a new existence, and another individual who is not familiar with the family's culture tells the child that this individual is now in heaven, the child will most likely be very confused. The nurse who is unaware of a family's beliefs should avoid inadvertently imposing their own belief system on the child. Similarly, if the family has decided not to offer any explanation of an afterlife or lack thereof to the child, that is the parents' decision, and the nurse should not use spiritual beliefs to help the child work through the grief.

Collaboration

In most cases, childhood grief progresses naturally and in a healthy manner with the help of supportive family members and friends. Adults need to understand that children's grief processes vary based on factors such as developmental stage, support system, relationship of the deceased and cause of death, or if the child witnessed the trauma/death. If the death occurred (or is likely to occur) in a hospital, a child life specialist may be available to work with the child through the dying process and following grief. Nurses can also recommend to the family to consult with the funeral director or the local hospice program, as they are specialists in the grieving process. Finally, if signs and symptoms of grief are persistent, the child can be referred to a mental health provider (American Academy of Child and Adolescent Psychiatry, 2018).

Pharmacologic Therapy

In most cases involving a child who is having difficulty working through grief, nonpharmacologic options such as therapy or group counseling are effective. Few pediatric patients will require pharmacologic intervention. Few studies have been done on the effectiveness and safety of pharmacologic intervention for complicated grief in children and adolescents. If mental health therapy and other nonpharmacologic interventions are given a significant trial and still prove ineffective, a child psychiatrist should be consulted for further recommendations (American Academy of Child and Adolescent Psychiatry, 2018). Because the use of antidepressants may increase risk for suicidal ideation and behaviors in some children and adolescents, the child psychiatrist and parent/guardian should collaborate to make the best decision with the child (American Academy of Child and Adolescent Psychiatry, 2018; Potter & Moller, 2020). If the child is prescribed antidepressants, regular follow-up appointments should be scheduled for at least the first 12 weeks after beginning the medication. Antidepressants should also be used in combination with nonpharmacologic options to help the child work through grief and eventually move on to acceptance.

Nonpharmacologic Therapy

Individual sessions with a therapist or participation in a bereavement group can help children work through a difficult loss. Children's bereavement groups often include activities involving drawing, writing, or other forms of arts and crafts. During these activities, children may be encouraged to draw expressions depicting how they feel about the loss. They may also be given the option of creating a scrapbook or a memory box about the individual who has died (Walsh, 2012).

Older children and adolescents may be encouraged to practice forms of writing therapy, which can involve keeping a journal about their feelings or writing letters to the deceased. In these writings, individuals are encouraged to be entirely honest without any fear of judgment from others or from themselves. The main idea behind this form of therapy is that writing about intense feelings of grief, pain, or trauma will eventually cause the feelings to begin to subside. Many individuals are not comfortable talking about these emotions or thoughts and find it easier to express their emotions openly in writing. Therapeutic writing can also be suggested for terminally ill children to express their fears and uncertainties.

Nursing Care

The nurse assesses the child's and the family's history of previous losses, coping skills, psychosocial supports, and cultural and spiritual practices and preferences. In the case of a pediatric or adolescent child experiencing grief from a recent loss, the overall health and reactions of the child should be assessed. Some families have difficulty talking about death; for some, talking about death outside the family may go against cultural beliefs or practices. The nurse needs to assess the ability of family members to support the child's grief responses. Additional parent education and referral may be necessary to help parents support their child as they grieve the loss.

Nursing interventions for childhood grief include providing emotional support for both the patient and family as appropriate.

For a child who is dying, comfort measures are essential. Some comfort measures are:

- Provide pain medication as needed to keep the patient comfortable.
- Involve parents/family by suggesting measures to help the child, including massages, warm or cool blankets as needed, singing, and reading.
- Allow family to stay with the child as much as possible.
- Offer resources for any spiritual or cultural traditions requested by the child or family.

Some emotional support measures are:

- Encourage the child and family to ask any questions they may have.
- Educate the family about the signs of impending death.
- Provide information about the normal coping mechanisms generally displayed during the developmental stage of the child.
- Assist in helping the family find meaning in the child's death; this has been shown to help facilitate acceptance.

For more information, see Exemplar 3.B, End-of-Life Care, in Module 3, Comfort, particularly the section on End-of-Life Care for Children.

For a child who is grieving the loss of a loved one or friend, appropriate nursing interventions include the following:

- Encourage the child to honestly express any feelings about the loss.
- Assure the child that it is normal to feel angry, sad, and even confused when someone dies.

- Educate the child and family about some healthy outlets for childhood grief, such as drawing, painting, or writing to the deceased.
- Provide the family with information about explaining death in an honest and age-appropriate manner.

In either of these situations, the nurse can consult with a child life specialist who is often part of the healthcare team in many hospitals and healthcare systems.

Communicating with Families

Introductory Phase

Assessing for grief and discussing death can be difficult for the child, the family, and the nurse. After introducing yourself, consider asking such open-ended questions as:

- Tell me a story about (the dying or deceased person).
- What cultural or spiritual practices do you find helpful?

Perinatal Loss

Perinatal loss is the death of an infant or fetus at any time from the point of conception to 28 days after birth. Perinatal loss is a traumatic event for the infant's parents as well as other family members. In the past, some have proposed that perinatal loss results in less intense grief because the parents and family have not had time to form a close bond with the infant. This theory has since been proven incorrect. In fact, the grief associated with the loss of a child can be more intense than most other losses depending on the mental health of the mother prior to the loss and her ability to cope after the loss (Kokou-Kpolou, Megalakaki, & Nieuviarts, 2018).

Causes of Perinatal Loss

Perinatal loss can be difficult for the mother both physically and emotionally. If the fetus is lost during the first 20 weeks of gestation, it is referred to as a **miscarriage** or a **spontaneous abortion**. This is a significant loss for the mother and should not be discounted for any reason. Loss of the infant after 20 weeks' gestation is known as **intrauterine fetal death (IUFD)** but is more commonly referred to as **fetal demise** or **stillbirth**. It is typical to assume that a stillbirth will produce a more difficult grief reaction for mothers. However, a study that looked at mothers experiencing miscarriages, stillbirths, and neonatal death found that the grief responses in the mothers were essentially the same (Kersting & Wagner, 2012). The grief response of fathers in perinatal loss has not been as well researched as that of mothers. What research has shown is that fathers do grieve like mothers, but with less intensity and for a shorter duration (Kersting & Wagner, 2012). In all cases, parents and other family members benefit from nursing care that provides a therapeutic presence and values parent and family statements and emotions (Potter & Moller, 2020).

The loss of a fetus in the womb results from a variety of circumstances that can occur between conception and birth. These include biological conditions such as infection, an abnormality in the fetus, problems with the placenta, or accidents involving the umbilical cord. Environmental conditions also can contribute to, or cause, perinatal loss—for example, domestic abuse, motor-vehicle crashes, or other accidents, such as a fall.

Miscarriage

Miscarriages occur in approximately 10% of confirmed pregnancies and an estimated 26% of all pregnancies (Dugas & Slane, 2020). Approximately 80% of miscarriages occur in the first trimester (Dugas & Slane, 2020). While the cause of many miscarriages is not known, chromosomal abnormalities are to blame in most cases. Health conditions, such as infections, hormone dysfunction, obesity, high blood pressure, and unmanaged diabetes in the mother, along with increased age can also contribute to miscarriage. Other causes of miscarriage include drug and alcohol use, exposure to toxins, and smoking.

Stillbirth

It may be impossible to know the reason for a stillbirth, even in the later stages of pregnancy. Some known factors that may contribute to and/or cause fetal demise include maternal health, birth defects or chromosomal disorders, placental issues, slow fetal growth, and umbilical cord problems. **Placental abruption** occurs when the placenta detaches from the uterine wall before delivery. This condition does not always result in fetal demise, but the fetus's survival depends on the stage of development and prompt medical treatment. Umbilical cord abnormalities are relatively unusual, but a knot in the cord could cause oxygen deprivation in the fetus. Another rare cause of fetal demise is **Rh disease**, where the mother is Rh negative and the child is Rh positive. If this condition arises, the mother's body sees the Rh-positive cells in the fetus as foreign and produces antibodies to fight off the Rh-positive cells. Rh disease results in the death of the fetus only in extreme cases.

Risk Factors and Prevention

Risk factors for perinatal loss include age, health conditions, and previous instances of perinatal loss. Increased age at the time of conception, particularly for women age 40 and older, can increase the risk for complications during pregnancy. A woman's medical history also factors into the risk for complications. Generally having one past experience with a miscarriage or spontaneous abortion does not impact future pregnancies—depending on the cause—but past instances of multiple complications put a woman at higher risk (National Institutes of Health, 2017). Risk for perinatal loss is greater for non-Hispanic Black women than any other group (see Focus on Diversity and Culture: Perinatal Loss).

When fetal demise occurs and the mother does not go into labor naturally, labor is induced, or a cesarean delivery is performed. In cases of prolonged retention of the fetus, a condition known as **disseminated intravascular coagulation (DIC)** may occur. DIC is a disorder where the proteins controlling clotting of the blood become abnormally active, causing excessive clotting and then bleeding as available clotting factors are consumed. In addition to DIC, both infection and sepsis can set in if the dead fetus remains in the woman's womb for an extended period.

In the majority of cases, it is not possible to prevent perinatal loss. As mentioned in the previous sections, many cases are circumstantial and/or biological and often cannot be detected until the miscarriage or fetal demise has occurred. The best prevention for parents is knowledge of factors that can compromise the mother's health. Women who are pregnant should avoid drugs, chemicals, nicotine, alcohol, and infections, as they may cause perinatal loss or other health complications for the fetus. Proper maternal care is also important, as some pregnancy complications can be caught early and treated before any harm is done to the fetus or the mother.

Focus on Diversity and Culture

Perinatal Loss

Perinatal death is defined as death of the fetus at 20 weeks or greater. The neonatal period is considered as the first 28 days of life. Perinatal and neonatal deaths continue to remain steady in the United States, with an average of 6.0 fetal deaths per 1000 live births (Gregory, Drake, & Martin, 2018). Fetal mortality is highest in mothers who are either in their teens or older than age 35, in mothers who are unmarried, and in mothers carrying multiple fetuses (Gregory et al., 2018). Non-Hispanic Black mothers experience the highest incidence of fetal death, with 10.59 per 1000 births, a perinatal mortality rate twice as high as that experienced by non-Hispanic white and Hispanic mothers (Gregory et al., 2018). Although causative factors for the increase in perinatal deaths in non-Hispanic Black mothers compared to others have not been pinpointed, several possible causes include access to healthcare and prenatal care, maternal preconception health, stress, income, infection, and birth equity issues. See Module 24, Culture and Diversity, for a discussion of birth equity and Module 33, Reproduction, for more information on perinatal mortality.

Clinical Manifestations

The manifestations of perinatal loss involve both physical and emotional changes. The physical changes are either changes to the mother's body, including spotting, severe back pain, and cramping, or changes in fetal movement or heart rate. These manifestations indicate that something has occurred that could lead to fatal complications. After a perinatal loss, the parents and family of the infant experience various, and often intense, forms of grief.

Grief

The loss of an infant during any stage of pregnancy can be an extremely traumatic event for both parents, and intense feelings of grief are to be expected. The intensity and duration of this grief depend on the individual, but it should not be assumed that this form of grief resolves quickly simply because the parents have not yet established a direct relationship with their baby. Studies have shown very little difference between the intensity of grief felt when a close family member dies and the grief felt after a perinatal death (Kersting & Wagner, 2012).

Grief in cases of perinatal loss may be intensified by the circumstances involving the loss. Many factors impact the parents' ability to resolve their emotions, including how the loss occurred, how the parents learned about the loss, and if the loss could have been prevented. Perinatal loss may also have a stigma attached to it, as some believe that it is unnecessary to mourn the loss of a child whom the parents have never come to know or raise. Beliefs such as these may hinder the parents' grieving process. These emotions can be further complicated for the mother if she feels guilt associated with the loss and/or if postpartum depression becomes a factor. Additionally, mothers with trauma history, mental health conditions, or maladaptive cognitive coping may have prolonged grief (Brooks et al., 2019).

Disenfranchised Grief

The loss of an infant before or immediately following birth may result in disenfranchised grief. Perinatal loss is often not a socially recognized loss, particularly if that loss occurred in the early stages of pregnancy. Early miscarriages are generally

Clinical Manifestations and Therapies

Perinatal Loss

ETIOLOGY	CLINICAL MANIFESTATIONS	CLINICAL THERAPIES
Miscarriage	■ Spotting ■ Cramping ■ Lower back pain	■ Antibiotics if an infection results
Placental abruption	■ Back pain ■ Uterine contractions ■ Vaginal bleeding ■ Abdominal pain	■ IV fluids ■ Blood transfusion ■ Delivery of the fetus ■ Antibiotics if infection occurs
Disseminated intravascular coagulation as a result of a retained fetus	■ Bleeding ■ Blood clots ■ Drop in blood pressure	■ Delivery of the fetus ■ Treatment of clotting ■ Plasma transfusions, if needed ■ Antibiotics if sepsis occurs

not discussed except between the parents and healthcare professionals; in such a case, the grief is unacknowledged socially. Losses that occur in the early stages of pregnancy can be more difficult to grieve, as no funeral services or other formal mourning traditions are practiced (Kersting & Wagner, 2012). The result may be that the parents feel they have no right to mourn or feel grief over the loss of their child. Disenfranchised or complicated grief can also occur if the pregnancy had to be terminated for health reasons. Many parents in this situation choose to tell friends and family that the loss of the child was due to miscarriage or fetal demise.

Postpartum Depression

Postpartum depression is a form of depression that occurs in the first few weeks after a child is born. Many do not realize that postpartum depression can also occur in women who have sustained perinatal loss; in fact, two of the major risk factors for developing postpartum depression are experiencing complications during the pregnancy and sustaining a perinatal loss. The exact cause of postpartum depression is unknown, but the symptoms are similar to those of other forms of depression and may include anxiety, anger, difficulty concentrating, lack of enjoyment, feelings of inadequacy, sleeplessness or oversleeping, decreased or increased appetite, and suicidal thoughts (National Institute of Mental Health, n.d.). Experiencing these symptoms while trying to mourn the loss of a child can make both the grief and the depression worse. Women who are experiencing these emotions should be encouraged to discuss their thoughts and should be monitored closely for worsening of symptoms.

SAFETY ALERT Mothers who have lost a child and develop postpartum depression should be closely monitored for signs of serious depression and/or suicidal thoughts. Signs of depression include loss of interest in once-enjoyable activities, alterations in appetite, fatigue, and unexplainable crying spells. Suicidal thoughts may be evidenced by intense periods of depression accompanied by statements such as "Everyone would be better off without me" or "I wish I was dead/had died instead." Some mothers will make very frank statements like, "That child needs her mother." Individuals contemplating suicide may also begin to give away items once valued, explaining that the items are not needed anymore.

Spiritual and Cultural Considerations

Parents who have lost a child may desire to speak with a religious or spiritual leader. Nurses can call for the chaplain to meet with the parents or facilitate the presence of a spiritual leader of their choosing. If the infant is born alive but not expected to live long, the parents may want the child to be baptized or to receive a form of blessing as soon as possible, depending on their beliefs (**Figure 27.7** ›). Nurses facilitate the family's participation in these rituals.

Religious or spiritual beliefs may affect how the parents mourn the loss of a child. For example, most members of the Catholic Church believe the ritual of baptism allows entrance into Heaven. However, this ritual is only for the living. Catholic parents may have spiritual angst when their baby is stillborn. Some members of the Jewish faith observe the practice that parents and family members are not to mourn for a child who has been alive less than 30 days.

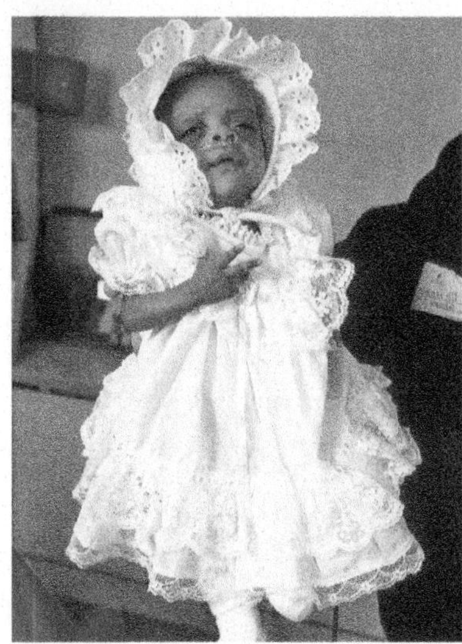

Figure 27.7 › Religious rituals such as baptism and the blessing of an ill infant may provide great comfort to the family. When the infant is stable, a traditional baptism may be performed in the home or church with family and friends present. When the infant has a life-threatening illness, baptism may be performed in the hospital by a chaplain or health professional.
Source: Pearson Education, Inc.

Parents of these babies are unable to hold any traditional services or burials (Dickstein, 1996; Tessler, 2014). Some traditions, such as Islam, believe the child is instantly admitted into Heaven. Others, such as Buddhism and Hinduism, believe the child's soul will be reincarnated. Nurses should be respectful of patients' beliefs and offer to meet any needs that arise.

Collaboration

After a perinatal loss, there may be an opportunity to test both the mother and the fetus to determine the cause of the fetal demise. Some parents refuse this testing for personal or religious reasons, and that decision must be honored. In the case of a first-trimester miscarriage that occurs in the home, products of conception may not be available for testing. Parents who have lost a child may also need additional support in the coming months. A large-scale epidemiologically based study found that women experiencing a stillbirth or early infant death (within the first 28 days of life) are 4 times as likely as live-birth mothers to exhibit symptoms of depression and 7 times as likely to exhibit symptoms of posttraumatic stress 9 months after the loss (Gold, Leon, Boggs, & Sen, 2016). Although many support groups and bereavement counselors can be recommended, this study suggests the need for follow-up after discharge, particularly for Black mothers, who were less likely to seek treatment for depressive or posttraumatic stress symptoms (Gold et al., 2016). Members of the interprofessional team caring for mothers experiencing perinatal loss should assess for resiliency factors, including support systems and access to follow-up care. Nurses should provide or ensure referrals for counseling and other resources are made before discharge.

Diagnostic Tests

A series of tests are available to determine the potential cause of fetal demise, but often it is impossible to determine the exact cause. After delivery, with the parents' consent, the fetus or stillborn baby will undergo an autopsy that will include chromosomal studies. Mothers may also undergo a series of testing for infection and other maternal factors that could have caused the demise. A Betke-Kleihauer test may also be performed to check the mother's Rh antibodies to determine if Rh disease was a contributing factor. These tests can help the parents to know of possible similar problems with future pregnancies.

Pharmacologic Therapy

Depending on the circumstances surrounding the fetal demise, medications may be administered to treat the mother for any infections or complications. If a placental abruption has occurred, the mother may need IV fluids as well as a blood transfusion if the blood loss is substantial. In cases where the fetal demise goes untreated and the dead fetus is retained, DIC may result, requiring treatment for the clotting, possible plasma transfusions, and treatment for sepsis, depending on how long the fetus has been retained. The mother may also need antibiotics if diagnostic tests indicate the presence of infection.

The mother is at risk for developing postpartum depression within the first 4 weeks after a perinatal loss. If this depression becomes overwhelming, especially in combination with the grief, two pharmacologic therapies may be recommended: antidepressants and hormone therapy. Antidepressants have been shown to be effective in the treatment of postpartum depression and can be used in combination with other forms of therapy and counseling. The U.S. Food and Drug Administration has approved one hormone replacement medication, brexanolone, for severe postpartum depression (National Institute of Mental Health, n.d.).

Nonpharmacologic Therapy

The grief resulting from perinatal loss can be intense and even overwhelming. Mothers may feel unnecessary guilt, believing that they, or their bodies, failed in some way and led to the infant's death. Intense grief and even feelings of guilt are entirely normal after the death of an infant and may last for a few weeks or possibly a few months. These emotions generally lessen on their own, but if they do not, or if the parents require further support, various forms of therapy can be helpful. Group therapy in cases of perinatal loss may be useful, or it may be more painful, depending on the patients. Some patients may find it therapeutic and reassuring to talk to other parents who have lost an infant, whereas others may see it as disorienting and painful to share others' experiences of such a traumatic event. In these cases, individual grief counseling is preferable.

Lifestyle changes may also assist mothers experiencing postpartum depression and grief. In place of isolation, mothers should seek out a strong support system after the loss; sharing their feelings about the loss as well as any trauma experienced has been proven to help prevent or alleviate any PTSD. Mothers who have trauma histories, high self-blame, and other negative thoughts are more likely to suffer from postpartum depression and develop PGD (Kokou-Kpolou et al., 2018). Physical activity and proper nutrition can also help to lessen the effects of depression.

Nursing Care

Perinatal loss can occur at any point in a pregnancy for a multitude of reasons. Mothers who are suspected of having sustained a perinatal loss should be evaluated immediately. A fetal heart monitor can be used to check the heart rate of the fetus. If a heartbeat cannot be found, an ultrasound should be done to determine if fetal demise has occurred. The safety of mother and fetus takes priority; if the assessment determines that the fetus is in distress, immediate action is necessary.

The nurse begins assessing the parents' needs and resources as well as planning for needs that will arise during delivery. The nurse assesses the parents' spiritual needs by asking if they would like to speak to the hospital chaplain or if they would like the presence of another spiritual leader. Nurses also collaborate with social workers or grief counselors to provide further assistance to the parents after the birth.

Caring for Parents

When parents are admitted with a possible perinatal loss, they should be put in a private room as far away from the other mothers as possible. If it is determined that perinatal loss has occurred, the privacy provided is likely to benefit both parents. Once tests are performed and perinatal loss is confirmed, parents are informed of the test results and encouraged to ask any questions they may have. Nurses should allow parents time to process their grief before asking about the mother's birthing preferences. When the parents have indicated that they are ready to discuss the birthing process, the nurse should explain what will happen in the delivery of a stillborn infant; the parents should also be informed about the methods of inducing labor, if induction is to occur. The mother's birthing preferences determine how the birth takes place. Nurses consult her regarding how the room should be lit, who she would like in the birthing room with her, if she would like relaxing music playing, and what position she would prefer to give birth in. The mother's comfort and understanding are an important priority for a nurse during the birthing process.

Before the child is born, the nurse should establish when and if the parents would like to see the infant. Parents should be gently encouraged to see the infant for their own sense of acceptance. If the parents wish to see the infant, the nurse should prepare them for how the child may look. For example, if the child is not fully developed, if the child is slightly blue or yellow from complications, or if the child is deformed in any way, the parents should be told before viewing the infant. It is important for nurses to respect parents' wishes if they would like time alone with the infant. The nurse also consults the parents to determine if they would like to take home keepsakes of the child, such as a picture, a lock of hair, or foot- or handprints.

After the birth has taken place and the parents have seen the infant, the nurse should again ask if they have any questions. The nurse assures both parents that any questions they may have are normal, even if the parents feel their questions are odd or morbid in some way. The nurse provides time and space for the parents to express their feelings, being careful to address feelings of guilt by explaining that most cases of perinatal loss cannot be prevented. Nurses provide information on discharge regarding the need to report any signs of infection, such as fever, chills, or dizziness. Nurses also make referrals for grief counseling and other sources of support the parents may require.

Communicating with Patients

Working Phase

Discussing death with parents who are experiencing perinatal loss requires compassion and supportive care. When addressing parents after the loss of a baby, consider offering condolences and provide time for reflective responses.

- I am at a loss for words other than I'm sorry this happened.
- Your baby is beautiful. What's his name?*
- How can I best support you during this time?

*Some cultures do not name deceased infants.

Caring for Siblings

If possible, the nurse should encourage parents to include siblings in the process of grieving for a stillborn baby. It is recommended that siblings meet their newborn brother or sister, even if the infant is dead. Studies have shown that siblings who are able to experience the deceased brother or sister are able to mourn the death with less traumatic results (Avelin, Erlandsson, Hildingsson, Bremborg, & Rådestad, 2012). In addition, having the older sibling create memories, such as taking pictures with or holding the deceased, also helps the older child cope with the loss. Children, however, should not be forced to hold, touch, or otherwise experience a deceased sibling. Rather, the parents and nurse should let the living sibling lead the encounter (Avelin et al., 2012).

Older Adults' Responses to Loss

Older adults' responses to grief and loss can be intricate because of inherent factors unique to this age demographic. Older adults are defined as anyone 65 years of age and older. At this point in life, the older adult has more than likely accumulated several losses, both symbolic and actual. This accumulation may compound any new grief felt by the individual: A new loss may bring up grief from one or more previous losses.

Sources of Loss

Grief and loss as experienced by older adults can be more complicated than at other ages. A single death may trigger a domino effect of losses. For example, a woman in the early stages of Alzheimer disease may be able to live in her home while her spouse is in good health. When the spouse dies and she moves in with one of her children, her loss of independence may accelerate or she may experience relocation syndrome and a worsening of her dementia (see Exemplar 23.A, Alzheimer Disease, in Module 23, Cognition, for more information on relocation syndrome). Older adults also begin to lose friends and acquaintances in their age group and, as that happens, they begin to anticipate their own death as well as the death of their partners (Walsh, 2012).

Losses associated with aging are varied and may include loss of independence, loss of mobility, loss of health, and loss of memory. Unfortunately, these create a misperception among some younger adults that aging brings frailty and deterioration of mental function. These misperceptions are considered a form of **ageism**, which involves forming stereotypes about older adults. Nurses must guard against such misperceptions. Many older adults live active, healthy, fulfilling lives.

Older adults are at greater risk of depression following significant real or symbolic losses. Depression in older adults is rarely the result of only one factor. Among the most common causes of depression in this population are the death of a loved one, loss of independence, illness, and isolation and loneliness. Untreated depression can worsen and is very serious. It can lead to the prolonging of other illnesses, and even to suicide. Unfortunately, death by suicide continues to be a factor in the aging population. Statistics show significant increase of suicide in both males and females 65 to 74 years old between the years 2000 and 2016, although suicide among older adults in more common in males (25.9 deaths by suicide per 100,000 deaths) than females (6.2 deaths per 100,000 deaths) (Hedegaard, Curtin, & Warner, 2018).

SAFETY ALERT Suicide in older adults may result from untreated depression. In the past, the chronic underdiagnosis of minor depression in older adults led to high suicide rates—particularly in men (Potter & Moller, 2020). Nurses in all settings should assess for signs of depression, even if it appears minor, and then assess for increased risk of suicide.

Clinical Manifestations

Manifestations of grief in older adults may be more profound than those observed in younger patients. Accumulating losses in combination with existing health conditions and medication side effects may contribute to a complicated grief reaction. As a result, grief in older adults that may present as a response to the loss of a single person, object, or freedom may actually be a reaction to numerous losses that have accumulated over time. How older adults handle loss depends on the circumstances of the loss, as well as the overall health of the individual—both physically and mentally.

Grief initially presents in older adults much as it presents in younger adults; anger, sadness, longing, disbelief, and depression may be present. The duration and intensity of these emotions vary from patient to patient. Older adults may seem to experience the emotional aspects of grief more acutely than younger adults; for example, older adults may show pronounced and overwhelming feelings of anger or sadness in response to a death. It also is common for older adults—particularly those living alone—to respond to intense grief by neglecting their own needs. Eating habits, personal hygiene, and health maintenance may fluctuate during periods of bereavement. Nurses need to be particularly observant of these changes in regular nutrition, hygiene, and health, as they indicate that patients are not taking care of themselves and may need additional support.

Patient's History

In working with older adults who are experiencing grief, it is important to inquire about other recent losses, as well as any present health concerns such as dementia, Alzheimer disease, or a history of depression or suicide attempts. If a patient has recently experienced a series of losses, a common experience for older adults, the accumulation of these losses can be overwhelming. When assessing the span of loss in older adults, it is important to consider all losses. For example, the loss of mobility, the loss of independence, and even the loss of a beloved pet can all contribute to feelings of overwhelming grief.

For persons with dementia or Alzheimer disease, the death of a loved one is very complicated. For example, a man in a memory care facility with dementia may respond to news of his spouse's death with great emotion, crying and mourning, only to ask when the spouse is coming to visit the next day. Even in the early stages of Alzheimer disease, newly learned information is often forgotten quickly. A patient's loss of memory of a loved one's death can be hard on the nurse and/or the patient's caretaker, as the individual may ask to see the loved one who has died. Similarly, the patient may become very upset because the deceased has not come to visit. If the patient were to be reminded daily of the loss, then he would experience fresh grief for the individual who has died. With the progression of Alzheimer disease, the grieving process becomes virtually impossible as it constantly requires time to accept and process the loss.

Prolonged Grief Disorder

Prolonged grief disorder in older adults manifests in feelings of unrelenting preoccupation and yearning resulting from the loss, experienced over an increased duration of time (at least 6 months or more). Memories, even those that are happy, elicit strong emotions, which may be coupled with an avoidance of familiar places or individuals who trigger thoughts of the deceased or regret for the loss. Patients may also manifest trust issues, suspecting once close friends and family members of judging their pain or not understanding their emotions. Because of these feelings of judgment or betrayal, the patients may appear distant and even uncaring. This may be especially true of older adults who have experienced a loss of independence or mobility. Nurses need to be observant of the progression of grief in older adults. If symptoms intensify or affect the patient's overall health, appropriate assessments and interventions need to be made.

Spiritual and Cultural Considerations

Many older adults find deep meaning in their religious or spiritual beliefs and practices, possibly because they grew up during a time when religious practices were more widespread than they are today. Religious and spiritual practices can provide comfort for patients and their families. If the patient is in a nursing home, hospital, hospice, or an extended care facility and is working through grief, nurses should inquire if the patient would like to participate in any specific form of religious practice. Nurses should assist patients in meeting these needs when possible. See Focus on Diversity and Culture: Loss Among Older Adults.

Sometimes, patients experience a disruption of their spiritual beliefs and/or values. This is known as spiritual distress. Rather than turning to religion in times of grief or loss, the patient may question or express anger toward the higher power or faith base as to why the loss occurred. Nurses can encourage patients to regain a sense of spirituality. Nurses can guide patients to address their spiritual distress, refer patients to a spiritual leader or chaplain, and meet patients' spiritual need requests when feasible. Those patients with a strong sense of spirituality have better coping mechanisms with serious illness, including less depression and better quality of life (Kunsmann-Leutiger, Loetz, Frick, Petersen, & Müller, 2018; Puchalski, 2012).

Focus on Diversity and Culture

Loss Among Older Adults

Nurses practice culturally sensitive care by assessing patients' cultural and spiritual beliefs and practices and incorporating them into the care plan appropriately. This aspect of nursing is particularly important in work with older adults experiencing loss. Culturally sensitive care requires assessing each individual patient's and family's beliefs and practices. Examples of cultures and beliefs regarding older adults include (Purnell & Fenkl, 2019; Spector, 2017):

- Many of those who uphold traditional Asian cultural beliefs have a great respect for older adults and are expected to take care of their parents if they need assistance in later life.
- Muslims are instructed by the Qur'an to honor, respect, and care for their parents as they age. It might be considered dishonorable for an older Muslim adult to be placed in a retirement or nursing home if a child or grandchild is still available to see to the patient's care.
- In many American Indian traditions, elders are considered the keepers of wisdom and knowledge. In some tribes, the care of older adults is not just by immediate family, but also by extended family and community members.

Families are often scattered throughout the United States and beyond. Family members are sometimes faced with having to place an elderly relative in an assisted living or nursing home situation to provide care. Some families bring the elderly family member into the home, but many times the older adult is placed in a long-term care facility.

Collaboration

Older adults experiencing significant losses may require support in a variety of areas. Nurses must assess their need for support carefully. Patients might find it helpful to talk to others who have had similar losses, or they might want to speak individually with a therapist. Some patients may need referral to a social worker to learn more about means of financial support, including financial assistance with groceries or housing. Some patients may require pharmacologic therapy.

Pharmacologic Therapy

Two conditions involving grief may require pharmacologic therapies: depression and PGD. While many studies have been done regarding antidepressants in older adults, studies regarding the use of antidepressants for treatment of complicated grief in the elderly are sparse (Shear, 2015). Treatment of depression begins with assessment to determine its underlying cause. Most of the time depression can be treated quite effectively through nonpharmacologic therapies, but if these prove ineffective, antidepressants may be used.

Antidepressants should be used with caution in older adults, however, as various other medications have adverse reactions with some forms of antidepressants. Similarly, some conditions that are particularly prevalent in older adults—such as diabetes, dementia, and heart problems—can be made worse by antidepressants (Wiese, 2011; Wilson, Shannon, & Shields, 2017). Older adults who are prescribed antidepressants for grief should be monitored closely for any side effects or complications.

Nonpharmacologic Therapy

Treatment of grief in older adults can be successful without medications. Group therapies and support groups can be quite effective, providing support the individual may be lacking in a judgment-free setting. Both group therapy and support groups introduce the patient to other individuals who have experienced the same loss and who may be having similar grief responses. For patients who are uncomfortable sharing with a group of people, individual therapy may be preferred, especially if PGD is present and the patient may benefit from CGT.

Nursing Care

Nursing care for older adults who are working through loss and grief requires a certain amount of sensitivity and understanding. Older adults may be reluctant to admit difficulty coping with grief, in part due to ageism and the stigma attached to conditions such as depression and dementia and mental health treatment. It is important for nurses to remember that, because of a patient's history with previous losses, a current loss that does not seem significant to the nurse may be very significant to the patient. Careful, holistic assessment is necessary for nurses to gain an accurate picture of the patient's care needs.

Nurses working with older adults who have experienced a loss and are subsequently grieving should complete a full assessment of the patient's history—both physical and mental health—as well as an assessment of the patient's coping mechanisms. Older adults, especially men, are at a particularly high risk for both depression and suicide, so the nurse should assess for signs of depression. The patient's support system should also be evaluated. Studies have found that the stronger the support of the patient, the quicker the return to normalcy. If the patient has been grieving for 6 months or more and the grief has not lessened, or has significantly increased, then the nurse should assess for signs of PGD. Collaboration with social workers can be quite helpful when working with patients who are grieving.

The nurse should provide the patient with assistance involving spiritual or cultural needs. If the patient would like to attend religious services or talk to a pastor, rabbi, or other spiritual leader, then the nurse should help to facilitate these needs. Similarly, the nurse should try to help the patient who mentions finding comfort in religious or spiritual texts, but not having access to them. Nursing interventions to assist older adults in coping with loss and grief are outlined in the Independent Interventions section earlier in the module.

Nursing Care Plan

Loss of a Parent by a Pediatric Patient

Ajay Patel, an 8-year-old boy, is brought to his primary care provider's office by his father. Since Ajay's mother died 8 months ago after a motor-vehicle crash, Ajay has been very withdrawn and quiet. In the last 2 weeks, he has stopped eating regularly, and his sleeping habits have been irregular.

ASSESSMENT	DIAGNOSES	PLANNING
Mr. Patel tells Ajay's primary care nurse, Fatima Forez, that Ajay has been acting very strangely since his mother died. He has stopped playing with his regular friends or with anyone else. He has also been very quiet, only speaking to others if he is required to. The school has reported that Ajay's grades have been declining. At first, Mr. Patel thought he was experiencing normal grief reactions, but 2 weeks ago he stopped eating almost entirely, and he has been sleeping only a few hours a night. Ms. Forez checks Ajay's vitals and discovers that his blood pressure and temperature are both normal. When she checks his weight, Ms. Forez notices that he has lost 7 pounds since his last visit 2 months ago. When Ms. Forez asks Ajay why he has been having trouble eating and sleeping, he refuses to answer the question and looks down at the floor instead. After discussing Ajay's case with his primary care provider, Ms. Forez recommends that Ajay start seeing a grief counselor once a week for help working through a probable complicated grief reaction.	■ Complicated grieving related to psychosocial conflicts associated with coping with the loss of a parent ■ Undernutrition related to loss of appetite secondary to grief and feelings of guilt ■ Sleep disturbance related to unexpressed emotions ■ Inadequate coping skills related to complicated grief reaction	Goals for Ajay's care include: ■ The patient will keep weekly appointments with grief counselor. ■ The patient will eat at least one full meal per day and eat whenever he feels hungry. ■ The patient will regain a relatively normal sleep schedule.

Nursing Care Plan *(continued)*

IMPLEMENTATION

- Teach about complicated grief reactions.
- Emphasize the importance of eating to maintain and increase weight.
- Explain the benefits of grief counseling.

EVALUATION

Ajay begins going to grief counseling every week. His therapist works with him to develop healthy coping mechanisms to work through his emotions and grief. Ajay starts to get his appetite back, and his sleeping habits begin to improve. After 2 months of grief counseling, Ajay goes to his follow-up appointment; his weight and disposition have returned to normal.

CRITICAL THINKING

1. If Ajay had not improved after 2 months with a grief counselor, how would you change the nursing care plan?
2. What resources could the nurse provide to Ajay's father other than individual grief counseling to help with Ajay's needs?
3. What role could a school nurse play in this patient's recovery in collaboration with the primary care nurse?

REVIEW The Concept of Grief and Loss

RELATE Link the Concepts

Linking the concept of grief and loss with the concept of violence:

1. You are caring for a 25-year-old woman who has sustained a perinatal loss as the result of domestic abuse. Describe at least four factors that put this patient at a high risk for a prolonged grief disorder.
2. A 6-year-old boy has been physically abused by his father until 2 months ago, when the father died suddenly. What nursing interventions would be appropriate for this boy's grief? How could his history of abuse make the grief more difficult?

Linking children's response to loss with the concept of development:

3. While assessing a 4-year-old whose mother died 2 years ago, you find the child has some small delays in developmental milestones. Why might this have happened?
4. What interventions can you initiate to help this child meet future developmental milestones?

Linking older adults' response to loss with the concept of mobility:

5. What are your goals for the older adult patient who has lost the use of their legs?
6. Create a plan of care for an older adult patient who lives alone and uses a wheelchair.

READY Go to Volume 3: Clinical Nursing Skills

REFER Go to Pearson MyLab Nursing and eText

REFLECT Apply Your Knowledge

Carol Iverson, a 56-year-old woman, lives in a rural town with her husband, James. Their only child, James Iverson Jr., a Marine, was deployed in the Middle East, where he was killed by an explosive device. While his remains were able to be returned to the family for burial, his casket was sealed. The community provided a hero's funeral with a great amount of support for Mr. and Mrs. Iverson and their extended family. However, within a few weeks, the town went back to its normal routine. Mrs. Iverson comes to the town's one health clinic 8 months later, complaining of lack of energy, little motivation, and poor appetite. She relates to the nurse that she hasn't had much closure with James Jr.'s death, even with the town's outpouring of grief. Mrs. Iverson reports that while her husband has been supportive, he too has gone back to his routine. She tells the nurse, "It seemed like everyone was there for me, and then the next minute, everyone was gone, just like James. I can't get over the last time I saw him, when he told me not to worry, and that he would be home soon. I believed him."

1. What would be a priority nursing diagnosis for Mrs. Iverson? What goals of care would be appropriate for her?
2. What factors play a role in this patient's grief response and possible development of complicated grief?
3. What would be the impact of resources for Mrs. Iverson living in a rural area versus an urban setting?

References

American Academy of Child and Adolescent Psychiatry (2018, June). Grief and children. *Facts for Families*, No. 8. https://www.aacap.org/AACAP/Families_and_Youth/Facts_for_Families/FFF-Guide/Children-And-Grief-008.aspx

Avelin, P., Erlandsson, K., Hildingsson, I., Bremborg, A. D., & Rådestad, I. (2012). Make the stillborn baby and the loss real for the siblings: Parents' advice on how the siblings of a stillborn baby can be supported. *Journal of Perinatal Education, 21*(2), 90–98. http://doi.org/10.1891/1058-1243.21.2.90

Brooks, M., Graham-Kevan, N., Robinson, S., & Lowe, M. (2019). Trauma characteristics and posttraumatic growth: The mediating role of avoidance coping, intrusive thoughts, and social support. *Psychological Trauma: Theory, Research, Practice, and Policy, 11*(2), 232–238. https://doi.org/10.1037/tra0000372

Canadian Virtual Hospice. (2015). *Tips for talking with someone who is dying*. http://www.virtualhospice.ca/en_US/Main+Site+Navigation/Home/Topics/Topics/Communication/Tips+for+Talking+with+Someone+Who+is+Dying.aspx

Child Traumatic Stress Network. (n.d.). *Childhood traumatic grief for mental health professionals and providers*. http://www.nctsn.org/trauma-types/traumatic-grief/mental-health-professionals

Dickstein, S. (1996). *Jewish ritual practice following a stillbirth*. Committee on Jewish Law and Standards of the Rabbinical Assembly. https://www.rabbinicalassembly.org/sites/default/files/public/halakhah/teshuvot/19912000/dickstein_stillbirth.pdf

Dugas, C., & Slane, V.H. (2020, June). *Miscarriage*. StatPearls. https://www.ncbi.nlm.nih.gov/books/NBK532992/

Gold, K. J., Leon, I., Boggs, M. E., & Sen, A. (2016). Depression and posttraumatic stress symptoms after perinatal loss in a population-based sample. *Journal of Women's Health, 25*(3), 263–269.

Gregory, E. C. W., Drake, P., & Martin, J. A. (2018). *Lack of change in perinatal mortality in the United States, 2014–2016* (National Center for Health Statistics Data Briefs, No. 316). Centers for Disease Control and Prevention. https://www.cdc.gov/nchs/products/databriefs/db316.htm

Hedegaard, H., Curtin, S.C., & Warner, M. (2018). Suicide rates in the United States continue to increase (National Center for Health Statistics Data Briefs, No. 309). Centers for Disease Control and Prevention. https://www.cdc.gov/nchs/products/databriefs/db309.htm

Hospice and Palliative Nurses Association. (n.d.). *Home page*. http://hpna.advancingexpertcare.org

Kessler, D. (2019). *Finding meaning: The sixth stage of grief*. Scribner.

Kersting, A., & Wagner, B. (2012). Complicated grief after perinatal loss. *Dialogues in Clinical Neuroscience, 14*(2), 187–194.

Killikelly, C., & Maercker, A. (2018). Prolonged grief disorder for ICD-11: The primacy of clinical utility and international applicability. *European Journal of Psychotraumatology, 8*(Suppl. 6), 1476441. https://doi.org/10.1080/20008198.2018.1476441

Kokou-Kpolou, K., Megalakaki, O., & Nieuviarts, N. (2018). Persistent depressive and grief symptoms for up to 10 years following perinatal loss: Involvement of negative cognitions. *Journal of Affective Disorders, 241*, 360–366. https://doi.org/10.1016/j.jad.2018.08.063

Kübler-Ross, E. (1969). *On death and dying*. Macmillan.

Kunsmann-Leutiger, E., Loetz, C., Frick, E., Petersen, Y., & Müller, J.J. (2018). Attachment patterns affect spiritual coping in palliative care. *Journal of Hospice & Palliative Nursing, 202*(4), 385–391. https://doi.org/10.1097/NJH.0000000000000455

Lunderhoff, M., Holmgren, H., Zachariae, R., Farver-Vestergaard, I., & O'Connor, M. (2017). Prevalence of prolonged grief disorder in adult bereavement: A systematic review and meta-analysis. *Journal of Affective Disorders, 212*, 138–149. https://doi.org/10.1016/j.jad.2017.01.030

National Institute of Mental Health. (n.d.). *Postpartum depression facts*. https://www.nimh.nih.gov/health/publications/postpartum-depression-facts/index.shtml

National Institutes of Health. (2017). *Pregnancy loss: Other FAQs*. https://www.nichd.nih.gov/health/topics/pregnancyloss/conditioninfo/Pages/faqs.aspx#health

Perregrini, M. (2019). Combating compassion fatigue. *Nursing 2020, 49*(2), 50–54. https://doi.org/10.1097/01.NURSE.0000552704.58125.fa

Peters, L., Cant, R., Payne, S., O'Connor, M., McDermott, F., Hood, K., et al. (2013). How death anxiety impacts nurses' caring for patients at the end of life: A review of literature. *Open Nursing Journal, 7*, 14–21. http://doi.org/10.2174/1874434601307010014

Pham, S. Porta, G., Biernesser, C. Walker Payne, M. Iyengar, S., Melhem, N. & Brent, D. (2018). Sudden parental death in a 7-year prospective study. *American Journal of Pyschiatry, 175*(9), 887–896. https://doi.org/10.1176/appi.ajp.2018.17070792

Potter, M. L., & Moller, M. D. (2020). *Psychiatric–mental health nursing care: From suffering to hope* (2nd ed.). Pearson.

Puchalski, C. M. (2012). Spirituality in the cancer trajectory. *Annals of Oncology, 23*(Suppl. 3), 49–55. https://doi.org/10.1093/annonc/mds088

Purnell, L. D., & Fenkl, E. A. (2019). *Handbook for culturally competent care*. Springer.

Robinson, C., & Pond, R. (2019). Do online support groups for grief benefit the bereaved?: Systematic review of the quantitative and qualitative literature. *Computers in Human Behavior, 100*, 48–59. https://doi.org/10.1016/j.chb.2019.06.011

Scherer, Z. (2019). *Parental mortality is linked to a variety of socio-economic and demographic factors*. U.S. Census Bureau. https://www.census.gov/library/stories/2019/05/when-do-we-lose-our-parents.html

Shear, K., Frank, E., Houck, P. R., & Reynolds, C. F. (2005). Treatment of complicated grief: A randomized controlled trial. *Journal of the American Medical Association, 293*(21), 2601–2608. http://jama.jamanetwork.com/article.aspx?articleid=200995

Shear, M. K. (2015). Complicated grief. *New England Journal of Medicine, 372*, 153–160. https://doi.org/10.1056/NEJMcp1315618

Shear, M. K., Reynolds, C. F. III, Simon, N. M., Zisook, S., Wang, Y., Mauro, C., et al. (2016). Optimizing treatment of complicated grief: A randomized clinical trial. *JAMA Psychiatry, 73*(7), 685–694. https://doi.org/10.1001/jamapsychiatry.2016.0892

Spector, R. E. (2017). *Cultural diversity in health and illness* (9th ed.). Pearson.

Stroebe, M., & Schut, H. (2010). The dual process model: A decade on. *Omega: Journal of Death & Dying, 61*, 273–291.

Szuhany, K. L., Young, A., Mauro, C., Garcia de la Garza, A., Spandorfer, J., Lubin, R., et al. (2020). Impact of sleep on complicated grief severity and outcomes. *Depression and Anxiety, 37*(1), 73–80. https://doi.org/10.1002/da.22929

Tessler, I. (2014, October 8). New procedure allows parents to bury stillborn babies. Ynetnews.com. http://www.ynetnews.com/articles/0,7340,L-4557158,00.html

Thompson, N. (2012). *Grief and its challenges*. Palgrave Macmillan.

U.S. Department of Veterans Affairs. (2020). *Managing healthcare workers' stress associated with the COVID-19 virus outbreak*. https://www.ptsd.va.gov/covid/COVID_healthcare_workers.asp

Utz, R. L., Caserta, M., & Lund, D. (2012). Grief, depressive symptoms, and physical health among recently bereaved spouses. *The Gerontologist, 52*(4), 460–471. https://doi.org/10.1093/geront/gnr110

Walsh, K. (2012). *Grief and loss: Theories and skills for the helping professions* (2nd ed.). Pearson.

Weir, K. (2018). *New paths for people with prolonged grief disorder*. https://www.apa.org/monitor/2018/11/ce-corner

Wiese, B. S. (2011). Geriatric depression: The use of antidepressants in the elderly. *BC Medical Journal, 53*(7), 341–347. http://www.bcmj.org/articles/geriatric-depression-use-antidepressants-elderly

Wilson, B. A., Shannon, M. T., & Shields, K. M. (2017). *Pearson nurse's drug guide 2017*. Pearson.

Worden, J. W., & Silverman, P. R. (1996). Parental death and the adjustment of school-age children. *Omega: Journal of Death and Dying, 29*, 219–230.

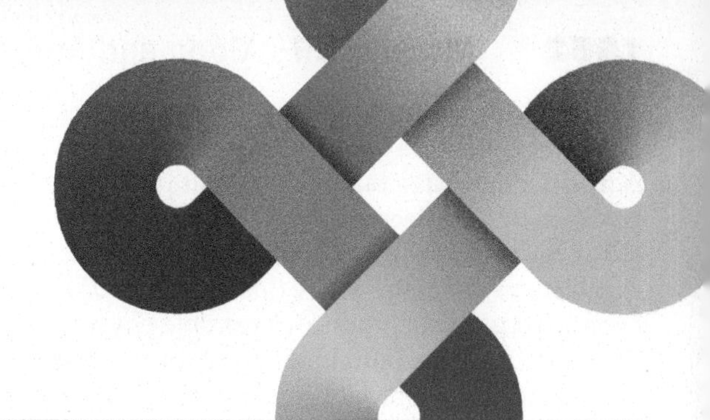

Module 28
Mood and Affect

Module Outline and Learning Outcomes

The Concept of Mood and Affect

Normal Mood and Affect

28.1 Summarize the characteristics of normal mood and affect.

Alterations to Mood and Affect

28.2 Differentiate alterations in mood and affect.

Concepts Related to Mood and Affect

28.3 Outline the relationship between mood and affect and other concepts.

Health Promotion

28.4 Explain the promotion of healthy mood and affect.

Nursing Assessment

28.5 Differentiate common assessment procedures and rating scales used to assess mood and affect.

Independent Interventions

28.6 Analyze independent interventions nurses can implement for patients with alterations in mood and affect.

Collaborative Therapies

28.7 Summarize collaborative therapies used by interprofessional teams for patients with alterations in mood and affect.

Lifespan Considerations

28.8 Differentiate considerations related to the assessment and care of patients with alterations in mood and affect throughout the lifespan.

Mood and Affect Exemplars

Exemplar 28.A Depression

28.A Analyze depressive disorders and relevant nursing care.

Exemplar 28.B Bipolar Disorders

28.B Analyze bipolar disorders and relevant nursing care.

Exemplar 28.C Peripartum Depression

28.C Analyze peripartum depression and relevant nursing care.

Exemplar 28.D Suicide

28.D Analyze the nurse's role in preventing and responding to patient suicide attempts.

›› The Concept of Mood and Affect

Concept Key Terms

Adjustment disorder with depressed mood, **1956**
Affect, **1952**
Aggressive behavior, **1964**
Anhedonia, **1953**
Anxious distress, **1953**
Assertive behavior, **1964**
Bipolar disorder, **1956**
Circadian rhythms, **1955**
Cognitive modification, **1967**
Depressive disorder with peripartum onset, **1956**
Dysthymia, **1956**
Electroconvulsive therapy (ECT), **1967**
Emotions, **1951**
Euthymia, **1952**
Hypomania, **1953**
Major depressive disorder (MDD), **1956**
Mania, **1953**
Mental health, **1952**
Mental illness, **1952**
Mindfulness, **1967**
Mood, **1952**
Mood stabilizers, **1966**
Passive behavior, **1964**
Persistent depressive disorder, **1956**
Postpartum blues, **1956**
Postpartum depression, **1956**
Postpartum psychosis, **1957**
Seasonal affective disorder (SAD), **1955**
Serious mental illness, **1952**
Serotonin syndrome, **1964**
Somatization, **1955**
Unipolar depression, **1956**

Emotions, mood, and affect are critical elements of the human experience in that they shape and reflect our perceptions of and interactions with the world around us. Although often used interchangeably, each of these terms refers to unique psychosocial attributes (Joseph et al., 2020). **Emotions** are an individual's feeling responses to a wide variety of stimuli. An emotion is reactionary and linked to a specific event or object that can be identified by the person who is experiencing the emotion (Joseph et al., 2020). Emotions tend to be intense, focused, and relatively short-lived. Examples include joy, surprise, fear, anger, and disgust (Joseph et al., 2020). Frequently, an individual's emotions precipitate certain physiologic responses, such as smiling, frowning, clenching fists, pacing, sweating, and increased heart rate. Although an individual may choose not to verbally communicate emotions to others, it is difficult to prevent nonverbal expression of emotions.

Moods are similar to emotions but are typically longer lasting, less focused on a particular object or event, and less intense. A mood might have one trigger, multiple triggers, or no specific cause at all. Because **mood** is an enduring state of mind rather than a discrete reaction, it can shape a person's general expectations about the future (Joseph et al., 2020). Unlike emotions, moods do not produce observable physiologic reactions. Therefore, only the individual is capable of describing mood; nurses and other clinicians must be careful not to assume they know a patient's mood based solely on their observations.

Affect refers to an individual's automatic reaction to an event or situation—the immediate, observable expression of mood. Like emotion, affect is evidenced by verbal and nonverbal responses; however, emotion involves a person's *conscious* reaction to an object or event, whereas affect involves a person's *unconscious* response to something as either good or bad. Affective reactions occur faster than emotional reactions, sometimes within a few microseconds. Individuals do not need to understand or even be familiar with something in order to have an affective response to it (Potter & Moller, 2020).

Together, mood and affect play a large part in determining an individual's **mental health**, defined as a state of well-being in which an individual is able to work productively, cope with change and adversity, engage in meaningful relationships, and realize their own potential. Alterations in mood and affect can disrupt an individual's ability to accomplish one or more of these tasks. When these alterations are severe enough to have lasting detrimental effects on a person's life, they may rise to the level of mental illness. **Mental illness** can be defined as a condition that affects emotions, thinking, behavior, or any combination of the three. Mental illness is not typically confirmed until the individual experiences serious and lengthy impairment in the ability to function (American Psychiatric Association [APA], 2013).

This module explores the concept of mood and affect and provides exemplars that facilitate an understanding of impaired mood and affect. Both depression and bipolar disorder are classified as **serious mental illnesses** that increase the possibility the individual will experience serious dysfunction related to daily functioning and ability to achieve life goals (McCallum, Batterham, Calear, Sunderland, & Carragher, 2019; Potter & Moller, 2020). Information related to assessment of individuals with alterations in mood and affect, collaborative therapies, and nursing care is also provided.

Normal Mood and Affect

Defining or describing normal mood and affect can be challenging for a number of reasons. For one, standards of desired or acceptable attitudes and behavior vary widely among cultures as well as among individuals. Also, nearly all individuals experience ongoing fluctuations in mood and affect in response to various biological, psychologic, sociologic, and cultural events and experiences (Potter & Moller, 2020).

In light of these complicating factors, mental health professionals typically describe mood and affect in terms of certain qualities rather than in terms of concrete categories of "normal" and "abnormal." Mood, as depicted in **Figure 28.1** », is said to exist on a continuum ranging from *depression* (an abnormally lowered mood characterized by sadness, emptiness, and irritability) to *mania* (an abnormally elevated mood that impairs functioning). Between these two extremes lies **euthymia**, or a stable range of mood that is neither elevated nor depressed. Although individuals who are euthymic experience occasional fluctuations in mood (for example, happiness at achieving a life goal or frustration associated with a temporary injury), these fluctuations are appropriate to the situation, are typical of the individual's usual pattern of response, and do not impair functional ability. Accordingly, an individual's mood is said to be "normal" if it falls somewhere in the central or euthymic portion of the continuum (Fava & Guidi, 2020; Linden, 2020).

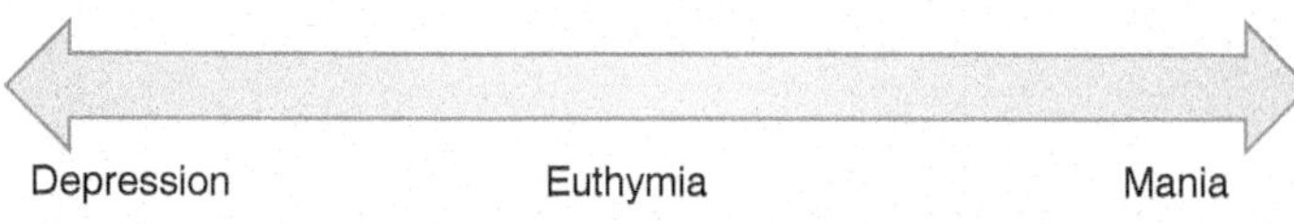

Figure 28.1 » Range of mood states.

When evaluating a person's affect, healthcare providers (HCPs) focus on several characteristics. *Appropriateness*, or *congruence*, refers to affect that matches the individual's emotional state and the immediate situation (Potter & Moller, 2020). *Range* refers to the variety of feelings an individual conveys through affect. Most people exhibit a broad or full range of affect, meaning they are able to convey many different feelings using verbal and nonverbal responses. *Broad affect* is therefore considered normal. In contrast, individuals with *restricted affect* express only a limited range of feelings. For example, a patient who weeps when describing his wife's illness but shows no sign of happiness or excitement when discussing the birth of his child may have a restricted affect.

Intensity describes the degree of emotion displayed in a person's affect. Normal intensity means that the level of emotion expressed in an individual's affect is proportionate to the situation. In contrast, individuals with flat affect display no visible cues to their feelings whatsoever. Intensity may be described as:

- ***Moderate.*** The individual displays a level of emotion that is appropriate to the situation.
- ***Overreactive.*** The individual's level of emotion is disproportionate or extreme given the situation.
- ***Blunted.*** The individual displays a level of emotion that is dulled or muted given the situation.
- ***Flat.*** The individual's affect provides no visible cues to their emotions.

Stability refers to how often and how rapidly an individual's affect fluctuates. A stable affect, or one that remains consistent when there is no provocation in the environment, is considered normal. Conversely, a labile or rapidly changing affect that is out of proportion to the stimulus or situation is often suggestive of disease or disorder (Potter & Moller, 2020).

Factors Contributing to Mood and Affect

Mood and affect are shaped by a number of internal and external factors, including neurologic function, personality, stress level, social interactions, and illness status. Each of these factors is briefly discussed below, and several are visited in greater depth later in the module in the section describing various theories of depression. Other factors that may influence mood and affect are identified in the Concepts Related to Mood and Affect section and within the specific exemplars.

Neurologic Function

Emotions, mood, and affect all originate deep within the brain, in an interconnected set of structures called the limbic system. Three structures of the limbic system—the hippocampus, the hypothalamus, and the amygdala—appear to be particularly important in the production and regulation of mood and affect. Under normal circumstances, limbic system activity is regulated by a nearby area of the brain called the medial prefrontal cortex (MPFC). If the MPFC fails to function properly, the limbic system may become overactive, and alterations in mood and affect may result. This is evidenced by brain imaging studies that show increased activity in the limbic systems of individuals with alterations in mood. Studies also reveal that these individuals tend to have decreased gray-matter volume and lower metabolic activity in the MPFC, which helps explain why this structure is unable to properly control the limbic system (He et al., 2017; Xia et al., 2019).

The exact cellular mechanisms of normal function within the MPFC and limbic system remain unclear. The prevailing theory is that alterations in neurotransmitter activity and/or neuronal receptivity to neurotransmitters contribute to the development of mood disorders such as depression and bipolar disorder (as described later in this module). Thus, normal neurotransmitter and neuronal function appears to be a key contributor to normal mood. Emerging research also suggests that proper glial cell function is necessary for normal mood and affect (Almeida, Nani, Oses, Brietzke, & Hagashi, 2019).

Personality

Temperament and personality play a large role in shaping an individual's mood and affect. In general, high levels of emotional instability and introversion and low levels of conscientiousness and agreeableness predispose individuals to negative affect, greater affect variability, and depressed mood. Conversely, emotional stability and high levels of extraversion, conscientiousness, and agreeableness are associated with greater likelihood of positive affect, lower affect variability, and elevated mood (Boson, Wennberg, Fahlke, & Berglund, 2019; Bucher, Suzuki, & Samuel, 2019).

Stress

Excessive stress and/or maladaptive coping responses are well-known contributors to alterations in mood and affect. When stress is chronic, it can lead to hormonal imbalances that disrupt normal brain function, especially in the hippocampus (McEwen, 2020). Stress also appears to have a negative effect on the reward circuitry within the MPFC (Stanton, Holmes, Chang, & Joormann, 2019). In addition, chronic stress increases a person's likelihood of inadequate sleep, poor dietary intake, and physical disease, which are themselves risk factors for altered mood and affect (as described later in this section).

Social Interactions

Social support and positive social interactions are clearly connected to stable, positive mood and affect: Multiple studies indicate that high-quality, positive social interactions themselves contribute to enhanced mood (Fernández-Theoduloz et al., 2019). Similarly, an individual's overall level of social support is often an important predictor of mood. Generally speaking, individuals who have greater levels of perceived support and larger, more diverse social networks tend to be at lower risk for depression and other alterations in mood and affect, which suggests that these factors offer a protective effect (Seddigh et al., 2020).

Illness Status

In some cases and for some individuals, physical disease or injury can alter mood and affect. For example, conditions that affect the brain tissue or that cause alterations in hormone levels may be directly responsible for alterations in affect or unusually high or low mood. Research has also found a link between autoimmune diseases and mood disorders, which suggests that some alterations in mood may have an immunologic basis (Rainville, Tsyglakova, & Hodes, 2018).

Individuals who have chronic conditions such as heart disease, diabetes, and cancer often face ongoing stress, physical limitations, alterations in self-concept, decreased quality of life, and/or concerns about mortality that contribute to negative mood. In fact, depression is one of the most common complications of chronic disease, and it can actually worsen the course of the disease if not promptly identified and addressed (Airaksinen, Gluschkoff, Kivimäki, & Jokela, 2020; Han et al., 2018; Lotfaliany et al., 2018).

Alterations to Mood and Affect

An elevation or decrease in mood and affect may impair an individual's ability to cope with typical daily life stressors. Prolonged alterations may progress into a depressive or bipolar disorder and require professional intervention.

Individuals with depressive disorder exhibit depressed mood characterized by feelings of sadness or emptiness. Other core symptoms include **anhedonia** (a loss of interest or inability to experience pleasure with activities), fatigue and sleep disturbances, and somatic complaints. In children and adolescents, irritability is a common symptom of depression. In contrast, individuals with bipolar disorder typically experience a major depressive episode alternating with a period of mania or hypomania. **Mania** is an abnormal, persistent, expansive, elevated mood that lasts at least 1 week and that significantly impairs functioning, potentially requiring hospitalization. **Hypomania** is a similar impairment of mood that lasts at least four consecutive days; its symptoms, although significant, do not necessitate hospitalization (APA, 2013). Because of the degree to which mood disorders may impact daily functioning, they can affect individuals across a wide variety of systems and situations (see Concepts Related to Mood and Affect).

Anxious distress is associated with depressive and bipolar disorders with sufficient frequency that the fifth edition of the *Diagnostic and Statistical Manual of Mental Disorders* (DSM-5; APA, 2013), includes it as a specifier clinicians may add to a diagnosis of depression or bipolar disorder. **Anxious distress** is a combination of symptoms associated with high anxiety, including restlessness, impaired concentration due to worry, fear of impending doom, and fear of losing control.

SAFETY ALERT Patients who experience anxious distress in combination with a depressive or bipolar disorder are typically harder to treat and are at greater risk for suicide (APA, 2013).

The National Institute of Mental Health (NIMH; 2017a) reports that mood disorders affect nearly 10% of adults, with 45% of cases classified as severe. Mood disorders impact individuals of every race and age. Treatment is critical; without it, patients are at increased risk for suicide. Mood disorders also carry economic costs. For example, depression is associated with lower rates of productivity, increased absenteeism, and increased rates of short-term disability (McCallum et al., 2019). Patients with depressive and bipolar disorders are found in the community and in all clinical settings, and they frequently experience difficulties with their communication skills, family relationships, and ability or motivation to adhere to a treatment plan.

Pathophysiology of Altered Mood

As mentioned earlier, both the limbic system and the MPFC play a central role in normal mood and affect, so disruptions in either portion of the brain may result in altered mood. The cellular mechanisms that underlie these disruptions are an area of intense interest to researchers, although they are widely believed to involve alterations in neurotransmitter activity and/or neuronal receptivity to neurotransmitters.

Alterations and Therapies

Mood and Affect

ALTERATION	DESCRIPTION	THERAPIES
Depression (including major depressive disorder and persistent depressive disorder)	Depressed mood that varies from mild to severe with severe phases lasting longer than 6 weeks. Symptoms include: ▪ Feelings of sadness, hopelessness, powerlessness, apathy, or guilt ▪ Changes in sleep and/or appetite ▪ Anhedonia ▪ Inability to concentrate ▪ Psychomotor retardation or agitation	▪ Antidepressant medications: selective serotonin reuptake inhibitors (SSRIs), serotonin–norepinephrine reuptake inhibitors (SNRIs), bupropion, tricyclic antidepressants (TCAs), monoamine oxidase inhibitors (MAOIs) ▪ Antidepressants may be combined with low-dose antipsychotic medication in resistant cases ▪ Nonpharmacologic therapy: cognitive-behavioral therapy (CBT); electroconvulsive therapy (ECT); transcranial magnetic stimulation; vagus nerve stimulation
Bipolar disorders	Extreme alterations in mood (mood swings) with intermittent periods of normal mood	▪ Mood-stabilizing medication ▪ Psychotherapy ▪ Hospitalization or partial hospitalization during severe episodes
Depressive disorder with peripartum onset (includes postpartum depression)	Severe depression that appears during pregnancy or within the first year following the birth of a child. Symptoms include: ▪ Sleep disturbances ▪ Fatigue ▪ Crying ▪ Feelings of despair ▪ Anxiety ▪ Mood swings	Combination of antidepressants and psychosocial interventions is most effective.
Adjustment disorder with depressed mood (situational depression)	Hyperreaction to an identifiable, life-altering (but not life-threatening) stressor that occurs within 3 months after the onset of the stressor and persists for no more than 6 months after termination of the stressor; symptoms are similar to but less severe than those of major depressive disorder	Psychotherapy alone may be sufficient to relieve symptoms and return patient to premorbid level of functioning
Suicide	Self-injurious behaviors resulting in death	Inpatient hospitalization for safety and stabilization. Stabilization will include therapies for the diagnosed depressive disorders and any comorbid disorders, such as substance use disorder

Abnormal variations to biological rhythms also appear to play a role in altering mood.

Alterations in Neurotransmission

Thus far, the so-called neurotransmitter hypothesis has largely focused on two monoamine neurotransmitters: serotonin and norepinephrine. Serotonin (5-HT) is involved in the regulation of aggression, mood, anxiety, impulsivity, appetite, sleep, and sex drive, whereas norepinephrine (NE) is involved in the regulation of attention, arousal, and behavior. Given that alterations in all of these areas are characteristic of mood disorders, dysregulation of both 5-HT and NE is thought to be a contributing factor to depression and bipolar disorder. This conclusion is supported by research showing decreased levels of both neurotransmitters in the brains of individuals with mood disorders (Boku, Nakagawa, Toda, & Hishimoto, 2018; Duman, Sanacora, & Krystal, 2019).

More recently, scientists have also begun to investigate the potential contribution of other neurotransmitters, including dopamine (DA), acetylcholine (ACh), gamma-aminobutyric acid (GABA), and glutamate. DA is an essential component of the brain's reward circuitry, and ACh helps regulate the sleep–wake cycle. GABA reduces the ability of nerve cells to transmit information, whereas glutamate causes the opposite effect. Although all of these neurotransmitters—along with 5-HT and NE—appear to be involved in the pathophysiology of mood disorders, the exact nature of their roles remains unclear. Some studies suggest that abnormal levels of these substances contribute to depressive and bipolar disorders, whereas other studies suggest that altered neuronal receptivity to one or more neurotransmitters may be to blame. It is also likely that the systems interact with one another in a variety of ways that scientists have yet to discover (Almeida et. al., 2019; Duman et al., 2019). As research continues to tease out the connections between these neurotransmitters and the cells on which they act, the underlying pathophysiology of mood disorders will no doubt become clearer.

Disruption of Biological Rhythms

Biological rhythms are the body's natural cycle of biochemical and hormonal changes within a given period of time. When these fluctuations occur on a 24-hour cycle, they are known as **circadian rhythms**. Research indicates that many individuals with affective disorders experience abnormal variations in their circadian rhythms. Dysregulation in the hypothalamus is thought to be a major contributing factor to circadian rhythm disruption (Palagini et al., 2019). These rhythm disruptions are observed as abnormalities in physiologic and behavioral processes within a 24-hour period, such as disturbances in daily activities, altered sleep/wake patterns, and fluctuations in hormones. Alterations in circadian rhythms have been linked to symptoms of bipolar disorder, such as mood swings, insomnia, and suicidality (Palagini et al., 2020; Wirz-Justice & Benedetti, 2020). Although much research has been conducted on the correlation of circadian rhythms to affective disorders, the direct cause-and-effect relationships are still unknown. (See Module 7, Health, Wellness, Illness, and Injury, for a more detailed discussion of circadian rhythms.)

Disruptions in the body's seasonal rhythms may also be problematic. For example, many people are at greater risk of depression during a specific time of year (typically, the winter months). This increased correlation between depressive symptoms and time of year is commonly referred to as **seasonal affective disorder (SAD)**, although the actual DSM-5 diagnosis is *major depressive disorder with seasonal pattern*. Common manifestations of SAD include decreased energy, increased periods of sleep, increased appetite, overeating, and weight gain (APA, 2013).

Common Manifestations

As mentioned earlier, an individual's mood is considered altered if it is excessively elevated (manic) or excessively depressed. Similarly, affect is said to be altered if it is inappropriate (incongruent), narrowed, overreactive, blunted, and/or excessively labile. Beyond these basic indicators of abnormality, a number of other manifestations are common in individuals who are experiencing altered mood and affect.

Maladaptive Coping Responses

As previously described, high stress levels and maladaptive coping responses are well-known contributors to altered mood and affect, but they can also be manifestations of such alterations. Some of the most commonly observed maladaptive coping responses include avoidance (i.e., refusal to confront stressors), escape, rumination (i.e., persistent mental focus on stressful situations or symptoms and their implications), denial, helplessness, isolation, self-pity, self-blame, excessive dependency, and aggression. Note, however, that a wide range of other responses may also be considered maladaptive if they impair an individual's ability to function effectively when faced with life's demands (Silveira et al., 2020; van Wijk-Herbrink et al., 2018).

Altered Thought Processes

Altered thought processes can also be a manifestation of disrupted mood and affect. Decreased concentration, poor memory, impaired problem-solving ability, indecisiveness, and poor decision making are among the most common alterations. Less common but more drastic alterations in thought include paranoid thinking, hallucinations, and other forms of psychosis, all of which are associated with unstable mood (Albert, Potter, McQuoid, & Taylor, 2018).

Sleep Disturbances

Changes in sleep patterns are often observed in patients with altered mood and affect. In fact, sleep disturbances are a defining characteristic of nearly all mood disorders. People with manic or elevated mood tend to have difficulty sleeping, whereas individuals with low or depressed mood may experience either insomnia or excessive sleepiness. Even when patients with mood alterations are able to fall and remain asleep, they may not feel adequately rested or refreshed upon awakening (Potter & Moller, 2020).

Somatization

Somatization is the phenomenon in which individuals experience or express psychologic distress through physiologic (or somatic) responses, such as head or stomachache, nausea, fatigue, or dizziness. Although somatization may occur in the absence of mood disruptions, it is commonly associated with alterations in mood and affect.

Between 65 and 80% of individuals with depression report pain as a symptom. For some patients, pain may be an expression of their illness; for others, altered mood and affect may result from pain. Regardless of the exact circumstance, the complicated and likely bidirectional connection between mood and pain highlights the need to assess all patients with chronic pain for signs and symptoms of depression (Potter & Moller, 2020; Yang et al., 2019).

Difficulties with Adaptive Functioning

Adaptive functioning refers to the ability to safely and independently participate in the demands of daily life—such as activities of daily living, maintaining home or living space, obtaining proper nutrition and medical care, managing finances, completing occupational tasks, planning for the future, and engaging in social interactions. Individuals with altered mood and affect commonly experience difficulties in one or more of these areas.

Disorders of Mood and Affect

When of sufficient duration and intensity, alterations in mood and affect may constitute a diagnosable disorder. Common mood disorders include depressive disorders, adjustment disorder with depressed mood, bipolar disorders, and postpartum mood disorders.

Depressive Disorders

Mental health practitioners recognize several types of depressive disorders, the most common of which is **major depressive disorder (MDD)**, also called **unipolar depression**. MDD is what most people think of when they hear the term *depression*. MDD is diagnosed when the patient experiences either depressed mood or anhedonia most of the day, almost every day, during the same 2-week period. The depression or loss of interest must be accompanied by at least four of the following core symptoms:

- Sleep disturbances
- Significant weight change (5% or greater in either direction) or change in appetite
- Fatigue or loss of energy
- Feelings of worthlessness or guilt
- Change in activity level (either psychomotor agitation or retardation)
- Poor concentration
- Suicidal ideation or attempt.

MDD may involve just a single depressive episode, although most affected individuals experience multiple recurring episodes over the course of their lives (APA, 2013).

Persistent depressive disorder (**dysthymia**) is sometimes also referred to as depression, but the diagnostic criteria differ from those for MDD. Dysthymia may be diagnosed when a depressed mood is present for most of the day, more days than not, for at least 2 years. Symptoms of dysthymia are similar to but less severe than those of MDD (APA, 2013).

Adjustment Disorder with Depressed Mood

Individuals often experience dramatic life changes related to events such as death of a loved one, relocation, loss of autonomy, illness, and financial stress. One or more life changes or stressors may contribute to the development of **adjustment disorder with depressed mood**, also known as *situational depression*. Adjustment disorder with depressed mood is a maladaptive reaction to an identifiable psychosocial stressor (or stressors) that occurs within 3 months after the stressor occurs and persists for no longer than 6 months after termination of the stressor (APA, 2013). Symptoms of adjustment disorder with depressed mood are similar to those of the other depressive disorders but are less severe, although a higher level of anxiety may be present.

Bipolar Disorders

Bipolar-related disorders include bipolar I, bipolar II, cyclothymic disorder, and other related disorders. The medical diagnosis of **bipolar disorder** is given when an individual's mood alternates between the extremes of depression and mania or hypomania, interspersed with periods of normal mood. *Bipolar I disorder* is characterized by the occurrence of one or more manic episodes and one or more depressive episodes. *Bipolar II disorder* is characterized by one or more hypomanic episodes (less severe) and one or more depressive episodes. Bipolar disorders may be further classified as follows (APA, 2013):

- ***With mixed features.*** The individual experiences symptoms of depression (e.g., depressed mood, anhedonia, and suicidal ideation or attempt) during episodes of mania or hypomania; or the individual experiences manic/hypomanic symptoms during the depressive episode.
- ***With rapid cycling.*** The individual experiences four or more mood episodes of illness (mania, hypomania, or depression) within a 12-month period, with at least 2 months between each episode *OR* with alternating episodes (e.g., a period of mania followed by a depressive episode). There is a higher risk of rapid cycling, cycle acceleration, and severity of mood episodes in women (Aedo et al., 2019; Gan et al., 2019).

Peripartum Mood Disorders

Peripartum depression is defined as moderate to severe depression experienced during pregnancy and/or up to a year after giving birth. In up to 50% of cases, the depression begins during pregnancy. Many women experience **postpartum blues** after childbirth, which includes symptoms such as mood swings, tearfulness, sleep disruptions, and increased anxiety. These symptoms usually occur within the first 2 to 3 days postpartum and may last up to a couple of weeks (Mayo Clinic, 2018b). When these symptoms are more severe and of longer duration, the woman may be diagnosed with **depressive disorder with peripartum onset**, often referred to as *peripartum* or **postpartum depression**.

When postpartum depression arises after delivery, it usually starts within a few weeks after giving birth; however, sometimes the symptoms may present up to 12 months after birth (APA, 2013). Women who give birth to multiple children and/or to preterm children also are at higher risk for postpartum depression.

It is important to identify depression occurring during or following pregnancy as early as possible in order to try to prevent increasing duration and severity of symptoms. Symptoms of postpartum depression are outlined in the

Alterations and Manifestations feature and the exemplar that appears later in this module. Symptoms may escalate to severe anxiety, panic attacks, and thoughts of suicide (suicidal ideation) or causing harm to the baby (Mayo Clinic, 2018b).

Contributing factors include hormonal changes, family history of depression, feelings of being overwhelmed by parenting tasks, changes in family dynamics, and inadequate support.

Postpartum mood episodes accompanied by psychotic features occur in between 1 in 500 and 1 in 1000 deliveries. **Postpartum psychosis** is characterized by psychotic features associated with peripartum or (more commonly) postpartum depression. These episodes frequently involve command hallucinations or delusions. The command hallucinations may direct the mother to harm the infant, while the delusions may cause the mother to feel that the baby is possessed (APA, 2013).

Suicide

Suicide is itself a mood disorder and may be triggered by one event or a series of events in individuals not previously diagnosed with a mood disorder. However, all major depressive episodes include the possibility of suicidal behavior. Suicide is the extreme of negative coping, leading to self-injurious behaviors causing death. The most reliable predictor of risk is a past history of suicidal threats or attempts. Other risk factors include gender (males are at higher risk), living alone, and persistent feelings of hopelessness (American Foundation for the Prevention of Suicide, 2019a; APA, 2013). It is critical that the nurse obtain a thorough history so that risk factors are identified and an appropriate plan of care can be developed. An individual who is actively suicidal requires inpatient hospitalization for safety and stabilization.

Prevalence

According to the National Institute of Mental Health (NIMH; 2019), an estimated 17.3 million adults in the United States have had at least one major depressive episode. NIMH also indicates that 13.3% of the U.S. population age 12 to 17, and 7.1% of all U.S. adults age 18 and over experienced a major depressive episode. Women experience depression at higher rates than men, with the highest rate (16.6%) occurring among women age 18–25 (Substance Abuse and Mental Health Services Administration [SAMHSA], 2017). (See Focus on Diversity and Culture: Influence of Culture and Gender on Depressive Disorders.) In contrast, prevalence of bipolar disorder is about similar for males (2.9%) and females (2.8%).

Not surprisingly, a study conducted early in the COVID-19 pandemic found that prevalence rates of depressive symptoms were three times higher than they were before the pandemic began (Ettman et al., 2020). Participants with fewer economic resources and fewer social supports reported more severe symptoms than their counterparts with greater resources. Factors cited as associated with greater symptom burden included having less than $5000 in savings, being single or widowed, and experiencing multiple COVID-related stressors (such as job loss, financial stress, and death of a loved one due to COVID-19) (Ettman et al., 2020).

Focus on Diversity and Culture

Influence of Culture and Gender on Depressive Disorders

Throughout the world, women experience more depression than men. Certainly, there are cross-cultural similarities in the way women are socialized and in the inferior status they experience in many societies. Psychosocial stressors—including multiple work and family responsibilities, poverty, sexual and physical abuse, gender discrimination, unequal pay, lack of social supports, and traumatic life experience—may contribute to women's increased vulnerability to depression (Hyde & Mezulis, 2020; Moorkath, Vranda, & Naveenkumar, 2019).

Gender socialization differences may also be a factor in the higher rate of depression in women. In many cultures, children are socialized to believe that girls are more influenced by emotions while boys are more influenced by reason. Similarly, girls are taught that it is acceptable to share their thoughts and feelings with others, while boys are encouraged to keep their emotions to themselves. Many societies also promote the idea that girls should be submissive and "nice" while boys should be tough and aggressive. Various disciplines—including psychology, sociology, nursing, and psychiatry—continue to study the effects that these differing messages have on children and adolescents and how expectations related to gender roles impact men and women into adulthood. Many researchers have theorized that these messages create an environment in which women feel devalued, thus increasing their risk of depression. It is also likely that internalization of these societal messages has created a healthcare system in which both patients and practitioners are more likely to view depression as a "women's disorder," whether consciously or not. As a result, women are more likely to be diagnosed with depression even in the absence of severe symptoms, whereas men are less likely to be diagnosed and indeed less inclined to seek help for their symptoms in the first place (Hyde & Mezulis, 2020; Vigod & Rochon, 2020).

Genetic Considerations and Nonmodifiable Risk Factors

Increasingly, genetics and neurobiology have been found to play a role in the development of depressive and bipolar disorders. However, all individuals operate within the context of their environments. Genetics and neurobiology inform nursing care and treatment for individuals with mood disorders, but nurses and clinicians must not overlook other determinants when providing care.

First-degree family members of an individual with major depressive disorder have a two- to fourfold increase in risk of being diagnosed with a similar disorder. Heritability is approximately 40% (APA, 2013; Corfield, Yang, Martin, & Nyholt, 2017). For bipolar disorder, a family history of bipolar disorder is one of the most reliable indicators of increased risk. Individuals have a tenfold increase in risk of developing bipolar disorder if a relative has been diagnosed with bipolar disorder.

Case Study » Part 1

Jason is a 22-year-old college student. He has missed several classes and did not turn in a major paper. When contacted by his professor, Jason admits to feeling so depressed that he has not been able to concentrate on his coursework and has not left his apartment for several days. His professor expresses concern and suggests Jason go to the campus health center, which takes walk-ins. He agrees to go to the campus health center as a condition of getting an extension on the paper. Once there, he tells the nurse he has no appetite and complains of difficulty falling asleep. Jason says he feels guilty for not getting his assignments done and is not doing well in any of his classes. He states he doesn't know what is wrong with him, he just can't seem to get motivated and he doesn't know why. Jason looked forward to going to college and was excited to be accepted and move away from home for the first time. He did very well last semester and in the beginning of this semester. He was active in several clubs and was thinking of running for the student senate and joining the track team, but recently things just seemed to fall apart. Although Jason has many acquaintances through his classes and activities, he has no close friends in the area. During the intake interview, the nurse observes that Jason sits hunched forward in his chair with his eyes downcast. He becomes tearful at times and never smiles.

Clinical Reasoning Questions Level I

1. What is the most important issue the nurse should assess? Explain the rationale for your prioritization.
2. How would you describe Jason's affect?
3. What are the physical health priorities for Jason at this time? If those physical needs are met by changes in lifestyle, for example, would Jason experience a sense of well-being?

Clinical Reasoning Questions Level II

4. What additional information would the HCPs need to determine the most likely cause of Jason's depressed mood? What is a good approach to obtaining relevant additional information?
5. What are the considerations in contacting Jason's family regarding his situation?
6. What sociocultural factors or stressors might be contributing to this patient's distress?

Concepts Related to Mood and Affect

Mood and affect are related to so many concepts and systems that a full discussion of these relationships is beyond the scope of this text. Selected examples of related concepts include addiction; cognition; health, wellness, illness, and injury; healthcare systems; stress and coping; and trauma.

The rate of comorbidity between mood disorders and substance use disorders is high. McHugh and Weiss (2019) indicate that depressive disorders are the most common psychiatric disorders among people with alcohol use disorder. Furthermore, individuals with alcohol dependence are 3.7 times more likely to also have major depressive disorder. Similarly, bipolar disorders are associated with some of the highest rates of alcohol and substance abuse (Gold et al., 2018). Suicide is the leading cause of death among individuals with substance use disorders (SAMHSA, 2016).

As mentioned earlier in the module, disturbances in mood and affect frequently lead to alterations in an individual's normal thought processes. Individuals who are experiencing mania often have racing thoughts, whereas individuals who are experiencing depression are more likely to report that their thinking feels slow or cloudy. Other alterations in thought processes that may occur include decreased concentration and memory and impaired problem-solving and decision-making ability. Although far less common, hallucinations, delusions, and other forms of psychosis may also be manifestations of mood disorders (Potter & Moller, 2020; van Bergen et al., 2019).

Depressive and bipolar disorders impact functioning and overall wellness on a number of levels. Both categories of illness can manifest sleep disturbances. Numerous studies show a direct link between decreased amount and/or quality of sleep and negative mood and affect (Baroni, Bruzzese, Di Bartolo, Ciarleglio, & Shatkin, 2018; Wirz-Justic & Benedetti, 2020; Yorgason et al., 2018). On the other hand, regular physical activity appears to have a protective effect against depression and negative affect (Morgan et. al., 2019; Paolucci, Loukov, Bowdish, & Heise, 2018; Szuhany & Otto, 2020). Individuals with moderate to severe alterations in mood and affect may neglect their physical health and personal hygiene and experience changes in eating patterns and weight gain or loss. Poor health outcomes can affect overall functioning.

Patients with mental illness may not have insurance to pay for health services; therefore, providing a list of free community resources (such as support groups) as well as scheduling appointments with community mental health centers may be necessary to assist the patient in securing increased access to care.

Individuals with depressive or bipolar disorder often have a history of trauma. Similar to trauma, prolonged and overwhelming stress can result in depression or trigger a manic episode. Anxiety disorders often occur along with depression, and poorly managed anxiety can use up the coping reserves needed to prevent the onset of a depressive or manic episode.

The Concepts Related to Mood and Affect feature links some, but not all, of the concepts integral to mood and affect. They are presented in alphabetical order.

Health Promotion

There is no definitive way to prevent depression due to causative and contributing genetic and biological factors that cannot be modified. Some strategies can be useful, however, for modifying stressors and environmental factors that can contribute to depressive illnesses. For instance, research demonstrates that certain lifestyle choices can help protect individuals against the onset of mood disorders. Patients should be encouraged to reduce their intake of sugar, saturated fat, and refined foods and increase their consumption of fruits, vegetables, legumes, fish, and whole grains. Research also suggests that increased intake of certain nutrients—including omega-3 fatty acids, folic acid, vitamin D, selenium, and calcium—may play a protective role (Davison et al., 2019; Dhami, Pandey, Kaur, & Kaur, 2018; Lee et al., 2019; Opie, O'Neil, Jacka, Pizzinga, & Itsiopoulos, 2018). Similarly, multiple studies emphasize the importance of adequate sleep and regular exercise in preventing mood alterations (Baroni et al., 2018; Lowe et al., 2019). Additional research indicates that smoking cessation may decrease the risk of various mental disorders, including depression (Lowe et al., 2019).

Concepts Related to
Mood and Affect

CONCEPT	RELATIONSHIP TO MOOD AND AFFECT	NURSING IMPLICATIONS
Addiction	Addiction → depression Mood disorders → addiction Mood disorders + addiction = ↑severity of both Mood disorders + addiction = ↑suicidal behavior	■ Assess for suicidal ideation. ■ Assess for substance use. ■ Provide concurrent treatment for mood disorders and substance abuse. ■ Refer to community resources. ■ Assess and educate family regarding codependency issues. ■ Anticipate patient denial of substance use.
Cognition	Mood disorders → ↓ concentration, memory, problem solving, and decision making; ↑ risk of psychosis Depression → ↓ clarity and speed of thought processes Mania → ↑ flight of ideas and racing thoughts	■ Conduct mental status examination. » **Skills:** See Skill 1.1 in Volume 3. ■ Provide patients who demonstrate slowed thinking adequate time to respond. ■ Because patients may have trouble concentrating, simplify the communication process by offering limited choices. ■ Do not challenge the patient's belief systems or values. ■ Provide a safe environment and seek immediate medical intervention for patients with signs of psychosis.
Health, Wellness, Illness, and Injury	Depression = ↓ sleep/nutrition/wellness → physical illness and ↓ functional status → ↑ depression	■ Promote self-care, adequate rest and sleep, and exercise as appropriate. ■ Assess for signs of physical illness and for somatic symptoms of depression (e.g., pain in the absence of injury). » **Skills:** See Skill 3.1 in Volume 3. ■ Promote routine health maintenance, screening, healthy lifestyle, and preventive care.
Healthcare Systems	↓ Access to healthcare → ↑ risk for depression and ↑ risk of suicide Depressive and/or manic symptoms ↑ individual use of healthcare systems Healthcare systems often ill-equipped to respond to comorbid psychiatric illness	■ Conduct routine screenings for depression and suicidal ideation as recommended. ■ Collaborate with interprofessional team to address psychologic needs of patients. ■ Refer patient to a mental health professional for follow-up. ■ Provide list of community services, including contact information. ■ Make first appointment for the patient.
Stress and Coping	↑ Stress → depression or triggers mania Ineffective coping → depression and/or anxiety	■ Assist patient in developing effective coping mechanisms. ■ Assess for symptoms of anxiety. ■ Assist patient in identifying triggers for anxiety symptoms. ■ Teach stress reduction techniques.
Trauma	Experiencing violence → depression Exposure to trauma → depression and/or posttraumatic stress disorder	■ Assess for suicide risk. ■ Assess for history of violence. ■ Assess for exposure to traumatic event. ■ Provide safe environment. ■ Educate regarding community resources.

Additional primary prevention strategies focus on psychosocial factors rather than biological factors: Education about stress management, coping strategies, or positive parenting is a primary strategy that may be helpful to many individuals. Other strategies may need to be more community- or situation-specific: For example, parents and children who are going through divorce or another stressful situation may benefit from facilitated discussion and use of coping strategies (Potter & Moller, 2020). Research also indicates that children of depressed parents are less likely to develop depression themselves after participating in family-based cognitive-behavioral interventions (Bettis, Forehand, Sterba, Preacher, & Compas, 2018; Hulgaard, Dehlholm, & Rask, 2019).

Secondary and tertiary prevention strategies are similar to primary strategies that focus on psychosocial factors. Notable secondary approaches include regular screening (described in greater detail below), referring individuals with suspected mood disorders for accurate diagnosis and treatment, and counseling patients about their relative risks for developing mood disorders. Useful tertiary prevention measures include establishing collaborative care programs for patients with mood disorders, employing clinic- and home-based approaches to reducing depression among older adults and individuals with chronic health problems, and developing community-based programs that provide mental health services to individuals experiencing homelessness or poverty (Potter & Moller, 2020).

Screenings

The U.S. Preventive Services Task Force (USPSTF) recommends that all adults, including pregnant and postpartum women, be screened for depression by their primary care providers (USPSTF, 2019). A similar screening approach is recommended for adolescents between the ages of 12 and 18, (USPSTF, 2016b). According to the USPSTF (2019), research indicates that screening patients age 12 and up presents little to no risk of harm. Moreover, there is adequate evidence that early detection of depression followed by use of appropriate pharmacologic and/or psychotherapy decreases clinical morbidity and improves clinical outcomes.

A number of different instruments may be used when screening for depression and other mood disorders (**Table 28.1** »). For example, the Patient Health Questionnaire (PHQ-9) is one of the most common instruments and can be used in a variety of settings to screen individuals to determine whether referral is necessary. The questionnaire is freely available in more than 30 languages (American Psychological Association, 2020; Maurer et al., 2018). Other screening tools are outlined in Table 28.1. Regardless of which instrument is used, patients who score in the range indicative of depression or another mood disorder should be referred to a mental health professional for a thorough diagnostic evaluation.

» **Stay Current:** Visit www.brightfutures.org/mentalhealth/pdf/professionals/bridges/ces_dc.pdf to see the CES-DC and http://cesd-r.com to see or take the CESD-R.

Care in the Community

Most people with mental illness are treated in the community. Deinstitutionalization has required more services to be available to the public at a lower level of care. Community services may include outpatient, intensive outpatient (part-day programs approximately 4 hours in duration), and partial hospitalization (typically services are provided at the hospital daily or near daily for a full day and the patient goes home in the evenings). There are also a multitude of support groups and hotlines available for the public. Group homes (residences for individuals who are functional but chronically mentally ill) and halfway houses (usually a step down from rehabilitation) are also part of community services.

TABLE 28.1 Common Instruments Used to Screen for Depression and/or Bipolar Disorder

Screening Tools	Description
Children	
Children's Depression Inventory (CDI-2)	Short and long forms are available. The child or adolescent completes the self-report scale; parents or caregivers and teachers complete separate forms.
Patient Health Questionnaire for Adolescents (PHQ-A)	41-question self-report scale assesses indicators of anxiety and depression.
Mood and Feelings Questionnaire (MFQ)	Short and long forms available; requires both child and parent(s) to complete a series of questions.
Center for Epidemiological Studies–Depression Scale for Children (CES-DC)	20-item self-report scale that screens for depression.
Mood Disorder Questionnaire (MDQ)	Brief self-report form used to screen adolescents for bipolar disorder.
Adults	
Patient Health Questionnaire (PHQ-9)	Commonly used, 10-question self-report scale used to screen adults for depression; may be used to monitor depression levels throughout treatment.
Beck Depression Inventory (BDI)	21-question self-report scale to screen adults for depression.
Center for Epidemiological Studies Depression Scale–Revised (CESD-R)	20-item self-report scale to screen adults for depression.
Older Adults	
Geriatric Depression Scale (GDS)	Individuals may complete the scale themselves or have a HCP read it to them and score their answers. Long and short forms available.
Cornell Scale for Depression in Dementia (CSDD)	Clinicians use the CSDD to screen individuals with dementia for depression; clinicians use the scale with the caregiver and briefly interview the patient.
Postpartum Depression	
Edinburgh Postnatal Depression Scale (EPDS)	Self-report form that may be used in any setting to screen postpartum mother for depression.
Beck's Postpartum Depression Screening Scale (PDSS)	35-item response scale for use during routine care with all postpartum women to identify those who might be experiencing postpartum depression.

Nursing Assessment

The first and most important aspect in conducting an assessment is to establish a therapeutic relationship based on mutual trust. The nurse should ask open-ended questions and allow adequate time for patient response. It is important that the nurse remain nonjudgmental and validate the patient's feelings. It may be necessary to reduce the patient's anxiety. The nurse should communicate with brief, clear statements, verify the patient's understanding, and clarify areas that may not be understood. Refer to Exemplar 38.B, Therapeutic Communication, in Module 38, Communication, for additional information.

The nurse conducting an assessment of the patient who reports feelings of sadness and irritability or exhibits symptoms of mania must remember that these disorders affect individuals in a variety of ways. More detail is provided below and in the exemplars that follow.

Observation and Patient Interview

Patients experiencing alterations in mood and affect may exhibit a variety of behavioral changes that will suggest the need for further assessment. For example, patients experiencing severe depressive or manic symptoms may exhibit poor hygiene. Other behavioral cues include incongruent verbal and nonverbal communication, irritability, exhaustion, lack of motivation, excitability, grandiosity, altered thought processes, pressured speech, and psychosis. Assess energy level, psychomotor symptoms such as agitation or retardation, and dietary and fluid intake.

During the patient interview, assess for previous diagnosis of mental illness, family history of mental illness, sleep quality, eating patterns, cognition, presence of chronic illness, and substance use.

Assess mood and affect, cognition and thought content, communication patterns, and pain and pain history. Obtain information about any mood fluctuations that may have occurred in the past. Assess the patient's perception of wellness and functioning. Is the patient's perception of health and mental health status congruent with the report of family members or caregivers? What is the patient's priority for care?

Assess coping patterns, home environment, and financial status as well as cultural beliefs and practices. These factors have important implications for treatment planning and patient adherence to treatment regimens.

Self-reporting scales are among the most common instruments used to screen for depression (see **Table 28.1** »). These scales may be used as part of the assessment process but should not be used alone or out of context. Manifestations of altered mood may have their origins in other areas (such as physical illness or adverse effects of medications), and nurses must screen for the presence of these as well.

Cultural Considerations

Culture influences expressions of mood and affect, and it affects the way individuals perceive and understand mental illness. To effectively assess and care for patients with diverse backgrounds, it is important to learn and understand their societal norms related to thoughts, emotions, and behaviors and what specific cultural or societal factors may increase patients' risk for depression (see Focus on Diversity and Culture: Depression in Recent Immigrants). Help-seeking behaviors also can be culturally determined. For example, many African Americans and Latinos often look to their family and faith communities for help before considering seeing

> ## Focus on Diversity and Culture
> ### Depression in Recent Immigrants
>
> Recent immigrants are at higher risk for depression as they cope with multiple stressors, such as long-distance family relationships, unemployment or underemployment, discrimination, language problems, and a new environment. Immigrant children are at risk for depression as they are often expected to interpret the concerns of adult family members to outside authority figures such as physicians, nurses, teachers, and government officials (American Psychological Association, 2018; Ramos-Sánchez, Pietrantonio, & Llamas, 2020).
>
> Currently there are approximately 11.1 million undocumented immigrants in the United States (Ramos-Sánchez et al., 2020). Deportation impacts individuals, families, and communities both physically and psychologically. Individuals facing deportation have reported a credible fear of persecution if they were to be forced to return to the countries from which they migrated. Many of those who are deported return to dangerous, turbulent environments, in which they are at risk of kidnapping, torture, rape, and murder (American Psychological Association, 2018). Additionally, those who have been removed and detained faced psychological trauma, mental deterioration, despondency, and in some cases, suicidality (Ramos-Sánchez et al., 2020).
>
> Psychosocial impacts of deportation and separation from family include economic hardship, with families losing 40–90% of their income, housing instability, and food insecurity. The American Psychological Association (2018) indicates that children who are left behind experience numerous emotional and behavioral issues, such as eating and sleeping changes, anxiety, sadness, anger, aggression, fear, withdrawal, and depression. Lovato et al. (2018) found that separation trauma puts children at greater risk for depression, behavioral problems, and poor educational outcomes. Even if the family is eventually reunited, the trauma of family separation often remains (American Psychological Association, 2018; Lovato et al., 2018; Ramos-Sánchez et al., 2020).
>
> Interventions provided to recent immigrants should be culturally aware and community based. For example, small talk groups known as *pláticas* can encourage relationship building and many communities offer counseling services to assist in processing family trauma (Ramos-Sánchez et al., 2020). Nurses must be knowledgeable about available resources, as undocumented immigrants are still eligible for some assistance programs, such as emergency Medicare, public health programs that provide immunizations or care for communicable diseases, school lunch programs, and the Special Supplemental Nutrition Program for Women, Infants, and Children (WIC) (Ramos-Sánchez et al., 2020).

a professional. There is a strong fear of hospitalization and involuntary commitment, both of which are more likely for African American and Latino populations than for white populations. Both African Americans and American Indians have reported greater distrust of the medical community and greater communication challenges (James et al., 2018; Smirnoff et al., 2018).

Although nurses need to take cultural factors into account during assessment (e.g., ensuring careful assessment that includes access to financial resources and attitudes toward the healthcare community), nurses must be careful not to stereotype patients during the assessment process. When nurses engage in stereotyping, they risk failing to assess for important indicators and are likely to increase barriers to trust and understanding when they should be building the therapeutic alliance and gaining patient trust.

Physical Examination

When conducting a physical examination of patients with diagnosed or suspected mood disorders, obtain a complete set of vital signs, including pain. Obtain a baseline weight and body mass index (BMI) to allow for the possibility of weight monitoring if the treatment plan includes an antidepressant or mood stabilizer. Also be sure to assess sleep, nutrition, activity, and elimination patterns.

A thorough physical examination is necessary to rule out any medical or drug-related causes of presenting signs and symptoms and to identify any comorbid medical illnesses that require treatment. Some chronic medical conditions, especially those that cause pain and/or fatigue, increase the risk of depressive symptoms. Furthermore, patients with depressive and bipolar disorders may be at greater risk of experiencing a comorbid medical illness because their mental illness may impair functioning in the areas of self-care and nutrition.

Diagnostic Tests

Although no diagnostic laboratory or medical tests exist for mood disorders, a thorough workup is necessary to rule out any underlying medical conditions that could mimic or cause symptoms of mood disorders, as well as to detect comorbid medical illness that could contribute to symptoms and functional abnormalities. Diagnostic and laboratory tests may include hormone levels and thyroid function tests to rule out endocrine disorders, which can mimic depression or hypomania; electrolyte panels, urinalysis, and toxicology to rule out substance abuse; and liver function tests because antidepressants are metabolized in the liver. Other tests may be ordered on the basis of the patient's individual symptoms and history (e.g., tests for specific nutritional deficiencies, presence of infection, or medication toxicity). A pregnancy test may be done in women of reproductive age because antidepressants may affect fetal development (Campagne, 2019; Mitchell & Goodman, 2018).

Case Study » Part 2

Following a clinical interview and administration of the Beck Depression Inventory, the HCP at the campus health center diagnosed Jason with major depressive disorder and prescribed extended-release venlafaxine (Effexor XR). One month later, he comes to the health center for his follow-up appointment. The nurse notes that Jason's behavior is nearly the opposite of what she observed at the initial visit. He describes his current mood as "fabulous." He states he is only sleeping about 2 hours a night but that "it's OK"—he feels great and is getting so much done in the extra hours of wakefulness. Jason also reports a heightened sexual desire and urges and attributes this to his decreased need for sleep. He tells the nurse that he completed his required paper and that it is so good he is turning it into a book about the secret to the meaning of life, although he has not yet received a grade. Jason is running for student senate, tried out for the track team, and volunteered at the campus tutoring center. The increased participation in activities has resulted in making new friends with whom he goes drinking two or three nights a week. Jason is considering taking five accelerated courses during the summer.

During the interview, Jason's speech is loud, rapid, and pressured. He is restless, unable to sit still for more than 5 minutes. He offers to give the nurse his autograph because he is convinced his intended book will win a Pulitzer Prize. Jason denies side effects of the medication and considers it a miracle drug because he feels better than he ever has in his entire life. When questioned about thoughts of suicide, Jason denies them, stating, "A person as special as I am needs to be cloned, not killed!"

Clinical Reasoning Questions Level I

1. What else should the nurse assess?
2. How would you describe Jason's affect during this visit?
3. What are the priority health and safety considerations for this patient?

Clinical Reasoning Questions Level II

4. What could be responsible for Jason's remarkable change in mood, affect, and behavior?
5. What are the priority topics to address in this patient's healthcare teaching plan during this visit?
6. How would you rate Jason's risk for suicide? Given your assessment, what would be an effective care plan suggestion?

Independent Interventions

Nurses are in the singular position to provide a number of caring interventions for patients with depressive or bipolar disorders and their families. The most important of these are preventing patient suicide and promoting patient and family safety.

Although treatment of patients with depressive and bipolar disorders is best accomplished by an interprofessional team that includes nurses, mental health professionals, and primary providers, of those individuals who seek and receive treatment, many see only one provider. Nurses working in any setting should consider the following points of treatment management outlined in the *Clinical Practice Guideline for the Treatment of Depression Across Three Age Cohorts* (American Psychological Association, 2019). These points are valid for any patient with any alteration of mood and affect:

- Establish safety
- Promote treatment adherence
- Coordinate care
- Monitor responses to treatment
- Provide education to patients and families.

Prevent Suicide and Promote Safety

Patients experiencing alterations in mood are at increased risk for suicide. When the risk for self-directed violence is high, immediate intervention is necessary. The risk of suicide increases as patients in the severest stage of depression begin to improve; it is then that patients have sufficient energy and cognitive ability to plan and successfully implement a suicide plan. When a patient expresses suicidal ideation, confidentiality does *not* apply. It is the nurse's duty to report suicidal thoughts or actions to the treatment team, or take necessary steps to have the patient transported via ambulance or police to a community crisis screening center, hospital emergency department, or other appropriate facility according to state guidelines. See **Box 28.1** » for guidelines to help prevent inpatient suicide and promote safety.

Communicating with Patients

Introductory Phase

Widespread stigma around suicide can make the patient and the nurse uncomfortable with openly discussing this major safety concern. Paying close attention to nonverbal cues such as downcast eyes, slumped posture, monotone speech, and decreased attention to hygiene and other activities of daily living can alert the nurse to a depressed mood and the need for follow-up questions about suicide. Using empathy, maintaining eye contact, and using direct invitations to explore feelings can help the patient reveal suicidal thoughts. Begin by making open-ended statements such as:

- I notice that you seem to be upset and sad today.
- Something more seems to be bothering you.
- Can you tell me more about how you are feeling today?

Nurses should assist in the transition from hospital to home by helping patients identify situations or events that trigger feelings of altered moods and to learn to use coping methods they find helpful. Nurses also assist in the transition by helping patients develop a safety plan that includes these strategies as well as information on how to contact family members or their mental health professional if they are unable to return to a stable mood without help from someone else.

Monitor Patient Response to Treatment

Nurses must closely monitor how patients with depressive or bipolar disorders respond to treatment. Close monitoring can help reveal whether patients are actually adhering to their treatment regimen. If they are not, the nurse should investigate the reasons for nonadherence. When barriers to treatment are identified (e.g., financial constraints, trouble obtaining and/or taking medication, uncomfortable side effects), the nurse can work with the patient to develop strategies to overcome these barriers or possibly to seek another means of treatment. If the patient is adhering to the treatment plan but is not improving, the nurse, patient, and other members of the healthcare team can collaborate to identify potential adjustments to the therapeutic regimen.

Monitoring the treatment response is also important for patients whose symptoms appear to be improving. In these cases, the nurse should consider whether the patient's recovery is occurring at an appropriate pace, whether any supplementary treatment approaches may be helpful, and/or whether any therapeutic measures are no longer necessary.

Support Family Functioning

The family members of an individual diagnosed with mental illness play an important role in treatment. The family member(s) also take responsibility for the patient's care, which can cause frustration and exhaustion, especially with

Box 28.1

Preventing Inpatient Suicide and Promoting Safety

Check the policy and procedures of the individual inpatient treatment facility and implement those guidelines. For patients who express intent to kill themselves (with or without a plan) or who have made a suicide attempt within the past week, institute safety precautions and request a psychiatric consult as well (Columbia University Medical Center, n.d.).

- Evaluate the patient's level of suicide intent regularly and institute the appropriate level of staff supervision following unit protocol. Patients may deny suicidal ideation or underestimate their own risk (Navin, Kuppili, Menon, & Kattimani, 2019).
- Let suicidal patients know that the environment is safe for them. Remove sharp objects, razors, breakable glass items, mirrors, matches, and straps or belts and explain why these objects are being removed. Monitor the use of scissors, razors, and other potential weapons.
- Do not leave patients at risk for suicide alone. In acute care hospitals or residential settings, one-to-one observation must be instituted until a psychiatrist or qualified physician determines the patient is no longer at risk. Family members cannot substitute for staff in performing one-to-one observation. Some facilities use 15-minute checks, but these are not recommended for use with patients who are seriously suicidal or whose risk level is uncertain (Kleiman & Nock, 2020; Navin et al., 2019).
- Be particularly alert during change of shifts and on holidays or other times when staffing is limited and during times of distraction, such as mealtimes and visiting hours.
- Examine items brought by visitors and monitor for safety. Many units have policies regarding what can and cannot be brought into the unit. Most prohibit food of any kind from outside of the facility.
- Facilitate the development of the therapeutic alliance and maintain a nonjudgmental attitude. Staff members' attitudes toward patients with mental illness can lead to breakdown of the therapeutic alliance and may indirectly increase patients' risk for attempting suicide (Kleiman & Nock, 2020; Navin et al., 2019).
- Use a calm, reassuring approach and encourage patients to discuss all of their feelings. Patients need to know that all feelings are valid and that it benefits them to express their emotions appropriately.

repeated episodes. This care can lead to role strain as the family member(s) often have to care for children, work, and compensate for the mentally ill person's inability to perform usual tasks. It is important to involve the family member(s) as early in treatment as possible. They will be able to assist with maintaining the treatment plan while the nurse lends support when needed. Family, along with the affected individual, will need to have coping skills reinforced and will require education regarding the nature of the patient's illness and the treatment plan.

Teach Assertive Behavior

Nurses working with patients can model, encourage, and teach assertive behavior. Assertiveness is a learned behavior. Everyone has the potential to be assertive, but not everyone instinctively knows how. Children learn patterns of communicating from the adults around them. Individuals can unlearn poor communication patterns that do not work and learn new ones, which is the idea behind assertiveness training. The goal is to help individuals express themselves without fear of disapproval from others. Being assertive does not guarantee that others will agree, but it does provide an individual the satisfaction of offering a personal opinion without ignoring the opinions of others.

Aggressive behavior is directed toward getting what one wants without considering the feelings of others. Aggressive communicators want to get their own way at any cost and may use intimidation to do so. An example of aggressive behavior is insisting on going to a certain movie even though you know your companion does not enjoy that type of movie. The outcome of aggressive behavior is that although you may get what you want in the short run, others feel discredited and tend to avoid you.

Passive behavior consists of avoiding conflict at any cost, even at the expense of one's own happiness. An example of passive behavior is agreeing to go to a movie you do not want to see because your friend pressures you to go. Passive communicators hold their feelings in and allow anger to build up. Anger can explode suddenly or can be expressed in passive–aggressive behavior. An example of passive–aggressive behavior is taking a long time to get ready to go out while your friend is waiting because you are angry that you are going to a movie you do not want to see. The outcome is that the passive person gives up control and is left with resentment, which usually emerges in other ways that damage relationships.

Assertive behavior consists of expressing one's wishes and opinions, or taking care of oneself, but not at the expense of others. An example of assertive communication is saying, "I really don't care for violent movies. Let's look at the movie listings and see if there is something playing that we can both enjoy." The outcome of assertive behavior is self-confidence and self-esteem.

Maintain Professional Boundaries

Patients who are hopeless have a tendency to form dependent relationships. Nurses must work from the first contact with these patients to minimize the likelihood that maladaptive dependence occurs in the nurse–patient relationship. Strategies to minimize maladaptive dependence include the following:

- Emphasize the short-term nature of the relationship.
- Recognize that a patient who singles out one staff member exclusively and refuses to relate to others is developing dependence.
- Avoid giving patients the hope that the nurse–patient relationship can continue after therapy has ended.
- Refuse (kindly but firmly) requests for your address or telephone number.
- Remind patients that social contact will not be allowed.

If you find yourself wanting to continue relationships with certain patients, discuss these feelings with your instructor (if you are a student), your supervisor, or a respected professional peer (if you are a practicing nurse). It is essential that you separate your professional life from your social life.

Collaborative Therapies

Collaborative therapies for patients with mood disorders include pharmacotherapy, CBT and other psychotherapies, and complementary health approaches. Often, combining therapies leads to greater success. Nurses help patients determine what combination of therapies may be most helpful for them, encourage adherence to the treatment plan, and suggest alternatives if a sufficient trial of a treatment or therapy (typically at least 6 weeks) proves ineffective.

Pharmacologic Therapy for Depressive Disorders

Antidepressants are the first-line treatment for depressive disorders and some anxiety disorders. Antidepressants are thought to exert changes to certain neurotransmitters in the brain, including norepinephrine, dopamine, and serotonin. The two basic mechanisms of action are blocking the enzymatic breakdown of norepinephrine and slowing the reuptake of serotonin (see **Figure 28.2** »). Nurses working with patients taking antidepressants must be alert to the symptoms of **serotonin syndrome**, which can occur in individuals taking two or more medications that increase serotonin levels. Serotonin syndrome exhibits as an altered mental status (e.g., anxiety, disorientation, agitation); neuromuscular abnormalities (e.g., tremor, muscle rigidity); and autonomic hyperactivity (e.g., gastrointestinal [GI] distress, hypertension, tachypnea, tachycardia, diaphoresis) (Francescangeli, Karamchandani, Powell, & Bonavia, 2019; Takata, Arashi, Abe, Arai, & Haruyama, 2019). Supportive measures and discontinuing the medications involved will usually resolve the patient's symptoms.

Nursing considerations for all antidepressants include:

- Assess health history, including history of sexual dysfunction.
- Monitor for suicidal ideation and behaviors throughout treatment. As patients begin to recover, their energy levels rise, which may increase their suicide risk.
- Obtain a baseline body weight to monitor weight gain.

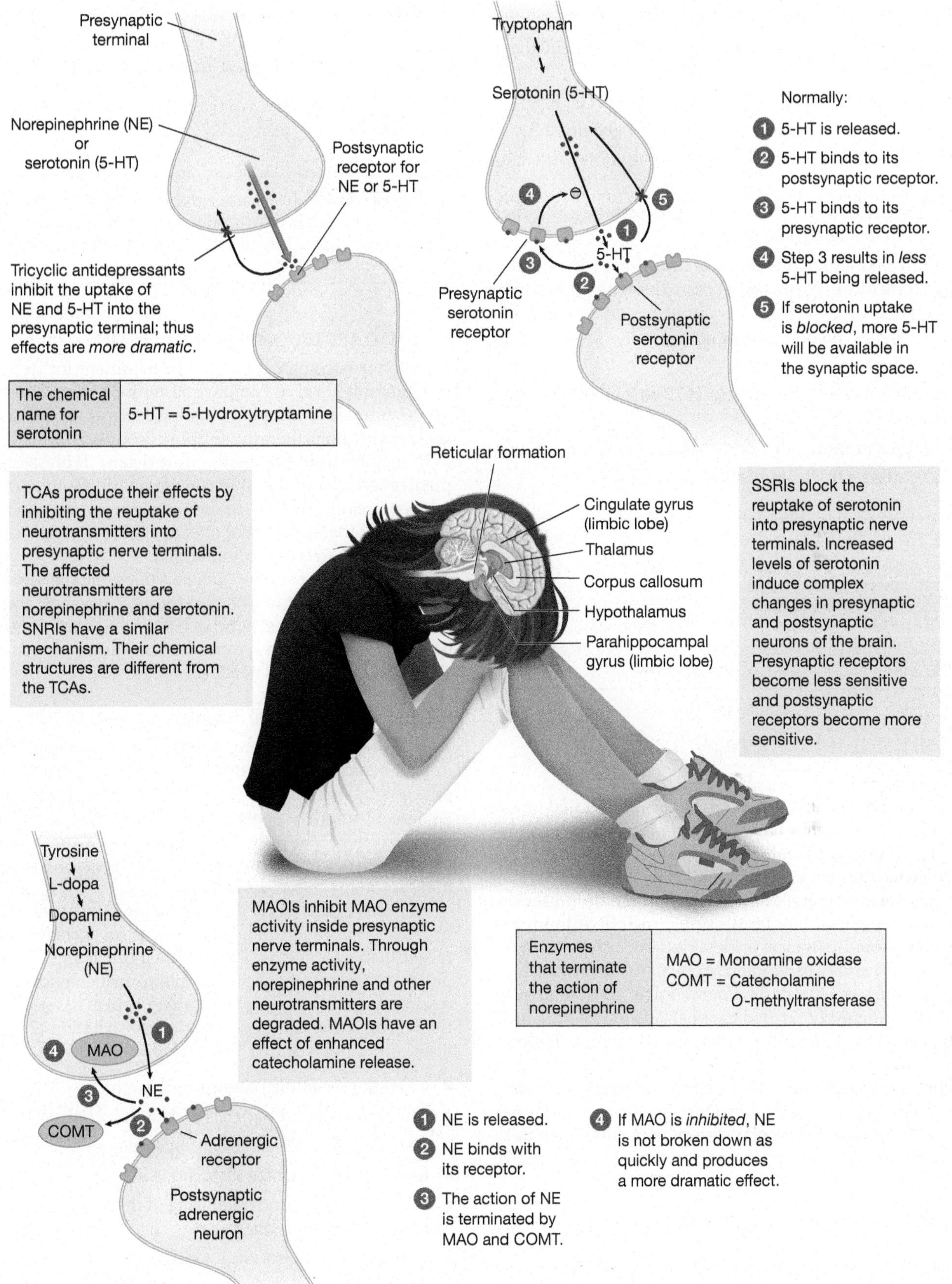
Presynaptic terminal
Norepinephrine (NE) or serotonin (5-HT)
Postsynaptic receptor for NE or 5-HT
Tricyclic antidepressants inhibit the uptake of NE and 5-HT into the presynaptic terminal; thus effects are *more dramatic*.
The chemical name for serotonin
5-HT = 5-Hydroxytryptamine
Tryptophan
Serotonin (5-HT)
5-HT
Presynaptic serotonin receptor
Postsynaptic serotonin receptor
Normally:
1 5-HT is released.
2 5-HT binds to its postsynaptic receptor.
3 5-HT binds to its presynaptic receptor.
4 Step 3 results in *less* 5-HT being released.
5 If serotonin uptake is *blocked*, more 5-HT will be available in the synaptic space.
Reticular formation
Cingulate gyrus (limbic lobe)
Thalamus
Corpus callosum
Hypothalamus
Parahippocampal gyrus (limbic lobe)
TCAs produce their effects by inhibiting the reuptake of neurotransmitters into presynaptic nerve terminals. The affected neurotransmitters are norepinephrine and serotonin. SNRIs have a similar mechanism. Their chemical structures are different from the TCAs.
SSRIs block the reuptake of serotonin into presynaptic nerve terminals. Increased levels of serotonin induce complex changes in presynaptic and postsynaptic neurons of the brain. Presynaptic receptors become less sensitive and postsynaptic receptors become more sensitive.
Tyrosine
L-dopa
Dopamine
Norepinephrine (NE)
MAO
NE
COMT
Adrenergic receptor
Postsynaptic adrenergic neuron
MAOIs inhibit MAO enzyme activity inside presynaptic nerve terminals. Through enzyme activity, norepinephrine and other neurotransmitters are degraded. MAOIs have an effect of enhanced catecholamine release.
Enzymes that terminate the action of norepinephrine
MAO = Monoamine oxidase
COMT = Catecholamine *O*-methyltransferase
1 NE is released.
2 NE binds with its receptor.
3 The action of NE is terminated by MAO and COMT.
4 If MAO is *inhibited*, NE is not broken down as quickly and produces a more dramatic effect.

Figure 28.2 ›› The mechanism of action of TCA, SSRI, and MAOI antidepressive drugs.

Patient education for all antidepressant medications includes:

- It may take several weeks or more to achieve the full therapeutic effect of the drug.
- Risk of suicide increases as therapeutic effect begins.
- Report increased suicidal thoughts and behaviors.
- Keep all scheduled follow-up appointments with your HCP.
- Report side effects, including nausea, vomiting, diarrhea, sexual dysfunction, and fatigue.
- Do not take other prescription drugs, over-the-counter (OTC) medications, or herbal remedies without notifying your HCP.
- Avoid using alcohol and other central nervous system (CNS) depressants.
- Immediately discuss with your HCP an intention or desire to become pregnant.
- Exercise and monitor caloric intake to avoid weight gain.
- Do not discontinue medication abruptly.

SAFETY ALERT The U.S. Food and Drug Administration (FDA) requires a "black box warning" on all antidepressants related to the increased risk for suicidal thoughts and behaviors associated with taking antidepressant medications. The nurse must be aware of this and educate patients and families to monitor for suicidal ideation and provide 24-hour emergency center contact numbers for use if it occurs. Patients age 24 and younger are especially at risk.

Pharmacologic Therapy for Bipolar Disorders

Drugs used to treat bipolar disorders are called **mood stabilizers** because they have the ability to moderate extreme shifts in emotions between mania and depression. Some anticonvulsive drugs are used for mood stabilization in patients with bipolar disorders. Medications commonly prescribed for the treatment of bipolar disorders include lithium carbonate (Lithobid); atypical antipsychotics, such as aripiprazole (Abilify) and olanzapine (Zyprexa) (see Exemplar 23.C, Schizophrenia, in Module 23, Cognition, for additional information on antipsychotic medications); and antiseizure medications, such as carbamazepine (Epitol, Equetro, Tegretol) and valproic acid (Depakote). Side effects and adverse effects of these drugs are many and varied. Generally speaking, however, nursing considerations for patients receiving pharmacologic therapy for bipolar disorders include the following (Bahji, Ermacora, Stephenson, Hawken, & Vazquez, 2020; Mannapperuma et al., 2019; Yatham et al., 2018):

- Monitor drug levels (especially lithium), blood glucose levels, and electrolyte panels periodically. (Note that older adults require more frequent monitoring for drug toxicity.)
- Monitor for and report increased signs of suicidality and suicidal ideation. (Children and adolescents may need more frequent monitoring.)
- Monitor for and report changes in cardiovascular status, particularly orthostatic hypotension. (Older adults require more frequent monitoring.)
- Monitor for and report signs of extrapyramidal symptoms or neuroleptic malignant syndrome.
- Monitor neurologic and neuromuscular status in older adults.

›› **Skills:** See Skill 1.22 in Volume 3.

SAFETY ALERT Patients with bipolar disorders who are in the depressive phase and prescribed only an antidepressant are at high risk for switching to a manic episode. For that reason, mood stabilizers are always prescribed at the same time.

Nonpharmacologic Therapy

A nonpharmacologic approach to treatment for depression is commonly used in conjunction with pharmacologic therapy. Examples of nonpharmacologic therapies include psychotherapy, light therapy, support groups, and meditation. ECT may be used for treatment-resistant depression. Both medication and psychotherapy alone are effective in treating depression; however, the combination of both medication and psychotherapy is most effective. Therefore, psychotherapy is almost always recommended.

One of the most successful forms of psychotherapy is CBT. However, a number of different forms of psychotherapy can be considered. The best approach to psychotherapy is chosen based on the cause and symptoms of the depressive condition as well as the patient's needs and personality.

Cognitive-Behavioral Therapy

Cognitive-behavioral therapy, which focuses on how thoughts impact behaviors and actions, has been demonstrated to be effective by many research studies. CBT has been linked to significant improvements and outcomes in functioning and quality of life. Many studies indicate that a combination of pharmacologic interventions and CBT is an effective treatment for many mood disorders.

Cognitive-behavioral therapy features skills training and problem-solving techniques that focus on current situations rather than past events. The therapist practicing CBT assists patients to identify specific problems or behaviors and the related flawed thought patterns and beliefs associated with them. The American Psychological Association (2020) outlines core aspects of CBT that include:

- Changing negative patterns of thought
- Changing learned patterns of unhelpful behaviors
- Learning more effective coping strategies
- Learning to recognize distortions in thinking
- Gaining a better understanding of the behavior and motivation of self and others
- Using problem-solving skills to cope with difficult situations
- Learning to develop a greater sense of confidence is one's own abilities.

Techniques in CBT sessions involve the therapist exploring current issues that the patient is experiencing by asking such questions as: *What is the current problem you are facing?*

What automatic thoughts arise when this problem happens? What evidence is there that this thought is true/untrue? Is there an alternative way of thinking about this situation? What can be done differently for a better outcome?

Another technique often used is **cognitive modification**. This technique focuses on automatic thoughts that may or may not be true of the situation. Cognitive modification assists the patient with identifying and changing negative thought patterns. An example is that of a wife whose husband has not called her after work and is late coming home. The wife's automatic thoughts may include:

- "He doesn't care about me or he would have called me so I don't worry."
- "He doesn't love me anymore and is probably having an affair."

Cognitive-behavioral therapists help patients reframe these automatic thoughts into more rational, logical, and fact-based ways of thinking. For example, a woman experiencing depression may automatically think the worst in situations involving her partner. CBT helps her rethink and reprocess these situations by helping her reevaluate her expectations. For example, she can reframe the automatic thought of "my partner didn't call, so they must be having an affair" to a more realistic perception that "they usually call when they leave, so they must be working late."

Mindfulness training is another specific technique used in CBT that has been proven to help patients with depression and anxiety. **Mindfulness** focuses on being acutely aware of what sensations and feelings are present in the current moment. Mindfulness takes practice and self-discipline. Stress and a busy lifestyle hinder the practice of mindfulness, as most people do not actively and consciously reflect on how they feel in most situations. By practicing and engaging in mindfulness, individuals can learn to recognize negative patterns of thinking, clearly identify them as such, and allow them to leave their thoughts.

Electroconvulsive Therapy

Electroconvulsive therapy (ECT) is a treatment procedure that passes an electric current through the brain to induce a seizure. It has been used clinically since the 1930s. It is usually given 2 to 3 times weekly for 3 to 4 weeks until a course of 6 to 12 treatments is completed. Research suggests that twice-weekly ECT is preferable, as it is roughly as effective as thrice-weekly administration, but frequently requires fewer treatments and may be associated with longer-lasting therapeutic effects (Bahji, Hawken, Sepehry, Cabrera, & Vazquez, 2019). ECT is typically considered a second-line therapy for both treatment-resistant MDD and bipolar disorder, and it produces similar overall remission rates in patients with either condition (Bahji et al., 2019). Current scholarly literature reviewing ECT (Bahji et al., 2019; Diermen et al., 2018; Dong et al., 2018) cites the following findings:

- ECT is effective in treating depression, with responses of over 80%.
- Response is even higher in patients who have depression with psychotic features.
- Response is relatively rapid (greater than 60% within 3 weeks).
- ECT is associated with improved mood, functional status, anxiety, and quality of life.
- Individuals of all ages, even older adults with cognitive impairment, tolerate and respond well to ECT.
- It does not cause a switch to mania when used to treat bipolar depression, and it may also be used in patients with bipolar disorder with mixed features.
- It is especially useful for patients with severe depression who are resistant to other treatments, those who are severely suicidal, and those with severe psychomotor retardation.

A review of ECT in pregnancy demonstrated its effectiveness in treating depression; however, it is linked with potential fetal and maternal complications such as premature labor, decreased fetal heart rate, and uterine contractions (Ward, Fromson, Cooper, De Oliveira, & Almeida, 2018). Risks and benefits of ECT must be weighed carefully on an individual basis before deciding to treat a pregnant woman with ECT.

ECT is typically an outpatient procedure and is administered while the patient is under anesthesia. A thorough medical examination is required prior to the procedure to clear the patient for anesthesia. Muscle relaxants are usually administered. The patient is ventilated during the procedure. Electroencephalogram and electrocardiogram (ECG), oxygen saturation via pulse oximetry, and vital signs are monitored during the procedure, which only takes 5 to 10 minutes. Mild confusion following the procedure (a postictal state) is typical. Vital signs must be monitored frequently for several hours afterward. During a course of ECT, a transient short-term memory loss (anterograde amnesia) is expected. This is distressing to some patients, and they need to be reassured that memory is usually restored. In rare cases, however, retrograde amnesia occurs and may be permanent. There are the usual risks associated with anesthesia. It is essential that all the potential risks and benefits of ECT be explained to and understood by the patient. A written, informed consent form must be signed by the patient before the procedure. Patients have the right to refuse treatment at any time during the course of therapy.

Transcranial Magnetic Stimulation

Repetitive transcranial magnetic stimulation (rTMS) is an FDA-approved treatment for depression and anxiety that has been used since 1985. r-TMS uses an electromagnetic coil that is placed against the forehead to target and stimulate the left prefrontal cortex region of the brain, the area that is thought to be implicated in depressive disorders. In cases of mania, the focus of treatment is on the right prefrontal cortex, which has been shown to produce therapeutic effects. Much like ECT, rTMS has been noted to have a faster onset (1 to 2 weeks) and quicker response rate than that of psychotropic medications. Although rTMS produces fewer short-term adverse cognitive effects than ECT, numerous studies have found that its benefits are fewer and of shorter duration than those associated with ECT (Chen, Zhao, Liu, Fan, & Xie, 2017; Svensson, Khaldi, Engström, Matusevich, & Nordenskjöld, 2018).

Complementary Health Approaches

In community surveys, depression, fatigue, insomnia, and anxiety are among the most commonly reported reasons for the use of alternative therapies. The following are some complementary therapies used for mood disorders. Note that these types of therapies should be used as complementary, rather than alternative, therapies in patients experiencing significant disruption in functioning related to mood disorders. Patients taking pharmacologic therapy should be encouraged to consult their prescribing provider before trying herbal or dietary supplements.

Exercise

Research indicates that exercise can reduce anxiety and promote healthy behaviors and overall health (Dhami et al., 2018; Morgan et al., 2019). These benefits alone make exercise a key part of health promotion and patient teaching in patients with alterations in mood and affect. However, research indicates that although exercise can improve symptoms in people with depression, it is not a cure-all and may have varying results (Belvederi-Murri et al., 2019; Schuch & Stubbs, 2019). Due to these findings, nurses should emphasize the overall health benefits of exercise rather than its use as a complementary or alternative therapy to patients with alterations in mood and affect. Still, exercise is recommended for people with mild to moderate depression, provided they are physically able to participate (Belvederi-Murri et al., 2019; Dhami et al., 2018; Morgan et al., 2019). Although some reviews indicate that no one form of exercise is best, others suggest that individuals with depressive symptoms should engage in moderate-intensity aerobic exercise three times a week for a minimum of 9 weeks. Exercise also appears to be most beneficial when used in combination with antidepressant medications (Kandola, Ashdown-Franks, Hendrikse, Sabiston, & Stubbs, 2019; Paolucci et al., 2018).

SAFETY ALERT St. John's wort is not a proven therapy for depression (National Center for Complementary and Integrative Health [NCCIH], 2017) and should not be used to postpone or replace conventional treatment. It should *not* be combined with prescription antidepressants. It also may interfere with the action of antiseizure medications. St. John's wort has been found to reduce the effectiveness of birth control pills and HIV medications, among others (NCCIH, 2017). If taken with SSRIs, TCAs, or some atypical antidepressants, serotonin syndrome may result.

Vitamin B

Low levels of the B vitamins have been linked to depression, as vitamin B plays a role in the development of serotonin and norepinephrine (Dhami et al., 2019). A systematic review found that short-term increase of folate or vitamin B_{12} is not helpful in the treatment of depression but may be helpful if taken for the long term (Dome, Tombor, Lazary, Gonda, & Rihmer, 2019; Jamilian et al., 2019). There is inconsistent evidence that folic acid may improve the action of some antidepressants (Dome et al., 2019).

Omega-3 Fatty Acids

A number of meta-analyses (including a Cochrane review) found that it is difficult to formulate concrete conclusions about the efficacy of omega-3 fatty acids in improving depression (Dome et. al., 2019). However, two meta-analyses did provide evidence that omega-3 fatty acids in combination with antidepressant medications have a greater antidepressant effect than either used alone (Dome et al., 2019).

Acupuncture

Acupuncture is best known for pain relief but may be coupled with SSRI antidepressants for increased benefit. In a systematic review of 29 studies of acupuncture for depression, which included 2268 participants, acupuncture was found to be associated with reducing the severity of depression (Armour et al., 2019). Clinical trials indicate that acupuncture, when used with SSRI antidepressants, enhances the therapeutic response, has an early onset of action, and is well tolerated compared to the use of SSRIs alone (Armour et al., 2019). Furthermore, patients who are treated with acupuncture coupled with SSRIs demonstrate a faster response time and decreased side effects (Armour et al., 2019; Smith, Shewamene, Galbally, Schmied, & Dahlen, 2019). There is also some evidence that acupuncture may be beneficial in the treatment of depression in pregnant women when it is targeted toward treatment of depression and not generalized (Smith et al., 2019).

Case Study » Part 3

Jason was admitted to the short-term acute care psychiatric unit of the local hospital. He was diagnosed with bipolar I disorder and started on aripiprazole (Abilify). Jason reports feeling as if he has to keep moving all the time, and he has mild dystonic symptoms involving muscle twitches in his hands. He is currently taking 20 mg of aripiprazole daily. He is attending individual and group therapy sessions. He is sleeping and eating more normally; his speech is no longer rapid and pressured. Jason no longer believes he has special talents. He says he now feels stupid about his previous behavior and ashamed that he ended up being hospitalized. He states, "I can't face anyone I know now that they know I am crazy. I don't want to live the rest of my life like this. What's the point?"

Clinical Reasoning Questions Level I

1. What cues or symptoms should be reported to the physician and therapist?
2. Based on the information provided, what does the nurse need to assess immediately?
3. What is the probable cause of Jason's feelings of restlessness and muscle twitches? What additional treatments might be indicated to address them?

Clinical Reasoning Questions Level II

4. What do Jason's statements indicate and how should the nurse respond?
5. What is the priority nursing diagnosis for this patient at this time?
6. Why do you think Jason was not prescribed an antidepressant?

Lifespan Considerations

Mood and Affect in Children and Adolescents

Determinants of normal mood and affect in children and adolescents are generally the same as those for adults; however, a greater level of emotional lability is common in younger patients and should not necessarily be considered suggestive of a mood disorder. Causes of "mood swings" among children and adolescents include anxiety about the physical changes they are experiencing, hormonal fluctuations associated with the onset of puberty, immaturity of the prefrontal cortex, and the pressures of adjusting to new roles and expectations (Casey, Heller, Gee, & Cohen, 2019; Ladouceur et al., 2019; Schweizer, Gotlib, & Blakemore, 2020). As adolescents progress toward adulthood, the mood swings typical of the teenage years become progressively less common (Casey et al., 2019; Ladouceur et al., 2019).

When children's mood and affect fall outside the normal range for members of their age group, the possibility of a mood disorder should be considered. According to the Centers for Disease Control and Prevention (CDC; 2020d), 3.2% of children age 3 to 17 years (approximately 1.9 million) have diagnosed depression. Girls are affected nearly twice as often as boys (NIMH, 2017a). Children experience depression, although onset typically occurs sometime between puberty and young adulthood; hence, depression rates rise during the later teenage years. In fact, according to the NIMH (2019), 13.3% of adolescents age 12 to 17 experience depression. Bipolar disorder is rarely observed in this population because onset nearly always occurs in late adolescence or when individuals are in their 20s (APA, 2013).

Initially, many parents choose to try psychotherapy alone to treat depressive disorders in their children and adolescents. However, if this proves unsuccessful, medication is indicated. Currently, fluoxetine (Prozac) is the only antidepressant that is FDA-approved for use in children. Most prescribers will start children on a lower dose of antidepressant than is normally prescribed for adults and titrate up to a dose that is effective in symptom relief.

In 2004, the FDA issued a public warning regarding increased risk of suicidal thoughts or behavior in children and adolescents treated with SSRI antidepressant medications. However, several newer studies indicate that the benefits associated with taking antidepressants may be greater than the risk of suicide (Goodyer & Wilkinson, 2019; Hayes, Lewis, & Lewis, 2019).

SAFETY ALERT Note that the FDA does not recommend paroxetine (Paxil) to treat depression in children and adolescents. Due to reports of increased suicidal thinking and behavior among children and adolescents during initial treatment with paroxetine, the FDA issued a "black box" warning about its use in this population.

Mood and Affect in Pregnant Women

Manifestations and potential causes of depressive disorder with peripartum onset are detailed in Exemplar 28.C, Peripartum Depression, in this module. Generally speaking, new onset of depression during pregnancy appears to be related to anxiety about the fetus's health and the birth process, concern about relationship changes and adapting to the maternal role, and the many physical and hormonal changes of pregnancy. It is also important to note that many women who previously experienced depression either continue to experience symptoms or have a recurrence of symptoms during pregnancy (Osman & Bahri, 2019). When both women with existing mood disorders and women with new-onset depression are considered, experts estimate that between 12 and 20% of women experience depression during the antepartum period. Many of these women remain undiagnosed or untreated, often because they feel ashamed to be depressed during a time in life when society expects them to be filled with joy and anticipation. Unfortunately, failure to seek treatment during pregnancy can have detrimental effects on both mother and child, including elevated likelihood of pregnancy complications, premature birth, high-risk maternal behavior, postpartum depression, intrauterine growth restriction, and developmental difficulties during childhood (Jordan, Davies, Thayer, Tucker, & Humphreys, 2019; Mitchell & Goodman, 2018; Sunnqvist, Sjöström, & Finnbogadóttir, 2019).

Several treatment options are available for women who experience mood disorders during pregnancy. Many women opt for group therapy or psychotherapy, often because they are hesitant to pursue or continue pharmacologic treatment. A major reason for this hesitation is that, to date, no psychotropic drug has been assigned a Category A rating by the FDA. (A Category A rating indicates that there are no known fetal risks associated with a medication.) Research indicates, however, that many women and prescribers alike overestimate the risk associated with pharmacologic therapy during pregnancy. For example, SSRIs are among the most studied drugs in pregnant women, and substantial evidence exists that these drugs (with the exception of paroxetine [Paxil]) present low risk of major birth defects. Nonetheless, babies of mothers who took SSRIs during pregnancy do have a slightly elevated risk of persistent pulmonary hypertension in the newborn (PPHN) and neonatal withdrawal. TCAs are also considered low risk, although use of MAOI antidepressants is not recommended (Campagne, 2019; Cepeda, Kern, & Nicholson, 2019; Niethe & Whitfield, 2018). For more information on the care and treatment of pregnant women with mood disorders, see the exemplars in this module.

Mood and Affect in Older Adults

Depression is not a normal part of aging; research suggests that older adults generally have a more positive mood and affect than younger adults (Emery, Sorrell, & Miles, 2020; Machado, Thompson, & Brett 2019). Thus, when older adults present with symptoms of depression, these symptoms need to be addressed. In many cases, these symptoms may be related to life changes, such as retirement; loss of aging friends, family, or spouse to death; downsizing or placement in assisted care; and loss of physical function. Major life-changing events can overwhelm coping mechanisms, leading to increased risk of depression (Potter & Moller, 2020). The presence of a chronic illness elevates the older adult's risk for depression.

When working with older patients, a thorough evaluation is necessary to rule out any underlying medical cause of mood alterations before medication is prescribed. As with most medications in older adults, the cardinal rule is to start with the lowest dose and increase slowly as tolerated and as needed to achieve therapeutic effect. Older adults may respond to a lower drug dose, but it is important to treat to remission. Also, because the majority of psychotropic medications are metabolized in the liver, caution must be taken in older adults with liver disease. For patients with depression, SSRIs are usually the drug of choice. Because psychotropic drugs lead to increased risk of orthostatic hypotension in older adults, patients should be educated to sit before standing and stand before walking to reduce their likelihood of falls. The patient and family should also be educated on fall risk-reduction strategies. In addition, a thorough medication history and periodic medication reconciliation should be conducted because of the risk of medication interactions and polypharmacy (Drahota & Revell-Smith, 2019; Krause et al., 2019). Most older adults with mood disorders respond well with antidepressants, psychotherapy, or a combination of the two (Potter & Moller, 2020).

SAFETY ALERT Atypical antipsychotics, often used to treat bipolar disorder, all have an FDA "black box" warning that they may increase mortality from pneumonia in older adults with dementia-related psychosis. Older adults taking these medications for bipolar disorder should be monitored carefully.

REVIEW The Concept of Mood and Affect

RELATE Link the Concepts

Linking the concept of mood and affect with the concept of development:

1. Explain how failure to master the developmental tasks of older adulthood could contribute to the development of depression (refer to developmental theories).
2. How can resiliency theory be applied to the development or prevention of depression?

Linking the concept of mood and affect with the concept of family:

3. How can the burden of having a family member with a severe mental illness such as bipolar disorder affect the family system?
4. How does the stage that the family is in affect family recovery from a mood disorder?

Linking the concept of mood and affect with the concept of self:

5. How would you assess self-esteem in a patient suspected of having a mood disorder?
6. What are some strategies that can be used to enhance the low self-esteem often experienced by patients with mood disorders?

READY Go to Volume 3: Clinical Nursing Skills

REFER Go to Pearson MyLab Nursing and eText

REFLECT Apply Your Knowledge

Gerald Hanes is a 72-year-old widowed man who is brought into his primary care provider's office by his daughter, who is worried about his unexplained weight loss. Gerald lives independently and is in good general health. Since Gerald's regular checkup 2 months ago, he has lost 20 pounds. He denies any concerns at this time. Gerald's daughter reports that he has not been attending church, which he used to do weekly. She further reports that ever since his wife died 3 months ago, he has not been maintaining his relationships with the family. She states that he still has most of the groceries left in the kitchen that she purchased for him 2 weeks ago. When asked if he is eating, Gerald states, "I'm just not hungry anymore." Gerald presents with a flat to sad affect and depressed mood. All laboratory test results are reported as negative or within normal limits.

1. What additional questions should the nurse ask Gerald during the assessment?
2. In further discussion with the daughter, she states that she knows that this is typical for the aging population. How should the nurse respond to this statement?
3. What are three appropriate care priorities for Gerald at this time?

Exemplar 28.A Depression

Exemplar Learning Outcomes

28.A Analyze depressive disorders and relevant nursing care.

- Describe the pathophysiology of depressive disorders.
- Describe the etiology of depressive disorders.
- Compare the risk factors and prevention of depressive disorders.
- Identify the clinical manifestations of depressive disorders.
- Summarize diagnostic tests and therapies used by interprofessional teams in the collaborative care of an individual with a depressive disorder.
- Differentiate care of patients with depressive disorders across the lifespan.
- Apply the nursing process in providing culturally competent care to an individual with a depressive disorder.

Exemplar Key Terms

Adjustment disorder with depressed mood, *1975*
Anhedonia, *1974*
Depression, *1970*
Dysthymia, *1974*
Hypersomnia, *1974*
Insomnia, *1974*
Learned helplessness, *1971*
Major depressive disorder (MDD), *1973*
Major depressive episode, *1973*
Persistent depressive disorder, *1974*
Psychomotor retardation, *1974*
Seasonal affective disorder (SAD), *1974*
Situational depression, *1975*

Overview

Depression is a mental health disorder that affects an estimated 264 million people of all ages worldwide (World Health Organization [WHO], 2020). Approximately 7.2% of adults (17.7 million adults) had at least one depressive episode within a year (SAMHSA, 2018). During a depressive episode, an individual experiences a sad or depressed mood accompanied by a loss of pleasure or interest in daily activities for a period of at least 2 weeks. Other symptoms may include difficulty sleeping, changes in appetite, poor concentration, low energy, and a decreased feeling of self-worth. Suicidal thoughts are common in more severe cases of depression. Up to 10% of individuals experiencing a depressive episode will attempt suicide (McConnell, Carter, & Patterson, 2019; SAMHSA, 2018).

Depression is associated with increased physical impairment and decreased quality of life. The financial burden of depression in the United States is considerable: It is estimated to be more than $2 billion annually in lost wages and associated healthcare costs (Wu et al., 2019). Because nurses will encounter patients with depression in all practice settings, they need to be aware of proper assessment methods for depression as well as collaborative care and treatment options.

Pathophysiology

As described in the Concept section of this module, the exact pathophysiology of depression has yet to be determined. As described in the concept, depression also appears to be at least partially rooted in a person's genetics. Still, structural, functional, and genetic variations may not be the only biological contributors to depressive disorders.

As mentioned earlier, individuals with depression often have increased limbic system activity, along with decreased gray-matter volume and lower metabolic activity in the MPFC (Arnone, 2018; Duman et al., 2019; van den Bosch & Meyer-Lindenberg, 2019). Specific reasons for these findings remain unclear, although the working theory is that they involve alterations in neurotransmitter activity and/or neuronal receptivity to neurotransmitters. Several different neurotransmitters have been implicated in the pathophysiology of depression, including 5-HT, NE, DA, ACh, GABA, and glutamate (Duman et al., 2019; Wray et al., 2018).

More recent studies have focused on a potential connection between depression and inflammation, based on the fact that many depressed individuals have increased levels of inflammatory biomarkers called cytokines; however, there does not appear to be a direct correlation (Sun, Drevets, Turecki, & Li, 2020; Wray et al., 2018). These findings have led to the hypothesis that some people with depression may have a genetic predisposition toward elevated cytokine production when faced with external stressors, as well as the hypothesis that others may have genetic factors that protect them against the potentially mood-lowering effects of cytokines (Duman et al., 2019; Sun et al., 2020; Wray et al., 2018).

Hormonal factors also continue to be investigated as a possible cause of depression. Researchers have noted that individuals with depression tend to have increased levels of cortisol and corticotropin-releasing hormone, both of which are produced in the brain's hypothalamic–pituitary–adrenal (HPA) axis. High levels of cortisol and corticotropin-releasing hormone are indicative of HPA and limbic system hyperactivity, which is commonly observed in individuals with depression (Caroleo et al., 2019; Sun et al., 2020; Wray et al., 2018). Research has not yet determined whether depression precipitates HPA hyperactivity and excess hormone production or whether HPA hyperactivity and excess hormone production precipitate depression. However, recent studies suggest that variations in the genes that code for corticotropin-releasing hormone may lead to increased susceptibility to major depression following negative life events (Caroleo et al., 2019; Rubinow & Schmidt, 2019).

The fact that women experience higher rates of depression than men indicates a connection between estrogen and depression. Decreased estrogen levels in particular seem to play a role, as evidenced by women's greater likelihood of depressive symptoms at certain points in the menstrual cycle, as well as at the onset of menopause. The exact nature of the estrogen–depression relationship remains unclear, however (Rubinow & Schmidt, 2019; Stanikova et al., 2019).

Etiology

Depression has been linked to multiple possible causes. Genetics clearly plays some role, although the exact nature of this role remains unclear. Other potential causative mechanisms (many of which may have a genetic component) include hormonal imbalances, disruptions in biological rhythms, high stress levels, poor coping mechanisms, traumatic life events, unhealthy or insufficient interpersonal relationships, and internalization of unhealthy or unrealistic gender-based expectations.

Theory of Learned Helplessness

The theory of **learned helplessness** asserts that as individuals are exposed to discomfort, pain, and suffering and fail to resolve their pain or discomfort, they eventually stop trying to find a solution and give up, even if an escape is later presented. These beliefs and traits are not innate; rather, they are a learned behavior and develop over time as individuals are conditioned to believe that they have no control over what is happening to them. Theorists believe that three deficits occur in individuals with learned helplessness: motivational, cognitive, and emotional. The cognitive deficit happens when the person believes that present circumstances are uncontrollable. The motivational deficit refers to a person's perception that escaping the negative stimuli is not possible. Emotional deficits are observed as the person expresses depressive symptoms in relation to feeling out of control of the situation (Smallheer, Vollman, & Dietrich, 2018).

Cognitive Theory

According to cognitive theory, which comes largely from the work of Aaron Beck (1967), individuals with depression have skewed core views of themselves, of their environment, and of the future. Moreover, their characteristically negative way of thinking makes it impossible for these individuals to alter their behavior or even see the possibility for change at some point in the future. Consequently, people with depression have deeply held negative life views that tend to be based on cognitive distortions rather than reality (e.g., "I am a bad parent because I yelled at my child yesterday") (Potter & Moller, 2020).

Sociocultural Theory

Sociocultural theory emphasizes the role that social stressors play in the development of depression. These stressors take a variety of forms. Some are economic, such as poverty and job insecurity (Hyde & Mezulis, 2020). Others involve a disruption in the family system, such as divorce, children leaving home, or the death of a loved one. Many individuals experience stressful life events without developing a disorder. However, stressful events may trigger onset or relapse in an individual who is already at risk (Potter & Moller, 2020).

A number of factors influence the degree of stress that accompanies significant life events. **Figure 28.3 ››** illustrates the relationship between life events and depression. Factors that protect against the onset of a mood disorder include healthy coping behaviors and communication skills as well as the ability to access and use resources. Difficulties with problem solving, inability to use resources, negative self-perception, and a negative interpretation of significant events can increase an individual's risk for developing a mood disorder. Perception and interpretation of events may be informed by cultural or gender norms (Miller & Kirschbaum, 2019; Moorkath et al., 2019).

SAFETY ALERT Childhood sexual abuse (CSA) is a significant risk factor for depression during both childhood and adulthood, as well as for self-harming behaviors (e.g., cutting), posttraumatic stress disorder (PTSD), and suicide (Angelakis, Gillespie, & Panagioti, 2019; Humphreys et al., 2020). Depressed patients with a history of CSA should be assessed and closely monitored for self-harming and suicidal behaviors.

Risk Factors

Risk factors for depression include family history of depression or other mental illness, female gender, history of child abuse or trauma, unemployment, poverty, lower education, lack of social supports, and bullying (Kwong et al., 2019). Ksinan and Vazsonyi (2019) noted that genetics as well as environmental influences play a critical role in the development of depression. However, a genetic risk for developing depressive symptoms does not necessarily guarantee an individual will develop depression. Rather, genetics interacting with environmental stimuli (such as bullying or trauma) may result in the manifestation of depression.

›› **Skills:** See Skill 15.1 in Volume 3.

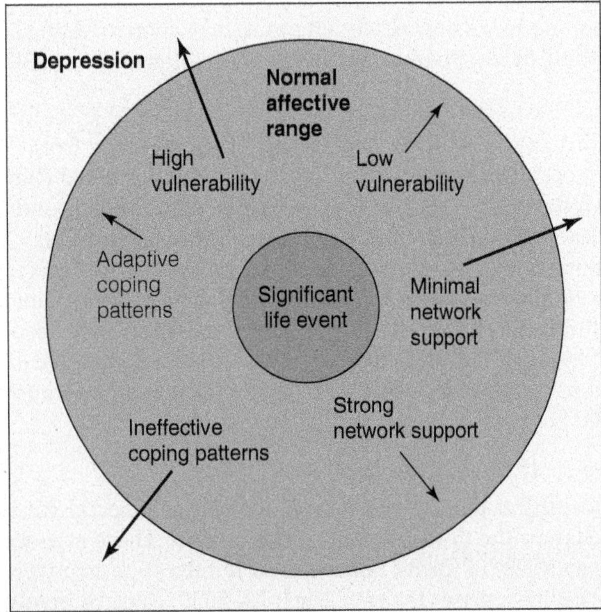

Figure 28.3 ›› The relationship between life events and depression.

Poverty and discrimination appear to increase risk for depression. Non-Hispanic Black adults experience depression at greater rates (9.2%) than other populations, with Asian adults experiencing the lowest rates of depression (3.1%) (CDC, 2018b). Adults living below the federal poverty level experience depression at almost five times the rate of those whose incomes are at or above 400% of the poverty level (15.8% vs. 3.5%) (CDC, 2018b).

Prevention

As discussed at the beginning of this module, there is no definitive way to prevent depression, because of causative and contributing genetic and biological factors that cannot be modified. However, a number of approaches can be useful in controlling these factors. Health promotion and primary prevention strategies include:

- Encouraging patients to eat a healthy diet, exercise regularly, obtain adequate sleep, and avoid smoking
- Educating patients about stress management and healthy coping
- Encouraging patients to participate in meaningful social relationships
- Providing targeted teaching and support to individuals who have experienced trauma or life-altering events
- Using family-based cognitive-behavioral interventions to reduce the likelihood of depression in children with depressed parents.

Secondary prevention strategies include regular screening, counseling patients about their relative risks for depression, and referring individuals with suspected depression for accurate diagnosis and treatment. Finally, tertiary prevention focuses on provision of collaborative care and establishment of community-focused programs that target depressed and high-risk individuals. For a detailed discussion of all of these prevention approaches, refer to the Health Promotion section within this module.

Clinical Manifestations

Some of the clinical manifestations of depression seem fairly obvious: sleep disturbances and feelings of sadness and despair, for example. Others may not be as obvious, such as anger and physical complaints. Manifestations of depression also can differ according to culture, especially if mental illness is stigmatized within the culture. Mental illness is often manifested by somatic symptoms such as headaches, GI discomfort, or sleep disturbances that may require assessment by a HCP. Some studies indicate that patients of Chinese heritage are more likely to report somatic symptoms when depressed than are European American patients (Chentsova-Dutton, Gold, Gomes, & Ryder, 2019). Depression is seen worldwide and is especially increased in conflict-affected populations. In conflict settings, such as countries at war, prevalence of depression and anxiety appears to increase with age (Charlson et al., 2019). It is important for nurses involved with patients with depression to know and recognize the symptoms.

Clinical Manifestations and Therapies

Depressive Disorders

DISORDER	CLINICAL MANIFESTATIONS	CLINICAL THERAPIES
Major depressive disorder	Symptoms must last 14 days or longer and may include: ▪ Feelings of sadness and hopelessness ▪ Somatic complaints such as pain, stomachaches ▪ Anxiety, anger, irritability ▪ Loss of interest in pleasurable activities ▪ Sleep disturbances	▪ Pharmacologic therapies include: • SSRIs, except fluvoxamine • TCAs, except clomipramine • Atypical antidepressants ▪ Electroconvulsive therapy (most often used for those who are resistant to treatment with medications) ▪ CBT
Adjustment disorder with depressed mood	Symptoms develop within 3 months in response to an identifiable stressor and may include: ▪ Insomnia, hypersomnia ▪ Crying ▪ Avoiding pleasurable activities ▪ Avoiding family and friends ▪ Ignoring financial responsibilities ▪ Performing poorly at work and school ▪ Fighting, behaving recklessly	▪ Improved sleep hygiene ▪ Short-term sedative ▪ CBT alone may be sufficient to help the individual return to normal ▪ Alternative therapies such as massage therapy may provide relief ▪ Antidepressant therapy ▪ CBT ▪ Family therapy
Persistent depressive disorder (dysthymic disorder)	Symptoms are not as severe as those of major depressive disorder, but last beyond 2 years with period of relief lasting less than 2 months.	▪ Pharmacologic therapies are the same as for MDD ▪ Electroconvulsive therapy (most often used for those who are resistant to treatment with medications) ▪ CBT
Seasonal affective disorder	Depressive symptoms occur in relation to the seasons; usually during the winter months, when days are shorter.	▪ Bupropion extended release ▪ Light therapy ▪ CBT

Major Depressive Disorder

A **major depressive episode** is characterized by a change in several aspects of an individual's emotional state and functioning consistently over a period of 14 days or longer. The most important factor is the patient's mood, which the patient may not describe in terms of "depression." Instead, the patient may describe feelings of sadness, discouragement, or hopelessness. Some patients may report vague somatic (physical) complaints such as aches and pains; other patients may report increased anger, frustration, and irritability, with uncharacteristic outbursts over minor matters. It is not difficult to imagine that someone who looks and feels sad or empty is depressed. A diagnosis of depression is more likely to be missed when an individual simply seems anxious or irritable.

Major depressive disorder (MDD) may consist of a single episode or may exhibit as recurrent major depression at various points in life. Signs and symptoms of single-episode and recurrent major depression are found in **Box 28.2** ». Onset of MDD generally occurs gradually, with symptoms progressing

Box 28.2

Symptoms of Major Depressive Disorder

- Significant distress or impairment of functioning
- Feelings of despair, hopelessness
- Sadness, crying
- Feelings of worthlessness, guilt
- Loss of self-esteem
- Loss of interest or pleasure in activities
- Substantial changes in weight or appetite over a short period of time
- Impairments in executive functioning (e.g., ability to plan, organize, solve problems, concentrate)
- Visible psychomotor agitation or retardation
- Aches and pains
- Excessive sleep loss or excessive sleeping
- Recurrent thoughts of death or suicide

Sources: Albert, Potter, Boyd, Kang, and Taylor (2019); American Psychiatric Association (2013); National Institute of Mental Health (2020a).

from anxiety and mild depression to a major depressive episode over a period of days, weeks, or months. The course of MDD is extremely variable, with some individuals experiencing remission for a period of months and others experiencing many years between episodes (APA, 2013). Individuals who experience MDD in the context of another disorder, such as substance use or borderline personality disorder, often experience symptoms that are more difficult to treat (APA, 2013). A diagnosis of MDD requires that the individual not have any previous episodes of mania or hypomania (which suggest a bipolar rather than a depressive disorder) and be free of any medical disorder that might otherwise explain the symptoms the individual is experiencing (e.g., dementia) (APA, 2013).

Individuals with a history of manic or hypomanic episodes are considered to have a bipolar disorder and are not classified under the categories of depressive disorders.

Individuals experiencing MDD often no longer enjoy activities that previously brought pleasure, such as hobbies, sports, and sex. This is a condition known as **anhedonia**. Changes in appetite, usually experienced as a reduction or loss of interest in food, are often seen, although increased appetite and cravings are also reported.

Sleep disturbances, particularly **insomnia** (inability to fall or stay asleep or, in some individuals, early-morning awakening), are common in individuals with depression. Two types of insomnia are most often experienced by people having a major depressive episode. *Middle insomnia* refers to waking up during the night and having difficulty falling asleep again. *Terminal insomnia* refers to waking at the end of the night and being unable to return to sleep. Depressed patients also may report **hypersomnia**, in which the individual sleeps for prolonged periods at night as well as during the day but still wakes up tired or fatigued. These sleep disturbances are discussed at length in Module 3, Comfort.

Fatigue and decreased energy are characteristic symptoms of depression. Individuals with depression may report being tired upon awakening regardless of how long they have slept. Even the smallest task seems insurmountable, and routine activities require substantial effort and take longer to accomplish. Decreased energy may be manifested in **psychomotor retardation**, in which thinking and body movements are noticeably slowed and speech is slowed or absent. Psychomotor agitation also may occur, in which the individual cannot sit still; paces; wrings the hands; and picks at the fingernails, skin, clothing, bedclothes, or other objects.

Other common symptoms in individuals with moderate to severe depression include guilt or a sense of worthlessness, self-blame, impaired concentration and decision-making ability (even about trivial things), and suicidal ideation (**Figure 28.4** »).

Persistent Depressive Disorder

The term **persistent depressive disorder**, also known as **dysthymia** or *dysthymic disorder*, describes chronic depression for the majority of most days for at least 2 years (1 year for children and adolescents). Throughout those 2 years, no more than 2 months can be described as symptom-free. The symptoms of dysthymic disorder, while distressing, tend to be less severe than those of MDD, with fewer physiologic symptoms, but the degree of impact on individual functioning can be as great or greater than that of MDD. Individuals with persistent depressive disorder are at higher risk for developing other mental health disorders than those with MDD (APA, 2013; Patel & Rose, 2019).

Persistent depressive disorder often occurs in childhood, adolescence, or early adulthood and tends to be chronic. Whereas both girls and boys are equally affected as children, there are two to three times as many adult women as men with dysthymic disorder. Factors that contribute to poorer long-term outcomes and increased risk for suicide include the presence of a comorbid anxiety or conduct disorder, greater symptom severity, and greater impairment in functioning (APA, 2013).

Seasonal Affective Disorder

Seasonal affective disorder (SAD) is not an official DSM diagnosis, but rather a specifier of MDD "with seasonal pattern." Individuals with SAD typically experience symptoms, including sadness and low energy, during the winter months, when daylight is shorter. Factors that increase a person's risk for SAD include female gender, age (with younger people being affected more often), and personal or family history of depression or bipolar disorder. Not surprisingly, the condition is also more common among people who live farther from the equator, where winters are longer (Forneris et al., 2019).

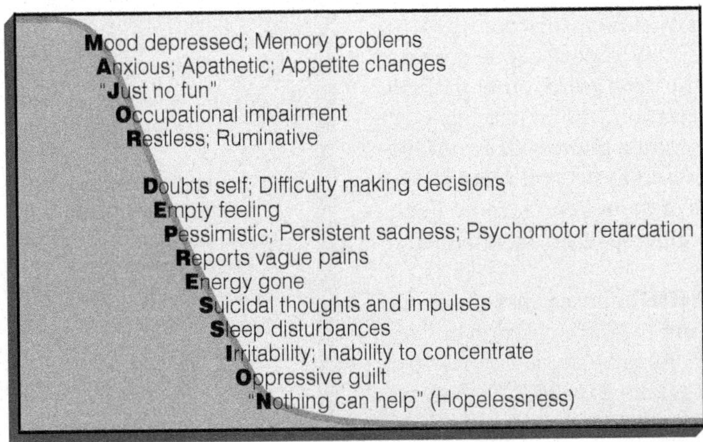

Mood depressed; Memory problems
Anxious; Apathetic; Appetite changes
"Just no fun"
Occupational impairment
Restless; Ruminative
Doubts self; Difficulty making decisions
Empty feeling
Pessimistic; Persistent sadness; Psychomotor retardation
Reports vague pains
Energy gone
Suicidal thoughts and impulses
Sleep disturbances
Irritability; Inability to concentrate
Oppressive guilt
"Nothing can help" (Hopelessness)

Figure 28.4 » Characteristics of major depression.

Seasonal affective disorder arises due to biological fluctuations triggered by decreased exposure to natural light. People with SAD have elevated levels of SERT, a protein involved in serotonin transport in the brain. SERT binds with serotonin, so higher SERT levels lead to lower serotonin activity. SERT levels are naturally suppressed by exposure to sunlight, so when days grow shorter during the winter months, affected individuals' SERT levels rise, causing their serotonin activity to decline and their depressive symptoms to increase. Evidence also indicates that individuals with SAD overproduce melatonin. Melatonin is a hormone secreted by the pineal gland that causes sleepiness. Melatonin production increases in all people in response to darkness, but levels are particularly elevated in patients with SAD. Together, decreased serotonin and increased melatonin cause disruptions in affected individuals' circadian rhythms (Menculini et al., 2018).

Pharmacologic approaches to the treatment of SAD generally involve extended-release bupropion (Aplenzin, Wellbutrin XL). Another common treatment approach is light therapy, also called phototherapy. With this approach, patients are exposed to a bright light that replicates natural outdoor lighting for 20 to 60 minutes each day. Light therapy is frequently the first-line treatment for SAD, as it generally has fewer adverse effects than drug therapy. Beyond pharmacologic and light therapy, counseling can also be useful in the treatment of SAD (Menculini et al., 2018).

Adjustment Disorder with Depressed Mood

Adjustment disorder with depressed mood represents a change in mood and affect following a stressor, such as the end of a relationship, or multiple stressors; it may also be called **situational depression**. Symptoms generally begin 3 months after the event and typically last no more than 6 months. Adjustment disorder with depressed mood is differentiated from an appropriate change in mood following a sad or stressful event in that the distress experienced by the patient is out of proportion to the event and results in significant impairment in functioning (APA, 2013).

Any life-altering event can create risk for the occurrence of adjustment disorder with depressed mood. This risk is further increased by a preexisting mental health issue, ineffective or unhealthy coping mechanisms, or lack of a support network. Patients with these preexisting conditions may find that adjustment disorder with depressed mood has exacerbated their condition. For example, in an attempt to diminish feelings of depression, a patient who has remained sober after a history of alcohol abuse may resume drinking as a coping mechanism following a stressful event.

Differentiating Depression from Grief

In some patients, depression and grief may present similarly on initial assessment. Nurses must distinguish whether a patient who exhibits sadness and anhedonia is depressed or grieving (**Table 28.2** »). Although this may appear to be easy, it can be difficult when working with new patients with whom the nurse has not yet developed a therapeutic relationship. Careful assessment includes determining if the feelings described by the patient were triggered by a loss or losses (such as the death of a family member).

Collaboration

Approximately 35% of people with depression do not seek treatment (NIMH, 2019). For those who do, many are treated in the community by a primary care provider or may go directly to a mental health provider for counseling but elect not to use prescription medications. In inpatient settings, nurses play an important role as a member of the interprofessional team that includes psychiatrists, social workers, occupational therapists, and other healthcare professionals. In outpatient settings, nurses may be the first HCP to screen or assess an individual for depression. In any setting, nurses play an important role in providing patient education about therapies, in answering questions, and in encouraging patients to follow their treatment regimens.

Diagnostic Tests

Although there is no diagnostic test to determine depression, primary care clinicians typically perform a complete medical history and thorough physical exam to rule out the possibility of an underlying medical condition causing the patient's depressive symptoms. If no physical causes are found, the clinician can start the patient on the depression "treatment cascade": recognizing the clinical illness, initiating treatment, and evaluating the patient's response to treatment (Jha et al., 2019). Existing medical conditions, such as diabetes, may inform selection of medication therapy if determined appropriate.

TABLE 28.2 Differences Between Depression and Grief[a]

Characteristic	Depression	Grief
Onset	May be gradual unless there is a specific trigger (e.g., trauma, change in medication)	Onset follows one or more losses
Affect/emotions	General feelings of hopelessness Sustained loss of pleasure, self-worth	General feelings of emptiness May come in waves Capacity to experience positive feelings remains Self-worth intact
Recovery	Will likely need clinical intervention to improve	Feelings may lessen, subside over time, and by participating in meaningful mourning or celebration practices, by returning to normal family and work life

[a]This table distinguishes depression from the experience of normal grieving. Prolonged grief disorder is described in Module 27, Grief and Loss.

Pharmacologic Therapy

Although SSRIs are the mainstay of treatment for depression due to their efficacy and safety, they may not work for some patients, and a period of trial and error may be necessary to find a medication that is effective for the patient. This can be a time of great frustration for patients who expect to "feel better" a few days after taking a drug, as many psychotropic medications take several weeks to reach efficacy. See **Medications 28.1**, Drugs Used to Treat Depression, for an overview of commonly used antidepressants.

A new approach for treatment-resistant depression is the use of esketamine. Current research indicates that esketamine given intranasally is a rapidly acting antidepressant for patients with treatment-resistant depression (Gautam, Mahajan, Sharma, Singh, & Singh, 2019; NIMH, 2019; Popova et al., 2019; Slomski, 2019). Twenty-four hours after administration, clinically significant improvements in depressive symptoms, including suicidality, were seen in the patients using esketamine (NIMH, 2019). These results lasted 4 to 7 days on average (Slomski, 2019). Gautam and colleagues (2019) note that, due to safety concerns such as a potential for abuse, esketamine is only administered through a restricted distribution system. When it is administered, a HCP must be present and the patient must be monitored, including blood pressure measurements, for at least 2 hours afterward, due to the risk of sedation and dissociation.

Medications 28.1

Drugs Used to Treat Depression

CLASSIFICATION AND DRUG EXAMPLES	MECHANISM OF ACTION	NURSING CONSIDERATIONS
Selective Serotonin Reuptake Inhibitors (SSRIs) ***Drug examples:*** citalopram (Celexa) escitalopram (Lexapro) fluoxetine (Prozac) fluvoxamine paroxetine (Paxil) sertraline (Zoloft) vilazodone (Viibryd) vortioxetine (Trintellix)	Slow the reuptake of serotonin into presynaptic nerve terminals. Increase the availability of serotonin in the synaptic cleft for postsynaptic receptors. ***Also used for:*** ■ Anxiety disorders (escitalopram, paroxetine) ■ Eating disorders (bulimia nervosa) (fluoxetine) ■ Obsessive–compulsive disorder (OCD) (fluoxetine, fluvoxamine, paroxetine, sertraline)	Take most SSRIs in the morning or evening, with or without food, except vilazodone (Viibryd), which should be taken with food to avoid GI upset. If the patient complains of feeling sedated or tired, the SSRI may be taken in the evening. St. John's wort and *Ginkgo biloba* may cause serotonin syndrome when taken with SSRIs. Provide patient teaching related to suicidal ideation and serotonin syndrome.
Atypical Antidepressants ***Drug examples:*** bupropion (Aplenzin, Wellbutrin)	Bupropion inhibits the uptake of dopamine and norepinephrine and elevates mood by increasing the levels of these neurotransmitters in the CNS. ***Also used for:*** ■ Smoking cessation	Bupropion should be used with caution in patients with seizure disorders because it lowers the seizure threshold. Monitor for increased suicidal thoughts or behavior.
nefazodone	Nefazodone inhibits the reuptake of serotonin and norepinephrine and blocks alpha$_1$ receptors.	Nefazodone is not for use in pediatric patients.
trazodone	Trazodone inhibits the reuptake of serotonin and blocks histamine and alpha$_1$ receptors.	Monitor for increased suicidal thoughts or behavior.
Serotonin–Norepinephrine Reuptake Inhibitors (SNRIs) ***Drug examples:*** desvenlafaxine (Pristiq) duloxetine (Cymbalta) levomilnacipran (Fetzima) venlafaxine (Effexor)	Inhibit the reabsorption of serotonin and norepinephrine and elevate mood by increasing the levels of serotonin, norepinephrine, and dopamine in the CNS. ***Also used for:*** ■ Anxiety disorders (duloxetine, venlafaxine) ■ Fibromyalgia, chronic musculoskeletal pain (duloxetine) ■ Neuropathic pain (duloxetine)	Monitor for serotonin syndrome and neuroleptic malignant syndrome–like reactions. Increased risk of hepatotoxicity. Instruct patient on changing positions slowly secondary to potential for orthostatic hypotension. Monitor for increased suicidal thoughts or behavior. Monitor for serotonin syndrome or neuroleptic malignant syndrome-like reactions.

Medications 28.1 *(continued)*

CLASSIFICATION AND DRUG EXAMPLES	MECHANISM OF ACTION	NURSING CONSIDERATIONS
Tricyclic Antidepressants (TCAs) ***Drug examples:*** amitriptyline amoxapine clomipramine (Anafranil) desipramine (Norpramin) doxepin (Silenor) imipramine nortriptyline (Pamelor) protriptyline trimipramine	Inhibit reuptake of both norepinephrine and serotonin at presynaptic nerve terminals. ***Also used for:*** ■ Anxiety (doxepin) ■ Childhood enuresis (imipramine) ■ Insomnia (doxepin) ■ OCD (clomipramine)	Enhance or reduce the effect of many different drugs. Monitor the patient's medication list for possible drug–drug interactions. Avoid eating grapefruit or grapefruit juice as it may prolong TCA effect and cause toxicity. Cause anticholinergic side effects of dry mouth, constipation, blurred vision, urinary retention. and increased heart rate. For patients over the age of 40, an ECG may be ordered prior to initiation of treatment to detect preexisting arrhythmias. TCAs are contraindicated in patients in the acute recovery phase of a myocardial infarction, with heart block, or with a history of dysrhythmias. TCAs lower the seizure threshold, so patients with epilepsy should be closely monitored. Patients with urinary retention, prostatic hypertrophy, or narrow-angle glaucoma may not be good candidates for TCAs.
Tetracyclic Antidepressants ***Drug examples:*** maprotiline mirtazapine (Remeron)	Work in different ways to affect norepinephrine, serotonin, and histamine.	Take mirtazapine at bedtime because it usually causes excessive drowsiness, especially at lower doses.
Monoamine Oxidase Inhibitors (MAOIs) ***Drug examples:*** isocarboxazid (Marplan) phenelzine (Nardil) selegiline (Zelapar) tranylcypromine (Parnate)	Inhibit monoamine oxidase, the enzyme that breaks down the neurotransmitters of dopamine, norepinephrine, epinephrine, and serotonin.	Monitor for increased suicidal thoughts or behavior. MAOIs interact with a number of foods and other medications—sometimes with serious effects. Hypertensive crisis can occur when an MAOI is used concurrently with other antidepressants or sympathomimetic drugs or with certain foods containing tyramine. MAOIs also potentiate the hypoglycemic effects of insulin and oral noninsulin drugs. Advise patient to wear a medic alert bracelet.

Source: Adapted from Adams, Holland, and Urban (2020).

Psychotherapy

Psychotherapy often is used in combination with medications to treat major depression. Some of the psychosocial problems associated with depression (e.g., ability to relate to others, motivation, problem-solving ability) cannot be resolved with medications. Psychotherapy promotes effective coping skills and positive, helpful patterns of thinking and behavior. Patients with mild depression may benefit from therapy alone. CBT is the most effective type of psychotherapy for depression.

Other Therapies

As discussed earlier in this module, ECT and integrative therapies may be appropriate for the patient diagnosed with depression. Another therapy, magnetic seizure therapy (MST), is being studied for efficacy. This treatment uses a magnetic pulse to stimulate the brain to induce a seizure, similar to ECT, but early results show fewer side effects than ECT and reduced recovery time. MSTs are shorter in duration and are thought to cause less cognitive loss after treatment (Daskalakis et al., 2020).

The nurse's role when working with patients receiving any type of therapy includes assessing for safety, assessing for potential contraindications, encouraging patient communication with all HCPs (e.g., primary care provider and mental health provider or therapist), and providing patient teaching related to types of therapies and the importance of adhering to the treatment plan.

Lifespan Considerations

Symptoms of depression can vary among age groups, although sadness and anhedonia are common at all ages. Treatment considerations also may vary.

Depressive Disorders in Children and Adolescents

Careful and thorough assessment of a child suspected of having depression is necessary to rule out physical illness that can be linked to depressive symptoms. Other tests, such as hearing and vision tests, may be indicated as well. It is essential to question parents, caregivers, or guardians regarding their observations of the child's behavior and recent changes or precipitating factors. Diagnostic evaluation must be performed by a child psychiatrist, psychiatric nurse practitioner, or other mental health professional experienced in the diagnosis and treatment of children and adolescents. A variety of scales and techniques are used; however, very little guidance is available relating to evaluation of children under 6 years of age. See the Concept section of this module for commonly used screening tools. Thorough assessment for both physical and mental health disorders is necessary because comorbidities (appearance with other disorders) are common. Examples of these include a history of bullying or substance abuse.

Depressive symptoms may vary with each age group:

Toddlers

May regress from independence to dependence in some activities (such as toileting)

Preschoolers

Increased irritability, whining

Destructive play themes

Lack of interest, lack of confidence related to activities

School-age children

Decreased academic performance

Changes in physical activity

Somatic complaints

Boredom

Talk of running away

Adolescents

Changes in peer groups, activities

Poor school performance

Decreased self-care

Increasing conflict with parents, teachers

See the section Lifespan Considerations: Mood and Affect in Children and Adolescents for additional information on treatment for depression in this population.

Depressive Disorders in Pregnant Women

Depression can occur at any time during or after the course of a woman's pregnancy. See Exemplar 28.C, Peripartum Depression, for a detailed outline of manifestations and treatment of women with peripartum depression.

Depressive Disorders in Older Adults

Depression is common among older adults, and it is important to note that it is not a normal part of aging. Manifestations of depression in older adults may include memory problems, social withdrawal, sleep disturbances, loss of appetite, and irritability. Some individuals may experience delusions or hallucinations. Depression in older adults can complicate treatment of other conditions because impairment of functioning due to depression may impair the individual's ability or motivation to participate in treatment. Other medical conditions can complicate treatment of depression if nurses and clinicians dismiss symptoms as related to another medical condition (or side effects of treatment) without doing a full assessment for depression.

Older adults are especially at risk for a depressive episode when they experience two or more stressors in proximity. Development of a disabling illness (whether cognitive, physical, or otherwise), loss of a loved one, retirement, moving out of the home, or another stressful event may result in a depressive episode in the older adult (NIMH, 2020a; Wei et al., 2019). Even those older adults who "see the glass as half full" are challenged by these types of stressors. The loss of driving privileges (due to physical or cognitive changes) is a huge loss to older adults, often putting a great deal of strain on family members who must accommodate the older adult who can no longer drive as well provide support as the individual learns to cope with this loss of independence.

Because of the increased risk older adults have for medical illness, careful assessment of the older adult is critical. Polypharmacy issues may make prescribing for older adults a challenge, and older adults taking psychotropic medications often require more frequent monitoring and laboratory tests (e.g., blood glucose levels). Lower starting doses are often recommended because older adults metabolize and excrete drugs at slower rates than younger adults. The Geriatric Depression Scale can be useful in screening older adults for depression and determining the need for further evaluation (Krishnamoorthy, Rajaa, & Rehman, 2020).

NURSING PROCESS

Priorities of nursing care focus on safety and meeting functional needs until the patient's condition improves. Risk of suicide must always be a consideration when caring for patients who are depressed. Patients with depression may not meet their daily hygiene, sleep, nutrition, or other needs. They are also at increased risk for accidental injury and medical illness. The nurse can initiate strategies to help them until they are able to function autonomously.

Assessment

Observation and Patient Interview

Assessment of patients with suspected depression begins with a thorough history and interview. Inquire about any past depressive, manic, or hypomanic episodes or behavior, as well as family history of mood disorders. Ask about and observe for the signs and symptoms discussed throughout the Concept section. Patients with depressive disorders may articulate any number of changes in mood and behavior: feelings of sadness, lack of interest in relationships and activities that previously brought pleasure, feelings of worthlessness or guilt, anxious distress, withdrawal, and/or social isolation. Patients may also articulate tearfulness and emotional outbursts.

Cognitive alterations are another frequent feature of depression. Be alert for signs or descriptions of problems such as impaired concentration, difficulty making decisions, poor memory, and impaired problem-solving ability. In severe cases, patients might also report or demonstrate paranoid thinking, delusions, and other forms of psychosis.

The interview and history portion of the assessment is also a good time to observe for difficulties with adaptive functioning. Patients will often describe how long it takes them to complete activities that they formerly accomplished easily, such as preparing a simple meal. They may also neglect regular grooming and hygiene tasks, either skip meals or eat excessively, and/or respond inappropriately to social cues.

Physical Examination

The next step in assessment is to consider the patient's physical manifestations; in fact, somatic concerns are often the presenting complaint. Among the most common problems are fatigue, sleep disturbances or excessive sleep, and changes in appetite and/or weight. Patients with depression may complain of abdominal pain, headaches, and vague body aches. A problem with sexual functioning or lack of desire also may be a presenting complaint. Constipation is a common result of the general slowing of metabolism due to inactivity. Patients from some cultures are more likely to express symptoms of depression through complaints about body function and discomfort. See **Box 28.3** ›› for information on how depression evidenced by somatic concerns can be detected in other settings. Possible medical problems that could be the cause of the patient's physical symptoms should always be investigated and ruled out before a diagnosis of depression is made.

Suicide Assessment

Assess all patients for suicide risk by using direct questioning. Ask whether the patient has thoughts of committing suicide (*suicidal ideation*), how often these thoughts occur, and whether or not the patient would act on these thoughts (intent). Inquire whether or not the patient has a plan regarding carrying out suicide (*plan/method*). If a plan exists, it is crucial to assess the lethality of the plan: degree of effort required, specificity of the plan, and accessibility of means to carry out the plan. Assess for history of prior suicide attempts or family history of suicide, as this signals increased risk. Note that asking about suicide will not "plant the idea" in the patient's mind. Rather, it is often a relief for the patient to be able to openly discuss these feelings and thoughts. See the Independent Interventions section and Exemplar 28.D, Suicide, in this module for more information.

Assess for Comorbidities

Assess for the presence of medical illnesses. This is important not only to rule out the possibility of an underlying medical condition causing the patient's symptoms of depression, but also to identify illnesses that may trigger depression. These include autoimmune, oncologic, metabolic, and endocrine disorders. Chronic illnesses, such as asthma and diabetes, are associated with increased risk of depression. A diagnosis of a chronic or life-threatening illness may also trigger a depressive episode.

Assessment of comorbidities includes assessing for substance use. Alcohol and other substances that act as CNS depressants can complicate depression. Co-occurring depression and substance use can complicate recovery from both conditions.

Assess use of prescription and OTC medications and supplements to determine if the patient is taking anything that may have depression as a side effect (such as corticosteroids or beta adrenergic blockers).

Diagnosis

Care priorities that may be appropriate for patients with depression, include the following:

- Risk of suicide, self-harm
- Situational or chronic low self-esteem
- Hopelessness
- Social isolation
- Inadequate health maintenance
- Inadequate coping skills.

Planning

When planning care, the nurse's immediate priority should be to ensure that patients with depression remain free from injury and refrain from attempts to hurt themselves or others. Other high-priority goals include alleviating any acute symptoms, ensuring adequate nutritional intake, and promoting restful sleep. Then, together with the patient, the

Box 28.3

Physical Complaints and Depression

There is a strong correlation between physical complaints (i.e., headaches, back and neck pain, and abdominal pain) and depression. The specific cause of pain experienced in depressive disorders is unknown; however, physical issues are often exacerbated when depression is present, and depression and chronic illnesses have a direct impact on functional disability (Ferenchick, Ramanuj, & Pincus, 2019; Yanartaş et al., 2019). Research suggests that somatic pain is related to both psychological and neurobiological factors (Yanartaş et al., 2019). Somatic symptoms in depression can cause poorer patient outcomes, leading to higher healthcare utilization and increased healthcare costs (Yanartaş et al., 2019). More than two-thirds of patients diagnosed with depression express concerns with somatic symptoms and reports of pain (Yanartaş et al., 2019). Approximately 69-percent of patients experiencing physical complaints from undiagnosed depression are seen in the primary care setting (Yanartaş et al., 2019). It is important for providers to pay careful attention to physical complaints and screen for depressive symptoms.

›› **Skills:** See Skill 3.1 in Volume 3.

nurse should design a plan of care that may include any of the following objectives:

- The patient will engage in necessary daily self-care activities (e.g., eating three meals a day, wearing clean clothes, and bathing regularly).
- The patient will resume normal activities.
- The patient will seek and engage in meaningful social interactions.
- The patient will articulate taking steps to restore health and well-being, such as returning to previously enjoyed activities or engaging in exercise once feeling better, or engaging in recreational activities or exercise *before* beginning to feel better.
- The patient will adhere to the treatment regimen.
- The patient will report a reduction in depressive symptoms, a reduction in thoughts of suicide, and increasing feelings of hopefulness and positivity.

Implementation

When providing nursing care for patients with depression, nurses must recognize that an overly cheerful attitude can be unhelpful, as patients may perceive this as the nurse minimizing their feelings or complaints. Maintaining a confident but emotionally neutral attitude will promote patients' trust in the nurse. Similarly, working with patients with depression can bring down the nurse's mood, an effect called *emotional contagion*. Nurses should engage in critical self-awareness and take appropriate actions to reduce burnout.

Interventions to address risk for suicide and self-harm are detailed in Exemplar 28.D. For patients with severe depression who manifest acute symptoms and altered thought processes, the nurse will facilitate pharmacologic and collaborative therapies as ordered; assess and facilitate orientation to person, place, time, and circumstance; promote adequate nutrition and rest; and take other actions to promote recovery such as reducing environmental stimuli and other potential triggers of anxiety.

Many patients with depression experience problems with self-esteem and social interaction as a result of their illness. Progression toward recovery requires that patients address these areas. Nursing interventions to promote self-esteem and social interaction follow.

Promote Healthy Self-Esteem

Nursing actions to improve self-esteem can reduce negative thinking and promote patient empowerment.

- Encourage patient participation in social and recreational activities. Be sure that activities are appropriate for the patient's cognitive and physical abilities. As the patient engages in the activities, negative thoughts will be interrupted. Promote activities that will allow the patient to experience success. See the Patient Teaching feature for more information.
- Make positive, general observations while interacting with the patient, such as "I notice that you got out of bed and showered today," rather than overly energetic compliments such as, "You look great today!" Generalized recognitions and observances increase the probability that the patient will continue with these behaviors. Avoid excessive praise and enthusiasm, as these comments can be perceived as infantizing.
- Allow the patient to express negative emotions and be accepting of them but set limits on the amount of time the patient dwells on and discusses negativity. Attempt to redirect negative thought and conversation patterns and replace them with more neutral ones.
- Teach assertiveness techniques. Patients with low self-esteem can have difficulty advocating for themselves and therefore tend to be taken advantage of. Patients who use assertive communication techniques can feel empowered and improve self-esteem. Allow patients to practice these techniques and provide feedback to patients, allowing them to express their feelings about utilizing assertiveness in communication.

Instill Hope

Instilling hope is an important part of the nurse–patient therapeutic relationship. The nurse can assist the patient to identify personal aspects that *cannot* be changed to bring about positive change and overcome feelings of hopelessness. Other interventions to help patients overcome hopelessness include the following:

- Assist patients to identify personal strengths. Although patients may find this task difficult at first, be patient with them and allow time for self-reflection. Some patients find it helpful to make a list of their identified strengths. Patients who identify strengths can better engage in care planning and take an active approach to their recovery process.
- Help patients be independent with decision making. Patients can increase self-esteem by actively making decisions and taking responsibility for their choices.
- Assist patients to problem-solve (**Table 28.3** »). Help patients identify a situation that was problematic. Ask open-ended questions to foster alternative solutions to the problem. For example: "You said that you locked your keys in the car and called your husband and started to yell

Patient Teaching

Increasing Self-Esteem

Patients often believe that *when* they feel better, they will want to engage in activities. For patients who express this belief, implement patient teaching and explain that the patient must begin doing things *in order* to feel better. Being active promotes a more balanced feeling state. Encourage the patient to acknowledge that it takes self-discipline and energy to do something when he does not really feel like it. Other strategies that may help the patient increase self-esteem include helping the patient to set daily, weekly, and monthly goals that are easily achievable, which is likely to improve the patient's self-esteem as each goal is met. As self-esteem improves, the goals should become increasingly harder to meet but still achievable.

TABLE 28.3 Promoting Patient Problem-Solving Skills

Patient Statement	Nurse Response	Rationale
"I feel like I am a failure. I lost my job, and I know I'll never find a new one. I will be homeless and living on the streets."	"You seem anxious about being unemployed right now. Have you ever lost a job before?"	Recognizing feelings and identifying similar past experiences. Patients can often relate current negative situations to past experiences. The nurse helps the patient explore how past stressors were overcome and apply techniques that worked previously to the current situation.
"Yes. About 5 years ago, my company was downsized."	"Can you tell me what you did after that job loss?"	The nurse uses open-ended questions and explores patient actions to deal with past negative experiences.
"Well, I felt terrible, but I looked online for jobs and sent out my resumé to a couple of different places."	"What was the result of that?"	The nurse helps the patient identify outcomes of past actions.
"After a few days, I got called in for an interview, and then I was offered the job."	"So you were able to find another job before by looking online and sending out your resumé. Do you think those actions would work for you again?"	The nurse restates the outcome and asks the patient to reflect on the current situation.
"I don't know. Maybe. I could try. It did work before."	"I believe that based on your previous experiences with finding a job, you will be able to find another. What can you do right now to help you feel better about losing your job?"	The nurse instills hope and assists the patient to develop a plan based on past experiences and past positive coping behaviors. The patient can explore with the nurse further steps to take to deal with the current situation.
"I think I could start to look online for jobs I could apply for."		

at him, and then he hung up on you. What could you do differently next time that could have a better outcome?"

- Help patients to identify support sources. Family, friends, and community connections can assist patients to overcome problems.

Because hopeless patients can be dependent on others for many needs, it is important to begin discharge planning immediately, upon first contact with the patient. Helping patients and family members identify support systems such as community, social, and therapy groups can ease anxieties and help the patient become more independent upon discharge.

Evaluation

Evaluation is based on the patient's ability to meet predetermined outcomes. These outcomes should be individualized to meet each patient's specific circumstances. Examples of goal-based outcomes for patients with depression include:

- The patient does not express suicidal ideation or a desire to harm self or others.
- The patient is free from acute symptoms.
- The patient obtains adequate nutrition and sleep.
- The patient meets daily self-care needs.
- The patient resumes normal activities.
- The patient participates in meaningful social interactions.
- The patient adheres to the treatment regimen.

Secondary interventions will need to be initiated if goals are not met with the current plan of care. Explore reasons that goals were not met, such as unresolved stressors, lack of adherence to the treatment regimen, or the possibility that a comorbid mental illness or an underlying medical condition has not been identified. If there are no identifiable causes of poor response to treatment, then secondary interventions will need to be implemented. These may include giving the patient additional time to allow the medication to take effect or to meet a goal or working with the treatment team to find a different medication or treatment approach.

REVIEW Depression

RELATE Link the Concepts and Exemplars

Linking the exemplar of depressive disorders with the concept of addiction:

1. Why might dependence on alcohol promote depression?
2. What impact might dependence on nicotine have on mood and affect?

Linking the exemplar of depressive disorders with the concept of elimination:

3. What aspects of depression increase the risk for constipation?
4. How might alterations in elimination put an older patient at risk for depression?

READY Go to Volume 3: Clinical Nursing Skills

REFLECT Apply Your Knowledge

Melvin Thomas is a 14-year-old boy whose mother brings him to their family physician's office because this is the third day in a row that Melvin "hasn't felt well." He has been getting in trouble at school for arguing with teachers, and he has missed a lot of school, complaining of stomachaches. Melvin's mother says that he rarely sees his dad but that her second husband tries to spend time with him when he can. When they do spend time together, they go shooting at the gun range or play video games. Melvin's expression at the physician's office is sullen, and he keeps his arms crossed in front of him. He answers the nurse by giving one-syllable responses or by nodding or shaking his head.

1. What assessment findings would make you suspect Melvin is depressed?
2. What priority teaching would you want to provide Melvin's mother if the diagnosis of depression is confirmed?
3. What impact is depression having on Melvin's ability to meet developmental milestones?

›› Exemplar 28.B Bipolar Disorders

Exemplar Learning Outcomes

28.B Analyze bipolar disorders and relevant nursing care.

- Describe the pathophysiology of bipolar disorders.
- Describe the etiology of bipolar disorders.
- Compare the risk factors and prevention of bipolar disorders.
- Identify the clinical manifestations of bipolar disorders.
- Summarize diagnostic tests and therapies used by interprofessional teams in the collaborative care of an individual with bipolar disorder.
- Differentiate care of patients with bipolar disorder across the lifespan.
- Apply the nursing process in providing culturally competent care to an individual with bipolar disorder.

Exemplar Key Terms

Bipolar disorders, *1982*
Cyclothymic disorder, *1984*
Flight of ideas, *1983*
Hypomania, *1983*

Overview

The **bipolar disorders** are a group of mood disorders that are characterized by manic, hypomanic, and depressive episodes. Cyclothymic disorder, a related disorder, is characterized by alternating periods of hypomanic and depressive symptoms that are not significant enough to meet the criteria for hypomania or depression. Although only about 2.8% of the population is diagnosed with bipolar disorders, these types of disorders can have a tremendous impact on patients and those closest to them (NIMH, 2017b).

Pathophysiology

No definitive cause or specific pathophysiology has been identified for bipolar spectrum disorders. Rather, they are thought to arise from a complex combination of genetic, physiologic, environmental, and psychosocial factors, with genetics being a strong predisposing factor (Kalman et al., 2019). Studies have not found significant evidence proving that bipolar disorder is localized to a specific area of the brain. However, studies in adults have found that there is a connection between bipolar disorder and cerebellar dysfunctions in emotion and motor processing regions of the brain (Johnson et al., 2018). Furthermore, Johnson and colleagues (2018) noted that altered function and/or structure in the basal ganglia and cerebellum, along with altered metabolic functioning in these regions, could possibly contribute to manifestations of different mood states in bipolar disorder.

Children of parents with bipolar disorders have an increased risk of having a bipolar disorder. Stressful life events (especially suicide of a family member), sleep-cycle disruptions, family or caregivers with high expressed emotion, and an emotionally overinvolved, hostile, and critical communication pattern are factors associated with heritability. Bipolar disorders, schizophrenia, and major depressive disorders share biological susceptibility and inheritance patterns. Several genes and loci have been discovered that may be associated with bipolar disorders (Kalman et al., 2019; Khanzada, Butler, & Manzardo, 2017; Medline Plus, 2020).

Bipolar I disorder consists of one or more manic or mixed episodes, and the course of illness is usually accompanied by major depressive episodes. *Bipolar II disorder* consists of one or more major depressive episodes accompanied by at least one hypomanic episode.

Etiology

Age of onset varies. Many individuals with bipolar disorder may go undiagnosed in the absence of a documented manic episode. Later diagnosis, more severe depressive symptoms, comorbid psychiatric conditions, and irritability are associated with greater functional impairment and poor quality of life (Singh, 2019; Sylvia et al., 2017). This supports the need to examine the patient's history over time, not just the history of the current exacerbation or presenting problem. Early assessment for history of manic symptoms in a patient presenting with depression may lead to more accurate and timely diagnosis of bipolar disorder (Ozten & Erol, 2019; Singh, 2019).

Risk Factors and Prevention

Risk factors for bipolar disorders include family history of bipolar disorder or other mental illness; history of adverse childhood experiences, especially abuse or neglect; prenatal viral infections; and substance use or abuse (especially cannabis) (Rowland & Marwaha, 2018). The risk for developing bipolar disorder is similar in men and women. Women tend to experience more rapid cycling and depressive symptoms, whereas men are more at risk for comorbid substance abuse (Mahmound et al., 2019; Ragazan, Eberhard, Ösby, &

Clinical Manifestations and Therapies

Bipolar Disorders

SYMPTOM CATEGORY	CLINICAL MANIFESTATIONS	CLINICAL THERAPIES
Mania/manic episode	Characterized by elevated, expansive, or irritable mood and increased activity or energy that significantly impairs social or occupational functioning and is accompanied by at least three of the following: ■ Increased self-esteem ■ Decreased need for sleep ■ Pressured speech ■ Flight of ideas ■ Distractibility ■ Increased involvement in goal-directed activities ■ Psychomotor agitation ■ Excessive involvement in pleasurable activities that carry a high risk of painful consequences	■ Assess for safety. ■ Administer mood stabilizers such as lithium. ■ Remove or limit environmental stimuli. ■ Set limits; teach limit setting. ■ Orient to self, place, and time.
Hypomania	■ Less extreme than mania; individuals describe themselves as feeling "wonderful" and do not recognize changes in their behavior, although friends and family can observe changes	■ Assess for safety. ■ Administer mood stabilizers such as lithium. ■ Remove or limit environmental stimuli. ■ Set limits or teach limit setting.
Depressed episode	■ Symptoms of depression	■ Assess for safety. ■ Administer antidepressant with mood stabilizer.

Berge, 2019). There is no prevention for bipolar disorders. As mentioned previously, early identification and treatment are associated with better quality of life and greater overall functionality.

Clinical Manifestations

Manifestations vary by type of bipolar disorder. Nurses in all settings should be able to recognize these manifestations, understand and differentiate between manic or hypomanic and depressive periods, and provide patient and family teaching about symptoms and treatments.

Key Diagnostic Criteria

The DSM-5 diagnostic criteria for bipolar disorder include criteria for manic, hypomanic, and major depressive episodes. At least one manic episode is necessary to make a diagnosis of bipolar disorder. The criteria for major depressive episodes are the same as the criteria for diagnosing major depressive disorder (see Box 28.2). The DSM-5 characterizes manic episodes as (APA, 2013):

- Lasting most of the day, every day, for at least 1 week, or any duration if hospitalization is required
- Including symptoms and behaviors that impair functioning in one or more domains (e.g., cognitive, social, occupational). Symptoms commonly seen in periods of mania include pressured speech, altered thought processes (such as racing thoughts), psychomotor agitation, grandiosity, increased goal-directed activity, and sleep disturbances (unable to sleep).

As with MDD (and any other mental disorder), the symptoms cannot be attributed to an underlying medical illness or to a substance or toxin. An individual experiencing hypomania does not experience impairment in functioning or require hospitalization. In the absence of mania, the individual with hypomania may be diagnosed with bipolar II disorder if other criteria are met (APA, 2013).

Mania and Hypomania

Mania is characterized by an abnormal and persistently elevated, expansive, or irritable mood and increased energy (or activity) present for most of the time, nearly every day, for a week or more and accompanied by specific symptoms as articulated in the DSM-5 and summarized above. **Flight of ideas** (rapidly changing, fragmented thoughts), pressured speech patterns, and increasing goal-directed activities are common during manic episodes. Psychotic symptoms such as delusions or hallucinations may be a feature of severe mania.

Hypomania refers to a mood that is "hypo" or under mania, meaning that the mood state is not as high or elated as mania, but more elevated than normal, or euthymic, mood. In hypomania, individuals express feeling good, having increased energy and focus, and can become easily irritated. While behavioral changes are obvious to others around them, those with hypomania do not recognize these changes. The behaviors in hypomania are not severe enough to require hospitalization and do not have any psychotic symptoms.

Stressors, such as going off to college or facing severe disappointments, can trigger manic episodes. The age of onset is typically late adolescence or early 20s. Patients who experience mania will have high, euphoric moods, flight of ideas, and pressured speech. Their behaviors may be very impulsive and risky and include delusional thinking, such as believing that they are invincible. This type of delusional thinking is known as grandiosity. Patients with mania may engage in many projects that are religious, political, or social in nature and can easily become irritated when they believe someone is interfering with these projects. Hypersexual behaviors are also common during a manic episode. The patient may be involved in flirting, dressing in a seductive manner, wearing heavy makeup, or having high-risk, inappropriate sexual relationships. Poor financial decisions and reckless spending are also characteristics of mania. Typically, patients exhibit poor insight and judgment and do not believe they are sick or need treatment. The characteristics of a manic episode are illustrated in **Figure 28.5** ».

Depressive Episodes

A diagnosis of bipolar disorder does not always mean that manic or hypomanic behaviors will be manifested in the current episode of illness. Bipolar I and bipolar II disorder are characterized by periods of mania/hypomania alternating with major depressive episodes. Mood stabilizers are the drug of choice, so it is important when assessing patients who present with depression to determine if the patient has ever had a manic or hypomanic episode. Antidepressant medications should be used with care, at low doses, and only during the severe depressive episode to reduce the chance of switching to a manic state.

Mixed Features

An individual who has bipolar disorder *with mixed features* may experience depression accompanied by mania or hypomania or may experience some depressive symptoms during a manic or hypomanic episode.

Rapid Cycling

Rapid cycling refers to four or more periods of alternating mania/hypomania and depression within a year. Some individuals may experience episodes more than once a week or even more than once in the same day (Aedo et al., 2018). Rapid cycling is associated with greater functional impairment (Aedo et al., 2018).

Cyclothymic Disorder

Cyclothymic disorder, or *cyclothymia*, is defined as a persistent mood disorder characterized by numerous periods of depressive symptoms alternating with periods of hypomania (APA, 2013). Cyclothymia has an early onset, and anxious and impulsive behaviors are common, as is labile mood (Perugi et al., 2017). These symptoms persist for at least 2 years but do not have the severe symptoms that qualify for the diagnosis of mania or major depressive disorder. **Figure 28.6** » compares mood in MDD, bipolar disorders, dysthymia, and cyclothymia. The incidence is mostly equal between males and females; however, females typically seek treatment more than males (APA, 2013; NIH, 2018).

Collaboration

Bipolar disorders are among those disorders classified as serious mental illnesses, and interprofessional, collaborative care is necessary for most patients to achieve stability. Patients will benefit from care that includes a nurse case manager, a nurse or nurses, the primary care provider, a mental health specialist, and other providers as appropriate. The nurse should work with the patient to track changes in feelings or behaviors, especially when starting a new medication or treatment. Early identification of triggers as well as helping the patient and family determine healthy ways to expend energy during manic episodes can be helpful and promote safety. Treatment focus goes beyond symptom reduction: the interprofessional team works together to help the patient on the path to recovery, which includes greater quality of life, better overall physical and mental health, and greater ability to function independently.

Unfortunately, functional recovery takes time for many patients. Many patients continue to experience symptoms between episodes. Interepisode (or residual) depression is associated with more frequent relapse, greater disability, and increased risk for suicide (Roux et al., 2017; Serafini et al., 2018). Nonadherence is common due to a variety of factors,

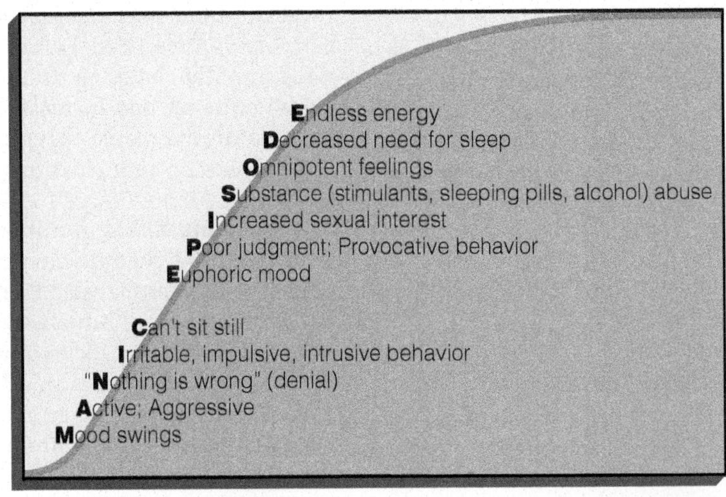

Figure 28.5 » Characteristics of a manic episode.

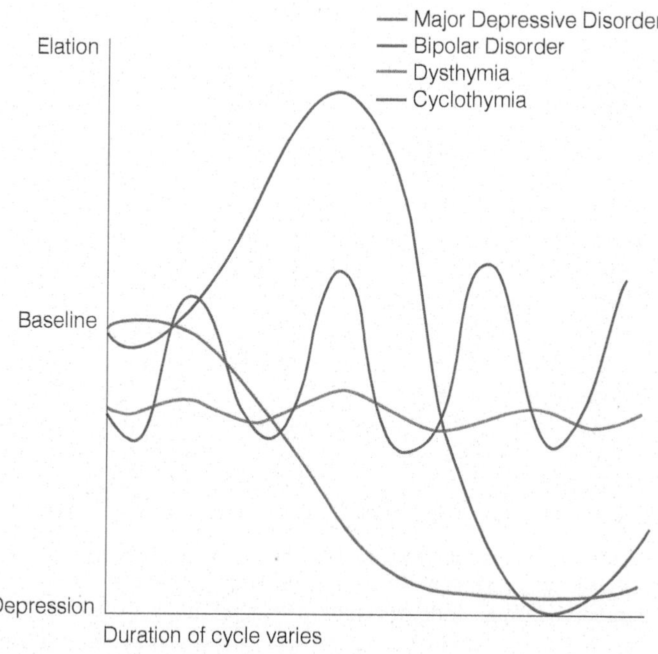

Figure 28.6 » Comparison of affect (mood) in major depressive disorder, bipolar disorder, dysthymia, and cyclothymia.

including access to appropriate care, severity of illness, poor insight into the illness, medication side effects, poor social and family support, and cognitive disturbances characteristic of bipolar disorders (Potter & Moller, 2020). Nurses play an important role in identifying barriers and solutions to issues of adherence.

Diagnostic Tests

There is no diagnostic test to determine bipolar and related disorders. Diagnosis is made on the basis of clinical manifestations and patient history. A physical examination, which may include drug testing, assists in ruling out the possibility of an underlying medical condition or substance as the source of the patient's symptoms.

Pharmacologic Therapy

Mood stabilizers and antipsychotics are the first-line treatments for mania (see **Medications 28.2,** Drugs Used to Treat Bipolar Disorders). Lithium, aripiprazole (Abilify), risperidone (Risperdal), and olanzapine (Zyprexa) are commonly used. Because lithium can take up to 3 weeks to take effect, administering an atypical antipsychotic can help manage symptoms until the lithium starts working. Antidepressant use in general is controversial, and current research indicates

Medications 28.2

Drugs Used to Treat Bipolar Disorders

CLASSIFICATION AND DRUG EXAMPLES	MECHANISM OF ACTION	NURSING CONSIDERATIONS
Mood Stabilizers ***Drug example:*** lithium (Lithobid)	Lithium's precise mechanism of action is not fully understood. It reduces excitatory neurotransmitters (dopamine and glutamate) but increases the inhibitory neurotransmitter (GABA), leading to mood stabilization.	Monitor blood levels because of narrow therapeutic range (0.6–1.2 mEq/dL). Initially, monitor levels weekly and then every 1–3 months once stabilized. Monitor for signs and symptoms of toxicity: *Mild toxicity:* GI upsets, thirst, fatigue, polyuria, fine hand tremors *Moderate toxicity:* Confusion, poor coordination, coarse tremors, persistent vomiting, diarrhea *Severe toxicity:* Extreme polyuria, blurred vision, tinnitus, ataxia, seizures, severe hypotension; may lead to coma and possible death Baseline labs prior to treatment: renal function, thyroid function, ECG, and (in women) pregnancy test. Subsequently, renal and thyroid function should be checked every 6 months. It may take 2–3 weeks to see improvement of symptoms. Weight gain is common; promote healthy eating and regular exercise. Do not use concurrently with NSAIDs, as this can increase absorption of lithium and cause toxicity. Thiazide diuretics are contraindicated with lithium, as they cause sodium excretion, which can lead to toxicity. Educate patients to avoid any change in their sodium intake, as this can cause lithium levels to fluctuate. Strenuous, constant exercise and sweating can lead to toxicity. Notify HCP immediately if pregnant or thinking about becoming pregnant. Emphasize the importance of adhering to blood work to check lithium levels.

(continued on next page)

Medications 28.2 *(continued)*

CLASSIFICATION AND DRUG EXAMPLES	MECHANISM OF ACTION	NURSING CONSIDERATIONS
Antiseizure Drugs ***Drug examples:*** carbamazepine (Equetro, Tegretol) lamotrigine (Lamictal) valproic acid (Depakote)	Block sodium channels and suppress the release of glutamate and aspartate, two of the main excitatory neurotransmitters in the CNS. Also increase GABA, leading to decreased neuronal excitation.	Monitor bloodwork to ensure a therapeutic level. Weight gain is common; promote a healthy diet and exercise. Can cause a serious skin rash (Stevens-Johnson syndrome). Report signs of a rash immediately. Each of these drugs can cause leukopenia, thrombocytopenia, and/or anemia. Baseline labs should be drawn. Report signs of infection and/or bruising. Patient should notify HCP immediately if pregnant or thinking about becoming pregnant. Carbamazepine can decrease the effects of oral contraceptives; alternative forms of contraception should be advised. Each of these drugs can cause hepatotoxicity. Baseline labs should be done and periodically monitored. Report signs of anorexia, fatigue, abdominal pain, and jaundice. Avoid drinking grapefruit juice with carbamazepine. Taking warfarin with carbamazepine can increase the metabolism of warfarin. Dosages may need to be adjusted.
Atypical Antipsychotic Drugs ***Drug examples:*** aripiprazole (Abilify) asenapine (Saphris) olanzapine (Zyprexa) quetiapine (Seroquel) risperidone (Risperdal) ziprasidone (Geodon)	Block dopamine D_2 receptors in the dopaminergic pathways of the brain. These drugs also act as serotonin antagonists. ***Also used for:*** ▪ Treatment-resistant depression (aripiprazole, olanzapine, quetiapine) ▪ Psychosis/psychotic disorders (including schizophrenia) (aripiprazole, asenapine, brexpiprazole(Rexulti), clozapine (Clozaril), paliperidone (Invega), quetiapine, risperidone, ziprasidone) ▪ Irritability with autism (aripiprazole, risperidone) ▪ Tourette disorder (aripiprazole)	Obtain a baseline weight and abdominal circumference as weight gain is common (50–100 lb), especially with olanzapine. Encourage a healthy diet and exercise. A baseline ECG is needed. Risperidone and quetiapine can cause QT prolongation. Obtain a baseline prolactin level for patients taking risperidone, as it may increase the prolactin level. Sexual dysfunction is common and can be managed by dosage adjustments. Orthostatic hypotension can occur. Teach the patient to change positions slowly to avoid falls. Concurrent use of anticholinergic medications like antihistamines can increase these side effects (dry mouth, urinary retention, blurry vision, agitation).

Source: Adapted from Adams et al. (2020).

that older classes of antidepressants like TCAs may have more risk to potentiate mania (Gitlin, 2018).

Nursing interventions include monitoring patients for adverse side effects of antipsychotic medications. These include extrapyramidal effects such as Parkinson-like symptoms (e.g., rigidity, tremor, or "pill rolling" movements of the fingers); dystonia, which is abnormal tonic contractions of the muscles (muscle spasms); and akathisia (subjective need to move, "jumping out of my skin"). Extrapyramidal symptoms should be reported and are usually treated by administration of an anticholinergic medication such as benztropine (Cogentin), diphenhydramine (Benadryl), or trihexyphenidyl (Artane). Acute dystonic reactions may be severe and require immediate medical intervention. These side effects can be distressing to the patient. The nurse must reassure the patient and explain what is occurring.

SAFETY ALERT For patients with bipolar disorder, the orally disintegrating form of olanzapine may be prescribed to reduce instances of "med cheeking," where patients hide the tablet in their mouth or cheek until they can dispose of it. Valproic acid comes in liquid form, which can also assist with prevention of "med cheeking."

Several psychopharmacologic agents have proven effective in the long-term treatment of mania. One effective and widely used agent is lithium carbonate.

Lithium Carbonate

Lithium is an inorganic compound. Also referred to as lithium salts, lithium is very similar to potassium and sodium as it interacts on the cellular level to alter the production and reuptake of certain neurotransmitters. The exact mechanism of action of lithium is unknown. The FDA approved lithium carbonate in 1970 for managing bipolar disorder and, until recently, it was the first-line drug of choice. However, due to many side effects and the need for continual bloodwork, other medications have replaced lithium as first-line treatments for patients with more depressive types of bipolar disorder (Mandal, Mamidipalli, Mukherjee, & Hara, 2019; Woo et al., 2020). It is still highly considered as a drug of choice for those who experience euphoria and mania, as seen in bipolar I disorder (Woo et al., 2020).

There are many factors to consider when prescribing lithium to patients. Lithium should not be considered for those who are pregnant or breastfeeding, have significant renal or cardiovascular disease, are on sodium-restricted diets or take diuretics, regularly take NSAIDs, or have untreated hypothyroidism. Typically, it takes 1 to 3 weeks to see the effects of lithium. During these first weeks, it is important to have bloodwork done to carefully monitor the levels, as there is a narrow therapeutic range (0.6 to 1.2 mEq/L).

Patients who take lithium are at high risk for toxicity because the difference between harmful and therapeutic lithium levels is quite small. Thus, patients' serum lithium levels should be determined prior to beginning drug therapy. Symptoms of lithium toxicity can begin at blood levels of 1.5 mEq/L. Due to this narrow therapeutic window, serum concentrations must be monitored frequently until stabilized and then regularly throughout treatment.

Note also that what is considered a therapeutic level for one patient might produce toxic effects in another patient. Accordingly, individual responses to specific lithium doses must be carefully documented (Bozkurt et al., 2018). For example, individuals of Asian descent may respond to lower doses and blood levels of lithium and therefore may experience toxicity at lower dosages than white patients (Quan et al., 2015). Monitor therapeutic effect as well as side effects. See the Patient Teaching feature for an overview of guidance for patients taking lithium.

Patient Teaching

Lithium

The nurse should provide patients who take lithium with information related to their medication, including:

Take medication as ordered.

Keep all scheduled laboratory appointments to check lithium levels.

Check with the HCP before changing your diet or decreasing your fluid intake, as this can affect lithium levels.

Consult with your HCP before taking any other prescription drugs, OTC medications, or supplements.

Do not discontinue use except under the guidance of your HCP.

Antiseizure Medications

Medications used to treat seizures are often prescribed in combination with lithium or antipsychotic medications. Agents commonly used in the treatment of mania include valproic acid (Depakote), lamotrigine (Lamictal), and carbamazepine (Tegretol). Side effects associated with antiseizure medications include drowsiness, fatigue, and weight gain. Typically, these side effects will decrease over time, but blood levels for some drugs must be regularly monitored to ensure that the patient is not experiencing toxicity. Pregnant women should not take these medications unless under the care of a HCP. Caution patients not to discontinue these medications abruptly, but to consult with their prescribing provider regarding how to taper off gradually.

Atypical Antipsychotics

Aripiprazole (Abilify), olanzapine (Zyprexa), quetiapine (Seroquel), risperidone (Risperdal), asenapine (Saphris), and ziprasidone (Geodon) are among the atypical antipsychotics approved for bipolar mania and are becoming first-line treatments for bipolar mania. Aripiprazole, olanzapine, and risperidone come in injectable forms for use in acute agitation. These agents, especially the injectable forms, work quickly to calm the patient.

Lifespan Considerations

The rate of attempted suicide in those with bipolar disorders is high, as is co-occurrence with other disorders such as attention-deficit/hyperactivity disorder (ADHD), anxiety, and substance abuse, all of which complicate diagnosis. At any age, patients suspected of having a bipolar disorder should receive thorough screening, including screening for suicidal ideation.

Bipolar Disorders in Children

Children with bipolar disorders present with mood changes (such as being overly silly or joyful when that is unusual for the child) and behavioral changes (such as sleeping little but not feeling tired and talking a lot and having racing thoughts) (American Psychological Association, 2019). Some children may exhibit lengthy, violent temper tantrums. Older children may take on multiple tasks simultaneously and develop grandiose plans for their projects (APA, 2013). Children must be assessed based on their personal baseline because children of the same age may be at different developmental stages. Taking this into consideration, it is difficult to define "normal" and "abnormal" behaviors.

Diagnosis of bipolar disorder may be made after other possibilities have been ruled out. Treatment of children with bipolar disorders may include medications to reduce severity of symptoms and psychotherapy to learn how to adapt to stressors and build relationships (American Psychological Association, 2019). It is important that children be prescribed the fewest medications possible at the lowest effective doses.

Bipolar Disorders in Adolescents

The average age of onset of the first episode of mania, hypomania, or major depression is approximately 18 (APA, 2013), and the lifetime prevalence of bipolar disorders in adolescents is approximately 1.8% (American Psychological

Association, 2019). Treatment for adolescents will follow the same guidelines as those used for children. Because teenagers commonly show mood changes, including changes in sleeping and eating patterns, it is important not to mistake typical mood swings for bipolar disorder.

Bipolar Disorders in Pregnant Women

Current research suggests that recurrence rates of bipolar disorder and depression are substantial in pregnancy, with about 19% of women who have bipolar disorder experiencing recurrence of symptoms. Depressive symptoms are more common than mania or hypomania. Risk for recurrence increases when women with a diagnosis of mood disorder discontinue their medication (Stevens et al., 2019). Stopping medications can worsen symptoms; therefore, some HCPs will slowly taper the woman off medications, decrease the dose, or change the medication. If lithium is continued, serum lithium levels must be monitored frequently to prevent toxicity. The fetus should be assessed for potential heart defects, as risk for them increases with lithium use during the first trimester. In addition, lithium doses should be decreased at the onset of labor to avoid maternal toxicity at delivery. Women taking divalproex (Depakote) or carbamazepine (Tegretol) should be switched to another mood stabilizer before conception because of the higher-than-average risk for neural tube, cardiac, and craniofacial defects (Yildizhan, Ozdemir, Miray Aytac, & Tomruk, 2019). Lamotrigine (Lamictal) can also be used for pregnant women, although it has more of an effect on the depressive symptoms than the manic symptoms (Yildizhan et al., 2019).

Close monitoring is necessary for pregnant women with bipolar disorder throughout the pregnancy and during the postpartum period. Ultimately, the decision of whether to continue, begin, or adjust pharmacologic treatment for mood disorders is up to the patient herself. However, HCPs have a duty to educate pregnant women about the potential risks and benefits of both drug use and untreated mental illness (Stevens et al., 2019).

Bipolar Disorders in Older Adults

Onset of bipolar disorder may occur at any time during life, including in older adulthood. As with any patient, first episodes of manic symptoms presenting during midlife or late life indicate a need to perform medical testing to verify that there is not a medical or substance-related etiology. Treatment will be the same for older adults as for adults, although doses of medications may be lower. Older adults are also prone to experience more side effects and toxicity, requiring them to be monitored very closely. For example, lithium is contraindicated in older patients with kidney disease and should be used cautiously in patients with thyroid disease.

NURSING PROCESS

Nursing care of patients with depressive symptoms is covered in Exemplar 28.A, Depression, in this module. This section focuses on hypomania and mania, which constitute the other half of the bipolar continuum of behaviors. For all patients, assess personal history of cyclical patterns and triggers. Common triggers include changes in sleep patterns, negative life events (such as breaking up with a partner or losing a job) and use of alcohol or drugs. Early identification of triggers can assist with early identification of helpful interventions and improve patient outcomes (Wu et al., 2019).

Assessment

- ***Observation and patient interview.*** Assessment of patients with known or suspected bipolar disorder begins with a thorough history and interview. Inquire about any past manic or depressive episodes or behavior, as well as family history of mood disorders. Ask about and observe for the signs and symptoms discussed throughout the Concept section of this module, taking note of their severity, as they may range from mild (in hypomania) to extreme (in a frank manic episode). The nurse should also investigate the speed of onset for any symptoms, noting whether it is gradual or dramatic.

  Patients who are experiencing their first manic episode are most likely to be young people in their late teens or early 20s, although adolescents are sometimes affected. Affected individuals may demonstrate or articulate any number of changes in mood and behavior, including:

  - Rapid changes in affect, such as going from elation in one moment to anger and irritability in the next.
  - Inflated self-esteem, sometimes to the extent of having delusions of grandeur. Delusions of persecution also may be a feature.
  - Ignorance or denial of fatigue, hunger, and even hygiene; being too involved in activity to focus on physiologic sensations.
  - Rapid, loud, pressured speech.
  - Unusual appearance (e.g., dressing inappropriately and using garish makeup or being disheveled and unkempt).
  - A surprising sense of well-being. Individuals who are hypomanic and those early in manic episodes feel wonderful and do not understand why people are upset with their behavior.

  Cognitive alterations are another frequent feature of mania. Be alert for changes in the patient's thought processes, evidenced by statements such as "I feel like my thoughts are racing." In addition to racing thoughts, other symptoms frequently common during manic episodes include an inability to concentrate and being easily distracted by the slightest stimulus in the environment. Some patients also experience hallucinations, delusions, and other forms of psychosis. Family members may report poor judgment and impulsivity, as evidenced by shopping sprees, drug use, or sexual activity that is out of character with the patient's usual behavior.

  With bipolar I disorder, impairments in adaptive functioning are common. This includes difficulties in occupational function, which may result in being laid off from work, being placed on a leave of absence, or being fired because the behavior is disruptive in the workplace. Individuals who have mania cause interpersonal chaos by behaving manipulatively, testing limits, and playing one person against another. If their attempts at manipulation fail, they become irritable or hostile, and such behavior further alienates others.

- ***Physical examination.*** Assessment of the patient's physical manifestations is also critical. The hallmark of mania is constant motor activity. During a manic episode, patients may not stop to eat. Individuals in a manic state do not rest, have disordered sleep patterns, and may go for days without sleep. Bruises and other injuries sometimes result from the constant activity.

  Patients experiencing mania are usually not able to cooperate fully during assessment. Nurses may need to hold some aspects of assessment until the patient is more fully able to participate, or may need to collaborate with secondary sources, such as family members. Even for patients able to participate fully, family members may be able to provide important information and better insight into the patient's illness.

Diagnosis

Patient needs and nursing care priorities will vary by patient but may typically include:

- Risk of injury
- Altered thought processes
- Inadequate social skills
- Poor impulse control
- Elevated mood
- Undernutrition
- Poor self-care
- Sleep disturbance
- Risk of suicide.

Planning

The overall goal of nursing care and treatment overtime is a return to normal functioning. Appropriate outcomes for patients experiencing a manic or hypomanic episode include:

- The patient will remain free of injury.
- The patient will demonstrate logical thought processes.
- The patient will report improved and greater sleep duration.
- The patient will maintain self-care.

Implementation

Building a trusting, therapeutic relationship with all patients is important. The nurse's reassuring presence and communication can help patients who are feeling out of control to gain a sense of security. When patients are in a manic or hypomanic state, it is important to set therapeutic boundaries while still being calm and relaxed. A matter-of-fact approach to limit setting is best.

Often when patients are manic, they unintentionally violate boundaries of others and engage in inappropriate and manipulative behaviors. Therefore, it is important for nurses to apply appropriate limit setting to ensure the safety of the manic patient as well as the safety of others in the milieu. It is also important for the nurse to self-reflect to be sure that they are maintaining their own emotions and boundaries.

Nurses should promote appropriate interactions between patients in the milieu by arranging activities and identifying behaviors that need to be modified. When inappropriate behaviors are observed, the nurse may need to be a mediator between patients to ensure safety for all in the milieu. Assigning activities that promote positive interactions between patients is important. Nursing actions should focus on promoting patient dignity and the rights of others.

Building rapport and forming a therapeutic alliance with the patient helps to encourage positive interpersonal interactions that explore patient perspectives and needs. These therapeutic relationships have been linked with better long-term outcomes for patients with bipolar disorders.

Promote Patient Safety

Providing safety is the priority focus for patients who experience mania.

- Community support is important to maintain safety. Giving the patient community support contacts such as local crisis hotlines and the National Suicide Hotline can greatly assist the patient in times of uncertainty and crisis.
- To ensure that the patient has access to follow-up care, the nurse can assist in scheduling appointments and arranging transportation, if needed.
- Monitor activities. Create an activity schedule that includes quiet times and periods of rest to ensure that the patient does not become exhausted. Collaborating with an activity therapist and choosing appropriate activities like walking, journaling, music, or dancing can help release tension. Highly competitive interactions such as sports and board games should be avoided, as these activities can result in hostility and aggression.
- When patients have difficulty controlling impulses, the nurse must set and enforce rules and limits. The most effective approach to limit setting is being matter-of-fact rather than becoming angry and using a scolding tone with the patient. Often, a patient may need to be reminded of rules and be redirected to a more appropriate social activity. Verbally recognizing appropriate behaviors and offering praise can help promote positive interactions and lasting behavioral change. Make statements such as: "I enjoyed listening to the radio with you because you shared and allowed us both to listen to music we enjoyed."
- Ensure that the environment is safe by reducing extraneous stimuli and providing a simply furnished room with all unnecessary objects removed. While patients are experiencing mania, a private room with low lighting and reduced noise may be necessary. Close monitoring is also necessary, so room placement should be considered. Although a room at the end of the hallway is quiet, it may not be best for a patient with mania who is constantly engaging in inappropriate behaviors.
- Monitor for safety hazards. Agitated patients are more apt to forget or disregard safety considerations such as safe use of smoking materials.

Promote Reality-Based Thinking

The patient in a state of mania may demonstrate thinking that is out of touch with reality. It is important to use reality orientation to assist the patient into reality-based thinking.

- Orient the patient to reality by identifying yourself; stating the date, time, and location; and offering other pertinent information. Spending time with the patient and keeping conversations grounded in concrete subjects such as local events and the weather can help present reality to them.
- Stability and consistency can reassure patients with altered thought processes. Establish a consistent schedule and, if possible, keep staff assignments consistent. This can help patients better understand what is expected of them.
- Use the therapeutic communication technique of reflection when patients communicate perceptions of altered reality. For example, asking, "Are you telling me that your boss is trying to have you murdered because he doesn't want you to be promoted?" can assist a patient to understand how her perceptions and thoughts sound to others. A patient making statements like "I know this sounds crazy, but . . . " can be a good indication that the patient is becoming less delusional.

Communicating with Patients

Working Phase

Do not engage in arguments with the patient who is experiencing delusions and altered thought processes. This is not therapeutic and often leads to the patient only holding more firmly to the delusion. Arguing with the patient can break trust and rapport. Instead, use phrases that can lead to instilling reasonable doubts, such as:

- That sounds very unlikely.
- I find that difficult to believe. Can you tell me what makes you believe that?

Promote Improved Self-Care

Self-care may become deficient during an exacerbation of symptoms of bipolar disorder. This includes activities of daily living such as nutrition, hygiene, rest, and elimination.

- During extended periods of mania and hyperactivity, patients are at risk for compromised nutrition. For patients in the psychiatric hospital setting, ensure that foods are convenient and can be consumed on the go because patients will often not want to sit down for a meal. Finger foods and high-calorie nutritional beverages are good options. For patients in the community setting, collaborate with the patient to determine preferences and create a list of easily prepared foods that the patient can make or eat on the go.
- Assist patients with activities of daily living. Often, patients who are experiencing mania are unwilling or unable to bathe, brush their teeth, change clothes, or use the toilet. Allow the patient to do as much as possible on their own and promote independence. Offer verbal redirection as needed and reinforce any self-care attempts with recognition; for example, "Mrs. Smith, I see that you did your laundry and put on clean clothes today."
- Incontinence of urine or feces is often seen in patients who experience severe mania and regression. This can be disturbing to staff and other patients in the milieu. Preserving patient dignity is important. The nurse should establish a toileting schedule and accompany the patient to the bathroom at least every hour until accidents no longer happen. Constipation is a more frequently occurring problem because hyperactive and manic patients often suppress the urge to defecate and become severely constipated.

Set Limits

The consistent enforcement of rules and limits as well as consequences for breaking those rules must be followed by all staff who work on the milieu. Patients must know what the behavioral expectations are on the unit and what consequences will result if they cannot comply with the expectations. Inconsistent approaches to following rules and limits and lack of enforcing consequences will result in a failure to decrease manipulative behavior.

Patients will often give creative and charming rationales for why they do not need to follow the rules and limits, and nurses should be prepared for these interactions and not be disarmed by them. Nurses must be matter-of-fact and enforce limits to promote adaptive behaviors.

Enhance Rest and Sleep

Patients in the manic phase of bipolar disorder can become exhausted and seem to be full of energy. In many cases, patients may remain awake for days at a time, increasing their risk for injury and further cognitive impairment.

- Provide a schedule that promotes good sleep hygiene and helps to maintain regular sleep–wake cycles. Assess patients for signs of fatigue and schedule rest periods. Limit daytime naps to help promote nighttime sleeping.
- Sleep can help rapidly resolve first episodes of mania. Encourage good bedtime rituals that promote relaxation such as decreasing light and noise, listening to soothing music, taking a warm bath, or having a bedtime snack. Administer prescribed medications that do not suppress rapid-eye-movement (REM) sleep, such as zolpidem tartrate (Ambien).
- For patients who have difficulty falling asleep, avoid engaging them in excessive conversations or overly stimulating activities like watching television and playing games. Use limit setting and reassure patients that staying in their darkened rooms quietly will help them fall asleep. If they will not stay in their room, provide a dull uninteresting task such as counting objects or sorting laundry to help encourage drowsiness.
- Do not wake patients who are able to sleep for nonessential care. Optimal sleep cycles last 90 minutes or more.

Evaluation

Outcomes that indicate the patient has improved include:

- The patient remains free from injury.
- The patient exhibits logical thought processes.
- The patient is performing adequate self-care.
- The patient is able to sleep through the night.
- The patient is behaving appropriately in social settings.

Secondary interventions will need to be implemented if goals are not met. As with depression, the time frame may need to be extended. Combination pharmacologic therapy may need to be implemented by administering both antiseizure medications (mood stabilizers) and atypical antipsychotic medications. The initiation of clozapine (Clozaril) or ECT may be effective when first-line therapies are not successful. It is important for patients to understand that finding the medication regimen that is effective for them is a process and not to become frustrated when adjustments need to be made.

Nursing Care Plan

A Patient with Bipolar Disorder

Mr. Goebel, a 48-year-old videographer, is brought to the emergency psychiatric clinic by his longtime partner, Ms. Henderson, at 2:00 a.m. She reports that he has not slept in 3 days and instead has been working on editing a new movie for Disney. She says she manages all the contracts for their videography business and there is no movie contract.

ASSESSMENT

Ms. Henderson reports that Mr. Goebel has had three prior episodes of manic behavior, beginning when he was in college many years ago. He was stabilized on lithium carbonate for years but stopped taking it about 3 months ago because he felt so good. The current episode began about 1 week ago, after he caused a car accident that sent the family in the other car to the hospital, fortunately only with minor injuries. Since then, he has been spending increasing amounts of time in his studio. Any attempt by his partner to talk him out of the "Disney" project has been met with anger and renewed resolve. Mr. Goebel angrily tells the admitting nurse, "I don't know why she brought me here. I need to get back to work! This is going to be a franchise! I'm going to make millions!"

DIAGNOSES

- Sleep disturbance
- Caregiver burden
- Disturbed thought processes
- Nonadherence

PLANNING

Goals for care include:

- The patient will adhere with instructions for taking medications as ordered.
- The patient will sleep through the night.
- The patient will be oriented to time and place.
- Patient and partner will return to normal activities.
- Partner will support medication administration.

IMPLEMENTATION

- With Mr. Goebel and his partner, develop a plan of activity that will help Mr. Goebel disperse energy at appropriate times.
- Help Ms. Henderson set and enforce limits. For example, "From 8:00 p.m. until 6:00 a.m., Mr. Goebel will remain indoors, engaged in sleep-promoting activities or sleeping."
- Refer Mr. Goebel and Ms. Henderson to a therapist who can help them learn how to orient Mr. Goebel to reality when his mind begins to stray.
- Help Mr. Goebel and his partner learn how to promote sleep by decreasing environmental stimuli in the bedroom and engaging in good sleep hygiene.

EVALUATION

Expected outcomes to evaluate the patient's care include:

- The patient adheres to the treatment regimen, including scheduled appointments to evaluate lithium levels.
- The patient and partner report that Mr. Goebel obtains 6 to 8 hours of sleep per night.
- The patient demonstrates logical thought processes.
- The partner reports a return to normal daily routine.

CRITICAL THINKING

1. What patient teaching can the nurse provide to reduce the risk of medication nonadherence once Mr. Goebel feels well and is no longer symptomatic?
2. What teaching will the nurse provide Ms. Henderson to help her cope with the patient's diagnosis?
3. How can the nurse assist the patient to meet his nutritional needs during manic phases of the illness?

REVIEW Bipolar Disorders

RELATE Link the Concepts and Exemplars

Linking the exemplar of bipolar disorders with the concept of family:

1. How might bipolar disorder affect parenting styles?
2. How might different family processes affect a child's treatment for bipolar disorder?

Linking the exemplar of bipolar disorders with the concept of nutrition:

3. How might bipolar disorder affect a patient's nutritional status?

Linking the exemplar of bipolar disorders with the concept of health, wellness, and illness:

4. What consumer education resources are available to patients with bipolar disorders and their families to help them maintain their health during periods of relapse?

READY Go to Volume 3: Clinical Nursing Skills

REFER Go to Pearson MyLab Nursing and eText

REFLECT Apply Your Knowledge

Sherry Goodman is a 19-year-old who has a full-time job at a retail store. She was recently diagnosed with bipolar I disorder and is currently experiencing mania. In one week, she spent $7,000 on her credit card doing online shopping and believed that the FBI was trying to ger her fired from her job. Since she was admitted to the inpatient psychiatric unit 72 hours ago, she has been averaging 3 hours of sleep a night. When she is awake, she sings loudly in the hallways and tells staff that she is on a singing competition TV show. She has been observed going into male patients' rooms and flirting with them. She wears short mini-skirts and low-cut halter tops that revel her midsection, and she refuses to wash her hair because "that's what my stylist tells me to do!" Every few hours she applies excessive eye makeup and bright red lipstick.

1. What safety risks should the nurse prioritize in caring for Ms. Goodman? What nursing actions should be implemented to ensure the safety of Ms. Goodman?
2. What health risks does Ms. Goodman have in the manic phase of bipolar? How should the nurse plan care based on these risks?

›› Exemplar 28.C Peripartum Depression

Exemplar Learning Outcomes

28.C Analyze peripartum depression and relevant nursing care.

- Describe the processes of maternal role attainment and attachment.
- Identify the clinical manifestations of peripartum depression and psychosis.
- Summarize diagnostic tests and therapies used by interprofessional teams in the collaborative care of an individual with peripartum depression.
- Apply the nursing process in providing culturally competent care to an individual with peripartum depression.

Exemplar Key Terms

Major depressive disorder with peripartum onset, *1993*
Postpartum blues, *1993*
Peripartum depression, *1993*
Postpartum psychosis, *1995*
Puerperium, *1993*

Overview

The postpartum period is a time of readjustment and adaptation for the entire family, but especially for the mother. The woman experiences a variety of responses as she adjusts to a new family member, postpartum discomforts, changes in her body image, and the reality that she is no longer pregnant. Alterations in mood may occur at any time during pregnancy.

According to the CDC (2020b), approximately 12.5% of women will experience a major depressive episode during pregnancy or within the first few months following pregnancy. Almost half of these women will begin experiencing depressive symptoms while pregnant. Therefore, clinical recommendations indicate that all pregnant women be assessed early in pregnancy for personal and family history of depressive disorders, bipolar disorders, peripartum or postpartum depression, and postpartum psychosis (see **Figure 28.7** ››) (American College of Obstetricians and Gynecologists,

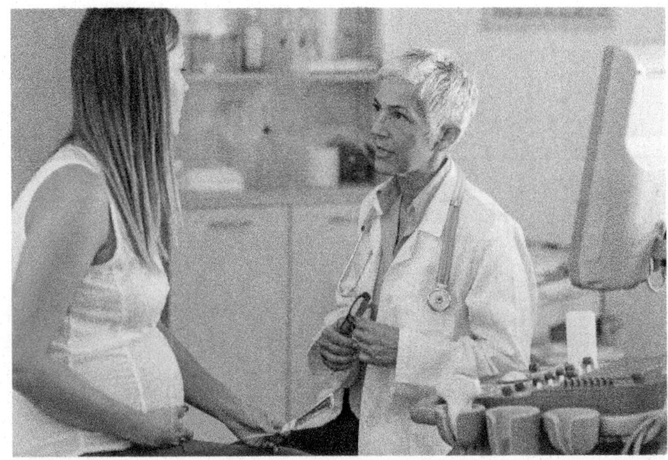

Figure 28.7 ›› All women should be assessed for depression during their pregnancies.
Source: Vgajic/E+/Getty Images.

2015; Earls, Yogman, Mattson, Rafferty, & Committee on Psychosocial Aspects of Child and Family Health, 2019).

The **puerperium** is that time immediately following childbirth when physiologic changes that occurred during pregnancy begin to return to normal. **Postpartum blues**, often referred to as "baby blues," are a common occurrence after childbirth and may affect up to 80% of women after giving birth. Symptoms include mood swings; feeling sad, anxious, or overwhelmed; crying spells (often for no reason); decreased appetite; and problems sleeping. These symptoms are not severe and do not require treatment. They usually resolve within a few days or a week (NIMH, 2020a). **Peripartum depression**, a depressive disorder associated with pregnancy, begins *during* pregnancy approximately 50% of the time and is formally called **major depressive disorder with peripartum onset** in the DSM-5. Women who experience a depressive episode during pregnancy typically experience severe anxiety, and panic attacks are not uncommon. Mood and anxiety during pregnancy and postpartum blues are both associated with greater risk for postpartum depression (APA, 2013). This exemplar discusses the psychologic struggles that women face during pregnancy and after giving birth and how nurses can support them during this critical time.

Postpartum Blues

As stated previously, the postpartum blues represent a transient period of depression that occurs in as many as 80% of women during the first few days following labor (NIMH, 2020a). A woman may experience postpartum blues while still in the hospital or birthing center, but it may occur afterward at home. Mood swings, anger, irritability, weepiness, sleep disturbance, loss of appetite, and a feeling of "letdown" are characteristic of postpartum blues. Potential reasons for postpartum blues include changing hormone levels, an unsupportive environment, and feelings of insecurity. If symptoms last beyond 10 to 14 days, the woman may need screening for postpartum depression. Depression screenings should be conducted on all women at least once during the perinatal period. Women with risk factors for perinatal depression should be monitored more closely (Earls et al., 2019). For women whose screenings indicate possible depression, mental health treatment should be encouraged and provided (Earls et al., 2019).

Common features of postpartum blues are feelings of worry, unhappiness, tearfulness, and exhaustion. Typically, when the woman is asked about why she is tearful or worrying, she will not be able to give a specific reason. Bass and Bauer (2018) identify possible factors that can contribute to the blues:

- Pregnancy complications and other obstetric issues (such as gestational diabetes)
- Depression prior to or during pregnancy, or episodes of postpartum depression with previous births
- Maternal age (both adolescent and advanced maternal age put the woman at greater risk).

It is important to encourage the mother's support system to watch for and report symptoms that may indicate that the woman is going into a deeper depression. Validate to the woman that the symptoms she is feeling are real and can be a normal part of adjusting to the postpartum period. This can reassure the mother that what she is experiencing is not her fault or something she could have prevented. Assist with planning good self-care and care for the infant and identify support systems that can be used at home. Proper rest, sufficient nutrition, accurate information, and family support aids recovery.

Strong support networks are vital to creating positive psychologic outcomes during the postpartum period. Women and their partners may rely more on their family relationships at this time, but they can also realize that increased family interactions can create additional stressors. New parents may increase their contact with other parents of small children and discover that contact with coworkers and other friends declines. New parents who lack social and family support have a greater tendency to have feelings of isolation and extreme stress. These negative feelings can result in situations of postpartum depression or infant neglect or abuse. Encouraging the woman to attend a support group for mothers can help build these important social support systems.

Postpartum doulas can be a supporting resource during this time. Doulas are trained professionals who provide continuous physical, emotional, and informational support to a mother. Doula services are designed to assist the new mother in making a healthy transition during the postpartum period. Areas of focused care include rest, nutrition, home care, and care of the infant.

Peripartum Mood Disorders

Peripartum Depression

Peripartum depression, or major depressive disorder with peripartum onset, is major depression that occurs during pregnancy or in the first 4 weeks following birth. It has an overall prevalence of approximately 12.5% of pregnant or postpartum women (CDC, 2020a). Peripartum depression occurs across all cultures and societies (see the Focus on Diversity and Culture feature). Peripartum depression may or may not be accompanied by psychotic symptoms.

Major depressive disorder with peripartum onset is very similar to major depression, and both disorders have nearly the same symptomatology. Peripartum depression presents as a combination of depressed mood, loss of interest, loss of pleasure, sleep and appetite disturbance, impaired concentration, psychomotor disturbance, fatigue, feelings of guilt or worthlessness, and suicidal thoughts. Additional symptoms can include mood lability, anxiety, irritability, feeling overwhelmed, and obsessional worries or preoccupations with the general health and care of the baby. Suicidal thoughts are common, affecting about 20% of women in the postpartum period. At times, women with postpartum depression may have thoughts of harming their baby. For some women, these thoughts are very disturbing and are part of the obsessional thought process and extreme anxiety. Concerns about self or infant harm should be evaluated and proper referrals to a mental health provider should be made (Stewart & Vigod, 2019).

Clinical Manifestations and Therapies

Peripartum Depression

DEGREE OF SEVERITY	CLINICAL MANIFESTATIONS	CLINICAL THERAPIES
Postpartum blues	■ Mood swings ■ Feeling sad ■ Feeling anxious or overwhelmed ■ Crying spells for no reason ■ Decreased appetite ■ Problems sleeping	■ May occur in the first days following birth; usually resolves without treatment within 3 to 14 days
Peripartum depression	■ Severe depression that occurs during pregnancy or within the first year of giving birth, with increased incidence at about the fourth week postpartum, just before menses resumes, and upon weaning	■ Antidepressants may be prescribed cautiously following a risk–benefit analysis with the individual patient based on patient clinical characteristics and personal history. ■ Support groups ■ Assistance with care of the newborn, taking care to promote self-confidence in mothering ■ Mental health counseling ■ Assistance with building self-esteem and self-confidence in mothering skills
Postpartum psychosis	■ Agitation ■ Hyperactivity ■ Insomnia ■ Mood lability ■ Confusion ■ Irrationality ■ Difficulty remembering or concentrating ■ Delusions and hallucinations that tend to be related to the infant	■ Lithium or antipsychotics ■ Should be supervised at all times when caring for infant or other children ■ Support groups ■ Short-term institutionalization may be required

Focus on Diversity and Culture

Peripartum Depression

Peripartum depression is a universal phenomenon and is not restricted to specific cultures. It is seen in both industrialized and nonindustrialized countries (Shorey et al., 2018).

The gender of an infant may influence the development of postpartum depression. In parts of Asia and some Middle Eastern countries, male offspring are highly preferred over female offspring (Arifin, Cheyne, & Maxwell, 2020; Li et al., 2020). However, practices in both cultures emphasize the support of the mother and offer extended support systems to aid in postpartum care (Shorey et al., 2020). Despite these practices, Shorey and colleagues (2020) reported that the Middle East had a higher prevalence of postpartum depression compared to other countries. In the Middle East and Asia, girls are known to marry as young as 16 years old, which has been shown to be a significant predictor of PPD, as well as cultural preferences for male children (Arifin et al., 2020).

An alarming cultural consideration in the United States is the disparity of healthcare for postpartum depression in low-income women. A study of more than 29,000 New Jersey Medicaid recipients found that Black and Latina women were significantly less likely than white women to initiate treatment for postpartum depression. Among those who did, Black and Latina women were less likely than white women to receive follow-up care, continue care, or refill antidepressant prescriptions (Ponting, Mahrer, Zelcer, Dunkel Schetter, & Chavira, 2020).

Risk Factors and Prevention

Risk factors for peripartum depression include the following:

- A history of mood or anxiety disorder (perinatal or otherwise), especially if symptomatic in pregnancy
- A family history of peripartum depression
- Poor social support and/or family support
- Persistent health problems of the infant or difficult infant temperament
- Intimate partner violence or prior sexual abuse
- Ambiguity about wanting a baby or an unplanned pregnancy
- Young age of the mother
- Marital or partner dissatisfaction.

As with major depressive disorder, safety is of great concern for women with peripartum depression. Thoughts of suicide can be common during this period. Although acting on suicidal thoughts is unlikely in deep depression, it should be carefully assessed when symptoms begin to improve and the mother's energy level is higher. In cases of postpartum psychosis, the woman may attempt suicide due to illogical thought processes. However, during depression, suicidal thoughts are connected to significant psychological distress and suffering, making death seem like a better choice than living with pain. Suicidal thoughts can also be linked to the mother's illogical perceptions that she will do something to harm the baby, so in dying, she will protect the child. Risk factors for suicide include previous attempts, a plan that is detailed and specific, and having lethal means available identified in the plan. More specific suicidal plans increase the likelihood of an attempt. Strategies to help prevent postpartum depression are outlined in the Patient Teaching feature.

Patient Teaching

Primary Prevention Strategies for Peripartum Depression

Nurses can encourage pregnant women, new mothers, and parents to participate in a number of strategies to help prevent peripartum depression. Providing education to the woman's partner and primary support persons assists in the prevention or early identification of peripartum depression. Suggestions include the following:

- Identify and use support systems. Receiving social support through friends and family during stressful times is thought to be a protective factor against developing peripartum depression.
- Communicate needs with your partner. Parents must decide how their new roles will affect their home life, work life, and relationships. Organize and plan new schedules and how household tasks will be done. Do not be afraid to ask for guidance or help from support systems.
- Encourage the expression of feelings and talk openly about them. Do not hide or suppress feelings. This can exacerbate feelings of anxiety and hopelessness.
- Get adequate sleep and do not overengage in activities. Sleep when the baby is sleeping. Adequate sleep and rest are important for healthy emotional functioning.
- Engage in light exercise three to five times a week. Studies show that mothers feel better emotionally and are more social when they have an exercise routine. Taking a brisk walk, getting fresh air, and enjoying nature can improve moods and perspectives.
- Do not focus on perfection (i.e., having a perfectly clean house, making a perfect meal).
- Make time to go out, visit friends, or spend time alone with your partner.
- Socialize with other mothers or join a support group. Isolation can cause anxiety. Meeting with other mothers and knowing that they are experiencing the same types of issues can help lessen feelings of inadequacy and stress. Additionally, support groups for couples can teach coping strategies and offer encouragement

Genetic Considerations

There is increasing support for the gene–environment interaction theory of depression and peripartum depression. Variants in genes that code enzymes affecting serotonin, dopamine, and noradrenalin (neurotransmitters affecting mood) were associated with development of depression in the peripartum period (Elwood et al., 2019). Several studies implicated a serotonin-related transporter genotype in postpartum depression (Elwood et al., 2019; Osman & Bahri, 2019; Payne & Maguire, 2019). Other studies implicated monoamine oxidase–related genes in postpartum depression (Osman & Bahri, 2019). More research is needed to definitively identify the role of specific genes in peripartum depression.

Postpartum Psychosis

Postpartum psychosis (postpartum mood episodes with psychotic features) is a medical emergency because the woman experiencing psychosis may have delusions or hallucinations that suggest the baby should not be allowed to live. Other characteristic symptoms include agitation, sleep disturbance, mood lability, irrational guilt, and confusion (Mohamied, 2019). Prompt treatment, usually with medication and additional supervision, is necessary to ensure the safety of both mother and infant (Mohamied, 2019). Postpartum psychosis is rare—about 1 in every 500 to 1000 deliveries (APA, 2013). The risk is greater in first deliveries, in women with prior postpartum depression, and in those with a history of depressive or bipolar disorder. Although relatively rare, postpartum psychosis gains considerable national attention when an incident of infanticide occurs.

Collaboration

It is not enough to simply refer women with a history of postpartum psychosis or peripartum depression or who are otherwise at high risk to a mental health professional for evaluation, counseling, and treatment between the second and sixth week postpartum. Clinical guidelines indicate these women require a detailed plan for psychiatric management during late pregnancy and during the early postpartum period. This plan should be shared (with consent) with the entire maternity team (e.g., obstetricians, nurses, and midwives). The plan should detail supports, contact information, and treatment considerations, including medications and breastfeeding (Forde, Peters, & Wittkowski, 2020; SA Maternal, Neonatal, & Gynaecology Community of Practice, 2019). In addition to more typical treatments for depressive symptoms, such as medication and psychotherapy, assistance with childcare and activities of daily living are commonly included in the treatment plan until the woman regains stability.

Diagnostic Tests

The routine use of a screening tool in a matter-of-fact approach significantly improves the diagnosis. The Edinburgh Postnatal Depression Scale (**Box 28.4** »)) and the Postpartum Depression Screening Scale (PDSS) are appropriate tools for use in assessing patients for peripartum depression. The PDSS is a 35-item scale that screens signs of depression such as cognitive impairment, sleeping and eating disturbances, emotional lability, guilt and shame, and thoughts of self-harm or suicide.

Box 28.4

Edinburgh Postnatal Depression Scale

In the past 7 days:

1. I have been able to laugh and see the funny side of things.
As much as I always could
Not quite so much now
Definitely not so much now
Not at all

2. I have looked forward with enjoyment of things.
As much as I ever did
Rather less than I used to
Definitely less than I used to
Hardly at all

***3.** I have blamed myself unnecessarily when things went wrong.
Yes, most of the time
Yes, some of the time
Not very often
No, never

4. I have been anxious or worried for no good reason.
No, not at all
Hardly ever
Yes, sometimes
Yes, very often

***5.** I have felt scared or panicky for no very good reason.
Yes, quite a lot
Yes, sometimes
No, not much
No, not at all

***6.** Things have been getting on top of me.
Yes, most of the time I haven't been able to cope at all
Yes, sometimes I haven't been coping as well as usual
No, I have been coping quite well
No, I have been coping as well as ever

***7.** I have been so unhappy that I have had difficulty sleeping.
Yes, most of the time
Yes, sometimes
Not very often
No, not at all

***8.** I have felt sad or miserable.
Yes, most of the time
Yes, quite often
Not very often
No, not at all

***9.** I have been so unhappy that I have been crying.
Yes, most of the time
Yes, quite often
Only occasionally
No, never

***10.** The thought of harming myself has occurred to me.
Yes, quite often
Sometimes
Hardly ever
Never

Note: Response categories are scored 0, 1, 2, and 3 according to increased severity of the symptoms. Items marked with an asterisk are reverse-scored (3, 2, 1, 0). The total score is calculated by adding together the scores for each of the 10 items. A score above the threshold of 12 to 13 out of 30 indicates with 86% sensitivity that the woman is experiencing postpartum depression.

Source: From Cox, J. L., Holden, J. M., & Sagovsky, R. (1987). Detection of postnatal depression: Development of the 10-item Edinburgh Postnatal Depression Scale. *British Journal of Psychiatry, 150*, 782–786. Users may reproduce the scale without further permission provided they respect copyright by quoting the names of the authors, the title, and the source of the paper in all reproduced copies.

Clinical Therapies

Treatment of postpartum psychosis is typically based on the types of symptoms that the patient displays. Lithium, antipsychotics, or electroconvulsive therapy in conjunction with psychotherapy have been proven effective in treating psychotic symptoms. Depending on severity of symptoms, it may be necessary to remove the infant from the mother's care.

Nurses must be aware of pharmacotherapy and how it could potentially impact breastfeeding mothers. Many of the medications used to treat postpartum psychiatric conditions are contraindicated. However, systematic reviews have concluded that the pharmacologic profile of a drug is not always useful in a risk-versus-benefit analysis and that generally speaking:

- Fluoxetine must be used with caution
- Doxepin (a tricyclic antidepressant) and nefazodone (an atypical antipsychotic) are not recommended
- Lithium, traditionally considered contraindicated, may be safer than once thought for postpartum mothers but is not recommended during breastfeeding by most clinicians (Davanzo, Copertino, De Cunto, Minen, & Amaddeo, 2011; Imaz, Torra, Soy, Garcia-Esteve, & Martin-Santos, 2019; Raza & Raza, 2019).

A combination of antidepressants and psychosocial supports are recommended, regardless of breastfeeding. It is important to provide education regarding the time it takes for antidepressants to be effective, in most cases it can be several weeks. In order for blood levels of antidepressants to reach a therapeutic level, providers may recommend starting the woman on them before the birth of the baby, typically around 36 weeks' gestation.

Brexanolone (Zulresso) is a new medication recently approved by the FDA for treating postpartum depression. It is administered via continuous IV infusion over 60 hours and is available only under a specialized program called the

Zulresso Risk Evaluation and Mitigation Strategy (REMS). Common side effects of brexanolone are sedation, drowsiness, and dizziness. Future recommendations for brexanolone focus on combining it with antidepressants to produce rapid symptom relief (Burval, Kerns, & Reed, 2020).

Limited research has been conducted about the use of ECT in postpartum depression and psychosis. ECT is considered safe and effective in treating both postpartum depression and psychosis and, in some cases, it is the preferred treatment method over antipsychotic medications. For severe depression and psychosis, ECT treatment is often quicker and more effective than pharmacotherapies (Lundberg, Nordanskog, & Nordenskjöld, 2019). The current literature indicates that ECT has a higher response rate during the postpartum period than outside of it. Furthermore, the most significant predictor of response to treatment was symptom severity (i.e., more severe symptoms were associated with greater probability of response to ECT), indicating that postpartum psychosis was highly responsive to this treatment (Grover et al., 2018; Lundberg et al., 2019; Rundgren et. al., 2018).

Support Groups

In addition to pharmacologic treatment, support groups have been proven to be highly effective in managing peripartum depression. Support groups offer many benefits to mothers and their partners, including providing a sense of community, helping to normalize feelings due to shared experiences, sharing informational resources about parenting and stress reduction, and openly expressing emotions in a safe and supportive environment. Lack of childcare can discourage participation in support groups, so offering safe childcare can encourage attendance. If a support group is not available locally, the mother and her partner can be encouraged to utilize online support groups such as Depression After Delivery (DAD) or Postpartum Support International.

NURSING PROCESS

Nursing care of the woman with peripartum or postpartum depression focuses on the safety of both the woman and her family, especially the infant and any other children in the home. Nurses especially may be reluctant to ask about feelings of self-harm or thoughts of harming the infant, for fear of introducing the idea. On the contrary, asking these questions in a nonjudgmental, therapeutic way can help the patient begin to articulate feelings she may have been too afraid to share with others and begin to identify threats to safety.

Assessment

Because depression may occur during pregnancy, assessment of risk factors for depression and psychosis should be made early in the pregnancy and to encourage women who are at risk to seek professional mental health care (Hutchens & Kearney, 2020). In addition, pregnant women should be reassessed for manifestations of depression throughout the pregnancy and for up to 3 to 4 months following delivery. Assessing for a personal or family history of mood disorders or postpartum disorders can be included in the prenatal history. Additional questionnaires to detect risks for peripartum issues can also be used (see the Evidence-Based Practice feature). Educate the woman and her partner about signs and symptoms of depression and provide referral resources as appropriate. If a history was not done previously, the nurses should include this in the assessment during labor and the postpartum stay.

It is important for the nurse to assess for both subjective and objective signs of depression while performing routine care. Objective signs of depression can include anxiety, irritability, poor concentration, forgetfulness, sleep difficulties, appetite changes, fatigue, and tearfulness. Listen for subtle cues and statements that can be more subjective, which can include feelings of failure, guilt, and low self-esteem. It is also important to note and report the severity of symptoms and how long they have persisted. Include in the assessment and immediately report any behaviors that are bizarre or that indicate that the woman may harm herself or the baby. Normal physiologic changes during the peripartum period may be similar to symptoms of depression (lack of sexual interest, appetite change, fatigue, anergia, issues with concentration). During assessment and documentation, the nurse should be as specific and as objective as possible.

According to Fallon and colleagues (2018), postpartum anxiety is among the most understudied, underdiagnosed, and undertreated complications of childbirth. Assessing the woman's level of anxiety and presenting symptoms is important because a primary source of anxiety is often attributed to care of the infant (Fallon et al., 2018). Lack of quality sleep and increased levels of fatigue impact mental health and can predispose the woman to depression (Doering & Dogan, 2018). Restorative sleep improves cognition and helps with decision making and coping. Assessing the level of fatigue at 2 weeks postpartum by telephone may be helpful in identifying early risk factors for depression.

A central challenge for nursing is identifying women at risk of suicide. Asking the patient directly if she has thoughts of self-harm is best. If the patient responds "yes," she must be screened by a qualified mental health professional as soon as possible and not left alone until this has been accomplished. Family members also should be alert to signals that she may be intent on self-harm and advised that threats are to be taken seriously. Contact information for community mental health and crisis resources should be given to both the patient and family, along with the National Suicide Hotline toll-free number. Family members should be told to be especially vigilant for suicide when the woman seems to be feeling better.

Diagnosis

As stated previously, the nursing care priority is the safety of the woman and baby. Additional priorities for care may include:

- Risk of suicide
- Risk of violence to self or others
- Inadequate parenting (due to obtrusive thoughts and depressive symptoms)
- Disturbed thought processes
- Inadequate coping skills.

Planning

Appropriate goals for the woman experiencing peripartum depression may include the following:

- The patient and family will remain free of injury.
- Family members and support persons will provide appropriate care for the newborn.
- The patient will articulate feelings and concerns.
- The patient will adhere to the plan of care.

Implementation

Helping prospective parents appreciate all the demands, responsibilities, and role changes of parenthood is an important task of the nurse working in the antepartum setting. The nurse should offer anticipatory guidance and provide parents with realistic expectations of infant care, such as debunking myths about being the perfect mother or father and having the perfect baby. Providing this type of education can help prevent peripartum depression. Social support teaching guides are available, and nurses should utilize them to help peripartum women identify specific social support needs during this time.

- Discuss the possibility of postpartum blues with the mother and her partner. Reassure them that these feelings are common and normal in the early days after birth and should last only a short time.
- Provide education about peripartum depression and inform the mother and her partner to notify the HCP if symptoms become severe, if they persist, or if at any time she feels she is unable to effectively cope.

SAFETY ALERT Make an immediate referral for a mental health evaluation if the mother rejects the infant or makes a threat or an act of aggression against the infant. If any of these occurs, ensure that the infant is not left alone with the mother.

A diagnosis of peripartum depression or other psychiatric disorder poses major problems for the family. Depression interferes with the mother's ability to bond with the baby, which can cause the baby to have problems sleeping and eating and may precipitate future behavioral issues. The woman's partner may have a difficult time adjusting. Symptoms of peripartum depression are harder to witness and are more difficult to comprehend than the physical issues associated with childbirth. The partner may experience feelings of being hurt and offended by the pregnant woman's anger and negativity, or may worry that she is losing touch with reality. Mood swings and lack of care for herself, the home, or the newborn may be extremely confusing and troubling to him. Furthermore, the

Evidence-Based Practice

Prevention of, Identification of, and Interventions for Peripartum Depression

How can the risk of peripartum depression be identified early in a pregnancy? What is the most effective way to prevent peripartum depression? When it occurs, how can it be treated?

Evidence

Peripartum depression is a serious condition that occurs in up to 14% of women during pregnancy or in the first 4 weeks following delivery (APA, 2021). It often goes undetected, as symptoms may be hidden or misinterpreted. Untreated, the condition may have consequences for mothers, infants, and their families.

But what are the best methods for the prevention, detection, and/or treatment of postpartum depression? As of 2016, an evidence report and systematic review for the U.S. Preventative Service Task Force (USPSTF) found that in 6 trials of 11,869 pregnant and postpartum women 18 years and older, between 18 and 59% showed relative reductions with screening programs in the risk of depression at follow-up (3 to 5 months) after participation in programs involving depression screening compared with usual care. These trials utilized the Edinburgh Postnatal Depression Scale (EPDS) and confirmed that this scale is effective in screening for peripartum depression. Based on the evidence, the reviewers (2016) concluded that screening pregnant and postpartum women for depression may reduce symptom severity in women with depression and reduce the prevalence of depression.

In 2019, the USPSTF issued recommendations for preventive interventions. These recommendations included the referral of pregnant and postpartum persons who are at increased risk of peripartum depression to counseling interventions. The USPSTF (2019) cited convincing research indicating that cognitive-behavioral therapy and interpersonal therapy are effective in preventing peripartum depression in those at increased risk. Furthermore, the task force suggested that although there is not a "correct time" for referring women to counseling, most referrals were initiated during the second trimester of pregnancy; however, referral could occur at any time.

Implications

Nurses are in a particularly good position to identify mothers at high risk for peripartum and postpartum depression. The EPDS should be an important part of these screening efforts. Once high-risk patients and/or patients who present with signs and symptoms of depression have been identified, they should be referred for additional support—ideally in the form of individually based interventions initiated postpartum. In-person interventions are most effective when delivered by a trained professional, whereas telephone interventions are effective when delivered by peers (Dennis & Dowswell, 2013). Other research supports that long-distance counseling through sending text messages to patients with depression can be an effective treatment along with other current treatments (Niksalehi, Taghadosi, Mazhariazad, & Tashk, 2018).

Critical Thinking Application

1. Why do you think prenatal classes have little impact in preventing peripartum depression?
2. What advantages might peer-based peripartum support via telephone offer?
3. Why does peripartum care need to be individualized?

partner may notice that communication and intimacy are negatively impacted. These concerning observations can cause the partner or another family member to reach out to the HCP to seek help for the mother. At times, the mother may not want to admit her need for help, or she may be too ill to know that she is experiencing emotional complications. Often, during these times, additional household responsibilities are placed on the partner. Even the most supportive and resourceful families can experience relationships that suffer during these times.

When the need for further education, emotional support, and additional care for the infant are identified, the nurse can assist the family by making referrals to community resources. The nurse can provide contact information for public health nursing services and social services and emergency services that the mother and family may need. Postpartum follow-up is especially important, and referrals to mental health services such as a visiting psychiatric nurse can be made.

Evaluation

Expected outcomes of nursing care include the following:

- The patient reports reduced severity and frequency of symptoms.
- The newborn is effectively cared for by another parent or support person until the mother is able to provide care.
- The mother and newborn remain safe.

Similar to major depressive disorder, peripartum depression may take time to resolve. The healthcare team will need to provide ongoing care for the mother, infant, and support persons, including integrating a mental health assessment into every postpartum follow-up appointment (Hutchens & Kearney, 2020). Regardless of the treatment provided, the safety of the infant, mother, and family must remain a priority for the healthcare team.

Nursing Care Plan

A Patient with Postpartum Depression

Salma al-Hussein, a 30-year-old woman who was born in Jordan but has lived in the United States for nearly 20 years, is brought to her primary care provider's office by her mother. Mrs. al-Hussein gave birth to her third child nearly 6 weeks ago. Her mother is worried because her daughter is showing almost no interest in the baby and very little interest in her older children. Mrs. al-Hussein's mother and sister have been providing most of the care for the children. Mr. al-Hussein is a small business owner who works 10 to 12 hours per day, 6 days a week.

ASSESSMENT	DIAGNOSES	PLANNING
At first, Mrs. al-Hussein is slow to answer the nurse's questions and keeps her eyes on the floor during the assessment. Mrs. al-Hussein's mother says that her daughter is not normally like this, that she is usually full of life and outgoing and polite with others, even those she does not know well. With the encouragement of her mother, Mrs. al-Hussein becomes more cooperative. The nurse uses the Edinburgh Postnatal Depression Scale; Mrs. al-Hussein scores 14 out of 30.	■ Ineffective parenting ■ Powerlessness ■ Potential for injury ■ Impaired coping	■ The patient will commit to safety. ■ The patient will express her feelings. ■ The patient will agree to participate in mental health counseling. ■ The family will continue to provide care for the children and support Mrs. al-Hussein as she begins the treatment process.

IMPLEMENTATION

- Refer to mental health professional.
- Attempt to persuade Mrs. al-Hussein to commit to safety for both herself and the children.
- Teach family to supervise mother's interaction with the infant and other children at all times to promote safety.
- Explain impact of postpartum depression to the family and help them cope with the impact on the family.
- Identify community resources for assisting with treatment.
- Encourage family to continue providing care for the infant and other children.
- Help Mrs. al-Hussein recognize the signs of depression and accept the diagnosis of postpartum depression.
- Explain to both Mrs. al-Hussein and her family members that postpartum depression is not uncommon and can be successfully treated, but risk for reoccurrence is high if she has additional children.

EVALUATION

Mrs. al-Hussein's care is evaluated based on the following expected outcomes:

- The patient begins treatment with a mental health counselor and is taking her medications as prescribed.
- Family members continue to provide supervision and care of the children until Mrs. al-Hussein's condition improves.
- The patient commits to safety for herself and her children.

CRITICAL THINKING

1. How would you persuade Mrs. al-Hussein to commit to safety for herself and her children?
2. What specific questions would you ask to determine if Mrs. al-Hussein is thinking about harming herself or her children?
3. If Mrs. al-Hussein admitted having fantasies of harming her children, how could you advocate for the family?

REVIEW Peripartum Depression

RELATE Link the Concepts and Exemplars

Linking the exemplar of peripartum depression with the concept of development:

1. How might a mother's peripartum depression impact the development of her 3-year-old daughter?
2. What is your priority developmental concern for the newborn when the mother has severe postpartum depression?

Linking the exemplar of peripartum depression with the concept of comfort:

3. What are your concerns for the mother who has peripartum depression regarding sleep and rest?
4. How will fatigue impact postpartum depression and the care of the newborn?

READY Go to Volume 3: Clinical Nursing Skills

REFER Go to Pearson MyLab Nursing and eText

REFLECT Apply Your Knowledge

Jessica Riley is a single 17-year-old new mother of a 1-month-old infant son named Ryan whose father ended his relationship with Jessica when she was 4 months pregnant. Jessica's relationship with her mother has been strained for the past few years and worsened when she became pregnant. Because she was constantly fighting with her mother, Jessica moved to a small apartment when she was 6 months pregnant. Jessica's father left the family when Jessica was 7 years old. She recently completed her GED and is now trying to go to school part time for an associate's degree in cosmetology. She also works nearly full time as a waitress, but because she is supporting herself and her baby, she struggles financially.

1. What information in Jessica's history puts her at risk for postpartum depression?
2. How would you assess Jessica for potential postpartum depression?
3. What interventions can you implement to reduce Jessica's risk of postpartum depression?

» Exemplar 28.D Suicide

Exemplar Learning Outcomes

28.D Analyze the nurse's role in preventing and responding to patient suicide attempts.

- Describe the pathophysiology of suicide.
- Describe the etiology of suicide.
- Compare risk and protective factors for suicide.
- Identify the clinical manifestations of suicidal ideation.
- Summarize diagnostic tests and therapies used by interprofessional teams in the collaborative care of an individual at risk for suicide.
- Differentiate care of patients at risk for suicide across the lifespan.
- Apply the nursing process in providing culturally competent care to an individual at risk for suicide.

Exemplar Key Terms

Nonsuicidal self-injury (NSSI), *2008*
Suicide, *2000*
Suicidal ideation, *2000*
Suicide attempt, *2000*

Overview

Suicide is the act of inflicting self-harm that results in death. When the act is not fatal, but the intent of the act was to cause death, it is referred to as a **suicide attempt**. Cases of an individual constantly considering, planning, or thinking about suicide are considered **suicidal ideation**. In the United States, suicide has become the 10th leading cause of death, even higher than homicide. In 2018, more than 47,000 individuals took their own lives, approximately 3.3 million made a detailed plan, 1.4 million attempted suicide, and more than 10.7 million adults considered suicide (CDC, 2020b).

Depression is considered to play a role in many instances of suicide. Between 30 and 70% of those who attempt suicide have underlying depression (Mental Health America, 2020). Recent statistics show that health disparities exist in the treatment of depression: Between 76 and 85% of people in low- and middle-income countries receive no treatment for their disorder (WHO, 2019). Lack of access to mental health care may result in underestimating the relationship between depression and suicide.

Influencing Factors

The majority of individuals who attempt or succeed at taking their own lives often cite a reason for wanting to die. However, suicide is generally influenced by a number of factors, not just one. By understanding the underlying causes of suicide, nurses can better recognize potential warning signs for suicidal behavior as well as identify individuals who are at greater risk.

Genetics and Neurobiology

Studies conducted over the past 15 to 20 years have indicated a familial aspect to suicidal tendencies in a number of cases. For example, an individual's risk for suicide is five times higher if a biological relative has committed suicide. Parental suicide attempts appear to be among the most important factors contributing to suicidal tendencies, although there are inherent difficulties in teasing out how much of the increased risk is due to genetics and how much is due to dysfunctional family processes (Miklin, Mueller, Abrutyn, & Ordonez, 2019). Evidence also suggests that early traumatic experiences can lead to changes in gene expression (via epigenetic mechanisms) in the brain that render a person at increased risk for suicidal ideation (Angelakis et al., 2019).

The most commonly studied neurotransmitter thought to be connected with suicide is serotonin, which is also believed to play a central role in major depression. Suicidal individuals have been found to have decreased levels of serotonin, which can cause increased impulsivity and suicidal behavior (De Berardis et al., 2018).

Interpersonal Factors

Individuals contemplating suicide can be influenced by a number of interpersonal factors, such as a history of trauma or a significant loss (e.g., the loss of a child). Any significant emotional disturbance can cause an individual to become depressed, and if the depression becomes unmanageable, that may lead to suicidal thoughts and behaviors. Loss and grief can be profound influencing factors for suicidal behavior, especially if the loss is of significant importance. Individuals who have lost a partner—especially those without other close family ties—should be monitored closely for warning signs of dangerous behavior.

With over a decade of empirical research, Joiner's (2009) interpersonal theory of suicide has helped provide a better understanding about suicide and the prevention of suicidal behavior. Joiner states that an individual will not die by suicide unless he has both the desire to die by suicide and the ability to do so. The interpersonal theory suggests that suicide results from the combination of (1) a perception of burdening others, (2) social alienation and isolation leading to a low sense of belongingness, and (3) possessing the capability for lethal injury. The perception of being a burden to others can lead to the fatal misperception that "if I die, it will make it easier for my family and friends." A low sense of belongingness can be described as feelings linked to isolation and disconnection from others (Joiner, 2009). Joiner concluded that the element of "acquired ability for lethal self-injury" must be present in addition to these factors to lead individuals to attempt to take their life. Furthermore, the acquired ability for lethal self-injury accumulates over time with repeated exposure to significant experiences: With more painful experiences comes greater capacity for suicide.

Comorbid Disorders

Of the people dying by suicide, about 50% have a co-occurring mood disorder and a history of psychiatric hospitalization. Approximately 90% of those who attempt or die by suicide have a comorbid psychiatric disorder. Research suggests that half of individuals who succeed at taking their own lives were either experiencing depression at the time or were in the recovery phase of depression (Aaltonen, Isometsä, Sund, & Pirkola, 2019; Ballard et al., 2019). The most common comorbid disorders for suicide are bipolar disorders, borderline personality disorders, conduct disorders, schizophrenia, and drug and alcohol dependency. All of these disorders have aspects of impaired impulse control, depression, and altered consciousness, thus making them the primary disorders associated with suicide attempts and completion (Aaltonen et al., 2019; Ballard et al., 2019).

Individuals with bipolar disorders are 15 to 20 times more likely to commit suicide than the general population. It is estimated that 25–50% of those with the disorder will attempt suicide at some point in their lives. Note that the risk for suicide among individuals with bipolar disorders decreases considerably with active treatment. The most commonly studied treatment associated with decreased suicide risk was administration of lithium (Maina, Quarato, & Bramante, 2019).

Other psychiatric disorders that carry a significant risk of suicide include schizophrenia, borderline personality disorder and alcohol use disorder (Aaltonen et al., 2019; Ballard et al., 2019; Maina et al., 2019).

Social Factors

Recession, bullying, and/or dominant social beliefs can have an impact on individuals' mental health. Economic recessions can cause financial strain and job loss, which are both stressful events often cited as potential indicators of suicidal behavior. Economic recessions and high unemployment rates often lead to individuals defaulting on mortgages and losing their homes. Research indicates that there is a considerable stigma related to mortgage strain, leading to feelings of shame and worthlessness. Concealing the mortgage strain due to the stigma leads to isolation, and isolation appears to increase the person's depression, anxiety, and emotional stress (Farré, Fasani, & Mueller, 2018).

Bullying is another social factor that increases suicide risk. Bullies in schools or in the workplace are emotionally abusive toward their victims, harassing them to the point where the victims feel worthless or hopeless about life in general. Despite greater awareness and prevention programs, bullying is still widespread in many schools and workplaces. Dominant social beliefs can also play a role. For example, bullying and discrimination have been linked to an increased risk for suicide among transgender and gender-nonconforming individuals (Wolford-Clevenger, Frantell, Smith, Flores, & Stuart, 2018). Another study found that female refugees from areas sustaining genocide need preventive suicide measures (Ingabire & Richters, 2020). Additional groups that the CDC reports at risk include individuals in the justice and child welfare settings; lesbian, gay, bisexual, and transgender (LGBT) populations; and members of the armed forces and veterans (CDC, 2020b).

Etiology

A common theme reported by many survivors of suicide attempts is that suicidal behavior comes from a feeling that death is the only option that will successfully solve the individual's current emotional strain (CDC, 2020b). It is commonly said that suicide is a "cry for help," and while that may be true some of the time, suicide is a desire for a permanent solution to whatever catalyst has prompted the individual's behavior. Some who attempt suicide do so with the mindset that they would like to die, but if they do not, then at least others will realize how truly unhappy, or lonely, or desperate they feel. In cases such as these, a mild overdose of pharmaceuticals will often be used, or they will cause an injury that would be life-threatening if no one found them in time.

Individuals who have only death in mind will generally use a gun, hang themselves, or jump from a tall building because these methods are more likely to cause mortal injuries. Assessing lethality is important in determining patient suicide risk. The use of a scale to assist in determining lethality of attempts is an important component of suicide assessment. The Suicide Assessment Five-Step Evaluation and Triage (SAFE-T) and the Columbia Suicide Severity Rating Scale (C-SSRS) are two clinically researched and proven rating scales for assessment of suicide and lethality. These tools include components of severity and intensity of suicidal ideation, types of suicidal behaviors, and lethality of suicide attempts (King, Horwitz, Czyz, & Lindsay, 2017; National Action Alliance for Suicide Prevention, 2020).

Risk and Protective Factors

Risk factors for suicide in the United States include depression or other mental disorders; previous suicide attempt; a family history of abuse, violence, or suicide; substance use disorders; exposure to suicidal behavior; and firearms in the home.

» **Skills:** See Skills 15.1 and 15.4 in Volume 3.

Other factors contributing to suicide risk include (CDC, 2020b; WHO, 2019):

- Social isolation; lack of support systems
- Recent unemployment
- Recent loss of a significant relationship
- Feelings of failure and hopelessness
- Access to lethal means (e.g., presence of a gun in the home)
- History of trauma or abuse
- Chronic physical illness, including chronic pain.

Other risk factors include gender and age. Men in the United States are more likely to die from suicide, whereas women are twice as likely to attempt suicide. Suicide is currently the seventh leading cause of death in males (Choo, Harris, & Ho, 2019; WHO, 2019). In 2017, the rate of suicide was highest in middle-aged white men. Men died by suicide 3.54 times more often than women. Suicide was the second leading cause of death for individuals age 15 to 34 and the fourth leading cause of death for those age 35 to 54 (American Foundation for the Prevention of Suicide, 2019b). Protective factors are biological, psychologic, social, or environmental factors that make it less likely an individual will develop a disorder (WHO, 2019). Examples of factors that are protective against the risk for suicide include the following:

- Strong family connections
- Community support
- Access to mental health providers
- Young children to care and provide for
- Strong ties to religions that denounce suicide.

Additional protective factors include caring for pets and use of healthy coping and decision-making skills (CDC, 2020b).

Clinical Manifestations

Although the clinical manifestations of suicidal ideation and behavior vary by age, culture, individual psychology, and life history, a few common factors underlie most suicidal behavior. Experts frequently cite impulsivity, aggression, pessimism, and an overall negative affect as personality traits associated with the condition. As stated earlier, negative events such as interpersonal crisis, trauma, or financial catastrophe can play a role. The sense of a loss of meaning in life produces the painful, hopeless mental state conducive to suicide. Factors that predict suicidal behavior in the short term include major depression, psychic anxiety, delusions, and alcohol abuse. The fundamental clinical manifestation of suicidal ideation is the domination of the patient's consciousness by an unrelenting stream of painful thoughts. The suicidal person feels that death is the only possible solution to escape a mental life of unrelenting stress, anxiety, and depression (Abbas, Mohanna, Diab, Chikoore, & Wang, 2018).

Behavior

Behavioral cues provide a window into the mind of an individual who may be contemplating suicide. Though not all people who commit suicide behave abnormally beforehand, many people provide clues that an attempt is imminent. An individual contemplating suicide may mention feeling helpless in the face of stress and may discuss life after death. He may also provide verbal cues such as "It won't matter for long" or "I can't take this much longer." Some behaviors may also demonstrate suicidal ideation, such as giving away personal possessions, withdrawing from relationships, and obtaining a means to end life such as purchasing a gun (American Foundation for the Prevention of Suicide, 2019a). It is important to note that some individuals may not demonstrate overt behaviors when suicidal. For example, data suggests that older adults may not report suicidal ideation (Schmutte & Wilkinson, 2020).

The American Association of Suicidology (2016) developed a mnemonic device for the short-term indications of suicidal intent with the phrase IS PATH WARM. The letters in the phrase indicate the following terms:

Ideation	Purposelessness	Withdrawal
Substance abuse	Anxiety	Anger
	Trapped	Recklessness
	Hopelessness	Mood changes

All of these terms are indicators of possible suicidal behavior, and concern for the patient's condition should increase if the individual exhibits more than one of these behaviors. An individual at immediate risk for suicide will often display the warnings signs of acute risk. These include talking of wanting to hurt oneself; looking for access to firearms, pills, or other means of suicide; and talking or writing about death. If these symptoms are observed, the individual should not be left alone and a mental health professional should be contacted.

Cognition

Individuals who attempt suicide are more likely than their peers to experience distortions in cognition. Common distortions include (but are not limited to) unusually rigid thinking, dichotomous thinking, magnification, overgeneralization, externalization of self-worth, and "fortune telling," or predicting negative outcomes without considering the possibility of other, more positive outcomes (Hughes et al., 2019).

Clinical Manifestations and Therapies
Suicide

CUES	CLINICAL MANIFESTATIONS	CLINICAL THERAPIES
Behavioral changes	■ Verbal cues indicating a desire to die or to "make it all stop" ■ Planning to commit suicide, including buying a gun, knife, or pills ■ Not participating in once-loved activities ■ Loss of interest in school or work ■ Participating in dangerous behavior such as drug use, driving too fast, or not taking safety precautions	■ Treat underlying condition ■ Behavioral therapy ■ Medication therapy ■ If a plan for suicide has been formed, make sure the person is not left alone ■ Educate about therapy options
Affect	■ Depression ■ Hopelessness ■ Loneliness ■ Anger ■ Anxiety	■ Treat underlying condition ■ Behavioral therapy ■ Medication therapy ■ Express a sincere desire to help the individual
Cognitive changes	■ Rigid thinking ■ Fantasies about death or dying ■ Thought disorders ■ Preoccupation with death ■ "Fortune telling" and extreme negativity	■ Treat underlying condition ■ Behavioral therapy ■ Medication therapy
Social isolation	■ Life stressors ■ Poor support systems ■ Social pressure ■ Feeling as though there is no one to ask for help ■ Feeling alienated from society ■ End of a relationship ■ Death of a close friend, spouse, or family member	■ Behavioral therapy ■ Medication therapy ■ Group therapy to recognize that other individuals are experiencing similar issues
Biophysical changes	■ Sleep disturbances ■ Relapse or exacerbation of coexisting mental disorder ■ Potential physical evidence of self-harm (e.g., scars from cutting)	■ Address any immediate physical needs ■ Consider possible medical contributors to reoccurrence or exacerbation of mental disorder ■ Behavioral therapy ■ Medication therapy

After an unsuccessful suicide attempt, an easing of emotional stress typically takes place, especially if the attempt was expected to be lethal, and cognitive distortions often abate. Without appropriate treatment, however, this reduction in stress and distorted thinking is only temporary, and suicidal behavior frequently recurs.

Rehospitalization for suicidal ideation or suicide attempt within a year of the first attempt ranges from 7.96 to 11.24%, with the highest risk occurring within the first month of the initial hospitalization. Almost 50% of rehospitalizations for suicidal ideation or suicidal behavior occur during the first 3 months. There is an increased likelihood that the second or third attempt will be fatal. Long-term studies have shown that 7–10% of individuals who seriously attempt suicide will eventually kill themselves, a risk that is about 5 times greater than the average risk of 1.4% (Cepeda, Schuemie, Kern, Reps, & Canuso, 2020; Gvion, 2018; Hooley, Butcher, Nock, & Mineka, 2017).

Social Isolation

A common precipitant to suicidal behavior is social stress or isolation. Individuals may become suicidal when they become alienated from family and friends, or even when they have difficulty adapting to the demands of new social roles. Loss of a loved one is a contributing factor related to suicide, as well as the loss of the ability to participate in once enjoyable activities. For older adults, the loss of autonomy, including a reliance on others to get around (e.g., loss of a driver's license or loss of mobility) and feeling like they are a burden to others, contributes to the sense of social isolation and increases suicide risk (SAMHSA, 2019).

Cultural Considerations

Within the United States, the various ethnic groups exhibit substantial differences in suicide rates. For example, American Indians and Alaska Natives have the highest

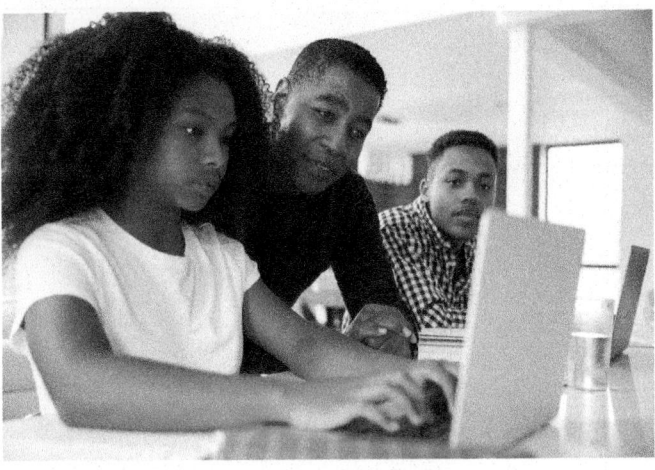

Figure 28.8 ⟫ What risk factors contribute to increased risk for suicide attempts among Black adolescents? What protective factors and nursing interventions might help reduce risk among young Black patients?
Source: Shutterstock.

rate of suicide, followed by non-Hispanic whites. African Americans have the second lowest suicide rate, and the lowest rate is in the Hispanic population (NIMH, 2020b). In 2019, researchers discovered that suicide attempts among white adolescents *decreased* by 7.5% from 1991 to 2017, but the rate of suicide attempts for Black adolescents *increased* by 73% during the same time period (Lindsey, Sheftall, Xiao, & Joe, 2019) (**Figure 28.8** ⟫). Researchers suggest that the increase in suicide attempts by Black adolescents can be attributed to a number of factors, including disparities in access to mental health treatment, stigma and discrimination, mistrust of mental health providers and the healthcare system generally, and adverse childhood experiences (Lindsey et al., 2019). Stigma and discrimination are also linked to increased risk for suicide among the LGBT population (see the Focus on Diversity and Culture feature).

Another cultural difference in the prevalence of suicide worldwide is gender disparity. Women are more likely to attempt suicide and men are more likely to complete suicide in the United States, but in India, Poland, and Finland, men are more likely to engage in nonfatal attempts. In China, India, and Papua New Guinea, women are more likely to complete suicide than men (Martinez, 2019; WHO, 2014; Zhang et al., 2019).

Adherence to religious beliefs is considered to be a protective factor for suicide. Faiths such as Catholicism and Islam strongly forbid suicide, and rates of suicide in nations that follow these religions are accordingly low. Many societies have strong cultural taboos against suicide in addition to formal declarations. However, some nations provide cultural exceptions to the rule outlawing suicide. Japanese culture is one of the few societies in which suicide has been approved as a socially acceptable solution to certain problems of disgrace or social cohesion. The suicidal zeal for a political and religious cause has found a new form in the suicide bombings of Muslim extremists in the Middle East. Across cultures, suicide can be a violent expression of inner turmoil or an act motivated by national or religious fervor (Dhungel, Sugai, & Gilmour, 2019; Mason et al., 2018; Ward, 2018).

Focus on Diversity and Culture

Suicide and LGBT Culture

Lesbian, gay, bisexual, and transgender (LGBT) individuals are at higher risk for suicide, in part, due to discrimination that they experience regularly from family, friends, colleagues, and society. Fear of nonacceptance may be a precipitant to depression and, if severe enough, has been known to lead to suicide.

- LGBT individuals are two times more likely to attempt suicide than heterosexual individuals.
- Gay and bisexual men are four times as likely to attempt suicide compared to heterosexual men.
- LGBT individuals are more likely to participate in suicide attempts and ideation compared to completed suicides.
- Increased risk for suicide in this population can be attributed to the presence of prejudice, stigmas, and discrimination.
- Adolescent LGBT individuals demonstrate a particularly high rate of suicide, attempted suicide, and suicidal ideation (CDC, 2017).

Collaboration

Suicide attempts and suicidal ideation, if caught early enough, can be addressed in a number of ways. The most common and effective method of treatment is to combine pharmaceutical interventions with talk or group therapy or counseling. For individuals who are also experiencing a comorbid disorder, the underlying disorder will need to be treated in addition to the suicidal behavior because the two conditions may exacerbate each other. Nurses will work with the patient, physicians, and therapists to create an effective plan of care.

Pharmacologic Therapy

Depending on the individual patient's manifestations and the presence of comorbid disorders, pharmacologic therapy may be appropriate for patients who are suicidal. The most likely choices of medications are antidepressants and mood stabilizers.

Antidepressants

The antidepressants most often used to treat depression (the underlying cause of the majority of suicide attempts) are fluoxetine (Prozac), citalopram (Celexa), sertraline (Zoloft), paroxetine (Paxil), and escitalopram (Lexapro). All five of these drugs are SSRIs and are used to balance and stabilize the neurotransmitters in the brain that affect mood and emotional responses. Although all of these medications are used to treat depression, they also have the potential side effect of causing suicidal tendencies. The use of antidepressants after a patient has attempted or seriously considered suicide should be combined with nonpharmacologic therapy.

Mood Stabilizers and Antipsychotics

Mood stabilizers commonly prescribed for bipolar disorder have the ability to moderate extreme shifts in emotions between mania and depression. Some antiseizure drugs are also used for mood stabilization in patients with bipolar disorders. For more on drugs for bipolar disorders, see Exemplar 28.B earlier in this module.

Antipsychotics (medications used in the treatment of schizophrenia) may be prescribed for patients who experience hallucinations and delusions or those with major depressive disorder with psychotic features. The treatment of these symptoms of the disease can help the suicidal patient immensely by eliminating one of the underlying causes of self-destructive thoughts. For more information about schizophrenia and antipsychotic medications, see Exemplar 23.C, Schizophrenia, in Module 23, Cognition.

It is important to note that medications can take up to 6 weeks to see full effects. Electroconvulsive therapy has been used in the past to treat acutely suicidal patients, with varying results. Currently, treatment for suicidal patients relies heavily on close monitoring or hospitalization along with medication and therapy (Witt et al., 2020). A new approach to treatment with internasal or intravenous ketamine is currently being investigated. Some research suggests that ketamine may accelerate the effect of ECT in patients with treatment-resistant depression and decrease suicidality. In a study of 572 participants, a single treatment of ketamine reduced suicidal ideation in adult psychiatric patients predominantly diagnosed with unipolar depression, with effects lasting up to 72 hours (Bartoli & Wlkinson, 2020; Gautam et al., 2020; Witt et al., 2020). Furthermore, some evidence suggests that the antisuicidal effect of ketamine is independent from the antidepressant effect, but more research is needed to make definite conclusions (Gautam et al., 2020; Witt et al., 2020). One recommendation for the use of ketamine to treat acute suicidality is combining brief psychological therapy with ketamine treatment, although more research is still needed to make concrete recommendations and guidelines (Bartoli & Wlkinson, 2020; Witt et al., 2020). However, as of 2020, ketamine is only approved by the FDA for use as a drug to induce and maintain general anesthesia.

Nonpharmacologic Therapy

Therapeutic approaches to suicide prevention can be quite effective in many cases. The type of therapy employed will depend on both the patient and the therapist, but the three most common forms of therapy used for suicidal patients are group therapy, individualized therapy, and family therapy. All three of these forms can be combined to further help the patient work through suicidal thoughts and behaviors. Family therapy will generally be used in tandem with either group or individualized therapy. The presence of the family can be very helpful in supporting the patient, especially because most individuals who are truly contemplating suicide will work to isolate themselves from friends and family before the event. Family therapy can also help the patients' families to understand what they are feeling and why they considered suicide, which can ultimately aid families in taking an active role in supporting patients' recovery.

Cognitive-behavioral therapy for suicide prevention (CBT-SP) is sometimes used with adolescents who display serious suicidal ideation or have recently attempted suicide. CBT-SP works to help the individual develop skills to prevent suicidal behavior in the future. The therapist works with the adolescent patient to develop and employ healthy coping mechanisms and avoid all forms of self-harm (Huntjens et al., 2020; Witt et al., 2020).

Patients who are at risk for suicide or who have attempted suicide often benefit from therapeutic interventions addressing healthy coping mechanisms. Writing therapy can be employed to help the patient work through any suicidal thoughts or fantasies; similarly, a preoccupation with death and dying can be addressed through writing and keeping a journal. The journal will also serve to allow the patient to see the progress that has been made from the start of therapy until its completion, with the goal that the writing will change tone from potentially hopeless at the start to more positive and hopeful at the end.

Lifespan Considerations

In the United States in 2018, males were 3.7 times more likely to commit suicide than females. Suicide rates among adult females were highest for those age 45 to 64; among males, the rates were highest for those age 75 and over (CDC, 2020b). Suicide rates for other age groups are provided in the following sections.

Firearms, suffocation, and poisoning are used for over 90% of all suicides. However, the preferred method of suicide differs between males and females. For the years in which the most recent data is available, 31.4% of females chose poisoning, 31.2% chose firearms, and 27.9% chose suffocation. In contrast, males predominantly used firearms (56%) compared to suffocation (27.7%) or poisoning (9%) (CDC, 2017).

Suicide in Children

In 2018, boys between the ages of 10 and 14 committed suicide at a rate of 3.7 per 100,000 individuals, and girls in this age range committed suicide at a rate of 2.0 per 100,000 individuals. Children are at an increased risk for suicidal ideation if they have lost a parent, have been physically or sexually abused, have an unstable family, experience humiliation in school, or have lost a loved one. Psychopathology in childhood—including depression, antisocial behavior, ADHD, and impulsivity—is a strong predictor of childhood suicide. Suicide is the third leading cause of death in children age 10 to 14 (CDC, 2020b). The most common means is hanging or strangulation. Statistics indicate that suicide is more common among Black children, especially Black females, than members of other ethnic and racial groups. Furthermore, more than a quarter of children who committed suicide discussed their intent to do so with someone else prior to their death. These findings highlight the importance of targeted prevention efforts, as well as not discounting the words of children who mention a desire to die (Ruch et al., 2019; Shain, 2019).

Suicide in Adolescents and Young Adults

In 2018, males between the ages of 15 and 24 committed suicide at a rate of 22.7 per 100,000 individuals, and females in this age range committed suicide at a rate of 5.8 per 100,000 individuals (CDC, 2020b). Suicidal cognition increases dramatically in adolescents, most likely because of the collision of depression, anxiety, drug use, and conduct disorders in the teenage years. Adolescents and young adults may also attempt suicide because of a lack of meaningful relationships, sexual problems, and/or acute problems with parents or significant others. Exposure to the dramatic suicides of role-model celebrities also plays a role in the cognition of adolescents, who are highly susceptible to imitative behavior (Musci et al., 2019; Paul, 2018). Similarly, suicide has an element of "contagion" among teenagers, meaning that adolescents are more likely to attempt suicide after learning of the suicide of a friend or acquaintance. In recent years, bullying and harassment via text messaging and social media has also been linked to a rise in suicide attempts (Baiden & Tadeo, 2020). As stated earlier, suicide attempts among Black adolescents have reached alarming rates. College students have additional risk factors, including anxiety about academics, new social situations and responsibilities, and anxiety about their place in the world. Suicide is the second leading cause of death among individuals age 15 to 34 (CDC, 2018a).

Suicide in Pregnant Women

Suicide during pregnancy is not a common occurrence, despite the fact that pregnant women are at risk for depression with peripartum onset. Pregnancy was previously thought to be a protective factor against suicide; however, research suggests that suicidal ideation during pregnancy is more common than once thought. One study found that the prevalence of suicidal ideation among pregnant women was as high as 33% (Gelaye, Kajeepeta, & Williams, 2016). Rodriguez and colleagues (2018) concluded that up to 20% of maternal deaths during pregnancy are due to suicide. Relationship issues appeared to be contributing factors to more than half of suicides in pregnant women. Older, white women were reported to be at greatest risk. Women are far more likely to attempt suicide in the postpartum period than during pregnancy, especially if they are experiencing postpartum depression or psychosis or if they have a history of mood disorders. In fact, suicide is believed to account for about 20% of deaths in women during the first year postpartum (Adu, Brown, Asaolu, & Sanderson, 2019).

Suicide in Older Adults

For older adults, men between the ages of 65 and 74 committed suicide at a rate of 27.8 deaths per 100,000 individuals, and this increased to 39.9 deaths per 100,000 men age 75 and older. Women between the ages of 65 and 74 committed suicide at a rate of 6.2 deaths per 100,000 individuals, and this decreased to 4.0 deaths per 100,000 women age 75 and older (CDC, 2020b). Men age 75 and older had the highest suicide rate of any other age group, and though older adults attempt suicide less often than individuals in other groups, they have a higher rate of completion because they use more lethal means. Furthermore, many are not as resilient as younger adults. White men over the age of 75 have the highest rates of suicide compared to all other age groups and ethnicities (CDC, 2020b; O'Rourke, Jamil, & Siddiqui, 2019). One of the leading causes of suicide in the older population is depression, often undiagnosed, and the negative events that frequently come with long life: death of loved ones, illness, and isolation. Although most of the suicide attempts in this population are associated with mental illness, terminal illness increases the risk of depression and suicidal ideation or suicide. Terminal illness that causes pain and suffering is known to be a precursor to successful suicides. Interestingly, although older adults have higher suicide rates than younger populations, they are less likely to mention suicidal ideation to their HCP (Troya et al., 2019).

NURSING PROCESS

Appropriate, nonjudgmental nursing care of the patient who is suicidal is imperative. Nurses will work to ensure the patient's safety while helping empower the patient's need to refrain from self-harm. Every situation involving suicide is different, and nurses evaluate patients based on their individual cases and without any personal judgment or biases.

Assessment

Nurses working with patients who are considering suicide, or who have recently attempted suicide, should be direct but respectful when evaluating the patient and asking questions. It is a common misconception that talking about suicide directly can cause the patient to act in a suicidal manner. Individuals who are experiencing suicidal ideation respect direct acknowledgment of the situation as opposed to a restrained approach.

During assessment, obtain a full patient and family history, focusing in particular on any personal or family history of mood disorders. Inquire whether the patient has a history of suicide attempts or ideation and if anyone in the patient's family has ever committed suicide.

Next, a thorough assessment to determine suicidality will need to occur. During this assessment, the nurse should evaluate the patient's mood and affect, behavior, cognition, and patterns of social interaction, looking specifically for the manifestations of suicidality described earlier. The nurse should also consider the various risk factors and protective factors outlined near the start of the exemplar. Questions to ask to assess suicidality may include (Columbia University Medical Center, n.d.; NIMH, 2020b):

- Have you wished you were dead or that you could go to sleep and not wake up?
- Have you had any thoughts of killing yourself?
- Have you been thinking of how you might do this?
- Do you have any intent of acting on these thoughts?
- Have you started to work out the details of how you intend to carry out this plan?
- Do you have access to a means of suicide (e.g., gun, pills, vehicle)?
- Have you told anyone of your plan?
- Have you attempted to end your life in the past?
- What is happening in your life that makes you feel like you don't want to live?
- Has anyone in your family ever attempted or succeeded with suicide?

Once the presence of suicidality has been established, the nurse must assess the patient's level of intent and lethality. One frequently used tool in this area is the Columbia-Suicide Severity Rating Scale (C-SSRS), which has been administered to millions of individuals and has demonstrated success in reducing rates of patient suicide (Matarazzo et al., 2019). The scale comes with a list of questions, many of which appear above, and recommendations for triage depending on the severity of the individual's suicidality. For example, a patient who has thought about killing himself or wished he was dead but does not express any intent to harm himself requires, at minimum, mental health referral at discharge. However, the patient who expresses intention to kill himself, with or without a plan, requires immediate safety monitoring and psychiatric consultation. For patients with a history of previous suicide attempt, interventions are determined by the amount of time that has lapsed since the previous attempt. These range from immediate monitoring for safety with a psychiatric consultation for the patient who attempted suicide within the last week to a referral to a mental health provider for the patient who attempted suicide more than a year ago (Columbia University Medical Center, n.d.). See Box 28.1 for an overview of safety precautions to reduce the risk of patient suicide in inpatient settings.

>> Stay Current: To download a copy of the C-SSRS and for more information, go to http://cssrs.columbia.edu.

Another valuable tool for evaluating suicidality is the Suicide Assessment Five-Step Evaluation and Triage (SAFE-T). This assessment helps the nurse both determine the patient's risk level and select appropriate care interventions. The five steps involved in SAFE-T assessment are as follows:

1. Assess the patient's risk factors.
2. Assess the patient's protective factors.
3. Directly ask the patient about intent to commit suicide. This means the nurse should pose specific questions regarding the patient's thoughts, plans, behaviors, and intent.
4. Determine the patient's risk level and intervention. This determination should be based on the nurse's clinical judgment after completion of steps 1 to 3. Use of C-SSRS can also be helpful. Ultimately, the nurse should assign a risk level of low, moderate, or high.
5. Document the patient's risk level and treatment plan, along with the rationales for both.

Low-risk patients can be treated in an outpatient setting, while high-risk patients require immediate hospitalization and support. Following evaluation, individuals with a moderate level of risk can usually be treated in an outpatient setting or with partial hospitalization, but only if they can elaborate a plan for seeking immediate help should their desire to commit suicide increase. Note that the SAFE-T assessment should be conducted upon first contact with the patient and in subsequent contacts as appropriate, but particularly with any additional suicidal behaviors, increase in suicidal ideation, or pertinent clinical change. In addition, patients in inpatient settings should be assessed before increasing unit privileges and at discharge (O'Rourke et al., 2019).

Communicating with Patients

Working Phase

In working with patients who are at risk for suicide, safety is priority. It is important to openly ask about suicide and specific plans that the patient may have. Using empathy, maintaining eye contact, and asking direct questions to assess safety is critical in this phase. The nurse can ask questions such as:

- Enduring this much stress is difficult. Have you ever had thoughts of hurting yourself?
- Have you ever thought of killing yourself?
- How long have you been feeling this way?
- Have you ever made a plan to kill yourself?

It is important to note that during these conversations, the nurse should not invalidate the patient's feelings by making such statements as "You have a lot to live for." It is more important for the nurse to actively listen and offer general leads such as "Tell me more" and "That must have been very difficult."

Diagnosis

The priority of care for the patient who has made a suicide attempt or who expresses suicidal ideation or intent is safety. The assessment will determine the patient's more specific needs. Identified needs and care priorities may include the following:

- Risk of suicide
- Potential for violence against self
- Potential for trauma
- History of trauma
- Hopelessness
- Powerlessness
- Low self-esteem.

Planning

Involving the patient in the planning process can be beneficial depending on the individual's current emotional outlook. Empowering the patient to take control of care goals can be a small step in working toward those goals. Some potential goals are:

- The patient will remain free from injury.
- The patient will ask for help when needed.
- The patient will discuss any extreme feelings of depression or hopelessness.
- The patient will participate in regularly scheduled meetings with the therapist.
- The patient will demonstrate healthy coping mechanisms.
- The patient will begin to demonstrate a desire to live.

Implementation

The majority of suicidal individuals are also depressed. Nurses will need to develop a therapeutic rapport with the patient, which will assist with adherence to the treatment plan. Prioritization of interventions is extremely critical, given the potentially lethal nature of the patient's condition.

This means the nurse's first actions should focus on reducing the patient's risk for self-directed violence. After that, other interventions may be carried out as appropriate. These include encouraging patients to verbalize emotions and concerns; encouraging patients to attend individual, family, and group therapy sessions as scheduled; teaching effective coping skills; and teaching patients how to seek help when needed. Some agencies use no-harm contracts as an intervention (see **Box 28.5** »).

Many patients at risk for suicide lack help-seeking behaviors, and feelings of hopelessness can skew perceptions and prevent patients from asking for help. Nurses can help patients identify sources for help and support and then provide opportunities for practice through role playing with the nurse, peers, or family members.

Promote Immediate Safety

- Ensure that patients who are actively experiencing suicidal ideation do not have access to any sharp objects, weapons, or modes that could be used to harm themselves.
- Ensure that the patient at high risk for suicide is never left alone. A nurse, healthcare professional, or other healthcare worker should be with the patient at all times until the risk for suicide decreases.
- Within the healthcare setting, instruct guests as to what objects they cannot have while visiting the patient, including knives, razor blades, and large quantities of pills.
- In home, outpatient, or community settings, if a patient is considering suicide, alert the appropriate people per agency protocols and applicable state laws: that can be the patient's family, the patient's primary HCP, or a mental health service provider.

Increase Patient Knowledge

- Provide patient and family teaching about symptoms of depression, including feelings of helplessness, worthlessness, and lack of energy. Reassure patients that it takes time for feelings associated with depression to dissipate.
- Provide education to patients who have other comorbid disorders, especially bipolar disorder and schizophrenia.
- Provide medication education, including how the medication works; its intended purpose; how long it may take to experience the full, intended effect; and potential side effects.
- Education of family members and concerned individuals should include the telephone numbers of the National Suicide Prevention Lifeline: 1-800-273-TALK (8255) (veterans press 1), 1-800-799-4TTY (4889). Links to state websites can be found through the Suicide Prevention Resource Center at http://www.sprc.org.

SAFETY ALERT An individual who is contemplating suicide will generally not ask for help in obvious ways. However, the person's behavior may include clues associated with suicide, such as talking about wanting to die, giving away prized possessions, or saying that he will not be around much longer. These warning signs are the patient's way of asking for help, and nurses should be able to recognize them and respond effectively.

Assess and Monitor for Self-Injury Behaviors

Patients may present with **nonsuicidal self-injury behaviors (NSSI)**. These are intentional self-inflicted acts of harm to body tissue without the intent of suicide. Self-mutilation and self-injury are used synonymously; however, currently, the preferred term is *self-injury* or *NSSI* (Shahwan et al., 2020). NSSI generally occurs during periods of painful moods, including guilt, sorrow, flashbacks, and depersonalization to physical pain. Additional reasons attributed to NSSI include self-punishment, attention seeking, imposing guilt, and adaptation to peers who also participate in NSSI (Kiekens et al., 2020; Shahwan et al., 2020). Patients demonstrating NSSI will need to be monitored closely and may be asked to sign a no-harm contract. Examples of NSSI include cutting, bruising, burning of the skin, interfering with wound healing, and extreme nail biting or hair pulling (Kiekens et al., 2020; Shahwan et al., 2020).

Box 28.5

Safety Plan Interventions

Some agencies employ the use of no-harm contracts (sometimes referred to as behavioral contracts or individualized safety plans) to assist patients in identifying options other than self-harm when they experience feelings of suicide. However, there is a lack of evidence to support the use of no-harm contracts (Bryan et al., 2017; Jobes & Chalker, 2019), and many practice guidelines now recommend the use of safety plan interventions (SPIs) as stabilization interventions for suicidal patients. These plans have been proven to be more effective than no-harm contracts (Jobes & Chalker, 2019; O'Connor et al., 2019; Stanley, Hom, Sachs-Ericsson, Gallyer, & Joiner, 2020). The SPI is an emergency safety plan collaboratively developed by the patient and provider. The SPI has been extensively utilized in the U.S. Department of Veterans Affairs and the U.S. Department of Defense healthcare systems, as well as in the public and private sectors in lieu of the no self-harm contract. Unlike the no self-harm contract that focuses on what a patient promises *not to do* (i.e., kill themselves), the SPI emphasizes planning for what the patient *will do* during a suicidal crisis (O'Connor et al., 2019; Stanley et al., 2020). SPIs guide patients through trigger identification, self-care and coping strategies, redirection activities, identifying and using support groups, reaching out for professional help, and securing lethal means (O'Connor et al., 2019; Stanley et al., 2020).

Individualized SPIs may help nurses and other clinicians to empower the patient, manage the suicidal crisis, strengthen the therapeutic alliance, provide an opportunity to educate the patient about warning signs and review coping strategies, and provide options for help and support (Jobes & Chalker, 2019; O'Connor et al., 2019). It is important for nurses and other providers to recognize that SPIs may be useful in these areas, but that they may not in and of themselves reduce a patient's risk for suicide. There is no guarantee that a patient who enters into a no-harm agreement will not attempt suicide. Furthermore, SPIs should be used alongside, and not be substituted for, other essential nursing and clinical interventions.

Evaluation

The outcomes for patients demonstrating suicidal behavior can be varied. If the patient is responsive to treatment, then the outcome has a chance of being favorable. Some potential outcomes for the patient who is receiving treatment for suicidal ideation or attempted suicide include the following:

- The patient remains free from injury.
- The patient verbalizes emotions and concerns.
- The patient participates in all scheduled meetings with therapists and counselors.
- The patient demonstrates effective coping skills.
- The patient seeks help when needed.
- The patient demonstrates a desire to live.

If the patient remains actively suicidal, extreme caution must be taken, including the aforementioned steps to prevent self-directed violence.

Although many interventions can be employed when a patient demonstrates an unwillingness to live, none of these will prove successful if one does not have the desire to help oneself. If a patient dies while in a nurse's care and there is an emotional or guilt response, then the nurse should find someone with whom to discuss feelings in regard to this event. Other nurses, physicians, therapists, or counselors are good sources of support for nurses who have lost a patient.

Nursing Care Plan

A Patient Who Is Suicidal

Brandon Lewis, age 45, is admitted to the behavioral health unit after having threatened to attempt suicide. He was severely intoxicated at the time of his admission. Mr. Lewis is withdrawn and hesitant to speak to anyone who approaches him.

ASSESSMENT	DIAGNOSIS	PLANNING
Danielle Serrano, an RN in the psychiatric department, enters Mr. Lewis's room to obtain a health history and suicide risk assessment. A nursing assistant is sitting in the room with Mr. Lewis. The hospital initiated suicide precautions when Mr. Lewis arrived because his daughter reported that she had walked in on him trying to kill himself. Mr. Lewis does not readily respond to the nurse's questions, so Ms. Serrano waits and begins talking to the patient about mundane topics such as the weather, a documentary she saw on television the evening before, and the lunch menu at the hospital for today. Eventually Ms. Serrano notices that Mr. Lewis seems to be more relaxed, so she asks him again if he would like to talk about what happened. When he does not reply, Ms. Serrano calmly explains that the patient's daughter told the nurse she found him with a large knife and a bottle of painkillers, and then called 911. Mr. Lewis asks if his daughter is still at the hospital, and the nurse responds that she will be back this evening. The patient begins to explain that his wife left him 2 months ago, and then shortly after that he lost his job. Mr. Lewis has been drinking heavily for the past month. The night of his suicide attempt, he wanted all of the pain to stop, so he tried to kill himself. Mr. Lewis's daughter walked in and got the knife away from him, then called for help. The patient claims that he probably would not have tried to kill himself if he had not been intoxicated. Mr. Lewis has no previous history of suicide, depression, or any other comorbid disorders. Mr. Lewis denies any current thoughts of or intent to kill himself.	■ Risk of suicide ■ Potential for self-injury ■ Hopelessness	Identified outcomes for Mr. Lewis include: ■ The patient will remain free from injury. ■ The patient will discuss emotions and concerns. ■ The patient will ask for help. ■ The patient will demonstrate healthy coping mechanisms. ■ The patient will participate in treatment for alcohol dependence.

IMPLEMENTATION

- Assist Mr. Lewis to decrease or eliminate self-abusive behaviors.
- Facilitate development of a positive outlook for the future.
- Provide for safety, stabilization, recovery, and maintenance until Mr. Lewis's depression improves.
- Administer antidepressants as ordered.
- Teach visitors about restricted items (razors, scissors, and so forth).
- Involve family, as patient allows, in discharge planning. Encourage creation of a family safety plan.
- Educate patient and family about signs of increased suicidality, as well as available resources (e.g., suicide prevention hotlines, emergency psychiatric care).
- Initiate a multidisciplinary patient care conference to develop a plan of care.
- Refer to mental health provider.
- Initiate suicide precautions (e.g., do not leave patient alone; make sure patient does not have access to potentially dangerous objects).

(continued on next page)

Nursing Care Plan *(continued)*

- Encourage Mr. Lewis to verbalize feelings.
- Develop an individualized safety plan to help Mr. Lewis recognize and cope with triggers and warning signs using strategies other than self-harming.
- Limit access to windows.
- Consider strategies to decrease isolation.

EVALUATION

Mr. Lewis agrees that he needs help to abstain from alcohol and agrees to be admitted to an alcohol rehabilitation facility. He says he probably would never have tried to harm himself if he had not been drinking, but agrees counseling is required and talks with a psychologist.

CRITICAL THINKING

1. If you are the nurse caring for Mr. Lewis on the behavioral health unit, what actions will you take to keep the patient safe?
2. Will you notify Mr. Lewis's wife of his admission? Explain your answer.
3. What strategies would you promote to Mr. Lewis to reduce hopelessness and have hope for the future?

REVIEW Suicide

RELATE Link the Concepts and Exemplars

Linking the exemplar of suicide with the concept of health, wellness, illness, and injury:

1. Explain the relationship between suicide and disrupted sleep pattern.
2. Explain the relationship between suicide and terminal illness.

Linking the exemplar of suicide with the concept of comfort:

3. Explain why the patient with chronic pain should be assessed for risk of suicide.
4. How will you assess the patient living with chronic pain for suicide risk?

READY Go to Volume 3: Clinical Nursing Skills

REFER Go to Pearson MyLab Nursing and eText

REFLECT Apply Your Knowledge

Jenny Vasquez, age 14, presents to the emergency department (ED) after having consumed a box of diphenhydramine (Benadryl) tablets. Her left wrist has also been cut horizontally; the amount of blood loss is unknown. Upon ED arrival, Jenny is lethargic. A security guard is present in the examination room. The physician begins to perform a physical assessment on Jenny.

Jenny's vital signs include temperature 96.2°F tympanic; pulse 118 bpm; and blood pressure 152/96 mmHg. Respirations are 14 per minute, and Jenny does not appear to be in any acute respiratory distress. The ED physician quickly assesses Jenny's left wrist wound; there is no active bleeding and the wound is superficial with no deep tissue damage. A dressing is applied to the wound. Gastric lavage is performed immediately to remove the drugs from Jenny's stomach. Afterward, her wrist laceration is cleaned and sutured, and a sterile dressing is applied to the site.

Upon reassessment of Jenny, she speaks quietly and makes eye contact with the nurse. She explains that the teenagers at school have been bullying her for the past year. Jenny is unsure about her sexual orientation but was seen kissing another girl at the winter formal last year. Ever since then, she has been ostracized and teased constantly at school. The day of the suicide attempt, Jenny arrived at her locker to find that someone had spray-painted the words "queer," "freak," and "spic" in red paint. Seeing no other way to stop the abuse, Jenny tried to kill herself.

1. Based on the information provided about Jenny's situation, do you believe she is at especially high risk for attempting suicide again? Please explain your answer.
2. Do you believe that Jenny was actually trying to kill herself, or was this incident more of a "cry for help"? Justify your answer with evidence from the case study.
3. Identify three patient priorities that are appropriate for inclusion in Jenny's plan of care.

References

Aaltonen, K. I., Isometsä, E., Sund, R., & Pirkola, S. (2019). Risk factors for suicide in depression in Finland: First-hospitalized patients followed up to 24 years. *Acta Psychiatrica Scandinavica, 139*(2), 154–163.

Abbas, M. J., Mohanna, M. A., Diab, T. A., Chikoore, M., & Wang, M. (2018). Why suicide?: The analysis of motives for self-harm. *Behavioural and Cognitive Psychotherapy, 46*(2), 209–225.

Adams, M., Holland, L. N., & Urban, C. Q. (2020). *Pharmacology for nurses: A pathophysiologic approach* (6th ed.). Pearson.

Adu, A., Brown, S. V., Asaolu, I., & Sanderson, W. (2019). Understanding suicide in pregnant and postpartum women, using the National Violent Death Reporting System data: Are there differences in rural and urban status? *Open Journal of Obstetrics and Gynecology, 9*(5), 547–565.

Aedo, A., Murru, A., Sánchez, R., Grande, I., Vieta, E., & Undurraga, J. (2019). Clinical characterization of rapid cycling bipolar disorder: Association with attention deficit hyperactivity disorder. *Journal of Affective Disorders, 240*, 187–192.

Airaksinen, J., Gluschkoff, K., Kivimäki, M., & Jokela, M. (2020). Connectivity of depression symptoms before and after diagnosis of a chronic disease: A network analysis in the U.S. Health and Retirement Study. *Journal of Affective Disorders, 266*, 230–234.

Albert, K., Potter, G., Boyd, B., Kang, H., & Taylor, W. (2019). Brain network functional connectivity and cognitive performance in major depressive disorder. *Journal of Psychiatric Research, 110*, 51–56. https://doi.org/10.1016/j.jpsychires.2018.11.020

Albert, K. M., Potter, G. G., McQuoid, D. R., & Taylor, W. D. (2018). Cognitive performance in antidepressant-free recurrent major depressive disorder. *Depression and Anxiety, 35*(8), 694–699.

Almeida, P. G., Nani, J. V., Oses, J. P., Brietzke, E., & Hayashi, M. A. (2019). Neuroinflammation and glial cell activation in mental disorders. *Brain, Behavior, & Immunity-Health, 2*, 100034. https://www.sciencedirect.com/science/article/pii/S2666354619300353

American Association of Suicidology. (2016). *Warning signs.* https://suicidology.org/resources/warning-signs/

American College of Obstetricians and Gynecologists (ACOG). (2015). *Committee Opinion No. 630: Screening for perinatal depression.* https://www.acog.org/clinical/clinical-guidance/committee-opinion/articles/2018/11/screening-for-perinatal-depression

American Foundation for the Prevention of Suicide. (2019a). *Risk factors and warning signs.* https://afsp.org/risk-factors-and-warning-signs

American Foundation for the Prevention of Suicide. (2019b). *Suicide facts.* https://afsp.org/suicide-statistics/

American Psychiatric Association (APA). (2013). *Diagnostic and statistical manual of mental disorders* (5th ed.). Author.

American Psychiatric Association. (APA). (2021). *What is postpartum depression?* https://www.psychiatry.org/patients-families/postpartum-depression/what-is-postpartum-depression

American Psychological Association. (2018). A policy statement by the Society for Community Research and Action: Division 27 of the American Psychological Association. Statement on the effects of deportation and forced separation on immigrants, their families, and communities. *American Journal of Community Psychology, 62*(1/2), 3–12.

American Psychological Association. (2019). *Clinical practice guideline for the treatment of depression across three age cohorts.* https://www.apa.org/depression-guideline/guideline.pdf

American Psychological Association. (2020). *Patient Health Questionnaire (PHQ-9 & PHQ-2).* https://www.apa.org/pi/about/publications/caregivers/practice-settings/assessment/tools/patient-health

Angelakis, I., Gillespie, E. L., & Panagioti, M. (2019). Childhood maltreatment and adult suicidality: a comprehensive systematic review with meta-analysis. *Psychological Medicine, 49*(7), 1057–1078.

Arifin, S. R. M., Cheyne, H., & Maxwell, M. (2020). Cross-cultural experience of maternal postnatal depression. *International Journal of Psychosocial Rehabilitation, 24*(3), 147–156.

Armour, M., Smith, C. A., Wang, L. Q., Naidoo, D., Yang, G. Y., MacPherson, H., et al. (2019). Acupuncture for depression: A systematic review and meta-analysis. *Journal of Clinical Medicine, 8*(8), 1140. https://www.mdpi.com/2077-0383/8/8/1140/htm

Arnone, D. (2018). Functional MRI findings, pharmacological treatment in major depression and clinical response. *Progress in Neuro-Psychopharmacology and Biological Psychiatry, 91*(20), 28–37. https://doi.org/10.1016/j.pnpbp.2018.08.004

Bahji, A., Ermacora, D., Stephenson, C., Hawken, E. R., & Vazquez, G. (2020). Comparative efficacy and tolerability of pharmacological treatments for the treatment of acute bipolar depression: A systematic review and network meta-analysis. *Journal of Affective Disorders, 269*, 154–184.

Bahji, A., Hawken, E. R., Sepehry, A. A., Cabrera, C. A., & Vazquez, G. (2019). ECT beyond unipolar major depression: Systematic review and meta-analysis of electroconvulsive therapy in bipolar depression. *Acta Psychiatrica Scandinavica, 139*(3), 214–226.

Baiden, P., & Tadeo, S. K. (2020). Investigating the association between bullying victimization and suicidal ideation among adolescents: Evidence from the 2017 Youth Risk Behavior Survey. *Child Abuse & Neglect, 102*, 104417. https://doi.org/10.1016/j.chiabu.2020.104417

Ballard, E. D., Cui, L., Vandeleur, C., Castelao, E., Zarate, C. A., Preisig, M., & Merikangas, K. R. (2019). Familial aggregation and coaggregation of suicide attempts and comorbid mental disorders in adults. *JAMA Psychiatry, 76*(8), 826–833. https://jamanetwork.com/journals/jamapsychiatry/fullarticle/2729443

Baroni, A., Bruzzese, J.-M., Di Bartolo, C. A., Ciarleglio, A., & Shatkin, J. P. (2018). Impact of a sleep course on sleep, mood and anxiety symptoms in college students: A pilot study. *Journal of American College Health, 66*(1), 41–50.

Bartoli, F., & Wlkinson, S. T. (2020). Ketamine and esketamine for suicidal ideation: Recent progress and practical issues. *Australian & New Zealand Journal of Psychiatry, 54*(2), 206–207.

Bass III, P. F., & Bauer, N. S. (2018). Parental postpartum depression: More than "baby blues." *Contemporary Pediatrics, 35*(9), 35–38.

Beck, A. (1967). *Depression: Clinical, experimental, and theoretical aspects.* Harper & Row.

Belvederi Murri, M., Ekkekakis, P., Magagnoli, M., Zampogna, D., Cattedra, S., Capobianco, L., et al. (2019). Physical exercise in major depression: Reducing the mortality gap while improving clinical outcomes. *Frontiers in Psychiatry, 9*, 762. https://www.frontiersin.org/articles/10.3389/fpsyt.2018.00762/full

Bettis, A. H., Forehand, R., Sterba, S. K., Preacher, K. J., & Compas, B. E. (2018). Anxiety and depression in children of depressed parents: Dynamics of change in a preventive intervention. *Journal of Clinical Child and Adolescent Psychology, 47*(4), 581–594.

Boku, S., Nakagawa, S., Toda, H., & Hishimoto, A. (2018). Neural basis of major depressive disorder: Beyond monoamine hypothesis. *Psychiatry and Clinical Neurosciences, 72*(1), 3–12.

Boson, K., Wennberg, P., Fahlke, C., & Berglund, K. (2019). Personality traits as predictors of early alcohol inebriation among young adolescents: Mediating effects by mental health and gender-specific patterns. *Addictive Behaviors, 95*, 152–159.

Bozkurt, H. T., Erbasan, V., Eğilmez, Ü., Şen, B., Aydın, M., & Altınbaş, K. (2018). Clinical, biological and genetic predictors of lithium treatment response. *Current Approaches in Psychiatry, 10*, 395–416.

Bryan, C. J., Mintz, J., Clemans, T. A., Leeson, B., Burch, T. S., Williams, S. R., et al. (2017). Effect of crisis response planning vs. contracts for safety on suicide risk in US Army soldiers: A randomized clinical trial. *Journal of Affective Disorders, 212*, 64–72.

Bucher, M. A., Suzuki, T., & Samuel, D. B. (2019). A meta-analytic review of personality traits and their associations with mental health treatment outcomes. *Clinical Psychology Review, 70*, 51–63.

Burval, J., Kerns, R., & Reed, K. (2020). Treating postpartum depression with brexanolone. *The Peer-Reviewed Journal of Clinical Excellence, 50*(5), 48–53.

Campagne, D. M. (2019). Antidepressant use in pregnancy: Are we closer to consensus? *Archives of Women's Mental Health, 22*(2), 189–197.

Caroleo, M., Carbone, A. Primerano, A., Foti, D., Brunetti, A., & Segura-Garcia, C. (2019). The role of hormonal, metabolic and inflammatory biomarkers on sleep and appetite in drug free patients with major depression: A systematic review. *Journal of Affective Disorders, 250*, 249–259. https://doi.org/10.1016/j.jad.2019.03.015

Casey, B. J., Heller, A. S., Gee, D. G., & Cohen, A. O. (2019). Development of the emotional brain. *Neuroscience Letters, 693*, 29–34.

Centers for Disease Control and Prevention (CDC). (2017). *Suicide statistics.* https://www.nimh.nih.gov/health/statistics/suicide.shtml

Centers for Disease Control and Prevention (CDC). (2018a). *Leading cause of death reports.* https://webappa.cdc.gov/cgi-bin/broker.exe

Centers for Disease Control and Prevention (CDC). (2018b). *Prevalence of depression among adults aged 20 and over: United States, 2013–2016.* https://www.cdc.gov/nchs/products/databriefs/db303.htm

Center for Disease Control and Prevention (CDC). (2020a). *Depression among women.* https://www.cdc.gov/reproductivehealth/depression/index.htm#Postpartum

Center for Disease Control and Prevention (CDC). (2020b). *Increase in suicide mortality in the United States, 1999–2018.* https://www.cdc.gov/nchs/products/databriefs/db362.htm

Center for Disease Control and Prevention (CDC). (2020c). *Preventing suicide: A technical package of policy, programs, and practice.* https://www.cdc.gov/violenceprevention/pdf/suicideTechnicalPackage.pdf

Center for Disease Control and Prevention (CDC). (2020d). *Statistics on children's mental health.* https://www.cdc.gov/childrensmentalhealth/data.html

Cepeda, M. S., Kern, D. M., & Nicholson, S. (2019). Treatment resistant depression in women with peripartum depression. *BMC Pregnancy and Childbirth, 19*, Article No. 323. https://bmcpregnancychildbirth.biomedcentral.com/articles/10.1186/s12884-019-2462-9

Cepeda, M. S., Schuemie, M., Kern, D. M., Reps, J., & Canuso, C. (2020). Frequency of rehospitalization after hospitalization for suicidal ideation or suicidal behavior in patients with depression. *Psychiatry Research, 285*, 112810. https://doi.org/10.1016/j.psychres.2020.112810

Charlson, F., van Ommeren, M., Flaxman, A., Cornett, J., Whiteford, H., & Saxena, S. (2019). New WHO prevalence estimates of mental disorders in conflict settings: A systematic review and meta-analysis. *Lancet, 394*(10194), 240–248. https://doi.org/10.1016/S0140-6736(19)30934-1

Chen, J., Zhao, L., Liu, Y., Fan, S., & Xie, P. (2017). Comparative efficacy and acceptability of electroconvulsive therapy versus repetitive transcranial magnetic stimulation for major depression: A systematic review and multiple-treatments meta-analysis. *Behavioural Brain Research, 320*, 30–36.

Chentsova-Dutton, Y. E., Gold, A., Gomes, A., & Ryder, A. G. (2019). Feelings in the body: Cultural variations in the somatic concomitants of affective experience. *Emotion.* Advance online publication. https://doi.org/10.1037/emo0000683

Choo, C. C., Harris, K. M., & Ho, R. C. (2019). Prediction of lethality in suicide attempts: Gender matters. *Omega: Journal of Death & Dying, 80*(1), 87–103.

Columbia University Medical Center. (n.d.) *Columbia-Suicide Severity Scale.* http://cssrs.columbia.edu/

Corfield, E. C., Yang, Y., Martin, N. G., & Nyholt, D. R. (2017). A continuum of genetic liability for minor and major depression. *Translational Psychiatry, 7*(5), e1131. https://www.nature.com/articles/tp201799

Cox, J. L., Holden, J. M., & Sagovsky, R. (1987). Detection of postnatal depression: Development of the 10-item Edinburgh Postnatal Depression Scale. *British Journal of Psychiatry, 150*, 782–786.

Daskalakis, Z. J., Dimitrova, J., McClintock, S. M., Sun, Y., Voineskos, D., Rajji, T. K., et al. (2020). Magnetic seizure therapy (MST) for major depressive disorder. *Neuropsychopharmacology, 45*(2), 276–282. https://doi.org/10.1038/s41386-019-0515-4

Davanzo, R., Copertino, M., De Cunto, A., Minen, F., & Amaddeo, A. (2011). Antidepression medications and breastfeeding: A review of the literature. *Breastfeeding Medicine, 6*(2), 89–98.

Davison, K. M., Lung, Y., Lin, S. (Lamson), Tong, H., Kobayashi, K. M., & Fuller-Thomson, E. (2019). Depression in middle and older adulthood: the role of immigration, nutrition, and other determinants of health in the Canadian longitudinal study on aging. *BMC Psychiatry, 19*(1), 329. https://doi.org/10.1186/s12888-019-2309-y

De Berardis, D., Fornaro, M., Valchera, A., Cavuto, M., Perna, G., Di Nicola, M., et al. (2018). Eradicating suicide at its roots: Preclinical bases and clinical evidence of the efficacy of ketamine in the treatment of suicidal behaviors. *International Journal of Molecular Sciences, 19*(10), 2888.

Dennis, C. L., & Dowswell, T. (2013). Psychosocial and psychological interventions for preventing postpartum depression. *Cochrane Database of Systematic Reviews*, Issue 2, Article No. CD001134. doi: 10.1002/14651858.CD001134.pub3

Dhami P., Pandey P., Kaur, A., & Kaur K. (2018). A review on synergistic relationship between nutrition and exercise in treating depression. *Indian Journal of Health & Wellbeing, 9*(4), 653–658.

Dhungel, B., Sugai, M. K., & Gilmour, S. (2019). Trends in suicide mortality by method from 1979 to 2016 in Japan. *International Journal of Environmental Research and Public Health, 16*(10), 1794. https://www.mdpi.com/1660-4601/16/10/1794

Diermen, L., Hebbrecht, K., Schrijvers, D., Sabbe, B. C. G., Fransen, E., & Birkenhäger, T. K. (2018). The Maudsley Staging Method as predictor of electroconvulsive therapy effectiveness in depression. *Acta Psychiatrica Scandinavica, 138*(6), 605–614.

Doering, J. J., & Dogan, S. (2018). A postpartum sleep and fatigue intervention feasibility pilot study. *Behavioral Sleep Medicine, 16*(2), 185–201.

Dome, P., Tombor, L., Lazary, J., Gonda, X., & Rihmer, Z. (2019). Natural health products, dietary minerals and over-the-counter medications as add-on therapies to antidepressants in the treatment of major depressive disorder: A review. *Brain Research Bulletin, 146*, 51–78.

Dong, M., Zhu, X., Zheng, W., Li, X., Ng, C. H., Ungvari, G. S., & Xiang, Y. (2018). Electroconvulsive therapy for older adult patients with major depressive disorder: A systematic review of randomized controlled trials. *Psychogeriatrics, 18*(6), 468–475.

Drahota, A., & Revell-Smith, Y. (2019). *Continuation and maintenance treatments for depression in older people.* Cochrane

Nursing Care. https://researchportal.port.ac.uk/portal/files/13130033/Continuation_and_maintenance.pdf

Duman, R. S., Sanacora, G., & Krystal, J. H. (2019). Altered connectivity in depression: GABA and glutamate neurotransmitter deficits and reversal by novel treatments. *Neuron, 102*(1), 75–90. http://dx.doi.org/10.1016/j.neuron.2019.03.013

Earls, M. F., Yogman, M. W., Mattson, G., Rafferty, J., & Committee on Psychosocial Aspects of Child and Family Health. (2019). Incorporating recognition and management of perinatal depression into pediatric practice. *Pediatrics, 143*(1), e20183259. https://pediatrics.aappublications.org/content/143/1/e20183259

Elwood, J., Murray, E., Bell, A., Sinclair, M., Kernohan, W. G., & Stockdale, J. (2019). A systematic review investigating if genetic or epigenetic markers are associated with postnatal depression. Journal of Affective Disorders, 253, 51–62. https://doi.org/10.1016/j.jad.2019.04.059

Emery, L., Sorrell, A., & Miles, C. (2020). Age differences in negative, but not positive, rumination. *Journals of Gerontology Series B: Psychological Sciences & Social Sciences, 75*(1), 80–84.

Ettman, C. K., Abdalla, S. M., Cohen, G. H., Sampson, L., Vivier, P. M., & Galea, S. (2020). Prevalence of depression symptoms in US adults before and during the COVID-19 pandemic. *JAMA Network Open, 3*(2), e2019686. https://doi.org/10.1001/jamanetworkopen.2020.19686

Fallon, V., Halford, J. C. G., Bennett, K. M., & Harrold, J. A. (2018). Postpartum-specific anxiety as a predictor of infant-feeding outcomes and perceptions of infant-feeding behaviours: New evidence for childbearing specific measures of mood. *Archives of Women's Mental Health, 21*(2), 181–191.

Farré, L., Fasani, F., & Mueller, H. (2018). Feeling useless: The effect of unemployment on mental health in the Great Recession. *IZA Journal of Labor Economics, 7*(1), 8. https://link.springer.com/article/10.1186/s40172-018-0068-5

Fava, G. A., & Guidi, J. (2020). The pursuit of euthymia. *World Psychiatry, 19*(1), 40–50. https://onlinelibrary.wiley.com/doi/full/10.1002/wps.20698

Ferenchick, E. K., Ramanuj, P., & Pincus, H. A. (2019). Depression in primary care: Part 2-managment. *British Medical Journal, 365*, l835. https://doi.org/10.1136/bmj.l835

Fernández-Theoduloz, G., Paz, V., Nicolaisen-Sobesky, E., Pérez, A., Buunk, A. P., Cabana, Á., & Gradin, V. B. (2019). Social avoidance in depression: A study using a social decision-making task. *Journal of Abnormal Psychology, 128*(3), 234–244.

Forde, R., Peters, S., & Wittkowski, A. (2020). Recovery from postpartum psychosis: A systematic review and metasynthesis of women's and families' experiences. *Archives of Women's Mental Health, 23*, 597–612. https://link.springer.com/article/10.1007/s00737-020-01025-z

Forneris, C., Nussbaumer-Streit, B., Morgan, C., Greenblatt, A., Van Noord, M., Gaynes, B., et al. (2019). Psychological therapies for preventing seasonal affective disorder. *Cochrane Database of Systematic Reviews*, Issue 11, Article No. CD011270. https://doi.org/10.1002/14651858.CD011270.pub2.

Francescangeli, J., Karamchandani, K., Powell, M., & Bonavia, A. (2019). The serotonin syndrome: From molecular mechanisms to clinical practice. *International Journal of Molecular Sciences, 20*(9), 2288. https://www.mdpi.com/1422-0067/20/9/2288/htm

Gan, Z., Wu, X., Chen, Z., Liao, Y., Wu, Y., He, Z., et al. (2019). Rapid cycling bipolar disorder is associated with antithyroid antibodies, instead of thyroid dysfunction. *BMC Psychiatry, 19*(1), 378. https://doi.org/10.1186/s12888-019-2354-6

Gautam, C., Mahajan, S., Sharma, J., Singh, H., & Singh, J. (2020). Repurposing potential of ketamine: Opportunities and challenges. *Indian Journal of Psychological Medicine, 42*(1), 22–29.

Gelaye, B., Kajeepeta, S., & Williams, M. (2016). Suicidal ideation in pregnancy: An epidemiologic review. *Archives of Women's Mental Health, 19*(5), 741–751. h

Gitlin, M. J. (2018). Antidepressants in bipolar depression: An enduring controversy. *International Journal of Bipolar Disorders, 6*(1), 25. https://doi.org/10.1186/s40345-018-0133-9

Gold, A. K., Otto, M. W., Deckersbach, T., Sylvia, L. G., Nierenberg, A. A., & Kinrys, G. (2018). Substance use comorbidity in bipolar disorder: A qualitative review of treatment strategies and outcomes. *American Journal on Addictions, 27*(3), 188–201.

Goodyer, I. M., & Wilkinson, P. O. (2019). Practitioner review: Therapeutics of unipolar major depressions in adolescents. *Journal of Child Psychology and Psychiatry, 60*(3), 232–243.

Grover, S., Sahoo, S., Chakrabarti, S., Basu, D., Singh, S., & Avasthi, A. (2018). ECT in the postpartum period: A retrospective case series from a tertiary health care center in India. *Indian Journal of Psychological Medicine, 40*(6), 562–567.

Gvion, Y. (2018). Aggression, impulsivity, and their predictive value on medical lethality of suicide attempts: A follow-up study on hospitalized patients. *Journal of Affective Disorders, 227*, 840–846.

Han, K.-M., Ko, Y.-H., Yoon, H.-K., Han, C., Ham, B.-J., & Kim, Y.-K. (2018). Relationship of depression, chronic disease, self-rated health, and gender with health care utilization among community-living elderly. *Journal of Affective Disorders, 241*, 402–410.

Hayes, J. F., Lewis, G., & Lewis, G. (2019). Newer-generation antidepressants and suicide risk. *Psychotherapy and Psychosomatics, 88*(6), 371–372.

He, H., Sui, J., Du, Y., Yu, Q., Lin, D., Drevets, W., et al. (2017). Co-altered functional networks and brain structure in unmedicated patients with bipolar and major depressive disorders. *Brain Structure and Function, 222*(9), 4051–4064.

Hooley, J. M., Butcher, J. N., Nock, M. K., & Mineka, S. M. (2017). *Abnormal psychology* (17th ed.). Pearson.

Hughes, C. D., King, A. M., Kranzler, A., Fehling, K., Miller, A., Lindqvist, J., & Selby, E. A. (2019). Anxious and overwhelming affects and repetitive negative thinking as ecological predictors of self-injurious thoughts and behaviors. *Cognitive Therapy and Research, 43*(1), 88–101.

Hulgaard, D., Dehlholm, L. G., & Rask, C. U. (2019). Family-based interventions for children and adolescents with functional somatic symptoms: A systematic review. *Journal of Family Therapy, 41*(1), 4–28.

Humphreys, K. L., LeMoult, J., Wear, J. G., Piersiak, H. A., Lee, A., & Gotlib, I. H. (2020). Child maltreatment and depression: A meta-analysis of studies using the Childhood Trauma Questionnaire. *Child Abuse & Neglect, 102*, 104361. https://doi.org/10.1016/j.chiabu.2020.104361

Huntjens, A., van den Bosch, L. M. C. W., Sizoo, B., Kerkhof, A., Huibers, M. J. H., & van der Gaag, M. (2020). The effect of dialectical behaviour therapy in autism spectrum patients with suicidality and/ or self-destructive behaviour (DIASS): Study protocol for a multicentre randomised controlled trial. *BMC Psychiatry, 20*, Article No. 127. https://doi.org/10.1186/s12888-020-02531-1

Hutchens, B. F., & Kearney, J. (2020). Risk factors for postpartum depression: An umbrella review. *Journal of Midwifery and Women's Health, 65*(1), 96–108. https://doi.org/10.1111/jmwh.13067

Hyde, J. S., & Mezulis, A. H. (2020). Gender differences in depression: Biological, affective, cognitive, and sociocultural factors. *Harvard Review of Psychiatry, 28*(1), 4–13.

Imaz, M. L., Torra, M., Soy, D., Garcia-Esteve, L., & Martin-Santos, R. (2019). Clinical lactation studies of lithium: A systematic review. *Frontiers in Pharmacology, 10*, 1005. 10.3389/fphar.2019.01005

Ingabire, C. M., & Richters, A. (2020). Suicidal ideation and behavior among Congolese refugees in Rwanda: Contributing factors, consequences, and support mechanisms in the context of culture. *Frontiers in Psychiatry, 11*, 299. https://doi.org/10.3389/fpsyt.2020.00299

James, R. D., West, K. M., Claw, K. G., EchoHawk, A., Dodge, L., Dominguez, A., et al. (2018). Responsible research with urban American Indians and Alaska Natives. *American Journal of Public Health, 108*(12), 1613–1616.

Jamilian, H., Amirani, E., Milajerdi, A., Kolahdooz, F., Mirzaei, H., Zaroudi, M., et al. (2019). The effects of vitamin D supplementation on mental health, and biomarkers of inflammation and oxidative stress in patients with psychiatric disorders: A systematic review and meta-analysis of randomized controlled trials. *Progress in Neuro-Psychopharmacology and Biological Psychiatry, 94*, 109651. https://doi.org/10.1016/j.pnpbp.2019.109651

Jha, M. K., Grannemann, B. D., Trombello, J. M., Clark, E. W., Eidelman, S. L., Lawson, T., et al. (2019). A structured approach to detecting and treating depression in primary care: VitalSign6 Project. *Annals of Family Medicine, 17*(4), 326–335. https://doi.org/10.1370/afm.2418

Jobes, D. A., & Chalker, S. A. (2019). One size does not fit all: A comprehensive clinical approach to reducing suicidal ideation, attempts, and deaths. *International Journal of Environmental Research and Public Health, 16*(19), 3606. https://www.mdpi.com/1660-4601/16/19/3606

Johnson, C. P., Christensen, G. E., Fiedorowicz, J. G., Mani, M., Shaffer, J. J., Magnotta, V. A., & Wemmie, J. A. (2018). Alterations of the cerebellum and basal ganglia in bipolar disorder mood states detected by quantitative T1ρ mapping. *Bipolar Disorders, 20*(4), 381–390.

Joiner, T. (2009). *The interpersonal-psychological theory of suicidal behavior: Current empirical status.* American Psychological Association. https://www.apa.org/science/about/psa/2009/06/sci-brief

Jordan, S., Davies, G. I., Thayer, D. S., Tucker, D., & Humphreys, I. (2019). Antidepressant prescriptions, discontinuation, depression and perinatal outcomes, including breastfeeding: A population cohort analysis. *PLoS One, 14*(11), e0225133. https://doi.org/10.1371/journal.pone.0225133

Joseph, D. L., Chan, M. Y., Heintzelman, S. J., Tay, L., Diener, E., & Scotney, V. S. (2020). The manipulation of affect: A meta-analysis of affect induction procedures. *Psychological Bulletin, 146*(3), 355–375.

Kalman, J. L., Papiol, S., Forstner, A. J., Heilbronner, U., Degenhardt, F., Strohmaier, J., et al. (2019). Investigating polygenic burden in age at disease onset in bipolar disorder: Findings from an international multicentric study. *Bipolar Disorders, 21*(1), 68–75.

Kandola, A., Ashdown-Franks, G., Hendrikse, J., Sabiston, C. M., & Stubbs, B. (2019). Physical activity and depression: Towards understanding the antidepressant mechanisms of physical activity. *Neuroscience & Biobehavioral Reviews, 107*, 525–539.

Khanzada, N. S., Butler, M. G., & Manzardo, A. M. (2017). GeneAnalytics pathway analysis and genetic overlap among autism spectrum disorder, bipolar disorder and schizophrenia. *International Journal of Molecular Sciences, 18*(3), 527. https://doi.org/10.3390/ijms18030527

Kiekens, G., Hasking, P., Nock, M. K., Boyes, M., Kirtley, O., Bruffaerts, R., et al. (2020). Fluctuations in affective states and self-efficacy to resist non-suicidal self-injury as real-time predictors of non-suicidal self-injurious thoughts and behaviors. *Frontiers in Psychiatry, 11*, 214. https://doi.org/10.3389/fpsyt.2020.00214

King, C., Horwitz, A., Czyz, E., & Lindsay, R. (2017). Suicide risk screening in healthcare settings: Identifying males and females at risk. *Journal of Clinical Psychology in Medical Settings, 24*(1), 8–20.

Kleiman, E. M., & Nock, M. K. (2020). New directions for improving the prediction, prevention, and treatment of suicidal thoughts and behaviors among hospital patients. *General Hospital Psychiatry, 63*, 1–4. https://doi.org/10.1016/j.genhosppsych.2019.06.002

Krause, M., Gutsmiedl, K., Bighelli, I., Schneider-Thoma, J., Chaimani, A., & Leucht, S. (2019). Efficacy and tolerability of pharmacological and non-pharmacological interventions in older patients with major depressive disorder: A systematic review, pairwise and network meta-analysis. *European Neuropsychopharmacology, 29*(9), 1003–1022. https://www.sciencedirect.com/science/article/pii/S0924977X19304237

Krishnamoorthy, Y., Rajaa, S., & Rehman, T. (2020). Diagnostic accuracy of various forms of geriatric depression scale for screening of depression among older adults: Systematic review and meta-analysis. *Archives of Gerontology and Geriatrics, 87*, 104002. https://doi.org/10.1016/j.archger.2019.104002

Ksinan, A., & Vazsonyi, A., (2019). Genetic and environmental effects on the development of depressive symptoms from adolescence to adulthood in a nationally representative sample. *Journal of Affective Disorders, 245*, 163–173. https://doi.org/10.1016/j.jad.2018.10.085

Kwong, A., López-López, J., Hammerton, G., Manley, D., Timpson, N., Leckie, G., & Pearson, R. (2019). Genetic and environmental risk factors associated with trajectories of depression symptoms from adolescence to young adulthood. *Journal of the American Medical Association, 2*(6), e196587. doi:10.1001/jamanetworkopen.2019.6587

Ladouceur, C. D., Kerestes, R., Schlund, M. W., Shirtcliff, E. A., Lee, Y., & Dahl, R. E. (2019). Neural systems underlying reward cue processing in early adolescence: The role of puberty and pubertal hormones. *Psychoneuroendocrinology, 102*, 281–291.

Lee, J.-E., Kim, Y. J., Park, H. J., Park, S., Kim, H., & Kwon, O. (2019). Association of recommended food score with depression, anxiety, and quality of life in Korean adults: The 2014–2015 National Fitness Award Project. *BMC Public Health, 19*(1), 956. https://doi.org/10.1186/s12889-019-7298-8

Li, Q., Yang, S., Xie, M., Wu, X., Huang, L., Ruan, W., et al. (2020). Impact of some social and clinical factors on the development of postpartum depression in Chinese women. *BMC Pregnancy and Childbirth, 20*, 226.

Linden, M. (2020). Euthymic suffering and wisdom psychology. *World Psychiatry, 19*(1), 55–56. https://doi.org/10.1002/wps.20718

Lindsey, M. A., Sheftall, A. H., Xiao, Y., & Joe, S. (2019). Trends of suicidal behaviors among high school students in the United States: 1991–2017. *Pediatrics, 144*(5), e20191187. https://doi.org/10.1542/peds.2019-1187

Lotfaliany, M., Bowe, S. J., Kowal, P., Orellana, L., Berk, M., & Mohebbi, M. (2018). Depression and chronic diseases: Co-occurrence and communality of risk factors. *Journal of Affective Disorders, 241*, 461–468.

Lovato, K., Lopez, C., Karimli, L., & Abrams, L. S. (2018). The impact of deportation-related family separations on the well-being of Latinx children and youth: A review of the literature. *Children and Youth Services Review, 95*, 109–116.

Lowe, H., Haddock, G., Mulligan, L. D., Gregg, L., Fuzellier-Hart, A., Carter, L.-A., & Kyle, S. D. (2019). Does exercise improve sleep for adults with insomnia?: A systematic review with quality appraisal. *Clinical Psychology Review, 68*, 1–12. https://doi.org/10.1016/j.cpr.2018.11.002

Lundberg, J., Nordanskog, P., & Nordenskjöld, A. (2019). Rehospitalization of postpartum depression and psychosis after electroconvulsive therapy. *Journal of ECT, 35*(4), 264–271.

Machado, L., Thompson, L. M., & Brett, C. H. (2019). Visual analogue mood scale scores in healthy young versus older adults. *International Psychogeriatrics, 31*(3), 417–424.

Mahmoud, D. R., Yang, A., Ciolino, J. D., Fisher, S. D., Sit, D., Pinheiro, E., et al. (2019). Validity of the WHIPLASHED as a tool to identify bipolar disorder in women. *Journal of Affective Disorders, 246*, 69–73. https://doi.org/10.1016/j.jad.2018.12.038

Maina, G., Quarato, F., & Bramante, S. (2019). Risk factors for suicide in bipolar disorder. *Journal of Psychopathology, 25*(3), 149–154. https://www.jpsychopathol.it/wp-content/uploads/2019/09/04_Maina-1.pdf

Mandal, S., Mamidipalli, S. S., Mukherjee, B., & Hara, S. (2019). Perspectives, attitude, and practice of lithium prescription among psychiatrists in India. *Indian Journal of Psychiatry, 61*(5), 451–456. https://doi.org/10.4103/psychiatry.IndianJPsychiatry

Mannapperuma, U., Galappatthy, P., Jayakody, R. L., Mendis, J., de Silva, V. A., & Hanwella, R. (2019). Safety monitoring of treatment in bipolar disorder in a tertiary care setting in Sri Lanka and recommendations for improved monitoring in resource limited settings. *BMC Psychiatry, 19*(1), 194. https://doi.org/10.1186/s12888-019-2183-7

Martinez, A. A. B. (2019). A critical literature review of the research on suicide from a gender perspective. *Social Medicine, 12*(2), 119–225.

Mason, K., Hu, Y., Kim, E., Korver, D., Xia, L., & Coniglio, N. (2018). Unique experiences in religious groups, in the US and China—a qualitative study. *Mental Health, Religion and Culture, 21*(6), 609–624.

Matarazzo, B. B., Brown, G. K., Stanley, B., Forster, J. E., Billera, M., Currier, G. W., et al. (2019). Predictive validity of the Columbia-Suicide Severity Rating Scale among a cohort of at-risk veterans. *Suicide & Life-Threatening Behavior, 49*(5), 1255–1265.

Maurer, D. M., Raymond, T. J., & Davis, B. N. (2018). Depression: Screening and diagnosis. *American Family Physician, 98*(8), 508–515. https://www.aafp.org/afp/2018/1015/p508.html

Mayo Clinic. (2018b). *Postpartum depression: Symptoms and causes.* https://www.mayoclinic.org/diseases-conditions/postpartum-depression/symptoms-causes/syc-20376617

McCallum, S. M., Batterham, P. J., Calear, A. L., Sunderland, M., & Carragher, N. (2019). Reductions in quality of life and increased economic burden associated with mental disorders in an Australian adult sample. *Australian Health Review, 43*(6), 644–652.

McConnell, V. L., Carter, S. L., & Patterson, K. (2019). Major depressive disorder: Treatment-resistant depression and augmentation of other medication classes. *MEDSURG Nursing, 28*(4), 251–256.

McEwen, B. S. (2020). Hormones and behavior and the integration of brain-body science. *Hormones and Behavior, 119*, 104619. https://doi.org/10.1016/j.yhbeh.2019.104619

McHugh, R. K., & Weiss, R. D. (2019). Alcohol use disorder and depressive disorders. *Alcohol Research: Current Reviews, 40*(1). https://doi.org/10.35946/arcr.v40.1.01

Medline Plus. (2020). *Bipolar disorder.* U.S. National Library of Medicine. https://ghr.nlm.nih.gov/condition/bipolar-disorder#inheritance

Menculini, G., Verdolini, N., Murru, A., Pacchiarotti, I., Volpe, U., Cervino, A., et al. (2018). Depressive mood and circadian rhythms disturbances as outcomes of seasonal affective disorder treatment: A systematic review. *Journal of Affective Disorders, 241*, 608–626. https://doi.org/10.1016/j.jad.2018.08.071

Mental Health America. (2020). *Suicide.* https://www.mhanational.org/conditions/suicide

Miklin, S., Mueller, A. S., Abrutyn, S., & Ordonez, K. (2019). What does it mean to be exposed to suicide?: Suicide exposure, suicide risk, and the importance of meaning-making. *Social Science and Medicine, 233*, 21–27.

Miller, R., & Kirschbaum, C. (2019). Cultures under stress: A cross-national meta-analysis of cortisol responses to the Trier social stress test and their association with anxiety-related value orientations and internalizing mental disorders. *Psychoneuroendocrinology, 105*, 147–154.

Mitchell, J., & Goodman, J. (2018). Comparative effects of antidepressant medications and untreated major depression on pregnancy outcomes: A systematic review. *Archives of Women's Mental Health, 21*(5), 505–516.

Mohamied, F. (2019). Postpartum psychosis and management: A case study. *British Journal of Midwifery, 27*(2), 77–84.

Moorkath, F., Vranda, M., & Naveenkumar, C. (2019). Women with mental illness – An overview of sociocultural factors influencing family rejection and subsequent institutionalization in India. *Indian Journal of Psychological Medicine, 41*(4), 306–310.

Morgan, J. A., Singhal, G., Corrigan, F., Jaehne, E. J., Jawahar, M. C., Breen, J., et al. (2019). Ceasing exercise induces depression-like, anxiety-like, and impaired cognitive-like behaviours and altered hippocampal gene expression. *Brain Research Bulletin, 148*, 118–130.

Musci, R. J., Kharrazi, H., Wilson, R. F., Susukida, R., Gharghabi, F., Zhang, A., et al. (2018). The study of effect moderation in youth suicide-prevention studies. *Social Psychiatry and Psychiatric Epidemiology, 53*(12), 1303–1310.

National Action Alliance for Suicide Prevention. (2020). *Zero Suicide: Screening for and assessing suicide risk.* https://zerosuicide.edc.org/toolkit/identify/screening-and-assessing-suicide-risk#footnote6_6i1y9r1

National Center for Complementary and Integrative Health. (2017). *St. John's wort and depression: In depth.* https://nccih.nih.gov/health/stjohnswort/sjw-and-depression.htm

National Institute of Mental Health. (2017a). *Any mood disorder.* https://www.nimh.nih.gov/health/statistics/any-mood-disorder.shtml

National Institute of Mental Health. (2017b). *Bipolar disorder.* https://www.nimh.nih.gov/health/statistics/bipolar-disorder.shtml

National Institute of Mental Health. (2019). *Major depression.* https://www.nimh.nih.gov/health/statistics/major-depression.shtml

National Institute of Mental Health. (2020a). *Depression.* https://www.nimh.nih.gov/health/topics/depression/index.shtml

National Institute of Mental Health. (2020b). *Suicide safety assessment guide.* https://www.nimh.nih.gov/research/research-conducted-at-nimh/asq-toolkit-materials/outpatient/brief-suicide-safety-assessment-guide.shtml

Navin, K., Kuppili, P., Menon, V., & Kattimani, S. (2019). Suicide prevention strategies for general hospital and psychiatric inpatients: A narrative review. *Indian Journal of Psychological Medicine, 41*(5), 403–412.

Niethe, M., & Whitfield, K. (2018). Psychotropic medication use during pregnancy. *Journal of Pharmacy Practice and Research, 48*(4), 384–391.

Niksalehi, S., Taghadosi, M., Mazhariazad, F., & Tashk, M. (2018). The effectiveness of mobile phone text massaging support for mothers with postpartum depression: A clinical before and after study. *Journal of Family Medicine and Primary Care, 7*(5), 1058–1062.

O'Connor, E., Rossom, R. C., Henninger, M., Groom, H. C., & Burda, B. U. (2016). Primary care screening for and treatment of depression in pregnant and postpartum women: Evidence report and systematic review for the U.S. Preventive Services Task Force. *JAMA, 315*(4), 388–406.

O'Connor, R. C., Lundy, J. M., Stewart, C., Smillie, S., McClelland, H., Syrett, S., et al. (2019). SAFETEL randomized controlled feasibility trial of a safety planning intervention with follow-up telephone contact to reduce suicidal behaviour: Study protocol. *BMJ Open, 9*(2), e025591. https://bmjopen.bmj.com/content/bmjopen/9/2/e025591.full.pdf

Opie, R. S., O'Neil, A., Jacka, F. N., Pizzinga, J., & Itsiopoulos, C. (2018). A modified Mediterranean dietary intervention for adults with major depression: Dietary protocol and feasibility data from the SMILES trial. *Nutritional Neuroscience, 21*(7), 487–501.

O'Rourke, M. C., Jamil, R. T., & Siddiqui, W. (2019). *Suicide screening and prevention.* StatPearls. https://www.ncbi.nlm.nih.gov/books/NBK531453/

Osman, N. N., & Bahri, A. I. (2019). Impact of altered hormonal and neurochemical levels on depression symptoms in women during pregnancy and postpartum period. *Journal of Biochemical Technology, 10*(1), 16–23.

Ozten, M., & Erol, A. (2019). Impulsivity differences between bipolar and unipolar depression. *Indian Journal of Psychiatry, 61*(2), 156–160.

Palagini, L., Cipollone, G., Moretto, U., Masci, I., Tripodi, B., Caruso, D., & Perugi, G. (2019). Chronobiological dis-rhythmicity is related to emotion dysregulation and suicidality in depressive bipolar II disorder with mixed features. *Psychiatry Research, 271*, 272–278.

Palagini, L., Miniati, M., Caruso, D., Massa, L., Novi, M., Pardini, F., et al. (2020). Association between affective temperaments and mood features in bipolar disorder II: The role of insomnia and chronobiological rhythms desynchronization. *Journal of Affective Disorders, 266*, 263–272.

Paolucci, E. M., Loukov, D., Bowdish, D. M. E., & Heisz, J. J. (2018). Exercise reduces depression and inflammation but intensity matters. *Biological Psychology, 133*, 79–84.

Patel, R. K., & Rose, G. M. (2019). *Persistent depressive disorder (dysthymia).* StatPearls. https://www.ncbi.nlm.nih.gov/books/NBK541052/

Paul, E. (2018). Proximally-occurring life events and the first transition from suicidal ideation to suicide attempt in adolescents. *Journal of Affective Disorders, 241*, 499–504.

Payne, J. L., & Maguire, J. (2019). Pathophysiological mechanisms implicated in postpartum depression. *Frontiers in Neuroendocrinology, 52*, 165–180.

Perugi, G., Hantouche, E., & Vannucchi, G. (2017). Diagnosis and treatment of cyclothymia: The "primary" of temperament. *Current Neuropharmacology, 15*(3), 372–379.

Ponting, C., Mahrer, N. E., Zelcer, H., Dunkel Schetter, C., & Chavira, D. A. (2020). Psychological interventions for depression and anxiety in pregnant Latina and Black women in the United States: A systematic review. *Clinical Psychology and Psychotherapy, 27*(2), 249–265. https://doi.org/10.1002/cpp.2424

Popova, V., Daly, E. J., Trivedi, M., Cooper, K., Lane, R., Lim, P., et al. (2019). Efficacy and safety of flexibly dosed esketamine nasal spray combined with a newly initiated oral antidepressant in treatment-resistant depression: A randomized double-blind active-controlled study. *American Journal of Psychiatry, 176*(6), 428–438.

Potter, M. L., & Moller, M. D. (2020). *Psychiatric-mental health nursing: From suffering to hope* (2nd ed.). Pearson.

Quan, W., Wang, H., Jia, F., & Zhang, X.-H. (Purpura associated with lithium intoxication. *Chinese Medical Journal, 128*(2), 284.

Ragazan, D. C., Eberhard, J., Ösby, U., & Berge, J. (2019). Gender influence on the bipolar disorder inpatient length of stay in Sweden, 2005–2014: A register-based study. *Journal of Affective Disorders, 256*, 183–191. https://doi.org/10.1016/j.jad.2019.05.052

Rainville, J. R., Tsyglakova, M., & Hodes, G. E. (2018). Deciphering sex differences in the immune system and depression. *Frontiers in Neuroendocrinology, 50*, 67–90.

Ramos-Sánchez, L., Pietrantonio, K., & Llamas, J. (2020). The psychological impact of immigration status on undocumented Latinx women: Recommendations for mental health providers. *Peace and Conflict, 26*(2), 149–161.

Raza, S. K., & Raza, S. (2019). *Postpartum psychosis.* StatPearls. https://www.ncbi.nlm.nih.gov/books/NBK544304/

Rodriguez, V. J., Mandell, L. N., Babayigit, S., Manohar, R. R., Weiss, S. M., & Jones, D. L. (2018). Correlates of suicidal ideation during pregnancy and postpartum among women living with HIV in rural South Africa. *AIDS and Behavior, 22*(10), 3188–3197. https://doi.org/10.1007/s10461-018-2153-y

Roux, P., Raust, A., Cannavo, A-S., Aubin, V., Aouizerate, B., Azorin, J.-M., et al. (2017). Associations between residual depressive symptoms, cognition, and functioning in patients with euthymic bipolar disorder: Results form the FACE-BD cohort. *British Journal of Psychiatry, 211*(6), 381–387.

Rowland, T. A., & Marwaha, S. (2018). Epidemiology and risk factors for bipolar disorder. *Therapeutic Advances in Psychopharmacology, 8*(9), 251–269.

Rubinow, D. R., & Schmidt, P. J. (2019). Sex differences and the neurobiology of affective disorders. *Neuropsychopharmacology, 44*(1), 111–128. https://www.nature.com/articles/s41386-018-0148-z

Ruch, D. A., Sheftall, A. H., Schlagbaum, P., Rausch, J., Campo, J. V., & Bridge, J. A. (2019). Trends in suicide among youth aged 10 to 19 years in the United States, 1975 to 2016. *JAMA Network Open, 2*(5). https://jamanetwork.com/journals/jamanetworkopen/fullarticle/2733430

Rundgren, S., Brus, O., Båve, U., Landén, M., Lundberg, J., Nordanskog, P., & Nordenskjöld, A. (2018). Improvement of postpartum depression and psychosis after electroconvulsive therapy: A population-based study with a matched comparison group. *Journal of Affective Disorders, 235*, 258–264.

SA Maternal, Neonatal, & Gynaecology Community of Practice. (2019). *South Australian Perinatal Practice Guideline: Psychotic disorders in the perinatal period.* https://www.sahealth.sa.gov.au/wps/wcm/connect/8fbf20004eeda373b123b36a7ac0d6e4/psychosis+in+pregnancy+and+postpartum_27042016.pdf?MOD=AJPERES&CACHEID=ROOTWORKSPACE-8fbf20004eeda373b123b36a7ac0d6e4-n5iYVYw

Schmutte, T. J., & Wilkinson, S. T. (2020). Suicide in older adults with and without known mental illness: Results from the National Violent Death Reporting System, 2003–2016. *American Journal of Preventive Medicine, 58*(4), 584–590.

Schuch, F. B., & Stubbs, B. (2019). The role of exercise in preventing and treating depression. *Current Sports Medicine Reports, 18*(8), 299–304. https://journals.lww.com/acsm-csmr/fulltext/2019/08000/the_role_of_exercise_in_preventing_and_treating.6.aspx

Schweizer, S., Gotlib, I. H., & Blakemore, S. J. (2020). The role of affective control in emotion regulation during adolescence. *Emotion, 20*(1), 80. https://psycnet.apa.org/fulltext/2020-03346-014.html

Seddigh, M., Hazrati, M., Jokar, M., Mansouri, A., Bazrafshan, M.-R., Rasti, M., & Kavi, E. (2020). A comparative study of perceived social support and depression among elderly members of senior day centers, elderly residents in nursing homes, and elderly living at home. *Iranian Journal of Nursing and Midwifery Research, 25*(2), 160–165.

Serafini, G., Vazquez, G. H., Gonda, X., Pompili, M., Rihmer, Z., et al. (2018). Depressive residual symptoms are associated with illness course characteristics in a sample of outpatients with bipolar disorder. *European Archives of Psychiatry and Clinical Neuroscience, 268*(8), 769.

Shahwan, S., Lau, J. H., Abdin, E., Zhang, Y., Sambasivam, R., Lin, T. W., et al. (2020). A typology of non-suicidal self-injury in a clinical sample: A latent class analysis. *Clinical Psychology and Psychotherapy.* https://onlinelibrary.wiley.com/doi/full/10.1002/cpp.2463

Shain, B. N. (2019). Increases in rates of suicide and suicide attempts among Black adolescents. *Pediatrics, 144*(5), e20191912. https://doi.org/10.1542/peds.2019-1912

Shorey, S., Chee, C. Y. I., Ng, E. D., Chan, Y. H., Tam, W. W. S., & Chong, Y. S. (2018). Prevalence and incidence of postpartum depression among healthy mothers: A systematic review and meta-analysis. *Journal of Psychiatric Research, 104*, 235–248.

Silveira, É. M., Passos, I. C., Scott, J., Bristot, G., Scotton, E., Teixeira Mendes, L. S., et al. (2020). Decoding rumination: A machine learning approach to a transdiagnostic sample of outpatients with anxiety, mood and psychotic disorders. *Journal of Psychiatric Research, 121*, 207–213.

Singh, M. K. (2019). Using screening tools and diagnosing bipolar disorder in pediatric patients. *Journal of Clinical Psychiatry, 80*(1). https://www.cmeinstitute.com/Psychlopedia/Pages/BipolarDisorder/14ocid/sec1/section.aspx

Slomski, A. (2019). Esketamine nasal spray effective in treatment-resistant depression. *Journal of the American Medical Association, 322*(4), 296.

Smallheer, B. A., Vollman, M., & Dietrich, M. S. (2018). Learned helplessness and depressive symptoms following myocardial infarction. *Clinical Nursing Research, 27*(5), 597–616.

Smirnoff, M., Wilets, I., Ragin, D. F., Adams, R., Holohan, J., Rhodes, R., et al. (2018). A paradigm for understanding trust and mistrust in medical research: The Community VOICES study. *AJOB Empirical Bioethics, 9*(1), 39–47. h

Smith, C. A., Shewamene, Z., Galbally, M., Schmied, V., & Dahlen, H. (2019). The effect of complementary medicines and therapies on maternal anxiety and depression in pregnancy: A systematic review and meta-analysis. *Journal of Affective Disorders, 245*, 428–439.

Stanikova, D., Zsido, R. G., Luck, T., Pabst, A., Enzenbach, C., Bae, Y. J., et al. (2019). Testosterone imbalance may link depression and increased body weight in premenopausal women. *Translational Psychiatry, 9*(1), 160. https://www.nature.com/articles/s41398-019-0487-5

Stanley, I. H., Hom, M. A., Sachs-Ericsson, N. J., Gallyer, A. J., & Joiner, T. E. (2020). A pilot randomized clinical trial of a lethal means safety intervention for young adults with firearm familiarity at risk for suicide. *Journal of Consulting and Clinical Psychology, 88*(4), 372–383.

Stanton, C. H., Holmes, A. J., Chang, S. W. C., & Joormann, J. (2019). From stress to anhedonia: Molecular processes through functional circuits. *Trends in Neurosciences, 42*(1), 23–42.

Stevens, A. W., Goossens, P. J., Knoppert-van der Klein, E. A., Draisma, S., Honig, A., & Kupka, R. W. (2019). Risk of recurrence of mood disorders during pregnancy and the impact of medication: A systematic review. *Journal of Affective Disorders, 249*, 96–103.

Stewart, D. E., & Vigod, S. N. (2019). Postpartum depression: Pathophysiology, treatment, and emerging therapeutics. *Annual Review of Medicine, 70*, 183–196. https://doi.org/10.1146/annurev-med-041217-011106

Substance Abuse and Mental Health Services Administration (SAMHSA). (2016). *Substance use and suicide: A nexus requiring a public health approach.* https://store.samhsa.gov/sites/default/files/d7/priv/sma16-4935.pdf

Substance Abuse and Mental Health Services Administration (SAMHSA). (2017). *Results from the 2017 National Survey on Drug Use and Health: Detailed tables.* https://www.samhsa.gov/data/sites/default/files/cbhsq-reports/NSDUHDetailedTabs2017/NSDUHDetailedTabs2017.htm#tab8-56A

Substance Abuse and Mental Health Services Administration (SAMHSA). (2018). *Key substance use and mental health indicators in the United States: Results from the 2018 National Survey on Drug Use and Health.* Retrieved from: https://www.samhsa.gov/data/sites/default/files/cbhsq-reports/NSDUHNationalFindingsReport2018/NSDUHNationalFindingsReport2018.pdf

Substance Abuse and Mental Health Services Administration (SAMHSA). (2019). *The treatment of depression in older adults: EPB toolkit.* https://store.samhsa.gov/product/Treatment-Depression-Older-Adults-Evidence-Based-Practices-EBP-Kit/SMA11-4631

Sun, Y., Drevets, W., Turecki, G., Li, Q., (2020). The relationship between plasma serotonin and kynurenine pathway metabolite levels and the treatment response to escitalopram and desvenlafaxine. *Brain, Behavior and Immunity, 87*, 404–412. https://doi.org/10.1016/j.bbi.2020.01.011

Sunnqvist, C., Sjöström, K., & Finnbogadóttir, H. (2019). Depressive symptoms during pregnancy and postpartum in women and use of antidepressant treatment–a longitudinal cohort study. *International Journal of Women's Health, 11*, 109–117. https://doi.org/10.2147/IJWH.S185930

Svensson, A. F., Khaldi, M., Engström, I., Matusevich, K., & Nordenskjöld, A. (2018). Remission rate of transcranial magnetic stimulation compared with electroconvulsive therapy: A case-control study. *Nordic Journal of Psychiatry, 72*(7), 471–476.

Sylvia, L. G., Montana, R. E., Deckersbach, T., Thase, M. E., Tohen, M., Reilly-Harrington, N., et al. (2017). Poor quality of life and functioning in bipolar disorder. *International Journal of Bipolar Disorder, 5*(1), 10. https://journalbipolardisorders.springeropen.com/articles/10.1186/s40345-017-0078-4

Szuhany, K. L., & Otto, M. W. (2020). Assessing BDNF as a mediator of the effects of exercise on depression. *Journal of Psychiatric Research, 123*, 114–118.

Takata, J., Arashi, T., Abe, A., Arai, S., & Haruyama, N. (2019). Serotonin syndrome triggered by postoperative administration of serotonin noradrenaline reuptake inhibitor (SNRI). *JA Clinical Reports, 5*, 55. https://doi.org/10.1186/s40981-019-0275-5

Troya, M. I., Babatunde, O., Polidano, K., Bartlam, B., McCloskey, E., Dikomitis, L., & Chew-Graham, C. A. (2019). Self-harm in older adults: Systematic review. *British Journal of Psychiatry, 214*(4), 186–200.

U.S. Food and Drug Administration. (n.d.). Paxil: Prescribing information. Retrieved from: https://www.accessdata.fda.gov/drugsatfda_docs/label/2012/020031s067,020710s031.pdf

U.S. Preventive Services Task Force (2016a). Screening for depression in adults. *Journal of the American Medical Association, 315*(4), 380–387. https://www.uspreventiveservicestaskforce.org/uspstf/document/evidence-summary-primary-care-screening-for-and-treatment-of/depression-in-adults-screening

U.S. Preventive Services Task Force. (2016b). Screening for depression in children and adolescents. *Annals of Internal Medicine, 161*(5), 360–367. https://www.uspreventiveservicestaskforce.org/uspstf/recommendation/depression-in-children-and-adolescents-screening

U.S. Preventive Services Task Force. (2019). *Interventions to prevent perinatal depression: U. S. Preventive Services Task Force recommendation statement.* https://www.uspreventiveservicestaskforce.org/uspstf/recommendation/perinatal-depression-preventive-interventions

van Bergen, A. H., Verkooijen, S., Vreeker, A., Abramovic, L., Hillegers, M. H., Spijker, A. T., et al. (2019). The characteristics of psychotic features in bipolar disorder. *Psychological Medicine, 49*(12), 2036–2048.

van den Bosch, M., & Meyer-Lindenberg, A. (2019). Environmental exposures and depression: Biological mechanisms and epidemiological evidence. *Annual Review of Public Health, 40*(1), 239–259. https://doi.org/10.1146/annurev-publhealth-040218-044106

van Wijk-Herbrink, M. F., Bernstein, D. P., Broers, N. J., Roelofs, J., Rijkeboer, M. M., & Arntz, A. (2018). Internalizing and externalizing behaviors share a common predictor: The effects of early maladaptive schemas are mediated by coping responses and schema modes. *Journal of Abnormal Child Psychology, 46*(5), 907–920.

Vigod, S. N., & Rochon, P. A. (2020). The impact of gender discrimination on a woman's mental health. *EClinicalMedicine, 20*, 100311. https://www.thelancet.com/journals/eclinm/article/PIIS2589-5370(20)30055-9/fulltext

Ward, H. B., Fromson, J. A., Cooper, J. J., De Oliveira, G., & Almeida, M. (2018). Recommendations for the use of ECT in pregnancy: Literature review and proposed clinical protocol. *Archives of Women's Mental Health, 21*(6), 715–722.

Ward, V. (2018). What do we know about suicide bombing?: Review and analysis. *Politics and the Life Sciences, 37*(1), 88–112. h

Wei, J., Hou, R., Zhang, X., Xu, H., Xie, L., Chandrasekar, E. K., Ying, M., et al. (2019). The association of late-life depression with all-cause and cardiovascular mortality among community-dwelling older adults: Systematic review and meta-analysis. *British Journal of Psychiatry, 215*(2): 449–455.

Wirz-Justice, A., & Benedetti, F. (2020). Perspectives in affective disorders: Clocks and sleep. *European Journal of Neuroscience, 51*(1), 346–365. https://onlinelibrary.wiley.com/doi/full/10.1111/ejn.14362

Witt, K., Potts, J., Hubers, A., Grunebaum, M. F., Murrough, J. W., Loo, C., et al. (2020). Ketamine for suicidal ideation in adults with psychiatric disorders: A systematic review and meta-analysis of treatment trials. *Australian & New Zealand Journal of Psychiatry, 54*(1), 29–45.

Wolford-Clevenger, C., Frantell, K., Smith, P. N., Flores, L. Y., & Stuart, G. L. (2018). Correlates of suicide ideation and behaviors among transgender people: A systematic review guided by ideation-to-action theory. *Clinical Psychology Review, 63*, 93–105.

Woo, Y. S., Yoon, B. H., Song, J. H., Seo, J. S., Nam, B., Lee, K., et al. (2020). Clinical correlates associated with the long-term response of bipolar disorder patients to lithium, valproate or lamotrigine: A retrospective study. *PloS One, 15*(1), e0227217. https://doi.org/10.1371/journal.pone.0227217

World Health Organization (WHO). (2014). *Preventing suicide: A global imperative.* https://appsa.who.int/iris/bitstream/handle/10665/131056/9789241564779_eng.pdf

World Health Organization. (2019). *Suicide: Key facts.* https://www.who.int/news-room/fact-sheets/detail/suicide

World Health Organization (2020). *Depression: Key facts.* https://www.who.int/news-room/fact-sheets/detail/depression

Wray, N. R., Ripke, S., Mattheisen, M., Trzaskowski, M., Byrne, E. M., Abdellaoui, A., et al. (2018). Genome-wide association analyses identify 44 risk variants and refine the genetic architecture of major depression. *Nature Genetics, 50*(5), 668–681. http://dx.doi.org/10.1038/s41588-018-0090-3

Wu, B., Cai, Q., Sheehan, J. J., Benson, C., Connolly, N., & Alphs, L. (2019). An episode level evaluation of the treatment journey of patients with major depressive disorder and treatment-resistant depression. *PLoSne, 14*(8), e0220763. https://doi.org/10.1371/journal.pone.0220763

Xia, M., Womer, F. Y., Chang, M., Zhu, Y., Zhou, Q., Edmiston, E. K., et al. (2019). Shared and distinct functional architectures of brain networks across psychiatric disorders. *Schizophrenia Bulletin, 45*(2), 450–463.

Yanartaş, Ö., Kani, H. T., Kani, A. S., Akça, Z. N. D., Akça, E., Ergün, S., et al. (2019). Depression and anxiety have unique contributions to somatic complaints in depression, irritable bowel syndrome and inflammatory bowel diseases. *Psychiatry and Clinical Psychopharmacology, 29*(4), 418–426. https://www.tandfonline.com/doi/full/10.1080/24750573.2019.1589177

Yang, L., Liu, X., Yao, K., Sun, Y., Jiang, F., Yan, H., et al. (2019). HCN channel antagonist ZD7288 ameliorates neuropathic pain and associated depression. *Brain Research, 1717*, 204–213.

Yatham, L. N., Kennedy, S. H., Parikh, S. V., Schaffer, A., Bond, D. J., Frey, B. N., et al. (2018). Canadian Network for Mood and Anxiety Treatments (CANMAT) and International Society for Bipolar Disorders (ISBD) 2018 guidelines for the management of patients with bipolar disorder. *Bipolar Disorders, 20*(2), 97–170. https://doi-org.ezproxy.hacc.edu/10.1111/bdi.12609

Yildizhan, E., Ozdemir, A., Miray Aytac, H., & Tomruk, N. B. (2019). Prepartum relapses or treatment resistance: A case of unipolar mania. *Journal of Psychiatry and Neurological Sciences, 32*(2), 161. https://dusunenadamdergisi.org/storage/upload/pdfs/1585144040-en.pdf

Yorgason, J. B., Godfrey, W. B., Call, V. R. A., Erickson, L. D., Gustafson, K. B., & Bond, A. H. (2018). Daily sleep predicting marital interactions as mediated through mood. *Journals of Gerontology Series B: Psychological Sciences & Social Sciences, 73*(3), 421–431.

Zhang, Y. Y., Lei, Y. T., Song, Y., Lu, R. R., Duan, J. L., & Prochaska, J. J. (2019). Gender differences in suicidal ideation and health-risk behaviors among high school students in Beijing, China. *Journal of Global Health, 9*(1), 010604. https://doi.org/10.7189/jogh.09.010604

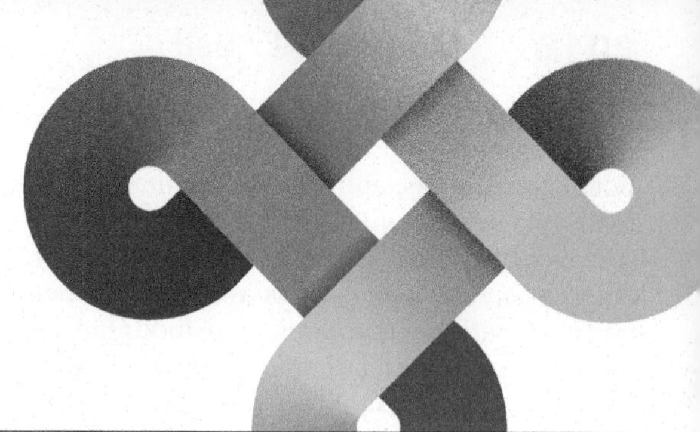

Module 29
Self

Module Outline and Learning Outcomes

The Concept of Self

Normal Presentation

29.1 Analyze the psychosocial processes related to self-concept.

Psychosocial Development Across the Lifespan

29.2 Differentiate considerations related to the development of self across the lifespan.

Alterations from Normal

29.3 Differentiate alterations in self-concept.

Concepts Related to Self

29.4 Outline the relationship between self-concept and other concepts.

Health Promotion

29.5 Explain the promotion of healthy self-concept.

Nursing Assessment

29.6 Differentiate common assessment procedures used to examine the individual's self-concept.

Independent Interventions

29.7 Analyze independent interventions nurses can implement for patients with alterations in self-concept.

Collaborative Therapies

29.8 Summarize collaborative therapies used by interprofessional teams for patients with alterations in self-concept.

Self Exemplars

Exemplar 29.A Feeding and Eating Disorders

29.A Analyze feeding and eating disorders and how they relate to self.

Exemplar 28.B Personality Disorders

29.B Analyze personality disorders and how they relate to self.

» The Concept of Self

Concept Key Terms

Anorexia nervosa (AN), **2022**
Body image, **2018**
Bulimia nervosa (BN), **2022**
Erik Erikson, **2020**
Feeding and eating disorders, **2022**
Global evaluative dimension of the self, **2020**
Global self-esteem, **2020**
Ideal body image, **2019**
Ideal self, **2018**
Introspection, **2020**
Personal identity, **2018**
Personality disorder (PD), **2024**
Prader-Willi syndrome (PWS), **2024**
Psychoanalytic theory, **2020**
Public self, **2018**
Purging, **2024**
Real self, **2018**
Role, **2019**
Role ambiguity, **2019**
Role conflicts, **2019**
Role development, **2019**
Role mastery, **2020**
Role performance, **2019**
Role strain, **2019**
Self-awareness, **2020**
Self-concept, **2018**
Self-esteem, **2020**
Specific self-esteem, **2020**

At the simplest level, caring for patients requires the nurse to be physically present in the care setting. Physical presence in the workplace requires adhering to a work schedule and honoring a commitment to an employer and to patients. However, the energy needed to maintain employment and to care for others requires that the nurse obtain adequate nutrition and rest. Likewise, the knowledge needed to apply the nursing process first requires education in the field of nursing.

On a deeper level, to assess and care for patients from a holistic perspective and to establish therapeutic relationships, the nurse must draw from psychosocial resources that include caring, empathy, and compassion—psychosocial resources whose attainment is far more personal than the attainment or use of time, energy, or knowledge. Nurses recognize that caring for others is not one-dimensional in nature; that is, caring for a patient extends beyond the treatment of injury or illness. For example, treatment of a pediatric patient who has sustained a forehead laceration incorporates far more than ensuring physiologic stability and providing wound care. Along with these priority concerns, other facets of nursing care include addressing the wounded child's pain, anxiety, and fear, as well as recognizing and addressing the concerns of the injured child's family or loved ones. Just as patients are not one-dimensional beings, neither are nurses. Needs of nurses also extend beyond the physiologic domain.

To promote health and wellness in others, nurses must first recognize and understand their own thoughts, emotions, perceptions, abilities, and limitations. Recognition of their own needs requires an understanding of the concept of self. *Self* can be described as the entirety of an individual's being as well as a conscious awareness of being, including body, sensations, emotions, and thoughts. Within the self are all personal traits, characteristics, beliefs, and behaviors. Accurate assessment of a patient's degree of psychosocial health requires that nurses be capable of recognizing signs and symptoms of impairments and alterations. In addition, nurses must be able to identify evidence-based interventions that are effective in the promotion of psychosocial well-being.

Both personally and professionally, wellness promotion requires the nurse to understand and apply principles related to the concept of self, which includes an individual's overall self-image and self-perception. This module explores the concept of self, as well as its various components.

Normal Presentation

Physiologic alterations often produce visible or measurable cues—manifestations or findings that can be discerned through laboratory and diagnostic tests. The use of established parameters or guidelines can simplify the process of identifying abnormal findings.

In contrast, identification of abnormal psychosocial function requires a different approach. Rather than following objective algorithms and guidelines, normal parameters within the psychosocial realm often range along a continuum. Moreover, to identify what is normal or abnormal, the nurse must assess the degree to which the psychosocial concern is affecting the patient. *Normal* is more easily defined within the physiologic realm, whereas *healthy* is the term that more readily applies to the psychosocial realm.

Development of self is a dynamic process that is influenced by interpersonal interactions throughout an individual's lifetime. Numerous theorists, including famed psychologists Erik Erikson and Jean Piaget, proposed theories to describe the processes of human growth and development, including specific stages and tasks associated with each phase of life. From a broad standpoint, principles of growth and development apply to mastery of numerous tasks, as well as to achievement of milestones related to physiologic, cognitive, psychosocial, spiritual, and moral development. For many developmental tasks throughout the lifespan, successful task completion is rooted in interpersonal interaction.

Although this module offers an overview of the development of self, the primary focus includes exploring and describing the impact of self on patient health, as well as its importance to nursing care. (For in-depth discussion of theories related to psychosocial development, see Module 25, Development.)

Self-concept

Self-concept, which is integral to psychosocial development, is the personal perception of self that forms in response to interactions with others and the environment throughout the course of an individual's lifetime. Self-concept affects an individual mentally, physically, and spiritually. A negative self-concept can lead to struggles with adapting to change and building interpersonal relationships. In addition, a negative self-concept can increase an individual's susceptibility to physical and psychologic illnesses. Within the psychosocial domain, effective nursing care includes assessing patients' self-concept and assisting them with the development of a healthy, positive self-perception (Shpigelman & HaGani, 2019). Because each individual's self-concept impacts the nature and efficacy of interpersonal interactions, including nurse–patient relationships, nurses are responsible for exploring and optimizing their own self-concept. In nursing, components of self-concept are often considered to include personal identity, body image, role performance, self-esteem, and self-awareness.

Personal Identity

Personal identity can be evaluated from the standpoint of three aspects of self: the ideal self, the real self, and the public self. The **ideal self** reflects qualities individuals believe they should possess, as well as those they aspire to develop. The **real self** represents the perceived true self (Behmaneshpour, Irandegani, & Miandoab, 2019). The real self may include observations about self or self-perceived qualities that individuals hide from others or do not readily share. For example, the real self may house perceptions such as "I am greedy" or "I am judgmental." The **public self** is formed on the basis of how individuals wish to be perceived by others. For example, in the workplace, individuals' public self may lead to behaviors that inspire others to deem them as being friendly, competent, and team oriented. While the ideal self reflects "who I should be and who I want to be," the real self represents "who I really am." The public self reflects "who I believe others think I am."

Characteristics that make up personal identity include objective descriptors, such as name, age, gender, marital status, and occupation. In addition, personal identity can include an individual's cultural background and ethnic origin. Values, beliefs, and self-expectations also shape personal identity. When individuals choose values that they believe to be important and act accordingly, their personal identity becomes stronger. This has a direct impact on nursing care, as congruence of nurses' behavior with their own personal character and values impact the extent to which patients and coworkers find them to be trustworthy (Behmaneshpour et al., 2019).

Body Image

Body image is individuals' mental picture of their physical self. How individuals perceive the appearance and size of their bodies and emotional reactions to those perceptions are components of body image. However, the impact of body image extends far beyond these two components. Elements of body image include those within the perceptual, cognitive, behavioral, affective, and subjective satisfaction dimensions (see **Table 29.1** ») (Glashouwer, van der Veer, Adipatria, de Jong, & Vocks, 2019). Body image takes into account prosthetic devices, including hairpieces and artificial limbs, as well as assistive devices, such as wheelchairs, walkers, eyeglasses, and hearing aids (see **Figure 29.1** »). The individual's perception of the need to use assistive devices is also part of body image.

TABLE 29.1 Elements of Body Image

Element	Description
Perceptual	Mental image of the body; includes perception of physical appearance and how someone perceives their body when viewing it in a mirror.
Cognitive	Includes beliefs and attitudes about one's body, as well as the degree to which body image is valued and the individual's level of investment in physical appearance.
Behavioral	Encompasses behavioral manifestations that may reveal cues about an individual's feelings and perceptions about their body; for example, indicators may include wearing revealing clothing and engaging in activities that require physical exposure (e.g., wearing a swimsuit to the swimming pool).
Affective	Represents feelings about one's body, in terms of both appearance and function. May be negative (e.g., shame or embarrassment) or positive (e.g., pride or satisfaction).
Subjective satisfaction	Reflects an individual's degree of satisfaction with their body, both as a whole and in terms of individual parts or regions.

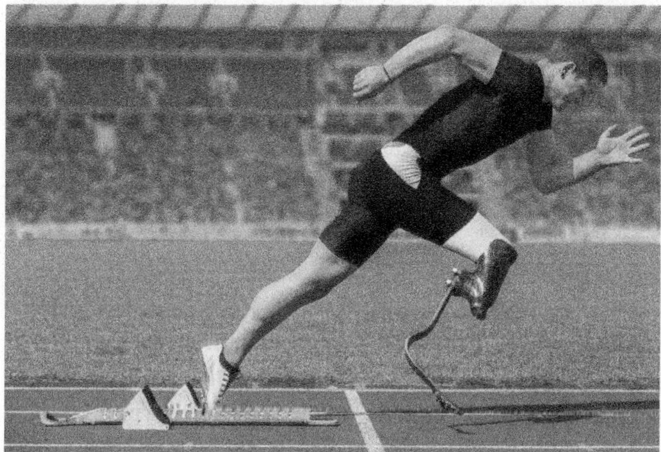

Figure 29.1 » Body image is the sum of individuals' conscious and unconscious attitudes about their bodies. How do you think the runner pictured here views his body image?

Source: mezzotint123rf/123RF.

Culture and society significantly impact body image, including the **ideal body image**, which is a mental representation of what individuals believe their body should look like. In particular, visual media—such as movies and magazine images—are viewed by some as promoting an unrealistic ideal body image. For example, in the United States, the modeling and advertising industries often feature women who are extremely thin, which is an issue that has sparked cultural debate with regard to the effects of this practice on the development of ideal body image among young females. Typically, the more congruent an individual's perceived body image is with their ideal body image, the greater their level of satisfaction with body image will be.

Role Performance

A nursing student is also someone's child, perhaps a sibling or a cousin, and may be a parent or caregiver as well. Each of these positions or roles—student, offspring, sibling, and parent—is associated with certain behavioral expectations. A **role** encompasses a grouping of behavioral expectations associated with a specified societal or organizational position. Role expectations may be defined by numerous entities, including society, culture, religion, tribal leadership, an employer, or any organization of which the individual is a member. The demonstration of behaviors or actions associated with a given role is called **role performance**.

Teaching and modeling the behaviors needed to successfully assume a role are part of **role development**, which is essential for effective role performance. Role development also includes socialization of the individual who is preparing to assume a given role. For example, a graduate nurse who accepts a position in a medical–surgical hospital unit will most often complete an orientation program, which includes exposure of the newly employed nurse to basic aspects related to working in that clinical setting, such as institutional protocols and charting requirements. After orientation, the nurse will usually be assigned a preceptor who models expected nursing behaviors and assists the nurse with continued role development.

Ineffective role development can lead to **role ambiguity**, which occurs when an individual lacks clarity regarding the expectations, behaviors, or demands associated with fulfilling a given role. Individuals who feel incapable of fulfilling a role may experience **role strain**. In some cases, role strain may be the result of sexual stereotyping. For example, a female firefighter who is told or given the impression by male colleagues that she is physically incapable of handling the rigorous demands associated with a male-dominated occupation may experience role strain. Both role ambiguity and role strain can negatively impact self-concept.

When role-related expectations clash or are incongruent, **role conflicts** may occur. If needs for recognition, accomplishment, and independence are not met, the role conflict can produce embarrassment, increased stress, and decreased self-esteem (Karkkola, Kuittinen, & Hintsa, 2019). Conflicts may occur between one or more individuals (interpersonal) or within one individual (intrapersonal), as well as between groups and organizations. Forms of role conflict include the following:

- ***Interpersonal conflict.*** Occurs when individuals hold varying or conflicting expectations about tasks and behaviors associated with a specific role; for example, a husband and wife may have conflicting expectations about who is responsible for completing household chores and preparing meals.
- ***Inter-role conflict.*** Occurs when roles create competing demands; for example, in the case of an individual who is balancing college courses with parenting, the demands associated with being a student may impinge on the demands of raising a child.
- ***Person–role conflict.*** Occurs when role expectations are in opposition to the values and beliefs of the one who fills the role; for example, despite the Western healthcare practice of promoting truth telling and autonomy, in some instances a family may ask that their family member not be informed when diagnosed with a terminal illness (Frögéli, Rudman, & Gustavsson, 2019).

Role mastery occurs when an individual's behaviors within a role meet or exceed predetermined expectations. The inability to achieve role mastery can lead to stress, internal conflict, and impaired self-esteem (Frögéli et al., 2019).

Self-Esteem

Self-esteem, which is separate from self-concept, is an individual's opinion of themself. In essence, self-esteem describes the degree to which an individual approves of, values, or likes themself (Fiorilli, Grimaldi Capitello, Barni, Buonomo, & Gentile, 2019).

While self-concept reflects how an individual perceives themself, self-esteem, which is the evaluative component of self-concept (Kawamoto, 2020), describes the individual's judgments and opinions about those perceived characteristics. Positive or high self-esteem is associated with greater levels of achievement, increased financial prosperity, and decreased incidence of depression (Fiorilli et al., 2019).

Researchers have proposed two categories of self-esteem: global and specific. **Global self-esteem**, or the **global evaluative dimension of the self**, is the degree to which an individual likes themself overall, as a whole being. **Specific self-esteem**, however, reflects an individual's positive regard for certain aspects of self (Kawamoto, 2020; Rentzsch & Schröder, 2018), such as physical appearance, athletic ability, parenting skills, or academic achievement.

Specific self-esteem influences global self-esteem (Kawamoto, 2020; Rentzsch & Schröder, 2018). For example, if an individual who highly values athletic ability possesses exceptional athletic skills, that individual's athletic performance will impact their global self-esteem. However, if that same individual assigns little value to academic achievement, their global self-esteem will be minimally influenced by failing a college course.

Many studies indicate that parent–child relationships are strongly related to adolescents' self-esteem (Gittins & Hunt, 2019; Keizer, Helmerhorst, & van Rijn-van Gelderen, 2019; Krauss, Orth, & Robins, 2020). Young adult children who reported exposure to greater levels of parental nurturing also reported higher self-esteem, whereas parental overprotectiveness was linked to lower self-esteem (Gittins & Hunt, 2019; Kawamoto, 2020). In addition, both behavioral and neural studies (using functional MRI) have identified a link between an individual's perceived experience of rejection and the expression of a sense of low self-esteem (Peng et al., 2019; van Schie, Chiu, Rombouts, Heiser, & Elzinga, 2018). A meta-analysis of self-esteem across the lifespan (participants ranging from 10 to 94 years of age) indicated that self-esteem impacts a person's life especially in the areas of social relationships, school and education, and physical and mental health. From early childhood to adolescence, gains in personal autonomy and in the general sense of mastery can increase self-esteem. Furthermore, the study identified that there was significant decline in self-esteem after the age of 90, possibly due to overall health and other physical issues (Orth, Erol, & Luciano, 2018).

Self-Awareness

For an individual to develop a reality-based perception of real self requires **self-awareness**. Development of self-awareness begins when infants learn to distinguish themselves from other individuals and objects in their environment. With the ability to differentiate their own voice and body from the voices and bodies of others, infants' self-awareness increases (Rasheed et al., 2019). Developing self-awareness is an ongoing process that requires intense examination of one's personal perspectives, beliefs, and values. Moreover, self-awareness includes identifying relationships that connect actions to self. By establishing connections between past experiences and current actions or choices, individuals who are self-aware gain insight into the meaning of their behaviors. As opposed to viewing life experiences as being isolated events, many of which are perhaps inexplicable, development of self-awareness requires that actions and behaviors are viewed within the context of individuals' deep-seated values and beliefs (Rasheed et al., 2019). Essentially, individuals who are self-aware understand why they do what they do, and their behaviors and actions can be linked to their core beliefs and values.

The process of developing self-awareness requires **introspection**, which is personal exploration and evaluation of one's own thoughts, emotions, behaviors, and values. Introspection also incorporates both verbal and nonverbal feedback from others (Rasheed, Younas, & Sundus, 2019). While the process of introspection is intimate and personal in nature, the outcome of this process is greatly influenced by a number of external factors. In many ways, individuals' view of themselves is significantly shaped by how others perceive them.

Development of Personality

Numerous behavioral theorists and scientists have proposed theories to describe the development of personality as a component of self. Among the most famous developmental theories are those originated by Sigmund Freud and Erik Erikson. Freud (1856–1939) is considered the founder of **psychoanalytic theory**, which provided the earliest framework for personality development and emphasized the presence of unconscious impulses and their influence on behaviors and the formation of self. Whereas Freud's theory is grounded in psychosexual elements and the human response to impulses, Erikson's theory incorporates social, cultural, and interpersonal components (Gündoğdu & Turan, 2018).

The theory of psychosocial development originated by German-born psychologist and psychoanalyst **Erik Erikson** (1902–1994) is still widely taught today. Erikson (1950, 1963) developed the primary theory on psychosocial development in humans. His ideas were greatly influenced by Freud's theory regarding personality (Zock, 2018). Whereas Freud concentrated on internal conflicts, Erikson emphasized the role of culture and society and the conflicts that can influence personality. According to Erikson, the self develops as it successfully resolves crises that are distinctly social in nature. Three overriding themes in Erikson's theory are establishing trust in others, developing a sense of identity in society, and helping the next generation prepare for the future. Erikson extended Freudian theory by focusing on the adaptive and creative characteristics of the self and by expanding the notion of the stages of personality development to include the entire lifespan (Zock, 2018). For more discussion of Erikson's developmental theory, see Table 25.2 in Module 25, Development.

Psychosocial Development Across the Lifespan

Early childhood experiences and brain circuitry development influence the child's developing central nervous system and have been linked to both risk and resiliency for mental illness in adulthood (Potter & Moller, 2020). Environmental factors, such as toxins, early childhood maltreatment, diet, and stress, can change gene activity and increase the risk for developing psychopathology later in life. Because approximately 75% of adult psychiatric disorders have their onset in childhood and adolescence, mental health promotion interventions that target these factors can change the course of development for children at risk and alter the course of development along the psychologic, biological, sociologic, cultural, and spiritual domains (Potter & Moller, 2020). For example, interventions that promote healthy nutrition in pregnant women and in young children can reduce the risk for disorders or dysfunction in multiple areas of growth and development.

An important influence on psychosocial development is the occurrence of trauma at any life stage. The frequency and number of abusive and traumatic events, referred to as *complex trauma*, influence the severity of psychologic distress and can hinder development. Emotional experiences of trauma can be particularly overwhelming for children, especially if the home environment is the source of maltreatment (Potter & Moller, 2020). Interpersonal violence is the primary source of trauma in adult women. Trauma can affect people of every race, ethnicity, age, sexual orientation, gender, psychosocial background, and geographic region (Substance Abuse and Mental Health Services Administration, 2019).

Other key considerations at each developmental stage are discussed below.

Newborns and Infants (Birth to 1 Year)

During the first year of life, infants are uncertain about their environment and look to the primary caregiver for stability and consistency of care as they adjust to life outside the womb. If infants receive consistent, predictable, and reliable care, they will develop a sense of trust, which they will expect to occur in other relationships (Chung, 2018; Rũgendo, 2019). They will feel secure even in threatening situations and develop a sense of hope that other people will provide support.

Infants who do not feel secure will become fearful when dealing with new people and situations. They may mistrust others and lack confidence in the world around them or in their abilities to influence events. Lack of trust may result in anxiety, heightened insecurities, and a pervasive feeling of uneasiness (Rũgendo, 2019). Three influential theorists were Erikson (discussed below), who advanced strong views on the importance of trust for infants, and Bowlby (1969) and Ainsworth (1973), both of whom outlined how the quality of the early experience of attachment can affect relationships with others in later life.

Toddlers (1 to 3 Years)

During this period, children are developing physically and becoming more mobile. Children will begin to assert their independence, develop skills, and engage in activities that promote growing independence and autonomy. Parents need to allow toddlers active exploration within an encouraging environment that is tolerant of failure, such as allowing children to don their own clothes without interference unless assistance is requested. The primary parental task at this stage is to foster independence while avoiding criticism of failures. By bolstering toddlers' self-esteem, parents will help children be supported in acquiring increased independence, thus becoming more confident and secure in their own ability to navigate in the world (Chung, 2018; Rũgendo, 2019).

Preschool Children (3 to 6 Years)

Around age 3 and continuing to age 5, children begin to assert themselves more frequently. They begin regularly interacting with other children and playing, which provides them with the opportunity to explore their interpersonal skills through initiating activities (Chung, 2018; Rũgendo, 2019). Children begin to plan activities, create games, and initiate activities with others, which help them begin to develop a sense of initiative and feel secure in their abilities to lead others and make decisions. However, if during this period children are overcontrolled or overcriticized, they may develop a sense of guilt and lack self-initiative (Rũgendo, 2019).

Children also begin to ask many questions to grow their knowledge base. If parents and caregivers do not allow children to question and treat them as a nuisance, children may develop a sense of guilt that will influence interpersonal interactions and inhibit creativity. The parental balance at this point is to impose enough restriction on children that they begin to develop a conscience and self-control (Chung, 2018).

School-Age Children (6 to 12 Years)

At age 6 to 12 years, the primary tasks of children are learning to read and write, to do math, and to perform activities on their own. Teachers begin to take an important role as they teach the specific skills (Rũgendo, 2019). At this stage, the child's peer group will gain greater significance and will become a major source of the child's self-esteem. The child now feels compelled to win approval by demonstrating specific competencies that are valued by society and begins to develop a sense of pride in acquired accomplishments (Rũgendo, 2019). Children age 5 to 9 exhibit increased control of emotions, form peer groups, and begin to understand how their actions affect others (Rũgendo, 2019).

Preteen adolescents (age 10 to 12) commonly have emotional swings (feeling wonderful one minute, and sad or irritable the next). They begin to believe peer acceptance means being liked. They still rely on bonds with their parents but may not demonstrate closeness. They question rules and values, often saying things are "unfair." They may begin to focus more on their looks and dress (Fiorilli et al., 2019). For preteens, it is important for parents, caregivers, and teachers to support their interests and their desire to acquire abilities and achieve goals. If this initiative is not encouraged or if it is restricted by parents or teachers, then preteens begin to feel inferior, doubting their own abilities, and therefore may not reach their full potential.

Adolescents (12 to 18 Years)

The major task of this life stage is to learn the roles required to become an adult. During this stage, the adolescent will reexamine personal identity, including sexual orientation and occupational roles (Chung, 2018). Adolescents explore possibilities and begin to form their own identities based on the outcome of their explorations. Failure to establish a sense of identity within society can lead to role confusion, where adolescents are uncertain regarding their place in society. In response to role confusion or identity crisis, adolescents may begin to experiment with different lifestyles in such areas as work, education, drugs/alcohol, or political views (Chung, 2018). Adolescents who are pressured into an identity have the potential to become unhappy and often rebel by establishing a negative identity.

Adolescents struggle with their sense of identity, worrying about being normal or "fitting in." They feel awkward about themselves and their body image and maintain high expectations for themselves. Although adolescents still rely on connectedness with their parents, they may complain that their parents interfere with their independence or behave rudely to their parents in front of others. Young teens begin testing rules and limits. As they develop more friendships with peers of both genders, they try to find a group of peers with whom they fit in and are accepted. Exposure to sex and drugs increases in adolescence. Moodiness is common, and young teens may return to childish behaviors when stressed. Intellectual efforts become more important (Chung, 2018).

Adults

In young adulthood (age 18 to 40 years), adults begin to share themselves more intimately with others, exploring relationships that lead toward longer-term commitments with someone other than a family member. Successful completion of this stage can lead to comfortable relationships and a sense of commitment, safety, and care within a relationship (Pusch et al., 2019). Avoidance of intimacy and fear of commitment and relationships can lead to isolation, loneliness, and sometimes depression.

Recent research has developed the term "emerging adulthood" (age 18 to 30) and suggests that this is a critical time for personality development (Chung, 2018; Pusch, Mund, Hagemeyer, Finn, & Wrzus, 2019; Schwaba & Bleidorn, 2018). During this period, people are most likely to be free to follow their own interests and desires, leading them in many different directions. Emerging adults vary so much in life experiences, some of which may affect personality development. Furthermore, emerging adults have shown greater personality change and diversity in change than young adults (Chung, 2018; Pusch et al., 2019).

During middle adulthood (age 40 to 65 years), adults establish careers, settle down within relationships, begin their own families, and develop a sense of being a part of the bigger picture. Adults give back to society through raising children, being productive at work, and becoming involved in community activities and organizations (Chung, 2018). If adults fail to achieve these objectives, they become stagnant and feel unproductive.

von Soest et al. (2018) conducted a study of over 5500 participants (age 40 to 80) during a 5-year time frame to examine how personality and self-esteem changed during late adulthood. They found that physical health, social relationships, and personality factors were associated with self-esteem and its development later in life. Furthermore, results showed that self-esteem peaked around age 50 and declined thereafter, especially in those age 70 and older (von Soest et al., 2018). Older adults (age 65 and older) with higher self-esteem were more likely to demonstrate emotional stability, extraversion, conscientiousness, and openness (von Soest et al., 2018). Overall, results suggested that declining self-esteem reported by older adults is primarily caused by changes in physical health and socioeconomic status (von Soest et al., 2018). If older adults see their lives as unproductive, feel guilty about the past, or perceive that they did not accomplish their life goals, they may become dissatisfied with life and develop despair, often leading to depression and hopelessness (Schwaba & Bleidorn, 2018).

Alterations from Normal

Alterations in self may stem from a variety of factors, including issues pertaining to the primary components of self-concept, self-esteem, and self-awareness. Within the component of self-concept, some researchers suggest that conflicts related to body image may lead to the development of feeding and eating disorders. Alterations in one or more components of self may manifest through the development of personality disorders.

Feeding and Eating Disorders

Feeding and eating disorders are marked by chronic disturbances in eating or eating-related practices that result in impairment in food consumption or absorption to the extent that daily functioning is affected and physical and psychologic health are significantly impaired (American Psychiatric Association [APA], 2013). Feeding and eating disorders cause low self-esteem, self-hatred, fear, and hopelessness, and they put the individual at risk for a variety of physiologic problems. Although the average age of onset is between 18 and 25 years old, eating disorders has been reported in children as young as 11 (National Institute of Mental Health [NIMH], 2017b; Yilmaz, Gottfredson, Zerwas, Bulik, & Micali, 2019). Affected individuals often also have other mental disorders such as anxiety disorders, substance abuse, or depression (K. E. Smith et al., 2019). Feeding and eating disorders can be fatal. Nurses should not underestimate the significance of these disorders.

The most common feeding and eating disorders include **anorexia nervosa**, **bulimia nervosa**, and binge-eating disorder, each of which is discussed in detail in the exemplar later in this module. The characteristic features of these three disorders are presented in **Table 29.2** ». Other disorders that may impact body image include nocturnal sleep-related eating disorder and Prader-Willi syndrome. Additional disorders often clustered with the more prevalent feeding and eating disorders include pica, rumination disorder, and avoidant/restrictive food intake disorder.

Nocturnal sleep-related eating disorder (NSRED) is characterized by an initial period of insomnia, followed by an episode of sleepwalking or semiconsciousness, during which time the affected individual consumes unusual foods or

Alterations and Therapies

Feeding and Eating Disorders and Personality Disorders

ALTERATION	DESCRIPTION	MANIFESTATIONS	INTERVENTIONS AND TREATMENTS
Feeding and Eating Disorders			
▪ Body image distortion	Impaired perception of body size and/or shape (e.g., a thin individual perceiving themself to be obese when they are excessively thin)	▪ Refusal to eat ▪ Verbalized self-perception of obesity ▪ Verbalized negative perception of body image	▪ Cognitive-behavioral therapy (CBT) ▪ Pharmacologic therapy for management of comorbid disorders or to treat acute symptoms of depression or anxiety
▪ Absence or loss of appetite	Extreme restriction or prohibition of oral intake through self-imposed starvation	▪ Absence of appetite ▪ Emaciation ▪ Potential nutritional deficiencies, dehydration, and electrolyte imbalances ▪ Potential death	▪ CBT ▪ In extreme cases, forced nutritional supplementation and hydration (e.g., through nasogastric feeding tube)
▪ Binge eating	Unrestrained consumption of excessive amounts of food within a 2-hour time period; eating continues even after sensing satiation	▪ Weight exceeds recommended guidelines ▪ If obesity is present, may have secondary physiologic alterations	▪ CBT ▪ Nutritional counseling and weight management programs
▪ Purging	Self-induced expulsion of food and/or products of digestion through use of forced vomiting, laxatives, enemas, and/or diuretics	▪ Dental caries (cavities) and damage to tooth enamel due to caustic effects of stomach acid if frequent vomiting is occurring ▪ Potential nutritional deficiencies, dehydration, and electrolyte imbalances; potassium and chloride levels due to frequent vomiting can lead to metabolic alkalosis ▪ Relatively stable weight patterns ▪ Relatively normal weight and body mass index (BMI)	▪ CBT ▪ Nutritional counseling, including encouragement to eat foods that provide replacement of electrolytes lost through vomiting (e.g., bananas, nuts, dried cereals, and potatoes for potassium replacement)
Personality Disorders			
▪ Absence or reduction of insight as to effects of behaviors ▪ Externalized stress response ▪ Failure to accept consequences of behaviors ▪ May include egocentricity, grandiosity, or perfectionism	▪ Pervasive pattern of behaviors, personal perceptions, and internal experiences that are significantly incongruent with an individual's cultural expectations ▪ Behaviors, perceptions, and experiences are relatively inflexible and cause distress or functional impairment	▪ Impaired function and disruption within personal, social, and professional realms ▪ Impulsivity with disregard for consequences of actions ▪ Outbursts of emotion, including anger and frustration ▪ Attempts to control external environment, including other individuals ▪ Potential self-directed violence ▪ Potential suicidal ideations and suicide attempts ▪ Potential other-directed violence ▪ Potential psychosis	▪ CBT ▪ Dialectical behavioral therapy (DBT) ▪ Schema-focused therapy (SFT) ▪ Family-focused therapy ▪ Expressive therapy ▪ Pharmacologic treatment with antidepressants (e.g., selective serotonin reuptake inhibitors [SSRIs], such as fluoxetine) for management of obsessive–compulsive, aggressive, and self-destructive behaviors ▪ Antipsychotics for cognitive-perceptual symptoms ▪ Pharmacologic mood stabilizers for control of impulsive behavior and anger

Sources: Based on Potter and Moller (2020); Shields, Fox, and Liebrecht (2019).

TABLE 29.2 Characteristic Manifestations of Common Feeding and Eating Disorders

Eating Disorder	Characteristics
Anorexia nervosa	▪ Obsessive focus on weight and body size ▪ Abnormally low body weight (usually 85% or less of the normal/expected weight) ▪ Extreme fear of weight gain ▪ May include **purging** behaviors (e.g., vomiting, diuretic use, laxative abuse)
Bulimia nervosa	▪ Obsessive focus on weight and body size ▪ Classified by presence or absence of purging behaviors ▪ *Purging type:* includes episodes of binge eating followed by purging through self-induced vomiting or use of diuretics or laxatives ▪ *Nonpurging type:* includes episodes of binge eating followed by fasting, intense and frequent exercise, or restrictive dieting
Binge-eating disorder	▪ Episodic compulsive consumption of excessive amounts of food within a 2-hour time period ▪ Overeating typically conducted in private/secrecy ▪ Not associated with purging behaviors

Sources: Based on National Institute of Mental Health (2019); Potter and Moller (2020).

nonfood items. Primary manifestations associated with NSRED include obesity and difficulty losing weight. This sleep-related eating disorder is more common in women and typically starts when individuals are in their 20s. It often occurs in those who have restless leg syndrome and may be a related condition. NSRED may also be linked to other sleep disorders, such as obstructive sleep apnea, and has been associated with use of short-acting sleep medications, such as zolpidem (Mayo Clinic, 2018). For these patients, interventions include referral to a nutritionist, evaluation of mood and stress, and screening for sleep-related disorders.

Pica refers to a continuing pattern of behavior in which the individual consumes nonnutritive, nonfood substances (e.g., chalk, paper, soap, dirt, metal, string, hair). Pica is more commonly reported in children, although it may appear in adults with intellectual disability or mental disorders. Pica may manifest in pregnancy related to cravings for nonfood substances (APA, 2013).

Rumination disorder describes the repeated regurgitation of food outside the presence of a medical condition (e.g., pyloric stenosis, gastroesophageal reflux). Onset may occur at any age, but if rumination begins in the first year of life, it may result in a medical emergency if it does not resolve spontaneously or if treatment is not initiated (APA, 2013).

Avoidant/restrictive food intake disorder is characterized as a disturbance in eating patterns manifested by failure to meet nutritional needs. Significant weight loss, nutritional deficiency, and dependency on enteral feeding or nutritional supplements may be observed along with impairment of psychosocial functioning. This disorder is seen more commonly in children and may result in impaired family functioning because of the increased stress related to meals and around functions including meals (APA, 2013).

Prader-Willi syndrome (PWS) is a chromosomal disorder that usually manifests at about 2 years of age. The characteristic features include intellectual disability, poor muscle tone, and an incessant desire to eat (Muscogiuri et al., 2019). Obesity occurs as a result of indiscriminate and excessive food consumption (Muscogiuri et al., 2019). Because individuals with PWS have a constant sense of hunger and desire to eat, treatment includes ensuring good nutritional habits and providing the patient with the proper amount of food intake. Because of hormonal deficiencies, these patients exhibit impaired physical growth and hypogonadism (underdevelopment of the sex organs). Treatment for patients with PWS may include hormonal therapies, as well as mental health services to address comorbid conditions. Speech, physical, and occupational therapy may also be of benefit to these patients (Muscogiuri et al., 2019).

Personality Disorders

A **personality disorder (PD)** manifests as a pervasive pattern of behaviors, personal perceptions, and internal experiences that are significantly incongruent with an individual's cultural expectations. This persistent pattern of behaviors, perceptions, and experiences is relatively inflexible and causes distress or functional impairment (see **Figure 29.2** »). Manifestations frequently lead to disruption of the individual's personal, social, and professional interactions. Typically, the onset of PDs occurs during adolescence or early adulthood (APA, 2013). At present, the American Psychiatric Association (2013) recognizes the following 10 forms of PD, each of which is discussed in Exemplar 29.B, Personality Disorders, in this module. Of these, borderline personality disorder (BPD) and antisocial personality disorder (ASPD) are the most challenging for patients, family members, and clinicians.

See the Alterations and Therapies feature for a summary of the manifestations and therapies for feeding and eating disorders and personality disorders.

Prevalence

Although feeding and eating disorders can impact individuals at any age, from the standpoint of patients who are officially diagnosed with an eating disorder, these conditions are reportedly more common among adolescents and young adults. In the United States, among adolescents between the ages of 13 and 17, an estimated 2.7% have an eating disorder. Bulimia nervosa is most prevalent among Hispanic adolescents, whereas anorexia nervosa is most prevalent among non-Hispanic white adolescents (National Eating Disorder

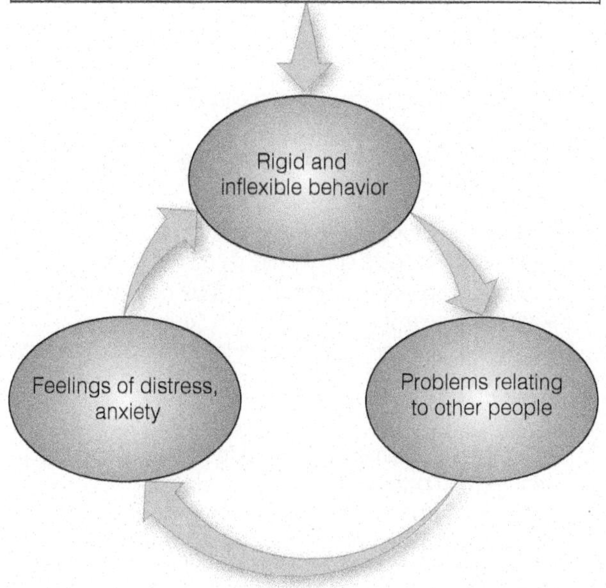
A person with a personality disorder has:
• Few strategies for relating to others
• Poor impulse control
• Different thought patterns and ways of perceiving
• Different range and intensity of affect from others in the culture.
Rigid and inflexible behavior
Problems relating to other people
Feelings of distress, anxiety

Figure 29.2 » Vicious cycle of personality disorders.

Association [NEDA], 2018). Bulimia nervosa is more common than is anorexia nervosa (APA, 2013). Lesbian, gay, and bisexual (LGB) identity has been associated with substantially elevated odds of purging and diet pill use in both male and female high school students, while bisexual females and males were also at elevated odds of obesity compared to same-gender heterosexuals (NEDA, 2018).

Among individuals 18 years and older, an estimated 15% of all adults in the United States have at least one personality disorder (APA, 2013). Prevalence rates vary, with borderline and antisocial personality disorders being among the most prevalent.

Genetic Considerations and Nonmodifiable Risk Factors

Compared to boys, girls are more than twice as likely to develop an eating disorder (NEDA, 2018). Prevalence varies with regard to specific PDs.

Research suggests there is a genetic component in PDs, and selected PDs with paranoid and delusional features may have a link with schizophrenia (APA, 2013). Certain personality characteristics can reflect the development of PDs, such as pervasive anxiety, fear, and aggression. Being a victim of childhood trauma or sexual abuse may promote the development of BPD. Adverse socioeconomic and sociocultural factors such as poverty or migration can influence the development of a PD. A PD may be exacerbated following the loss of a significant support person, such as a spouse, or previously stabilizing social situations such as a job (APA, 2013).

Case Study » Part 1

Jocelyn LeMandre, a 28-year-old woman, is transported to the emergency department (ED) by a friend. Although she is alert, oriented, and denies any complaints, her friend reports that Ms. LeMandre "passed out during an aerobics class" and also notes she has been complaining of being light-headed for the past few weeks. Ms. LeMandre reports she is finishing her doctoral degree in chemistry and currently teaches university courses.

When questioned about her symptoms, Ms. LeMandre admits to "feeling a little light-headed" but also notes that she hasn't been drinking enough fluids lately. She reports that she exercises daily for 2 hours prior to teaching her first course and occasionally exercises for another hour before going to bed. When asked about her dietary habits, Ms. LeMandre quietly replies, "I eat almost anything I want to eat. I might as well—I'm still going to be fat," and then looks away. When asked, Ms. LeMandre reports her height and weight as 5′7″ tall and 154 pounds. By observation, her weight is relatively proportionate to her height. Upon assessment, Ms. LeMandre's vital signs, which are within normal limits, include temperature 97.8°F oral; pulse 89 bpm; respirations 20/min; and blood pressure 92/52 mmHg.

Clinical Reasoning Questions Level I

1. Considering the report provided by Ms. LeMandre's friend and Ms. LeMandre's statements, what may be the cause of her light-headedness?
2. Based on this patient's educational background, occupation, and exercise regimen, what aspects of her personality are apparent?

Clinical Reasoning Questions Level II

3. At this time, what nursing diagnoses may be appropriate for inclusion in Ms. LeMandre's plan of care?
4. Based on the available information, what additional assessment data might you expect the primary healthcare provider (HCP) to order for Ms. LeMandre?

Concepts Related to Self

An individual's self-concept and self-esteem may be affected by alterations in other systems. For example, someone who is challenged by alterations in mobility may experience difficulty with accomplishing simple tasks associated with daily living. Loss of independence and autonomy may negatively impact self-concept or self-esteem. Similarly, a positive self-concept and high self-esteem may help motivate the individual to move beyond the impairment and learn to adapt and function independently.

As discussed earlier, family plays a role in the development of healthy self-esteem. Overprotective parenting has been associated with lower self-esteem (Rũgendo, 2019). Authoritative parenting, interfamilial violence, and the loss of a close family member may also impact an individual's self-esteem.

Decreased self-esteem has been associated with an increased risk for depression. Alterations in mood and affect influence an individual's level of resilience and coping abilities. Patients with personality disorders who have difficulty adhering to treatment regimens may experience negative consequences, including shame and stigmatization, as a result of their behaviors.

The Concepts Related to Self feature links some, but not all, of the concepts related to self. They are presented in alphabetical order.

Concepts Related to
Self

CONCEPT	RELATIONSHIP TO SELF	NURSING IMPLICATIONS
Advocacy	Being a member of a vulnerable and underserved population (e.g., the chronically mentally ill, the poor, LGBT populations, the homeless, certain ethnic groups) → ↓ access to healthcare services → ↓ quality of life and ↓ health outcomes	■ Educate yourself on vulnerable and underserved populations in your region. ■ Join professional and community groups that try to address these issues. ■ As a nurse, advocate for outreach efforts to include these populations in healthcare services. ■ Advocate for increased funding and research to better serve these populations.
Development	Missed development stages → ↓ fulfillment of life roles and ↓ cognitive, physical, and psychosocial development → ↓ self-esteem	■ Screen patients for developmental delays and refer to appropriate healthcare community resources. ■ Develop appropriate accommodations for nonmodifiable disorders or presentations. ■ Educate the family on how to assist the family member with developmental delays and refer to appropriate community agencies for support.
Ethics	Nurses are required to administer self-care that is at the same level as that which they provide to others	■ Perform self-assessment and strive for self-awareness both personally and professionally. ■ Identify and meet personal needs in order to promote optimal physical, psychosocial, and spiritual self-wellness.
Family	↑ Parental nurturing → ↑ self-esteem ↑ Parental overprotectiveness → ↓ Self-esteem	■ Interview the patient regarding perception of familial style of parenting. ■ Assess patient's level of self-esteem.
Mobility	Mobility → independence in daily living → ↑ self-esteem Impairment of mobility → increased dependence on others → may ↓ self-esteem and negatively impact self-concept High self-esteem and positive self-concept → greater resilience → increased likelihood for adaptation and achievement of optimal independence despite impairment	■ Assess self-concept and self-esteem in the patient with alterations in mobility. ■ Collaborate with other HCPs, including physical therapists and occupational therapists, to assist the patient with achieving maximum independence and autonomy. ■ Encourage the patient to focus on strengths and abilities as opposed to limitations.
Mood and Affect	↓ Self-esteem linked to ↑ risk for depression	■ Assess patients who exhibit low self-esteem for presence of signs and symptoms of depression. ■ In the clinical setting, report signs and symptoms of depression to the patient's primary care provider. ■ Facilitate referrals to mental health professionals for patients at risk for depression.
Stress and Coping	↑ Stress → biogenic and psychosocial manifestations of stress → impaired physical and mental health	■ Assess patients for signs and symptoms of ineffective coping. ■ Refer patients for short-term pharmacologic interventions and CBT. ■ Refer patients to appropriate resources in the community.

Health Promotion

Promotion of healthy self-concept varies according to the individual. Early recognition of negative self-concept and poor self-esteem can assist nurses in identifying strategies that may promote healthy self-concept and self-esteem in individual patients. Because eating disorders and personality disorders have complex and multifactorial etiologies, there is no single way to prevent their development.

School-Based Interventions

With eating disorders, some experts recommend implementation of school-based interventions because schools play a vital role in promoting the intellectual, physical, social, and emotional development and well-being of children and adolescents (National Eating Disorders Collaboration [NEDC], 2020). Some of the suggested interventions include providing a body image–friendly environment and celebrating diversity; prohibiting appearance-related teasing, including cyber-bullying, in school policy; ensuring no weighing, measuring, or anthropometric assessment of students in any context; providing an opportunity for all students to engage in regular physical activity in a noncompetitive, non-weight-loss-focused, and safe environment; providing a balance of food options in the cafeteria; and displaying public material/posters including a wide diversity of body shapes, sizes, and ethnicities (NEDC, 2020).

Other school-based interventions include training all relevant teaching staff in the early identification and referral of students with serious body image concerns and suspected eating disorders. Training teachers, especially athletic coaches, on risk factors that are reinforced by social environments and to use body-friendly language in their interactions with students is also recommended (NEDC, 2020).

Promoting Healthy Self-Esteem

The promotion of healthy self-esteem throughout childhood and adolescence is helpful in creating a stronger sense of self. Children with low self-esteem see temporary setbacks as permanent, intolerable conditions and maintain a sense of pessimism, which can increase their risk for experiencing stress, mental health problems, and difficulty with problem solving and meeting challenges (NEDA, 2018). Children with healthy self-esteem tend to enjoy interacting with others and are comfortable in social settings. When challenges arise, they can work toward finding solutions and voice discontent without belittling themselves or others (NEDA, 2018). These children are more likely to accept their strengths and weaknesses and are more optimistic.

Strategies nurses can offer to parents and caregivers to promote healthy self-esteem in children include the following (Tian, Liu, & Shan, 2018):

- Praise children not only for a job well done but also for effort.
- When children lack certain skills, help them to use learning these skills as an opportunity to learn about themselves and appreciate what makes them unique.
- Be a role model by not being excessively harsh on yourself or pessimistic. Children mirror what they see.
- Identify and redirect inaccurate beliefs children have about themselves.
- Be spontaneous about giving affection, hugs, and praise. Give praise honestly without overdoing it. By praising children when they make good choices, you reinforce the good choices and encourage them to continue making good choices.
- Create a safe, loving home environment. Children exposed to parents and caregivers who fight and argue repeatedly may feel they have no control over their environment and become helpless or depressed.
- Encourage children to participate in activities that require cooperation with others.

Screenings

Screening for eating disorders may include administration of the SCOFF questionnaire (Lichtenstein, Hemmingsen, & Støving, 2017). The SCOFF questionnaire was developed in England and has been found to reliably identify core elements of early-stage anorexia nervosa and bulimia nervosa (Lichtenstein et al., 2017; Tavolacci, Gillibert, Zhu Soubise, Grigioni, & Déchelotte, 2019).

S Do you make yourself **S**ick because you feel uncomfortably full?

C Do you worry you have lost **C**ontrol over how much you eat?

O Have you recently lost more than **O**ne stone (14 pounds) in a 3-month period?

F Do you believe yourself to be **F**at when others say you are too thin?

F Would you say that **F**ood dominates your life?

Score one point for every "yes"; a total score of 2 or higher indicates a likely case of anorexia nervosa or bulimia and the need for referral to a mental health specialist.

Identification of manifestations and diagnosis of personality disorders are guided by the fifth edition of the *Diagnostic and Statistical Manual of Mental Disorders* (DSM-5; APA, 2013).

Nursing Assessment

Assessment of the patient with suspected impairments related to self requires giving priority consideration to establishing and maintaining a safe environment. Because certain PDs are associated with impulsive or aggressive behavior, the nurse should ensure that the patient, the nurse, or anyone else in the area is not at risk for physical injury throughout the patient's care. The second priority is establishing a therapeutic relationship, which requires the nurse to build trust and apply principles of therapeutic communication.

After establishing trust, the nursing assessment begins by tactfully interviewing the patient regarding components related to self-concept, self-esteem, and self-awareness. Although it is important to complete a thorough assessment, the nurse should avoid asking personal questions that are unlikely to substantially add to the assessment data. For examples of basic components of a psychosocial assessment, see **Table 29.3** ».

Observation and Patient Interview

For many patients with alterations of self, observation may not yield visible clues. Exceptions do occur with patients who have eating disorders. For example, a patient with a restrictive eating disorder such as anorexia nervosa may appear skeletal, with downy hair (lanugo) on the face and limbs. Conversely, a patient who has bulimia or binge-eating disorder (BED) may present as overweight (BMI $>$ 25 to 30) or meet criteria for obesity (BMI $>$ 30) (Potter & Moller, 2020). When performing a patient history, the nurse may note that patients with anorexia display signs of reduced alertness and concentration and cognitive deficits as well as multiple physiologic characteristics, including poor sleep, sensitivity to the cold, and decreased energy (Potter & Moller,

TABLE 29.3 Sample Psychosocial Assessment Criteria

Dimension	Sample Assessment Criteria
Personal identity	Name Age Gender Marital status Occupation Cultural background, practices Ethnic origin Religious or spiritual affiliation, practices Self-perception: "How do you describe yourself?" Perceived image viewed by others: "How do others describe you?" Values: "In your life, what is most important to you?"
Physical history	Current physical illness History of physical illness Level of energy Disabilities
Communication skills and behaviors	Emotional tone Ability to follow conversation Verbal expression of emotion Verbal and nonverbal cues
Role performance	Current roles Presence of role conflicts or recent changes (e.g., retirement, death of spouse) Level of congruence between current developmental life stage and role performance Past behaviors used in management of role conflict
Body image	*Perceptual:* "What do you think when you look at your body in a mirror?" *Cognitive:* "How important is physical appearance to you?" *Behavioral:* "Are you comfortable in clothing that exposes more of your body, such as a swimsuit?" *Affective:* "In one or two words, how do you feel about your body?" *Subjective satisfaction:* "Overall, how satisfied are you with your body? Which is your favorite body part or region? Which is your least favorite body part or region?"
Self-esteem	(Global) "How satisfied are you with yourself?" (Global) "Overall, do you feel you're the person you should be?" (Specific) "What do you like most about yourself?" (Specific) "What do you like least about yourself?"

Sources: Based on Berman, Snyder, and Frandsen (2021); Cagle, Osteen, Sacco, and Frey (2017); Potter and Moller (2020).

2020). These signs and symptoms are discussed more fully in Exemplar 25.A, Feeding and Eating Disorders, in this module.

During the patient history, the nurse will assess the content of the patient's thinking patterns. In particular, patients with eating disorders exhibit distorted thinking regarding eating, calories, exercise, and body image. Patients with higher acuity will be unable to engage in normal activities and maintain productive relationships. A comprehensive nursing assessment also should determine the level of impairment and functioning within the family, relationships with peers, and performance in school or work (Potter & Moller, 2020). Any evidence of pica should be further investigated. In women, pica can lead to iron deficiency anemia. Ice pica may be indicative of an obsessive–compulsive or developmental disorder (Rajput, Kumar, & Moudgil, 2020).

It is less likely that a nurse will observe visible signs of a personality disorder upon initially meeting a patient. Because of the nature of PDs, clinicians are cautioned not to hurry a diagnosis. Although a single interview may confirm a prior assessment of a PD in a patient, clinicians are urged to assess the stability of personality traits over time across different situations (APA, 2013). Furthermore, assessment is complicated because patients often do not see personality characteristics reflecting psychopathology as problematic (APA, 2013).

Despite these considerations, some features of PDs may be apparent during an initial conversation. For example, patients with Cluster A traits, which include paranoid, schizoid, and schizotypal PDs, may appear odd or eccentric. Patients with Cluster B traits, which include antisocial, borderline, histrionic, and narcissistic PDs, may display dramatic, emotional, and erratic behaviors. Finally, patients with Cluster C traits, which include avoidant, dependent, and obsessive–compulsive PDs, may appear as anxious or fearful (APA, 2013). During the assessment, careful attention to cultural considerations is necessary to prevent inadvertent mislabeling of behaviors (see the Focus on Diversity and Culture feature).

As part of the assessment, it may be necessary to interview family members or coworkers (with the patient's permission) to more fully assess the patient's perceptions of reality and behaviors as well as what manifestations or behaviors family members or coworkers find most challenging.

Physical Examination

When caring for patients with eating disorders, the nurse should always remember that even though the etiologies of eating disorders are often psychologic, eating disorders have serious physiologic complications. For example, morbidity and mortality rates of anorexia are among the highest for all mental disorders (Potter & Moller, 2020). Thus, the assessment of patients with feeding and eating disorders requires thorough and ongoing medical monitoring. This includes frequently assessing vital signs, measuring height and weight, and repeating diagnostic tests such as complete blood count (CBC) and electrolytes and cardiac studies (e.g., electrocardiogram [ECG]).

A physical examination of a patient with a suspected PD is less likely to yield valuable clues, especially given that the treatments are primarily psychologic. If the patient has had a recent physical exam and any medical comorbidities are being managed by a HCP, mental health clinicians will likely defer to the physical exam. If a physical exam is conducted, it will include vital signs, assessment of the patient's appearance, and evidence of self-injurious

Focus on Diversity and Culture

Culture and Personality Disorders

Behaviors influenced by sociocultural contexts or specific life circumstances may be erroneously labeled as abnormal during the mental health assessment phase. For example, immigrants and political and economic refugees may display guarded or defensive behaviors that are interpreted as paranoid because of the HCP's unfamiliarity with the language or customs in the United States and/or because of previous negative experiences with the U.S. healthcare system (Ronningstam, Keng, Ridolfi, Arbabi, & Grenyer, 2018; Spector, 2017). In cultures with strong family values, like some Asian and Italian cultures, personality problems tend to be less pronounced, whereas in cultures where there is much social and political unrest, more severe behaviors such as aggression can tend to prevail (Ronningstam et al., 2018). Diagnostic criteria for personality disorders must be considered in light of an individual's cultural background. For example, a criterion for borderline personality disorder includes fear of abandonment, which is not acceptable or recognized in the Chinese culture, where values are placed upon collectivistic identities and enmeshed relationships (Ronningstam et al., 2018).

behaviors (e.g., cutting), which are indicative of some Cluster B diagnoses.

Diagnostic Tests

In the diagnosis and treatment of patients with alterations in self, there are no specific laboratory diagnostics that can be used to conclusively confirm a diagnosis. For these patients, laboratory and diagnostic tests are initially used to rule out physiologic causes that might be the source of associated signs and symptoms.

For patients diagnosed with feeding and eating disorders, laboratory and diagnostic testing may be used to assess for additional impairments that have occurred as a result of the primary disorder. For example, in the care of a patient with anorexia nervosa who is severely dehydrated and malnourished, laboratory studies may include a CBC and electrolyte studies, as well as tests to assess kidney function, such as blood urea nitrogen (BUN) and creatinine, and liver function tests. Other diagnostic exams may include ECG, thyroid screening, arterial blood gas (ABG), and urinalysis.

Case Study » Part 2

After assessing Ms. LeMandre, the ED physician orders a CBC and serum electrolytes, as well as administration of intravenous fluids for treatment of acute dehydration. When you return to insert Ms. LeMandre's IV catheter, she asks if she can first use the restroom. You respond that she is welcome to use the restroom; however, because of her recent loss of consciousness and history of light-headedness, policy dictates that she must be transferred to the restroom by wheelchair. Ms. LeMandre replies, "That's ridiculous. I'm perfectly capable of walking to the restroom!" Against your wishes, she quickly rises from the ED gurney and proceeds to ambulate to the restroom with you following at her side. She staunchly refuses to allow you to assist her. As you wait outside the restroom door, you hear water running, followed by retching sounds. When you knock on the door and ask if she is okay, Ms. LeMandre replies, "I'm fine—I'll be out shortly."

Less than a minute later, Ms. LeMandre emerges with what appears to be a small amount of emesis on the front of her hospital gown. When you ask if she vomited, she replies, "I just ate too much before I worked out this morning. Sometimes, when I eat too much, I get an upset stomach."

Ms. LeMandre denies any further complaints and, at your insistence, she agrees to allow you to return her to her ED room via wheelchair. You insert her IV catheter without incident and begin infusion of 500 mL of lactated Ringer solution, as ordered. Per Ms. LeMandre's request, you provide her with magazines to read while she awaits her lab draw and further assessment.

Clinical Reasoning Questions Level I

1. How does Ms. LeMandre's initial refusal to allow you to assist her to the restroom coincide with other aspects of her personality?
2. Does Ms. LeMandre's vomiting episode seem congruent with her explanation? How might her vomiting contribute to her light-headedness?

Clinical Reasoning Questions Level II

3. Based on all available data, including nursing observations, what nursing diagnoses may be appropriate for inclusion in Ms. LeMandre's plan of care?
4. What actions should the nurse take next? What information should be reported to the primary care physician?

Independent Interventions

In the promotion of psychosocial wellness, nurses have the unique opportunity to build trusting relationships with patients and to create a safe environment in which patients can openly discuss both positive and negative aspects of themselves as holistic beings. Through assessment of patient psychosocial wellness, the nurse can assist them with identifying areas of strength and weakness, which enhances patients' level of self-awareness.

Establishing the Therapeutic Relationship

Establishment of trust and application of therapeutic communication techniques require the nurse to exercise authenticity. The principle of authenticity includes remaining committed to promoting the patient's health and well-being (Flora, 2018). Particularly for patients with alterations in self, trust and respect are keys to both assessment and treatment. When caring for these patients, building a therapeutic relationship can be especially challenging. Patients with PDs may already be impacted by the stigma and shame often associated with mental illness, and they may have limited social support systems. For patients with feeding and eating disorders, many of whom maintain their condition and behaviors in secrecy, speaking openly about their self-perceptions and eating patterns may be especially difficult. Recovery rates are poor and dropout rates are high among patients who receive inpatient treatment for feeding and eating disorders (MacDonald & Trottier, 2019).

Interventions for Patients with Eating Disorders

Interventions that focus on reducing stress and not specifically addressing the problematic eating behaviors may help initially to create a therapeutic nurse–patient relationship. At this stage, patient education about possible stressors that contribute to eating disorder behavior is also appropriate. While this approach does not directly confront the problem behavior, it does address the stressors that can lead to problem behaviors (MacDonald & Trottier, 2019; Serin & Şanlıer, 2018). Nursing interventions include decreasing exposure to environmental stress; decreasing anxiety by eliminating caffeine and other stimulants; helping patients increase social and familial connectedness through improving communication skills; and assessing and teaching coping strategies. As patients' stress lowers and they become more trusting and open to change, they can be referred to treatment using established methods such as CBT (Serin & Şanlıer, 2018).

Patients with eating disorders often are paralyzed by low self-esteem. Nurses can promote self-worth and positive self-regard in these patients through a variety of interventions. When nurses provide positive reinforcement to patients who adhere to treatment and make efforts to meet goals, patients begin to view their efforts more optimistically (Serin & Şanlıer, 2018). Assisting patients to set short-term, realistic goals helps them to see and measure their treatment progress. Encouraging patients to reconnect with activities and experiences that they enjoy helps them begin to regain control over their own behaviors and begin to reexperience positive emotions (Serin & Şanlıer, 2018).

Interventions for Patients with Personality Disorders

For patients with PDs, the priority interventions are directed to safety. Once safety is ensured, the nurse turns the focus toward building the therapeutic relationship, which, in turn, supports other nursing interventions in the areas of medication management, facilitating coping skills, strengthening reality orientation, maintaining professional boundaries, and milieu management (Acford & Davies, 2019; Sheppard & Duncan, 2018). These interventions help patients begin to feel hopeful that they can progress in their treatment and improve their ability to function on a daily basis.

Regarding safety, the nurse will assess patients for suicidal ideation, history of suicide attempts, and desire and history of self-injurious behaviors (for detailed information, see Exemplar 28.D, Suicide, in Module 28, Mood and Affect). If a patient does self-injure in some way, it is important for the nurse to remain objective and matter-of-fact. The nurse responds first with the necessary medical attention. Then, when the crisis is over, the nurse will process the event with the patient, looking for cues and feelings that may have contributed to or triggered the patient's desire to self-harm (Acford & Davies, 2019; Potter & Moller, 2020; Sheppard & Duncan, 2018).

Self-awareness is an essential component of the therapeutic relationship when working with patients with PDs. Nurses must have a strong sense of identity, be willing to set limits and reinforce boundaries, and should have supervision or collaborative relationships with colleagues with whom they can process their relationships with patients (Acford & Davies, 2019; Potter & Moller, 2020). Nurses working with these patients should frequently examine their patient relationships in order to maintain a consistent and therapeutic effect.

Nurses working with patients who have PDs should help reconnect patients with coping behaviors they have employed successfully in the past and teach patients new adaptive coping skills. For example, patients who act impulsively and aggressively may be taught to count until less angry, employ deep-breathing exercises, and eventually to express anger verbally (Acford & Davies, 2019). Self-management, taking responsibility for one's own behavior and well-being, is another coping technique that can help bring a sense of order and empowerment to patients. Self-management behaviors promote social interaction and reduce disruptive behaviors and include adhering to the treatment plan and using appropriate social skills (Acford & Davies, 2019; Sheppard & Duncan, 2018).

Collaborative Therapies

One problem among collaborative providers, especially when dealing with patients with personality disorders, is creating a therapeutic relationship that provides firm, consistent boundaries. Individuals diagnosed with PDs, especially BPD, often require limit setting to reinforce those boundaries (Nathan, 2018; Potter & Moller, 2020; Stone, 2019). A consistent, firm approach reinforcing elements of the care plan and institutional policies is necessary. If reinforcement is inconsistent, a patient will often engage in splitting by playing one staff person against another (Acford & Davies, 2019; Ilagan & Choi-Kain, 2020; Potter & Moller, 2020). Therefore, nurses and other members of the treatment team need to consistently enforce interventions and boundaries and confront patients who are testing them. Specific interventions nurses and other members of the interprofessional team can take toward developing a therapeutic relationship include maintaining consistent staffing, following through on all agreements and promises, setting limits on inappropriate behavior, maintaining appropriate professional boundaries, and processing patient interactions with trusted colleagues (Acford & Davies, 2019; Ilagan & Choi-Kain, 2020; Potter & Moller, 2020). These are helpful strategies when working with patients with any type of mental illness, and not just personality disorders.

Pharmacologic Therapy

Pharmacologic therapy normally is not the primary course of treatment for alterations in self, although it may be used to treat specific manifestations and/or comorbid conditions. For example, antipsychotic medications may be indicated in the care of patients with PDs who are experiencing delusions, hallucinations, or other manifestations associated with psychosis. Similarly, patients with feeding and eating disorders who experience comorbid anxiety or depression may also benefit from pharmacologic therapy.

Nonpharmacologic Therapy

For many patients with feeding and eating disorders or PDs, counseling and therapy are the mainstays of treatment. In particular, CBT, which emphasizes focusing on immediate problems and developing solutions through activities such as repatterning the patient's thinking or developing healthy coping behaviors to replace maladaptive ones, has been deemed useful in the treatment of patients with feeding and eating disorders (Little, Tickle, & das Nair, 2018; NIMH, 2017b; Potter & Moller, 2020). Other forms of therapy include DBT and SFT; these are discussed in Exemplar 29.B, Personality Disorders, in this module.

Case Study » Part 3

You report Ms. LeMandre's vomiting episode to the ED physician. Shortly thereafter, her CBC and serum electrolyte findings become available. All findings are within normal limits, although both her potassium level (3.7 mEq/L) and chloride level (99 mmol/L) are on the low end of the normal range. The physician diagnoses Ms. LeMandre with dehydration. However, in light of her laboratory results, rigorous exercise regimen, statements about her eating patterns, expressed body image, and vomiting episode, the physician is concerned that Ms. LeMandre's signs and symptoms may be manifestations of an eating disorder. He asks you to accompany him while he speaks with her. After speaking with her for several minutes about her dietary patterns and what she now describes as "occasionally getting sick when my stomach is too full," the physician asks Ms. LeMandre if he may ask her a few questions about her overall physical health and her views about food. Reluctantly, she agrees.

The physician proceeds to administer the SCOFF Questionnaire. Ms. LeMandre responds "yes" to two of the questions contained in the questionnaire: "Do you make yourself sick because you feel uncomfortably full?" and "Do you worry you have lost control over how much you eat?" Subsequently, the ED physician requests that Ms. LeMandre speak with the on-call psychiatrist. Once again, she reluctantly agrees. Following the consultation, the psychiatrist diagnoses Ms. LeMandre with bulimia nervosa and schedules her for a follow-up appointment in 3 days for further evaluation and treatment.

Clinical Reasoning Questions Level I

1. What is the SCOFF Questionnaire? What criteria suggest the potential presence of anorexia nervosa or bulimia nervosa?
2. If Ms. LeMandre does have an eating disorder, why do you think her weight is within normal limits?
3. How does anorexia nervosa differ from bulimia nervosa?

Clinical Reasoning Questions Level II

4. Based on all available data, including nursing observations, what nursing diagnoses may be appropriate for inclusion in Ms. LeMandre's plan of care?
5. What is the most likely cause of this patient's near-hypokalemia (low serum potassium) and near-hypochloremia (low serum chloride)? In light of these deficiencies, what dietary recommendations might be appropriate for her?
6. What long-term risks are associated with feeding and eating disorders? How might Ms. LeMandre's personality traits affect her willingness to follow treatment protocols?

REVIEW The Concept of Self

RELATE Link the Concepts

Linking the concept of self with the concept of fluids and electrolytes:

1. Explain how alterations in self may affect fluid and electrolyte balance. Which personality disorders might lead the patient to be most vulnerable to alterations in fluid and electrolyte balance?
2. Describe at least three independent and collaborative nursing interventions that are appropriate for implementation in the plan of care for a patient with an alteration in fluid and electrolyte balance due to an eating disorder. Include discussion of diagnostic testing that may be useful for evaluating fluid and electrolyte balance in these patients.

Linking the concept of self with the concept of ethics:

3. Describe ethical considerations related to the nurse's self-care. How might a nurse's self-concept affect the ethical aspects of the nurse's behavior, both personally and professionally?
4. Describe ethical considerations that impact the care of a patient who is known or believed to be at risk for self-injury.
5. In the course of caring for a patient with an eating disorder who refuses to eat, what ethical considerations might the nurse face?

READY Go to Volume 3: Clinical Nursing Skills

REFER Go to Pearson MyLab Nursing and eText

REFLECT Apply Your Knowledge

The family nurse practitioner (FNP) is seeing Caitlin Smith, a 26-year-old woman, who has come in for her annual checkup, primarily to renew her prescription for birth control pills. Caitlin is very well dressed and obviously overweight. She is 5′4″ tall and weighs 188 pounds. The exam goes routinely until the FNP addresses Caitlin's weight, pointing out that her BMI of 32.3 makes her technically obese. Caitlin angrily explodes, saying loudly to the FNP, "When I want your opinion, I will ask for it!" The FNP soothes Caitlin by saying she needs to discuss the weight because of the possible adverse health effects. Caitlin then starts crying. During additional questioning when Caitlin has calmed, the FNP finds out that she has a high-stress job in real estate management. She enjoys her job but feels that clients unfairly judge her because of her weight. Caitlin is vague about her dietary habits, but she admits to being a stress-eater and having a weakness for chocolate and sweets. "I can eat an entire chocolate cake at one sitting and not even be aware of it," she says. Sometimes after a stressful day, she goes home from work and eats snack foods continually until bedtime. She denies vomiting or overuse of laxatives. Caitlin also admits that her boyfriend recently broke up with her "because of my moods and anger. . . . I just think it is raging hormones." However, this is the fourth romantic relationship that has broken off abruptly since Caitlin graduated from college. Caitlin also worries about losing control or becoming angry at work.

1. Given Caitlin's statements and findings, she likely has which eating disorder?
2. The FNP will probably make which referrals for Caitlin's weight issue?
3. In a later visit, Caitlin discloses that she was sexually abused by an uncle during her preteen and early teen years. Caitlin's mother stopped the abuse when she found out about it, but it was never reported and Caitlin never received any counseling. Given her history of emotional lability, Caitlin may have or be at risk for developing which personality disorder?

Exemplar 29.A Feeding and Eating Disorders

Exemplar Learning Outcomes

29.A Analyze feeding and eating disorders and how they relate to self.

- Describe the pathophysiology of feeding and eating disorders.
- Describe the etiology of feeding and eating disorders.
- Compare the risk factors and prevention of feeding and eating disorders.
- Identify the clinical manifestations of feeding and eating disorders.
- Summarize diagnostic tests and therapies used by interprofessional teams in the collaborative care of an individual with a feeding and eating disorder.
- Differentiate care of patients with feeding and eating disorders across the lifespan.
- Apply the nursing process in providing culturally competent care to an individual with a feeding and eating disorder.

Exemplar Key Terms

Overview

Food is essential to life. The body requires an adequate supply of **nutrients** to meet energy requirements such as thermoregulation, cellular regulation, and metabolism. Feeding and eating disorders are complex conditions that stem from myriad social, cultural, and psychologic causes and that culminate in the disruption of the body's nutrient supply. These disorders can cause either under- or overnutrition, both of which have negative physiologic effects. In the absence of a food source to use for energy, the body digests body fat and muscles. When it has excess food in proportion to energy use, weight gain and obesity result. Feeding and eating disorders produce biochemical and physiologic interruptions of the metabolism that endanger the whole body. **Metabolism** is the complex process by which the body breaks down and converts food and fluids into energy sources.

The three disorders discussed in this exemplar are anorexia nervosa, bulimia nervosa, and binge-eating disorder. Anorexia nervosa (AN) is a condition characterized by an extreme aversion to gaining weight, as well as physiologic and mental consequences associated with food restriction. Bulimia nervosa (BN) is characterized by a pernicious cycle of bingeing and purging. Binge-eating disorder (BED) is characterized by the consumption of large amounts of food and a feeling of loss of control during binges. These three conditions create biological, physiologic, and social imbalances that ravage an individual's health and self-concept. For individuals with feeding and eating disorders, the irregular supply of the nutrients necessary for physical health is compounded by psychologic states such as depression, isolation, and self-destructive tendencies.

Other feeding and eating disorders include pica, rumination, avoidant/restrictive food intake disorder, and night eating syndrome (NES). See the Clinical Manifestations and Therapies feature for an overview of feeding and eating disorders.

Feeding and eating disorders are not defined by body weight and external appearance but, rather, by the psychologic states that cause the resulting changes in eating behaviors and nutrition status. There are many causes for feeding and eating disorders that are outcomes of biological, psychologic, and social processes. At present, researchers believe that an individual's family, social context, and culture provide triggers, but that hormones, brain chemicals, and genetics cause individuals to push themselves to starvation or obesity.

Pathophysiology

The biological aspects of eating disorders are complex and not fully understood. During active illness, there are known disturbances in neuroendocrine, neurochemistry, and neurotransmission circuitry and signal pathways (Gianni, De Donatis, Valente, De Ronchi, & Atti, 2020). Investigators have found disturbances in serotonin and neuropeptide systems that modulate appetite, mood, cognitive function, impulse control, energy metabolism, and hormonal systems. As a result of their malnourished and emaciated state, individuals with AN have alterations of brain structure that are related to the course of the illness, metabolism, and neurochemistry (Duncan et al., 2017; Gianni et al., 2020). In contrast, those with BN have shown brain atrophy in imaging studies (Gianni et al., 2020).

The genetic heritability of feeding and eating disorders is comparable to other biologically based mental illnesses. Twin studies in AN, BN, and BED estimate that 40–60% of the variance is accounted for by genetic factors (Duncan et al., 2017; Hübel, Leppä, Breen, & Bulik, 2018; Potter & Moller, 2020). Furthermore, these studies revealed that puberty has a powerful impact in activating the genes of etiologic importance in feeding and eating disorders (Hübel et al., 2018). Duncan et al. (2017) found that eating disorders, especially anorexia nervosa, have a complex heritable phenotype with significant genetic correlations to both psychiatric disorders such as obsessive–compulsive disorder and neuroticism and multiple metabolic traits.

The regulation of feeding behavior involves a complex integrative signaling network system of positive and negative feedback mechanisms that work to maintain energy homeostasis (Gianni et al., 2020). In the case of binge eating, if there is a dysregulation in the relative potency of the negative feedback signaling mechanism, meal size and eating duration can be increased.

Ghrelin, a gut peptide that increases appetite, acts on the vagus nerve and stimulates neurons in the hypothalamus. Short-acting satiation signals from the gut to the hindbrain also interact with the long-acting adiposity hormones, leptin and insulin, which are then released and circulate in the blood (Berner et al., 2018; Potter & Moller, 2020). These hormones gain access to the hypothalamus in response to the amount of fat stores and energy needs to maintain weight regulation, metabolism, and homeostasis. This higher-order integration evaluates inhibitory signals and metabolic state to determine energy storage needs for regulation, whereas the nucleus tractus solitarius in the caudal brainstem primarily controls the amount of food eaten. During food deprivation or restriction, the sensitivity of the short-acting satiation signals decreases. Therefore, it takes larger amounts of food to generate adequate signaling to terminate a meal (Brambilla, Santonastaso, Caregaro, & Favaro, 2018; Potter & Moller, 2020). These hormones can affect satiety by either increasing or decreasing the amount of food eaten.

Research has shown that in comparison to individuals without weight issues, those with feeding and eating disorders experience blunted or attenuated functioning in both the short- and long-acting signaling processes responsible for appetite and weight regulation. When individuals cease eating-disordered behaviors, these hormones may return to a normalized state. However, in some individuals these hormones may remain dysfunctional, indicating a trait-related phenomenon. Therefore, it remains to be determined whether these dysfunctions are a cause, consequence, or maintenance factor in eating disorders (Potter & Moller, 2020). When individuals who stop engaging in eating-disordered behaviors experience normalization of a hormone (such as cholecystokinin), this may indicate an adaptive response (Berner et al., 2018; Fetissov & Hökfelt, 2019).

It may be that a recalibration begins to effectively regulate and control the input of neuronal and hormonal signals necessary to restore homeostasis and stability of hormone system feedback loops. The resulting responses are the absence of debilitating behaviors, such as bingeing or vomiting.

What is unclear is which adaptive mechanism(s) must be present and properly functioning for hormonal response to return to normal and for disordered eating behaviors to cease. The lack of research data about which biological adaptations must occur to achieve remission and how nurses and HCPs can promote them is one reason why the treatment of individuals with feeding and eating disorders is so challenging.

Etiology

Although many studies on the causes of feeding and eating disorders have been performed and published, there is no medical consensus on the etiology of these conditions. Biological and cognitive-behavioral theories are relevant to the development of these alterations. An understanding of these theories allows the nurse to take a holistic approach when caring for patients with feeding and eating disorders.

It seems clear that biology—including genetic and neurologic factors—plays a large part in the development of feeding and eating disorders. Research shows that relatives of patients with feeding and eating disorders are 5 to 10 times more likely to develop a disorder. Studies of twins have demonstrated that feeding and eating disorders occur for both twins at a rate of 40–60%, indicating that a genetic predisposition may play into the development of these conditions. Neurologic factors include neurotransmitter dysregulation. The neurotransmitter in question is 5-HT, or serotonin, which is synthesized partially of carbohydrates. A low level of 5-HT typically reduces an individual's satiety and increases the consumption of nutrients; a high level of the neurotransmitter increases satiety and decreases food intake. A current theory of binge eating holds that repeated binge episodes may result from a deficiency in serotonin and that the tendency of individuals with bulimia to binge carbohydrate-rich foods is a manifestation of the body's attempt to replenish serotonin. However, 5-HT is not the only neurotransmitter involved in feeding and eating disorders. Norepinephrine and neuropeptide Y increase food consumption, while dopamine inhibits eating. In addition, endogenous opioids, such as endorphins, increase food intake and elevate mood. Individuals who are significantly underweight typically have significantly lower endorphin levels than individuals of normal weight. The fact that endorphin levels return to normal when weight returns to normal outlines the complex relationship between biology, nutrition, and psychology in feeding and eating disorders (Fetissov & Hökfelt, 2019; Gianni et al., 2020).

Cognitive-behavioral theories view feeding and eating disorders as learned patterns of behavior based on irrational thought and beliefs. These theories look at the affected individual's cognition and behavior to stimuli, whether physiologic, psychologic, or social, and attempt to help the patient with the disorder by changing the maladaptive behavior and replacing it with a healthier response. An essential element of cognitive-behavioral theory is that the individual's thought patterns give rise to destructive behavioral patterns and that irrational thoughts are at the heart of the network of problems that leads to feeding and eating disorders (Forrest, Jones, Ortiz, & Smith, 2018; Potter & Moller, 2020).

Risk Factors

Because the origination of feeding and eating disorders is so complex, the risk factors for feeding and eating disorders are closely related to their etiologies. In addition to biological and genetic factors, sociocultural factors and family systems can contribute to the psychologic conditions that prime an individual for an eating disorder.

Sociocultural risk factors are elements of an individual's social and cultural context that exert the pressure that initiates an eating disorder. In the United States, portrayals of men's and women's bodies in the media and a pervasive cultural understanding of a trim body as the "ideal" lead to the unrealistic expectation that everyone should have a low weight. In addition to glamorizing an unrealistically trim body shape, the cultural obsession with thinness leads to a bias against those who are overweight. These social factors diminish the self-esteem of those who believe they do not fit the "ideal" body shape and enhance self-worth for those who are deemed attractive. Girls and women are hardest hit by the cultural emphasis on thin bodies. Magazines targeted at adolescent girls present dieting as a sensible solution to the crises of adolescents and contain 90% more articles promoting weight control than magazines targeted at teenage boys.

For many young women, self-esteem becomes centered on concerns about weight (Potter & Moller, 2020).

In recent years, the American ideal of male attractiveness has also shifted toward the unhealthy. Men and boys are confronted every day with images of male beauty that center on muscle-bound figures defined by their strength. The use of anabolic steroids is common among men with feeding and eating disorders because in addition to seeking thinness they also seek improved muscle tone (Carrard, Rothen, & Rodgers, 2020; Limbers, Cohen, & Gray, 2018). Because of the pressure that the media, social, and cultural expectations exert, feeding and eating disorders like anorexia and bulimia can be considered culture-reactive syndromes in the United States and the rest of the Western world. Negative body image, degraded self-worth, and body dissatisfaction create the stress that leads to feeding and eating disorders (Carrard et al., 2020; Potter & Moller, 2020).

Family systems theories do not necessarily hold that harmful family patterns cause feeding and eating disorders, but rather that the family enables maladaptive behaviors. Some individuals with feeding and eating disorders are survivors of childhood and adolescent abuse—including sexual abuse—much of which occurs in immediate and extended family systems. In addition to abuse, many families of patients with eating disorders have impaired conflict resolution skills. Another factor that enables the development of feeding and eating disorders is a family-wide emphasis on achievement and performance, with ambition for the family's success being one of the principal goals of the parents. Body shape is frequently related to success in these families, and an emphasis on fitness combined with a desire for control may become obsessive.

In addition to the family system impacting the development of an eating disorder, the appearance of a disorder can disrupt the fragile order of a family unit. After the diagnosis or appearance of a disorder such as anorexia, certain families become enmeshed: The boundaries between members become weak, interactions intensify, members become more dependent, and autonomy decreases. When these patterns occur, each family member becomes less stable and more involved with the other members' private concerns. The parents become overprotective, and food can take on extreme importance. A family's system of interpersonal relations influences the development of an eating disorder, and the presence of an eating disorder impacts the way a family conducts itself in a harmful cycle (Erriu, Cimino, & Cerniglia, 2020; Potter & Moller, 2020).

Prevention

Prevention is a systematic attempt to change the circumstances that facilitate feeding and eating disorders. Prevention can involve reducing negative risk factors such as body dissatisfaction and depression and basing self-esteem on appearance. Prevention also involves increasing protective factors such as basing self-esteem on factors other than appearance and replacing unhealthy dieting with an appreciation for the body's natural functionality. A broad-based cultural emphasis on prevention is essential for the global reduction of the suffering associated with feeding and eating disorders (NEDA, 2018).

Healthcare providers should target two types of audiences when implementing eating disorder prevention. Universal prevention, the first type, should be aimed at the general public, even at those individuals who show no signs of feeding and eating disorders. This type of prevention aims to promote healthy development and understanding of the many complex issues that cause these disorders, as a way of spreading the information that can cut them off before they begin. Targeted prevention, the second type of prevention, educates individuals who are beginning to show symptoms of feeding and eating disorders. These individuals may have high levels of body dissatisfaction. The goal of targeted prevention is to provide enough information to stop an eating disorder from developing (NEDA, 2018). Both universal and targeted programs have had success in preventing feeding and eating disorders, though targeted programs seem to be more effective.

Instruction and interventions interwoven and scaffolded by age throughout all years of K–12 education also seem to hold promise because teachers and coaches play an important

Patient Teaching

Sports and Eating Disorders: Warning Signs

Competitive sports that overemphasize body type and physique have been associated with disordered eating behaviors (DE) and eating disorders (EDs). The reported prevalence of DE and EDs in athletic populations ranges from 35 to 58% in female athletes and up to 38% of male athletes (NEDA, 2018). The most common sports-related ED is *anorexia athletica*, a condition in which individuals engage in excessive exercise and calorie restriction to achieve a lean body type, which is thought to be more prevalent among women gymnasts and dancers. However, Stanford Children's Health (2020) and other organizations emphasize that any competitive sport that focuses on appearance, diet, weight requirements, and personal performance may create an environment or culture that promotes the development of DEs/EDs.

Some of the warning signs of EDs associated with sports participation include the following findings (NEDA, 2018; Smoll, 2018). The child or adolescent may exhibit:

- Excessive and compulsive concern with appearance and exercise; engaging in extra workouts beyond what is required
- Decreased concentration, energy, muscle function, coordination, and/or speed
- Longer recovery time needed after workouts, games, or races
- More frequent muscle strains, sprains, and/or fractures
- Slowed heart rate and low blood pressure
- Reduced body temperature and being sensitive to cold (cold hands and feet)
- Complaints of light-headedness and dizziness, abdominal pain
- Poorer interaction with coaches/teammates
- Perfectionism; irritability
- Avoidance of water or excessive water intake
- Dieting that approaches self-starvation or unusual eating habits (including excessive or secretive food intake)
- Excessive concern with body aesthetic.

role in promoting health and well-being within the school environment (see the Patient Teaching feature). Education about body image, disordered eating, and the risks of dieting and eating disorders are all important topics that should be addressed to help prevent an eating disorder from developing, ease the suffering of a young person in the early stages of an eating disorder, and reduce the stigma and misconceptions that surround eating disorders (NEDA, 2018). Proactive efforts to promote positive body image and healthy lifestyle choices should be integrated across the curriculum with the aim of helping to prevent eating disorders rather than simply responding reactively to existing issues (NEDA, 2018).

Clinical Manifestations

Clinical manifestations of the different feeding and eating disorders vary, but similarities include body image disturbance, anxiety, and ineffective coping skills. Commonly occurring feeding and eating disorders include anorexia nervosa, bulimia nervosa, and binge-eating disorder. These and less prevalent feeding and eating disorders are outlined in the Clinical Manifestations and Therapies feature.

Anorexia Nervosa

Anorexia nervosa (AN) is a potentially deadly ED that compels individuals to lose more weight than is healthy for their age and height. Patients with anorexia have an intense fear of gaining weight, even when they show the symptoms of being dangerously underweight. Individuals with anorexia engage in dieting and exercising to the point of dangerous malnutrition to avoid gaining weight (MentalHealth.gov, 2017; NEDA, 2018). Information related to the severity of anorexia nervosa and criteria for hospitalization are summarized in **Box 29.1** ».

Anorexia nervosa typically begins during the teen years, and it is more commonly diagnosed in females. In particular, AN is more prevalent among white females with a history of high academic achievement. See the Evidence-Based Practice feature in the Collaboration section for a discussion of how those with feeding and eating disorders are affected by the internet. These women frequently have goal-oriented families or personalities, and they develop rigid "rules" that they use to control weight. These rituals can be simple, such as cutting food into tiny pieces, or elaborate, such as preparing lavish dinners for friends or family without consuming any food themselves. Criteria for diagnosis of AN include possessing an intense fear of weight gain, refusing to maintain a healthy weight, and perceiving a distorted body image. In previous years, amenorrhea (absence of menstruation for 3 or more months) was also a diagnostic criterion for AN; however, this is no longer the case. In order to maintain low body weight, individuals with anorexia severely limit food consumption and offset consumption with excessive exercise. Other behaviors include self-induced vomiting; refusing to eat in the presence of others; using diuretics, laxatives, and diet pills; and cutting food into small pieces as a way of pretending to eat (MentalHealth.gov, 2017; Potter & Moller, 2020).

Anorexia nervosa takes a toll on the entire body (see the Multisystem Effects feature). As an individual loses body weight and becomes malnourished, hair and nails become brittle, skin becomes dry and yellow, and a fine layer of hair called *lanugo* appears on previously hairless parts of the body. Individuals with anorexia may constantly feel cold, as the body loses its ability to retain heat. The starvation resulting from anorexia can cause damage to vital organs such as the brain, kidneys, and heart. Pulse rate and blood pressure drop, and irregular heart rhythms can cause heart failure. Loss of nutrients can lead to brittle bones and even changes in the brain, which in turn lead to impaired thinking. In the worst cases of anorexia, patients can starve themselves to death. The condition has the highest mortality rate of any mental illness, due to the complications of malnutrition and the high rate of suicide in the population (National Association of Anorexia Nervosa and Associated Disorders [ANAD], 2020).

Box 29.1

Severity of Anorexia Nervosa and Criteria for Hospitalization

Clinical signs are important indicators of the severity of anorexia nervosa for two reasons: (1) Patients with anorexia nervosa often hide their symptoms and behaviors, and therefore may not always report reliably about the extent to which symptoms interfere with function or the duration of the symptoms and (2) as the illness becomes more acute, the patient is at increased risk for physiologic dysfunction and even organ damage.

The DSM-5 identifies BMI (the weight in kilograms divided by the square of the height in meters) as an important clinical indicator of the severity of AN (APA, 2013):

Mild: BMI $\geq$ 17

Moderate: BMI 16–16.99

Severe: BMI 15–15.99

Extreme: BMI $<$ 15

Healthcare providers with patients who have symptoms of anorexia nervosa with severe to extreme BMI deficits may determine a need for hospitalization based on the patient's BMI and other clinical signs, such as arrhythmia, systolic BP $<$ 90 mmHg, and heart rate below 40 to 50 beats per minute (Buchman, Attia, Dawson, & Steinglass, 2019; Khalifa & Goldman, 2019; Potter & Moller, 2020). Although specific clinical markers may vary by clinician or healthcare agency, the following indicators will likely necessitate admission (Buchman et al., 2019; Potter & Moller, 2020):

- Acute medical complication(s) requiring stabilization
- Refusal to eat
- Risk of self-harm or suicide
- Failure to respond to outpatient treatment.

In addition to these markers, guidelines for admission of adolescents include temperature below 35.5°C (95.9°F) (Khalifa & Goldman, 2019).

Bulimia Nervosa

Bulimia nervosa (BN) is a condition in which individuals binge on food or have episodes of overeating in which they feel a loss of control. After periods of bingeing, the individuals use methods such as vomiting or laxative abuse to prevent weight gain. Bingeing may also be followed by periods of extreme exercise. Many individuals who have bulimia also have anorexia nervosa. Individuals with bulimia are obsessed with their body appearance and engage in the destructive

Clinical Manifestations and Therapies

Feeding and Eating Disorders

DISORDER	CLINICAL MANIFESTATIONS	CLINICAL THERAPIES
Anorexia nervosa	▪ Obsession over body shape and food ▪ Extreme perfectionism ▪ Rigidity, overcontrol, obsessive rituals ▪ Significant weight loss ▪ Body disturbances ▪ Strenuous exercise ▪ Reductions in heart rate, blood pressure, metabolic rate, and in production of estrogen or testosterone ▪ Extreme sensitivity to cold ▪ Feelings of depression	▪ Antidepressants ▪ Cognitive-behavioral therapy (CBT) ▪ Group therapy ▪ Family therapy
Avoidant/restrictive food intake disorder	▪ Avoidance of food or restriction of food intake ▪ Inadequate nutrition resulting in significant weight loss and nutritional deficiencies ▪ Disruptive behaviors, conflict surrounding meals	▪ Enteral feeding/nutrition supplements ▪ Refeeding in hospital setting may be a necessary first step ▪ CBT ▪ Family therapy ▪ Anxiety management strategies, cognitive restructuring
Bulimia nervosa	▪ Cycle of bingeing and purging food ▪ Body image disturbances ▪ Abuse of laxatives, enemas, and diuretics ▪ Extreme exercise to compensate for bingeing ▪ Hoarding food ▪ Secretive behaviors	▪ Antidepressants ▪ CBT ▪ Family therapy
Binge-eating disorder	▪ Bingeing once a week for at least 3 months ▪ Absence of purging ▪ Sense of loss of control ▪ Allowing eating and weight to interfere with personal relationships ▪ Sense of embarrassment, disgust after overeating	▪ Antidepressants ▪ CBT
Night eating syndrome	▪ Recurrent episodes of night eating (eating after awakening or excessive food consumption after the evening meal) ▪ Night eating usually involves consumption of carbohydrates ▪ Sense of guilt and shame	▪ Stress-reduction programs ▪ CBT, DBT
Pica	▪ Persistent eating of substances other than food, such as paper, soap, cloth, hair, paint, gum, and pebbles ▪ Usually begins in childhood and typically lasts for just a few months ▪ Potential medical complications associated with ingestion of foreign substances (e.g., mechanical intestinal and bowel obstruction, perforation, parasitic infections, and poisoning)	▪ No specific way to prevent pica. ▪ Pay careful attention to eating habits and close supervision of children with pica to help prevent complications ▪ Nutrition assessment to rule out vitamin or mineral deficiencies ▪ If appropriate, antidepressants and CBT ▪ Group therapy ▪ Family therapy
Rumination	▪ Repeated regurgitation of food after eating ▪ Food may be rechewed and then ejected from mouth or reswallowed ▪ Occurs more frequently in individuals with intellectual disability	▪ Habit reversal behavioral therapy (for those without intellectual disability) ▪ Mild aversive therapy or other behavioral strategies ▪ Proton pump inhibitors may be described if rumination is damaging the esophagus

Multisystem Effects of
Anorexia Nervosa

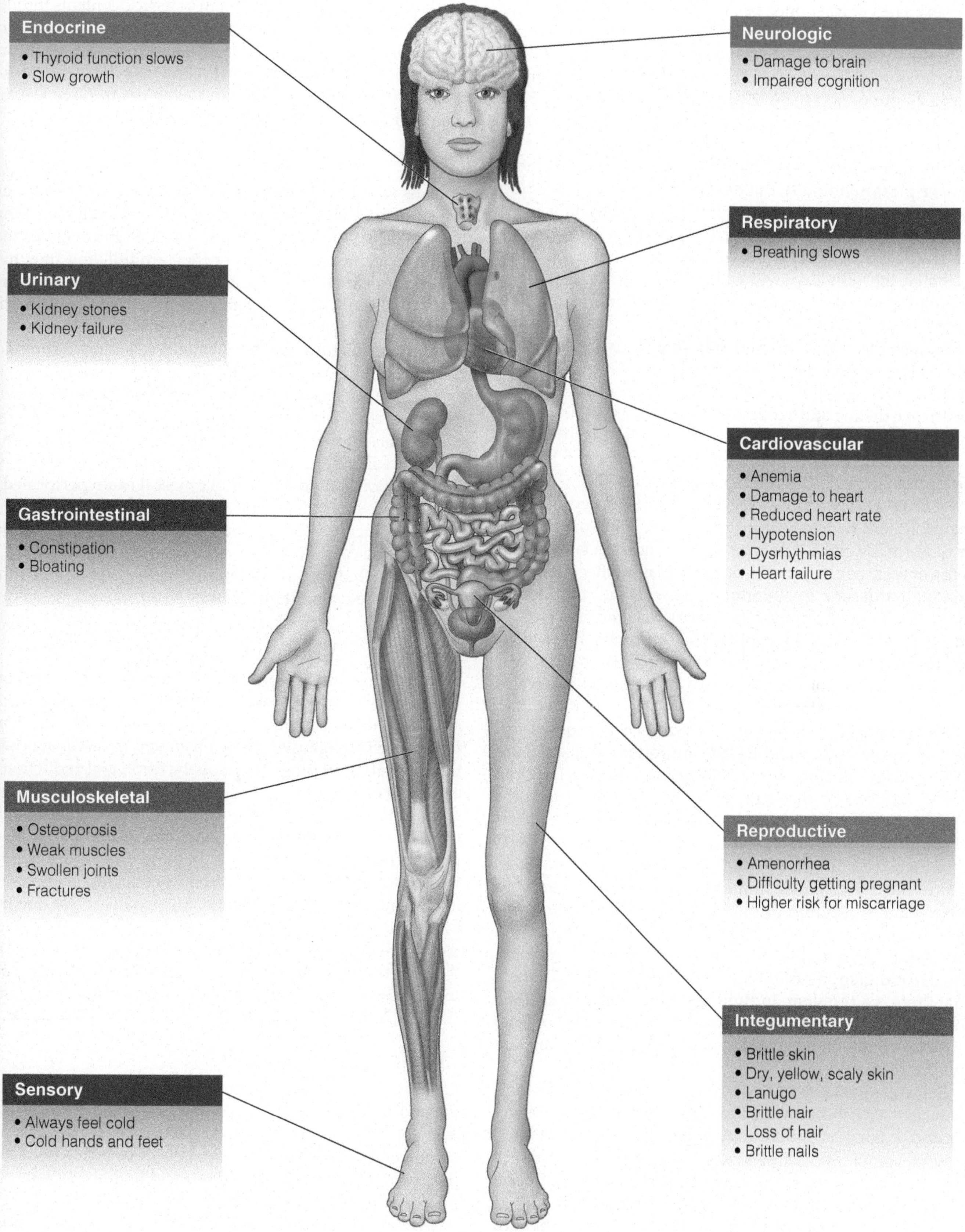

Endocrine
- Thyroid function slows
- Slow growth

Neurologic
- Damage to brain
- Impaired cognition

Respiratory
- Breathing slows

Urinary
- Kidney stones
- Kidney failure

Cardiovascular
- Anemia
- Damage to heart
- Reduced heart rate
- Hypotension
- Dysrhythmias
- Heart failure

Gastrointestinal
- Constipation
- Bloating

Musculoskeletal
- Osteoporosis
- Weak muscles
- Swollen joints
- Fractures

Reproductive
- Amenorrhea
- Difficulty getting pregnant
- Higher risk for miscarriage

Integumentary
- Brittle skin
- Dry, yellow, scaly skin
- Lanugo
- Brittle hair
- Loss of hair
- Brittle nails

Sensory
- Always feel cold
- Cold hands and feet

pattern of bingeing and purging to control weight (ANAD, 2020; NIMH, 2017b). For diagnosis of bulimia nervosa, the individual must demonstrate binge eating in association with unhealthy compensatory behaviors (e.g., purging or excessive exercise) at least once per week over a 3-month period (APA, 2013).

Binge eating is the rapid consumption of an uncommonly large amount of food in a short amount of time, for example, over a 2-hour period (APA, 2013). Individuals who binge-eat feel out of control during the episode, and although eating binges may involve any kind of food, they usually consist of junk foods, fast foods, and high-calorie foods. Bingeing may be pleasant initially, but the individual who is bingeing quickly becomes distressed. A binge usually ends only when abdominal pain becomes powerful, when the individual is interrupted, or when the individual runs out of food. After the binge, the individual with bulimia feels guilt and engages in purging activities to rid the body of excess calories (NAMI, 2020; NIMH, 2017b).

Purging behaviors are frequently dangerous and include a wide variety of activities that are meant to remove all food from the body, such as self-induced vomiting, enemas, or diuretics. Restrictive dieting and extreme exercise also are common. For many with bulimia, purging becomes a purification ritual and a means of regaining self-control in addition to a mechanism for emptying the body of nutrients (NAMI, 2020).

Bulimia nervosa is frequently underdiagnosed because many of those who have the condition are either overweight or of normal weight. The typical age at onset is late adolescence or early adulthood. The disorder mainly affects females, although at least 1 in 10 individuals with the condition is male. BN is more common than anorexia, and it occurs in approximately 1% of the population. In addition, BN is often comorbid with other psychiatric disorders, such as mood disorders, anxiety disorders, substance abuse, and disorders of self-injurious behavior (NIMH, 2017b).

The principal indicator of BN is an incessant obsession with food and body weight. Other important indicators are physical signs of bingeing and purging. These include the trash produced by the large quantity of food required for bingeing, and the products—enemas and laxatives—used in purging. Individuals affected by BN may also experience menstrual irregularity and depressed mood, in addition to the unexplained stomach pain and sore throat that bingeing and purging produce. The signs of self-induced vomiting—unexplained damage to teeth, scarring on the backs of fingers, and swollen cheeks due to the damage to the parotid glands—often indicate to doctors and dentists that there is a problem. Individuals who engage in chronic ingestion of emetics (available over the counter and online) can experience toxicity with serious side effects such as dysrhythmias.

Behaviors associated with BN can lead to severe physiologic damage, even if the individual's weight remains normal. Bingeing and purging cause unhealthy nutritional patterns, and self-induced vomiting can cause serious injury to the digestive tract. Tooth decay, esophageal and stomach injury, and acid reflux are all common in individuals with the condition.

Purging behaviors can lead to dehydration and changes in the body's electrolytes. Because stomach acid contains potassium and chloride, electrolyte disturbances associated with purging include low potassium (hypokalemia) and low chloride (hypochloremia). Frequent vomiting, diuretic use, or laxative abuse may cause hypokalemia; in each case, metabolic alkalosis may result (Potter & Moller, 2020). Bloating and slowed peristalsis (movement of gastric contents through the intestines) also may accompany BN. Complications stemming from electrolyte disturbances, severe dehydration, and undernutrition associated with BN may include cardiac dysrhythmias, heart failure, and even death (U.S. Department of Health and Human Services [DHHS], 2018).

Binge-Eating Disorder

Persons with **binge-eating disorder (BED)** experience periods of rapid food consumption, episodes during which they are unable to stop eating. Individuals with the disorder may continue to eat until long after they are full, and they may experience embarrassment about their behavior. For some individuals with BED, bingeing can produce a sense of relief or fulfillment that gives way as the episode progresses into feelings of disgust, guilt, worthlessness, and depression (NIMH, 2017b).

There is no specific test that can diagnose someone with BED. Rather, a diagnosis is made by a mental health practitioner based on an assessment that includes a formal history and collateral information. Any patient diagnosed with the condition should have a full physical exam performed in order to screen for complications of the illness. These complications include obesity, high cholesterol, type 2 diabetes, and heart disease. In cases of extreme weight gain, complications can include arthritis, obstructive sleep apnea, and other weight-related conditions (DHHS, 2018).

Collaboration

Feeding and eating disorders are diagnosed through a combination of laboratory tests to detect the effects of irregular nutrition and consultation with a medical professional. Once a disorder is diagnosed, reestablishment of adequate nutrition, cessation of binge–purge behaviors, and reduction of excessive exercise are the essential points of treating feeding and eating disorders. These goals are accomplished through a combination of pharmacologic and nonpharmacologic therapies, including psychotherapy. Treatment plans are tailored to individual needs but include counseling, medication, and, in extreme cases, hospitalization. Some patients require hospitalization to treat problems caused by severe malnutrition. An inpatient stay at a hospital can also be used to ensure that the patients are eating if they are severely underweight and to establish new eating patterns in a supportive environment (DHHS, 2018).

Diagnostic Tests

Laboratory tests can reveal the physiologic hallmarks of feeding and eating disorders. Screening for anorexia may include tests for albumin, total protein, electrolyte levels, CBC, and a bone density test to check for signs of osteoporosis. Other diagnostic exams include an electrocardiogram; kidney, thyroid, and liver function tests; and urinalysis. These exams determine whether there is a severe deficiency of any nutrients or any wasting of the body as a result of malnutrition (DHHS, 2018).

Evidence-Based Practice

Eating Disorders and the Internet

Problem

For a patient coping with an ED, the internet can be perilous territory. Not only does the internet offer websites dedicated to encouraging and celebrating feeding and eating disorders, but some research suggests that sites provide erroneous diagnostic criteria that can be detrimental to patients and their families. Especially for adolescent patients who spend hours every day engaged with media, information on the internet can both prompt and exacerbate disordered eating behaviors.

Evidence

Approximately 45% of teens say they use the internet "almost constantly." Another 44% say they go online several times a day. On average, 9 in 10 teens go online at least multiple times per day (Anderson & Jiang, 2018). Almost 95% of teens report owning a smartphone (Anderson & Jiang, 2018).

In a 2018 study, approximately 80% of teens reported using the internet for health-related searches, and 65% stated that the internet was their primary source for health information (Park & Kwon, 2018). Teens report using online sources to learn more about puberty, drugs, sex, depression, and other issues.

Digital media has become an important source of the social pressure, cultural expectations, and health misinformation that contribute to the development of feeding and eating disorders in adolescents. Park and Kwon (2018) also found that 61.2% of teens preferred to use an online support group instead of an in-person support group. The researchers reported that unfortunately only 10.9% of teens accessed the health-related websites recommended by experts, and 10.6% looked to social media for mental health issues such as anxiety or depression (Park & Kwon, 2018).

With the prevalence of adolescent internet use, it is essential to consider that *more than 100* pro-eating-disorder websites not only encourage feeding and eating disorders but also offer specific advice on anorexic and bulimic techniques, with pro-anorexia content composing almost 30% of the content on certain social media platforms (Holland, Dickson, & Dickson, 2018). These pro-eating-disorder websites offer advice on bingeing, purging, and extreme forms of weight control and they provide interactive resources such as message boards. Research indicated that the sites are alarmingly easy to access and understand (Holland et al., 2018). Pro-eating-disorder websites are readily accessible communities with dynamic, user-distributed content.

In addition to sites that provide information that explicitly promotes feeding and eating disorders, websites that purport to provide medical information can spread damaging information to individuals of all ages. Research shows that the quality of medical content related to the diagnosis and treatment of feeding and eating disorders is relatively low. Few sites fully describe the criteria for diagnosis, complications, and treatment options of any ED, and some provide a good deal of erroneous information. Some sites use inaccurate "diagnostic" terms—"bulimerexia," for example—as well as multiple "optimal" treatment options for each of the feeding and eating disorders. Inaccurate information is particularly dangerous for adolescents with disordered eating, and it may interfere with the family's decision to seek medical treatment (Holland et al., 2018).

Implications

The fact that almost all adolescents have easy access to the internet and its variety of viewpoints creates a new set of problems for parents and nurses. The Web offers an interactive way for impressionable adolescents and young adults to engage with unhealthy cultural expectations of thinness. In addition, the myriad viewpoints expressed online include pathologic websites that support the damaging behaviors associated with anorexia and bulimia. Even sites that purport to present medical information and treatment options for EDs often contain flawed and medically inadequate information.

Critical Thinking Application

Consider a consultation with an adolescent female patient who has been exhibiting the behaviors associated with AN for the past 3 years. This patient has also been taking part in pro-anorexia message boards online for the past 2 years. She knows that anorexia is unhealthy but embraces the damage she deals her body by fasting and exercising, partly because she learned most of what she knows about the condition from websites full of incorrect "information." Identify a communication strategy that will enable you to correct her misconceptions about AN while attempting to communicate the grim reality of her disorder.

Diagnostic tests for bulimia nervosa consider many more visible symptoms of disease than do the tests for anorexia because of the physical damage induced by purging. The dentist is often the first medical professional to identify signs of bulimia, including cavities and gum infections. The enamel of teeth may be worn or pitted because of exposure to the acid in vomit. Loss of stomach acid can lead to metabolic alkalosis. A physical exam may discover broken blood vessels in the eyes (from the stress of vomiting), a dry mouth, pouchlike cheeks, rashes and pimples, and cuts and calluses on the finger joints. Laboratory tests may show an electrolyte imbalance or dehydration from purging (Cost, Krantz, & Mehler, 2020).

In order to diagnose a BED, a clinician typically conducts a physical exam, followed by blood and urine tests. A psychologic evaluation is necessary to complete the evaluation, including a discussion of the patient's eating habits. Following diagnosis, other tests should be performed to check for the common health implications of BED, including heart problems and gallbladder disease (Mayo Clinic, 2018).

Pharmacologic Therapy

There is currently no surgical treatment, aside from bariatric surgeries for extremely overweight patients, indicated as primary treatment for any of the feeding and eating disorders. Treating AN involves restoring the patient to a healthy weight, treating underlying psychologic issues, and eliminating behaviors that might lead to malnutrition and relapse. Research suggests that antidepressants, antipsychotics, or mood stabilizers may be modestly effective in treating patients with anorexia. Medications can treat some of the psychologic states that undergird the ED, but it is not yet clear whether medications are effective in preventing relapse. No medication has yet been shown to be effective in assisting weight gain.

The antidepressant fluoxetine (Prozac) is the only medication approved by the U.S. Food and Drug Administration for treating bulimia. This and other antidepressants may help individuals for whom depression and anxiety are at the root of bulimic behavior. Fluoxetine appears to lessen bingeing and purging behaviors, reduce the likelihood of relapse, and improve attitudes toward eating.

SAFETY ALERT Selective serotonin reuptake inhibitors, such as fluoxetine, which can be prescribed to treat underlying depression in patients with EDs, carry an FDA-mandated black box warning regarding increased suicidality. The risk of suicide is especially increased in pediatric, adolescent, and young adult patients age 18 to 24. Parents should be made aware of this risk, know the symptoms of suicidal ideation, and know to contact the prescribing clinician immediately if symptoms present.

The pharmacologic options for treating BED are similar to the treatments for bulimia nervosa. Antidepressants, particularly fluoxetine, have been found to reduce binge-eating episodes and help ease depression (NIMH, 2017b).

Nonpharmacologic Therapy

Although pharmacologic treatments may play a role in the treatment of feeding and eating disorders, therapies that do not make use of medication have proven to be more consistently effective. In the treatment of AN, individual, group, and family-based psychotherapy can address the psychologic reasons for the illness. A therapy called the *Maudsley approach* has been shown to be particularly effective in the treatment of adolescents with anorexia. In the Maudsley approach, the parents of the affected adolescent take responsibility for feeding the patient. Research shows that for patients with anorexia, a combined approach of medical attention and psychotherapy produces more complete recoveries than psychotherapy alone. There is no cure-all approach for AN, but evidence indicates that individualized treatment programs frequently achieve success and that specialized treatment may help reduce the risk of death.

The nonpharmacologic treatment of bulimia nervosa frequently involves a combination of options and depends on the needs of the individual patient. The most effective psychotherapy for patients with bulimia is CBT, which helps individuals focus on their present problems and how to solve them. CBT may be individualized or group based, and it is effective in changing binge-and-purge behaviors and attitudes to eating. Systemic family therapy and family-based therapy are family-systems approaches that focus on family strengths and narratives (Linardon, Wade, de la Piedad Garcia, & Brennan, 2017). Family-based therapies are often used with adolescent patients with anorexia, mobilizing the family as the primary resource in feeding and restoring health to an undernourished child.

Nonpharmacologic treatment options for BED are very similar to the options for bulimia nervosa. Psychotherapy, especially CBT that is individualized, has been shown to be effective in many cases with adolescent and adult patients (NIMH, 2017b).

Treatment Settings

Day-patient programs are considered to be the first-line treatment approach when a more structured program is needed for a patient with anorexia. Day programs have advantages over inpatient programs in allowing continued engagement with the patient's educational, occupational, and social contexts. Day-patient settings are also more conducive to the active involvement of family members (including siblings) in treatment (O'Mara, VanDine, Tarescavage, & Ben-Porath, 2020; Stewart et al., 2019).

Patients with high acuity must be treated with inpatient therapy. An inpatient stay provides a structured and contained environment in which patients have access to clinical support at all times. The close proximity of medical help reduces the chance of relapse while improving the chances of recovery. Inpatient programs are now frequently affiliated with daytime programs so that patients can move back and forth to the correct level of care. The majority of inpatient programs treat only patients with anorexia, bulimia, and BED so that the symptoms can be isolated and treated as effectively as possible (Academy for Eating Disorders, 2020). Inpatient settings also allow sufficient monitoring for *refeeding syndrome*, a dangerous and potentially fatal condition that can occur when patients who are severely malnourished begin eating again.

Criteria for admission include patients at immediate risk or for whom previous treatments have failed. Further indicators for hospital admission include less than 75% ideal body weight, ongoing weight loss despite intensive management, rapid or persistent decline in oral intake, and decline in weight despite maximally intensive outpatient intervention. Other considerations include physical parameters, such as hemodynamic instability, cardiovascular risk, and electrolyte abnormalities, as well as psychiatric assessment of such factors as risk of harm to self and others (Buchman et al., 2019; Potter & Moller, 2020).

Complementary Health Approaches

For individuals with feeding and eating disorders, a variety of complementary health approaches can help improve recovery outcomes. However, those with feeding and eating disorders sometimes use alternative medical techniques to achieve the unhealthy goals of disordered eating. For example, some individuals use herbal dietary substances as appetite suppressants or weight loss aids. Herbal supplements can be dangerous when they interact with other products, such as laxatives and diuretics, which are frequently used by those with feeding and eating disorders. Health professionals have not determined conclusively that any complementary or alternative therapies are helpful for individuals with anorexia, bulimia, or BED, but some research indicates that some therapies may help reduce anxiety. Acupuncture, massage, yoga, and meditation have been shown to improve mood and reduce the stress associated with feeding and eating disorders (NEDA, 2018).

Mindfulness-based approaches are growing in popularity as interventions for disordered eating and weight loss. Mindful meditation instructs the practitioner to become mindful of thoughts, feelings, and sensations and to observe them in a nonjudgmental way. Many alternative practitioners believe that mindfulness-based interventions, combined with other traditional weight loss strategies, have the potential to offer a long-term, holistic approach to wellness (Sala, Shankar Ram, Vanzhula, & Levinson, 2020). One study found that mindfulness meditation effectively decreased binge eating and emotional eating in populations engaging in this behavior, with results lasting up to 6 months after the intervention (Pinto-Gouveia et al., 2019). Another study that explored the effect of mindfulness on binge-eating impulses showed that mindfulness was negatively associated with the total number of binge-eating episodes. Mindfulness was correlated with better control over eating impulses as well as an improved ability to express sensations, thoughts, and feelings (V. M. Smith et al., 2019).

Lifespan Considerations

Feeding and eating disorders are often thought of as conditions limited to adolescent and teen populations, but anorexia, bulimia, BED, and other feeding/eating disorders frequently affect other populations as well. BED differs from AN and BN in terms of age at onset, gender and racial distribution, psychiatric comorbidity, and association with obesity (NIMH, 2017b). The *avoidant/restrictive food intake disorder (ARFID)* diagnosis addresses patients who struggle with impaired and distressing eating behaviors and symptoms and who lack the weight and body image–related concerns associated with AN and BN (NEDA, 2018; Thomas et al., 2017). Typically, patients with ARFID require the expertise of an interprofessional treatment team to provide the nutritional rehabilitation, medical management, and psychologic treatment characteristic of anorexia.

Some of the considerations related to EDs at various stages of the lifespan are discussed in the following section.

Feeding and Eating Disorders in Children

Of all the EDs, ARFID is the most significant diagnosis among this age group (Zimmerman & Fisher, 2017). Note that the diagnosis of ARFID is carefully distinguished from the "picky eating" often characteristic of infants and young children. Picky or fussy eating often includes limitations in the variety of foods eaten, unwillingness to try new foods (known as food "neophobia"), and aberrant eating behaviors, such as rejecting foods of a particular texture, consistency, color, or smell (Zimmerman & Fisher, 2017). Prevalence rates for picky eating range from 14 to 50% in preschool children and from 7 to 27% in older children. The ARFID diagnosis eliminates picky eaters by identifying only those children with clinically significant restrictive eating problems that result in persistent failure to meet the child's nutritional and/or energy needs (APA, 2013).

Despite their high prevalence, associated morbidity and mortality, and available treatment options, EDs continue to be underdiagnosed by pediatric professionals (Oakley, Dey, Discombe, Fitzpatrick, & Paul, 2017). Higher rates of EDs are seen now in younger children, boys, and people of color; EDs are increasingly recognized in patients with previous histories of obesity. Furthermore, younger patients diagnosed with EDs, specifically ARFID, are more likely to be male. Recently, it has been estimated that up to 67% of AFRID cases are preadolescent males and up to 50% of all clinically diagnosed eating disorders are males (Murray et al., 2017).

Feeding and Eating Disorders in Adolescents and College-Age Adults

According to NEDA (2018), the 12-month prevalence of anorexia among young females is approximately 0.4%. For bulimia, the prior-year prevalence for young females was estimated to be 1–1.5%, with the highest prevalence occurring among young adults because the disorder peaks in late adolescence and young adulthood (Jagielska & Kacperska, 2017; NEDA, 2018). The 12-month prevalence rate for binge eating among females was 3.5% (NEDA, 2018).

Young females at risk for developing anorexia often have co-occurring anxiety disorders or display obsessional traits in childhood (APA, 2013). Young women who develop bulimia often have temperamental traits such as weight concerns, low self-esteem, depressive symptoms, social anxiety disorder, and overanxious disorder of childhood. Risk factors for bulimia include thin body ideal; childhood sexual or physical abuse; and childhood obesity and early pubertal maturation. BED has the same psychopathology as AN and BN, but co-occurring disorders commonly associated with BED also include bipolar disorder, depressive disorders, anxiety disorders, and substance use disorders (APA, 2013). For all eating disorders, the severity of co-occurring psychiatric disorders will predict worse long-term outcomes.

Feeding and Eating Disorders in Adults

Eating disorders, especially bulimia and binge-eating behaviors, that are developed in adolescence and young adulthood often persist into adulthood. The risk factors and associated behaviors remain intact with one exception: Adults who have developed obesity from an eating disorder are now more likely than ever to undergo bariatric surgery as an intervention. Overall, the prevalence of BED in bariatric surgery candidates can be almost 50% (Cella et al., 2019; Tess, Maximiano-Ferreira, Pajecki, & Wang, 2019). Cella et al. (2019) found that these patients report experiencing a sense of lack of control over eating and inappropriate compensatory behaviors that were correlated with low self-esteem; emotional dysfunction; impulse behaviors, including substance use and self-injury; self-destructiveness; distress; and reticence in social situations.

Whereas patients with obesity are having some success with bariatric surgery, adults with AN have notoriously poor outcomes, and treatment evidence is limited (Jagielska & Kacperska, 2017). There has been some limited clinical success with these patients with the Maudsley Model of Anorexia Nervosa Treatment for Adults, in which patients receive 20 to 30 weekly therapy sessions focusing on concerns specific to AN, including a need to avoid intense emotions; personality traits such as perfectionism; pro-anorexia beliefs (believing that the illness will help manage difficult emotions and the relationships that arouse them); and the response of families to the illness (National Institute for Health and Care Excellence, 2017).

Feeding and Eating Disorders in Pregnant Women

Pregnancy and childbirth are major life events accompanied by profound biological, social, and psychologic changes. Research has indicated that disordered eating in pregnancy persists in a substantial proportion of women who have pre-pregnancy eating disorders. The presence of an eating disorder in this period may negatively affect the pregnancy (e.g., weight gain), delivery (e.g., cesarean delivery, preterm delivery), or offspring (e.g., birth weight) (Mantel, Hirschberg, & Stephansson, 2020).

Pregnancy may also influence the course of eating disorders. For the majority of women with AN and BN, pregnancy appears to lead to adaptive changes in eating behaviors, with the disorders often remitting during and after pregnancy. However, for some, pregnancy may lead to maladaptive changes in eating behavior. Research has found that pregnancy poses a risk for the onset of BED in vulnerable individuals, occurring in nearly 1 in every 20 women (dos Santos, 2017; Silvani et al., 2020). Obstetricians/gynecologists and clinicians need training to detect eating disorders and devise interventions to enhance pregnancy and neonatal outcomes.

Pica, the practice of eating nonfood items during pregnancy, has been documented in health literature for many years. One recent study of women of Hispanic origin in the United States associated pica with iron deficiency, not anemia as customarily reported. Furthermore, there was also an association with pica and food insecurity. Over half the women in the study reported engaging in pica (Roy, Fuentes-Afflick, Fernald, & Young, 2018). Finally, a large meta-analysis of pica found that the prevalence was higher in Africa compared with elsewhere in the world, increased as the prevalence of anemia increased, and decreased as educational attainment increased (Fawcett, Fawcett, & Mazmanian, 2016). Other, more recent studies also supported this finding and emphasized the importance of providing nutrition education to women during pregnancy (Ayano & Amentie, 2018; Rono, Kombe, & Makokha, 2018).

Feeding and Eating Disorders in Men

In the past, it has been believed that men have eating disorders less frequently than women. According to the APA (2013), anorexia and bulimia occur less frequently among males than females, with a 1:10 male-to-female ratio. However, some studies have contradicted this statistic, reporting up to 25% of ED patients being male (Jagielska & Kacperska, 2017; Matsumoto & Rodgers, 2020; Murray et al., 2017). The APA has estimated that BED occurs in males at half the rate in females (0.8% and 1.6%, respectively). However, one ED study found that BED was more common among males than previously believed (Erskine & Whiteford, 2018). Recent studies have attempted to better quantify prevalence in this population and to discover factors that distinguish male ED behaviors from that of females.

Research has found that men with EDs differ from women in their weight histories. Men frequently reported being mildly to moderately obese at some point in their lives before developing an eating disorder and were particularly susceptible if they were obese in childhood (Murray et al., 2017). In contrast, most women with EDs typically had a normal weight history. Furthermore, research indicated that males with EDs are more likely to report a wider variety of psychiatric comorbidities such as substance use and psychotic symptoms (Murray et al., 2017). Males who present with AN focus more on leanness, thus enhancing the visibility of one's musculature, whereas females with AN focus on thinness and emaciation (Matsumoto & Rodgers, 2020; Murray et al., 2017).

As is the case with women, many men with EDs have a history of sexual abuse. Research has demonstrated a strong correlation between sexual abuse and eating disorders, with an estimated 30% of eating-disordered patients having a history of sexual abuse (Jagielska & Kacperska, 2017; Murray et al., 2017). For men, sexual abuse has likely been underreported because of a disproportionate amount of shame and stigmatization that accompanies abuse for men versus women.

Factors predicting a male ED include childhood bullying; being gay or bisexual, which some studies have suggested may increase the likelihood of an ED by tenfold; depression and shame; excessive exercise coupled with increased diet success ("manorexia"); comorbid substance abuse, including the use of stimulants to lose weight; and media pressures resulting in male body dissatisfaction (Jagielska & Kacperska, 2017; Murray et al., 2017).

Feeding and Eating Disorders in Older Adults

The most common concern regarding older adults and disordered eating is the physiologic anorexia of aging. This process is characterized by a decrease in appetite and energy intake that occurs even in healthy people and is possibly caused by changes in the digestive tract, gastrointestinal hormone concentrations and activity, neurotransmitters, and cytokines (Cox, Ibrahim, Sayer, Robinson, & Roberts, 2019). Unintentional weight loss in older people may be a result of protein-energy malnutrition, cachexia, the physiologic anorexia of aging, or any combination of these factors.

However, recent research has found that typical ED symptoms are also common in older adults. A large sample of males age 40 to 75 revealed that 12% and 9.5% indicated dissatisfaction with their weight and shape, respectively, and 23% reported that their self-evaluation was dependent on their weight and shape (Matsumoto & Rodgers, 2020). In another large community-based study, 62% of women age 50 and over reported that eating, weight, and shape "occasionally" to "often" negatively affected their lives (Goodman et al., 2018). Bingeing and purging are both prevalent among women in their early 50s but occur in women older than 75 as well. Research participants reported using unhealthy methods to lose weight and maintain thinness, including diet pills, excessive exercise, diuretics, laxatives, and vomiting. Feeding and eating disorders are detrimental to the health of individuals of all ages, but they can be particularly damaging to the bodies of older adults. The damaging effects of bulimia and anorexia exacerbate preexisting osteoporosis, cardiovascular problems, and gastroesophageal reflux disease (Mangweth-Matzek & Hoek, 2017).

NURSING PROCESS

When assessing the patient with a known or suspected eating disorder, keep in mind that denial is often inherent to these conditions. Recognize that deceit and manipulation are characteristics of the disorder and not necessarily consciously chosen behaviors on the part of the patient.

Assessment

For the patient with an eating disorder, assessment combines a thorough review of both physiologic and psychosocial functioning as well as careful observations for the physiologic manifestations associated with feeding and eating disorders.

When a patient presents with a significant weight gain or loss, do not automatically assume the patient has an eating disorder. Numerous physiologic conditions can lead to muscle wasting and weight loss, including cancer, hyperthyroidism, and impaired gastrointestinal function. Likewise, weight gain may occur due to a variety of causes, including endocrine disorders and medication side effects. Before the primary care provider establishes the diagnosis of an eating disorder, other causes for weight alteration must be ruled out (Potter & Moller, 2020; Serin & Şanlıer, 2018).

Focused assessment of the patient's nutritional status incorporates data obtained through the patient interview, physiologic assessment findings, and review of laboratory and diagnostic test results. Assessment of nutritional status includes height, weight, BMI, mid-arm circumference, and waist-to-hip ratio. It also includes assessment of the skin, the oral mucosa and tongue, the shape of the abdomen, and the nature and presence of bowel sounds. Assess the teeth and gums for any irregularities.

On physical assessment, patients with anorexia nervosa will appear emaciated. Their skin may be dry and covered by a fine layer of hair called *lanugo*, and they also may appear jaundiced (yellow-orange in color). As a result of malnourishment, hair and nails will appear to be brittle. Undernutrition may impair the function of any body system, including the brain, musculoskeletal system, kidneys, and heart. In particular, cardiovascular manifestations may include bradycardia, hypotension, and cardiac dysrhythmias (Potter & Moller, 2020). Because the potential effects of undernutrition are numerous, these patients require a complete physical assessment.

Assessment of patients with known or suspected bulimia nervosa usually includes completion of a physical exam by the primary HCP, followed by psychologic evaluation and laboratory diagnostics. Patients with BN typically maintain a body weight that meets or exceeds normal weight limits. For these patients, focused assessment of the oral cavity can be very revealing. If purging behaviors include vomiting, patients' teeth may demonstrate pitting and enamel erosion, as well as an increased incidence of dental caries. Patients who purge by vomiting may also exhibit ruptured blood vessels in the eyes, as well as a hoarse voice due to throat irritation. Laboratory tests may reveal electrolyte imbalances or dehydration due to purging (Serin & Şanlıer, 2018). In particular, patients with BN are susceptible to metabolic acidosis. If dehydrated, they may demonstrate a variety of manifestations, including hypotension, dry mouth, poor skin turgor, complaints of light-headedness or dizziness, general weakness, decreased urine production, and concentrated urine.

Diagnosis

Priorities for nursing care are based on the results of an individualized, holistic assessment. The plan of care for the patient with an eating disorder may include the following:

- Risk of injury related to orthostatic hypotension, fluid volume deficiency, and electrolyte imbalances
- Fluid volume deficiency
- Undernutrition
- Decreased cardiac output
- Disrupted integrity of oral mucous membranes
- Poor dentition
- Disturbed body image
- Inadequate coping skills
- Chronic low self-esteem
- Anxiety.

Planning

Primary long-term goals of care for the patient with an eating disorder include restoring nutritional status and fluid and electrolyte balance, maintenance of body weight within an acceptable range, and development of a healthy body image. Because these patients face significant psychosocial barriers, including body image distortion and rigid behavioral patterns, intensive psychologic care is often necessary for achieving long-term outcomes. Examples of short-term patient goals that may be applicable to the nursing plan of care for the patient with an ED include the following:

- The patient will remain free from injury.
- The patient will demonstrate manifestations of fluid volume balance, including adequate urine production, vital signs that range within normal limits, and absence of symptoms such as light-headedness or dizziness.
- The patient's laboratory testing will demonstrate electrolyte levels that are within normal limits.
- The patient will remain free of purging behaviors.
- The patient will actively participate in individual and/or group therapy.
- The patient will remain free of nonsuicidal self-injurious (NSSI) behaviors, such as cutting, and will report any suicidal ideation.

SAFETY ALERT Suicide attempts and repeated attempts are common among patients with eating disorders. For a number of years, anorexia nervosa has been consistently associated with high rates of suicide among adolescents and young adults. Findings also support that suicide risk appears elevated in bulimia nervosa and is perhaps even higher than individuals with anorexia. There seems to be an association with self-injurious behaviors, with a higher risk among individuals who binge and purge. Suicide risk should be routinely assessed in all patients with eating disorders (Serin & Şanlıer, 2018).

Implementation

Care of the patient who is diagnosed with an eating disorder is highly complex. Priorities of care include protecting the patient from physiologic effects of the ED. However, the ultimate goal is identification and treatment of the cause of the alterations, which is the ED itself. For these patients, the primary intervention involves intensive therapy provided by a mental health professional who is specially trained in the treatment of patients with feeding and eating disorders. While recognizing the complexity of the origin and treatment of feeding and eating disorders, the nurse can promote wellness through preventing patient injury and encouraging healthy patient behaviors and thought patterns.

Prevent Injury

Patients with feeding and eating disorders are at constant or near-constant risk for injury due to undernutrition and its consequences. The effects of purging behaviors also keep the patient at risk for injury.

Behavioral contracts that outline prohibited actions and their consequences may prove effective in the care of patients who are at risk for injurious behaviors. However, especially early in the course of treatment, behavioral contracts may have adverse effects, particularly as asking patients to promise to control compulsive behaviors is unrealistic. For these patients, many of whom are already struggling with shame, the inability to adhere to the contract could serve to heighten the sense of shame and further diminish self-esteem. For patients in the clinical setting, constant monitoring and supervision may be necessary to ensure adequate nutritional intake and prevent purging behaviors.

Additional interventions include the following:

- Teach the patient to decrease exposure to environmental stress.
- Teach the patient to decrease anxiety by eliminating caffeine and other stimulants, such as energy drinks.
- Help the patient increase social and familial connectedness through improving communication skills.
- Teach methods of self-soothing, such as watching TV, reading a book, listening to energizing music, calling a friend, or creating art.
- Encourage the patient to eliminate drugs or alcohol, which can increase impulsivity (Potter & Moller, 2020).

In extreme cases, inpatient intake of nutrients and fluids may be medically ordered and administered to patients whose lives are at risk. For all patients, such issues raise ethical concerns and require the nurse to be aware of legal considerations related to forced care. Among experts in the field of feeding and eating disorders, the practice of forcing patient interventions to prevent injury (including death) is the subject of intense debate (Blikshavn, Halvorsen, & Ro, 2020). If the patient is hospitalized for medical stabilization, the following interventions may be employed:

- Limit the patient's activity and energy expenditure (e.g., no excessive exercise).
- Monitor vital signs, food and fluid intake/output, and electrolyte levels.
- Observe for signs of fluid overload, which may indicate refeeding syndrome.
- Monitor trips to the bathroom and look for food hoarding (e.g., the patient has hidden food rather than eating it).
- Assess/monitor gastrointestinal and cardiac functioning as necessary (Potter & Moller, 2020).

Promote a Therapeutic Relationship and Positive Self-Regard

Many patients with feeding and eating disorders have maintained secrecy with regard to their nutritional habits and purging behaviors. Treatment requires patients to be open about their behaviors, as well as to discuss sensitive topics and issues that may be psychologically painful. Transitioning from secrecy to openness is a major challenge that requires great courage on the part of the patient, as well as establishment of trust between the patient and the HCP. With these patients, respect, consistency, and patience are keys to establishing trust, which is part of the foundation of a therapeutic relationship. Other interventions, which are equally appropriate in outpatient and inpatient settings, may include the following:

- Help the patient to identify triggers, such as troubling interpersonal relationships and turbulent internal emotional states, that promote disordered eating behaviors.
- Help the patient to reframe the feelings of purging behavior that contribute to a sense of empowerment, control, and relief from tension.
- Provide positive reinforcement when patients adhere to treatment and make efforts to meet goals.
- Help patients set short-term, realistic goals that they can easily achieve to foster opportunities for success and allow patients to see and measure their treatment progress.
- Encourage patients to reconnect with activities and experiences that they enjoy to help them begin to regain control over their own behaviors and to reexperience positive emotions (Potter & Moller, 2020; Serin & Şanlıer, 2018).

Promote Family Communication

Dysfunctional family patterns and relationships play a role in eating disorders. It is important for the nurse to establish rapport and a therapeutic relationship with the patient and family and promote effective communication. Strategies for promoting family communication include (Serin & Şanlıer, 2018):

- Help the patient and family understand and clarify the perception and impact of the disorder.
- Encourage open expression of concerns among family members.
- Assist the family to change unrealistic expectations and review inaccurate perceptions.
- Help the patient to set limits among family members and respond to negative criticism in a positive way.

Communicating with Patients and Families

Working Phase

It can be difficult for family members who have been communicating poorly with each other to embrace healthy communication strategies. By asking clarifying questions and facilitating open communication, the nurse can promote successful communication between family members.

- Can you describe how you think your eating has impacted you and your family?
- What do you (as the family), find most concerning right now?
- Can you tell me how you can rephrase the statement "Mom, just stop nagging me" to help your mother see your perspective?

Evaluation

Evaluation is a dynamic, ongoing feature of the nursing process that includes identifying the degree to which patients have achieved the goals and outcomes established in conjunction with each nursing diagnosis. While goals and outcomes for the patient with an eating disorder will vary based on patient individuality and the patient's nursing diagnoses, examples of potential outcomes relevant to the care of these patients may include the following:

- The patient remains free from injury.
- The patient's vital signs remain within normal limits.
- The patient's serum electrolytes remain within normal limits.
- The patient demonstrates production of nonconcentrated urine.
- The patient denies light-headedness or dizziness.
- The patient does not demonstrate purging behaviors.
- The patient actively participates in individual and/or group therapy.

Many clinicians view recovery from eating disorders to be a cyclical rather than a linear process. Because eating disorders are complex with multifactorial influences, the care plan may need to be modified periodically if patients are not responding to planned interventions. Nurses and clinicians may need to reevaluate triggers and treatment regimens as well as help patients identify alternative methods of coping.

Nursing Care Plan

A Patient with Anorexia Nervosa

Angelina Santos is the 16-year-old daughter of first-generation Filipino immigrants. She has been admitted as an inpatient to the local municipal hospital because of a weight loss from 118 pounds to 83 pounds (37.7 kg). Angel (as she is known by her family) is 5′6″; her BMI is 13.4, well under the BMI of 18.5 considered to be underweight. She was a high-achieving student at her charter school until a few weeks ago, when she became too fatigued to go to school. Her father was an engineer in the Philippines and, because of language issues, struggled very hard to be recertified as a professional engineer in the United States when the family arrived 20 years ago. Angel's mother never attended college and has stayed home with their children. Her mother's English is not as good as her father's. Although Angel and her two siblings, a 13-year-old boy and a 7-year-old girl, speak excellent English, the family speaks Tagalog at home. Both of Angel's parents value education and have expectations that their children will be high academic achievers. Angel has a 4.0 grade point average at high school and has taken several advanced placement courses to enhance her chances of getting into a good college so she can study cellular biology.

Angel also is a member of a local gymnastics squad, attends practice several days a week, and works out regularly. She competes in gymnastics competitions and usually finishes middle of the pack. Her gymnastics work has been criticized as "too mechanical," and she has tried very hard to become more relaxed and spontaneous in her performances. Angel is the president of the French club at school, volunteers at a local food pantry at the Catholic church she attends with her family and participates as a member of her school's soccer team. When asked about their daughter's food restriction, Mrs. Santos said that it started when Angel was 13 and was playing soccer. An older boy remarked about Angel's "thunder thighs and bubble booty" when she was running off the field. Her weight has spiraled downward since that time. For the last 6 months, Angel has been treated as an outpatient in an eating disorders program but has since lost an additional 8 pounds. She has been admitted for weight stabilization.

ASSESSMENT	DIAGNOSIS	PLANNING
When Angel arrives in the ED for admission, a CBC with differential and erythrocyte sedimentation rate and comprehensive metabolic panels (CMP) are drawn stat. She is attached to a 12-lead electrocardiogram (ECG). Liver function tests (LFTs) and an arterial blood gas are also drawn. The CBC shows low WBCs with slightly elevated hemoglobin, indicating dehydration. An elevated BUN and creatinine from the CMP support the diagnosis of dehydration. The CMP also shows that Angel has hyponatremia (123 mEq/L), hypokalemia (2.8 mEq/L), and hypoglycemia (70 mg/dL). The ECG shows sinus bradycardia with ST-segment elevation and T-wave flattening. Her vital signs are T 97.7, RR = 20, HR = 54, and BP 102/64. LFTs are minimally elevated. The ABG shows metabolic acidosis. While the activity is going on, Angel says, "I just want the fuss to go away. I just want to rest." Angel's parents seem very surprised when the ED physician and the hospitalist tell them that their daughter, who is in the extreme stage of anorexia, is in imminent danger of dying without emergency interventions and treatment.	■ Undernutrition ■ Fluid volume deficiency ■ Decreased cardiac output ■ Fatigue ■ Disturbed body image ■ Inadequate coping skills ■ Inadequate family coping skills/resources ■ Denial	■ With insertion of a percutaneous endoscopic gastrostomy (PEG) tube and regular administration of enteral nutrition and vitamin supplements, weight gain will start. ■ Electrolyte levels will return to within normal limits. ■ Fluid volume balance will be restored to normal limits. ■ ECG strips will show a normal rhythm. ■ ABGs will return to normal limits. ■ The patient will be monitored for indications of refeeding syndrome. ■ The patient will actively collaborate in her plan of care. ■ The patient will address her overvaluation of shape and weight. ■ Both the patient and family will be reeducated regarding the dangers of anorexia.

(continued on next page)

Nursing Care Plan *(continued)*

IMPLEMENTATION

- Provide nutrition support as ordered.
- Monitor patient labs and physical manifestations for signs and symptoms of refeeding syndrome.
- Monitor telemetry readings while patient is in acute care.
- When the patient begins oral intake of food, monitor the patient closely after meals, especially during restroom use.
- Provide educational counseling to both the patient and parents regarding the seriousness of anorexia.
- Address underlying psychological issues by encouraging the patient to participate in enhanced CBT (CBT-E) to address the behavioral and psychological symptoms characteristic of anorexia.
- Focus on reducing patient stress.

EVALUATION

Angel stays on the inpatient unit and participates in therapy for 4 weeks. During that time, her tube feedings are titrated downward and eventually cease as her oral intake increases. Her intake started at 1200 kcal per day, and then was advanced slowly by adding 200 kcal every other day to a maximum of 2200 kcal. During her hospitalization, Angel experienced no weight gain during the first 6 days of treatment, but then gained an average of 1.5 pounds per week for a total of 4.5 pounds gained by discharge. During her stay, the plan of care included individual and group therapy, treatment of anxiety and depression with a prescription for fluoxetine (Prozac), and family education and therapy including instruction on Maudsley family therapy. Because family approaches are most effective with adolescents, the social worker and a nursing discharge planner assigned to the case include Angel's parents in the treatment planning from the beginning. They bring in an interpreter to ensure successful communication with Mrs. Santo. Family participation is an important aspect of the Maudsley treatment model, with the parents assuming direction and coaching responsibilities to help stabilize Angel's eating patterns and weight until Angel begins to reach her treatment goals.

At the end of her hospitalization, Angel is discharged to a day program for four additional weeks. She attends 3 days a week, learning how to prepare meals and eat in social settings, restaurants, and cafeterias.

Despite the intensive therapy she receives, Angel relapses 6 months after her treatment ended and starts purging and overexercising again. After she started losing weight again, Angel was readmitted to the day program at the local university hospital, this time with partial hospitalization to provide more structure to her treatment. Angel is very dejected about her illness, saying, "I am so ashamed. I have let down my family and I am costing them so much. I will never be able to go to college! I just want to stop this now."

CRITICAL THINKING

1. What aspects of Angel's history indicates that she could be at risk for developing anorexia nervosa?
2. Is it unusual for individuals being treated for anorexia nervosa to relapse?
3. What would cause Angel to relapse into her former anorexic habits?
4. Are Angel's concerns regarding causing her family financial hardship valid?
5. After Angel's second admission, the nurse finds Mrs. Santos sobbing in a waiting room. When asked about her concerns, Mrs. Santos states, "She's dying, I know it and we can't stop it!" Are Mrs. Santos's concerns regarding Angel's mortality realistic?

REVIEW Feeding and Eating Disorders

RELATE Link the Concepts and Exemplars

Linking the exemplar on feeding and eating disorders with the concept of teaching and learning:

1. In the context of caring for a patient diagnosed with an eating disorder, describe the barriers the nurse faces with regard to teaching about nutrition.
2. The nurse is caring for a 17-year-old female patient who is diagnosed with anorexia nervosa. The patient's father states, "Once she starts eating regularly, she'll get better. She's just being stubborn." To effectively teach the father about the basis of AN, how should the nurse respond?

Linking the exemplar on feeding and eating disorders with the concept of acid–base balance:

3. How does purging by way of self-induced vomiting most often affect the individual's acid–base balance? How does purging through laxative abuse most often affect acid–base balance?
4. What potential cardiac complications may arise as a result of acid–base imbalances associated with feeding and eating disorders?

READY Go to Volume 3: Clinical Nursing Skills

REFER Go to Pearson MyLab Nursing and eText

REFLECT Apply Your Knowledge

Anisha Robinson is an 18-year-old college student who received a full scholarship for gymnastics. At 5′2″ and 101 pounds, she is tiny, but she frequently complains about being overweight. When she is not practicing with the gymnastics team, she spends much of her time studying. Although Anisha's grades are outstanding, she worries that she will not be admitted into pharmacy school. Sometimes she is so anxious at night that she can't sleep. In order not to keep her roommate up, she'll go out and run 2 to 3 miles in the middle of the night. Her friends worry about her because they don't know how she can keep her strength up when she eats so little, despite the fact that she'll exercise for an hour or more after every meal. Her roommate becomes worried when they return from Thanksgiving break and she hears the gymnastics coach complaining that Anisha has gained 3 pounds over the holiday. She tearfully resolves to eat less and work out more.

1. What are the priority nursing diagnoses for Anisha?
2. What nursing interventions may be appropriate for inclusion in this patient's nursing plan of care?
3. What assessment findings may indicate that Anisha's health is deteriorating?

Exemplar 29.B Personality Disorders

Exemplar Learning Outcomes

29.B Analyze personality disorders and how they relate to self.

- Describe the pathophysiology of personality disorders.
- Describe the etiology of personality disorders.
- Compare the risk factors and prevention of personality disorders.
- Identify the clinical manifestations of personality disorders.
- Summarize diagnostic tests and therapies used by interprofessional teams in the collaborative care of an individual with a personality disorder.
- Differentiate care of patients with personality disorders across the lifespan.
- Apply the nursing process in providing culturally competent care to an individual with a personality disorder.

Exemplar Key Terms

Antisocial personality disorder (ASPD), *2049*
Avoidant personality disorder, *2050*
Borderline personality disorder (BPD), *2052*
Dependent personality disorder, *2051*
Disinhibition, *2049*
Ego-syntonic, *2047*
Histrionic personality disorder, *2050*
Impulsiveness, *2047*
Manipulation, *2047*
Narcissism, *2047*
Narcissistic personality disorder, *2053*
Obsessive–compulsive personality disorder, *2051*
Paranoid personality disorder, *2050*
Personality, *2047*
Personality disorder (PD), *2047*
Personality traits, *2047*
Schizoid personality disorder, *2050*
Schizotypal personality disorder, *2050*
Splitting, *2052*

Overview

The American Psychological Association (2020) defines **personality** as enduring characteristic patterns of thinking, feeling, and behavior that make an individual unique. These patterns begin to take shape in childhood and are set by early adulthood. Character and temperament constitute two important aspects of a person's personality. *Character* refers to moral and ethical value judgments, whereas *temperament* refers to innate characteristics, such as nervousness or sensitivity.

The elements that make up an individual's personality are called **personality traits**. They number in the hundreds, and examples include affability, impulsiveness, and honesty. In the field of psychology, however, special emphasis has been placed on the five-factor model: neuroticism, extraversion, openness, agreeableness, and conscientiousness (Barańczuk, 2019). Psychologists generally use these traits to describe an individual's personality, as they are considered to be universal; however, recent research raises questions as to their universality in all cultures, especially outside North America and Western Europe (Boudouda & Gana, 2020).

An individual's personality determines how that individual interacts with others. When established personality patterns result in repeated conflicts with others and impair the individual's ability to function in society, that individual is said to be experiencing a **personality disorder (PD)**. PDs affect all aspects of an individual's life and are marked by overly rigid and maladaptive behaviors that make it difficult for the individual to adapt to social demands and change. PDs are independent of mental disorders and substance abuse and are generally consistent over time and across varying situations.

Personality disorders typically manifest themselves during adolescence and continue throughout the lifespan, although in some cases symptoms diminish with age. Symptoms include interpersonal difficulties, identity problems that result in a weak sense of self, a lack of intimate relationships, and clumsy social skills that hinder cooperation. Individuals with PDs exhibit behaviors that may include **manipulation** (controlling and taking advantage of others); **narcissism** (believing oneself superior and worthy of special treatment); and **impulsiveness** (acting without regard to potential consequences) (Barańczuk, 2019).

Pathophysiology

The nature of these dysfunctions is not fully understood. The American Psychiatric Association has described a number of PDs, but because clinical definitions lack precision, there is often overlap. Consequently, individuals experiencing a PD are usually diagnosed with more than one. That said, all individuals with PDs demonstrate three common behaviors:

- Managing stress by attempting to change the environment rather than themselves
- Failing to take responsibility for the consequences of their actions
- Failing to understand how their behavior affects others.

In effect, individuals with PDs are **ego-syntonic**, meaning that they behave according to the beliefs, desires, and values that concur with their disorder. In other words, they see themselves and their behavior as normal and view the problems that arise with others as external to themselves, often believing they are being victimized (Hart, Tortoriello, & Richardson, 2018).

Personality disorders are also characterized by deficits in the areas of cognition, affect, interpersonal relationships, and impulse control; individuals with PDs manifest problems and difficulties in at least two of these areas of functioning (Potter & Moller, 2020). In addition to this impairment, developing healthy coping strategies proves to be a challenge as individuals with PDs are typically inflexible. This lack of adaptability feeds into a continual negative cycle in which the same behaviors are consistently exhibited, sabotaging opportunities to gain new skills, and ultimately leading to social isolation.

Etiology

Much about PDs remains unknown, and studies on PDs are hampered by several factors. For example, the lack of diagnostic uniformity makes it difficult for researchers to define samples and replicate previous studies. Another problem is that most individuals experiencing PDs do not come to the attention of mental health professionals. Many individuals with PDs fail to recognize their beliefs or behaviors as abnormal and see no need to seek out treatment (Potter & Moller, 2020). Consequently, mental health professionals often do not encounter individuals with PD unless behaviors are severe enough to warrant intervention by family members or the court system.

What is known is that the inflexible personality and behavioral patterns that characterize PDs appear to develop gradually, often with origins in childhood (Potter & Moller, 2020). PDs do not appear to be the result of any one cause. Instead, they seem to be the result of an interaction between biological and environmental factors.

Genetics

There does appear to be a genetic causal relationship with certain PDs. According to the Mayo Clinic (2020), a family history of schizotypal PD and/or schizophrenia increases the likelihood of an individual developing schizotypal PD. However, many research studies indicate that both genetics and environmental factors are linked to the development of PDs. One large-scale study of twins indicated that neither genetics nor environmental factors alone caused the development of PDs; rather, personality disorders are significantly influenced by genetic factors and there is a gene–environment interplay in the etiology (Czajkowski et al., 2018; Kendler et al., 2019; South & Reichborn-Kjennerud, 2017). Another study that focused on antisocial personality disorder (ASPD), concluded that a unidimensional ASPD phenotype exists and strongly supports both genetic and environmental influences (Wesseldijk et al., 2018). During childhood, genetic and environmental factors shared by children in families explained up to 44% of the variance of conduct problems; the remaining variance was due to environmental factors. During adolescence and adulthood, genetic and environmental factors equally explained the variation (Wesseldijk et al., 2018).

Neurobiology

Research points to several neurobiological factors as contributors to the development of PDs, including gene plasticity and vulnerability and the role of gene–environment interactions (Cattane, Rossi, Lanfredi, & Cattaneo, 2017). Trait anxiety may also play a role; a neuroimaging study found that trait anxiety may disrupt cognitive processing and cause emotional interference in individuals with borderline personality disorder (Krause-Utz et al., 2018).

Trauma History

Early life stress, including sexual abuse, physical abuse, emotional abuse, physical neglect, and emotional neglect, has been associated with the onset and severity of psychiatric disorders in adults. One study showed that emotional abuse and physical neglect were demonstrated to be strongly associated with the development of personality disorders (Naismith, Zarate Guerrero, & Feigenbaum, 2019). Another study showed a strong correlation between childhood sexual abuse and the development of borderline personality disorder (BPD) (Cattane et al., 2017). A systematic review of literature showed that the link is stronger among females, although this may reflect more self-reporting of abuse among females than males (de Aquino Ferreira, Queiroz Pereira, Neri Benevides, & Aguiar Melo, 2018). In summary, early life stress triggers aggravate, maintain, and increase the recurrence of PDs and other psychiatric diagnoses.

Exposure to interpersonal and accidental traumatic events and/or repeated episodes of trauma that result in posttraumatic stress disorder (PTSD) are also strongly linked to the development of PDs and other mental illnesses. The link between PTSD and development of BPD was significantly stronger than the link between PTSD and other psychiatric comorbidities (Beck et al., 2019; de Aquino Ferreira et al., 2018). Although PTSD is a factor in the development of BPD, trauma also is strongly correlated with the development of avoidant, obsessive–compulsive, and dependent personality disorders (Naismith et al., 2019).

Intrapersonal Factors

Individuals with different PDs interact with others in a variety of ways. They may project their feelings onto those around them, demonstrate problems in developing genuine intimate relationships, lack a sense of guilt, or behave childishly, depending on their personality dysfunction (Potter & Moller, 2020).

As discussed earlier in the concept, parent–child interactions can significantly affect a person's developing sense of self, and as a result, a child's perception of reality may become distorted if parents are insensitive to the child's needs. Individuals with a family background of criminality and parental separation, or a childhood marked by continually changing caregivers or care institutions, show a higher propensity for PDs. In a meta-analysis, Wilson, Stroud, and Durbin (2017) found that all PD dimensions were significantly related to various forms of family and school problems as well as child abuse. Hock et al. (2018) found correlations between childhood adversities and PDs. Malnutrition in childhood was associated with the development of paranoid, schizoid, schizotypal, and avoidant personality disorders. Furthermore, Hock et al. noted associations between childhood maltreatment and ASPD and emotional abuse and BPD.

Malnutrition in the first year of life is associated with increased neuroticism and decreased levels of openness, agreeableness, and conscientiousness in adulthood, suggesting that early child malnutrition is a risk factor for traits associated with personality disorders (Hock et al., 2018). Last, although mood and anxiety disorders are distinct from PDs, overlapping features among the three types of disorders exist, which makes the correlation between childhood verbal abuse by a parent and the later development of mood and anxiety disorders and PTSD noteworthy (Gardner et al., 2019).

Sociocultural Factors

The influence of social and cultural factors in personality disorders is not fully understood, yet it is known that they contribute to personal development. For example, when certain groups are discriminated against in a society, it is difficult for the members of that group to develop a healthy self-image.

In traditional cultures, such as those found in Japan, there is societal pressure to conform and adhere to group norms. In the United States, on the other hand, emphasis is placed on the personal versus the communal, leading to the prevalence of a "me-first" mentality. Thus, individuals from different parts of the world have a greater propensity for certain kinds of PDs according to their sociocultural backdrop.

Personality disorders are expressed differently and have variations in presentations in some cultures. Gawda (2018) noted significantly lower prevalence of PDs among Black as compared to white populations. Prevalence of PDs in Asian cultures is generally lower than in white populations. Latin American populations are thought to be more frequently misdiagnosed with histrionic or narcissistic PD traits. However, it does not mean that the disorders are highly prevalent in these populations; rather, cultural expressions tend to be more outgoing and vibrant, which is culturally acceptable (Gawda, 2018). Gawda also noted that the overall rate for any PD in Mexico was 6.10%, compared to 14.4% in North America.

Risk Factors

As discussed in the concept section of this module, both genetic and environmental factors are believed to influence the development of a PD. According to the American Psychological Association (2020), notable risk factors include genetics, such as having relatives diagnosed with a PD or another mental illness; family life, such as an unstable home life or parental loss via death or divorce; childhood abuse, such as verbal, physical, and sexual abuse or neglect; diagnosis of other disorders, such as childhood conduct disorder; and low socioeconomic status. That said, diagnosing PDs in children can prove to be challenging because the behavioral and thinking patterns that may indicate such a disorder could actually be the consequence of a developmental phase or the experimentation that often occurs during adolescence.

Prevention

PDs can be prevented if the developing patterns of behavior, feeling, and thought are identified before they become set. This generally requires intervention during childhood and early adolescence. Consequently, prevention programs have been created to address both developmental and environmental risk factors and to break the cycle of repeating problematic patterns by providing interventions at school and in the home. Screening programs have been implemented in schools and primary care settings to help detect risk factors and identify patterns that indicate a PD may be forming (Chanen & Thompson, 2018).

In terms of interventions, there are several programs in the United States focused on imparting parenting skills to address aggressive and antisocial behaviors. The Nurse–Family Partnership Program is one of them. Under this program, registered nurses visit at-risk families with newborn children starting at the prenatal period and lasting through the child's second birthday. The nurses impart parenting skills and work with family members to change poor habits, such as smoking and unhealthy eating choices (Eckenrode et al., 2017; Nurse–Family Partnership, 2019).

Barriers to these preventive measures include competing priorities, lack of infrastructure for implementation, lack of public education regarding mental health, the effectiveness of prevention, stigma, and a paucity of facilitating factors (Eckenrode et al., 2017; Nurse–Family Partnership, 2019). Facilitators include leadership, flexible resources, linkage to healthcare reform or other legislation, coordination across agencies and governmental levels, and additional research.

Clinical Manifestations

The fifth edition of the *Diagnostic and Statistical Manual of Mental Disorders* (APA, 2013) specifies that individuals with PDs must exhibit dysfunctional behavior toward self and others, and they must also maintain persistent, rigid thoughts and beliefs that are incongruent with sociocultural norms. Although each of the 10 PDs is viewed as being a clinically distinct syndrome, the American Psychiatric Association outlines criteria that are characteristic of PDs in general. These include that the individual exhibits a stable pattern of perceptions and behaviors that are out of line with cultural expectations and that occur in two or more areas: cognition, affect, impulse control, and personal relationships (APA, 2013). These patterns must not be consistent with any other psychiatric disorder or with any underlying medical illness or use or abuse of medications or substances.

The 10 personality disorders are categorized into three clusters: Cluster A includes those PDs that may be characterized by odd or eccentric behaviors; Cluster B includes the PDs characterized by dramatic, erratic, or emotional behaviors; and Cluster C includes those PDs typified by avoidant, dependent, or obsessive–compulsive behaviors (APA, 2013). This text focuses primarily on two of the most challenging personality disorders: antisocial PD and borderline PD. All of the primary personality disorders are described in **Table 29.4** » and in the Clinical Manifestations and Therapies table.

Antisocial Personality Disorder

One of the first named PDs was **antisocial personality disorder (ASPD)**, which is distinguished by the individual's propensity to manipulate or violate others' rights with a disregard for their feelings and/or the consequences (Skodol, 2019). Risk factors include having a caregiver who has antisocial PD or alcoholism and being a victim of child abuse. An estimated 3–4% of the U.S. population has ASPD, with approximately four times as many men having the disorder than women (Potter & Moller, 2020). Because of the lack of remorse and inclination for risk-taking behavior associated with ASPD, many individuals with this PD are found in prison and substance abuse treatment centers.

To confirm diagnosis of antisocial PD, an individual must illustrate dysfunction as illustrated by egocentric behaviors, including pleasure-seeking and unlawful behaviors. In addition, impairments must exist in interpersonal functioning either via a lack of empathy and remorse for wrongdoings or the inability to form and maintain intimate relationships, which often includes deceptive or coercive behaviors. Two trait domains are associated with antisocial PD: antagonism and **disinhibition**. In addition to the other general criteria for PDs, an individual with antisocial PD must be at least 18 years of age (APA, 2013). Often individuals younger than age 18 who demonstrate behaviors typical of antisocial PD have

TABLE 29.4 Personality Disorders and Associated Characteristics

Behavioral Traits	Affective Traits	Cognitive Traits	Social Traits
Paranoid Personality Disorder			
■ Suspicious and mistrusting of others ■ Rigid, fixed worldview	■ Inflexible about beliefs, perceptions, and suspicions ■ Argumentative	■ Generally intelligent and highly capable of arguing in support of personal beliefs	■ Extreme jealousy may impair intimate relationships with significant others ■ Tends to believe every action by others is driven by malevolent intent or ulterior motive
Schizoid Personality Disorder			
■ Loners; tend to prefer solitary activities ■ Uninterested in socialization	■ Generally appear apathetic ■ Flat (emotionless) affect	■ Generally indifferent to situations and circumstances ■ May appear to be cognitively impaired	■ Uninterested in intimate relationships ■ Prefers social isolation and avoids roles that require socialization
Schizotypal Personality Disorder			
■ Bizarre behaviors, appearance, and speech ■ Prefers solitary activities ■ Frequent lack of eye contact	■ Indifferent ■ Nonreactive or inappropriate in emotional situations	■ Extreme suspicion of others ■ Paranoid fears of persecution ■ Odd or distorted thoughts	■ Excessive anxiety in social situations ■ Fears intimate relationships ■ Alienation ■ Lacks the desire to form close relationships ■ Introverted
Antisocial Personality Disorder			
■ Impulsive; difficulty in delaying gratification ■ Dishonest ■ Irresponsible ■ Risk taking ■ Criminal behavior	■ Has no problems with self-expression yet remains detached in interactions ■ Lack of guilt and remorse for committing harmful acts ■ Callous ■ Easily agitated ■ Hostile ■ Failure to empathize	■ Egocentric ■ Grandiose ■ Despite lack of long-term planning, exhibits confidence in future success	■ Cannot form intimate relationships ■ Exploits others as form of interaction ■ Exhibits controlling and abusive behaviors ■ Aggressive
Borderline Personality Disorder			
■ Impulsive ■ Dangerous risk taking ■ Can self-mutilate and have suicidal tendencies ■ Unpredictable	■ Intense anxiety ■ Difficulty empathizing and feeling guilt ■ Psychotic episodes are common ■ Reactive moods ■ Difficulty in controlling anger ■ Consistently low mood; rarely experiences satisfaction or happiness	■ Unstable perception of self, ranging from grandiosity to self-loathing	■ Highly unstable relationships ■ Manipulative ■ Intense fear of abandonment ■ Mistrust ■ Behavior swings from all-encompassing interest in another individual to complete withdrawal
Histrionic Personality Disorder			
■ Flamboyant ■ Dramatic ■ Seeks to be the center of attention	■ Appears inconsiderate and incapable of empathy ■ Pervasive craving for excitement	■ Egocentric ■ Tends to prefer creative and artistic endeavors as opposed to academic achievement	■ May use sexual behaviors to manipulate others ■ May engage in high-risk sexual behaviors
Narcissistic Personality Disorder			
■ Very competitive in search for power, fame, and love ■ Arrogant ■ Manipulates others to achieve own ends	■ Difficulty in expressing emotions ■ Empathy is a challenge ■ Anxiety and fear in relation to failure	■ Grandiosity ■ Believes is better than others ■ Spends much time fantasizing about being powerful, famous, loved, and beautiful	■ Balanced reciprocal relationships are rare ■ Seeks out relationships as a way to boost own self-esteem
Avoidant Personality Disorder			
■ Intense discomfort in social situations ■ Avoids social contact unless feels will be fully accepted	■ Timid ■ Fearful of rejection ■ Intense worry and anxiety, especially with regard to forming relationships	■ Hypersensitive to others' opinions of self ■ Acceptance of others' negative evaluations	■ Wants to have intimate relationships but an extreme fear of being embarrassed, judged, or rejected by others often prevents it ■ Possesses very few close relationships that are not familial

TABLE 29.4 Personality Disorders and Associated Characteristics (*continued*)

Behavioral Traits	Affective Traits	Cognitive Traits	Social Traits
Dependent Personality Disorder			
■ Passive by nature ■ Seeks out others who are dominant and who will control the relationship	■ Strives to appear friendly and helpful ■ Will subordinate personal desires and needs and instead prioritize the desires and needs of others	■ Insecure with personal decision making ■ Pervasive sense of inferiority	■ Intense fear of rejection ■ Separation from the dominant other may produce extreme anxiety and depression
Obsessive–Compulsive Personality Disorder			
■ Perfectionist ■ Inflexible ■ Hardworking ■ High achiever ■ Compulsive; engages in repetitive or ritualistic checking	■ Difficulty in expressing emotions ■ Empathy is a challenge ■ Anxiety and fear in relation to failure	■ Extreme fear of making mistakes; may procrastinate or avoid tasks because of fear of failure	■ Tends to be controlling in relationships, which limits intimacy

Sources: Based on Mental Health America (2020); Potter and Moller (2020); Skodol (2019).

Clinical Manifestations and Therapies

Personality Disorders

DISORDERS	CLINICAL MANIFESTATIONS	CLINICAL THERAPIES
CLUSTER A		
Paranoid	■ Unable to trust others ■ Rigid, fixed worldview that often is conspiratorial in nature ■ Believes others' actions are based on ulterior motives	■ Psychotherapy ■ If accepted by the patient, pharmacologic therapy may include antidepressants, anxiolytics, and antipsychotic medications
Schizoid	■ Prefers solitude, uninterested in interpersonal relationships ■ Generally unable to perceive or express strong emotions	■ CBT ■ Group therapy with others who are also learning interpersonal skills ■ Pharmacologic treatment may include antidepressant and antipsychotic medications
Schizotypal	■ Odd mannerisms and speech patterns ■ Cold demeanor, inappropriate responses ■ Lack of affect ■ Distorted thoughts ■ Intense anxiety in social situations ■ Paranoid fears of persecution	■ CBT ■ Family-focused therapy (FFT) ■ Pharmacologic therapy (antidepressants, antianxiety medications, antipsychotics) ■ Alternative therapy
CLUSTER B		
Antisocial	■ Impulsive ■ Lack of remorse ■ Failure to empathize ■ Easily agitated, aggressive, and controlling	■ Group therapy ■ Anger management therapy ■ Psychodynamic therapy ■ Psychoeducation ■ Pharmacologic therapy (antidepressants, mood stabilizers, antianxiety medications, antipsychotics)
Borderline	■ Extreme risk taking ■ Impulsive ■ Self-injury, suicidal ■ Intense anxiety ■ Consistently low mood ■ Unstable relationships due to intense mistrust of others	■ SFT ■ DBT ■ CBT ■ Pharmacologic therapy (antidepressants, antianxiety medications, antipsychotics, mood stabilizers) ■ Group therapy (e.g., STEPPS) ■ Alternative therapy

(continued on next page)

Clinical Manifestations and Therapies *(continued)*

DISORDERS	CLINICAL MANIFESTATIONS	CLINICAL THERAPIES
Histrionic	■ Flamboyant, highly seductive in behavior and/or appearance ■ May be sexually manipulative ■ Demands to be center of attention ■ Constantly seeks excitement and activity	■ Psychotherapy may be effective ■ Group therapy not recommended because of attention-seeking behaviors
Narcissistic	■ Grandiosity ■ Rage ■ Depression, anxiety ■ Manipulative ■ Lack of empathy	■ CBT ■ FFT ■ Pharmacologic therapy (antidepressants, antianxiety medications)
CLUSTER C		
Avoidant	■ Extreme discomfort socially ■ Hypersensitive ■ Intense anxiety related to social contact ■ Easily internalizes negative comments by others	■ Social skills training ■ CBT ■ Group therapy ■ Pharmacologic therapy (antidepressants, antianxiety medications) ■ Alternative therapy
Dependent	■ Pervasive need to be under control by a dominant other ■ Insecure about making decisions ■ Chronic sense of inadequacy	■ Psychotherapy ■ Pharmacologic treatment of symptoms with antidepressants or anxiolytics; caution to monitor for dependence on medications
Obsessive-compulsive	■ Inflexible, controlling ■ Anxiety ■ Difficulty with empathy ■ Perfectionist	■ CBT ■ Pharmacologic therapy (SSRIs) ■ Alternative therapy

been diagnosed with a conduct disorder, such as oppositional defiant disorder, or attention-deficit/hyperactivity disorder (Skodol, 2019; Potter & Moller, 2020).

Borderline Personality Disorder

In 1938, psychoanalyst Adolf Stern established the label of **borderline personality disorder (BPD)**, as he believed the symptoms of BPD sat on the dividing line or "border" between psychosis and neurosis. Currently, many mental healthcare professionals take exception with Stern's use of the term *borderline* because it can reinforce already existing negative perceptions of individuals with BPD (Stoffers-Winterling et al., 2018).

Impulsivity, unstable emotions, and depression are key symptoms of BPD; self-harm is also common (see **Figure 29.3** ⟫), with suicide occurring in 8–10% of those with this disorder (NIMH, 2017a). **Splitting**, the inclination to perceive people or situations as one extreme or the other (e.g., all good or all bad), is also commonly found among individuals with BPD; this feature contributes to their frequent extreme shifts in mood (Potter & Moller, 2020). Other core characteristics include identity disturbances; frantic attempts to prevent abandonment (real or perceived); impulsive behaviors; chronic feelings of emptiness; transient paranoia; and difficulty managing anger (APA, 2013).

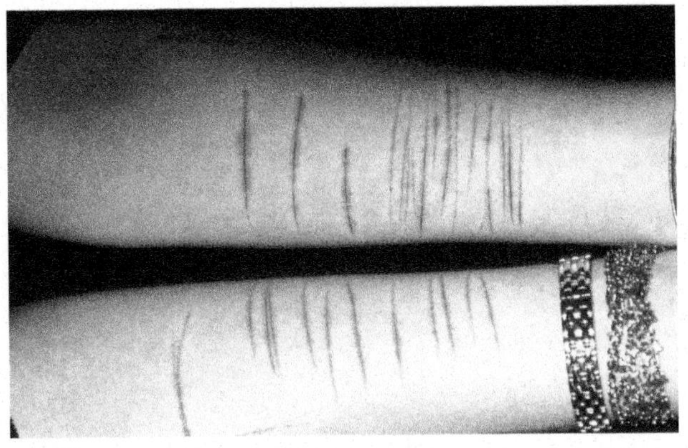

Figure 29.3 ⟫ Some individuals with borderline personality disorder engage in self-mutilating behavior, such as cutting.
Source: Dr. P. Marazzi/Science Source.

Gender plays a significant role in that 75% of diagnosed cases are in women (APA, 2013; Stoffers-Winterling et al., 2018). Approximately 20% of psychiatric inpatients have BPD and 1.6% of the general population is affected; some estimates have ranged as high as 5.9% of the general population (APA, 2013). Risk factors include childhood abuse and abandonment and a strong genetic link: Individuals are five times more likely to be diagnosed with BPD if a first-degree relative also has the disorder. Antisocial personality disorder, mood disorders, and substance abuse disorders are also much more probable in families where individuals are affected with BPD (APA, 2013).

SAFETY ALERT Borderline personality disorder is often associated with self-mutilation, which can include cutting or carving into the skin (see Figure 29.3), burning, pulling out hair, and head banging, all known as nonsuicidal self-injury (NSSI). Nurses must be extremely cognizant of the signs of self-injury and demonstrate sensitivity when conducting an assessment. Patients often hide their injuries by wearing long sleeves or pants, even in warm weather (Mental Health America, 2020; Skodol, 2019).

Low self-esteem, intense self-criticism, and disassociation are associated with BPD. Interpersonal functioning is marked by the tendency to take offense easily or an intense fear of abandonment, which creates conflict-ridden and unstable relationships. The dysfunctional personality traits in BPD fall within the trait domains of negative affectivity (including emotional lability), disinhibition, and antagonism (APA, 2013). More information on borderline personality disorder can be found in **Box 29.2** ».

Borderline personality disorder carries a great deal of stigma, even among mental health professionals. Day et al. (2018) found that a large portion of mental health providers hold negative attitudes toward those with borderline personality disorder. Often, these attitudes become manifested through the use of stigmatizing language to describe patient behavior, such as "manipulative" and "attention seeking." Furthermore, Florence (2020) noted countertransference reactions to BPD to be more negative than with any other disorder.

Dickens et al. (2019) and Stacey et al. (2018) have recommended improved nurse training and education aimed at fostering a holistic view of BPD in order to better understand its causes and resulting behaviors. They cite CBT and BPD workshops as possible models. Day et al. (2018) voiced concerns on how stigmatizing language and attitudes affect the relationship between patient and clinician and how such language impacts recovery, and suggested self-governance measures that clinicians could use to improve patient interactions.

» **Stay Current:** In addition to the American Psychiatric Association's website, additional information about PDs can be found at www.MayoClinic.org and the National Institute for Mental Health at www.nimh.nih.gov.

Narcissistic Personality Disorder

Narcissistic personality disorder (NPD) features a sense of grandiosity, an inability to empathize with others, and attention-seeking behaviors. Substance abuse disorders (especially cocaine abuse), eating disorders (particularly anorexia nervosa), and depression, dysthymia, and social withdrawal are commonly found in conjunction with NPD (APA, 2013). More men than women are diagnosed, with 50–75% of the diagnoses being made in males. It is estimated that up to 6.2% of the general population experiences the disorder (APA, 2013; Skodol, 2019).

Narcissistic personality disorder is characterized by extreme reliance on other individuals' perceptions and/or an inflated sense of self or by approval seeking and either an extremely low or high set of personal standards. A failure to identify with others and their emotions or a hypersensitivity to others creates difficulty in developing meaningful relationships. NPD aligns with the trait domain of antagonism, specifically the trait facets of grandiosity and attention seeking (APA, 2013; Potter & Moller, 2020).

Box 29.2

Characteristics of Borderline Personality Disorder

Classified as a serious mental illness, borderline personality disorder impairs functioning in multiple areas because of the instability in mood, behavior, and self-image associated with the disorder. Characteristics of borderline PD include impulsive and often reckless behaviors, chronic feelings of emptiness, feelings of shame and guilt, and labile mood ranging from fear of abandonment to rage, as well as the increased risk for suicide or self-injurious behavior (APA, 2013; Stoffers-Winterling et al., 2018). Symptoms must occur over time and not be attributed to another mental disorder or to substance use or medication side effects. In addition, individuals with borderline PD often have co-occurring mental illness. Participation in pharmacotherapy and more intensive treatment modalities (i.e., inpatient and day treatment programs associated with psychiatric hospitals) is higher with patients with borderline PD than with patients with other personality disorders. Stoffers-Winterling et al. (2018) reported that 79.7% of patients with borderline PD were taking antidepressant medications, 46.6% were taking anxiolytics, 38.6% were taking antipsychotics, and 35.9% were taking mood stabilizers. The authors also note that about 71% of people with borderline PD were using standing medications at 6-year follow-up and that they were still more likely than any other personality disorder to be using pharmacological treatments at 16-year follow-up. It is also important to note that, to date, any drug used in borderline PD is considered off-label (if not targeted at specific symptoms such as depression or anxiety).

Family members of patients with borderline PD need support and resources to learn how to help their loved one as well as to take care of themselves. The National Alliance on Mental Illness (2017) recommends several strategies for family members to follow:

- Find emotional support.
- Take care of yourself—eat right, exercise, and avoid alcohol and drugs.
- Encourage your loved one to continue treatment.
- Learn and model techniques your loved one can use as coping strategies.

Nurses can help family members by encouraging them to participate in their loved one's treatment plan, find local or online support groups, and maintain their own physical and mental health.

Cultural Considerations

As environmental influences play a part in the development of personality, nurses and other healthcare professionals must take care not to deem a personality trait or behavior maladaptive or dysfunctional without first considering the influence of culture. For example, individuals who are new to the United States may present as paranoid or overly suspicious of others when in fact their behavior could simply be a result of their unfamiliarity with American customs and some cultures condition girls and women to avoid social situations. Cultural competence and being aware of one's own biases are crucial in providing quality care for patients. For additional examples, see the Focus on Diversity and Culture feature.

Collaboration

The treatment of PDs requires a collaborative effort that includes the patient, the interprofessional team responsible for the patient's care, and the patient's family. The team working with the patient may include a primary medical care provider; a psychiatrist or psychologist; a licensed mental health professional; an advanced practice nurse who specializes in psychiatric mental healthcare; a registered nurse; and other professionals. The registered nurse can fill several important functions, including providing education and follow-up related to the therapeutic regimen and instilling hope in the patient and family that achieving a more normal level of functioning is possible.

Focus on Diversity and Culture

Mental Health and Religious Beliefs

When caring for patients with personality disorders, nurses should be aware that some patients may interpret their condition in the context of deeply held religious and spiritual beliefs. More specifically, the symptoms of delusions and hallucinations may be viewed not as mental health issues but, rather, as demonic possession or the work of evil spirits (Cheng, 2017; Spector, 2017).

In both the distant and recent past, the medical community viewed religious and spiritual influences as more likely to be harmful than helpful in patient care. As a consequence, individuals with personality disorders who maintained a strong spiritual or religious practice often chose not to enter the mental health system, either because of shame or fear of how their beliefs would be perceived, or because of their conviction that only religious and spiritual healing could help them (Ayvaci, 2017). Today, the role of religion is viewed much differently. Partly because of a greater awareness of the need for cultural competence in mental healthcare, professional caregivers are more willing to integrate religious and spiritual elements into treatment (Ayvaci, 2017). Many clinicians have realized that for some patients, religion instills hope, purpose, and meaning in their lives and also influences treatment compliance and outcomes (Ayvaci 2017; Potter & Moller, 2020). Some therapists have begun to incorporate religious contexts and accommodations into CBT and other therapies with good results (Correa & Sandage, 2018).

Treating PDs is a considerable challenge and can generate frustration and try the patience of healthcare workers. All those involved, including nurses, must understand that an individual's personality developed over that person's lifetime, reflecting learned experiences, and is therefore unlikely to change drastically. The aim instead should be realistic, short-term outcomes. Eventually, patients should be encouraged to seek long-term therapy, which is considered the most effective in the treatment of PDs. Long-term therapy demands time, dedication, and buy-in from the patient (Potter & Moller, 2020). Nurses should also be especially cognizant of establishing and maintaining firm, consistent boundaries with patients.

Diagnostic Tests

There is no one test mental health professionals use to diagnose PDs. Instead, PDs are typically diagnosed through an interview with the patient that covers issues such as symptoms, family history, and thoughts of violence, suicide, or self-injury. Although a single interview may be sufficient for an experienced clinician to make a diagnosis, it is more often necessary for the clinician to conduct more than one interview spaced over time to arrive at a definitive diagnosis (APA, 2013). A physical exam and laboratory tests (such as a toxicology screen) also help rule out other factors that could be the cause of abnormal behavior, such as drug and alcohol abuse (Cleveland Clinic, 2020).

Although mental health professionals refer to the specific diagnostic criteria for each PD found in the most recent version of the DSM, identifying the specific PD that a patient is experiencing can be complicated because of the frequent overlap of symptoms across disorders. The subjectivity of the patient's descriptions and the care provider's interpretation of those descriptions also pose a challenge (Leising, Scherbaum, Packmohr, & Zimmerman, 2018). In this respect, there are a number of psychologic tests that can help mental health professionals arrive at a more definitive diagnosis, including personality inventories such as the Standardized Assessment of Personality: Abbreviated Scale (SAPAS). This scale is brief and easy to use to screen for personality disorders and can be used in routine psychiatric assessments (Ball, Tully, & Egan, 2017; Olajide et al., 2018).

If the disorder becomes so pronounced that an individual is unable to provide self-care or is in imminent jeopardy of causing harm to self or others, especially with dangerous self-injurious behaviors or suicidal ideation, then the individual should be hospitalized. Different inpatient options exist, such as day hospitalization or residential treatment (Skodol, 2019).

Pharmacologic Therapy

Individuals with PDs often are prescribed medications to control their symptoms. Obsessive–compulsive, aggressive, and self-destructive behaviors may be held in check with the use of SSRIs such as fluoxetine (Prozac). Symptoms associated with avoidant and borderline disorders may be minimized with antidepressants, just as acute psychosis may be ameliorated with antipsychotic drugs. Medications, however, should be used to complement a comprehensive treatment plan that includes therapy (ideally long-term) that incorporates various approaches (Potter & Moller, 2020).

Psychotherapy

Long-term psychotherapy is the most highly recommended treatment for individuals with PDs. There are different types of psychotherapy, some more suitable to certain types of PDs than others. Medical professionals usually draw from and combine elements of the different types of psychotherapy to meet a particular patient's needs (Mayo Clinic, 2020; Skodol, 2019). All of the therapies described here are generally available as both outpatient and inpatient services.

Cognitive-Behavioral Therapy

CBT combines cognitive aspects to change thoughts and beliefs with behavioral aspects to alter problematic action patterns. It focuses on skill training and problem solving. Typically, the therapist serves as a guide to assist the patient in recognizing harmful ways of thinking and erroneous beliefs and works with the individual to purge them by analyzing and reinterpreting both past and current experiences, thus helping the patient adopt positive behaviors and interactions with others.

If trauma has occurred, exposure therapy can be used. This is a behavioral therapy in which patients, guided by the therapist, repeatedly approach trauma-related thoughts, feelings, and situations that they have been avoiding because of the distress they cause. Repeated exposure to these thoughts, feelings, and situations helps reduce the power they have to cause distress (Nenadić, Lamberth, & Reiss, 2017). These therapies aim to reduce symptoms by offering patients the chance to develop concrete coping strategies in conjunction with the therapist. CBT can also help individuals with mood disorders recognize when their mood is about to shift, thus giving them the foresight to apply coping strategies to deal with these changes (APA, 2013; Nenadić et al., 2017).

Dialectical Behavioral Therapy

A combination of cognitive and behavior therapy, DBT originally was developed to treat individuals with suicidal thoughts. *Dialectical* refers to striking a balance between two extremes; the therapist displays understanding and validates the patient's behaviors and feelings while at the same time imposing limits and making the patient responsible for changing unhealthy patterns. It has proven effective in treating BPD, showing lower dropout rates than other therapies and decreasing the frequency of suicide attempts. Through DBT, patients learn to accept things as they are and apply techniques to control strong emotions that might otherwise overwhelm them. Mindfulness is one such technique, where patients learn to become aware of and explore emotions without reacting to them. DBT also teaches patients emotional regulation and distress tolerance. This type of therapy usually relies on individual sessions to teach new skills and strategies, and then group sessions to apply them. Traditional and cognitive approaches are also used in conjunction with DBT to help patients foster better relationships with others (APA, 2013; O'Sullivan, Murphy, & Bourke, 2017).

Schema-Focused Therapy

Schema-focused therapy combines aspects of CBT with other forms of psychotherapy to change a patient's self-perception. This is often applied to personality disorders, where the individual typically has a poor self-image. SFT aims to help patients view themselves differently so they can create new and more effective ways of interacting with their environment and others (Nenadić et al., 2017; Skodol, 2019). Research has shown that SFT is an extremely effective treatment option for individuals with BPD, sometimes leading to recovery (Nenadić et al., 2017).

Group Therapy

Group therapy is also important to the treatment of certain PDs. For example, it can be helpful in strengthening empathic skills for individuals with ASPD in that it allows for feedback about the perceptions of the other group members (Potter & Moller, 2020). Another example of group therapy is Systems Training for Emotional Predictability and Problem Solving (STEPPS), consisting of 20 two-hour sessions led by a social worker. According to the Mayo Clinic (2020), the STEPPS program, when combined with other approaches, such as pharmacologic treatments and psychotherapy, has alleviated depression and improved the quality of life of individuals with BPD.

Family-Focused Therapy

Family-focused therapy can help family members of patients with PD cope with the stress of living with a loved one with a personality disorder and avoid behaviors that might worsen the patient's condition. FFT educates family members about their loved one's disorder, giving them the necessary knowledge to improve interactions and play an active role in supporting the patient. For example, the patient's family can develop a course of action in case warning signs of a relapse appear. In addition, family therapy programs such as Family Connections address the needs and concerns of the patient's family members. DBT family therapy helps family members understand and support relatives with PD by teaching the family members skills and strategies and having them participate in the patient's treatment sessions (Bateman & Fonagy, 2019).

Complementary Health Approaches

Although there is not a specific form of integrative therapy that is recommended for patients with PDs, complementary health approaches may provide some relief from certain symptoms, such as anxiety and depression. For instance, yoga, meditation, breathing exercises, and chamomile tea can help individuals with anxiety to relax, while vitamin B12 and omega-3 fatty acids can ease depression (National Center for Complementary and Integrative Health [NCCIH], 2018). Studies indicate that omega-3 fatty acids may also serve to prevent psychosis from fully emerging in young individuals who show signs of developing such a disorder (NCCIH, 2018).

Lifespan Considerations

Personality traits are enduring patterns of perceiving, relating to, and thinking about the environment that are exhibited in many social and personal contexts and that exhibit in at least two of the following areas: cognition, affectivity, interpersonal functioning, and impulse control (APA, 2013). Characteristics of personality disorders at different ages during the lifespan are discussed below.

Personality Disorders in Childhood

Many times, traits of a PD that appear in childhood do not persist into adult life. However, a PD may be diagnosed in children or preadolescents in relatively unusual cases where the child's particular maladaptive personality traits appear to be pervasive, persistent, and unlikely to be limited to a specific development stage or another mental disorder (APA, 2013). For a PD to be diagnosed in childhood, the features must have been present for at least 1 year.

The exception is ASPD, which cannot be diagnosed in someone under age 18. Often younger patients with similar behaviors are diagnosed with more age-appropriate disruptive, impulse-control, or conduct disorders (APA, 2013). Research in this area has been focusing on the genetic, cognitive, emotional, biological, environmental, and personality characteristics of callous and unemotional traits displayed early in life by children with conduct disorders (Wesseldijk et al., 2018). Research has also been conducted to determine whether borderline personality–related characteristics observed in children are associated with increased risk for the development of BPD. The research found that BPD-related characteristics measured in the early adolescent years were highly heritable; were more common in children who had exhibited poor cognitive function, impulsivity, and more behavioral and emotional problems at 5 years of age; and co-occurred with symptoms of conduct disorder, depression, anxiety, and psychosis (Winsper, Hall, Strauss, & Wolke, 2017).

The avoidant behavior characteristics of Cluster C (avoidant and dependent personality disorders) often start in infancy or childhood, with display of shyness, isolation, and fear of strangers and new situations (APA, 2013). Although these behaviors are not uncommon in young children, they do tend to dissipate as most children age.

Personality Disorders in Adolescence and Early Adulthood

The features of a personality disorder become recognizable typically during adolescence or early adulthood. Cluster A disorders, such as paranoid, schizoid, and schizotypal PDs, may present in childhood and adolescence. These individuals will display characteristics such as solitariness, poor peer relationships, social anxiety, underachievement in school, hypersensitivity, peculiar thoughts and language, and idiosyncratic fantasies (APA, 2013).

Individuals diagnosed with Cluster B disorders, such as BPD, often overuse health- and mental health–related resources. Individuals with BPD frequently display chronically unstable behaviors in early adulthood, with a serious lack of affective and impulse control. Impairment from the disorder and the risk for suicide are highest during the young adult years (APA, 2013).

Individuals who will be later diagnosed with a Cluster C disorder (avoidant or dependent) will become increasingly shy during adolescence and early adulthood and avoid developing the social relationships characteristic of that developmental age (APA, 2013). However, mental health providers caution against diagnosing children with dependent and avoidant disorders when the behaviors may actually be developmentally appropriate.

Personality Disorders in Pregnant Women

Little is known about the relationship of personality disorders and pregnancy. Crowley et al. (2020) reported the prevalence of personality disorder symptomology during pregnancy to be 6.4%. Furthermore, they noted that higher levels of PD symptomatology were associated with other current self-reported psychiatric symptoms such as depression and anxiety. In a review of literature, Crowley et al. found that pregnant women with a clinical diagnosis of borderline PD were more likely to experience adverse birth outcomes such as newborns with low Apgar scores. Overall, research is limited in this area. Nurses caring for pregnant women with diagnosed or suspected personality disorders should focus on promoting healthy behaviors during the peripartum period, including healthy mother–newborn attachment behaviors, described in Exemplar 33.D, Newborn Care, in Module 33, Reproduction.

Personality Disorders in Older Adults

Although by definition personality disorders have an onset no later than early adulthood, individuals with PDs may escape clinical attention until they are middle-aged or in later life. Often, loss of a significant support person or a stabilizing social situation, such as a job, exacerbates display of the disorder, and associated symptoms cause the individual to seek treatment (APA, 2013). Accurate evaluation of personality changes in middle or older adulthood requires ruling out potential causative medical conditions or previously undiagnosed substance use issues (APA, 2013; Bangash, 2020). Some types of personality disorders, such as antisocial and borderline PDs, become less evident or remit with age (APA, 2013). The risk of suicide also gradually wanes with age.

NURSING PROCESS

Just as the care of patients with personality disorders will be specific to each patient and the manifestations of the disorder, certain features of the nursing assessment will vary as well. Nurses working with patients with personality disorders should remember that some of the symptoms (e.g., labile affect and impairments in social skills) make it difficult to develop the nurse–patient relationship, especially when the patient denies the presence of symptoms or problems.

Assessment

Assessment data serves as the basis for application of the nursing process. However, assessment of the patient with a personality disorder may be complicated by a number of factors, including lack of insight or self-awareness, denial of the existence or manifestations of a disorder, inability to trust, and ineffective communication skills.

Within the realm of psychosocial assessment, the primary goals of assessment include identification of behaviors, beliefs, or thought patterns that disrupt the patient's social, professional, and personal life. When the patient lacks insight about the existence or effects of a PD, pertinent information may be gleaned from reports by family members or others who are closely associated with the patient. However, because maintenance of patient confidentiality is essential, the nurse must avoid overstepping the patient's personal and legal boundaries during data collection.

Data collection should include assessing work history; history of behavior problems, including violence directed at self or others; history of suicidal ideation; methods of resolving conflicts; alcohol and drug use; and nature of relationships with family members, coworkers, and friends. The nurse should ask questions that encourage the patient to describe aspects of self:

- When was the last time you were upset? What upset you? How did you handle it?
- How do others describe you?
- How would you describe yourself?
- What do you like about yourself? What would you like to change?
- How do you usually relate to others?

Assess for signs of self-directed violence, such as cutting (see Figure 29.3); assess for evidence of alcohol or drug use.

Diagnosis

Priorities for nursing care are based on patient-specific needs and strengths, as well as on functional capability. For example, high-functioning patients who have insight into the nature and effects of their PD may be well suited for patient teaching, whereas patients who demonstrate significant functional impairment and lack of insight may not benefit from teaching. Some care needs that may be appropriate for inclusion in the plan of care for the patient with a PD may include the following:

- Risk of injury
- Potential for violence (against self or others)
- Potential for self-mutilation, NSSI
- Inadequate coping skills
- Social isolation
- Anxiety
- Disturbed personal identity
- Impaired family functioning.

Planning

Patient goals are measurable, patient-specific outcomes that allow for evaluation of the efficacy of nursing interventions. Goals of care should be realistic and tailored to the patient. Examples of patient goals that may be applicable to the nursing plan of care for the patient with a PD include the following:

- The patient will remain free from injury.
- The patient will refrain from violent behaviors.
- The patient will report a reduction in anxiety.
- The patient will verbalize emotions to staff.
- The patient will adhere to established rules and guidelines.
- The patient will actively participate in one-on-one and/or group therapy sessions.

Implementation

As with assessment and planning, implementation of the nursing plan of care will vary based on the manifestations and effects of the patient's PD. In addition to promoting the safety of the patient and others with whom the patient interacts, promoting comfort—both physical and psychosocial—is a priority of care. Psychosocial aspects of comfort promotion include building a therapeutic relationship with the patient and effectively managing conflicts. In a respectful, professional manner, the nurse establishes clear boundaries and limits for the patient. For patients who are amenable to socialization, the nurse identifies patient-specific interventions that will afford the patient the opportunity to learn and practice social skills.

Promote Safety

With all patients, priorities of care include injury prevention and safety promotion. For patients with PDs, some of whom are prone to self-destructive and impulsive behavior, the emphasis on injury prevention is heightened. Behavioral contracts that outline prohibited actions and the consequences of those actions may be used to establish clear guidelines and expectations with regard to any form of behavior, including that related to injuring self or others. Basic precautions for patients in hospital settings include:

- Ensuring that the patient's environment is free from items that may be used to harm self or others
- Providing close supervision and monitoring
- Encouraging patients to seek assistance from members of the healthcare team when they need to process their feelings, including when they perceive that their stress levels are rising
- Encouraging patients to participate actively in therapy and groups.

In the community setting, nurses and clinicians monitor patients for safety. Some considerations include the following points on medication safety and self-monitoring of mood and environment:

- Provide medication teaching regarding dosage and intervals, anticipated side effects, potential adverse reactions, and when to contact the HCP for follow-up care.
- With adolescents and young adult patients, make sure that the patient and the family or support persons know that SSRIs carry an FDA black box warning regarding increased suicidality for that age group and are aware of the warning signs of increased suicidal ideation.
- Ensure that patients who engage in NSSI know to contact their HCPs if they experience an increase in the occurrence or severity of these behaviors.

- Make sure that patients live in a safe environment where they will not be exposed to violence or be financially or emotionally exploited. Patients who receive disability payments for their mental health disorders are often isolated and can be preyed on by coercive family or individuals in the community.

Promote the Therapeutic Relationship

The ineffective social skills and impaired perceptions that often accompany PDs can create unique challenges in the establishment of a therapeutic nurse–patient relationship. Moreover, for patients who struggle with trust issues, unplanned admission to a hospital or treatment center can exacerbate their anxiety and sense of mistrust. Consistency with patient care—including demonstration of respect for the patient at all times—is one of the first steps to building trust.

- Avoid stigmatizing the patient because of the illness. Individuals with PDs have a neurobiological imbalance in the brain, not a defective personality. Also, consider that many patients also have medical conditions and have experienced stress, trauma, severe childhood abuse, prolonged substance abuse, and exposure to toxins and have genetically inherited traits.
- Balance flexibility with firmness. Patients may be unwilling to accept responsibility and unable to remember agreements, and they may be difficult to understand, inconsistent with discipline, poor at keeping appointments, and unpredictable emotionally. However, missed appointments, lying, and dangerous behaviors cannot be accepted. Precise oral and written communication is the best way to avoid misunderstandings.
- Focus on the strengths of individuals and their family systems. Clinicians will have more success and reduce stress and stigmatization if they match interventions with patient strengths.

Establish Boundaries

Boundaries are limits that define what is acceptable to an individual in every facet of life, including the physical, mental, emotional, sexual, relational, spiritual, and professional realms. A breach of boundaries occurs when those limitations are ignored or exceeded. In many ways, definition of boundaries occurs during childhood, beginning in infancy, through experiencing interactions with others.

In the context of the nurse–patient relationship, establishing and maintaining healthy boundaries promotes a sense of safety and predictability for the patient. As the result of past experiences, including a history of abuse and a sense of shame that may accompany the stigmatization often associated with mental illness, the patient with a PD may have unhealthy, unclear, or nonexistent boundaries. The nurse can help the patient to understand and set healthy boundaries through interventions such as teaching, as well as through role playing with the patient. In helping the patient establish healthy boundaries, the nurse can use role play to simulate situations in which the patient is faced with potential boundary violations, assess the patient's coping skills, and teach the patient about healthy responses to attempted boundary violations (Potter & Moller, 2020).

Regardless of the patient's behaviors, the nurse is responsible for maintaining healthy professional boundaries. Provision 2 of the American Nurses Association's Code of Ethics (2015) requires the nurse to establish and maintain boundaries and to effectively set limits with patients. Establishing professional boundaries includes choosing which of the nurse's personal information is appropriate for sharing with the patient. Especially because of the intimate nature of the nurse–patient relationship, the patient also may ask personal questions—for example, whether or not the nurse is married or has children. Sharing some degree of background information in an appropriate, professional manner can strengthen the nurse–patient relationship; however, the oversharing of personal information is detrimental and nontherapeutic. Through sharing details of personal problems and struggles with the patient, the nurse can create an unnecessary—and unethical—burden for the patient, who is the one seeking care. Boundary violations occur when meeting the nurse's needs takes precedence over meeting the patient's needs. For further illustration of maintaining professional boundaries in nursing, see **Table 29.5** ».

Communicating with Patients

Working Phase

Patients with antisocial personality disorder can have symptoms of impulsivity, extreme negative emotions, aggression, and poor adherence to rules and social norms, which can lead to a wide range of interpersonal and social issues and behaviors. The nurse working with these patients should implement limit setting to establish a therapeutic milieu and promote safety.

1. Identify the unacceptable behavior(s).
2. Clearly outline the consequences of breaking rules.
3. Clearly state the expected behaviors.

For example, if the patient asks for the nurse's phone number, an appropriate response would be to restate the limits of the relationship and focus the patient's attention on a therapeutic issue:

- It is not acceptable to ask me for my phone number. Our relationship will remain professional, as nurse and patient. We need to refocus and discuss how you have been having some issues today with your peers.

Cursing or violations of other guidelines of the care setting must also be addressed professionally and objectively:

- Using bad language is not permitted on the unit. If you cannot follow this rule, you will not be allowed in the TV room until you can control your behavior.

» **Stay Current:** The National Council of State Boards of Nursing offers additional guidance and strategies regarding professional boundaries at https://www.ncsbn.org/professionalboundaries.htm.

Evaluation

Evaluation is a dynamic, ongoing feature of the nursing process that includes identifying the degree to which patients have achieved the goals and outcomes established in relationship to each nursing diagnosis. While goals and outcomes for

TABLE 29.5 Maintaining Professional Boundaries in Nursing

Boundaries Maintained	Boundaries Breached
Keeping one's personal life private and focusing on the patient's needs	Sharing details of personal life, issues, and/or problems with a patient
Sharing limited details about basic background information when asked, such as marital status, number of children, educational background, and professional nursing background	Discussing the state of one's marriage (e.g., marital separation or currently in the process of divorce); sharing about one's children's behavioral problems or medical challenges; discussing personal, emotional, or legal problems or setbacks
Maintaining all patient-related information as confidential, and discussing only relevant aspects of the patient's condition and care with the necessary healthcare team members in the workplace	Revealing patient-related information to anyone who is not involved in planning or administering care to the patient
Limiting discussion of patients and their care to within the clinical setting	Discussing patients and their care in the hospital cafeteria, hallways, or other nonclinical areas; sharing any patient-related information through any format, including via social media
Interacting with the patient only during scheduled duty hours for professional intents and purposes	Visiting the patient during off-duty hours, in or away from the clinical setting; communicating with the patient by any means for purposes other than those directly related to the patient's plan of healthcare
Demonstrating respect for one's institution or organization, work policies, and other members of the healthcare team and declining to discuss workplace-related conflicts or criticisms	Venting to the patient about issues or concerns regarding one's employer, work policies, or other members of the healthcare team
Facilitating referrals for patients with financial needs to appropriate organizations or assisting the patient in connecting with official agencies who can provide assistance	Giving patients personal items or financial assistance
Identification and referral to appropriate healthcare team members for resolution of the patient's personal conflicts	Choosing to side with a patient during conflict between patients and their spouses, family members, or significant others

Sources: Based on Go (2017); Potter and Moller (2020).

the patient with a PD will vary based on patient individuality and the nursing diagnoses included in the nursing plan of care, examples of achieved outcomes relevant to the evaluation of patient care may include the following:

- The patient remains free from injury.
- The patient does not demonstrate violent behaviors toward self or others.
- The patient verbalizes understanding of the concept of boundaries.
- The patient verbalizes understanding of the principles of respecting boundaries related to self and others.
- The patient actively participates in individual and/or group therapy.

Given that many of the personality disorders discussed in this section are resistive to treatment and the therapies are challenging and lengthy even for motivated patients, treatment failures do occur. In these cases, the clinician should reevaluate the plan of care. This includes conducting a strengths-based assessment of patients and their supports: Has the patient's financial situation changed, necessitating more community services? Has a lifelong support died or disappeared from a patient's life, affecting the ability to cope? Are additional community services available that were not in place when the patient's last plan of care was constructed? Is the patient enthusiastic about the new plan of care and capable of participating in the interventions proposed?

Nursing Care Plan

A Patient with Borderline Personality Disorder

Kathryn Harrison is a 20-year-old female patient transported to the ED by law enforcement. Officer Rick Natami, the attending police officer, reported that she broke a window with her fist while arguing with her boyfriend. Subsequently, Ms. Harrison told her boyfriend she was going to kill herself. At that point, her boyfriend called 911. In addition to law enforcement, emergency medical personnel also responded to the call. Officer Natami reported that Ms. Harrison was combative at the scene and would not allow the paramedics to assess her injuries, nor would she permit them to transport her to the ED by ambulance. Her boyfriend had handed her a dish towel to wrap her hand, and while there is blood visible on the towel, the bleeding does not appear to be copious. As a result of her injuries and her threat to commit suicide, Officer Natami handcuffed and transported Ms. Harrison in his squad car for physical and psychiatric evaluation.

Upon arrival to the ED, Ms. Harrison is cursing at Officer Natami, as well as anyone with whom she makes eye contact, including her attending nurse. When the ED physician asks if he can assess her injuries, she replies, "Yeah, if you tell the cop to take these handcuffs off me and make him leave! You're cool, but he's a total jerk!" The ED physician tells Ms. Harrison he will ask the police officer to remove the handcuffs and stand outside the examination room, but only if she agrees to remain calm and noncombative. She agrees, and the officer removes her handcuffs and steps outside the room. Because Ms. Harrison has previously been treated at the facility, her electronic medical record (EMR) is accessible. Based on her EMR, her past medical history includes BPD and previous treatment for self-inflicted superficial leg lacerations. Before the ED physician evaluates Ms. Harrison's lacerations, he quietly asks the nurse to order a psychiatric consultation for the patient.

Nursing Care Plan *(continued)*

ASSESSMENT	DIAGNOSES	PLANNING
Following closure of her lacerations, Ms. Harrison agrees to allow the nurse to assess her vital signs and auscultate her heart and lungs. Vital signs include temperature 97.3°F oral, pulse 90 bpm, respirations 20/min, and blood pressure 133/71 mmHg. Ms. Harrison's heart tones are normal; however, the nurse hears faint, bibasilar wheezes in her lungs. When the nurse asks if Ms. Harrison has had any recent respiratory problems, she replies, "I have no idea. I don't have health insurance, and nobody cares anyway. I'm just a piece of garbage." Ms. Harrison begins to cry and states, "I don't know why I get so mad. I'm such an idiot! My boyfriend should dump me, just like everybody else does." The nurse verbally reassures her that she is safe and will receive the best possible care. Ms. Harrison replies, "I'm sorry I called you names earlier—you're the nicest nurse I've ever met. The nurses on the psych floor are mean. They're only going to make me take a bunch of pills. I wish I could stay here, with you."	■ Risk for injury ■ Potential for violence (against self or others) ■ Compromised skin integrity ■ Potential for self-mutilation ■ Inadequate coping skills ■ Risk of suicide	■ The patient will sustain no further physical injury. ■ The patient will not injure others. ■ The patient's wound will be closed and protected from further injury or contamination. ■ The patient will express her emotions to members of the healthcare team in a nondestructive manner. ■ The patient contracts for safety by agreeing to notify staff if she experiences any thoughts of NSSI or suicide.

IMPLEMENTATION

- Maintain or delegate a team member to maintain constant observation of the patient to assess for and prevent injurious behavior.
- Outline behavioral guidelines for the patient, including the requirement that she cannot injure herself or attempt to injure others.
- Follow institutional guidelines for the application of physical restraints as needed.
- Seek to establish rapport with the patient through demonstrating respect and establishing therapeutic communication patterns.
- Enforce firm boundaries with the patient to prevent staff splitting.
- Encourage the patient to verbalize her emotions and use active listening techniques.
- Educate the patient about dressing changes and basic principles of wound care.

EVALUATION

Following evaluation by the on-call psychiatrist, Ms. Harrison was admitted to the psychiatric unit and hospitalized for 3 days. During her stay, she was argumentative with several of the staff nurses and patient care technicians, but she appeared to favor one of the nurses, Jim. When Jim was on duty, she first insisted that he be assigned to care for her but later refused to allow him to be her nurse, stating, "He's a jerk, just like my boyfriend." In meetings with the clinical psychologist, Ms. Harrison reported a history of physical abuse during childhood, including sexual abuse by an uncle, as well as several physically abusive dating relationships. When asked about abuse in her current relationship, she denied any abuse and reported that her boyfriend was "the only person who ever cared" about her. The psychologist referred Ms. Harrison to a counselor who specialized in DBT, but she declined and stated, "I don't want to keep talking about stuff that happened when I was a kid. I just need to stop getting so mad at my boyfriend." She sustained no further injury during her hospitalization and was not physically abusive toward staff. Upon discharge, Ms. Harrison agreed to return to the ED in 7 days for suture removal.

CRITICAL THINKING

1. What other nursing interventions might be appropriate for inclusion in the plan of care for Ms. Harrison?
2. Describe two instances in which Ms. Harrison demonstrated splitting. How should the nurse address patients who demonstrate splitting behaviors?
3. Why did the psychologist recommend DBT for Ms. Harrison? How is DBT believed to be beneficial to patients diagnosed with BPD?

REVIEW Personality Disorders

RELATE Link the Concepts and Exemplars

Linking the exemplar on personality disorders with the concept of stress and coping:

1. In relationship to personality disorders (PDs), describe three behaviors that reflect impaired coping.

2. How does manipulation, which is a behavior associated with several PDs, affect the nurse's morale and stress level? Explain how the nurse can effectively cope with manipulation in the course of a therapeutic relationship.

Linking the exemplar on personality disorders with the concept of safety:

3. Which PDs are associated with a high risk for injury? How does impulsiveness increase the risk for injury?

4. A patient who is diagnosed with schizotypal personality disorder tells her nurse she hears voices that are ordering her to cut her wrists. How should the nurse respond? To protect the patient from injury, what actions should the nurse take?

READY Go to Volume 3: Clinical Nursing Skills

REFER Go to Pearson MyLab Nursing and eText

REFLECT Apply Your Knowledge

Steffan Richter, a 32-year-old man, was recently diagnosed with avoidant personality disorder. The psychiatrist who made the diagnosis recommended that he begin psychotherapy, but he declined after learning that group therapy may be indicated at some point during treatment. To Mr. Richter, psychotherapy would be almost unbearable, but talking about his issues in a group setting would be impossible.

Since graduating from college 10 years ago, Mr. Richter has worked as a mailroom clerk. Having earned a bachelor's degree in accounting, he is qualified to apply for other, higher-paying positions within the company. However, he chooses to maintain his current position, as his present job responsibilities greatly limit his need to interact with other individuals. Several years earlier, Mr. Richter was offered a supervisory position; however, he declined the offer. The promotion would have increased his salary significantly, but the job responsibilities included a great deal of interaction with the mailroom team and administrators.

During lunchtime, the mailroom shuts down operations so all employees can eat their meals together in the staff lounge. Because he finds the lunchtime social interaction in the staff lounge to be forced, unpleasant, and overwhelming, Mr. Richter remains in the quiet mailroom and reads a book during his break. Company policy restricts employees from eating in any areas other than the staff lounge, and employees are forbidden to leave the building during their work shift. Therefore, Mr. Richter never eats lunch during the week.

Because Mr. Richter is extremely shy and quiet, several of his coworkers refer to him as "the invisible man." He is also very underweight, and some of his coworkers tease him about his size. Although he finds his nickname and the teasing to be cruel and humiliating, Mr. Richter does not share his feelings; instead, he resolves to stay as far away as possible from the group. Several of his coworkers have invited him to join the group for social activities outside of work; however, he declines their invitations, as he knows his coworkers will only further demean and embarrass him. To avoid being humiliated or rejected, Mr. Richter does not build friendships at or away from his workplace.

1. How are the effects of avoidant personality disorder impacting Mr. Richter's occupational and professional advancement?
2. In what ways does avoidant personality disorder impact this patient socially, both in and out of his workplace?
3. How does avoidant personality disorder affect Mr. Richter's nutritional habits?

References

Academy for Eating Disorders. (2020). *Resources: Treatment options*. https://www.aedweb.org/resources/about-eating-disorders/treatment-options

Acford, E., & Davies, J. (2019). Exploring therapeutic engagement with individuals with a diagnosis of personality disorder in acute psychiatric inpatient settings: A nursing team perspective. *International Journal of Mental Health Nursing, 28*(5), 1176–1185. https://doi.org/10.1111/inm.12629

Ainsworth, M. D. S. (1973). The development of infant–mother attachment. In B. Cardwell & H. Ricciuti (Eds.), *Review of child development research* (Vol. 3, pp. 1–94). University of Chicago Press.

American Nurses Association (ANA). (2015). *Code of ethics for nurses with interpretive statements*. Retrieved from http://nursingworld.org/Document-Vault/Ethics-1/Code-of-Ethics-for-Nurses.html

American Psychiatric Association (APA). (2013). *Diagnostic and statistical manual of mental disorders* (5th ed.). Author.

American Psychological Association. (2020). *What causes personality disorders?* https://www.apa.org/topics/personality/disorders-causes

Anderson, M., & Jiang, J. (2018). *Teens, social media, & technology 2018*. https://www.pewresearch.org/internet/2018/05/31/teens-social-media-technology-2018/

Ayano, B., & Amentie, B. (2018). Assessment of prevalence and risk factors for anemia among pregnant mothers attending ANC clinic at Adama Hospital Medical College, Adama, Ethiopia, 2017. *Journal of Gynecology and Obstetrics, 6*(3), 31–39.

Ayvaci, E. M. (2017). Religious barriers to mental healthcare. *American Journal of Psychiatry Residents' Journal*. https://ajp.psychiatryonline.org/doi/full/10.1176/appi.ajp-rj.2016.110706

Ball, L., Tully, R. J., & Egan, V. (2017). The SAPAS, personality traits, and personality disorder. *Journal of Personality Disorders, 31*(3), 385–398. https://doi.org/10.1521/pedi_2016_30_259

Bangash, A. (2020). Personality disorders in later life: epidemiology, presentation and management. *BJPsych Advances, 26*(4), 208–218.

Barańczuk, U. (2019). The five factor model of personality and alexithymia: A meta-analysis. *Journal of Research in Personality, 78*, 227–248. https://doi.org/10.1016/j.jrp.2018.12.005

Bateman, A., & Fonagy, P. (2019). A randomized controlled trial of a mentalization-based intervention (MBT-FACTS) for families of people with borderline personality disorder. *Personality Disorders: Theory, Research, and Treatment, 10*(1), 70–79.

Beck, J. G., Woodward, M. J., Pickover, A. M., Lipinski, A. J., Dodson, T. S., & Tran, H. N. (2019). Does a history of childhood abuse moderate the association between symptoms of posttraumatic stress disorder and borderline personality disorder in survivors of intimate partner violence? *Journal of Clinical Psychology, 75*(6), 1114–1128.

Behmaneshpour, F., Irandegani, F., & Miandoab, N. Y. (2019). Relationship between the nurses' observance of professional ethics and quality of nursing care from the patients' point of view. *Drug Invention Today, 12*(12), 2876–2880.

Berman, A., Snyder, S. J., & Frandsen, G. (2021). *Kozier and Erb's fundamentals of nursing: Concepts, process, and practice* (11th ed.). Pearson.

Berner, L. A., Brown, T. A., Lavender, J. M., Lopez, E., Wierenga, C. E., & Kaye, W. H. (2019). Neuroendocrinology of reward in anorexia nervosa and bulimia nervosa: Beyond leptin and ghrelin. *Molecular and Cellular Endocrinology, 497*, 110320. https://doi.org/10.1016/j.mce.2018.10.018

Blikshavn, T., Halvorsen, I., & Rø, Ø. (2020). Physical restraint during inpatient treatment of adolescent anorexia nervosa: frequency, clinical correlates, and associations with outcome at five-year follow-up. *Journal of Eating Disorders, 8*, 20. https://doi.org/10.1186/s40337-020-00297-1

Boudouda, N. E., & Gana, K. (2020). Neuroticism, conscientiousness and extraversion interact to predict depression: A confirmation in a non-Western culture. *Personality & Individual Differences, 167*, 110219. https://doi.org/10.1016/j.paid.2020.110219

Bowlby, J. (1969). *Attachment and loss: Vol. 1. Loss*. Basic Books.

Brambilla, F., Santonastaso, P., Caregaro, L., & Favaro, A. (2018). Growth hormone and insulin-like growth factor 1 secretions in eating disorders: Correlations with psychopathological aspects of the disorders. *Psychiatry Research, 263*, 233–237.

Buchman, S., Attia, E., Dawson, L., & Steinglass, J. E. (2019). Steps of care for adolescents with anorexia nervosa-A Delphi study. *International Journal of Eating Disorders, 52*(7), 777–785.

Cagle, J. G., Osteen, P., Sacco, P., & Frey, J. J. (2017). Psychosocial assessment by hospice social workers: A content review of instruments from a national sample. *Journal of Pain and Symptom Management, 53*(1), 40–48.

Carrard, I., Rothen, S., & Rodgers, R. F. (2020). Body image and disordered eating in older women: A Tripartite Sociocultural model. *Eating Behaviors, 38*, 101412. https://doi.org/10.1016/j.eatbeh.2020.101412

Cattane, N., Rossi, R., Lanfredi, M., & Cattaneo, A. (2017). Borderline personality disorder and childhood trauma: exploring the affected biological systems and mechanisms. *BMC Psychiatry, 17*, 1–14.

Cella, S., Fei, L., D'Amico, R., Giardiello, C., Allaria, A., & Cotrufo, P. (2019). Binge eating disorder and related features in bariatric surgery candidates. *Open Medicine (Warsaw, Poland), 14*, 407–415.

Chanen, A. M., & Thompson, K. N. (2018). Early intervention for personality disorder. *Current Opinion in Psychology, 21*, 132–135.

Cheng, K. (2017). "My husband is possessed by a jinn": A case study in transcultural mental health. *Australasian Psychiatry, 25*(5), 471–473.

Chung, D. (2018). The eight stages of psychosocial protective development: Developmental psychology. *Journal of Behavioral and Brain Science, 8*(6), 369. https://doi.org/10.4236/jbbs.2018.86024

Cleveland Clinic. (2020). *Personality disorders: Diagnosis and treatment*. https://my.clevelandclinic.org/health/diseases/9636-personality-disorders-overview/diagnosis-and-tests

Correa, J. K., & Sandage, S. J. (2018). Relational spirituality as scaffolding for cognitive-behavioral therapy. *Spirituality in Clinical Practice, 5*(1), 54.

Cost, J., Krantz, M., & Mehler, P. (2020). Medical complications of anorexia nervosa. *Cleveland Clinic Journal of Medicine, 87*(6), 361–366.

Cox, N. J., Ibrahim, K., Sayer, A. A., Robinson, S. M., & Roberts, H. C. (2019). Assessment and treatment of the anorexia of aging: A systematic review. *Nutrients, 11*(1), 144. h4

Crowley, G., Molyneaux, E., Nath, S., Trevillion, K., Moran, P., & Howard, L. M. (2020). Disordered personality traits and psychiatric morbidity in pregnancy: a population-based study. *Archives of Women's Mental Health, 23*, 43–52.

Czajkowski, N., Aggen, S. H., Krueger, R. F., Kendler, K. S., Neale, M. C., Knudsen, G. P., et al. (2018). A twin study of normative personality and DSM-IV personality disorder criterion counts: evidence for separate genetic influences. *American Journal of Psychiatry, 175*(7), 649–656.

Day, N. J., Hunt, A., Cortis-Jones, L., & Grenyer, B. F. (2018). Clinician attitudes towards borderline personality disorder: A 15-year comparison. *Personality and Mental Health, 12*(4), 309–320.

de Aquino Ferreira, L. F., Queiroz Pereira, F. H., Neri Benevides, A., & Aguiar Melo, M. C. (2018). Borderline personality disorder and sexual abuse: A systematic review. *Psychiatry Research, 262*, 70–77.

Dickens, G. L., Lamont, E., Stirling, F. J., Mullen, J., & MacArthur, N. (2019). Mixed-methods evaluation of an educational intervention to change mental health nurses' attitudes to people diagnosed with borderline personality disorder. *Journal of Clinical Nursing, 28*(13/14), 2613–2623.

dos Santos, A. M., Benute, G. R. G., dos Santos, N. O., Nomura, R. M. Y., de Lucia, M. C. S., & Francisco, R. P. V. (2017). Presence of eating disorders and its relationship to anxiety and depression in pregnant women. *Midwifery, 51*, 12–15.

Duncan, L., Yilmaz, Z., Gaspar, H., Walters, R., Goldstein, J., Anttila, V., et al. (2017). Significant locus and metabolic genetic correlations revealed in genome-wide association study of anorexia nervosa. *American Journal of Psychiatry, 174*(9), 850–858.

Eckenrode, J., Campa, M. I., Morris, P. A., Henderson Jr., C. R., Bolger, K. E., Kitzman, H., & Olds, D. L. (2017). The prevention of child maltreatment through the nurse family partnership program: Mediating effects in a long-term follow-up study. *Child Maltreatment, 22*(2), 92–99.

Erriu, M., Cimino, S., & Cerniglia, L. (2020). The role of family relationships in eating disorders in adolescents: A narrative review. *Behavioral Sciences, 10*(4), 71. https://doi.org/10.3390/bs10040071

Erskine, H. E., & Whiteford, H. A. (2018). Epidemiology of binge eating disorder. *Current Opinion in Psychiatry, 31*(6), 462-470.

Fawcett, E. J., Fawcett, J. M., & Mazmanian, D. (2016). A meta-analysis of the worldwide prevalence of pica during pregnancy and the postpartum period. *International Journal of Gynecology & Obstetrics, 133*(3), 277–283. https://doi.org/10.1016/j.ijgo.2015.10.012

Fetissov, S. O., & Hökfelt, T. (2019). On the origin of eating disorders: Altered signaling between gut microbiota, adaptive immunity and the brain melanocortin system regulating feeding behavior. *Current Opinion in Pharmacology, 48*, 82–91.

Fiorilli, C., Grimaldi Capitello, T., Barni, D., Buonomo, I., & Gentile, S. (2019). Predicting adolescent depression: The interrelated roles of self-esteem and interpersonal stressors. *Frontiers in Psychology, 10*, 565. https://doi.org/10.3389/fpsyg.2019.00565/full

Flora, K. (2018). The therapeutic relationship in borderline personality disorder: A cognitive perspective. *Journal of Evidence-Based Psychotherapies, 18*(2), 19–33.

Florence, S. A. (2020). *Understanding the distinctive presentations of therapist countertransference with Cluster B personality disorders.* Unpublished doctoral dissertation, Nova Southeastern University. https://nsuworks.nova.edu/cps_stuetd/140/

Forrest, L. N., Jones, P. J., Ortiz, S. N., & Smith, A. R. (2018). Core psychopathology in anorexia nervosa and bulimia nervosa: A network analysis. *International Journal of Eating Disorders, 51*(7), 668–679.

Frögéli, E., Rudman, A., & Gustavsson, P. (2019). The relationship between task mastery, role clarity, social acceptance, and stress: An intensive longitudinal study with a sample of newly registered nurses. *International Journal of Nursing Studies, 91*, 60–69. https://doi.org/10.1016/j.ijnurstu.2018.10.007

Gardner, M. J., Thomas, H. J., & Erskine, H. E. (2019). The association between five forms of child maltreatment and depressive and anxiety disorders: A systematic review and meta-analysis. *Child Abuse and Neglect, 96*, 104082.

Gawda, B. (2018). Cross-cultural studies on the prevalence of personality disorders. *Current. Issues in Personality Psychology, 6*(4), 318–329.

Gianni, A. D., De Donatis, D., Valente, S., De Ronchi, D., & Atti, A. R. (2020). Eating disorders: Do PET and SPECT have a role?: A systematic review of the literature. *Psychiatry Research: Neuroimaging Section, 300*, 111065. https://doi.org/10.1016/j.pscychresns.2020.111065

Gittins, C. B., & Hunt, C. (2019). Parental behavioural control in adolescence: How does it affect self-esteem and self-criticism? *Journal of Adolescence, 73*, 26–35.

Glashouwer, K. A., van der Veer, R. M. L., Adipatria, F., de Jong, P. J., & Vocks, S. (2019). The role of body image disturbance in the onset, maintenance, and relapse of anorexia nervosa: A systematic review. *Clinical Psychology Review, 74*, 101771. https://doi.org/10.1016/j.cpr.2019.101771

Go, R. A. (2017). Maintaining professional boundaries in nursing. *Nursing Bulletin.* https://www.ncbon.com/myfiles/downloads/course-bulletin-offerings-articles/bulletin-article-winter-2018-maintaining-professional-boundaries.pdf

Goodman, E. L., Baker, J. H., Peat, C. M., Yilmaz, Z., Bulik, C. M., & Watson, H. J. (2018). Weight suppression and weight elevation are associated with eating disorder symptomatology in women age 50 and older: Results of the gender and body image study. *International Journal of Eating Disorders, 51*(8), 835–841.

Gündoğdu, Y. B., & Turan, Y. (2018). Evaluation of critical periods during the development of the personality in terms of religious education. *Ordu University Journal of Social Science Research, 8*(1), 229–239.

Hart, W., Tortoriello, G. K., & Richardson, K. (2018). Are personality disorder traits ego-syntonic or ego-dystonic?: Revisiting the issue by considering functionality. *Journal of Research in Personality, 76*, 124–128.

Hock, R. S., Bryce, C. P., Fischer, L., First, M. B., Fitzmaurice, G. M., Costa, P. T., & Galler, J. R. (2018). Childhood malnutrition and maltreatment are linked with personality disorder symptoms in adulthood: Results from a Barbados lifespan cohort. *Psychiatry Research, 269*, 301–308.

Holland, K., Dickson, A., & Dickson, A. (2018). "To the horror of experts": Reading beneath scholarship on pro-ana online communities. *Critical Public Health, 28*(5), 522–533.

Hübel, C., Leppä, V., Breen, G., & Bulik, C. M. (2018). Rigor and reproducibility in genetic research on eating disorders. *International Journal of Eating Disorders, 51*(7), 593–607. https://doi.org/10.1002/eat.22896

Ilagan, G. S., & Choi-Kain, L. W. (2020). General psychiatric management for adolescents (GPM-A) with borderline personality disorder. *Current Opinion in Psychology, 37*. https://doi.org/10.1016/j.copsyc.2020.05.006

Jagielska, G., & Kacperska, I. (2017). Outcome, comorbidity and prognosis in anorexia nervosa. *Psychiatria Polska, 51*(2), 205–218.

Karkkola, P., Kuittinen, M., & Hintsa, T. (2019). Role clarity, role conflict, and vitality at work: The role of the basic needs. *Scandinavian Journal of Psychology, 60*(5), 456–463.

Kawamoto, T. (2020). The moderating role of attachment style on the relationship between self-concept clarity and self-esteem. *Personality and Individual Differences, 152*, 109604. https://doi.org/10.1016/j.paid.2019.109604

Keizer, R., Helmerhorst, K. O. W., & van Rijn-van Gelderen, L. (2019). Perceived quality of the mother–adolescent and father–adolescent attachment relationship and adolescents' self-esteem. *Journal of Youth & Adolescence, 48*(6), 1203–1217.

Kendler, K. S., Aggen, S. H., Gillespie, N., Krueger, R. F., Czajkowski, N., Ystrom, E., & Reichborn-Kjennerud, T. (2019). The structure of genetic and environmental influences on normative personality, abnormal personality traits, and personality disorder symptoms. *Psychological Medicine, 49*(8), 1392–1399.

Khalifa, I., & Goldman, R. D. (2019). Anorexia nervosa requiring admission in adolescents. *Canadian Family Physician, 65*(2), 102–108.

Krause-Utz, A., Winter, D., Schriner, F., Chiu, C.-D., Lis, S., Spinhoven, P., et al. (2018). Reduced amygdala reactivity and impaired working memory during dissociation in borderline personality disorder. *European Archives of Psychiatry and Clinical Neuroscience, 268*(4), 401–415.

Krauss, S., Orth, U., & Robins, R. W. (2020). Family environment and self-esteem development: A longitudinal study from age 10 to 16. *Journal of Personality and Social Psychology, 119*(2), 457–478.

Leising, D., Scherbaum, S., Packmohr, P., & Zimmermann, J. (2018). Substance and evaluation in personality disorder diagnoses. *Journal of Personality Disorders, 32*(6), 766–783.

Lichtenstein, M. B., Hemmingsen, S. D., & Støving, R. K. (2017). Identification of eating disorder symptoms in Danish adolescents with the SCOFF questionnaire. *Nordic Journal of Psychiatry, 71*(5), 340–347.

Limbers, C. A., Cohen, L. A., & Gray, B. A. (2018). Eating disorders in adolescent and young adult males: prevalence, diagnosis, and treatment strategies. *Adolescent Health, Medicine and Therapeutics, 9*, 111–116. https://doi.org/10.2147/AHMT.S147480

Linardon, J., Wade, T. D., de la Piedad Garcia, X., & Brennan, L. (2017). The efficacy of cognitive-behavioral therapy for eating disorders: A systematic review and meta-analysis. *Journal of Consulting and Clinical Psychology, 85*(11), 1080–1094.

Little, H., Tickle, A., & das Nair, R. (2018). Process and impact of dialectical behaviour therapy: A systematic review of perceptions of clients with a diagnosis of borderline personality disorder. *Psychology & Psychotherapy: Theory, Research & Practice, 91*(3), 278–301.

MacDonald, D. E., & Trottier, K. (2019). Rapid improvements in emotion regulation predict eating disorder psychopathology and functional impairment at 6-month follow-up in individuals with bulimia nervosa and purging disorder. *International Journal of Eating Disorders, 52*(8), 962–967.

Mangweth-Matzek, B., & Hoek, H. W. (2017). Epidemiology and treatment of eating disorders in men and women of middle and older age. *Current Opinion in Psychiatry, 30*(6), 446–451.

Mantel, Ä., Hirschberg, A. L., & Stephansson, O. (2020). Association of maternal eating disorders with pregnancy and neonatal outcomes. *JAMA Psychiatry, 77*(3), 285–293.

Matsumoto, A., & Rodgers, R. F. (2020). A review and integrated theoretical model of the development of body image and eating disorders among midlife and aging men. *Clinical Psychology Review, 81*, 101903. https://doi.org/10.1016/j.cpr.2020.101903

Mayo Clinic. (2018). *Binge eating disorder.* https://www.mayoclinic.org/diseases-conditions/binge-eating-disorder/symptoms-causes/syc-20353627

Mayo Clinic. (2020). *Schizotypal personality disorder.* https://www.mayoclinic.org/diseases-conditions/schizotypal-personality-disorder/symptoms-causes/syc-20353919?p=1

MentalHealth.gov. (2017). *Anorexia nervosa.* https://www.mentalhealth.gov/what-to-look-for/eating-disorders/anorexia

Mental Health America. (2020). *Personality disorder.* https://www.mhanational.org/conditions/personality-disorder

Murray, S. B., Nagata, J. M., Griffiths, S., Calzo, J. P., Brown, T. A., Mitchison, D., et al. (2017). The enigma of male eating disorders: A critical review and synthesis. *Clinical Psychology Review, 57*, 1–11. https://doi.org/10.1016/j.cpr.2017.08.001

Muscogiuri, G., Formoso, G., Pugliese, G., Ruggeri, R. M., Scarano, E., & Colao, A. (2019). Prader-Willi syndrome: An uptodate on endocrine and metabolic complications. *Reviews in Endocrine and Metabolic Disorders, 20*(2), 239–250.

Naismith, I., Zarate Guerrero, S., & Feigenbaum, J. (2019). Abuse, invalidation, and lack of early warmth show distinct relationships with self-criticism, self-compassion, and fear of self-compassion in personality disorder. *Clinical Psychology & Psychotherapy, 26*(3), 350–361.

Nathan, J. (2018). The use of benign authority with severe borderline patients: A psychoanalytic paradigm. *British Journal of Psychotherapy, 34*(1), 61–77.

National Alliance on Mental Illness. (2017). *Borderline personality disorder.* https://www.nami.org/About-Mental-Illness/Mental-Health-Conditions/Borderline-Personality-Disorder/Support

National Alliance on Mental Illness. (2020). *Eating disorders.* https://www.nami.org/About-Mental-Illness/Mental-Health-Conditions/Eating-Disorders

National Association of Anorexia Nervosa and Associated Disorders (ANAD). (2020). *Eating disorder statistics.* https://anad.org/education-and-awareness/about-eating-disorders/eating-disorders-statistics/

National Center for Complementary and Integrative Health (NCCIH). (2018). *Complementary, alternative, or integrative health: What's in a name?* https://www.nccih.nih.gov/health/complementary-alternative-or-integrative-health-whats-in-a-name

National Eating Disorder Association (NEDA). (2018). *Statistics & research on eating disorders: Anorexia.* https://www.nationaleatingdisorders.org/statistics-research-eating-disorders

National Eating Disorder Collaboration (NEDC). (2020). *Early intervention.* https://www.nedc.com.au/eating-disorders/early-intervention/

National Institute for Health and Care Excellence. (2017). *Eating disorders: Recognition and treatment.* https://www.nice.org.uk/guidance/ng69/ifp/chapter/Anorexia-nervosa-treatment-for-adults

National Institute of Mental Health (NIMH). (2017a). *Borderline personality disorder.* https://www.nimh.nih.gov/health/topics/borderline-personality-disorder/index.shtml

National Institute of Mental Health (NIMH). (2017b). *Eating disorders.* https://www.nimh.nih.gov/health/statistics/eating-disorders.shtml

National Institute of Mental Health. (2019). *Eating disorders: About more than food.* https://www.nimh.nih.gov/health/publications/eating-disorders-new-trifold/index.shtml

Nenadić, I., Lamberth, S., & Reiss, N. (2017). Group schema therapy for personality disorders: A pilot study for implementation in acute psychiatric in-patient settings. *Psychiatry Research, 253*, 9–12.

Nurse–Family Partnership. (2019). *Proven effective through extensive research.* https://www.nursefamilypartnership.org/about/proven-results/

Oakley, T. J., Dey, I., Discombe, S., Fitzpatrick, L., & Paul, S. P. (2017). Recognition and management of eating disorders in children and young people. *Nursing Standard, 32*(9), 52–63.

Olajide, K., Munjiza, J., Moran, P., O'Connell, L., Newton-Howes, G., Bassett, P., et al. (2018). Development and psychometric properties of the Standardized Assessment of Severity of Personality Disorder (SASPD). *Journal of Personality Disorders, 32*(1), 44–56.

O'Mara, S., VanDine, L., Tarescavage, A. M., & Ben-Porath, D. (2020). Examining DBT day treatment in treating mood dysregulation expectancy and anxiety in women diagnosed with eating disorders. *Journal of Contemporary Psychotherapy*. https://doi.org/10.1007/s10879-020-09475-3

Orth, U., Erol, R. Y., & Luciano, E. C. (2018). Development of self-esteem from age 4 to 94 years: A meta-analysis of longitudinal studies. *Psychological Bulletin, 144*(10), 1045–1080. http://dx.doi.org/10.1037/bul0000161

O'Sullivan, M., Murphy, A., & Bourke, J. (2017). The cost of dialectic behaviour therapy (DBT) for people diagnosed with borderline personality disorder (BPD): A review of the literature. *Value in Health, 20*(9), PA714. https://doi.org/10.1016/j.jval.2017.08.1895

Park, E., & Kwon, M. (2018). Health-related internet use by children and adolescents: Systematic review. *Journal of Medical Internet Research, 20*(4), e120. https://doi.org/10.2196/jmir.7731

Peng, M., Wu, S., Shi, Z., Jiang, K., Shen, Y., Dedovic, K., & Yang, J. (2019). Brain regions in response to character feedback associated with the state self-esteem. *Biological Psychology, 148*, 107734. https://doi.org/10.1016/j.biopsycho.2019.107734

Pinto-Gouveia, J., Carvalho, S. A., Palmeira, L., Castilho, P., Duarte, C., Ferreira, C., et al. (2019). Incorporating psychoeducation, mindfulness and self-compassion in a new programme for binge eating (BEfree): Exploring processes of change. *Journal of Health Psychology, 24*(4), 466–479.

Potter, M. L., & Moller, M. D. (2020). *Psychiatric–mental health nursing: From suffering to hope* (2nd ed.). Pearson.

Pusch, S., Mund, M., Hagemeyer, B., Finn, C., & Wrzus, C. (2019). Personality development in emerging and young adulthood: A study of age differences. *European Journal of Personality, 33*(3), 245–263.

Rajput, N., Kumar, K., & Moudgil, K. (2020). Pica an eating disorder: An overview. *Pharmacophore, 11*(4), 11–14.

Rasheed, S., Younas, A., & Sundus, A. (2019). Self-awareness in nursing: A scoping review. *Journal of Clinical Nursing, 28*, 762–774. https://doi.org/10.1111/jocn.14708

Rentzsch, K., & Schröder, A. M. (2018). Stability and change in domain-specific self-esteem and global self-esteem. *European Journal of Personality, 32*(4), 353–370.

Ronningstam, E. F., Keng, S. L., Ridolfi, M. E., Arbabi, M., & Grenyer, B. F. (2018). Cultural aspects in symptomatology, assessment, and treatment of personality disorders. *Current Psychiatry Reports, 20*(4), 22.

Rono, B. C., Kombe, Y., & Makokha, A. (2018). Multiple micronutrients versus iron folic acid on pica and hemoglobin levels among pregnant women in Kenya. *Central African Journal of Public Health, 4*(4), 95–101.

Roy, A., Fuentes-Afflick, E., Fernald, L. C., & Young, S. L. (2018). Pica is prevalent and strongly associated with iron deficiency among Hispanic pregnant women living in the United States. *Appetite, 120*, 163–170.

Rūgendo, F. G. (2019). A discussion on basic virtues and crisis in the child's developmental stages. *European Journal of Research in Social Sciences, 7*(4), 26–32.

Sala, M., Shankar Ram, S., Vanzhula, I. A., & Levinson, C. A. (2020). Mindfulness and eating disorder psychopathology: A meta-analysis. *International Journal of Eating Disorders, 53*(6), 834–851.

Schwaba, T., & Bleidorn, W. (2018). Individual differences in personality change across the adult life span. *Journal of Personality, 86*(3), 450–464.

Serin, Y., & Şanlıer, N. (2018). Emotional eating, the factors that affect food intake, and basic approaches to nursing care of patients with eating disorders. *Journal of Psychiatric Nursing, 9*(2), 135–146. https://doi.org/10.14744/phd.2018.23600

Sheppard, K., & Duncan, C. (2018). Borderline personality disorder: Implications and best practice recommendations. *Nurse Practitioner, 43*(6), 14–17.

Shpigelman, C. N., & HaGani, N. (2019). The impact of disability type and visibility on self-concept and body image: Implications for mental health nursing. *Journal of Psychiatric and Mental Health Nursing, 26*(3–4), 77–86. https://doi.org/10.1111/jpm.12513

Shields, K. M., Fox, K. L., & Liebrecht, C. (2019). *Pearson nurse's drug guide*. Hoboken, NJ: Pearson Education, Inc.

Silvani, J., Schmidt, M. I., Zajdenverg, L., Galliano, L. M., & Antunes Nunes, M. A. (2020). Impact of binge eating during pregnancy on gestational weight gain and postpartum weight retention among women with gestational diabetes mellitus: LINDA-Brasil. *International Journal of Eating Disorders, 53*(11), 1818–1825. https://doi.org/10.1002/eat.23361

Skodol, A. (2019). *Overview of personality disorders*. Merck Manual Professional Version. https://www.merckmanuals.com/professional/psychiatric-disorders/personality-disorders/overview-of-personality-disorders

Smith, K. E., Mason, T. B., Crosby, R. D., Cao, L., Leonard, R. C., Wetterneck, C. T., et al. (2019). A comparative network analysis of eating disorder psychopathology and co-occurring depression and anxiety symptoms before and after treatment. *Psychological Medicine, 49*(2), 314–324.

Smith, V. M., Seimon, R. V., Harris, R. A., Sainsbury, A., & da Luz, F. Q. (2019). Less binge eating and loss of control over eating are associated with greater levels of mindfulness: Identifying patterns in postmenopausal women with obesity. *Behavioral Sciences, 9*(4), 36. https://doi.org/10.3390/bs9040036

Smoll, F. L. (2018). 5 warning signs for detecting eating disorders in athletes. *Psychology Today*. https://www.psychologytoday.com/us/blog/coaching-and-parenting-young-athletes/201809/5-warning-signs-detecting-eating-disorders-in

South, S. C., & Reichborn-Kjennerud, T. (2017). Genetics of personality disorders. *eLS*. https://doi.org/10.1002/9780470015902.a0022415.pub2

Spector, R. E. (2017). *Cultural diversity in health and illness* (9th ed.). Pearson.

Stacey, G., Baldwin, V., Thompson, B. J., & Aubeeluck, A. (2018). A focus group study exploring student nurse's experiences of an educational intervention focused on working with people with a diagnosis of personality disorder. *Journal of Psychiatric & Mental Health Nursing, 25*(7), 390–399.

Stanford Children's Health. (2020). *Eating disorders and young athletes*. https://www.stanfordchildrens.org/en/topic/default?id=eating-disorders-and-young-athletes-160-28

Stewart, C. S., Baudinet, J., Hall, R., Fiskå, M., Pretorius, N., Voulgari, S., et al. (2019). Multi-family therapy for bulimia nervosa in adolescence: A pilot study in a community eating disorder service. *Eating Disorders, 23*(4), 345–355.

Stoffers-Winterling, J. M., Storebø, O. J., Völlm, B. A., Mattivi, J. T., Nielsen, S. S., Kielsholm, M. L., et al. (2018). Pharmacological interventions for people with borderline personality disorder. *Cochrane Database of Systematic Reviews*, Issue 2, Article No. CD005653. https://doi.org/10.1002/14651858.CD005653

Stone, M. H. (2019). Borderline personality disorder: Clinical guidelines for treatment. *Psychodynamic Psychiatry, 47*(1), 5–26.

Substance Abuse and Mental Health Services Administration. (2019). *Trauma and violence*. https://www.samhsa.gov/trauma-violence

Tavolacci, M. P., Gillibert, A., Zhu Soubise, A., Grigioni, S., & Déchelotte, P. (2019). Screening four broad categories of eating disorders: Suitability of a clinical algorithm adapted from the SCOFF questionnaire. *BMC Psychiatry, 19*(1). https://doi.org/10.1186/s12888-019-2338-6

Tess, B. H. , Maximiano-Ferreira, L., Pajecki, D., & Wang, Y.P. (2019). Bariatric surgery and binge eating disorder: should surgeons care about it?: A literature review of prevalence and assessment tools. *Arquivos de Gastroenterologia, 56*(1), 55–60.

Thomas, J. J., Lawson, E. A., Micali, N., Misra, M., Deckersbach, T., & Eddy, K. T. (2017). Avoidant/restrictive food intake disorder: A three-dimensional model of neurobiology with implications for etiology and treatment. *Current Psychiatry Reports, 19*(8), 54.

Tian, L., Liu, L., & Shan, N. (2018). Parent–child relationships and resilience among Chinese adolescents: The mediating role of self-esteem. *Frontiers in Psychology, 9*, 1030. https://doi.org/10.3389/fpsyg.2018.01030

U.S. Department of Health and Human Services (DHHS). (2018). *Eating disorders*. https://www.womenshealth.gov/mental-health/mental-health-conditions/eating-disorders/bulimia-nervosa

van Schie, C. C., Chiu, C.-D., Rombouts, S. A. R. B., Heiser, W. J., & Elzinga, B. M. (2018). When compliments do not hit but critiques do: An fMRI study into self-esteem and self-knowledge in processing social feedback. *Social Cognitive & Affective Neuroscience, 13*(4), 404–417.

von Soest, T., Wagner, J., Hansen, T., & Gerstorf, D. (2018). Self-esteem across the second half of life: The role of socio-economic status, physical health, social relationships, and personality factors. *Journal of Personality & Social Psychology, 114*(6), 945–958.

Wesseldijk, L. W., Bartels, M., Vink, J. M., Beijsterveldt, C. E. M., Ligthart, L., Boomsma, D. I., & Middeldorp, C. M. (2018). Genetic and environmental influences on conduct and antisocial personality problems in childhood, adolescence, and adulthood. *European Child and Adolescent Psychiatry, 27*(9), 1123–1132.

Wilson S., Stroud, C., & Durbin, C. (2017). Interpersonal dysfunction in personality disorders: A meta-analytic review. *Psychology Bulletin, 143*(7), 677–734.

Winsper, C., Hall, J., Strauss, V. Y., & Wolke, D. (2017). Aetiological pathways to borderline personality disorder symptoms in early adolescence: Childhood dysregulated behaviour, maladaptive parenting and bully victimisation. *Borderline Personality Disorder and Emotion Dysregulation, 4*, 10. https://doi.org/10.1186/s40479-017-0060-x

Yilmaz, Z., Gottfredson, N. C., Zerwas, S. C., Bulik, C. M., & Micali, N. (2019). Developmental premorbid body mass index trajectories of adolescents with eating disorders in a longitudinal population cohort. *Journal of the American Academy of Child and Adolescent Psychiatry, 58*(2), 191–199.

Zimmerman, J., & Fisher, M. (2017). Avoidant/restrictive food intake disorder (ARFID). *Current Problems in Pediatric and Adolescent Health Care, 47*(4), 95–103.

Zock, H. (2018). Human development and pastoral care in a post-modern age: Donald Capps, Erik H. Erikson, and beyond. *Journal of Religion and Health, 57*(2), 437–450.

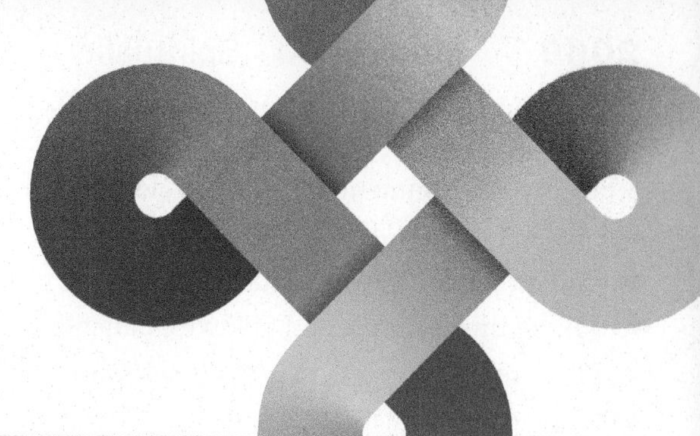

Module 30
Spirituality

Module Outline and Learning Outcomes

The Concept of Spirituality

Spiritual Health

30.1 Distinguish between spiritual wellness and spiritual discomfort.

Religion

30.2 Discuss how religious practices may impact nursing and healthcare.

Concepts Related to Spirituality

30.3 Outline the relationship between spirituality and other concepts.

Spiritual Care Resources

30.4 Identify spiritual care resources available within hospitals and communities.

Lifespan Considerations

30.5 Summarize the development of spirituality across the lifespan.

Nursing Process

30.6 Analyze the nurse's role in supporting the spiritual health of patients.

›› The Concept of Spirituality

Concept Key Terms

Faith community nurse, **2075**
Holistic nursing, **2065**
Meditation, **2070**
Mindfulness, **2066**
Religion, **2065**
Resilience, **2066**
Spiritual care actions, **2079**
Spiritual distress/ discomfort, **2067**
Spiritual health, **2066**
Spiritual wellness, **2067**
Spirituality, **2065**
Stereotyping, **2069**

For many people, **spirituality** is a personal but universal human experience that connects them to something bigger than themselves, something that transcends time and space and assists them in their search for meaning and purpose in life (Fitch & Bartlett, 2019). Spirituality is not the same as **religion**, which can be described as an organized framework for a group of believers with similar beliefs, moral values, and spiritual practices to express their faith and worship for God or their spiritual higher power. However, spirituality may have elements of religion, such as faith in a higher power. An individual can be spiritual without being religious; that is, without adhering to or belonging to any one organized religion. Spirituality is more of an individual's search for peace, purpose, transcendence, and connection with God or another spiritual higher power, with others, and, in some cases, with nature through spiritual practices (ReachOut, 2020). Some individuals define spirituality according to religious values, whereas others find expression of spirituality through personal relationships or through nature.

Spirituality includes the range of spiritual health, from spiritual wellness and well-being to spiritual discomfort or distress. When the spiritual needs of individuals are not being met, it can have a major impact on spiritual health, resulting in increased despair, symptoms of unhealthiness and poor health outcomes, feeling less connected with others, and even spiritual pain. The World Health Organization recognizes the provision of spiritual care that addresses the spiritual needs of patients as a core domain of patient care (Fitch & Bartlett, 2019). Guidelines and standards of palliative care emphasize the need to include spiritual care in daily nursing care.

Providing care that promotes patients' spirituality and interconnectedness with others is within the scope of practice of every nurse. In any setting, nurses should work to provide holistic nursing care for all patients.

Holistic nursing is a form of whole-health nursing grounded in forming caring relationships with patients and developing interconnectedness with them. It involves providing individualized care for the whole patient, including the mind, body, and spirit of the patient, and not just care for the patient's presenting symptoms or medical diagnosis. Florence Nightingale is credited with making the first connection between patients and their environment by focusing on changing the environment to improve the outcomes of the patients instead of focusing solely on their physical care (Practical Nursing, 2020).

Holistic nursing is recognized as a nursing specialty by the American Holistic Nurses Association (AHNA). The AHNA defines holistic nursing and standards of practice, supports research studies, and offers educational programs for integrative healthcare therapies. Registered nurses can obtain certification as holistic nurses by meeting certain education and experience requirements. Holistic nursing care takes the effects of illness on the mind, body, spirituality, and emotions of patients into consideration. Nursing actions that promote a healthy environment and the development of the nurse–patient relationship include:

- Calling patients by their stated names
- Taking time to smile and talk with patients
- Encouraging patients to provide self-care
- Using nonpharmacologic pain relief methods that patients use at home, such as relaxation techniques or imagery (» **Skills:** See Chapter 3, Clinical Nursing Skills, in Volume 3, for more information)
- Assisting patients with complementary health treatments routinely used at home, such as massage
- Asking patients about spiritual practices they would like to continue while in the healthcare facility.

In addition to learning basic nursing knowledge, skills, and behaviors, holistic nurses learn complementary and integrative health therapies. A holistic approach is supported by the understanding that a healthy mind helps to have a healthy body, and a healthy body promotes a healthy mind. Healing the mind can influence healing of the body (Silver, 2020). Performing a holistic comprehensive assessment on patients on admission provides important data that nurses can compare to expected norms for various developmental stages (see the section Holistic Health Assessment Across the Lifespan, in Module 34, Assessment).

Nurses in every setting act to promote patients' health and well-being and respond to patient expressions of discomfort and distress. This includes promoting patient spiritual health and intervening in times of spiritual discomfort. It is also necessary for nurses to attend to their own spiritual health (see **Box 30.1** »).

Spiritual Health

Health is a broad concept that refers to the status of well-being. Wellness describes harmony and balance of all areas of health contributing to wellness lifestyles. Areas of health and wellness, sometimes referred to as components or dimensions, overlap, interconnect, and work together for the overall health and well-being of individuals. They include physical health, mental health, spiritual health, emotional health, social health, and environmental health (Nishat, 2020).

Individuals can take action to improve their overall health, wellness, and sense of well-being for a satisfying life (see Module 7, Health, Wellness, Illness, and Injury, for more information). For example, physical health may be improved by following exercise and dietary wellness guidelines; emotional and environmental health may be improved by volunteering to help in community improvement projects; and mental and social health may be improved by joining a local hobby club.

Spiritual health supports a person's efforts to lead a fulfilling life, with purpose, transcendence, and self-actualization of what that person can accomplish (Ghaderi,

Box 30.1

Spiritual Self-Care for Nurses

Nurses provide physical, mental, emotional, and spiritual care for patients and their families in highly stressful healthcare environments. Because of this, nurses are at risk for stress-induced conditions such as compassion fatigue, burnout, moral injury, spiritual discomfort, mental fatigue, and secondary or vicarious traumatization. Today's patients are more complex with higher acuity, which puts greater demands on nurses. Specialties such as critical care nursing demand special knowledge, skills, and behaviors to coordinate compassionate care as well as to implement nursing interventions to promote healing.

Extended time caring for more complex patients can reduce nurses' mental and physical capacity as they exhaust themselves caring for others. In addition to physical and mental exhaustion, nurses can experience a spiritual disconnect within themselves. A spiritual disconnect within the nurse may result in an inability to provide spiritual care to patients and their families. An imbalance may develop in which nurses are providing more care, compassion, and empathy for patients than for themselves.

When they neglect their own needs, nurses can develop thoughts and feelings of depression, self-doubt, anxiety, irritability, and spiritual, physical, and mental exhaustion. In a recent American Nurses Association Health Risk Appraisal report, 82% of nurses thought they were at risk for illness due to workplace stress (Penque, 2019). To minimize or avoid these stress-induced conditions, nurses can adopt coping strategies and self-care practices to maintain their mental/emotional, physical, and spiritual health.

- Adopting healthy coping strategies, including healthy eating and regular exercise
- Avoiding unhealthy coping strategies, such as use of alcohol, tobacco, or other drugs
- Engaging in their own spiritual practices regularly
- Practicing mindfulness.

Mindfulness is a cognitive method of paying attention and building awareness of thoughts, emotions, and actions in the present moment. Mindfulness can include a form of meditation that contains deep breathing for relaxation. Using mindfulness has the potential to help nurses reframe challenging situations and promote positive stress-free responses to them. Other activities that have been linked to mindfulness include gardening and cooking, both of which require attention in the present moment.

Another important self-care practice for nurses to develop and demonstrate is resilience. **Resilience** is the ability to respond positively and adapt to change, while gaining strength in the process.

Resilience can help prevent stress-induced conditions and physical complaints of stress such as headache, exhaustion, chest pain, and inability to sleep restfully. Nurses who engage in activities that promote resilience may experience increased work satisfaction, best patient outcomes, and a healthier mind, body, and spirit.

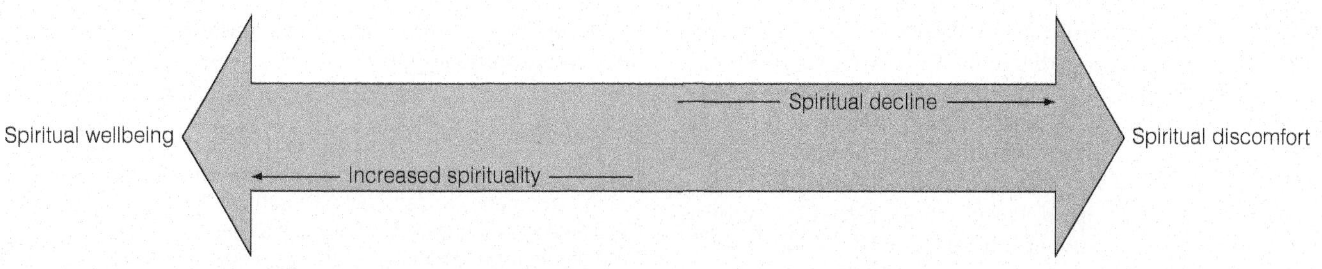

Figure 30.1 ››› The continuum of spiritual health may be influenced by an individual's life experiences, coping skills, social support, and belief system.

Tabatabaei, Nedjat, Javadi, & Larijani, 2018). Spiritual health is characterized by an overall feeling of strength, hope, and well-being that contributes to the healing processes of physical and mental health. Wellness is enhanced by participating in life-sustaining and enriching wellness opportunities. Individuals who maintain a high level of spiritual health typically have a clear set of beliefs and live life following their morals, values, and ethics. Spiritual health often, but not always, encompasses religious and natural elements. Each individual's spiritual health and sense of well-being is influenced by a number of factors, including personal spiritual beliefs and practices, coping strategies, life events, family and community supports, and environmental and social determinants of health.

As with other aspects of health, spiritual health occurs along a continuum, from spiritual wellness to spiritual discomfort or distress (**Figure 30.1 ›››**). When individuals achieve a high degree of spiritual, physical, and emotional health, they are experiencing an optimal level of health and wellness. On the other end of the continuum, poor physical, emotional, and spiritual health signal the need for prompt holistic nursing care based on a thorough assessment of the patient's needs.

Spiritual Wellness

Individuals define and describe spiritual wellness in different ways. To many people, **spiritual wellness** is feeling a sense of peace with life, of optimism, and the sensation of comfort from their spirituality when hardships come along. For many, spiritual wellness provides a sense of value, a deeper meaning in life and in relationships with others, and feelings of purpose in life (American Association of Equine Practitioners, 2020). To help meet their spiritual needs and promote their spiritual health to reach higher levels of wellness, individuals can perform a variety of physical and mental spiritual practices (**Box 30.2 ›››**). Brief spiritual practices performed daily—such as meditation, prayer, or taking a short time out to reconnect with oneself during the day—bring many people comfort and a positive sense of well-being (Dienstman, 2019). Greater spiritual wellness and well-being is associated with decreased illness, injury, and disease; better immune responses; shorter recovery times; and increased longevity (Centers for Disease Control and Prevention, 2018).

When individuals achieve spiritual wellness, they report feelings of hopefulness, positiveness, happiness, and usefulness. They have an interest in helping others, as shown by volunteering to help others, participating in worthwhile causes, connecting with others, having a sense of belonging, and taking care of themselves physically, mentally, emotionally, socially, and spiritually. When individuals are spiritually healthy, they feel more connected not only to their spiritual higher power, but also to those around them. They have more clarity when it comes to making everyday choices, and their actions become more aligned with their beliefs and values.

Box 30.2
Selected Practices for Promoting Spiritual Health

- Explore your spiritual self. Ask yourself who you really are and what your purpose is in life. Who or what matters to you most? What footprint in life do you want to leave behind?
- Try yoga as a relaxation exercise to help decrease physical strain, lower anxiety, reduce depression, and lower stress.
- Look for a deeper meaning in life and think about your patterns of behavior. Think about what you want in life and how you can control making it happen.
- Find a spiritual community or group of friends who can support you on your spiritual journey and provide a sense of belonging and connection.
- Spend time outside. Find a quiet place and reflect on your surroundings or take a long walk and engage in mindfulness and connection with nature.
- Try meditation to practice quietness and inner self peace and relaxation while sitting quietly. This can be done in a quiet space, outside in a peaceful setting, or even near a piece of art that speaks to you.
- Get in touch with your inner creativity. Inspire yourself to sing, write, play a musical instrument, draw, paint, work with clay, or whatever brings you joy.
- Because you are what your thoughts are, think positive, beneficial thoughts. Redirect your mind to be kindhearted, reframe how you think about situations. Relax your muscle groups one at a time until your whole body is relaxed.
- Take care of your physical body by giving it what it needs; good nutrition, plenty of exercise, a balance of work and play, and enough relaxation and sleep time.

Sources: University of Kansas (2020); University of Minnesota (2016).

Spiritual Distress

Patients who experience **spiritual distress** (sometimes referred to as *spiritual pain* or *spiritual discomfort*) are challenged or unable to find meaning in life, peace, comfort, strength, connection to God or a higher power, or with friends and family, resulting in feelings of distress or suffering. Some may feel a disconnection from themselves. *Spiritual distress* is a term widely used in nursing, in palliative and end-of-life care, and by chaplains and spiritual leaders (ACEP et al., n.d.; Herdman & Kamitsuru, 2018; Smith & Jackson, 2013).

Spiritual distress or discomfort can develop when patients have very low levels of spiritual health and decreased or impaired overall health and wellness. Patients may experience physical, mental, or emotional pain and feelings of isolation or loss of control. In turn, this spiritual suffering or distress can lengthen physical and mental health healing processes and slow recovery times. In some cases, spiritual discomfort arises when individual spiritual and religious practices are disrupted or challenged. Any number of events can cause patients to experience decreased participation in spiritual practices, including (Crossroads Hospice & Palliative Care, 2018):

- Onset of a meaningful loss, such as the death of a family member
- Life-threatening or life-altering illness
- Deteriorating mental or cognitive health
- Separation from their spiritual community due to hospitalization or relocation
- General physical or functional decline

For example, patients diagnosed with a terminal illness may question their spiritual beliefs by trying to answer the question, "Why did this happen to me?" Even though patients express spiritual discomfort with a variety of symptoms, the following are common manifestations characteristic of spiritual discomfort (Crossroads Hospice & Palliative Care, 2018; Smith & Jackson, 2013):

- Expressing a fear of dying
- Depression or withdrawal; feelings of loneliness and isolation
- Changes in eating and sleeping patterns
- Expressing anger, bitterness, shame, and hopelessness
- Feeling disconnected from their spiritual higher power
- Questioning spiritual or religious beliefs
- Feeling anxious, regretful, guilty, or confused
- Ineffective or impaired decision making.

Nurses can provide effective interventions to help relieve spiritual discomfort and, in turn, increase the patient's energy level to support physical, mental, and spiritual healing. Compassionate, attentive listening and providing a quiet and calm setting that supports peaceful interactions are critical when working with patients experiencing spiritual distress.

Nurses can take time to listen to patients, sitting at the same level as the patients with appropriate eye contact, and giving them opportunities to talk about their thoughts and feelings. If patients have questions about spirituality and would like to speak with a chaplain, nurses can arrange a chaplain to visit them. Sometimes journaling (writing down feelings and thoughts on paper) can help patients who are afraid to say their thoughts out loud "get them out." Nurses can use open-ended questions when talking with patients to encourage dialogue, express empathy about the patient's situation, and offer comfort and support.

Case Study » Part 1

Ryan Owens, a 42-year-old male and Jehovah's Witness, is brought into the emergency department (ED) with acute upper gastrointestinal (GI) bleeding secondary to peptic ulcer disease. He is vomiting blood, hypotensive, pale, diaphoretic, and has a weak and thready pulse. He is alert enough to hear Sharon Hynes, the ED physician, order a type and cross for four units of blood. Mr. Owens interrupts and states that he does not want the blood transfusion because of personal religious beliefs as a Jehovah's Witness follower. Dr. Hynes orders 2 liters isotonic NaCl solution to be given IV instead. Mr. Owens's wife Sandra arrives not long before he loses consciousness, and they discuss the use of IV isotonic fluids versus blood transfusions. She agrees with his decision and tells him she loves him. He tells her he loves her also.

Clinical Reasoning Questions Level I

1. What are the primary concerns for Mr. and Mrs. Owens?
2. How are the staff and others likely to react to the couple's decision? Why?
3. How do the principles of autonomy affect this scenario?

Clinical Reasoning Questions Level II

4. If Dr. Hynes had written a PRN order for blood "just in case Mr. or Mrs. Owens change their mind," what would be your role as a nurse advocate?
5. If Sandra had disagreed with Ryan regarding this matter, how could an RN facilitate open and helpful communication between them?

Religion

As described earlier, a religion is an organized framework with a group of believers who share similar beliefs, moral values, and spiritual practices to express their faith and worship for God or a spiritual higher power. Many of the religions around the world have subgroups, called denominations or branches, each with their own distinct differences in beliefs, traditions, and organization. While religion is usually practiced in a community setting, many religious individuals also maintain their religious beliefs and behaviors in everyday life. *Religiosity* is a general term that refers to an individual's devotion to a particular religion. Although there are many differences among religions, there are also many similarities. Characteristics common among most religions include:

- Belief in God or a spiritual higher power.
- Belief in values of compassion, love, forgiveness, faith, and charity.
- Belief that God or a spiritual higher power has influence over people.
- Belief that followers can communicate and interact directly with God or a spiritual higher power through prayer, meditation, or fellowship with other believers.
- A sense of community or congregation cohesion.
- Identified places of worship (such as a church, synagogue, temple, or mosque).
- Identified times of worship, whether scheduled times for prayer or holy days that mark an important religious event.

- Ethical or moral codes for followers to obey.
- Belief in a moral standard of treating others as you would like to be treated (the "Golden Rule").

More than 6 billion people around the world participate in one of the estimated 4200 active religions. Some religions, such as Taoism (a religion that originated in Japan), have relatively few followers. Among the major religions—Christianity, Islam, Hinduism, Buddhism, Shintoism, and Judaism—Christianity is the most practiced, followed by Islam, Hinduism, Buddhism, and Judaism (Waltner, 2020). Many American Indian and indigenous populations practice independent systems of spirituality (see Focus on Diversity and Culture: American Indian Spirituality). Among individuals who consider themselves "religious," degree of religiosity varies. Worldwide, many people consider themselves "religious" but are unaffiliated with any single religion.

Focus on Diversity and Culture

American Indian Spirituality

In the United States, 573 American Indian tribes have been recognized by state and federal levels of government (PowWows.com, 2019). Each tribe has its own system of spirituality that includes spiritual beliefs, ceremonies, and practices used in everyday living. One spiritual practice common among many tribes is the sweat lodge. Rocks are heated up in a fire outside the lodge and brought inside it to create a steamy setting used for purification, a process of physical and spiritual cleansing and renewal of the self. A sweat lodge can also be part of a vision quest and place to offer prayers. Traditional beliefs are passed down either as or alongside historic accounts of significant events. Traditional beliefs and practices are also passed down through the cultural practice of the *pow wow*, a meeting of tribes that features traditional dancing, singing, drumming, food, costumes, and crafts.

Some American Indian tribes worship a single spirit, whereas others have many spirits. Animals, plants, rivers, and weather are perceived as living beings by many tribes. Many tribes view poor health as a result of failure to live in harmony with nature and sacred places and other people (Swihart, Yarrarapu, & Martin, 2020). Most tribes have sacred areas for native rituals and prayers and where offerings to the spirits or the ancestors may be made.

Unfortunately, the United States as a nation has not always recognized the legitimacy of American Indian religious and spiritual practices. For more than a century, the United States government actively promoted Christianity among American Indians, even to the extent of permitting religious groups to force native children to attend Christian boarding schools far away from their homes and by banishing traditional Indian dances, feasts, and other cultural observances. American Indian religious practices were not protected under federal law until the American Indian Religious Freedom Act passed in 1970. Additional protections were provided in the Religious Freedom Restoration Act, which was passed in 1993 (PowWows.com, 2019; Zotigh, 2018).

Religious Traditions

Religions have similarities and differences related to how to think about health, illness, suffering, and death. The very brief descriptions included in this module are mere snapshots intended to raise awareness of some important areas of health and healthcare that can be influenced by an individual's religion. These beliefs and traditions often pertain to how patients relate to holy days, scriptures, symbols, and to God or a spiritual higher power through prayer, meditation, singing, chanting, and other religious practices. Note that these are practices commonly recognized in many religions, but that how and to what extent individuals practice them varies greatly. Learning about a patient's spiritual and religious beliefs and practices is an important part of the nursing assessment. Nurses should avoid **stereotyping**, the act of generalizing that all people in a group are the same or believe the same things.

Holy Days

Holy days are times of reflection and celebration of significant spiritual events. Religions around the world recognize various holy days. For many believers, it is a time for them to set their faith as a priority and worship with others participating in holy day activities. Sometimes one or more religions with similar beliefs observe the same holy days. For example, traditionally, the Sabbath, or "the Lord's day" in Christianity, is observed on Sunday. In Judaism, the Sabbath is observed on Saturday, and in the Islamic religion, followers (called Muslims) may gather together on Friday.

Depending on the religion, participation in observance of holy days may include fasting, extended praying, giving up an indulgence of something, avoiding specific foods on certain days, or completing other ritual practices. In contrast, some holy days are observed through festivals. For example, in India, people celebrate the festival of Diwali (the festival of lights, an important Hindu festival) by decorating their homes with clay lamps and gathering for feasts and fireworks. Because holy days are usually viewed as a day dedicated to religious practices or service to others, patients may refuse medical treatments or diagnostic tests scheduled on their holy days. In these situations, nurses can advocate for their patients by notifying the healthcare provider (HCP) of the patient's refusal and exploring if the treatment or diagnostic test can be rescheduled to another day.

Sacred Scriptures

Most major religions have sacred scriptures that provide guidance for followers' beliefs, behaviors, and rules for living, as well as cautions against disobedience. In addition, these writings frequently serve to record the history of the religion through informative accounts of its kings, heroes, and major events throughout its past. In most religions, these scriptures are thought to be the word of God or a spiritual higher power as written down by prophets or other holy people. Sacred scriptures are often combined into a single text, such as the Bible of Christianity, the Torah of Judaism, and the Quran, which is the sacred text of Islam. Sacred texts are often a source of comfort to patients and family members in illness or crisis, especially passages that describe historical or holy individuals with physical or mental illness who were comforted or healed through faith.

Religious Symbols

Religious symbols are emblems, shapes, or drawings that represent or stand for a religion, such as the cross of Christianity, the Jewish Star of David, and the yin and yang of Taoism. Other objects such as jewelry, medals, amulets, altars, figures, totems, or clothing may be used as symbolic representations of religions. Many people wear or carry religious objects or keep them in their homes or workplaces as a personal reminder of their faith or as a source of comfort and strength.

Some patients may wear religious medals at all times, and therefore want to wear them when they are undergoing diagnostic studies, medical treatments, or surgery. Individuals who are Roman Catholic may carry a rosary for prayer; an individual who is Muslim may carry a mala, or string of prayer beads (see **Figure 30.2** »). Hospitalized patients or long-term care residents may wish to have spiritual objects with them as a source of comfort.

Prayer and Meditation

Prayer is a form of direct communication between religious followers and God or the spiritual higher power they worship. Prayers can be made privately or publicly in community with other followers or during a religious ceremony. Prayers may be made for many reasons, such as proclaiming praise, asking for forgiveness, speaking on behalf of others, asking for something specific (such as healing from illness or favorable weather for crops), and giving thanks. Prayer continues to be a prevalent practice in the United States, with 55% of survey participants (nearly 6 in 10 people) reporting that they pray daily (Feldman, 2019).

Meditation is the practice of focusing the mind on inner deep thoughts instead of what is happening outside the body. Some individuals use a mantra—a repeated word, phrase, or chant—to help block outside thoughts during meditation, whereas others may use music or silence. Because meditation is used for spiritual purposes and also helps induce relaxation, it is commonly associated with spiritual well-being and balance in life. An increasing body of evidence indicates that meditation can be a helpful tool in fighting chronic illnesses, including depression, heart disease, and chronic pain (Welch, 2019).

There are many different forms of meditation, such as mindfulness meditation, guided meditation or guided imagery, and yoga meditation. The practice of using meditation in the United States is increasing across all age groups (Welch, 2019). Hospitalized patients may ask nurses for a quiet time during the day in which they can pray or meditate.

Prayer guidelines vary according to religions and individualized prayer experiences. Examples of practices around prayer include:

- Use of prayer books that contain prescribed prayers for use at different times or for specific reasons
- Use of a prayer rug or mat when sitting or kneeling on the ground for prayer (**Figure 30.3** »)
- Observance of specific times for prayers or meditation.

When patients desire to continue their prayer practices while hospitalized, nurses can assist in creating a quiet space and time for prayer or meditation.

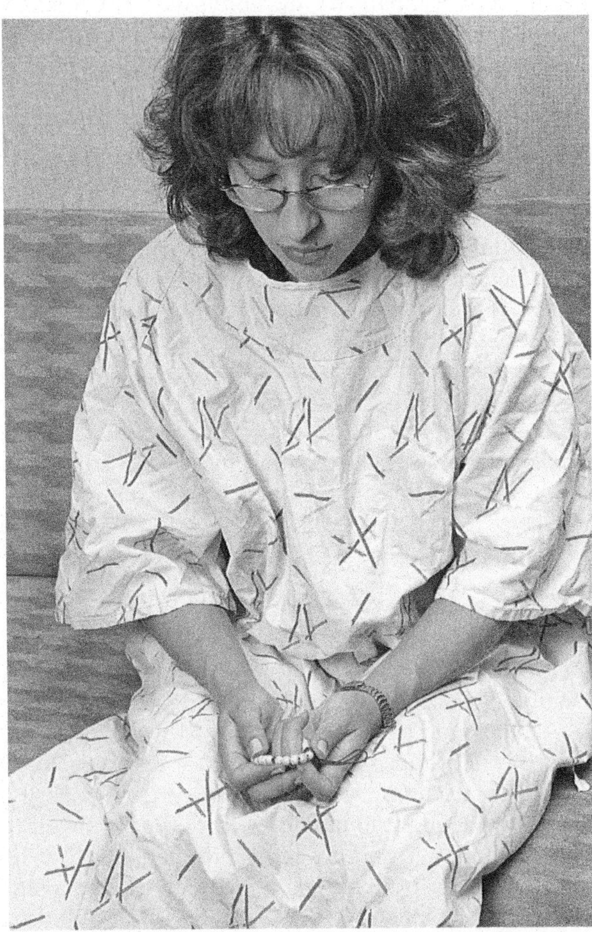

Figure 30.2 » Patients may bring objects to the hospital to use in prayer or other religious rituals. Caregivers should respect these objects because they usually have great significance to patients.
Source: Pearson Education, Inc.

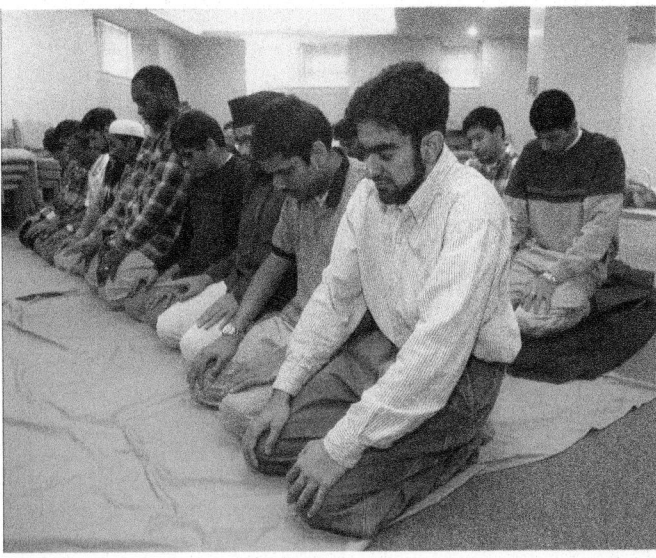

Figure 30.3 » Muslim students at Johns Hopkins University at their weekly prayer meeting.
Source: John Gillis/AP Images.

Communicating with Patients

Be respectful and sensitive when discussing a patient's religious practices. Maintain a relaxed body posture, use attentive listening, speak compassionately, and maintain appropriate eye contact.

- Maria told me you were not able to read your prayer book this morning. Can you share with me what's going on?
- I imagine it must be very difficult for you not to be able to read your prayer book.

Religious Practices

When patients enter healthcare systems, they bring with them a variety of cultural, social, and religious differences. For example, for medical treatment, some patients prefer Eastern medicine, other patients prefer Western medicine, and some patients prefer a combination of both. *Eastern medicine* uses a holistic approach to maintain health in a balanced state with treatments including diet therapy, acupuncture, massage, herbal remedies, meditation, and t'ai chi. *Western medicine* uses a scientific approach, focusing on the patient's signs and symptoms to diagnose the pathology and treat the disease or medical condition with medications, diet therapy, exercise, radiation, and surgery (Medibank, 2019). Nurses need to be culturally competent and sensitive to the spiritual needs of patients and their families during the stresses of receiving necessary medical care (see Module 24, Culture and Diversity, for more information about cultures and cultural competence). Nurses should provide holistic nursing care to patients and maintain patient's rights and best practices when providing consistent, quality care to all patients (see Module 44, Ethics, for more information about patients' rights). Religion and spirituality can influence patients' medical decisions based on their spiritual beliefs.

Patients are asked about religious preferences as part of the assessment process. Diets, medications, modesty behaviors, and rituals such as prayer times may conflict with treatments or diagnostic tests. Early discussion of these considerations with the patient or family member can help clarify and build the nurse's awareness of specific spiritual, mental, and physical preferences and health practices. As appropriate, the nurse can then attempt to accommodate the patient's religious and spiritual needs (Swihart et al., 2020). Additional strategies for promoting religious practices are outlined in **Box 30.3** ».

Clothing

Many religions have strict guidelines or traditions about clothing. Guidelines may address wearing head coverings (**Figure 30.4** ») or covering parts of the body (by wearing sleeves or long pants or skirts). For some, such as the Church of Jesus Christ of Latter-Day Saints, guidelines may speak to what kind of undergarments to wear. Both women and men accustomed to following religious dress codes may find wearing hospital gowns uneasy and uncomfortable.

Diet

Many religions have traditional dietary guidelines. There may be rules about which foods and beverages are allowed and which are prohibited. Religious laws may also dictate how food is prepared. The spiritual practice of fasting may

Box 30.3

Supporting Religious Practices

- Create a trusting relationship with the patient so that any religious concerns or practices can be openly discussed and addressed.
- If unsure of the patient's religious needs, ask how nurses can assist in having these needs met. Avoid relying on personal assumptions when caring for patients.
- Do not discuss personal spiritual beliefs with a patient unless it is requested. Be sure to assess whether such self-disclosure contributes to a therapeutic nurse–patient relationship.
- Inform patients and family caregivers about spiritual support available at your institution (e.g., chapel or meditation room, chaplain services).
- Allow time and privacy for, and provide comfort measures prior to, private worship, prayer, meditation, reading, or other spiritual activities.
- Respect and ensure safety of the patient's religious articles (e.g., icons, amulets, clothing, jewelry).
- If desired by the patient, facilitate clergy or spiritual care specialist visitation. Collaborate with the chaplain (if available).
- Prepare the patient's environment for spiritual rituals or clergy visitations as needed (e.g., have a chair near the bedside for clergy, create private space).
- Make arrangements with the dietitian so that dietary needs can be met. If the institution cannot accommodate the patient's needs, ask the family to bring food. (Most religions have some recommendations about diet, such as espousing vegetarianism or rejecting alcohol.)
- Acquaint yourself with the religions, spiritual practices, and cultures of the area in which you are working.
- Facilitating/supporting a patient's religious practice does not require that you share the same beliefs or must participate in it yourself.
- Ask another nurse to assist if a particular religious practice makes you uncomfortable.
- All spiritual interventions must be done within agency guidelines.

Source: Berman, Snyder, and Frandsen (2016), p. 963. Pearson Education, Inc., Hoboken, NJ.

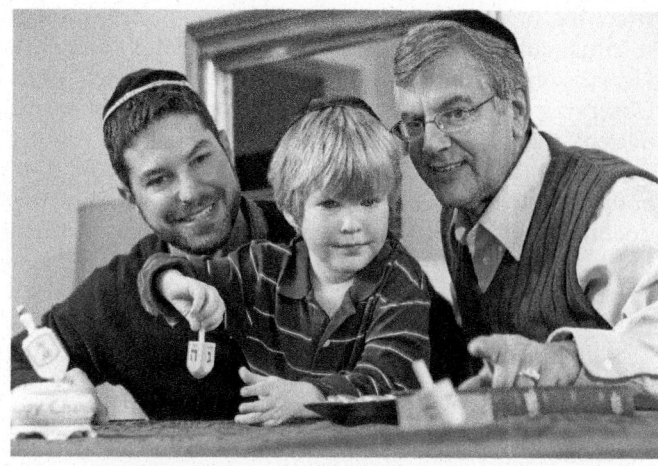

Figure 30.4 » Conservative and Orthodox Jewish men may wear a yarmulke at all times, even in the hospital. Reform Jews may wear yarmulkes only while praying and on religious occasions, such as this family celebrating Hanukkah.

Source: GoldenKB/iStock/Getty Images.

include total abstinence of consuming any food or just a specified food. Fasting may or may not include restrictions on beverages. The nurse can arrange for a dietician to meet with the patient to discuss food and beverage options included in the prescribed diet that would support the patient's spiritual dietary routines.

Healing

Some religious traditions view illness and suffering as tests of faith, as opportunities to grow spiritually. In contrast, some religions view illness as punishment, reflections of a spiritual weakness, or as the result of an evil force, such as "If I hadn't been so wild as a youth, I wouldn't have this problem now" (Farran, 2019). Careful assessment is necessary to determine if a patient's religious views affect their understanding of illness, as this can affect the patient's views of treatment and recovery.

In addition to beliefs around health and illness, many religions have healing rituals that symbolize turning over the outcome of an individual's illness to God or a spiritual higher power. For example, many Christian religions incorporate prayers for healing of the sick into their weekly services and have chaplains available to pray with patients at the bedside. Despite the diversity of healing rituals and traditions patients may use, they all reflect a desire for healing and good health.

Birth

Many religions have specific ritual ceremonies to dedicate newborns to God or a spiritual higher power. These ceremonies may include chanting, praying, singing, reading sacred scriptures, and baptism with water. Different religions have their own guidelines about the circumcision of male infants. Some ceremonies incorporate naming of the newborn.

Death

Many religions believe life doesn't end when the physical body dies, but that life transforms to a better, solely spiritual existence in what is often referred to as the afterlife or heaven (Uzell, 2018). Other religions, such as Judaism, reject the notion of an afterlife. Religions have different spiritual guidelines and religious rituals related to an individual's end-of-life care and care of the body after death. Observing these rituals can provide comfort to the dying patient and family members. Many patients are making decisions about their end-of-life care and care of their body postmortem in their living will or advance directive document (see Module 49, Legal Issues, for more information about healthcare advance directives). Nurses can also gather this information with other assessment data when patients are admitted to healthcare facilities.

Religious rituals practiced during end-of-life care may include singing, chanting, reciting special prayers, and reading sacred scriptures. These may be performed by the family or a religious leader. Some religions, such as Islam and Judaism, specify how the body should be cleansed and prepared for burial, whether the body may be buried or cremated, and the amount of time after death to wait for burial of the body. The nurse can help to support family members of the deceased by providing a quiet and peaceful place for them to perform their traditional death rituals as appropriate.

Religious Beliefs and Healthcare

The following is an alphabetical list of the world's major religions and selected beliefs and practices related to healthcare. The information provided is general and should not take the place of a thorough, individualized nursing assessment of patient spiritual needs and religious practices.

Buddhism

Some Buddhist patients and patients of Asian background believe most illnesses can be cured through the mind. They may use traditional Chinese Medicine in addition to Western medicine therapies prescribed by a HCP. Buddhists may be vegetarian and practice one of several types of meditation.

Christianity

Christian practices affecting healthcare often depend on the denomination to which the individual belongs. The following examples are general and may not apply to every member of a particular denomination. They can, however, serve to illustrate the wide-ranging beliefs among different denominations of Christianity. For example, Christian denominations generally leave the decision of circumcising male infants to the parents or primary caregivers.

- Christians in the United States (Catholics, Orthodox, and Protestants) generally embrace Western medicine, but may differ in their views about birth control, abortion, same-sex marriage, and end-of-life care. Some denominations administer a symbolic anointing of the sick ritual or laying-on of hands ritual for healing (United States Conference of Catholic Bishops [USCCB], 2020). The season of Lent, the 40 days extending from the holy day of Ash Wednesday to Easter, may involve some degree of abstention from certain foods, such as red meat.
- The Amish rely on their religious community for support and may not carry medical insurance coverage. They may refuse expensive healthcare, believing it is poor stewardship.
- Christian Scientists oppose Western medical interventions, relying instead on lay and professional Christian Science practitioners. Faith and a positive attitude are paramount to them.
- Jehovah's Witnesses refuse most blood products. Alternative treatments to increase blood volume can be discussed with the patient (see Module 17, Perioperative Care, for more information). When a baby is born, a Jehovah's Witness will request that placental or umbilical cord blood be disposed of rather than extracted (Victoria Angel, 2020).
- Seventh-Day Adventists likely will avoid unnecessary treatments on Sabbath, which begins on Friday at sundown and ends on Saturday at sundown. They are often vegetarian and may abstain from caffeinated beverages, as well as tobacco products and alcohol.
- Many Roman Catholics believe that abortion, euthanasia, and birth control are sinful. Confession of one's sins to a priest and accepting absolution from the priest is an important healing sacrament. Older Catholics may choose not to eat meat on Fridays because it was prohibited in years past, and abstinence from meat is still required on some days during Lent. A patient who is a member of the

Roman Catholic faith and who is seriously ill, about to have a major surgical procedure, or dying may want to call for a priest to administer the Sacrament of the Anointing of the Sick, which is given by a Catholic priest for the patient's spiritual healing (USCCB, 2020).

- Orthodox Christians often prefer the services of their local priest rather than a hospital chaplain. They may follow the practice of fasting on Holy Days, although fasting rules may be relaxed for those who are ill or for whom fasting may cause a risk to their health.

Hinduism

Hinduism is a religion practiced by individuals from India and other parts of southern Asia. Hindus embrace Western medicine, but they may also use culturally based therapies such as yoga, massage, herbal medicine, and acupuncture. Many Hindus eat little or no meat and may prefer not to use medications that are derived from animals. Hindu women accustomed to wearing saris often prefer to cover all of the body except their arms and feet (**Figure 30.5** »). Many Hindus value cleanliness, and nurses may need to offer assistance for specific cleansing rituals at the start of the day or before a meal. As with many other religions, Hinduism has ceremonial rites that are practiced at the time of dying and immediately after death. The body is then cremated.

Islam

Many individuals who practice Islam view illness or death as the will of Allah (the Islamic word for God) and, therefore, believe that healing can take place only through Allah's will. Cleanliness and modesty are of great importance to many.

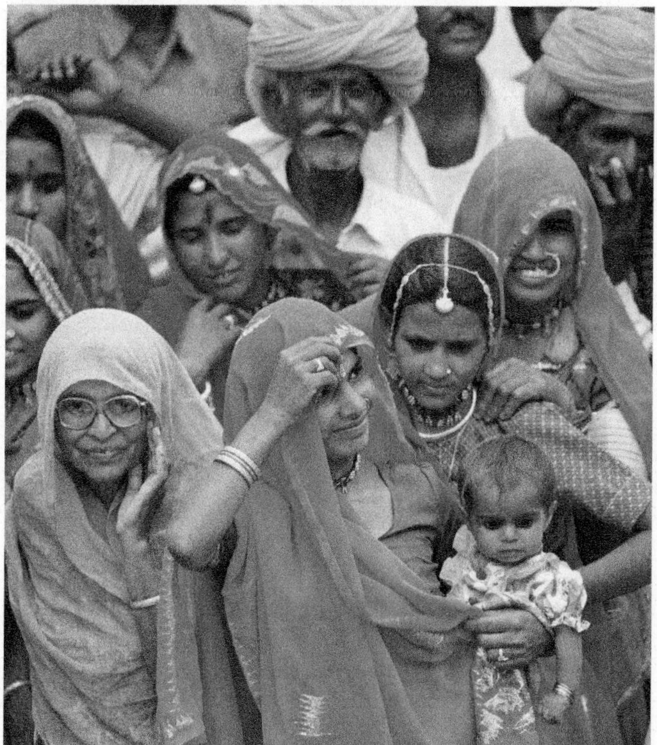

Figure 30.5 » Many Hindu women cover all of their bodies except for their face, arms, and feet.
Source: Charlie Westerman/Photodisc/Getty Images.

Many Muslim women choose to keep hands, face, and feet covered, although Islamic modesty rules are open to a wide range of interpretations (Arthur, 2020). When possible, a nurse of the same gender should care for the patient. A male family member may request to remain present when a woman or girl is being examined or treated, but the extent to which a family insists on this will vary (Attum, Hafiz, Malik, & Shamoon, 2018). Male infants are circumcised. Most practicing Muslims avoid overeating, alcohol, and pork products. The patient may request *halal* food, meaning food that has been prepared according to Islamic law. A central tenant—or belief— of Islam is ritual prayer at five specific times each day, so nurses working with Muslim patients should take prayer times into consideration. Prior to prayer, cleansing rituals are performed. Whenever possible, prayers are made while facing the direction of Mecca, the Muslim holy city in Saudi Arabia. Following a death, Muslims will bury the body within 24 hours (Uzell, 2018).

Judaism

Jewish individuals typically participate actively in their medical care and seek treatment from modern Western physicians. Some Jewish people observe a Kosher diet, which refrains from mixing dairy and meat and avoids pork and shellfish. Most Orthodox and Conservative Jewish men believe that it is important to have their heads covered at all times and wear yarmulkes. Most Orthodox Jewish women cover their hair with a wig or scarf as a sign of respect to God (Arthur, 2020). Orthodox Jewish people avoid using electronic appliances and lights on the Sabbath. Male infants are circumcised.

If a Jewish patient asks the nurse to pray with him, the nurse may use "God" or "Lord" to address the divine. Because there are prescribed Jewish rituals for individuals who are near death, dying, and after death, Jewish families will often request the presence of a rabbi, a Jewish spiritual leader, when they know a loved one is near death. Jewish burial customs require the dead to be buried as soon as possible, preferably within 24 hours, except on the Sabbath.

Case Study » Part 2

Mr. Owens has slipped into a coma. Mrs. Owens is crying and begging her husband not to leave her. The staff members continue to treat the patient with the isotonic NaCl IV solution, but there is no significant improvement. Dr. Hynes speaks to Mrs. Owens and asks whether she has changed her mind.

Clinical Reasoning Questions Level I

1. What would be an empathic and spiritually supportive comment the RN could offer to Mrs. Owens?
2. Who could be called to help Mrs. Owens during this time?
3. What resources are available to help Mrs. Owens?

Clinical Reasoning Questions Level II

4. How should the nurse assess the needs of Mr. and Mrs. Owens at this time?
5. Does Dr. Hynes have the right to ask Mrs. Owens this question? Why or why not?
6. What would be characteristics of a healing environment for a patient in a coma?

Concepts Related to Spirituality

In today's busy healthcare environment, it can be easy for nurses and other healthcare professionals to overlook a patient's spirituality even when a spiritual assessment is a component of the initial patient assessment performed on admission. Patients often depend on their religious and spiritual beliefs when making medical decisions related to their physical, mental, and emotional health and safety (Swihart et al., 2020). For example, religious practices may include certain dietary restrictions or practices that can affect prescribed diets. Spirituality may affect sexuality and reproduction if the patient adheres to sexual practices outlined by a religion. Spiritual practices can reduce stress and promote healthy coping, but at times, practices may also negatively impact a patient's ability to cope with stress.

The Concepts Related to Spirituality feature links some, but not all, of the concepts integral to spirituality. They are presented in alphabetical order.

Spiritual Care Resources

Patients who are an active part of a spiritual or religious community may not need referrals to be part of their discharge plan. Others may benefit from the nurse helping them to connect with resources once they are discharged home or to the next stage of care. Religious or spiritual congregations, spiritual leaders, members, and other resources may provide support for a patient member and family in various ways whether the patient is in a healthcare facility or at home. In addition to providing spiritual care when the patient returns home to recover, members may organize meals and a visitation schedule, volunteer respite care time for family members, take up an offering to give to the patient or family, or help with household chores.

When healthcare facilities do not provide culturally and spiritually competent care, there is a potential for patients to experience adverse health outcomes, receive poor quality care, or be unhappy with the care they receive (Swihart et al., 2020). Patients' perceptions of the quality of patient–nurse and patient–provider interactions influence patients' overall satisfaction with care. Low-quality interactions are associated with lower facility satisfaction scores. Facilities that are accredited by The Joint Commission are accountable for maintaining the accommodation of cultural, religious, and spiritual values in patient rights (Swihart et al., 2020). State and federal guidelines also support responsiveness to population diversity in healthcare facilities.

Hospitals and long-term care facilities typically provide access to a variety of spiritual care resources. These may include one or a combination of the following: chaplains, critical incident stress management programs; spiritual care departments; and faith community nurses.

Chaplain

Chaplains are the professional, board-certified spiritual care specialists on the healthcare team. They are based in large

Concepts Related to **Spirituality**

CONCEPT	RELATIONSHIP TO SPIRITUALITY	NURSING IMPLICATIONS
Comfort	Spiritual/religious beliefs may dictate how to interpret and relieve pain and discomfort.	Assess how patients give meaning to pain and suffering. Consider complementary health approaches to manage discomfort if the patient wants to avoid opioids and other pharmaceuticals.
Culture and Diversity	Religion, an expression of spirituality, is often intertwined with culture.	Assess religious beliefs and practices of patients (e.g., "Please tell me about any religious beliefs or practices that may affect your healthcare").
Legal Issues	Western cultures, such as those in North America, have federal laws protecting personal religious liberties.	Clarify, advocate, and seek legal support as necessary when a patient's or colleague's religious liberties are being threatened.
Nutrition	Spiritual/religious beliefs often have specific guidelines for dietary foods and beverages (e.g., vegetarianism, abstinence from alcohol). Some religious holidays are observed with fasting from all or certain specified foods and beverages.	Assess dietary foods and beverages the patient prefers.
Sexuality	Practices related to sexuality, such as family planning/birth control, may be influenced by spirituality.	When appropriate, assess the influence of spirituality on sexuality and associated practices. Provide care that is congruent with patients' spiritual/religious beliefs and practices.
Stress and Coping	People can use positive and negative religious coping strategies. Negative religious coping is associated with spiritual discomfort and poor outcomes.	Observe for expressions of negative religious coping (e.g., "God is punishing me" or "God/my church isn't there for me anymore"); offer patient spiritual support (e.g., chaplain) as appropriate.

healthcare facilities and may make visits in smaller healthcare facilities. Sometimes they are also ordained clergy or recognized religious/spiritual leaders. Many take interfaith clinical pastoral education courses to learn interpersonal and interprofessional skills necessary to help patients of all faiths during crises (HealthCare Chaplaincy Network, 2018).

Chaplains can help patients, family members, visitors, and medical staff who are experiencing spiritual discomfort to find and use inner sources of spiritual strength and courage, regardless of their religious preference or beliefs. Chaplains are sometimes asked to visit with patients experiencing life-threatening illnesses. Nurses can be instrumental in making referrals to chaplains and collaborating with them to support patients' spiritual well-being at any stage of illness. In addition to being on call as requested, chaplains also may make rounds through visitor waiting areas and nursing units asking if they can be of help. They can also assist in having religious resources and dietary foods available to patients, help patients participate in religious observances, and help schedule quiet times for prayer or meditation.

Spiritual Care Department

Some healthcare facilities have a spiritual care department that oversees spiritual and pastoral care services for patients and their families, visitors, and facility staff who need spiritual care (Atlantic Health System, 2020). Spiritual support may be available 24 hours a day, 7 days a week or available during daytime hours, with a chaplain on call during the evening and night hours. There may be chaplains in a variety of religions or interfaith chaplains available.

Larger facilities may hold scheduled services, communion, or prayer times for anyone wanting to attend. The facility may have special quiet rooms for personal prayer and meditation practices in designated areas. Special foods congruent with dietary laws for specific religions are made available working together with the nutrition services department.

Faith Community Nurse

A nursing specialty that focuses on spiritual care is that of the faith community nurse (parish nurse), which requires completion of a certification program approved by the American Nurses Association. Different religions may use other titles for faith-based or parish nurses, such as Crescent nurse, Shabbat nurse, congregational nurse, or church nurse. These registered nurses have received additional training in spiritual care. **Faith community nurses** work in affiliation with houses of worship, social service agencies, and nonprofit organizations, or they can work independently, providing holistic nursing care, healing, and spiritual care to members of the community, including those that are uninsured and low-income families.

Faith community nurses operate from a holistic health perspective focusing on the needs of members of a faith community. They can provide educational health programs, health screenings, lead support groups, visit members of the community in their homes, provide preventive health screenings, and volunteer in community service projects to promote wellness and minimize illness for those in the community. They have strong faith-based caring leadership skills to be effective in helping those in the community that are feeling hopeless and helpless. They advocate for those who need their assistance and, because they are familiar with the community and health resources, they can network throughout their community to find resources and make connections to meet patients' needs.

Critical Incident Stress Management

Many larger healthcare facilities have critical incident stress management (CISM) programs to help first responders in the community and employees of healthcare facilities cope with traumatic situations that may occur in the community or in the facility itself. Chaplains, counselors, first responders, and nurses trained in crisis intervention can be members of this team of professionals. CISM teams offer crisis intervention in an effort to reduce psychological casualties among public safety personnel and hospital staff. They also support those involved in emergent operations under conditions of extreme stress with the goal of preventing posttraumatic stress disorder. CISM debriefings, which often include spiritual care, are scheduled and sometimes mandated for professionals involved in or responding to traumatic incidents (Substance Abuse and Mental Health Services Administration, 2018).

Lifespan Considerations

Patients may participate in age-appropriate spiritual practices and religious rituals to enhance their spiritual health and promote overall health and wellness. Nurses can assist patients to continue personal spiritual practices and traditions while hospitalized, arrange chaplain visits, or make patients and families aware of spiritual resources available in the healthcare facility. Good health habits for all the dimensions of health listed earlier in this module can help patients be healthier at all ages.

Young Children

Young children learn to identify with spiritual traditions when parents provide them opportunities to participate and interact with others in a spiritual community that shares the same spiritual beliefs. As they share in their family's practices and rituals, children acquire a sense of connectiveness and feelings of belonging (Oswalt, Reiss, & Dombeck, 2020). Most young children are very "hands-on," and by actively engaging in spiritual practices, they can learn about religious holy days, dress, foods, behaviors, and symbols. They also can learn to sing songs, recite chants, say prayers and lines from scriptures, and participate in many other spiritual practices. As children grow, they can move from imitating group spiritual practices to developing their own individual spiritual practices and beliefs.

When children are patients in a healthcare facility, nurses can ask the parents about any spiritual practices the child may find comforting or need time to do. For newborns and infants in an intensive care unit, it is especially important that nurses support parent–child bonding so that trust and a secure attachment can be encouraged. Some parents may wish to go ahead and baptize or otherwise welcome the newborn into their religious faith, or to perform healing prayers or rituals. Nurses can assist parents in modifying religious observances while ensuring the safety and health of the newborn or infant.

Adolescents

Adolescence is a time of searching for purpose and wanting to belong or feel connected to others while exploring and maintaining individuality. Many adolescents choose to remain in religious groups to which their parents belong, continuing their spiritual practice and participating in faith-based social groups that support a sense of well-being or sense of religious service. Some, however, may choose to explore their spirituality outside the religion of their childhood. A few adolescents may move in an opposite direction, toward gangs or antisocial groups, ending their participation in religious traditions and adapting new behaviors and habits (Dollahite & Marks, 2019).

Adolescents often demonstrate a commitment to their faith through more personal spiritual actions such as mindfulness, meditation, and development of a relationship with God or their spiritual higher power. They develop caring and nurturing altruistic thoughts and behaviors oriented toward family, friends, and others. When participating in social activities with others, many make decisions that support their religious beliefs instead of "going along with the crowd," although this can vary considerably from one young person to the next and according to the situation.

Adults

Studies show that there is a decline in adult attendance for all religions: 54% of American adults report attending religious services a few times a year or less, while only 45% report attending at least monthly (Pew Research Center, 2019). Many young adults and millennials (those born between 1981 and 1996) have nontraditional approaches to religion. Only one-third of millennials report attending religious services at least once or twice a month (Pew Research Center, 2019). More people than ever are leaving organized religions and describing themselves as unaffiliated: In 2019, 26% of adults described themselves as unaffiliated with any religion, an increase of 17% over the previous 10 years (Pew Research Center, 2019).

Many young adults prefer nontraditional religious belief systems that allow more freedom and less conventional structured teaching and obedience. One study showed that most young adults stay true to their spiritual self and want genuine religious experiences in a worship community. These individuals say they are spiritual more than religious but in nontraditional ways that are flexible and supportive of learning with friends and others in a worship community (Greenthal, 2020).

Despite the increasing trend away from organized religion, many adults continue to describe spirituality as an integral, meaningful part of their lives. Findings from a study of the transcendent (rising above the self and realizing one is a part of a greater whole) nature of spirituality experienced by adults indicate that participants experienced spirituality as part of their identity or sense of self, which shaped the way they lived and how they made decisions. They also described spirituality as providing a general sense of joy, peace, and meaning in life (Kavar, 2020).

Older Adults

Statistics show that 90% of older adults identify themselves as being religious or spiritual and represent the most religious demographic group in the United States (Intriago, 2020). However, there is no scientific evidence to support the trend of most people becoming more spiritual as they age. Instead, it is generally accepted that the older generation of adults are continuing to participate in organized religion as they learned to do when they were younger (Jacobs, 2019).

Evidence shows that religion and spirituality are associated with better physical and mental health and longevity in older adults (Intriago, 2020). Their religious or spiritual community gives them opportunities for socialization, which can provide a sense of family, hope, resilience, and coping strategies for life stresses. Instead of being isolated and adjusting to a slow physical decline with aging, many older adults participate in religious or spiritual practices and communities. Communities can provide networks that help older adults share meals, transportation, and provide emotional and mental support. Spiritual older adults report being happier and finding purpose in life. They also experience less anxiety and have a lower risk of suicide and depression than older adults who report not being affiliated with a religious or spiritual community (American Seniors Housing Association, 2020). Spirituality in older adulthood is associated with improved diet and healthy behaviors, including use of safety measures (such as seat belts) and participation in health promotion activities (Intriago, 2020). Older adults with dementia may find peace and comfort from listening to sacred texts, poetry, and songs. Senior living options often network with faith-based communities to support the traditions and values of their patients.

Case Study » Part 3

An elder from Mr. Owens's congregation arrives, and Mrs. Owens and the elder discuss the situation. They agree that the situation has been handled according to Mr. Owens's beliefs. Mr. Owens dies, and Mrs. Owens states, "He remained faithful to his beliefs to honor God." Members of the ED staff are overheard saying things like "He was too young to die" and "If only they had allowed him to have a blood transfusion."

Clinical Reasoning Questions Level I

1. What should the nurse do to help Mrs. Owens at this time?
2. How can the nurse support community-based spiritual caregivers such as ministers?
3. What could the staff members do to help deal with their own feelings?

Clinical Reasoning Questions Level II

4. If the patient in the case study had been 10 years old and the parents had made the decision not to treat with blood transfusions, with the same results, what would have been the staff's responsibility?
5. What ethical and legal issues would be involved in the decision-making process in this situation?
6. What end-of-life care would be appropriate before and after Mr. Owens's death?

NURSING PROCESS

Nurses using a holistic approach provide nursing care that promotes healing of the whole patient including their physical, spiritual, mental, and emotional needs. Many patients experiencing spiritual discomfort are stressed from coping with a physical or mental illness that is causing them to feel fatigued, hopeless, separated from their spiritual beliefs, and as though they are losing their faith. The spiritually competent nurse can provide patient care to support their spiritual needs and nurture them to a higher level of spiritual wellness in addition to addressing physical and mental healthcare needs.

Religious patients and their families may observe a number of religious practices at home that are an essential part of their everyday lives. Patients may experience an interruption in family processes if an illness or injury interferes with their ability to practice their religion beyond a few days or weeks, or if the unfamiliar healthcare setting is not accommodating to their needs. Because an individual's sense of self may be closely bound to religious practices, nurses should be alert for cues that patients are experiencing a decline in spiritual health, such as restless sleeping, a change in eating habits, or feelings of despair, and advocate for patients to be able to participate in their religious practices.

In certain situations, medical conditions may require decisions that conflict with the patient's or family's religious beliefs and values. Consider the example of the pregnant woman who discovers at 20 weeks' gestation that she will not be able to carry the baby to term, and that attempting to do so will most likely result in her death. How might she feel when her care team offers her the opportunity to terminate her pregnancy? How will she decide what to do? If she had been trying for years to get pregnant without success, how would that influence her decision? How would her decision be affected if she had two small children at home? There are many complex and difficult situations in which medical conditions present complications and moral decisions that may conflict with patient beliefs. In situations such as these, patients may experience moral conflict or spiritual discomfort.

The spiritually competent nurse can support patients and families in spiritual discomfort by doing assessment of the patient's spiritual needs, making referrals to a chaplain or spiritual leader of the patient's choice, arranging private quiet times for prayer and meditation, showing respect for the patient's beliefs, being compassionate to the patient and family, and being an active listener.

These are strategies that promote spiritual health and promote the therapeutic nurse–patient relationship. In contrast, a number of actions can have detrimental consequences on the nurse–patient relationship and serve as barriers to promoting spiritual health. Examples of these are outlined in **Box 30.4** ».

Box 30.4

Inappropriate Nurse Actions That Hinder the Nurse–Patient Relationship

- Presenting oneself as a spiritual expert or talking about religious or spiritual topics about which the nurse is unfamiliar
- Debating spiritual or religious beliefs with a patient
- Moralizing by making such statements as "If you'd followed your beliefs, you might not be in this situation"
- Fabricating answers to a patient's questions in an attempt to "fix" the problem or make the patient feel better
- Giving inappropriate responses such as "You'll be fine" or "Everything will work out; it always does"
- Giving opinions or advice with such statements as "If I were you, I would do as the doctor suggests"
- Trying to force the nurse's own beliefs or religious viewpoint onto a patient
- Dismissing or devaluing a patient's religious beliefs or views because the nurse disagrees with them.

Sources: Freeman (2018); Potter and Moller (2020).

Assessment

Spiritual needs commonly thought to be universal to everyone are defined as the human needs for finding meaning, purpose, and value in life. Spiritual needs can also include the needs of belonging, hopefulness, creativity, feeling love, safety, and having relationships and communications with others and God or a spiritual higher power. Nurses can perform a spiritual assessment to identify individual needs of patients. This gives patients the opportunity to discuss their specific needs and how the nurse or healthcare team can best assist them in meeting their spiritual needs while in care. Once spiritual needs are identified, they can be integrated into the patient's nursing care plan. Satisfying an individual's spiritual needs can improve physical and mental health as well as spiritual health.

Initial Assessment

Patient assessments include observing for cues while gathering data about patient spiritual beliefs and practices and discussing with them how best to support them to continue their spiritual beliefs and practices while they are in a healthcare facility. When asking patients about their spiritual or religious histories, there are some common mnemonic assessment tools that can be used to help guide nurses and other professionals such as HOPE, FICA, and SPIRIT (Rindfleisch, 2020). For example, the **SPIRIT** assessment tool assesses the following areas (Rindfleisch, 2020):

Spiritual belief system
Personal spirituality
Integration and involvement in a spiritual community
Ritual practices and restrictions
Implications for medical care
Terminal events planning (advance directives).

These tools focus on inquiries about the patient's belief system, spiritual community, spiritual or religious practices, and how they may relate to medical care. Building a therapeutic nurse–patient relationship is encouraged by showing respect for the patient's responses, using attentive listening, and exploring any responses for better understanding, such as a patient stating, "I feel so lost not being able to attend my church while I'm here."

Fitch and Bartlett (2019) studied spirituality and spiritual care of patients with advanced disease to better understand their thoughts about spiritual care and the role of healthcare professionals in providing their care. Results of the study showed spiritual distress was about separation, whereas spiritual care was about connecting. Participants stated HCPs should be able to recognize patients having spiritual discomfort and connect them to appropriate spiritual care resources (Fitch & Bartlett, 2019).

Gathering assessment data from patients about spiritual and religious beliefs and practices that influence daily routines and medical decisions provides an opportunity to discuss accommodations necessary to meet patient needs while in the healthcare facility. In addition, patients with illnesses or injuries that may become life-threatening should be asked about end-of-life spiritual needs and postmortem religious rituals. Nurses can observe for cues about common religious practices in the patient's environment while exploring preferences related to:

- Dietary preferences, specific foods or drinks the patient believes promote healing (such as chicken soup or herbal tea) or avoids due to religious beliefs (such as pork products)
- Prayer, devotion, or worship times; nursing staff can assist the patient with any religious practices the patient wants to participate in while in care
- Favorite sacred objects or religious books that nursing staff can help the patient keep safe while in the healthcare facility
- Any medical procedures or treatments the patient prohibits and would refuse to have done.

Recognizing Spiritual Health Decline

When patients are stressed by physical or emotional pain or other medical circumstances, they may become fatigued and unable to find strength, comfort, or meaning from their spiritual beliefs and religious practices. Alongside their physical or mental decline, they may experience a decline in their spiritual health (Zarzycka & Zietek, 2019). Nurses need to be attentive when providing patient care for characteristics of spiritual health decline. These include decreased appetite, questions about life's purpose, refraining from usual religious practices, despondent facial expressions, fatigue, feeling like God has forgotten them, and observed irritability (Crossroads Hospice & Palliative Care, 2018). Nursing interventions in response to spiritual decline or discomfort include:

- Give the patient and family members information about spiritual support in the healthcare facility, including chaplain visits and locations of the public chapel or prayer room.
- Offer to call the chaplain or the patient's spiritual leader to visit the patient to answer questions and listen to the patient's spiritual concerns.
- Provide a calm and quiet environment in the patient's room.
- Be available as time allows to attentively listen and answer questions the patient may have about their hospitalization.

Communicating with Patients

When a patient experiencing spiritual distress asks a question about religious practices, nurses need to be empathetic to what they are hearing. While nurses actively listen to the patient, they can provide support with calm and understanding facial expressions. They encourage patients to express thoughts, feelings, and concerns freely.

The patient states, "I used to enjoy playing hymns on my piano, but now I don't feel I can play hymns, and I don't know why."

- I have some time now if you would like to talk about this. I'd like to hear more about you playing hymns.
- So what I'm hearing is that you used to enjoy playing hymns, but something's different now, and you feel you can't play them.

Diagnosis

Not all patients will experience spiritual discomfort. Some may be healthy spiritually but in need of help in maintaining their spiritual wellness. Continuing spiritual practices such as prayer and meditation may require arranging a quiet calm time and place for patients. Nurses can provide support and referrals as appropriate. For example, in hospital settings and long-term care settings, nurses may ensure patients have access to religious materials that provide comfort and can schedule appointments around religious observances as appropriate.

Illness or injury that disrupts religious practices can impair the patient's religiosity and result in emotional distress. An example of impaired religiosity might be the Roman Catholic patient who normally attends daily Mass but is on enforced bedrest or requires an extended hospitalization.

Planning

In the planning phase, interventions are prioritized that will assist patients to move from spiritual discomfort to a higher level of spiritual health and reconnect to spiritual beliefs and practices. Outcomes of care may include the following:

- The patient will resume personal spiritual practices while hospitalized.
- The patient will verbalize acceptance of and start to make peace with the medical diagnosis before being discharged.
- The patient will state feeling a sense of hope and purpose.
- The patient will participate in religious observances as desired.
- The patient will participate in prayer at prescribed times without interruption.
- The patient will receive meals in keeping with religious dietary guidelines and within the prescribed diet.
- The patient will have access to religious resources, including ministers, prayer partners, sacred texts, and sacred objects.

Implementation

When selecting interventions to support patients moving toward spiritual wellness, nurses can ask patients what they have done in the past to reconnect with their spiritual beliefs and which spiritual practices helped bring them feelings of fulfillment and purpose. Treating patients experiencing spiritual discomfort with dignity and respect can improve their self-worth. When nurses provide spiritual care, it can influence the patient's sense of well-being, help them to have positive feelings, and regain hope and energy to manage their illness (Clarke & Baume, 2019).

Patients do not routinely expect nurses to be experts in spirituality, to be able to provide answers to their spiritual questions, or to have lengthy conversations with them. Nurses may feel unsure of their ability to answer patient's spiritual questions, such as discussing after-death issues. Although everyone on the interprofessional healthcare team can provide many of the spiritual care actions listed above, some patients may benefit from the nurse making a referral to the chaplain's office (Clarke & Baume, 2019).

Provide Spiritual Care Actions

Spiritual care actions are interventions that support spiritual wellness, such as a sense of humor, which can promote a connection between the nurse and patient through laughter. There are many spiritually nurturing activities that nurses can teach to patients, such as observing nature through the window, performing small acts of kindness, and smiling at people who go by. Nurses can integrate the following spiritual care actions while providing daily nursing care to patients:

- Attentive listening
- Respecting privacy and dignity
- Making eye contact, if appropriate
- Offering choices to the patient
- Giving support and reassurance
- Using a gentle, therapeutic touch, if appropriate
- Encouraging motivation and self-determination.

Another significant spiritual care action occurs when nurses are completely present with patients in ways that communicate, "I hear you; I am with you; you are important; I will not judge you." When nurses are being completely present with patients, they are giving them their full attention, listening to them, and encouraging them to express their feelings (Clarke & Baume, 2019). Being present with a patient does not always include talking; sometimes it means offering to sit with the patient quietly even if only for a short amount of time. By doing this, the patient is not alone and can feel the presence, comfort, and connection with another person.

Nurses can help patients meet their needs by scheduling quiet times during the day for prayer or meditation; helping patients connect with family, friends, or a chaplain to talk with; or listening and showing empathy to patients talking about their concerns. Sometimes patients may not want to wait for a chaplain to come talk with them, so nurses can listen to patients talk when providing other care, such as while assisting them to ambulate down a hallway. Examples of how nurses can provide other spiritual interventions to support patients include:

- Attentively listening to patients talk about what they are wondering or concerned about.
- Asking patients about good and bad times in their life and helping them reflect and remember the mix of both in their past and how they felt.
- Using appropriate humor and laughter to lighten conversations.
- Providing inspirational reading or music to comfort patients as needed.

Support Religious Practices

For patients whose spirituality informs their medical decisions or provides comfort in times of illness, continuing religious traditions and practices while hospitalized supports their spiritual health. The longer patients are hospitalized, the more important it becomes for nurses to periodically assess their spiritual health and ability to follow religious practices. Older adult patients may need assistance with some religious routines. Nursing interventions include those outlined in Box 30.3.

When a patient asks for prayer, the nurse may need to ask about the patient's prayer preferences and what the patient would like the nurse to pray for. If policy at the healthcare facility allows a nurse to pray with the patient when the patient requests it and if the nurse is comfortable praying, the nurse can say a simple and short prayer using everyday words. If the nurse is uncomfortable saying a prayer with a patient, the nurse can make a referral to a chaplain or ask a nurse who is comfortable praying with patients to meet the patient's request. Patients sometimes may want the nurse to stay with them while they are praying either out loud or silently.

Evaluation

Expected outcomes of nursing care related to the patient's religious needs include the following:

- The patient has been able to practice religious rituals, including prayers.
- The dietary staff made the patient appropriate food choices within dietary restrictions.
- The patient successfully maintained connection with the community of faith.
- The patient resumed spiritual practices while hospitalized.
- The patient verbalizes a sense of hope and purpose.

Nursing Care Plan

A Patient with Spiritual Discomfort

Sally Horton is a 60-year-old woman post-op from a right radical mastectomy. Her surgeon told her he found her breast cancer was not well differentiated, which means the prognosis is poor. In the evening, her nurse finds her tearful, refusing to eat supper and not wanting to take her medications because as Sally told the nurse, "What's the use?"

(continued on next page)

Nursing Care Plan *(continued)*

ASSESSMENT	DIAGNOSES	PLANNING
■ Sally Horton, post-op today from a right radical mastectomy, was told by her surgeon her prognosis was poor. ■ Currently, 6 hours later, she is crying, refusing to eat supper or take her medications, because as she stated, "What's the use?" ■ She asks the nurse, "Why has God done this to me? I think God's mad at me for not going to church all these years. Is there somewhere I can go to pray? I'm afraid to die."	■ Manifesting spiritual discomfort due to impact of hearing poor prognosis and realization of her future, expressing distress from grief, hopelessness of her diagnosis, guilt and regret of past discord with God, and feeling fear and aloneness because of a disconnect with God.	■ Patient will express emotions and feelings about her diagnosis and prognosis before discharge. ■ Patient will begin doing two spiritual practices, such as reading scriptures, praying, or meditating before discharge. ■ Patient will connect with others to share thoughts, feelings, and beliefs by discharge.

IMPLEMENTATION

- Plan time each shift to sit with patient and attentively listen to her concerns and feelings.
- Offer to contact the chaplain to visit and answer any questions the patient may have.
- Ask patient what spiritual resources she would like to read or have in her room and, as able, bring them to her or ask her who could bring them to her while hospitalized.
- Integrate spiritual care actions when providing nursing interventions to patient.
- Maintain a quiet, calm environment in the patient's room.

EVALUATION

- Ms. Horton is able to talk about her diagnosis and prognosis.
- She has begun to read scriptures and say short prayers at bedtime.
- She is sometimes able to smile and laugh when talking with her friends that come to visit her.

CRITICAL THINKING

1. What spiritual resources might be helpful for this patient?
2. If Ms. Horton asks you to pray with her, what would you do?
3. What are four spiritual care actions you could do when providing care to Ms. Horton?

REVIEW The Concept of Spirituality

RELATE Link the Concepts

Linking the concept of spirituality with the concept of development:

1. How might a nurse address the spiritual needs of an 8-year-old child who has leukemia?

2. How might a nurse address the spiritual needs of a teenager with cystic fibrosis?

Linking the concept of spirituality with the concept of culture and diversity:

3. What could a nurse say to a Muslim patient who wants to fast during the day because it is the month of Ramadan, even though the HCP has ordered a clear liquid diet?

4. How would you preoperatively prepare a Khalsid Sikh man for surgery requiring shaving of body hair when this man has vowed to never cut his hair?

Linking the concept of spirituality with the concept of oxygenation:

5. Describe the risk for spiritual discomfort faced by the parents of a child who has just died from sudden infant death syndrome.

6. What caring interventions would you offer to the child's parents?

Linking the concept of spirituality with the concept of stress and coping:

7. How might the patient's inability to perform customary religious rituals during times of illness result in anxiety?

8. How does helping patients meet their religious needs, thus reducing anxiety, help them to recover more quickly?

REFER Go to Pearson MyLab Nursing and eText

REFLECT Apply Your Knowledge

Terry Mears is a 32-year-old man who owns a small farm. He is recovering from a spider bite to his left thumb 6 days ago, but a purple ring is developing around the bite site that looks like a blister. Despite having chills and body aches, he refuses to go to the community health clinic for "just a little spider bite." Mr. Mears asks several people who attend his church to pray that his hand will heal quickly so he can take care of his farm. He becomes very discouraged, despondent, and angry when, after 10 more days, his hand has not healed and he is having trouble getting things done around the farm.

1. Would it have made a difference if Mr. Mears had gone to the health clinic for medical treatment when he was first bitten by a spider? Why or why not?
2. What symptoms suggest that Mr. Mears may be experiencing spiritual discomfort?
3. How might prolonged healing affect an individual's spiritual beliefs?

References

ACEP, Association of Professional Chaplains, Canadian Association for Spiritual Care/Association, National Association of Catholic Chaplains, and Neshama: Association of Jewish Chaplains. (n.d.). *The impact of professional spiritual care*. https://www.professionalchaplains.org/Files/resources/The%20Impact%20of%20Professional%20Spiritual%20Care_PDF.pdf

American Association of Equine Practitioners. (2020). *Spiritual wellness*. https://aaep.org/wellness/spiritual-wellness

American Seniors Housing Association. (2020). *Spirituality and aging*. https://www.whereyoulivematters.org/spirituality-and-aging/

Arthur, L. B. (2020). *Religion and dress*. LoveToKnow. https://fashion-history.lovetoknow.com/fashion-history-eras/religion-dress

Atlantic Health System. (2020). *Pastoral care*. https://www.atlantichealth.org/patients-visitors/hospital-stays-visits/pastoral-care.html

Attum, B., Hafiz, S., Malik, A., & Shamoon, Z. (2018). *Cultural competence in the care of Muslim patients and their families*. StatPearls. https://pubmed.ncbi.nlm.nih.gov/29763108/

Berman, A., Snyder, S., & Frandsen, G. (2016). *Kozier & Erb's fundamentals of nursing: Concepts, process, and practice*, (10th ed.). Pearson.

Centers for Disease Control and Prevention (CDC). (2018). *Well-being concepts*. https://www.cdc.gov/hrqol/wellbeing.htm

Clarke, J., & Baume, K. (2019). Embedding spiritual care into everyday nursing practice. *Nursing Standard*. https://doi.org/10.7748/ns.2019.e11354

Crossroads Hospice & Palliative Care. (2018). Signs and symptoms of spiritual distress. https://www.crossroadshospice.com/hospice-palliative-care-blog/2018/october/10/signs-and-symptoms-of-spiritual-distress/

Dienstman, A. M. (2019). *8 simple, everyday spiritual practice ideas*. Goodnet. https://www.goodnet.org/articles/8-simple-everyday-spiritual-practice-ideas

Dollahite, D. C., & Marks, L. D. (2019). Positive youth religious and spiritual development: What we have learned from religious families. *Religions*, *10*, 548. https://doi.org/10.3390/rel10100548

Farran, K. (2019). *10 reasons God entrusts us with trials*. ABWE International. https://www.abwe.org/blog/10-reasons-god-entrusts-us-trials

Feldman, S. (2019). *How does daily prayer differ around the world?* Statista. https://www.statista.com/chart/17865/daily-prayer-worldwide/

Fitch, M. I., & Bartlett, R. (2019). Patient perspectives about spirituality and spiritual care. *Asia-Pacific Journal of Oncology Nursing*, *6*(2), 111–121.

Freeman, S. (2018). What causes spiritual distress? *HomeCare Magazine*. https://www.homecaremag.com/december-2018/spiritual-distress-care

Ghaderi, A., Tabatabaei, S. M., Nedjat, S., Javadi, M., & Larijani, B. (2018). Explanatory definition of the concept of spiritual health: A qualitative study in Iran. *Journal of Medical Ethics and History of Medicine*, *11*, 3.

Greenthal, S. (2020). *How young adults are finding religion*. VeryWell Mind. https://www.verywellmind.com/how-young-adults-are-finding-religion-4128793

HealthCare Chaplaincy Network. (2018). *What is a professional health care chaplain?* http://chaplainsonhand.org/cms/about/what-is-chaplain.html

Herdman, T. H., & Kamitsuru, S. (2018). *Nursing diagnoses: Definitions and classification 2018–2020*. Thieme.

Intriago, J. (2020). Religion and spirituality in older people. SeniorsMatter. https://www.seniorsmatter.com/religion-spirituality-older-people/2492159

Jacobs, M. (2019). *What spirituality means to older people*. Silver Century Foundation. https://www.silvercentury.org/2019/01/what-spirituality-means-to-older-people/

Kavar, L. F. (2020, January). *The experience of spirituality: Adults and millennials*. Paper presented at the Qualitative Report Conference, Fort Lauderdale, FL.

Medibank. (2019). *The origins of Western and Eastern medicine*. https://www.medibank.com.au/livebetter/health-brief/health-insights/the-origins-of-western-and-eastern-medicine/

Monroe, S. (2020). *The difference between health and wellness*. International Association of Wellness Professionals. https://iawpwellnesscoach.com/difference-between-health-and-wellness/

Nishat, N. (2020). Types of health. *The World Book*. https://theworldbook.org/types-of-health/

Oswalt, A., Reiss, N. S., & Dombeck, M. (2020). *Cultural and spiritual nurturing in early childhood*. Gracepoint. https://www.gracepointwellness.org/462-child-development-parenting-early-3-7/article/14347-cultural-and-spiritual-nurturing-in-early-childhood

Penque, S. (2019). Mindfulness to promote nurses' well-being. *Nursing Management*, *50*(5), 38–44.

Pew Research Center. (2019). *In U.S., decline of Christianity continues at rapid pace*. https://www.pewforum.org/2019/10/17/in-u-s-decline-of-christianity-continues-at-rapid-pace/

Potter, M. L., & Moller, M. D. (2020). *Psychiatric–mental health nursing: From suffering to hope* (2nd ed.). Pearson.

PowWows.com. (2019). *Native American religion and spirituality – Common threads, unique beliefs, and too many misconceptions*. https://www.powwows.com/native-american-religion-and-spirituality-common-threads-unique-beliefs-and-too-many-misconceptions/

PracticalNursing.org. (2020). *The importance of holistic nursing care: How to completely care for your patients*. https://www.practicalnursing.org/importance-holistic-nursing-care-how-completely-care-patients

ReachOut. (2020). *What is spirituality?* https://au.reachout.com/articles/what-is-spirituality

Rindfleisch, J. A. (2020). *Whole health: Change the conversation*. University of Wisconsin–Madison School of Medicine. http://projects.hsl.wisc.edu/SERVICE/modules/11/M11_Spiritual_Assessment_Tools.pdf

Silver, V. (2020). *The mind, body, spirit connection*. Holistic MindBody Healing. https://www.holistic-mindbody-healing.com/mind-body-spirit-connection.html

Smith, L. N., & Jackson, V. A. (2013). How do symptoms change for patients in the last days and hours of life? In N. E. Goldstein & R. S. Morrison (Eds.), *Evidence-based practice in palliative medicine* (pp. 218–227). Elsevier Saunders.

Substance Abuse and Mental Health Services Administration. (2018). First responders: Behavioral health concerns, emergency response, and trauma. *Disaster Technical Assistance Center Supplemental Research Bulletin*. https://www.samhsa.gov/sites/default/files/dtac/supplementalresearchbulletin-firstresponders-may2018.pdf

Swihart, D. L., Yarrarapu, S. N. S., & Martin, R. L. (2020). *Cultural religious competence in clinical practice*. StatPearls. https://www.ncbi.nlm.nih.gov/books/NBK493216/?report=printable

United States Conference of Catholic Bishops (USCCB). (2020). *Anointing of the sick*. https://www.usccb.org/prayer-and-worship/sacraments-and-sacramentals/anointing-of-the-sick

University of Kansas. (2020). *Seven ways to improve your spiritual health*. https://wellness.ku.edu/seven-ways-improve-your-spiritual-health

University of Minnesota. (2016). *Develop your spiritual resources*. https://www.takingcharge.csh.umn.edu/develop-your-spiritual-resources

Uzell, J. (2018). Death/funeral rituals in world religions. Religion Media Centre. https://religionmediacentre.org.uk/factsheets/death-funeral-rituals-in-world-religions/

Victoria Angel Public Cord Blood Bank. (2020). *Cord blood use*. https://victoriaangel.org/donate-cord-blood/faqs/

Waltner, A. (2020). *Largest religions in the world (2020)*. Swedish Nomad. https://www.swedishnomad.com/largest-religions-in-the-world/

Welch, A. (2019). *A guide to 7 different types meditation*. Everyday Health. https://www.everydayhealth.com/meditation/types/

Zarzycka, B., & Zietek, P. (2019). Spiritual growth or decline and meaning-making as mediators of anxiety and satisfaction with life during religious struggle. *Journal of Religion and Health*, *58*(4), 1072–1086.

Zotigh, D. (2018). Native perspectives on the 40th anniversary of the American Indian Religious Freedom Act. *Smithsonian Magazine*. https://www.smithsonianmag.com/blogs/national-museum-american-indian/2018/11/30/native-perspectives-american-indian-religious-freedom-act/

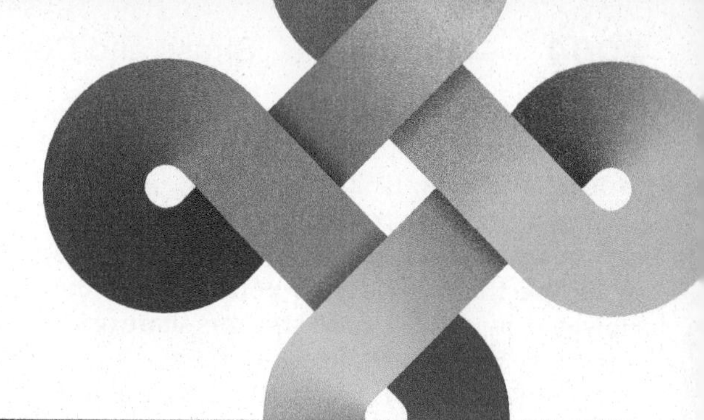

Module 31
Stress and Coping

Module Outline and Learning Outcomes

The Concept of Stress and Coping

Stress and Homeostasis

31.1 Contrast stress and homeostasis.

Stressors and the Coping Process

31.2 Explain types of stressors and the psychodynamics of coping.

Manifestations of Stress

31.3 Outline the manifestations and indicators of stress.

Concepts Related to Stress and Coping

31.4 Outline the relationship between stress and coping and other concepts.

Alterations from Normal Coping Responses

31.5 Differentiate alterations in coping.

Health Promotion

31.6 Explain the promotion of healthy coping and the prevention of stress-related illness.

Nursing Assessment

31.7 Differentiate among common assessment procedures and tests used to examine levels of stress and coping mechanisms.

Independent Interventions

31.8 Analyze independent interventions nurses can implement for patients with alterations in stress and coping.

Collaborative Therapies

31.9 Summarize collaborative therapies used by interprofessional teams for patients with stress-related illness and alterations in coping.

Lifespan Considerations

31.10 Differentiate considerations related to the care of patients with stress throughout the lifespan.

Stress and Coping Exemplars

Exemplar 31.A Anxiety Disorders

31.A Analyze anxiety disorders as they relate to stress and coping.

Exemplar 31.B Crisis

31.B Analyze crisis as it relates to stress and coping.

Exemplar 31.C Obsessive–Compulsive Disorder

31.C Analyze obsessive–compulsive disorder (OCD) as it relates to stress and coping.

>> The Concept of Stress and Coping

Concept Key Terms

Adaptation, **2088**
Allostasis, **2084**
Allostatic load, **2084**
Anger, **2092**
Anxiety, **2092**
Approach coping, **2088**
Avoidance coping, **2088**
Burnout, **2094**
Cognitive appraisal, **2087**
Cognitive-behavioral therapy (CBT), **2100**
Coping, **2084**
Countershock phase, **2089**
Daily hassles, **2086**
Depression, **2092**
Diseases of adaptation, **2089**
Distress, **2084**
Ego defense mechanisms, **2092**
Emotion-focused coping, **2088**
Eustress, **2084**
External environmental stressors, **2086**
Fear, **2092**
General adaptation syndrome (GAS), **2089**
Homeostasis, **2083**
Internal environment, **2086**
Local adaptation syndrome (LAS), **2089**
Maslow's hierarchy of needs, **2087**
Meaning-focused coping, **2088**
Nursing transactional model, **2090**
Primary appraisal, **2087**
Problem-focused coping, **2088**
Problem solving, **2092**
Reappraisal, **2088**
Secondary appraisal, **2087**
Shock phase, **2089**
Stage of exhaustion, **2089**
Stage of resistance, **2089**
Stimulus-based stress model, **2088**
Stress, **2084**
Stress mediators, **2084**
Stress response, **2084**
Stressor, **2083**

Although everyone experiences stress, what triggers stress in one individual may not cause stress in another. These triggers are known as stressors. A **stressor** is an external influence that threatens to disrupt the equilibrium necessary to maintain homeostasis. **Homeostasis** is classically described as the body's ability to maintain a stable, balanced internal environment despite the constant challenges posed by external influences (Cannon, 1932). When healthy and functioning properly, the body adapts to these external influences, or stressors, and promotes maintenance or restoration of homeostasis. Homeostasis is demonstrated by the body's ability to maintain fluid and electrolyte balance, oxygenation, and thermoregulation (the control of heat production and heat loss to maintain a steady body temperature).

In particular, physiologic maintenance of the body's delicate acid–base balance provides a classic example of homeostasis in action (Cannon, 1932).

Stressors may be physical, mental, or emotional; they also may be positive or negative, depending on several variables, including the individual's perception of the experience. However, by definition, all stressors share one commonality: They have the capacity to cause stress.

In *Stress In America™ 2020*, the American Psychological Association reported that Americans were overwhelmed by "multiple sources of stress and associated symptoms," with nearly 8 in 10 adults surveyed reporting the COVID-19 pandemic as a "significant source of stress" and two-thirds reporting increased stress since the pandemic began (2020, p. 2). To a certain degree, pandemic-related stress reflected individual life stage, with 7 in 10 parents reporting significant stress related to family responsibilities and between 51 and 67% of the Gen Z population reporting disruptions to their ability to plan for the future as a major source of stress. Additional sources of stress included work and financial disruptions, discrimination, and the presidential election, among others. According to the American Psychological Association, the combination of multiple stressors across domains of living has led to a "national mental health crisis that could yield serious health and social consequences for years to come" (p. 1).

Widespread stress resulting from the pandemic means that nurses in every setting will face patients and families struggling to cope with additional financial and social burdens, possibly without meaningful supports, for the foreseeable future. This module provides information about how individuals respond to stress and anxiety generally and how nurses can promote healthy coping in patients across the lifespan; priority considerations for caring for those experiencing a major crisis; and nursing care of patients with diagnosed anxiety and obsessive–compulsive disorders.

Stress and Homeostasis

The term *stress* has appeared in the literature since approximately the 14th century, when it was used in reference to hardship, adversity, or some form of affliction (Lumsden, 1981). However, the present-day understanding of the concept of stress was initially developed through the research and publications of Dr. Hans Selye (1907–1982). Selye was an endocrinologist and a pioneer in the study of stress and the stress response. Selye (1956) defined **stress** as the body's general, nonspecific response to the demands placed on it by a stressor. Selye further asserted that not all stress is bad; in some cases, stress can help an individual achieve desired goals or exceed self-imposed limitations (Cherry, 1978; Selye, 1956, 1976). Good stress, which Selye called **eustress**, is associated with accomplishment and victory. The opposite of eustress is **distress**, which is stress that is associated with inadequacy, insecurity, and loss (Cherry, 1978; Selye, 1956).

In further refining Cannon's conceptualization of homeostasis from a more holistic standpoint, Sterling and Eyer (1988) originated the term **allostasis**, which refers to the changes necessary to achieve the characteristic stability of homeostasis. During homeostasis, the body maintains vital functions such as heart and respiratory rates and oxygen and glucose levels within an ideal range. In contrast, more current literature describes allostasis as the process the body uses to maintain a pathophysiologic deviation from the normal homeostatic operating level in the presence of stressors (Fava et al., 2019). This deviation from normal homeostasis allows the body to function as optimally as possible in the presence of major stressors. The process of allostasis includes the psychosocial and physiologic changes that occur in response to stress, many of which are triggered by activation of the sympathetic nervous system (SNS).

In addition to other functions, the SNS triggers the body's "fight-or-flight" response, which is necessary for survival. Activation of the SNS causes release of hormones such as epinephrine, which increases the heart rate and blood pressure to help deliver oxygen to tissues and organs. Epinephrine also causes bronchial dilation, which allows for increased oxygen uptake. This increase in oxygen uptake and delivery is intended to meet the increased metabolic demands associated with facing (fight) or escaping (flight) the stressor.

Formally referred to as the **stress response**, physiologic changes triggered by stress include activation of the neural, neuroendocrine, and endocrine systems as well as activation of target organs (Everly & Lating, 2019). The two primary stress mediators are glucocorticoids (e.g., cortisol) and catecholamines (e.g., epinephrine). These hormonal **stress mediators** promote adaptation (e.g., by triggering an increase in heart rate and blood pressure) when faced with physical danger.

Under ideal conditions, the stress response permits the body to compensate for the impact of stressors and ensure survival by either maintaining or regaining homeostasis. However, repeated activation of the stress response takes a toll on the individual. The physical cost of adaptation to physiologic or psychosocial stressors is referred to as the **allostatic load**. In addition to hormonal changes, the allostatic load also includes behavioral responses to stress. These can be favorable, as in participating in yoga or exercise, or unfavorable—for example, smoking or drinking alcohol. Chronic, prolonged overexposure to stress mediators, as well as inefficiency of the stress response and unhealthy behavioral responses to stress, can lead to illness and other negative sequelae (see the Evidence-Based Practice feature) (Fava et al., 2019).

How an individual responds to stress varies and depends on both the individual and the stressor. **Coping** is a dynamic process through which an individual applies cognitive and behavioral measures to handle internal and external demands that the individual perceives as exceeding available resources (Lazarus & Folkman, 1984). Individuals cope by integrating environmental and cognitive measures to mitigate or reduce the stress response (Everly & Lating, 2019). For example, a nursing student who is studying for final exams might cope with stress through environmental measures such as taking a walk or meeting a friend for coffee. Cognitively, the nursing student might alter the appraisal of the upcoming examination, choosing not to see it as an insurmountable problem, but rather as a challenge for which the student can prepare and successfully master.

When an individual is unable to adapt to stress sufficiently to maintain homeostasis, functional impairment may occur. For example, a young child may become irritable and not be able to sit in the circle during morning carpet time at preschool and may strike out at a classmate. An adult who fears the consequences of exposure to germs may perform handwashing or clean the house compulsively, disrupting the ability to participate in normal activities. Individuals who experience impairment in functioning related to stress and coping may develop one of several stress or anxiety disorders. This module provides a discussion of stress and coping as well as a more detailed picture of anxiety disorders, crisis, and obsessive–compulsive disorder.

Stressors and the Coping Process

When patients in distress present to clinics, emergency departments (EDs), or mental health centers, nurses assist by assessing the source of the stress and the patient's response and by helping to cope with the stressor. To be able to respond appropriately, nurses must have a working knowledge of types of stressors; how human beings respond to or cope with stress; and theoretical models of stress and coping that provide insight into how nurses can support patients during times of stress.

How people perceive stressors varies. For example, one person may view bungee jumping as a terrifying, life-threatening event that should be avoided, but another may consider it an exhilarating form of stress release. Identification of a stressor depends on the individual's personal perception of the event or circumstance. However, certain stressors naturally evoke the physiologic stress response in all individuals, without regard to personal perception.

Types of Stressors

Stressors may be categorized using a variety of methods. From a broad standpoint, stressors often are categorized as being either biogenic or psychosocial (Everly & Lating, 2019).

Biogenic stressors directly trigger the stress response without any necessary cognitive process on the part of the individual; that is, the individual does not need to recognize the experience or circumstance as being stressful. Common examples of biogenic stressors include caffeine, amphetamines, and extreme temperatures (Everly & Lating, 2019). *Psychosocial stressors* may be either real or imagined. Rather than directly triggering the stress response, psychosocial stressors can facilitate its activation, depending on how the individual perceives the stressor (a process called *cognitive appraisal*, discussed later in this module) (Everly & Lating, 2019). For example, an individual who has a fear of heights may respond to cleaning the gutters on the house differently than an individual who is not afraid of heights.

Just as the severity (or perceived severity) of a stressor impacts the magnitude of the stress response, so does the length of time to which the individual is exposed to the stressor. This is true regardless of whether the stressor is biogenic or psychosocial in nature—both can be equally powerful. In fact, anticipation of a stressor can produce the same physiologic response that occurs when faced with the stressor in reality (Neubauer, Smyth, & Sliwinski, 2017). For example, anticipating or imagining a potential physical attack

Evidence-Based Practice

Parenting Stress during a Pandemic

Problem

The COVID-19 global pandemic caused increased stress on parents and guardians due to the closing of schools, working from home, role conflict, social isolation, lost income and related housing insecurity, food insecurity, overcrowding, and worry about catching the virus (Swedo et al., 2020). According to a report by the World Health Organization (WHO, 2020), approximately 1.5 billion children around the world lost time in school due to the pandemic. This increased stress on families, coupled with the inability to access normal support services that schools offer, increased the potential for child abuse.

Evidence

Brown and colleagues (2020) studied the effects of the pandemic on perceived stress in parents and the potential for child abuse. Perceived stress is the thoughts and feelings a person has about the amount of stress experienced and is related to control, predictability, the number of irritating hassles, and confidence in the ability to deal with these issues (Cohen, Kamarck, & Mermelstein, 1983).

The researchers found that high levels of anxiety, manifestations of depression, and a higher number of stressors related to COVID-19 were associated with greater perceived stress by parents (Brown et al., 2020). Parents who received government assistance (such as EBT/food stamps, childcare subsidy, or Medicaid) or other financial assistance (such as child support) and those who had greater levels of anxiety or depression were at greater risk for engaging in child abuse. They also found that parents who had higher levels of support within the home or through family networks and who felt a degree of control over life events experienced lower levels of perceived stress and had a lower potential for child abuse.

Implications

Brown et al. concluded that the accumulation of stressors from COVID-19 in the parents they studied did not directly increase the potential for child abuse, even though cumulative stress is highly connected with child abuse. Some parents even reported that being home with their children for an extended time period was a constructive experience that positively impacted their parenting. This indicates more research is needed to understand the long-term effects of cumulative stress on families and children. The researchers recommended that parents should receive additional social and emotional support to lower their perceived levels of stress and to support their parenting when usual sources of support, such as school-based supports, are not available.

Critical Thinking Application

1. Consider the relationship between high levels of perceived stress and the increased potential for child abuse. During a pandemic or a community or regional disaster, how can nurses provide support to parents?
2. What interventions can nurses take to reduce parents' perceived levels of stress?
3. How can nurses provide anticipatory guidance on stress reduction during a pandemic and increase parents' feelings of control over life?

TABLE 31.1 Classifications and Examples of Stressors

Classification of Stressors	Examples
1. Acute and time limited	Ankle sprain Nursing licensure exam
2. Sequential events following an initial stressor	Losing a job and subsequently filing for bankruptcy
3. Chronic intermittent	Strained relationship with in-laws Shared caregiving for an elderly parent
4. Chronic permanent	Paralysis Death of a child

can evoke the release of the same stress hormones as those released during an actual physical fight.

From the standpoint of duration of exposure, stressors may be classified into four categories:

1. Acute and time limited
2. Sequential events following an initial stressor
3. Chronic intermittent
4. Chronic permanent.

See **Table 31.1** >> for examples of each classification.

To understand the reciprocal and dynamic relationship between the individual and the environment, it is necessary to consider sources of stress and types of stressors. The degree of a stressor's impact ranges from the benign (nonthreatening) hassles of daily living to traumatic events within an individual, family, and society. Examples of traumatic events include rape, life-threatening illness or injury, and natural disasters such as hurricanes. **Box 31.1** >> lists some common stressors. Additional stressors related to lifespan and development are discussed in the section Lifespan Considerations.

Box 31.1

Types of Stressors

Daily Hassles

- Roles of living
- Caring for children
- Pets
- Work responsibility
- Paying bills
- Traffic
- Neighbors

Internal Stressors

- Cognition (thoughts)
- Spirituality
- Emotions

Environmental Stressors

- Major cataclysmic changes affecting a large number of people (natural disasters, war, floods, hurricanes)
- Major changes affecting one or a few people (divorce, bereavement)

Daily Hassles

The individual day-to-day tensions that people face are commonly referred to in stress and coping research as **daily hassles**. Examples of daily hassles include making it through a workday or having to care for a small child after a poor night's sleep. The seminal work of DeLongis and colleagues (1982) indicated that hassles can be more strongly correlated with somatic health and symptoms than more eventful stressors. A person's physical, emotional, and spiritual health affects whether the individual views a hassle as a minor inconvenience or a major strain. Alterations of health in any of these areas may overwhelm an individual's ability to cope with a specific stimulus or event, no matter how mild.

Internal Stressors

The **internal environment** includes the physical, spiritual, cognitive, emotional, and psychologic well-being of an individual and depends on the satisfaction of basic human needs. According to Lazarus and Folkman (1984), the drive to fulfill human needs internally sparks the stimulus to produce energy to seek gratification. When these internal needs are not met, individuals find it harder to cope with changes to their circumstances, including dealing with daily hassles, developmental stressors, or external stressors.

Dossey and Keegan view the spiritual dimension of the human condition as part of the individual's internal environment and define *spirituality* as the essence of who we are and how we relate to the world (Blaszko, Shields, Avino, & Rosa, 2022). They incorporate elements of spirituality that include individual values, our place or fit in the world, and a sense of peace. Recent research has identified interconnectedness with the self, individuals, and the world around us as important components of spirituality. (See Module 30, Spirituality.)

The impact of chronic, life-threatening, or debilitating illness has been identified as a significant stressor. For example, the term *diabetes distress* describes a negative emotional state caused by the burden and worry of living with the complex, chronic condition of diabetes and is associated with negative health outcomes. The stress of managing the delicate balance of dosing and timing of medications with blood glucose levels, meals, and activity as well as coping with debilitating complications and the financial impact of dealing with the illness can lead to diabetes distress. Diabetes distress is associated with elevated A1C levels and less adherence with treatment and activity recommendations (American Diabetes Association, 2019).

Environmental Stressors

External environmental stressors include triggers outside of the individual that necessitate change or disrupt homeostasis. Positive stressors, such as graduation from college, generally produce eustress. Negative stressors, such as the inability to find employment, tend to cause distress. Stressors also may be simultaneously positive and negative, as with the combination of pending college graduation and imminent lack of employment. An event is a stressor if it creates a change in individuals or their circumstances. **Table 31.2** >> outlines specific individual and environmental factors that affect individuals' response to a stressor.

TABLE 31.2 Factors Affecting Stress Response

Individual Factors	Environmental Factors
Genetic predisposition	Family support and connectedness
Past experience coping with stressors	Community support
Ability to meet own basic human needs	Financial resources
Cultural beliefs and customs	Community resources
Holistic health and well-being	Access to healthcare and education
Personal worldview and appraisal	Family appraisal
Coping mechanisms and history of coping successes	Social support

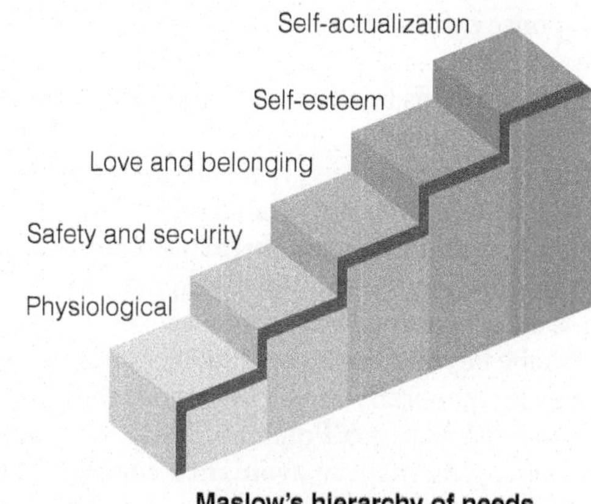

Figure 31.1 » Maslow's hierarchy of needs.

The Coping Process

As stated earlier, *coping* is the process by which individuals can control or modify their responses to stressors. Successful coping allows individuals to maintain or return to homeostasis within a reasonable amount of time. Individuals who are unable to cope successfully may experience a range of symptoms requiring intervention from nurses and other healthcare professionals.

Cognitive Appraisal

Cognitive appraisal is a key factor in the ability to cope with stressors. As an individual experiences exposure to a stressor, the person appraises it—mentally sorting, assessing, categorizing, evaluating, and framing the significance of an event or stressor with respect to well-being. The **primary appraisal** is the "first impression" that occurs immediately on exposure to a stressor. Based on the transactional model (described in detail later in this module), there are three ways in which an individual categorizes a stimulus or stressor: (1) irrelevant, (2) benign-positive, or (3) stressful. Irrelevant stressors are appraised as having no meaningful effect on the individual or circumstance and are disregarded. Benign-positive stressors are demands for change that are perceived as preserving or enhancing well-being, such as taking a driver's education class. Stressors or stimuli categorized as stressful include those viewed as harmful, threatening, or disturbing, such as the death of a family member or a threat to life or safety.

During the **secondary appraisal**, the individual attempts to predict the impact, intensity, and duration of the coping behavior necessary to respond to the stressor. At this time, the individual selects a coping response.

In some cases, the intensity of an individual's stress response may appear to be incongruent with the stressor. For example, for some individuals, the loss of a family pet may be devastating and elicit an extreme stress response, whereas other individuals may demonstrate a response that is mild in intensity when faced with a similar loss. Likewise, some students may view earning a grade of "C" on an examination as being successful because it is a passing grade; for others, earning anything less than an "A" is distressing. Keeping in mind that each individual is unique, Maslow's hierarchy of needs offers a model that is useful for understanding the significance of stressors within the context of human needs.

Maslow's Hierarchy of Needs

Maslow's hierarchy of needs refers to five categories of human need proposed by Abraham Maslow in 1943: physiological, safety, love and belonging, self-esteem, and self-actualization (see **Figure 31.1** »), listed in order of importance. Although Maslow later expanded his model to include self-transcendence as a sixth level of need (Koltko-Rivera, 2006; Maslow, 1968, 1987), the five-stage model is widely used to assist nurses and other professionals in identifying and prioritizing patient needs and interventions. According to Maslow, unmet lower-order needs will dominate the individual and prohibit higher-order needs from emerging. As each category of needs is met, the individual's focus shifts to meeting higher-order needs. For example, for a parent who has just lost their job, the primary focus will be to find new employment so they can continue to feed and shelter their family. Once the family's lower order needs are met, the parent may be able to focus on higher order needs. When both physiologic and safety needs are met, needs related to love and belonging emerge. This process continues as the individual is able to meet each stage of needs (Maslow, 1987).

It is important to note that individual traits and variations lead to flexibility with regard to the sequencing of Maslow's hierarchy of needs. As a result, the prioritization of needs may vary, depending on the person (Maslow, 1987). As an example, for an individual who demonstrates an extremely powerful drive to achieve professional success, esteem needs (e.g., respect from others, empowerment, competence) may supersede needs related to love and belonging. Likewise, mental illness may lead to the exclusion of certain categories of needs (Maslow, 1987). For example, antisocial personality disorder is characterized by a lack of concern for the safety needs of self or others.

Effective Coping

Effective coping is a learned process, not an inherent personality trait. It includes all efforts an individual mobilizes to manage stressors. Coping involves constant change by the individual and includes spiritual, emotional, cognitive, and behavioral efforts to manage the demand. Lazarus and Folkman's (1984) transactional model describes coping as a means to manage or alter the problem causing the distress. The appraisal process allows the individual to inform the coping response by incorporating the person's own spiritual, cognitive, affective, and inherent vulnerability. In essence, every person responds to a stressor according to their unique worldview and condition.

Two forms of coping are (1) **problem-focused coping**, which is aimed at managing or altering the stressor, event, or circumstance, and (2) **emotion-focused coping**, which is directed at regulating the emotional response to the distress. Emotion-focused coping is used most when the stressor is perceived to be beyond the individual's control. In problem-focused coping, generally the perception is that the stressor can be changed (Lazarus & Folkman, 1984). Additional subcategories of coping include **avoidance coping** (using both behaviors and cognitive processes to avoid the stressor) and **approach coping** (confronting and trying to change the stressor by taking direct action). Finally, there is also **meaning-focused coping**, which involves re-evaluation to reduce the appraisal of a threat.

It is crucial for nurses to understand that any form of coping is an individual process influenced by the number of stressors; their source, type, intensity, and duration; and the individual's support, experience, and vulnerability. Nurses need to be aware of their own coping styles and maintain a nonjudgmental attitude about the coping mechanisms of individuals experiencing stressors. **Table 31.3** » depicts various forms and examples of coping with stressors.

Healthcare professionals and researchers have clearly established the strong and complex relationship among stress, coping, and physical and psychologic illness (Boullier & Blair, 2018). Lazarus and Folkman (1984) note that it is the reaction to the demand, not the stimulus itself, that causes stress. The nursing transactional model allows the nurse to consider individual patient preferences, resources, culture, and environment in the assessment of the patient's abilities to respond to stress and to assist the patient in returning to homeostasis.

Reappraisal and Adaptation

Following attempts to cope with the stressor, the individual engages in a **reappraisal** process. During this time, the individual evaluates which coping mechanisms were successful and which were not. Ideally, the person begins another attempt to respond to the stressor and return to homeostasis. In terms of its effects on the body, stress is not viewed as "good" or "bad," but merely according to how much, what kinds, and under what conditions is it harmful or helpful (Lazarus & Folkman, 1984). **Adaptation** refers to the use of physiologic and psychologic processes to come to terms with the implications and outcomes of stressors (Biesecker et al., 2013). Adaptation and the development of health alterations are influenced by personal variables, including cognitive appraisal of the stressor, genetic predisposition to illness, and behavioral responses to stress.

Theoretical Models of Stress and Coping

Several theories and models exist to explain the phenomenon of stress. This section outlines stimulus- and response-based stress models before presenting the transactional model in more detail.

Stimulus-Based Stress Models

Stimulus-based stress models view "stress" as being synonymous with "stressor." These models define stress as a life event that requires change or adaptation on the part of the person who is experiencing the life event. Exposure to such life events leads to physiologic and psychologic "wear and tear" and can increase the individual's susceptibility to illness (Holmes & Rahe, 1967). In their classic work, Holmes and Rahe (1967) proposed the Social Readjustment Rating Scale (SRRS), which quantified the impact of 43 significant life events—with none of the events classified as being either positive or negative—by assigning a numerical value to each individual experience. Examples of life events identified by Holmes and Rahe include death of a spouse or child, marriage, divorce, change of residence, and loss of a job. Variations of the SRRS questionnaire are still in use today.

When considering the validity of the SRRS and similar scales, note that perception of a life event will vary among individuals, particularly with regard to cognitive appraisal of the event as being a stressor. Likewise, the impact of significant events must be considered from the standpoint of the individual's simultaneous exposure to routine stressors. According to Lazarus and Folkman (1984), in comparison to experiencing significant life events, exposure to life's daily hassles was more likely to lead to stress-related alterations.

TABLE 31.3 Examples of Types of Coping

Types	Emotion-Focused Coping (Defensive)	Problem-Focused Coping	Avoidance	Approach	Meaning
Cognitive	Minimizing the event: "Oh, it's not that bad!"	Information gathering: "What are my odds of surviving?"	Denial of a situation or limiting information about stressful situations: "This is a bad dream!"	Confronting the situation	Identifying positive changes associated with stressful events; for example, personal illness that leads to increased family bonding
Behavioral	Performing physical activity to avoid thinking about a stressful situation	Adhering to a healthcare plan	Refusing to get a mammogram when a history of breast cancer runs in the family	Seeking means to exercise control	Attempting to fit into the environment: "I'll make the best of the situation."
Affective	Hoping for a miracle	Keeping feelings from interfering	Dealing with feelings later	Using feelings to motivate change	Seeking control of environment; regulating the emotional response to stress

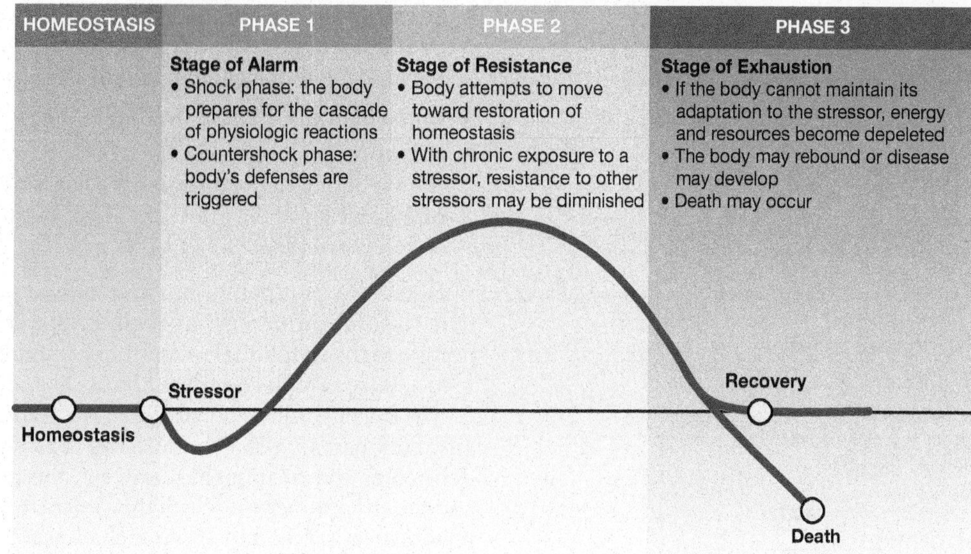
HOMEOSTASIS
PHASE 1
PHASE 2
PHASE 3
Stage of Alarm
• Shock phase: the body prepares for the cascade of physiologic reactions
• Countershock phase: body's defenses are triggered
Stage of Resistance
• Body attempts to move toward restoration of homeostasis
• With chronic exposure to a stressor, resistance to other stressors may be diminished
Stage of Exhaustion
• If the body cannot maintain its adaptation to the stressor, energy and resources become depeleted
• The body may rebound or disease may develop
• Death may occur
Stressor
Homeostasis
Recovery
Death

Figure 31.2 ›› The three stages of adaptation to stress: the alarm reaction, the stage of resistance, and the stage of exhaustion.

Response-Based Stress Models

In response-based stress models, stress is considered to be a *response* to a stressor. According to Selye, stress is "the nonspecific response of the body to any kind of demand made upon it" (1976, p. 1). Selye's model described the stress response as a three-stage chain of events called the **general adaptation syndrome (GAS)** or *stress response*. Selye used the term *stressor* to distinguish between the stimulus and the response. Within the context of GAS, stressors are any stimuli that evoke the stress response. Selye (1974) also proposed that not every instance of disruption of homeostasis qualifies as an occurrence of stress. For example, a close-flying insect that stimulates an individual to blink excessively may disturb the body's equilibrium, but this event does not necessarily trigger the GAS.

The stress response may be global (generalized) or local. A global response typically provokes physiologic changes that include hormone production and release and alterations in organs and structures. A local stress response, during which one organ or body system reacts to stress, may produce **local adaptation syndrome (LAS)**. For example, local inflammation in response to a scrape or minor laceration is an example of LAS. However, according to Selye (1976), both GAS and LAS produce a three-stage response: alarm reaction, resistance, and exhaustion (see **Figure 31.2** ››).

Alarm Reaction

The body's initial response is the two-part alarm reaction, which begins with the **shock phase**. During the shock phase, as the body prepares for the cascade of physiologic reactions to the stressor, the SNS is suppressed and the individual may experience manifestations such as hypotension, decreased body temperature, and decreased muscle tone. During the second part of the alarm reaction, which is referred to as the **countershock phase**, SNS stimulation triggers the body's defenses, which in turn stimulates the hypothalamus. The hypothalamus releases corticotropin-releasing hormone (CRH), which stimulates the anterior pituitary gland to release adrenocorticotropic hormone (ACTH). This sympathetic stimulation, known as the hypothalamic–pituitary–adrenal (HPA) axis, results in secretion of catecholamines (epinephrine and norepinephrine) and glucocorticoids (cortisol) (see **Figure 31.3** ››). Significant body responses to epinephrine include increased myocardial activity, bronchial dilation, and increased fat mobilization. This adrenal hormonal activity prepares the individual for *fight or flight*. This primary response is short lived, lasting from 1 minute to 24 hours.

Stage of Resistance

During the second stage of the GAS, the **stage of resistance**, the body attempts to move toward restoration of homeostasis while continuing to respond to the stressor. With chronic exposure to a stressor, the body may maintain resistance to the primary stressor while resistance to other stressors decreases. For example, an individual who is going through the divorce process may become emotionally and psychologically stable, giving an outward appearance of effectively coping with the emotional impact of the divorce. However, the prolonged physiologic stress response—which includes increased production of catecholamines (such as epinephrine and norepinephrine), glucose, and cortisol—may lead to increased susceptibility to physical illness, including sleep disturbance and hypertension (HTN). Selye (1946) called stress-related illnesses **diseases of adaptation**.

Stage of Exhaustion

During the third stage, the **stage of exhaustion**, if the body cannot maintain its adaptation to the stressor, the stressor will overwhelm the individual's ability to cope or mount a continued defense, resulting in the depletion of energy and resources. Without sufficient rest or recovery, disease and even death may develop. How this stage ends depends largely on the adaptive energy resources of the individual, the severity of the stressor, and the external adaptive resources

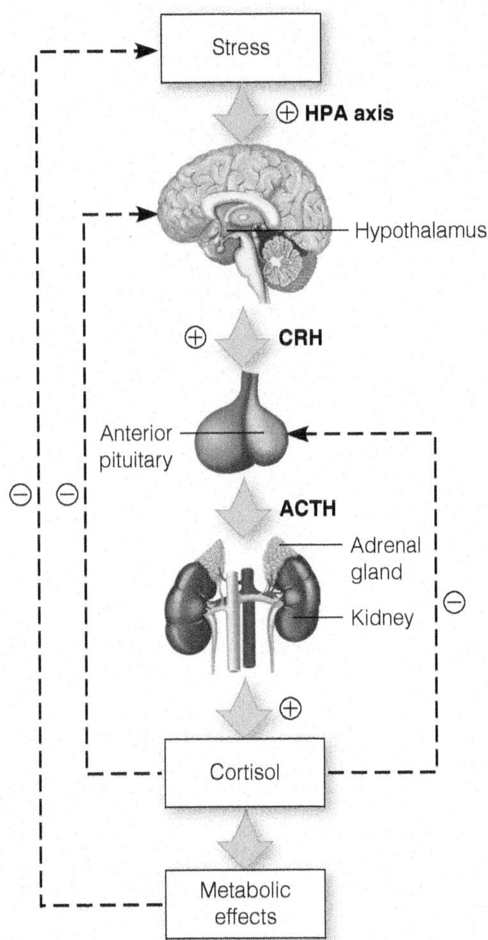

Figure 31.3 ›› Chronic stress results in overactivity of the hypothalamus–pituitary–adrenal axis, which results in excessive release of cortisol, which results in more stress.

that are provided. An example of this can be seen in the patient who lives with chronic pain. The patient may be able to tolerate the pain during the day, but at night finds the pain far more stressful because energy resources are diminished to the point that the pain is intolerable.

Transactional Model

The transactional model of stress and coping emphasizes the individual's perception, or cognitive appraisal, of a given threat as being the most significant factor in the process. Proposed by Lazarus and Folkman (1984) in their landmark book *Stress, Appraisal, and Coping*, this model incorporates variations among individuals in terms of the perception of stressors and the response to stress. Within the context of the transactional model, a perceived threat or stressor is an event or circumstance that has the ability to negatively impact well-being or that is appraised by the individual as exceeding the individual's coping resources. The primary danger posed by a stressor is that it threatens the individual's primary values and goals (Monat & Lazarus, 1991). The process of cognitive appraisal includes the following steps:

- ***Primary appraisal:*** evaluation of the transaction, which is the event or circumstance in terms of its potential to harm, benefit, threaten, or challenge the individual
- ***Secondary appraisal:*** evaluation of the individual's available coping resources and potential options for responding to the event or circumstance
- ***Coping:*** application of available coping resources
- ***Reappraisal:*** ongoing evaluation and reinterpretation of the event or circumstance, as well as continued evaluation of the efficacy of the individual's coping strategies (Lazarus & Folkman, 1984).

Culturally competent nursing care requires recognizing that cultural influences, as well as characteristics that are unique to the individual (including personality and temperament), impact both cognitive appraisal and coping styles.

The nursing transactional model is an adaptation of Lazarus and Folkman's work. The **nursing transactional model** is defined as the relationship between the nurse, the patient, and the environment in which they interact. This interaction or relationship is dynamic—with each transaction, the individual and the stressor engage to form a new transaction with a particular meaning. This model has numerous implications for the profession of nursing and care of patients experiencing stress. The emphasis is on the relationship among stress, the patient, the nurse, and both the internal and external environment.

The nursing transactional model emphasizes communication and the development of the therapeutic relationship with the intent of decreasing the patient's anxiety and increasing or improving the patient's coping resources. This perspective and approach are largely based on the work of nursing theorist Hildegard Peplau, who is widely considered to be the mother of psychiatric nursing. In 1952, Peplau published her classic text *Interpersonal Relations in Nursing*. As opposed to the task-oriented focus traditionally associated with nursing practice, Peplau viewed nursing as a therapeutic interpersonal process. As described in Peplau's theory, although the nurse begins as a stranger to the patient, during the course of the nurse–patient relationship, the nurse proceeds to assume several roles, including teacher, resource person, counselor, surrogate, and leader (Peplau, 1952).

Manifestations of Stress

Just as each individual is unique in their cognitive appraisal and coping methods, individuals also may vary in terms of the internal and external manifestations of stress. In addition to the physiologic domain, stress also may yield manifestations in various other domains, including psychologic and cognitive.

Physiologic Indicators

Physiologic manifestations of stress primarily result from stimulation of the sympathetic and neuroendocrine systems. As previously discussed, the individual's perception of the potential stressor triggers physiologic manifestations of stress. Prolonged exposure to perceived stressors and chronic activation of the stress response can lead to disease and may even be fatal. The relationship between this mind–body connection is illustrated in the Multisystem Effects of Stress feature.

Psychologic Indicators

Individual manifestations of stress within the psychologic domain may include fear, anxiety, anger, depression, and a variety of other responses.

Multisystem Effects of
Stress

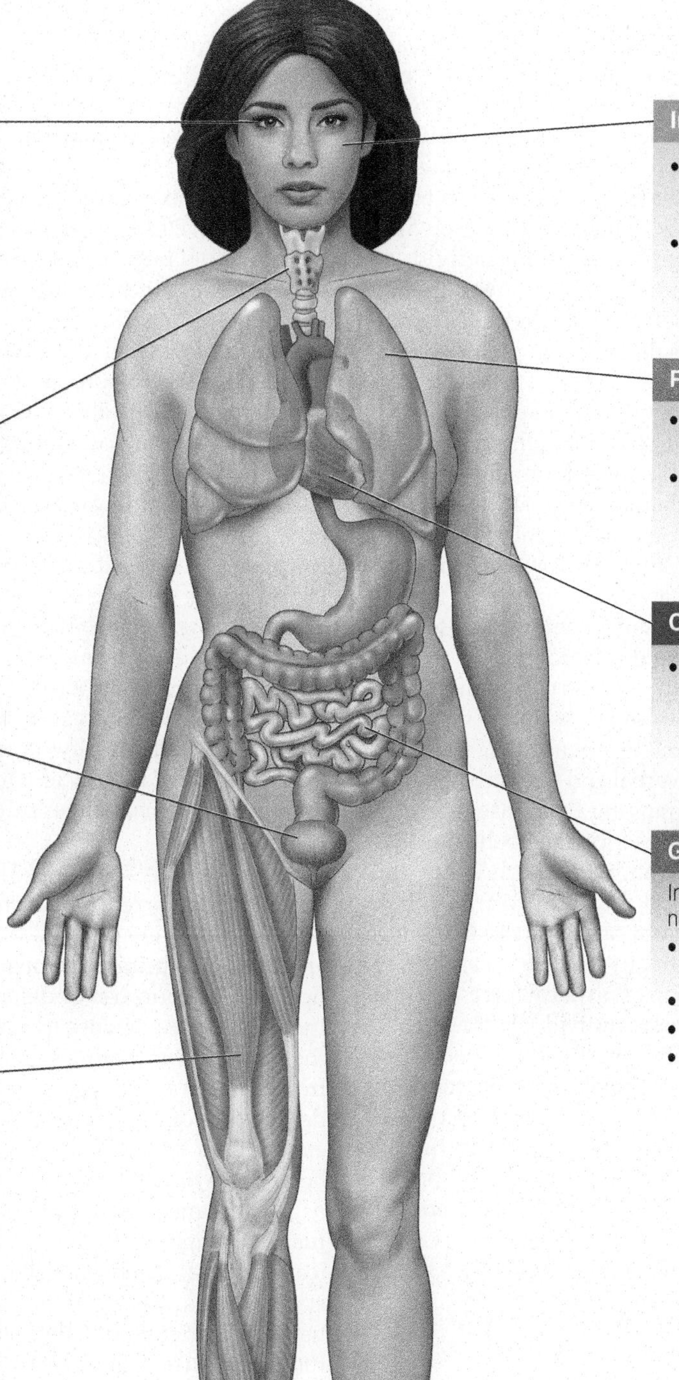

Sensory

- Pupillary dilation allows entrance of more light and enhanced visual perception
- Enhanced awareness and alertness in response to severe threats

Endocrine

- ↑ release of glucocorticoids and increased gluconeogenesis, which leads to increased serum glucose

Urinary

- ↑ sodium and water retention due to mineralocorticoid release, which leads to ↓ urine output and ↑ blood volume

Musculoskeletal

- ↑ muscular tension in preparation for fight or flight

Other Disorders

- Cancer
- Accident proneness
- Decreased immune response

Integumentary

- Diaphoresis to offset increased body temperature secondary to increased metabolism
- Skin pallor secondary to vasoconstrictive effects of norepinephrine

Respiratory

- ↑ respiratory rate and depth of respirations
- Dilation of bronchioles to facilitate increased oxygenation

Cardiovascular

- ↑ heart rate and cardiac output to promote transport of oxygen and nutrients throughout the body

Gastrointestinal

Inhibition of the parasympathetic nervous system leads to:

- ↓ peristalsis and possible constipation
- ↑ flatus
- ↓ salivation
- ↑ serotonin levels in the gut which leads to feelings of nausea

Fear is a sense of apprehension triggered by a perceived threat to safety or well-being, including a painful stimulus or dangerous event. Fear may be aroused by memories of an actual past experience, exposure to a present threat, or anticipated exposure to an event or circumstance. Events that trigger fear may be real or perceived. For example, an individual who has never experienced a motor-vehicle accident but who fears the possibility of one may fear driving a car. Even when the origin of fear is not based in reality or founded on an individual's actual experience, fear usually can be tied to a specific source.

Anxiety is characterized by apprehension, dread, mental uneasiness, and a sense of helplessness in response to an actual or perceived threat to the well-being of self or others. The degree of anxiety experienced by an individual may yield effects that range from minimal to debilitating. Unlike fear, an individual's anxiety may not have an apparent identifiable cause. Anxiety is discussed in greater detail in Exemplar 31.A in this module.

Anger is a subjective sense of intense displeasure, irritation, or animosity. For those individuals who are taught that this emotion is unacceptable, development of anger may trigger a sense of guilt or shame. However, processing and expressing anger through constructive communication methods may lead to conflict resolution and personal growth. Constructive communication of anger requires clear identification of the source of the anger and a commitment to preventing escalation of anger during discussions.

Escalation of anger may lead to destructive emotions and behaviors, including hostility, aggression, or violence. Generally, hostility is characterized by open antagonism and may be expressed through both verbal and nonverbal means in combination with behaviors ranging from insensitive to destructive in nature. *Aggression* describes any behavior that is intended to harm another person, particularly when the other person is motivated to avoid the harm (Warburton & Anderson, 2015). The intended harm can be physical or emotional. Aggression associated with physical harm can lead to violence. *Violence* is the application of physical force with the intent to abuse or injure one or more individuals.

Depression is a persistent, abnormally low mood characterized by feelings of emptiness, hopelessness, sadness, or despair. It is often accompanied by a loss of interest (apathy) in activities, including those related to daily living. Manifestations of depression include behavioral, emotional, and physical signs and symptoms. Chronic, recurrent, or extended periods of depression signal the need for evaluation and potential treatment (see Exemplar 28.A, Depression, in Module 28, Mood and Affect).

Cognitive Indicators

In response to stress, cognitive indicators include changes in mental processes such as problem solving and cognitive structuring. When under stress, impairments in cognitive abilities may manifest as suppression, diminished or impaired self-control, and fantasizing.

Problem solving incorporates evaluating a challenging situation, identifying potential steps to resolve the situation, and then implementing those steps. In addition, problem solving includes evaluating the efficacy of solutions and identifying and implementing alternative approaches to adequately resolve a problem or challenge.

Cognitive structuring refers to the mental processes used to interpret and make sense of environmental stimuli. For example, through cognitive structuring, a nurse working in the hospital environment interprets the sound associated with an activated nursing call light to mean that a patient needs assistance. More complex application of cognitive structuring includes drawing from previous experiences with problem solving and its associated outcomes and then, through general application of those past experiences, forming a plan for resolving a present challenge.

Suppression, which is a defense mechanism, is the active, conscious process of denying unacceptable thoughts or emotions (Costa, 2020). Suppression can be healthy; for example, an individual may suppress anger related to a disagreement with their significant other in order to effectively perform work-related duties and demonstrate a positive attitude toward coworkers. However, suppression may also lead to avoidance of facing problems or challenges.

Self-control is the ability to refrain from acting on impulse or to behave in such a manner as to delay gratification. In an extreme example, exercising self-control may prevent fear or panic from overriding logic when faced with a stressful situation. However, attempts at exercising self-control—or a desire to appear to have self-control—can lead to ignoring or denying emotions and neglecting to ask for needed assistance.

Fantasizing, or *daydreaming*, is imagining the fulfillment of desires or wishes or mentally picturing the resolution of a situation in a manner that is more favorable than the resolution that occurred in reality. Fantasizing can be healthy and may even lead to identifying solutions to problems. However, excessive use of fantasy as a form of coping or in an attempt to avoid facing challenges can delay problem resolution.

Ego Defense Mechanisms

Frequently referred to as *defense mechanisms*, **ego defense mechanisms** were proposed and defined by Sigmund Freud (1946) as being unconscious psychologic processes developed for the purpose of defending the personality (or self). Individuals use defense mechanisms to balance the tensions that emerge during times of stress and to protect themselves from anxiety and its adverse effects. See **Table 31.4** >> for a description of the primary defense mechanisms, as well as examples of their functional purpose and effects, which may be positive or negative.

Defense mechanisms are essential to psychologic survival. Just as the fight-or-flight response supports individual physical survival, defense mechanisms protect our psychologic state. Nurses must not only identify the defense mechanisms used by patients, but they also must recognize how they themselves use defense mechanisms to gain insight into their own defensive coping patterns. It is important to remember that defenses protect the individual and the ego. Providing a safe and nonjudgmental environment helps patients let go of protective defenses and begin to cope with reality.

Concepts Related to Stress and Coping

Stress and coping are integrally linked to all aspects of nursing care. Patients who experience illness and disease are exposed to increased physical and emotional stress compared

TABLE 31.4 Ego Defense Mechanisms

Defense Mechanism	Example(s)	Use/Purpose
Compensation: covering up weaknesses by emphasizing a more desirable trait or by overachievement in a more comfortable area	A high school student too small to play football becomes the star long-distance runner for the track team.	Allows an individual to overcome weakness and achieve success
Denial: attempting to screen or ignore unacceptable realities by refusing to acknowledge them	A woman, though told her father has metastatic cancer, continues to plan a family reunion 18 months in advance.	Temporarily isolates an individual from the full impact of a traumatic situation
Displacement: transferring or discharging emotional reactions from one object or person to another object or person	A husband and wife are fighting, and the husband becomes so angry that he hits a door instead of his wife. A student gets a C on a paper she worked hard on and goes home and yells at her family.	Allows for feelings to be expressed through or to less dangerous objects or people
Identification: attempting to manage anxiety by imitating the behavior of someone feared or respected	A student nurse imitates the nurturing behavior she observes one of her instructors using with patients.	Helps an individual avoid self-devaluation
Intellectualization: evading the emotional response that normally would accompany an uncomfortable or painful incident by using rational explanations that remove from the incident any personal significance and feelings	The pain over a parent's sudden death is reduced by saying, "He wouldn't have wanted to live disabled."	Protects an individual from pain and traumatic events
Introjection: a form of identification that allows for the acceptance of others' norms and values into oneself, even when contrary to one's previous assumptions	A 7-year-old tells his little sister, "Don't talk to strangers." He has introjected this value from the instructions of parents/caregivers and teachers.	Helps an individual avoid social retaliation and punishment; particularly important during child development
Minimization: not acknowledging the significance of one's behavior	An individual says, "Don't believe everything my wife tells you. I wasn't so drunk I couldn't drive."	Allows an individual to decrease responsibility for behavior
Projection: blaming others or the environment for unacceptable desires, thoughts, shortcomings, and mistakes	A mother is told her child must repeat a grade in school, and she blames this on the teacher's poor instruction. A husband forgets to pay a bill and blames his wife for not giving it to him earlier.	Allows an individual to deny the existence of shortcomings and mistakes; protects self-image
Rationalization: justifying certain behaviors by faulty logic and ascription of motives that are socially acceptable but did not in fact inspire the behavior	A mother spanks her toddler too hard and says it was all right because he couldn't feel it through the diapers anyway.	Helps an individual cope with the inability to meet goals or certain standards
Reaction formation: a mechanism that causes people to act exactly opposite to the way they feel	An executive resents his bosses for calling in a consulting firm to make recommendations for change in his department, but verbalizes complete support of the idea and is exceedingly polite and cooperative.	Aids in reinforcing repression by allowing feelings to be acted out in a more acceptable way
Regression: resorting to an earlier, more comfortable level of functioning that is characteristically less demanding and responsible	A person throws a temper tantrum when she does not get her own way. A critically ill patient allows the nurse to bathe and feed him.	Allows an individual to return to a point in development when nurturing and dependency were needed and accepted with comfort
Repression: an unconscious mechanism by which threatening thoughts, feelings, and desires are kept from becoming conscious; the repressed material is denied entry into consciousness	A teenager, seeing his best friend killed in a car crash, becomes amnesic about the circumstances surrounding the accident.	Protects an individual from a traumatic experience until they have the resources to cope
Sublimation: displacing energy associated with more primitive sexual or aggressive drives into socially acceptable activities	An individual with excessive, primitive sexual drives invests psychic energy into a well-defined religious value system.	Protects an individual from behaving in irrational, impulsive ways
Substitution: replacing a highly valued, unacceptable, or unavailable object with a less valuable, acceptable, or available object	A woman wants to marry a man exactly like her dead father and settles for someone who looks a little bit like him.	Helps an individual achieve goals and minimizes frustration and disappointment
Undoing: performing an action or using words designed to cancel some disapproved thoughts, impulses, or acts in which the person relieves guilt by making reparation	A father spanks his child and the next evening brings home a present for him. A teacher writes an examination that is far too difficult, then constructs a grading curve that makes it easy to earn a high grade.	Allows an individual to appease guilty feelings and atone for mistakes

to their healthy counterparts, and this stress may extend to their caregivers (American Psychological Association, 2017a). Individuals who have been exposed to personal loss or trauma are also susceptible to increased stress. Even on the joyful occasion of a new baby, new parents and siblings experience stress related to disrupted sleep patterns, exhaustion, caregiving demands, and decreased attention to self. This stress is heightened even more for the family if the infant has health problems, especially if it is a chronic illness that will affect the child long term (Pinquart, 2018).

Individuals exposed to high levels of stress due to personal health problems, caregiving responsibilities, or daily life struggles are more susceptible to emotional and physical health problems such as depression, obesity, and cardiovascular disease. This is because stress is intricately linked to physiologic function. The stress response triggers activation of the SNS, which in turn prompts the release of numerous neurotransmitters and hormones, with the primary stress mediators being catecholamines and glucocorticoids. The development of glucocorticoid receptor resistance associated with chronic stress may produce an environment that fails to downregulate the inflammatory response, thus leading to disease susceptibility (Walsh et al., 2018).

Nursing professionals are not exempt from the stress related to caregiving duties. Left unmanaged, what initially manifests as stress can translate into something far more serious. Because of occupation-specific demands, including irregular work schedules and increased workloads due to staffing shortages, nurses are at particularly high risk for **burnout**. In addition to adverse emotional and physical effects on the nurse, burnout is also associated with reduced quality of care and decreased patient satisfaction with nursing care (Bakhamis, Paul, Smith, & Coustasse, 2019).

Although stress may not be a primary diagnosis for all patients, every patient who seeks medical attention and requires nursing care will benefit from knowledge about coping techniques related to their unique situation. Individuals who experience chronic stress are more likely to engage in unhealthy coping behaviors. Nurses can support healthy coping behaviors by implementing caring interventions, using therapeutic communication, and providing patient teaching. In addition, they can advocate for patients, caregivers, and other nursing professionals when collaborative care is needed. The Concepts Related to Stress and Coping feature lists some, but not all, of the related concepts. They are presented in alphabetical order.

Concepts Related to
Stress and Coping

CONCEPT	RELATIONSHIP TO STRESS AND COPING	NURSING IMPLICATIONS
Addiction	High chronic stress → unhealthy coping behaviors → ↑ alcohol, nicotine, or substance abuse	■ Assess all patients and caregivers for signs of addiction. ■ Educate patients and caregivers about the harmful effects of substance use and addictive behaviors. ■ Refer patients and caregivers to counseling or support groups as needed.
Collaboration	Multiple health issues → ↑ stress for the patient → ↑ need for collaboration between healthcare providers (HCPs) Conflict between family members or between patients and HCPs → ↑ stress for all parties involved → ↑ need for collaboration with a neutral third party	■ Assess stress levels and coping habits of patients with multiple health issues. ■ Identify HCPs who may be able to collaborate and provide information or patient teaching that will help reduce the patient's stress level and increase the use of healthy coping techniques. For example, a patient with high stress levels related to obesity, diabetes mellitus, and cardiovascular disease may benefit from collaboration with a nutritionist. ■ Assess families for signs of family conflict that may be increasing the stress level for patients and caregivers. ■ Refer patients and families struggling with family conflict to family therapists or mediators.
Mood and Affect	Depression → ↑ stress → ↑ depression ↑ depression → ↑ risk for suicide	■ Assess coping techniques of patients with mood and affective disorders and their caregivers. ■ Use therapeutic communication to encourage patients to engage in positive coping and adhere to their recommended treatment regimen. ■ Refer patients and caregivers to counseling or support groups as needed.
Perfusion	Stress response → release of catecholamines epinephrine and norepinephrine → ↑ blood pressure and ↑ heart rate	■ Assess patients for HTN and tachycardia. ■ Be aware that prolonged exposure to stress can lead to long-term HTN and secondary complications, including cardiovascular disease, cerebrovascular accident (CVA; or stroke), and renal damage. ■ Educate patients about stress management techniques, including regular physical exercise. ■ Facilitate referrals to counselors as ordered.

Concepts Related to *(continued)*

CONCEPT	RELATIONSHIP TO STRESS AND COPING	NURSING IMPLICATIONS
Reproduction	Changing hormone levels associated with pregnancy and childbirth → ↑ feelings of being overwhelmed → ↓ ability to cope Responsibilities associated with caring for a newborn → ↑ stress	■ Assess pregnant women for self-care activities and emotional health. ■ Assess mothers with newborns for self-care activities, sleep patterns, and emotional health. ■ Assess mothers with newborns for postpartum depression. ■ Assess parents and caregivers of premature newborns for signs of stress and inadequate coping techniques. ■ Provide patient teaching on newborn care techniques, breastfeeding, infant sleeping patterns, and other topics that may be contributing to stress in new parents.
Self	Stress → ↑ incidence of feeding and eating disorders	■ Assess individuals with stress for abnormal weight gain or loss. ■ Assess patients' eating habits, including whether stress makes them eat more or less than normal. ■ Provide patient teaching about healthy eating habits to individuals who use unhealthy eating habits to cope with stress. ■ Refer patients and caregivers to counseling or support groups as needed.
Teaching and Learning	Patient teaching about coping techniques → ↓ stress → ↑ healthy coping behaviors → ↑ overall health Mentoring less experienced HCPs → ↓ stress → ↑ job performance → ↑ patient satisfaction and health	■ Teach patients and family members struggling with high levels of stress about healthy coping techniques, including relaxation techniques and therapeutic communication. ■ Provide mentoring and encouragement to other HCPs to reduce stress. ■ Teach coping techniques to other HCPs, which can reduce on-the-job stress, prevent burnout, and increase job performance.

Alterations from Normal Coping Responses

When an individual experiences stress so disabling that functioning is adversely affected, the individual is highly susceptible to the development of a disorder of anxiety, stress, or trauma. The fifth edition of the *Diagnostic and Statistical Manual of Mental Disorders* (DSM-5; American Psychiatric Association, 2013) recognizes three different classifications of disorders related to stress and coping:

- ***Anxiety disorders***, which include separation anxiety disorder, selective mutism, specific phobia, social anxiety disorder (social phobia), panic disorder, agoraphobia, generalized anxiety disorder, substance/medication-induced anxiety disorder, anxiety disorder due to another medical condition, other specified anxiety disorder, and unspecified anxiety disorder. Anxiety disorders and phobias are discussed in detail in Exemplar 31.A in this module.
- ***Obsessive–compulsive and related disorders***, which include obsessive–compulsive disorder, body dysmorphic disorder, hoarding disorder, trichotillomania (hair-pulling disorder), excoriation (skin-picking disorder), substance/medication-induced obsessive–compulsive and related disorder, obsessive–compulsive and related disorder due to another medical condition, other specified obsessive–compulsive and related disorder, and unspecified obsessive–compulsive and related disorder. Obsessive–compulsive disorder (OCD) is discussed in detail in Exemplar 31.C in this module.
- ***Trauma- and stressor-related disorders***, which include reactive attachment disorder, disinhibited social engagement disorder, posttraumatic stress disorder, acute stress disorder, adjustment disorders, and other specified trauma- and stressor-related disorder. Posttraumatic stress disorder is discussed in Exemplar 32.C in Module 32, Trauma.

Prevalence

According to the Anxiety and Depression Association of America (ADAA, 2020a), anxiety disorders are the most common mental health disorders in the United States. The prevalence of anxiety disorders is approximately 18%, impacting 40 million individuals (ADAA, 2020a). Generalized anxiety disorder (GAD) affects 6.8 million adults in the United States, and twice as many women as men. The disorder can develop at any time in the life cycle, although individuals between childhood and middle age are at greatest risk for developing it (ADAA, 2020b). Additional U.S. prevalence rates for disorders that are discussed in this module's exemplars include the following (ADAA, 2020a):

- Obsessive–compulsive disorder affects approximately 2.2 million individuals or an estimated 1.0% of the population.
- Phobias affect an estimated 19 million individuals, which is approximately 8.7% of the population.

Genetic Considerations and Risk Factors

Gender is a significant risk factor associated with anxiety and stress-related disorders. Overall, women are about twice as

Alterations and Therapies

Stress and Coping

ALTERATION	DESCRIPTION	MANIFESTATIONS	INTERVENTIONS AND THERAPIES
Generalized anxiety disorder	Excessive worry about everyday problems for at least 6 months, with anxiety that is more intense than the situation warrants	▪ Anticipation of disaster and preoccupation with health issues, money, familial problems, or challenges at work ▪ Difficulty relaxing, tendency to startle easily, trouble concentrating and falling asleep ▪ Various somatic complaints, which may include fatigue, headache, muscle tension and aches, digestive issues, irritability, shortness of breath or dyspnea, and hot flashes	▪ Psychotherapy, including cognitive-behavioral therapy (CBT) ▪ Pharmacotherapy, which includes antidepressants (e.g., selective serotonin reuptake inhibitors [SSRIs] and serotonin/norepinephrine reuptake inhibitors [SNRIs]) and anxiolytic medications (e.g., benzodiazepines) ▪ Relaxation techniques, such as massage and guided imagery ▪ Mental health counseling
Phobias	An intense, persistent, irrational fear or dread of an object, situation, or activity that elicits panic and automatic avoidance of or compelling urge to stay away from it	▪ Fear and anxiety in response to exposure (or, in some cases, imagined exposure) to the phobia-related object, situation, or activity	▪ Pharmacotherapy, which may include short-term use of benzodiazepines or administration of SSRIs ▪ CBT ▪ Desensitization and implosion therapy for specific phobias
Panic disorder	A sudden attack of terror that can produce a sense of unreality, impending doom, or a fear of losing control	▪ Somatic manifestations may include pounding heart, rapid heart rate (tachycardia), rapid respirations (tachypnea), weakness, sweatiness, light-headedness, or dizziness	▪ Reduced environmental stimuli or placement in a quiet, nonstimulating environment ▪ CBT ▪ Pharmacotherapy, which may include antidepressants (e.g., SSRIs or SNRIs) or anxiolytic medications (e.g., benzodiazepines) ▪ Relaxation techniques, such as massage and guided imagery ▪ Mental health counseling
Obsessive–compulsive disorder	Characterized by obsessive thoughts and compulsive repetitive behaviors formed in response to the obsessive thoughts to lower the level of anxiety experienced	▪ Signs and symptoms vary depending on the theme of the specific obsessions and compulsions (see Exemplar 31.C in this module). For example, OCD that features a theme of excessive cleanliness may include a fixation on the need to clean oneself and/or the environment (and fear of contamination), along with repetitive behaviors related to cleaning.	▪ CBT ▪ Tricyclic antidepressants, SSRIs

likely as men to develop an anxiety disorder. This may be because women are more sensitive to low levels of the stress hormone corticotropin-releasing factor (ADAA, 2020e). However, women are not more susceptible to every type of anxiety disorder. For example, OCD and social anxiety disorder are equally common in men and women (ADAA, 2020a).

Both genetic factors and life experiences contribute to anxiety disorders. Anxiety disorders tend to run in families, a trend related partially to genetics and partially to environment. For example, an estimated 43% of those with panic disorder have a close relative with the disorder (Memon, 2018). In addition, many children develop fears and anxiety that are similar to those of their parents or primary caregivers. For some patients, exposure to trauma or a significant event may trigger an anxiety disorder in individuals who are genetically susceptible (Cleveland Clinic, 2020).

Other factors that influence the development of anxiety disorders include personality-related characteristics; for example, shy children are at an increased risk (Mayo Clinic, 2017a). Traumatic events, including a history of spousal or childhood abuse and being bullied, also increase the risk of impairment. Social factors, especially limited or absent socialization and living in a threatening environment, increase an individual's susceptibility to developing an anxiety disorder.

Case Study » Part 1

Kevin DeLarno is a 23-year-old student who is completing his second year of graduate school in the study of anatomy and physiology. He presents to the university student health services center with complaints of frequent headaches, including a current headache that he describes as "a throbbing in the front of my head." He rates his pain as 7 on a scale of 0 to 10, with 10 being the worst imaginable pain. During his patient interview, he denies any past medical history or any additional complaints, including trauma, visual disturbances, dizziness, weakness, or neurologic changes. According to Mr. DeLarno, his headaches are "interfering with my study schedule. I have exams every week and I can't concentrate on studying. If I don't get these headaches under control, I'm going to end up failing at least one class this semester." He reports that he drinks "about a pot of coffee a day" and occasionally smokes a cigar when he is socializing with his friends.

Upon arrival, Mr. DeLarno's vital signs include temperature 97.9°F oral; pulse 92 beats/min; respirations 18/min; and blood pressure 153/82 mmHg. Auscultation of his heart and lungs reveals no abnormal findings. Mr. DeLarno insists he is "fine, except for these stupid headaches. I'm sure it's just stress. I need something to help me get them under control so I can get my work done." During his assessment interview, the nurse asks if Mr. DeLarno has made any recent changes to his daily routine or health habits. He replies, "There aren't any recent changes, but soon, there will be. I'm getting married in 3 months and my fiancé and I will be moving off campus." Mr. DeLarno further states that he is "excited about getting married," but feels the wedding planning has gotten out of hand, as he and his fiancé have already exceeded their wedding budget. When asked what activities he engages in for enjoyment and recreation, he replies, "I don't have time for anything except classes and studying. I used to work out and play racquetball three times a week, but I don't have the time for that right now."

Clinical Reasoning Questions Level I

1. Based on Mr. DeLarno's statements, what are his current potential sources of stress?
2. In addition to his complaints of recurrent headaches, which cues in his assessment data reflect manifestations of the stress response?
3. Describe the effects of coffee and nicotine intake, including how these effects are similar to those evoked by the stress response.

Clinical Reasoning Questions Level II

4. Do positive stressors and negative stressors differ in terms of physiologic effects? Explain your answer.
5. Presuming Mr. DeLarno's headaches are stress related, what priorities for care would be appropriate for him at this time?
6. What nursing interventions could be implemented to promote stress reduction for Mr. DeLarno?

Health Promotion

Health promotion for individuals experiencing anxiety focuses on decreasing exacerbation of symptoms and identifying healthy coping behaviors that the patient is motivated to use. It is important to note that patients who are experiencing severe or panic levels of anxiety will not be able to retain new information and will require different interventions. For those who are able to focus on new information, topics for patient teaching can be found in the Patient Teaching feature.

Family wellness promotion is also essential to enhancing physiologic and psychosocial outcomes for patients of all ages (see Module 26, Family). The link between the development of mental illness and childhood abuse and neglect serves to emphasize this point. Research suggests that childhood abuse is associated with an increased risk for physical and psychologic disorders, including depression and anxiety.

Patient Teaching

Wellness Promotion for Patients with Stress-Related Disorders

Nurses should provide patient teaching to patients with stress-related disorders to promote wellness and healthy coping techniques. Topics for teaching may include:

- ***Physical exercise.*** Educate the patient about the benefits of physical exercise (see Module 7, Health, Wellness, Illness, and Injury). Physiologic benefits of regular physical exercise include improved cardiac and pulmonary function, enhanced muscle tone and joint mobility, and weight control. Psychologic benefits include tension relief, stress reduction, enhanced sense of well-being, and promotion of relaxation following activity.
- ***Sleep/rest patterns.*** Promote a healthy balance between sleep/rest and activity and teach relaxation techniques to promote relaxation and sleep. Adequate sleep and rest are essential to survival, allow for physical healing and restoration, and enhance cognitive function. Sleep also helps remove free radicals, which are believed to be associated with illness and disease. Promote good sleep hygiene (see Box 3.1, Guidelines for Sleep Hygiene, in Module 3, Comfort). Consider providing patient teaching about breathing exercises, imagery, muscle relaxation, movement techniques, and biofeedback.
- ***Nutrition.*** Provide education related to balanced nutrition and facilitate referrals to dietary professionals and nutritionists. Teach patients that inadequate nutrition reduces physical resistance to illness and increases susceptibility to disease and illness (see Module 14, Nutrition). Teach patients that the excessive intake of caffeine and use of nicotine may interfere with sleep/rest patterns.
- ***Time management.*** Teach patients how to balance fulfilling personal responsibilities (e.g., work, family, school) with time for rest, socialization, and extracurricular activities. Teach patients that effective time management is associated with an increased sense of control and decreased sense of stress.
- ***Boundary setting.*** Teach patients how to identify potential stressors and how to implement personal boundaries. Setting up personal boundaries can aid the patient in determining the appropriateness of requests/demands made by others and can allow the individual to identify which requests/demands can be fulfilled while still maintaining wellness.

These increased risks remain in effect decades after the abuse occurs (Lippard & Nemeroff, 2020). Even when overt abuse and neglect are not factors, family dynamics and parenting styles can pose serious threats to a child's psychosocial well-being. For example, frequent changes in caregivers may predispose a child to the development of separation anxiety disorder or reactive attachment disorder (American Psychiatric Association, 2013; Mayo Clinic, 2017a).

Nursing Assessment

Just as individuals evaluate (appraise) and prioritize stressors, the nurse assesses and prioritizes health concerns. During the assessment, the nurse will help patients identify stressors that trigger unhealthy coping responses and the potential effects of those responses.

Many patients with anxiety will present complaining of physical symptoms. In the case study example, Mr. DeLarno's presenting complaint is a headache, which he then attributes to "just stress." Some patients, however, will be unable to articulate anxiety because of a lack of either awareness or understanding of the source of their symptoms or because of a reluctance to disclose what they consider very personal information. Through developing the therapeutic nurse–patient relationship, the nurse may be able to encourage reluctant patients to disclose necessary information or come to an awareness of how stress and anxiety are impacting their health.

During the nursing assessment, the nurse acknowledges and affirms the patient's concerns. **Box 31.2** ›› describes application of the nursing transactional model with regard to specific communication strategies that may be appropriate for use during assessment of the patient with anxiety.

Box 31.2

Application of the Nursing Transactional Model to Assessment of the Patient with Anxiety

In the nursing transactional model, the nurse is part of the anxious patient's environment and can influence changes in the patient with both verbal and nonverbal cues. From the very first interaction with the patient, the nurse's demeanor conveys a great deal of information to the patient about how the individual can expect to be treated. Initial nursing actions that inspire confidence and that may help calm anxiety in patients include the following:

- Focus on the person: Make eye contact as appropriate and minimize distractions.
- Assume a nonthreatening demeanor.
- Validate the patient's feelings: "I know you are very uncomfortable; we will do everything we can to help you feel better."
- Determine and address the patient's immediate concerns: "What can I do right away to help you?"
- Remember to address the patient by name. Some patients find terms of endearment such as "Honey" or "Sweetie" impersonal or demeaning. Using the patient's first name may be seen as patronizing if the patient is expected to use the nurse's last name. On the other hand, some patients respond positively to the informality of first-name use. Ask patients how they would like to be addressed, and never use the first name of anyone over age 18 without permission.

Observation and Patient Interview

The patient interview should include collection of data related to the patient's current and past illnesses, specific physical complaints, general health history, patient-perceived stressors or stressful incidents, manifestations of stress, and past and present coping strategies. In addition to an assessment interview, the nurse may use a simple checklist while talking with and observing the patient to note indications of stress (see **Box 31.3** ›› for a sample checklist). The first step in mediating the effect of a stressor is conscious awareness of the manifestations of stress. Review the symptom checklist to increase your awareness of and assess your own stress reactions and behaviors.

SAFETY ALERT Legal requirements to maintain patient confidentiality do not apply in the event of a patient's threat to harm self or others. If a patient indicates an intention to injure self or others, the nurse has the responsibility to report this information to the proper authorities.

Screening tests are available for use in the identification of many anxiety and stress-related disorders, including GAD, OCD, and specific phobias.

›› **Stay Current:** To view a sample of these screening tools, visit the Anxiety and Depression Association of America's online library at https://adaa.org/find-help/treatment-help/self-screening.

Physical Examination

Physical assessment of the patient should include observation and testing of body systems for physical manifestations of stress. GI indicators of stress may include constipation, diarrhea, dry mouth, and nausea. Integumentary signs may include diaphoresis and pallor. Neurologic symptoms may include insomnia, fatigue, headaches, and restlessness. Cardiovascular and respiratory cues may include tachycardia and hyperpnea. Endocrine and urinary signs may include hyperglycemia and urinary frequency. Motor symptoms may include sluggish or stiff movements and muscle tension. Stress and anxiety may also manifest in behavioral habits that can be observed, such as cutting, fingernail biting, or evidence of crying. Remember that physical manifestations of distress may not be apparent when cognitive coping is effective.

Diagnostic Tests

For identification of disorders of anxiety and stress-related disorders, diagnostic criteria are collected primarily through patient interviews and reports of subjective symptoms. Medical testing may be conducted to rule out a medical etiology such as cardiovascular dysfunction or an adverse response to a medication. Patients with disorders related to stress and coping, particularly children, may present with somatic (physical) complaints and may not initially articulate any anxiety or trauma. Although patients may present to primary care providers with complaints that appear to be related to exposure to stress or due to impaired coping mechanisms, diagnosis of associated psychiatric disorders requires evaluation by a trained mental health professional, such as a psychiatrist, physician assistant, nurse practitioner, or advanced practice psychiatric nurse.

Box 31.3
Stress Assessment Checklist

BEHAVIORAL	COGNITIVE	EMOTIONAL	PHYSICAL
Always doing too much	Ambivalence	Agitation/anger	Constipation
Argumentativeness	Difficulty concentrating or listening	Anxiety and feeling pressured	Diaphoresis
Grinds teeth during sleep	Fear of the unknown	Crying	Diarrhea
Increase in compulsive behaviors (eating, drinking, nail biting, sexual activity, smoking)	Forgetfulness	Defensiveness	Difficulty falling asleep
Looks at watch or clock often	Lack of creativity	Easily annoyed	Dry mouth
Loud voice	Lack of initiative	Fear	Fatigue
Pacing	Lack of a sense of humor	Feeling overwhelmed	Gastrointestinal (GI) upsets or "butterflies"
Talks too fast	Memory lapses/loss	Feeling powerless	Headaches
Vigilance	Short attention span	Hostility	Increase in blood glucose levels
Withdrawal	Trouble thinking	Irritability	Increase in respiration rate
Work on multiple projects simultaneously	Wanting to run away	Isolation	Insomnia
	Worrying	Jumpiness and nervousness	Muscular stiffness and tension
		Sadness	Pallor
		Suspiciousness	Racing or pounding heart
			Restlessness
			Shakiness
			Sweaty palms
			Urinary frequency

Assessing Patients from Different Cultures

When working with patients from different cultures, nurses must take care not to inadvertently attribute a normal, healthy cultural response as inappropriate or maladaptive behavior. Cultural expressions of distress vary. Therefore, a thorough assessment of stressors, the individual patient's perception of the stressors and cultural background, and the patient's efforts to seek help or reduce distress will help distinguish each patient's individual stress responses.

The Cultural Formulation Interview (CFI) outlined in the DSM-5 may be used to assist HCPs in interviewing patients as part of a comprehensive mental health assessment. The CFI is a series of 16 questions designed to assess patients in four areas (American Psychiatric Association, 2013):

- Cultural definition of the problem
- Cultural perceptions of cause and support
- Cultural factors affecting coping and past help-seeking behaviors
- Cultural factors affecting current help-seeking behaviors.

Case Study » Part 2

Mr. DeLarno is awaiting evaluation by the university healthcare clinic's nurse practitioner. He agrees to dimming of his room lights while he waits. After resting quietly for 10 minutes, he falls asleep. When the nurse awakens Mr. DeLarno to reassess him, he states, "I'm surprised I fell asleep. Usually, I can't fall asleep no matter how hard I try to relax. I'm only sleeping a couple of hours each night." He reports his headache "feels quite a bit better, but I know it's going to come back with a vengeance as soon as I start studying again." He rates his pain as 3 on a scale of 0 to 10. His blood pressure has decreased to 128/72 mmHg and his pulse is now 78 beats/min.

Upon arriving to assess Mr. DeLarno, the nurse practitioner introduces herself and asks the patient to describe his current complaints, as well as any similar problems he has experienced in the past. Mr. DeLarno states, "My headache is better, but I need something to help me control it when I'm studying. I think alprazolam would help—I have a friend who takes that when he gets stressed." The nurse practitioner responds by noting that she would like to further assess Mr. DeLarno, as well as ask him a few questions, before making any treatment recommendations. He replies, "The nurse I saw earlier already listened to my heart and lungs, and she already asked me a bunch of questions. Headaches are my only problem—I don't need any additional workup. I can't stay here all day. Are you able to help me or not?"

Clinical Reasoning Questions Level I

1. Explain the most likely reasons for Mr. DeLarno's decreased headache and decrease in blood pressure and heart rate.
2. What is the significance of this patient's reported sleep habits?

Clinical Reasoning Questions Level II

3. In the event that Mr. DeLarno's complaints are related to anxiety, is a prescription for alprazolam a preferable first approach to treatment? Why or why not?
4. How should the nurse practitioner respond to Mr. DeLarno's seeming frustration with the need for additional assessment?

Independent Interventions

Nursing care of patients with alterations in stress and coping includes independent interventions such as using therapeutic communication, encouraging the patient to maintain or achieve optimal health, and assisting the patient with identifying strategies that will promote coping and reduce feelings of anxiety and the allostatic load.

Additional independent nursing interventions include implementing cognitive-behavioral interventions, such as teaching nonpharmacologic relaxation techniques and encouraging patient and family participation in support groups. Validating the patient's feelings is essential to building self-esteem and fostering healthy coping. Reinforcing positive coping efforts, offering hope and reassurance to the patient about the ability to cope, and helping the patient identify successes in life can provide a sense of personal power and hope. Spiritual distress occurs when an individual loses hope of ever resolving the problem or coping more adaptively. The chronic nature of anxiety disorders can be devastating and can erode an individual's sense of power and self-worth.

In the care of patients diagnosed with mental illness, one of the nurse's most crucial roles is patient advocacy. Covert discrimination against individuals with mental illness still exists today in society and in the healthcare system. According to the U.S. Department of Housing and Urban Development (2019), an estimated 20% of homeless individuals experience mental illness. Every individual and nurse who cares enough about the plight of people living with mental illness has the ability to impact public policy. Organizations such as the National Alliance on Mental Illness (NAMI) provide a platform for individuals to work collaboratively.

>> **Stay Current:** To learn more about advocating for individuals with mental illness, visit NAMI's website, www.nami.org. NAMI is the nation's largest organization for individuals experiencing mental illness and their families. NAMI has affiliates in every state and in many communities across the country.

Collaborative Therapies

Collaborative interventions for patients experiencing moderate to severe difficulty coping with stressors include administration of prescribed pharmacologic therapies and facilitation of counseling, psychotherapy, and other therapies as ordered. In addition to being well informed about various interventions and treatment options, such as psychotherapy, nurses should be able to recognize and manage their own responses to stress.

Psychotherapy

Psychotherapy is a preferred method of treating anxiety and other psychiatric disorders. Psychotherapy involves talking with a mental health professional, such as a psychiatrist, mental health nurse, advanced practice psychiatric nurse, psychologist, social worker, or counselor, to explore the nature and symptom management of the disorder (American Psychological Association, 2017b). Severe symptoms may warrant hospitalization in a safe therapeutic milieu or treatment setting. Such an intervention provides needed protection from environmental stressors and the additional support of group therapy. The impact of overwhelming and disabling anxiety can create vulnerability to depression, suicidal thoughts, or self-harm.

Cognitive-Behavioral Therapy

Cognitive-behavioral therapy (CBT) combines cognitive techniques and behavior modification to change detrimental beliefs and thought patterns. The goals of CBT include enhancing problem-solving and coping skills. Usually, the therapist guides the patient in identifying distorted thought patterns and assists with restructuring those thoughts and beliefs. Through analysis and reinterpretation of past and current experiences, the patient is able to learn and apply new skills that promote healthy behaviors and positive interpersonal interactions (American Psychiatric Association, 2013). One such technique is thought stopping, in which the therapist guides the individual to practice strategies to stop or interrupt intrusive or recurrent negative thoughts (Melton, 2017).

Different types of CBT have been developed to address different symptoms or disorders. For example, exposure-based CBT combines the techniques used in CBT with exposure of the patient to a controlled version of the situation that triggers the anxiety. By inducing mild anxiety under the supervision of a mental health expert, exposure-based CBT can help an individual with panic disorder learn that panic attacks are not heart attacks, for example (National Institute of Mental Health [NIMH], 2018). Cognitive-behavioral therapy for insomnia (CBT-I) can help patients with insomnia replace thoughts or behaviors that impede sleep with strategies that promote sleep (Martin, 2021).

Pharmacologic Therapy

The therapeutic goal of psychopharmacology is to manage symptoms and alleviate distress. Generally speaking, pharmacologic therapies are most successful when used in combination with psychotherapy. Many patients require medication for only short periods of time. Some patients, however, may require longer courses of medication. Many patients with anxiety or obsessive–compulsive disorders can lead normal, fulfilling lives if they receive proper treatment (NIMH, 2018).

Medications used in the treatment of anxiety-related disorders include benzodiazepines. These medications are used for short-term treatment during an acute phase of an anxiety disorder. Patients experiencing anxiety prior to undergoing medical or surgical procedures find benzodiazepines helpful to relieve anxiety. The benzodiazepines diazepam, lorazepam, and midazolam can be given IM or IV when the patient has been NPO prior to a procedure. Midazolam may also be given intranasally. Benzodiazepines are generally not recommended for use beyond a few weeks because of their addictive properties. Patients should consult with their prescribing provider about the potential side effects of long-term benzodiazepine use.

For long-term management of certain anxiety-related disorders, prescribers may consider using certain antidepressants, such as SNRIs, SSRIs, and TCAs. The serotonin/norepinephrine reuptake inhibitors (SNRIs) duloxetine and venlafaxine are used to treat GAD; venlafaxine is also used to treat panic disorder and social anxiety disorder. The selective serotonin reuptake inhibitors (SSRIs) fluoxetine and paroxetine are helpful in the treatment of phobias, OCD, and panic disorder. The tricyclic antidepressant clomipramine is indicated for the treatment of OCD.

The beta-blocker propranolol was used in the past to treat performance anxiety, but that is no longer a medically acceptable indication. Hydroxyzine (Vistaril), an antihistamine, has a side effect of sedation that is indicated for decreasing the anxiety associated with asthma. See **Medications 31.1** for more information about medications used to treat anxiety-related disorders.

Herbal supplements, including valerian, kava, and passionflower, are used by some individuals in the treatment of anxiety. However, these medications have not been conclusively proven to be effective and may cause various side effects (Mayo Clinic, 2018b). The nurse should caution patients to consult with their primary HCPs before taking herbal supplements.

Medications 31.1

Drugs Used to Treat Anxiety-Related Disorders

CLASSIFICATION AND DRUG EXAMPLES	MECHANISMS OF ACTION/ INDICATIONS FOR USE	NURSING CONSIDERATIONS
Antidepressants **Serotonin/Norepinephrine Reuptake Inhibitors (SNRIs)** ***Drug examples:*** duloxetine (Cymbalta, Drizalma Sprinkle) venlafaxine (Effexor XR)	Inhibit the reuptake of both serotonin and norepinephrine, resulting in increased levels in the brain.	■ Monitor for development of suicidal ideation or worsening of symptoms. ■ Assess for adverse effects, including dizziness or drowsiness. ■ Counsel patients to avoid alcohol in combination with SSRIs or TCAs. ■ Periodically obtain complete blood count with differential, serum electrolyte panel, and liver and kidney function studies. ■ Do not start SSRIs within 14 days of discontinuing an monoamine oxidase inhibitor drug. ■ Women who are pregnant or breastfeeding should not take SSRIs or TCAs.
Selective Serotonin Reuptake Inhibitors (SSRIs) ***Drug examples:*** escitalopram (Lexapro) fluoxetine (Prozac) fluvoxamine paroxetine (Brisdelle, Paxil) sertraline (Zoloft)	Inhibit reuptake of the neurotransmitter serotonin in the brain, resulting in circulation of an increased level of serotonin. Although primarily used for treatment of depression, certain SNRIs and SSRIs, as listed, are also effective in the treatment of patients with GAD, OCD, and panic disorder.	
Tricyclic antidepressants (TCAs) ***Drug example:*** clomipramine (Anafranil)	Block presynaptic neuronal reuptake of serotonin and norepinephrine, resulting in increased circulating levels of these neurotransmitters. Clomipramine is used in the treatment of patients with OCD.	
Benzodiazepines ***Drug examples:*** alprazolam (Xanax) chlordiazepoxide clonazepam (Klonopin) clorazepate (Tranxene-T) diazepam (Valium) lorazepam (Ativan) oxazepam	Potentiate the effect of the naturally occurring inhibitory neurotransmitter gamma aminobutyric acid (GABA), leading to relaxation and a decrease in the subjective experience of anxiety. These drugs are used to treat GAD and panic disorder.	■ Not recommended for long-term use because of habit-forming properties (these are Schedule IV drugs). ■ Monitor patient for excess sedation and dizziness. ■ Use cautiously in patients with impaired hepatic function and monitor liver function studies. ■ Counsel patient to avoid alcohol or opioids in combination with benzodiazepines.
Nonbenzodiazepines ***Drug examples:*** buspirone meprobamate	Buspirone acts as a dopamine agonist in the brain and also inhibits serotonin reuptake (leading to increased circulating serotonin), producing an antianxiety effect. Meprobamate affects the thalamus and limbic system and emotions. Used to treat GAD.	■ Assess for side effects, including nausea, headaches, and dizziness. ■ Use with caution in individuals with impaired liver or kidney function. ■ Advise patient this medication requires daily administration for several weeks to produce antianxiety effect.

Source: Based on Adams, Holland, and Urban (2020).

SAFETY ALERT The antihistamine diphenhydramine (Benadryl) is not suitable for use in the long-term treatment of anxiety-related disorders. Although diphenhydramine does produce sedation, its effects do not help patients achieve anxiolysis (reduction of anxiety). Moreover, cessation of diphenhydramine after long-term use can cause withdrawal symptoms. Of even greater concern is a report published in *JAMA Internal Medicine* that showed a link between dementia and the long-term use of diphenhydramine because the drug blocks acetylcholine, a neurotransmitter in the brain that is important for learning and memory (Gray et al., 2015). Taking an anticholinergic drug for 3 years or more was associated with a 54% higher risk of dementia. Patients with anxiety-related signs and symptoms should seek professional evaluation and guidance rather than try to self-medicate with an over-the-counter drug.

Case Study » Part 3

Following Mr. DeLarno's assertion that he cannot "stay here all day" and his prompting for rapid treatment, the nurse practitioner replies, "I can imagine that your headaches are interfering with every aspect of your life, Mr. DeLarno. In particular, it must be miserable to try to study while you have a pounding headache, much less to take an exam. I want to help you find the best solution, which means I'll need some more information from you." She further explains to Mr. DeLarno that additional assessment is needed to accurately identify the cause of his headaches, as well as to choose the appropriate treatment approach. Initially, Mr. DeLarno is disappointed about not receiving a prescription for alprazolam, which he again suggests will fully resolve his headaches. However, after talking with the nurse practitioner, he agrees with the plan for further assessment.

The nurse practitioner performs a focused neurologic assessment, including assessing Mr. DeLarno's pupillary response to light and his extremity strength. She also interviews him as to the presence of any alterations in sensory perception, including numbness, tingling, or other unusual sensations. With the exception of his headache and sleep disturbances, which Mr. DeLarno reports began about 8 months earlier, his assessment findings reveal no abnormalities.

Based on assessment findings, the nurse practitioner suspects Mr. DeLarno may have developed GAD. For further evaluation and treatment, she refers him to a mental health specialist affiliated with the university clinic. She further instructs Mr. DeLarno to avoid caffeine and nicotine and to contact the clinic if his headaches worsen or if he experiences any alterations in sensory perception. In addition, she offers to refer him to a local massage therapist who offers one free massage to students referred by the university student health services center. The patient agrees to follow up with the student wellness center and pleasantly accepts the referral for massage, stating, "I'm calling the massage therapist as soon as I walk out of here."

Clinical Reasoning Questions Level I

1. Which of the nurse practitioner's statements represent validation of the patient's complaints? Explain how validation can serve to diffuse a tense verbal interaction with a patient.
2. How could the staff nurse support and facilitate the interventions prescribed by the nurse practitioner?

Clinical Reasoning Questions Level II

3. Identify three nursing care priorities that are appropriate for Mr. DeLarno.
4. What additional recommendations could be offered by the staff nurse to promote healthy sleep/rest patterns for this patient?

Lifespan Considerations

Each stage of the lifespan comes with its own developmental stressors (see **Box 31.4** »). The individual's response to those stressors and the coping mechanisms used to deal with each stressor will differ on the basis of the developmental stage, personality, and environment.

Box 31.4
Developmental Stressors Across the Lifespan

Infants and Toddlers
- Separation from primary caregiver
- Cold stress, heat exposure
- Premature birth
- Maternal consumption of substances, toxins
- Feeding issues
- Impaired maternal bonding or attachment

Children
- Starting school
- Playing with peers/making friends
- Separation from parents/caregivers
- Conflict with parents/siblings

Adolescents
- Puberty
- Performance (sports, academics, arts)
- Independence (driving, job, social life)
- Relationships (peers, friends, dating, teachers, parents, caregivers)
- Peer pressure
- Spiritual development

Adults
- Dating/marriage
- Birth or death of children
- Career
- Purchasing a house
- Health changes
- Divorce or death of spouse

Pregnant Women
- Hormone changes
- Body changes
- Childbirth
- Financial fears
- Fear of having miscarriage or an unhealthy baby

Older Adult
- Aging
- Retirement
- Loss of independence
- Terminal illness or multiple chronic illnesses
- Loneliness and isolation
- Death of peers or spouse

Stress and Coping in Children and Adolescents

Stressors in children and adolescents can be divided into normative and non-normative stressors. Normative stressors that are common to all children include separation from parents or caregivers, starting school, and making new friends. Normative stressors change as the child ages. For example, the transition from childhood to adolescence involves stressors such as navigating relationships with peers and completing performance-related tasks, such as academic assignments that require public speaking.

In contrast, non-normative stressors are those that very few children and adolescents face but that produce higher stress levels. Non-normative stressors may include serious illness of the child or a close family member, death of a parent, child abuse, natural disasters, or homelessness. Non-normative stress can become "toxic" if the child or adolescent does not receive necessary adult support. Toxic stress can influence a child's health into adulthood, increasing the risk for developing chronic diseases such as cardiovascular disease, cancer, asthma, and depression. Prevention of toxic stress often requires intervention at the family, community, and federal levels rather than at the biological level (Boullier & Blair, 2018).

In the early stages of development, some degree of anxiety is normal, particularly when children are separated from their parents or caregivers. Stranger anxiety is most pronounced during the first 2 years of life. Many young children have not yet developed normal coping processes, so they frequently cry or throw a temper tantrum when faced with stressful situations. However, as a result of normal cognitive development, usually around the toddler stage, children become better able to distinguish between dangerous and nonthreatening situations, and fears begin to abate. Along with this developing sense of discernment, toddlers also begin to learn how to cope with fear.

As children learn to cope with stressors, they face new stressors such as starting school, making new friends, and feeling pressured to get good grades. Later in childhood, especially during adolescence, stressors often include changes related to puberty, performance, and conflict with parents. If the child does not learn how to cope with these stressors or does not receive appropriate support from a parent or other caregiver, anxiety disorders may develop. A child or adolescent whose anxiety or fear persists beyond the expected age of resolution or endures for 6 months or longer may have developed an anxiety disorder and will benefit from referral to a mental health specialist (American Psychiatric Association, 2013).

When working with children and adolescents, the challenge for the nurse is to differentiate between true anxiety disorders and normal developmental stressors and fears. Therefore, it is vital to assess not only the presence of emotional and behavioral cues related to stress but also the duration, severity, and timing of symptoms. Psychosocial assessment of the pediatric patient should be age and developmentally specific (see Module 25, Development) and should take into consideration that children may exhibit manifestations of disorders in ways that vary significantly from those demonstrated by adult patients. Signs of stress or anxiety in children may include irritability, withdrawal from pleasurable activities, clinging to a parent, frequent complaints of feeling ill, new or recurring fears, crying, sleeping or eating too much or too little, bedwetting, and declining grades at school (American Psychological Association, 2019a). Signs of stress or anxiety in adolescents may include excessive tiredness, anger and defiance, refusing to participate in favorite activities, becoming involved in substance abuse or criminal activities, sudden drops in grades at school, and social withdrawal.

When assessing children, nurses need to be aware of the language children use to express their stress or anxiety because they often use terms different from those used by adults. Children may not understand the concept of stress, so they may use terms such as "worry," "confused," or "mad" to describe their feelings. They may also convey stressful feelings by expressing negative thoughts about themselves or their environment (American Psychological Association, 2019a). In addition, nurses should be aware that children and adults have different views of what types of circumstances are stressful to children. Nurses should also assess how the child's parents cope with stress because children often mimic what they see.

When performing a nursing assessment on adolescents, the nurse should interview both the patient and the guardian individually with the approval of the guardian. Adolescents may feel more comfortable discussing stressful situations when their parents are not present. The nurse should encourage adolescents to be truthful about stressors they are exposed to, including peer pressure to participate in sexual activities, criminal activities, and substance or alcohol abuse. Because adolescents may feel more comfortable discussing these issues with a HCP of the same gender, the nurse should always ask the patient and the guardian whether a provider of the same gender is preferred.

Several tools are available to assess the stress levels of children and adolescents. The most widely used diagnostic tool is the Anxiety Disorders Interview Schedule for Children and Parents (ADIS-C/P; Freidl et al., 2017). The Pediatric Anxiety Rating Scale (PARS) is a shorter interview schedule that is administered to children and parents. Some tools, such as the Revised Children's Anxiety and Depression scale, are aimed directly at children. Other tools are geared toward specific syndromes, such as the Penn State Worry Questionnaire for Children and the Panic Disorder Severity Scale for Children. Tools are available that measure the extent that anxiety impacts family, social, and school life, such as the Child Anxiety Impact Scale and the Strengths and Difficulties Questionnaire (Freidl et al., 2017).

If a child or adolescent is experiencing elevated levels of stress, the nurse can teach coping strategies to both the child and the parents or primary caregivers. Strategies that may be beneficial for children to practice include:

- Talking about their problems with a parent or other trusted adult
- Practicing relaxation exercises such as listening to calm music, taking deep breaths, or practicing a hobby or favorite activity
- Participating in physical activity
- Setting realistic expectations
- Asking for help to manage stress.

Strategies that may be beneficial for parents to practice to help their children cope with stress include providing a safe and secure home environment, being selective about television programming that young children can watch (to decrease their exposure to violence and potential fears), spending time with their child, listening to their child and encouraging the child to talk about fears or worries, building the child's sense of self-worth, and keeping the child informed during potentially stressful changes (MedlinePlus, 2021).

In addition to teaching coping strategies, the nurse, along with the provider, may recommend CBT as a treatment method for childhood and adolescent anxiety. Treatment of children and adolescents with CBT is often based on Kendall's "Coping Cat," a method that involves psychoeducation, modification of negative thoughts, exposure to feared stimuli, and training in coping skills (California Evidence-Based Clearinghouse, 2018).

When discussing treatment methods for children and adolescents with alterations in stress and coping, treatment should focus on teaching multiple coping strategies rather than on pharmacologic intervention. Many antianxiety and antidepressant medications are not approved for children and adolescents, and some medications increase the risk of depression and suicide (ADAA, 2020d). Therefore, medications are used only in severe cases of anxiety in children and adolescents. If the patient is prescribed an anxiolytic medication or antidepressant, the nurse should teach the patient and guardian about the risks associated with medication use.

Stress and Coping in Older Adults

Stressors for older adults are often related to changes associated with aging: loss of mobility, loss of independence, retirement, loss of peers or a spouse, or being diagnosed with a terminal illness or multiple chronic illnesses. Older adults who experience a loss of mobility or who have lost friends or a spouse to death may also feel a sense of isolation or loneliness, which can cause additional stress. Even the advancement of everyday technology can be a stressor for older adults who may not understand how to use computers or smartphones.

Signs and symptoms of stress in older adults include alterations in sleep patterns, eating habits, and self-care; headaches or other pains; tachycardia; GI problems; negative feelings or attitudes; mood swings; social isolation; frequent crying; poor judgment; and lack of concentration. Older adults are more likely to report physical discomforts before they will report mental or cognitive problems. However, the diagnosis of anxiety-related disorders can be complicated by preexisting physical illness or cognitive changes in this population. For example, changes in self-care habits may be in response to stress, or they may be in response to cognitive changes that decrease the patient's ability to remember how to use basic grooming tools. Fear of stigmatization is also a significant consideration. Because many older adults were raised during a time when mental illness carried a heavy stigma, they may be especially resistant to reporting any symptoms of mental disorders (ADAA, 2020c). Alterations due to anxiety and stress may also be difficult to identify in older adults because they often have better emotional control and coping strategies than younger adults (Miller, 2019).

When faced with stressors, older adults tend to use more passive emotion-focused coping strategies, including denial or acceptance. Older adults often carefully select the events or situations that they worry about because they are attempting to conserve energy for the most important situations. Thus, they may tend to avoid some problems or withdraw from normal activities rather than face the situation that causes anxiety (Miller, 2019). For example, an older adult who has anxiety related to incontinence will often avoid leaving the house in order to prevent potential embarrassment related to the incontinence. This can lead to isolation and depression.

Older adults who maintain their social circles and remain physically active have better mental and physical health than those who isolate themselves (Miller, 2019). Nurses can promote wellness in older adults by encouraging them to remain socially and physically active and pursue activities that bring them joy and fulfillment. Older adults will benefit from spending time with family and friends or by participating in religious practices or volunteering. This support system can help them maintain their mental health and feel a sense of well-being rather than a sense of anxiety or stress.

Depending on the individual and the level of stress, some older adults may also be candidates for CBT or medication. However, medications should be used carefully because of potential drug interactions that may occur in older adults who are taking multiple other medications.

REVIEW The Concept of Stress and Coping

RELATE Link the Concepts

Linking the concept of stress and coping with the concept of communication:

1. Describe the application of therapeutic communication in the nursing care of patients with disorders related to stress and coping.
2. Particularly during the care of patients with disorders related to stress and coping, why is giving advice contraindicated? What specific communication strategies are recommended for these patients?

Linking the concept of stress and coping with the concept of ethics:

3. What is patient confidentiality, and how does this principle pertain to patients who seek treatment for alterations related to stress and coping? Under what circumstances is the requirement to maintain patient confidentiality not applicable?
4. While in the hospital cafeteria, a nurse overhears a nursing colleague discussing a patient's recent hospital admission for treatment related to an unusual phobia. Although the nursing colleague does not specify the patient's name, she includes a detailed discussion of the patient's complaints. How should this situation be addressed?

READY Go to Volume 3: Clinical Nursing Skills

REFER Go to Pearson MyLab Nursing and eText

REFLECT Apply Your Knowledge

Martina Carrillo is a sixth-grader at Longview Middle School. She speaks Spanish and English. Over the past month, she has been to see the school nurse several times with complaints of a stomachache. She has not complained about any other physical symptoms, and her stomachache has not led to vomiting. However, the school nurse notes that her heart rate and respiratory rate have increased slightly over the month. Based on school records and talking with Martina, the school nurse knows that she is the oldest of four children in an immigrant family. Her father is still in Mexico, and her mother works a shift from 3:00 p.m. to 11:00 p.m. at a local factory. Martina is on the free lunch program at school. Normally a good student, her grades have been declining over the past 3 months. When asked about this, Martina states that she often doesn't understand her homework and doesn't have time to do it because she is caring for her younger siblings in the evenings after school.

1. What potential stressors might Martina be facing each day in addition to those listed in the case study that the nurse might need to ask Martina about?
2. What physiologic processes might be leading to her complaint of a stomachache?
3. What coping strategies may be advantageous for the school nurse to teach Martina?
4. How can the school nurse be an advocate for Martina during this time?

Exemplar 31.A Anxiety Disorders

Exemplar Learning Outcomes

31.A Analyze anxiety disorders as they relate to stress and coping.

- Describe the pathophysiology of anxiety disorders.
- Describe the etiology of anxiety disorders.
- Compare the risk factors for and prevention of anxiety disorders.
- Identify the clinical manifestations of anxiety disorders.
- Summarize diagnostic tests and therapies used by interprofessional teams in the collaborative care of individuals with anxiety disorders.
- Differentiate considerations for care of patients with anxiety disorders across the lifespan.
- Apply the nursing process in providing culturally competent care to an individual with an anxiety disorder.

Exemplar Key Terms

Anxiety, *2105*
External locus of control, *2109*
Free-floating anxiety, *2105*
Generalized anxiety disorder (GAD), *2108*
Internal locus of control, *2109*
Panic disorder, *2108*
Phobia, *2109*
Vulnerability, *2106*

Overview

Anxiety is a response arising in anticipation of a perceived or actual threat to oneself or significant relationships. Anxiety is characterized by feelings of mental uneasiness, apprehension, dread, foreboding, and feelings of helplessness. Generally, anxiety helps people cope; it is a reaction to a stressor and is part of daily living. Anxious energy is a productive force for most people, and the experience of anxiety is influenced by an individual's genetic makeup as well as emotional, developmental, physical, cognitive, sociocultural, and spiritual factors.

Anxiety disorders may occur when normal feelings of anxiety get out of control and begin to impair individual functioning. Anxiety disorders are mental illnesses characterized by feelings of distress or fear during everyday situations. Fear is typically a heightened physical and emotional response to imminent danger, real or perceived (American Psychiatric Association, 2013). Left untreated, anxiety disorders can damage personal relationships and the ability to work. Anxiety disorders impair daily activity and can lead to low self-esteem, substance misuse or abuse, and social isolation. Anxiety disorders are the most common mental illnesses in the United States, typically affecting around 18% of the population (ADAA, 2020a). Effective treatments exist for anxiety disorders, but many people do not seek treatment because they fail to realize how severe their symptoms are or because family, friends, and even physicians have difficulty recognizing the symptoms.

The ability to differentiate healthy and expected stress responses from those that are harmful is an essential psychosocial competency for all nurses. Every individual experiences anxiety at times. The individual's anxiety is no longer healthy when the anxiety level reaches the point at which it prevents the individual from returning to homeostasis through healthy coping and adaptation.

Pathophysiology

Research suggests that people are more likely to experience anxiety disorders if their parents have anxiety disorders (Cleveland Clinic, 2020). However, it is not clear whether biological or environmental factors play a greater role in the development of these conditions. In any case, scientists have found that certain areas of the brain, including the amygdala, function differently in people with anxiety disorders (Babaev, Piletti Chatain, & Kreuger-Burg, 2018).

The appearance of an anxiety disorder in an individual of any age requires attention by both healthcare professionals and caregivers. Family and friends may be the first to notice anxiety symptoms. Healthcare professionals recognize that many medical problems—including hormonal and neurologic conditions—may cause symptoms of anxiety. The primary symptom of anxiety disorders is what psychiatrists sometimes refer to as **free-floating anxiety**. This is characterized by excessive worry that is hard to control and whose focus may shift from moment to moment. Free-floating anxiety is anxiety that is not connected to a specific stimulus (Gerlach & Gloster, 2020). Examples of anxiety disorders are listed in the Concept section earlier in this module. This exemplar discusses three of them: generalized anxiety disorder, panic disorder, and phobias.

Etiology

Across the range of anxiety disorders, there are some important similarities in the basic causes of the anxiety response. Biological causes seem to play a significant role in the development of anxiety disorders. Abnormal function of structures in the limbic system and certain parts of the cortex appear to be involved. The neurotransmitters most closely involved with the anxiety response are GABA, norepinephrine, and serotonin. Genetic contributions play a role as well, with at least part of the genetic vulnerability being nonspecific, or common across the disorders. Psychosocial and behavioral factors include the classical conditioning of fear and a perception of lack of control over one's environment, an attitude that begins in childhood (Hooley, Butcher, Nock, & Mineka, 2017).

Vulnerability refers to the individual's susceptibility to react to a specific stressor. Individual vulnerability stems from biological and environmental sources, both of which have been the subjects of etiologic research. (See Focus on Diversity and Culture: Anxiety Disorders in Immigrant Populations.) Current explanations of the origin of anxiety disorders include neurobiological, neurochemical, psychosocial, behavioral, genetic, and humanistic theories.

Neurobiological Theories

Several areas of the brain orchestrate the experience of anxiety and the expression of its symptoms (see **Figure 31.4** ››). The amygdala is known as the "emotional brain" and is the focus of much research related to feelings of anxiety, fear, and anger, which are elicited in this area. The hippocampus stores memory related to fear. The locus coeruleus stimulates arousal and contains almost half of all the neurons that use norepinephrine as a neurotransmitter. Stimulating an animal's locus coeruleus produces anxious behaviors. Heart rate and respirations are regulated by the brainstem, and the hypothalamus activates the entire response. The frontal cortex assists with appraisal of a threat and is the center of cognitive processes. The thalamus integrates all sensory stimuli, and the basal ganglia are responsible for the tremors associated with anxiety (Morris, McCall, Charney, & Murrough, 2020). Individual differences in the structure of or injury to the brain will also alter the anxiety response.

Neurochemical Theories

Communication within the brain occurs between neurons through the transmission of electrical stimuli (see **Figure 31.5** ›› and **Figure 31.6** ››). To transmit a signal, a neuron releases chemicals called neurotransmitters. These chemicals deliver messages by binding to the receptors on the surface of another neuron, causing the neuron to fire and transmit the electrical impulse. Once the message is delivered, the neurotransmitter is taken back to a vesicle in the presynaptic cell (National Institute of Neurological Disorders and Stroke, 2020). Any disruption in these transporters,

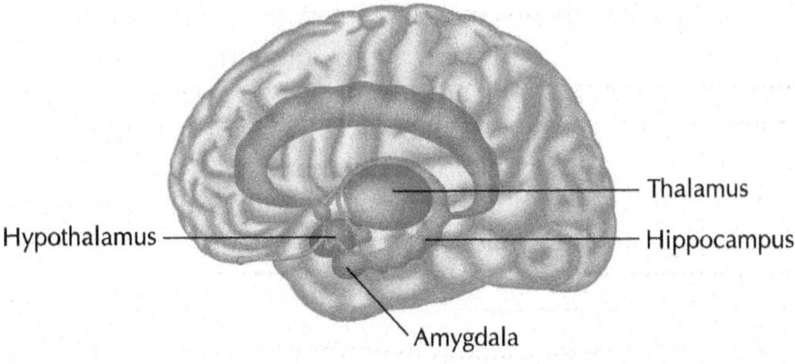

Figure 31.4 ›› Areas of the brain that orchestrate the experience and expressions of anxiety.

Source: From Manson (2015) Copyright © 2015 by Pearson Education

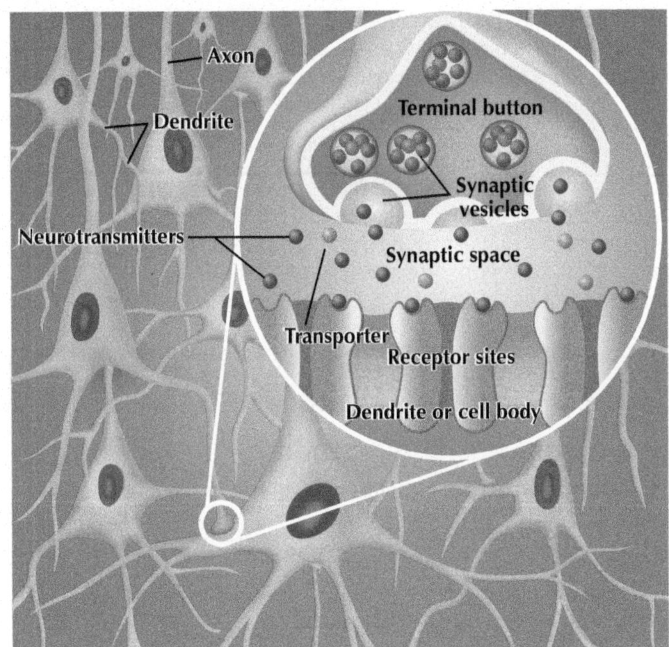

Figure 31.5 ›› Neurotransmission: How neurons communicate.

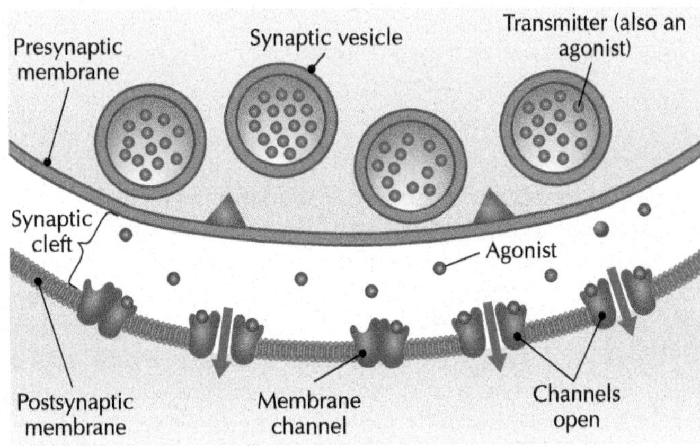

A, Strong agonist activates receptors without transmission.

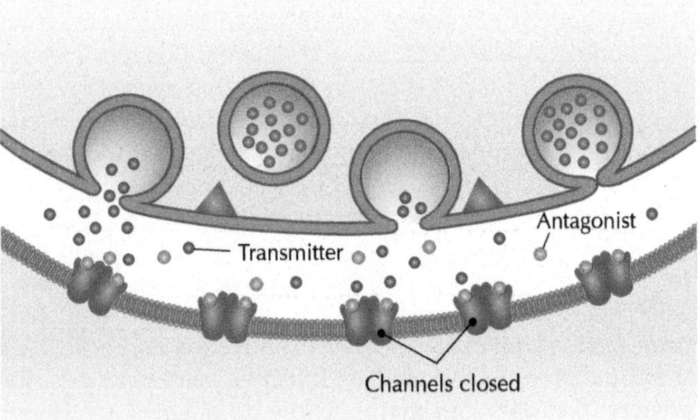

B, Antagonist blocks receptors. Agonist cannot act.

Figure 31.6 ›› Agonists and antagonists bind to the same binding site as transmitters. ***A***, Agonists have potency, so they activate the cell biologically, while ***B***, antagonists bind and have no potency. Antagonists produce their effect by blocking the binding site, preventing a transmitter from binding and producing its biological effect.

binding sites, or cell structure can cause an alteration in cell functioning, leading to misfiring.

Structural anatomic differences, dysregulation of neurotransmitters, sensitivity of neuronal receptor sites, and the balance of neurotransmitters in the synaptic cleft all have an effect on the anxiety reaction. The brain's benzodiazepine receptor system enhances the activity of GABA, an inhibitory neurotransmitter that "shuts down" or slows excitability in the cell. It is present in the locus coeruleus, where norepinephrine is produced. Norepinephrine is an excitatory neurotransmitter that signals arousal and hyperarousal. Researchers believe that an imbalance in the regulation of these two neurotransmitters produces anxiety disorders: When GABA is decreased and norepinephrine is increased, anxiety results (Kaur & Singh, 2017). Serotonin is also implicated in the pathology of anxiety. It is thought to produce a feeling of well-being and is believed to be correlated with a decrease in anxiety (Hooley et al., 2017).

Psychosocial Theories

Psychoanalytic theory views anxiety as a sign of internal conflict resulting from the threatened emergence of repressed emotions into consciousness. An individual fears expressing forbidden emotions and so becomes anxious. In contrast, psychosocial theory as proposed by Erik Erikson (1969) emphasizes the interactions of the individual with other people as essential to individuals mastering developmental tasks, and that failure to master these tasks can give rise to anxiety and cause individuals to regress in their development. See Module 25, Development, for an overview of Erikson's theory of development.

Behavioral Theories

Behaviorists believe that faulty thinking and behavior are learned dysfunctional responses to stressors. They believe individuals can unlearn unhealthy behaviors by engaging in behavior modification, a treatment approach that teaches patients new ways to behave in response to stress. Behavior modification therapies use conditioning techniques—positive and negative reinforcements—in order to produce systematic desensitization, a process in which the patient builds up tolerance to anxiety through gradual exposure to a series of anxiety-provoking stimuli.

Genetic Theories

As stated earlier, research suggests that genetic predisposition may play a part in the development of anxiety disorders. According to twin and family studies, panic disorder, phobic disorders, and GAD all have a genetic component, with twins and first-order family members of individuals having a higher risk of developing the same disorder compared to more distant relatives. Overall, the estimated heritability of anxiety disorders is between 30 and 50% (Smoller, 2020). Genetic predisposition can produce the biological conditions necessary for an anxiety disorder to develop, priming an individual for anxious behavior.

Humanistic Theories

A humanistic, holistic explanation of anxiety disorders argues that biological, psychologic, behavioral, and genetic causes do not exist in isolation—they interact with one another to produce the complex of symptoms known as anxiety disor-

Focus on Diversity and Culture

Anxiety Disorders in Immigrant Populations

Evidence suggests that the migration experiences of first-generation immigrant parents contribute to the risk for depression and anxiety in first- and second-generation immigrant children (Klein et al., 2020). Unique migration stressors such as discrimination, lack of cultural resources, and lack of social acceptance give rise to acculturative stress. *Acculturative stress* is a term used to describe the experiences and reactions involved in adjusting to and integrating into a new culture (Waldman et al., 2019). High levels of acculturative stress in first-generation immigrant parents are correlated with anxiety symptoms in their children but are not necessarily linked to anxiety symptoms in parents. Separation of immigrant families due to federal immigration policies and enforcement can result in mental health issues including lower academic achievement in children, toxic stress, and symptoms of posttraumatic stress disorder (Vesely, Bravo, & Guzzardo, 2019).

approach to patient care that integrates psychotherapeutic interventions, steps to develop social support systems, techniques to reduce external stress, and psychopharmacologic therapy.

Risk Factors

Risk factors for anxiety disorders include the dysregulation of neurotransmitters such as serotonin, norepinephrine, GABA, and a neuropeptide known as cholecystokinin. Other risk factors include the following (Cabral & Patel, 2020):

- Childhood adversity, including witnessing traumatic events
- Family history of anxiety disorders
- Social factors, such as lack of social connection
- Serious or chronic illness
- Traumatic events
- Personality factors such as shyness and worrying
- Multiple stressors, such as chronic illness concurrent with loss of employment.

Prevention

Prevention of anxiety disorders depends on the ability of individuals to recognize their own growing anxiety. Individuals at risk for anxiety disorders should seek medical help early because these conditions become harder to treat as they progress. Keeping track of patterns of worrying can also help stop anxiety before it grows out of control. Mental health professionals advise that individuals at risk for anxiety disorders keep journals to catalog stressors and sources of relief and to manage priorities. Finally, individuals with multiple risk factors should avoid unhealthy substance use, including the misuse or abuse of alcohol, illegal drugs, and even nicotine and caffeine. These drugs can stimulate anxiety, and for people who are addicted, quitting can worsen anxiety

TABLE 31.5 Summary of Criteria for Anxiety Disorders

The following are summaries of the criteria for the anxiety disorders discussed in this exemplar. Refer to the DSM-5 for the complete diagnostic criteria.

Disorder	Summary
Generalized anxiety disorder	■ Characterized by intense tension and worry, even in the absence of external stressors. ■ May demonstrate anticipation of disaster and/or preoccupation with health issues, money, familial problems, or work-related challenges. ■ Affected individuals usually recognize that their anxiety is disproportionate to the circumstances. ■ Manifestations include difficulty relaxing, pronounced startling, trouble concentrating, and difficulty falling asleep. ■ Somatic symptoms include fatigue, headache, muscle tension and aches, digestive issues, irritability, feeling out of breath, and hot flashes. ■ Diagnostic criteria include excessive anxiety about everyday problems for at least 6 months.
Panic disorder	■ Recurrent unexpected panic attacks, when at least one of the attacks has been followed by 1 month of persistent concern about having more attacks, worry about the implications of the attack, or a significant change in behavior related to the attacks. ■ The attacks are not due to the physiologic effects of a substance. ■ The attacks are not better accounted for by another mental disorder.
Phobias Specific phobia Agoraphobia Social anxiety disorder	■ Intense, persistent, irrational fear of an object or situation that compels the individual to avoid the stressor that elicits the fear. ■ Exposure to the stressor produces an anxiety response that may take the form of a panic attack. ■ Anxiety about the stressor is out of proportion to the actual threat of danger posed by the object or situation, after accounting for cultural contextual factors. ■ Symptoms must last at least 6 months for patients regardless of age.

Sources: Based on American Psychiatric Association (2013); National Institute of Mental Health (2018); Substance Abuse and Mental Health Services Administration (2016).

Clinical Manifestations

Anxiety disorders are clustered around a range of physiologic, psychologic, behavioral, and cognitive manifestations. Although each of the disorders is distinct (e.g., GAD is completely distinct from acute stress disorder), the symptoms of all the disorders cluster around excessive, irrational fear and dread (NIMH, 2018). Worry is a major component of each of the anxiety disorders. Individuals in anxiety states experience the emotion both as a subjective condition and as a range of physical symptoms resulting from muscular tension and autonomic nervous system activity. Chronic anxiety can lead to physical manifestations and disabilities, including constipation, diarrhea, epigastric distress, and heartburn, as well as musculoskeletal aches and pains. Anxiety can develop suddenly or gradually, and it may be expressed as relatively mild physiologic symptoms or as an incapacitating episode of acute anxiety. See **Table 31.5** » for an overview of three types of anxiety disorders; each is discussed in more detail in the following sections.

Generalized Anxiety Disorder

Individuals with **generalized anxiety disorder (GAD)** go through their days filled with intense tension and worry, even if no external stressors are present. They anticipate disaster and are preoccupied with health issues, money, familial problems, or challenges at work. GAD may be diagnosed when excessive worrying is out of proportion to stressors (perceived or actual), interferes with daily functioning, and occurs for a period of at least 6 months (American Psychiatric Association, 2013). Individuals with GAD cannot rid themselves of their anxious state, although they can usually recognize that their anxiety is more intense than the situation requires. They have difficulty relaxing, startle easily, and have trouble concentrating and falling asleep. Somatic symptoms of GAD include fatigue, headache, muscle tension and aches, digestive issues, irritability, feeling out of breath, and hot flashes. Sleep disturbances are common. Adults with mild or well-controlled GAD can function in social situations and at work, but those with severe, poorly controlled GAD have great difficulty carrying out daily tasks. GAD affects 2.7% of adults in the United States, and more women (3.4%) than men (1.9%). The disorder can develop at any time in the life cycle, although people are at highest risk for the condition in early adulthood, between childhood and middle age (NIMH, 2017a).

Generalized anxiety disorder can manifest in children with all the same symptoms as in adults. Children with GAD feel significantly distressed and, as with adults, the principal sign of GAD is intense worry over a long period of time. GAD in children may have physical manifestations, including headache, muscle tension, restlessness, palpitations, and GI issues. GAD is common among children and adolescents and is treated mostly with psychotherapy, the goal of which is to build up healthy and constructive responses to anxiety (Boston Children's Hospital, n.d.).

Panic Disorder

Panic disorder is characterized by sudden attacks of terror, sometimes accompanied by a pounding heart, sweating, fainting, or dizziness. Manifestations of a panic attack include feeling flushed or chilled; tingling or numbness in the hands; nausea, chest pain, and a sense of breathlessness in addition to a sense of unreality; a fear of impending death; and a terror of losing control. A fear of one's own unexplained symptoms is itself a symptom of panic disorder. Individuals in the grip of a panic attack sometimes believe they are dying or losing their minds; between episodes, they may worry intensely about the next panic attack (American Psychiatric Association, 2013). Attacks can occur at any time of day and even during sleep. An attack usually lasts only around 10 minutes, but some symptoms may last much longer. The disorder affects around 2.7% of adults in the United States and is twice as common in women as in men (NIMH, 2017c).

People who have full-fledged panic disorder can become incapacitated by their condition and should seek treatment before they start to avoid situations in which attacks have occurred. In severe cases, people who have panic attacks avoid normal activities. Some people who have panic disorder become housebound and are able to confront a feared situation only when accompanied by a loved one or trusted friend. Panic disorder may be treated with psychotherapy and medications (NIMH, 2018).

SAFETY ALERT Panic attacks and heart attacks have many common symptoms, making it difficult to discern one from the other. Any patient experiencing sudden, severe chest pain should be assessed and treated as though they are having a cardiac event.

Phobias

Individuals with **phobias** experience intense, persistent fear or anxiety associated with a particular object or situation, called a *stressor*, and tend to avoid that stressor at all costs. Contact with the stressor produces severe panic. Stressors can be anything; needles and syringes, airplanes, spiders, dogs, closed areas, performing, and social activities are a few examples. Phobias adversely impact quality of social, occupational, and academic function and also interfere with activities of daily living (American Psychiatric Association, 2013). An estimated 8.7% of the U.S. population is affected by a specific phobia, and women are twice as likely to develop a specific phobia as men (ADAA, 2020a).

Individuals with phobias and other forms of anxiety may exhibit an external locus of control. Lazarus and Folkman (1984) describe *locus of control* as the extent to which individuals believe they have control over life events. Individuals with an **internal locus of control** believe their actions, choices, and behaviors impact life events. Those with an **external locus of control** believe that powers outside of themselves, such as luck or fate, determine life events.

There are three primary categories of phobias: specific phobia, agoraphobia, and social anxiety disorder. Specific phobia is intense or extreme fear with regard to a particular object or situation such as spiders, snakes, flying, or heights. *Agoraphobia* is characterized by anxiety associated with two or more of the following situations: being in enclosed spaces, being in open spaces, using public transportation, being in a crowd or standing in a line of people, or being alone outside the home environment (American Psychiatric Association, 2013). Social anxiety disorder is characterized by pervasive, extreme fear of one or more social situations that may lead to scrutiny by others.

Phobias are frequently comorbid with other psychiatric alterations, including depressive disorders, anxiety disorders, bipolar disorders, and substance-related disorders. Treatment focuses on teaching coping strategies and may be paired with pharmacologic interventions and psychotherapy.

Levels of Anxiety

Levels of anxiety range from mild to panic. The patient's level of anxiety greatly impacts nursing care. For patients experiencing panic or severe anxiety, safety is a priority. Because the individual will be unable to take in any new information during these stages, interventions focus on reducing the anxiety level prior to providing any new

Clinical Manifestations and Therapies

Anxiety Disorders

LEVEL OF SEVERITY OF ANXIETY	CLINICAL MANIFESTATIONS	CLINICAL THERAPIES
Mild	▪ Increase in sensory perception and arousal ▪ Increase in alertness ▪ Sleeplessness insomnia ▪ Increase in motivation ▪ Restlessness and irritability Hyperactivity	▪ Mild anxiety is typically resolved by an individual's coping mechanisms. Mild anxiety may be helpful to the patient to accentuate focus and concentration. ▪ Patients who are distressed by mild anxiety may benefit from: Improved sleep hygiene Relaxation techniques Behavior therapy Massage Aromatherapy. complementary
Moderate	▪ Narrowing of perceptual field and attention span (a process called "selective inattention") ▪ Reduction in alertness and awareness of surroundings ▪ Feeling of discomfort and irritability with others ▪ Self-absorption ▪ Increased restlessness ▪ Increase in respirations, heart rate, and muscle tension ▪ Increase in perspiration ▪ Rapid speech, louder tone, and higher pitch	▪ Cognitive and behavior therapy to identify triggers and learn improved coping techniques ▪ Relaxation techniques ▪ Integrative therapies such as yoga, acupuncture, massage ▪ Short-term use of antianxiety medications if symptoms do not improve with other therapies

(continued on next page)

Clinical Manifestations and Therapies *(continued)*

LEVEL OF SEVERITY OF ANXIETY	CLINICAL MANIFESTATIONS	CLINICAL THERAPIES
Severe	▪ Perceptual field greatly reduced ▪ Difficulty following directions ▪ Feelings of dread, horror ▪ Need to relieve anxiety ▪ Headache ▪ Dizziness ▪ Nausea, trembling, insomnia ▪ Palpitations, tachycardia, hyperventilating, diarrhea	▪ Cognitive and behavior therapy to learn to identify triggers and to learn better coping techniques ▪ Short-term antianxiety medications ▪ Relaxation techniques ▪ Integrative therapies such as yoga, acupuncture, massage ▪ Hospitalization may be required initially to manage severe anxiety until improved coping mechanisms are developed.
Panic	▪ Inability to focus ▪ Perception distorted ▪ Terror ▪ Feelings of doom ▪ Bizarre behavior ▪ Dilated pupils ▪ Trembling, sleeplessness, palpitations, pallor, diaphoresis, muscular incoordination ▪ Immobility or hyperactivity, incoherence	▪ Immediate, structured intervention required ▪ Immediate therapies include the following: Placing patient in a quiet, less stimulating environment Use of repetitive or physical task to diffuse energy Administration of antianxiety medications; use of sedative drugs for severe agitation. ▪ Long-term therapies include the following: Psychotherapy (cognitive, behavioral, or CBT) Relaxation techniques Improved sleep hygiene Integrative health therapies such as massage, acupuncture, yoga, hydrotherapy Nutrition consultation Mental health counseling.

information. Immediate interventions include reducing exposure to stimuli and providing comfort measures to assist in reducing symptom severity. Distractions and relaxation techniques may be helpful. Once the patient's anxiety level decreases, additional interventions to reduce anxiety, such as beginning a course of medication and starting psychotherapy, may be introduced. Patients who experience mild anxiety may benefit from nonpharmacologic interventions, such as yoga, deep breathing, and journaling.

Collaboration

With the exception of panic disorder, the treatment of anxiety disorders occurs more frequently in the home and community than in the hospital. Considering the level of distress that accompanies anxiety disorders, it is not difficult to understand the vulnerability of individuals with anxiety to substance abuse and/or depression. This combination is a threat to treatment success and positive outcomes for the individual. Because the individual is part of a family and a larger community, nurses need to support positive outcomes for individuals by involving both the individual and the family in the treatment process. Such treatment is multimodal and involves the assessment of age, education, health and health practices, spirituality, and culturally specific needs (NIMH, 2016).

Diagnostic Tests

Evaluation of an individual with symptoms of an anxiety disorder includes a complete medical history and physical exam. Currently no laboratory tests are available to diagnose any of the anxiety disorders, but various diagnostic tests may be used to rule out physical illness as the cause of the symptoms. If no physical illness is found, the patient may be referred to a mental health professional trained to diagnose and treat mental illnesses. Mental health providers use specially designed interview and assessment tools to evaluate an individual for an anxiety disorder. The mental health professional bases the diagnosis on the patient's subjective report of the duration and intensity of symptoms, including any interference with daily functioning. The diagnosis is typically made according to the criteria in the DSM-5 (American Psychiatric Association, 2013).

Pharmacologic Therapy

Medication does not cure anxiety disorders, but it can control or diminish the severity of the associated signs and symptoms while the patient enters psychotherapy. Medication may be prescribed by a psychiatrist, advanced practice psychiatric/mental health nurse, or primary HCP (e.g., physician, physician's assistant, nurse practitioner). The medications usually used for anxiety disorders are antianxiety drugs (anxiolytics) and some antidepressants. See Medications 31.1 in this module's Concept section for more information.

Antidepressants were developed to treat depression, but some have been found to be effective for anxiety disorders. Although they begin to alter brain chemistry after the first dose, their full effect requires a few weeks because a series of neurobiological changes must take place before antidepressants achieve efficacy. SSRIs alter the level of the neurotransmitter serotonin in the brain and are commonly prescribed for some anxiety disorders. These drugs are generally started at low doses and then increased as their effectiveness becomes apparent. SSRIs have fewer side effects than previous generations of antidepressants, but they sometimes cause nausea, agitation, and sexual dysfunction. Examples of these drugs include escitalopram, fluoxetine, paroxetine, and sertraline. Related to the SSRIs, serotonin/norepinephrine reuptake inhibitors (SNRIs) inhibit the reabsorption of both serotonin and norepinephrine to treat some anxiety disorders. Examples of SNRIs include duloxetine and venlafaxine. One tricyclic antidepressant, clomipramine (Anafranil), has also been found useful in treating anxiety disorders.

The most commonly used drugs to treat anxiety disorders are certain benzodiazepines. When used for a short time, these drugs have few side effects other than drowsiness. However, higher and higher doses may be necessary over a long period of time, so benzodiazepines are typically not prescribed for long-term use. Because they take only hours to reach efficacy, they often are prescribed for patients experiencing severe or panic levels of anxiety. Patients with panic disorder can typically take benzodiazepines for up to a year without harm. Examples of benzodiazepines used in the treatment of anxiety include alprazolam (Xanax), clonazepam (Klonopin), clorazepate (Tranxene-T), diazepam (Valium), and lorazepam (Ativan) (Adams et al., 2020).

Some patients experience withdrawal symptoms if they stop taking benzodiazepines abruptly, and anxiety can return immediately after cessation of the drug. Their potential for tolerance and withdrawal (they are Schedule IV drugs) have led some providers to avoid prescribing them. Nonbenzodiazepine drugs, such as buspirone (Buspar) and meprobamate, are used to treat GAD. These drugs have the benefit of no risk of dependence. Possible side effects include nausea, headaches, and dizziness. Unlike benzodiazepines, buspirone must be taken consistently for at least 2 weeks to achieve an antianxiety effect.

SAFETY ALERT Because they are Schedule IV drugs, benzodiazepines can be habit forming and should be used cautiously in individuals with a history of addiction. Abruptly discontinuing use of benzodiazepines can result in withdrawal and seizures. Patients discontinuing these drugs should slowly taper down following their HCP's instructions. In addition, benzodiazepine use in older adults is linked to an increased incidence of dementia, so they should be used with caution in this population (He, Chen, Wu, Li, & Fei, 2019).

Monoamine oxidase inhibitors (MAOIs) are used rarely in the treatment of generalized anxiety disorder when patients do not respond to more conventional treatments (Andrews et al., 2018; Bhatt, 2019; Potter & Moller, 2020). MAOIs inhibit the action of monoamine oxidase, which is responsible for terminating the action of neurotransmitters such as serotonin, norepinephrine, and dopamine. These drugs have a high side effect profile (e.g., insomnia, hypertensive crisis, sexual dysfunction, respiratory and circulatory collapse, and serotonin syndrome). MAOIs also have several drug–drug interactions and food–drug interactions that make their use more complicated in patients with multiple diseases.

Nonpharmacologic Therapy

Nonpharmacologic therapy is very effective in the treatment of anxiety disorders. Integrative health practices can be used in conjunction with pharmacotherapy to bring relief to patients with anxiety disorders, but the most effective nonpharmacologic therapy is psychotherapy, including CBT. Psychotherapy involves talking with a mental health professional (e.g., psychiatrist, psychologist, advanced practice psychiatric nurse, social worker, counselor) to uncover what triggers the anxiety disorder and to determine how to work through its symptoms. The most effective treatment strategy for most people with anxiety disorders is a combination of CBT and medication (NIMH, 2018).

Cognitive-Behavioral Therapy

Cognitive-behavioral therapy is a useful nonpharmacologic intervention for treating anxiety disorders. The cognitive aspect of this treatment helps patients recognize and change the thought patterns that support their fears, and the behavioral aspect helps patients change the way they react to anxiety-provoking situations. This intervention has been proven to reduce the symptoms of all types of anxiety disorders. For additional discussion of CBT, refer to the Concept section of this module.

Integrative Health

Although conventional medical therapies have been consistently shown to ease the symptoms of anxiety disorders, integrative therapies also have been shown to ease the symptoms of anxiety. These therapies include herbal preparations, massage and touch, and yoga and meditation.

Herbal Preparations

Overall, herbal preparations show little promise as potential therapies for the symptoms of anxiety. However, a few different plant species seem to have moderate effects on anxiety disorders. Scientific studies provide evidence that kava, a member of the pepper family, may be beneficial for anxiety management, but the U.S. Food and Drug Administration (FDA) has warned that kava supplements have been linked to a risk of severe liver damage. In addition, kava has been associated with cases of dystonia, drowsiness, and scaly, yellowed skin. It is also suspected to interact with drugs used to treat Parkinson disease.

Lavender is commonly used for aromatherapy, in which the essential oil from the flowers is inhaled. Dried lavender flowers can be used to make teas or liquid extracts that can be taken orally. Small studies on lavender show mixed results, and topical use of diluted lavender and the use of the oil for aromatherapy is considered safe for adults. However, the undiluted oil irritates skin, is poisonous by mouth, and may cause drowsiness (National Center for Complementary and Integrative Health [NCCIH], 2020b).

Chamomile is a traditional remedy in widespread use, and some data indicate that it has modest benefits for some people with mild to moderate GAD. Chamomile is generally well tolerated. However, it may increase the risk of bleeding for patients taking blood thinners and there are reports of allergic reactions in people who are allergic to plants in the daisy family, including ragweed, chrysanthemums, marigolds, and daisies (Mayo Clinic, 2018b; NCCIH, 2020a).

Mind and Body Practices

In addition to being a state of mind, relaxation physically changes the way the body functions, relieving stress in the process. When the body relaxes, breathing slows, blood pressure and oxygen consumption decrease, and well-being increases. Being able to produce the relaxation response by using relaxation techniques may counteract the long-term stress that can lead to anxiety disorders. Relaxation techniques often combine breathing and focused attention to calm the mind and body, and usually only require brief instruction from a practitioner before they can be done without assistance. Common relaxation techniques include autogenic training, biofeedback, deep breathing, guided imagery, progressive relation, and self-hypnosis.

Yoga, a tradition linked to Indian spiritual practice, can also be used to produce a relaxation response. Yoga is currently widely used as an integrative health practice and for exercise purposes. Many people who practice yoga do so to maintain well-being, improve fitness, and relieve stress, in addition to addressing specific health conditions such as back pain, arthritis, and anxiety (NCCIH, 2019).

Evidence also suggests that religious or secular meditation can be used to combat the effects of anxiety. Several studies have found that transcendental meditation (TM) helped participants decrease psychologic distress and increase coping ability. One recent study showed that TM produced changes in the brain leading to reduced perceived anxiety and stress (Avvenuti et al., 2020).

Lifespan Considerations

Anxiety is common in every age group, but stressors, coping mechanisms, and treatment options are different depending on the patient's developmental level. For children, adolescents, pregnant women, and older adults, specific knowledge of their unique situations is required in order to provide appropriate care.

TABLE 31.6 Symptoms of Anxiety in Children and Adolescents

Symptoms common to both children and adolescents	■ Excessive worrying ■ Headaches and body aches ■ Stomachaches ■ Muscle tension
Symptoms common in children	■ Frequently missing school or social activities ■ Tiredness/exhaustion/fatigue ■ Declining grades at school ■ Trouble sleeping/nightmares ■ Restlessness ■ Trouble concentrating ■ Irritability ■ Extreme homesickness when away from family ■ Shyness ■ Frequent crying
Symptoms common in adolescents	■ Withdrawal from social activities ■ Inner restlessness ■ Continual nervousness ■ Perform poorly in school ■ Dependency ■ Easily startle, sweat, blotch, or flush ■ Engage in substance abuse ■ Impulsive sexual behavior ■ May also have depression or an eating disorder ■ Interferes with their ability to function ■ Suicidal ideations ■ Changes in eating habits and sleeping patterns ■ Self-injury/cutting ■ Trembling ■ Frequent need to urinate

Anxiety in Children

Anxiety disorders affect approximately 8% of children and adolescents, making them the most prevalent mental health concern for this age group (American Academy of Pediatrics, 2021). Similar to adults, children with anxiety disorders run the risk of developing other anxiety disorders, depression, and substance abuse. Common signs and symptoms of anxiety in children are listed in **Table 31.6** ».

One of the most common anxiety disorders in children is separation anxiety disorder (SAD). Children with SAD fear being lost from their family or fear something bad happening to a loved one. They may have inappropriate or excessive worry about being apart from people to whom they are most attached, may refuse to sleep alone or have repeated nightmares with a theme of separation, may worry excessively about family members, and may refuse to go to school. Other manifestations may include a reluctance to be alone, frequent physical complaints, muscle aches, and excessive "clinginess" even when at home. Symptoms of fear must be powerful enough to interfere with everyday life and must last for at least 4 weeks to be considered SAD.

Symptoms of SAD are more severe than those of normal separation anxiety, which is a developmental phase that most children experience between the ages of 18 months and 3 years. SAD is also distinct from stranger anxiety, which is normal for children between 7 and 11 years old. In children, SAD occurs equally in boys and girls, and the first indications of the condition often occur between the ages of 7 and 9. Up to 4% of children age 7 to 11 have SAD (The Recovery Village, 2020). In some cases, separation anxiety can persist or recur in adulthood as adult separation anxiety disorder (ASAD), though ASAD may have its first onset in adulthood (Feriante & Bernstein, 2020). Some phobias also develop during childhood. Social anxiety disorder, for example, typically develops between the ages of 11 and 15 and almost never after the age of 25. Situational phobias, on the other hand, generally develop by the mid-20s. Unlike adults with phobic disorders, children are not always able to understand that the fear created by a phobic stressor is irrational.

Anxiety in children is often treated with CBT, medication, or a combination of both. SSRIs are the medications of choice for children with anxiety, and evidence indicates a combination of an SSRI with CBT is most likely to achieve favorable results (Dwyer & Block, 2019). Other forms of therapy, including acceptance and commitment therapy and dialectical behavioral therapy, may be used in children in place of CBT (ADAA, 2020d). Children may also benefit from family therapy and parent education.

Anxiety in Adolescents

An estimated 8% of adolescents between ages 13 and 18 have an anxiety disorder, with symptoms often manifesting in childhood. However, less than 60% of them receive treatment (Ghandour et al., 2019). The difficulty in distinguishing anxiety from the normal developmental challenges of adolescence contributes to this low rate of treatment. Girls are more than twice as likely as boys to be diagnosed with anxiety during adolescence (Child Mind Institute, 2017).

Issues of social acceptance and independence are common stressors for adolescents, as is dissatisfaction with physical changes to the body during the teen years. Adolescents with anxiety disorders may appear shy or withdrawn in social situations and may refuse to engage in new experiences. They may also avoid activities that they previously enjoyed. Extremes of emotion may occur, with responses being either overly emotional or overly restrained. In an attempt to lessen feelings of anxiety, individuals may engage in dangerous or uncharacteristic behaviors. Anxiety tends to be comorbid with other mental health problems (Centers for Disease Control and Prevention, 2020). Adolescents believed to have an anxiety disorder should be assessed for depression, developmental conditions, and language problems. Treatment of anxiety in adolescents is similar to treatment of anxiety in children.

SAFETY ALERT Studies have indicated that adolescents, as well as some children, have an increased risk of developing suicidal ideations when taking SSRIs (FDA, 2018b), so medical professionals should discuss the risks and rewards of pharmacologic therapy with adolescents and their parents or caregivers before prescribing these drugs.

Anxiety in Pregnant Women

Psychologic stress is common during pregnancy, with mild anxiety presenting frequently both before and after giving birth (American Academy of Pediatrics, 2019). Maternal anxiety leads to negative physical outcomes for mother and child and inhibits parental bonding. Maternal anxiety is often accompanied by depression.

Common stressors during pregnancy include concerns about resources, employment, and personal responsibilities, as well as fears related to the birth process and pregnancy complications. Risk factors associated with anxiety during pregnancy may be environmental, physiological, social, and biological (Araji et al., 2020). Common symptoms of anxiety such as fatigue and sleep disturbance are not reliable predictors of anxiety in pregnancy because they are commonly experienced during pregnancy; other symptoms such as panic attacks and muscle tension may be indicative of maternal anxiety.

Pregnant women must be very careful about treating anxiety with medication because of the risk of birth defects. They should work closely with their HCPs to develop a treatment plan during pregnancy. The use of SSRIs can increase the risk of respiratory distress, pulmonary HTN, apnea, feeding difficulties, and other problems in the newborn (FDA, 2018a). However, abruptly stopping SSRI use could be harmful for both mother and baby, so women with mild anxiety who are considering getting pregnant should taper off antianxiety medications several months before attempting to become pregnant. Untreated anxiety in a pregnant woman is also hazardous, potentially leading to low birth weight, premature birth, and difficulty adapting to life outside the womb for the infant and to pregnancy termination, postpartum depression, impaired attachment to the baby, substance misuse or abuse, and other complications for the mother. Therefore, nonpharmacologic approaches such as CBT and relaxation techniques are a high priority for treatment of anxiety in pregnant women. In addition, women with severe anxiety may decide to continue their medication after discussing all options with their HCP because even though the risk of birth defects is higher for women who take SSRIs and other antianxiety medications, the risk is still low.

Anxiety in Older Adults

Older adults with cognitive impairments or one or more chronic physical impairments are at increased risk for developing anxiety. Significant emotional loss, such as the death of a spouse, also increases the older adult's risk for anxiety. In older adults, manifestations of anxiety may overlap with medical illness, resulting in their presenting first to their primary care provider. Although the prevalence rates of anxiety disorders in older adults are lower than in the general population, this may be due to misdiagnosis rather than to an actual lower rate of anxiety. Risk factors for anxiety disorders in older adults include physical illness, disability, cognitive decline, living alone, social isolation, and loss of spouse and friends (Hellig & Domschke, 2019).

Older adults have differences in drug absorption, action, metabolism, and excretion compared with younger adults. They also are more likely to experience side effects associated with antianxiety medications, especially if they take other medications for physical illnesses that may have drug–drug interactions with medications prescribed for anxiety. Pharmacologic treatment should begin with low doses in this population and be titrated to higher doses based on effectiveness and occurrence of side effects. In addition, long-term use of benzodiazepines should be avoided in the older population because of harmful side effects such as a decrease in cognition. Similar to other age groups, older adults may find that CBT is effective for treating their anxiety.

NURSING PROCESS

Nursing interventions are focused on reducing the severity of anxiety symptoms. Specific interventions include establishing a rapport, communicating therapeutically, supporting and enhancing coping skills, assessing and identifying maladaptive coping, fostering mental health, maintaining a therapeutic milieu, minimizing the deleterious effects of anxiety, and promoting the health of the individual. The generalist nurse provides case management, home healthcare, psychoeducation, and medication administration.

Assessment

- ***Observation and patient interview.*** Assessment of patients with anxiety includes interviewing the patient with regard to current and previous illnesses, medication (and supplement) regimen, and past and present stressors. In addition, the nurse should tactfully interview the patient about current and previous methods of coping, including the use of alcohol and drugs, particularly because certain coping methods may actually compound the individual's sense of anxiety and may predispose the patient to developing an illness or other health alteration.

  In particular, the nursing assessment for individuals experiencing mild anxiety should focus on appraisal. To gain understanding about the individual, the nurse acquires information about how the person appraises and prioritizes stressors. To facilitate the adaptive coping process, the nurse critically evaluates thoughts that may be increasing the person's anxiety. In addition, the nurse should do the following when appraising the patient's anxiety or fear:

  - Observe for physical symptoms associated with anxiety. Muscle tension or twitching, trembling, body aches and soreness, cold or clammy hands, dry mouth, and sweating are common in individuals with anxiety disorders. Nausea, diarrhea, and urinary frequency may also occur.
  - Review the patient's family history and past medical history for diagnosis of mental illness. Depression, bipolar disorders, substance abuse, and eating disorders may occur in addition to anxiety disorders.
  - Assess the patient's emotional and psychologic well-being, level of life satisfaction, and happiness. Determine how self-acceptance, new experiences, personal relationships, hopefulness, and sense of purpose are impacted by anxiety.
  - Consider socioeconomic pressures the patient is facing. Pressures such as unemployment or financial loss pose risks to individual mental health and create anxiety (WHO, 2018).
  - Assess the patient's home and work conditions. Stressful or violent home life, high-pressure work conditions, and rapid change in either the home or workplace contribute to anxiety (WHO, 2018).
- ***Physical examination.*** Physical assessment should include a general assessment, as well as a focused assessment of any body systems that are relevant to the patient's current complaints.

Diagnosis

Selection of nursing care priorities should be patient-specific and depends on numerous factors, including the degree to which anxiety is impacting the patient's daily life and social interaction. Examples of patient needs that may be appropriate for inclusion in the plan of care for the individual with an anxiety or a phobic disorder may include the following:

- Anxiety
- Fear
- Lack of knowledge about illness or healthy coping mechanisms
- Inadequate coping skills
- Sleep disturbance
- Ineffective health maintenance.

Planning

The nursing plan of care, designed in collaboration with the patient, may include the following goals:

- The patient will report a decrease in level of anxiety and frequency and severity of symptoms.
- The patient will articulate successful coping mechanisms.
- The patient will report increasing use of successful coping mechanisms.
- The patient will verbalize healthy ways of responding to fear.
- The patient will demonstrate effective implementation of relaxation techniques.
- The patient will participate in psychotherapy or group counseling activities as outlined by the HCP.

Implementation

Interventions appropriate for patients with anxiety symptoms vary depending on the severity of the individual's symptoms. Patients with severe anxiety or panic require immediate intervention and close supervision. The safety of the individual is at risk because of the narrowing of perception and inability to process information and think rationally. Patients with mild or moderate anxiety can benefit from several nursing interventions, including helping them identify triggers for their anxiety, providing patient teaching, and promoting effective coping

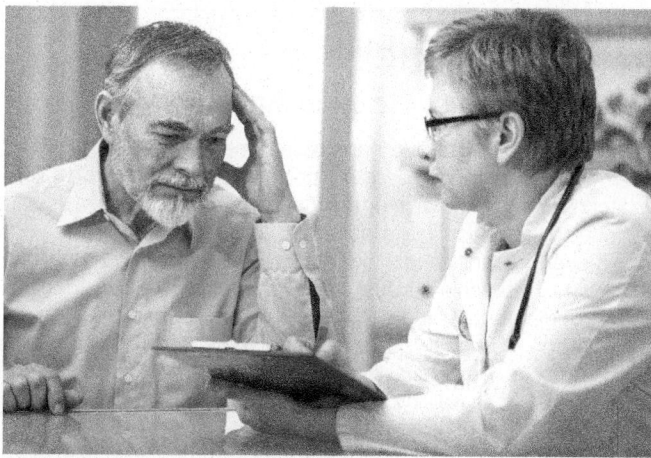

Figure 31.7 ›› Nurses can help patients cope with anxiety through a number of interventions.

Source: Alexander Raths/Shutterstock.

and healthy behaviors (see **Figure 31.7 ››**). Patients with severe anxiety or panic will also benefit from these interventions once their anxiety has subsided to a manageable level.

Interventions for Mild Anxiety

Patients experiencing mild anxiety are often able to learn information and acquire new behaviors easily. The nurse is able to provide valuable information to these patients, teaching them ways to manage stress and modify thinking processes and behaviors. The nurse should review the following when teaching the patient about anxiety disorders:

- How to recognize triggers and symptoms of anxiety. Early recognition of triggers can help patients respond with healthy coping strategies before anxiety levels rise.
- How to identify anxiety levels. Mild levels of anxiety can sometimes improve motivation and learning, whereas moderate and severe anxiety impact concentration and perception. Differentiating among the various levels helps patients determine if they are having a useful, appropriate anxiety response or an inappropriate anxiety response with potentially negative effects.
- Self-management and diversion techniques for coping with anxiety. Stepping back from a situation in order to reassess it and learning to accept that some things cannot be controlled are important self-management skills. Exercising, engaging in hobbies, and spending time with friends or family are often effective diversions. These techniques help the patient refocus the mind away from stressors to lessen anxiety (Mayo Clinic, 2018a).
- Introducing the concept of positive self-talk for coping with anxiety. Positive self-talk helps patients replace anxious thoughts with more rational and realistic ones. Self-talk typically involves patients repeating a set of statements to themselves in an effort to curtail anxiety. The first statement is generally a firm but gentle admonition designed to stop anxious thoughts. This may be followed by one or more positive coping statements.
- Encouraging the use of muscle relaxation and mental visualization to refocus attention away from anxiety. Meditation, deep breathing, and yoga are popular relaxation techniques that patients can do in their own homes.
- The importance of taking medications as prescribed. The majority of medications used to treat anxiety disorders influence activity of neurotransmitters and typically take up to several weeks to achieve efficacy. Skipping a dose on days when anxiety levels are low will negatively impact a medication's overall effectiveness. It may also increase the patient's risk for relapse of anxiety symptoms. Medication should only be discontinued as instructed by a HCP.
- The importance of attending therapy sessions as prescribed. The goal of psychotherapy and CBT is the reduction of anxiety symptoms. Throughout the therapy process, symptoms improve as initial successes are built upon. Failure to participate in therapy sessions hinders the building process.
- Information about community resources for everyday and emergency situations. Everyday resources include support groups, message boards, and local and national organizations dedicated to anxiety disorders. Emergency resources include crisis hotlines, EDs, and trusted mental health professionals familiar with the patient's disorder.

For additional information, see the Patient Teaching feature.

Communicating with Patients

Working Phase

The nurse can help the patient cope with mild anxiety through positive self-talk. This technique can be used to break negative thoughts and replace them with positive thinking. Self-talk can have a major influence on the way people see themselves. Explain to the patient that positive self-talk is speaking to, reassuring, and having faith in oneself. Teach the patient that the first statement should be a gentle but firm one to stop anxious thoughts. For example:

- These thoughts are not helpful. I need to stop them and think differently about myself.

Then, provide the patient with examples of positive self-talk, such as:

- I can do this job; I am a smart person.
- I am proud of myself for trying, it took courage.
- I am strong and capable and can make changes in my eating.
- I can learn from my mistakes; I can do this.
- I am anxious right now, but I will not be overwhelmed.

Interventions for Moderate Anxiety

Patients with moderate anxiety need appropriate intervention to prevent escalation of symptoms. Interventions may include:

- Encourage participation in diversional activities, such as exercise, to reduce stress. For example, walking briskly, running, or working out large muscle groups assists individuals to manage their own physical responses to anxiety.

- Help the patient identify current stressors. When the patient knows and can identify the situations that cause anxiety, he can develop a systematic approach to addressing or eliminating the stressor. Eliminating the stressor rather than simply avoiding it reduces the anxiety associated with it in the long term.
- Help the patient identify what coping strategies have been successful in the past. When the patient knows and can identify strategies used successfully in the past, the patient may be able to return to earlier patterns that are helpful in reducing anxiety.
- Encourage the patient to adhere to the treatment regimen and discuss the addition of integrative therapies with the primary care provider. Patients can become discouraged while waiting for pharmacologic interventions to take full effect or while learning new strategies for coping in psychotherapy. Adding one or more integrative therapies as adjuvant treatment may help relieve symptoms of anxiety until medications or psychotherapy begin to take effect.

Interventions for Severe Anxiety

Patients with severe anxiety benefit from clear, direct communication and simple questions rather than questions or instructions that require the patient to process more than one thing at a time. Some interventions for moderate anxiety, such as identifying triggers and determining helpful strategies that have worked in the past, are also appropriate when working with patients with severe anxiety. As always, the nurse should administer medications as ordered and encourage patients to adhere to the therapeutic regimen (including therapy, exercise, and use of previously identified integrative therapies such as yoga). Some patients may require inpatient hospitalization until they are able to reduce their anxiety level and develop new strategies for coping.

Interventions for Panic

Patients who are at a panic level of anxiety require active supervision and clear, direct communication. Remain with patients to ensure their own and others' safety. Patients at this stage may require assistance from the nurse to meet basic needs, such as nutrition and fluids, pain relief, elimination, or rest.

- Maintain a calm demeanor. Speak slowly using a low-pitched voice. High-pitched voices can increase anxiety, and the nurse's calm presence may help reduce patient anxiety and fear.
- Reduce environmental stimuli. A calm environment promotes calmness in the patient.
- Reinforce reality when thought processes are altered because of fear. Help the patient focus on what is real.

Patient Teaching

Techniques to Reduce Anxiety

Essential teaching for the individual experiencing an anxiety disorder or phobia includes deep breathing and progressive relaxation techniques to lower anxiety responses. Avoidance of stimulants, caffeine, and nicotine is essential. Instructing the patient on the use of cognitive techniques can be helpful in lowering the individual's response to the threat. Strategies such as thought blocking, self-talk, and conversation with a support person all assist the individual to manage and empower more adaptive coping skills. Physical exercise that makes use of large muscle groups, such as walking, running, weight-lifting, hiking, and various sports activities, can dissipate pent-up energy. Exercising also releases natural chemicals such as endorphins, improving mood and natural pain relief.

- Set limits as necessary to ensure safety. Use simple statements and speak in an authoritative voice.
- Allow pacing or harmless repetitive physical tasks, as these can help diffuse negative energy.
- Administer medications as ordered.

Evaluation

Evaluation of the patient experiencing anxiety is based on the symptoms presented and the patient's strengths and weaknesses. Suggested expected outcomes may include:

- The patient's anxiety has diminished as reflected by vital signs returning to baseline and report of a decreased level of anxiety.
- The patient demonstrates new or improved coping measures to reduce anxiety.
- The patient self-moderates the anxiety response when stressors occur.
- The patient engages in healthy behaviors related to sleep, exercise, and nutrition.
- The patient demonstrates a desire to overcome anxiety and a willingness to follow the treatment regimen.

If the patient is still experiencing anxiety during the evaluation phase, the nurse should provide secondary interventions. In all cases of unresolved anxiety, the nurse should provide patient teaching related to additional nonpharmacologic coping techniques that the patient may use. For example, if the patient was taught only relaxation exercises, the nurse may advocate for CBT or teach deep-breathing exercises. If the patient has tried CBT with little success, the nurse may advocate with the physician to prescribe an antianxiety medication. Using multiple coping strategies in addition to nonpharmacologic and pharmacologic therapies may be needed to successfully reduce anxiety over the long term in patients with anxiety disorders.

Nursing Care Plan

A Patient with Agoraphobia

LaChell Randolph is 43 years old, married, and the mother of four daughters in their late teens and early 20s. She is referred to the psychiatric outpatient clinic from the local ED following an acute panic attack with symptoms of racing heartbeat, sweating, feeling faint, and the belief that she was dying.

ASSESSMENT

Ms. Randolph could not identify any events, thoughts, or feelings that precipitated the incident; it seemed to occur "out of the blue." She felt unable to cope with the severity of the symptoms of the attack: "I tried to talk myself out of it; to tell myself it would go away, but it only got worse." Ms. Randolph reports she has had similar attacks lasting from 2 minutes to 2 hours in the past with no physical cause found by her family physician. Her daily routine has become restricted, and she will not leave the house without a family member. She is not comfortable alone in her home and can't sleep if any family member is still out. Ms. Randolph is ashamed and angry about her growing disability and often tries to cover up her fears to friends and family. Recent life events include a hysterectomy 4 weeks ago and loss of employment resulting from hospitalization; the second anniversary of her father's sudden death is upcoming. She has no other history of mental health issues. She saw a therapist for her panic disorder when the attacks first started, "about the time I left home to marry," but did not follow up because she felt ashamed ("I've always been a strong and effective person!") because the episodes were not so severe then and because she found relief from the panic attacks after she had children. Her mother rarely left the house, never participating in social events unless they were in the home. Ms. Randolph described her relationship with her husband as emotionally warm and supportive. She dreads seeing her daughters move from home.

Assessment findings:

- Is a carefully groomed woman who looks her stated age.
- Appears somewhat tense.
- Answers questions cooperatively, but at times with some hesitation, as if expecting criticism or judgment from the interviewer.
- Oriented to time, place, and person.
- Memory intact, good recall, no difficulty with calculations.
- Affect appears normal, with occasional evidence of anger in the form of irritability or sarcasm. Mood is within normal limits.
- Speech normal in flow and volume, pressured at times when she corrects an impression.
- Posture rigid at times, but she relaxes as she becomes more comfortable with the interview.

DIAGNOSES

- Inadequate role performance related to fear and anxiety level
- Inadequate coping related to overwhelming fears
- Disturbed thought processes related to high level of anxiety

PLANNING

Goals of care include:

- The patient will describe specific changes in role function.
- The patient will demonstrate appropriate decision making.
- The patient will demonstrate effective coping as evidenced by employing behaviors to reduce stress and reporting fewer negative feelings.

IMPLEMENTATION

- Maintain a calm manner.
- Stay with the patient.
- Use short, simple sentences.
- Direct patient's attention to a repetitive or physical task.
- Administer pharmacologic agents as ordered.
- Encourage patient to identify previous coping skills.
- Help patient identify coping resources (including social supports).
- Teach patient relaxation techniques.
- Encourage patient to verbalize feelings.

(continued on next page)

Nursing Care Plan *(continued)*

EVALUATION

Expected outcomes to evaluate the patient's response to care include:

- The patient demonstrates role performance as evidenced by the ability to meet role expectations, knowledge of role transition periods, and reported strategies for role changes.
- The patient demonstrates ability to choose between two or more alternatives.
- The patient uses actions to manage stressors that tax personal resources.

CRITICAL THINKING

1. What factors may be contributing to Ms. Randolph's agoraphobia?
2. What interview questions would you like to ask this patient's family?
3. What strategies would you recommend to help Ms. Randolph overcome her fear of leaving her house alone?

REVIEW Anxiety Disorders

RELATE Link the Concepts and Exemplars

Linking the exemplar of anxiety disorders with the concept of perfusion:

1. What impact does anxiety have on perfusion?
2. What medications normally prescribed for anxiety would be contraindicated for an individual with a history of heart disease?

Linking the exemplar of anxiety disorders with the concept of acid–base balance:

3. How might anxiety impact acid–base balance?
4. What nursing interventions might the nurse recommend for the patient with anxiety that is altering acid–base balance?

READY Go to Volume 3: Clinical Nursing Skills

REFER Go to Pearson MyLab Nursing and eText

REFLECT Apply Your Knowledge

Heather O'Malley is a 34-year-old woman who is newly separated from her husband. She has been a stay-at-home mother of children ages 7, 5, and 4, along with a 3-month-old infant. Her days are very busy caring for her young children, and she wonders how she will manage on her own, especially because she will need to find a job in order to provide for the financial needs of the household now that her husband has moved out. Although he is paying court-ordered child support, it is not enough to meet the living expenses of Ms. O'Malley and all four children. Her attempts to work with a lawyer to get additional money in the form of alimony are on hold because she does not have money to pay the lawyer.

Ms. O'Malley worked as a nurse before quitting when the oldest child was born. She looks into taking a refresher course so she can return to nursing and learns that several hospitals provide the course free of charge if she agrees to work for them after successful completion. She applies to one of these hospitals and is called for an interview. Ms. O'Malley wakes up early on the morning of the interview, feeds the older children and sends them to school, then takes the youngest child to the house of a neighbor who has agreed to babysit. She returns home to dress for her interview, thinking about how she will find good child care if she takes a full-time job and trying to figure out what salary she will need to meet her financial obligations if they are to stay in their home. As she is starting the car, Ms. O'Malley suddenly finds she can't catch her breath, feels light-headed and dizzy, and has acute chest pressure. She sits in the car concentrating on her breathing until the feeling subsides and then returns to the house to cancel her interview. She reschedules twice, and each time the same physical symptoms begin before she can get to the interview. When she calls to reschedule a third time, the hospital declines to set up another interview.

1. What stressors are impacting Ms. O'Malley at this time?
2. If Ms. O'Malley came to the clinic and you were admitting her to the office, what assessment questions would you ask to explore her methods of coping?
3. Describe three care priorities that may be appropriate for Ms. O'Malley.
4. For each nursing care priority, list at least two relevant nursing interventions.

» Exemplar 31.B Crisis

Exemplar Learning Outcomes

31.B Analyze crisis as it relates to stress and coping.

- Describe the characteristics of crisis.
- Describe factors that affect individual response to crisis.
- Identify the clinical manifestations of a crisis response.
- Summarize diagnostic tests and therapies used by interprofessional teams in the collaborative care of an individual in crisis.
- Differentiate considerations for care of patients in crisis across the lifespan.
- Apply the nursing process in providing culturally competent care to an individual in crisis.

Exemplar Key Terms

Crisis, *2119*
Crisis counseling, *2122*
Crisis intervention, *2123*
Crisis intervention centers, *2123*
Maturational crisis, *2119*
Resilience, *2119*
Scaling, *2125*
Situational crisis, *2119*

Overview

By necessity, human experiences of life include the experience of crisis. A **crisis** refers to any acute incident that can evolve from a situation or event and that overwhelms an individual's normal coping process. Such a situation or event may involve a developmental, biological, psychosocial, environmental, or spiritual stressor. When the typical or normal methods an individual uses to cope with stressful situations no longer reduce the anxiety or resolve the situation, an acute state of anxiety can result. Adaptation and successful resolution of a crisis may involve a number of adjustments and may result in a change in the individual's coping process. A crisis also affords the individual an opportunity to grow and change as a result of successful adaptation to the crisis.

Characteristics of Crisis

A crisis is, by definition, an acute situation and is precipitated by an event that creates disequilibrium. Crises occur in the lives of all individuals. The experience of crisis is an individual event. What is a crisis for one person may not constitute a crisis for someone else. The characteristics of a crisis are:

- Something all individuals will experience as a part of living
- Presence of a specific stimulus or event
- Defined individually
- Acute event that will resolve (usually within 4 to 6 weeks)
- Affords the opportunity for growth or deterioration.

All crises provide opportunities for growth or deterioration (Townsend, 2018). Typically, an individual resolves a crisis in one of three ways: (1) adapt to the crisis and return to the previous level of functioning, (2) use the opportunity to improve as an individual and cope with life more effectively, or (3) deteriorate to a lower level of functioning. The first possible resolution preserves the individual's status quo, the second changes it for the better, and the third changes it for the worse.

The contributions of Caplan (1964) to the prevention of mental illness have long provided the groundwork on which to build what is known today as *crisis theory*. Individuals interact constantly with the environment; internally, they struggle to meet Maslow's hierarchy of needs (see Figure 31.1). These needs—physical, psychologic, social, and spiritual—manifest differently as an individual progresses through the lifespan. The individual's ability to fulfill needs, maintain homeostasis, regulate affect, mobilize resources, and maintain reality testing affects the individual's capability for adaptation. The individual's perception of the crisis, resources, support, and ego strength all influence the capacity to return to prior levels of functioning after crisis.

Types of crises include both situational and maturational crises. A **situational crisis** involves an unexpected stressor or circumstance that occurs in the course of daily living (see **Figure 31.8** »). Acute stressors may arise from the external environment, such as tornadoes or earthquakes; the internal environment, such as critical illness or disfigurement; and interpersonal sources, such as the death of a loved one or a lost relationship. **Maturational crisis** occurs normally as individuals progress through the life cycle. Everyone experiences

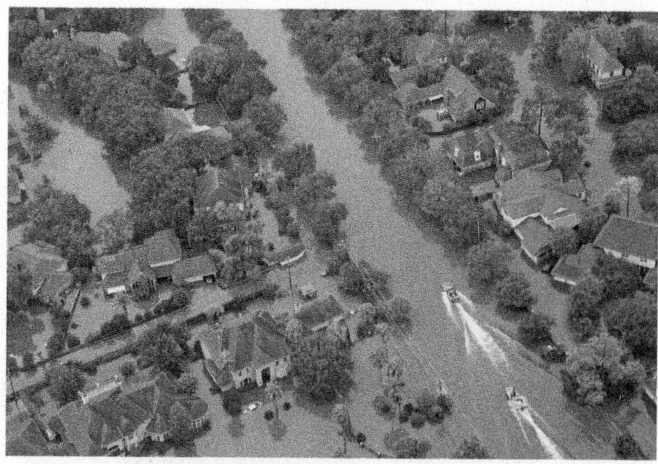

Figure 31.8 » In August and September 2017, Hurricane Harvey hit the Houston area of Texas (shown here) and Hurricane Irma hit lower Florida. Winds, rain, and storm surges damaged and/or flooded hundreds of thousands of homes, creating crises for many families.

Source: DIIMSA Researcher/Shutterstock.

predictable stages of human growth and development as outlined by Erikson (1968) (see Table 25.2 in Module 25, Development). During each stage, the individual is subject to unique stressors. A failure at any one stage compromises the next stage of development.

Holistically, achievement of growth and developmental milestones requires a tremendous amount of energy. Unexpected life events may alter the person's ability to adapt successfully to either a maturational or a situational crisis. This increases an individual's vulnerability, often requiring supportive interventions from HCPs.

Resilience

The American Psychological Association defines **resilience** as "the process of adapting well in the face of adversity, trauma, tragedy, threats or significant sources of stress" (American Psychological Association, 2012). Although resilience may be thought of variously as a trait, a process, or an outcome, it involves numerous biological, psychologic, social, and cultural factors and determinants (Unger & Theron, 2020). As a process, resilience is the way in which individuals adapt successfully to crisis events to develop positive outcomes. Resilience exists on a continuum, manifesting in varying degrees at different times depending on the event and the individual (Vella & Pai, 2019). Resilience is dynamic in nature. That is, an individual may demonstrate varying degrees of resilience when exposed to the same or similar stressors throughout the lifespan. Individuals may also be more or less resilient in different domains of life—better able to adapt to stress in their professional life than in their personal life, for example.

Individual resilience is strongly influenced by the person's optimistic sense of perceived self-efficacy (see **Figure 31.9** »). Psychologist Dr. Albert Bandura posited that individuals must have a strong feeling of personal efficacy to successfully persevere in the face of adversity (Bandura, 1994). Optimism refers to a sense of confidence and hope with regard to positive or favorable resolution of a situation or set of circumstances.

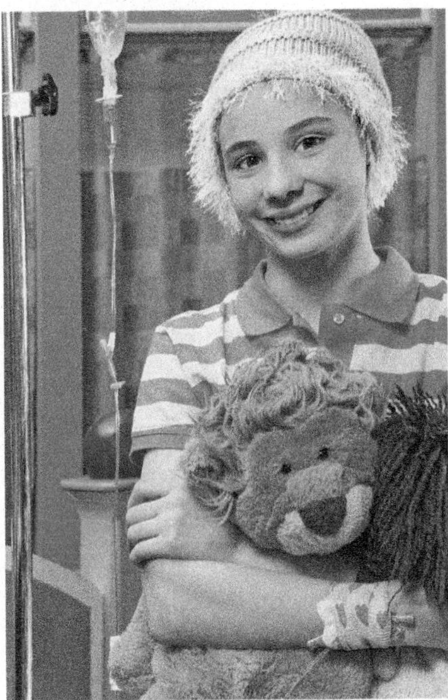

Figure 31.9 » Resilience is the ability to adapt successfully in the face of adversity.
Source: XiXinXing/iStock/Getty Images.

Perceived self-efficacy refers to an individual's beliefs concerning their own capability to influence and exercise control over the events that shape their life (Bandura, 1994).

Bandura, whose contributions to the field of psychology include his famous *social learning theory*, conducted in-depth research in the area of self-efficacy. According to Bandura (1994), an individual's perception of self-efficacy is shaped by the following influences:

- ***Mastery experiences:*** Personal experiences with conquering obstacles through tenacious efforts and perseverance; a pattern of easy achievement of success may lead individuals to expect victory and then be easily discouraged by failure.
- ***Vicarious experiences:*** When observing the success or failure of someone similar to themselves performing a task, individuals will tend to believe that they will perform similarly given the same task.
- ***Social persuasion:*** The extent to which individuals are verbally persuaded by others to believe they are capable of achieving success and to accomplish given tasks.
- ***Somatic and emotional states:*** Incorporates self-judgments regarding individuals' stress response and physical abilities, as well as mood state. Individuals may be self-critical of their stress response or when faced with stressors; in turn, these same individuals may perceive their physical response to stress as rendering them susceptible to failure. In comparison to a negative mood, a positive mood is associated with greater perceived self-efficacy (Bandura, 1994).

Resilience, along with factors such as cognitive appraisal and coping style (as discussed in the Concept section of this module), affects both the physical and psychologic manifestations of an individual's response to crisis.

Coping with Crisis Over Time

By definition, the term *crisis* calls to mind an acute, potentially life-changing but usually time-limited event, such as a hurricane. But many times, a crisis can extend over months or even years. Following hurricanes Harvey in the Gulf Coast and Florence on the Atlantic coast, many families were displaced from their homes for months, even more than a year, waiting for repairs and restoration. The COVID-19 pandemic created numerous crises as families lost jobs, time in school, and access to numerous resources associated with quality of life. Nurses and HCPs faced increased risk of infection, bringing fears of exposing loved ones to the virus and even necessitating separate living quarters for some families of healthcare workers. Other COVID-related stressors for nurses and providers included caring for many patients at critical levels of acuity at once, caring for many who were dying, helping loved ones say goodbye over video apps, and reduced time off.

When a crisis extends over months and even into the next year, the loss of routine combines with the specific stressors of the event to increase the individual's allostatic load (the cumulative cost of adapting to the crisis), impacting mental health and well-being. In the wake of the pandemic, a number of sources offered suggestions for ways to cope with the loss of routines and manage or reduce the allostatic load created by the pandemic (**Box 31.5** »). Many of these are strategies nurses can offer to patients and follow themselves.

Box 31.5
Promoting Healthy Coping During a Crisis

Strategies to promote coping and manage or reduce chronic burdens associated with crisis include:

- *Adapt routines.* Encourage finding ways to adapt routines, such as using online support groups and workout videos at home.
- *Try something new.* Recommend taking up a new hobby or learning a new language. If there are children at home, suggest a new family activity.
- *Talk to someone.* Speak with a friend or a professional by phone or video. Being heard promotes connectedness with the person who is listening and can create a sense of safety.
- *Follow personal values.* Following personal values and interests helps maintain a sense of belonging and continuity through times of loss or crisis. For example, an individual who volunteered at a homeless shelter can make food or run errands for a neighbor.
- *Engage in positive self-talk.* Reframing thoughts to believe you can handle the crisis and be able to manage change can be empowering and reduce anxiety. (See the Communicating with Patients feature in Exemplar 31.A, Anxiety Disorders, in this module for examples of positive self-talk.)
- *Limit viewing of the news.* Encourage turning off the news if it is contributing to increased stress and anxiety.
- *Focus on what is possible.* Suggest that families who are unable to visit a loved one stay in contact by video or phone.
- *Find and use available resources.* Provide referrals to resources such as local food banks, nonprofits, and other agencies that can help bridge gaps and provide resources for people in need.

Sources: From Mayo Clinic (2020a); New York Presbyterian (2020); Penn Medicine News (2020).

Clinical Manifestations

Individuals in crisis need immediate assistance and support. The Clinical Manifestations and Therapies feature outlines the common clinical symptoms and manifestations of individuals in crisis.

The goal in crisis is to stabilize the reactions of the individual, thereby initiating the process of adaptation and reducing the disruption created by the crisis. To facilitate adaptive coping, it is essential that nurses encourage patients to express their feelings and listen attentively and supportively. The nurse is an active participant in the intervention process. The generalist nurse serves as communicator, facilitator, and resource expert for the patient.

Collaboration

Caring for patients during times of crisis may include facilitating counseling referrals, connecting patients and families with community agencies, and implementing crisis interventions. For some patients, an extended or severe response to crisis may warrant pharmacologic intervention.

Diagnostic Tests

The patient interview and physical assessment provide the most valuable data for use in planning patient care. In addition, tools are available for use in evaluating the impact of a crisis event. For example, the Horowitz Impact of Event Scale (IES) allows for measurement of an individual's stress response following traumatic or impactful life experiences (Horowitz, Wilner, & Alverez, 1979; Weiss & Marmer, 1997). Some researchers have found the IES-R to be especially useful in helping to identify signs and symptoms associated with posttraumatic stress disorder.

Pharmacologic Therapy

Pharmacologic therapies may be prescribed to address immediate medical needs, which vary widely depending on the nature of the crisis. Immediate needs that may require pharmacologic treatment include:

- Pain following injury (e.g., associated with a motor-vehicle crash or injury from a power tool following a natural disaster)
- Threat of infection following injury or exposure to a bacterial infection (e.g., prophylactic treatment for tuberculosis following a lengthy stay in a disaster shelter)
- Sleep disturbance
- Anxiety or depression.

For additional discussion about medications used in the treatment of patients with manifestations such as anxiety and depression, see Medications 31.1 in the Concept section of this module.

Nonpharmacologic Therapy

Nursing care of patients in crisis includes:

- Establishing a therapeutic relationship
- Ensuring patient safety from the first moment of contact
- Mobilizing support through the significant other, family, relatives, friends, religious support groups, healthcare institutions, and organizations such as the American Red Cross
- Collaborating with mental health professionals.

Directive suggestion may be helpful, such as gently advising caregivers of critically sick family members to go home and sleep while assuring them that they will be called immediately if conditions change. Offering time, attention, and direction is most critical during a crisis. An arrangement for a follow-up care appointment suggests concern for the individual's well-being. The opportunities to offer care in crisis are endless and may involve only a moment of time.

Clinical Manifestations and Therapies

Crisis

ETIOLOGIES	CLINICAL MANIFESTATIONS	CLINICAL THERAPIES
▪ Physical trauma (including rape, assault, and exposure to violence) ▪ Emotional trauma (including psychologic and verbal abuse) ▪ Exposure to violence, including in the school or workplace settings ▪ Illness- and health-related alterations ▪ Significant loss (including death of a loved one or significant other) ▪ Exposure to natural and environmental disasters ▪ Exposure to acts of terrorism ▪ Financial stressors ▪ Legal stressors (including divorce, child custody disputes, and identity theft)	▪ Difficulty problem solving ▪ Disorganized thought processes with difficulty processing information ▪ Disorientation ▪ Vulnerability ▪ Increased tension and helplessness ▪ Fearfulness and sense of being overwhelmed ▪ Intense emotional reactions ▪ Increased sensory input and bombardment ▪ Hypervigilance ▪ Intense physical reactions depicted in the fight-or-flight response ▪ By definition, event usually is time limited and resolves within 6 weeks	▪ Counseling ▪ Crisis intervention ▪ Inpatient hospitalization and intensive counseling ▪ Couple, family, and/or group therapy ▪ Pharmacologic treatment for specific stress-related manifestations, if indicated (e.g., short-term administration of benzodiazepines for treatment of anxiety) or as indicated based on patient-specific needs (e.g., prophylactic antibiotics)

Therapeutic Communication

Communicating with individuals in crisis requires frequent, brief, simple, and often directive communication. Biologically, the brain of the individual in crisis is in the process of being bombarded with electrochemical reactions. Concentration and the ability to remember and retain information can be impaired. The nurse must continually reassess what the individual has heard or interpreted. In applying the transactional model, it is important to remember primary appraisal. What does the individual believe is happening? How can the nurse add resources and information to the reappraisal process to facilitate adaptive coping? Continual observation of patterns of communication within the family and/or group is essential. Because of the hyperarousal that occurs during the crisis, the nurse must monitor and assess nonverbal communication, tone, inflection, and mannerisms while communicating. See **Box 31.6** >> for guidelines concerning how to conduct effective therapeutic communication with patients. For more information, see Module 38, Communication.

In times of crisis, the nurse may be the one responsible for communicating bad news regarding injury or death of loved ones. As in all care settings, the nurse uses therapeutic communication strategies to impart this information and to provide support to family or friends as they process the information (see **Box 31.7** >>).

Box 31.7

Communicating Painful Information

One of the uncomfortable roles of the nurse is to communicate painful information to individuals. This task can be unnerving. A few simple guidelines convey a professional attitude of concern and care for those receiving dire news:

1. Greet individuals with warmth, kindness, and an introduction.
2. Inform them that you are there and will assist during this difficult time.
3. Provide privacy, go to a place to sit down to discuss the information, and offer tissues and drinks.
4. Inquire about what they know, answer questions, and provide support.
5. Apprise them of the current circumstances in terms that they can understand.
6. Respond to their feelings and offer support.
7. Ask what they need from you and what has helped them in the past to cope with difficult situations.
8. Incorporate cultural and religious practices of the individuals in crisis to provide comfort.
9. Inform them you will facilitate communication and provide direction about the best means of accessing information.
10. Focus on the immediate reaction and needs of the individuals in crisis.
11. Write down specific contact numbers and instructions.
12. Check back with them as needed to see how they are doing and update them with any new information.

Crisis Counseling

Crisis counseling offers brief solutions, focused interventions, and supportive care. During the course of a crisis, nurses should consider each individual's physical vulnerability and degree of emotional stability, with special emphasis on determining the patient's risk for self-harm or potential for harming others. While prioritizing the safety of the patient and others, the nurse should assess the patient's perception of and response to the crisis while also ensuring that the patient's basic needs are met. The alarm reaction, anxiety, and fear may prevent the person from resting, sleeping, or eating. In the hospital and other clinical settings, important members of the healthcare team during a crisis may include the hospital chaplain or family minister, a grief counselor, a social worker, a child and family therapist, and a teacher. However, crisis counseling is often performed in a community context. For example, the Federal Emergency Management Agency's (2020) Crisis Counseling Program emphasizes that crisis counseling should be:

- ***Outreach oriented***, delivering counseling services in the communities affected instead of waiting for survivors to seek out the services themselves
- ***Conducted in nontraditional settings***, contacting survivors in their homes and communities, outside of clinical or office settings
- ***Designed to strengthen existing community support systems***, supplementing and supporting existing community response systems

See **Box 31.8** >> for an overview of the components of crisis counseling.

Box 31.6

Guidelines for Therapeutic Communication in Crisis

- Incorporate verbal and nonverbal communication.
- Maintain eye contact or nod as appropriate, and avoid distractions to signal genuine concern for the patient.
- Maintain congruence between verbal and nonverbal messages communicated to the patient (Wanko Keutchafo, Kerr, & Jarvis, 2020).
- Paraphrase and repeat the patient's statements to validate your understanding of the patient and seek clarification; for example, "I hear you saying that you feel like everything's a mess" and "Tell me what that means to you."
- Avoid making statements or comments that invalidate or judge the patient's experience instead of listening to and trying to understand it. Examples include statements such as "That doesn't sound important" or "I doubt it happened like that."
- Although encouraging the expression of emotions is important, when appropriate, silence is also an effective communication tool. In addition to demonstrating respect for the patient's privacy and willingness to share, periods of silence also allow the patient to reflect on thoughts and emotions in order to more effectively express them.

Communicating Difficult News with Patients and Families

Working Phase

Prepare for the conversation. Think about what you will say and how you will say it. Start with asking what the individual or family already know. Let them know the news is not good so they can emotionally prepare for it. Empathize after delivering the news and ask what questions they have. The shape of your conversation may go as follows:

- Hello, I am [name], and I work in the emergency department on the team taking care of your loved one. I'm here to give you an update. Let's go sit in the conference room. (Give a warm introduction and go to a private area)
- Tell me what you already know about your loved one's condition. (Find out what the family knows)
- I'm afraid I have difficult news. (Prepare them emotionally for bad news)
- Here is what is happening. (Let them know what is happening)
- I am sure this is very upsetting for you. (Acknowledge their feelings)
- What questions do you have for me about what I have told you? (Ask if they have questions)
- I will update you every 30 minutes. Please let the desk know if you need me sooner. (Let them know you will communicate with them regularly and how to reach you)
- Is there anything you need right now? (Focus on the family's needs)

Crisis Intervention

A **crisis intervention** is an emergent approach to care that is intended to assist patients with recognizing a crisis situation and identifying and implementing an immediate, short-term solution. For the patient, the ultimate goal of crisis intervention is restoration to a level of functioning that is at or above the level of the pre-crisis state. This approach often incorporates the patient's family members and loved ones as well as those individuals who are significant to the patient in terms of providing social support. Depending on the circumstances, a crisis intervention also may include professionals from a variety of specialties, such as school guidance counselors, law enforcement or probation officers, rescue workers, and clergy members. Successful completion of a crisis intervention depends on the patient's needs; for example, some crisis interventions may culminate in the patient's receiving outpatient counseling or guidance, whereas others may require immediate hospital admission or transfer to a facility that provides treatment for patients with substance use disorders. Crisis interventions may happen in a community setting outside of a hospital context if that is what an individual patient's particular needs dictate. For example, the Minnesota Department of Human Services (2019) lists potential mobile crisis intervention services as:

- Coping with immediate stressors to lessen suffering
- Identifying and using available resources as well as the strengths of the individual receiving the intervention
- Avoiding unnecessary hospitalization and the loss of the ability to live independently
- Developing action plans
- Returning the individual to a pre-crisis level of functioning.

Crisis intervention centers provide telephone consultation for patients in crisis. Some organizations also offer consultation by way of email and online chatting or texts. In most cases, call-in crisis intervention centers, also known as crisis hotlines, are staffed by trained volunteers who follow protocols to assist the patient and who have professional consultation available to them, such as mental health

Box 31.8

ABCs of Crisis Counseling

Achieve Rapport

In the first stage of crisis counseling, the nurse or therapist works to achieve rapport with the patient by using therapeutic communication. Helping patients clarify feelings and perceptions of the event first will assist them in venting initial emotions, lower their anxiety levels, and create an environment that will support building of the therapeutic relationship and development of a plan of care. Additional goals at this stage include assessing immediate needs and ensuring the patient's immediate physical and emotional safety.

Boil Down the Problem (Identify, Validate, and Intervene)

At this stage, the nurse or therapist helps the patient identify the problem, providing validation and intervention. Communication with the patient at this stage focuses on identifying the problem, assessing how the individual is thinking and feeling about the problem, and evaluating the patient's functional ability since the crisis event. Goals at this stage include helping patients identify their most pressing problems, encouraging them to talk about the present, and assessing and addressing ongoing safety concerns, such as risk for suicide, interpersonal violence, or substance abuse.

In some situations, patients may not have previous experience and coping mechanisms that they can articulate. Giving patients small choices, such as asking what they would like to drink or if they would like to make a phone call, can help build their confidence.

Assessment and intervention will vary greatly depending on the patient and the crisis. The safety assessment of a patient with asthma following a natural disaster will be very different from the safety assessment of a patient who is being abused by a partner.

Cope with the Problem (Resolution and Referral)

At this stage, the nurse or therapist determines what is necessary to help the patient cope with the problem. Using Maslow's hierarchy of needs to focus on the patient's basic needs of shelter, food, water, and physiologic safety is a good framework to use when prioritizing care for patients in crisis. For patients who are victims of violence, physiologic and emotional safety needs will be very closely related. Consider both short- and long-term needs for resolution and referral. Goals at this stage include determining what the patient wants to happen and what will help the individual to meet needs and to support the need for validation and hope for the future.

Sources: From Ahmad (2019); Jones (1968); Kanel (2019).

Box 31.9

Crisis Connection

1. Make contact and connect with the individual.
2. Assess immediate safety needs.
3. Determine thought processes.
4. Scan for physical distress.
5. Listen intently, supporting emotional reactions.
6. Explore perceptions of the crisis.
7. Identify coping strengths.
8. Develop a support plan and a follow-up plan.

counselors and psychologists. These 24-hour services allow callers to remain anonymous. For individuals who use crisis hotline services, primary goals include preventing the caller from inflicting harm directed at self or others, giving the caller an opportunity to share emotions and conflicts, and encouraging follow-up care with a local mental health professional, if needed.

A step-by-step intervention is outlined in **Box 31.9** ». A crisis connection provides a lifeline for the patient in crisis and allows the nurse to determine immediate needs.

Temporary Relocation

Patients in crisis—in particular, those who are homeless and those who are subject to abuse—may require assistance with meeting one of the most basic needs: finding shelter. Nurses should be aware of community organizations and representatives who can assist patients with finding emergency living arrangements.

Lifespan Considerations

The response to trauma varies throughout the lifespan. For all age groups, nurses should carefully assess the particular cultural, social, and family factors that may influence how each patient speaks about their feelings and needs. Nurses may also identify and recommend community resources and organizations that can assist patients in crisis in their area.

Children and Adolescents in Crisis

Children and adolescents are highly susceptible to crisis. Because of their developmental level and lack of experience dealing with crises, they are less able to cope with extreme circumstances than are adults. This is especially true for children with disabilities. Types of crises to which children and adolescents may be exposed include bullying, divorce or separation of parents, child abuse, school shootings, death of a parent or sibling, nonfatal suicide attempts, friends dying by suicide, unexpected pregnancy, and trauma from accidents, natural disasters, sports, and other events.

Children and adolescents will respond to and cope with crisis events differently depending on their age, developmental maturity, support resources, life experiences, and association with the event. Nurses should work closely with parents and caregivers to assess and care for children and adolescents after a crisis because they know their children best and can report changes in behavior that may signal a poor coping response to the crisis that requires additional intervention.

All children and adolescents dealing with crisis should receive emotional support from parents and healthcare professionals. Nurses can provide support by reassuring the safety of the child; encouraging the child to express feelings; telling the child that it is appropriate to feel emotions such as sadness, anger, grief, or fear; and keeping the child informed about what is happening in the crisis situation. Nurses should encourage parents to spend extra time with their child, talk to the child about the event at a developmentally appropriate level, monitor the child for changes in behavior, limit their child's television viewing about the event, and help the child maintain a normal routine. Nurses should teach parents that behavior changes often associated with crisis events that may signal a poor coping response include clinginess, nightmares, bedwetting, irritability, a decrease in normal play activity, changes in eating patterns, reporting headaches or stomachaches, aggression, and behavior problems at school. Adolescents should be monitored carefully for signs of depression and risk for suicide.

If a child or adolescent continues to respond to the crisis event with abnormal behavior and poor coping beyond a reasonable time for the severity of the event, the nurse should advocate for the child and family to receive additional counseling from a child or family mental health professional. The nurse may also encourage the child and family to find creative ways to respond to the crisis. For example, the death of a sibling or friend may be commemorated by planting a tree in their honor or making a donation to their favorite charity.

Pregnant Women in Crisis

In addition to crises that other adults face, pregnant women may face crises related to unexpected pregnancy, miscarriage, having a child with a disability or other chronic illness, and preterm birth. Some pregnant women may experience a crisis if they are pregnant as the result of a rape, and teen mothers may experience crisis related to social isolation from family and friends and the fear of raising a child while still in school. Other women may experience a crisis if they decide to have an abortion or give up the baby for adoption. These crises may take on an even greater magnitude if the pregnant woman does not receive support from her partner or support system.

Nurses can provide a safe and calming environment in which the pregnant woman can express her fears and other emotions. Nurses should validate the pregnant woman's emotions and correct any misconceptions the woman might have. Nurses should provide pregnant women with information specific to their situation. For example, if a pregnant woman has been told she will have a child with Down syndrome, the nurse can provide the woman with literature about what to expect when caring for such a child and referral information for early childhood intervention services in her community. Nursing interventions that increase knowledge about the crisis situation will increase the woman's ability to cope with the stressor.

For women who are pregnant as a result of rape, the nurse can encourage the woman to work with law enforcement and court personnel and provide support and a listening ear as the woman expresses her distress over the situation. If the pregnant woman is a teenager, the nurse can ensure that the teen's support system will provide a stable environment for the teen and baby or work with the teen and social system to find a stable home for the new family.

If a pregnant woman must deal with a crisis unrelated to her pregnancy, she may need encouragement to maintain her emotional and physical health. Pregnant women experience many hormonal changes during pregnancy that can affect their moods and their ability to deal with crisis situations. Behavioral and physical changes, especially changes that affect the pregnant woman's health, can affect the development of the baby. For example, high blood pressure from high levels of stress increases the potential for preterm labor or a low-birth-weight infant (National Institute of Child Health and Human Development, 2017). Coping with a crisis situation by drinking alcohol or smoking can lead to fetal alcohol spectrum disorders or problems with placental attachment (American College of Obstetricians and Gynecologists, 2020). Therefore, pregnant women in crisis should be monitored carefully, and the nurse should provide support for the mother and baby throughout the pregnancy and after birth.

Older Adults in Crisis

Older adults are often more susceptible to injury during crisis events such as natural disasters, motor-vehicle accidents, and home fires. Older adults also have higher incidence of chronic disorders such as diabetes and heart disease, so they are more susceptible to changes in health related to lack of access to medications and nutrition. Older adults may be more susceptible to confusion and disorientation.

The nurse caring for an older adult during a crisis should begin by orienting the older adult to person, time, and place and asking what the patient remembers about the crisis event. The nurse should provide any emergency care needed and begin a physical and mental assessment. An emotional assessment can be performed if the older adult is oriented. In particular, the nurse should determine the older adult's health history and gain access to any medications that may be needed during the time they are in the nurse's care. The nurse should encourage the older adult's family and friends to provide support during and after the crisis, as isolation and loneliness can lead to further deterioration of the patient's physical and mental health.

NURSING PROCESS

Initially, the primary focus of crisis intervention is to ensure safety. Once safety is established, the ideal goals include helping the patient acknowledge and manage the crisis and assisting the patient to identify and access resources needed to achieve resolution.

Assessment

The nurse systematically assesses the patient in crisis, beginning with making contact and connecting with the patient. Assess and identify patient safety issues such as:

- Safe and adequate shelter
- Access to food and healthcare
- Feelings of hopelessness or threat to self or others
- Risk for harm or violence (to/from self or others).

To ensure the patient's safety, emergent admission to a hospital or treatment center may be necessary. Ideally, assessment also includes interviewing the patient's family or significant others.

Individual Assessment

During the assessment process, the nurse must determine the patient's thought processes, orientation, and ability to process information. Assessment of the patient's physical condition includes any physical complaints and determining if the patient is able to fulfill basic needs such as eating, resting, sleeping, and self-care. Because of the intensity of the fight-or-flight reaction, vulnerable individuals may be at risk for physical illness during a crisis.

Psychosocial assessment includes assessing the patient's perception of the precipitating event, impact of the crisis, and ability to cope with the crisis. The nurse should also interview the patient regarding current and past coping methods, as well as the patient's support system. Particularly for individuals who survive disasters, the issue of survivor's guilt should be explored. For these patients, guilt may stem from the act of surviving while knowing others have died. They may also harbor guilt as a result of the actions they took to survive.

Scaling assessment questions involve asking the patient to rate the severity of symptoms or problems. This allows the nurse to determine the patient's perceptions. For example, the nurse may ask, "Mr. Smith, on a scale of 0 to 10, with 10 being absolutely intolerable, how would you score your distress right now?" Assessment information is prioritized based on input from the individual.

It is important to remember that the expression of feelings about and interpretations of an event are culturally influenced and must be considered within the context of the individual's life (see Focus on Diversity and Culture: Expression of Emotion). Sociocultural factors greatly impact an individual's interpretation of a crisis or traumatic event, as well as the response to the event. For example, among members of some cultures, persistent anxiety is considered to be a sign of weakness, as opposed to being a potential sign of a stress-related disorder. This belief is particularly prevalent among Pacific Islander and Asian cultures, who may not reach out for help until they enter a crisis stage (NAMI, n.d.).

Cultural competence extends beyond the identification of a patient's cultural and ethnic background; it encompasses being aware of a patient's health practices and beliefs and demonstrating respect for the individual's preferences. However, the nurse also has a responsibility to identify health practices that may be detrimental to the patient's well-being. Identification and evaluation of the patient's culturally based health practices requires sensitive, nonjudgmental exploration of the topic. For example, the patient interview may include statements such as "I want to try to understand how this experience may be affecting you; please tell me more about how you feel" and "How would you expect your family or close friends to react to a similar experience?"

Focus on Diversity and Culture

Expression of Emotion

Cultural factors may influence how an individual expresses emotions. In certain cultures, expressions of pain, sorrow, or fear are viewed as signs of weakness. The nurse should be aware of patients' cultural background and, while maintaining respect for their privacy, gently offer patients the opportunity to express themselves.

Emotional expression tends to be congruent with what the culture values. In a study of the cultural differences in emotional regulation (Deng, An, & Cheng, 2019), researchers found that Chinese individuals viewed expression of emotion as more negative and emotional control as more positive than European American persons. Therefore, nurses need to be aware of cultural differences in values and how these may affect the expression of emotions during a time of crisis.

Some individuals may openly express their feelings, whereas others may interpret their emotions in terms of physical symptoms and fail to show an emotional response at all. In some cases, lack of an emotional response or failure to engage with a HCP may be a result of previous negative experiences with the healthcare system (Spector, 2017). Taking the time to understand each patient's emotions through their cultural viewpoint can help provide a supportive and calming environment.

Family Assessment

House fires, motor-vehicle crashes, serious illness or injury or death of an immediate family member, and natural disasters are just a few of the crises that families can experience. Emotional crises such as divorce, bankruptcy, and abuse also affect families. Each individual family member's response to a crisis will impact family functioning. Family communication patterns may promote or hinder family members' response to crises. Nurses working with families in crisis situations will benefit from assessing how family members have coped in previous crises as well as assessing immediate individual and family needs. If the crisis results in serious injury or illness to one or more family members, nurses can assist by offering a variety of interventions, including:

- Obtaining and providing information regarding the health status of the loved one
- Facilitating communication between the family and the healthcare team
- Ensuring access to and promoting communication with the loved one
- Providing privacy and emotional support (Ball, Bindler, Cowan, & Shaw, 2022).

Community Assessment

Nurses may be among the first civilians called on to offer assistance in the wake of a disaster. For the community faced with crisis, assessment begins with triage and treatment of patients in need. Next follows assessment of living conditions and availability of basic resources, such as food, water, and shelter. Identification of the community's mental health and support resources, as well as the availability of financial and organizational resources (such as disaster assistance organizations), is also essential.

Diagnosis

Identifying needs to incorporate into the nursing plan of care depends on the patient's crisis response and associated manifestations. Examples of nursing care priorities that may be appropriate for inclusion in the nursing plan of care for a patient in a state of crisis may include the following:

- Risk of injury
- Anxiety
- Self-neglect
- Compromised coping skills
- Confusion.

Planning

Planning involves the selection of realistic goals and identified outcomes that promote resolution of the selected care priorities. Examples of patient goals and outcomes that may be relevant to the nursing care of a patient in crisis may include the following:

- The patient will remain free from injury.
- The patient will identify and use necessary resources and social support.
- The patient will engage in self-care activities such as proper hygiene, adequate nutrition, and sufficient sleep.
- The patient will report a reduction in perceived anxiety.
- The patient will actively participate in counseling and group therapy activities as outlined by the primary care provider.
- The patient will express understanding of coping techniques that can be used during times of crisis.
- The patient will respond appropriately to questions and conversation and show no signs of confusion.

Implementation

Implementation involves assisting patients with meeting needs identified in the assessment phase. Establishment of trust and application of therapeutic communication techniques serve as the foundation for building a relationship with the patient in crisis. The nurse should avoid minimizing the patient's feelings or offering false reassurances of hope.

Reduce Risk of Injury

Patients may be at greater risk of injury during a crisis because they are overwhelmed and unable to properly cope with or respond to changes in their environment. Depending on the type of crisis, patients may be at risk for injury directly due to the crisis, or they may be at risk for injury inflicted by self or others. For example, a woman who has been beaten by her husband may be at risk for further injury from her husband either at the hospital or when she returns home. Similarly, that same woman may be at risk for self-inflicted injury if she decides to attempt suicide. To reduce the risk for injury:

- Identify risk factors for injury in the patient's home environment that the individual can control and remove. Depending on the patient's situation, this may include fixing stairs, installing lights, removing hazardous materials, and removing weapons, among other interventions. Discuss potential risk factors with patients to make them aware of ways to reduce their risk for injury.
- Assess the patient's community for ongoing threats and changes that could produce new risk factors. Especially in a crisis situation affecting the community at large when the crisis and the response to it are ongoing, the situation on the ground could change rapidly.
- Isolate patients from any potential sources of injury. If the potential injury is from another person, isolate the patient from the threatening individual. If the potential injury is from self, remove any potential weapons from the patient's immediate surroundings. If the potential source of injury is the environment, remove the patient from the environment and place the individual in a safe location.
- If the patient is in a hospital environment and is a source of risk for injury to self, a patient companion may be assigned, the patient may be moved to a location easily observed by nursing staff, or restraints may be used as a last resort. Use of restraints should always be consistent with the level of risk and the patient's need to be kept from harm.

SAFETY ALERT Nurses need to be constantly aware of the potential dangers and risk of injury involved in responding to patients in crisis. These threats may come from the environment, particularly if the crisis is a natural disaster or community crisis, or threats may come from other people involved in the crisis, and even from the patients themselves. Also, nurses must be careful to ensure that in responding to crises they are aware of the possibility of becoming overwhelmed psychologically, emotionally, or physically themselves, to the point where they are no longer able to monitor effectively for risks to their safety.

Decrease Anxiety

Anxiety may accompany the patient's feeling of being overwhelmed by the crisis and unable to properly cope and make recovery from the crisis difficult. Almost all patients who are dealing with a crisis will experience anxiety at some point, although when they experience anxiety, the magnitude of anxiety that they experience and how they cope with it will differ with each individual. To learn more about nursing interventions associated with anxiety, see Exemplar 31.A in this module.

Promote Self-Care

A crisis creates a strong potential for patients to fall into habits of self-neglect, with individuals who are overwhelmed falling out of established routines of self-care. Patients may ignore self-care activities such as bathing and other hygiene rituals, neglect home responsibilities such as caring for family or paying bills, or neglect work responsibilities that could result in loss of a job and further crisis. To promote patient self-care and reduce the risk for self-neglect:

- Encourage family members to assist the patient in meeting self-care needs. Monitor for signs of self-neglect such as unwashed hair or clothing the patient has worn for several days or that is mismatched, inadequate, or inappropriate.
- Encourage family and friends to help with home responsibilities such as providing child care or making sure bills are paid to prevent further crisis for the patient.
- Ensure the patient is eating and drinking enough at home and has support from family or friends in ensuring proper routines of hydration and nutrition. If needed, recommend community nutrition resources such as Meals on Wheels.
- Ensure that the patient is getting sufficient sleep. In a crisis, the patient may need reminders to go to bed or support in maintaining routines.
- Help patients reduce stress associated with returning to work during a time of crisis.
- Encourage patients to research family leave, vacation, and other work resources that may allow them to be away from work for an extended period of time without losing their jobs.
- In a hospital setting, encourage patients to follow routines of self-care that are within their control. Also ensure that they are taking in appropriate nutrition and hydration. Arrange care, if possible, to provide for uninterrupted sleep.

Promote Effective Coping

Depending on the type of crisis, the patient or the patient's family members and friends may display ineffective coping. Ineffective coping is often evidenced by blank emotions, shock, a lack of appetite, self-neglect, ineffective communication, ineffectual learning, excessive crying, or hysteria. The nurse can promote effective coping by:

- Providing information about community resources that may help the patient return to independence after a crisis. This may include resources for housing, furniture and clothing, transportation, food, jobs, physical therapy, counseling, and support groups (see Patient Teaching feature). Resources needed will vary depending on the patient's situation.
- Presenting a calm and collected demeanor to the patient and family at all times. Seeing others display calmness can help calm individuals who are anxious or upset.
- Removing the patient or the patient's family from visual reminders of the crisis situation. For example, the patient whose house has burned down should be taken to a hotel or hospital rather than being allowed to stay at the site. Similarly, nurses may encourage the patient or the patient's family to find a quiet environment and minimize external stimuli to help them achieve a sense of calmness.

- Encouraging the patient or the patient's family members to drink water and eat small snacks to sustain nutrition and hydration.
- Encouraging the patient or the patient's family members to participate in self-care activities such as sleeping and bathing. The nurse may need to encourage family members of hospitalized patients to go home to get some sleep or a change of clothing.
- Contacting next of kin for the patient to reduce isolation and provide a support system.
- Providing patients or their family members with small, simple tasks that they can perform. Completing simple tasks may help them feel like they are helping or achieving some control over the situation.
- Keeping patients informed about their medical status or the medical status of their loved one using therapeutic communication techniques. See Boxes 31.6 and 31.7. Consider also providing written information about the patient's situation or status so that patients or family members with ineffective learning can review the information when they are more emotionally stable. Offer to answer any questions and be available to talk with the family as needed.

Decrease Acute Confusion

Patients who have had a head injury or a major shock associated with a crisis may display acute confusion. This confusion may pertain to disorientation about location, events, time and date, or even personal identity. The nurse can decrease a patient's confusion by:

- Providing orienting information, such as a reminder about the events that caused the crisis or a reminder of the individual's location and the time and date.
- Providing written instructions related to treatments and care.
- Helping patients remember who they are (if their identity is known by the nurse). This may include showing patients their own ID card, such as a driver's license, or allowing them to see family and friends.
- Repeating information as needed in a calm and soothing manner until the patient begins to feel oriented to the situation and less confused.

Evaluation

Expected outcomes that may be appropriate for the patient experiencing a crisis include:

- The patient has identified and removed risk factors for injury from the environment.
- The patient reports using community resources and sources of social support such as family and friends.
- The patient reports feeling less anxiety associated with the crisis.
- The patient maintains proper hygiene, nutrition, hydration, and other self-care tasks, as evidenced by lack of fatigue, maintenance of appropriate weight, and clean clothes and body.
- The patient displays effective coping techniques that are appropriate to the situation and expresses a regained sense of control over the crisis.
- The patient is independently oriented to self, time, and place and can describe the precipitating event.

The nurse may have to evaluate the patient in crisis multiple times before the situation is resolved and the patient appears to be in good health again. Each time, the nurse should reevaluate the patient for safety, adequate self-care, anxiety levels, coping techniques, and social support. Any areas that still require improvement to stabilize the patient should be prioritized to promote the individual's physical and mental health. Once the patient is stabilized, additional nursing interventions for milder symptoms or needs can be implemented.

Patient Teaching

Benefits of Support Groups

Nurses should be ready to provide patients with information and recommendations regarding support groups that may be helpful for people coping with their particular crisis. Potential benefits of support groups include:

- Participation in regular, judgment-free contact with people whose needs are similar to the patient's
- Empowerment and a feeling of being in control
- Improved coping skills and better adjustment increases the chance of moving forward from the crisis
- Freedom to speak openly and honestly
- A support network and sounding board for emotional responses to crisis
- A reduction in feelings of distress, depression, anxiety, or fatigue caused by putting problems in perspective
- An increase in feelings of self-worth and self-esteem, improved assertiveness, and improved personal relationships
- A reduction in feelings of isolation caused by realizing that others are struggling with the same problems, leading to increased social reconnection
- Development of a better understanding of the patient's situation, including providing a space for the patient to break down misconceptions and reduce harmful self-talk
- Practical advice and information about treatment options, including integrative treatments
- Diversity within the group gives new perspectives on how to approach the problem
- Comparison of notes regarding resource and physician options.

Sources: Data from American Psychological Association (2019b); Graham, Powell, and Karam (n.d.); Mayo Clinic (2020c).

Nursing Care Plan

A Patient in Crisis

ASSESSMENT

Deborah Smith is a 30-year-old woman who comes to the ED following a fall down the stairs outside her apartment. She breaks down in tears during the assessment. Not only is her ankle painful and swollen, but the father of her two small children has recently been arrested for nearly killing his girlfriend. She has no idea when he will be able to pay child support again, and she is afraid she will not be able to return to work at her job as a waitress if her ankle is sprained. The physical assessment reveals the following:

- Vital signs include temperature 99.0°F oral; pulse 96 bpm; respirations 18/min; and blood pressure 136/86 mmHg.
- Hands are trembling, patient is tearful and crying
- Circular scars noted on both forearms the size of pencil erasers
- Left ankle is edematous and painful to touch, unable to perform range of motion in ankle
- Abrasions on the palm of the right hand, left elbow, and both knees.

DIAGNOSES

- Pain
- Anxiety
- Potential for caregiver burden
- Potential for inadequate resilience

PLANNING

- Identify community resources that can provide assistance until Ms. Smith can return to work.
- Identify Ms. Smith's strengths in terms of available resources and family support.
- Manage pain to allow Ms. Smith to maintain comfort.
- Teach patient crutch walking and self-care for injured ankle.

IMPLEMENTATION

- Encourage Ms. Smith to express her feelings.
- Ask Ms. Smith whom she can look to for help. Are the children's grandparents supportive? Does she have a supportive spiritual community? Does her workplace have a sick leave policy? Are there resources within the community that can provide support and assistance?
- Provide referral to the hospital's department of social services to determine potential community resources.
- Encourage Ms. Smith to identify her strengths that can help her resolve her current crisis.
- Establish a follow-up plan for this patient's physical as well as psychosocial needs.
- Provide teaching on care of ankle injury, symptoms to report to provider immediately, crutch-walking, and wound care.

EVALUATION

Social services assisted Ms. Smith in obtaining unemployment insurance during her medical leave of absence and provided anticipatory guidance to help her retain her job until she was able to return. Ms. Smith developed a stronger relationship with her church community, whose members assisted in picking up the children from school, delivered meals, and helped to perform tasks such as laundry that Ms. Smith could not perform with limited mobility.

CRITICAL THINKING

1. If you were the nurse caring for Ms. Smith and lived in the same community, would it be appropriate for you to offer to provide home care for her and the children when you had time available? Why or why not?
2. Is it appropriate for you, as the nurse caring for this patient, to solve problems for her? Explain your answer.
3. What functions can social service provide to help patients in crisis like Ms. Smith?

REVIEW Crisis

RELATE Link the Concepts and Exemplars

Linking the exemplar of crisis with the concept of addiction:

1. When a crisis results from addiction behavior, what is the nurse's priority intervention? Explain your answer.
2. When a patient's spouse is demonstrating addiction behavior that has caused the individual's crisis, what community referrals might you consider suggesting to help the patient?

Linking the exemplar of crisis with the concept of culture and diversity:

3. Why might one series of events trigger a crisis for one patient but not another?
4. How do coping strategies differ during times of crisis for patients from vulnerable populations versus those who are less vulnerable? How would your nursing interventions differ for each patient?

READY Go to Volume 3: Clinical Nursing Skills

REFER Go to Pearson MyLab Nursing and eText

REFLECT Apply Your Knowledge

Carol Holland is a 51-year-old mother of three. She is a nurse educator and works full time at a community college. Her son Paul recently moved back to live with her to attend college full time. Along with Paul, Mrs. Holland lives with her husband Tom and their other son Mike. Her oldest and only daughter Angela lives in an apartment nearby. The Hollands receive a call in the wee hours of the morning. One of Mike's friends tells them that Mike has been in a terrible accident, and they need to come to the hospital immediately. Arriving at the trauma unit at 3:00 a.m., the Hollands and their son Paul enter the satellite unit. Mike is intubated and requires mechanical ventilation. Mrs. Holland scans Mike's body for signs of independent life, but he is motionless. His face is so swollen that he is nearly unrecognizable to her. What appears to be a blue cable cord holds together a laceration that encompasses most of his head. His left arm is swollen three times its size and is blue and seeping from lacerations. As Paul collapses in a nearby chair and begins weeping, the nurse quietly gathers vital information from Mrs. Holland. She directs Mike's family to the lounge where they will wait during a procedure to insert an external ventricular drain (EVD). The neurosurgeon is unsure Mike will survive the night.

1. What type of crisis is this family experiencing?
2. Given the information presented thus far, what are Mike's priorities for care?
3. What are some possible psychosocial interventions for the patient and the family?
4. What basic needs might this family have throughout the night?

» Exemplar 31.C Obsessive–Compulsive Disorder

Exemplar Learning Outcomes

31.C Analyze obsessive–compulsive disorder (OCD) as it relates to stress and coping.

- Describe the pathophysiology of OCD.
- Describe the etiology of OCD.
- Compare the risk factors for and prevention of OCD.
- Identify the clinical manifestations of OCD.
- Summarize diagnostic tests and therapies used by interprofessional teams in the collaborative care of an individual with OCD.
- Differentiate considerations for care of patients with OCD across the lifespan.
- Apply the nursing process in providing culturally competent care to an individual with OCD.

Exemplar Key Terms

Compulsion, *2130*
Obsession, *2130*
Obsessive–compulsive disorder (OCD), *2130*

Overview

Obsessive–compulsive disorder (OCD) is a disabling condition characterized by obsessive thoughts and compulsive, repetitive behaviors that dominate an individual's life (see **Figure 31.10 »**). An **obsession** is a recurrent, unwanted, and often distressing thought or image that leads to feelings of fear and anxiety. A **compulsion** is a repetitive behavior or mental activity (such as counting) used in an attempt to mitigate the obsessive thoughts and reduce feelings of anxiety (American Psychiatric Association, 2013). To be diagnosed with OCD, the individual must experience distress and lose time (more than 1 hour a day) due to the consuming rituals and repetitive behaviors associated with the disorder (American Psychiatric Association, 2013).

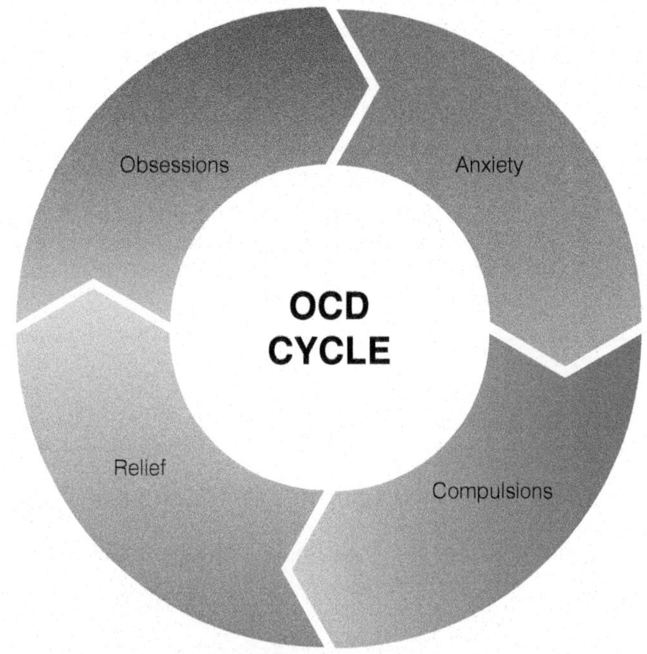

Figure 31.10 » Individuals with OCD experience anxiety-inducing obsessions and engage in compulsive behaviors in an attempt to reduce feelings of anxiety.

Pathophysiology

A malfunction in the cortico-striato-thalamo-cortical (CSTC) circuit in the brain is the possible cause for OCD (see **Figure 31.11 »**); the neurotransmitters serotonin, dopamine, and glutamate are all involved in OCD (Graat, Figee, & Denys, 2017). A specific gene has not yet been isolated, but research has identified many candidate genes and found that some regions of the genome might include disease genes (Arnold, 2017). The neurobiology of OCD involves several areas of the brain: the orbitofrontal

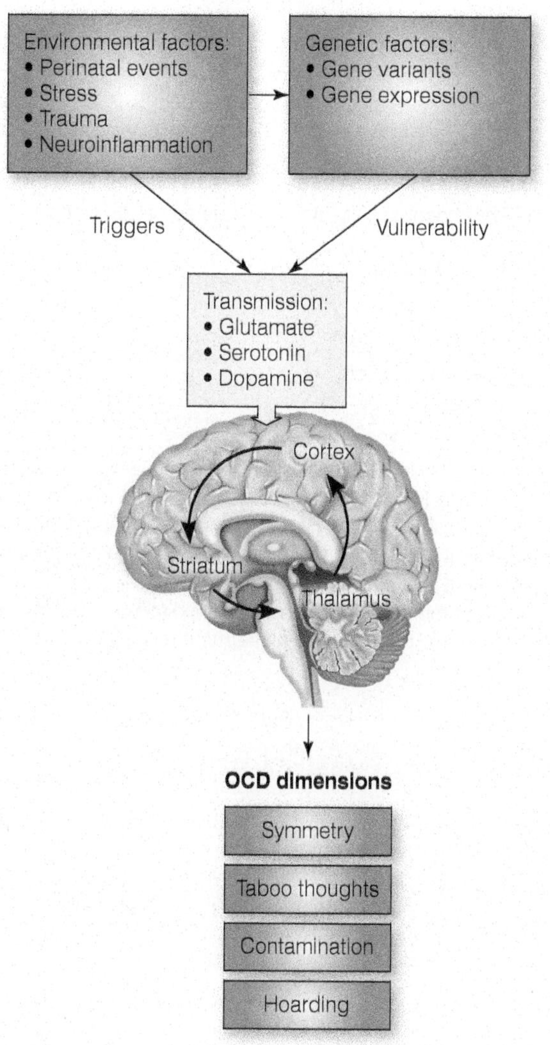

Figure 31.11 ›› A combination of environmental and genetic factors can result in a malfunction in the CSTC circuit in the brain. This malfunction is thought to play a role in the development of OCD.

cortex, anterior cingulate gyrus, and basal ganglia (Liu et al., 2020). Neuroimaging of individuals with OCD shows abnormalities in the basal ganglia and the orbitofrontal cortex. Imaging data, genomic studies, and animal models of aberrant grooming behavior have contributed to the idea that the glutamatergic system plays a role in OCD. These findings are compatible with circuit-based theories of OCD and have driven interest in testing the efficacy of pharmacologic treatments that modulate glutamate function (Karthik, Sharma, & Narayanaswamy, 2020). Studies of OCD's pathogenesis have produced mounting evidence that increased immune system activation plays an important role (Renna et al., 2018).

Diagnosis of OCD may be challenging for those who are untrained or uninformed about the disease. Variances that occur in the disorder, and that are explained in detail in the Clinical Manifestations section, also contribute to difficulty in diagnosing OCD. Contamination obsessions combined with washing and cleaning compulsions are probably the best-known variant of the disorder.

Etiology

Approximately 1.2% of the U.S. population has OCD within a 12-month span, and this number increases to 2.3% for lifetime prevalence (NIMH, 2017b). OCD typically begins in adolescence or early adulthood, although some cases do begin in childhood. OCD affects men and women equally, but men develop the disorder earlier. Among males, approximately 25% of those with OCD demonstrate onset before 10 years of age (American Psychiatric Association, 2013). Without treatment, the rate of remission is estimated to be low. However, for individuals who experience childhood-onset OCD, approximately 40% may experience remission by the time they reach early adulthood (American Psychiatric Association, 2013).

Risk Factors

Risk factors for OCD include having a first-degree relative with the disorder. A history of childhood sexual or physical abuse also increases the risk, as does exposure to other stressful or traumatic events during childhood (American Psychiatric Association, 2013).

Clinical Manifestations

Obsessive–compulsive disorder is not to be confused with *obsessive–compulsive personality disorder*. The clinical manifestations of the personality disorder involve more of a preoccupation with perfection and are characterized by inflexibility. See Exemplar 29.B, Personality Disorders, in Module 29, Self, for more information.

The most frequently reported obsessions in OCD are repeated thoughts about contamination from shaking hands; repeated doubts with fear of having hurt someone or leaving a door unlocked; and a need to have things in a certain order. Common themes of the associated intrusive, repetitive thoughts include thoughts that the individual considers to be forbidden or taboo; for example, religious or sexual obsessions and fears related to self-harm or injury of others (American Psychiatric Association, 2013). Aggressive impulses are often of a sexual nature or obscene. The obsessions are not rational or real-life problems. The patient with OCD is, at some point, aware that the obsessions are not real (American Psychiatric Association, 2013).

Compulsions are also part of OCD. Commonly reported repetitive behaviors include handwashing, ordering, checking, and counting. Note that hoarding, a behavior associated with OCD in DSM-IV, is recognized in DSM-5 as a distinct and separate disorder, hoarding disorder, within the category of Obsessive–Compulsive and Related Disorders (American Psychiatric Association, 2013). For additional examples of commonly occurring obsessions and their related compulsions, see the Clinical Manifestations and Therapies feature.

Compulsive behavior does not produce a sense of pleasure for the patient with OCD. Rather, the individual feels driven to perform the compulsion to reduce the anxiety produced by the obsession.

Clinical Manifestations and Therapies

Obsessive–Compulsive Disorder

ETIOLOGY (OBSESSIONS)	CLINICAL MANIFESTATIONS (COMPULSIONS)	CLINICAL THERAPIES
Aggressive, sexual, and religious obsessions with checking compulsions	▪ Checks doors, locks, appliances, written work ▪ Confesses frequently (to anything) ▪ Needs to ask others repeatedly for assurance	▪ Pharmacologic therapies include some SSRIs and TCAs. SSRIs: fluoxetine (Prozac) fluvoxamine paroxetine (Paxil) sertraline (Zoloft) TCAs: clomipramine (Anafranil) ▪ CBT may include exposure therapy, in which the person is carefully exposed over a period of time to an object that promotes fear. For example, the therapist and patient may, at an appropriate time, agree that the patient will touch a doorknob. ▪ Other therapies such as deep brain stimulation may be helpful to those who are treatment resistant.
Symmetry obsessions with ordering, arranging, and repeating compulsions	▪ Needs to have objects in fixed and symmetrical positions ▪ Repeats movements, such as going in and out of doorways, getting in and out of chairs, touching objects ▪ Counts or spells silently or aloud	
Contamination obsessions with washing and cleaning compulsions	▪ Repeatedly washes hands, showers, bathes, brushes teeth ▪ Cleans personal space frequently	

Collaboration

Diagnosis of OCD is made by a licensed clinical mental health professional. Care often occurs in the community and may include the nurse in collaboration with the patient's mental health provider, primary care provider, and school counselor or social worker. Because the impact of OCD can range from mild to disabling, the patient's needs will vary. The most common therapy for OCD is pharmacotherapy, followed by psychotherapies. Guidelines for treatment of OCD are summarized in **Box 31.10** ». Note that most research on treatment for OCD has been limited in its scope with regard to diversity (see Focus on Diversity and Culture: Lack of Diversity in OCD Research).

Diagnostic Tests

No definitive laboratory findings have been identified for diagnosing OCD.

Pharmacologic Therapy

For the patient with OCD, SSRI antidepressants are often prescribed as part of the treatment regimen, as well as clomipramine, a TCA (Mayo Clinic, 2020b). While SSRIs tend to have fewer side effects than TCAs, all medications carry risks and potential adverse effects. The nurse's role includes educating the patient about the safe administration of medications, as well as the potential side effects.

Box 31.10

Guidelines for the Treatment of Individuals with OCD

- ***Psychiatric management.*** OCD is usually a chronic illness. Treatment is necessary when the symptoms interfere with functioning or cause significant distress. Therapeutic management consists of a variety of therapeutic interventions throughout the course of the illness.
- ***Psychiatric assessment.*** The psychiatrist or psychiatric nurse practitioner will usually consider a medical evaluation and assessment of common comorbid conditions, such as depression, bipolar symptoms, other anxiety disorders, tics, impulse-control disorders, anorexia nervosa, bulimia nervosa, alcohol use, attention-deficit/hyperactivity disorder, and a history of panic attacks.
- ***Pharmacotherapy.*** Successful medication treatment should be continued for 1 to 2 years before gradually tapering and while observing for symptom exacerbation. The antidepressant SSRIs fluoxetine (Prozac), fluvoxamine, paroxetine (Paxil), and sertraline (Zoloft) and the TCA clomipramine (Anafranil) are approved by the FDA specifically for treatment of OCD. The SSRIs have fewer side effects than clomipramine and are recommended for the first medication trial.
- ***Psychotherapy.*** CBT that relies primarily on behavioral techniques such as exposure and response prevention is recommended because it has the best evidentiary support. Family therapy may reduce interfamily tensions due to the individual's OCD symptoms.

Sources: From Del Casale et al. (2019); Greenberg (2018); Mayo Clinic (2020b).

Focus on Diversity and Culture

Lack of Diversity in OCD Research

Evaluation of clinical studies on OCD shows that the majority of studies focus on white populations. The Black population is underrepresented in many clinical studies, even though prevalence rates and many manifestations of OCD in Black people are similar to those experienced by white populations (American Psychiatric Association, 2017). Limited studies on cultural differences between groups indicate that Black populations are less likely to receive treatment for OCD based on the negative stigma associated with mental health conditions and socioeconomic barriers (Williams, Rouleau, La Torre, & Sharif, 2020). However, Black patients report contamination symptoms more frequently than white patients and are twice as likely to report excessive concerns about animals (George, Pittenger, Kelmendi, Lohr, & Adams, 2018). In addition, religious differences often have a role in the development of OCD: Individuals who adhere to religions that practice rituals, such as people of the Jewish, Catholic, and Islamic faiths, are more likely to develop OCD signs and symptoms and have a higher severity of those manifestations (Nicolini et al., 2017).

Nonpharmacologic Therapy

Psychotherapy is an integral component of treatment for the patient with OCD. In addition to focusing on the patient, therapy and counseling sessions may include the patient's family members or significant others. In particular, a kind of CBT called exposure and response prevention (ERP) has proven to be most effective for patients with OCD. Using ERP, the patient is gradually exposed to the object of the obsession or fear and is taught healthy methods of coping with the associated anxiety (Mayo Clinic, 2020b). Other CBT therapies, especially those that involve restructuring thought patterns and behavior, have been found effective for these patients. For a discussion of CBT, refer to the Concept section of this module.

Lifespan Considerations

Obsessive–compulsive disorder most commonly begins in childhood or young adulthood. Understanding the differences in younger and older populations of individuals with OCD is essential to the proper care of these individuals.

OCD in Children and Adolescents

The mean age of onset of OCD symptoms in children is around age 7.5, but it is often not recognized or diagnosed until much later. Diagnosis of OCD generally peaks in prepubescent children and then again in early adulthood. An estimated 2–3% of children have OCD. In children and adolescents, boys appear to develop symptoms of OCD earlier than girls (Brasic, 2019).

Symptoms of OCD in children are often hidden or ill defined, causing them to be missed by parents and clinicians. Younger children in particular are not able to articulate their fears, which often relate to fear of a major disaster such as the loss of a parent (Kelly, 2021). Obsessions and compulsions are often similar to those experienced by adults, but they may change over time, with the same individuals experiencing different obsessions or compulsions as they age. Compulsions are often related to sensory stimuli, including the perception of both physical (tactile, musculoskeletal) and mental (tactile, auditory, visual) sensations. Children and adolescents are also more likely than adults to experience rage attacks in relation to their OCD, a phenomenon that is enhanced if their family accommodates or reinforces their OCD behaviors (Brasic, 2019).

Controversy exists about whether the development of OCD in some children may be linked to streptococcal infection (Wilbur et al., 2019). Initially referred to by the acronym PANDAS, which stands for pediatric autoimmune neuropsychiatric disorders associated with streptococcal infections, researchers have proposed revision of this condition to pediatric acute-onset neuropsychiatric syndrome (PANS). Its hallmark is a sudden and abrupt exacerbation of OCD symptoms after a strep infection. The cause of this form of OCD appears to be antibodies mistakenly attacking a region of the brain. Another major risk factor for the development of OCD in children is association with a first-order relative (parent or sibling) who also has OCD (Zai et al., 2019).

Many children with OCD will spontaneously resolve their symptoms as they age. However, a shorter duration of illness, less severe symptoms, fewer comorbid conditions, no previous pharmacological treatment, and a strong response to initial treatment were associated with a higher rate of remission (Sharma & Math, 2019). When possible, CBT and ERP therapy should be used as a first-line treatment for OCD in children. For more severe cases, such as children with declining grades and stronger compulsions in a school setting, medication may be needed. SSRIs appear effective in alleviating symptoms of OCD in children.

OCD in Older Adults

Older adults are more likely to report their physical complaints and avoid discussing their mental complaints (ADAA, n.d.). As a result, it is commonly thought that symptoms of anxiety and related disorders decrease with age. In those over 65 years of age, OCD symptoms tend to improve, however, they may still experience new or subclinical symptoms (Dell'Osso et al., 2017).

Because older adults are less likely to discuss their mental symptoms, a general assessment of older adults should include assessment for changes in mental status, including obsessive and compulsive symptoms. Older adults with one or more mental or anxiety disorders should be given a thorough psychiatric assessment because OCD is often comorbid with other mental disorders. This comorbidity may interfere with responsiveness to treatment and increase the time it takes for medications to be effective in older adults.

NURSING PROCESS

The primary nursing goals for the patient with OCD are to ensure patient safety and to alleviate anxiety and distress. Care must be taken not to prevent the performance of rituals that the patient uses to reduce anxiety but rather to promote new behavioral patterns and coping mechanisms to make the rituals unnecessary while maintaining the safety of the patient.

Assessment

Observation and Patient Interview

The nursing assessment interviews of patients with OCD share many similarities to those used with patients who have anxiety disorders. Suggested interview questions include:

Current and Past Medical History

- Does anyone in your family experience an anxiety disorder?
- Have you experienced intrusive or unwanted thoughts? Please describe the nature of the unwanted thoughts.
- Do you find yourself performing repetitive actions and behaviors to alleviate your anxiety? Please describe.
- Describe how these actions interfere with your life.
- How old were you when you first experienced these thoughts and behaviors? Age at diagnosis?
- Approximately how much time out of your day is spent dealing with these thoughts and behaviors?
- On a scale of 0 to 10, please rate your current level of distress (0 = no distress, 10 = intolerable anxiety).
- What have you tried in the past to alleviate the anxiety? What do you think was successful?
- Describe any repetitive or ritualistic behaviors.
- Do you use counting when feeling anxious?
- Have you experienced depression? Have you considered suicide? If yes, please rate on a scale from 0 to 10 how likely you are to act on these thoughts or impulses (0 = not at all, 10 = I will kill myself).
- Do you drink or use illicit drugs to manage your anxiety? If so, please list name, frequency, and amount.

Activities of Daily Living

- Is your health at risk as a result of the compulsive behaviors?
- Describe a typical day (sleep, eating, activities, employment).
- How have these behaviors affected your relationships?
- How has your spirituality been affected?
- How is your emotional well-being and mental health affected?

Physical Examination

A thorough examination may determine physical problems resulting from manifestations associated with OCD. For example, excessive handwashing or the use of irritating cleansing agents may result in loss of tissue integrity.

Diagnosis

Appropriate nursing priorities for OCD may vary depending on the nature of the obsessive thoughts and compulsive behaviors and the severity of the illness. In addition to anxiety, possible care priorities for OCD patients include the following:

- Fear
- Inadequate coping skills
- Inadequate role performance
- Potential for impaired tissue integrity
- Social isolation.

Planning

Planning in collaboration with the patient should be prioritized according to what the patient identifies as most important and may include the following goals:

- The patient will verbalize reduced fears associated with contamination or causing harm to others.
- The patient will identify triggers for obsessive–compulsive behaviors.
- The patient will experience reduced anxiety without performing associated compulsive behaviors.
- The patient will incorporate coping techniques to decrease the need to perform compulsive behaviors.
- The patient will perform skin care to hands to prevent cracking and bleeding.
- The patient will decrease time spent performing compulsive behaviors so that they no longer interfere with everyday role performance.
- The patient will participate in appropriate social activities previously avoided because of obsessive or compulsive tendencies.

Implementation

A supportive and nonjudgmental demeanor is essential when working with patients with OCD. Often the individual is aware that the compulsive behaviors are unreasonable and feels embarrassed. Compulsive behaviors serve as coping mechanisms to lower the level of anxiety or defensively "undo" the obsessive thoughts. Interrupting an individual during a ritual or compulsive behavior creates more anxiety and frequently leads to the individual redoing or repeating the behavior to reduce the anxiety. If a patient with OCD is admitted to the hospital, the hospital staff may need to collaborate with the patient to accommodate the rituals until the patient experiences relief from anxiety. Administration of medications to lower anxiety and reevaluation of the patient's response to the medication are the responsibility of the nurse in collaboration with the HCP and the patient.

Alleviate Fear

Patients with OCD often perform ritualistic behaviors to help alleviate fears associated with contamination or causing harm to others. These fears are often based on distortions of reality that the patient believes. Most of the time, the patient is aware that the compulsions are unnecessary. The patient's mental health professional will help the patient work to alter beliefs and correct perceptions. However, the nurse can implement several nursing interventions to help reduce a patient's fears:

- Provide a calm presence for the patient that will encourage verbalization of fears. Validate the patient's feelings without encouraging the belief in a distorted reality.

- Provide facts related to the patient's fears that are based in reality. For example, a patient who is afraid of contamination may benefit from knowledge about the immune system and the benefit of limited exposure to germs.
- For patients who are hospitalized for treatment of their OCD or for any other reason, take steps to reduce environmental stimulation. Remove or hide items associated with any triggers associated with the patient's obsession or compulsion. Teach patients to remove triggers from their home or work environment as much as possible.

Communicating with a Patient with OCD

Working Phase

When communicating with patients who are engaging in compulsive behaviors, reflect on the behavior, be nonjudgmental, and offer support. Confronting them or trying to talk them out of their behavior will only alienate, frustrate, and increase their anxiety. Consider that being in the hospital may accentuate OCD tendencies, so you might be seeing an exaggerated rendition of what patients' normal experiences are. Sensitively observing the behavior has the potential to engage patients in a dialogue that will allow them to observe their own behavior and change these maladaptive tendencies. For example, upon walking into a patient's room and finding the patient lining up and rearranging the sheets and blankets on the bed, you might say:

- I notice that you keep rearranging the sheets.
- You seem preoccupied with this task.
- It seems very important for you for everything to be orderly.
- Is there something about your bedding that I can help with?

Promote Effective Coping

When patients with OCD experience fears or obsessions, they are unable to use normal coping strategies to prevent the practice of compulsive behaviors. Instead, they perform compulsive behaviors as a coping mechanism. This often disrupts the performance of normal roles and may cause them to feel embarrassed or isolated from society. Nurses can teach patients effective coping behaviors, as described in the Patient Teaching feature.

Patient Teaching

Adaptive Coping

Establishing a therapeutic relationship provides the nurse with an opportunity to promote healthy adaptive coping. Patient teaching about the nature of obsessive thinking is critical to lowering the patient's feelings of shame and anxiety. The nurse can help the patient realize that fears arise from the disease, not from any real threat. Nurses can help patients reframe how they think about their disease and help them reframe thought processes in order to reduce ritual performance, such as helping the patient meditate instead of performing a ritual and then recognizing that nothing bad happened as a result of the absence of the ritual. The nurse has an essential role in helping patients with OCD understand that they can decrease anxiety and gain control over the disease through pharmacologic and behavior therapies.

Promote Effective Role Performance

The ritualistic behaviors and shame associated with OCD often interfere with the ability of the patient to perform normal roles, including family, home, and work responsibilities. OCD behaviors may also interfere with the patient's ability to perform self-care activities. The nurse can help patients adequately perform their roles by:

- Encouraging patients to have healthy conversations with their family members about the disorder.
- Listening to patients describe how the ritualistic behaviors are disrupting their ability to perform normal roles. This includes having patients describe normal roles that they are not performing because of the disorder. This may help patients discover why they feel compelled to perform compulsive behaviors and to discuss ways in which they can begin to perform normal roles again in the future.
- Promoting self-awareness for patients to understand their reaction to environmental triggers. Understanding their own thought processes and the reasons behind those thoughts can promote changes in thought patterns necessary to decrease disruptive behaviors and increase performance of normal roles.
- Encouraging patients to participate in individual or family behavioral therapy or counseling. In addition to medication, therapy or counseling is one of the most effective ways to help patients with OCD regain control over their life and behaviors. The nurse can provide references to therapists or counselors who specialize in the treatment of OCD.

SAFETY ALERT Patients who perform excessive washing rituals are at a high risk for impaired skin integrity, especially on the hands. Excessive handwashing with soaps and antibacterial gels can dry the skin and leave it susceptible to cracking and bleeding. Teach the patient about consequences of excessive handwashing and techniques to help maintain skin integrity, including the regular use of lotions.

Promote Social Interaction

Patients with OCD who spend hours each day performing ritualistic behaviors may find that they are no longer able to participate in social activities. Performing rituals or checking behaviors often delays the patient's arrival at an event or prevents the individual from leaving home altogether. Friends may avoid spending time with the patient because of odd behaviors and time-wasting. As patients progress through treatment, nurses can promote social interaction of patients by teaching time management techniques so they can plan to arrive at social events on time and encouraging them to be open with their friends about the disorder and to enlist their support during social interactions. The nurse may also encourage patients to invite close friends and family to a counseling session so they can be a part of the healing process.

Evaluation

About 70% of patients with OCD improve with treatment, however, about 15% have symptoms that progressively get worse over time (Greenberg, 2018). Therefore, the nurse will need to continually evaluate the patient and adjust the care plan and interventions. Successful response to nursing care may be evaluated by using the following expected outcomes:

- The patient verbalizes a reduction in anxiety associated with the compulsive need to perform ritualistic behaviors.
- The patient demonstrates an understanding of appropriate coping behaviors and verbalizes successful use of healthy coping behaviors to reduce the need to perform compulsive behaviors.
- The patient demonstrates an ability to effectively perform expected roles, including family, home, and work roles.
- The patient verbalizes increased social interaction and a decrease in missed events due to the performance of ritualistic behaviors.
- The skin on the patient's hands does not show signs of breakdown, such as cracking or bleeding.

The nurse should understand that complete healing from OCD will likely take many years for most patients. During this time, the nurse should continually reevaluate the patient and suggest changes in treatment modalities depending on the success or failure of previous treatment plans. The nurse may need to teach additional coping strategies or advocate for the patient to receive different medication or to add CBT or family counseling to the treatment plan. Importantly, the nurse should encourage the patient to continue treatment, not give up, and not accept the disorder as normal or inevitable.

REVIEW Obsessive–Compulsive Disorder

RELATE Link the Concepts and Exemplars

Linking the exemplar of obsessive–compulsive disorder with the concept of mood and affect:

1. How might mood be impacted in the patient who is unable to control his ritualistic compulsive disorders?
2. Is assessment for suicidal ideation important when admitting a new patient with OCD? Why or why not?

Linking the exemplar of obsessive–compulsive disorder with the concept of advocacy:

3. If a patient's rituals involve an act that places her in danger, what actions can the nurse take to advocate for the patient while not causing increased anxiety that can result from not being able to perform the ritual?
4. While working on a medical unit in a local hospital, you admit an adult patient for surgery. While collecting the admission assessment, you note what you suspect is ritualistic compulsive behavior. How can you best advocate for this patient?

READY Go to Volume 3: Clinical Nursing Skills

REFER Go to Pearson MyLab Nursing and eText

REFLECT Apply Your Knowledge

Karleen Lassiter, a married, 40-year-old mother of three children, is admitted to a hospital psychiatric unit with complaints of anxiety, inability to relax, and intrusive thoughts that she states are "horrific." When asked to describe her thoughts, she states, "I'm afraid I'm going to hell as punishment for what goes through my mind sometimes. It's really dark stuff." In conjunction with her intrusive thoughts, Ms. Lassiter recites the same prayer up to 50 times daily. She is trained as a respiratory therapist, but she has not practiced in the clinical setting for the past 5 years. In part, she reports that her departure from her position was related to her need to complete her prayer rituals. Ms. Lassiter explains that her employment was terminated due to her being late for work on several occasions because "I needed to finish praying before I could leave for work." She is aware that her behavior is irrational and that it is negatively impacting her life; however, she is unable to control or cease the behavior.

Ms. Lassiter's medical history includes panic attacks between the ages of 18 and 21, during college enrollment. She denies suicidal ideation; however, she states, "I don't think I can handle living like this. My husband and kids think I'm crazy, and they're right."

1. Based on the available assessment data, identify Ms. Lassiter's apparent obsessions and compulsions.
2. Describe appropriate communication strategies for encouraging this patient to further describe her intrusive thoughts.
3. Based on the patient's statements, identify the priority nursing diagnosis for Ms. Lassiter.

References

Adams, M. P., Holland, L. N., & Urban, C. (2020). *Pharmacology for nurses: A pathophysiologic approach* (5th ed.). Pearson.

Ahmad, N. S. (2019). Crisis intervention: Issues and challenges. *Advances in Social Sciences, Education and Humanities Research, 304*, 452–455.

American Academy of Pediatrics. (2019). *Depression and anxiety during pregnancy and after birth: FAQs*. https://www.healthychildren.org/English/ages-stages/prenatal/Pages/Depression-and-Anxiety-During-Pregnancy-and-After-Birth-FAQs.aspx

American Academy of Pediatrics. (2021). *Anxiety fact sheet*. https://www.aap.org/en-us/advocacy-and-policy/aap-health-initiatives/resilience/Pages/Anxiety-Fact-Sheet.aspx

American College of Obstetricians and Gynecologists. (2020). *Tobacco, alcohol, drugs, and pregnancy*. http://www.acog.org/Patients/FAQs/Tobacco-Alcohol-Drugs-and-Pregnancy

American Diabetes Association. (2019). 5. Lifestyle management: Standards of Medical Care in Diabetes-2019. *Diabetes Care, 42*(Suppl. 1), S46–S60.

American Psychiatric Association. (2013). *Diagnostic and statistical manual of mental disorders* (5th ed.). Author.

American Psychiatric Association. (2017). *Mental health facts for African Americans*. https://www.psychiatry.org/psychiatrists/cultural-competency/education/mental-health-facts

American Psychological Association. (2012). *Building your resilience*. https://www.apa.org/topics/resilience

American Psychological Association. (2017a). *Stress in America: Coping with change*. https://www.apa.org/news/press/releases/stress/2016/coping-with-change.pdf

American Psychological Association. (2017b). *What is the difference between psychologists, psychiatrists and social workers.* https://www.apa.org/ptsd-guideline/patients-and-families/psychotherapy-professionals

American Psychological Association. (2019a). *Identifying signs of stress in your children and teens.* https://www.apa.org/topics/stress/children

American Psychological Association. (2019b). *Psychotherapy: Understanding group therapy.* https://www.apa.org/topics/group-therapy

American Psychological Association. (2020). *Stress in America™ 2020: A national mental health crisis.* https://www.apa.org/news/press/releases/stress/2020/sia-mental-health-crisis.pdf

Andrews, G., Bell, C., Boyce, P., Gale, C., Lampe, L., Marwat, O., et al. (2018). Royal Australian and New Zealand College of Psychiatrists clinical practice guidelines for the treatment of panic disorder, social anxiety disorder and generalised anxiety disorder. *Australian and New Zealand Journal of Psychiatry, 52*(12), 1109–1172.

Anxiety and Depression Association of America (ADAA). (2020a). *Facts & statistics.* http://www.adaa.org/about-adaa/press-room/facts-statistics

Anxiety and Depression Association of America (ADAA). (2020b). *Generalized anxiety disorder (GAD).* http://www.adaa.org/generalized-anxiety-disorder-gad

Anxiety and Depression Association of America (ADAA). (2020c). *Living and thriving with anxiety or depression means conquering your symptoms: Older adults—Symptoms.* http://www.adaa.org/living-with-anxiety/older-adults/symptoms

Anxiety and Depression Association of America (ADAA). (2020d). *Treatment.* https://adaa.org/living-with-anxiety/children/treatment

Anxiety and Depression Association of America (ADAA). (2020e). *Women: Facts.* http://www.adaa.org/living-with-anxiety/women/facts

Anxiety and Depression Association of America (ADAA). (n.d.). *Older adults.* https://adaa.org/finding-help/older-adults#Anxiety

Araji, S., Griffin, A., Dixon L, Spencer, S.-K., Peavie, C., & Wallace, K. (2020). An overview of maternal anxiety during pregnancy and the post-partum period. *Journal of Mental Health and Clinical Psychology, 4*(4), 47–56.

Arnold, P. (2017). Genetics of OCD. In C. Pittenger (Ed.), *Obsessive–compulsive disorder: Phenomenology, pathophysiology, and treatment.* Oxford University Press. https://oxfordmedicine.com/view/10.1093/med/9780190228163.001.0001/med-9780190228163-chapter-19

Avvenuti, G., Leo, A., Cecchetti, L., Franco, M. F., Travis, F., Caramella, D., et al. (2020). Reductions in perceived stress following Transcendental Meditation practice are associated with increased brain regional connectivity at rest. *Brain and Cognition, 139,* 105517.

Babaev, O., Piletti Chatain, C., & Krueger-Burg, D. (2018). Inhibition in the amygdala anxiety circuitry. *Experimental and Molecular Medicine, 50*(4), 18.

Bakhamis, L., Paul, D. P., Smith, H., & Coustasse, A. (2019). Still an epidemic: The burnout syndrome in hospital registered nurses. *The Health Care Manager, 38*(1), 3–10.

Ball, J. W., Bindler, R. C., Cowen, K., & Shaw, M. R. (2022). *Principles of pediatric nursing: Caring for children* (8th ed.). Pearson.

Bandura, A. (1994). Self-efficacy. In V. S. Ramachandran (Ed.), *Encyclopedia of human behavior* (Vol. 4, pp. 71–81). Academic Press.

Bhatt, N. V. (2019). *Which medications in the drug class monoamine oxidase inhibitor (MAOI) are used in the treatment of anxiety disorders?* Medscape. https://www.medscape.com/answers/286227-18359/which-medications-in-the-drug-class-monoamine-oxidase-inhibitor-maoi-are-used-in-the-treatment-of-anxiety-disorders

Biesecker, B. B., Erby, L. H., Woolford, S., Adcock, J. Y., Cohen, J. S., Lamb, A., et al. (2013). Development and validation of the Psychological Adaptation Scale (PAS): Use in six studies of adaptation to a health condition or risk. *Patient Education and Counseling, 93*(2), 248–254.

Blaszko, M. A., Shields, D. A., Avino, K. M., & Rosa, W. E. (2022). *Dossey & Keegan's holistic nursing: A handbook for practice* (8th ed.). Jones & Bartlett.

Boston Children's Hospital. (n.d.). *Generalized anxiety disorder (GAD).* https://www.childrenshospital.org/conditions-and-treatments/conditions/g/generalized-anxiety-disorder-gad

Boullier, M., & Blair, M. (2018). Adverse childhood experiences. *Paediatrics and Child Health, 28*(3), 132–137.

Brasic, J. D. (2019). *Pediatric obsessive–compulsive disorder.* Medscape. https://emedicine.medscape.com/article/1826591-overview#a6

Brown, S. M., Doom, J. R., Lechuga-Peña, S., Watamura, S. E., & Koppels, T. (2020). Stress and parenting during the global COVID-19 pandemic. *Child Abuse and Neglect, 110*(Pt. 2), 104699.

Cabral, M. D., & Patel, D. R. (2020). Risk factors and prevention strategies for anxiety disorders in childhood and adolescence. In Y. K. Kim (Ed.), *Anxiety disorders* (*Advances in Experimental Medicine and Biology,* Vol. 1191, pp. 543–559). Springer.

California Evidence-Based Clearing House (CEBC). (2018). *Coping cat.* https://www.cebc4cw.org/program/coping-cat/detailed

Cannon, W. B. (1932). *The wisdom of the body.* Norton.

Caplan, G. (1964). *Principles of preventive psychiatry.* Basic Books.

Centers for Disease Control and Prevention (CDC). (2020). *Data and statistics on children's mental health.* https://www.cdc.gov/childrensmentalhealth/data.html

Cherry, L. (1978). On the real benefits of eustress: An interview with Hans Selye. *Psychology Today, 11*(10), 60–70.

Child Mind Institute. (2017). *Anxiety and depression in adolescence.* https://childmind.org/report/2017-childrens-mental-health-report/anxiety-depression-adolescence/

Cleveland Clinic. (2020). *Anxiety disorders.* http://my.clevelandclinic.org/services/neurological_institute/center-for-behavorial-health/disease-conditions/hic-anxiety-disorders

Cohen, S., Kamarck, T., & Mermelstein, R. (1983). A global measure of perceived stress. *Journal of Health and Social Behavior,* 24, 385–396.

Costa, R. M. (2020). Suppression (defense mechanism). In V. Zeigler-Hill & T. K. Shackelford (Eds.), *Encyclopedia of personality and individual differences.* Springer.

Del Casale, A., Sorice, S., Padovano, A., Simmaco, M., Ferracuti, S., Lamis, D. A., et al. (2019). Psychopharmacological treatment of obsessive–compulsive disorder (OCD). *Current Neuropharmacology, 17,* 710–736.

Dell'Osso, B., Benatti, B., Rodriguez, C. I., Arici, C., Palazzo, C., Altamura, A. C., et al. (2017). Obsessive–compulsive disorder in the elderly: A report from the International College of Obsessive–Compulsive Spectrum Disorders (ICOCS). *European Psychiatry, 45,* 36–40.

DeLongis, A., Coyne, J. C., Dakof, G., Folkman, S., & Lazarus, R. (1982). Relationship of daily hassles, uplifts, and major life events to health status. *Health Psychology, 1*(2), 119–136.

Deng, X., An, S., & Cheng, C. (2019). Cultural differences in the implicit and explicit attitudes toward emotion regulation. *Personality and Individual Differences, 149,* 220–222.

Dwyer, J. B., & Block, M. H. (2019). Antidepressants for pediatric patients. *Current Psychiatry, 18*(9), 26–42F.

Erikson, E. H. (1968). *Identity: Youth and crisis.* Norton.

Erikson, E. H. (1969). *Childhood and society.* Penguin Books.

Everly, G. S., & Lating, J. M. (2019). *A clinical guide to the treatment of the human stress response* (4th ed.). Springer.

Fava, G. A., McEwen, B. S., Guidi, J., Gostoli, S., Offidani, E., & Sonino, N. (2019). Clinical characterization of allostatic overload. *Psychoneuroendocrinology, 108,* 94–101.

Federal Emergency Management Agency. (2020). *Crisis counseling assistance & training program.* https://www.fema.gov/sites/default/files/documents/fema_crisis-counseling-program_2020.pdf

Feriante, J., & Bernstein, B. (2020). *Separation anxiety.* StatPearls. https://www.ncbi.nlm.nih.gov/books/NBK560793/

Freidl, E. K., Stroeh, O. M., Elkins, M., Steinberg, E., Albano, A. M., & Rynn, M. (2017). Assessment and treatment of anxiety among children and adolescents. *Focus, 15,* 144–156.

Freud, S. (1946). *The ego and mechanisms of defense.* International Universities Press.

George, J. R., Pittenger, C., Kelmendi, B., Lohr, J. M., & Adams, T. G. (2018). Disgust sensitivity mediates the effects of race on contamination aversion. *Journal of Obsessive–Compulsive and Related Disorders, 19,* 72–76.

Gerlach, A. L., & Gloster, A. T. (2020). Worry, generalized anxiety disorder (GAD), and their importance. In A. L. Gerlach & A. T. Gloster (Eds.), *Generalized anxiety disorder and worrying: A comprehensive handbook for clinicians and researchers* (pp. 1–8). Wiley.

Ghandour, R. M., Sherman, L. J., Vladutiu, C. J., Lynch, S. E., Bitsko, R. H., & Blumberg, S. J. (2019). Prevalence and treatment of depression, anxiety, and conduct problems in U.S. children. *Journal of Pediatrics, 206,* P256–267, E3.

Graat, I., Figee, M., & Denys, D. (2017). Neurotransmitter dysregulation in OCD. In C. Pittenger (Ed.), *Obsessive–compulsive disorder: Phenomenology, pathophysiology, and treatment.* Oxford University Press. https://oxfordmedicine.com/view/10.1093/med/9780190228163.001.0001/med-9780190228163-chapter-25

Graham, L., Powell, R., & Karam, A. (n.d.). *The power of social connection.* National Sexual Violence Resource Center. http://www.nsvrc.org/sites/default/files/the-power-of-social-connection.pdf

Gray, S. L., Anderson, M. L., Dublin, S., Hanlon, J. T., Hubbard, R., Walker, R., et al. (2015). Cumulative use of strong anticholinergics and incident dementia: A prospective cohort study. *JAMA Internal Medicine, 175*(3), 401–407.

Greenberg, W. M. (2018). *Obsessive-compulsive disorder treatment & management.* Medscape. http://emedicine.medscape.com/article/1934139-treatment#showall

He, Q., Chen, X., Wu, T., Li, L., & Fei, X. (2019). Risk of dementia in long-term benzodiazepine users: evidence from a meta-analysis of observational studies. *Journal of Clinical Neurology, 15*(1), 9–19.

Hellig, S., & Domschke, K. (2019). Anxiety in late life: A update of pathomechanisms. *Gerontology, 65,* 465–473.

Holmes, T. H., & Rahe, R. H. (1967). The social readjustment rating scale. *Journal of Psychosomatic Research, 11,* 213–218.

Hooley, J. M., Butcher, J. N., Nock, M. K., & Mineka, S. (2017). *Abnormal psychology* (17th ed.). Pearson.

Horowitz, M. J., Wilner, M., & Alverez, W. (1979). Impact of events scale: A measure of subjective stress. *Psychosomatic Medicine, 41*(3), 209–218.

Jones, W. L. (1968). The A-B-C method of crisis management. *Mental Hygiene, 52*(1), 87–89.

Kanel, K. (2019). *A guide to crisis intervention* (6th ed.). Cengage Learning.

Karthik, S., Sharma, L., & Narayanaswamy, J. C.(2020). Investigating the role of glutamate in obsessive–compulsive disorder: Current perspectives. *Neuropsychiatric Disease and Treatment, 16,* 1003–1013.

Kaur, S., & Singh, R. (2017). Role of different neurotransmitters in anxiety: A systematic review. *International Journal of Pharmaceutical Sciences and Research, 8*(2), 411–421.

Kelly, O. (2021). *How to recognize signs of OCD in children.* Verywellmind. https://www.verywellmind.com/parenting-children-with-ocd-2510563

Klein, E. M., Müller, K. W., Wölfling, K., Dreier, M., Ernst, M., & Beutel, M. E. (2020). The relationship between acculturation and mental health of 1st generation immigrant youth in a representative school survey: Does gender matter? *Child and Adolescent Psychiatry and Mental Health, 14,* 29.

Koltko-Rivera, M. E. (2006). Rediscovering the later version of Maslow's hierarchy of needs: Self-transcendence and opportunities for theory, research, and unification. *Review of General Psychology, 10*(4), 302–317.

Lazarus, R. S., & Folkman, S. (1984). *Stress, appraisal, and coping.* Springer.

Lippard, E. T. C., & Nemeroff, C. B. (2020). The devastating clinical consequences of child abuse and neglect: Increased disease vulnerability and poor treatment response in mood disorders. *American Journal of Psychiatry, 177*(1), 20–36.

Liu, W., Hua, M., Qin, J., Tang, Q., Han, Y., Tian, H., et al. (2020). Disrupted pathways from frontal-parietal cortex to basal ganglia and cerebellum in patients with unmedicated obsessive compulsive disorder as observed by whole-brain resting-state effective connectivity analysis – a small sample pilot study. *Brain Imaging and Behavior.* https://link.springer.com/article/10.1007/s11682-020-00333-3

Lumsden, D. P. (1981). Is the concept of "stress" of any use, anymore? In *Contributions to primary prevention in mental health: Working papers.* Toronto National Office of the Canadian Mental Health Association.

Mansen, T. (2015). *Patient focused assessment: The art and science of clinical data gathering.* Pearson.

Martin, J. L. (2021). *Cognitive behavioral therapy for insomnia in adults.* UpToDate. https://www.uptodate.com/contents/cognitive-behavioral-therapy-for-insomnia-in-adults

Maslow, A. (1943). A theory of human motivation. *Psychological Review, 50*(4), 370–396.

Maslow, A. H. (1968). *Toward a psychology of being* (2nd ed.). Van Nostrand Reinhold.

Maslow, A. H. (1987). *Motivation and personality* (3rd ed.). Harper & Row.

Mayo Clinic. (2017a). *Diseases and conditions: Anxiety*. http://www.mayoclinic.org/diseases-conditions/anxiety/basics/symptoms/con-20026282

Mayo Clinic. (2018a). *Anxiety*. https://www.mayoclinic.org/diseases-conditions/anxiety/diagnosis-treatment/drc-20350967

Mayo Clinic. (2018b). *Is there an effective herbal treatment for anxiety?* https://www.mayoclinic.org/diseases-conditions/generalized-anxiety-disorder/expert-answers/herbal-treatment-for-anxiety/faq-20057945

Mayo Clinic. (202a). *Coronavirus grief: Coping with the loss of routine during the pandemic*. https://www.mayoclinic.org/diseases-conditions/coronavirus/in-depth/coping-with-coronavirus-grief/art-20486392

Mayo Clinic. (2020b). *Obsessive-compulsive disorder (OCD)*. Retrieved from https://www.mayoclinic.org/diseases-conditions/obsessive-compulsive-disorder/diagnosis-treatment/drc-20354438.

Mayo Clinic. (2020c). *Support groups: make connections, get help*. http://www.mayoclinic.org/healthy-lifestyle/stress-management/in-depth/support-groups/art-20044655

MedlinePlus. (2021). *Stress in childhood*. https://medlineplus.gov/ency/article/002059.htm

Melton, L. (2017). Brief introduction to cognitive behavioral therapy for the advanced practitioner in oncology. *Journal of the Advanced Practitioner in Oncology, 8*(2), 188–193.

Memon, M. A. (2018). *What are the genetic factors that contribute to panic disorder?* Medscape. https://www.medscape.com/answers/287913-95578/what-are-the-genetic-factors-that-contribute-to-panic-disorder

Miller, C. A. (2019). *Nursing for wellness in older adults* (8th ed.). Wolters Kluwer.

Minnesota Department of Human Services. (2019). *Mobile crisis mental health services*. https://mn.gov/dhs/people-we-serve/adults/health-care/mental-health/programs-services/mobile-crisis.jsp

Monat, A., & Lazarus, R. S. (1991). *Stress and coping* (3rd ed.). Columbia University Press.

Morris, L. S., McCall, J. G., Charney, D. S., & Murrough, J. W. (2020). The role of the locus coeruleus in the generation of pathological anxiety. *Brain and Neuroscience Advances, 4*.

National Alliance on Mental Illness (NAMI). (n.d.). *Identity and cultural dimensions: Asian American and Pacific Islander*. https://www.nami.org/Your-Journey/Identity-and-Cultural-Dimensions/Asian-American-and-Pacific-Islander

National Alliance on Mental Illness (NAMI). (2017). *Mental illnesses: Anxiety disorders*. https://www.nami.org/About-Mental-Illness/Mental-Health-Conditions/Anxiety-Disorders

National Center for Complementary and Integrative Health (NCCIH). (2019). *Yoga for health*. https://nccih.nih.gov/health/yoga/introduction.htm

National Center for Complementary and Integrative Health (NCCIH). (2020a). *Chamomile*. https://www.nccih.nih.gov/health/chamomile

National Center for Complementary and Integrative Health (NCCIH). (2020b). *Lavender*. https://www.nccih.nih.gov/health/lavender

National Institute of Child Health and Human Development. (2017). *Will stress during pregnancy affect my baby?* National Institutes of Health. https://www.nichd.nih.gov/health/topics/preconceptioncare/conditioninfo/pages/stress.aspx

National Institute of Mental Health (NIMH). (2016). *Psychotherapies*. Retrieved from https://www.nimh.nih.gov/health/topics/psychotherapies/index.shtml

National Institute of Mental Health (NIMH). (2017a) *Generalized anxiety disorder*. Retrieved from https://www.nimh.nih.gov/health/statistics/generalized-anxiety-disorder.shtml

National Institute of Mental Health (NIMH). (2017b). *Obsessive–compulsive disorder*. https://www.nimh.nih.gov/health/statistics/obsessive-compulsive-disorder-ocd.shtml

National Institute of Mental Health (NIMH). (2017c). *Panic disorder*. http://www.nimh.nih.gov/health/topics/panic-disorder/index.shtml

National Institute of Mental Health (NIMH). (2018). *Anxiety disorders*. http://www.nimh.nih.gov/health/topics/anxiety-disorders/index.shtml

National Institute of Neurological Disorders and Stroke. (2020). *Brain basics: Know your brain*. https://www.ninds.nih.gov/Disorders/Patient-Caregiver-Education/Know-Your-Brain

Neubauer, A. B., Smyth, J. M., & Sliwinski, M. J. (2017). When you see it coming: Stressor anticipation modulates stress effects on negative affect. *Emotion, 18*(3), 342–354.

New York Presbyterian. (2020). *How to cope with grief amid COVID-19*. https://healthmatters.nyp.org/how-to-cope-with-grief-amid-covid-19/

Nicolini, H., Salin-Pascual, R., Cabrera, B., & Lanzagorta, N. (2017). Influence of culture in obsessive–compulsive disorder and its treatment. *Current Psychiatry Reviews, 13*(4), 285–292.

Penn Medicine News. (2020). *How coronavirus complicates the grieving process*. https://healthmatters.nyp.org/how-to-cope-with-grief-amid-covid-19/

Peplau, H. (1952). *Interpersonal relations in nursing*. Putnam.

Pinquart, M. (2018). Parenting stress in caregivers of children with chronic physical condition-A meta-analysis. *Stress and Health, 34*, 197–207.

Potter, M. P., & Moller, D. (2020). *Psychiatric–mental health nursing: From suffering to hope* (2nd ed.). Pearson.

The Recovery Village. (2020). *Separation anxiety facts and statistics*. https://www.therecoveryvillage.com/mental-health/separation-anxiety/related/separation-anxiety-statistics/

Renna, M. E., O'Toole, M. S., Spaeth, P. E., Lekander, M., & Mennin, D. S. (2018). The association between anxiety, traumatic stress, and obsessive–compulsive disorders and chronic inflammation: A systematic review and meta-analysis. *Depression and Anxiety, 35*, 1081–1094.

Selye, H. (1946). The general adaptation syndrome and the diseases of adaptation. *Journal of Clinical Endocrinology, 6*(1), 117–231.

Selye, H. (1956). *The stress of life*. McGraw-Hill.

Selye, H. (1974). *Stress without distress*. Lippincott.

Selye, H. (1976). *The stress of life* (revised ed.). McGraw-Hill.

Sharma, E., & Math, S. B. (2019). Course and outcome of obsessive-compulsive disorder. *Indian journal of psychiatry, 61*(Suppl. 1), S43–S50.

Smoller, J. W. (2020). Anxiety genetics goes genomic. *American Journal of Psychiatry, 177*(3), 190–194.

Spector, R. E. (2017). *Cultural diversity in health and illness* (9th ed.). Pearson.

Sterling, P., & Eyer, J. (1988). Allostasis: A new paradigm to explain arousal pathology. In S. Fisher & J. Reason (Eds.), *Handbook of life stress, cognition and health* (pp. 629–649). Wiley.

Substance Abuse and Mental Health Services Administration. (2016). *Impact of the DSM-IV to DSM-5 changes on the National Survey on Drug Use and Health*. https://www.ncbi.nlm.nih.gov/books/NBK519697/

Swedo, E., Idaikkadar, N., Leemis, R., Dias, T., Radhakrishnan, L., Stein, Z., et al. (2020). Trends in U.S. emergency department visits related to suspected or confirmed child abuse and neglect among children and adolescents aged <18 years before and during the COVID-19 pandemic—United States, January 2019–September 2020. *Morbidity and Mortality Weekly Report, 69*, 1841–1847.

Townsend, M. (2018). *Psychiatric mental health nursing: Concepts of care in evidence based practice* (9th ed.). Davis.

Ungar, M., & Theron, L. (2020). Resilience and mental health: how multisystemic processes contribute to positive outcomes. *Lancet Psychiatry, 7*, 441–448.

U.S. Department of Housing and Urban Development. (2019). *HUD 2019 continuum of care homeless assistance programs: Homeless populations and subpopulations*. Author.

U.S. Food & Drug Administration (FDA). (2018a). *FDA safety communication: Selective serotonin reuptake inhibitor (SSRI) antidepressant use during pregnancy and reports of a rare heart and lung condition in newborn babies*. https://www.fda.gov/drugs/drug-safety-and-availability/fda-drug-safety-communication-selective-serotonin-reuptake-inhibitor-ssri-antidepressant-use-during

U.S. Food and Drug Administration (FDA). (2018b). *Suicidality in children and adolescents being treated with antidepressant medications*. https://www.fda.gov/drugs/postmarket-drug-safety-information-patients-and-providers/suicidality-children-and-adolescents-being-treated-antidepressant-medications

Vella, S. L. C., & Pai, N. B. (2019). A theoretical review of psychological resilience: Defining resilience and resilience research over the decades. *Archives of Medicine and Health Sciences, 7*, 233–239.

Vesely, C. K., Bravo, D. Y., & Guzzardo, M. T. (2019). *Immigrant families across the life course: Policy impacts on physical and mental health*. National Council on Family Relations. https://www.ncfr.org/resources/research-and-policy-briefs/immigrant-families-across-life-course-policy-impacts-physical-and-mental-health

Waldman, K., Koyanagi, A., Wang, J. S. H., Ko, J., DeVylder, J., & Oh, H. (2019). Acculturative stress, disability, and health treatment utilization among Asian and Latin American immigrants in the United States. *Social Psychiatry and Psychiatric Epidemiology, 54*, 1275–1284.

Walsh, C. P., Ewing, L. J., Cleary, J. L., Vaisleib, A. D., Farrell, C. H., Wright, A., et al. (2018). Development of glucocorticoid resistance over one year among mothers of children newly diagnosed with cancer. *Brain, Behavior, and Immunity, 69*, 364–373.

Wanko Keutchafo, E. L., Kerr, J., & Jarvis, M. A. (2020). Evidence of nonverbal communication between nurses and older adults: a scoping review. *BMC Nursing 19*, 53.

Warburton, W. A., & Anderson, C. A. (2015). Aggression, social psychology of. In J. D. Wright (Ed.), *International encyclopedia of the social and behavioral sciences* (2nd ed., Vol. 1, pp. 373–380). Elsevier.

Weiss, D. S., & Marmer, C. R. (1997). The impact of event scale—Revised. In J. P. Wilson & T. M. Keane (Eds.), *Assessing psychological trauma and PTSD: A handbook for practitioners* (pp. 399–411). Guilford Press.

Wilbur, C., Bitnun, A., Kronenberg, S., Laxer, R. M., Levy, D. M., Logan, W. J., et al. (2019). PANDAS/PANS in childhood: Controversies and evidence. *Paediatrics and Child Health, 24*(2), 85–91.

Williams, M. T., Rouleau, T. M., La Torre, J. T., & Sharif, N. (2020). Cultural competency in the treatment of obsessive–compulsive disorder: Practitioner guidelines. *The Cognitive Behaviour Therapist, 13*, e48.

World Health Organization (WHO). (2018). *Mental health: Strengthening our response*. http://www.who.int/mediacentre/factsheets/fs220/en/

World Health Organization (WHO). (2020). *Global status report on preventing violence against children 2020*. https://www.unicef.org/media/70731/file/Global-status-report-on-preventing-violence-against-children-2020.pdf

Zai, G., Barta, C., Cath, D., Eapen, V., Geller, D., & Grünblatt, E. (2019). New insights and perspectives on the genetics of obsessive-compulsive disorder. *Psychiatric Genetics, 29*(5), 142–151.

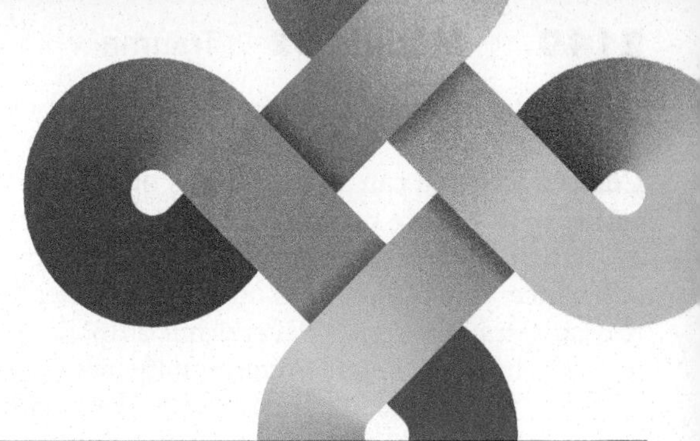

Module 32
Trauma

Module Outline and Learning Outcomes

The Concept of Trauma

Intentional Causes of Trauma

32.1 Analyze intentional trauma.

Community and Systemic Violence

32.2 Analyze community and systemic violence.

Unintentional Causes of Trauma

32.3 Analyze unintentional trauma.

Concepts Related to Trauma

32.4 Outline the relationship between trauma and other concepts.

Health Promotion

32.5 Summarize health promotion as it relates to trauma.

Nursing Assessment

32.6 Differentiate common assessment procedures and tests used to examine trauma.

Independent Interventions

32.7 Analyze independent interventions nurses can implement for patients who have experienced trauma.

Collaborative Therapies

32.8 Summarize collaborative therapies used by interprofessional teams for patients who have experienced trauma.

Trauma Exemplars

Exemplar 32.A Abuse

32.A Analyze abuse as it relates to trauma.

Exemplar 32.B Multisystem Trauma

32.B Analyze multisystem trauma as it relates to trauma.

Exemplar 32.C Posttraumatic Stress Disorder

32.C Analyze posttraumatic stress disorder (PTSD) as it relates to trauma.

Exemplar 32.D Sexual Violence

32.D Analyze sexual violence as it relates to trauma.

» The Concept of Trauma

Concept Key Terms

ABCDEs, **2150**
Adverse childhood experiences (ACEs), **2140**
Aggravated assault, **2143**
Blunt trauma, **2142**
Complex trauma, **2139**
Community violence, **2144**
Cycle of violence, **2142**
Interpersonal violence, **2141**
Major trauma, **2141**
Minor trauma, **2141**
Multisystem trauma, **2141**
Penetrating trauma, **2142**
Physical abuse, **2142**
Precipitating factors, **2148**
Predisposing factors, **2148**
Protective factors, **2148**
Risk factors, **2148**
Sexual abuse, **2142**
Simple assault, **2143**
Trauma, **2139**
Trauma-informed care, **2151**
Triage, **2152**
Vicarious trauma, **2151**
Youth violence, **2145**

According to the Substance Abuse and Mental Health Services Administration (SAMHSA; 2019), **trauma** "results from an event, series of events, or set of circumstances that is experienced by an individual as physically or emotionally harmful or life threatening and that has lasting adverse effects on the individual's functioning and mental, physical, social, emotional, or spiritual well-being."

Traumatic injuries (whether physical, psychologic, or emotional) are associated with intentional or unintentional causes. Intentional causes of trauma include abuse, sexual violence, and human-caused disaster, whereas unintentional causes of trauma include falls, motor-vehicle collisions, and natural disasters. When referring to individuals who have experienced trauma, sometimes the word *survivor* is used and sometimes the word *victim* is used. For the purposes of this concept, *victim* will be used when referring to the victimization of a person or when referring to exact language from research or crime statistics sources. *Survivor* will be used when referring to individuals and patients outside those circumstances. This is consistent with the terms of use of the Rape, Abuse, & Incest National Network (RAINN; 2020a) and other professional organizations.

Trauma can be classified as acute, chronic, or complex. *Acute trauma* occurs when a person experiences a single traumatic event, such as a motor-vehicle crash or a sexual assault. *Chronic trauma* occurs when a person experiences repeated and/or prolonged exposure to traumatic events, such as child abuse. **Complex trauma** results from exposure to multiple traumatic events or an accumulation of traumatic events throughout a lifetime.

Complex traumas result from interrelated forms of traumatic experiences and are often interpersonal in nature. Complex trauma can affect persons of any age and is associated with a wide range of adverse health outcomes such as mental health disorders, posttraumatic stress disorder, substance abuse disorders, and chronic health problems (Complextrauma.org, 2019; Perzichili, 2018). Complex trauma in adults has been linked to community violence, civil unrest, and war (Blue Knot Foundation, 2021). Complex trauma experienced in childhood is often the result of direct, prolonged, or recurrent exposure to harm (abuse, neglect, and exploitation), which can affect brain development and neurochemistry (Blue Knot Foundation, 2021). **Adverse childhood experiences (ACEs)** can contribute to complex trauma. ACEs are traumatic events that occur in childhood that are linked to chronic health problems, mental illness, and substance abuse in adulthood (Centers for Disease Control and Prevention [CDC], 2020a).

Nurses are an integral part of the healthcare team for victims of trauma and must know the fundamentals of trauma care. Each trauma patient will present differently with unique needs based on individual experience; the nursing care plan will need to be person-centered to meet the needs of each patient. A common nursing intervention for all trauma patients is to provide a supportive and safe environment for care.

For patients experiencing physical trauma, interventions will include the following: Assess the patient, identify injuries sustained, and prioritize care of each injury; assess and monitor pain level; assess and monitor mental status; and document clearly and precisely, including all specifics about wounds, as the documentation may be used for legal purposes at a later date.

Interventions appropriate for patients experiencing emotional trauma include the following: Assess and monitor mental status; prioritize mental health needs; validate expressed feelings; and provide community support services information, including a crisis hotline number.

Nursing implications for all criminally related situations (e.g., abuse, neglect, sexual violence) include reporting to proper authorities per established facility protocol and state guidelines; verifying that the patient has a safety plan established; ensuring that the patient has a safe environment to go to following discharge; and, as stated earlier, documenting wounds and injuries clearly and precisely, as the documentation may be used later as evidence.

Alterations and Therapies

Trauma

ALTERATION	DESCRIPTION	MANIFESTATIONS	INTERVENTIONS AND THERAPIES
Physical injury	■ Physical injuries include minor and major intentional and unintentional injuries and medical (sudden and catastrophic or terminal/life threatening) injuries.	■ Lacerations and contusions ■ Sprains, strains, dislocations, and fractures ■ Amputations ■ Puncture wounds ■ Internal injuries or bleeding (laceration of spleen) ■ Shock ■ Hypovolemia ■ Head trauma ■ Loss of senses ■ Respiratory impairment ■ Exposure (chemical, radiation)	■ Assess patient, identifying injuries sustained. ■ Prioritize care of each injury. ■ Assess and monitor pain level. ■ Assess and monitor mental status.
Emotional injury	Emotional stress that evolves after exposure to a traumatic or overwhelming event in which an individual's physical and mental health are endangered. Although most people show resiliency after a traumatic event, some may have symptoms that evolve into exaggerated stress responses.	Immediately following event: ■ Feeling numb or dazed ■ Confusion or disorientation ■ Disbelief and despair ■ Anxiety, nervousness, and fear of the event reoccurring ■ Unresolved emotional responses that evolve into acute stress disorder or PTSD ■ May include flashbacks, nightmares, and recurrent, intrusive memories of the adverse event(s); hypervigilance; avoidance of stimuli associated with the traumatic event	■ Support groups ■ Community support ■ Individual therapy ■ Cognitive-behavioral therapy (CBT) ■ Eye movement desensitization and reprocessing (EMDR) ■ Pharmacologic treatments, which may include antipsychotic agents, antidepressants, and anxiolytics ■ Relaxation techniques, such as massage and guided imagery ■ Mental health counseling

Alterations and Therapies *(continued)*

ALTERATION	DESCRIPTION	MANIFESTATIONS	INTERVENTIONS AND THERAPIES
		▪ May include intense physiologic reactions when exposed to cues that are similar to or representative of some part of the traumatic experience ▪ Manifestations may include some form of dissociation; for example, viewing oneself from the perspective of another individual or being unable to recall certain events related to the traumatic event (American Psychiatric Association, 2013)	
Loss of community	▪ Displaced from home due to any cause that was not by choice (e.g., natural disaster, war, forced immigration, and interpersonal violence) ▪ Loss of ability to communicate secondary to destruction of means of communication or congestion of telephone service ▪ Destruction of roadways ▪ Destruction of stores or markets resulting in a loss of availability of required supplies, food, water, and medicines	▪ Feelings of helplessness and complete loss of control ▪ Anger ▪ Confusion, disorientation ▪ Anxiety, nervousness ▪ Feeling vulnerable, lack of shelter or safety ▪ Basic needs not being met (food, water, shelter, hygiene)	▪ Ensure safety and shelter. ▪ Provide method of communication when available. ▪ Provide food, water, and medications as available. ▪ Offer support. ▪ Refer to community services (Red Cross or other organizations providing aid). ▪ Assist with disaster registries to help reunite separated loved ones.
Complicated grief/traumatic grief	▪ Grief response that is severe, long term, and debilitating. Often related to a sudden loss of life due to unexpected illness, accident, or violent event. ▪ Suicide survivors also experience trauma-related grief. ▪ A risk factor associated with traumatic grief includes being the survivor of disaster. Survivors may experience traumatic grief because they know that their loved one has died or their loved one may be missing and presumed dead	▪ Intense sorrow ▪ Focus is on the death of the loved one ▪ Numbness or detachment ▪ Bitterness, agitation, and irritability ▪ Lack of trust in others ▪ Anhedonia (inability to feel pleasure) and inability to think of positive experiences with the loved one	▪ Psychotherapy (similar to what is used for PTSD) ▪ CBT ▪ Pharmacologic treatments, which may include antidepressants

Intentional Causes of Trauma

Intentional causes of trauma are directly related to **interpersonal violence**. Interpersonal violence occurs within relationships, such as between family members (*family violence*), intimate partners (*intimate partner violence [IPV]*), and acquaintances or strangers (*community violence*). Violence of this nature may include abuse, homicide, physical assault, and sexual violence.

All types of violence are considered violent crime. According to the Federal Bureau of Investigation (FBI; n.d.-a), approximately 1,203,808 violent crimes occurred nationwide in 2019, with aggravated assaults accounting for 68.2% and homicide accounting for 1.4%.

Violence may result in minor or major trauma. **Minor trauma** involves minor injury to a single part or system of the body. A fracture of the clavicle, a small second-degree burn, and a laceration requiring sutures are examples of minor trauma. **Major trauma** involves serious single-system injury (such as the amputation of a leg) or multiple-system injuries (simultaneous injuries such as a punctured lung, traumatic brain injury, and crushed bones in the arms and legs; also called **multisystem trauma**). Multisystem trauma commonly occurs as a result of a motor-vehicle crash but may also be seen with falls, physical assaults, poisonings, and other forms of injury.

Violence may also result in blunt or penetrating trauma. **Blunt trauma** occurs when there is no communication between the damaged tissues and the outside environment. For example, a baseball batter being hit by a pitch may cause damage to the underlying vascular tissue, muscles, and bones. Blunt trauma is frequently caused by motor-vehicle crashes, falls, assaults, and sports activities. **Penetrating trauma** occurs when a foreign object enters the body, causing damage to body structures. Examples of penetrating trauma are gunshot wounds, stab wounds, and impalement.

Violence may occur with a patterned frequency, generally referred to as the **cycle of violence**. The cycle of violence consists of three phases and tends to occur among families and intimate partners. In the first phase, tension builds between individuals in a relationship as communication fails or expectations are not met. During this phase, victims may feel like they are walking on eggshells (Peace Over Violence, n.d.). An abusive or threatening incident occurs in the second phase. During this phase, victims feel traumatized and aggressors blame victims for the incident. The third phase of the cycle is known as the honeymoon period, a time during which aggressors may show love and affection and may also promise to change. During the honeymoon phase, victims may feel responsible for the abuse, consider reconciliation, and recant or minimize the incident. However, tension tends to build again, continuing the cycle (Peace Over Violence, n.d.). When the cycle of violence occurs within families, intergenerational transmission of child abuse and neglect, also known as the *cycle of abuse*, can occur (VanWert, Anreiter, & Fallon, 2019). Through the cycle of abuse, the children who experienced violence at home have an increased likelihood of subjecting their own children to maltreatment.

Violence in the United States is a complex problem and a cause for concern that impacts both the law enforcement community and the healthcare community. The healthcare community may encounter victims of violent acts as they seek treatment at emergency departments, urgent care centers, or physician's offices. For injuries that are psychologic in nature, individuals may seek treatment from counselors, therapists, or other mental health specialists.

Abuse and Neglect

Abuse and neglect occur within all ages, races, and socioeconomic groups. Vulnerable populations such as children, older adults, and people with disabilities experience higher rates of abuse. Nurses should be acutely aware and assess for abuse in all patients, especially vulnerable populations.

Generally, child abuse involves any intentional mistreatment of a child under the age of 18 by someone in a custodial role. Each state has established definitions of what constitutes child abuse. Most states recognize four types of child abuse: physical, neglect, sexual, and emotional. Child abuse is a significant source of ACEs.

Elder abuse is the abuse and neglect of individuals 65 years of age and older. The perpetrator is typically a trusted caregiver. Failure of the caregiver to provide care or protect an older adult from harm also constitutes maltreatment. Types of elder abuse include physical abuse, sexual abuse, emotional or psychologic abuse, neglect, abandonment, and financial or material exploitation (National Council on Aging [NCA], n.d.).

Another group of individuals vulnerable to abuse and neglect are people with physical and developmental disabilities. People with disabilities experience abuse at a much higher rate than people without disabilities. According to Disability Justice (2020), people with disabilities are up to 10 times more likely to be abused than their peers. Children with disabilities are two times more likely to experience abuse or neglect than children without disabilities (Disability Justice, 2020).

Physical Abuse

Common recognizable symptoms of **physical abuse** include unexplained injuries, bruising, and fractures, as well as multiple injuries in different stages of healing. An important cue indicating physical abuse is incongruence between the explanation of an injury and the injury itself. Some signs of physical abuse are less overt and include behavioral changes, depression, withdrawal from friends or family, and suicide attempts.

Neglect

Symptoms of neglect may present differently based on the age group and population. For example, a child who lives in an area with cold winters may be wearing a coat that is not warm enough or may not have warm clothing at all. Poor hygiene, lack of medical or dental care, poor growth and development of a child, or unexplained weight loss in a dependent or older adult are indicative of neglect. Behavioral issues, such as inability to focus or pay attention, stealing food, and apathy, may also be observed.

Sexual Abuse

Sexual abuse differs from sexual assault. With **sexual abuse**, an individual who has perceived power over the victim (e.g., parent, teacher, coach, family friend, or relative) takes advantage of the trust established, luring the victim into sexual activity. In contrast, sexual assault is a nonconsensual act of violence in which physical force or coercion is used to force a victim into sexual activity (RAINN, 2020c). Overt symptoms of sexual abuse may include knowledge about sexually related topics that are inappropriate for the child's age, minors or older adults who present with sexually transmitted infections (STIs), pain upon sitting or walking, and blood in underwear. Because overt symptoms of sexual abuse are not always present, the nurse must also observe for covert manifestations including depression, anxiety, fear, shame, guilt, nightmares, eating disorders, self-neglect, withdrawal, and mistrust of adults. Sexual promiscuity and substance abuse are also common behaviors for victims of sexual abuse.

Emotional Abuse

Symptoms of emotional abuse may be difficult to identify, as they are not as easily observable. Social withdrawal, apathy, and diminished self-confidence and self-esteem may be noted. Psychosomatic issues, such as complaints of not feeling well or unexplained headaches or stomachaches, may also be reported. A pattern of these behaviors warrants assessment.

Physical Assault

Assault is a physical attack or threat of attack that ranges from minor threats to nearly fatal incidents (Bureau of Justice Statistics [BJS], n.d.). Assaults may be classified as aggravated or simple. **Simple assault** is generally considered a physical attack by an individual against another in which a weapon is not used and the attack does not result in serious physical injury. In contrast, **aggravated assault** is a physical attack or attempted attack in which a weapon is used, with or without resulting injury, and also an attack without a weapon that results in serious injury (BJS, n.d.).

Sexual Violence

The CDC (2020l) contends that sexual violence is a serious public health problem that impacts every community and affects people of all ages, genders, and sexual orientations. Sexual violence results in various forms of traumatic injuries (physical and emotional) and includes sexual assault, human trafficking, and online enticement. *Sexual assault is any type of sexual contact without consent of the victim.*

Human sex trafficking is a major domestic and international concern that has come to the attention of authorities, healthcare providers (HCPs), policymakers, and the public. In the decade that the FBI (n.d.-a) has been collecting human-trafficking data, there has been a steady increase in reported incidents. In 2019, the state of Texas had the highest occurrence of sex trafficking, with 337 reported cases. Sex trafficking is a profitable criminal industry, based on supply and demand, that has had rapid expansion, as evidenced by the increase in cases (National Human Trafficking Hotline, n.d.).

Online enticement is the use of the internet to communicate with a child with the intent to exploit. Often there is sexual intent, in which a perpetrator entices or persuades a child to participate in sexual acts (National Center for Missing and Exploited Children ([NCMEC], 2020a). Online enticement occurs in a variety of ways to children of all ages and genders. See Exemplar 32.D, Sexual Violence, later in this module for more information.

Self-Directed Violence

Self-directed violence, often referred to as *nonsuicidal self-injury (NSSI)*, is any action a person takes intentionally to harm or injure the self. Suicide and NSSI are types of self-directed violence. Suicide includes attempted and completed suicides. Common types of NSSI include self-mutilation (cutting), head banging, self-biting (including extreme nail biting), and self-scratching (including interfering with wound healing). According to the CDC (2019), behaviors such as head banging, self-biting, and self-scratching are more common in youth with disability.

Homicide

Homicide occurs when the unlawful acts of a perpetrator result in the death of a victim. According to the FBI (n.d.-a), there were an estimated 16,425 homicides in 2019, a slight increase over the previous year. In addition to caring for the victims of assault and attempted homicide, nurses may also be responsible for caring for perpetrators. Nurses provide the same high quality of care for all patients regardless of the events that have led them to seek medical treatment.

SAFETY ALERT In situations in which patients have the potential to become violent toward the healthcare professionals working to treat their injuries, nurses should take appropriate precautions. In the clinical setting, security personnel or police officers should be present when needed.

Prevalence

In the United States, violence and accompanying trauma-related events are widespread and affect people of all ages. Alarmingly, in 2017 more than 1.7 million people were treated for an assault-related injury and 19,000 people were victims of homicide (CDC, 2020m). The CDC (2020m) identifies homicide as the third leading cause of death in young people ages 10 to 24. Cases of child maltreatment reported to local and state agencies indicate that nearly 700,000 children are abused and neglected in the United States each year (National Children's Alliance, 2019b). Data about maltreatment of older adults is harder to assess, largely because it is extremely underreported and often occurs at the hands of the person's caregiver. CDC (2020j) data from the years 2002 to 2016 indicate that more than 643,000 older adults were treated for nonfatal assaults and over 19,000 homicides occurred during that time period.

Genetic Considerations and Risk Factors

To better understand the causes and risk factors of the occurrence of trauma, specifically related to violence, researchers have conducted studies about the influence that genetic predisposition, age, and gender have on people who commit violent acts. Each of these lenses explores the scope of violent behavior.

Genetic Predispositions Toward Violence

Epigenetics is the study of how behaviors and environment can cause changes in genes. Through investigation of epigenetics, researchers study whether a genetic predisposition toward violent behavior exists. Epigenetic changes begin before birth and continue throughout life (CDC, 2020t). For example, exposure to traumatic conditions, such as interpersonal violence in childhood, can increase an individual's risk of developing violent behaviors (CDC, 2020t).

Genetic disorders that relate to social and mental health are often discussed in conjunction with studies that look at the genetic predisposition toward violence. The presence of a mental health disorder is not a predictor of violence but may be a contributing factor, especially if it goes untreated (Harvard Health Publishing, 2021). Zhang-James et al. (2019) suggest that violent behavior is the result of multiple interacting factors, including genetics, environment, and culture. For instance, human aggression and antisocial behaviors may be learned from environmental exposure to the same and are also heritable traits associated with the *monoamine oxidase A (MAOA)* gene (Clukay, 2019).

Age

Violence and associated trauma affect people at all ages from infant to elderly. For youth, ACEs are associated with experiencing or witnessing violence and are contributing factors to experiencing or perpetrating violence in the future. In a survey conducted by the CDC (2020a), approximately 61% of adults reported that they had experienced at least one ACE. In a study examining the trajectory of violence, Fahlgren et al. (2020) found that perpetration of violence peaks in young adulthood and then decreases across the lifespan.

A number of behaviors displayed in youth are considered risk factors for becoming a violent perpetrator. These include a history of being a victim of violence, low IQ, substance use or abuse, history of early aggressive behaviors, deficits in social-cognitive or information-processing abilities, and exposure to violence and conflict in the family (CDC, 2020g).

Gender

Gender is a contributing factor to violence and is connected to both perpetrators and victims of violence. Fahlgren et al. (2020) found that violence was more prevalent among males. According to the CDC (2020l), several factors are associated with an increased risk for violent behavior in males, including impulsiveness, aggression, substance abuse, and unemployment. Although individuals of any gender may become victims of violence, females are victims of IPV more frequently than males. Physical violence and resulting traumatic injury at the hands of an intimate partner affected 35% of female victims versus 11% of male victims (CDC, 2020k).

Gender-based violence (GBV) is a global pandemic (World Bank, 2019). GBV is violence that is directed against people because of their gender identity. The prominent victims of GBV are women and girls, with one in three women being affected by violence in their lifetime (World Bank, 2019). GBV also disproportionately affects the transgender and gender-nonconforming population (Roberts, 2020). The Human Rights Campaign has been tracking violence against transgender and gender non-conforming persons since 2013. The year 2020 marked a grim milestone, with 37 transgender and gender-nonconforming people being violently killed, more than any other year recorded (Roberts, 2020).

Case Study » Part 1

A gunshot victim is en route to the emergency department (ED) by ambulance. You will be the patient's admitting nurse. At present, you have minimal information about the patient. The paramedics report that the bleeding is controlled and the patient is alert with temperature 97.0°F oral; pulse 92 beats/min; respirations 22/min; and blood pressure 105/75 mmHg. It is currently unclear how much blood loss the patient has sustained. The ambulance's ETA (estimated time of arrival) is 5 minutes.

Clinical Reasoning Questions Level I

1. How would severe blood loss affect the patient's blood pressure?
2. What are the primary nursing considerations for this patient?

Clinical Reasoning Questions Level II

3. Consider your perceptions of this patient, knowing only that this individual is a gunshot victim. What is your initial response?
4. How would your perceptions change if the patient is a victim of IPV? An alleged perpetrator or criminal assailant? Someone who was injured while protecting another individual from harm? Explain your perceptions for each category.
5. Describe the symptoms of severe blood loss and shock. Describe the nursing interventions for a patient who presents with severe blood loss.

Community and Systemic Violence

Although violence often occurs between two individuals, violence can also occur at a community level and within organizations such as the workplace or school. Community and systemic violence often involve multiple victims with varying degrees of trauma. This can put a strain on ED resources and healthcare workers because of the rapid influx of a large number of patients, some of whom will likely have life-threatening injuries.

Community Violence

The Violence Policy Center (2017, p. 4) defines **community violence** as "Exposure to intentional acts of interpersonal violence committed in public areas by individuals who are not intimately related to the victim." Community violence encompasses various types of violence, including shootings, gang violence, bullying, bias-motivated violence (hate crimes), and social unrest (see the Focus on Diversity and Culture feature). Community violence can take place in any community setting, including neighborhoods, clinics and businesses (workplaces), and schools.

Workplace Violence

Workplace violence (WPV) is prevalent in healthcare settings. Healthcare workers are four times more likely to be victimized than workers in private industry (The Joint Commission, 2018). Locke, Bromley, and Federspiel (2018) note

Focus on Diversity and Culture

Extremists and Gangs

Some cultural groups, such as extremists and gangs, hold beliefs or ideologies that legitimize the ability to commit acts of violence upon others. Extremists such as the Islamic State of Iraq and Syria (ISIS) and white supremacist groups such as the Aryan Brotherhood are similarly known for their propensity for violent acts (FBI, n.d.-b). As an act of homage to their belief systems, these groups commit crimes against a person or property with the underlying motivation of bias against ethnicity, race, religion, gender identity, or sexual orientation (FBI, n.d.-b).

Political extremists have used violence as an act of revenge against political decisions that do not align with their belief system. For example, on January 6, 2021, a mob of political extremists who believed the 2020 U.S. presidential election results were fraudulent rioted at the U.S. Capitol. They subsequently breached security and stormed the chambers of the U.S. Congress. Their violent attack on the nation's capital targeted members of Congress and resulted in injuries to well over 100 capitol police officers and five deaths (National Public Radio, 2021).

The presence of gangs in a community creates significant challenges to community safety. As reported by the FBI (n.d.-c), there are 33,000 violent street gangs, motorcycle gangs, and prison gangs active in both urban and rural areas in the United States today. Typically, gangs use violence to control neighborhoods and support illegal money-making activities including drug and gun trafficking as well as prostitution and human trafficking (FBI, n.d.-c). Street gangs target teens for recruitment, which supports findings that there is a high propensity for violence in youth (Fahlgren et al., 2020).

that 67% of all non-fatal WPV injuries occur in healthcare settings, yet healthcare represents only 11.5% of the U.S. workforce. Furthermore, one in four nurses is assaulted at work (American Nurses Association [ANA], 2020). Most incidents of WPV in healthcare are verbal in nature and commonly involve patients and/or visitors. Other incidents involve assault, battery, stalking, and sexual harassment. Contributing factors for violent episodes included long wait times, patients with psychiatric problems, patients under the influence of drugs or alcohol, and patients with a history of violent behavior (Locke et al., 2018).

The Joint Commission (2018) captured sentinel event data that revealed 68 incidents of homicide, rape, or assault of hospital staff members over an 8-year period. Incidents of WPV are likely underreported as nurses may minimize their importance, viewing the incidents as part of the job. The American Nurses Association warns that violence is not just part of the job and that ED and psychiatric nurses are most at risk to experience violence from a patient (Locke et al., 2018).

Incivility and bullying in nursing practice are forms of workplace violence that exist in the healthcare setting. Incivility and bullying are often directed horizontally (horizontal violence) by employee against employee but can also occur between employee and employer. Incivility and bullying violate professional nursing standards of practice, including the ethical code that underpins nursing practice. In a position statement, the ANA (2015) advises that even when incivility is not necessarily directed at a specific person or persons, that does not render it inconsequential, as incivility of any kind can negatively impact individuals, peers, clients, and organizations. Moreover, incivility can be a precursor to bullying. Incivility is often evidenced by discourteous actions, use of a condescending tone, gossiping, name-calling, and refusing to assist a coworker (ANA, 2015).

In contrast, bullying is repeated behavior, often directed toward a specific person, with the intent to undermine, humiliate, offend, degrade, and cause distress or harm (ANA, 2015). Bullying is evidenced by actions similar to those as incivility but with greater frequency and intensity (ANA, 2015). With bullying, intense actions such as hostile remarks, threats, and intimidation may be evident.

The negative impacts of incivility and bullying can be significant and may progress to more violent acts or situations if left unaddressed. Nurses who experience incivility or bullying may experience a barrage of symptoms that mimic posttraumatic stress disorder, including headaches, sleep disruptions, intestinal problems, anxiety, irritability, and depression (ANA, 2015). When nurses feel insecure and unsafe at work, it can affect their ability to care for patients and ultimately can negatively impact patient well-being and outcomes. All nurses are susceptible to incivility and bullying but novice nurses, within their first few years of practice, may be at higher risk. The ANA (2015) calls for both novice and experienced nurses to respect each other and treat each other fairly.

SAFETY ALERT Nurses will encounter violent patients at times; therefore, it is important to monitor for and identify warning signs that a patient may be escalating so that nurses and other staff can act to deescalate the patient's behaviors. Some indications that a patient may become aggressive include pacing, loud voice, reddened face, clenched fists, and rigid posture.

Youth Violence

Youth violence is an ACE that occurs in minors and may continue into young adulthood. Youth violence may include being a victim of violence, a person who commits violence, or a witness to violence. Every day, approximately 14 young people ages 10 to 24 die from homicide and more than 1,300 are treated for violence-related injuries (CDC, 2020u).

Violence, whether perpetrated by an adult or a youth, is associated with risk factors such as truancy and failure in school, substance abuse, involvement in gangs, and toxic (prolonged and recurrent) stress (CDC, 2020u). Witnessing violence in the family, being abused, and prolonged exposure to a community culture of violence can all condition children and adolescents to view violence as an acceptable means of solving problems (CDC, 2020u). Violence has a negative effect on communities, increases healthcare costs, decreases property values, and disrupts social services (CDC, 2020u).

School Violence

School violence is a form of youth violence that negatively affects students, schools, and the communities in which they reside. Violent behaviors linked to the school setting include bullying, fighting, and gang violence. A survey conducted in 2019 that evaluated occurrences of school violence within the past year found that 8% of high school students experienced a physical fight on school property and more than 7% had been threatened or injured with a weapon on school property (CDC, 2020u). According to the CDC (2020u), 1–2% of all homicides happen on school grounds or on the way to or from a school-sponsored event.

Bullying

Bullying is a form of youth violence and is defined as "any unwanted aggressive behavior(s) by another youth or group of youths, who are not siblings or current dating partners, involving an observed or perceived power imbalance that is repeated multiple times or is highly likely to be repeated" (CDC, 2020u). Bullying occurs frequently in the high school setting, with one in five students reporting being bullied (CDC, 2020u). Youth who are lesbian, gay, bisexual, or unsure of their sexual orientation experience bullying more frequently than their heterosexual peers (CDC, 2020u). Bullying can be overt, where perpetrators use physical aggression, tease, and call the victim names. However, more passive bullying methods may be prevalent, such as spreading rumors, intentionally leaving the victim out of a group activity, and encouraging others to exclude the victim. Bullying may result in physical injuries, psychologic injuries, and emotional distress and may disturb academic progress.

Cyberbullying, in which technology (i.e., text messages, chat rooms, and social media) is used to bully, has become common. Youth can use technology to threaten, embarrass, and harass their peers. Reports on bullying indicate that one in six high school students has experienced cyberbullying (CDC, 2020u). Cyberbullying allows for anonymity of the bully, which makes it difficult for parents, caregivers, or authorities to address the behavior.

Youth who experience bullying (victim, perpetrator, or witness) have an increased risk for suicidal behaviors as well as increased negative physical and emotional outcomes (Duan et al., 2020). Current research suggests that students who experience bullying are almost two times as likely to attempt suicide (Hinduja & Patchin, 2018). Due to the relationship between bullying and suicide, all 50 states have enacted legislation or policies within educational districts to both prevent bullying and respond to bullying when it occurs (CDC, 2020u).

SAFETY ALERT Screenings of all youth at school and healthcare settings should include questions related to bullying to identify risk factors and occurrences early so that intervention can be planned.

Human-Caused Disasters

Intentional trauma can be caused by human action or inaction. Often intentional trauma that is human caused results in a *disaster*, which is an event that causes great damage or loss of life. Human causes of intentional trauma include mass shootings, chemical spills, terrorist attacks, and war. Deployment to and events experienced in war can cause trauma-related stress for military personnel and their families. Military personnel who return from deployment may experience posttraumatic stress disorder (PTSD), a debilitating constellation of symptoms (including intrusive thoughts, flashbacks, anxiety) that may result from exposure to a traumatic event.

Firearm Violence and Mass Shooter Incidents

Firearm violence is a persistent and frequent problem within communities the United States that has a devastating impact. Firearm-related injuries affect people of all stages of life and are one of the five leading causes of homicide in people age 1 to 64. Firearm suicide rates are highest among people age 75 years and older, whereas firearm homicide rates are highest among teens and young adults age 15 to 34 years (CDC, 2020e). Firearm violence disproportionately affects Black, American Indian/Alaskan Native, and Hispanic populations as they experience the highest homicide rates (CDC, 2020e). Firearm violence in schools tends to mirror firearm violence nationally, with a higher incidence among Black students (Everytown Research & Policy, 2019a). In 2019 there were approximately 130 incidents of gunfire on school grounds resulting in 32 deaths, including 4 suicide deaths and 77 injuries (Everytown Research & Policy, 2019a).

The FBI (2020, p. 3) describes mass-shooting incidents as those that involve an "active shooter" where "one or more individuals actively engage in killing or attempting to kill people in a populated area." Of the shooting incidents that occurred in 2019, 28 were designated as active-shooter incidents (FBI, 2020). Active-shooter incidents often result in mass shootings, which are defined as the killing of three or more people in a single incident; 12 of the 28 designated active-shooter incidents in 2019 were deemed mass shootings (FBI, 2020). These mass shootings resulted in 247 casualties, with 97 killed and 150 injured (FBI, 2020). The devastation and impact of mass-shooting incidents reach far beyond persons killed or injured to negatively influence the health and well-being of survivors and the community.

One of the most devastating mass shootings in modern U.S. history occurred on October 1, 2017, when an active shooter opened fire upon a large crowd in attendance at a music festival on the Las Vegas strip. The mass shooting resulted in 58 deaths and more than 400 injuries (Everytown Research & Policy, 2019b). Mass shootings occur all too frequently in educational environments, including at Marjory Stoneman Douglas High School in Parkland, Florida, on February 14, 2018, where a former student killed 17 students and staff members and injured another 17 (Everytown Research & Policy, 2019b).

Systemic Violence

Systemic violence, also known as structural violence, refers to the trauma people experience due to issues within social structures (i.e., education, legal, politics, and religion), deliberate social injustices, or inequality (Lewis, 2020). Some examples of systemic violence include health, economic, gender, and racial disparities. Systemic violence often violates human rights, prevents persons from satisfying their basic needs, perpetuates poverty, causes injury or homicide, and potentiates mass murders and war.

Systemic violence is linked with historical trauma. *Historical trauma* describes the cumulative emotional and psychologic injuries that result from traumatic experiences spanning generations in a community. It is often associated with racial or ethnic groups that have experienced widespread oppression in the form of violence, slavery, persecution, and discrimination. Historical trauma is also associated with living in areas of war or conflict, especially for persons forcefully displaced from their homes to become refugees or to immigrate to other areas.

Long-term effects of historical trauma can include poor health outcomes, substance abuse, and a propensity for violent behavior (U.S. Department of Health and Human Services [DHHS], n.d.-b). Additionally, high rates of suicide are observed in persons who have experienced historical trauma (DHHS, n.d.-b).

Unintentional Causes of Trauma

Unintentional trauma or unintentional injury is caused by unplanned actions. It is one of the 10 leading causes of death in the United States and the leading cause of death in children and in adults younger than age 45 (Herron, 2019). Injuries from unintentional trauma are commonly caused by falls, motor-vehicle collisions, and drug overdoses. Unintentional injury from firearm violence and drug overdose (most involving opioids) have been on the rise (Herron, 2019; Scholl, Seth, Kariisa, Wilson, & Baldwin, 2019).

Serious accidents, injuries, and catastrophic events can have a major physical and emotional impact on patients. Traumatic injuries are often complex and not isolated to one body system. Multisystem trauma occurs when injury involves multiple body systems, such as to the cardiac, respiratory, integumentary, or musculoskeletal systems, and are frequently associated with motor-vehicle crashes (see Exemplar 32.B, Multisystem Trauma, in this module) but may also be seen in the form of direct injuries occurring during or following natural disasters (see **Box 32.1** »).

Concepts Related to Trauma

Trauma is related to various nursing practices, among them the concepts of communication, sexuality, and stress and coping.

Communication is vital in all areas of nursing, especially when violence is a contributing factor. Patients who have been exposed to a traumatic situation are likely to be experiencing pain (both physical and emotional) and significant amounts of stress. Nurses need to employ therapeutic communication to help patients work through the stress.

In addition, the concepts of comfort, development, grief, and ethics are associated with trauma. Comfort measures will need to be employed to address the physical discomfort and emotional trauma. If tragedy strikes a child, development could be altered. Traumatic events may cause such strong responses that they may impair emotional development.

Grief is the powerful, normal response that people experience following a painful or traumatic event such as the death of a loved one. Grief manifests itself physically, emotionally, mentally, and spiritually. Each person grieves in a unique way. There is no specific timetable for how long someone experiences grief, although most survivors gradually feel grief dissipating within weeks to months (Kraybill, 2019). Some, however, experience traumatic grief, which is severe and prolonged grief that can interfere with daily functioning. Traumatic grief often occurs in response to being diagnosed with a terminal disease or if an unexpected violent death occurs (Kraybill, 2019). Traumatic grief can lead to exaggerated reactions and even PTSD.

Ethical principles will guide practice related to trauma victims. Treatment requires informed consent; however, trauma victims are often unable to give consent, so the HCP will need to obtain alternative consent, such as from a parent, caregiver, spouse, or designated healthcare advocate. Some, but not all, of the concepts related to trauma are outlined in the Concepts Related to Trauma feature. They are presented in alphabetical order.

Box 32.1
Natural Disasters

Natural disasters—such as earthquakes, floods, tornadoes, hurricanes, and wildfires—affect thousands of people every year. Natural disasters have the ability to cause severe emotional and physical trauma, major destruction, and death. Survivors of natural disasters may experience a range of mental and physical reactions, including a mild to moderate stress response during and immediately after the disaster. Some survivors exhibit resiliency after disasters, whereas others may experience chronic or debilitating stress responses, such as PTSD, that will require medical intervention (U.S. Department of Veterans Affairs [VA], 2019a). Individuals who are displaced (unable to return home due to extensive damage) appear to experience greater symptom burden than those who are able to remain in their homes in the aftermath of a disaster (Makwana, 2019; Schwartz, Liu, Lieberman-Cribbin, & Taioli, 2017). Physical injuries vary according to the nature of the disaster and disaster-related behaviors. For example, chainsaw injuries are a common result of tree removal following hurricanes and other windstorms (CDC, 2017). See Exemplar 32.B, Multisystem Trauma, in this module for information on nursing care of individuals during and immediately after a crisis.

Impact from natural disasters is seen across communities, necessitating a multilayered response by emergency personnel. In August 2020, a derecho (intense, widespread, and fast-moving windstorm or thunderstorm) tracked across eastern Iowa and northern Illinois, bringing wind gusts between 100 and 126 mph and two tornadoes, causing extensive damage to homes across several midwestern states. The devastating storm caused widespread displacement, numerous injuries, and death (National Weather Service, 2020). See Exemplar 46.A, Emergency Preparedness, in Module 46, Healthcare Systems, for information about emergency management.

Concepts Related to
Trauma

CONCEPT	RELATIONSHIP TO TRAUMA	NURSING IMPLICATIONS
Comfort	Physical needs will need to be met so that psychologic needs may be addressed. Pain will need to be assessed and controlled. Assistance with meeting basic needs such as food, shelter, and the ability to maintain personal hygiene may be necessary.	■ Assess and monitor pain; administer analgesics as prescribed. ■ Employ comfort measures to decrease stress, such as warm blankets, relaxation techniques, and reassurance of safety. ■ Provide supplies and opportunity to tend to basic hygiene.
Communication	Clear and therapeutic communication with patients after a violent or traumatic experience can help alleviate stress and facilitate acceptance.	■ Use therapeutic communication to facilitate healing and acceptance. ■ Encourage the patient to ask questions. ■ Explain any procedures or tests suggested to the patient. ■ Use appropriate nonverbal communication (body language) to encourage open communication.
Development	The neurobiological impact of a traumatic event is contingent on the developmental stage of a child having experienced a traumatic event or a series of traumatic events.	■ Use therapeutic communication to promote trust and feelings of safety; use age-appropriate terminology. ■ Provide reassurance. ■ Encourage child to ask questions. ■ Explain any procedures or tests suggested to the patient. ■ Maintain therapeutic environment with decreased stimulation to assist in feelings of safety.

(continued on next page)

Concepts Related to *(continued)*

CONCEPT	RELATIONSHIP TO TRAUMA	NURSING IMPLICATIONS
Ethics	Traumatic situations require principles of ethical nursing care so that effective treatment may be obtained by the victims; this promotes the most positive outcomes possible.	Promote principles of ethical nursing care: ■ Autonomy—allow patients to make decisions for themselves; informed consent. ■ Beneficence—compassionate care such as administering analgesics to control physical pain. ■ Nonmaleficence—Follow institutional guidelines and established best practice while administering care. ■ Justice—Equal and fair treatment; prioritizing victims' injuries accurately (Haddad & Geiger, 2020).
Grief and Loss	Trauma-related incidents, especially related to disasters and sudden unexpected death of a loved one, are risk factors associated with traumatic grief.	■ Assess for safety. ■ Use therapeutic communication. ■ Promote trust. ■ Validate patient feelings. ■ Assess spiritual needs. ■ Assist with disaster registries to find missing loved ones.
Sexuality	Sexual trauma is a form of violence that can cause both psychologic and physical trauma. Sexual trauma can also result in diseases, infections, and unwanted pregnancy.	■ For victims of sexual assault, assessment may include use of a sexual assault evidence collection kit. ■ Educate about options regarding the possibility of unwanted pregnancy (e.g., emergency contraception). ■ Educate about tests for STIs. ■ Facilitate referrals to resources such as support groups, therapy, and counseling.
Stress and Coping	All forms of trauma can cause stress, potentially leading to exacerbation of the injury and increased emotional strain.	■ Communicate with the patient regarding needs and wants, especially those in relation to stress relief (e.g., the presence of a family member or friend). ■ Answer questions regarding treatment and injuries calmly and honestly.

Health Promotion

Health promotion methods to reduce morbidity and mortality must address trauma prevention. To implement preventive measures, factors that cause trauma need to be examined. Trauma often results from a combination of predisposing, precipitating, and protective factors in several areas. **Predisposing factors** increase an individual's risk of being a victim of a traumatic experience or causing a traumatic experience for others (i.e., perpetrating violence). **Precipitating factors** trigger an event or incident. **Protective factors** reduce the risk of perpetration and victimization.

Many factors influence an individual's response to traumatic events, in terms of both vulnerability factors and **risk factors**. Influencing factors do not cause destructive behavior, nor do they wholly determine that an individual will become a victim; rather, factors such as these can define trends and warning signs. For example, an individual may have a childhood history of being abused, reacting with anger, and experiencing academic failures from a young age. All of these elements are predisposing factors to violent behavior, but they are not determining factors (CDC, 2020c).

Predisposing Factors

Predisposing factors for trauma include environmental, psychologic, cultural, and behavioral variables. Geographical and environmental factors can deeply affect other aspects of an individual's life. Living in an impoverished community, especially one with a strong presence of gangs and drugs, puts an individual at increased risk for witnessing, experiencing, or even committing acts of violence (CDC, 2020c). These environmental situations can also become cyclical, with multiple generations feeling trapped in the same community with the same high levels of violence.

Families themselves can be a predisposing factor to violence, especially if there is a history of abuse and neglect within the family or if family members are involved in drug or alcohol abuse. Other influencing variables are individual or behavioral in nature, such as a preoccupation with danger or violence, a history of abusing or torturing animals, or a history of bullying (either as the bully or as the bullied). Psychologic predisposing factors include aggressive tendencies, uncontrolled anger, extreme emotional distress, emotional instability, and depression (CDC, 2020k).

Protective Factors

In contrast to predisposing factors to violence and trauma, protective factors reduce the risk of becoming a perpetrator or experiencing debilitating responses to traumatic situations. Many of these protective factors apply to adolescents. For example, connectedness to school has been found to be a protective factor for youth violence (CDC, 2020v) (**Figure 32.1** »).

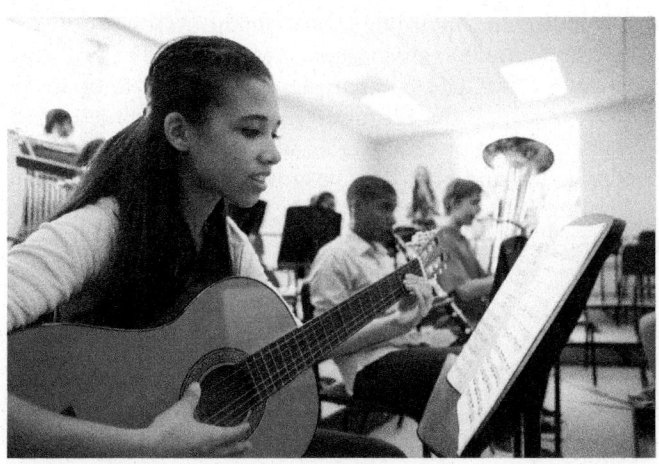

Figure 32.1 >> Connectedness and success in school decrease risks associated with violence and promote resilience to trauma.
Source: Shutterstock

According to the CDC (2020v), some variables that decrease risks associated with violence include:

- Determination and success in school
- Healthy and positive social relationships
- Parents who show interest in their child's experiences
- Involvement in the community
- Participation in family activities
- Participation in cultural or religious practices
- Strong emotional support from friends and family.

Over time, most people will recover from trauma and move forward with their lives without having severe, chronic mental health issues. Factors that can increase resiliency include a strong, well-developed support system; effective coping skills and the positive belief that one can survive; hope, including feelings of optimism; spiritual beliefs; and practical resources (VA, 2019a).

Promoting Safety

Anyone can become a perpetrator or victim of violence or abuse, and anyone can develop chronic mental health issues following traumatic situations. Knowing the warning signs of violent behavior can help promote safety. Warning signs of potentially violent behavior include uncontrolled anger, threatening language, and aggression.

Promoting a healthy community and reducing violence involves changing the roots of negative behavior in individual homes, in schools, and within the community. Community programs should focus on education regarding abuse, bullying, and neighborhood violence. Middle and high schools should include a curriculum about dating violence, bullying, and overall safety. Youth centers devoted to healthy recreational and educational activities can help prevent youth violence.

Nurses can help promote safety by educating patients about high-risk situations, such as IPV, drug-facilitated sexual assault, and violence. Assessing the signs of abuse and offering interventions can also help establish safety. Nurses working in schools or other community settings can help dispel myths about aggression and abuse, reinforcing that it is never acceptable for someone to control or injure another person. Assessing for inadequate coping mechanisms, signs of inadequate anger management, or inappropriate behavior can help identify risk factors and implement behavior therapy before someone is victimized.

Promotion of safety has been addressed through the political advocacy measures of nurses. In 2019, the U.S. House of Representatives passed the Workplace Violence Prevention for HealthCare and Social Service Workers Act and sent it to the U.S. Senate for action. The act, if approved by the Senate and signed into law, would promote safety as it requires employers to implement comprehensive plans that protect healthcare professionals from violence in the workplace (ANA, 2020).

Community safety can be promoted through disaster prevention measures. Natural disasters happen in predictable ways and people living in susceptible regions should be educated on how to prepare. In example, communities on the West Coast should be educated on wildfires and tropical storms whereas people in the Midwest should be educated on tornados and derechos. Community education should include making preparations and gathering supplies, implementing a communication plan, and choosing a family meeting place if separated. Nurses must remain current with new, evidence-based practice initiatives to help promote safety for individuals, patients, facilities, and the community during and after traumatic events.

Trauma Prevention

Promoting safe behaviors and prevention measures can have a large impact on decreasing trauma-related injuries and death. Nurses must demonstrate a proactive role in safety and prevention of trauma. Areas of health promotion and trauma prevention interventions for individuals and communities include the following:

- ***Motor-vehicle safety.*** Teach individuals and families on the use of seat belts and helmets as appropriate, have properly functioning air bags, avoid driving under the influence of alcohol or drugs, refrain from reckless driving, test for visual or cognitive deficits in older adults, avoid cell phone use while driving, avoid driving while fatigued, and reduce distraction of young drivers by limiting the number of passengers.
- ***Relationships.*** Teach communities how to recognize IPV, child abuse, elder abuse, abuse of developmentally delayed persons, or neglect.
- ***Communities.*** Promote gun control, reduce participation in gangs, improve the condition of streets, promote neighborhood safety, and review child abuse and fatalities for trends.

One example of a community trauma prevention strategy or intervention is the CDC's STOP SV technical package. The package provides evidence-based strategies and programs to help communities prevent and reduce sexual violence (CDC, 2020l). Many of the strategies are proactive and are targeted at reducing the likelihood that sexual violence will be perpetrated. Community health nurses, school nurses, and visiting nurses are important members of the community team focusing on preventing sexual violence.

Nursing Assessment

Conducting an ACEs screen to determine a patient's history of trauma can be an important aspect of assessment. ACEs are strong predictors of health outcomes (CDC, 2020a; Tribie, 2019). Screening for ACEs, via a survey questionnaire, can inform the patient's plan of care and allow nurses to provide more holistic care.

Assessment of a trauma patient will depend on the nature and extent of the injuries. Manifestation of injuries from trauma will vary depending on the patient's overall disposition, experience, age, and history. Because both acute trauma and chronic trauma can lead to long-standing mental health issues such as depression, anxiety, and PTSD, the nurse not only must address the physical injuries identified but also should perform a mental health assessment. During the assessment phase, it is imperative for nurses to consider the patient's cultural and spiritual practices because these can have a bearing on further treatment, interventions, and outcomes.

Abuse Assessment

When conducting assessment, the nurse is responsible to be alert for signs and symptoms of abuse including IPV. The nurse who suspects abuse must ensure privacy and safety for the patient. Furthermore, the nurse must follow state regulations and organizational policies regarding mandatory reporting. Victims of physical abuse may sustain a variety of injuries, some of which may be in various stages of healing. During a head-to-toe assessment, the nurse may observe for indications of abuse, such as contusions, open wounds, cuts, hematomas, scars, edema, fractures or evidence of previous fractures, and genital/anal injury (including bruising and bleeding).

Trauma Assessment

Violence- or disaster-related events result in traumatic injury that may involve multiple systems that may require a variety of nursing interventions. Because of the serious consequences of trauma, it is important to identify the patient's injuries and institute appropriate interventions immediately. When caring for the trauma patient, the nurse must prioritize assessments and rapidly intervene for life-threatening injuries. The **ABCDE** mnemonic helps the nurse identify the highest-priority concerns (American College of Surgeons Committee on Trauma [ACSCOT], 2017; Emergency Nurses Association [ENA], 2020):

- Airway with cervical spine protection and alertness. Assess for airway patency and ability of the patient to maintain the airway. The cervical spine is protected with manual stabilization or immobilization with a cervical collar. The **AVPU** mnemonic is used to assess alertness: **A**, alert; **V**, responds to verbal stimuli; **P**, responds to pain; **U**, unresponsive.
- Breathing and ventilation. Assess chest by inspection, auscultation, and palpation to identify signs of breathing inadequacy or chest trauma (i.e., pneumothorax).
- Circulation with hemorrhage control. Assess skin color, capillary refill, and palpate central and peripheral pulses. If signs of external bleeding are noted, the ABC may be reprioritized to CAB to control hemorrhage.
- Disability and neurologic assessment. Assess pupillary function and level of consciousness (LOC). The Glasgow Coma Scale (GCS) is a scoring system used to quantify LOC in which the score ranges between 1 and 15 (for more information on the GCS, see Module 11, Intracranial Regulation and Skill 7.1, Glasgow Coma Scale: Using, in Volume 3).
- Exposure and environmental control. Assess for obvious injuries and uncontrolled bleeding. The patient is completely undressed for thorough inspection and therefore must be protected from hypothermia by using warming devices, warmed covers, and warm fluids.

If lifesaving interventions are identified in the assessment of any of the ABCDEs, the nurse will treat the injury to stabilize the patient before moving on with the assessment. Once the priority assessments have been conducted and needs have been met, the nurse will then conduct a more complete assessment or a focused assessment on an identified injury. In further assessment a detailed history and description of current symptoms should be obtained to ensure that mental and emotional injuries are identified along with physical injuries. See the Focus on Diversity and Culture feature for an overview of considerations of patients' cultural and religious practices when providing trauma care.

Diagnostic Tests

The diagnostic tests ordered once the patient reaches the hospital depend on the type of injury the patient has sustained. Tests that may be ordered for victims of trauma include the following (ENA, 2020; Family Practice Notebook, 2021):

- ***Blood type and crossmatch*** in the event blood transfusion may be necessary
- ***Blood alcohol level*** to screen for the amount of alcohol in the patient's blood, which may alter consciousness and pain response

Focus on Diversity and Culture

Religious Practice Considerations for Trauma

Assessment of patients' religious preferences regarding treatment and rehabilitation is critical.

Cultural and spiritual considerations in treatments for trauma are numerous and will vary based on the incident (e.g., abuse vs. extensive trauma). For example, Christian Scientists believe that healing is a matter of faith and find that they can live happy and healthy lives without drugs and traditional medical interventions (Christian Science, 2021). Jehovah's Witnesses (2021) believe it is in defiance of their religious scripture to accept blood transfusions, even as a lifesaving procedure. If a patient participates in a religion that prohibits blood transfusions or any lifesaving procedure, nurses and physicians should explain the dangers and potential outcomes of not accepting the procedure, as well as educate the patient and family on alternative options, but ultimately the care team must honor the patient's decision.

- ***Urine drug screen***, which may be ordered to assess for the presence of drugs or toxins
- ***Pregnancy test*** to rule out pregnancy in women of child-bearing age
- ***Focused assessment by sonography in trauma (FAST)*** exam to assess for the presence of blood in body cavities, primarily in the peritoneum, pleura, and pericardium.
- ***Electrocardiogram*** to monitor heart activity and assess for damage to the heart.
- ***CT scans*** to assess for injuries to the brain, skull, spine, spinal cord, chest, and abdomen.
- ***MRI scans*** to confirm or rule out injuries to the brain and spinal cord.
- ***X-rays*** to evaluate bone fractures.

Case Study » Part 2

The ambulance arrives at the ED and paramedics emerge with the patient, Mark Alvarez, a 32-year-old police officer. Officer Alvarez was shot during a routine traffic stop, sustaining a bullet wound to his right shoulder. Upon arrival, the patient is awake and alert. His clear speech suggests a patent airway. His respirations are regular and nonlabored. His skin is pink, warm, and dry. You obtain another set of vital signs, which include temperature 97.2°F oral; pulse 90 beats/min; respirations 20/min; and blood pressure 100/72 mmHg. Following a thorough medical assessment by the ED physician, Officer Alvarez is declared stable. He will require surgical intervention to explore and treat his shoulder injury. The ED physician orders laboratory diagnostics, including complete blood count, serum electrolytes, and type and crossmatch for possible administration of blood products.

Following assessment and evaluation by the trauma surgeon, Officer Alvarez is scheduled for immediate surgical exploration of his right shoulder.

You remain with Officer Alvarez while he is waiting to be taken to surgery. The patient seems slightly anxious. When you ask if he has any questions about his surgery, he responds by asking if his wife has arrived yet. You report that she has not. Officer Alvarez seems disappointed to hear this; he asks you to make sure she is told he is going into surgery and you assure him she will be informed as soon as she arrives. A nurse from the operating room arrives to transport Officer Alvarez to surgery.

Clinical Reasoning Questions Level I

1. Explain two possible reasons for the patient's decrease in blood pressure.
2. Why do you think the patient seems more concerned about his wife's absence than his impending surgery?
3. How would the case have changed if the patient's airway had not been patent?

Clinical Reasoning Questions Level II

4. Would the patient's injury have been worse had he been shot in the left shoulder? Explain your answer.
5. Describe three long-term interventions for patient care after surgery.
6. Describe two possible complications that could arise during the patient's surgery.

Independent Interventions

Caring for patients who have experienced traumatic events may evoke strong emotional responses from the nurse. However challenging the situation, the nurse must maintain focus on the patient to provide effective, high-quality care. Nurses, when providing medical care to perpetrators of trauma, must maintain a nonjudgmental and unbiased attitude. Interventions for all types of trauma-related care will be both independent and collaborative, but the nurse may have first contact with the patient, during which time several independent interventions can be employed. Nurses providing care to patients who have experienced trauma, either recently or in the past, promote patient recovery and resiliency by practicing trauma-informed care (see the Evidence-Based Practice feature).

Evidence-Based Practice

Trauma-Informed Care

Problem

Trauma is a widespread, pervasive health concern that impacts all populations and contributes to both acute and chronic health conditions. Trauma is a result of violence and has become more prevalent in the United States as rates of violence have increased (CDC, 2020r). Trauma directly impacts persons who experience it and can also have a secondary, indirect impact on the HCPs that care for survivors of trauma. HCPs are at risk for experiencing **vicarious trauma** from exposure to and caring for survivors of firsthand trauma (Perzichilli, 2018).

At times the systems in place to assist and protect people may cause trauma or re-traumatization. An example of system-induced trauma is when a child welfare department has to abruptly remove children from their home, causing separation of siblings and placement in foster care. Another example would be the use of seclusion or mechanical restraints on a previously traumatized patient (i.e., victim of human trafficking), which may cause traumatic memories to surface or potentiate a relapse of an existing mental illness.

Evidence

The need to effectively address trauma and its varied impacts is a vital aspect of healthcare. Addressing trauma requires a multilevel and collaborative approach, including prevention through public education, early identification, and trauma-specific assessment and treatment (SAMHSA, 2014; Schulman & Menschner, 2019). **Trauma-informed care** is a framework for recognizing and responding to trauma and its effects and preventing retraumatization. It is an approach that emphasizes the need to understand the impact of trauma and provide physical and psychological safety for both the patient and the HCP. Schulman and Menschner (2019) emphasize that a trauma-informed approach to care enhances patient outcomes and improves HCP wellness.

Implications

Implementing a trauma-informed care approach has positive implications for the health of patients and HCPs. Through trauma-informed care, patients may develop a more trusting rapport with their provider, take an active role in their care, and experience

(continued on next page)

Evidence-Based Practice *(continued)*

improved long-term health outcomes (Schulman & Menschner, 2019). This approach supports mental health and resiliency in HCPs, thereby combating burnout (Center for Health Care Strategies [CHCS], 2021). Trauma-informed care interventions are person centered and are anchored in the principles of (CHCS, 2021; SAMHSA, 2014):

- Safety (physical and emotional)
- Trustworthiness and transparency
- Peer support
- Collaboration and mutuality
- Empowerment
- Cultural, historical, and gender issues.

Strategies for providing trauma-informed care range from simple interventions such as reducing environmental stimuli to more integrated efforts. For example, the Montefiore Medical Group in Bronx, New York, has a team of mental health specialists that can respond to any of its clinics within 24 hours of a violent crime or traumatic event within the community to support working healthcare staff. The team assists staff by providing psychological debriefings and support sessions and offering referrals for staff needing counseling (CHCS, 2021). In this way, Montefiore's efforts at providing trauma-informed care extend beyond its patients to its own healthcare team, reducing team members' risk for developing an acute or chronic trauma response.

Critical Thinking Application

1. Describe an ethical principle that aligns with the trauma-informed care approach of preventing and avoiding retraumatization.
2. Identify ways in which nurses can implement trauma-informed care practices that correlate with the principles listed above.
3. Consider how patient and HCP outcomes are affected by trauma-informed care.

Interventions for Victims of Abuse

When caring for victims of abuse it is essential to provide safety, validate the patient's decision to disclose abuse, and emphasize that the patient is not to blame. Nursing interventions for patients who have been abused is multifaceted, including both physical and emotional care. Physical care may include cleaning wounds, applying dressings, and administering medications for pain. Emotional care may include use of listening skills, contacting a survivor advocate for support, and offering a referral to counseling services.

The nurse must use a person-centered approach, avoid a judgmental attitude, and support the patient's choices. If an older adult or person who is experiencing IPV chooses to return to the home with the abuser, the nurse should assist in creating a safety plan (see Exemplar 32.A, Abuse, later in this module). If a patient wants help leaving an abuser, the nurse should assist in exploring alternative living arrangements and supportive services.

Nurses need to follow organizational protocols for mandatory reporting, documentation, and use of available support services (e.g., the police department, social service agencies, and child welfare agencies). Nurses should know the laws associated with reporting abuse. In the United States and Canada, nurses are required to report any suspected child abuse. Adult victims of IPV generally will make the decision whether they want to report the violent episode(s) to law enforcement. It is important that the nurse educate patients who have been abused on all options and resources available so that an informed decision can be made.

Interventions for Victims of Trauma

Interventions and treatment for trauma vary depending on the specific injury and its severity. Victims of trauma often present in the ED with life-threatening injuries, including hypovolemia due to blood loss, organ damage, and multisystem complications. Traumatic injuries can cause psychologic and physiologic shock. Medical care for the patient in shock focuses on treating the underlying cause, increasing arterial oxygenation, and improving tissue perfusion. Depending on the cause and type of shock, interventions include emergency care measures, oxygen therapy, fluid replacement, and medication administration.

The nurse's role in trauma care begins with **triage**, the process of determining which patient most urgently needs medical intervention. Triage is based on the ABCDEs of trauma care. The nurse begins the triage process by performing a rapid general assessment, including vital signs, LOC, and a head-to-toe review looking for obvious physical alterations (ACSCOT, 2017; ENA, 2020).

When caring for a patient who has experienced trauma, maintaining a patent airway and monitoring breathing and circulation are ongoing responsibilities. If the patient has experienced blood loss, is in shock, or is in unstable condition, the initiation of an IV line is often a high priority because it allows for administration of medications, fluid, and blood products. Changes in the patient's condition can be marked by subtle alterations, so the nurse's primary role is in performing ongoing assessments in order to correct problems before they become more acute. Nurses must also consider and provide referrals for long-term consequences that trauma patients may experience such as issues with mobility, cognition, and appearance.

Trauma care is consistent across the lifespan, with variations related to the trauma experienced and the patient's age and developmental level. Refer to exemplars contained within this module for specific lifespan considerations related to abuse and neglect, multisystem trauma, and sexual violence.

Collaborative Therapies

Care of the trauma patient is approached in an integrated, collaborative, interprofessional way that can optimize delivery of care and reduce morbidity and mortality (Bach et al., 2017). A team of professionals experienced in trauma deliver care from the prehospital setting to discharge and rehabilitation services. The initial focus of the trauma team is physiologic stabilization through identifying and treating physical injuries. Physiologic treatment is addressed by paramedics, nurses, nurse practitioners, and physicians. To provide optimal care during physiologic treatment, nurses may call upon foreign language interpreters and supportive services such as a hospital chaplain. Once a patient is physiologically stable, psychosocial and rehabilitation treatment is addressed by nurses, physicians, social workers, survivor advocates, counselors, protective agencies, and law enforcement. Nurses may need to draw upon their role as patient advocate and intervene within organizational protocols if law enforcement officers, during their investigations, become an obstacle to providing effective care.

The nurse plays a critical role on the interprofessional trauma team, especially in regard to working with families involved in traumatic injuries. The nurse is often the healthcare worker who spends the most time with patients and forms a trusting nurse–patient relationship. As a result, the patient may feel most comfortable when talking with the nurse and be more likely to relate details of the traumatic event. The nurse should assess the family for a variety of needs, including counseling, social, spiritual, and financial support.

Surgery

Surgical intervention may be required to treat injuries related to trauma. Some injuries require emergency surgery to stop bleeding or repair organ damage, and others may require orthopedic surgery. Nurses will work to keep patients stable while preparing them for surgery, diagnostic testing, or other treatments to repair their injuries. Whereas some injuries sustained from trauma will require basic surgical interventions, other injuries will require more complex surgery.

Pharmacologic Therapy

Pharmacologic treatment for trauma patients may include administering analgesics for pain, depending on the severity of the injury. Inotropic agents and vasopressors also may be indicated.

Opioid analgesics such as morphine are commonly used to treat pain. The effects of opioid pain medications may cause respiratory depression or alter patient responses to injury, thereby masking potential injuries. For this reason, patient assessment is generally performed prior to administration of opioids or other medications that may produce sedative effects. When administering opioid analgesics, nurses must monitor for respiratory depression and administer a reversal agent (naloxone), if needed. See Exemplar 3.A, Acute and Chronic Pain, in Module 3, Comfort, for information on opioid analgesics.

Vasopressors (vasoconstrictors) and inotropes are used to create vasoconstriction or increase cardiac contractility to increase cardiac output and improve tissue perfusion in trauma patients with shock (VanValkinburgh, Kerndt, & Hashmi, 2020). Vasopressors include phenylephrine, norepinephrine, epinephrine, vasopressin, and dopamine (which has inotropic properties). When administering vasopressors, nurses monitor for cardiovascular response (heart rate/rhythm and blood pressure) to medications. Inotropes include dopamine, dobutamine, and isoproterenol. Nurses administer inotropic drugs after fluid volume restoration and monitor for signs of local tissue necrosis (from extravasation), pain, irregular heartbeat, or rise in diastolic pressure. See Exemplar 16.L, Shock, and Medications 16.8, Drugs Used to Treat Shock, in Module 16, Perfusion, for more information.

Nonpharmacologic Therapy

A common issue with physical trauma is pain control. A patient who does not have effective pain management may require longer hospitalization, experience additional complications, and have poor outcomes. Along with pharmacologic pain management, the nurse will also need to employ nonpharmacologic pain management techniques such as guided imagery, breathing exercises, and distraction. For more information on nonpharmacologic pain control, see Module 3, Comfort.

Complementary Health Approaches

Complementary health approaches may be added to the traditional treatment to assist in symptom management. Patients with a long treatment trajectory (e.g., those needing extensive physical therapy and rehabilitation) may benefit from complementary strategies such as stress reduction techniques or acupuncture to help alleviate pain. Patients who face long-term disability will benefit from referrals to organizations that provide education and support in obtaining assistive devices, including service animals. Nurses should educate patients to inform their providers if they use any herbal remedies or supplements due to the possibility of contraindication with prescription medications.

Case Study » Part 3

One month following his right shoulder injury and surgery, Officer Alvarez presents to the clinic for his post-op visit. His surgery was successful; the bullet was excised, and damage to the surrounding tissues was minimal. Officer Alvarez has been attending physical therapy sessions, which he describes as "sort of helpful, but my shoulder swells a little bit after my therapy appointments." He reports that he is gaining range of motion in his right shoulder. On a scale of 0 to 10 (with 10 being extreme pain), Officer Alvarez rates his pain as 2.

When asked about his anticipated return to work, Officer Alvarez becomes very quiet. After a pause, he tells you he is expected to return to work in 3 days. He explains that he will be on light duty, which entails working in an administrative role inside the police department until he has fully recovered. You notice that Officer Alvarez seems uncomfortable discussing this, so you tactfully explore the topic. You begin by asking how he feels about returning to work. Officer Alvarez reports that he feels fine physically; however, he has been having nightmares about the shooting. When you ask if he has discussed his nightmares or the actual shooting with anyone, he replies, "It's not something I really want to talk about. I have an appointment with the department shrink tomorrow, though. They're making me see her before I can go back to work." When you ask if he would like to speak with a counselor outside his department, Officer Alvarez replies, "I really don't want to talk about anything with anybody. I just want my shoulder to heal up."

Clinical Reasoning Questions Level I

1. What nursing interventions could you suggest to Officer Alvarez to promote comfort in his shoulder following the therapy sessions?
2. What concerns might this patient have in regard to his return to work, both in the psychosocial and physical realms?

Clinical Reasoning Questions Level II

3. Is Officer Alvarez at risk for developing PTSD? Explain your answer.
4. In light of Officer Alvarez's statements, should the nurse proceed with exploring psychosocial considerations related to his injury? Why or why not?

REVIEW The Concept of Trauma

RELATE Link the Concepts

Linking the concept of trauma with the concept of cognition:

1. Describe how untreated schizophrenia could lead to instances of violence and/or violent behavior.
2. How would you assess and diagnose abuse in a patient with advanced Alzheimer disease? What signs and symptoms would you look for in particular?

Linking the concept of trauma with the concept of mood and affect:

3. What assessment questions would you want to ask the patient who was admitted after sustaining injuries from IPV whose mood appears sad with a tearful affect?
4. Could a woman experiencing postpartum depression be at increased risk for abusing her children or spouse? Explain your answer.

Linking the concept of trauma with the concept of clinical decision making:

5. You are working in the ED when several ambulances arrive simultaneously because of a nearby apartment fire. When triaging the patients, you find that there are patients with fractures, second- and third-degree burns, and respiratory distress. Another patient is unconscious. Which of the patients require priority care? Explain your answer.
6. A patient has been admitted to the ED following a motor-vehicle crash. The patient has an open fracture of the femur, deep facial lacerations, and broken ribs coupled with a pneumothorax. What priority nursing interventions would you implement first? Explain your answer.

READY Go to Volume 3: Clinical Nursing Skills

REFER Go to Pearson MyLab Nursing and eText

REFLECT Apply Your Knowledge

A family of four was vacationing on the West Coast when a major earthquake occurred. The destruction where their hotel was located was severe, and many buildings were damaged, including their hotel. The parents and 13-year-old daughter were unharmed; however, the 9-year-old son, James, sustained severe physical trauma with obvious open fractures and profuse bleeding from the head. James was unconscious when the rescue team found him. The disaster response team triaged James and immediately transported him, via ambulance, to Los Angeles, the nearest city that remained operational, for medical care. Upon arrival, James's respirations were 26 per minute, blood pressure was 78/40 mmHg, and pulse was 140 beats/min. James has regained consciousness and is being sent for x-rays and a CT scan of the brain. Test results show fractures of the left femur and tibia, the left humerus, radius and ulna, and a skull fracture. The CT scan shows a contusion of the brain with no other anomalies. James will need to have surgery to correct placement of the open, complete fractures. After surgery, he will need to remain in the hospital for additional tests, stabilization, and monitoring. The parents and sister have arrived and are displaced. The entire family is traumatized (crying, confused, and in a state of disbelief) and the nurse noted that the mother was clenching her prayer beads.

1. What three priority nursing diagnoses would you select for James?
2. Whom should the nurse contact regarding arrangements that can be made for the family so that they can remain close to James during his stay in the hospital? What might these arrangements include?
3. What other healthcare professionals and ancillary staff members should the nurse involve in the care of James and his family?

Exemplar 32.A Abuse

Exemplar Learning Outcomes

32.A Analyze abuse as it relates to trauma.

- Describe the pathophysiology of abuse.
- Describe the etiology of abuse.
- Compare the risk factors and prevention of abuse.
- Identify the clinical manifestations of abuse.
- Summarize diagnostic tests and therapies used by interprofessional teams in the collaborative care of an individual who has been abused.
- Apply the nursing process in providing culturally competent care to an individual who has been abused.

Exemplar Key Terms

Child abuse, *2155*
Elder abuse, *2155*
Intimate partner violence (IPV), *2155*
Neglect, *2155*
Psychologic abuse, *2157*

Overview

Abuse is a public health problem in the United States that affects people in all stages of life and from any demographic or sociocultural background (CDC, 2020a). Abuse can break down an individual's self-confidence and self-worth and instill feelings of shame that, along with fear of the abuser, can lead to underreporting. The CDC (2020a) identifies four common types of abuse as physical abuse, sexual abuse, emotional abuse, and neglect.

Types of Abuse

Types of abuse can overlap and coexist, yet each has unique characteristics and requires individual approaches to diagnosis and management (Magana & Kaufhold, 2018).

Abuse sometimes starts as emotional (i.e., name-calling, rejection) and escalates over time to physical or even sexual abuse (CDC, 2020i). The American Psychological Association (2020) and other professional organizations define sexual abuse as unwanted sexual activity forced upon another person. Definitions of sexual abuse include threats, sexual activity with those who are unable to give consent, and exposure of minor children to sexual activities either directly or through witnessing sex or sexual violence. Many childhood sexual abuse survivors are also exposed to forms of emotional abuse whereby the perpetrator will use the child's need for love and approval against them in order to force the child to submit (American Psychiatric Association, 2013).

Child Abuse

According to the Child Abuse Prevention and Treatment Act (CAPTA), **child abuse** and **neglect** are defined as "any recent act or failure to act on the part of a parent or caretaker which results in death, serious physical or emotional harm, sexual abuse or exploitation" of a child or "an act or failure to act which presents an imminent risk of serious harm" to a child (DHHS, 2019b). Child abuse and neglect are common in the U.S., with children living in families of low socioeconomic status (SES) experiencing higher rates (CDC, 2020c). In 2018, one in seven children experienced child abuse or neglect, resulting in nearly 1,770 deaths. The CDC (2020c) indicates child abuse cases are likely underreported.

Intimate Partner Violence

Intimate partner violence (IPV) is the act of inflicting sexual, emotional, or physical harm on a current or previous partner or spouse (CDC, 2020k). Stalking is a form of IPV resulting in a person fearing for safety due to a pattern of repeated, unwanted attention or contact (CDC, 2020k). IPV can occur in any couple, including same-sex couples, adolescent couples (identified as teen dating violence), and older adult couples. IPV is often related to one person in the relationship feeling entitled to power and control (see **Figure 32.2** ») and using violence or the threat of violence to maintain control (National Coalition Against Domestic Violence [NCADV], n.d.).

One in four women and one in ten men have experienced some form of IPV in their lifetimes; most report first experiences of IPV occurring before the age of 18 (CDC, 2020k). Incidence of IPV in same-sex couples is comparable to heterosexual couples (Rollè, Giardina, Caldarera, Gerino, & Brustia, 2018). The potential for fatality from IPV is high: One in five homicide victims is killed by an intimate partner (CDC, 2020k). Survivors of IPV often have long-lasting physical and emotional negative health outcomes such as chronic cardiac disease, depression, and PTSD (CDC, 2020k).

Elder Abuse

Elder abuse includes physical abuse, emotional abuse, sexual abuse confinement, financial exploitation, and neglect of an

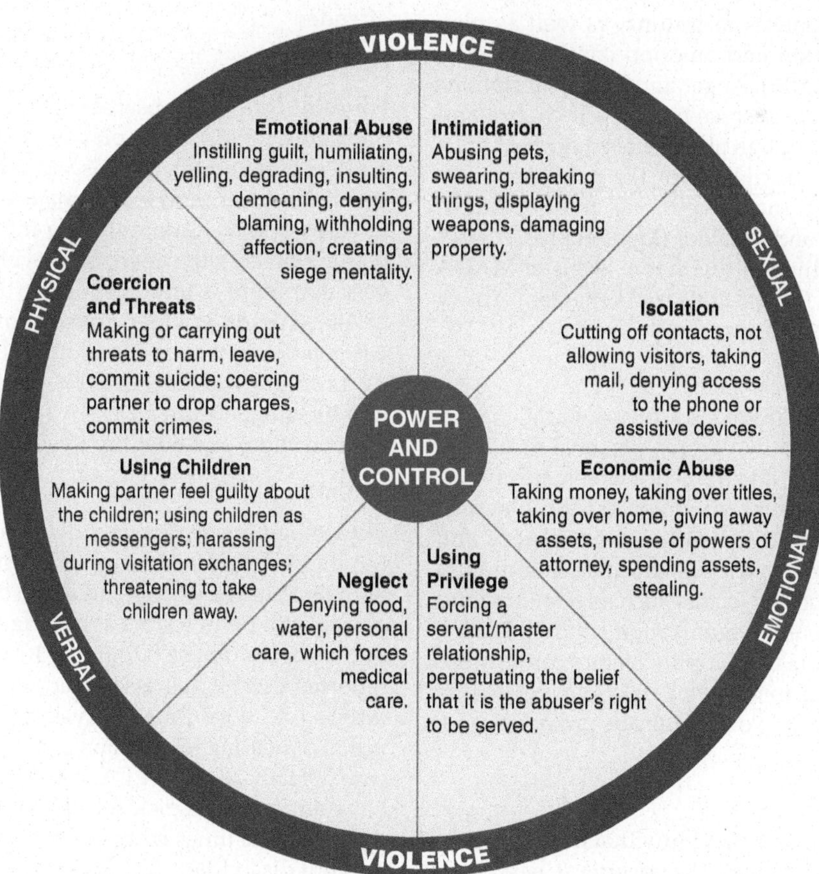

Figure 32.2 » The power and control wheel illustrates the strategies one partner may use to intimidate, control, and harm another.
Source: Potter and Moller (2020). Pearson Education, Inc., New York, NY.

individual 60 years of age and older (NCA, n.d.). Approximately one in ten older adults have experienced abuse, with fewer than 10% reporting it (NCA, n.d.). A multitude of reasons exist for underreporting (NCA, n.d.):

- Unwillingness to report family members (often the perpetrators of the abuse)
- Physical or mental inability to report
- Fear of the abuser retaliating if they report.

Additionally, older adults may fear they will not have a place to live or that they will be sent to a residential nursing facility if they report the abuse. The nurse will need to assure patients who report abuse that they will be protected and that safety is a priority.

Etiology

Many theories exist concerning the underlying causes for violent and abusive behaviors. Some theories propose that individuals are genetically predisposed to violence, whereas other theories discuss the influences of society and family structure. A number of theories have developed to explain the development of abuse and neglect in a family or a relationship. Although no single cause has been isolated, neurobiology, the social ecologic model, and social learning theory highlight some factors that contribute to abusive behavior.

Neurobiology

Neurobiology is the study of how the nervous system mediates behavior. Neurobiologic studies indicate that genetic variations influence responses to trauma, as well as play a role in anger modulation and emotion control (Clukay et al., 2019; Klasen et al., 2019). Anger and its manifestations vary among individuals, with some having self-control and others expressing anger through abusive behaviors. MAOA is a genetic enzyme that breaks down the neurotransmitters serotonin, epinephrine, norepinephrine, and dopamine, which influence emotion and behavior (MedlinePlus, 2020a). Gene studies suggest individuals with low levels of MAOA are more prone to aggressive and antisocial behavior (Clukay et al., 2019).

Social-Ecologic Model

The Social-Ecologic Model (SEM) is a theory-based framework used to understand how various personal and environmental factors interrelate and influence violent behaviors. The SEM holds that interpersonal violence is an outcome of the interaction among individual (personal history and biology), relationship (family, friends, partner), community (context/settings), and societal factors such as economic and social policies (World Health Organization [WHO], 2020a), The model depicts how the overlapping factors can contribute to some people having an increased risk for experiencing or perpetrating violence while others may be protected from it (CDC, 2020s).

Social Learning Theory

Social learning theory explains that individuals learn behaviors by observing and imitating other people (Chesworth, Lanier, & Rizo, 2019). Children are especially susceptible to this form of learning because they model the behaviors of those around them. This theory provides a rationale for why a child who experiences violence later perpetrates violence, furthering a cycle of family abuse (DHHS, n.d.-a).

Risk Factors

Understanding risk factors can assist the nurse in recognizing abuse. Risk factors associated with perpetration of abuse include individual (e.g., parents' history of child maltreatment), family (e.g., family disorganization, dissolution, and violence), and community. Risk factors associated with victimization include very young children, older adults, and individuals with special needs (CDC, 2020c).

Age

Younger children and older adults comprise the age groups that are more vulnerable and, therefore, at increased risk for abuse. Research indicates that children age 3 and younger are the most frequent victims of maltreatment, accounting for 71% of child fatalities; abuse and neglect accounts for approximately 46.6% of fatalities in children under the age of 1 (DHHS, 2019c). In cases of elder abuse, it is virtually impossible to know the full extent of instances of abuse because many are not reported (National Center on Elder Abuse [NCEA], n.d.-b). Abuse of older adults is commonly in the form of financial exploitation and neglect (NCEA, n.d.-b; Weissberger et al., 2020). The NCEA (n.d.-b) reports that older adults who have experienced abuse have a 300% higher risk of death as compared to older adults who have not experienced abuse and that between 30 and 40% of abused older adults experience more than one form of abuse by the same offender.

Sex

For some forms of abuse, sex can be a risk factor, whereas for other forms it does not play an active role. For example, in cases of child abuse, there is virtually no difference between the numbers of female and male survivors (DHHS, 2019c). In cases of IPV, figures show a higher incidence of women being abused than men; however, some arguments suggest that there is underreporting by male survivors (CDC, 2020k). Trends in elder abuse show a clear delineation of women being abused more often than men (NCEA, n.d.-b). According to the CDC (2020k), risk factors for IPV perpetration include belief in strict sex roles (i.e., male dominance in relationships) and hostility toward women.

Physiologic Development

Physiologic disorders and disabilities may present one of the highest risk factors for all forms of abuse. Individuals with disabilities are more likely to be seen as easy targets for abuse, with perpetrators assuming that they will not, or cannot, report the abuse (Disability Justice, 2020). Some common reported disabilities associated with cases of abuse include intellectual disabilities, physical and learning disabilities, visual or hearing impairments, dementia, and Alzheimer disease (DHHS, 2019c; NCEA, n.d.-a). Children with disabilities have an increased risk for abuse; one study indicates that they are three times more likely to be abused than their peers without disabilities (Disability Justice, 2020). It has also been discovered that IPV among individuals with disabilities is increasingly prevalent and even disproportionate (Breiding & Armour, 2015).

Cultural Factors

Culture encompasses a group's social behaviors, traditions, and norms. Behaviors considered abusive in one culture may not be in another.

An individual's culture can also be a risk factor for abuse, with some cultures condoning acts that Western culture considers to be abusive. For example, some Asian cultures use shame as a method of teaching children respect or for controlling individuals within the family unit (Louie, 2020). Shame in these instances could be considered a form of **psychologic abuse**, as individuals being shamed may be continually verbally confronted with supposed their shortcomings and mistakes. Parents from Asian cultures that use honor and shame for control may continue the practice even when they migrate to the United States and, in many cases, it is passed down from generation to generation (Louie, 2020).

Within cultures that are strictly patriarchal (in which the husband or male partner is the head of the family with responsibility for all major decisions), IPV may be more prevalent as traditional beliefs and practices that influence power relations create tension that could lead to physical or psychologic violence (Asian Pacific Institute on Gender-Based Violence [APIGBV], n.d.). Patriarchal cultures tend toward abusive relationships when the husband or male head of household maintains strict control of all members of the family, giving them the right to use punishments that he considers necessary (APIGBV, n.d.).

Pregnancy

The risk for IPV can increase with pregnancy (American College of Obstetricians and Gynecologists [ACOG], 2019). For individuals in an abusive relationship, the abuse can often escalate during pregnancy (ACOG, 2019). Abuse during pregnancy has the potential to affect both the woman and the fetus.

Intimate partner violence during pregnancy can be associated with fatal and nonfatal adverse health outcomes such as placental abruption, preterm delivery, low birth weight, and stillbirth (ACOG, 2019). The World Health Organization (2011) released a cardinal resource that indicates nurses have an opportunity for identifying women who experience IPV in the antenatal care period. Interventions when caring for a woman in the antenatal period include conducting assessment to measure risk and implementing prevention measures such as education and developing a safety plan (WHO, 2011).

Social Risk Factors

Social determinants of health (SDOH) and family circumstances can increase risk of abuse or neglect, including interpersonal violence. Examples include living in poverty, substance abuse, and at least one partner being in the military.

Socioeconomic status, specifically poverty, is a risk factor for and predictor of child abuse and interpersonal violence. Living in poverty or an economically depressed area contributes significantly to rates of child abuse fatalities (Farrell et al., 2017). Despite the well-recognized associated between low SES and poorer child health outcomes (including risk for violence and injury), child abuse and neglect may also occur in families regardless of socioeconomic status.

Abuse of alcohol and/or drugs has been correlated with and is a leading risk factor for abusive behavior (American Addiction Centers, 2020). Substance abuse can contribute to aggressive and violent behaviors by reducing inhibitions and limiting self-control (American Addiction Centers, 2020). Substance abuse also impairs healthy family systems and communication. When use of drugs or alcohol are combined with an already abusive situation, the abuse can become intensified. For example, if an individual is already being emotionally abusive, the use of drugs or alcohol may escalate the abuse to physical or sexual abuse. Substance abuse alone does not create the abusive situation; other factors such as the personality of the individual using the substances also needs to be considered.

SAFETY ALERT A patient who is under the influence of an illegal substance and/or alcohol is highly unpredictable, which increases the risk for violent behavior. The nurse will need to monitor the patient at all times and assess for signs of escalating behavior. If there is potential for violence, it is important that the healthcare team and security be made aware for safety purposes.

Although statistics related to IPV in military families are considered to be low due to underreporting, several factors related to being in the military increase risk for the development of IPV. Frequent relocation adds a layer of stress and instability to the partner relationship and separates families from established social networks, increasing social isolation and reducing access to support systems. This can reduce available options for relief, such as the potential for moving in with other family or friends to escape the abuse (Congressional Research Service, 2019).

Firearms in the Home

It is controversial and extremely difficult to assign statistics for an increased risk for mortality in cases of abuse when a gun is present in the home because these statistics depend on too many variables such as the type of firearm, the storage of the firearm, and the location of the incident. However, according to the FBI (n.d.-a), in 2019:

- 62.1% of weapons used during murders were handguns.
- 43.2% of murder victims were killed during arguments.
- 28.3% of murder victims were killed by someone known to them (including boyfriend/girlfriend) and 13.0% were killed by family members (including husband/wife).

A seminal study of data from 11 cities sought to identify risk factors for homicide in abusive relationships (Campbell et al., 2003). Although this study looked only at data on heterosexual couples in which the man was the abuser, the findings indicate that physical violence is the primary risk factor for intimate partner homicide, with access to a firearm making it five times more likely that the abused partner will be killed.

Prevention

The social-ecological model presents an approach to violence prevention that considers the multiple factors of the model simultaneously (CDC, 2020v). Prevention measures aim to address abusive behavior before it happens, Targeted prevention measures include individual counseling programs, parenting classes, family-focus programs, community education, and societal campaigns.

Nurses can help prevent IPV by being observant for its manifestations (see the Clinical Manifestations section below) and helping to empower the survivor. Furthermore, when assessing an individual for IPV, nurses must remain nonjudgmental regardless of the sex, sexual orientation, culture, or SES of the patient. Individuals who have experienced IPV may fear cultural or societal judgment, which can hinder efforts to seek support or escape (NCADV, n.d.).

Nurses can help prevent abuse and IPV by observing for the signs and symptoms of abuse and taking action to address the situation. When children are involved, nurses must report abuse per facility protocol and state regulations. In cases of IPV, the decision to report is made by the survivor. When a patient does desire help to stop a violent and abusive situation, nurses can work to facilitate referrals to domestic violence shelters, other HCPs, law enforcement, and lawyers. For patients who want to leave an abusive home or relationship, nurses can provide patient teaching regarding the development of a safety plan (see the Patient Teaching feature).

SAFETY ALERT Sudden unemployment or other forms of financial stress can greatly increase an individual's stress and, in turn, increase risk of participating in abusive behavior toward another individual.

Clinical Manifestations

The signs of abuse can vary based on the population being abused as well as the type of abuse. IPV, for example, will often manifest with signs of intense fear and control, such as the person being abused not having access to cash and losing all contact with friends and family. The signs of physical and emotional abuse vary among populations, with children reacting to psychologic abuse differently than adults. In cases of sexual abuse, however, the signs are primarily consistent across age demographics. Nurses should be vigilant in assessing for signs of abuse in all patients. Many of the manifestations of physical abuse are apparent, such as broken or fractured bones in different stages of healing, abusive head trauma (AHT) or shaken baby syndrome, excessive bruising, and burns or scars in specific shapes (**Figure 32.3** »). More of these physical indicators are outlined in the Clinical Manifestations and Therapies table.

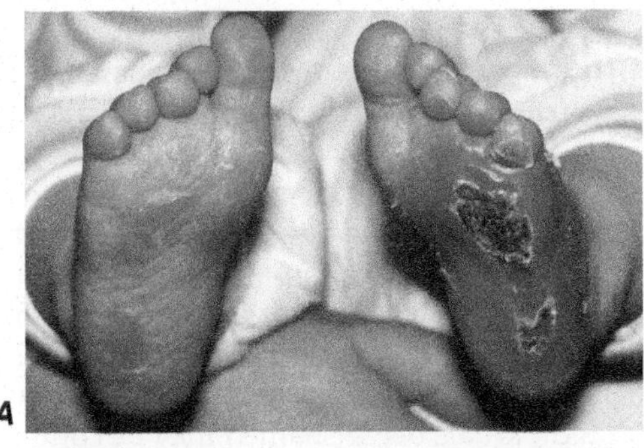

A

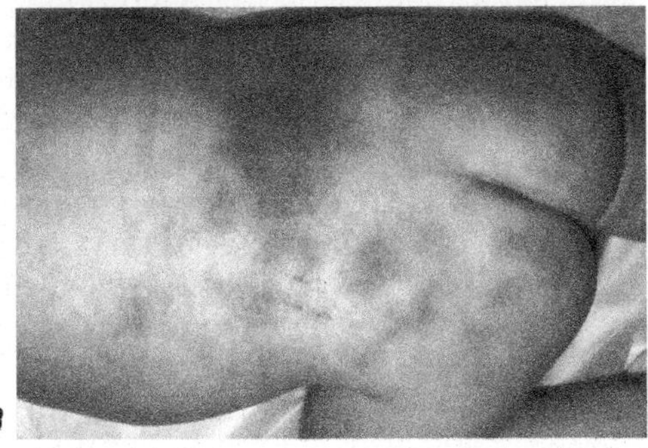

B

Figure 32.3 » Examples of child abuse. ***A***, This child's feet were burned when the parent held the feet against a heater. ***B***, Battered child showing bruises and lacerations.

Source: ***A***, SPL/Science Source. ***B***, Biophoto Associates/Science Source.

Patient Teaching

Developing a Safety Plan

Developing a safety plan will help an individual who lives in an abusive environment to plan an escape. Elements of a safety plan may include:

- Keep purse or wallet and keys easily accessible at all times.
- Keep an extra cell phone and a set of house and car keys in a safe (and secret) location.
- Have a designated contact person available who can be notified to call police.
- Teach children to call police or 911 and consider having emergency phones hidden throughout the home.
- Have a code word to indicate a violent situation so that friends, family, or children know to call police.
- Move to a low-risk area in the event of an argument (rooms with access to outside door and not in bathroom, kitchen, or room with weapons).
- Practice how to get out safely. Know the easiest escape route from the current location (exiting through doors, windows, fire escapes).
- Take photos of injuries, record threatening phone calls, and save threatening voice mail or text messages.
- Use judgment. If the situation is serious, give the partner what is being demanded to calm the individual down.

Sources: Center for Family Justice (n.d.); Domestic Violence Resource Center (2020).

Manifestations of Child Abuse and Neglect

Infants have the highest prevalence of fatality due to physical abuse, which is likely related to the infant's small body. AHT can occur in as little as 5 seconds of violent shaking. Shaking a newborn or infant causes the brain to bounce back and forth against the skull, leading to bruising, swelling, pressure, and bleeding in the brain, all of which may lead to permanent brain damage. Shaking an infant may also lead to other injuries, including damage to the neck, spine, and eyes (National Institute of Neurological Disorders and Stroke, 2019). If an infant falls or is accidentally dropped, it will cause a different type of brain trauma than that associated with AHT.

Some signs of neglect of an infant include untreated diaper rash, dirty diapers, poor hygiene, poor eye contact or detachment, and failure to thrive. HCPs need to be mindful

Clinical Manifestations and Therapies
Abuse

ETIOLOGY	CLINICAL MANIFESTATIONS	CLINICAL THERAPIES
Infant abuse	▪ Untreated diaper rash; lengthy time spent in soiled diapers; poor hygiene ▪ Poor eye contact; detachment ▪ Frequent ear infections (from bottle propping) ▪ Failure to thrive ▪ Sores; rashes; flea bites ▪ Fractures (multiple or in various stages of healing, inconsistent with explanations of injury); bruises; welts ▪ AHT (shaken baby syndrome)	▪ Treat physical injuries. ▪ Give antibiotics for any infections as prescribed. ▪ Reporting of the abuse is mandatory. ▪ Ensure the safety and security of the child.
Child abuse	▪ Bruises or welts in unusual places or in several stages of healing; distinctive shapes ▪ Wary of physical contact with adults ▪ Behavioral extremes of withdrawal or aggression ▪ Burns (especially cigarette burns; immersion burns of hands, feet, or buttocks; rope burns; or distinctively shaped burns) ▪ Apprehensive when other children cry ▪ Fractures (multiple or in various stages of healing, inconsistent with explanations of injury) ▪ Joint swelling or limited mobility ▪ Long-bone deformities ▪ Lacerations and abrasions to the mouth, lip, gums, eye, genitalia ▪ Human bite marks ▪ Signs of AHT ▪ Deformed or displaced nasal septum ▪ Bleeding or fluid drainage from the ears or ruptured eardrums ▪ Broken, loose, or missing teeth ▪ Difficulty in respirations, tenderness or crepitus over ribs ▪ Abdominal pain or tenderness ▪ Recurrent urinary tract infection ▪ Emotional and/or behavioral problems ▪ Frequent absenteeism from school	▪ Treat physical injuries. ▪ Give antibiotics for any infections as prescribed. ▪ Therapy may be behavioral, cognitive, group, or play therapy depending on developmental stage. ▪ Reporting of the abuse is mandatory. ▪ Ensure the safety and security of the child.
Sexual abuse	▪ Torn, stained, or bloody underwear ▪ Pain or itching in genital areas ▪ Bruises or bleeding from external genitalia, vagina, rectum ▪ Poor peer relationships ▪ Withdrawal ▪ STI ▪ Unwilling to participate in physical activities ▪ Swollen or red cervix, vulva, or perineum ▪ Wears long sleeves and several layers of clothing even in hot weather ▪ Semen around the mouth or genitalia or on clothing ▪ Pregnancy ▪ Delinquency or running away ▪ Inappropriate sexual behavior or mannerisms ▪ Regressive behaviors	▪ Treat physical injuries. ▪ Test for STIs. ▪ Administer pregnancy test. ▪ Take DNA swabs for identification of the perpetrator. ▪ Treat for depression and/or suicidal behavior. ▪ Therapy may be behavioral, cognitive, group, or play, depending on developmental stage. ▪ Educate on rights and ability to report to authorities. ▪ Consider behavioral therapy for perpetrators.

(continued on next page)

Clinical Manifestations and Therapies *(continued)*

ETIOLOGY	CLINICAL MANIFESTATIONS	CLINICAL THERAPIES
Intimate partner violence	▪ Chronic fatigue ▪ Casual response to serious pain ▪ Vague complaints, aches, and injury or excessively emotional response to a relatively minor injury ▪ Frequent injuries ▪ Recurrent STIs ▪ Frequent ambulatory or ED visits ▪ Muscle tension ▪ Nightmares ▪ Facial lacerations ▪ Depression ▪ Injuries to chest, breasts, back, abdomen, or genitalia ▪ Anorexia or other eating disorder ▪ Bilateral injuries of arms or legs ▪ Anxiety ▪ Symmetric injuries ▪ Drug or alcohol abuse ▪ Obvious patterns of belt buckles, bite marks, fist or hand marks ▪ Suicide attempts ▪ Poor self-esteem ▪ Burns of hands, feet, or buttocks or with distinctive patterns ▪ Headaches ▪ Gastrointestinal or stress ulcers	▪ Treat physical injuries and physiologic conditions. ▪ Treat psychologic effects such as depression with medication or therapy. ▪ Suggest substance abuse counseling for perpetrator and survivor as needed. ▪ Provide referrals for community services, support groups, and shelters.
Elder abuse	▪ Constant hunger or malnutrition ▪ Listlessness ▪ Poor hygiene ▪ Social isolation ▪ Inappropriate dress for the weather ▪ Chronic fatigue ▪ Unattended medical needs ▪ Poor skin integrity or decubiti ▪ Contractures ▪ Urine burns/excoriation ▪ Dehydration ▪ Fecal impaction ▪ Bruises and welts ▪ Withdrawal ▪ Burns ▪ Confusion ▪ Fractures ▪ Fear or suspicion of caretaker, family members, HCPs ▪ Sprains or dislocations ▪ Lacerations or abrasions ▪ Evidence of oversedation ▪ Failure to meet financial obligations	▪ Treat physical injuries. ▪ Treat dehydration and malnutrition with increased fluids and food intake. ▪ Treat psychologic effects such as depression with medication or therapy. ▪ Arrange for respite services. ▪ Consider adult daycare. ▪ Reporting of the abuse is mandatory. ▪ Ensure the safety and security of the older adult. ▪ Refer perpetrators to treatment or therapy. ▪ Arrange transfer of legal authority.

Source: Adapted from Blais and Hayes (2016).

when assessing infants, as some of the signs of neglect may be attributed to other factors. For example, failure to thrive can be the result of an inborn error of metabolism or other organic disorder.

Signs of long-term physical abuse in children can be evidenced by poor language, cognitive, and emotional development as well as visual and motor impairments. A child who is being abused may present with behavioral changes, such as trouble sleeping, changes in eating habits, bedwetting, and high-risk behaviors (CDC, 2020i; Mayo Clinic, 2020a). Children may display signs of neglect in various ways including poor hygiene, dirty clothing, clothing that is too small or inappropriate for conditions, and appearing hungry or presenting with no money for lunch at school. Health and developmental problems may present as untreated medical or dental issues, not reaching developmental milestones, and poor language development.

Manifestations of Sexual Abuse

Survivors of sexual abuse may be withdrawn or combative, acting out in various situations. Emotions such as guilt, anxiety, depression, suicidal thoughts, and fear are quite common. In children who have experienced sexual abuse, one of the most pronounced indicators is early knowledge about or early interest in sexual acts (National Child Traumatic Stress Network [NCTSN], n.d.-b). Other children may instead regress, demonstrating behavioral difficulties, bedwetting, and insomnia. Physical manifestations of sexual abuse at any age include injuries to genitals or anus, swollen genitals, bladder or kidney infections, STIs, unintended pregnancies, and pelvic inflammatory disease (NCTSN, n.d.-b).

In addition, there are warning signs that may be suggestive of a perpetrator of sexual abuse. Some examples of these behaviors include ignoring social, emotional, or physical boundaries; oversharing adult issues with a child; being overly interested in the sexuality of a teen; frequently walking in on children/teens in the bathroom; and exposing a child to adult sexual interactions (National Sex Offender Public Website, n.d.). If the nurse observes any of these behaviors in an older teen or adult, the nurse should assess the situation further.

Neglect of Older Adults

Neglect is a common form of abuse of the older adult (CDC, 2020j). Similar to that in children, neglect of an older adult comprises needs not being met or care being intentionally withheld. The needs of an older adult include physical, emotional, and social needs. Manifestations of neglect of older adults may include unexplained weight loss, dehydration, poor hygiene, unsanitary conditions, untreated medical issues, decubiti, and unsafe living conditions (National Institute on Aging, n.d.).

SAFETY ALERT Claims of abuse from an older adult should not be dismissed because of a history of confusion or dementia. The nurse must explore and report any complaint related to any form of abuse. It is not the job of the nurse to determine whether abuse is occurring, but rather to advocate for the patient by obtaining as much information as possible and reporting the potential abuse per institution protocol and state regulations.

Cultural Considerations

Cultural considerations in cases of abuse are twofold, with some acts or traditions presenting as signs of abuse (such as cupping or coining), and other cultures partaking in acts that Western culture considers abusive (hitting one's wife for disobedience or hitting children with objects as a form of punishment). In cases of suspected abuse due to marks on the patient's body, nurses must take cultural healing practices into consideration. The practices of cupping and coining (generally practiced by many Asian cultures as well as individuals who participate in holistic healing) can create marks on the body that could be misinterpreted as signs of abuse (**Figure 32.4** ») (Killon, 2017). *Cupping* is the act of placing a glass cup on the skin and then using heat to create suction and is performed to promote blood flow and overall healing. Cupping can cause circular red welts or even dark bruising, which are often found along the individual's back. *Coining* is used to treat a multitude of ailments from headaches and fevers to minor illnesses, and it also leaves marks on the skin. In this treatment, warm oil is rubbed on the skin and then a coin is rubbed in a diagonal line until long marks appear. If these marks are seen without knowledge of their origin, they may look almost like marks from a whip. Neither of these treatments are abusive in nature but instead are traditional healing practices.

What is considered acceptable physical punishment of a child may vary among cultures (see the Focus on Diversity and Culture feature). In cases of suspected culturally influenced abuse, nurses practicing with cultural awareness

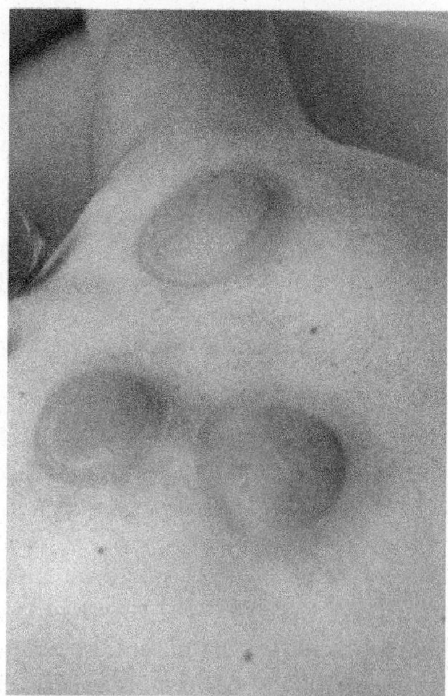

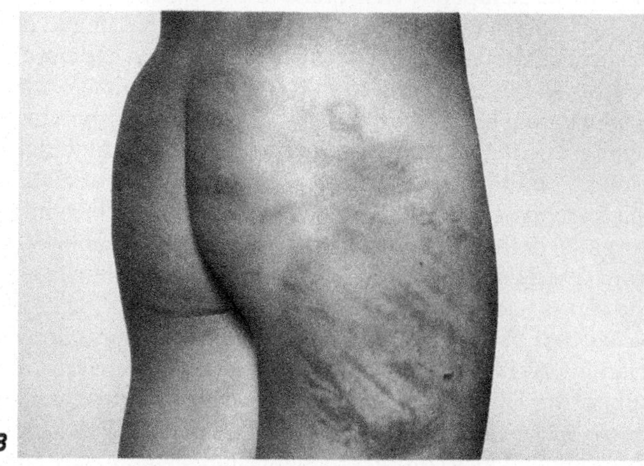

Figure 32.4 » It is important to differentiate cultural practices such as ***A***, cupping, and ***B***, coining, from signs of child abuse.

Source: Used with permission of the American Academy of Pediatrics, "Visual Diagnosis of Child Abuse Slide Kit." Copyright © AAP/Kempe. ***A***, Norbert Reismann/doc-stock/Alamy Stock Photo ***B***, Clinical Photography, Central Manchester University Hospitals NHS Foundation Trust, UK/ Science Source.

Focus on Diversity and Culture

Cultural Interpretations of Abuse

- Disciplining children by having them kneel on uncooked rice for a short period of time (Pennsylvania Family Support Alliance, 2020).
- Use of corporal (physical) punishment varies widely. In a longitudinal study of nine countries, Lansford et al. (2015) found that 93% of parents in Syria believed in using corporal punishment, whereas only 4% of parents in Albania reported physical punishment as a necessary component of childrearing. Use of severe forms of physical punishment (such as beating a child with an object or hitting a child on the head) also varied widely.
- In some South Asian, North African, and Middle Eastern cultures, reporting IPV or sexual abuse would dishonor or shame the family (Beller, Kröger, & Hosser, 2019).

will recognize that parents or caregivers may not see the injuries to their child as inappropriate or even abusive but rather as an unfortunate result of the child's behavior. It is not a nurse's place to judge; however, nurses are mandated reporters of child abuse and should follow state regulations and facility protocol on reporting, even if the abuse is a cultural form of discipline.

Collaboration

Usually, the best way to treat abusive families is to use an interprofessional approach involving nurses, physicians, social workers, protective services personnel, law enforcement, and, often, lawyers.

The nurse plays an important role in the interprofessional team providing treatment to the patient who is the survivor of abuse. The nurse should ensure that the team creates a safe environment in which the patient feels supported at home and in the therapeutic environment.

For patients who are children, safety at school should also be a consideration. Survivors of abuse are often deprived of control, so it is important to shift control back to them while helping them feel empowered. Building trust is also imperative because it will help the nurse develop a rapport with the patient. Building trust should never involve lying or making false promises; for example, do not promise that the child's parent(s) or the older adult's son will not get in trouble—that is for Child Protective Services, Elder Protective Services, and the courts to decide.

As part of the interprofessional team, the nurse should plan interventions that will encourage affective release in a supportive environment. Play therapy helps children explore traumatic themes, fears, and distorted beliefs. It is a nonthreatening way to process thoughts and feelings associated with abuse. Art therapy provides an opportunity to express feelings for which the patients have no words, and it can be useful in working with both children and adults. Therapeutic stories can be used to present the traumatic issues of abuse, link survivors' feelings to their behaviors, and describe new coping methods. Journal writing can help patients cope with intrusive thoughts and feelings.

Diagnostic Tests

Diagnostic tests cannot prove that an individual is being abused, but some tests, such as x-rays, MRIs, and CT scans, can show evidence of possible abuse. In most cases, tests are used to diagnose the full extent of the damage in order to properly treat the patient. In cases of physical abuse, an ultrasound or a CT scan of the abdomen can check for abdominal or organ injuries, CT scans of the head will show hemorrhage or skull fractures, and an MRI of the spine will show any spinal injuries. For sexual abuse, swabs for DNA are needed to provide the abuser's identity, and urine samples will show bladder or kidney infections. Tests for STIs should be conducted. Pregnancy tests should be administered to females of childbearing age who are survivors of sexual abuse. The range of testing to be conducted will depend on the type of abuse, injuries, and consent of the survivor.

Pharmacologic Therapy

Because injuries associated with abuse vary greatly depending on the situation and type of abuse, pharmacologic therapies also vary. Physical injuries such as broken bones and dislocations will require pain medication, sedatives, and anti-inflammatories while setting the injury and for resultant pain. Stabbings, gunshot wounds, or other penetrating injuries will require immediate action to address bleeding and wound care, as well as medications to prevent or heal infections and fluids to correct fluid volume deficit. Tetanus boosters or vaccines will be needed for most deep penetrating wounds. In cases of physical and emotional abuse, the patient may experience PTSD, which will require mental health interventions (see Exemplar 32.C, Posttraumatic Stress Disorder, in this module).

Nonpharmacologic Therapy

The physical effects of abuse will often heal long before the emotional effects begin to fade. Therapy, counseling, and support groups are the most commonly prescribed forms of treatment in cases of abuse. The type of therapy will depend on the personality, needs, and desires of the patient.

Children's Advocacy Centers

Children's Advocacy Centers (CACs) offer comprehensive services and support for children who have been abused. CACs are agencies, available throughout the United States and in 34 countries throughout the world, that facilitate an interprofessional approach to child abuse interventions including forensic interviewing, examination, and therapy (National Children's Advocacy Center, 2020). The overarching goal of a CAC is to provide a safe and supportive environment for children while they recover from abuse.

Domestic Violence Shelters

Domestic violence shelters offer a broad array of services for patients of all ages, including immediate shelter for survivors and their children and referrals to agencies that provide group therapy for parents and children, advocacy, and parent training. Some shelters may be sex specific, but most offer shelter regardless of sex. Many shelters have lists of attorneys and other professionals who offer services with sliding-scale fees. Many programs offer outreach services, including education and training on workplace violence and elder abuse. Nurses working in all settings should have contact information available for community domestic violence shelters.

NURSING PROCESS

Care of an individual who has been abused will vary depending on the type of abuse and the age of the individual. A patient's reaction to the abuse will also affect care, especially if fear, shame, and/or self-blaming are present. Nurses treat individuals from a person-centered approach, assessing the needs of a specific individual.

Assessment

The nurse's assessment in cases of abuse will be in order of the severity of the injuries. Life-threatening injuries will be assessed first, and other injuries will be assessed after the patient's safety is ensured. A complete medical history will be performed to determine if the patient has a history of injuries that could be the result of abuse. Nurses need to consider the patient's emotional state: Survivors of abuse could be scared of their abuser or of being blamed for the abuse. Similarly, some patients may be more nervous around staff of the same gender as the abuser. If possible, make adjustments to the staff directly caring for that patient.

Communicating with Patients and Families

Working Phase

Upon assessment of an elderly patient who lives with her adult son, the visiting nurse notes the patient has poor hygiene, dirty clothing, and a strong body odor. The patient nervously whispers, "I know I'm dirty and stinky. I wish my son would help me like he is supposed to." The nurse uses paraphrasing to convey the patient's statement was understood and uses open-ended questions that invite the patient to elaborate.

- You are having difficulty taking care of yourself?
- Tell me more about your relationship with your son.

Diagnosis

Priorities for care depend on the patient's current physical and psychosocial status and can vary considerably among patients. Patient care priorities relevant to actual or suspected survivors of child abuse, elder abuse, or interpersonal violence may include, but are not limited to:

- Acute pain
- Powerlessness
- Posttrauma syndrome
- Sexual dysfunction
- Social isolation.

Planning

Goals for a patient who has experienced abuse will change according to priorities of care, with the patient's immediate safety being a consistent focus of care. The age of the patient will also affect care planning. Examples of goals for the patient who has experienced abuse include:

- The patient will be safe and free from harm.
- The patient will report mild to no pain.
- The patient will ask for help in safely resolving the abusive situation.
- The patient will honestly convey feelings of fear, helplessness, anger, or depression.
- The patient will report any suicidal ideation.
- The patient will acknowledge that they are not responsible for the abuse.
- The patient will practice healthy coping mechanisms.

Implementation

The nurse's ability to implement care measures will depend on the patient's willingness to accept help in receiving care and in leaving or reconciling the abusive situation. Interventions vary depending on the individual's age and circumstances. Nurses have a responsibility to protect patients who cannot protect themselves and therefore have been designated, in the United States, as mandated reporters (Child Welfare Information Gateway, 2019). As mandatory reporters, nurses must follow facility protocols and state requirements related to reporting of suspected abuse or neglect of children, older adults, and vulnerable individuals (including adults with intellectual disabilities).

Promote Safety

In cases of abuse, the patient's safety is the primary concern. When mandatory reporting is not indicated, it is imperative for nurses to provide the patient with information about resources for seeking help. Adults who have experienced a form of abuse can be gently encouraged to seek assistance in promoting their own safety. If the patient chooses not to seek assistance, then information should be provided in case assistance is ever needed. Resources can be in the form of the patient's friends and family members or community liaisons who can work to help the individual find a secure living environment. Other resources can be offered, such as police, lawyers, and agencies that can provide ongoing assistance for survivors. Nurses encourage the patient to accept help in seeking an abuse-free living situation, but the decision ultimately lies with the patient. Some individuals will not be ready to seek help, and while nurses may disagree with this decision, they must refrain from judgment and be respectful of the patient's decision. The primary action for the nurse is to offer assistance and resources; this lets the survivor know how to access support if it is needed in the future.

Establish a Therapeutic Relationship

Establishing appropriate trust with a patient who has been abused is vital. Many cases of physical abuse involve psychologic abuse, which often belittles an individual's sense of self-worth and self-love, sometimes to the point of feeling it is impossible to do anything correctly. Nurses promote trust, in part, by providing nonjudgmental care, promoting patient self-confidence, and encouraging patients to make choices. For example, by offering the patient a choice of beverages or asking if the patient would like to complete toileting before going for an x-ray.

In contrast, a nurse who appears angry or disappointed in a patient for refusing care or not choosing to seek assistance in leaving an abusive situation will shatter all forms of trust that have been established with that patient and may inhibit the patient's trust in the healthcare system altogether. Nurses need to work to establish a trusting relationship with adults who have been abused, assuring them that they are in a judgment-free and safe setting.

Nurses who suspect child abuse must provide developmentally appropriate support and care. The child needs to feel safe and secure, particularly from the potential abuser. All early conclusions about the situation should be dismissed because it is unwise to assume knowledge of a situation until all the details are presented.

When assessing a child who may have been abused, nurses should avoid all forms of leading questions. For example, asking "How did you hit your head?" is an appropriate question for assessment. But asking, "Did your mother hit you?" is a leading question. Children in high-stress situations will sometimes work to tell an adult what they think that individual wants to hear. With this in mind, nurses should ask open-ended questions with no indication of the answer they expect to receive. It is imperative for nurses to follow organizational protocols with regard to suspected child abuse interviews.

Facilitate Communication

Survivors of abuse may be guarded and initially not want to discuss their experiences with or feelings about being abused. Additionally, survivors may not be ready to leave their abuser. Nurses should facilitate communication by demonstrating patience, empathy, and remaining nonjudgmental while offering support (Power, 2020). Nurse communication behaviors can facilitate survivor disclosure of experiences. One way is to use a scripted statement to investigate the possibility of violence without being suggestive: "Are you in a relationship where you feel unsafe? We ask every patient about the safety of their relationships because unhealthy relationships can have a significant impact on health." If the survivor discloses being in an unsafe relationship or being unsafe at home, the nurse should communicate belief and validate the decision to disclose (Power, 2020).

Promote Empowerment

A survivor may experience difficulty in accepting help due to fear of the abuser, lack of social support, decreased financial resources, and a sense of hopelessness. Nurses need to understand these fears to better assist the patient. Helping patients achieve a sense of control within the situation is one of the first steps in helping them accept assistance. All forms of abuse include an element of control on the part of the perpetrator and generally result in taking control away from the survivor.

In working to help patients regain a sense of control, nurses reassure patients that options and resources are available to help them leave the abusive situation being experienced. Nurses can also foster connections with social workers, counselors, and community liaisons to find safe housing and assist with social and financial support. Additionally, the patient can be put in contact with local law enforcement to file an order of protection against the abuser, which will prohibit the individual from making contact with the patient. Collaborating with the patient to develop a safety plan will also aid in empowerment (see Patient Teaching: Developing a Safety Plan).

Evaluation

All forms and cases of abuse are different depending on the age of the survivor and the circumstances of the abuse; therefore, the outcomes in these cases will vary. It is important to set realistic goals for patients. Some desired outcomes include the following:

- The patient remains free from injury or harm.
- The patient has a safety plan in place.
- The patient seeks assistance when needed.
- The patient demonstrates knowledge of the resources available to individuals in abusive situations.
- The patient verbalizes awareness of not being responsible for or deserving of abuse.
- The patient openly communicates fears with regard to the abusive situation.

Individuals with severe injuries related to abuse may need additional evaluation and follow-up, including potential surgical interventions. The nurse should treat these patients like any other patients undergoing surgery, including prepping the patient for surgery and providing aseptic care of the surgical wound. In addition, nurses may need to continue to suggest counseling or group therapy or other types of emotional support to individuals who seem reluctant to get help for emotional trauma. When a nurse sees a patient repeatedly because of injuries from abuse, the nurse should continue to advocate for patient safety and encourage the patient to seek help. The patient may not be receptive to help after a first or second instance of abuse, but the patient may be more likely to want help if the abuse has happened repeatedly. Continued evaluation and support of the patient sustaining abuse is necessary to promote the most positive outcome possible.

REVIEW Abuse

RELATE Link the Concepts and Exemplars

Linking the exemplar of abuse with the concept of development:

1. What protective factors would indicate a child probably has not experienced abuse? At age 3? At age 15?
2. What factors would put a child at risk for abuse?

Linking the exemplar of abuse with the concept of mood and affect:

3. What mood and affect would you anticipate a survivor of abuse might display?
4. What nursing assessment regarding mood and affect would be a priority when admitting a patient who was abused by a family member?

READY Go to Volume 3: Clinical Nursing Skills

REFER Go to Pearson MyLab Nursing and eText

REFLECT Apply Your Knowledge

Savannah Preston, a 26-year-old woman who is 24 weeks pregnant, comes to the ED. She says she fell and hit her head at home and is having headaches. During the assessment, the nurse notices multiple bruises in various stages of healing over her body and asks Savannah how she got them. She says that she is just clumsy and falls a lot. While the nurse is assessing her, another nurse enters the room to tell Savannah that her boyfriend is there to take her home. At that point, Savannah becomes frightened and tells the nurse that her boyfriend has been hitting her almost daily, and this last time he knocked her head against a wall. She says he has threatened to kill her if she tells anyone, and she does not want to leave with him.

1. Identify questions that the nurse could use in continuing the assessment and in documenting the discussion with Savannah.
2. What other people in the ED should participate in Savannah's care?
3. Who should make the decision about where Savannah should go?

›› Exemplar 32.B Multisystem Trauma

Exemplar Learning Outcomes

32.B Analyze multisystem trauma as it relates to trauma.

- Describe the etiology of multisystem trauma.
- Compare the risk factors and prevention of multisystem trauma.
- Identify the clinical manifestations of multisystem trauma.
- Summarize diagnostic tests and therapies used by interprofessional teams in the collaborative care of an individual with multisystem trauma.
- Differentiate care of patients with multisystem trauma across the lifespan.
- Apply the nursing process in providing culturally competent care to an individual with multisystem trauma.

Exemplar Key Terms

Mass-casualty incident (MCI), *2166*
Motor-vehicle crash (MVC), *2166*
Multisystem trauma, *2166*
Traumatic brain injury (TBI), *2167*
Whiplash, *2167*

Overview

Multisystem trauma refers to injuries affecting multiple body systems, such as the neurologic, respiratory, and circulatory systems. Multisystem trauma results from intentional as well as unintentional injuries. Intentional injuries are caused by abuse, firearm violence, **motor-vehicle crashes (MVCs)**, and human-made disasters, whereas unintentional injuries are caused by falls, poisonings, and natural disasters. According to the Centers for Disease Control and Prevention (2020f), unintentional injuries are the leading cause of death in the United States among people age 1 to 44 years. Unintentional poisonings are the leading cause of injury-related deaths, followed by MVCs (CDC, 2020f).

Etiology

Poisonings are the leading cause of injury death in the United States, with 70,000 people losing their lives to drug poisoning in 2018 (CDC, 2020b) (see **Figure 32.5** ››). The CDC (2020b) indicates the majority of drug poisonings involved prescription as well as nonprescription opioids. Opioid drug poisoning is such a major concern in the United States that it has been identified as an epidemic (DHHS, 2020a).

Motor-vehicle crashes are also a major concern because of the significance of the injuries sustained. Distracted and impaired driving are leading causes of MVCs (CDC, 2020p). A report issued in 2020 found MVCs to be the leading cause of death among U.S. adolescents (Yellman, Bryan, Sauber-Schatz, & Brener, 2020). Furthermore, MVCs often result in multiple injured persons and have potential to be mass-casualty incidents.

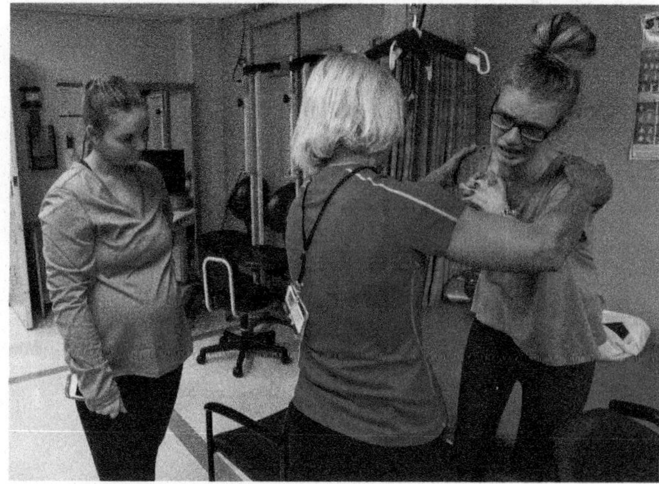

Figure 32.5 ›› A physical therapist works with a 19-year-old as she learns to walk after experiencing a heroin overdose 2 years earlier.

Source: Nikki Kahn/The Washington Post/Getty Images.

Mass-casualty incidents (MCIs) are not defined by a specific number of persons injured but as the number of casualties that exceed local capacity to respond or that exceed available resources. Available resources include both medical supplies and medical personnel (Ahmad, 2018). Disasters, whether natural or human made, have been on the rise over the past two decades and commonly result in MCIs.

In the year 2020, wildfires plagued California's landscape, with 9,639 incidents of wildfires resulting in 31 fatalities (State of California, 2020). Reports indicate that California's annual fire season is expanding in length, increasing by as much 75 days. An extended fire season can tax resources that have historically not been needed to manage the disastrous wildfires (State of California, 2020).

Human-made disasters, such as shooting incidents, are the basis for a multitude of MCIs. In 2019, the FBI recorded 28 shooting incidents that resulted in mass casualties (U.S. Department of Justice [DOJ], 2020). A shooting incident in El Paso, Texas, had the highest number of casualties that year, with 23 killed and 22 wounded. Following close behind was a shooting incident in Dayton, Ohio, in which 9 people were killed and 27 were wounded. Resources to respond to shooting incidents can quickly become overwhelmed when many people are injured. Traumatic injuries from shootings tend to be multisystem in nature, which can further tax resources.

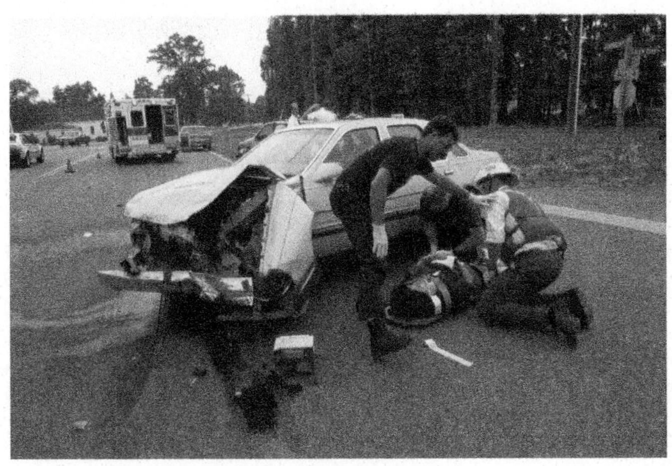

Figure 32.6 ›› Beginning drivers take more risks and are three times more likely to be involved in a crash.
Source: Tim Wright/Corbis Historical/Getty Images.

Risk Factors

A multitude of risk factors are associated with multisystem trauma. Some of the major causes of injury and death, associated with the etiologies of poisonings, MVCs, and MCIs are discussed in this section. Refer to the following sections in this module for additional information related to risk factors for multisystem trauma related to these etiologies: interpersonal violence, community and systemic violence, and accidental/incidental trauma.

Poison includes any substance that is harmful to the body with too much exposure (i.e., ingestion, inhalation, injection). While many of the poisonings in the United States are attributed to the opioid epidemic, poisoning related to environmental agents still remains. Poisoning in children is often associated with exploration in the environment; for example, by ingestion of household cleaners or prescription medications that were not secured. Conversely, adult poisonings are often related to misuse of drugs. In 2018 misuse of opioids accounted for 69.5% of all drug-related poisoning deaths (CDC, 2020d).

While some MVCs are influenced by forces of nature, such as bad weather or wildlife running across the road, the primary cause of accidents is human error. Risk factors associated with human error include speeding, distraction, aggressive driving, and impaired driving. Another factor that is commonly associated with MVCs is age.

People at all ages are at risk for MVCs, with an elevated incidence in younger and older drivers (CDC, 2020g, 2020q) (**Figure 32.6 ››**). Inexperience is associated with the elevated risk for MVC in the younger driver. Younger drivers are more likely to speed and underestimate dangerous driving situations or conditions than adult drivers (CDC, 2020g). Individuals age 16 to 19 are three times more likely to be involved in a crash than drivers age 20 and older (CDC, 2020g). Increased risk for MVCs in the older adult driver (age 65 and older) are in part associated with age-related decline in cognitive function and vision (CDC, 2020q).

Unsafe driving practices are major contributors to risk for MVCs and span every age group. For instance, when speeding it is difficult to stop effectively if there is a sudden incident —such as another car stopping suddenly or a pedestrian unexpectedly crossing the street. Impaired driving limits a driver's ability to react quickly, potentially leading to an accident due to delayed response time. Other driving traits that represent a risk for MVCs are driver distraction and aggressive driving. Distraction can result from using a phone, dropping a beverage or food item while driving, or even having a crying child in the car. Aggressive driving leads to tailgating and other dangerous driving habits that increase the risk for accidents.

Prevention

Trauma-related injuries and deaths are preventable. Knowledge of the causes of multisystem trauma and at-risk groups directs prevention efforts. Injury is the greatest health hazard for most age groups; therefore, injury prevention must be integrated into every health contact with all patients.

Poisonings can be prevented by ensuring that medications are taken as prescribed, keeping medications in a secure area out of reach of children, and monitoring medications taken by children, teenagers, and older adults to ensure that no errors occur in administration. Household cleaners and other substances should be kept out of reach of children. Substance abuse may also lead to poisoning; therefore, it is important to encourage the abuser to obtain substance abuse treatment.

MVCs can be prevented by teaching and following safe driving practices, including not texting while driving and using a designated driver. Prevention efforts among older adults can be in the form of regular eye and hearing examinations as well as considerations of side effects of any medications being taken.

Adolescents are at risk for sports-related injuries as well as MVCs. Prevention programs may center around sports safety, including concussion prevention education and use of safety equipment. Prevention efforts for MVCs can include driver education, public safety campaigns, and mitigation efforts to identify potential hazards and likelihood of their occurrence (see Exemplar 46.A, Emergency Preparedness, in Module 46, Healthcare Systems). Health promotion and injury prevention strategies for people of all ages are provided in Module 7, Health, Wellness, Illness, and Injury, and in Module 51, Safety.

SAFETY ALERT Older adults are frequently on multiple medications that may cause vertigo, drowsiness, or orthostatic hypotension. The patient should be educated on the side effects of the medications and be advised of the dangers of driving while taking them.

Patient Teaching

Poison Safety for Families with Children

Persons with children in the home should be educated on poison safety:

- Read the label before you give medicine to a child.
- Use the right dosing cup, measuring spoon, or syringe.
- Never refer to medications as "candy."
- Put medication caps on tightly and know that child-resistant closures are not childproof.
- Lock medicines and household products high, where children can't see or reach them.
- Store medications and household products in their original containers.
- Maintain working smoke and carbon monoxide detectors in the hallway near every sleeping area in the home.
- Learn first aid and CPR.
- If you use e-cigarettes, buy refills that use child-resistant packaging and keep refills locked away where children can't see or reach them.
- Know the names of all the plants in your house and yard and consider removing those that are poisonous to young children or pets.

Sources: American Academy of Pediatrics (2019); National Capital Poison Center (2020).

Clinical Manifestations

Motor-vehicle crashes, violence, abuse, and disaster-related events often result in a combination of physical and emotional injuries. Physical injuries can range from mild (minor scrapes and contusions) to severe (broken bones, head injuries, and even fatal injuries). When emotional injuries are present, they are often in the form of acute stress disorder (especially if other victims were severely or fatally injured) or a fear of exposure to the same event. Nurses will see a wide range of injuries as the result of trauma-related events.

Injuries are very common as the result of trauma, with some of the more prevalent injuries being whiplash, **traumatic brain injury (TBI)** (brain trauma that occurs from external physical force), spinal cord injuries, facial injuries, internal organ damage, and fractures. **Whiplash** results when a sudden impact to a motor vehicle causes an individual's head and neck to be forcibly contorted, resulting in injury to the spine. Spinal injuries are common in trauma and can result in partial or complete paralysis. Facial injuries and TBI often occur in trauma-related events due to the individual's head hitting the dashboard, steering wheel, or air bag; blunt trauma from a violent assault; or objects falling on the victim's head. Although wearing a seat belt can save a life, seat belts can also cause injuries during a crash. Common injuries from a seat belt are fractured ribs, fractured collarbone, internal injuries, and organ damage (e.g., cardiac contusion), as well as the potential for a punctured lung secondary to broken ribs.

Clinical Manifestations and Therapies

Multisystem Trauma

ETIOLOGY	CLINICAL MANIFESTATIONS	CLINICAL THERAPIES
Mild head injury	▪ Headache ▪ Sensitivity to light, blurred vision ▪ Nausea, dizziness, balance problems ▪ Changes in memory	▪ CT, MRI, and/or electroencephalogram (EEG) to determine the extent of the injury ▪ Stitches for open wounds ▪ Elevation of head of bed to 30 degrees ▪ Pharmacologic therapies such as analgesics and nonsteroidal anti-inflammatory drugs (NSAIDs)
Traumatic brain injury	▪ Loss of consciousness ▪ Headache; repeated nausea and vomiting ▪ Dilation of one or both pupils ▪ Confusion ▪ Seizures and coma	▪ CT, MRI, and/or EEG to determine the extent of the injury ▪ Stitches for open wounds ▪ Elevation of head of bed to 30 degrees ▪ Pharmacologic therapies such as diuretics, anticonvulsants, analgesics, and NSAIDs ▪ Surgery to remove hematomas, repair skull fractures, remove skull fragments from the brain, or cut out a section of the skull to allow for swelling of the brain, which diminishes the pressure on the brain ▪ Physical and/or speech therapy depending on the severity of the injury

(continued on next page)

Clinical Manifestations and Therapies *(continued)*

ETIOLOGY	CLINICAL MANIFESTATIONS	CLINICAL THERAPIES
Cervical spine injury (whiplash)	▪ Neck stiffness and pain ▪ Dizziness, blurred vision, headaches, ringing in the ears ▪ Concentration and memory problems	▪ Lidocaine injections into the affected muscle to relieve pain and muscle spasms ▪ Ice and heat therapy ▪ Physical therapy ▪ Immobilization collar to promote proper healing ▪ Pharmacologic therapies such as muscle relaxants, analgesics, and NSAIDs
Spinal cord injury, either incomplete or complete	▪ Loss of sensation and movement below affected area ▪ Pain if nerve damage is present ▪ Breathing difficulty ▪ Loss of bladder and bowel control ▪ Numbness and tingling in extremities	▪ Immobilization of the spine with a neck collar ▪ Sedation to prevent further damage to the spine, if necessary ▪ Surgery, if indicated ▪ Physical therapy and rehabilitation ▪ Pharmacologic therapies such as analgesics, NSAIDs, and methylprednisolone (Medrol) to decrease inflammation and nerve damage
Cardiovascular injury	▪ Pallor ▪ Tachycardia ▪ Dysrhythmia ▪ Dyspnea ▪ Hypotension ▪ Hemorrhage ▪ Pain	▪ X-ray, CT, electrocardiogram, ultrasound ▪ Control bleeding ▪ Cardiac enzymes ▪ Cardiac monitoring ▪ Treatment for arrhythmia ▪ Pharmacologic therapies such as analgesics, NSAIDs, and antiarrhythmics. ▪ Administration of blood products ▪ Surgical repair
Respiratory injury	▪ Cyanosis ▪ Dyspnea ▪ Tachypnea ▪ Hypotension ▪ Confusion ▪ Agitation ▪ Crepitus	▪ X-ray, CT ▪ Arterial blood gases ▪ Respiratory monitoring ▪ Oxygenation ▪ Assisted ventilation ▪ Pharmacologic therapies such as analgesics, NSAIDs, corticosteroids, and bronchodilators ▪ Surgical repair
Gastrointestinal injury	▪ Nausea ▪ Vomiting ▪ Hematemesis ▪ Diarrhea ▪ Pain ▪ Rigid abdomen ▪ Rebound tenderness	▪ CT, ultrasound, colonoscopy, endoscopy ▪ Nasogastric aspiration ▪ Pharmacologic therapies such as analgesics, NSAIDs, and antibiotics. ▪ Peritoneal wash ▪ Surgical repair
Musculoskeletal injury	▪ Deformity ▪ Numbness and tingling ▪ Crepitus ▪ Altered range of motion ▪ Pain ▪ Edema ▪ Bruising	▪ X-ray, CT, MRI ▪ Ice and heat therapy ▪ Immobilization/casting ▪ Physical therapy ▪ Surgical repair ▪ Pharmacologic therapies such as analgesics, NSAIDs, corticosteroids

Collaboration

Collaborative care of the patient who has sustained multisystem traumatic injury is guided by an organized and systematic team approach (**Figure 32.7** »). The team is comprised of an interprofessional group of individuals that may vary by institution, often including emergency medical technicians, nurses, physicians, surgeons, and allied health professionals. The primary focus of the team is rapid resuscitation and stabilization of the patient. Prompt delegation of tasks and responsibilities improves the patient's chances for survival and decreases the morbidity that may result from traumatic injuries.

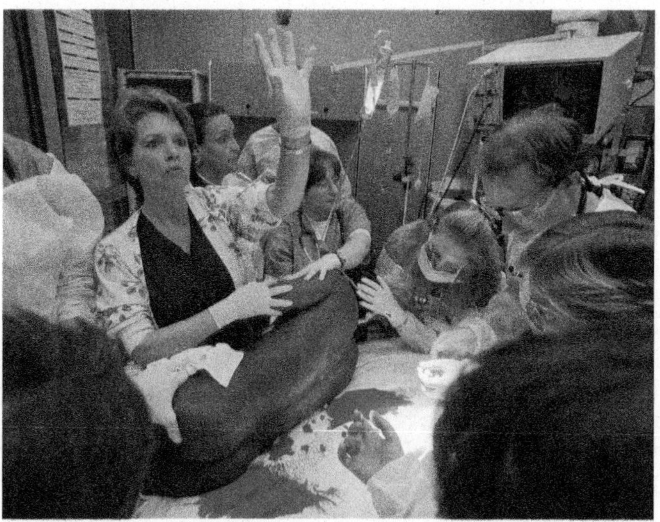

Figure 32.7 » A nurse in the emergency department asks for a wipe to clean off blood from the victim of a stabbing.
Source: Robert Tirey/Alamy Stock Photo.

Community awareness and health promotion efforts require collaboration as well. Healthcare institutions along with local fire departments, law enforcement, and health departments will often combine to offer awareness campaigns regarding issues related to MVCs, violence prevention, and disaster readiness. Communities create disaster or emergency readiness plans that train healthcare professionals and volunteers to improve capability of response.

» **Stay Current:** Many organizations such as the Society of Trauma Nurses and the American College of Surgeons offer courses in trauma care for nurses. For more information, visit the Advanced Trauma Care for Nurses page at http://www.traumanurses.org/atcn and the Advanced Trauma Life Support page at www.facs.org/trauma/atls/about.html.

Diagnostic Tests

Because trauma-related injuries vary widely, so do the diagnostic tests used to assess the severity of those injuries. Common diagnostic procedures include MRIs, CT scans, x-rays, ultrasound, and the focused abdominal sonography for trauma (FAST) that is conducted at the patient's bedside. These procedures can help to determine the severity of head, neck, and back injuries and to identify internal bleeding, broken bones, or torn muscles. An EEG can be used to diagnose changes in brain activity.

Surgery

The life-threatening nature of traumatic incidents will often lead to a patient needing surgery to repair damage and/or stop internal bleeding. If internal organ damage is indicated—due either to organ rupture or to a foreign object puncturing the abdominal cavity—emergency surgery will be needed to repair the damage and stabilize the patient.

Injuries involving severe head or spinal trauma may require surgery depending on the circumstances. Head injuries will not always need surgery; however, if an intracranial hemorrhage is present and the bleeding does not stop on its own, surgery may be the only solution. Intracranial pressure will be monitored when a head injury is present, and if the pressure rises to dangerous levels, surgery will be performed to release some of the pressure. Spinal injuries are often irreversible; in most cases surgery is needed to remove bone fragments and to stabilize the spine (Mayo Clinic, 2020e).

Pharmacologic Therapy

The majority of injuries sustained will be painful to patients and will require pain management. Less severe injuries involving sprains, minor cuts, and mild concussions may be treated with analgesics such as acetaminophen and ibuprofen. Deep cuts requiring sutures will usually be treated with lidocaine as a numbing agent. In cases of more severe injuries, particularly those that require surgery, stronger pain medications—most often opioids—are administered. Sedation may be necessary if the patient's reaction to the injuries or the pain puts the individual in danger of further injury.

Nonpharmacologic Therapy

Distraction has been identified as an effective nonpharmacologic therapy in the treatment of pain (Birnie, Chambers, & Spellman, 2017; Boles, 2018). Distraction may be used alone or in combination with pharmacologic interventions but may not be appropriate in cases of severe pain (University of Florida Health, 2020).

Physical therapy and rehabilitation are often required for severe injuries, including broken bones (especially compound fractures), spinal injuries, and some TBIs. Patients with impairments in neurologic, motor, speech, and/or language functioning may require speech therapy. Patients with TBI or another injury that impairs self-care and other abilities may work with an occupational therapist to relearn some of those activities. Individuals will be provided with a referral and resources for therapy and counseling to help with emotional trauma resulting from the accident.

Complementary Health Approaches

Complementary health approaches are normally not recommended for anything other than mild injuries, although some pain reduction strategies, such as mindfulness meditation, may be used in conjunction with pharmacologic therapy with provider approval. For patients requiring rehabilitation, therapists may use integrative therapy that is tailored to the patient's specific needs. Thorough assessment of patient preferences regarding the use of complementary health approaches is necessary at each stage of assessment and treatment for patients with multisystem trauma.

Lifespan Considerations

Infants and Toddlers with Multisystem Trauma

Traffic accidents are a leading cause of multisystem trauma in infants and toddlers (**Figure 32.8** »). Infants and children are more susceptible to multisystem trauma than adults because of their small body size and, with infants, open cranial sutures and fontanels; however, they recover better than adults, especially from head trauma (Kennedy, Scorpio, & Coppota, 2018). The open fontanels allow for increased intracranial mass or brain swelling, which may mask symptoms of injury until a rapid decompensation occurs; therefore, bulging fontanels indicate a severe injury and should be treated as such.

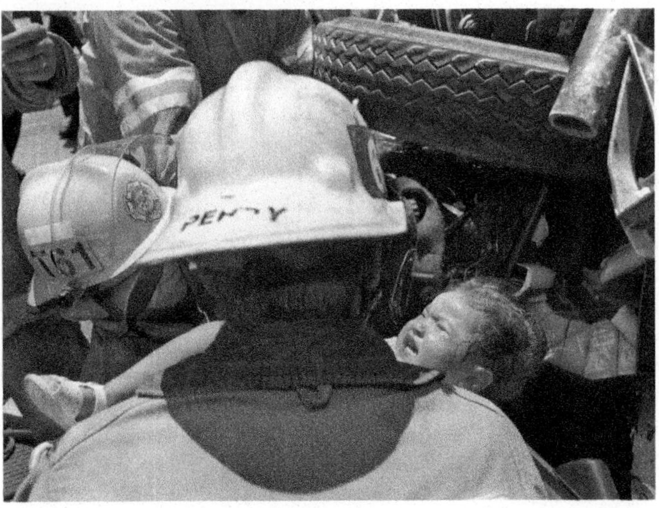

Figure 32.8 » Motor-vehicle crashes are the leading cause of multisystem trauma in infants and toddlers. This 2-year-old girl was trapped under a tractor-trailer and had to be extricated using the Jaws of Life. She was in a car seat strapped in the backseat of her mother's car, and she sustained moderate injuries.
Source: Kari Rene Hall/Los Angeles Times/Getty Images.

Nurses working in pediatric clinics and urgent and emergency settings need to be alert for signs of child abuse. Injuries such as fractured ribs, multicolored bruises, evidence of previous healed injuries, fractures of long bones in children younger than 3 years, and retinal hemorrhages may indicate maltreatment and warrant an intensive investigation.

Children and Adolescents with Multisystem Trauma

Assessment priorities for a child are the same as for an adult; however, there may be even more serious effects of trauma in the pediatric patient because of the anatomical and physical characteristics of the younger patient (Kennedy et al., 2018). Children are still growing, which means that after a traumatic injury, their bodies must not only heal from the injury but also continue to develop. The nurse also needs to be alert for signs of abuse.

Children are more likely to experience seizures after head trauma and require diagnostic testing with a CT scan (Bennett, DeWitt, Harlaar, & Bennett, 2017). Children often present with injuries to the pancreas, perforations to the small bowel, and bladder ruptures that are generally related to blunt impact such as from bicycle handlebars and seat belts worn during an MVC (Kennedy et al., 2018). When a child has a fractured bone, the bone will heal, but the bone's growth plate may be affected, causing that affected bone to quit growing. Thoracic trauma in children, while not as common as abdominal trauma, presents risk for pneumothorax (Kennedy et al., 2018). If a pneumothorax is identified, treatment is the same as for adults.

Pregnant Women with Multisystem Trauma

There are two patients when a pregnant woman sustains multisystem trauma—the mother and the fetus; however, treatment priorities are the same for a pregnant woman as for a nonpregnant woman (ACSCOT, 2017). The best treatment for the fetus is resuscitation of the mother. The mother should be assessed, followed by an assessment of the fetus, and then a secondary assessment of the mother. Abdominal examination is a priority in the pregnant patient.

An increase in blood volume occurs in the pregnant woman. In cases of severe blood loss, the fetus may be in distress and the placenta deprived of oxygen before symptoms (tachycardia, hypotension, and other signs of hypovolemia) occur in the mother. The mother's condition and vital signs may appear stable initially with hypovolemia. It is also important to keep uterine compression of the vena cava from occurring. This can be completed by manually displacing the uterus to the left side, which relieves pressure on the inferior vena cava.

Fetal demise is often a result of maternal shock or death. Fetal heart rate can indicate fetal distress and should be monitored closely in the pregnant woman who is being treated for injury (average fetal heart rate is 110 to 160 beats per minute). The main cause of fetal death from trauma during pregnancy is placental abruption (Mayo Clinic, 2020f). It is important to note that abruption of the placenta or other fetal demise does not always cause vaginal bleeding.

Older Adults with Multisystem Trauma

Older adults are more likely to have a fatal outcome from injury, with falls being the most common cause of multisystem trauma resulting in death (ACSCOT, 2017). Older adults wearing dentures, which can interfere with maintaining airway, should remove them or have them removed if broken or loose. Monitoring the respiratory system closely is critical secondary to the decreased respiratory reserve due to the aging process. Another consideration regarding the older adult includes obtaining a medication history, as the patient may be on one or more medications that may alter the response to the physiologic stress of trauma. For instance, patients taking beta blockers may not have the same tachycardic response to hypovolemia that most patients do, as beta blockers do not allow for the increased heart rate. The nurse should always be alert to the increased risk of abuse for this vulnerable population.

NURSING PROCESS

Nursing care of a patient who is injured begins with primary assessment of injuries. Life-threatening injuries require immediate, collaborative interventions per protocol. For MCIs an additional part of the nursing process assessment is to use reverse triage where the most severely injured patients, who may require the greatest amount of resources, are treated last (see Exemplar 46.A, Emergency Preparedness, in Module 46, Healthcare Systems).

Assessment

Airway maintenance and obstruction are given primary consideration. Any changes to breath sounds, breathing patterns, oxygen levels, or LOC require immediate assessment. Hemorrhage also requires immediate intervention. Cervical and spinal immobilization should be maintained to reduce risk of spinal cord injury. Cervical and spinal immobilization should be discontinued only by physician's order after determining that the patient has not sustained a spinal injury.

Diagnosis

Traumatic injuries can be complex and put the patient at risk for a variety of potential alterations in health, as well as psychological, financial, and family stress. Priorities for care include ongoing monitoring of the respiratory and circulatory status as well as monitoring LOC. Priorities for care will be patient and injury specific, but may include airway clearance and patency, tissue perfusion, fluid volume, risk for infection, mobility, pain, and stress and coping.

Planning

Goals are based on individualized patient needs and the type and amount of trauma sustained. Goals may include the following:

- The patient's airway will remain patent.
- The patient will demonstrate regular, nonlabored respirations and oxygen saturation level 95% or greater.
- The patient's blood pressure will be maintained within normal limits.
- The patient will not develop cardiac dysrhythmias.
- The patient will remain free of signs or symptoms of infection.
- The patient will remain free of sensory deficits.
- The patient will retain or regain mobility.

Implementation

Nursing interventions for the patient who has sustained trauma injuries follow the priorities of ABCDE: airway, breathing, circulation, disability (neurologic status), and exposure (tissue integrity, temperature). Once these areas have been addressed, the nurse can begin to assess other areas.

Maintain Airway Patency and Ventilation

Airway obstruction and apnea are risks for the patient with multiple injuries. Bleeding and vomiting increase risk for aspiration, while facial injuries and loose teeth can create an airway obstruction. Cerebral edema can alter the respiratory drive.

- For patients who do not require tracheal intubation and controlled or assisted ventilation, administer supplemental oxygen per hospital protocols by way of face mask or nasal cannula.
- Monitor and maintain oxygen saturation between 95 and 100%. Decreased oxygen saturation readings despite a patent airway may indicate inadequate ventilation or ineffective oxygen exchange.
- Monitor LOC. Changes in LOC can be an early sign of an ineffective airway. Restlessness, irritability, anxiety, or unresponsiveness indicate a need for immediate assessment of airway patency.

SAFETY ALERT Pulse oximetry is an unreliable indicator of oxygen status in cases of carbon monoxide exposure because it cannot differentiate between carboxyhemoglobin and oxyhemoglobin.

Assess for Neurologic Deficits and Expose Obscured Areas

For a trauma assessment, neurologic status and exposure are also assessed.

- Neurologic assessment includes identifying altered LOC, abnormal pupillary response to light, impaired or diminished mobility, and decreased or absent sensation.
- Exposure requires removal of the patient's clothing to allow for identification of injuries that may be obscured. Expose the patient only as needed for assessment and treatment.
- Full assessment requires that the patient be rolled to one side for inspection of the back and posterior of the body. When rolling the patient to one side, the trauma team will use a technique known as "logrolling," which allows for maintenance of neutral alignment of the spine.
- To prevent hypothermia, warm blankets may be used to cover the patient, and the room temperature may be increased during periods for which exposure is required.

Promote Fluid Volume Balance

Both blood loss and the shifting of fluid from the intravascular space can lead to hypovolemia, which, if left untreated, may progress to cardiovascular shock. Therefore, the plan of care for patients who sustain significant traumatic injuries includes:

- Insertion of a large-bore IV catheter (preferably two catheters 18 gauge or larger in diameter) for administration of fluids, medications, and blood products.
- Administration of IV fluid and blood products as per the physician's orders.
- Insertion of a Foley catheter for continued assessment of urine production, which is an indirect reflection of the patient's kidney function and fluid volume status.

Prevent Infection

Traumatic injuries are considered dirty wounds, especially if the skin has been punctured by external material or by an open fracture. Risk factors for wound infection include contamination, inadequate wound care, and the condition of the wound at the time of closure (Bauldoff, Gubrud, & Carno, 2020). Strict standard precautions and aseptic technique when providing wound care will reduce the risk of infection for both the patient and the nurse. Ongoing monitoring includes:

- Assessing wounds for signs of infection, such as redness, heat, swelling, or purulent drainage.
- Avoiding cross-contamination between wounds. Clean each wound separately.
- Assess vital signs frequently for indications of infection, such as elevated body temperature.
- Provide adequate fluids and nutrition to promote wound healing.
- Determine status of tetanus immunization and immunize patient as prescribed.
- Use strict aseptic technique when performing any invasive procedure, such as inserting a catheter or administering parenteral medications, to reduce the risk of infection.

SAFETY ALERT Following traumatic injury with serious tissue damage, patients have an increased risk of developing gangrene, which is the death of body tissue due to lack of blood flow or major bacterial infection (Mayo Clinic, 2020b). Manifestations of gangrene include fever, pain, swelling, and drainage with a foul odor. Gangrene that goes unnoticed and untreated can lead to sepsis and even death.

Promote Mobility

Patients with spinal injuries, multiple injuries, peripheral nerve injuries, or amputations are at the greatest risks for complications related to an inability to change positions independently. Complications can range from integumentary (e.g., pressure injuries) to respiratory complications (such as pneumonia) and complications in other organ systems. A collaborative approach with the nurse, physical therapist, and occupational therapist will be used to determine the most effective methods of promoting mobility to reduce complications, including:

- Provide active or passive exercises to extremities at least once every 8 hours as long as active bleeding and edema are not present.
- Encourage and help patients to change positions at least every 2 hours.
- Encourage patients to use the incentive spirometer at least every 2 hours and to engage in deep breathing and coughing.
- Monitor lower extremities daily for signs of deep venous thrombosis (heat, swelling, and pain). Measure and record thigh and calf circumference daily.
- Remove compression stockings for an hour each shift and assess the skin.

Promote Healthy Grieving

Death as a result of traumatic injury usually strikes quickly and without warning. Families may be overwhelmed by the need for decisions (such as whether to donate a loved one's organs) to be made quickly. Nursing care may include the following measures to assist families as they process their new reality:

- Give the family information about organ donation and stress that it is only an option and the choice is up to them.
- Encourage family members to ask questions and express their feelings about what happened, the nature of the trauma, and/or organ donation.
- Refer the family for follow-up care if they desire.
- Provide the family of a dying or deceased patient the opportunity to observe religious rituals, such as prayer, together. Provide an opportunity for the family to call for a minister or spiritual leader.
- Provide presence, ensuring the family that they and their loved one are valued.

More information on promoting healthy grieving can be found in Module 27, Grief and Loss. Information on providing care to patients and family members in spiritual distress can be found in Module 30, Spiritualty.

Communicating with Patients and Families

Working Phase

A family has just experienced the death of their loved one from a motor vehicle crash. The nurse is offering them information regarding organ donation. The patient's husband is tearful and states, "This is overwhelming." The nurse uses physical presencing and empathetic listening.

- Presencing is demonstrated as the nurse sits down to be in the moment with the patient's husband.
- Empathetic listening is demonstrated as the nurse sits still, silently giving the patient's husband time to collect his thoughts.

Promote Psychosocial Well-Being

Acute stress disorder is an immediate, intense, sustained emotional response to a disastrous event. It is characterized by intrusive distressing memories and emotions that range from anger to fear. The patient may be calm or may express feelings of anger, disbelief, terror, and shock, which may last from 3 days up to 1 month. Some individuals who witness or experience a traumatic event may develop PTSD, characterized by flashbacks and nightmares of the traumatic event (see the exemplar that follows). The patient may use ineffective coping mechanisms, such as alcohol or drugs, and withdraw from relationships. Appropriate nursing interventions include the following:

- Assess for psychological manifestations of acute stress disorder and PTSD. Observe for hyperarousal, exaggerated startle response, aggressive behaviors, sleep disturbances, and patient's description of intrusive thoughts.
- Create a quiet and calm environment. Reassure that the patient is safe and maintain an open presence, encouraging the patient to express feelings.
- Teach relaxation techniques, such as deep breathing or guided imagery, in response to stressors These techniques produce increased relaxation and are often useful in coping with exaggerated emotions and intrusive thoughts surrounding the trauma.
- Advocate for patients and their families by linking them to treatment resources needed for a successful recovery from trauma. Resources include counseling, psychotherapy, and support groups. Additionally, financial resources to ensure accessibility to treatment resources may be needed.

Facilitate Transitions

Whether a patient is discharged to a rehabilitation center or to home, the patient and family may have many questions about "what comes next." Provide patient and family teaching about services ordered (such as physical therapy), medications, and wound care. Help family members understand the extent of assistance the patient will need and whom to call for assistance, equipment, and supplies.

Evaluation

The care of each patient will vary based on the type and severity of injuries. In some cases, the patient will be discharged the same day as the injury occurred, whereas other patients will need treatment for a longer period. Some desired outcomes for patients include the following:

- The patient's airway remains free of obstruction.
- The patient's respiratory rate remains within normal limits

- The patient's oxygen saturation is maintained at 95% or greater.
- The patient develops no cardiac dysrhythmias.
- The patient's blood pressure is maintained within normal limits.
- The patient remains free of signs or symptoms of infection.
- The patient develops no neurovascular deficits.
- The patient retains mobility.
- The patient verbally expresses emotions and concerns.

If outcomes are not met, another assessment will need to occur to determine what is preventing the patient from meeting established goals. For example, if the patient is not able to bear weight in the set amount of time, there may be an unidentified injury or complications related to a postsurgical procedure. Another example would be that the patient's vital signs do not stabilize after surgery. An assessment will need to occur to determine the cause of the decompensation, which may be an unidentified internal hemorrhage.

Nursing Care Plan

A Patient with Multiple Injuries

Jane Souza is a 25-year-old married woman with two children who provides daycare for preschool children in her home. As she is driving the interstate at 65 miles per hour, a car crosses the median and strikes her vehicle head-on. Ms. Souza, who is not wearing a seat belt, is thrown forward against the steering wheel. The front of her car is pushed up against her by the car that struck her, entrapping her lower extremities. After extensive efforts to extricate her from the car, Ms. Souza is transported to the local trauma center. She is still conscious, is receiving high-flow oxygen by mask, and has one IV line in place. Her vital signs are a palpable systolic blood pressure of 80 mmHg, a pulse rate of 120 beats/min, and a respiratory rate of 36/min. On arrival, she states that she is having difficulty breathing.

ASSESSMENT	DIAGNOSES	PLANNING
■ *Airway:* Maintainable with high-flow oxygen in place. ■ *Breathing:* Respiratory rate of 36/min, multiple bruising and abrasions on right side of her chest, decreased breath sounds on the right side. ■ *Circulation:* No palpable radial pulses; palpable brachial pulses. Monitor shows sinus tachycardia. No active external bleeding noted. Skin color pale, cool to the touch, and diaphoretic. ■ *Neurologic:* Moved her fingers when asked; complains of difficulty breathing; denies that she is hurt. Pupils 4 mm, equal, and react to light. Has a fractured right arm and an open fracture of the left ankle; because of these injuries, extremity movement is limited. Because of Ms. Souza's respiratory distress, she is intubated and ventilated with 100% oxygen. Another IV line is inserted and O-negative is blood administered.	■ Ineffective breathing pattern related to multiple bruises and abrasions on the right side of the chest and respiratory difficulty ■ Potential for fluid volume deficiency related to acute internal blood loss (presumed as external source of bleeding was not identified) ■ Risk of injury related to trauma resuscitation	Patient goals include: ■ The patient will maintain adequate oxygenation. ■ The patient will maintain adequate circulating blood volume.

IMPLEMENTATION

- Monitor airway and assist in any needed airway management.
- Explain all procedures.
- Monitor the effects of fluid and blood administration, including any changes in blood pressure and pulse.
- Prepare for transfer to the operating room for emergency surgery.
- Keep family informed about her condition.

EVALUATION

Ms. Souza is transferred to the operating room, where it is determined that she has a ruptured spleen and a serious pelvic fracture.

Ms. Souza's treatment continues in the operating room.

CRITICAL THINKING

1. Is the priority of potential for fluid volume deficiency appropriate for Ms. Souza? Why or why not?
2. The assessment of a patient who has experienced trauma is ABCDE. What is the rationale for this sequence?
3. Following surgery, Ms. Souza is moved to the surgical intensive care unit. She is very anxious and restless. What assessments would you make to identify the cause of her restlessness?
4. Infection is a common complication for the trauma patient. Describe five risks for infection that are present from the time of injury to the time of hospital discharge.

REVIEW Multisystem Trauma

RELATE Link the Concepts and Exemplars

Linking the exemplar of multisystem trauma with the concept of intracranial regulation:

1. What is the priority of care when your patient who experienced a head injury in a MVC has a blood pressure of 90/60 mmHg and a heart rate of 51 bpm?
2. What nursing interventions would be appropriate for inclusion in the plan of care for the patient who has a head injury from a MVC to prevent the rise of intracranial pressure?

Linking the exemplar of multisystem trauma with the concept of perfusion:

3. Describe potential threats to a patient's perfusion as a result of a MVC. How would perfusion be impacted if the patient's mobility was altered because of traction or other immobilizing treatments?
4. How can you promote mobility for a patient involved in a MVC who has a casted left leg and right arm? How would this plan change if the patient were an older adult with diminished mobility prior to the trauma?

READY Go to Volume 3: Clinical Nursing Skills

REFER Go to Pearson MyLab Nursing and eText

REFLECT Apply Your Knowledge

Lilia Hoffman, age 25, was the driver of a vehicle that was struck by another vehicle at an intersection. The driver of the car that hit her ran a red light. Ms. Hoffman was extracted from her car using the Jaws of Life and was moaning when initially removed but did not respond to verbal commands. Her pupils were pinpoint and reactive to light. The paramedics at the scene provided initial emergent care. Her vital signs included temperature 96.2°F oral; pulse 110 beats/min; respirations 12/min; and blood pressure 90/50 mmHg. She had bleeding from facial and scalp lacerations as well as suspected rib fractures. Her lung sounds were clear and equal bilaterally, and her oxygen saturation was 97%. Ms. Hoffman's airway was determined to be patent and oxygen was administered via face mask at 10 liters per minute.

The air bag in Ms. Hoffman's car deployed. It was unknown whether she sustained a head or neck injury. One of the paramedics immediately administered manual stabilization of her cervical spine until a cervical collar (c-collar) was applied. In addition to c-spine immobilization, Ms. Hoffman was placed on a long spinal board to prepare for transport to the local ED. Circulatory status was assessed and an 18-gauge IV catheter was inserted in her left forearm, followed by IV administration of 0.9% normal saline at a rate of 150 mL/hr.

In the ED, Ms. Hoffman's vital signs were temperature 98°F oral; pulse 118 beats/min; respirations 14/min; and blood pressure 98/50 mmHg. An IV bolus of 250 mL of normal saline was administered and a Foley catheter inserted. Her airway remained patent and oxygen was continued.

1. What are three nursing care priorities for Ms. Hoffman?
2. What laboratory and diagnostic tests should the nurse anticipate being ordered?
3. Under what circumstances can Ms. Hoffman's spinal precautions (cervical collar and longboard spinal immobilization) be discontinued?

» Exemplar 32.C Posttraumatic Stress Disorder

Exemplar Learning Outcomes

32.C Analyze posttraumatic stress disorder (PTSD) as it relates to trauma.

- Describe the pathophysiology of PTSD.
- Describe the etiology of PTSD.
- Compare the risk factors and prevention of PTSD.
- Identify the clinical manifestations of PTSD.
- Summarize therapies used by interprofessional teams in the collaborative care of an individual with PTSD.
- Differentiate care of patients with PTSD across the lifespan.
- Apply the nursing process in providing culturally competent care to an individual with PTSD.

Exemplar Key Terms

Acute stress disorder, *2175*
Depersonalization, *2176*
Eye movement desensitization and reprocessing (EMDR), *2177*
Flashbacks, *2176*
Posttraumatic stress disorder (PTSD), *2174*

Overview

Each individual responds to traumatic events differently based on their own personal history, coping mechanisms, and the exact circumstances surrounding the nature of the traumatic event. For an individual to be diagnosed with a trauma or stressor-related disorder (e.g., acute stress disorder or PTSD), the individual must meet specific criteria for diagnosis, of which the first is exposure to a traumatic or stressful event (such as war, assault, childhood trauma, or natural or human-caused disaster). There is a close relationship between trauma-related disorders and anxiety, obsessive–compulsive, and dissociative disorders. Depending on the individual, emotional symptoms of trauma or stressor-related disorders can vary greatly from fear and anxiety to agitation and dysphoria (American Psychiatric Association, 2013). PTSD can affect any person from any background across the lifespan.

The American Psychiatric Association (2013) characterizes **posttraumatic stress disorder (PTSD)** as a disorder in which an individual who is exposed to a traumatic event develops intrusive symptoms, such as recurrent nightmares; patterns of persistent attempts to avoid stimuli associated with or reminiscent of the traumatic event; negative changes in cognition or mood; and marked changes in reactivity or arousal, such as hypervigilance or impaired concentration. For an individual to be diagnosed, these symptoms must occur for more than 1 month beyond the precipitating event. Acute stress disorder is similar to PTSD, but the symptoms only last from 3 days to 1 month following exposure to one or more traumatic events (American Psychiatric Association, 2013).

Pathophysiology

The pathophysiology of PTSD is unclear. What is known is that PTSD leads to changes in the anatomy and neurophysiology of the brain. MRI studies in individuals with PTSD have shown an overly reactive amygdala, which is involved in processing emotions and modulating fear response (Gore, 2018). Individuals with PTSD tend to have low circulating levels of cortisol, the hormone that fuels the "fight-or-flight" response (Gore, 2018).

Some individuals who experience trauma may experience acute stress during the immediate aftermath of the trauma. An acute stress or anxiety response sufficient to impair functioning may result in acute stress disorder, discussed in **Box 32.2** ». Acute stress disorder shares several aspects of PTSD but is of a much shorter duration.

Etiology

The etiology of PTSD is associated with exposure to an overwhelming stressor. Genetics may contribute to an individual's susceptibility to PTSD through an interaction with environmental factors (MedlinePlus, 2020b). Multiple or recurrent exposure to trauma further increases a person's risk of developing PTSD.

PTSD is commonly associated with military personnel who have returned from war and conflict. However, not all deployed military personnel will develop PTSD, and other events can trigger it, including violence (personal assault, sexual assault, mass shootings), natural disasters (hurricanes and wildfires), MVCs, and child abuse (American Psychiatric Association, 2013). Intentional infliction of harm or violence, such as torture or rape, are associated with a higher incidence of PTSD (American Psychiatric Association, 2013).

Childhood trauma, abuse, and molestation can create enduring effects and clinical symptoms that last into adulthood. Additional factors that contribute to the development of PTSD include individual history of a psychiatric disorder and a lack of emotional support or resources during the trauma. Approximately 8% of the population will have PTSD at some point in their lives, with women being more susceptible (VA, 2019b). Incidence of PTSD among veterans varies by service area; approximately 11–20% of veterans who have been exposed to combat have experienced PTSD (VA, 2019b).

Often individuals diagnosed with TBI have a concurrent diagnosis of PTSD (VA, 2019b). Bae et al. (2020) found that PTSD is an important consideration in veterans who have been diagnosed with TBI. Furthermore, evidence from the study of military populations correlating PTSD and TBI has informed care considerations for civilians (Qureshi et al., 2018). Co-occurrence of PTSD and TBI can complicate treatment of and recovery from both conditions.

Box 32.2

Overview of Acute Stress Disorder

The individual with **acute stress disorder** experiences symptoms for 3 days to 1 month immediately after exposure to a traumatic event (American Psychiatric Association, 2013). In contrast, patients with PTSD experience symptoms for more than 1 month, with the onset of symptoms usually occurring 3 months or more after exposure to the trauma (American Psychiatric Association, 2013).

Acute stress disorder stems from an individual experiencing, learning of, or witnessing an extremely stressful event that involves a threat to life, actual or threatened serious injury, the violent death of another, or physical or sexual violation. The individual is said to be having acute stress disorder if experiencing nine (or more) symptoms from any of five categories—intrusion (intrusive distressing memories), negative mood, dissociation (an altered sense of reality or dissociative amnesia), avoidance, and arousal (such as sleep disturbances, irritability, or poor concentration)—that begin or get worse after the traumatic event (American Psychiatric Association, 2013).

Focus on Diversity and Culture

Refugee Trauma

In 2019, a total of 29,916 refugees were admitted into the United States (Department of Homeland Security, Office of Immigration Statistics, 2019). *Refugee trauma* is a form of PTSD that is specific to trauma related to war or persecution (or the flight from war or persecution) that may have lifelong effects. Child refugees may exhibit symptoms such as nightmares, anxiety, psychosomatic symptoms, hopelessness, and disrupted sleep patterns (NCTSN, n.d.-a). One in ten adult refugees experience PTSD (McWhorter et al., 2020). In addition to the mental health effects of PTSD, refugees also need to be assessed for physical and sexual trauma secondary to possible torture and other forms of violence endured (see **Figure 32.9** »).

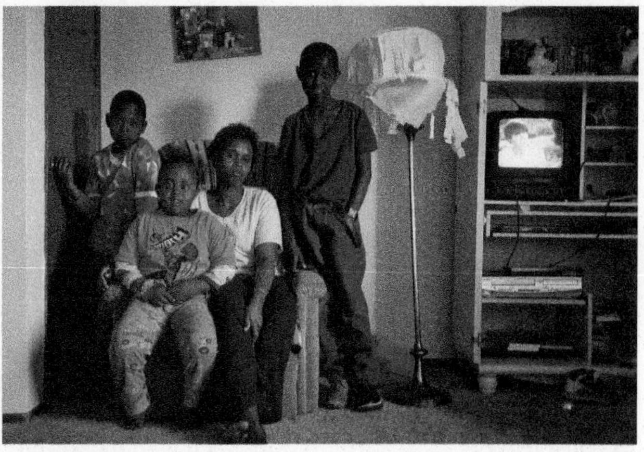

Figure 32.9 » This family, originally from the Democratic Republic of Congo, was living in a refugee camp in Burundi called Gatumba in 2004. One night, armed factions attacked the refugee camp, killed 166 people, and injured another 116. The oldest boy in this family had a leg amputated. Since that night, 525 Gatumba survivors have been relocated to North America. This family lives in Boise, Idaho, where the mother works cleaning rooms at a hotel.

Source: Christophe Calais/Corbis Historical/Getty Images.

Risk Factors

Individuals of any age and any cultural group may develop PTSD. In the United States, its incidence is higher among military veterans, law enforcement officers, firefighters, and emergency medical personnel (American Psychiatric Association, 2013). As described by the National Institute of Mental Health (NIMH; n.d.-a) other risk factors for PTSD include:

- The severity of the event itself, including whether the individual was harmed or watched others be harmed or killed
- Little or no social or psychologic support following the trauma
- Additional stressors immediately following the event, such as loss of a spouse or family member or loss of employment
- Presence of preexisting mental illness.

Prevention

The most effective way to prevent the development of PTSD is to seek and receive support as soon as possible after exposure to a traumatic event. Support may be from friends, family or professionals (MedlinePlus, 2020b). Early support is integral in preventing normal stress reactions from developing into acute stress disorder or PTSD. Obtaining support helps individuals engage in positive, effective coping skills and prevents them from relying on ineffective or harmful coping skills, such as self-medicating with drugs or alcohol (Mayo Clinic, 2020d).

Clinical Manifestations

Posttraumatic stress disorder is an intense physical and emotional response to thoughts and reminders of a traumatic event (NIMH, n.d.-b). Although manifestations may vary from one individual to another, they usually involve some reexperiencing of the event, physical and psychologic symptoms, and alterations in arousal or reactivity (American Psychiatric Association, 2013). Some patients will experience manifestations that predominantly reflect one category of alterations, whereas others will experience a combination of manifestations (American Psychiatric Association, 2013). For example, one patient may experience flashbacks as a primary symptom, whereas another may experience flashbacks, nightmares, hyperarousal, and bouts of extreme anger.

A **flashback** is a form of reexperiencing the traumatic event during which the individual experiences a recurrence of images, sounds, smells, or feelings from the traumatic event. Flashbacks may be so lifelike that they appear to be happening in reality. Flashbacks are often triggered by daily events, such as a car backfiring on the street or the smell of a perpetrator's cologne. Patients who experience flashbacks may lose touch with reality and may cognitively return to the traumatic incident as if it is happening again. Recurrent nightmares or intrusive memories related to the traumatic event, another form of reexperiencing, are common.

Physical manifestations may include palpitations and headaches. Psychologic reactions may exhibit as fear of harm, uncharacteristic irritability, aggression, and violence (NIMH, n.d.-b). Some may experience **depersonalization**, an emotional numbing, in which the individual feels detached from the body and loses the sense of reality and sense of self in relation to others (American Psychiatric Association, 2013). This emotional numbness can lead to difficulty trusting or being affectionate, and impairment in establishing or maintaining interpersonal relationships.

Hyperarousal associated with PTSD is a state of "high alert." The individual may experience sleep disturbances, restlessness, be easily startled, feel a strong sense of agitation, and have poor concentration. Dissociation, during which the individual blocks emotions related to the traumatic event, may occur, as can dissociative amnesia when certain elements of the traumatic event are blocked altogether (Choi et al., 2017). Individuals with PTSD may have accompanying depression and substance abuse disorder.

Although manifestations of PTSD usually emerge within 3 months following exposure to the traumatic event, years may pass before the individual's signs and symptoms meet the criteria needed for an official diagnosis of PTSD (American Psychiatric Association, 2013).

Collaboration

Caring for the patient with PTSD requires the skillful ability to assess and facilitate the care of patients, families, and communities. As a patient advocate, the nurse must effectively connect individuals with the resources they need to recover

Clinical Manifestations and Therapies

Acute and Posttraumatic Stress Disorders

DISORDER	CLINICAL MANIFESTATIONS	CLINICAL THERAPIES
Acute Stress Disorder Anxiety disorder that evolves from exposure to actual trauma or threat of physical harm. Recovery varies from 3 days to 1 month.	■ Intrusive distressing memories ■ Negative mood ■ Dissociation ■ Avoidance ■ Arousal problems	■ Ensure the safety of the patient and provide basic needs. ■ Promote support by family and friends. ■ Provide patient teaching related to coping mechanisms. ■ Provide emotional support. ■ Administer medications as prescribed to decrease arousal. ■ Holistic approach to treatment includes CBT

Clinical Manifestations and Therapies *(continued)*

DISORDER	CLINICAL MANIFESTATIONS	CLINICAL THERAPIES
Posttraumatic Stress Disorder Anxiety disorder that evolves from exposure to actual trauma or threat of physical harm. Recovery varies from 1 month to several years. Comorbidity may include depression, substance abuse, or other anxiety disorders.	■ Persistent frightening thoughts and memories or flashbacks of the event: images, sounds, smells, or feelings ■ Emotional numbing ■ Sleep disorders ■ Hypervigilance and exaggerated startle response ■ Reexperiencing the event ■ Trouble with affection ■ Irritability, aggressiveness, or violence ■ Avoidance of trauma-related situations or general social contacts ■ Drug and alcohol abuse ■ Depression ■ Suicidal thoughts or violence	■ Holistic approach to treatment includes CBT ■ Eye movement desensitization and reprocessing (EMDR) ■ Supportive therapy ■ Group therapy ■ Pharmacologic therapy, including antidepressants, antianxiolytics, and antipsychotic agents

successfully from trauma. These resources may include financial resources, such as social services; medical resources, such as free clinics and mental health providers who treat uninsured patients on a sliding-scale basis; and agencies that provide food and shelter. If support from a spiritual leader is requested, it should be provided.

Because of the all-encompassing impact of trauma on an individual's life, a holistic approach to treatment may be most effective. A combination of pharmacologic, nonpharmacologic, and integrative health therapies can be implemented to treat PTSD. The integration of therapies should be a collaborative approach with support from an interprofessional team of providers.

Pharmacologic Therapy

Depending on the severity and nature of a patient's PTSD manifestations, antidepressants may be used in conjunction with psychotherapy. Two selective serotonin reuptake inhibitors (SSRIs) approved by the U.S. Food and Drug Administration for the treatment of PTSD are sertraline (Zoloft) and paroxetine (Paxil). Prazosin, which is an antihypertensive medication, is effective in the reduction of nightmares associated with PTSD (Mayo Clinic, 2020c).

SAFETY ALERT SSRI medications may produce undesirable side effects; therefore, it is important to educate the patient that most side effects will diminish after the first few weeks. If the patient does not understand this, the risk of nonadherence to the medication regimen increases, leaving the patient untreated and susceptible to decompensation of illness.

Nonpharmacologic Therapy

Psychotherapy (such as CBT) is a treatment for PTSD that emphasizes education about symptoms and teaching skills to help identify and manage triggers of symptoms (NIMH, n.d.-b). Talking with a mental health professional individually or in a group setting is a form of psychotherapy. Talking through the trauma can assist patients in not being fearful of their memories.

Exposure therapy is a form of CBT that assists patients by gradual exposure to elements of the traumatic event, enabling them to face their fears. It uses writing, pictures, and possibly visiting the place where the traumatic event occurred (NIMH, n.d.-b). Exposure therapy allows patients to develop effective coping skills in a safe, controlled environment. The use of virtual reality in exposure therapy can assist patients in revisiting the site where the traumatic event occurred without physically having to return there (Mayo Clinic, 2020c).

Eye movement desensitization and reprocessing (EMDR) is a form of psychotherapy that contains elements of several types of therapy, including CBT and body-centered therapy. EMDR is a structured therapy that involves *dual-attention stimulus* in which the patient focuses on the traumatic event while also focusing on a second stimulus of eye movements, taps, or tones (EMDR Institute, 2020). This allows the patient to reprocess or reappraise the trauma by focusing internally on the traumatic event or another stressor while simultaneously focusing on a different external stimulus (EMDR Institute, 2020).

Collaborative Health Approaches

Integrative health therapies are used in the treatment of PTSD in conjunction with standard pharmacologic and nonpharmacologic therapies. Complementary health approaches appropriate for use with patients who have PTSD include acupuncture and relaxation techniques (VA, 2018a).

During acupuncture, a certified practitioner stimulates specific points on the body, usually by inserting needles through the skin. Research suggests that acupuncture may be effective in treating the mental and physical symptoms associated with PTSD (Moiraghi, Poli, & Piscitelli, 2019). Nurses working with patients who are interested in trying acupuncture as a treatment for PTSD should encourage patients to seek acupuncture as an adjunctive therapy in addition to primary therapies such as CBT.

Relaxation techniques include breathing methods to produce increased relaxation in response to stressors. Diaphragmatic breathing is a method that demands the conscious focus on the rise and fall of the abdomen while breathing deeply (Malaktaris & Lang, 2018). Breathing retention is another effective technique that teaches the patient how to control breathing while experiencing the stressful feelings. Breathing retention is a pattern of inhaling, holding the breath (retention), exhaling, and holding exhale (retention).

Lifespan Considerations

PTSD in Children

Manifestations of PTSD in young children vary significantly from those demonstrated by adult patients. For example, children with PTSD may reexperience the trauma through repetitive play or by drawing pictures that symbolize the trauma (CDC, 2020h). Children with PTSD may also behave recklessly or aggressively or they may withdraw from interacting with others. Because of their undeveloped ability to express thoughts or identify emotions, very young children with PTSD may exhibit increasingly frequent negative moods, including episodes of irritability, fear, anger, sadness, or confusion (American Psychiatric Association, 2013). Additional symptoms that may be seen in children may include hypervigilance, problems with concentration, nocturnal enuresis (bedwetting) after the child has already been toilet-trained, forgetting how to talk or not talking at all, acting out the traumatic event during activities with other children, and being exceptionally needy or clingy (American Psychiatric Association, 2013; CDC, 2020h).

PTSD in Adolescents

Older children and adolescents have manifestations similar to those that adults experience. Adolescents are more likely to demonstrate disruptive, disrespectful, or destructive behaviors (NIMH, n.d.-a). Adolescents may feel guilty for not preventing injury or death to others and engage in traumatic reenactment where aspects of the event are injected into their daily life (VA, 2019c). Adolescents with PTSD are at increased risk of substance abuse, social isolation, poor concentration, and poor physical health (NIMH, n.d.-a).

PTSD in Older Adults

PTSD can be a common issue in older adults because they have an increased likelihood of having experienced a traumatic event over the course of their lifetimes. PTSD in the older adult can be the result of a recent trauma or a traumatic event that occurred earlier in life that surfaces as an individual reflects on previous life experiences (Chopra, 2018). Older adults may report more somatic complaints and fewer emotional and psychologic symptoms than younger adults (Chopra, 2018).

Because of the higher incidence of cognitive impairment and dementia in the older adult, which may interfere with ability to communicate symptoms, a complete mental status exam is recommended when conducting assessment. There are no specific practice guidelines for treatment of PTSD in the older adult (Chopra, 2018). Treatment interventions are based on clinical experience and therapies that are well tolerated by the older adult patient.

NURSING PROCESS

Patients with PTSD experiencing hyperarousal and vigilance may exhibit unpredictable, aggressive, or bizarre behavior. The nursing priority for these patients is to ensure or reinforce the safety of the patient and others while quickly lowering patient anxiety levels (see the Communicating with Patients feature below). Patients with PTSD exhibiting extreme anxiety need immediate pharmacologic intervention, a quiet and calm environment, and reassurance that they are safe. Once anxiety levels are reduced, the healthcare team can help patients learn a new process of appraisal and coping mechanisms.

Families play a key role in the support of the individual experiencing PTSD. Because of the complexity of trauma, families may also experience PTSD and require the nurse's assistance and support. Evaluation of the impact on the family must also be included in the assessment, evaluation, and decision-making process. In the case of natural disasters, entire communities may be involved in the trauma.

Communicating with Patients

Working Phase

While caring for a hospitalized patient who is a combat veteran, the nurse recognizes the sound of thunder outside. As the thunder grows louder, the patient begins to visibly shake and says, "I can't focus, my mind is wandering." Then suddenly the patient yells, "Bomb! Bomb!" When a patient with PTSD is anxious and experiencing flashbacks, the nurse remains calm and supportive. The nurse uses paraphrasing to offer a clearer idea of what the patient has said and presents reality to help the patient differentiate between the real and the unreal.

- You're having difficulty concentrating?
- The sound you heard is thunder from the rainstorm outside.

Assessment

Assessing a patient for PTSD will involve both physical and psychologic approaches. Identify risk and protective factors and assess immediate and long-term safety concerns. Multiple tools are available for use in screening for PTSD; some have been developed for use with children. Specific interview questions to ascertain the diagnosis of PTSD are aimed at the following clinical manifestations: reexperiencing or flashbacks, hyperarousal and vigilance, an exaggerated startle response, and sleep disturbances. For example, an interview question might be: "Have you experienced painful images or memories of combat or other trauma that you couldn't get out of your mind, even though you may have wanted to? Have these been recurrent?" (VA, 2018b).

Identification of PTSD in children is improved when they are questioned directly about their experiences. Assessment of younger children involves questioning the child and/or the parents or caregivers about significant changes in behavior and sleep patterns. For children and vulnerable patients who are believed to be victims of abuse, the nurse should follow organizational protocols for reporting these situations. Questions may include:

- How would you describe your mood?
- When do you feel most content? When do you feel least content?
- What are your favorite activities?
- What activities help you relax?
- How often do you socialize or participate in activities with others?
- Describe your sleep habits. Do you sleep soundly through the night? Do you feel rested when you awaken?
- Do you have friends or other individuals with whom you can be open and honest about your thoughts and emotions?
- How important is being able to share your thoughts and feelings?
- Are you currently working? If so, what type of work are you engaged in?

Because of the traumatization experienced by these patients, as well as the subsequent potential for emotional and physical isolation, establishing trust can be especially challenging. During the assessment and throughout the care of all patients with PTSD, the nurse should be aware that direct questioning of the patient with regard to traumatic experiences may inhibit establishment of a trusting relationship and can even provoke frustration and anger in the patient. The nursing assessment should include interview questions that allow for assessment without pressuring patients to reveal information they are not ready or able to share. Through the inclusion of open-ended questions, the nurse affords patients the opportunity to express themselves to the degree with which they are comfortable while demonstrating respect for the patient's personal boundaries.

SAFETY ALERT Safety is always a priority. The nurse must remember that a patient diagnosed with PTSD may demonstrate agitation, aggressiveness, and even violence. The nurse will need to educate the family on the need for a safety plan in the event that the patient becomes violent.

Diagnosis

Evaluating assessment data for an individual with PTSD can be challenging. For some patients, manifestations of the disorder can be compounded by substance abuse, depression, and insomnia. Priority nursing considerations for the patient with PTSD may include any of the following:

- Potential for violence against self or others
- Anxiety
- Fear
- Inadequate coping skills or resources (patient or family)
- Sleep disturbance.

Planning

Planning includes identification of measurable, realistic patient goals that are relevant to the selected nursing diagnoses. Examples of patient goals that may be relevant to the care of the patient with PTSD include the following:

- The patient will remain free from injury or harm.
- The patient will report a decreased perception of anxiety.
- The patient will report a reduction or cessation of nightmares.
- The patient will discuss emotions related to traumatic experiences with at least one trusted mental health specialist or counseling professional.
- The patient will verbalize awareness of nonpharmacologic stress reduction techniques.

Implementation

The presence of PTSD is not an inevitable outcome of a traumatic event. Some individuals may require only limited interventions. Clinically significant indicators are the severity of the event itself and the severity of the individual's initial response. For patients who develop this disorder, in addition to the interventions described previously, it is important to recognize the profound impact PTSD exerts on multiple aspects of daily life, including an impact on the social, interpersonal, and occupational domains. Patients may benefit from being connected with organizations and community resources that can facilitate long-term assistance and can offer sensitive guidance to the process for building trusting relationships with others. The nurse should reinforce understanding of effective coping strategies and encourage their use, which may assist in decreasing anxiety (see Module 31, Stress and Coping).

SAFETY ALERT Compassion fatigue (CF) is an emotional strain that can be precipitated by providing care on a regular basis to people who are helpless, suffering, or traumatized. Symptoms of CF include mental, physical, and emotional exhaustion, including a reduced sense of meaning in work (American Institute of Stress, 2020). Once CF is identified, the nurse has already made the first step in overcoming the issue. Actions such as taking care of oneself, expressing needs, and clarifying boundaries will assist in eliminating these negative emotions.

Patient Teaching

Typical Human Responses to Traumatic Events

Patients with PTSD should be given ample information about the typical human responses to traumatic events. Education about the process helps patients normalize the experience and gain information for reappraisal. Information and resources can lead to adaptive coping; conversely, a lack of resources may induce maladaptive coping. It is the nurse's responsibility to provide information about recommended treatments, available support, and resources for PTSD to help the individual and family make informed choices.

Evaluation

The nurse evaluates the patient's response to treatment using these suggested expected outcomes:

- The patient uses self-calming techniques.
- The patient experiences fewer cognitive distortions and fewer repetitive thoughts (ruminations) or obsessions.
- The patient decreases time spent ruminating over worries, verbalizing more accurate predictions of future events.

If patient outcomes are not met, additional measures should be taken, including evaluation of medication efficacy and adherence to treatment regimen. The patient may need to journal daily events in order to identify triggers, allowing effective coping skills to be incorporated. The patient may need to be encouraged to avoid triggers while learning coping strategies.

Nursing Care Plan

A Patient with Posttraumatic Stress Disorder

Sarah Green is a 44-year-old nurse whose 14-year-old son was killed in a MVC just over 6 months ago. At the time of the MVC, she was driving her son to soccer practice when another vehicle crossed the interstate median and struck her vehicle. Her son died at the scene, and Ms. Green sustained serious injuries. She also has a 17-year-old daughter and a 19-year-old son.

ASSESSMENT

At present, Ms. Green attends a support group for grieving parents, which she finds to be therapeutic. However, she has been having flashbacks about the night of the accident and can barely control herself when she knows one of her children is driving or riding in a car. Usually, when one of the children asks to borrow the car, she just says no to avoid having to worry about them. Ms. Green knows she needs to see someone. She talks to a friend who is also a coworker, who recommends that she talk with an occupational health counselor at work. Ms. Green does not want anyone at work to know she is having trouble, but she agrees to see a mental health nurse that her friend recommended.

At her initial appointment, Ms. Green freely shares her experiences with the flashbacks, which happen two or three times a week, usually at night. She says that when she knows her children are going anywhere, she can feel her heart racing, her breathing speeding up, and her palms getting sweaty. She tells the mental health nurse that she gets through these episodes by lying down and saying the Lord's Prayer out loud.

DIAGNOSES

The mental health nurse develops the following nursing diagnoses:

- Posttrauma syndrome
- Anxiety
- Fear

PLANNING

Goals for Ms. Green's care include the following:

- The patient will use deep breathing to control escalating anxiety.
- The patient will express fears clearly.
- The patient will describe the symptoms associated with the various levels of anxiety.
- The patient will demonstrate breathing exercises to reduce anxiety.

IMPLEMENTATION

- Teach Ms. Green how to monitor her physiologic level of arousal.
- Teach use of abdominal breathing at the first sign of anxiety.
- Help patient to express fears that interfere with her life.
- Encourage patient to search for, confront, and relieve the source of the original anxiety.
- Teach distraction techniques that can control moderate levels of anxiety.
- Teach the use of positive imagery.
- Teach calming techniques such as muscle relaxation.
- Teach positive affirmations such as "I am calm and happy" or "I am very relaxed."
- Identify safe physical outlets for negative feelings, such as exercise.

EVALUATION

- The patient expresses feelings appropriately.
- The patient spends less time thinking about the accident and instead turns thoughts to more positive memories.
- The patient allows her adolescent children to borrow the car, setting reasonable limits to reduce her anxiety.

CRITICAL THINKING

1. What impact does Ms. Green's PTSD have on her children's development?
2. How would you teach Ms. Green relaxation techniques?

REVIEW Posttraumatic Stress Disorder

RELATE Link the Concepts and Exemplars

Linking the exemplar of posttraumatic stress disorder with the concept of development:

Explore the incidence of childhood abuse, molestation, and incest in the United States.

1. What impact does childhood abuse, molestation, and incest have on the growth and development of a child?
2. Childhood abuse, molestation, and incest can negatively affect the physical, emotional, spiritual, and cognitive processes of individuals. What alterations in health are associated with abuse later in life?

Linking the exemplar of posttraumatic stress disorder with the concept of mood and affect:

3. What questions should be asked of a patient who is experiencing manifestations of PTSD and expresses hopelessness?
4. What nursing interventions should be employed if the patient with PTSD is expressing suicidal ideation?

READY Go to Volume 3: Clinical Nursing Skills

REFER Go to Pearson MyLab Nursing and eText

REFLECT Apply Your Knowledge

Melinda Burns lives in northern California. Twenty-five years old, she is engaged to be married to a man she says she loves very much, and although this should be the happiest time of her life, she is feeling very anxious and stressed.

Last year, Ms. Burns's family had to evacuate her childhood home, where she was living while teaching at a local elementary school. All but her father evacuated in the face of wildfires raging nearby. Her father insisted on staying to try to defend their home. They weren't allowed to go home until several weeks later, when they returned to nothing but ash and debris. Ms. Burns's father perished in the fire. She says the worst part is that her father's body was never identified from the wreckage, so she feels like she has no closure or confirmation that her father is really dead.

Ms. Burns is seeking care because she is having trouble functioning and has difficulty performing activities of daily living (ADLs). She reports severe anxiety whenever she hears a siren, she has been waking from nightmares related to her home burning several times a week, and she can't bring herself to watch any television programs or movies showing any type of fire. Although the school at which Ms. Burns works is holding classes at a nearby church, she hasn't been able to return to work. She says lately she has been having trouble concentrating, even when planning her wedding, because she can't seem to think about anything other than the wildfires and what her father's final minutes must have been like.

1. What nursing care priorities are appropriate for Ms. Burns?
2. What collaborative actions can the healthcare team take to help this patient?
3. What independent nursing interventions would you initiate if Ms. Burns were your patient?

Exemplar 32.D Sexual Violence

Exemplar Learning Outcomes

32.D Analyze sexual violence as it relates to trauma.

- Distinguish different types of sexual violence.
- Describe the etiology of sexual violence.
- Compare the risk factors and prevention of sexual violence.
- Identify clinical manifestations of sexual violence.
- Summarize diagnostic tests and services used by interprofessional teams in the collaborative care of an individual who has experienced sexual violence.
- Differentiate care of patients across the lifespan with a history of sexual violence.
- Apply the nursing process in providing culturally competent care to an individual who has experienced sexual violence.

Exemplar Key Terms

Grooming, *2182*
Online enticement, *2182*
Sex trafficking, *2182*
Sexual assault, *2181*
Sexual violence, *2181*

Overview

Sexual violence (SV) is a significant problem across the world, affecting people of all genders and ages. A concise definition of SV is any type of unwanted sexual contact. In a seminal report, the World Health Organization (2002, p. 149) provided a comprehensive definition of **sexual violence**: "any sexual act, attempt to obtain a sexual act, unwanted sexual comments or advances, or acts to traffic, or otherwise directed against a person's sexuality using coercion, by any person regardless of their relationship to the victim, in any setting, including but not limited to home and work." All acts of SV can have a profound impact on the physical, psychological, and emotional health of a survivor.

Sexual assault is sexual contact or behavior that occurs without explicit consent of the victim, whereas the term *rape* is often used as a legal definition for sexual penetration without consent (RAINN, 2020c). Sexual assault is an act of violence that is obvious in situations in which a weapon, physical force, or threats are used to force a survivor into a sexual act. More subtle forms of sexual assault include coercion and manipulation, as when a person who is older or in a position of authority coerces or manipulates the survivor into a sexual act.

The majority of persons who are sexually assaulted know their perpetrators (CDC, 2020l). For instance, sexual assault can occur within a marriage or normally consenting relationship if one partner forces the other partner to have sex. Also, a person can be sexually assaulted by a familiar individual (acquaintance, friend, or peer) by force or by coercion into an unwanted sexual activity through use of incapacitating substances such as alcohol or drugs. Alcohol and drugs can make people confused about what is happening, render them unable to defend themselves from unwanted sexual contact, or create amnesia where they are unable to remember what happened (DHHS, 2019c).

Sex trafficking is a form of human trafficking that organizes the movement of people between and within countries by use of force, fraud, or coercion for the purpose of sexual exploitation or commercial sex acts (DHHS, 2020b). Human trafficking disproportionately affects women and girls, who are 71% of all victims worldwide (International Labour Organization [ILO], 2017). The WHO (2002) contends that women and children who are trafficked are often promised work in the service industry and instead are taken captive and their identification confiscated, they are confined, and they are promised their freedom if it is earned through prostitution.

According to the National Center for Missing and Exploited Children (NCMEC, 2020b) **online enticement** occurs when an individual communicates, via the internet, with someone believed to be a child with the intent to commit a sexual offense or abduction. Online enticement takes place across every platform where social spaces (e.g., Facebook, chat rooms, gaming rooms) can be used as tools or doorways to open up the opportunity to perpetrate SV. *Sextortion* is a form of online enticement in which a child is groomed to engage in a sexual conversation, take sexually explicit images (that will be sold or traded), or meet face-to-face with someone for sexual purposes (NCMEC, 2020a).

Grooming is the psychological and emotional manipulation of a child or adolescent with the goal to exploit or abuse. A perpetrator may build a relationship or emotional connection (grooming) with a child or adolescent over a short or long period of time. The NCMEC (2020a) lists various grooming tactics that perpetrators may use, such as pretending to be younger, developing a rapport through compliments or by "liking" their online posts, and engaging in role play to introduce sexual conversation.

Influencing Factors

Sexual violence is multifactorial in nature. Individual, community, and societal factors contribute to an increased risk of being a victim of SV. Furthermore, the factors influencing SV are similar to those influencing abuse and IPV.

Individual Factors

There is no single profile that fits a survivor of SV, but some contributing factors for risk have been identified, such as age and vulnerability. A large percentage of SV survivors report having been sexually assaulted before the age of 18 (CDC, 2020l). Individuals can be at a higher risk for being sexually assaulted if they are under the influence of drugs and/or alcohol, although being under the influence does not cause sexual assault to occur. Various online behaviors can increase risk for online enticement, including lying about being older to access platforms that allow for communication with adults, sending explicit photos or videos of oneself to another person online, and offering some type of exchange with offenders (such as requesting financial compensation or gifts for sexually explicit content of oneself) (NCMEC, 2020b).

Community Factors

Various characteristics within a community can influence the risk for SV. Communities that are impacted by poverty or have a seemingly increased tolerance for violence are more likely to have a higher percentage of SV (CDC, 2020o). Additionally, unsafe environments, such as workplaces that do not have a policy against sexual harassment or schools that employ individuals without background checks, pose an increased risk for the occurrence of SV (CDC, 2020l).

Societal Factors

Societal factors are a part of the context that surrounds SV. Various cultures follow social norms or traditions where women or men are seen as possessions. People who believe they have ownership over others may also believe that they have the right to force sexual acts on them despite objections (APIGBV, n.d.). Furthermore, some cultures have social norms related to ideals of male sexual entitlement where sex is considered a man's right in marriage or that sexual assault is a sign of masculinity (WHO, 2020b). The CDC (2020o) points to weak local or regional policies or legal sanctions as contributing factors for SV.

Etiology

The spectrum of SV includes sexual assault, sex trafficking, and online enticement each with their own set of causes and prevalence. Although anyone can be a victim of SV, some populations experience greater vulnerability (see the Focus on Diversity and Culture feature).

According to RAINN (2020d), every 73 seconds someone in the United States is sexually assaulted and (on average) there are 433,648 victims age 12 and older of sexual assault each year. Available statistics reveal that one in five women, one in six men, and nearly half of all transgender people have experienced sexual assault in their lifetime (James et al., 2016; RAINN, 2020b). Reports indicate that both female and male college students, ages 18 to 24, are three to five times more likely to experience sexual assault than nonstudents in the same age and gender group (RAIIN, 2020d). Transgender, genderqueer, and gender-nonconforming college students were identified as at higher risk for SV, comprising 21% of persons sexually assaulted as compared to 18% for cisgender females and 4% for cisgender males (RAINN, 2020d).

Sex trafficking is a pervasive problem that has been described as a modern-day form of slavery (CDC, 2020n). Globally, an estimated 3.8 million adults and 1 million children have been sexually trafficked or sexually exploited (ILO, 2017). In the United States, 8248 sex-trafficking cases were reported in 2019 (National Human Trafficking Hotline, n.d.). Furthermore, the NCMEC (2020b) estimated that one in six endangered runaways reported to them in 2019 were likely sex-trafficking survivors.

In 2019, NCMEC's CyberTipline received 16.9 million reports related to suspected child sexual exploitation, including online enticement (NCMEC, 2020b). Online enticement occurs in a variety of ways and involves boys and girls of all ages. Reports from NCMEC (2020b) indicate that the mean age of victims of online enticement in 2019 was 15 years old. The majority of reported victims were girls (78%) while boys accounted for 13% of reports; in 9% of reports gender was unknown (NCMEC, 2017).

Risk Factors for Perpetration of Sexual Violence

Multiple factors have been associated with an increased risk for committing SV. Some associated risk factors are environmental or social in nature, whereas others are relationship based or related to the individual's patterns of behavior and psychologic well-being (CDC, 2020o).

Focus on Diversity and Culture

Sexual Assault of Vulnerable Populations

A history of chronic homelessness is correlated with experiences of violence (Kuo, 2019). Fleeing a home where SV is occurring has been identified as a contributing factor to homelessness (Edmondson Baur, Bein, & Fribley, 2017; Kuo, 2019). An increased risk for sexual assault among homeless persons exists for those who may resort to "survival sex," engaging in sex acts in exchange for money or goods required to meet life's basic needs (Edmondson et al., 2017). A recent study found that 42% of homeless women had experienced sexual assault in their lifetime, with 27% experiencing SV within the past year (including women age 51 and older) (Kuo, 2019). Kuo (2019) further identified an intersection between homelessness and human trafficking, as 14.2% of the women reported they were survivors of sex trafficking.

According to the Indian Law Resource Center (n.d.), more than half of American Indian and Alaskan Native women have experienced SV. In particular, Alaskan Native women experience a disproportionate rate of forcible sexual assault than women in the rest of the United States.

American Indian populations are twice as likely to experience sexual assault compared to all races (RAINN, 2020d). On average, approximately 5,900 sexual assaults are reported annually by American Indian youth and adults age 12 and older (RAINN, 2020d). Additionally, recent data collected from the U.S. and Canada indicates that 40% of women who were victims of sex trafficking identified as American Indian or Alaskan Native (National Congress of American Indians Policy Research Center, 2016).

The disabled population is also at higher risk for SV. A review of data from the seminal 2010 National Intimate Partner and Sexual Violence Survey found that women who have a disability are three times more likely to experience SV than those without a disability (Smith et al., 2018). An investigation conducted by National Public Radio (2018) based on unpublished U.S. Department of Justice data found that men and women with intellectual disabilities face a rate of sexual assault that is seven times higher than that of individuals without disabilities.

Some of the risk factors linked with a greater likelihood of SV perpetration include alcohol and drug use, exposure to sexually explicit media, hypermasculine beliefs, childhood history of maltreatment or desensitization by exposure to exploitation or violence, involvement in an abusive intimate relationship, and community or societal tolerance for crime including SV.

Although both men and women commit SV, there is an increased prevalence of male perpetrators. For instance, of the persons who perpetrated online enticement of children, 82% were males, 9% were females, and in the remaining cases the sex of the perpetrator was unknown (NCMEC, 2020b). There is a large association with relationship-based risk factors for individuals who perpetrate sexual assault, as they often know the victim. Common relationships include spouse or partner/ex-spouse or ex-partner, acquaintance, friend, or relative.

What is clearly known about human traffickers is they target the vulnerable and use coercion, threats, and physical violence to exploit them for economic purposes. Less known are the contributing factors that increase likelihood of becoming a human trafficker. Long (2016) identified three main life events and experiences associated with increased risk of becoming a human trafficker: exposure, heritage, and opportunity. Exposure occurs when individuals grew up around sexual exploitation and become desensitized (Long, 2016). Heritage is associated with joining the family or community business of human trafficking (Long, 2016), Lastly, opportunity is linked with limited job opportunities and the quick money to be made via human trafficking (Long, 2016).

Although the risk factors are known to contribute to an increased likelihood of an individual perpetrating SV, they may not be causal, and often a combination of factors are evident in those who commit SV (CDC, 2020o). Understanding risk factors may help with treatment modalities for perpetrators. Moreover, understanding the risk factors can help identify various opportunities for prevention.

Prevention

Strategies to address SV are centered around primary prevention approaches. Primary prevention strategies are directed at the general population through educational awareness campaigns or programs, action-based programs, and public policy. An example of public policy is the Trafficking Victims Protection Act of 2000 (TVPA), which established a framework that addresses human trafficking through protection, prosecution, and prevention (DOJ, 2017a). Survivors are protected through access to health benefits and visa status, and sex trafficking is identified as a serious violation of federal law, with traffickers receiving harsh prosecution. Prevention efforts are aligned with international initiatives to improve opportunities for potential victims to deter trafficking (DOJ, 2017a).

Through protection, prevention, and prosecution, the TVPA addresses the societal influencing factors that contribute to SV. Another approach to preventing SV, aligned with societal influencing factors, that has been proposed is instituting mandatory reporting of suspected human-trafficking victims. Mandatory reporting would connect these individuals to social services and law enforcement agencies (English, 2017). A criticism of mandatory reporting of sex trafficking, in the case of adults, is the same as for cases of interpersonal violence: that reporting could discourage trafficked persons from seeking help and thereby limit the ability of healthcare professionals to gain trust and provide care (English, 2017).

The NCMEC (2020b) delivers an educational program that uses games, videos, and classroom-based lesson plans to help empower children to make safe online choices. It also offers an action-based program, the Child Victim Identification Program, which provides training of law enforcement and attorneys on how to identify child victims of sexual exploitation so they may be rescued (NCMEC, 2020b).

The CDC (2020l) created an evidence-based SV prevention package that presents several strategies individuals, communities, and legislators can use to reduce and prevent SV. The preventative programs focus on reducing the likelihood that a person will commit SV as well as creating knowledge and awareness about situations that could foster an environment that could lead to sexual assault. Many of the programs are based in education for the adolescent population surrounding reducing teen dating violence and bullying as well as strengthening positive relationships to change social norms and behaviors.

>> **Stay Current:** The National Center for Missing and Exploited Children offers a wealth of resources for families and professionals. For more information, go to the website https://missingkids.org.

Clinical Manifestations

The clinical manifestations of SV vary depending upon the type, context, or circumstances surrounding the SV. Furthermore, each survivor may react to the experience of SV in their own way. Manifestations of injury associated with SV may be acute, consisting mostly of the immediate traumatic physical injuries, and also long term, consisting more of the psychological injuries on negative chronic health outcomes.

Common manifestations include physical injury, concerns about pregnancy or contracting STIs, and psychologic symptoms such as fear, depression, and anxiety (National Sexual Violence Resource Center, n.d.). Some survivors experience psychologic symptoms so severe that their functioning is impacted to the extent that the survivor may develop PTSD (American Psychiatric Association, 2013). Although manifestations and reactions can vary, most survivors of SV experience significant impacts in multiple areas of health and need support to heal from the same. Clinical manifestations listed below are not entirely inclusive; any single manifestation or

Clinical Manifestations and Therapies

Sexual Violence

ETIOLOGY	CLINICAL MANIFESTATIONS	CLINICAL THERAPIES
Sexual assault	▪ Defensive injuries: bruises, lacerations, and/or fractured bones ▪ Edema ▪ Pain ▪ Genital trauma/injuries ▪ Knife and/or gunshot wounds ▪ Psychologic injuries: depression, stress-related disorders, thoughts of suicide, flashbacks ▪ Emotional injuries: detachment, fear, guilt, anxiety ▪ Substance abuse ▪ Death	▪ Ensure the safety and security of the patient. ▪ Treat physical injuries. ▪ Collect forensic evidence. ▪ Pharmacologic therapies such as analgesics, antianxiolytics, antidepressants, and antibiotic prophylaxis ▪ Mandatory reporting when a child, older adult, or disabled person is the survivor ▪ Arrange for/refer to survivor advocate for ongoing support. ▪ Educate on rights related to reporting to law enforcement. ▪ Provide referral for follow-up care with a medical professional, therapy, and/or counseling.
Sex trafficking	▪ Genital trauma/injuries ▪ Restraint injuries: bruising/abrasion/ligature marks found around the wrists, ankles, and neck ▪ Scars ▪ STIs ▪ Dehydration ▪ Multiple unwanted pregnancies ▪ Malnutrition ▪ Psychological injuries: depression, stress-related disorders, disorientation, confusion, phobias, panic attacks, and flashbacks ▪ Emotional injuries: detachment, fear, shame, humiliation, denial, and disbelief ▪ Death	▪ Ensure the safety and security of the patient. ▪ Treat physical injuries. ▪ Treat dehydration and malnutrition. ▪ Collect forensic evidence. ▪ Administer pregnancy test. ▪ Arrange for/refer to survivor advocate for ongoing support. ▪ Pharmacologic therapies such as analgesics, antianxiolytics, antidepressants, and antibiotics ▪ Mandatory reporting when a child, older adult, or disabled person is the survivor ▪ Collaborate with social services to determine housing options. ▪ Provide referral for follow-up care with a medical professional, therapy, and/or counseling.

Clinical Manifestations and Therapies *(continued)*

ETIOLOGY	CLINICAL MANIFESTATIONS	CLINICAL THERAPIES
Online enticement	■ Psychologic injuries: depression and stress-related disorders ■ Emotional injuries: embarrassment, shame, anxiety, and irritability ■ Withdrawal from parents and/or peer groups ■ Feelings of responsibility for being abused or deserving of the abuse that occurred—if present, may make it difficult for the child to disclose ■ Issues with trust causing long-term issues with relating to others ■ Substance abuse ■ Promiscuous sexual activity *If a child or adolescent is groomed into meeting a perpetrator in person:* ■ Physical injuries consistent with sexual assault ■ Death	■ Ensure the safety and security of the patient. ■ Treat physical injuries. ■ Collect forensic evidence. ■ Mandatory reporting ■ Provide referral for follow-up care with a medical professional, therapy, and/or counseling. ■ Pharmacologic therapies such as antidepressants and antianxiolytics

Patient Teaching

Drug-Facilitated Sexual Assault

Drug-facilitated sexual assault occurs when any type of drug is used to make a person vulnerable to sexual assault. The effects of the drug(s) may make a person physically helpless, unable to refuse sex, and unable to remember what happened (RAINN, 2020a). Drugs used to facilitate SV are often colorless, odorless, and tasteless and thereby easily added to beverages without a person's knowledge. Commonly used drugs are prescription or over-the-counter tranquilizers and sleeping aids, as well as rohypnol (or "roofies"), gamma-hydroxybutyric acid (GHB), and ketamine (DHHS, 2019a).

Prevention methods nurses should teach include safety steps that can be taken in social situations and what to do if a person suspects they have been drugged (DHHS, 2019a; MedlinePlus, 2021):

- Be aware of drinks in punchbowls or other containers that could be spiked with a drug.
- Do not accept premade or open drinks from other people.
- Watch your drink being made by the bartender and carry it yourself.
- Open your drink yourself and keep control of it at all times; never leave it unattended.
- Inspect drinks; if you see, smell, or taste something strange, stop drinking.
- Do not drink more than you want to, especially if being urged by someone else.
- Do not leave a location if you are alone or with someone that you do not know or explicitly trust.
- Keep your cell phone charged and with you.
- If you feel uncomfortable in a situation or location, try to leave as soon as possible.
- Always carry enough cash or a debit/credit card to be able to get a taxi or ride-share home.

Symptoms of being drugged include:

- Becoming dizzy, sleepy, or confused.
- Feeling drunk when you haven't consumed any alcohol.
- Feeling like the effects of consuming alcohol are stronger than usual.
- Feelings of weakness or loss of coordination.
- Feeling nauseous or vomiting.

Get help immediately if you feel drugged. Seek out a friend, security, or even a bartender to help you remain safe and pursue medical care. Go to a hospital ED for treatment.

combination of manifestations may indicate SV and should prompt the nurse to investigate further and identify priority actions for the situation (CDC, 2020l; DHHS, 2020b; Marchenko, 2017; NCMEC, 2020b).

Long-Term Manifestations

The impact of SV can be deep and long-lasting, affecting survivors in a multitude of ways. In the weeks following a SV incident, a variety of psychological and emotional manifestations may be present. Common manifestations include anger, flashbacks of the incident, avoidance of previously enjoyed activities, and sleep and eating disturbances (CDC, 2020l; DHHS, 2020b; Marchenko, 2017; NCMEC, 2020b). The common manifestations mirror the cluster of symptoms of PTSD, which may arise months and even years after the traumatic SV experience (ACOG, 2019).

Survivors can experience persistent long-term physical complications such as pelvic pain, back pain, frequent headaches, and gastrointestinal disorders. Some of the long-term symptoms can be caused by a mix of intense stress and injuries from sexual assault (RAINN, 2020b). Other long-term effects could be the presence of STIs, such as herpes or HIV, and reproductive complications associated with scar tissue from STIs or prior aborted unwanted pregnancies (DHHS, 2019d). Dealing with the emotional distress of experiencing SV can trigger the use of unhealthy coping mechanisms such as substance abuse (CDC, 2020l). Furthermore, many survivors of SV will have lifelong issues with trust that can alter the ability to build healthy relationships and intimacy (CDC, 2020l; DHHS, 2020b; NCMEC, 2020b).

SAFETY ALERT Survivors of SV may experience long-term effects that include depression and suicidal ideations. The nurse should be mindful of the warning signs of suicide (see Module 28, Mood and Affect) and employ appropriate intervention. Referrals should be provided for support groups and other community services, including crisis hotline numbers, which may assist the patient in coping effectively with the traumatic event.

Cultural Considerations

The cultural considerations surrounding SV often involve the culture's dominant definition of SV and what that act entails. For instance, in a study conducted by Ramiro et al. (2019) related to online child sexual exploitation and abuse, participation in online sex activities by teenagers in Metro Manila in the Philippines was viewed as a normal, if disgusting, activity by many. The lack of any physical contact and relative anonymity contribute to a sense of tolerance of the activity (Ramiro et al., 2019).

Marital and intimate partner SV are tolerated and not criminalized in many cultures around the world. Up until 1975, every U.S. state considered a husband's rape of his wife an exception to rape laws (Maclen, 2020). Currently, marital or spousal rape is illegal in all 50 states; however, laws and punishments vary (Maclen, 2020). A recent study contended the India legal system views wives as husbands' property and therefore does not recognize sexual assault within a marriage as criminal (Chattopadhyay, 2019). The failure to criminalize marital sexual assault leads to many incidents of nonconsensual SV within marriage being unreported, which may also be associated with women being socialized to believe that satisfying a husband's sexual desire is part of their marital obligation (Chattopadhyay, 2019).

Another cultural consideration is attributable to the perception of what constitutes a sexually violent crime within an intimate partnership. Findings from a recent study indicated an intimate relationship is a mitigating factor to what is considered criminal severity of sexual assault (Lynch, Golding, Jewell, Lippert, & Wasarhaley, 2019). Although participants in the study believed SV was not acceptable within an intimate relationship, there was hesitancy to issue severe criminal punishment for an intimate partner as would be for a stranger or acquaintance sexual assault (Lynch et al., 2019). The lack of legal implications for intimate partner perpetrators of sexual assault provides, in part, rationale for the underreporting that exists.

Individuals in the sex industry (e.g., sex workers or exotic dancers) may also experience sexual assault. Regardless of whether an individual's job includes having sexual relations with others, if someone states an unwillingness to continue with a sexual act and the other person does not stop, the forced act is sexual assault. Nurses must convey a nonjudgmental approach and provide quality care to all individuals regardless of the circumstance in which the sexual assault occurred.

Collaboration

Preventive approaches are best accomplished through collaborative efforts of individuals, communities (healthcare professionals, law enforcement, social services, schools, and workplaces), and legislators. A collaborative approach in the clinical setting is also best practice. The interprofessional team that cares for patients who have experienced SV includes nurses and other medical professionals, law enforcement personnel, and survivor advocates; mental health professionals are part of the long-term care team addressing ongoing treatment.

Many hospital EDs employ Sexual Assault Nurse Examiners (SANEs) who are specially trained in the clinical care of survivors of sexual assault. SANEs perform assessment and medical forensic evidentiary examinations consistent with the needs of the patient and the legal system (ACOG, 2019) (**Figure 32.10** »). A nurse may be certified as a SANE to treat the adult/adolescent population (SANE-A) and/or the pediatric population (SANE-P).

Children and adolescents are vulnerable and require competent pediatric medical professionals to provide medical-forensic examinations (DOJ, 2016). Pediatric patients may be referred to specialty centers, such as a Children's Advocacy Center (CAC), if a pediatric-certified SANE or other competent pediatric medical professional is not available within an acute care setting (DOJ, 2016). CACs provide comprehensive case management services, from an interprofessional approach, to respond holistically to the pediatric patient's needs. Services include therapy, advocacy, medical exams, and interviewers who are trained to conduct an interview without retraumatizing the child (National Children's Alliance, 2019a).

Any nurse may be involved in the care of a survivor of SV and should carefully follow policies and protocols for provision of care and documentation. As available, nurses should call upon survivor advocates to support the survivor.

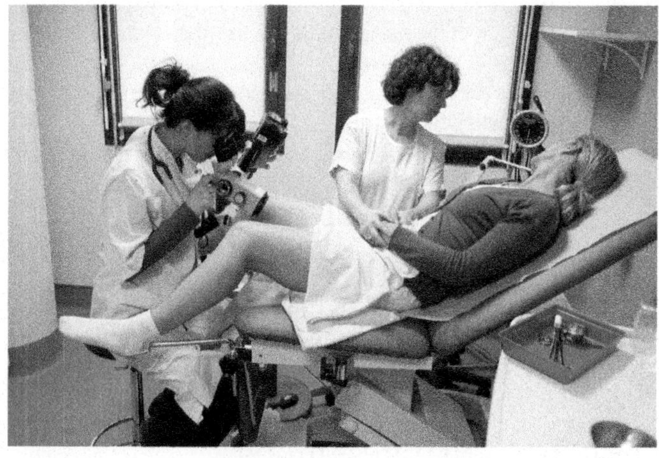

Figure 32.10 » A SANE examines a patient using a colposcope with camera while a survivor's advocate provides emotional support.

Source: BURGER/PHANIE/Alamy Images.

Many social services agencies have trained staff who serve as survivor advocates, guiding survivors through the medical-legal system and proving support or referral services such as for emergency housing.

>> **Stay Current:** Visit the website of the International Association of Forensic Nurses at www.iafn.org to learn more about becoming a Sexual Assault Nurse Examiner.

Diagnostic Tests

Although not diagnostic in nature, a sexual assault evidence collection kit (sometimes referred to as a rape kit) will be used, with consent of the survivor, to collect and preserve forensic evidence for use in legal criminal proceedings. Generally, it is best to collect forensic evidence within 72 hours after the sexual assault. Various sexual assault evidence collection kits are available for use; local and state policy requirements should be followed regarding what kit to use.

Though sexual assault evidence collection kits vary, each includes step-by-step instructions of how to collect forensic evidence with the goal of identifying DNA material from the perpetrator. The evidence commonly collected includes vaginal, oral, and anal swabs; fingernail scrapings; and clothing worn by the survivor. An aspect of education that a nurse can provide, if the opportunity presents, is the importance of not showering or bathing before the examination as doing so may remove evidence that could be collected and used to identify the perpetrator.

Nurses who collect sexual assault evidence must comply with local and state policies and requirements, including maintaining evidence integrity and a chain of custody. Adhering to chain of custody and maintaining integrity ensures there is no loss or alteration of evidence. The nurse maintains integrity and chain of custody through careful collection of evidence, being in constant control of the evidence until it is sealed, and limiting the transfer of evidence within the interprofessional team (e.g., from nurse to law enforcement).

Diagnostics include radiologic exams to identify various injuries such as fractures. Laboratory diagnostics include tests for drugs used to facilitate sexual assault, STIs, and pregnancy (in women). Rapid HIV diagnostic tests provide preliminary results but must be followed by additional testing to definitely rule out or diagnose HIV (CDC, 2015). Accordingly, the nurse must educate the patient on importance of follow-up HIV testing and provide referral to a healthcare professional who can prescribe testing.

Pharmacologic Therapy

Emergency contraception can be offered to women who have been sexually assaulted to prevent unwanted pregnancy. The contraceptive is more likely to be successful if taken within 3 days after the assault. The nurse should explain that the emergency contraceptive is optional and respect whatever decision the patient makes.

Numerous STIs can be contracted during a sexual assault. Commonly contracted and treatable infections are listed below, along with their prescribed pharmacologic treatment (CDC, 2015; St. Cyr et al., 2020):

- Syphilis, treated with penicillin
- Chlamydia, treated with a dose of azithromycin or a week of doxycycline
- Gonorrhea, treated with ceftriaxone
- Trichomoniasis, treated with metronidazole or tinidazole.

Nonpharmacologic Therapy and Resources

Psychotherapy (counseling) and/or support groups are recommended for patients who have experienced SV. Some patients will be more receptive to support groups, whereas others may prefer a more individualized private setting with a counselor. The overall goal of therapy is to help patients process their experience and develop healthy coping mechanisms.

A compilation of resources for survivors of SV, intended to help the survivor heal, are offered by nurses or social services. The resources link survivors to a wide range of services including survivor advocates, confidential helplines, counselors, peer support groups, emergency shelter, and legal aid. The National Center for Victims of Crime (NCVC) is a comprehensive national advocacy resource center that provides financial resources for follow-up care. The NCVC offers the Victim Connection Resource Center (n.d.), which provides referral to the most appropriate local or national resources. Connection to national resources helps bridge gaps in areas where local resources are limited.

When nurses offer resources, they should be survivor centered and best align with the needs and experience of the survivor. Various sexual assault crisis centers (also referred to as rape crisis centers) provide counseling and other intervention services; many have advocates available 24 hours a day (National Sexual Violence Resource Center, n.d.). Children's Advocacy Centers provide advocacy services and therapy for pediatric victims of SV including sexual assault, sex trafficking, and online enticement (National Children's Alliance, 2019a). The Freedom Network USA (2020) is a coalition that supports survivors of human trafficking in a variety of ways, including providing access to emergency, transitional, and affordable long-term housing.

Lifespan Considerations

Sexual violence can occur at any point in the lifespan. Although younger people age 12 to 34 are more likely to experience SV, it can happen to anyone at any age (RAINN, 2020d). Treatment includes many of the same elements regardless of age, however, a patient's reaction to SV may vary greatly in accordance with the situation and their developmental age. Some survivors may have unique needs, for example creating a safety plan for an older adult patient or placement in foster care for a child if they were sexually assaulted by a caregiver or family member. Online enticement, by definition, impacts children and nurses should be prepared to support the patient and the family. Key considerations regardless of age include ensuring safety, promoting autonomy, and empowering decision making.

When caring for a child or adolescent, it is essential to approach care in a developmentally appropriate way designed with the child's needs, abilities, and best interests in mind (DOJ, 2016), for instance, ensuring that nurses and clinicians use language the child can understand and the child's care team makes every effort to reduce the potentially traumatic effects of the exam process (e.g., by limiting exposure of the child's body, offering appropriate toys/electronic devices for distraction, providing comfortable furniture and lighting). Whether a child is being assessed for sexual assault, human trafficking, or online enticement, competent medical professionals, such as the pediatric SANE, should be responsible for the provision of care (DOJ, 2016).

NURSING PROCESS

Nursing care for a patient who has experienced SV depends on a number of factors, including the extent of any physical injuries, the patient's emotional state, and the patient's willingness to allow an examination. Nurses recognize that seeking help may itself put the patient in a dangerous situation, and therefore nurses must be supportive, patient, and understanding. Overall, nurses should employ a survivor-centered approach and find the best strategies for meeting patients' individualized needs. The survivor-centered approach empowers the survivor, promoting autonomy and dignity.

Communicating with Patients and Families

Working Phase

A nurse enters the exam room of a patient who has presented to the ED for reported sexual assault. The nurse offers self, which reflects the nurse values the patient and is willing to give their time and attention. The nurse gives information to promote patient decision making and decrease the patient's anxiety of the unknown.

- I will be with you while you are here today.
- The physician will be with us soon to talk with you about an examination. We will provide information and choices about your care throughout your time with us today.

Assessment

Assessment of any patient generally follows the parameters outlined in Module 34, Assessment. This section covers screening patients for SV and cues that indicate the patient may be a sex-trafficking victim.

Screening for Sexual Violence

A vital aspect of assessment of any patient is screening for SV. Screening, via scripted questions, should be completed at each healthcare interaction to identify SV or other safety needs and help prevent continued SV (ACOG, 2019; Hachey & Phillippi, 2017). Screening is especially important with sex trafficking; a study of 173 U.S. survivors of human trafficking found that 68% had been seen by a healthcare professional while they were being trafficked and their trafficking went unidentified (Chisolm-Straker et al., 2016). Screening questions to assess for SV may include (ACOG, 2019; Hachey & Phillippi, 2017):

- Are you safe at home?
- Has anyone ever touched you against your will or without your consent?
- Tell me about your living situation.
- Have you ever been forced or pressured to engage in sexual activities when you did not want to?

When conducting a nursing assessment for patients who have experienced SV, any severe or life-threatening injuries must be assessed and treated first. The vagina, anus, and throat may be locations of more severe injuries and should be assessed carefully. Minor injuries, psychologic injuries, and emotional needs are subsequently assessed and treated. During assessment of emotional needs, the nurse asks if patients would like a parent, friend, or survivor advocate to be with them and remain present during any examination. When caring for adult patients, the nurse further assesses whether they would like to speak with law enforcement.

Cues that Suggest Sex Trafficking

Many sex-trafficking victims who present for healthcare services while they are still in captivity come through emergency or urgent-care clinics. Through careful screening and observation for physical and emotional cues, nurses may identify a person who is being sex trafficked (Emergency Nurses Association & International Association of Forensic Nurses, 2018). Some indications that a person is a victim of sex trafficking include (Hachey & Phillippi, 2017):

- Lack of valid identification or unable to verify address
- Avoiding eye contact
- Presence of a controlling person (i.e., a person who answers questions on the patient's behalf rather than letting the patient answer)
- Withdrawn posture
- Appearing malnourished
- Poor physical or dental health
- Signs of physical injuries
- Multiple, recurrent, or untreated STIs.

Diagnosis

Nursing care priorities are contingent on the injuries and emotional state of the individual. Some potential nursing diagnoses include:

- Risk of infection
- Acute pain
- Impaired skin integrity
- Fear
- Anxiety
- Powerlessness
- Potential for low self-esteem.

Planning

It is critical for the patient who has experienced SV to have control over the planning process. The patient's input regarding short-term and long-term goals is essential to prevent re-victimization and to help the patient regain control over self and environment. Treatment and testing should be discussed with the patient and interventions should be planned accordingly. Appropriate short-term goals include:

- The patient will remain safe while receiving care.
- The patient will receive treatment for physical injuries.

- The patient will discuss the need for and participate in evidence collection and follow-up care for physical, psychologic, and emotional needs.
- The patient will help create and follow a safety plan.

Long-term goals may be difficult for the patient to establish immediately. In effort to empower patients and ensure readiness, establishing long-term goals and further planning may be best approached during follow-up care. Appropriate long-term goals include:

- The patient will experience hopefulness and confidence in continuing with life plans.
- The patient will increase the ability to trust and attach to others.
- The patient will use healthy coping mechanisms.
- The patient will have resolution of anger, guilt, fear, and depression.
- The patient will experience decreased flashbacks and nightmares.
- The patient will report physical traumatic injuries have healed and symptoms such as sleep disturbances and poor appetite have subsided.

Implementation

Patients who have experienced SV will require extensive nursing care. First, nurses must provide comfort for the patient, including providing privacy and ensuring safety. The nurse will assist in treatment of physical trauma and facilitate evidence collection. The nurse also helps empower the patient to recover emotionally and psychologically from the event.

Provide Safety

Upon admission, individuals who have experienced SV are placed in a private room. The patient's safety and emotional well-being are priority. Therefore, access to the patient is restricted to only necessary members of the interprofessional team and an individual, as selected by the patient, to provide support. Patients are assured of their safety and privacy, and nurses maintain a nonjudgmental approach respecting the patient's decisions involving evaluation and treatment. Nurses provide emotional support and administer analgesics as needed to promote patient comfort.

Treat Physical Injuries

Physical injuries are treated in order of severity. Some survivors sustain more extensive injuries that may require surgical intervention. Tests for STIs are performed, and patients are informed about appropriate treatments. Patients are educated on the importance of follow-up HIV testing and informed about potential outcomes. Emergency contraception is explained and offered to the patient.

Facilitate Evidence Collection

If a patient was sexually assaulted, the nurse will facilitate evidence collection. The nurse first ensures the patient is informed and has provided consent. The patient may choose to decline examination or collection of evidence, and the nurse should support the decision and empower the patient's control. If the patient chooses to have an examination and evidence collected, the nurse will clearly explain every step of the process with the understanding that the patient can choose to decline any portion of the exam at any time. If available, a SANE will typically conduct the evidentiary exam and collect forensic evidence.

Nurses are responsible to accurately and completely document what the patient relays about the sexual assault and findings of the exam. The patient is not required to make a report or even speak to law enforcement but should be offered the opportunity. If evidence was collected, the patient will be informed that the evidence will only be processed in a forensic lab if the patient chooses to make a report to law enforcement and wants to pursue legal proceedings. If the patient does not choose to make a report to law enforcement. the evidence will be safely stored for a designated period of time (determined by each state), generally by law enforcement or a forensic lab, should the patient decide to report at a later date (DOJ, 2017b).

Empower the Patient

Nurses work to empower patients by providing choices for examination and explaining options for seeking further help. Nurses provide referrals to social workers, counselors, support groups, and law enforcement. If a patient chooses not to use the referrals, the nurse continues to empower the patient by supporting the decision. The nurse should educate the patient on the importance of and assist in developing a safety plan *prior* to discharge from the hospital (see Patient Teaching: Developing a Safety Plan in Exemplar 32.A, Abuse, in this module).

Evaluation

Patients are encouraged to ask questions about the examination process or about future testing and resources. Nurses explore all options with the patient as appropriate. Some potential outcomes are as follows:

- The patient expresses emotions regarding the SV experienced.
- The patient is empowered to take control of the situation.
- The patient discusses any fears or questions about the examination.
- The patient employs healthy coping mechanisms.
- The patient asks for, and accepts, help when needed.
- The patient acknowledges that the SV experienced was not their fault.

If outcomes are not met, the nurse should reassess the patient to determine if the individual needs additional time to meet the outcomes or if the outcomes were unrealistic. Working with survivors of SV requires compassion and understanding because each person will cope differently. Due to the trauma of the SV experienced, the patient may have an altered ability to understand or retain information. The nurse should demonstrate patience and review information as necessary.

Nursing Care Plan

A Patient Who Has Been Sexually Assaulted

Renee Meyers, age 28, comes into the ED after having been sexually assaulted by her ex-boyfriend. She explains that the incident happened 4 hours ago, but she was hesitant to ask for help because she feels some responsibility for the attack.

ASSESSMENT

Camilla Wright, an RN in the ED, escorts Ms. Meyers to a private examination room. Ms. Meyers is resistant to talking about the events, repeating multiple times that she feels that the attack was her own fault and that she cannot believe this could have happened. Nurse Wright is patient and encourages Ms. Meyers to take her time in relaying the events as they occurred. The nurse also reassures the patient that she is safe in the hospital and that no action will be taken without her permission.

After approximately 30 minutes, Ms. Meyers begins to discuss the details of the sexual assault, reporting that her ex-boyfriend forced her to have sexual intercourse with him. When she tried to resist, the reported perpetrator struck her repeatedly in the face with his fists. Nurse Wright notices slight discoloration near the patient's right eye, and the left side of her face is moderately swollen. The patient is visibly shaking, and she is fighting back tears. Ms. Meyers explains that the reported perpetrator did not use a condom and says she is very worried about becoming pregnant.

Nurse Wright does not interrupt while Ms. Meyers is relaying the events; when she is finished, she asks if the patient has showered since the incident. She reports that she has not showered. Nurse Wright then explains the process of collecting evidence and testing for STIs and asks Ms. Meyers if she is willing to consent to the examination and completion of sexual assault evidence collection. At first, Ms. Meyers is hesitant. Nurse Wright does not try to pressure her into consent; instead, she asks Ms. Meyers if she would like some time alone to think it over.

Ms. Meyers takes some time alone and then informs Nurse Wright that she would like to have evidence collected. She also requests to be tested for STIs.

DIAGNOSES

- Risk of infection related to STIs
- Impaired tissue integrity
- Fear related to possible pregnancy
- Acute pain from physical trauma
- Powerlessness

PLANNING

Goals for Ms. Meyers's care include:

- The patient will be tested and treated for any potential infections.
- The patient will make an informed decision with regard to emergency contraceptive treatment.
- The patient will report physical pain as absent or tolerable, as evidenced by patient rating of pain as 3 or less on a scale of 0 to 10.
- The patient will make an informed decision with regard to reporting the sexual assault to law enforcement officials.
- The patient will make an informed decision with regard to evidence collection for potential future prosecution of the perpetrator.
- The patient will openly express emotions and concerns to trusted confidantes.
- The patient will seek follow-up counseling and psychosocial care.
- The patient will develop a safety plan prior to discharge.

IMPLEMENTATION

- Refer to a survivor advocacy program.
- Administer prescribed analgesics as needed for pain control.
- Administer medications to prevent STIs and as desired to prevent pregnancy.
- Support and educate about the physical examination and specimen collection process.
- Assist in collection of specimens following chain of custody using a sexual assault evidence collection kit.
- Inform of HIV testing.
- Educate about legal procedures available.
- Educate on importance of and assist with completion of safety plan.

EVALUATION

Ms. Meyers consented to collection of specimens and physical examination. She verbalizes pain as a 3 on a scale of 0 to 10. Ms. Meyers agreed to speak with the survivor advocate and was given community support phone numbers and addresses. She has verbalized understanding of the need for future HIV testing and has completed a safety plan. She has called her best friend to drive her home when discharged.

CRITICAL THINKING

1. How should the nurse respond to Ms. Meyers if she declined to have specimens collected or a physical examination completed at this time?
2. Explain how the nurse should describe emergency contraceptives and their actions.
3. How might this patient's emotional state change over the next 24 to 48 hours?

REVIEW Sexual Violence

RELATE Link the Concepts and Exemplars

Linking the exemplar of sexual violence with the concept of stress and coping:

1. What teaching would you provide a patient who has experienced SV about managing anxiety?
2. Describe the differences in communication strategy to assess for SV in a 12-year-old child versus a 30-year-old woman.

Linking the exemplar of sexual violence with the concept of self:

3. How will you plan to assist the victim of SV to regain self-esteem?
4. When collecting specimens for use by law enforcement during the investigation of a reported sexual assault, what nursing interventions can be implemented to help the patient maintain a positive self-concept?

READY Go to Volume 3: Clinical Nursing Skills

REFER Go to Pearson MyLab Nursing and eText

REFLECT Apply Your Knowledge

Dyani Chavos, a 13-year-old American Indian girl, was transported to the ED by local law enforcement after she was rescued in a sting operation that targeted sellers in a human sex-trafficking ring. Police are working to locate Dyani's parents. Upon observation, Dyani appears malnourished and dehydrated and her skin is pale, with abrasions and scar tissue noted circumferentially to her wrists and ankles. She is quiet and avoiding eye contact but tells the nurse she wants to describe how she was taken. The nurse sits quietly and listens. Dyani shares that she was contacted through Facebook by a man who said he was an agent for a modeling company. He would always compliment her on pictures she posted, and he talked her into meeting him at a local park so he could take photos of her to make a portfolio and then she could start getting paid to work as a model. When she met him at the park, he walked her over to his car because he said he needed to grab his camera. He lifted the trunk of his car and took out a big camera. The last thing Dyani remembers about being at the park was the man raising the camera above his head like he was going to hit her with it. Then she said she woke up in a dark room with her hands and feet tied together.

1. What are the three primary nursing interventions for this patient?
2. What resources should be provided for Dyani?
3. What are some survivor-centered interventions for this patient? Explain your answer.

References

Ahmad, S. (2018). Mass casualty incident management. *Missouri Medicine, 115*(5), 451–455.

American Academy of Pediatrics. (2019). *Poison prevention & treatment tips*. https://www.healthychildren.org/English/safety-prevention/all-around/Pages/Poison-Prevention.aspx

American Addictions Centers. (2020). *Understanding the connection between drug addiction, alcoholism, and violence*. https://americanaddictioncenters.org/rehab-guide/addiction-and-violence

American College of Obstetrics and Gynecologists (ACOG). (2019). *ACOG Committee Opinion 777 sexual assault*. https://www.acog.org/clinical/clinical-guidance/committee-opinion/articles/2019/04/sexual-assault

American College of Surgeons Committee on Trauma (ACSCOT). (2017). *Advanced trauma life support* (10th ed.). Author.

American Institute of Stress. (2020). *Compassion fatigue*. https://www.stress.org/military/for-practitionersleaders/compassion-fatigue

American Nurses Association (ANA). (2015). *Position statement on incivility, bullying, and workplace violence*. https://www.nursingworld.org/~49d6e3/globalassets/practiceand-policy/nursing-excellence/incivility-bullying-and-workplace-violence--ana-position-statement.pdf

American Nurses Association (ANA). (2020). Advocacy: Workplace violence legislation passes. *American Nurse 15*(1).

American Psychiatric Association. (2013). *Diagnostic and statistical manual of mental disorders* (5th ed.). Author.

American Psychological Association. (2020). *Sexual abuse*. https://www.apa.org/topics/sexual-assault-harassment

Asian Pacific Institute on Gender-Based Violence (APIGBV). (n.d.). *Patriarchy and power*. https://www.api-gbv.org/about-gbv/our-analysis/patriarchy-power/

Bach, J. A., Leskovan, J. J., Scharschmidt, T., Boulger, C., Papadimos, T. J., Russell, S., et al. (2017). The right team at the right time: Multidisciplinary approach to multi-trauma patient with orthopedic injuries. *International Journal of Critical Illness and Injury Science, 7*(1), 32–37. https://www.ncbi.nlm.nih.gov/pmc/articles/PMC5364767/

Bae, S., Sheth, C., Legarreta, M., McGlade, E., Lyoo, I. K., & Yurgelum-Todd, D. A. (2020). Volume and shape analysis of the hippocampus and amygdala in veterans with traumatic brain injury and posttraumatic stress disorder. *Brain Imaging and Behavior 14*, 1850–1864.

Bauldoff, G., Gubrud, P., & Carno, M. (2020). *LeMone & Burke's medical-surgical nursing* (7th ed.). Pearson.

Beller, J., Kröger, C., & Hosser, D. (2019). Disentangling honor-based violence and religion: The differential influence of individual and social religious practices and fundamentalism on support for honor killings in a cross-national sample of Muslims. *Journal of Interpersonal Violence*. https://doi.org/10.1177/0886260519869071

Bennett, K. S., DeWitt, P. E., Harlaar, N., & Bennett, T. D. (2017). Seizures in children with severe traumatic brain injury. *Pediatric Critical Care Medicine, 18*(1), 54–63.

Blais, K. K., & Hayes, J. S. (2016). *Professional nursing practice: Concepts and perspectives* (7th ed.). Pearson.

Blue Knot Foundation. (2021). *What is complex trauma?* https://www.blueknot.org.au/Resources/Information/Understanding-abuse-and-trauma/What-is-complex-trauma

Birnie, K. A., Chambers, C., Spellman, C. (2017). Mechanisms of distraction in acute pain perception and modulation. *Pain, 158*(6), 1012–1013.

Boles, J. (2018). The powerful practice of distraction. *Pediatric Nursing 44*(5), 247–253.

Breiding, M. J., & Armour, B. S. (2015). The association between disability and intimate partner violence in the United States. *Annals of Epidemiology, 25*(6), 455–457.

Bureau of Justice Statistics. (n.d.). *Violent crime*. https://www.bjs.gov/index.cfm?ty=tp&tid=31

Campbell, J. C., Webster, D., Koziol-McLane, J., Block, C., Campbell, D., Curry, M. A. . . . & Laughon, K. (2003). Risk factors for femicide in abusive relationships: Results from a multisite case control study. *American Journal of Public Health, 98*(7), 1089–1097.

Center for Family Justice. (n.d.). *What is a safety plan?* https://centerforfamilyjustice.org/faq/safety-plan/

Center for Health Care Strategies. (2021). *What is trauma-informed care?* https://www.traumainformedcare.chcs.org/what-is-trauma-informed-care/

Centers for Disease Control and Prevention (CDC). (2015). *2015 sexually transmitted diseases treatment guidelines, 2015*. https://www.cdc.gov/std/tg2015/default.htm

Centers for Disease Control and Prevention (CDC). (2017). *Preventing chain saw injuries during tree removal after a disaster*. https://www.cdc.gov/disasters/chainsaws.html

Centers for Disease Control and Prevention (CDC). (2019). *Self-directed violence and other forms of self-injury*. https://www.cdc.gov/ncbddd/disabilityandsafety/self-injury.html

Centers for Disease Control and Prevention (CDC). (2020a). *Adverse childhood experiences*. https://www.cdc.gov/violenceprevention/aces/fastfact.html?CDC_AA_refVal=https%3A%2F%2Fwww.cdc.gov%2Fviolenceprevention%2Facestudy%2Ffastfact.html

Centers for Disease Control and Prevention (CDC). (2020b). *America's drug overdose epidemic*. https://www.cdc.gov/injury/features/prescription-drug-overdose/index.html?CDC_AA_refVal=https%3A%2F%2Fwww.cdc.gov%2Ffeatures%2Fprescription-drug-overdose%2Findex.html

Centers for Disease Control and Prevention (CDC). (2020c). *Child abuse and neglect: Risk and protective factors*. http://www.cdc.gov/violenceprevention/childmaltreatment/riskprotective-factors.html

Centers for Disease Control and Prevention (CDC). (2020d). *Drug overdose deaths*. from https://www.cdc.gov/drugoverdose/data/statedeaths.html

Centers for Disease Control and Prevention (CDC). (2020e). *Firearm violence prevention*. https://www.cdc.gov/violenceprevention/firearms/fastfact.html

Centers for Disease Control and Prevention (CDC). (2020f). *Injury and violence are leading causes of death*. https://www.cdc.gov/injury/wisqars/animated-leading-causes.html

Centers for Disease Control and Prevention (CDC). (2020g). *Older adult drivers*. https://www.cdc.gov/transportationsafety/older_adult_drivers/index.html#riskgroups

Centers for Disease Control and Prevention (CDC). (2020h). *Post-traumatic stress disorder in children*. https://www.cdc.gov/childrensmentalhealth/ptsd.html

Centers for Disease Control and Prevention (CDC). (2020i). *Preventing child abuse and neglect*. https://www.cdc.gov/violenceprevention/pdf/can/CAN-factsheet_2020.pdf

Centers for Disease Control and Prevention (CDC). (2020j). *Preventing elder abuse*. https://www.cdc.gov/violence-prevention/elderabuse/fastfact.html

Centers for Disease Control and Prevention (CDC). (2020k). *Preventing intimate partner violence*. https://www.cdc.gov/violenceprevention/intimatepartnerviolence/fastfact.html

Centers for Disease Control and Prevention (CDC). (2020l). *Preventing sexual violence*. https://www.cdc.gov/violence-prevention/sexualviolence/fastfact.html

Centers for Disease Control and Prevention (CDC). (2020m). *Preventing youth violence*. https://www.cdc.gov/violence-prevention/youthviolence/fastfact.html

Centers for Disease Control and Prevention (CDC). (2020n). *Sex trafficking*. https://www.cdc.gov/violenceprevention/sexualviolence/trafficking.html

Centers for Disease Control and Prevention (CDC). (2020o). *Sexual violence risk and protective factors*. https://www.cdc.gov/violenceprevention/sexualviolence/riskprotectivefactors.html

Centers for Disease Control and Prevention (CDC). (2020p). *Transportation safety*. https://www.cdc.gov/transportationsafety/

Centers for Disease Control and Prevention (CDC). (2020q). *Teen drivers*. https://www.cdc.gov/transportationsafety/teen_drivers/index.html

Centers for Disease Control and Prevention (CDC). (2020r). *Violence prevention: A public health issue*. https://www.cdc.gov/violenceprevention/publichealthissue/social-ecologicalmodel.html

Centers for Disease Control and Prevention (CDC). (2020s). *Violence prevention: The social-ecological model: A framework for prevention*. https://www.cdc.gov/violenceprevention/publichealthissue/social-ecologicalmodel.html

Centers for Disease Control and Prevention (CDC). (2020t). *What is epigenetics?* https://www.cdc.gov/genomics/disease/epigenetics.htm

Centers for Disease Control and Prevention (CDC). (2020u). *Youth violence*. https://www.cdc.gov/violenceprevention/youthviolence/index.html

Centers for Disease Control and Prevention (CDC). (2020v). *Youth violence: risk and protective factors*. https://www.cdc.gov/violenceprevention/youthviolence/riskprotectivefactors.html

Chattopadhyay, S. (2019). The responses of health systems to marital sexual violence – A perspective from Southern India. *Journal of Aggression, Maltreatment and Trauma 28*(1), 47–67.

Chesworth, B., Lanier, P., & Rizo, C. F. (2019). The association between exposure to intimate partner violence and child bullying behaviors. *Journal of Child and Family Studies 28*(8), 2220–2231.

Child Welfare Information Gateway. (2019). *Mandatory reporters of child abuse and neglect*. U.S. Department of Health and Human Services, Children's Bureau.

Chisolm-Straker, M., Baldwin, S., Gaïgbé-Togbé, B., Ndukwe, N., Johnson, P. N., & Richardson, L. D. (2016). Health care and human trafficking: We are seeing the unseen. *Journal of Health Care for the Poor and Underserved, 27*(3), 1220–1233.

Choi, K. R., Seng, J. S., Briggs, E. C., Munro-Kramer, M. L., Graham-Bermann, S. A., Lee, R. C., & Ford, J. D. (2017). The dissociative subtype of posttraumatic stress disorder (PTSD) among adolescents: Co-occurring PTSD, depersonalization/derealization, and other dissociation symptoms. *Journal of the American Academy of Child and Adolescent Psychiatry, 56*(12), 1062–1072.

Chopra, M. (2018). PTSD in late life: Special Issues. *Psychiatric Times 35*(3). https://www.psychiatrictimes.com/view/ptsd-late-life-special-issues

Christian Science. (2021). *How can I be healed?* https://www.christianscience.com/christian-healing-today/how-can-i-be-healed

Clukay, C. J., Dajani, R., Hadfield, K., Quinlan, J., Panter-Brick, C., & Mulligan, C. J. (2019) Association of MAOA genetic variants and resilience with psychosocial stress: A longitudinal study of Syrian refugees. *PLoS One, 14*(7), e0219385. https://doi.org/10.1371/journal.pone.0219385.

Complextrauma.org. (2019). *Complex trauma: What is it and how does it affect people?* https://www.complextrauma.org/complex-trauma/complex-trauma-what-is-it-and-how-does-it-affect-people/

Congressional Research Service. (2019). *Military families and intimate partner violence: Background and issues for Congress*. https://crsreports.congress.gov/product/pdf/R/R46097

Department of Homeland Security, Office of Immigration Statistics (2019). *Refugees and asylees: 2019*. https://www.dhs.gov/sites/default/files/publications/immigration-statistics/yearbook/2019/refugee_and_asylee_2019.pdf

Disability Justice. (2020). *Abuse and exploitation of people with developmental disabilities*. https://disabilityjustice.org/justice-denied/abuse-and-exploitation/

Domestic Violence Resource Center. (2020). *Safety planning*. http://www.dvrc-or.org/safety-planning/

Duan, S., Duan, Z., Li, R., Wilson, A., Wang, Y., & Jia, Q., et al. (2020). Bullying victimization, bullying witnessing, bullying perpetration and suicide risk among adolescents: A serial mediation analysis. *Journal of Affective Disorders, 273*(1), 274–279.

Edmondson Baur, E., Bein, K., & Fribley, C. (2017). *College-aged but on the streets: Young adults who experience homelessness and sexual violence*. https://evawintl.org/wp-content/uploads/YoungAdultsWhoExperienceHomelessnessandSexualViolenceMay2017-1.pdf

EMDR Institute. (2020). *Dual attention stimuli*. http://www.emdr.com/?s=dual+stimulation

Emergency Nurses Association (ENA). (2020). *ESI emergency severity index: A triage tool for emergency department care*. Author.

Emergency Nurses Association & International Association of Forensic Nurses. (2018). *Human trafficking awareness in the emergency care setting* [Position statement]. https://www.ena.org/docs/default-source/resource-library/practice-resources/position-statements/humantraffickingpatientawareness.pdf

English, A. (2017). Mandatory reporting of human trafficking: Potential benefits and risks of harm. *American Medical Association Journal of Ethics 19*(1), 54–62.

Everytown Research & Policy. (2019a). *Gunfire on school grounds in the United States*. https://maps.everytownresearch.org/gunfire-in-school/#17152

Everytown Research & Policy. (2019b). *Mass shootings in America*. https://maps.everytownresearch.org/massshootingsreports/mass-shootings-in-america-2009-2019/

Fahlgren, M. K., Kleiman, E. M., Puhalla, A. A., & McCloskey, M. S. (2020). Age and gender effects in recent violence perpetration. *Journal of Interpersonal Violence 35*(17–18), 3513–3529.

Family Practice Notebook. (2021). *Diagnostic testing in trauma*. https://fpnotebook.com/er/trauma/DgnstcTstngInTrm.htm

Farrell, C. A., Fleeger, E. W., Monuteaux, M. C., Wilson, C. R., Christian, C. W., & Lee, L. K. (2017). Community poverty and child abuse fatalities in the United States. *Pediatrics, 139*(5). https://doi.org/10.1542/peds.2016-1616

Federal Bureau of Investigation (FBI). (n.d.-a). *2019 crime in the United States*. https://ucr.fbi.gov/crime-in-the-u.s/2019/crime-in-the-u.s.-2019/topic-pages/expanded-homicide

Federal Bureau of Investigation (FBI). (n.d.-b). *What are known violent extremist groups?* https://www.fbi.gov/cve508/teen-website/what-are-known-violent-extremist-groups

Federal Bureau of Investigation (FBI). (n.d.-c). *What we investigate: Gangs*. https://www.fbi.gov/investigate/violent-crime/gangs#The-Gang%20Threat

Federal Bureau of Investigation (FBI). (2020). *Active shooter incidents in the United States*. https://www.fbi.gov/file-repository/active-shooter-incidents-in-the-us-2019-042820.pdf/view

Freedom Network USA. (2020). *Housing project*. https://freedomnetworkusa.org/training/housing-project/

Gore, T. (2018). *What is the pathophysiology of the brain in post-traumatic stress disorder (PTSD)?* https://www.medscape.com/answers/288154-95784/what-is-the-pathophysiology-of-the-brain-in-posttraumatic-stress-disorder-ptsd

Hachey, L. M., & Phillippi, J. C. (2017). Identification and management of human trafficking victims in the emergency department. *Advanced Emergency Nursing Journal, 39*(1), 31–51.

Haddad L. M., & Geiger, R. A. (2020). *Nursing ethical considerations*. StatPearls. https://www.ncbi.nlm.nih.gov/books/NBK526054/

Harvard Health Publishing. (2021). *Mental illness and violence*. https://www.health.harvard.edu/newsletter_article/mental-illness-and-violence

Herron, M. (2019). *Deaths: Leading causes for 2017*. Centers for Disease Control and Prevention. https://www.cdc.gov/nchs/data/nvsr/nvsr68/nvsr68_06-508.pdf

Hinduja, S., & Patchin, J. (2018). Connecting adolescent suicide to the severity of bullying and cyberbullying. *Journal of School Violence, 18*(3), 333–346.

Indian Law Resource Center. (n.d.). *Ending violence against native women*. Retrieved from https://indianlaw.org/issue/ending-violence-against-native-women

International Labour Organization (ILO). (2017). *Global estimates of modern slavery*. Author.

James, S. E., Herman, J. L., Rankin, S., Keisling, M., Mottet, L., & Anafi, M. (2016). *The Report of the 2015 U.S. Transgender Survey*. National Center for Transgender Equality.

Jehovah's Witness. (2021). *Why don't Jehovah's Witness accept blood transfusions?* https://www.jw.org/en/jehovahs-witnesses/faq/jehovahs-witnesses-why-no-blood-transfusions/

The Joint Commission. (2018). *Physical and verbal violence against healthcare workers*. Sentinel Event Alert 59. https://www.jointcommission.org/-/media/documents/office-quality-and-patient-safety/sea_59_workplace_violence_4_13_18_final.pdf?db=web&hash=9E659237DBAF28F07982817322B99FFB

Kennedy, A., Scorpio, J., & Coppota, C. (2018). Assessment of the pediatric trauma patient: Differences in approach. *Journal of Emergency and Critical Care Medicine 2*(1).

Killon, C. M. (2017). Cultural healing practices that mimic child abuse. *Annals of Forensic Research and Analysis, 4*(2), 1042.

Klasen, M., Wolf, D., Eisner, P. D., Eggermann, T., Zerres, K., Zepf, F. D., et al. (2019). Serotonergic contributions to human brain aggression networks. *Frontiers in Neuroscience, 13*. https://doi.org/10.3389/fnins.2019.00042

Kraybill, O. G. (2019, September 29). Grief vs. traumatic grief. *Psychology Today*. https://www.psychologytoday.com/us/blog/expressive-trauma-integration/201909/grief-vs-traumatic-grief

Kuo, A. (2019). *Downtown Women's Center 2019 Los Angeles city women's needs assessment*. https://www.downtownwomenscenter.org/wp-content/uploads/2020/01/DWC-2019-Los-Angeles-Womens-Needs-Assessment.pdf

Lansford, J. E., Godwin, J., Uribe Tirado, L. M., Zelli, A., Al-Hassan, S. M., Bacchini, D., et al. (2015). Individual, family, and culture level contributions to child physical abuse and neglect: A longitudinal study in nine countries. *Development and Psychopathology, 27*, 1417–1428.

Lewis, E. (2020). *What is structural violence?* https://www.thoughtco.com/structural-violence-4174956

Locke, L., Bromley, G., & Federspiel, K. A. (2018, May 10). Patient violence: It's not all in a day's work. *American Nurse Today*. https://www.myamericannurse.com/patient-violence/

Long, M. (2016). *How someone becomes a trafficker*. https://www.endslaverynow.org/blog/articles/how-someone-becomes-a-trafficker

Louie, S. (2020), *How Asian shame and stigma contribute to suicide*. National Alliance on Mental Illness. https://www.nami.org/Blogs/NAMI-Blog/July-2020/How-Asian-Shame-and-Stigma-Contribute-to-Suicide

Lynch, K. R., Golding, J. M., Jewell, J. A., Lippert, A., & Wasarhaley, N. E. (2019). "She is his girlfriend—I believe this is a different situation": Gender differences in perceptions of the legality of intimate partner rape. *Journal of Family Violence, 34*, 213–230.

Maclen, S. (2020, May 15). The bizarre legal loopholes surrounding spousal rape. *Psychology Today*. https://www.psychologytoday.com/us/blog/making-sense-chaos/202005/the-bizarre-legal-loopholes-surrounding-spousal-rape

Magana, J., & Kaufhold, M. (2018). *Child abuse*. Medscape. from https://emedicine.medscape.com/article/800657-overview#a4

Makwana, N. (2019). Disaster and its impact on mental health: A narrative review. *Journal of Family Medicine and Primary Care, 8*(10), 3090–3095.

Malaktaris, A. L., & Lang, A. J. (2018). Complementary and integrative health approaches for PTSD. *Psychiatric Times 35*(8). https://www.psychiatrictimes.com/view/complementary-and-integrative-health-approaches-ptsd

Marchenko, S. (2017). *Web of darkness: Groomed, manipulated, coerced, and abused in minutes*. Biometrica. https://www.biometrica.com/icmec-online-grooming/

Mayo Clinic. (2020a). *Child abuse: Overview*. https://www.mayoclinic.org/diseases-conditions/child-abuse/symptoms-causes/syc-20370864

Mayo Clinic. (2020b). *Gangrene*. Retrieved from https://www.mayoclinic.org/diseases-conditions/gangrene/symptoms-causes/syc-20352567

Mayo Clinic. (2020c). *Post-traumatic stress disorder: Diagnosis and treatment*. https://www.mayoclinic.org/diseases-conditions/

post-traumatic-stress-disorder/diagnosis-treatment/drc-20355973

Mayo Clinic. (2020d). *Post-traumatic stress disorder: Symptoms and causes*. https://www.mayoclinic.org/diseases-conditions/post-traumatic-stress-disorder/symptoms-causes/syc-20355967

Mayo Clinic. (2020e). *Spinal cord injury*. https://www.mayoclinic.org/diseases-conditions/spinal-cord-injury/diagnosis-treatment/drc-20377895

Mayo Clinic. (2020f). *Trauma in pregnancy: A unique challenge*. https://www.mayoclinic.org/medical-professionals/trauma/news/trauma-in-pregnancy-a-unique-challenge/mac-20431356

McWhorter, L. G., Ortiz, P. M., Gurung, A., Saulinas, K., Walens, L., Anil, L., et al. (2020). *Effective treatment for refugee adults with post-traumatic stress disorder (PTSD): A summary of practice recommendations for clinicians*. https://policylab.chop.edu/reports-and-tools/effective-treatment-refugee-adults-post-traumatic-stress-disorder-ptsd-summary

MedlinePlus. (2020a). *MAOA gene*. U.S. National Library of Medicine. https://medlineplus.gov/genetics/gene/maoa/

MedlinePlus. (2020b). *Post-traumatic stress disorder*. U.S. National Library of Medicine. https://medlineplus.gov/posttraumaticstressdisorder.html

MedlinePlus. (2021). *Sexual assault prevention*. Retrieved from https://medlineplus.gov/ency/article/007461.htm

Moiraghi, C., Poli, P., & Piscitelli, A. (2019). An observational study on acupuncture for earthquake-related post-traumatic stress disorder: The experience of the Lombard Association of Medical Acupuncturists/Acupuncture in the World, in Amatrice, Central Italy. *Medical Acupuncture, 31*(2), 116–122. https://doi.org/10.1089/acu.2018.1329

National Capital Poison Center. (2020). *Prevent serious poisonings in children*. https://www.poison.org/~/media/files/poisonorg/public-ed-materials/pdfs/tip-card-to-prevent-poisonings-in-children.pdf?la=en

National Center for Missing and Exploited Children (NCMEC). (2017). *The online enticement of children: An in-depth analysis of cybertripline reports*. https://www.missingkids.org/content/dam/missingkids/pdfs/ncmec-analysis/Online%20Enticement%20Pre-Travel1.pdf

National Center for Missing and Exploited Children (NCMEC). (2020a). *Grooming in the digital age*. https://www.missingkids.org/blog/2020/grooming-in-the-digital-age

National Center for Missing and Exploited Children (NCMEC). (2020b). *The issues online enticement*. https://www.missingkids.org/theissues/onlineenticement

National Center on Elder Abuse. (n.d.-a). Research brief: Abuse of adults with a disability. https://ncea.acl.gov/NCEA/media/docs/Abuse-of-Adults-with-a-Disability-(2012).pdf

National Center on Elder Abuse. (n.d.-b). *Statistics/data*. https://ncea.acl.gov/About-Us/What-We-Do/Research/Statistics-and-Data.aspx#challenges

National Child Traumatic Stress Network (NCTSN). (n.d.-a). *Refugee trauma*. https://www.nctsn.org/what-is-child-trauma/trauma-types/refugee-trauma

National Child Traumatic Stress Network (NCTSN). (n.d.-b). *Sexual abuse*. https://www.nctsn.org/what-is-child-trauma/trauma-types/sexual-abuse/effects

National Children's Advocacy Center. (2020). *History*. https://www.nationalcac.org/multidisciplinary-team/

National Children's Alliance. (2019a). *How the CAC model works*. https://www.nationalchildrensalliance.org/cac-model/

National Children's Alliance. (2019b). *National statistics on child abuse*. https://www.nationalchildrensalliance.org/media-room/national-statistics-on-child-abuse/

National Coalition Against Domestic Violence. (n.d.). *Dynamics of abuse*. https://ncadv.org/dynamics-of-abuse

National Congress of American Indians Policy Research Center. (2016). *Human & sex trafficking: Trends and responses across Indian Country*. Tribal Insights Brief Spring 2016. https://www.courts.ca.gov/documents/BTB24-4L-6.pdf

National Council on Aging (NCA). (n.d.). *Elder abuse facts*. https://www.ncoa.org/public-policy-action/elder-justice/elder-abuse-facts/

National Human Trafficking Hotline. (n.d.). *Sex trafficking*. https://humantraffickinghotline.org/type-trafficking/sex-trafficking

National Institute on Aging (n.d.). Elder *abuse*. Retrieved from https://www.nia.nih.gov/health/elder-abuse#types

National Institute of Mental Health (NIMH). (n.d.-a). *Helping children and adolescents cope with disasters and other traumatic events: What parents, rescue workers, and the community can do*. https://www.nimh.nih.gov/health/publications/helping-children-and-adolescents-cope-with-disasters-and-other-traumatic-events/index.shtml#pub5

National Institute of Mental Health (NIMH). (n.d.-b). *Post-traumatic stress disorder*. https://www.nimh.nih.gov/health/topics/post-traumatic-stress-disorder-ptsd/index.shtml

National Institute of Neurological Disorders and Stroke. (2019). *Shaken baby syndrome information page*. https://www.ninds.nih.gov/Disorders/All-Disorders/Shaken-Baby-Syndrome-Information-Page

National Public Radio. (2018, January 8). The sexual assault epidemic no one talks about [Radio broadcast episode]. https://www.npr.org/2018/01/08/570224090/the-sexual-assault-epidemic-no-one-talks-about

National Public Radio. (2021, January, 7). Insurrection at the capitol live updates: Police confirm death of officer injured during attack on capitol [Radio broadcast episode]. https://www.npr.org/sections/insurrection-at-the-capitol/2021/01/07/954333542/police-confirm-death-of-officer-injured-during-attack-on-capitol

National Sex Offender Public Website (NSOPW). (n.d.). *Recognizing sexual abuse*. https://www.nsopw.gov/en/SafetyAndEducation/HowToIdentify

National Sexual Violence Resource Center. (n. d.). *About sexual assault*. https://www.nsvrc.org/about-sexual-assault

National Weather Service. (2020). *Mid-west derecho*. https://www.weather.gov/dvn/summary_081020

Peace Over Violence. (n.d.). *The cycle of violence and power and control*. https://www.peaceoverviolence.org/iii-the-cycle-of-violence-and-power-and-control

Pennsylvania Family Support Alliance. (2020). *Discipline, parenting styles and abuse*. https://www.pa-fsa.org/Parents-Caregivers/Preventing-Child-Abuse-Neglect/Discipline-Parenting-Styles-and-Abuse

Perzichilli, T. (2018). *Broadening our understanding of trauma: Why context matters*. GoodTherapy. https://www.goodtherapy.org/blog/broadening-our-understanding-of-trauma-why-context-matters-0723184

Potter, M. L., & Moller, M. D. (2020). *Psychiatric-mental health nursing: From suffering to hope* (2nd ed.). Pearson.

Power, C. (2020). *Domestic violence: What can nurses do?* https://www.crisisprevention.com/Blog/Domestic-Violence-What-Can-Nurses-Do

Qureshi, K. L., Upthegrove, R., Toman, E., Sawlani, V., Davies, D. J., & Belli, A. (2018). Post-traumatic stress disorder in UK civilians with traumatic brain injury: An observational study of TBI clinic attendees to estimate PTSD prevalence and its relationship with radiologic markers of brain severity. *British Medical Journal Open, 9*, e021675. https://doi.org/10.1136/bmjopen-2018-021675

Ramiro, L. S., Martinez, A. B., Tan, J. R. D., Mariano, K., Miranda, G. M. J., & Bautista G. (2019). Online child sexual exploitation and abuse: A community diagnosis using the social norms theory. *Child Abuse and Neglect, 96*. https://doi.org/10.1016/j.chiabu.2019.104080

Rape, Abuse, & Incest National Network (RAINN). (2020a). *Drug facilitated sexual assault*. https://www.rainn.org/articles/drug-facilitated-sexual-assault

Rape, Abuse, & Incest National Network (RAINN). (2020b). *Effects of sexual violence*. https://www.rainn.org/effects-sexual-violence

Rape, Abuse, & Incest National Network (RAINN). (2020c). *Key terms and phrases*. https://www.rainn.org/articles/key-terms-and-phrases

Rape, Abuse, & Incest National Network (RAINN). (2020d). *Victims of sexual violence: Statistics*. https://www.rainn.org/statistics/victims-sexual-violence

Roberts, M. (2020). *Marking the deadliest year on record, HRC releases report on violence against transgender and gender non-conforming people*. Human Rights Campaign. https://www.hrc.org/press-releases/marking-the-deadliest-year-on-record-hrc-releases-report-on-violence-against-transgender-and-gender-non-conforming-people

Rollè, L., Giardina, G., Caldarera, A. M., Gerino, E., & Brustia, P. (2018). When intimate partner violence meets same sex couples: A review of same sex intimate partner violence. *Frontiers in Psychology, 9*, 1506. https://doi.org/10.3389/fpsyg.2018.01506

Scholl, L., Seth, P., Kariisa, M., Wilson, N., & Baldwin, G. (2019). Drug and opioid-involved overdose deaths—United States, 2013–2017. *Morbidity and Mortality Weekly Report, 67*(5152), 1419–1427.

Schulman, M., & Menschner, C. (2019). *Laying the groundwork for trauma-informed care* [Brief]. Center for Health Care Strategies. https://www.traumainformedcare.chcs.org/wp-content/uploads/Brief-Laying-the-Groundwork-for-TIC_11.10.20.pdf

Schwartz, R. M., Liu, B., Lieberman-Cribbin, W., & Taioli, E. (2017). Displacement and mental health after natural disasters. *The Lancet Planetary Health, 1*(8), E314.

Smith, S. G., Zhang, X., Basile, K. C., Merrick, M. T., Wang, J., Kresnow, M., & Chen, J. (2018). *The National Intimate Partner and Sexual Violence Survey (NISVS): 2015 Data Brief – Updated Release*. National Center for Injury Prevention and Control, Centers for Disease Control and Prevention.

St. Cyr, S., Barbee, L., Workowski, K. A., Bachmann, L. H., Pham, C., Schlanger, K., et al. (2020). Update to CDC's treatment guidelines for Gonoccal infection, 2020. *Morbidity and Mortality Weekly Report 69*(50), 1911–1916.

State of California. (2020). *CalFire 2020 incident archive*. https://www.fire.ca.gov/incidents/2020/

Substance Abuse and Mental Health Services Administration (SAMHSA). (2019). *Trauma and violence*. https://www.samhsa.gov/trauma-violence

Substance Abuse and Mental Health Services Administration (SAMHSA). (2014). *SAMHSA's concept of trauma and guidance for a trauma-informed approach* (HHS Publication No. [SMA] 14-4884). Author.

Tribie, K. (2019). *Improving health outcomes for children requires us to look at the big picture*. https://www.kevinmd.com/blog/2019/08/improving-health-outcomes-for-children-requires-us-to-look-at-the-big-picture.html

University of Florida Health. (2020). *Pain assessment management initiative: Nonpharmacologic toolkit*. https://pami.emergency.med.jax.ufl.edu/resources/distraction-toolkit/

U.S. Department of Health and Human Services (DHHS). (n.d.-a). *Healthy People 2030: Injury prevention*. https://health.gov/healthypeople/objectives-and-data/browse-objectives/injury-prevention

U.S. Department of Health and Human Services (DHHS). (n.d.-b). *Trauma: What is historical trauma*. https://www.acf.hhs.gov/trauma-toolkit/trauma-concept

U.S. Department of Health and Human Services (DHHS). (2019a). *Date rape drugs*. https://www.womenshealth.gov/a-z-topics/date-rape-drugs

U.S. Department of Health and Human Services (DHHS). (2019b). *Definitions of child abuse and neglect in federal law*. https://www.childwelfare.gov/pubPDFs/define.pdf

U.S. Department of Health and Human Services (DHHS). (2019c). *Effects of domestic violence on children*. https://www.womenshealth.gov/relationships-and-safety/domestic-violence/effects-domestic-violence-children

U.S. Department of Health and Human Services (DHHS). (2019d). *Pelvic inflammatory disease*. Retrieved from https://www.womenshealth.gov/a-z-topics/pelvic-inflammatory-disease

U.S. Department of Health and Human Services (DHHS). (2020a). *Opioid crisis*. https://www.hrsa.gov/opioids

U.S. Department of Health and Human Services (DHHS). (2020b). *What is human trafficking*. https://www.acf.hhs.gov/otip/about/what-is-human-trafficking

U.S. Department of Justice (DOJ). (2016). *A national protocol for sexual abuse medical forensic examinations pediatric*. https://www.justice.gov/ovw/file/846856/download

U.S. Department of Justice (DOJ). (2017a). *Human trafficking key legislation*. https://www.justice.gov/humantrafficking/key-legislation

U.S. Department of Justice (DOJ). (2017b). *Sexual assault kit testing initiatives and non-investigative kits* [White paper]. https://www.justice.gov/ovw/page/file/931391/download

U.S. Department of Justice (DOJ). (2020). *Active shooter incidents in the United States in 2019*. https://www.fbi.gov/file-repository/active-shooter-incidents-in-the-us-2019-042820.pdf/view

U.S. Department of Veterans Affairs (VA). (2018a). *Complementary and integrative health*. https://www.research.va.gov/pubs/docs/va_factsheets/cih.pdf

U.S. Department of Veterans Affairs (VA). (2018b). *PTSD: National Center for PTSD: Structured interview for PTSD (SI-PTSD)*.

https://www.ptsd.va.gov/professional/assessment/adult-int/si-ptsd.asp

U.S. Department of Veterans Affairs (VA). (2019a). *Effects of disasters: Risk and resilience factors*. https://www.ptsd.va.gov/understand/types/disaster_risk_resilience.asp

U.S. Department of Veterans Affairs (VA). (2019b). *PTSD: National center for PTSD: Facts about how common PTSD is*. https://www.ptsd.va.gov/understand/common/common_adults.asp

U.S. Department of Veterans Affairs (VA). (2019c). *National Center for PTSD: Specific populations*. https://www.ptsd.va.gov/professional/treat/specific/index.asp

VanValkinburgh, D., Kerndt, C.C., & Hashmi, M.F. (2020). *Inotropes and vasopressors*. StatPearls. https://www.ncbi.nlm.nih.gov/books/NBK482411/

VanWert, M., Anreiter, I., & Fallon, B. (2019). Intergenerational transmission of child abuse and neglect: A transdisciplinary analysis. *Gender and the Genome*, *3*, 1–21.

Victim Connect Resource Center. (n.d.). *Confidential referrals for crime victims*. https://victimconnect.org

Violence Policy Center. (2017). *The relationship between community violence and trauma*. https://vpc.org/studies/trauma17.pdf

Weissberger, G. H., Goodman, M. C., Mosqueda, L., Schoen, J., Nguyen, A. L., Wilber, K. H., et al. (2020). Elder abuse characteristics based on calls to the national center on elder abuse resource line. *Journal of Applied Gerontology*, *39(10)*, 1078–1087.

World Bank. (2019). *Gender-based violence*. https://www.worldbank.org/en/topic/socialsustainability/brief/violence-against-women-and-girls

World Health Organization (WHO). (2002). *World report on violence and health*. https://www.who.int/violence_injury_prevention/violence/world_report/en/full_en.pdf?ua=1

World Health Organization. (2011). *Intimate partner violence during pregnancy*. https://www.who.int/reproductivehealth/publications/violence/rhr_11_35/en/

World Health Organization (WHO). (2020a). *Violence Prevention Alliance: The ecological framework*. https://www.who.int/violenceprevention/approach/ecology/en/

World Health Organization (WHO). (2020b). *Violence against women*. https://www.who.int/news-room/fact-sheets/detail/violence-against-women

Yellman, M. A., Bryan, L., Sauber-Schatz, E. K., & Brener, N. (2020). Transportation risk behaviors among high school students – Youth Risk Behavior Survey, United States, 2019. *Morbidity and Mortality Weekly Report*, *69*(1, Suppl.), 77–83.

Zhang-James, Y., Fernàndez-Castillo, N., Hess, J. L., Malki, K., Glatt, S. J., Cormand, B., & Faraone, S. V. (2019). An integrated analysis of genes and functional pathways for aggression in human and rodent models. *Molecular Psychiatry*, *24*, 1655–1667.

Part III

Reproduction Module

Part III consists of the module on reproduction, which falls within the individual domain. **Reproduction** is the process by which humans produce offspring. It encompasses the processes by which female and male gametes unite, conception, embryonic and fetal development, pregnancy, labor, and birth. This module presents the concept of reproduction, with exemplars designed to take the nursing student through the stages of pregnancy to caring for the newborn and the baby who is born prematurely. This module addresses care for newborn, mother, and family, including biophysical and psychosocial needs. Note that some aspects of care for the pregnant woman and the newborn are covered in other concepts and exemplars. For example, in Exemplar 28.C, Peripartum Depression, in Module 28, Mood and Affect, and Exemplar 16.H, Hypertensive Disorders of Pregnancy, in Module 16, Perfusion.

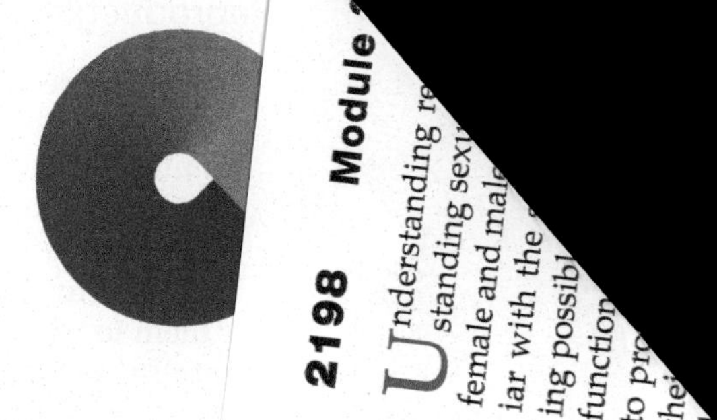

Module 33
Reproduction

Module Outline and Learning Outcomes

The Concept of Reproduction

Normal Presentation of the Female Reproductive System

33.1 Analyze the physiology of the reproductive system.

Conception and Embryonic Development

33.2 Explain the processes of conception and embryonic development.

Embryonic to Fetal Development

33.3 Explain the processes of embryonic to fetal development.

Physical and Psychologic Changes of Pregnancy

33.4 Analyze the physical and psychologic changes of pregnancy.

Sociocultural Factors and Pregnancy

33.5 Discuss implications of cultural differences and social determinants of health in the nursing care of pregnant women.

Concepts Related to Reproduction

33.6 Outline the relationship between reproduction and other concepts.

Health Promotion

33.7 Explain the promotion of healthy reproduction.

Nursing Assessment

33.8 Differentiate among common assessment procedures and tests used to examine reproduction.

Independent Interventions

33.9 Analyze independent interventions nurses can implement for patients with alterations in reproduction.

Collaborative Therapies

33.10 Summarize collaborative therapies used by interprofessional teams for patients with alterations in reproduction.

Lifespan Considerations

33.11 Differentiate considerations related to the care of patients with alterations in reproduction throughout the lifespan.

Reproduction Exemplars

Exemplar 33.A Antepartum Care

33.A Summarize antepartum care of the pregnant woman.

Exemplar 33.B Intrapartum Care

33.B Summarize intrapartum care of the pregnant woman.

Exemplar 33.C Postpartum Care

33.C Summarize postpartum care of the mother.

Exemplar 33.D Newborn Care

33.D Summarize care of newborns.

Exemplar 33.E Prematurity

33.E Summarize care of premature newborns.

» The Concept of Reproduction

Concept Key Terms

Acrosomal reaction, **2206**
Amnion, **2208**
Amniotic fluid, **2208**
Aortocaval compression, **2216**
Ballottement, **2221**
Blastocyst, **2207**
Braxton Hicks contractions, **2210**
Capacitation, **2206**
Chadwick sign, **2215**
Chloasma, **2217**
Chorion, **2207**
Corpus luteum, **2203**
Cotyledons, **2210**
Diastasis recti, **2218**
Ductus arteriosus, **2212**
Ductus venosus, **2212**
Embryo, **2213**
Embryonic membranes, **2207**
Estimated date of birth (EDB), **2212**
False pelvis, **2199**
Female reproductive cycle, **2200**
Fertilization, **2205**
Fetus, **2213**
Foramen ovale, **2212**
Gametes, **2198**
Gametogenesis, **2205**
Goodell sign, **2215**
Graafian follicle, **2203**
Hegar sign, **2220**
McDonald sign, **2220**
Meiosis, **2204**
Melasma gravidarum, **2217**
Mitosis, **2204**
Morning sickness, **2220**
Morula, **2206**
Nägele rule, **2245**
Oogenesis, **2205**
Ovulation, **2200**
Pelvic inlet, **2199**
Pelvic outlet, **2199**
Physiologic anemia of pregnancy, **2216**
Placenta, **2209**
Postconception age, **2212**
Prenatal education, **2248**
Quickening, **2220**
Risk factors, **2244**
Spermatogenesis, **2205**
Striae, **2215**
Supine hypotensive syndrome, **2216**
Teratogens, **2233**
Transverse diameter, **2199**
Trophoblast, **2207**
True pelvis, **2199**
Umbilical cord, **2208**
Vena caval syndrome, **2216**
Wharton jelly, **2208**
Zygote, **2205**

Also see Box 33.1 on page 2242 for additional key terms.

eproduction requires more than under- al intercourse or the process by which the sex cells unite. The nurse also must be famil- tructures and functions that make childbear- e and the phenomena that initiate it. The primary s of both female and male reproductive systems are duce sex cells and transport them to locations where r union can occur. The sex cells, called **gametes**, are pro- uced by specialized organs called *gonads*. A series of ducts and glands in both the male and female reproductive systems contribute to the production and transport of the gametes.

Normal Presentation of the Female Reproductive System

The female reproductive system is described in detail in Module 19, Sexuality. Two key components of the female reproductive system are discussed here in relation to their importance to conception and childbearing: the bony pelvis and the female reproductive cycle.

Bony Pelvis

The female bony pelvis has two unique functions:

- To support and protect the pelvic contents
- To form the relatively fixed axis of the birth passage.

The structure of the pelvis must be clearly understood because it is an essential component of the childbirth process.

Bony Structure

The pelvis is composed of four bones: two innominate bones, the sacrum, and the coccyx. The pelvis resembles a bowl or basin; its sides are the innominate bones, and its back is the sacrum and coccyx. Lined with fibrocartilage and held tightly together by ligaments, the four bones join at the symphysis pubis, the two sacroiliac joints, and the sacrococcygeal joints (**Figure 33.1** »).

The innominate bones, also known as the hip bones, are made up of three separate bones: the ilium, ischium, and pubis. These bones fuse to form a circular cavity, the acetabulum, which articulates with the femur.

The ilium is the broad, upper prominence of the hip. The iliac crest is the margin of the ilium. The ischial spines, the foremost projections nearest the groin, are the site of attachment for ligaments and muscles.

The ischium, the strongest bone, is under the ilium and below the acetabulum. The L-shaped ischium ends in a marked protuberance, the ischial tuberosity, on which the weight of a seated body rests. The ischial spines arise near the junction of the ilium and ischium and jut into the pelvic cavity. The shortest diameter of the pelvic cavity is between the ischial spines. The ischial spines serve as reference points during labor to evaluate the descent of the fetal head into the birth canal.

The pubis forms the slightly bowed front portion of the innominate bone. Extending medially from the acetabulum to the midpoint of the bony pelvis, each pubis meets the other to form a joint called the *symphysis pubis*. The triangular space below this junction is known as the *pubic arch*. The fetal head passes under this arch during birth. The symphysis pubis is formed by heavy fibrocartilage and the superior and inferior pubic ligaments. The mobility of the inferior ligament increases during a woman's first pregnancy and increases further in subsequent pregnancies.

The sacroiliac joints also have a degree of mobility that increases near the end of pregnancy as the result of an upward gliding movement. The pelvic outlet may be increased by 1.5 to 2 cm in the squatting and sitting positions. This relaxation of the joints is induced by *relaxin*, which is a pregnancy hormone.

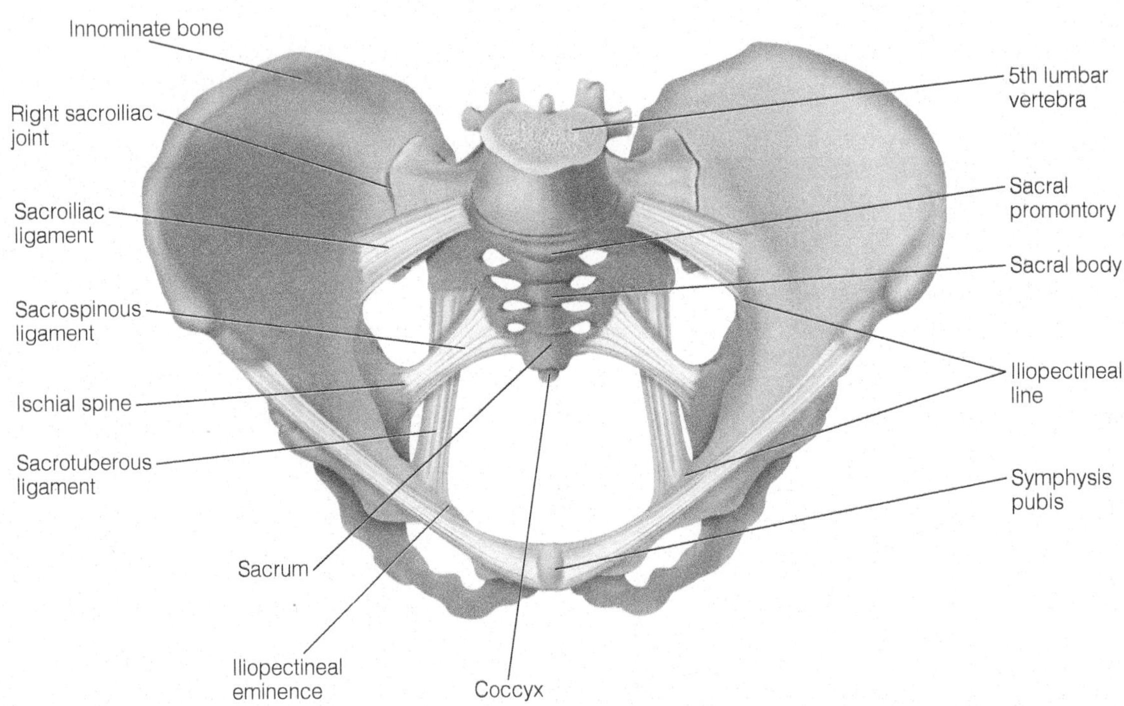

Figure 33.1 » Pelvic bones with supporting ligaments.

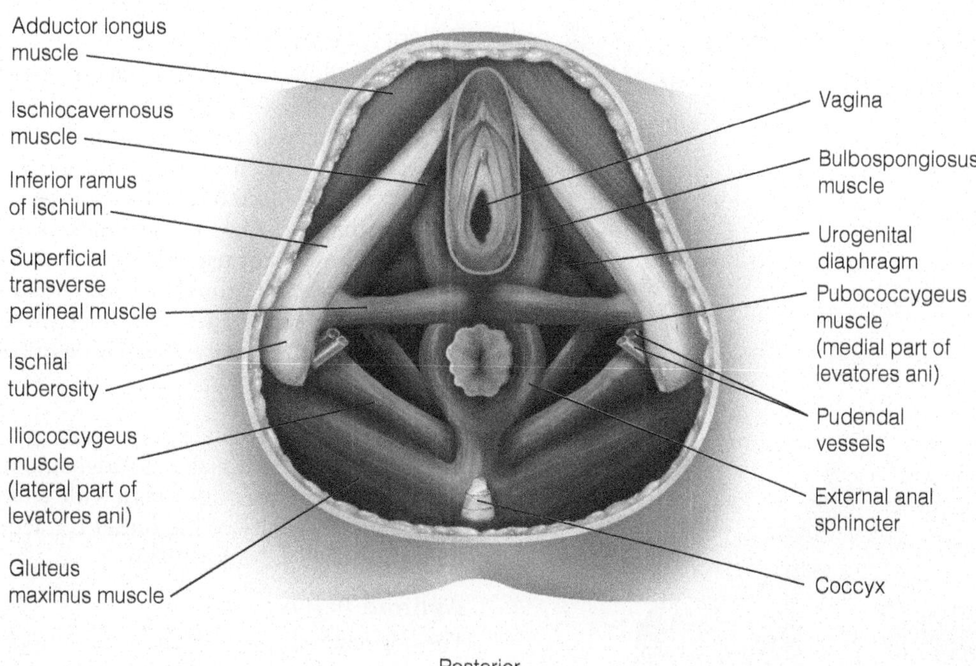

Figure 33.2 » Muscles of the pelvic floor. (The puborectalis, pubovaginalis, and coccygeal muscles cannot be seen from this view.)

The sacrum is a wedge-shaped bone formed by the fusion of five vertebrae. On the anterior upper portion of the sacrum is a projection into the pelvic cavity known as the *sacral promontory*. This projection is a guide in determining pelvic measurements.

The small triangular bone last on the vertebral column is the coccyx. It articulates with the sacrum at the sacrococcygeal joint. The coccyx usually moves backward during labor to provide more room for the fetus.

Pelvic Floor

The muscular pelvic floor of the bony pelvis is designed to overcome the force of gravity exerted on the pelvic organs. It acts as a supporting structure to the irregularly shaped pelvic outlet, providing stability and support for surrounding structures.

Deep fascia, the levator ani, and coccygeal muscles form the part of the pelvic floor known as the pelvic diaphragm. The components of the pelvic diaphragm function as a whole, yet they are able to move over one another. This physiology provides an exceptional capacity for dilation during birth and return to pre-pregnancy condition following birth. Above the pelvic diaphragm is the pelvic cavity; below and behind it is the perineum. The sacrum is located posteriorly.

The levator ani muscle makes up the major portion of the pelvic diaphragm and consists of four muscles: the iliococcygeus, pubococcygeus, puborectalis, and pubovaginalis. The iliococcygeal muscle, a thin muscular sheet underlying the sacrospinous ligament, helps the levator ani support the pelvic organs. Muscles of the pelvic floor are shown in **Figure 33.2** ».

Pelvic Division

The pelvic cavity is divided into the false pelvis and the true pelvis. The **false pelvis** (**Figure 33.3A** »), the portion above the pelvic brim, or linea terminalis, supports the weight of the enlarged pregnant uterus and directs the presenting fetal part into the true pelvis below.

The **true pelvis** is the portion that lies below the linea terminalis (pelvic brim). The bony circumference of the true pelvis is made up of the sacrum, coccyx, and innominate bones and represents the bony limits of the birth canal. The relationship between the true pelvic cavity and the fetal head is of paramount importance: The size and shape of the true pelvis must be adequate for normal fetal passage during labor and at birth. The true pelvis consists of three parts: the inlet, the pelvic cavity, and the outlet (**Figure 33.3B** »).

The **pelvic inlet** is the upper border of the true pelvis and is typically rounded. The **transverse diameter** is the largest diameter of the inlet.

The midpelvis or pelvic cavity (canal) is a curved canal with a longer posterior than anterior wall. A change in the lumbar curve can increase or decrease the tilt of the pelvis and influence the progress of labor because the fetus has to adjust itself to this curved path as well as to the different diameters of the true pelvis (see Figure 33.3B).

The **pelvic outlet** is at the lower border of the true pelvis. The anteroposterior diameter of the pelvic outlet increases during birth as the presenting part of the fetus pushes the coccyx posteriorly at the mobile sacrococcygeal joint. Decreased mobility, a large fetal head, and/or a forceful birth can cause the coccyx to break. As the fetus' head emerges, the long diameter of the head (occipital frontal) parallels the long diameter of the outlet (anteroposterior).

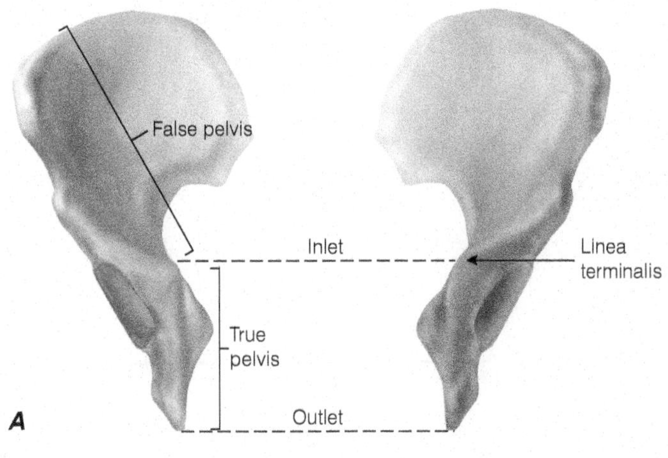

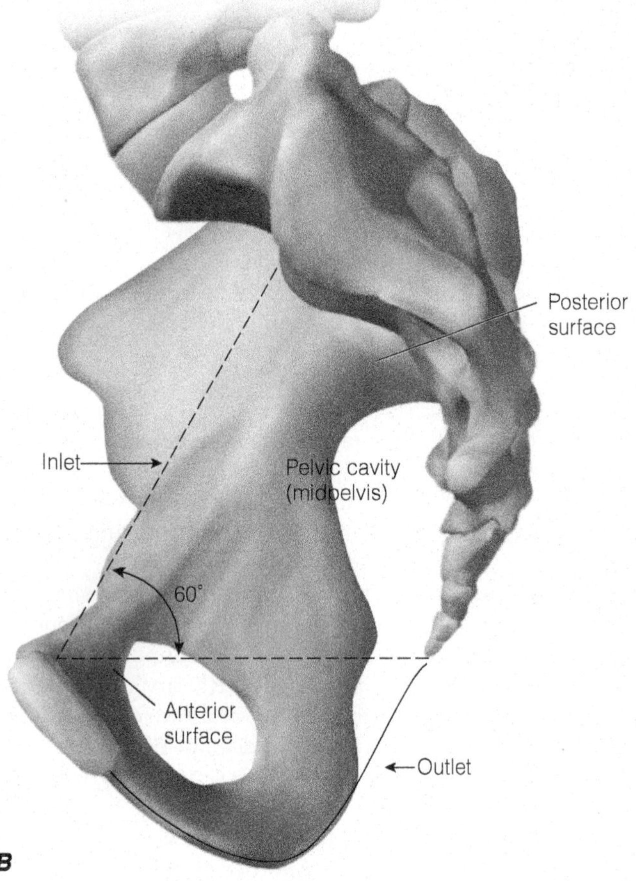

Figure 33.3 ››› Female pelvis. ***A***, The false pelvis is a shallow cavity above the inlet; the true pelvis is the deeper portion of the cavity below the inlet. ***B***, The true pelvis consists of the inlet, cavity (midpelvis), and outlet.

The transverse diameter (bi-ischial or intertuberous) extends from the inner surface of one ischial tuberosity to the other. It is the shortest diameter of the pelvic outlet and is even shorter in a woman who has a narrowed pubic arch. The pubic arch is of great importance because the fetus must pass under it during birth. If it is narrow, the baby's head may be pushed backward toward the coccyx, making extension of the head difficult. This situation, known as *outlet dystocia*, may require the use of forceps or a cesarean delivery. The shoulders of a large baby also may become wedged under the pubic arch, making birth more difficult.

Pelvic Types

The Caldwell–Moloy classification of the pelvis is still sometimes used to differentiate bony pelvic types (Caldwell & Moloy, 1933). The four basic types are gynecoid, android, anthropoid, and platypelloid, each with a characteristic shape and implications for birth (**Figure 33.4** ›››). However, a more recent study supports that variations in the female pelvis are so great that classic types are not usual (Delprete, 2017). The Caldwell–Moloy classification should be used with caution until further research has been conducted to either prove or disprove these classifications. The types are briefly described here.

Gynecoid Pelvis

The most common female pelvis is the gynecoid type. All of the inlet diameters are at least adequate for a vaginal birth. The gynecoid pelvic outlet has a wide and round pubic arch. The overall capacity of the outlet is adequate for a vaginal birth (Caldwell & Moloy, 1933).

Android Pelvis

The normal male pelvis is the android type; this type is occasionally seen in females. The inlet is heart shaped. The anteroposterior and transverse diameters are adequate for a vaginal birth, but the posterior sagittal diameter is too short and the anterior sagittal diameter is long. The capacity of the outlet is reduced. The structure of an android pelvis is not favorable for a vaginal birth. Cesarean delivery may be required.

Anthropoid Pelvis

The inlet of an anthropoid pelvis is oval, with a long anteroposterior diameter and an adequate but rather short transverse diameter. The midpelvic diameters are at least adequate, making its capacity adequate for a vaginal birth. The outlet capacity is adequate.

Platypelloid Pelvis

The platypelloid type refers to the flat female pelvis. The inlet is a distinctly transverse oval with a short anteroposterior and extremely short transverse diameter. The transverse diameter is wide, but the anteroposterior diameter is short. The outlet capacity may be inadequate for a vaginal birth. The platypelloid bones are similar to those of a gynecoid pelvis.

Female Reproductive Cycle

The **female reproductive cycle** is composed of the ovarian cycle, during which **ovulation**, the release of a mature egg from an ovary, occurs, and the uterine cycle, during which menstruation occurs. These two cycles take place simultaneously (**Figure 33.5** ›››).

Effects of Female Hormones

After menarche, a female undergoes a cyclic pattern of ovulation and menstruation, which is disrupted only by pregnancy, for a period of 30 to 40 years. This cycle is an orderly process under neurohormonal control. Each month multiple oocytes mature, with typically one, and sometimes more than one, rupturing from the ovary and entering the fallopian tube. The ovary, vagina, uterus, and fallopian tubes are major target organs for female hormones.

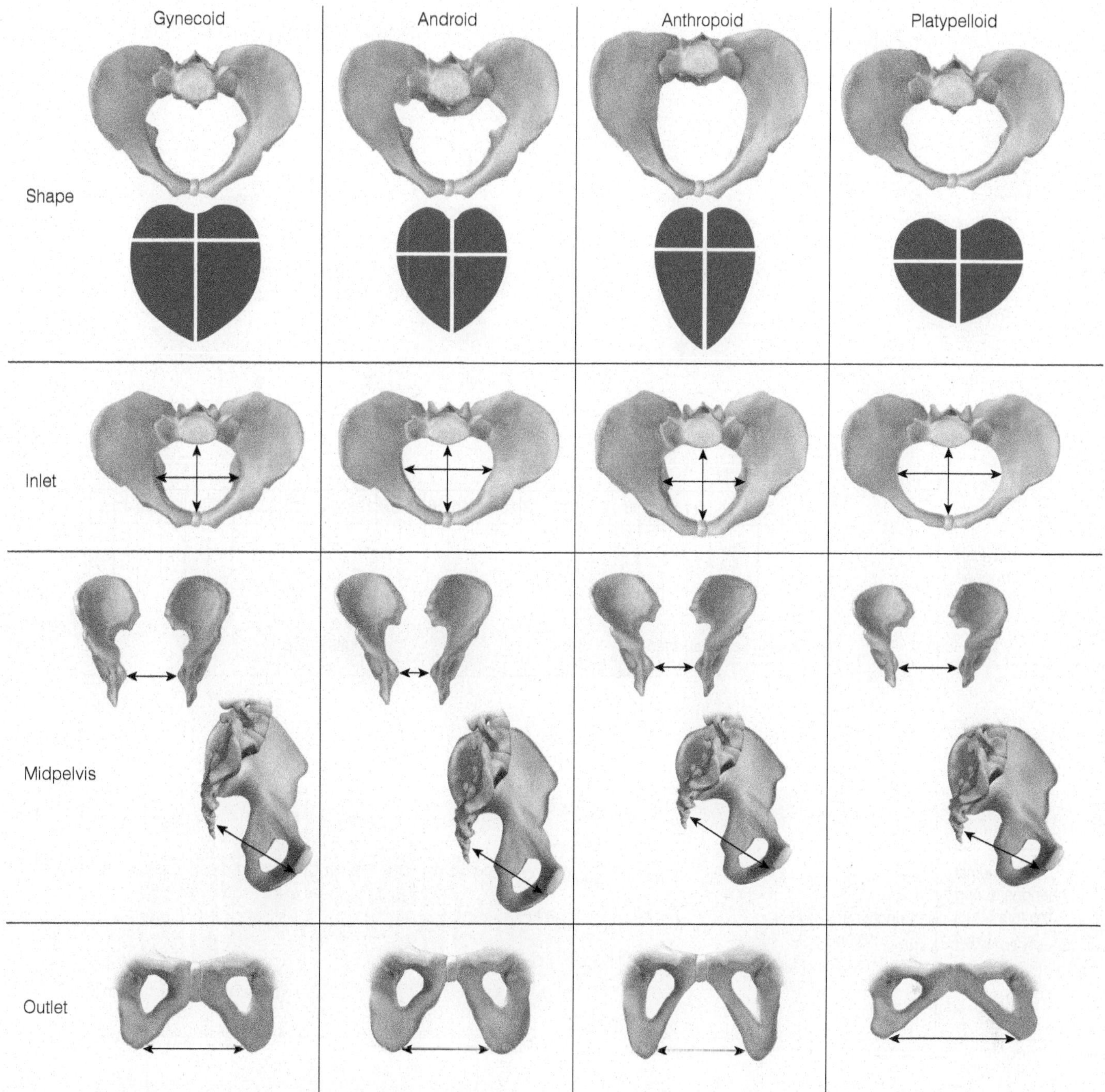

Figure 33.4 » Comparison of Caldwell–Moloy pelvic types.

Estrogen

The ovaries produce mature gametes and secrete hormones (estrogens, progesterone, and testosterone). Estrogens cause the uterus to increase in size and weight because of increased glycogen, amino acids, electrolytes, and water. Blood supply is expanded as well. Under the influence of estrogens, myometrial contractility increases in both the uterus and fallopian tubes. Uterine sensitivity to oxytocin also increases. Estrogens inhibit follicle-stimulating hormone (FSH) production and stimulate luteinizing hormone (LH) production.

Estrogens have effects on many hormones and other carrier proteins. For example, they contribute to the increased amount of protein-bound iodine in pregnant women and in women who use oral contraceptives containing estrogen. Estrogens decrease the excitability of the hypothalamus, which may cause an increase in sexual desire.

Progesterone

Progesterone is secreted by the corpus luteum and is found in greatest amounts during the secretory (luteal or progestational) phase of the menstrual cycle. Progesterone is often called the *hormone of pregnancy* because its effects on the uterus allow pregnancy to be maintained. Under the influence of progesterone, the vaginal epithelium proliferates, the cervix secretes thick, viscous mucus, and contractility of the uterus is suppressed. Breast glandular tissue increases in

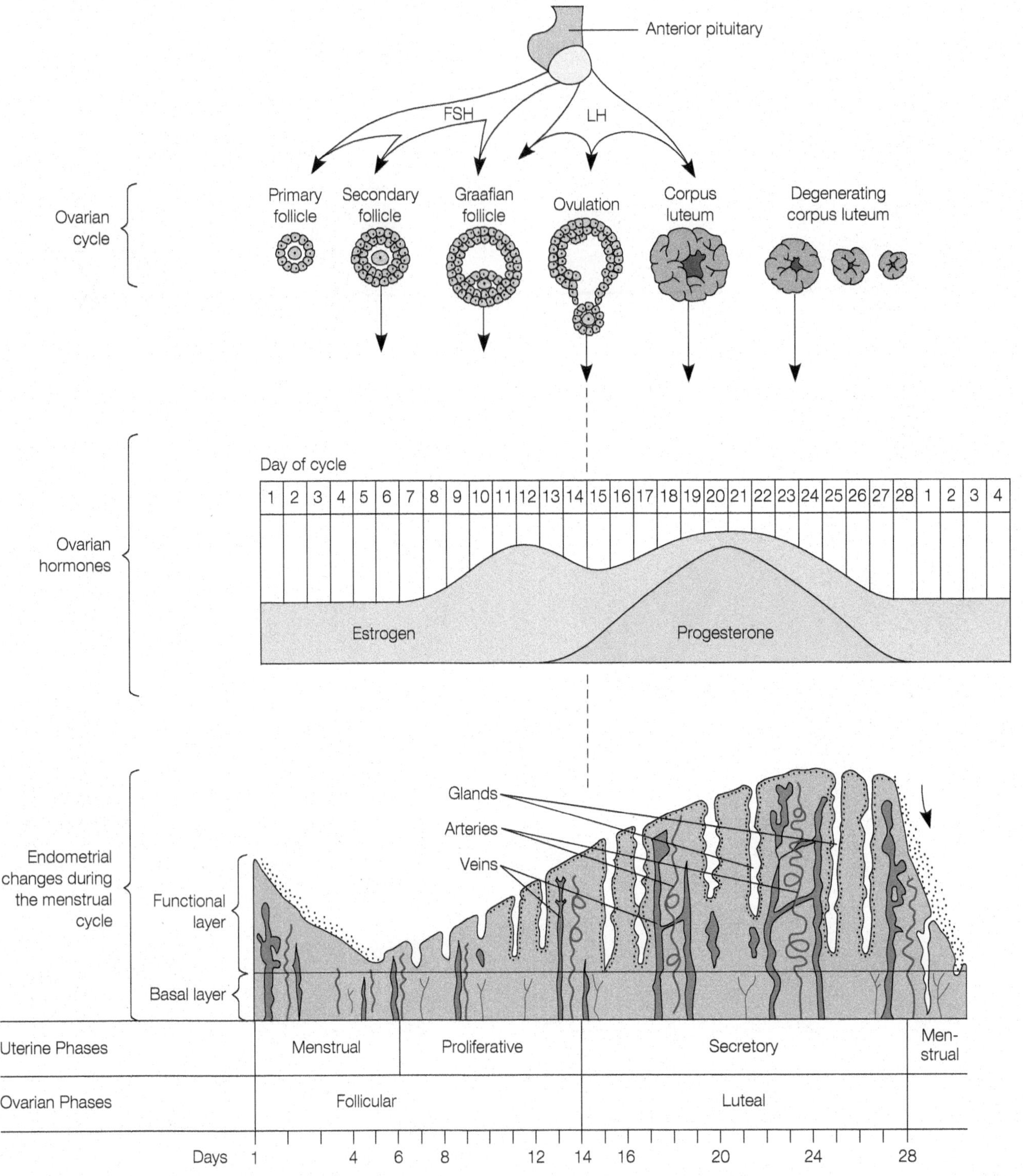

Figure 33.5 ›› Female reproductive cycle: interrelationships of hormones with the three phases of the uterine cycle and the two phases of the ovarian cycle in an ideal 28-day cycle.

Source: Ladewig, P. W., London, M. L., & Davidson, M. R. (2017). Contemporary Maternal-Newborn Nursing Care. 9e, p35. Hoboken, NJ: Pearson Education, Inc.

size and complexity. Progesterone also prepares the breasts for lactation and may contribute to constipation in pregnancy due to relaxation of smooth muscle, which results in decreased peristalsis.

Prostaglandins

Prostaglandins (PGs), which are oxygenated fatty acids, are produced by the cells of the endometrium. They are classified as hormones. Prostaglandins have varied action in the body. The two primary types of PGs are groups E and F. Generally, PGE relaxes smooth muscles and is a potent vasodilator; PGF is a potent vasoconstrictor and increases the contractility of muscles and arteries. Although the primary actions of PGE and PGF seem antagonistic, their basic regulatory functions in cells are achieved through an intricate pattern of reciprocal events.

Prostaglandin production increases during follicular maturation, is dependent on gonadotropins, and seems to be critical to follicular rupture (Cunningham et al., 2018). Significant amounts of PGs are found in and around the follicle at the time of ovulation.

Neurohumoral Basis of the Female Reproductive Cycle

The female reproductive cycle is controlled by complex interactions between the nervous and endocrine systems and their target tissues. These interactions involve the hypothalamus, anterior pituitary, and ovaries.

The hypothalamus secretes *gonadotropin-releasing hormone (GnRH)* to the pituitary gland in response to signals received from the central nervous system (CNS). This releasing hormone is also called *luteinizing hormone–releasing hormone (LHRH)* and *follicle-stimulating hormone–releasing hormone (FSHRH)* (Blackburn, 2018).

In response to GnRH, the anterior pituitary secretes the gonadotropic hormones FSH and LH. FSH is primarily responsible for the maturation of the ovarian follicle. As the follicle matures, it secretes increasing amounts of estrogen, which enhances the development of the follicle (Cunningham et al., 2018). This estrogen is also responsible for the rebuilding or proliferation phase of the endometrium after it is shed during menstruation.

Final maturation of the follicle cannot occur without the action of LH. The anterior pituitary's production of LH increases six- to tenfold as the follicle matures. The peak production of LH can precede ovulation by as much as 12 to 24 hours (Cunningham et al., 2018). The LH is also responsible for the increase in production of progesterone by the granulosa cells of the follicle, thereby stimulating ovulation. As a result, estrogen production is reduced and progesterone secretion continues. Although estrogen levels fall a day before ovulation, small amounts of progesterone continue to be present. Ovulation takes place following the very rapid growth of the follicle, as the sustained high level of estrogen diminishes and progesterone secretion begins.

The ruptured follicle undergoes rapid change, complete luteinization occurs, and the mass of cells becomes the **corpus luteum**. The lutein cells secrete large amounts of progesterone with smaller amounts of estrogen. Concurrently, the excessive amounts of progesterone are responsible for the secretory phase of the uterine cycle. On day 7 or 8 following ovulation, if pregnancy does not occur, the corpus luteum begins to involute, or decrease in size and functional activity. It loses its secretory function, severely diminishing the production of progesterone and estrogen. The anterior pituitary responds with increasingly large amounts of FSH, and LH production begins a few days later. As a result, new follicles become responsive to subsequent ovarian cycles and begin maturing.

Ovarian Cycle

The ovarian cycle has two phases. During a 28-day cycle, the *follicular phase* occurs during days 1 to 14 and the *luteal phase* occurs during days 15 to 28. **Figure 33.6** ⟫ depicts the changes the follicle undergoes during the ovarian cycle. In women whose menstrual cycles vary, usually only the length of the follicular phase varies because the luteal phase is of fixed length. During the follicular phase, the immature follicle matures as a result of FSH. Within the follicle, the oocyte grows.

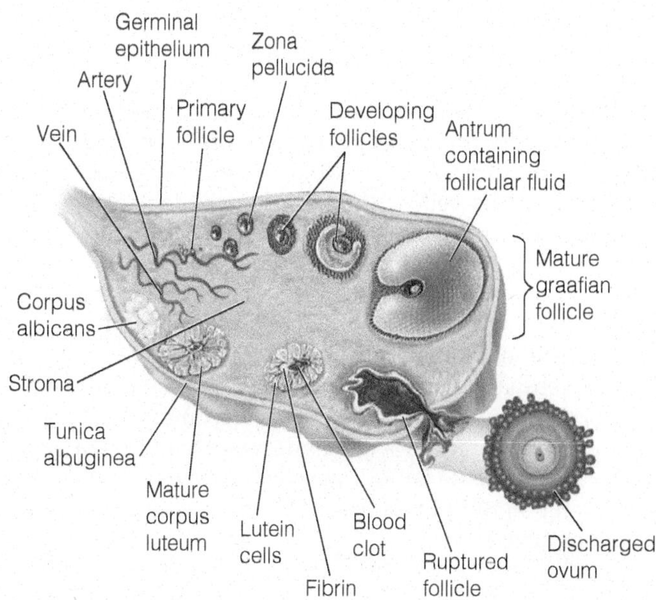

Figure 33.6 ⟫ Various stages of development of the ovarian follicles.

A mature **graafian follicle** appears at about the 14th day under dual control of FSH and LH. It is a large structure, measuring about 5 to 10 mm, that produces increasing amounts of estrogen. In the mature graafian follicle, the cells surrounding the fluid-filled antral cavity are called granulosa cells. The mass of granulosa cells surrounding the oocyte and follicular fluid is called the cumulus oophorus. In the fully mature graafian follicle, the zona pellucida, a thick elastic capsule, develops around the oocyte. Just before ovulation, the mature oocyte completes its first meiotic division. As a result of this division, two cells are formed: a small cell, called a *polar body*, and a larger cell, called a *secondary oocyte*. The secondary oocyte matures into the ovum.

As the graafian follicle matures and enlarges, it comes close to the surface of the ovary. The ovary surface forms a blister-like protrusion 10 to 15 mm in diameter, and the follicle walls become thin. The secondary oocyte, polar body, and follicular fluid are pushed out. The ovum is discharged near the fimbria of the fallopian tube and pulled into the tube to begin its journey toward the uterus.

In some women, ovulation is accompanied by midcycle pain known as *mittelschmerz*. This pain may be caused by a local peritoneal reaction to the expulsion of the ovum. Vaginal discharge may increase during ovulation, and a small amount of blood (midcycle spotting) may be discharged as well.

The body temperature increases about 0.3 to 0.6°C (0.5 to 1.0°F) 24 to 48 hours after ovulation. It remains elevated until the day before menstruation begins. There may be an accompanying sharp drop in basal body temperature before the increase. These temperature changes are useful clinically to determine the approximate time ovulation occurs (Blackburn, 2018).

Generally, the ovum takes several minutes to travel through the ruptured follicle to the fallopian tube opening. The contractions of the tube's smooth muscle and its ciliary action propel the ovum through the tube. The ovum remains in the ampulla, where, if it is fertilized, cleavage can begin.

The ovum is thought to be fertile for only 12 to 24 hours. It reaches the uterus 72 to 96 hours after its release from the ovary.

The luteal phase begins when the ovum leaves its follicle. Under the influence of LH, the corpus luteum develops from the ruptured follicle. Within 2 or 3 days, the corpus luteum becomes yellowish and spherical and increases in vascularity. If the ovum is fertilized and implants in the endometrium, the fertilized egg begins to secrete *human chorionic gonadotropin (hCG)*, which is needed to maintain the corpus luteum. If fertilization does not occur within about a week after ovulation, the corpus luteum begins to degenerate, eventually becoming a connective tissue scar called the corpus albicans. With degeneration comes a decrease in estrogen and progesterone. This decrease triggers the hypothalamus to release GnRH, which stimulates the synthesis and secretion of LH and FSH. This process initiates a new ovulatory cycle.

Menstrual Cycle

Menstruation is cyclic uterine bleeding in response to cyclic hormonal changes. Menstruation occurs when the ovum is not fertilized and begins about 14 days after ovulation in an ideal 28-day cycle. The menstrual discharge, also referred to as the menses or menstrual flow, is composed of blood mixed with fluid, cervical and vaginal secretions, bacteria, mucus, leukocytes, and other cellular debris. The menstrual discharge is dark red and has a distinctive odor.

Menstrual parameters vary greatly among individuals. Generally, menstruation occurs every 28 days, but the cycle varies from 21 to 35 days. Some women have longer cycles, which can skew standard calculations of the estimated date of birth. Emotional and physical factors such as illness, excessive fatigue, stress or anxiety, and vigorous exercise programs can alter the cycle interval. Certain environmental factors such as temperature and altitude also may affect the cycle. The duration of menses is from 2 to 8 days, with the blood loss averaging 25 to 60 mL and the loss of iron averaging 0.5 to 1 mg daily.

The uterine (menstrual) cycle has three phases: menstrual, proliferative, and secretory. Menstruation occurs during the *menstrual phase*. Some endometrial areas are shed, although others remain. Some of the remaining tips of the endometrial glands begin to regenerate. The endometrium is in a resting state following menstruation. Estrogen levels are low, and the endometrium is 1 to 2 mm deep. During this part of the cycle, the cervical mucus is scanty, viscous, and opaque.

The *proliferative phase* begins when the endometrial glands enlarge, becoming twisted and longer in response to increasing amounts of estrogen. The blood vessels become prominent and dilated, and the endometrium increases in thickness six- to eightfold. This gradual process reaches its peak just before ovulation. The cervical mucus becomes thin, clear, watery, and more alkaline, making the mucosa more favorable to spermatozoa. As ovulation nears, the cervical mucus shows increased elasticity, called *spinnbarkeit*. At ovulation, the mucus will stretch more than 5 cm. The pH of the cervical mucus increases from below 7.0 to 7.5 at the time of ovulation. On microscopic examination, the mucus shows a characteristic ferning pattern (**Figure 33.7** »). This fern pattern is useful in assessing ovulation time.

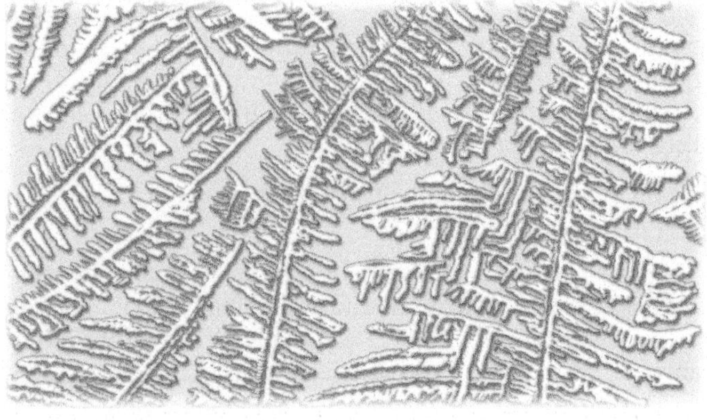

Figure 33.7 » Ferning pattern.

The *secretory phase* follows ovulation. The endometrium, under estrogenic influence, undergoes slight cellular growth. Progesterone, however, causes such marked swelling and growth that the epithelium is warped into folds. The amount of tissue glycogen increases. The glandular epithelial cells begin to fill with cellular debris, become twisted, and dilate. The glands secrete small quantities of endometrial fluid in preparation for a fertilized ovum. The vascularity of the entire uterus increases greatly, providing a nourishing bed for implantation. If implantation occurs, the endometrium, under the influence of progesterone, continues to develop and becomes even.

If fertilization does not occur, the *menstrual phase* begins. The corpus luteum begins to degenerate, and as a result, both estrogen and progesterone levels fall. Areas of necrosis appear under the epithelial lining. Extensive vascular changes also occur. Small blood vessels rupture, and the spiral arteries constrict and retract, causing a deficiency of blood in the endometrium, which becomes pale. This phase is characterized by the escape of blood into the stromal cells of the uterus. The menstrual flow begins, thus beginning the menstrual cycle again. After menstruation, the basal layer remains so that the tips of the glands can regenerate the new functional endometrial layer. (For more about the female reproductive cycle, see Module 19, Sexuality.)

Conception and Embryonic Development

Each human begins life as a single cell called a *fertilized ovum*, or *zygote*. This single cell reproduces itself and, in turn, each resulting cell reproduces itself in a continuing process. The new cells are similar to the cells from which they came. Cells are reproduced by mitosis or meiosis, two different but related processes.

Mitosis results in the production of diploid body (somatic) cells, which are exact copies of the original cell. Mitosis makes growth and development possible, and in mature individuals, it is the process by which the body's cells continue to divide and replace themselves. **Meiosis** is a process of cell division leading to the development of the eggs and sperm needed to produce a new organism. Unlike cells produced during mitosis, the cells produced during meiosis contain only half the genetic material or number of chromosomes (the haploid number).

Mitosis

During mitosis, the cell undergoes several changes, ending in cell division. As the last phase of cell division nears completion, a furrow develops in the cell cytoplasm, which divides it into two daughter cells, each with its own nucleus. Daughter cells have the same diploid number of chromosomes (46) and same genetic makeup as the cell from which they came. After a cell with 46 chromosomes goes through mitosis, the result is two identical cells, each with 46 chromosomes.

Meiosis

Meiosis is a special type of cell division by which diploid cells in the testes and ovaries give rise to gametes (sperm and ova) with the haploid number of chromosomes, which is 23.

Meiosis consists of two successive cell divisions. In the first division, the chromosomes replicate. Next, a pairing takes place between homologous chromosomes (Sadler, 2018). Instead of separating immediately, as in mitosis, the chromosomes become closely intertwined. At each point of contact, a physical exchange of genetic material takes place between the chromatids (the arms of the chromosomes). New combinations are provided by the newly formed chromosomes; these combinations account for the wide variation of traits in people (e.g., hair and eye color). The chromosome pairs then separate, and the members of the pair move to opposite sides of the cell. In contrast, during mitosis, the chromatids of each chromosome separate and move to opposite poles. The cell divides, forming two daughter cells, each with 23 double-structured chromosomes; thus, each contains the same amount of deoxyribonucleic acid (DNA) as a normal somatic cell. In the second division, the chromatids of each chromosome separate and move to opposite poles of each of the daughter cells. Cell division occurs, resulting in the formation of four cells, each containing 23 single chromosomes, identified as the haploid number of chromosomes. These daughter cells contain only half the DNA of a normal somatic cell (Sadler, 2018).

Mutations may occur during the second meiotic division if two of the chromatids do not move apart rapidly enough when the cell divides. The still-paired chromatids are carried into one of the daughter cells and eventually form an extra chromosome. This condition, called *autosomal nondisjunction* (chromosomal mutation), is harmful to the offspring that may result should fertilization occur. Another type of chromosomal mutation can occur if chromosomes break during meiosis. If the broken segment is lost, the result is a shorter chromosome—a situation known as deletion. If the broken segment becomes attached to another chromosome, a harmful mutation, called a *translocation*, results.

Gametogenesis

Meiosis occurs during **gametogenesis**, the process by which germ cells, or gametes (*ovum* and *sperm*), are produced. These cells contain only half the genetic material of a typical body cell. The gametes must have a haploid number (23) of chromosomes so that when the female gamete (egg or ovum) and the male gamete (sperm or spermatozoon) unite to form the **zygote** (fertilized ovum), the normal human diploid number of chromosomes (46) is reestablished.

Oogenesis

Oogenesis is the process that produces the female gamete, called an ovum (egg). The ovaries begin to develop early in the fetal life of the female. All of the ova that the female will produce in her lifetime are present at birth. The ovary gives rise to oogonial cells, which develop into oocytes. Meiosis begins in all oocytes before the female fetus is born but stops before the first division is complete and remains in this arrested phase until puberty. During puberty, the mature primary oocyte proceeds (by oogenesis) through the first meiotic division in the graafian follicle of the ovary.

The first meiotic division produces two cells of unequal size with different amounts of cytoplasm but with the same number of chromosomes. These two cells are the secondary oocyte and the first polar body. Both the secondary oocyte and the first polar body contain 22 double-structured autosomal chromosomes and one double-structured sex chromosome (X).

At ovulation, a second meiotic division begins immediately and proceeds as the oocyte moves down the fallopian tube. Division is again not equal, and the secondary oocyte moves into the metaphase stage of cell division, where its meiotic division is arrested until and unless the oocyte is fertilized.

When the secondary oocyte completes the second meiotic division after fertilization, the result is a mature ovum with the haploid number of chromosomes and virtually all of the cytoplasm. In addition, the second polar body (also haploid) forms at this time. The first polar body now has also divided, producing two additional polar bodies. Thus, at the completion of meiosis, four haploid cells have been produced: the three polar bodies, which eventually disintegrate, and one ovum (Sadler, 2018).

Spermatogenesis

During puberty, the germinal epithelium in the seminiferous tubules of the testes begins the process of **spermatogenesis**, which produces the male gamete (sperm). The diploid spermatogonium replicates before it enters the first meiotic division, during which it is called the primary spermatocyte. During this first meiotic division, the spermatogonium replicates and forms two haploid cells called secondary spermatocytes, each of which contains 22 double-structured autosomal chromosomes and either a double-structured X sex chromosome or a double-structured Y sex chromosome. During the second meiotic division, they divide to form four spermatids, each with the haploid number of chromosomes. The spermatids undergo a series of changes during which they lose most of their cytoplasm and become sperm (spermatozoa). The nucleus becomes compacted into the head of the sperm, which is covered by a cap called an acrosome that is, in turn, covered by a plasma membrane. A long tail is produced from one of the centrioles.

Fertilization

Fertilization is the process by which a sperm fuses with an ovum to form a new diploid cell, or zygote. The zygote begins life as a single cell with a complete set of genetic material, 23 chromosomes from the mother's ovum and 23 chromosomes from the father's sperm for a total of 46 chromosomes. The following events lead to fertilization.

Preparation for Fertilization

The mature ovum and spermatozoon have only a brief time to unite. Ova are considered fertile for about 12 to 24 hours after ovulation. Sperm can survive in the female reproductive tract for 48 to 72 hours, but they are believed to be healthy and highly fertile for only the first 24 hours.

The ovum's cell membrane is surrounded by two layers of tissue. The layer closest to the cell membrane is called the *zona pellucida*. It is a clear, noncellular layer whose thickness influences the fertilization rate. Surrounding the zona pellucida is a ring of elongated cells, called the *corona radiata* because they radiate from the ovum like the gaseous corona around the sun. These cells are held together by hyaluronic acid. The ovum has no inherent power of movement. During ovulation, high estrogen levels increase peristalsis in the fallopian tubes, which helps move the ovum through the tube toward the uterus. The high estrogen levels also cause a thinning of the cervical mucus, facilitating movement of the sperm through the cervix, into the uterus, and up the fallopian tube.

The process of fertilization takes place in the ampulla (outer third) of the fallopian tube. In a single ejaculation, the male deposits approximately 200 million to 500 million spermatozoa into the vagina, of which only approximately 1000 sperm actually reach the ampulla (Sadler, 2018). Fructose in the semen, secreted by the seminal vesicles, is the energy source for the sperm. The spermatozoa propel themselves up the female tract by the flagellar movement of their tails. Transit time from the cervix into the fallopian tube can be as short as 5 minutes but usually takes an average of 2 to 7 hours after ejaculation (Sadler, 2018). Prostaglandins in the semen may increase uterine smooth muscle contractions, which help transport the sperm. The fallopian tubes have a dual ciliary action that facilitates movement of the ovum toward the uterus and movement of the sperm from the uterus toward the ovary.

The sperm must undergo two processes before fertilization can occur: capacitation and the acrosomal reaction. **Capacitation** is the removal of the plasma membrane overlying the spermatozoa's acrosomal area and the loss of seminal plasma proteins. If the glycoprotein coat is not removed, the sperm will not be able to fertilize the ovum (Sadler, 2018). Capacitation occurs in the female reproductive tract (aided by uterine enzymes) and is thought to take about 7 hours. Sperm that undergo capacitation take on three characteristics: (1) the ability to undergo the acrosomal reaction, (2) the ability to bind to the zona pellucida, and (3) the acquisition of hypermotility.

The **acrosomal reaction** follows capacitation, whereby the acrosomes of the sperm surrounding the ovum release their enzymes (hyaluronidase, the protease acrosin, and trypsin-like substances) and thus break down the hyaluronic acid in the ovum's corona radiata (Sadler, 2018). Approximately a thousand acrosomes must rupture before enough hyaluronic acid is cleared for a single sperm to penetrate the ovum's zona pellucida successfully.

At the moment of penetration by a fertilizing sperm, the zona pellucida undergoes a reaction that prevents additional sperm from entering a single ovum. This is known as the block to polyspermy. This cellular change is mediated by release of materials from the cortical granules, organelles found just below the ovum's surface, and is called the *cortical reaction*.

The Moment of Fertilization

After the sperm enters the ovum, a chemical signal prompts the secondary oocyte to complete the second meiotic division, forming the nucleus of the ovum and ejecting the second polar body. Then the nuclei of the ovum and sperm swell and approach each other. The true moment of fertilization occurs as the nuclei unite. Their individual nuclear membranes disappear, and their chromosomes pair up to produce the diploid zygote. Because each nucleus contains a haploid number of chromosomes (23), this union restores the diploid number (46). The zygote contains a new combination of genetic material that results in an individual different from either parent and from anyone else.

The sex of the zygote is determined at the moment of fertilization. The two chromosomes (the sex chromosomes) of the 23rd pair—either XX or XY—determine the sex of an individual. The X chromosome is larger and bears more genes than the Y chromosome. Females have two X chromosomes, and males have an X and a Y chromosome. Whereas the mature ovum produced by oogenesis can have only one type of sex chromosome—an X—spermatogenesis produces two sperm with an X chromosome and two sperm with a Y chromosome. When each gamete contributes an X chromosome, the resulting zygote is female. When the ovum contributes an X and the sperm contributes a Y chromosome, the resulting zygote is male. Certain traits are termed *sex-linked* because they are controlled by the genes on the X sex chromosome. Two examples of sex-linked traits are color blindness and hemophilia.

Preembryonic Development

The first 14 days of development, starting the day the ovum is fertilized (conception), make up the preembryonic stage, or the stage of the ovum. Development after fertilization can be divided into two phases: cellular multiplication and cellular differentiation. These phases are characterized by rapid cellular multiplication and differentiation and establishment of the primary germ layers and embryonic membranes. Synchronized development of the endometrium and the embryo is a prerequisite for implantation to succeed (Moore, Persaud, & Torchia, 2019). These phases and the process of implantation (nidation), which occurs between them, are discussed next.

Cellular Multiplication

Cellular multiplication begins as the zygote moves through the fallopian tube toward the cavity of the uterus. This transport takes 3 days or more and is accomplished mainly by a weak fluid current in the fallopian tube resulting from the beating action of the ciliated epithelia that line the tube.

The zygote now enters a period of rapid mitotic divisions called cleavage, during which it divides into two cells, four cells, eight cells, and so on. These cells, called blastomeres, are so small that the developing cell mass is only slightly larger than the original zygote. The blastomeres are held together by the zona pellucida, which is under the corona radiata. The blastomeres eventually form a solid ball of 12 to 32 cells called the **morula**.

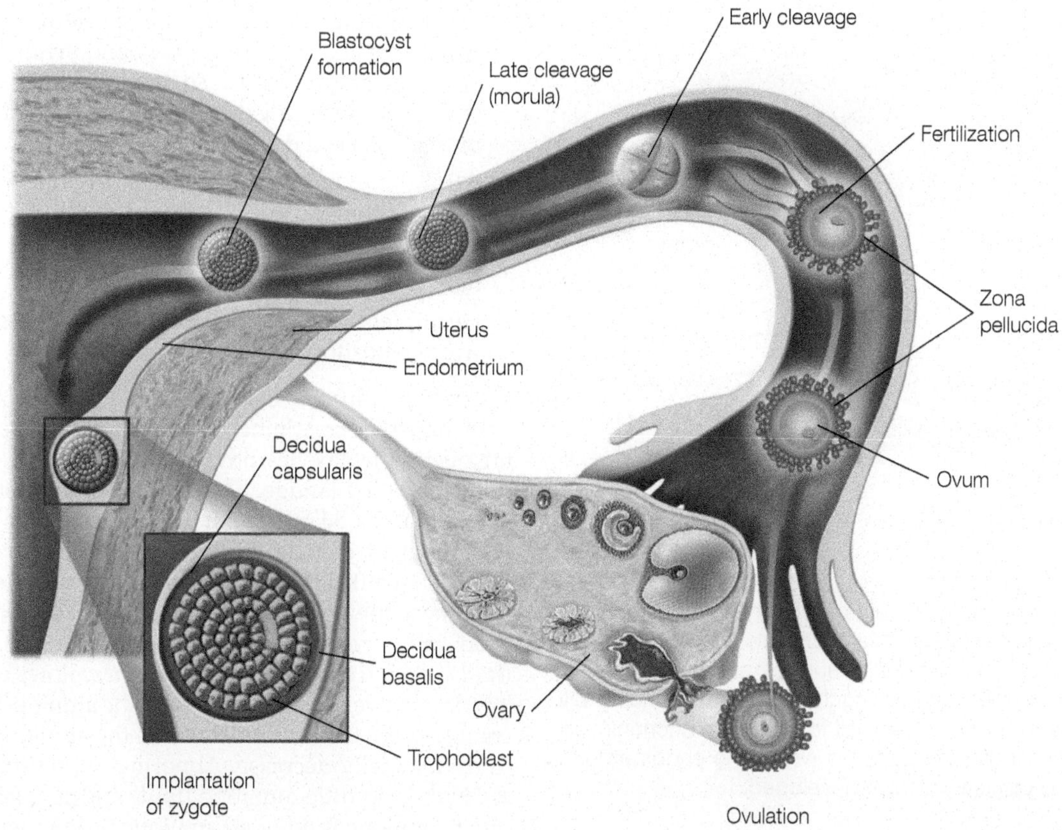

Figure 33.8 ⟫ During ovulation, the ovum leaves the ovary and enters the fallopian tube. Fertilization generally occurs in the outer third of the fallopian tube. The figure depicts subsequent changes in the fertilized ovum from conception to implantation.

As the morula enters the uterus, two things happen: The intracellular fluid in the morula increases, and a central cavity forms within the cell mass. Inside this cavity is an inner solid mass of cells called the **blastocyst**. The outer layer of cells that surrounds the cavity and replaces the zona pellucida is the **trophoblast**. Eventually, the trophoblast develops into one of two embryonic membranes, the **chorion**. The blastocyst develops into a double layer of cells called the embryonic disc, from which the *embryo* and the *amnion* (embryonic membrane) develop. The journey of the fertilized ovum to its destination in the uterus is illustrated in **Figure 33.8** ⟫.

Early pregnancy factor (EPF), an immunosuppressant protein, is secreted by the trophoblastic cells. This factor appears in the maternal serum within 24 to 48 hours after fertilization and forms the basis of a pregnancy test during the first 10 days of development (Caudle, 2019; Moore et al., 2019).

Implantation (Nidation)

While floating in the uterine cavity, the blastocyst is nourished by the uterine glands, which secrete a mixture of lipids, mucopolysaccharides, and glycogen. The trophoblast attaches to the surface of the endometrium for further nourishment. The most frequent site of attachment is the upper part of the posterior uterine wall. Between 7 and 10 days after fertilization, the zona pellucida disappears and the blastocyst implants itself by burrowing into the uterine lining and penetrating down toward the maternal capillaries until it is completely covered (Moore et al., 2019). The lining of the uterus thickens below the implanted blastocyst, and the cells of the trophoblast grow down into the thickened lining, forming processes that are called *chorionic villi*.

Under the influence of progesterone, the endometrium increases in thickness and vascularity in preparation for implantation and nutrition of the ovum. After implantation, the endometrium is called the decidua. The portion of the decidua that covers the blastocyst is called the decidua capsularis, the portion directly under the implanted blastocyst is the decidua basalis, and the portion that lines the rest of the uterine cavity is the decidua vera (parietalis). The maternal part of the placenta develops from the decidua basalis, which contains large numbers of blood vessels (London et al., 2017) (see magnified inset in Figure 33.8). The chorionic villi (discussed shortly) in contact with the decidua basalis will form the fetal portion of the placenta.

Cellular Differentiation

Primary Germ Layers

About the 10th to 14th day after conception, the homogeneous mass of blastocyst cells differentiates into the primary germ layers. These three layers—the ectoderm, mesoderm, and endoderm—are formed at the same time as the embryonic membranes. All tissues, organs, and organ systems will develop from these primary germ cell layers.

Embryonic Membranes

The **embryonic membranes** begin to form at the time of implantation (**Figure 33.9** ⟫). These membranes protect and support the embryo as it grows and develops inside the uterus.

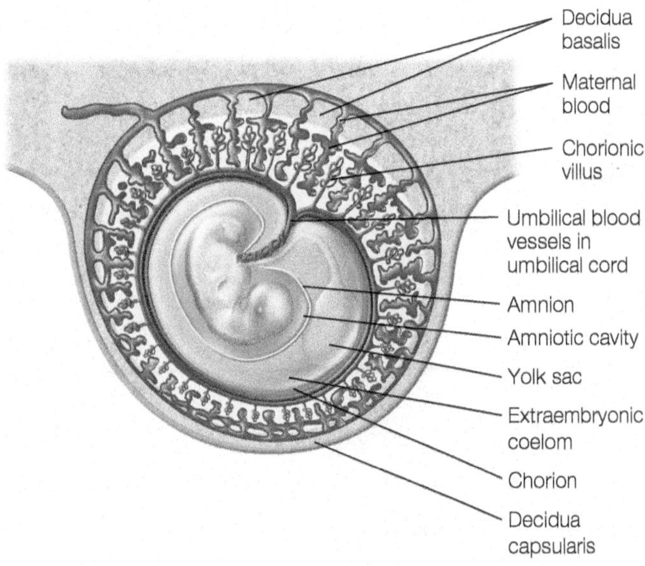

Figure 33.9 >> Early development of primary embryonic membranes. At 4½ weeks, the decidua capsularis (placental portion enclosing the embryo on the uterine surface) and decidua basalis (placental portion encompassing the elaborate chorionic villi and maternal endometrium) are well formed. The chorionic villi lie in blood-filled intervillous spaces within the endometrium. The amnion and yolk sac are well developed.

The first and outermost membrane to form is the chorion. This thick membrane develops from the trophoblast and has many fingerlike projections called chorionic villi on its surface. These chorionic villi can be used for early genetic testing of the embryo at 10 to 11 weeks' gestation by chorionic villus sampling (CVS). As the pregnancy progresses, the chorionic villi begin to degenerate, except for those just under the embryo, which grow and branch into depressions in the uterine wall, forming the fetal portion of the placenta. By the fourth month of pregnancy, the surface of the chorion is smooth except at the place of attachment to the uterine wall.

The second membrane to form, the amnion, originates from the ectoderm, a primary germ layer, during the early stages of embryonic development. The **amnion** is a thin protective membrane that contains amniotic fluid. The space between the membrane and the embryo is the amniotic cavity. This cavity surrounds the embryo and yolk sac, except where the developing embryo (germ-layer disc) attaches to the trophoblast via the umbilical cord. As the embryo grows, the amnion expands until it comes in contact with the chorion. These two slightly adherent membranes form the fluid-filled amniotic sac, which protects the floating embryo.

Amniotic Fluid

The primary functions of **amniotic fluid** are to:

- Act as a cushion to protect the fetus against mechanical injury during pregnancy and labor.
- Help control the embryo's temperature (the embryo relies on the mother to release heat).
- Permit symmetrical external growth and development of the embryo.
- Prevent adherence of the embryo–fetus to the amnion (decreases chance of amniotic band syndrome) to allow freedom of movement so that the embryo–fetus can change position (flexion and extension), thus aiding in musculoskeletal development.
- Allow the umbilical cord to be relatively free of compression.
- Act as an extension of fetal extracellular space (hydropic fetuses have increased amniotic fluid).
- Permit fetal swallowing and excretion, thus serving as a waste repository.

Amniotic fluid is slightly alkaline and contains albumin, urea, uric acid, creatinine, lecithin, sphingomyelin, bilirubin, fat, fructose, leukocytes, proteins, epithelial cells, enzymes, and fine hair called lanugo. The amount of amniotic fluid at 10 weeks is about 30 mL, and it increases to 210 mL at 16 weeks (Cunningham et al., 2018). After 28 weeks, the volume ranges from 700 to 1000 mL. As the pregnancy continues, the fetus influences the volume of amniotic fluid by swallowing the fluid and excreting lung fluid and urine into the amniotic fluid (London et al., 2017). The fetus swallows up to 262 mL/kg/day. Between 29 and 30 weeks, the amniotic fluid volume changes very little. After 39 weeks the amniotic fluid begins to dramatically decrease. Abnormal variations are *oligohydramnios* (too little amniotic fluid) and *polyhydramnios* (too much amniotic fluid or an amniotic fluid index greater than the 95th percentile; also called *hydramnios*).

Yolk Sac

In humans, the yolk sac is small, and it functions only in early embryonic life. It develops as a second cavity in the blastocyst on about day 8 or 9 after conception. It forms primitive RBCs during the first 6 weeks of development, until the embryo's liver takes over the process. As the embryo develops, the yolk sac is incorporated into the umbilical cord, where it can be seen as a degenerated structure after birth.

Umbilical Cord

As the placenta develops, the **umbilical cord** is being formed from the mesoderm and is covered by the amnion. The body stalk, which attaches the embryo to the yolk sac, contains blood vessels that extend into the chorionic villi. The body stalk fuses with the embryonic portion of the placenta to provide a circulatory pathway from the chorionic villi to the embryo. As the body stalk elongates to become the umbilical cord, the vessels in the cord decrease to one large vein and two smaller arteries. About 0.5% of umbilical cords have only two vessels: an artery and a vein. This condition may be associated with congenital malformations primarily of the genitourinary, musculoskeletal, central nervous, gastrointestinal, and cardiovascular systems. A specialized connective tissue known as **Wharton jelly** surrounds the blood vessels in the umbilical cord. This tissue, in addition to the high blood volume pulsating through the vessels, prevents compression of the umbilical cord in utero. The umbilical cord has no sensory or motor innervation, so cutting the cord after birth is not painful. At term (37 to 42 weeks' gestation), the average cord is 2 cm (0.8 in.) across and about 55 cm (22 in.) long. The cord can attach itself to the placenta at various sites. Central insertion into the placenta is considered normal.

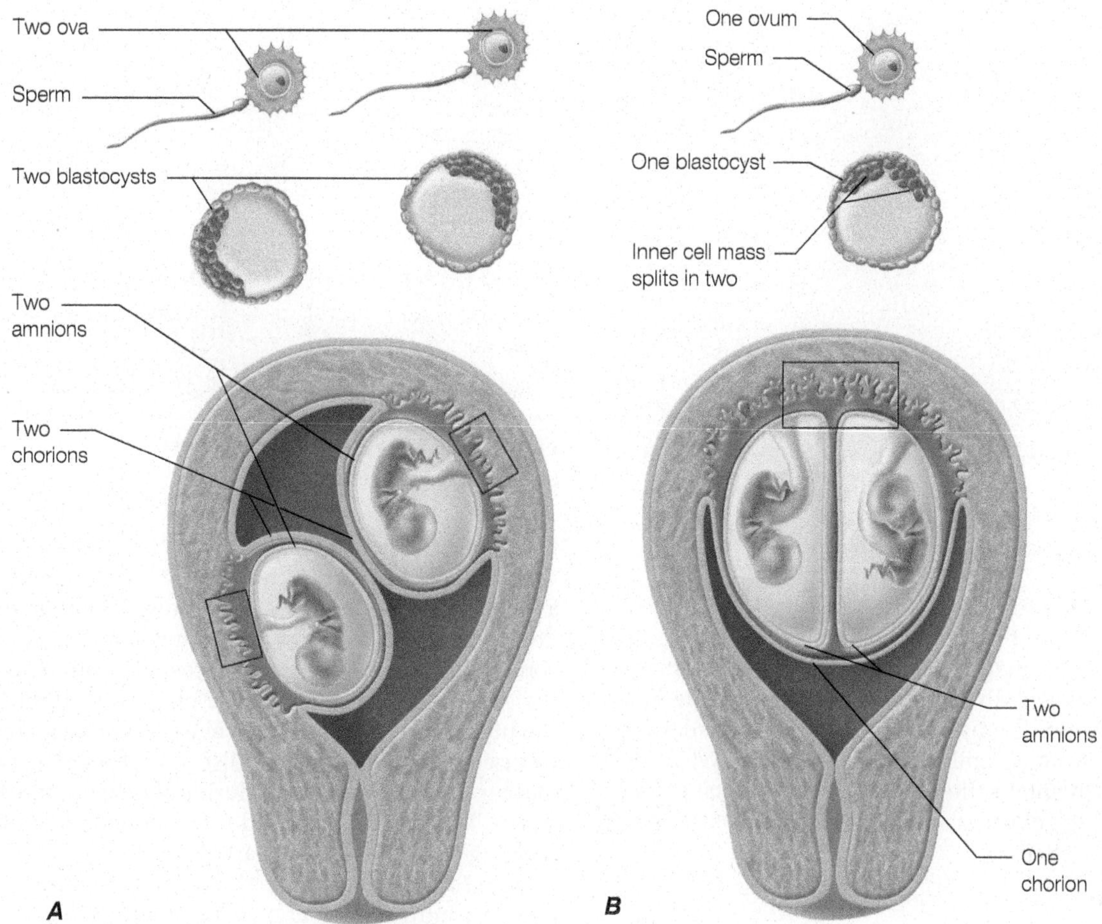

Figure 33.10 ›› ***A***, Dizygotic (fraternal) twins. (Note separate placentas.) ***B***, Monozygotic (identical) twins.

Umbilical cords appear twisted or spiraled, which is most likely caused by fetal movement. A true knot in the umbilical cord rarely occurs; if it does, the cord is longer than usual. More common are so-called false knots, caused by the folding of cord vessels. A *nuchal cord* is said to exist when the umbilical cord encircles the fetal neck.

Twins

Twins normally occur in approximately 33 of 1000 pregnancies, and triplets occur in 1 in 1000 pregnancies. The current rate of multiple-gestation pregnancies is attributed to delayed childbearing and the use of artificial reproductive treatments (London et al., 2017). Twins may be fraternal or identical (**Figure 33.10 ››**).

›› *Go to* ***Pearson MyLab Nursing and eText*** *for a MiniModule on twins.*

Development and Functions of the Placenta

The **placenta** is the means of metabolic and nutrient exchange between the embryonic and maternal circulations. Placental development and circulation do not begin until the third week of embryonic development. The placenta develops at the site where the embryo attaches to the uterine wall. Expansion of the placenta continues until about 20 weeks, when it covers approximately one-half of the internal surface of the uterus. After 20 weeks' gestation, the placenta becomes thicker but not wider. At 40 weeks' gestation, the placenta is about 15 to 20 cm (5.9 to 7.9 in.) in diameter and 2.5 to 3 cm (1 to 1.2 in.) in thickness. At that time, it weighs about 400 to 600 g (14 to 21 oz).

The placenta has two parts: the maternal and fetal portions. The maternal portion consists of the decidua basalis and its circulation. Its surface is red and fleshlike. The fetal portion consists of the chorionic villi and their circulation. The fetal surface of the placenta is covered by the amnion, which gives it a shiny gray appearance (**Figure 33.11 ››** and **Figure 33.12 ››**).

Development of the placenta begins with the chorionic villi. The trophoblastic cells of the chorionic villi form spaces in the tissue of the decidua basalis. These spaces fill with maternal blood, and the chorionic villi grow into them. As the chorionic villi differentiate, two trophoblastic layers appear: an outer layer, called the syncytium (consisting of syncytiotrophoblasts), and an inner layer, known as the cytotrophoblast. The cytotrophoblast thins out and disappears around the fifth month, leaving only a single layer of syncytium covering the chorionic villi. The syncytium is in direct contact with the maternal blood in the intervillous spaces. It is the functional layer of the placenta, and it secretes the placental hormones of pregnancy.

A third inner layer of connective mesoderm develops in the chorionic villi, forming anchoring villi. These anchoring

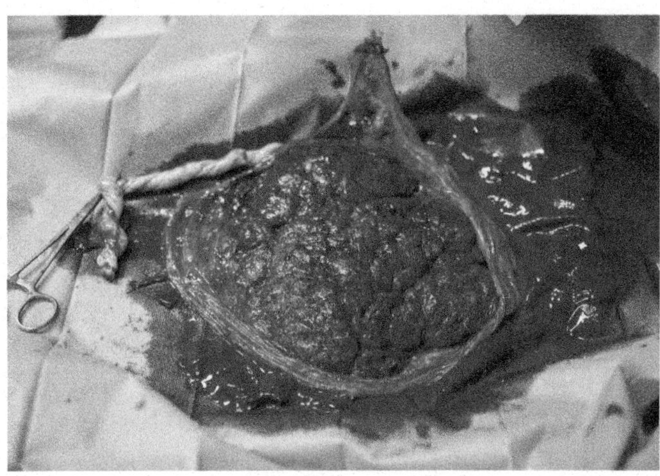

Figure 33.11 ›› Maternal side of placenta.
Source: fotowunsch/iStock/Getty Images.

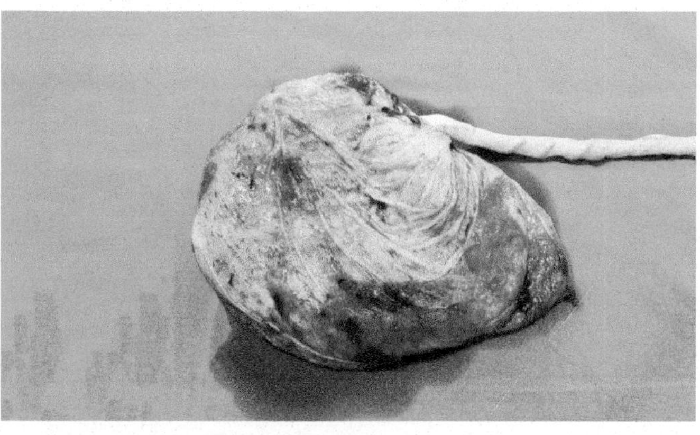

Figure 33.12 ›› Fetal side of placenta.
Source: ravipat/Shutterstock.

villi eventually form the septa (partitions) of the placenta. The septa divide the mature placenta into 15 to 20 segments called **cotyledons** (subdivisions of the placenta made up of anchoring villi and decidual tissue). In each cotyledon, the branching villi form a highly complex vascular system that allows compartmentalization of the uteroplacental circulation. The exchange of gases and nutrients takes place across these vascular systems.

Placental Circulation

After implantation of the blastocyst, the cells distinguish themselves into fetal cells and trophoblastic cells. The proliferating trophoblast successfully invades the decidua basalis of the endometrium, first opening the uterine capillaries and later opening the larger uterine vessels. The chorionic villi are an outgrowth of the blastocystic tissue. As these villi continue to grow and divide, the fetal vessels begin to form. The intervillous spaces in the decidua basalis develop as the endometrial spiral arteries are opened.

By the end of the fourth week, the placenta has begun to function as a means of metabolic exchange between embryo and mother. The completion of the maternal–placental–fetal circulation occurs about 17 days after conception, when the embryonic heart begins functioning (Moore et al., 2019). By 14 weeks, the placenta is a discrete organ. It has grown in thickness as a result of growth in the length and size of the chorionic villi and accompanying expansion of the intervillous space.

In the fully developed placenta's umbilical cord, fetal blood flows through the two umbilical arteries to the capillaries of the villi, becomes oxygen enriched, and then flows back through the umbilical vein into the fetus (**Figure 33.13** ››). Late in pregnancy a soft blowing sound (funic souffle) can be heard over the area of the umbilical cord. The sound is synchronous with the fetal heartbeat and fetal blood flow through the umbilical arteries.

Maternal blood, rich in oxygen and nutrients, moves from the arcuate artery to the radial artery to the uterine spiral arteries and then spurts into the intervillous spaces. These spurts are produced by the maternal blood pressure. The spurt of blood is directed toward the chorionic plate, and as the blood loses pressure, it becomes lateral (spreads out). Fresh blood enters continuously and exerts pressure on the contents of the intervillous spaces, pushing blood toward the exits in the basal plate. The blood then drains through the uterine and other pelvic veins. A uterine souffle, timed precisely with the mother's pulse, also is heard just above the mother's symphysis pubis during the last months of pregnancy. This souffle is caused by the augmented blood flow entering the dilated uterine arteries.

Braxton Hicks contractions are intermittent painless uterine contractions that may occur every 10 to 20 minutes; they occur more frequently near the end of pregnancy. These contractions are believed to facilitate placental circulation by enhancing the movement of blood from the center of the cotyledon through the intervillous space. Placental blood flow is enhanced when the woman is lying on her left side because venous return from the lower extremities is not compromised (Blackburn, 2018).

Placental Functions

Placental exchange functions occur only in those fetal vessels that are in intimate contact with the covering syncytial membrane. The syncytium villi have brush borders containing many microvilli, which greatly increase the exchange rate between maternal and fetal circulation (Blackburn, 2018; Sadler, 2018).

The placental functions, many of which begin soon after implantation, include fetal respiration, nutrition, and excretion. To carry out these functions, the placenta is involved in metabolic and transfer activities. In addition, it has endocrine functions and special immunologic properties. (See the discussion later in this section.)

Metabolic Activities

The placenta continuously produces glycogen, cholesterol, and fatty acids for fetal use and hormone production. The placenta also produces numerous enzymes, such as sulfatase, which enhances excretion of fetal estrogen precursors, and insulinase, which increases the barrier to insulin. These enzymes are required for fetoplacental transfer. The placenta breaks down

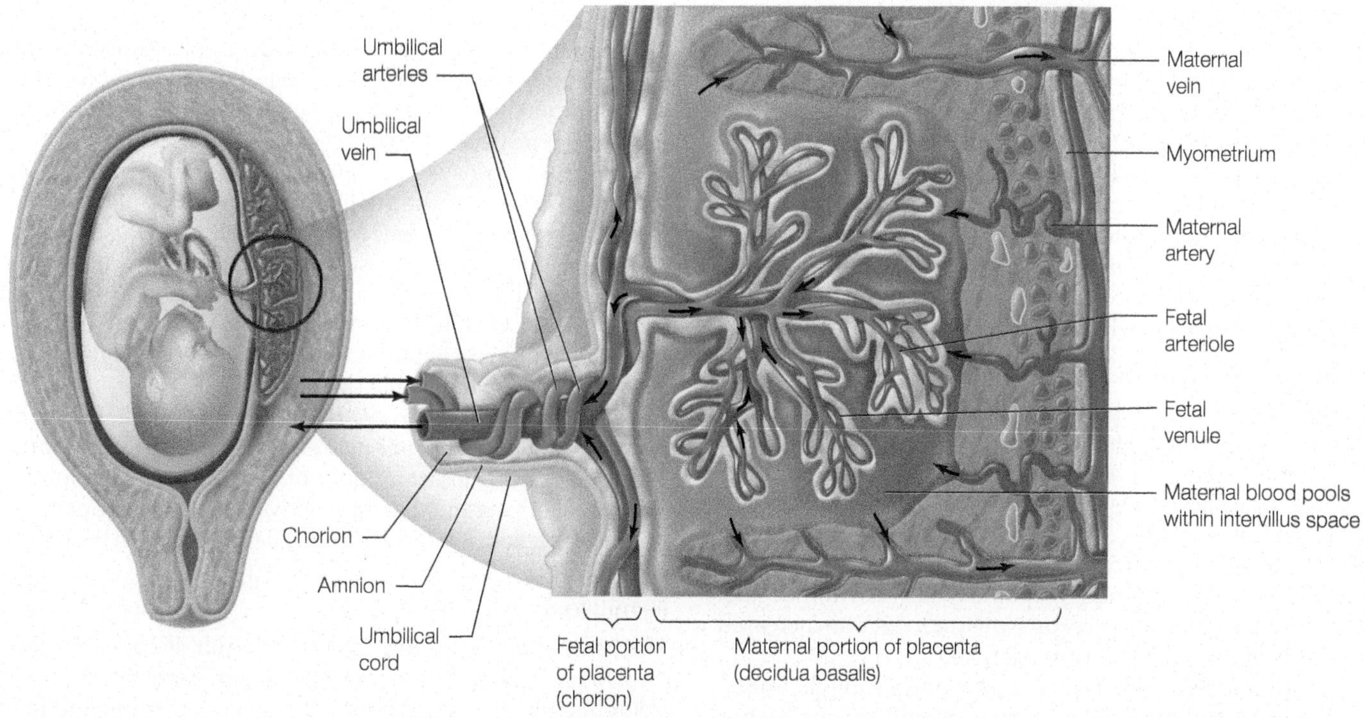

Figure 33.13 ⟫ Vascular arrangement of the placenta. *Arrows* indicate the direction of blood flow. Maternal blood flows through the uterine arteries to the intervillous spaces of the placenta and returns through the uterine veins to maternal circulation. Fetal blood flows through the umbilical arteries into the villous capillaries of the placenta and returns through the umbilical vein to the fetal circulation.

certain substances such as epinephrine and histamine (Blackburn, 2018). In addition, it stores glycogen and iron.

Transport Function

The placental membranes actively control the transfer of a wide range of substances by a variety of transport mechanisms.

- *Simple diffusion* moves substances from an area of higher concentration to an area of lower concentration. Substances that move across the placenta by simple diffusion include water, oxygen, carbon dioxide, electrolytes (sodium and chloride), anesthetic gases, and drugs. Insulin and steroid hormones originating from the adrenals, as well as thyroid hormones, also cross the placenta. However, this happens at a very slow rate. The rate of oxygen transfer across the placental membrane is greater than that allowed by simple diffusion, indicating that oxygen also is transferred by some type of facilitated diffusion transport. Unfortunately, many substances of abuse, such as cocaine and heroin, cross the placenta via simple diffusion.
- *Facilitated transport* involves a carrier system to move molecules from an area of greater concentration to an area of lower concentration. Molecules such as glucose, galactose, and some oxygen are transported by this method. Ordinarily, the glucose level in the fetal blood is approximately 20–30% lower than the glucose level in the maternal blood because the fetus is metabolizing glucose rapidly. This, in turn, causes rapid transport of additional glucose from the maternal blood to the fetal blood.
- *Active transport* can work against a concentration gradient and allows molecules to move from areas of lower concentration to areas of higher concentration. Amino acids, calcium, iron, iodine, water-soluble vitamins, and glucose are transferred across the placenta this way. The measured amino acid content of fetal blood is greater than that of maternal blood, and calcium and inorganic phosphate occur in greater concentration in fetal blood than in maternal blood (Blackburn, 2018).

In addition, fetal RBCs can pass into the maternal circulation through breaks in the capillaries and placental membrane, particularly during labor and birth. Certain cells (e.g., maternal leukocytes) and microorganisms such as viruses (e.g., HIV, which causes AIDS) and the bacterium *Treponema pallidum* (which causes syphilis) can cross the placental membrane under their own power (Moore et al., 2019). Some bacteria and protozoa infect the placenta by causing lesions and then entering the fetal blood system.

Reduction of the placental surface area, as with abruptio placentae (partial or complete premature separation of the placenta), lessens the area that is functional for exchange. Placental diffusion distance also affects exchange. In conditions such as diabetes and placental infection, edema of the villi increases the diffusion distance, thus increasing the distance the substance must be transferred.

Blood flow alteration changes the transfer rate of substances. Decreased blood flow in the intervillous space is seen in labor and with certain maternal diseases such as hypertension (HTN). Mild fetal hypoxia increases the umbilical blood flow, but severe hypoxia results in decreased blood flow.

As the maternal blood picks up fetal waste products and carbon dioxide, it drains back into the maternal circulation through the veins in the basal plate. Fetal blood is hypoxic in comparison to maternal blood; therefore, it attracts oxygen from the mother's blood. Affinity for oxygen increases as the fetal blood gives up its carbon dioxide, which also decreases its acidity.

Endocrine Functions

The placenta produces hormones that are vital to the survival of the fetus. These include hCG; human placental lactogen (hPL); and two steroid hormones, estrogen and progesterone.

The hormone hCG is similar to LH and prevents the normal involution of the corpus luteum at the end of the menstrual cycle. If the corpus luteum stops functioning before the 11th week of pregnancy, spontaneous abortion occurs. The hCG also causes the corpus luteum to secrete increased amounts of estrogen and progesterone.

After the 11th week, the placenta produces enough progesterone and estrogen to maintain pregnancy. In the male fetus, hCG also exerts an interstitial cell-stimulating effect on the testes, resulting in the production of testosterone. This small secretion of testosterone during embryonic development is the factor that causes male sex organs to grow. The hormone hCG may play a role in the trophoblast's immunologic capabilities (ability to exempt the placenta and embryo from rejection by the mother's system). This hormone is used as a basis for pregnancy tests. (Placental hormones are discussed further in the Endocrine System section.)

Development of the Fetal Circulatory System

The circulatory system of the fetus has several unique features that, by maintaining the blood flow to the placenta, provide the fetus with oxygen and nutrients while removing carbon dioxide and other waste products.

Most of the blood supply bypasses the fetal lungs because they do not carry out respiratory gas exchange. The placenta assumes the function of the fetal lungs by supplying oxygen and allowing the fetus to excrete carbon dioxide into the maternal bloodstream. **Figure 33.14** ›› shows the fetal circulatory system. The blood from the placenta flows through the umbilical vein, which enters the abdominal wall of the fetus at the site that, after birth, is the umbilicus (belly button). As umbilical venous blood approaches the liver, a small portion of the blood enters the liver sinusoids, mixes with blood from the portal circulation, and then enters the inferior vena cava via hepatic veins. Most of the umbilical vein's blood flows through the **ductus venosus** directly into the inferior vena cava, bypassing the liver. This blood then enters the right atrium, passes through the **foramen ovale** into the left atrium, and pours into the left ventricle, which pumps blood into the aorta. Some blood returning from the head and upper extremities by way of the superior vena cava is emptied into the right atrium and passes through the tricuspid valve into the right ventricle. This blood is pumped into the pulmonary artery, and a small amount passes to the lungs for nourishment only. The larger portion of blood passes from the pulmonary artery through the **ductus arteriosus** into the descending aorta, bypassing the lungs. Finally, blood returns to the placenta through the two umbilical arteries, and the process is repeated.

The fetus obtains oxygen via diffusion from the maternal circulation because of the gradient difference of 50 mmHg PO_2 (partial pressure of oxygen) in maternal blood in the placenta to 30 mmHg PO_2 in the fetus. At term, the fetus receives oxygen from the mother's circulation at a rate of 20 to 30 mL/min (Sadler, 2018). Fetal hemoglobin facilitates obtaining oxygen from the maternal circulation because it carries as much as 20–30% more oxygen than adult hemoglobin.

Fetal circulation delivers the highest available oxygen concentration to the head, neck, brain, and heart (coronary circulation) and a lesser amount of oxygenated blood to the abdominal organs and the lower body. This circulatory pattern leads to cephalocaudal (head-to-tail) development in the fetus.

Fetal Heart

The heart of the fetus, like that of the adult, is controlled by its own pacemaker. The sinoatrial (SA) node sets the rate and is supplied by the vagus nerve. Bridging the atrium and the ventricle is the atrioventricular (AV) node, also supplied by the vagus nerve. Baseline changes in the fetal heartbeat have been shown to be under the influence of this nerve. When the fetus is stressed, the sympathetic nervous system causes the release of norepinephrine, which increases the fetal heart rate (FHR). To counteract the increase in blood pressure, baroreceptors, which respond to the increase in pressure, are present in the vessel walls at the junction of the internal and external carotid arteries. When stimulated, these receptors, under the influence of the vagus and glossopharyngeal nerves, cause the heart rate to slow. Chemoreceptors in the fetal peripheral and central nervous systems respond to decreased oxygen tensions and to increased carbon dioxide tensions, leading to fetal tachycardia and an increase in blood pressure. The CNS also has control over heart rate. Increased activity of the fetus in a wakeful period is exhibited in an *increase* in the variability and accelerations of the fetal heart baseline. Sleep patterns involve a *decrease* in the baseline variability. In cases of severe hypoxia, the release of epinephrine and norepinephrine will cause an increase in the FHR.

Embryonic to Fetal Development

Pregnancy is calculated to last an average of 10 lunar months: 40 weeks, or 280 days. This period of 280 days is calculated from the onset of the last normal menstrual period to the time of birth. **Estimated date of birth (EDB)**, the date around which childbirth will occur, and sometimes referred to as the *estimated date of delivery (EDD)*, is usually calculated by this method. Most fetuses are born within 10 to 14 days of the calculated date of birth. The fertilization age (or **postconception age**) of the fetus is calculated to be about 2 weeks less, or 266 days (38 weeks) or 9.5 calendar months. The latter measurement is more accurate because it measures time from the fertilization of the ovum, or conception.

›› *Go to **Pearson MyLab Nursing and eText** for Chart 1: Organ Development in the Embryo and Fetus.*

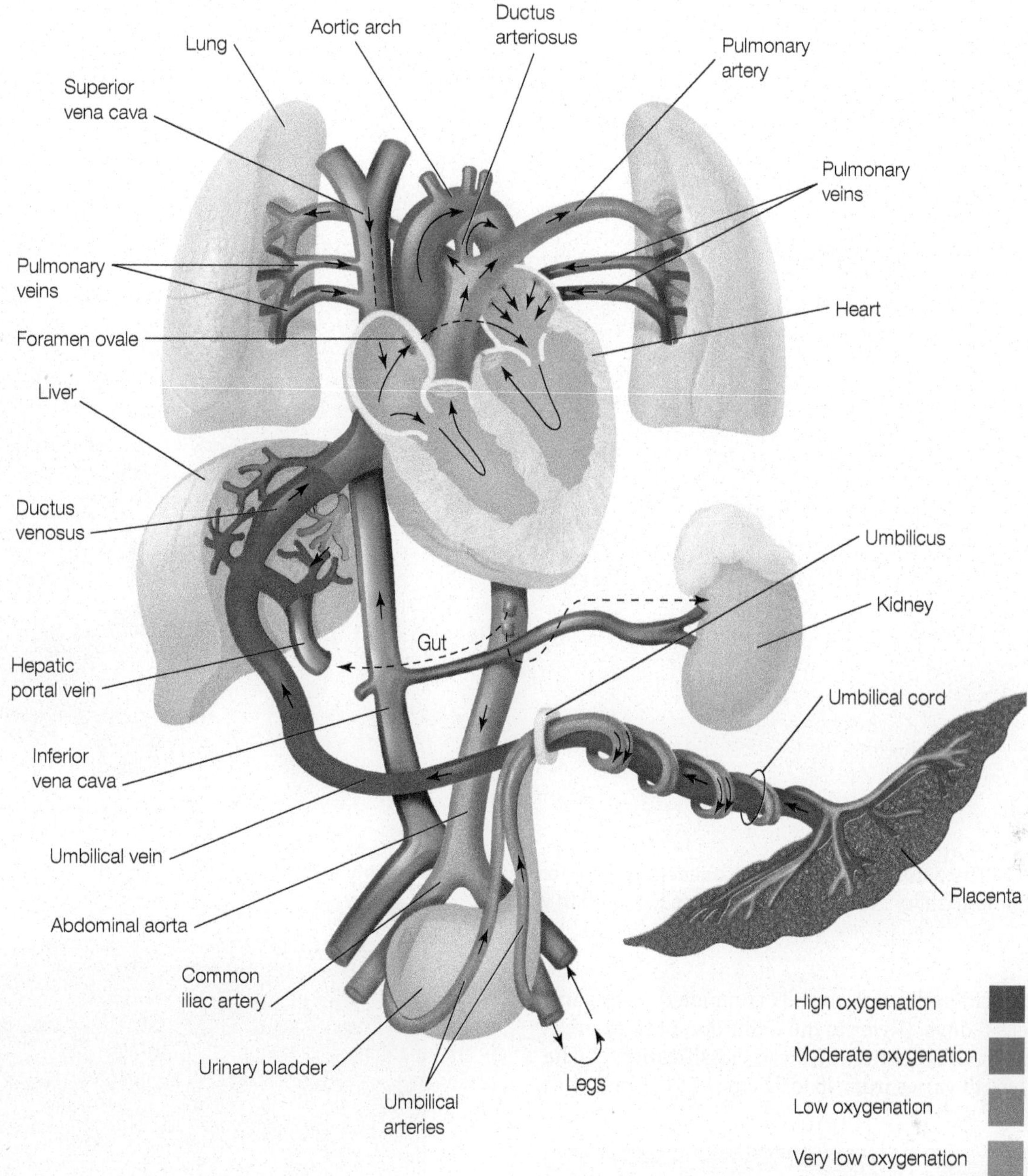

Figure 33.14 ›› Fetal circulation. Blood leaves the placenta and enters the fetus through the umbilical vein. After circulating through the fetus, the blood returns to the placenta through the umbilical arteries. The ductus venosus, the foramen ovale, and the ductus arteriosus allow the blood to bypass the fetal liver and lungs.

In review, human development follows three stages. The preembryonic stage, as discussed earlier in this module, consists of the first 14 days of development after the ovum is fertilized. The embryonic stage covers the period from day 15 until approximately the end of the eighth week, and the fetal stage extends from the end of the eighth week until birth (**Figure 33.15** ››).

Embryonic Stage

The stage of the **embryo** starts on day 15 (the beginning of the third week after conception) and continues until approximately the eighth week, or until the embryo reaches a crown–rump length of 3 cm (1.2 in.). This length is usually reached about 56 days after fertilization (the end of the eighth gestational week). During the embryonic stage, tissues differentiate into essential organs and the main external features develop. The embryo is most vulnerable to *teratogens* during this period (**Figure 33.16** ››).

Fetal Stage

By the end of the eighth week, the embryo is sufficiently developed to be called a **fetus**. Every organ system and external structure that will be found in the full-term newborn is present. The remainder of gestation is devoted to refining structures and perfecting function. **Figure 33.17** ›› shows the fetus at 20 weeks' gestation.

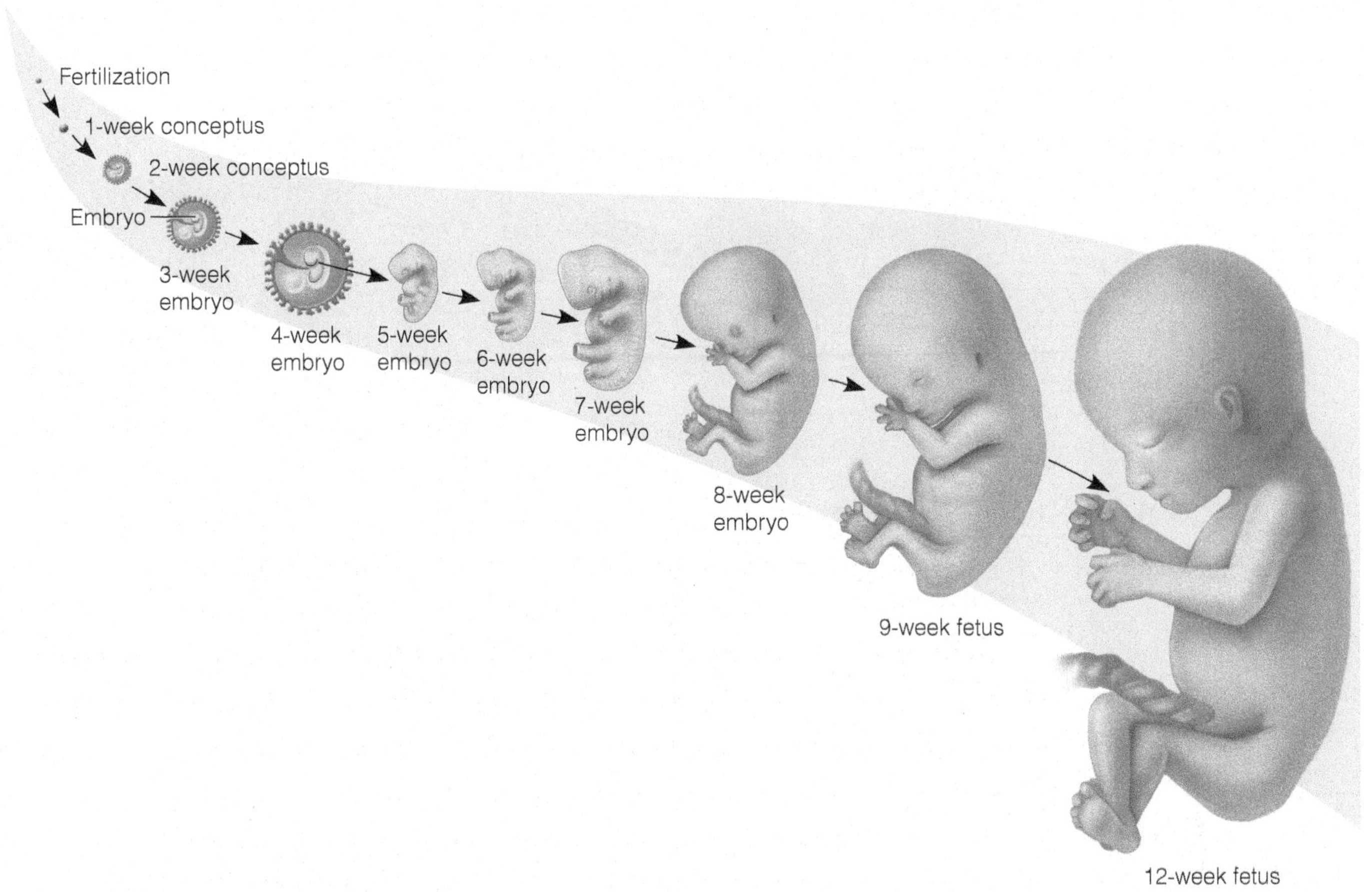

Fertilization
1-week conceptus
2-week conceptus
Embryo
3-week embryo
4-week embryo
5-week embryo
6-week embryo
7-week embryo
8-week embryo
9-week fetus
12-week fetus

Figure 33.15 ›› The actual size of a human conceptus from fertilization to the early fetal stage. The embryonic stage begins in the third week after fertilization; the fetal stage begins in the ninth week.

Full Term

The fetus is considered full term at 39 completed weeks and up to 40 weeks 6 days. (Refer to the definition of term pregnancy for further distinction of these classifications.) The crown–heel length varies from 48 to 52 cm (19 to 21 in.), with

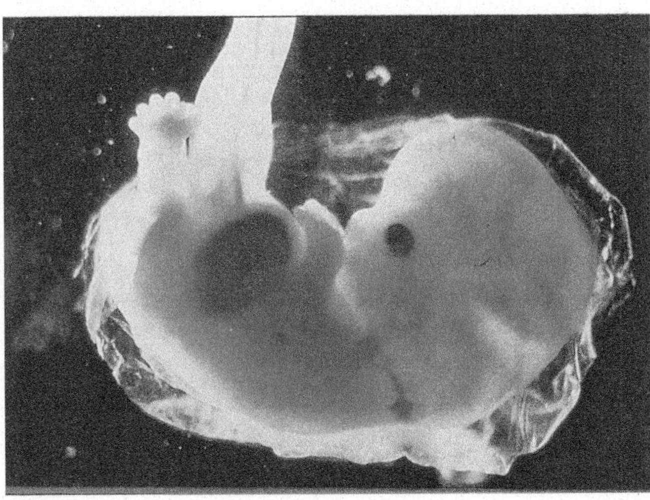

Figure 33.16 ›› The embryo at 7 weeks. The head is rounded and nearly erect. The eyes have shifted forward and closer together, and the eyelids begin to form.
Source: Petit Format/Science Source.

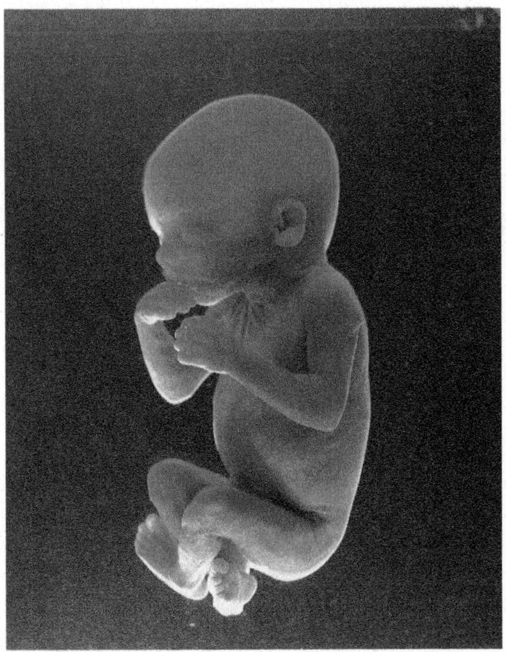

Figure 33.17 ›› The fetus at 20 weeks. The fetus now weighs 435 to 465 g (15.2 to 16.3 oz) and measures about 19 cm (7.5 in.). Subcutaneous deposits of brown fat make the skin a little less transparent. "Woolly" hair covers the head, and nails have developed on the fingers and toes.
Source: James Stevenson/Science Source.

males usually longer than females. Males also usually weigh more than females. The weight at term is about 3000–3600 g (6 lb 10 oz–7 lb 15 oz) and varies in different ethnic groups. Skin color also varies and has a smooth, polished look. The only lanugo left is on the upper arms and shoulders. The hair on the head is no longer woolly but is coarse and about 2.5 cm (1 in.) long. Vernix caseosa is present, with heavier deposits remaining in the creases and folds of the skin. The body and extremities are plump, with good skin turgor, and the fingernails extend beyond the fingertips. The chest is prominent but still a little smaller than the head, and mammary glands protrude in both sexes. In males, the testes are in the scrotum or are palpable in the inguinal canals.

As the fetus enlarges, amniotic fluid diminishes to about 500 mL or less and the fetal body mass fills the uterine cavity. The fetus assumes what is called its *position of comfort*, or *lie*. The head is generally pointed downward, following the shape of the uterus (and possibly because the head is heavier than the feet). The extremities, and often the head, are well flexed. After 5 months, patterns in feeding, sleeping, and activity become established; so at this gestation, the fetus has its own body rhythms and individual style of response.

Physical and Psychologic Changes of Pregnancy

The growth of the developing fetus and the physical and psychologic changes that occur in the pregnant mother continue to inspire feelings of awe and amazement, not to mention curiosity. First, it is nothing short of a miracle that the union of two microscopic entities—an ovum and a sperm—can produce a living being. Second, the woman's body must undergo extraordinary physical changes to maintain a pregnancy.

Pregnancy is divided into three trimesters, each approximately a 3-month period. Each trimester brings predictable changes for both mother and fetus. This section describes these physical and psychologic changes. It also presents the various sociocultural factors that can affect a pregnant woman's well-being.

Anatomy and Physiology of Pregnancy

The changes that occur in the pregnant woman's body may result from hormonal influences, the growth of the fetus, and the mother's physiologic adaptation to the pregnancy. Virtually every system must adapt to support the growing fetus and maintain the pregnant woman's body functions.

Reproductive System

Some of the most dramatic changes of pregnancy occur in the reproductive organs.

Uterus

The changes in the uterus during pregnancy are significant. Before pregnancy, the uterus is a small, semisolid, pear-shaped organ measuring approximately 7.5 × 5 × 2.5 cm and weighing about 60 g (2 oz). At the end of pregnancy, it measures about 28 × 24 × 21 cm and weighs approximately 1100 g (2.5 lb); its capacity also has increased from about 10 mL to 5000 mL (5 L) or more (Cunningham et al., 2018).

The enlargement of the uterus is primarily caused by the enlargement (hypertrophy) of the preexisting myometrial cells as a result of the stimulating influence of estrogen and the distention caused by the growing fetus. Only a limited increase in cell number (hyperplasia) occurs. The fibrous tissue between the muscle bands increases markedly, which adds to the strength and elasticity of the muscle wall. The enlarging uterus, developing placenta, and growing fetus require additional blood flow to the uterus. By the end of pregnancy, one-sixth of the total maternal blood volume is contained in the vascular system of the uterus.

Cervix

Estrogen stimulates the glandular tissue of the cervix, which increases in cell number and becomes hyperactive. The endocervical glands secrete a thick, sticky mucus that accumulates and forms a mucus plug, which seals the endocervical canal and prevents the ascent of microorganisms into the uterus. This plug is expelled when cervical dilation begins. The hyperactivity of the glandular tissue also increases the normal physiologic mucorrhea, at times resulting in profuse discharge. Increased cervical vascularity also causes both the softening of the cervix (**Goodell sign**) and its blue-purple discoloration (**Chadwick sign**).

Ovaries

The ovaries stop producing ova during pregnancy. During early pregnancy, hCG maintains the corpus luteum, which persists and produces hormones until weeks 6 to 8 of pregnancy. The corpus luteum secretes progesterone to maintain the endometrium until the placenta produces enough progesterone to maintain the pregnancy. The corpus luteum then begins to disintegrate slowly.

Vagina

Estrogen causes a thickening of the vaginal mucosa, a loosening of the connective tissue, and an increase in vaginal secretions. These secretions are thick, white, and acidic (pH 3.5 to 6.0). The acid pH helps prevent bacterial infection but favors the growth of yeast organisms. Thus, the pregnant woman is more susceptible to *Candida* infection than usual.

The supportive connective tissue of the vagina loosens throughout pregnancy. By the end of pregnancy, the vagina and perineal body are sufficiently relaxed to permit passage of the baby. Because blood flow to the vagina is increased, the vagina may show the same blue-purple color (Chadwick sign) as the cervix.

Breasts

Estrogen and progesterone cause many changes in the breasts. They enlarge and become more nodular as the milk-producing glands increase in size and number in preparation for lactation. Superficial veins become more prominent, the nipples become more erectile, and the areolas darken. Montgomery follicles (sebaceous glands) enlarge, and **striae** (reddish stretch marks that slowly turn silver after childbirth) may develop.

Colostrum, an antibody-rich yellow secretion, may leak or be expressed from the breasts during the last trimester. Colostrum gradually converts to mature milk during the first few days after childbirth.

Respiratory System

Many respiratory changes occur to meet the increased oxygen requirements of a pregnant woman. The volume of air breathed each minute increases 30–40%. In addition, progesterone decreases airway resistance, permitting a 15–20% increase in oxygen consumption as well as increases in carbon dioxide production and in the respiratory functional reserve.

As the uterus enlarges, it presses upward and elevates the diaphragm. The subcostal angle increases, so that the rib cage flares. The anteroposterior diameter increases, and the chest circumference expands by as much as 6 cm; as a result, there is no significant loss of intrathoracic volume. Breathing changes from abdominal to thoracic as pregnancy progresses, and descent of the diaphragm on inspiration becomes less possible. Some hyperventilation and difficulty in breathing may occur.

Nasal stuffiness and epistaxis (nosebleeds) also may occur because of estrogen-induced edema and vascular congestion of the nasal mucosa.

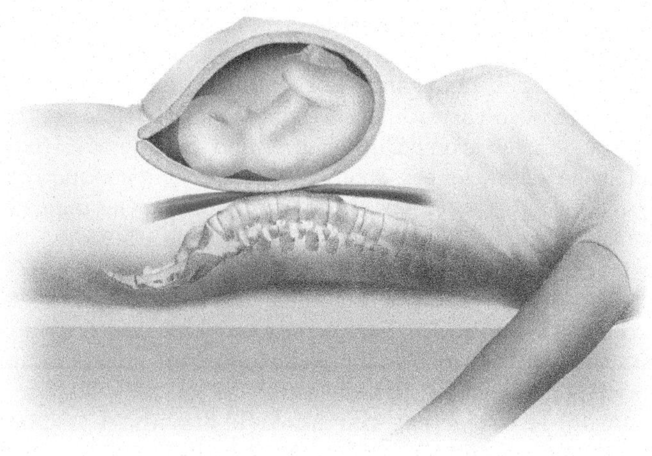

Figure 33.18 ›› Vena caval syndrome. The gravid uterus compresses the vena cava when the woman is supine. This reduces the blood flow returning to the heart and may cause maternal hypotension.

Cardiovascular System

During pregnancy, blood flow increases to organ systems with an increased workload. Thus, blood flow increases to the uterus, placenta, and breasts, whereas hepatic and cerebral flow remains unchanged. Cardiac output begins to increase early in pregnancy and peaks at 25 to 30 weeks' gestation at 30–50% above pre-pregnancy levels. It generally remains elevated in the third trimester.

The pulse may increase by as many as 10 to 15 beats/min at term. The blood pressure decreases slightly, reaching its lowest point during the second trimester. It gradually increases to near pre-pregnancy levels by the end of the third trimester.

The enlarging uterus puts pressure on pelvic and femoral vessels, interfering with returning blood flow and causing stasis of blood in the lower extremities. This condition may lead to dependent edema and varicosity of the veins in the legs, vulva, and rectum (hemorrhoids) in late pregnancy. This increased blood volume in the lower legs also may make the pregnant woman prone to postural hypotension.

When the pregnant woman lies supine, the enlarging uterus may press on the vena cava. This reduces blood flow to the right atrium; lowers blood pressure; and causes dizziness, pallor, and clamminess. Research indicates that the enlarging uterus also may press on the aorta and its collateral circulation (Cunningham et al., 2018). This condition is called **supine hypotensive syndrome**. It also may be referred to as **vena caval syndrome** or **aortocaval compression** (**Figure 33.18 ››**). It can be corrected by having the woman lie on her side, preferably on her left. Blood volume progressively increases beginning in the first trimester, increases rapidly until about 30 to 34 weeks' gestation, and then plateaus until birth at about 40–50% above nonpregnancy levels. This increase occurs because of increases in both erythrocytes and plasma (Cao & O'Brien, 2013).

The total erythrocyte (RBC) volume increases by about 25%. This increase in erythrocytes is necessary to transport the additional oxygen required during pregnancy. However, the increase in plasma volume during pregnancy averages about 50%. Because the plasma volume increase (50%) is greater than the erythrocyte increase (25%), the hematocrit, which measures the concentration of RBCs in the plasma, decreases slightly (Cao & O'Brien, 2013). This decrease is referred to as the **physiologic anemia of pregnancy** (pseudoanemia).

Iron is necessary for hemoglobin formation, and hemoglobin is the oxygen-carrying component of erythrocytes. Thus, the increase in erythrocyte levels results in the pregnant woman's increased need for iron. Even though the gastrointestinal (GI) absorption of iron is moderately increased during pregnancy, it is usually necessary to add supplemental iron to the diet to meet the expanded RBC and fetal needs. Women who are diagnosed with anemia prior to pregnancy may require more iron supplementation.

Leukocyte production increases slightly to an average of 8500 mm^3, with a range of 5600 to 12,200 mm^3. During labor and the early postpartum period, these levels may reach 25,000/mm^3 or higher (Antony, Racusin, Aagard, & Dildy, 2017). Although the cause of leukocytosis is not known, this increase is a normal finding (Cunningham et al., 2018).

Both the fibrin and plasma fibrinogen levels increase during pregnancy. Although the blood-clotting time of a pregnant woman does not differ significantly from that of a nonpregnant woman, clotting factors VII, VIII, IX, and X increase; thus, pregnancy is a somewhat hypercoagulable state. These changes, coupled with venous stasis in late pregnancy, increase the pregnant woman's risk of developing venous thrombosis.

Gastrointestinal System

Nausea and vomiting are common during the first trimester because of elevated hCG levels and changed carbohydrate metabolism. Gum tissue may soften and bleed easily. The secretion of saliva may increase and even become excessive (ptyalism).

Elevated progesterone levels cause smooth muscle relaxation, resulting in delayed gastric emptying and decreased peristalsis. As a result, the pregnant woman may complain of bloating and constipation. These symptoms are aggravated as the enlarging uterus displaces the stomach upward and the intestines are moved laterally and posteriorly. The cardiac sphincter also relaxes, and heartburn (pyrosis) may occur because of reflux of acidic secretions into the lower esophagus. Hemorrhoids frequently develop in late pregnancy from constipation and from pressure on vessels below the level of the uterus.

Only minor liver changes occur with pregnancy. Plasma albumin concentrations and serum cholinesterase activity decrease with normal pregnancy, as with certain liver diseases.

The emptying time of the gallbladder is prolonged during pregnancy as a result of smooth muscle relaxation from progesterone. This, coupled with the elevated levels of cholesterol in the bile, can predispose the woman to gallstone formation.

Urinary Tract

During the first trimester, the enlarging uterus is still a pelvic organ and presses against the bladder, producing urinary frequency. This symptom decreases during the second trimester, when the uterus becomes an abdominal organ and pressure against the bladder lessens. Frequency reappears during the third trimester, when the presenting part descends into the pelvis and again presses on the bladder, reducing bladder capacity, contributing to hyperemia, and irritating the bladder.

The ureters (especially the right ureter) elongate and dilate above the pelvic brim. The glomerular filtration rate (GFR) rises by as much as 50% beginning in the second trimester and remains elevated until birth. To compensate for this increase, renal tubular reabsorption also increases. However, glycosuria is sometimes seen during pregnancy because of the kidneys' inability to reabsorb all of the glucose filtered by the glomeruli. Glycosuria may be normal or may indicate *gestational diabetes mellitus* (diabetes mellitus with onset or first recognition during pregnancy), so it always warrants further testing.

Skin and Hair

Changes in skin pigmentation commonly occur during pregnancy. Increased estrogen, progesterone, and melanocyte-stimulating hormone levels are thought to stimulate these changes. Pigmentation of the skin increases primarily in areas that are already hyperpigmented: the areola, the nipples, the vulva, the perianal area, and the linea alba. The linea alba refers to the midline of the abdomen from the pubic area to the umbilicus and above. During pregnancy, this area darkens and is referred to as the *linea nigra* (**Figure 33.19** »). Facial **chloasma**, or **melasma gravidarum** (also known as the "mask of pregnancy"), a darkening of the skin over the cheeks, nose, and forehead, may develop. Chloasma or melasma is more prominent in dark-haired women and is aggravated by exposure to the sun. The condition fades or becomes less prominent soon after childbirth, when the hormonal influence of pregnancy subsides.

The sweat and sebaceous glands are often hyperactive during pregnancy. Some women may notice heavy perspiration, night sweats, and the development of acne even if they have never experienced these symptoms before.

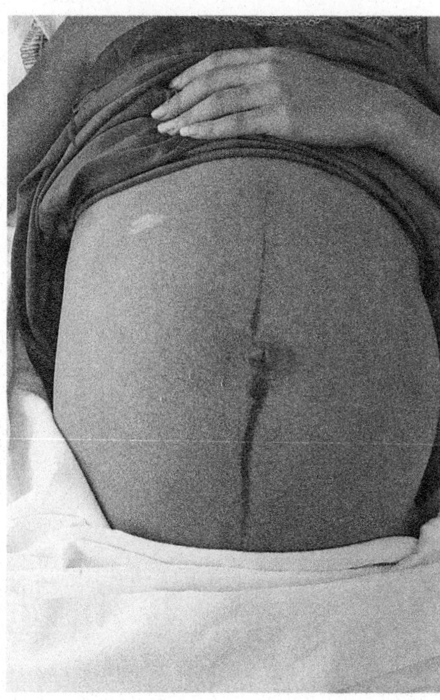

Figure 33.19 » Linea nigra.
Source: Pearson Education, Inc.

Striae may appear on the abdomen, thighs, buttocks, and breasts. They result from reduced connective tissue strength because of elevated adrenal steroid levels.

Vascular spider nevi—small, bright red elevations of the skin radiating from a central body—may develop on the chest, neck, face, arms, and legs. They may be caused by increased subcutaneous blood flow in response to elevated estrogen levels.

The rate of hair growth may decrease during pregnancy; the number of hair follicles in the resting or dormant phase also decreases. After birth, the number of hair follicles in the resting phase increases sharply and the woman may notice increased hair shedding for 1 to 4 months. However, practically all hair is replaced within 6 to 12 months (Cunningham et al., 2018).

Musculoskeletal System

No demonstrable changes occur in the teeth of pregnant women. The dental caries that sometimes accompany pregnancy are probably caused by inadequate oral hygiene and dental care, especially if the woman has problems with bleeding gums or nausea and vomiting.

The joints of the pelvis relax somewhat because of hormonal influences. The result is often a waddling gait. As the pregnant woman's center of gravity gradually changes, the lumbodorsal spinal curve becomes accentuated and her posture changes (**Figure 33.20** »). This posture change compensates for the increased weight of the uterus anteriorly and frequently results in low backache.

Pressure of the enlarging uterus on the abdominal muscles may cause the rectus abdominis muscle to separate,

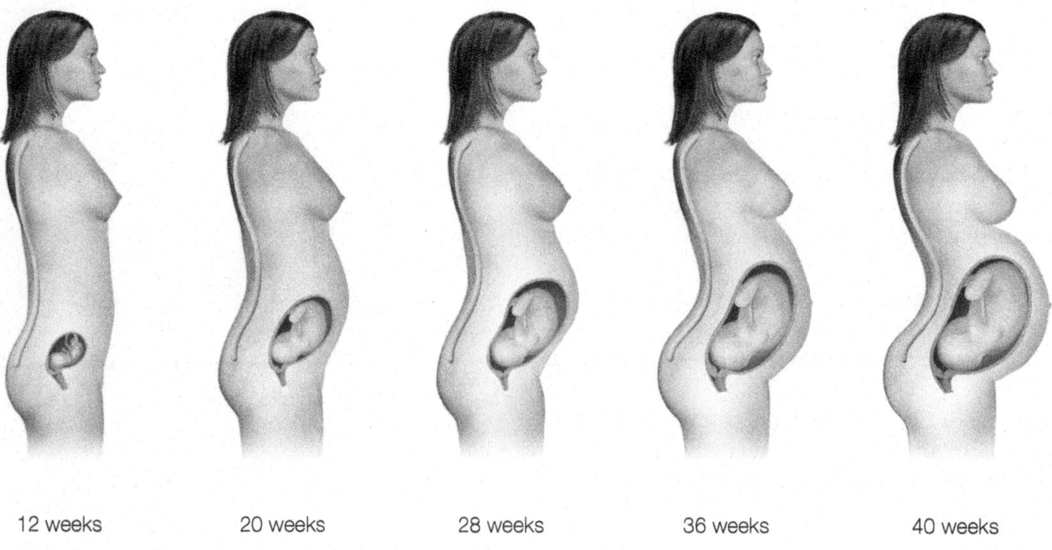

Figure 33.20 ›› Postural changes during pregnancy. Note the increasing lordosis of the lumbosacral spine and the increasing curvature of the thoracic area.

producing **diastasis recti**. If the separation is severe and muscle tone is not regained postpartum, subsequent pregnancies will not have adequate support and the woman's abdomen may appear pendulous.

Eyes

Two changes generally occur in the eyes during pregnancy. First, intraocular pressure decreases, probably as a result of increased vitreous outflow. Second, a slight thickening of the cornea occurs, which is generally attributed to fluid retention (Antony et al., 2017). Although these changes are not readily perceived, some pregnant women experience difficulty wearing previously comfortable contact lenses. The change in the corneas generally disappears by 6 weeks postpartum (Davidson, London, & Ladewig, 2020).

Central Nervous System

Pregnant women frequently describe decreased attention, concentration, and memory during and shortly after pregnancy, but few studies have explored this phenomenon. One study did compare a group of pregnant women and a control group, finding a decline in memory among the pregnant women that could not be attributed to depression, anxiety, sleep deprivation, or other physical changes of pregnancy. This memory loss disappeared soon after childbirth. Another study found that sleep problems are common in pregnancy. These include difficulty going to sleep, frequent awakenings, fewer hours of night sleep, and reduced sleep efficiency (Cunningham et al., 2018).

Metabolism

Most metabolic functions accelerate during pregnancy to support the additional demands of the growing fetus and its support system. The expectant mother must meet her own tissue replacement needs, those of the fetus, and tissue changes preparatory for labor and lactation. No other event in life induces such profound metabolic changes.

Weight Gain

Growth of the uterus and its contents, growth of the breasts, and increases in intravascular fluids account for most of the weight gain in pregnancy. In addition, extra water, fat, and protein are stored; these are called *maternal reserves.*

Adequate nutrition and weight gain are important during pregnancy. The recommended total weight gain during pregnancy for a woman of normal weight before pregnancy is 11.5 to 16 kg (25 to 35 lb); for women who were overweight before becoming pregnant (body mass index [BMI] of 25 to 29.9), the recommended gain is 6.8 to 11.5 kg (15 to 25 lb). Obese women (BMI 30 and greater) are advised to limit weight gain to 5 to 9 kg (11 to 20 lb). Underweight women (BMI less than 18.5) are advised to gain 12.7 to 18.1 kg (28 to 40 lb) (American College of Obstetricians and Gynecologists [ACOG], 2013a, reaffirmed 2016). Weight may decrease slightly during the first trimester because of nausea, vomiting, and food intolerances of early pregnancy. The lost weight is soon regained, and for normal women, the ACOG (2013a, reaffirmed 2016) recommends a gain of 0.5 to 2 kg (1.1 to 4.4 lb) during the first trimester, followed by an average gain of about 0.45 kg (1 lb) per week during the last two trimesters.

Water Metabolism

Increased water retention is a basic chemical alteration of pregnancy. Several interrelated factors cause this phenomenon. The increased level of steroid sex hormones affects sodium and fluid retention. The lowered serum protein also influences the fluid balance, as do the increased intracapillary pressure and permeability. The extra water is needed for the products of conception—the fetus, placenta, and amniotic fluid—and the mother's increased blood volume, interstitial fluids, and enlarged organs.

Nutrient Metabolism

The fetus makes its greatest protein and fat demands during the second half of gestation, doubling in weight in the last 6 to 8 weeks. The increased protein retention that begins in early pregnancy is initially used for hyperplasia and hypertrophy of maternal tissues, such as the uterus and breasts. Protein must also be stored during pregnancy to maintain a constant level within the breast milk and to avoid depletion of maternal tissues.

Fats are more completely absorbed during pregnancy, resulting in a marked increase in the serum lipids, lipoproteins, and cholesterol and decreased elimination through the bowel. Fat deposits in the fetus increase from about 2% at midpregnancy to almost 12% at term. The excess nitrogen and lipidemia are considered to be a preparation for lactation. In addition, the woman's body switches from glucose metabolism to lipid metabolism once glucose from food intake has been used up. This leads to an increased tendency to develop ketosis between meals and overnight. The demand for carbohydrate increases, especially during the last two trimesters. Intermittent glycosuria is not uncommon during pregnancy. When it is not accompanied by a rise in blood sugar levels, glycosuria is secondary to the increased GFR. Fasting blood sugar levels tend to fall slightly, returning to more normal levels by the sixth postpartum month. The oral glucose tolerance test shows no change with pregnancy.

The possibility of diabetes during pregnancy must not be overlooked. Plasma levels of insulin increase during pregnancy (probably because of hormonal changes that cause increased tissue resistance) and rapid destruction of insulin takes place within the placenta. The woman's insulin production must increase during the second trimester, and any marginal pancreatic function quickly becomes apparent. The woman with diabetes often experiences increased exogenous insulin demands during pregnancy.

The demand for iron during pregnancy is accelerated, and the pregnant woman needs to guard against anemia. Iron is necessary for the increase in erythrocytes, hemoglobin, and blood volume, as well as for the increased tissue demands of both woman and fetus. Iron transfer takes place at the placenta in only one direction: toward the fetus. It has been demonstrated that approximately five-sixths of the iron stored in the fetal liver is assimilated during the last trimester of pregnancy. This stored iron in the fetal liver compensates in the first 4 months of neonatal life for the normal inadequate amounts of iron available in breast milk and non-iron-fortified formulas.

The progressive absorption and retention of calcium during pregnancy have been noted. The maternal plasma concentration of bound calcium decreases as the levels of bindable plasma proteins fall. Approximately 30 g of calcium is retained in maternal bone for fetal deposition late in pregnancy.

Endocrine System

Hormonal changes during pregnancy may affect endocrine function in different ways. Most changes are temporary and resolve within 6 weeks of delivery. Nurses should anticipate common changes involving the thyroid, parathyroid, pituitary, and adrenal glands.

Thyroid

Pregnancy influences the thyroid gland's size and activity. Often a palpable change is noted, which represents an increase in vascularity and hyperplasia of glandular tissue. Total serum thyroxine (T_4) increases in early pregnancy, and thyroid-stimulating hormone (TSH) decreases. The elevated levels of total T_4 continue until several weeks postpartum, although the level of free serum T_4 returns to normal after the first trimester (Cunningham et al., 2018).

Increased thyroxine-binding capacity is evidenced by an increase in serum protein-bound iodine, probably due to the increased levels of circulating estrogens. The basal metabolic rate increases by as much as 20–25% during pregnancy. The increased oxygen consumption is due primarily to fetal metabolic activity.

Parathyroid

The concentration of the parathyroid hormone and the size of the parathyroid glands increase, paralleling the fetal calcium requirements. Parathyroid hormone concentration reaches its highest level of approximately twofold between 15 and 35 weeks of gestation, returning to a normal or even subnormal level before childbirth.

Pituitary

Pregnancy is made possible by the hypothalamic stimulation of the anterior pituitary gland. The anterior pituitary produces *FSH*, which stimulates follicle growth in the ovary, and *LH*, which affects ovulation. Stimulation of the pituitary also prolongs the ovary's corpus luteal phase, which maintains the secretory endometrium in preparation for pregnancy. *Prolactin*, another anterior pituitary hormone, is responsible for initial lactation.

The posterior pituitary secretes *vasopressin* (antidiuretic hormone) and *oxytocin*. Vasopressin causes vasoconstriction, which results in increased blood pressure; it also helps regulate water balance. Oxytocin promotes uterine contractility and stimulates ejection of milk from the breasts (the let-down reflex) in the postpartum period.

Adrenals

Little structural change occurs in the adrenal glands during a normal pregnancy. Estrogen-induced increases in the levels of circulating cortisol result primarily from lowered renal excretion. The circulating cortisol levels regulate carbohydrate and protein metabolism. A normal level resumes 1 to 6 weeks postpartum.

The adrenals secrete increased levels of aldosterone by the early part of the second trimester. The levels of secretion are even more elevated in the woman on a sodium-restricted diet. This increase in aldosterone in a normal pregnancy may be the body's protective response to the increased sodium excretion associated with progesterone (Cunningham et al., 2018).

Pancreas

The islets of Langerhans are stressed to meet the increased demand for insulin during pregnancy, and a latent deficiency may become apparent during pregnancy, producing symptoms of gestational diabetes.

Hormones in Pregnancy

Several hormones are required to maintain pregnancy. Most of these are produced initially by the corpus luteum; the placenta then assumes production.

- ***Human chorionic gonadotropin:*** The trophoblast secretes hCG in early pregnancy. This hormone stimulates progesterone and estrogen production by the corpus luteum to maintain the pregnancy until the placenta is developed sufficiently to assume that function.

- ***Human placental lactogen:*** Also called *human chorionic somatomammotropin*, this is produced by the syncytiotrophoblast. This hormone is an antagonist of insulin; it increases the amount of circulating free fatty acids for maternal metabolic needs and decreases maternal metabolism of glucose to favor fetal growth.
- ***Estrogen:*** Secreted originally by the corpus luteum, estrogen is produced primarily by the placenta as early as the seventh week of pregnancy. Estrogen stimulates uterine development to provide a suitable environment for the fetus. It also helps to develop the ductal system of the breasts in preparation for lactation.
- ***Progesterone:*** Progesterone, also produced initially by the corpus luteum and then by the placenta, plays the greatest role in maintaining pregnancy. It maintains the endometrium and also inhibits spontaneous uterine contractility, thus preventing early spontaneous abortion due to uterine activity. In addition, progesterone helps develop the ductal system of the breasts in preparation for lactation.
- ***Relaxin:*** Relaxin is detectable in the serum of a pregnant woman by the time of the first missed menstrual period. Relaxin inhibits uterine activity, diminishes the strength of uterine contractions, aids in the softening of the cervix, and has the long-term effect of remodeling collagen. Its primary source is the corpus luteum, but small amounts are believed to be produced by the placenta and uterine decidua throughout pregnancy.

Prostaglandins in Pregnancy

Prostaglandins (PGs) are lipid substances that can arise from most body tissues but occur in high concentrations in the female reproductive tract and are present in the decidua during pregnancy. Although their exact functions during pregnancy are still unknown, it has been proposed that PGs are responsible for maintaining reduced placental vascular resistance. Decreased PG levels may contribute to HTN and preeclampsia. Prostaglandins are also believed to play a role in the complex biochemistry that initiates labor, although their specific functions are still being defined.

Signs of Pregnancy

Changes that occur during pregnancy are often used to diagnose it. These changes, or signs, are categorized as subjective (or presumptive), objective (or probable), and diagnostic (or positive).

Subjective (Presumptive) Changes

Subjective changes, which include nausea and vomiting and an increase in urinary frequency, are those symptoms that the woman experiences and reports to the nurse or provider. They are not considered diagnostic because they can be caused by other conditions.

*>> Go to **Pearson MyLab Nursing and eText** for Chart 2: Differential Diagnosis of Pregnancy—Subjective Changes.*

Amenorrhea, or the absence of menses, is the earliest symptom of pregnancy. The missing of more than one menstrual period, especially in a woman whose cycle is ordinarily regular, is an especially useful diagnostic clue. Excessive fatigue may be noted within a few weeks after the first missed menstrual period and may persist throughout the first trimester. Urinary frequency is experienced during the first trimester as the enlarging uterus presses on the bladder. This improves during the second trimester when the enlarging uterus escapes the pelvis, and then recurs in the third trimester when the growing fetus presses on the bladder.

Nausea and vomiting in pregnancy (NVP) occur frequently during the first trimester and may be the result of elevated hCG levels and changed carbohydrate metabolism. Because these symptoms often occur in the early part of the day, they are commonly referred to as **morning sickness**. In reality, the symptoms may occur at any time and can range from a mere distaste for food to severe vomiting.

Changes in the breasts are frequently noted in early pregnancy. These changes include tenderness and tingling sensations, increased pigmentation of the areola and nipple, and changes in the Montgomery glands. The veins in the breasts also become more visible and form a bluish pattern beneath the skin.

Quickening, or the mother's perception of fetal movement, occurs about 18 to 20 weeks after the last menstrual period (LMP) in a woman pregnant for the first time, but may occur as early as 16 weeks in a woman who has been pregnant before. Quickening is a fluttering sensation in the abdomen that gradually increases in intensity and frequency.

Objective (Probable) Changes

Objective changes are signs that can be noted by the nurse or provider on examination. Because these changes also have other causes, they do not confirm pregnancy.

*>> Go to **Pearson MyLab Nursing and eText** for Chart 3: Differential Diagnosis of Pregnancy—Objective Changes.*

The only physical changes detectable during the first 3 months of pregnancy are caused by increased vascular congestion. These changes are noted on pelvic examination. As noted earlier, there is a softening of the cervix called the Goodell sign. The Chadwick sign is a bluish, purple, or deep red discoloration of the mucous membranes of the cervix, vagina, and vulva. (Some sources consider this a presumptive sign.) The **Hegar sign** is a softening of the isthmus of the uterus, the area between the cervix and the body of the uterus. The **McDonald sign** is an ease in flexing the body of the uterus against the cervix.

General enlargement and softening of the body of the uterus can be noted after the eighth week of pregnancy. The fundus of the uterus is palpable just above the symphysis pubis at about 10 to 12 weeks' gestation and at the level of the umbilicus at 20 to 22 weeks' gestation (**Figure 33.21 >>**).

Enlargement of the abdomen during the childbearing years is usually regarded as evidence of pregnancy, especially if it is continuous and accompanied by amenorrhea. Braxton Hicks contractions are palpable with abdominal palpation after week 28. As the woman approaches the end of pregnancy, these contractions may become uncomfortable.

Uterine souffle may be heard when the examiner auscultates the abdomen over the uterus. It is a soft blowing sound that occurs at the same rate as the maternal pulse. The funic souffle occurs at the same rate as the FHR.

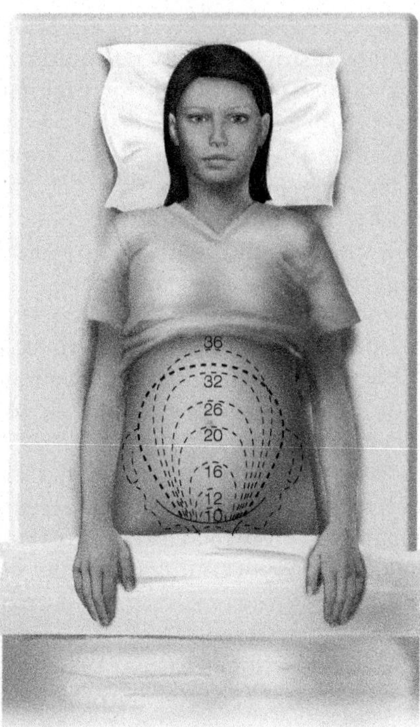

Figure 33.21 ›› Approximate height of the fundus at various weeks of pregnancy.

The fetal outline may be identified by palpation in many pregnant women after 24 weeks' gestation. **Ballottement** is the passive fetal movement elicited when the examiner inserts two gloved fingers into the vagina and pushes against the cervix. This action pushes the fetal body up, and as it falls back, the examiner feels a rebound.

Pregnancy tests are based on analysis of maternal blood or urine for the detection of hCG, the hormone secreted by the trophoblast. These tests are not considered positive signs of pregnancy because the similarity of hCG and the pituitary-secreted LH occasionally results in cross-reactions. In addition, certain conditions other than pregnancy can cause elevated levels of hCG.

Clinical Pregnancy Tests

The most commonly used assay for pregnancy diagnosis is measuring the beta subunit of hCG in either urine or serum. Currently four main hCG tests are used: (1) radioimmunoassay, (2) immunoradiometric assay, (3) enzyme-linked immunosorbent assay (ELISA), and (4) fluoroimmunoassay. False-negative or false-positive results can also occur. In pregnancy, levels normally peak at 10 to 12 weeks' gestation, and this initial rise is important in monitoring high-risk pregnancies where viability has not been documented. Failure to observe the expected rise may suggest an ectopic pregnancy or spontaneous abortion. An abnormally high level or accelerated rise can also prompt investigation into possible disorders such as molar pregnancy, multiple gestations, or chromosomal abnormalities. There is a rapid decline in the hCG levels from 12 to 22 weeks' gestation when another gradual rise occurs (Cunningham et al., 2018).

Diagnostic (Positive) Changes

The positive signs of pregnancy are completely objective, cannot be confused with a pathologic state, and offer conclusive proof of pregnancy.

The fetal heartbeat can be detected with a fetoscope by approximately weeks 17 to 20 of pregnancy. With an electronic Doppler device, the fetal heartbeat can be detected as early as weeks 10 to 12. The FHR is between 110 and 160 beats/min and must be counted and compared with the maternal pulse for differentiation. Auscultation of the abdomen may reveal sounds other than that of the fetal heart. The maternal pulse, emanating from the abdominal aorta, may be unusually loud, or a uterine souffle may be heard.

Fetal movement is actively palpable by a trained examiner after about 20 weeks' gestation. The movements vary from a faint flutter in the early months to more vigorous movements late in pregnancy.

Visualization of the fetus by ultrasound confirms a pregnancy. The gestational sac can be observed by 4 to 5 weeks' gestation (2 to 3 weeks after conception). Fetal parts and fetal heart movement can be seen as early as 8 weeks. A transvaginal ultrasound has been used to detect a gestational sac as early as 10 days after implantation (Cunningham et al., 2018).

Psychologic Response of the Expectant Family to Pregnancy

Pregnancy is a turning point in a family's life, accompanied by stress and anxiety, whether the pregnancy is desired or not. Especially with the first child, parents may not have any idea what to expect. New feelings and behaviors that providers know to be normal can be disconcerting to first-time parents. By providing timely and accurate information, nurses can help reduce parent anxiety and promote healthy coping behaviors that will, in turn, help ensure a healthy pregnancy.

Most parents experience significant role changes. Career goals, daily routines, and family dynamics may be altered by the pending arrival, whether this child is the first child, the only child, or a younger child.

Pregnancy is a time of decisions. Parents, whether single or in a relationship, face decisions about finances, child care, and how to maintain household and other responsibilities (for example, caring for an aging parent).

Women who are planning to relinquish a baby may face other challenges, such as decisional conflict, especially if they lack support systems or if the people in their support system don't agree with their decision.

In all cases, nurses work to understand the needs of the mother and family at each healthcare interaction. Parental concerns and priorities may change from one appointment to the next. Understanding the larger concerns of the parents can help nurses provide appropriate and timely information and support.

Developmental Tasks of the Expectant Couple

Pregnancy can be viewed as a developmental stage with its own distinct developmental tasks. For a couple, it can be a time of support or conflict depending on the amount of adjustment each is willing to make to maintain the family's equilibrium.

During a first pregnancy, the couple plans together for the child's arrival, collecting information on how to be parents. At the same time, each member of the couple continues to participate in some separate activities with friends or family members. The availability of social support is an important factor in psychosocial well-being during pregnancy. The social network is often a major source of advice for the pregnant woman; however, both sound and unsound information may be conveyed.

During pregnancy, the expectant parents face significant changes and must deal with major psychosocial adjustments. Other family members, especially other children of the woman or couple and the grandparents-to-be, also must adjust to the pregnancy.

» *Go to **Pearson MyLab Nursing and eText** to see Chart 4: Parental Reactions to Pregnancy.*

Pregnancy as Maturational Crisis

For some individuals or couples, pregnancy is a time of crisis, a disturbance of equilibrium. A *maturational crisis* is a crisis that is part of normal development in the life of an individual or family. During a maturational crisis, relationships and roles may change, and normal defense mechanisms and coping strategies may be insufficient to meet individual or family need. If the crisis is not resolved, the individual or family may experience long-term consequences. Individuals or families who are able to resolve the crisis can return to normal functioning and may, in some cases, grow in the process and strengthen their relationships with one another.

The Mother

Pregnancy is a condition that alters body image and necessitates a reordering of social relationships and changes in the roles of family members. The way each woman meets the stresses of pregnancy is influenced by her emotional makeup, her sociologic and cultural background, and her acceptance or rejection of the pregnancy. However, many women manifest similar psychologic and emotional responses during pregnancy, including ambivalence, acceptance, introversion, mood swings, and changes in body image.

A woman's attitude toward her pregnancy can be a significant factor in its outcome. Even if the pregnancy is planned, there is an element of surprise at first. Many women commonly experience feelings of ambivalence during early pregnancy. This ambivalence may be related to feelings that the timing is somehow wrong; worries about the need to modify existing relationships or career plans; fears about assuming a new role; unresolved emotional conflicts with the woman's own mother; and fears about pregnancy, labor, and birth. These feelings may be more pronounced if the pregnancy is unplanned or unwanted. Indirect expressions of ambivalence include complaints about considerable physical discomfort, prolonged or frequent depression, significant dissatisfaction with changing body shape, excessive mood swings, and difficulty in accepting the life changes resulting from the pregnancy.

Many pregnancies are unintended, but not all unintended pregnancies are unwanted. A pregnancy can be unintended and wanted at the same time. However, an unintended pregnancy can be a risk factor for depression. Because of the potential negative impact of depression on maternal and fetal health, all women should be screened for depression at regular intervals during pregnancy (ACOG, 2018f).

Conflicts about adapting to pregnancy are no more pronounced for older pregnant women (age 35 and over) than for younger ones. Moreover, older pregnant women tend to be less concerned about the normal physical changes of pregnancy and are confident about handling issues that arise during pregnancy and parenting. This difference may result because older pregnant women have more experience with problem solving. However, they may have fewer pregnant peers and thus may have fewer people with whom to share concerns and expectations.

Pregnancy produces marked changes in a woman's body within a relatively short period of time. Pregnant women experience changes in body image because of physical alterations and may feel a loss of control over their bodies during pregnancy and later during childbirth. These perceptions are related to a certain extent to personality factors, social network responses, and attitudes toward pregnancy. Although changes in body image are normal, they can be very stressful for the woman. Explanation and discussion of the changes may help both the woman and her partner deal with the stress associated with this aspect of pregnancy.

Fantasies about the unborn child are common among pregnant women. The themes of the fantasies (baby's appearance, sex, traits, impact on parents, and so on) vary by trimester and differ among women who are pregnant for the first time and women who already have children.

First Trimester

Feelings of disbelief and ambivalence are common early in the pregnancy—the baby does not yet seem real, and the mother may begin to adapt to the idea of a baby before feeling any early symptoms. When early symptoms first occur (nausea or breast tenderness, for example), they can be uncomfortable and unsettling.

During the first trimester, the mother may begin to exhibit normal behavioral changes, such as abrupt changes in mood, and become more introspective. Fantasies may extend to thinking about miscarriage, accompanied by feelings of guilt and concern that thinking about miscarriage may harm the baby.

Nursing responsibilities at this time include providing anticipatory guidance regarding the common symptoms and physical changes associated with pregnancy, helping the mother to identify coping strategies, and providing options and counseling for women experiencing symptoms of depression.

Second Trimester

During the second trimester, quickening occurs around 20 weeks. This perception of fetal movement helps the woman think of her baby as a separate individual, and she generally becomes excited about the pregnancy even if she had not been looking forward to the pregnancy earlier. The woman becomes increasingly introspective as she evaluates her life, her plans, and her child's future. This introspection helps the woman prepare for her new mothering role. Emotional lability, which may be unsettling to her partner, persists. In some instances, the partner may react by withdrawing. This withdrawal is especially distressing to the woman because she needs increased love and affection. Once the couple understands that these behaviors are characteristic of pregnancy, it is easier for the couple to deal with them effectively, although to some extent they may be sources of stress throughout pregnancy. As pregnancy becomes more noticeable, the woman's body image changes. She may feel great pride, embarrassment, or concern. Generally, women feel best during the second trimester, which is a relatively tranquil time.

Third Trimester

In the third trimester, the woman feels both pride about her pregnancy and anxiety about labor and birth. Physical discomforts increase, and the woman is eager for the pregnancy to end. She experiences increased fatigue, her body movements are more awkward, and her interest in sexual activity may decrease. During this time, the woman tends to be concerned about the health and safety of her unborn child and may worry that she will not cope well during childbirth. Toward the end of this period, the woman often experiences a surge of energy as she prepares for childbirth. Many women report bursts of energy, during which they vigorously clean and organize the home (called *nesting*).

Psychologic Tasks of the Mother

Rubin (1984) identified four major tasks that the pregnant woman undertakes to maintain her intactness and that of her family and at the same time to incorporate her new child into the family system. These tasks form the foundation for a mutually gratifying relationship with her baby:

1. ***Ensuring safe passage through pregnancy, labor, and birth.*** The pregnant woman feels concern for her unborn child and for herself. She looks for competent prenatal care to provide a sense of control. She may read literature and observe and seek advice from other pregnant women and new mothers. She also attempts to ensure safe passage by engaging in self-care activities related to diet, exercise, alcohol consumption, and the like. In the third trimester, she becomes more aware of external threats in the environment—a toy on the stairs, the awkwardness of an escalator—that pose a threat to her well-being. She may worry if her partner is late or if she is home alone. Sleep becomes more difficult, and she longs for birth even though it, too, is frightening.
2. ***Seeking acceptance of this child by others.*** The birth of a child alters a woman's primary support group (her family) and her secondary affiliate groups. The woman slowly and subtly alters her network to meet the needs of her pregnancy. In this adjustment, the woman's partner is the most important figure. The partner's support and acceptance help form a maternal identity. If there are other children in the home, the mother also works to ensure their acceptance of the coming child. Acceptance of the anticipated change is sometimes stressful, and the woman may work to maintain special time with her partner or older children. The woman without a partner looks to others, such as a family member or friend, for this support.
3. ***Seeking commitment and acceptance of herself as mother to the newborn (binding in).*** During the first trimester, the child remains a rather abstract concept. With quickening, however, the child begins to become a real individual, and the mother begins to develop bonds of attachment. The mother experiences the movement of the child within her in an intimate, exclusive way, and out of this experience, bonds of love form. This binding-in process, characterized by its strong emotional component, motivates the pregnant woman to become competent in her role and provides satisfaction for her in the role of mother. This possessive love increases her maternal commitment to protect her fetus now and her child after he or she is born.
4. ***Learning to give of oneself on behalf of one's child.*** Childbirth involves many acts of giving. A man "gives" a child to a woman; she in turn "gives" a child to her partner. Life is given to a baby; a sibling is given to older children of the family. The woman begins to develop a capacity for self-denial and learns to delay immediate personal gratification to meet the needs of another. Baby showers and gifts are acts of giving that increase the mother's self-esteem and help her recognize the separateness and needs of the coming baby.

Accomplishment of these tasks helps the expectant woman develop her self-concept as a mother. The expectant woman who was well nurtured by her own mother may view her mother as a role model and emulate her; the woman who views her mother as a poor mother may worry that she will make similar mistakes. A woman's self-concept as a mother expands with experience and continues to grow through subsequent childbearing and childrearing.

The Father or Partner

How couples view parenting and parenting roles varies from one family to the next, but many couples today see parenting as a shared responsibility, with the father or partner expected to be a nurturing, caring, and involved parent and provider.

Expectant fathers and partners experience many of the same feelings and conflicts experienced by expectant mothers when the pregnancy has been confirmed. Initials feelings may include both pride and ambivalence. The extent of ambivalence depends on many factors, including the father's (or partner's) relationship with the mother, previous experience with pregnancy, age, economic stability, and whether the pregnancy was planned. Expectant fathers and partners must first deal with the reality of the pregnancy and then struggle to gain recognition as a parent from the mother, family, friends, coworkers, society—and from the baby as well. The expectant mother can help her partner be a participant and not merely a helpmate to her if she has a definite sense of the experience as *their* pregnancy and *their* baby and not *her* pregnancy and *her* baby.

When a pregnancy follows a previous pregnancy loss, both the mother and her partner may experience a variety of emotions attributable to the loss. These emotions might include an increased sense of risk, feelings of increased concern about the outcome of the current pregnancy, the recognition that something could go wrong again, and the sense that increased vigilance is essential. The father or partner may call home more often to check on the mother's condition and the baby and may also feel an increased need to be involved more actively in the current pregnancy.

In general, the expectant father or partner faces psychologic stress making the transition from nonparent to parent or from parent of one to parent of two or more. Sources of stress include financial issues, unexpected events during pregnancy, concern that the baby will not be healthy and normal, worry about the pain the mother will experience in childbirth, and the father or partner's role during labor and birth. Other sources of stress include concern over the changing relationship with their partners, diminished sexual responsiveness in their partners or in themselves, changes in relationships with others (especially friends who are not parents), and concerns about being a good parent.

Nurses can promote fathers or partners in their new role by encouraging and welcoming their involvement during pregnancy. Patient education for fathers and partners includes how to support the mother and promoting healthy child development.

The expectant father or partner must establish a fatherhood or parenting role just as the expectant mother develops a motherhood role. The mother experiences biologic changes of pregnancy that aid in the transition to motherhood. Her partner may feel left out because they are unable to experience what their partner is experiencing. Those who are most successful at developing a comfortable role generally are excited about the prospect of becoming a parent, are eager to nurture a child, have confidence in their ability to be a parent, and share the experiences of pregnancy and childbirth with the mother. Fathers or partners who lack experience with children, came from dysfunctional families, or grew up without positive parenting role models may experience more anxiety about their ability to parent.

First Trimester

After the initial excitement of announcing the pregnancy to friends and relatives and receiving their congratulations, an expectant father or partner may begin to feel left out of the pregnancy. The father or partner is also often confused by their partner's mood changes and perhaps bewildered by their responses to her changing body. The partner may resent the attention given to the woman and the changes in their relationship as she experiences fatigue and a decreased interest in sex. The pregnancy itself may seem unreal until the woman shows more physical signs.

Second Trimester

The father's or partner's role in the pregnancy is still vague in the second trimester, but their involvement can be increased by watching and feeling fetal movement. It is helpful if both parents have the opportunity to hear the fetal heartbeat. That requires a visit to the healthcare provider's office. Involvement of fathers and partners in antepartum care is increasing and may even be expected by the mother. For many partners, seeing the fetus on an ultrasound is an important experience in accepting the reality of the pregnancy.

Like expectant mothers, expectant fathers and partners need to confront and resolve some of their own conflicts about the parenting they received, determining what parenting behaviors they want to imitate and what behaviors they wish to avoid using.

The anxiety experienced by the father or partner is lessened if both parents agree on the support role the father or partner is to assume during pregnancy and on the projected parental role. An open and honest discussion about the expectations each parent has about their roles will help the father or partner in the transition to parenthood (London et al., 2017).

As the woman's appearance alters over time, her partner may have different reactions to her physical changes, experiencing increased or decreased sexual interest. Both partners experience a multitude of emotions, and it continues to be important for them to communicate and accept each other's feelings and concerns. In situations in which the expectant mother's demands dominate the relationship, the expectant father's or partner's resentment may increase to the point of spending more time at work, involved in a hobby, or with friends. The behavior is even more likely if the expectant partner did not want the pregnancy or if the relationship was not a good one before the pregnancy.

Third Trimester

If the couple have communicated their concerns and feelings to one another and grown in their relationship, the third trimester is a special and rewarding time. A more clearly defined role evolves at this time for the expectant father or partner, and it becomes more obvious how the couple can prepare together for the coming event. They may become involved in childbirth education classes and make concrete preparations for the arrival of the baby, such as shopping for a crib, car seat, and other equipment. If the expectant father or partner has developed a detached attitude about the pregnancy before this time, however, it is unlikely that they will become a willing participant even though their role becomes more obvious.

Concerns and fears may recur. Many partners are afraid of hurting the unborn baby during intercourse. Some may also begin to have anxiety and fantasies about what could happen to the mother and the unborn baby during labor and birth and feel a great sense of responsibility. The questions asked earlier in pregnancy emerge again. *What kind of parents will we be? Will I really be able to be helpful during labor? Can we afford to have a baby?*

The nurse needs to be prepared to meet the needs of all type of families, including both married and unmarried couples and LGBTQ families. While all 50 states in the United States now recognize same-sex marriage, these couples may still face unique challenges in completing their developmental tasks, including discrimination by healthcare providers. Providing nonjudgmental care of the mother and her partner is essential at all stages throughout pregnancy, delivery, and postpartum care.

Siblings

The introduction of a new baby into the family often leads to sibling rivalry, which results from children's fear of change in the security of their relationships with their parents. Some of the behaviors demonstrating feelings of sibling rivalry may even be directed toward the mother during the pregnancy as she experiences more fatigue and less patience with her toddler, for example. Parents who recognize the situation early in pregnancy and make constructive responses can help minimize the problems of sibling rivalry.

Preparation of the young child for a new sibling should begin several weeks before the anticipated birth and is best designed according to the age and experience of the child. The mother may let the child feel the fetus moving in her uterus, explaining that this is "a special place where babies grow." The child can help the parents put the baby clothes in drawers or prepare the baby's room. Because they do not have a clear concept of time, young children should not be told too early about the pregnancy.

Consistency is important in dealing with young children. They need reassurance that certain people, special things, and familiar places will continue to exist after the new baby arrives. The crib is an important though transient object in a child's life. If it is to be given to the new baby, the parents should thoughtfully help the child adjust to this change. Any move from crib to bed or from one room to another should precede the baby's birth by several weeks or more. If the new baby is to share a room with one or more siblings, the parents must discuss this with them.

If the sibling is ready for toilet training, it is most effectively done several months before or after the baby's arrival. Parents should know that the older, toilet-trained child may regress to wetting or soiling because he or she sees the new baby getting attention for such behavior. The older, weaned child may want to drink from the breast or bottle again after the new baby comes. If the new mother anticipates these behaviors, they will be less frustrating during her early postpartum days.

During the pregnancy, older children should be introduced to a new baby for short periods to get an idea of what a new baby is like. This introduction dispels fantasies that the new arrival will be big enough to be a playmate. Pregnant women may also find it helpful to bring their children to a prenatal visit after they have been told about the expected baby. The children are encouraged to become involved in prenatal care and to ask any questions they may have. They are also given the opportunity to hear the fetal heartbeat, either with a stethoscope or with the Doppler device. This helps make the baby more real to them.

If siblings are school-age, the pregnancy should be viewed as a family affair. Teaching about the pregnancy should be based on the child's level of understanding and interest. Overeager parents may go into longer and more in-depth responses than the child is able to understand. Some children are more curious than others. Books at their level of understanding can be made available in the home. Involvement in family discussions, attendance at sibling preparation classes, encouragement to feel fetal movement, and an opportunity to listen to the fetal heart supplement the learning process and help make the school-age child feel part of the pregnancy. Sibling preparation classes assist in the transition process for both parents and children. After attending the classes, children often exhibit an increased ability to express their feelings and less anxiety.

Older children or adolescents may appear to have a sophisticated knowledge base, but it may be intermingled with many misconceptions. Thus, parents should make opportunities to discuss their concerns and should involve the children in preparation for the new baby.

Even after the birth, siblings need to feel that they are part of a family event. Changes in hospital regulations allowing siblings to be present at the birth or to visit their mother and the new baby facilitate this process. Participation in special programs for siblings may also help in this process. On arrival at home, siblings can share in "showing off" the new baby.

Sibling preparation for the arrival of a new baby is essential, but other factors are equally important. These include the amount of parental attention focused on the new arrival, the amount of parental attention given the older child after the birth of the new arrival, and parental skill in dealing effectively with regressive or aggressive behavior.

Grandparents

How involved grandparents are in the life of a family varies considerably. Grandparents who live in close proximity and are actively involved in their adult children's lives may take on a greater role within the family. If they are already grandparents, their current grandparenting relationships may continue to extend to the new child in the family, without many changes or conflicts. Grandparents who live further away or who do not have a good relationship with their adult children may play less of a role in the newborn and family's life.

Many communities offer classes for grandparents to help them learn about changes in parenting practices and practical issues such as car seat installation and regulations.

Sociocultural Factors and Pregnancy

Most humans share a universal need to create ceremonies or rituals to celebrate or observe important life events such as pregnancy, childbirth, marriage, and death. These rituals often have spiritual and/or cultural contexts and reflect shared values and beliefs. Although a general knowledge of different sociocultural values and beliefs can be helpful in nursing, generalization about sociocultural factors is difficult and not viewed as best practice because not every individual from a particular culture or geographical area may display these characteristics. Just as variations are seen between cultures, they are also seen within cultures. For example, because of their exposure to the American culture, a third-generation Chinese American family might have different values and beliefs from those of a Chinese family that has recently immigrated to America. For this reason, the nurse needs to supplement a general knowledge of cultural values and practices with a complete assessment of the individual's values and practices.

The effect of sociocultural factors on patient care is increasingly important when related to the delivery of quality care. A patient's sociocultural background can have a significant impact on values, beliefs, and behaviors regarding reproduction, pregnancy, and the care related to both.

Focus on Diversity and Culture: Culturally Competent Perinatal Care summarizes key actions to promote socially and culturally competent care of the pregnant woman and her family.

Cultural assessment is an important aspect of prenatal care. Increasingly, healthcare professionals know that they must address cultural needs during a prenatal assessment to provide culturally competent healthcare during pregnancy.

In many parts of the world, gender roles are specifically defined and enforced. Cultural differences in attitudes toward sexuality and gender should be approached and discussed with respect to ensure and maintain quality of care. For example, patients may have apprehension regarding genital or breast exams, or discussing issues related to reproduction, when the provider is a different (or, sometimes, the same) gender as the patient. To promote the therapeutic relationship, healthcare providers (HCPs) should be attentive to patient preferences regarding sexuality and gender roles when caring for patients of all cultures. The nurse needs to identify the prospective parents' main beliefs, values, and behaviors related to pregnancy and childbearing.

Culturally competent nursing assessment of the pregnant woman and her spouse or support people includes information about ethnic background, degree of affiliation with the ethnic group, patterns of decision making, religious preference, language, communication style, and common etiquette practices. The nurse also can explore the woman's (or family's) expectations of the healthcare system. Once this information has been gathered, the nurse can plan and provide care that is appropriate and responsive to a family's needs.

Sociocultural differences between patients and HCPs influence communication and clinical decision making. The communication and decision-making processes are directly correlated with patient satisfaction, compliance, and outcomes. A failure to recognize these differences can result in lower-quality care and adverse patient outcomes.

Case Study » Part 1

Emma Halleck is a 22-year-old woman who presented at the antepartum clinic on June 15. She suspects that she is pregnant: A home pregnancy test was positive. Her LMP began on April 10. Mrs. Halleck reports having urinary frequency, breast tenderness, fatigue, and occasional nausea and vomiting. She has begun to have some lightheadedness and dizziness when she first gets up after sitting or sleeping.

Mrs. Halleck tells you she is married and states that this is her second pregnancy. She miscarried at 10 weeks approximately 6 months ago. She denies any history of drug or alcohol use, sexually transmitted infections (STIs), multiple partners, family violence, medical–surgical disorders, or mental illness. Mrs. Halleck is excited about the pregnancy, and she reports that her husband is also. She does express concern over her ability to carry the pregnancy to term, although she feels relieved that she is beyond the time of her first pregnancy loss. This pregnancy was a planned pregnancy. Mrs. Halleck is a college graduate, is employed as a teacher, and has group health insurance through the local public school system.

Exam

Weight 122 lb (pre-pregnant weight usually between 115 and 120 lb)

Height 5′4″

BP 110/60 mmHg, P 82 beats/min, R 16/min

Hgb 12, Hct 33%, WBC 5000

UA, blood glucose, and protein all negative

Rubella titer—immune

Focus on Diversity and Culture

Culturally Competent Perinatal Care

According to the American College of Obstetricians and Gynecologists (2018d), it is essential that nurses and other HCPs "recognize that stereotyping patients based on presumed cultural beliefs can negatively affect patient interactions, especially when patients' behaviors are attributed solely to individual choices without recognizing the role of social and structural factors."

Patients and providers have their own values and beliefs, some of which may be influenced by their social and cultural backgrounds. To prevent the nurse's own cultural beliefs, expectations, or biases from interfering with patient care, the nurse must maintain self-awareness and always put the focus on the patient's preferences and needs. Nursing actions to promote culturally competent care of pregnant women and their families include those interventions mentioned in Module 24, Cultural and Diversity. They include self-examination of the nurse's own values, recognition of the limits of the nurse's knowledge of patient sociocultural factors, and showing respect for the cultures, values, and beliefs of those different from that of the nurse. Interventions specific to caring for the pregnant woman and her family include:

- Making social and cultural assessment a routine part of perinatal care.
- Using standardized screening tools to screen for social determinants of health (SDOH), such as inadequate access to fresh food, that can affect the course of the pregnancy and the health of both mother and baby.
- Using patient-centered communication, using open-ended questions, about the patient's culture, beliefs, and values.
- Exploring the reasons behind patient actions. For example, failure of a patient to follow the treatment plan for a chronic illness may be due to fear that a medication might harm the baby, inability to afford the medication, or another factor that may benefit from nurse intervention or referrals to community resources.
- Advocating for qualified interpreter services on-site when working with patients who speak another language.
- Accommodating patient's preferences related to sociocultural values and beliefs, including sexuality and gender roles.

General questions to screen for SDOH include:

- Do you ever eat less than you feel is healthy because you do not have enough money to buy food or can't get to the grocery store?
- Are you having any trouble maintaining your housing or paying your utility bills?
- Do you ever not see your doctor because of the cost or because you don't have a way to get there?
- Do you feel safe in your own home?

As always, the nurse maintains a nonjudgmental attitude toward the patient's beliefs, values, and socioeconomic situation.

Source: Adapted from American College of Obstetricians and Gynecologists (2018d).

HIV, STIs—negative
Hepatitis antibody—negative
Immunoassay pregnancy test—positive
Mother: O Rh negative; father: O Rh positive.

On pelvic exam, the physician determines that Mrs. Halleck's uterus is enlarged and at the top of the symphysis pubis. The lower uterine segment is soft; the cervix is soft and bluish in color. There is an increase in vaginal and cervical secretions. The HCP determines that Mrs. Halleck's pelvis is adequate for a normal vaginal birth. Vaginal ultrasound confirms pregnancy with fetal heart tones at 120 beats per minute.

Clinical Reasoning Questions Level I

1. Why is Mrs. Halleck experiencing urinary frequency?
2. Why is Mrs. Halleck having breast tenderness at this time?
3. Are light-headedness and dizziness normal? Why or why not? What nursing intervention should be taught to all pregnant women to avoid these symptoms?

Clinical Reasoning Questions Level II

4. Are the uterine changes assessed on examination considered normal? Why or why not?
5. How does the body maintain pregnancy during the first 12 weeks?
6. Which developmental stage of pregnancy is Mrs. Halleck in? How did you determine this?
7. How would you assess whether fetal attachment is occurring?

Concepts Related to Reproduction

Pregnancy and its related changes affect all body systems and many aspects of health and wellness. The Concepts Related to Reproduction feature outlines some, but not all, of the concepts that are integral to pregnancy. They are presented in alphabetical order.

Sexuality is a key concept in reproductive health, as intercourse is the means by which conception occurs. Anatomic and hormonal changes of pregnancy may alter sexual activity between partners, affecting intimacy and relationships. An additional concern is the potential for unprotected sex before or during pregnancy. Unprotected sex may lead to STIs, which could result in infertility, fetal loss, or complications for mother and fetus. Sexuality is considered as families plan the timing of pregnancies and consider future pregnancies.

Expected physiologic changes in pregnancy often result in discomfort. Anatomic adjustments occur over time as the fetus grows and maternal tissues and structures adapt to physical and hormonal changes. Chronic pain caused by existing diagnoses may increase as pregnancy progresses. During labor, contractions, cervical dilation, and vaginal distention cause pain that may be managed using nonpharmacologic and pharmacologic interventions. The source of postpartum pain varies depending on the length of labor and pushing, types of delivery, and potential perineal trauma. Cramping and discomfort that may accompany breastfeeding are also possible.

Antepartum monitoring includes methods to assess perfusion of mother and fetus. Because poor tissue perfusion decreases the amount of oxygen that reaches the tissues, it is important to maintain normal hemoglobin and hematocrit levels to promote the production and function of RBCs. In addition, screening allows for early identification of conditions that may impair perfusion, including congenital anomalies, abnormalities of the placenta, and nutritional deficits. Hypertensive disorders of pregnancy may decrease perfusion, resulting in poor fetal growth or neurologic risks for the mother. Conditions that threaten the viability of mother or fetus may require preterm delivery.

Concepts Related to **Reproduction**

CONCEPT	RELATIONSHIP TO REPRODUCTION	NURSING IMPLICATIONS
Comfort	Pregnancy discomforts Labor pain Postpartum pain	■ Pregnancy: provide comfort measures for common discomforts. ■ Labor: provide comfort measures for labor (relaxation, hot/cold, positioning, ambulating, birthing balls, hydrotherapy), medications for pain relief, including IVP and epidurals. ■ Postpartum: Provide instruction on Kegel exercises, provide information on pharmacologic and nonpharmacologic methods of pain relief.
Metabolism	Diabetes, gestational diabetes ↑ risks to both mother and baby	■ Assess for signs/symptoms of hypoglycemia and hyperglycemia. ■ Assess for and provide education regarding risk factors for gestational diabetes. ■ Encourage 30 minutes of exercise after each meal. ■ Conduct fetal kick counts twice daily beginning at 28 weeks. ■ Teach blood glucose monitoring. ■ Refer to dietitian. ■ Encourage frequent prenatal visits. ■ Encourage verbalization of feelings related to diabetes diagnosis.

(continued on next page)

Concepts Related to *(continued)*

CONCEPT	RELATIONSHIP TO REPRODUCTION	NURSING IMPLICATIONS
Nutrition	Prenatal nutrition is critical for a healthy fetus Breastfeeding	■ Educate patient on need to increase calories and fluid intake and on safe food consumption during pregnancy. ■ Provide health promotion strategies to enhance fetal/neonatal health: • Easily digested foods • Decreased allergies, risk for illness • Promotion of self-regulation of feedings.
Oxygenation	Untreated or undertreated respiratory disease ↑ risk of inadequate oxygenation to fetus	■ Educate patient regarding need to adhere to therapeutic regimen for respiratory conditions such as asthma. ■ Refer patients who need specialized care who do not already have a provider (e.g., pulmonologist). ■ Assess respiratory status and patient signs/symptoms at each healthcare interaction.
Perfusion	↓ Tissue perfusion creates oxygen deficit to organs	■ Assess for and provide education regarding risk factors for cardiovascular disease, HTN. ■ Assess perfusion, including pulses, nail beds, color, body position for comfort, orientation. ■ Be alert for tachycardia, then hypotension, cool clammy skin, altered level of consciousness. ■ Administer oxygen. ■ Replace IV fluids. ■ Weigh pads. ■ Administer pharmacotherapy to contract uterus.
Sexuality	Unprotected intercourse ↑ likelihood of pregnancy, ↑ risk for STIs Anatomic and hormonal changes	■ Educate patient regarding safe sex practices. ■ Assess risk factors. ■ Provide additional education related to risk factors. ■ Educate couple about normal alterations affecting intimacy.
Stress and Coping	Emotional and relational changes occur with growth of the family Responsibilities expand with incorporation of a new child. Expected physical changes may impact self-esteem Pregnancy, delivery, and recovery may not meet expectations (i.e., birth experience and idealized child)	■ Encourage expression of concerns. ■ Assess patient's and family's past coping strategies. ■ Reinforce adaptive coping. ■ Reinforce realistic expectations.
Teaching and Learning	Patient/couples education enhances pregnancy outcomes	■ Educate patient/couple about labor and comfort measures. ■ Inform patient about expected physiologic and psychologic changes associated with pregnancy. ■ Provide information about purpose and significance of findings.

Prenatal nutrition is crucial for adequate growth and development of fetal tissues. Nutritional assessment occurs throughout pregnancy via laboratory values and monitoring of weight gain. Nutritional deficits may occur in vulnerable populations or for those diagnosed with hyperemesis or other GI disorders. Adequate nutrition is also required for the production of nutrient-dense breast milk and continues to be a critical component of continued growth and development of the newborn.

Hormonal influences may alter carbohydrate metabolism during pregnancy, leading to the development of gestational diabetes mellitus (GDM). Increased maternal glucose levels may cause the fetus to become large for gestational age (LGA), leading to potential complications for mother and fetus during and after delivery. Patients with an existing diagnosis of diabetes mellitus may develop vascular changes that impair fetal perfusion, resulting in a newborn that is small for gestational age (SGA). Glucose tolerance tests occur during pregnancy to screen for and diagnose GDM. (GDM is discussed in detail in Exemplar 33.A, Antepartum Care, in this module.)

Oxygenation is essential for normal tissue growth and function. Alterations in oxygenation may cause fetal acidosis, which could result in impaired function in the newborn or fetal loss (see Module 1, Acid–Base Balance). Existing maternal diagnoses such as asthma may cause poor maternal oxygenation, which, in turn, disrupts placental gas exchange for the fetus. Assessment of fetal oxygenation occurs via monitoring of the FHR, and takes place in the clinic, antepartum testing unit, or the labor and delivery unit. Adequate maternal nutrition, avoidance of the supine position, and treatment of respiratory conditions help to maintain oxygenation of the mother and fetus.

The addition of a child to the family unit requires role transitions for each family member. Impaired coping may disrupt normal family processes and relationships as members adjust to pregnancy, prepare for delivery, and incorporate the new child into the family. Ineffective coping skills may result in alterations in family dynamics and relationships as members compare the reality of the birth experience with expectations. Negative responses to expected physical changes of pregnancy may also have an impact on body image, which could result in unhealthy behaviors involving nutrition and physical activity.

Effective teaching and learning are key factors that may improve patient outcomes. Pregnant women, especially those who are pregnant for the first time, require a great deal of education and support from HCPs. Patient understanding of the need for antepartum testing and regular clinic visits improves compliance and leads to better patient outcomes. Anticipation of expected changes of pregnancy may enhance the pregnancy experience, especially if both the mother and father/partner understand the physiology of pregnancy and normal changes that may occur. The labor process may be enriched if the mother and father/partner attend childbirth classes in preparation for the delivery.

Health Promotion

The nurse can help promote maternal and fetal well-being by providing expectant couples with accurate, complete information about health behaviors and issues that can affect pregnancy and childbirth. Health behaviors—such as breast care, rest, sexual activity, and exercise—help protect both the fetus and the mother and decrease the discomfort of the mother during both pregnancy and labor. Issues that can affect pregnancy range from clothing to employment to travel. The nurse working with pregnant women needs to be able to provide patient teaching in all of these areas.

Breast Care

Whether the pregnant woman plans to formula-feed or breastfeed her baby, support of the breasts is important to promote comfort and prevent back strain, particularly if the breasts become large and pendulous. The sensitivity of the breasts in pregnancy is frequently relieved by good support.

Wearing a well-fitting bra with good support that has the following qualities is essential:

- The straps are wide and do not stretch (elastic straps soon lose their tautness with the weight of the breasts and frequent washing).
- The cup holds all breast tissue comfortably.
- Tucks or other devices allow the bra to expand, thus accommodating the enlarging chest circumference.
- The bra supports the nipple line approximately midway between the elbow and shoulder but is not pulled up in the back by the weight of the breasts.

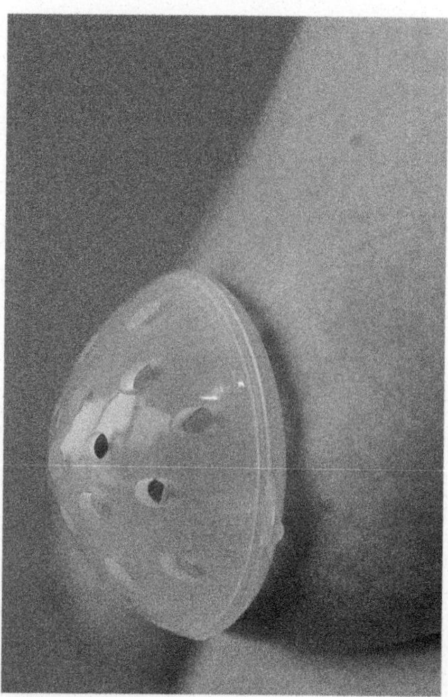

Figure 33.22 » This breast shell is designed to increase the protractility of inverted nipples. Worn the last 3 to 4 weeks of pregnancy, it exerts gentle pulling pressure at the edge of the areola, gradually forcing the nipple through the center of the shield. It may be used after birth, if necessary.

Source: Pearson Education, Inc.

Cleanliness of the breasts also is important, especially if they begin leaking colostrum, which may occur during the last trimester (or earlier in women pregnant with multiples). If colostrum crusts on the nipples, it can be removed with warm water. The woman planning to breastfeed is advised not to use soap on her nipples because of its drying effect.

Some women have flat or inverted nipples. True nipple inversion, which is rare, is usually diagnosed during the initial prenatal assessment. Breast shells designed to correct inverted nipples are effective for some women, but others gain no benefit from them (**Figure 33.22 »**).

Activity and Rest

Exercise during pregnancy helps maintain maternal fitness and muscle tone, leads to improved self-image, promotes regular bowel function, increases energy, improves sleep, relieves tension, helps control weight gain, and is associated with improved postpartum recovery. Pregnancy is an ideal time for the adoption of a healthy lifestyle, including exercise, because of the motivation and frequent assessment of maternal and fetal well-being. Normal participation in exercise can continue throughout an uncomplicated pregnancy and, in fact, is encouraged.

The pregnant woman should take care to avoid extremes of heat and to maintain adequate hydration during exercise. The woman can check with her certified nurse-midwife (CNM) or obstetrician about taking part in moderate- to high-intensity workouts or continuing participation in strenuous sports.

Certain medical or obstetric complications require thorough evaluation by the CNM or obstetrician prior to making recommendations on physical exercise in pregnancy. Activity restriction should not be routinely prescribed to reduce the risks to the mother or fetus without a thorough evaluation. All pregnant women should be educated to stop exercise if they experience any of the following warning signs (ACOG, 2020b):

- Vaginal bleeding
- Abdominal pain
- Regular painful contractions
- Amniotic fluid leakage
- Dyspnea before exertion
- Dizziness
- Headache
- Chest pain
- Muscle weakness affecting balance
- Calf pain or swelling.

See Patient Teaching: Pregnant Women and Exercise.

Sexual Activity

As a result of the physiologic, anatomic, and emotional changes of pregnancy, couples usually have many questions and concerns about sexual activity during pregnancy. Often, these questions are about possible injury to the baby or the woman during intercourse and about changes in the desire each partner feels.

In a healthy pregnancy, there is no medical reason to limit sexual activity. Intercourse is contraindicated for medical reasons, such as rupture of membranes, placenta previa, threatened spontaneous abortion, or the risk of preterm labor (Cunningham et al., 2018).

The expectant mother may experience changes in sexual desire and response. Often, these changes are related to the various discomforts that occur throughout pregnancy. For instance, during the first trimester, fatigue or nausea and vomiting may decrease desire, and breast tenderness may make the woman less responsive to fondling of her breasts. During the second trimester, many of the discomforts have lessened, and with the vascular congestion of the pelvis, the woman may experience greater sexual satisfaction than she experienced before pregnancy.

During the third trimester, interest in coitus may again decrease as the woman becomes more uncomfortable and fatigued. In addition, shortness of breath, painful pelvic ligaments, urinary frequency, leg cramps, and decreased mobility may lessen sexual desire and activity. If they are not already doing so, the heterosexual couple should consider coital positions other than male superior, such as side by side, female superior, and vaginal rear entry.

Sexual activity does not have to include intercourse. Many of the nurturing and sexual needs of the pregnant woman can be satisfied by cuddling, kissing, and being held. The warm, sensual feelings that accompany these activities can be an end in themselves. Her partner, however, may choose to masturbate.

The sexual desires of partners of pregnant women are also affected by many factors in pregnancy. These factors include the previous relationship with the partner, acceptance of the pregnancy, attitudes toward the partner's change of appearance, and concern about hurting the expectant mother or baby. Some find it difficult to view their partners as sexually appealing while they are adjusting to the concept of their partners as mothers. Others find their partners' pregnancies arousing and experience feelings of increased happiness, intimacy, and closeness.

The expectant couple should be aware of their changing sexual desires, the normality of these changes, and the

Patient Teaching

Pregnant Women and Exercise

The following guidelines are helpful in counseling pregnant women about exercise:

- Even mild to moderate exercise is beneficial during pregnancy. Regular exercise—at least 20 to 30 minutes of moderate exercise daily on most days—is preferred (ACOG, 2020b).
- After the first trimester, women should avoid exercising for long periods in the supine position. In most pregnant women, the supine position is associated with decreased venous return due to compression of the abdominal aorta and the inferior vena cava, leading to hypotension.
- Because decreased oxygen is available for aerobic exercise during pregnancy, women should modify the intensity of their exercise based on their symptoms, should stop when they become fatigued, and should avoid exercising to the point of exhaustion.
- Exercises that activate large muscle groups, such as walking, aerobic dance, swimming, cycling, rowing, and jogging, as well as exercises that maintain strength with weights or bands, are encouraged. Yoga in pregnancy can increase maternal strength and fitness as well as reduce stress. Women should avoid hot yoga and use their judgment about modifying or avoiding yoga positions that are uncomfortable or likely to result in loss of balance and falling (Babbar & Shyken, 2016).
- As pregnancy progresses and the center of gravity changes, especially in the third trimester, women should avoid exercises in which the loss of balance could pose a risk to mother or fetus. Similarly, women should avoid any type of exercise that might result in even mild abdominal trauma.
- A normal pregnancy requires an additional 300 kcal/day of nutritional intake. Women who exercise regularly during pregnancy should be careful to ensure that they consume an adequate diet.
- To augment heat dissipation, especially during the first trimester, pregnant women should wear clothing that is comfortable and loose while exercising, ensure adequate hydration, and avoid prolonged overheating. For the same reason, pregnant women are advised to avoid exposure to extreme heat and humidity, including exposure to hot tubs and saunas.
- As a result of the cardiovascular changes of pregnancy, heart rate is not an accurate indicator in pregnant women for the intensity of exercise. The use of the "talk-test" is a good measure of exertion. If the woman can maintain a conversation during exercise, she is not overexerting herself (ACOG, 2020b).

importance of communicating these changes to each other so that they can make nurturing adaptations. The nurse has an important role in helping the expectant couple adapt. The couple should feel free to express concerns about sexual activity, and the nurse should be able to respond and give anticipatory guidance in a comfortable manner. See Patient Teaching: Sexual Activity During Pregnancy.

Dental Care

Proper dental hygiene is important in pregnancy because ensuring a healthy oral environment is essential to overall health. Periodontal disease is a contributing factor to preterm labor (ACOG, 2013b, reaffirmed 2017). In spite of such discomforts as nausea and vomiting, gum hypertrophy and tenderness, possible ptyalism (excessive, often bitter salivation), and heartburn, pregnant women need to maintain regular oral hygiene by brushing at least twice a day and flossing daily.

The nurse should encourage the pregnant woman to have a dental checkup early in her pregnancy. Dentistry should proceed as needed in pregnancy. Local anesthesia is fine, but epinephrine should not be used. The woman should inform her dentist of her pregnancy so that she is not exposed to teratogenic substances. See Exemplar 7.B, Oral Health, in Module 7, Health, Wellness, Illness, and Injury.

Other Health Promotion Measures

A number of health promotion measures not directly related to pregnancy are necessary to ensure the health of the mother and fetus. Some of these measures relate to immunizations, clothing, bathing, maternal employment, and travel.

Immunizations

All women of childbearing age need to be aware of the risks of receiving certain immunizations if pregnancy is possible. The influenza and Tdap vaccines are recommended for pregnant women (Sukumaran et al., 2018). Immunizations with attenuated live viruses, such as rubella vaccine, should not be given in pregnancy because of the teratogenic effect of the live viruses on the developing embryo.

Patient Teaching

Sexual Activity During Pregnancy

Discussion about various sexual activities requires that nurses be comfortable with their sexuality and also be tactful. A discussion of sexuality and sexual activity should stress the importance of open communication so that the couple feels comfortable expressing feelings, preferences, and concerns. Nurses can assist the couple regarding sexual activity during pregnancy with the following patient teaching:

- Begin by explaining that the pregnant woman may experience changes in desire during the course of pregnancy. During the first trimester, discomforts such as nausea, fatigue, and breast tenderness may make intercourse less desirable for many pregnant women. Universal statements that give permission, such as "Many couples experience changes in sexual desire during pregnancy. What kind of changes have you experienced?" are often effective in starting discussion. Depending on the woman's (or couple's) level of knowledge and sophistication, part or all of this discussion may be necessary.
- In the second trimester, as symptoms decrease, desire may increase. In the third trimester, discomfort and fatigue may lead to decreased desire in the pregnant woman. If the partner is present, approach the partner in the same nonjudgmental way discussed previously. If not, ask the pregnant woman if she has noticed any changes in her partner or if her partner has expressed any concerns.
- Explain that partners of pregnant women may notice changes in their level of desire, too. Among other things, this change may be related to feelings about their partner's changing appearance, their belief about the acceptability of sexual activity with a pregnant woman, or concern about hurting the woman or fetus. Some partners find the changes of pregnancy erotic; others must adjust to the notion of their partners as mothers. Deal with any specific questions about the physical and psychologic changes that the couple may have.
- Explain that the woman may notice that orgasms are much more intense during the last weeks of pregnancy and may be followed by cramping. Because of the pressure of the enlarging uterus on the vena cava, the pregnant woman should not lie flat on her back for intercourse after about the fourth month. If the couple prefers that position, a pillow should be placed under the pregnant woman's right hip to displace the uterus. Alternative positions such as side by side, female superior, or vaginal rear entry may become necessary as her uterus enlarges.
- Stress that sexual activities both partners enjoy are generally acceptable. It is not advisable, however, for couples who favor anal sex to go from anal penetration to vaginal penetration because of the risk of introducing *Escherichia coli* into the vagina. The couple may be content with these approaches to meeting their sexual needs, or they may require assurance that such approaches are indeed "normal."
- Suggest that alternative methods of expressing intimacy and affection, such as cuddling, holding and stroking each other, and kissing, may help maintain the couple's feelings of warmth and closeness. If the partner feels desire for further sexual release, the pregnant woman may help her partner masturbate to climax, or the partner may prefer to masturbate in private.
- Advise the pregnant woman who is interested in masturbation as a form of gratification that the orgasmic contractions may be especially intense during later pregnancy.
- Stress that sexual intercourse is contraindicated once the membranes have ruptured or if bleeding is present. Pregnant women with a history of preterm labor may be advised to avoid intercourse because the oxytocin that is released with orgasm stimulates uterine contractions and may trigger preterm labor. Because oxytocin is also released with nipple stimulation, fondling the breasts may be contraindicated in those cases as well.
- Some couples are skilled at expressing their feelings about sexual activity. Others find it difficult and can benefit from specific suggestions. The nurse should provide opportunities for discussion throughout the talk. An explanation of the contraindications accompanied by their rationale provides specific guidelines that most couples find helpful. Specific handouts on sexual activity are helpful for couples and may address topics that were not discussed.

Pregnant women with COVID-19 are at increased risk for early delivery and severe illness requiring hospitalization compared to pregnant women who do not develop COVID-19. The CDC (2021) recommends COVID-19 vaccinations for all women who are pregnant or considering becoming pregnant, women who are breastfeeding, and anyone eligible to receive the vaccine who lives in the same household. The most current recommendations on vaccines related to pregnancy are available at the Centers for Disease Control and Prevention website (www.cdc.gov).

Clothing

Traditionally, maternity clothes have been constructed with fuller lines to allow for the increase in abdominal size during pregnancy. However, maternity wear has changed in recent years and now also includes clothes that are more fitted, with little attempt to hide the pregnant abdomen. Maternity clothing can be expensive, and it is worn for a relatively short time. Women can economize by sharing clothes with friends, sewing their own garments, or buying used maternity clothes.

High-heeled shoes tend to aggravate back discomfort by increasing the curvature of the lower back. They are best avoided if the woman experiences backache or has problems with balance. Shoes should fit properly and feel comfortable.

Bathing

Because perspiration and mucoid vaginal discharge increase during pregnancy, hygiene is important. Practices related to cleansing the body are often influenced by cultural norms; thus, a pregnant woman may choose to cleanse only some portions of her body daily or may elect to take daily showers or tub baths. Caution is needed during tub baths because balance becomes a problem in late pregnancy. Rubber mats and hand grips are important safety devices. Vasodilation caused by warm water may make the woman feel faint when she attempts to get out of the tub, so she may require assistance, especially during the last trimester. During the first trimester, pregnant women should avoid hyperthermia associated with the use of a hot tub or Jacuzzi because it may increase the risk for miscarriage or neural tube defects (Snijder et al., 2012).

Employment

Pregnant women who have no complications can usually continue to work until they go into labor (ACOG, 2018b). Although pregnant women who are employed in jobs that require prolonged standing (> 5 hours) do have a higher incidence of preterm birth, it has no effect on fetal growth (Snijder et al., 2012).

Fetotoxic hazards are always a concern to the expectant couple. The pregnant woman (or the woman contemplating pregnancy) who works in industry should contact her company physician or nurse about possible hazards in her work environment and do her own reading and research on environmental hazards as well. Similarly, a male partner can seek information about hazards in his workplace that might affect his sperm.

Travel

If medical or pregnancy complications are not present, there are no restrictions on travel. Pregnant women are advised to avoid travel if they have a history of bleeding or preeclampsia or if multiple births are anticipated. Availability of medical care at the destination is an important factor for the near-term woman who travels. It may be helpful to travel with a copy of the woman's medical record.

Travel by automobile can be especially fatiguing, aggravating many of the discomforts of pregnancy. The pregnant woman needs frequent opportunities to get out of the car and walk. (A good pattern is to stop every 2 hours and walk around for approximately 10 minutes.) She should wear both lap and shoulder belts; the lap belt should fit snugly and be positioned under the abdomen and across the upper thighs. The shoulder strap should rest comfortably between the woman's breasts. Seat belts play an important role in preventing fetal and maternal morbidity and mortality with subsequent fetal death (Cunningham et al., 2018). Fetal death in car crashes is related to placental separation (abruptio placentae) as a result of uterine trauma. Use of the shoulder belt decreases the risk of traumatic flexion of the woman's body, thereby decreasing the risk of placental separation.

As pregnancy progresses, long-distance trips are best taken by plane or train. Currently, flying is considered to be safe up to 36 weeks of gestation in the absence of any complications (ACOG, 2018a). Before flying, the woman should check with her airline to see if they have any travel restrictions. Prolonged air travel may lead to edema in the lower extremities and the development of venous thrombolytic events. To minimize complications, the traveler should consider wearing support stockings, maintain oral hydration, periodically move the lower extremities, change positions frequently, and move about the cabin at least every 2 hours when conditions are favorable (ACOG, 2018a).

SAFETY ALERT The Zika virus is transmitted directly from mother to fetus through the placenta, resulting in neural damage to the fetus.

Transmission of the Zika virus occurs via mosquito bites and through sexual contact. Only one in five people with Zika infection will exhibit symptoms. Once infected, individuals are protected from future infection.

Symptoms of Zika infection include mild fever, maculopapular rash, headache, arthralgia (joint pain), and myalgia (muscle pain). Prevention strategies include wearing long-sleeved shirts and pants, using window screens or mosquito bed nets, eliminating standing water where mosquitoes breed, and avoiding travel to areas where the virus is actively circulating.

Source: American College of Obstetricians and Gynecologists (2019b).

Complementary Health Approaches

Complementary health approaches (CHA) are increasingly popular among pregnant women and may include mind–body practices such as yoga, acupressure and acupuncture, and massage, as well as use of herbal medicine and supplements. Nurses should ask about use of CHA at each health-care interaction.

Patient teaching about CHA for pregnant women should include that herbs are considered to be dietary supplements and are not regulated through the U.S. Food and Drug Administration (FDA), as prescription or over-the-counter (OTC) drugs are. Because of limited scientific evaluation of potential harmful effects on the fetus, herbal supplements should be avoided, particularly in the first trimester (Romm, 2014).

Some yoga positions are contraindicated during pregnancy. Pregnant women should avoid extreme stretching positions and positions that put pressure on the uterus. Pregnant women should also avoid any positions that require lying on the stomach. After 20 weeks' gestation, pregnant women should lie on their side rather than on their back for floor positions. Pregnant women should immediately stop any position that is uncomfortable (Babbar & Shyken, 2016).

» **Stay Current:** Additional information about herbs, homeopathic remedies, and other alternative options may be accessed at the website of the National Center for Complementary and Integrative Health at http://nccih.nih.gov.

Teratogenic Substances

Evidence supports that exposure to teratogens and toxic substances can lead to significant reproductive and pregnancy risks. **Teratogens** are substances that cause an abnormality in the fetus, following exposure during pregnancy. Teratogens can be found in the home and in the workplace. The effect of the substance is directly related to type of agent, dose, and duration and time of exposure. The first half of pregnancy is the most vulnerable. The pregnant patient should be counseled to discuss the use of all medications, including prescription and OTC, with her HCP. If medications are indicated during pregnancy, the lowest dose possible should be used and patients should be encouraged to use a single pharmacy to reduce the risk of drug–drug interactions. Additionally, patients should be educated to avoid exposure to pesticides and x-rays in the first trimester.

The nurse who is caring for the pregnant woman, or for the woman who is trying to become pregnant, should teach her about teratogenic substances, including alcohol, and emphasize the need for the woman to discuss the use of any and all medications, including psychotropic drugs, with her obstetrician. Obstetricians and nurse-midwives are the most informed about the potential effects of medications on the fetus. The nurse should also instruct the patient with a chronic condition, such as asthma or diabetes, to inform her treating provider if she is (or is trying to become) pregnant. The pregnant woman with a chronic condition should be encouraged to use a single pharmacy and to inform the pharmacy staff that she is pregnant. Discussing potential hazards in the work and home environments, such as pesticides and radiologic exposure in the first trimester, is important for preventing teratogenic effects on the fetus.

For a more thorough discussion of the risks of substance abuse during pregnancy, see Exemplar 22.C, Substance Use Disorder, in Module 22, Addiction. An overview of the risks associated with tobacco use is provided here.

In the United States, smoking tobacco during pregnancy is one of the most significant, modifiable causes of poor pregnancy outcomes. Smoking during pregnancy has a strong association with low-birth-weight neonates. Mothers who smoke have an increased risk of preterm birth, premature rupture of the membranes, fetal demise, placenta previa, abruptio placentae, premature rupture of membranes, and preterm birth (Cunningham et al., 2018). Pregnant women who smoke tobacco and participate in other unhealthy behaviors, such as alcohol use, further increase their risk for low-birth-weight newborns (Barron, 2020). Research also links maternal tobacco smoking, both during and after pregnancy, with an increased risk of sudden unexpected infant death. Maternal smoking exposes young children to other risks of secondhand smoke, including middle ear infections, acute and chronic respiratory tract illnesses, and learning disabilities.

Nursing Assessment

During the initial prenatal assessment, the nurse's primary role centers around health promotion and patient education. The nurse is responsible for establishing open communication with the patient through the use of evidence-based interview techniques such as reflection, empathy, and the use of open-ended questions. This communication and assessment are necessary to screen for both maternal and fetal risks and to be able to minimize any complications that present and promote healthy outcomes for both mother and baby. The advanced practice nurse (APN or CNM) is a registered nurse who receives additional training through the completion of a master's degree, or higher level. The APN/CNM provides direct patient care through collaboration, consultation, and referral to physicians. In many states, APNs are able to practice without the direct supervision of a physician.

This section focuses on the initial prenatal assessment.

Prenatal Assessment

PHYSICAL ASSESSMENT/ NORMAL FINDINGS	ALTERATIONS AND POSSIBLE CAUSES*	NURSING RESPONSES TO DATA†
Vital Signs		
Blood pressure (BP): less than or equal to 140/90 mmHg	High BP (essential HTN; renal disease; apprehension or anxiety associated with pregnancy diagnosis, exam, or other crises; gestational HTN or preeclampsia if initial assessment not done until after 20 weeks' gestation)	BP greater than 140/90 mmHg requires immediate consideration; establish woman's BP; refer to HCP if necessary. Assess woman's knowledge about high BP; counsel on self-care and medical management.
	*Possible causes of alterations are identified in parentheses.	†This column provides guidelines for further assessment and initial nursing intervention.

(continued on next page)

Prenatal Assessment *(continued)*

PHYSICAL ASSESSMENT/ NORMAL FINDINGS	ALTERATIONS AND POSSIBLE CAUSES*	NURSING RESPONSES TO DATA†
Pulse: 60–100 beats/min; rate may increase 10 beats/min during pregnancy	Increased pulse rate (excitement or anxiety, cardiac disorders)	Count for 1 full minute; note irregularities.
Respirations: 12–20 breaths/min (or pulse rate divided by 4); pregnancy may induce a degree of hyperventilation; thoracic breathing predominant	Marked tachypnea or abnormal patterns	Assess for respiratory disease.
Temperature: 36.0–38.5°C (96.8–101.3°F)	Elevated temperature (infection)	Assess for infection process of disease state or ruptured membranes, if temperature is elevated; refer to HCP.
Body Mass Index (BMI)		
Between 18.5 and 24.9 based on pre-pregnant weight or weight on presentation to care if pre-pregnant weight is unknown	Less than 18.5 or greater than 25	Evaluate need for nutritional counseling; obtain information on eating habits, cooking practices, food regularly eaten, income limitations, need for food supplements, and pica and other abnormal food habits. Note initial weight to establish baseline for weight gain throughout pregnancy.
Skin		
Color: consistent with racial background; pink nail beds	Pallor (anemia); bronze, yellow (hepatic disease; other causes of jaundice) Bluish, reddish, mottled; dusky appearance or pallor of palms and nail beds in dark-skinned women (anemia)	The following tests should be performed: complete blood count (CBC), bilirubin level, urinalysis, and blood urea nitrogen (BUN). If abnormal, refer to HCP.
Condition: absence of edema (slight edema of lower extremities is normal during pregnancy)	Edema (possible preeclampsia); rashes, dermatitis (allergic response)	Counsel on relief measures for slight edema. Initiate preeclampsia assessment; refer to HCP.
Lesions: absence of lesions	Ulceration (varicose veins, decreased circulation)	Further assess circulatory status; refer to HCP if lesion is severe.
Spider nevi common in pregnancy	Petechiae, multiple bruises, ecchymosis (hemorrhagic disorders; abuse) Change in size or color (carcinoma)	Evaluate for bleeding or clotting disorder. Provide opportunities to discuss abuse if suspected. Refer to HCP.
Pigmentation: changes of pregnancy include linea nigra, striae gravidarum, melasma		Assure woman that these are normal manifestations of pregnancy and explain the physiologic basis for the changes.
Café-au-lait spots	Six or more (Albright syndrome or neurofibromatosis)	Consult with HCP.
Nose		
Character of mucosa: redder than oral mucosa; in pregnancy, nasal mucosa is edematous in response to increased estrogen, resulting in nasal stuffiness (rhinitis of pregnancy) and nosebleeds (epistaxis)	Olfactory loss (first cranial nerve deficit)	Counsel woman about possible relief measures for nasal stuffiness and nosebleeds; refer to HCP for olfactory loss.
	*Possible causes of alterations are identified in parentheses.	†This column provides guidelines for further assessment and initial nursing intervention.

Prenatal Assessment *(continued)*

PHYSICAL ASSESSMENT/ NORMAL FINDINGS	ALTERATIONS AND POSSIBLE CAUSES*	NURSING RESPONSES TO DATA†
Mouth		
May note hypertrophy of gingival tissue because of estrogen	Edema, inflammation (infection); pale in color (anemia)	Assess hematocrit for anemia; counsel regarding dental hygiene habits. Refer to HCP or dentist, if necessary. Routine dental care is appropriate during pregnancy (no epinephrine, no nitrous anesthesia). Dental x-rays can be done during the second trimester, if needed.
Neck		
Nodes: small, mobile, nontender nodes	Tender, hard, fixed, or prominent nodes (infection, carcinoma)	Examine for local infection; refer to HCP.
Thyroid: small, smooth, lateral lobes palpable on either side of trachea; slight hyperplasia by third month of pregnancy	Enlargement or nodule tenderness (hyperthyroidism)	Listen over thyroid for bruits, which may indicate hyperthyroidism. Question woman about dietary habits (iodine intake). Ascertain history of thyroid problems; refer to HCP.
Chest and Lungs		
Chest: symmetric, elliptic, smaller anteroposterior (AP) than transverse diameter	Increased AP diameter, funnel chest, pigeon chest (emphysema, asthma, chronic obstructive pulmonary disease [COPD])	Evaluate for emphysema, asthma, COPD.
Ribs: slope downward from nipple line	More horizontal (COPD) angular bumps (rachitic rosary) (vitamin C deficiency)	Evaluate for COPD. Evaluate for fractures. Consult HCP, nutritionist.
Inspection and palpation: no retraction or bulging of intercostal spaces (ICS) during inspiration or expiration; symmetric expansion	ICS retractions with inspirations, bulging with expiration; unequal expansion (respiratory disease)	Do thorough initial assessment. Refer to HCP.
Tactile fremitus	Tachypnea, hyperpnea, Cheyne-Stokes respirations (respiratory disease)	Refer to HCP.
Percussion: bilateral symmetry in tone	Flatness of percussion, which may be affected by chest wall thickness	Evaluate for pleural effusions, consolidations, or tumor.
Low-pitched resonance of moderate intensity	High diaphragm (atelectasis or paralysis), pleural effusion	Refer to HCP.
Auscultation: upper lobes: bronchovesicular sounds above sternum and scapula; equal expiratory and inspiratory phases	Abnormal if heard over any other area of chest	Refer to HCP.
Remainder of chest: vesicular breath sounds heard; inspiratory phase longer (3:1)	Rales, rhonchi, wheezes; pleural friction rub; absence of breath sounds; bronchophony, egophony, whispered pectoriloquy	Refer to HCP.
Breasts		
Supple: symmetric in size and contour; darker pigmentation of nipple and areola; may have supernumerary nipples Axillary nodes unpalpable or pellet-sized	"Pigskin" or orange-peel appearance, nipple retractions, swelling, hardness (carcinoma); redness, heat, tenderness, cracked or fissured nipple (infection) Tenderness, enlargement, hard node (carcinoma); may be visible bump (infection)	Encourage monthly self-examination; instruct woman how to examine her breasts. Refer to HCP if evidence of inflammation.
	*Possible causes of alterations are identified in parentheses.	†This column provides guidelines for further assessment and initial nursing intervention.

(continued on next page)

Prenatal Assessment *(continued)*

PHYSICAL ASSESSMENT/ NORMAL FINDINGS	ALTERATIONS AND POSSIBLE CAUSES*	NURSING RESPONSES TO DATA†
Pregnancy changes: 1. Size increase noted primarily in first 20 weeks. 2. Become nodular. 3. Tingling sensation may be felt during first and third trimester; woman may report feeling of heaviness. 4. Pigmentation of nipples and areolae darkens. 5. Superficial veins dilate and become more prominent. 6. Striae seen in multiparas. 7. Tubercles of Montgomery enlarge. 8. Colostrum may be present after 12th week. 9. Secondary areola appears at 20 weeks, characterized by series of washed-out spots surrounding primary areola. 10. Breasts less firm, old striae may be present in multiparas.		Discuss normalcy of changes and their meaning. Teach and/or institute appropriate relief measures. Encourage use of well-fitting bra with good support.
Heart		
Normal rate, rhythm, and heart sounds	Enlargement, thrills, thrusts, gross irregularity or skipped beats, gallop rhythm or extra sounds (cardiac disease)	Complete an initial assessment. Explain normal pregnancy-induced changes. Refer to HCP, if indicated.
Pregnancy changes: 1. Palpitations may occur due to sympathetic nervous system disturbance 2. Short systolic murmurs that increase in held expiration are normal due to increased volume		
Abdomen		
Normal appearance, skin texture, and hair distribution; liver nonpalpable; abdomen nontender	Muscle guarding (anxiety, acute tenderness); tenderness, mass (ectopic pregnancy, inflammation, carcinoma)	Assure woman of normalcy of diastasis. Provide initial information about appropriate prenatal and postpartum exercises. Evaluate woman's anxiety level. Refer to HCP, if indicated.
Pregnancy changes: 1. Purple striae may be present (or silver striae on a multipara) as well as linea nigra. 2. Diastasis of the rectus muscles late in pregnancy. 3. Size: flat or rotund abdomen; progressive enlargement of uterus due to pregnancy.	Size of uterus inconsistent with length of gestation (intrauterine growth restriction, multiple pregnancy, fetal demise, hydatidiform mole, polyhydramnios, inaccurate dating)	Reassess menstrual history regarding pregnancy dating. Use ultrasound to establish diagnosis.
	*Possible causes of alterations are identified in parentheses.	†This column provides guidelines for further assessment and initial nursing intervention.

Prenatal Assessment *(continued)*

PHYSICAL ASSESSMENT/ NORMAL FINDINGS	ALTERATIONS AND POSSIBLE CAUSES*	NURSING RESPONSES TO DATA†
10–12 weeks: fundus slightly above symphysis pubis *16 weeks:* fundus halfway between symphysis and umbilicus *20–22 weeks:* fundus at umbilicus *28 weeks:* fundus three finger breadths above umbilicus *36 weeks:* fundus just below ensiform cartilage		
4. Fetal heart rate: 110–160 beats/min may be heard with Doppler at 10–12 weeks' gestation; may be heard with fetoscope at 17–20 weeks.	Failure to hear fetal heartbeat with Doppler (fetal demise, hydatidiform mole)	Refer to HCP. Administer pregnancy tests. Use ultrasound to establish diagnosis.
5. Fetal movement palpable by a trained examiner after 18th week.	Failure to feel fetal movements after 20 weeks' gestation (fetal demise, hydatidiform mole)	Refer to HCP. Refer to HCP for evaluation of fetal status.
6. Ballottement: during fourth to fifth month, fetus rises and then rebounds to original position when uterus is tapped sharply.	No ballottement (oligohydramnios)	Refer to HCP for evaluation of fetal status.
Extremities		
Skin warm, pulses palpable, full range of motion; may be some edema of hands and ankles in late pregnancy; varicose veins may become more pronounced; palmar erythema may be present	Unpalpable or diminished pulses (arterial insufficiency); marked edema (preeclampsia)	Evaluate for other symptoms of heart disease; initiate follow-up if woman mentions that her rings feel tight. Discuss prevention and self-treatment measures for varicose veins; refer to HCP, if indicated.
Spine		
Normal spinal curves: concave cervical, convex thoracic, concave lumbar	Abnormal spinal curves; flatness, kyphosis, lordosis	Refer to HCP for assessment of cephalopelvic disproportion.
In pregnancy, lumbar spinal curve may be accentuated	Backache	May have implications for administration of spinal anesthetics.
Shoulders and iliac crests should be even	Uneven shoulders and iliac crests (scoliosis)	Refer very young women to HCP; discuss back-stretching exercise with older women.
Reflexes		
Normal and symmetric	Hyperactivity, clonus (preeclampsia)	Evaluate for other symptoms of preeclampsia.
Pelvic Area		
External female genitals: normally formed with female hair distribution; in multiparas, labia majora loose and pigmented; urinary and vaginal orifices visible and appropriately located	Lesions, hematomas, varicosities, inflammation of the Bartholin glands; clitoral hypertrophy	Explain pelvic examination procedure. Encourage woman to minimize her discomfort by relaxing her hips. Provide privacy.
	*Possible causes of alterations are identified in parentheses.	†This column provides guidelines for further assessment and initial nursing intervention.

(continued on next page)

Prenatal Assessment *(continued)*

PHYSICAL ASSESSMENT/ NORMAL FINDINGS	ALTERATIONS AND POSSIBLE CAUSES*	NURSING RESPONSES TO DATA†
Vagina: pink or dark pink, vaginal discharge odorless, nonirritating; in multiparas, vaginal folds smooth and flattened; may have episiotomy scar	Abnormal discharge associated with vaginal infections	Obtain vaginal smear. Provide understandable verbal and written instructions about treatment for woman and partner if indicated.
Cervix: pink color; os closed except in multiparas, in whom os admits fingertip	Eversion, reddish erosion, nabothian or retention cysts, cervical polyp; granular area that bleeds (carcinoma of cervix); lesions (herpes, human papillomavirus); presence of string or plastic tip from cervix (intrauterine device [IUD] in uterus)	Provide woman with a hand mirror and identify genital structures for her; encourage her to view her cervix if she wishes. Refer to HCP if indicated. Advise woman of potential serious risks of leaving an IUD in place during pregnancy; refer to HCP for removal.
Pregnancy changes: *1–4 weeks' gestation:* enlargement in AP diameter *4–6 weeks' gestation:* softening of cervix (Goodell sign); softening of isthmus of uterus (Hegar sign); cervix takes on bluish coloring (Chadwick sign) *8–12 weeks' gestation:* vagina and cervix appear bluish violet in color (Chadwick sign) Uterus: pear-shaped, mobile; smooth surface	Absence of Goodell sign (inflammatory conditions, carcinoma) Fixed (pelvic inflammatory disease [PID]); nodular surface (fibromas)	Refer to HCP. Refer to HCP.
Ovaries: small, walnut-shaped, nontender (ovaries and fallopian tubes are located in adnexal areas)	Pain on movement of cervix (PID); enlarged or nodular ovaries (cyst, tumor, tubal pregnancy, corpus luteum of pregnancy)	Evaluate adnexal areas; refer to HCP.
Anus and Rectum		
No lumps, rashes, excoriation, tenderness; cervix may be felt through rectal wall	Hemorrhoids, rectal prolapse; nodular lesion (carcinoma)	Counsel about appropriate prevention and relief measures; refer to HCP for further evaluation.
Laboratory Evaluation		
Hemoglobin: 12–16 g/dL; women residing in areas of high altitude may have higher levels of hemoglobin	Less than 11 g/dL (anemia)	*Note:* Wear nonlatex gloves when drawing blood. Hemoglobin less than 12 g/dL requires nutritional counseling; less than 11 g/dL requires iron supplementation.
ABO and Rh typing: normal distribution of blood types	Rh negative	If Rh negative, check for presence of anti-Rh antibodies. Discuss the need for measurement of antibody titers during pregnancy, management during the intrapartum period, and possible need for Rh immune globulin. Determine the father's Rh status, if possible.
CBC: Hematocrit: 38–47% physiologic anemia (pseudoanemia) may occur	Marked anemia or blood dyscrasias	Perform CBC and Schilling differential cell count. Consider iron studies and hemoglobin electrophoresis.
RBCs: 4.2–5.4 million/microliter		
WBCs: 5000–12,000/microliter	Presence of infection; may be elevated in pregnancy and with labor	Evaluate for other signs of infection.
	*Possible causes of alterations are identified in parentheses.	†This column provides guidelines for further assessment and initial nursing intervention.

Prenatal Assessment *(continued)*

PHYSICAL ASSESSMENT/ NORMAL FINDINGS	ALTERATIONS AND POSSIBLE CAUSES*	NURSING RESPONSES TO DATA†
Differential Neutrophils: 40–60% Bands: up to 5% Eosinophils: 1–3% Basophils: up to 1% Lymphocytes: 20–40% Monocytes: 4–8%		
Syphilis tests: serologic tests for syphilis (STS), complement fixation test, Venereal Disease Research Laboratory test—nonreactive	Positive reaction STS—tests may have 25–45% incidence of biologic false-positive results; false results may occur in individuals who have acute viral or bacterial infections, hypersensitivity reactions, recent vaccinations, collagen disease, malaria, or tuberculosis	Positive results may be confirmed with the fluorescent treponemal antibody-absorption test; all tests for syphilis give positive results in the secondary stage of the disease; antibiotic tests may cause negative test results.
First-trimester combined test	Abnormal fetal nasal bone and/or nuchal fold combined with abnormal lab values pregnancy-associated plasma protein A and/or hCG	Offered to all pregnant women at 11–13 weeks' gestation. If abnormal, further testing, such as CVS, is offered.
Full integrated screen	Abnormal fetal nasal bone and/or nuchal fold on ultrasound combined with abnormal lab values on the quad screen.	Offered to all pregnant women at the gestational age appropriate for each test. If abnormal, further testing such as ultrasound or amniocentesis is offered.
Serum integrated test		Offered to all pregnant women where the option for the expertise of a full integrated test is not available. If abnormal, further testing such as ultrasound and amniocentesis is advised.
Noninvasive prenatal testing / cell-free fetal DNA	Detection of abnormal fetal alleles in maternal serum	Refer to HCP.
Quad screen (evaluates four factors—maternal serum alpha-fetoprotein [MSAFP], unconjugated estriol [UE], hCG, and inhibin-A: normal levels)	Elevated MSAFP (neural tube defect, underestimated gestational age, multiple gestation); lower than normal MSAFP (Down syndrome, trisomy 18); higher than normal hCG and inhibin-A (Down syndrome); lower than normal UE (Down syndrome)	Refer to HCP for possible amniocentesis.
Indirect Coombs test: done on all pregnant women at the initial prenatal visit and repeated at 28 weeks for Rh-negative women	RBC antibodies present (either Rhesus or non-Rhesus)	A number of RBC antigens may cause isoimmunization and fetal and newborn hemolytic disease. The most common of these is the D antigen, which may occur when a Rh-negative mother carries a Rh-positive fetus. This may be prevented through prenatal administration of Rh immune globulin (RhoGAM).
Screening for group B streptococcus: Rectal and vaginal swabs obtained at 35–37 weeks' gestation for all pregnant women	Positive culture (maternal colonization)	Antibiotics administered during labor for infection prophylaxis in the neonate.
Glucose tolerance test: 50-g 1-hour glucose screen (done between 24 and 28 weeks' gestation)	Plasma glucose level greater than 130–140 mg/dL is considered abnormal, depending on provider preference; be aware of your institution's guidelines	Refer for a diagnostic 3-hour glucose tolerance test.
Urinalysis: normal color; specific gravity; pH 4.6–8.0	Abnormal color (porphyria, hemoglobinuria, bilirubinemia); alkaline urine (metabolic alkalemia, *Proteus* infection, old specimen)	Repeat urinalysis; refer to HCP.
	*Possible causes of alterations are identified in parentheses.	†This column provides guidelines for further assessment and initial nursing intervention.

(continued on next page)

Prenatal Assessment *(continued)*

PHYSICAL ASSESSMENT/ NORMAL FINDINGS	ALTERATIONS AND POSSIBLE CAUSES*	NURSING RESPONSES TO DATA†
Urinalysis: negative for protein, RBCs, WBCs, casts	Positive findings (contaminated specimen, kidney disease)	Repeat urinalysis; refer to HCP.
Urinalysis: glucose: negative (a small degree of glycosuria may occur in pregnancy)	Glycosuria (physiologic secondary to increased glomerular filtration of pregnancy for glucose, diabetes mellitus)	Assess blood glucose level; test urine for ketones.
Rubella titer: hemagglutination-inhibition (HAI) test—1:10 or above indicates woman is immune	HAI titer less than 1:10	Immunization will be given postpartum or within 6 weeks after childbirth. Instruct woman whose titers are less than 1:10 to avoid children who have rubella.
Hepatitis B screen for hepatitis B surface antigen: negative	Positive	If negative, consider referral for hepatitis B vaccine postpartum. If positive, refer to physician. Babies born to women who test positive are given hepatitis B immune globulin soon after birth, followed by first dose of hepatitis B vaccine.
Hepatitis C screen for hepatitis C antibody: nonreactive (Centers for Disease Control and Prevention [CDC], 2020d)	Reactive	If reactive, test for presence of hepatitis C virus ribonucleic acid (RNA) and refer for additional care or testing as appropriate.
HIV screen: offered to all women; encouraged for those at risk; negative	Positive	Refer to HCP.
Illicit drug screen: offered to all women; negative	Positive	Refer to HCP.
Hemoglobin screen for patients of African, Mediterranean, or south Asian descent: negative	Positive; test results would include a description of cells	Refer to HCP.
Pap smear: negative	Test results that show atypical cells	Refer to HCP. Discuss with the woman the meaning of the findings and the importance of follow-up.
Gonorrhea culture: negative	Positive	Refer for treatment.
CULTURAL ASSESSMENT	**VARIATIONS TO CONSIDER**	**NURSING RESPONSES TO DATA†**
Determine the woman's fluency in written and oral English	Woman may be fluent in language other than English	Work with a knowledgeable interpreter to provide information and answer questions.
Ask the woman how she prefers to be addressed	Some women prefer informality; others prefer to use titles	Address the woman according to her preference. Maintain formality in introductions if that seems preferred.
Determine customs and practices regarding prenatal care.	Practices are influenced by individual preference, cultural expectations, or religious beliefs. Some women believe they should perform certain acts related to sleep, activity, or clothing	Honor a woman's practices and provide for specific preferences unless they are contraindicated for safety reasons.
Ask the woman if there are any activities she cannot do while she is pregnant	Some women have restrictions or taboos they follow related to work, activity, sexual, environmental, or emotional factors	Provide alternative activities, if needed.
Ask the woman whether there are certain foods she is expected to eat or avoid while she is pregnant; determine whether she has lactose intolerance	Foods are an important cultural factor. Some women may have certain foods they must eat or avoid; many women have lactose intolerance and have difficulty consuming sufficient calcium	Respect the woman's food preferences, help her plan an adequate prenatal diet within the framework of her preferences, and refer to a dietitian, if necessary.
	*Possible causes of alterations are identified in parentheses.	†This column provides guidelines for further assessment and initial nursing intervention.

Prenatal Assessment *(continued)*

CULTURAL ASSESSMENT	VARIATIONS TO CONSIDER	NURSING RESPONSES TO DATA†
Ask the woman whether the sex of her caregiver is of concern	Some women are comfortable only with a female caregiver	Arrange for a female caregiver if it is the woman's preference.
Ask the woman about the degree of involvement in her pregnancy that she expects or wants from her support person, mother, and other significant people	A woman may not want her partner involved in the pregnancy. The role may fall to the woman's mother or a female relative or friend	Respect the woman's preferences about her partner's involvement; avoid imposing personal values or expectations.
Ask the woman about her sources of support and counseling during pregnancy	Some women seek advice from a family member or traditional healer	Respect and honor the woman's sources of support.
PSYCHOLOGIC AND SOCIAL HEALTH	**VARIATIONS TO CONSIDER**	**NURSING RESPONSES TO DATA†**
Excitement and/or apprehension, ambivalence	Marked anxiety (fear of pregnancy diagnosis, fear of medical facility)	Establish lines of communication. Active listening is useful. Establish trusting relationship. Encourage woman to take active part in her care.
	Apathy; display of anger with pregnancy diagnosis	Establish communication and begin counseling. Use active listening techniques.
Educational Needs		
May have questions about pregnancy or may need time to adjust to reality of pregnancy		Establish educational, supporting environment that can be expanded throughout pregnancy.
Social Determinants of Health		
Identifies 2+ individuals with whom she has healthy, supportive relationships	Reports lack of support by parents or close friends and/or isolation (no telephone, no access to reliable transportation)	Provide referrals to community resources. Help woman develop trusting relationships with HCPs.
Family Functioning		
Supportive family she can depend on during difficult times	Reports (or nurse observes) unrealistic expectations, pessimistic attitudes, inadequate support from close family members	Help identify the problems and stressors and encourage healthy communication and coping behaviors.
Economic Status		
Source of income is stable and sufficient to meet basic needs of daily living and medical needs	Limited prenatal care; poor physical health; limited use of healthcare system; unstable economic status	Discuss available resources for health maintenance and the birth. Institute appropriate referral for meeting expanding family's needs (e.g., food stamps).
Stability of Living Environment		
Adequate, stable housing for expanding family's needs	Crowded or unhealthy living conditions; inadequate or undependable child care for newborn following birth for working mothers; questionable supportive environment for newborn	Refer to appropriate community agency. Work with family on self-help ways to improve situation.
	*Possible causes of alterations are identified in parentheses.	†This column provides guidelines for further assessment and initial nursing intervention.

Source: Adapted from London et al. (2017).

Box 33.1
Definition of Terms

The following terms are used in recording the history of prenatal patients:

Abortion: Spontaneous loss or termination of pregnancy that occurs before the end of 20 weeks' gestation or the birth of a fetus–newborn who weighs less than 500 g (Cunningham et al., 2018)

Antepartum: Time between conception and the onset of labor; often used to describe the period during which a woman is pregnant; used interchangeably with ***prenatal***

Gestation: The number of weeks since the first day of the LMP

Gravida*: The number of pregnancies in the woman's lifetime, regardless of duration, including current pregnancy

Intrapartum: Time from the onset of true labor until the birth of the baby and placenta

Multigravida: A woman who is in her second or any subsequent pregnancy

Multipara: A woman who has had two or more births at more than 20 weeks' gestation

Nulligravida: A woman who has never been pregnant

Nullipara: A woman who has had no births at more than 20 weeks' gestation

Para*: Birth after 20 weeks' gestation regardless of whether the baby is born alive or dead

Postpartum: Time from birth until the woman's body returns to an essentially pre-pregnant condition

Postterm labor: Labor that occurs after 42 weeks' gestation

Prenatal: Time between conception and the onset of labor; antepartum

Preterm or premature labor: Labor that occurs after 20 weeks' gestation but before completion of 37 weeks' gestation

Primigravida: A woman who is pregnant for the first time

Primipara: A woman who has had one birth at more than 20 weeks' gestation, regardless of whether the baby was born alive or dead

Stillbirth: A baby born dead after at least 20 weeks' gestation

Term: A word that was formerly used to identify the normal duration of pregnancy. ACOG (2013c, reaffirmed 2017) recommends that the following definitions be used as an alternative:

- **Late preterm:** births that occur before 34 0/7 through 36 6/7 weeks' gestation
- **Early term:** births that occur between 37 weeks 0 days and 38 weeks 6 days
- **Full term:** births that occur between 39 weeks 0 days and 40 weeks 6 days
- **Late term:** births that occur between 41 weeks 0 days and 41 weeks 6 days
- **Postterm:** 42 weeks and 0 days and beyond

*The terms *gravida* and *para* are used in relation to pregnancies, not the number of fetuses. Thus, twins, triplets, and so on, count as one pregnancy and one birth.

Patient Interview

The course of a pregnancy depends on a number of factors, including the woman's pre-pregnancy health, the presence of disease states, the woman's emotional status, and her past healthcare. A thorough history is useful in determining the status of a woman's pre-pregnancy health, as well as identifying risk factors and associated interventions. Terms useful for recording the history of prenatal patients are listed in **Box 33.1** ».

Patient Profile

The history is essentially a screening tool that identifies factors that may place the mother or fetus at risk during the pregnancy. The following information is obtained for each pregnant woman at the first prenatal assessment:

1. ***Current Pregnancy***
   - First day of LMP (Is she sure or unsure of the date? Do her cycles normally occur every 28 days, or do her cycles tend to be longer?)
   - Presence of cramping, bleeding, or spotting since LMP
   - Woman's opinion about the time when conception occurred and when baby is due
   - Woman's attitude toward pregnancy (Is this pregnancy planned? Wanted?)
   - Results of pregnancy tests, if completed
   - Any discomforts since LMP (e.g., nausea, vomiting, urinary frequency, fatigue, or breast tenderness)
2. ***Past Pregnancies***
   - Number of pregnancies
   - Number of abortions, spontaneous or therapeutic
   - Number of living children
   - History of previous pregnancies, length of pregnancy, length of labor and birth, type of birth (vaginal, forceps- or vacuum-assisted, or cesarean), type of anesthesia used (if any), woman's perception of the experience, and complications (antepartum, intrapartum, and postpartum)
   - Neonatal status of previous children: Apgar scores (see Exemplar 33.D, Newborn Care, in this module for a discussion of Apgar scoring), birth weights, general development, complications, and feeding patterns (breast milk or formula)
   - Loss of a child (miscarriage, elective or medically indicated abortion, stillbirth, neonatal death, relinquishment, or death after the neonatal period) (What was the experience like for her? What coping skills helped? How did her partner, if involved, respond?)
   - If Rh negative, was Rh immune globulin received during pregnancy and/or after birth/miscarriage/abortion to prevent sensitization?
   - Prenatal education classes and resources (books)
3. ***Gynecologic History***
   - Date of last Pap smear; any history of abnormal Pap smear; any follow-up therapy completed

- Previous infections: vaginal, cervical, tubal, sexually transmitted (see Exemplar 19.E, Sexually Transmitted Infections, in Module 19, Sexuality)
- Previous surgery (uterine/ovarian)
- Age at menarche
- Regularity, frequency, and duration of menstrual flow
- History of dysmenorrhea
- Sexual history
- Contraceptive history (If birth control pills were used, did pregnancy occur immediately following cessation of pills? If not, how long after?)
- Any issues related to infertility or fertility treatments

4. ***Current Medical History***
   - Weight
   - Blood type and Rh factor, if known
   - General health, including nutrition (dietary practices such as vegetarianism) and regular exercise program (type, frequency, and duration)
   - Any medications currently being taken (including nonprescription, homeopathic, or herbal medications) or taken since the onset of pregnancy
   - Previous or present use of alcohol, tobacco, or caffeine (Ask specifically about the amount of alcohol, cigarettes, and caffeine [specify coffee, tea, cola, and chocolate] consumed each day)
   - Illicit drug use or abuse. (Ask about specific drugs such as cocaine, crack, methamphetamines, and marijuana.) Use of a validated screening tool for substance use or abuse is recommended. The nurse should appropriately refer screen-positive patients for evaluation and treatment.
   - Drug allergies and other allergies (Ask about latex allergies or sensitivities)
   - Potential teratogenic insults, such as viral infections, medications, x-ray examinations, surgery, or cats in the home (possible source of toxoplasmosis)
   - Presence of current physical or mental illness such as diabetes, HTN, cardiovascular disease, or depression
   - Record of immunizations
   - Presence of any abnormal symptoms

5. ***Past Medical History***
   - Childhood diseases
   - Past treatment for any disease condition
   - Surgical procedures
   - Presence of bleeding disorders or tendencies
   - Accidents requiring hospitalizations
   - Blood transfusions

6. ***Family Medical History***
   - Presence of diabetes, cardiovascular disease, cancer, HTN, hematologic disorders, tuberculosis, or preeclampsia–eclampsia
   - Occurrence of multiple births
   - History of congenital diseases or deformities
   - History of mental illness
   - Causes of death of deceased parents or siblings
   - Occurrence of cesarean births and cause, if known

7. ***Religious, Spiritual, and Cultural History***
   - Does the woman want to specify a religious preference on her chart? Does she have any spiritual beliefs or practices that might influence her healthcare or that of her child, such as prohibition against receiving blood products, dietary considerations, or circumcision rites?
   - What practices are important to maintaining her spiritual well-being?
   - Might practices in her culture or that of her partner influence her care or that of her child?

8. ***Occupational History***
   - Occupation
   - Physical demands (Does she stand all day, or are there opportunities to sit and elevate her legs? Any heavy lifting?)
   - Exposure to chemicals or other harmful substances
   - Opportunity for regular meals and breaks for nutritious snacks
   - Provision for maternity or family leave

9. ***Partner's History***
   - Presence of genetic conditions or diseases in partner's or partner's family history, if partner is biologically related to the child
   - Age
   - Significant health problems
   - Previous or current alcohol intake, drug use, or tobacco use
   - Blood type and Rh factor, if partner is biologically related to the child
   - Occupation
   - Educational level; methods by which the partner learns best
   - Attitude toward the pregnancy

10. ***Social History***
    - Age
    - Educational level; methods by which she learns best
    - Race or ethnic group (to identify need for prenatal genetic screening and racially or ethnically related risk factors)
    - Housing; stability of living conditions
    - Economic level
    - Acceptance of pregnancy, whether intended or unintended
    - Any history of emotional or physical deprivation or abuse of herself or children or any abuse in her current relationship (Ask specifically whether she has been hit, slapped, kicked, or hurt within the past year or since she has become pregnant. Ask whether she is afraid of her partner or anyone else. If yes, of whom is she afraid? *Note:* Ask these questions when the woman is alone.)
    - Support systems
    - Personal preferences about the birth (expectations of both the woman and her partner, presence of others, and so on)
    - Plans for care of child following birth
    - Feeding preference for the baby (breast milk or formula?)

Obtaining Data

In many instances, a questionnaire is used to obtain information. The woman should complete the questionnaire in a quiet place with a minimum of distractions. Many HCPs offer the option of the patient completing the questionnaire prior to the initial appointment, either online or through an intake phone call with a nurse. The nurse can obtain further information in an interview, which allows the pregnant woman to clarify her responses to questions and gives the nurse and the woman the opportunity to develop rapport.

The expectant father or partner can be encouraged to attend the prenatal examinations; the individual is often able to contribute to the history. The nurse should encourage partners to use the opportunity to ask questions or express concerns that are important to them.

Prenatal High-Risk Screening

Risk factors are any findings that suggest that the pregnancy may have a negative outcome, for either the woman or her unborn child. Screening for risk factors is an important part of the prenatal assessment. Many risk factors can be identified during the initial assessment; others may be detected during subsequent prenatal visits. It is important to identify high-risk pregnancies early so that appropriate interventions can be started promptly. Not all risk factors threaten a pregnancy equally; thus, many agencies use a scoring sheet to determine the degree of risk. Information must be updated throughout the pregnancy as necessary. A pregnancy may begin as low risk and change to high risk because of complications.

Providers need to be attentive to the signs and symptoms of cardiac disease, especially in women with risk factors. Maternal cardiovascular disease complicates 1–4% of pregnancies in the United States, and it is considered one of the leading causes of nonobstetric maternal death. Congenital heart disease is the most common form of maternal cardiovascular disease complicating pregnancy in the United States. The normal alterations in the circulatory and respiratory systems during pregnancy can have negative effects on the mother with cardiovascular disease and on her developing fetus. There are two major hemodynamic alterations: fall in systemic vascular resistance and increase in cardiac output. Because of the increased risks associated with cardiovascular disease in pregnancy, initial prenatal care should include cardiovascular risk assessment, education regarding the patient's responsibilities for monitoring of associated symptoms, activity modification (if applicable), follow-up with providers, and guidance regarding the anticipated course of pregnancy and delivery. Risk assessment includes history, physical examination, echocardiogram, and electrocardiogram. The frequency of follow-up visits, as well as co-management of the pregnancy, is dependent on the severity of the disease (Waksmonski & Foley, 2020; Waksmonski, LaSala, & Foley, 2019).

Obstetric History

The nurse interviews the patient regarding previous pregnancies to inform the woman's plan of care. A woman who has experienced previous miscarriages or complications of pregnancy may require increased monitoring and a greater level of support than a woman who has already had one or more successful pregnancies without complication.

The terms *gravida* and *para* are used in relation to pregnancies, not to the number of fetuses. Thus, twins, triplets, and other multiples count as one pregnancy and one birth. Miscarriages and fetal losses before viability at 24 weeks of gestation are called *fetal demise*. Those before 20 weeks are called *abortions*.

The following examples illustrate how these terms are applied in clinical situations:

1. Jean Sanchez has one child born at 38 weeks of gestation and is pregnant for the second time. At her initial prenatal visit, the nurse indicates her obstetric history as "gravida 2 para 1 ab 0." Her present pregnancy terminates at 16 weeks of gestation. She is now "gravida 2 para 1 ab 1."
2. Tracy Hopkins is pregnant for the fourth time. At home, she has a child who was born at term. Her second pregnancy ended at 10 weeks of gestation. She then gave birth to twins at 35 weeks of gestation. One of the twins died soon after birth. At her antepartum assessment, the nurse records her obstetric history as "gravida 4 para 2 ab 1."

To avoid confusion, it is best for practicing nurses to clarify the recording system used at their facilities.

GTPAL can be a helpful acronym for detailing the system (**Figure 33.23** »):

G Number of pregnancies (Gravida)

T Number of Term babies born—that is, the number of babies born after 37 weeks of gestation

P Number of Preterm babies born—that is, the number of babies born after 20 weeks but before the completion of 37 weeks of gestation

A Number of pregnancies ending in either spontaneous or therapeutic Abortion

L Number of currently Living children.

Name	Gravida	Term	Preterm	Abortions	Living Children
Jean Sanchez	2	1	0	1	1
Tracy Hopkins	4	1	2	1	2

Figure 33.23 » The **GTPAL** approach provides detailed information about a woman's pregnancy history.

Source: George Dodson/Pearson Education, Inc.

SAFETY ALERT It is recommended that assessment of previous pregnancies occurs while the partner is not present and to refrain from sharing that information. Some women may not disclose previous pregnancies to their partners. Revealing this information without permission would violate the woman's privacy and confidentiality.

Determining Due Date

Families generally want to know the "due date," or the date around which childbirth will occur. Historically, the due date has been called the estimated date of confinement. However, the concept of confinement is rather negative, and many caregivers avoid it by referring to the due date as the estimated date of delivery. Even then, childbirth educators often stress that babies are not "delivered" like a package; they are born. In keeping with a view that emphasizes the normalcy of the process, this text refers to the due date as the estimated date of birth, or EDB.

To calculate the EDB, it is helpful to know the date of the woman's LMP. However, some women have episodes of irregular bleeding or fail to keep track of menstrual cycles. Thus, other techniques also help determine how far along a woman is in her pregnancy—that is, at how many weeks of gestation she is. These techniques include evaluating uterine size, determining when quickening occurs, and auscultating FHR with a Doppler device or ultrasound and, later, with a fetoscope.

The most common method of determining the EDB is to use the **Nägele rule**. To use this method, one begins with the first day of the LMP, subtracts 3 months, and adds 7 days. For example:

First day of LMP	November 21
Subtract 3 months	−3 months
	August 21
Add 7 days	+7 days
EDB	August 28

It is simpler to change the months to numeric terms:

November 21 becomes	11-21
Subtract 3 months	−3
	8-21
Add 7 days	+7
EDB	8-28

A gestation calculator or wheel permits the caregiver to calculate the EDB even more quickly (**Figure 33.24** »).

If a woman with a history of menses every 28 days remembers her LMP and was not taking oral contraceptives before becoming pregnant, the Nägele rule may be a fairly accurate determiner of the EDB. However, ovulation usually occurs 14 days before the onset of the next menses, not 14 days after the previous menses. Consequently, if the woman's cycle is irregular or is more than 28 days long, the time of ovulation may be delayed. If she has been using oral contraceptives, ovulation may be delayed for several weeks following her last menses. Then, too, a postpartum woman who is breastfeeding may resume ovulating but be amenorrheic for a time, making calculation impossible. Thus, the Nägele rule, although helpful, is not foolproof.

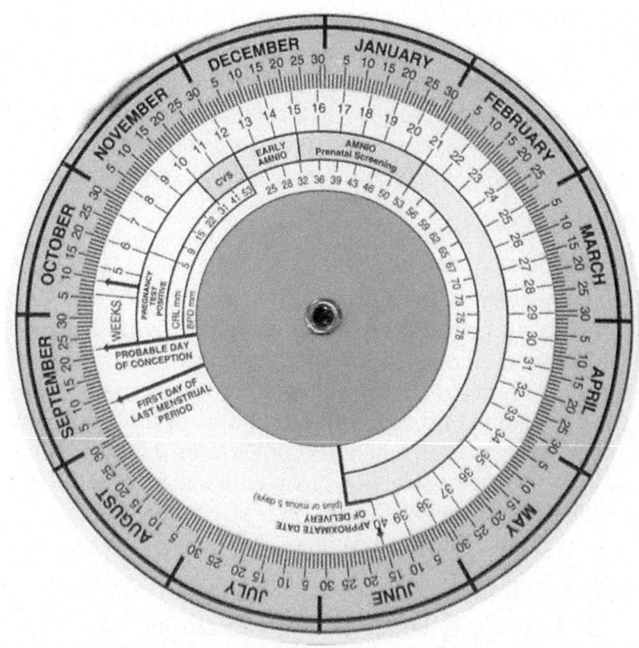

Figure 33.24 » The EDB wheel can be used to calculate the due date. To use it, place the arrow labeled "1st day of last period" on the date of the woman's last menstrual period. Then read the EDB at the arrow labeled "40." In this case, the LMP is September 8 and the EDB is June 16.

It is important to determine the EDB as accurately as possible, as the gestational age at which many prenatal screenings are done is extremely important. It is also essential for evaluating fetal growth and deciding on the timing of intervention for postterm pregnancies. The most accurate estimation of gestational age is a crown–rump length measurement, performed at less than 9 weeks, consistent with LMP dating. If there is a discrepancy of more than 5 days between early ultrasound and LMP, the pregnancy is dated by the ultrasound (ACOG, 2017e).

Physical Examination

The physical examination begins with assessment of vital signs; then the woman's body is examined. The pelvic examination is performed last. Before the examination, the woman should provide a clean urine specimen. When her bladder is empty, the woman is more comfortable during the pelvic examination and the examiner can palpate the pelvic organs more easily. After the woman has emptied her bladder, the nurse asks her to disrobe and gives her a gown and sheet or some other protective covering.

Increasing numbers of nurses (e.g., CNMs and other nurses in advanced practice) are prepared to perform complete physical examinations. The nurse who does not yet possess advanced assessment skills can assess the woman's vital signs, explain the procedures to allay apprehension, position her for examination, and assist the examiner as necessary. Nurses are responsible for operating at the expected standard for their skill and knowledge base.

Thoroughness and a systematic procedure are the most important considerations when performing the physical portion of a prenatal examination. To promote completeness, the

Prenatal Assessment feature is organized in three columns that address the areas to be assessed and the normal findings, the variations or alterations that may be observed and their possible causes, and nursing responses to the data. The nurse should be aware that certain organs and systems are assessed concurrently with others during the physical portion of the examination.

Uterine Assessment

Physical Examination

When a woman is examined in the first 10 to 12 weeks of pregnancy and her uterine size is compatible with her menstrual history, uterine size may be the single most important clinical method for dating her pregnancy. In many cases, however, women do not seek prenatal care until well into their second trimester, when it becomes more difficult to evaluate specific uterine size. In women with obesity, it is difficult to determine uterine size early in a pregnancy because the uterus is more difficult to palpate.

Fundal Height

Fundal height may be used as an indicator of uterine size, although this method is less accurate late in pregnancy. A centimeter tape measure is used to measure the distance abdominally from the top of the symphysis pubis to the top of the uterine fundus (the McDonald method) (**Figure 33.25** »). Fundal height in centimeters correlates well with weeks of gestation after 20 weeks. The normal variation is gestational weeks plus or minus 2 cm. Thus, at 26 weeks' gestation, fundal height is 24 to 28 cm, depending on fetal position and maternal body habitus. The woman should have voided within 30 minutes of the exam and should lie in the same position each time. In the third trimester, variations in fetal weight decrease the accuracy of fundal height measurements. A lag in progression of measurements of fundal height from month to month and from week to week may signal a fetus that is SGA. A sudden increase in fundal height may indicate twins or hydramnios.

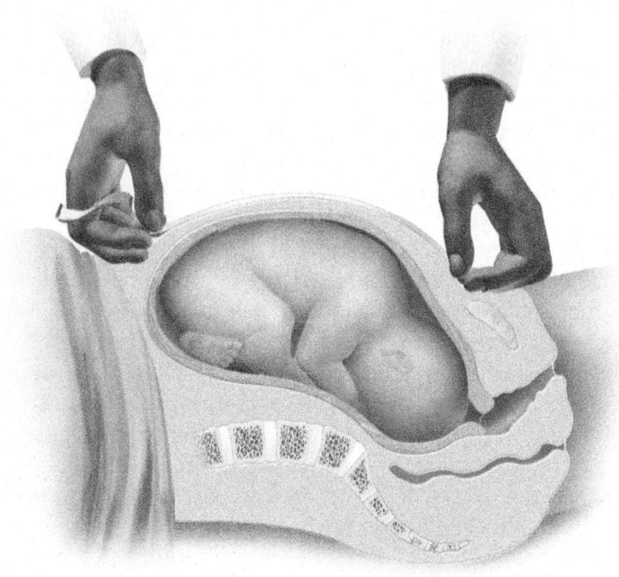

Figure 33.25 » A cross-sectional view of fetal position when the McDonald method is used to assess the fundal height.

Small for gestational age is defined as a fetal weight estimated by ultrasound or a baby's actual birth weight that is less than the 10th percentile for gestational age. When no cause for this can be identified and the fetus or newborn shows no evidence of compromise, it may be concluded that it is constitutionally small. When a fetus is SGA in the setting of some pathology, this is called *intrauterine growth restriction (IUGR)*. Causes include congenital anomalies, exposure to teratogens, maternal smoking and substance abuse, malnutrition, abnormal formation of the placenta, and decreased placental perfusion (King et al., 2019).

Leopold Maneuvers

Leopold maneuvers are a system of palpating the uterus externally, starting at the fundus and moving downward, to assess the baby's position and orientation. The accuracy of Leopold maneuvers can be impacted by maternal body habitus, the presence of uterine fibroids, multiple gestations, or polyhydramnios. Prior to performing the maneuvers, the HCP should instruct the mother to empty her bladder. The mother is then positioned supine, with her head slightly elevated. In the first maneuver, the examiner grips the fundus with both hands and identifies the fetal parts in the fundus. The second maneuver consists of palpating the sides of the uterus to locate the fetal back and legs. The third maneuver consists of grasping the lower portion of the uterus to identify the fetal part that is lowest in the pelvis, called the *presenting part*. It should be the head in the third trimester. The fourth maneuver consists of identifying the position of the fetal brow or occiput to determine the degree of flexion or extension of the head (Gabbe et al., 2016).

Assessment of Fetal Development

Assessment of fetal health and development is necessary at various points during pregnancy. Both suggestive findings (such as the mother reporting movement) and objective findings (such as fetal heartbeat and ultrasound) are used. Assessment findings are compared with gestational age and developmental milestones to develop a plan of care.

Quickening

The first perception of fetal movement by the mother is termed *quickening*. Quickening may indicate that the fetus is nearing 20 weeks' gestation. However, quickening may be experienced between 16 and 22 weeks' gestation, so this method is not completely accurate.

Fetal Heartbeat

A Doppler fetal monitor (**Figure 33.26** ») is a hand-held ultrasound device used to assess fetal heartbeat early in pregnancy, between 8 and 12 weeks' gestation. Fetoscopes, although rarely used, can assess fetal heartbeat between 16 and 20 weeks' gestation.

Ultrasound

In the first trimester, ultrasound scanning can detect a gestational sac as early as 5 to 6 weeks after the LMP, fetal heart activity by 6 to 7 weeks, and fetal breathing movement by 10 to 11 weeks of pregnancy. Crown-to-rump measurements can be made to assess fetal age until the fetal head can be visualized clearly. Biparietal diameter (BPD) can then be used. The BPD measures the diameter across the fetus's

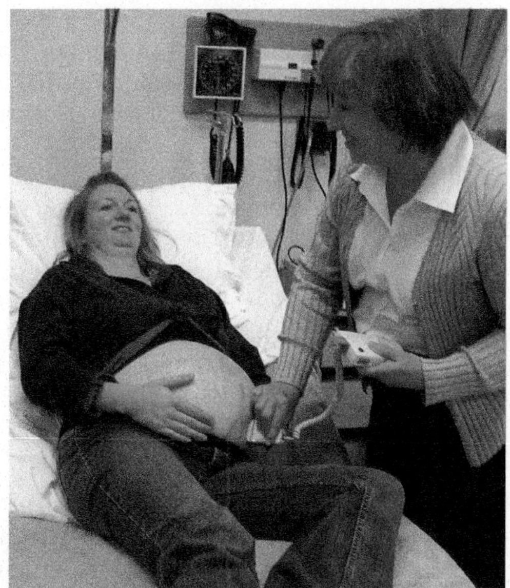

Figure 33.26 ›› Listening to the fetal heartbeat with a Doppler device.

Source: Pearson Education, Inc.

skull from one parietal bone to the other. BPD measurements can be made by approximately 12 to 13 weeks and are most accurate between 20 and 30 weeks, when rapid growth in the BPD occurs. Measurements and visualization of structures in the fetal body are used to determine appropriate growth, development, and function.

Assessment of Pelvic Adequacy (Clinical Pelvimetry)

Clinical pelvimetry is a vaginal examination that may be performed by a physician or advanced practice nurse to assess the pelvis on initial physical examination or later, when effects of hormones are greatest and the provider can evaluate fetal size. However, pelvic adequacy can be reliably determined only by a trial of labor. Both radiographic and physical assessments of pelvic adequacy are poor predictors of the course of labor and birth (World Health Organization [WHO], 2018a).

Prenatal Tests

A number of tests may be used to detect hCG during pregnancy and to monitor the safety of the pregnant woman and child. These tests are summarized in **Table 33.1 ››**. Some are discussed in greater detail in Exemplar 33.A, Antepartum Care, in this module. Nursing care of a woman undergoing prenatal testing includes making sure she understands the reasons for the test (and ensuring informed consent is obtained) and providing support for the woman during the test. The nurse also works with the healthcare team to promote the safety of both the woman and the fetus during all phases of the test.

TABLE 33.1 Summary of Selected Antenatal Surveillance and Screening

Goal	Test	Timing
To confirm intrauterine pregnancy and viability	Ultrasound: gestational sac volume	5 or 6 weeks after LMP by transvaginal ultrasound
To determine gestational age	Ultrasound: crown-to-rump length	6–10 weeks' gestation
	Ultrasound: BPD and fetal body measurement rations	Greater than or equal to 14 weeks
To detect congenital anomalies and problems	Nuchal translucency testing	11–13 weeks' gestation
	Ultrasound	Greater than or equal to 18 weeks
	Chorionic villus sampling	10–12 weeks' gestation
	Amniocentesis	After 15 weeks' gestation
	First-trimester combined test	11–13 weeks' gestation
	Full integrated screen	10–13 weeks' gestation; repeated at 15–18 weeks, if needed
	Cell-free fetal DNA	From 9 weeks onward
To determine placental location	Ultrasound	18–20 weeks initially; repeated at 28–32 weeks for reevaluation, if needed
To diagnose cardiac problems	Fetal echocardiography	Second and third trimesters
To assess fetal status	Biophysical profile	Approximately 23 weeks to birth
	Maternal assessment of fetal activity	Approximately 28 weeks to birth
	Nonstress test	Approximately 28 weeks to birth
To evaluate fetal growth	Ultrasound: BPD	Greater than or equal to 14 weeks
	Ultrasound: fetal body measurement ratios	About 23–42 weeks' gestation
	Ultrasound: estimated fetal weight	
To assess fetal lung maturity with amniocentesis or vaginal pool sampled amniotic fluid	L/S ratio	32–39 weeks
	Phosphatidylglycerol	32–39 weeks
	Phosphatidylcholine	32–39 weeks
	Lamellar body counts	32–39 weeks
To determine fetal presentation	Ultrasound	At term or on admission for labor and birth

Source: Adapted from London et al. (2017).

Case Study » Part 2

When Mrs. Halleck returns to the clinic at 32 weeks' gestation, she says, "I feel like I need to pee all the time." She also states that she doesn't feel like exercising as much as she used to. She used to go to the gym three or four times a week, but now she only goes on the weekends, saying "I just don't feel like it. I keep getting these dull headaches, and all I seem to be able to do is sit on the sofa and eat and go to the bathroom." On examination, Mrs. Halleck has gained 12 pounds since her last appointment and her current weight is 150 lb. Her vital signs are TO 98.6°F, BP 139/90 mmHg, P 84 beats/min, R 21/min. Otherwise, her examination is normal. When the nurse asks Mrs. Halleck how her family has responded to her pregnancy, she replies, "Everyone's been great except my mother. She's only 45. She says she's too young to have a grandchild, and that I'm too young to have a baby." Mrs. Halleck looks away as she says this, adding, "I really wish I had her support."

Clinical Reasoning Questions Level I

1. How should the nurse respond to Mrs. Halleck's statements about her mother?
2. What interventions can the nurse recommend to help this patient with her nausea?
3. What interventions can the nurse recommend to Mrs. Halleck in response to her complaint about urinary frequency?

Clinical Reasoning Questions Level II

4. Which findings should concern the nurse caring for Mrs. Halleck?
5. *Referring to Exemplar 16.H, Hypertensive Disorders of Pregnancy, in Module 16, Perfusion:* What other signs and symptoms of preeclampsia should the nurse assess in Mrs. Halleck?
6. *Referring to Exemplar 16.H, Hypertensive Disorders in Pregnancy, in Module 16, Perfusion:* What clinical therapies would be appropriate for Mrs. Halleck if the nurse observes edema in her extremities in addition to her high blood pressure?

Independent Interventions

Although the nurse's primary role in the first trimester centers around health promotion and patient education, the nurse assesses patients at each encounter. Assessment at each healthcare interaction is necessary to screen for any risks to the woman and fetus and to be able to minimize any complications that present and promote healthy outcomes for both mother and baby. Holistic care that is congruent with the mother's cultural beliefs and practices is important to promoting the therapeutic relationship and making the experience as easy and enjoyable as possible for the mother and her family. Interventions covered in this section relate to fetal safety and some of the more common discomforts of pregnancy. Additional interventions are discussed in Exemplars 33.A and 33.B in this module.

Prenatal Education

Prenatal education programs provide important opportunities to share information about pregnancy and childbirth and to enhance the parents' decision-making skills. The content of each class is generally directed by the overall goals of the program. For example, in classes that aim to provide preconception information, preparations for becoming pregnant and optimizing the woman's health status are the major topics. Other classes may be directed toward childbirth choices available today, preparation of the mother and her partner for pregnancy and birth, preparation for a vaginal birth after a previous cesarean birth, and preparation for the birth by specific people such as grandparents or siblings. The nurse who knows the types of prenatal programs available in the community can direct expectant parents to programs that meet their special needs and learning goals.

From the expectant parents' point of view, class content is best presented in chronology with the pregnancy. It is important to begin the classes by finding out what each parent wants to learn and including a discussion of related choices. Classes that provide an environment supportive of practicing newly learned techniques and the freedom to ask questions and receive explanations are beneficial in helping class participants obtain these goals (Davidson et al., 2020).

Relief of the Common Discomforts of Pregnancy

Common discomforts associated with pregnancy relate to physical changes that occur during each trimester. Table 33.2 in Exemplar 33.A in this module outlines common discomforts of pregnancy and helpful self-care measures. Discomforts associated with pregnancy can increase a woman's anxiety. The nurse's role is to help the pregnant woman understand the source and cause of the discomfort and to help ease it and any related anxiety.

Nausea and Vomiting

Many pregnant women experience nausea and vomiting as early symptoms that appear sometime after the first missed menstrual period and usually cease by the fourth missed menstrual period. Some women develop an aversion to specific foods, many experience nausea on arising in the morning, and others experience nausea throughout the day or in the evening.

The exact cause of nausea and vomiting in pregnancy (NVP) is unknown, but it is thought to be multifactorial. An elevated hCG level is believed to be a major factor, but changes in carbohydrate metabolism, fatigue, and emotional factors also may play a role. Research suggests that pregnant women should start taking a multivitamin before reaching 6 weeks' gestation to reduce the effects of NVP (ACOG, 2018e).

In addition to the self-care measures identified in Table 33.2, certain complementary therapies may be useful. For example, many women find that acupressure applied to pressure points in the wrists is helpful. Ginger also may relieve NVP (see Focus on Integrative Health: Ginger for Morning Sickness). Pyridoxine (vitamin B_6) or vitamin B_6 plus doxylamine (Unisom), an OTC antihistamine, is considered a first-line treatment. This is now available by prescription as a combined tablet under the brand name Diclegis. Antihistamine H1-receptor blockers, phenothiazines, and antinausea medications such as promethazine (Phenergan), metoclopramide (Reglan), and ondansetron (Zofran) are considered safe and effective for treating refractory cases. In severe cases, methylprednisolone, a steroid, may be used, but as a last resort because it poses a potential risk to the fetus (ACOG, 2018e).

Patient teaching for nausea and vomiting includes signs of dehydration (such as dry mouth and concentrated urine). The mother should be encouraged to call her provider if she is unable to keep food or fluids down for more than 12 hours or shows any signs of dehydration.

Focus on Integrative Health

Ginger for Morning Sickness

Women who experience NVP often try alternative approaches to relieve their symptoms because they are reluctant to take medication for fear of harming their fetus. Research supports that the use of ginger is comparable with vitamin B_6 for the treatment of mild to moderate nausea and vomiting (Sharifzadeh et al., 2018). It has few side effects when taken in small doses (National Center for Complementary and Integrative Health, 2016). Ginger is available in a variety of forms, including the fresh root, capsules, tea, candy, cookies, crystals, inhaled powdered ginger, and sugared ginger.

Urinary Frequency

Urinary frequency, a common discomfort of pregnancy, occurs in the first trimester and again during the third trimester because of pressure of the enlarging uterus on the bladder. Although frequency is considered normal during the first and third trimesters, the woman is advised to report to her HCP signs of bladder infection such as pain, burning with voiding, or blood in the urine. Fluid intake should never be decreased to prevent frequency. The woman needs to maintain an adequate fluid intake—at least 2000 mL (eight to ten 8-oz glasses) per day. The nurse should also encourage her to empty her bladder frequently (about every 2 hours while awake).

Backache

Nearly 70% of women experience backache during pregnancy (King et al., 2019). Backache is due primarily to exaggeration of the lumbosacral curve that occurs as the uterus enlarges and becomes heavier. Maintaining good posture and using proper body mechanics throughout pregnancy can help prevent backache. The pregnant woman is advised to avoid bending over at the waist to pick up objects and should bend from the knees instead. She should place her feet 12 to 18 inches apart to maintain body balance. If the woman uses work surfaces that require her to bend, the nurse can advise her to adjust the height of the surfaces.

Collaborative Therapies

Members of the interprofessional team collaborate to coordinate high-quality, safe, and patient-centered evidence-based care. Team members may include perinatologists, neonatologists, certified nurse-midwives, women's health practitioners, obstetricians, pediatricians, dietitians, social workers, mental HCPs, pharmacists, endocrinologists, cardiologists, lactation consultants, and registered nurses.

Pharmacologic Therapy

Careful assessment and use of medications play a role in protecting the safety of and promoting positive outcomes for the mother and fetus. Patients with chronic illnesses (especially diabetes, cardiovascular or respiratory disease, HIV, or serious mental illness) need to discuss their treatment and pregnancy with all members of their healthcare team. Nurses and other providers will need to provide additional teaching to pregnant women with chronic illness over the course of the pregnancy. Careful and consistent collaboration among all members of the interprofessional team is needed to ensure maternal and fetal health and well-being.

The use of medications during pregnancy, including prescriptions, OTC drugs, and herbal remedies, is of great concern because maternal drug exposure is associated with congenital anomalies. Many pregnant women need medication for therapeutic purposes, such as the treatment of infections, allergies, or other pathologic processes. In these situations, the problem can be complex. Known teratogenic agents are not prescribed and usually can be replaced with medications that are considered safe. Even when a woman is highly motivated to avoid taking any medications, she may have taken potentially teratogenic medications before her pregnancy was confirmed, especially if she has an irregular menstrual cycle.

The greatest potential for gross abnormalities in the fetus occurs during the first trimester of pregnancy, when fetal organs are first developing. Many factors influence teratogenic effects, including the specific type of teratogen and the dose, the stage of embryonic development, and the genetic sensitivity of the mother and fetus. For example, the commonly prescribed acne medication isotretinoin (Accutane) is associated with a high incidence of spontaneous abortion and congenital malformations if taken early in pregnancy.

To provide information for caregivers and patients, the FDA has developed a labeling system for medications administered during pregnancy. Medications were previously listed under a five-category system (Categories A, B, C, D, and X) to assist patients and caregivers to make informed decisions about the safety of medication to treat conditions during pregnancy. In 2014, the FDA amended its regulations governing the labeling to prescription drugs and biologic products for women who are pregnant or lactating. These regulations became effective in June 2015. According to the new requirements, three categories have been specified (FDA, 2014):

- ***Pregnancy.*** If the drug is absorbed systemically, labeling must include a risk summary of adverse developmental outcomes that includes data from all relevant sources, including human, animal, and/or pharmacologic information. The labeling must also contain relevant information to help HCPs counsel women about the use of the drug during pregnancy. In addition, if there is a pregnancy exposure registry for the drug, the labeling should include a specific statement to that effect followed by contact information needed to obtain information about the registry or to enroll.
- ***Lactation.*** For drugs that are absorbed systemically, labeling must include a summary of the risks of using a drug when the woman is lactating. To the extent that information is available, the summary should include relevant information about the drug's presence in human milk, the effects of the drug on milk production, and the effects of the drug on the breastfed child.
- ***Females and Males of Reproductive Potential.*** This section must include information when human or animal data suggests drug-associated effects on fertility. It should also specify when contraception or pregnancy testing is required or recommended, such as before, during, or after the drug therapy.

Although the first trimester is the critical period for teratogenesis, some medications are known to have a teratogenic effect when taken in the second and third trimesters. For example, tetracycline taken in late pregnancy is commonly associated with staining of teeth in children and has been shown to depress skeletal growth, especially in premature babies. Sulfonamides taken in the last few weeks of pregnancy are known to compete with bilirubin attachment of protein-binding sites, increasing the risk of jaundice in the newborn (Niebyl, Weber, & Briggs, 2016).

Pregnant women need to avoid all medications—prescribed, homeopathic, or OTC—if possible. If no alternative exists, it is wisest to select a well-known medication rather than a newer drug whose potential teratogenic effects may not be known. When possible, the oral form of a drug should be used, and it should be prescribed in the lowest possible therapeutic dose for the shortest time possible. The advantage of using a particular medication must outweigh the risk. Any medication with possible teratogenic effects is best avoided.

Nonpharmacologic Therapy and Complementary Health Approaches

Nonpharmacologic therapies are considered safe and effective for use during pregnancy for women with depression, chronic headaches, sleep disturbances, back pain, and NVP. Examples include relaxation therapy, physical therapy, massage therapy, cognitive-behavioral therapy, and hydrotherapy. Many women use complementary and alternative medicine (CAM)—such as homeopathy, herbal therapy, acupressure, acupuncture, biofeedback, therapeutic touch, massage, and chiropractic—as part of a holistic approach to their healthcare regimen. Nurses are in a unique position to bridge the gap between conventional therapies and CAM therapies. As patient advocates, nurses are able to provide patients with the information needed to make informed decisions about their health and healthcare. Using a nonjudgmental approach, the nurse should inquire about the use of CAM as part of a routine antepartum assessment. It is important that nurses working with pregnant women and their families develop a general understanding of the more commonly used therapies to be able to answer questions and provide resources as needed.

It is important for the pregnant woman to understand that herbs are considered to be dietary supplements and are not regulated as prescription or OTC drugs by the FDA. In general, it is best to advise pregnant women not to ingest any herbs, except ginger, during the first trimester of pregnancy. The website of the National Center for Complementary and Integrative Health is a reliable source for information about herbs, homeopathic remedies, and other alternative options.

Lifespan Considerations

Although pregnancy is a normal process for many women, it can carry increased risk for adolescents and women over age 35. These special populations require additional considerations throughout the childbearing process. Considerations may include additional testing, monitoring, and the assessment of psychosocial needs.

Adolescent Pregnancy

Over the past decade, U.S. adolescent birthrates have steadily decreased; however, the rate is substantially higher than in other Western industrialized countries (CDC, 2019a). As recently as 2017, a total of 194,377 babies were born to females age 15 to 19 years, for a birth rate of 18.8 (down from 24.2 in 2014) per 1000 women in this age group (CDC, 2019a). This represents a decrease of approximately 55,000 births per year.

Adolescent pregnancy is a health and social issue with no single cause or cure. For the adolescent, pregnancy comes at a time when her physical development and the developmental tasks of adolescence are incomplete. She may not be prepared physically, psychologically, or economically for parenthood. Thus, both she and her child are at high risk for a number of adverse outcomes. Compared with women of similar socioeconomic status (SES) who postpone childbearing, teen mothers are less likely to finish high school, less likely to go to college, more likely to be single, less likely to receive child support, and more likely to require public assistance. Babies of adolescent mothers are at an increased risk for preterm birth, low birth weight, and newborn/infant mortality. In addition, children of teen mothers tend to score lower on assessments of knowledge, language development, and cognition. They are also more likely to grow up without a father. In addition, children of adolescent mothers are at an increased risk for abuse and neglect (Udo, Lewis, Tobin, & Ickovics, 2016).

Pregnancy over Age 35

An increasing number of women are choosing to have their first baby after age 35. Many factors contribute to this trend, including the following:

- The availability of effective birth control methods
- The expanded roles and career options available to women
- The increased number of women obtaining advanced education, pursuing careers, and delaying parenthood until they are established professionally
- The increased incidence of later marriage and second marriage
- The high cost of living, which causes some young couples to delay childbearing until they are more secure financially
- The increased availability of specialized fertilization procedures, which offers opportunities for women who had previously been considered infertile.

There are advantages to having a first baby after the age of 35. Single women or couples who delay childbearing until they are older tend to be well educated and financially secure. Usually, their decision to have a baby was deliberately and thoughtfully made. Because of their life experiences, they are also more aware of the realities of having a child than younger women, and they recognize what it means to have a baby at their age. This delay in family allows for women to pursue advanced educational degrees and prepare financially for the impact children will have on their lives. Some women are ready to make a change in their lives, desiring to stay home with a new baby. Those who plan to continue working outside the home are typically able to afford good child care.

No matter what their age, most expectant individuals and couples have concerns regarding the well-being of the fetus and their ability to parent. The older couple has additional concerns related to their age, especially if they are over 40. Some couples are concerned about whether they will have enough energy to care for a new baby. Of greater concern is their ability to deal with the needs of the older child as they themselves age.

The financial concerns of an older couple are usually different from those of a younger couple. The older couple is generally more financially secure than the younger couple. However, when their "baby" is ready for college, the older couple may be near retirement and might not have the means to provide for their child.

While considering their financial future and future retirement, the older couple may be forced to face their own mortality. Certainly this is not uncommon in midlife, but instead of confronting this issue at 40 to 45 years of age or later, the older expectant couple may confront the issue several years earlier as they consider what will happen as their child grows.

The older couple facing pregnancy following a late or second marriage or after therapy for infertility may find themselves somewhat isolated socially. They may feel "different" because they are often the only couple in their peer group expecting their first baby. In fact, many of their peers are likely to be parents of adolescents or young adults and may be grandparents as well.

The response of older couples who already have children to learning that the woman is pregnant may vary greatly depending on whether the pregnancy was planned or unexpected. Other factors influencing their response include the attitudes of the couple's children, family, and friends to the pregnancy; the impact on their lifestyle; and the financial implications of having another child. Sometimes couples who had previously been married to other mates will choose to have a child together. The concept of blended family applies to situations in which "her" children, "his" children, and "their" children come together as a new family group.

The woman who has delayed pregnancy may be concerned about the limited amount of time that she has to bear children. When pregnancy does not occur as quickly as she hoped, the older woman may become increasingly anxious as time slips away on her "biological clock." When an older woman becomes pregnant but experiences a spontaneous abortion, her grief for the loss of her unborn child is exacerbated by her anxiety about her ability to conceive again in the time remaining to her.

Healthcare professionals may treat the older expectant couple differently than they would a younger couple. Older women may be offered more medical procedures, such as amniocentesis and ultrasound, than younger women. An older woman may be prevented from using a birthing room or birthing center even if she is healthy because her age is considered to put her at risk.

Medical risks for the pregnant woman over age 35 are discussed in Exemplar 33.A, Antepartum Care, in this module.

Case Study » Part 3

Mrs. Halleck is at the clinic for a weekly follow-up appointment. She reports that she has been taking her blood pressure at home, and her readings during the past 2 weeks have been consistently around 130/85 mmHg. On examination, her weight is 151 lb, TO 98.5°F, BP 131/84 mmHg, P 85 beats/min, R 20/min. Mrs. Halleck reports that she is very stressed about her blood pressure. She has already lost a baby and she is afraid she may lose this one. In addition, as a relatively young teacher, she does not have a lot of sick time built up and if she cannot return to work, she doesn't know how she and her husband will be able to pay their bills. "My parents won't help," she says, "My mother is still more worried about her image than she is about me." Mrs. Halleck begins to cry and states, "I cry all the time now. I can't sleep. My husband says he doesn't know what to do with me. I knew we should've waited before we tried to have another baby!"

Clinical Thinking Questions Level I

1. What is the priority for care for Mrs. Halleck at this time?
2. Based on the history of her pregnancy and the findings at this visit, what screenings do you anticipate the HCP will order for this patient?
3. What do you think the nurse's responsibility to Mr. Halleck is right now?

Clinical Thinking Questions Level II

4. What independent nursing interventions can the nurse implement to assist Mrs. Halleck at this time?
5. *Referring to Exemplar 28.C, Peripartum Depression, in Module 28, Mood and Affect:* What risk factors does Mrs. Halleck have for postpartum depression?
6. *Referring to Exemplar 28.C, Peripartum Depression, in Module 28, Mood and Affect:* What could the nurse do to assess Mrs. Halleck for possible depression with peripartum onset?

REVIEW The Concept of Reproduction

RELATE Link the Concepts

Linking the concept of reproduction with the concept of family:

1. Identify specific examples that demonstrate how the childbearing family is meeting developmental tasks of pregnancy.
2. Discuss family adaptation to pregnancy.
3. Describe the impact of family stressors on pregnancy.

Linking the concept of reproduction with the concept of nutrition:

4. Develop health promotion strategies to promote optimal nutrition during pregnancy, postpartum, and throughout the first year of life.
5. Analyze the impact of nutritional deficits on birth outcomes.
6. Identify motivational strategies to improve nutritional status throughout the childbearing period.

Linking the concept of reproduction with the concept of perfusion:

7. Analyze fetal assessments to determine placental perfusion and fetal well-being.
8. Discuss the impact of poor perfusion on maternal–fetal outcomes.
9. Prioritize nursing care according to severity of postpartum hemorrhage.

READY Go to Volume 3: Clinical Nursing Skills

REFER Go to Pearson MyLab Nursing and eText

- MiniModule: Twins
- Chart 1: Organ Development in the Embryo and Fetus
- Chart 2: Differential Diagnosis of Pregnancy—Subjective Changes
- Chart 3: Differential Diagnosis of Pregnancy—Objective Changes
- Chart 4: Parental Reactions to Pregnancy

REFLECT Apply Your Knowledge

Mrs. Patterson, 41, is a G1P0 with a history of infertility. She currently works as an account manager for a pharmaceutical company and has been promoted to International Sales Director. She typically works long hours and must travel on occasion. She and her husband, 43, married for 15 years, are anticipating the arrival of their first child, but have expressed some concerns. Mrs. Patterson's height is 167.6 cm (5′ 6″); weight, 64.9 kg (143 lb); and fundal height, 26 cm; ultrasound results show an intrauterine pregnancy at 25 weeks' gestation. No fetal abnormalities were noted. She has no existing medical diagnoses. Mrs. Patterson voices concerns about balancing motherhood with her career. She states that her husband is supportive but recognizes that a new child may alter their routine and lifestyle. Mrs. Patterson also states that she is worried that her busy schedule may compromise the pregnancy.

1. What are the priority concerns for Mrs. Patterson?
2. Given the current findings, what interventions would be most therapeutic?
3. What resources might be appropriate for this patient?
4. What independent nursing interventions can the nurse implement to assist Mrs. Patterson at this time?

» Exemplar 33.A Antepartum Care

Exemplar Learning Outcomes

33.A Summarize antepartum care of the pregnant woman.

- Summarize relief of the common discomforts of pregnancy.
- Describe commonly occurring alterations related to pregnancy.
- Summarize maternal and fetal risk factors related to pregnancy.
- Compare diagnostic tests used to assess fetal well-being.
- Describe factors that influence maternal nutrition and weight gain.
- Differentiate considerations related to the assessment and care of pregnant adolescents and women over age 35.
- Illustrate the nursing process in providing culturally competent care to the pregnant woman and her family.

Exemplar Key Terms

Amniocentesis, *2270*
Contraction stress test (CST), *2269*
Daily Nutritional Goals, *2271*
Dietary Reference Intakes (DRIs), *2277*
Fetal movement record, *2264*
Folic acid, *2260*
Gestational diabetes mellitus (GDM), *2261*
Kegel exercises, *2289*
Lactase deficiency, *2275*
Lacto-ovovegetarians, *2274*
Lactose intolerance, *2275*
Lactovegetarians, *2274*
Nonstress test (NST), *2267*
Pelvic tilt, *2287*
Penta screen, *2271*
Pica, *2273*
Quadruple screen, *2271*
Ultrasound, *2265*
Vegans, *2274*

Overview

Antepartum describes the period of pregnancy before childbirth. During this time, the woman experiences many physical and psychologic changes and adaptations. These changes, and the adjustment to them, causes the woman to have many questions. The priority role for the nurse is to have an understanding of the physiology of the adaptations associated with pregnancy and to provide the woman with education and anticipatory guidance.

Among these alterations are common discomforts of pregnancy, such as nausea and vomiting, fatigue, and urinary frequency. The nurse should understand the common causes of these discomforts and provide the woman with education and suggestions for relief of discomfort. Additionally, the nurse should be aware of potential alterations in pregnancy such as gestational diabetes, gestational HTN, and anemia. The nurse should educate the woman on the warning signs of these alterations and advise when to seek care from her provider. Common discomforts of pregnancy, alterations of pregnancy, and warning signs are covered in detail in the following sections.

Relief of the Common Discomforts of Pregnancy

Table 33.2 » provides an overview of common discomforts associated with each of the three trimesters. The level of discomfort varies, and HCPs should not dismiss any reports of discomfort from pregnant women. Some common discomforts (such as dyspnea and ankle edema) can, in some instances, signal something more serious. Women of color in particular are in danger of having their concerns dismissed. Black women are three to four times more likely to die from pregnancy-related complications than white women, contributing to the current high maternal mortality rates in the United States (American Heart Association, 2019; CDC, 2020c). Nurses who are responsive to their patients' concerns and who provide timely patient education and assessment promote positive health outcomes for both the mother and the fetus.

As the mother progresses through the pregnancy, patient teaching should focus on changes and potential discomforts that might be encountered in the next month or trimester. Inquire about what complementary therapies or traditional

TABLE 33.2 Self-Care Measures for Common Discomforts of Pregnancy

Discomfort	Influencing Factors	Self-Care Measures
First Trimester		
Nausea and vomiting	Increased levels of hCG Changes in carbohydrate metabolism Emotional factors Fatigue	Avoid odors or causative factors. Eat dry crackers or toast before arising in morning. Have frequent, small meals. Avoid greasy or highly seasoned foods. Take dry meals with fluids between meals. Drink caffeine-free carbonated beverages.
Urinary frequency	Pressure of uterus on bladder in both first and third trimesters	Void when urge is felt. Increase fluid intake during the day. Decrease fluid intake *only* in the evening to decrease nocturia.
Fatigue	Specific causative factors unknown May be aggravated by nocturia due to urinary frequency	Plan time for a nap or rest period daily. Go to bed early. Seek family support and assistance with responsibilities so that more time is available to rest.
Breast tenderness	Increased levels of estrogen and progesterone	Wear well-fitting bra with good support.
Increased vaginal discharge	Hyperplasia of vaginal mucosa and increased production of mucus by the endocervical glands due to the increase in estrogen levels	Promote cleanliness by daily bathing. Avoid douching, nylon underpants, and pantyhose; cotton underpants are more absorbent.
Nasal stuffiness and nosebleed (epistaxis)	Elevated estrogen levels	May be unresponsive, but cool-air vaporizer may help; avoid use of nasal sprays and decongestants.
Ptyalism (excessive, often bitter salivation)	Specific causative factors unknown	Use astringent mouthwashes, chew gum, or suck hard candy. Carry tissues or a small towel to spit into when necessary.
Second and Third Trimesters		
Heartburn (pyrosis)	Increased production of progesterone, decreasing GI motility and increasing relaxation of cardiac sphincter, and displacement of stomach by enlarging uterus, thus regurgitation of acidic gastric contents into the esophagus	Eat frequent, small meals. Use low-sodium antacids, if approved by HCP. Avoid overeating; acidic, fatty, and fried foods; lying down after eating; and sodium bicarbonate.
Ankle edema	Prolonged standing or sitting Increased levels of sodium due to hormonal influences Circulatory congestion of lower extremities Increased capillary permeability Varicose veins	Practice frequent dorsiflexion of feet when prolonged sitting or standing is necessary. Elevate legs when sitting or resting. Avoid tight garters or restrictive bands around legs. Consider wearing support stockings when sitting or standing for long periods of time.
Varicose veins	Venous congestion in the lower veins that increases with pregnancy Hereditary factors (weakening of walls of veins, faulty valves) Increased age and weight gain	Elevate legs frequently. Wear supportive hose. Avoid crossing legs at the knees, standing for long periods, garters, and hosiery with constrictive bands.
Hemorrhoids	Constipation (see following discussion) Increased pressure from gravid uterus on hemorrhoidal veins	Avoid constipation. Apply ice packs, topical ointments, anesthetic agents, warm soaks, or sitz baths; gently reinsert hemorrhoid into rectum as necessary.
Constipation	Increased levels of progesterone, which cause general bowel sluggishness Pressure of enlarging uterus on intestine Iron supplements Diet, lack of exercise, and decreased fluids	Increase fluid intake, fiber in the diet, and exercise. Develop regular bowel habits. Use stool softeners as recommended by HCP.
Backache	Increased curvature of the lumbosacral vertebrae as the uterus enlarges Increased levels of hormones, which cause softening of cartilage in body joints Fatigue Poor body mechanics	Use proper body mechanics. Practice the pelvic-tilt exercise. Avoid uncomfortable working heights, high-heeled shoes, lifting of heavy loads, and fatigue. Apply heat, cold, or massage to the area.

(continued on next page)

TABLE 33.2 Self-Care Measures for Common Discomforts of Pregnancy (*continued*)

Discomfort	Influencing Factors	Self-Care Measures
Leg cramps	Imbalance of calcium/phosphorus ratio Increased pressure of uterus on nerves Fatigue Poor circulation to lower extremities Pointing the toes	Practice dorsiflexion of feet to stretch affected muscle. Evaluate diet. Apply heat to affected muscles. Arise slowly from resting position. Consider magnesium supplement as recommended by provider.
Flatulence	Decreased GI motility leading to delayed emptying time Pressure of growing uterus on large intestine Air swallowing	Avoid gas-forming foods. Chew food thoroughly. Get regular daily exercise. Maintain normal bowel habits.
Faintness	Postural hypotension Sudden change of position causing venous pooling in dependent veins Standing for long periods in warm area Anemia	Avoid prolonged standing in warm or stuffy environments. Change positions slowly. Evaluate hematocrit and hemoglobin.
Carpal tunnel syndrome	Compression of median nerve in carpal tunnel of wrist Aggravated by repetitive hand movements	Avoid aggravating hand movements. Use splint as prescribed. Elevate affected arm.
Dyspnea	Decreased vital capacity from pressure of enlarging uterus on the diaphragm	Use proper posture when sitting and standing. Sleep propped up with pillows for relief if problem occurs at night.

Source: Adapted from Davidson et al. (2020), pp. 275–276.

cultural practices the mother may use to relieve discomforts. Assess and document social and structural determinants of health (SDOH) that may influence the patient's overall health and access to healthcare. Use standardized methods of assessing SDOH and recognize that discrimination based on race or culture can impact SDOH. Word questions sensitively, as it is common for women to fail to disclose this information for fear of being judged unfavorably. Encourage the use of support systems and spiritual aids that provide comfort for the pregnant woman. Encourage her to share information on any herbs she may be using to determine their safety. Examples of different cultural practices include (ACOG, 2018d; Miller, 2018; Spector, 2017):

- For prenatal and intrapartum care, some women of Mexican heritage may prefer to use a *partera* (midwife) who speaks their language and is familiar with traditional birthing customs.
- Many Native American women may prefer to follow traditional methods of caring for and birthing their babies. In some cases, they may not live near a medical center that provides services to pregnant women.
- Middle Eastern, African, and South Asian women may prefer care from a female provider. Accommodations should be made when feasible.

Women from some cultures may not be aware of the importance of prenatal care. Others may face barriers such as poverty and lack of transportation to services. Culturally competent nursing assessment can help identify and address these issues early in the pregnancy.

Alterations of Pregnancy

Although pregnancy is normally a healthy process for most women, some women experience life-threatening complications during pregnancy, labor, or after delivery. Factors such as SES, preexisting medical and psychiatric conditions, parity, age, and blood type can threaten the outcomes of both mother and fetus. Alterations or complications may occur due to pregestational factors. Other conditions may arise during pregnancy and increase risk for preterm delivery, perinatal loss, or maternal mortality. Effective antepartum nursing care includes identifying risks to mother and fetus and developing a care plan that promotes optimal health for both patients.

Anemia During Pregnancy

Anemia indicates inadequate levels of hemoglobin (Hb) in the blood. Anemia is defined as Hb less than 12 g/dL in nonpregnant women and less than 11 g/dL in pregnant women (ACOG, 2008, reaffirmed 2019). Ethnicity, altitude, smoking, nutrition, and medications can affect the normal limits of hemoglobin. The lower limit of normal tends to be higher for women who smoke and those who live at higher altitudes because their bodies require a greater quantity of RBCs to maintain their tissue oxygen levels. The common anemias of pregnancy are due either to insufficient hemoglobin production related to nutritional deficiency in iron or folic acid during pregnancy or to hemoglobin destruction in inherited disorders, specifically sickle cell disease and thalassemia.

Iron Deficiency Anemia

The most common medical complication of pregnancy, iron deficiency anemia results when iron stores are low and intake of iron is insufficient to meet the demands for RBC production (Means, 2020). This generally occurs because of expansion of plasma volume without normal expansion of maternal hemoglobin mass (ACOG, 2008, reaffirmed 2019). The greatest need for increased iron intake occurs in the second half

Alterations and Therapies

Pregnancy

ALTERATION	DESCRIPTION	THERAPY
Pregestational Factors		
Prenatal substance use or abuse	Use of tobacco, alcohol, or illegal substances, including cocaine, methamphetamines, narcotics, or abuse of prescription medications. Such use can be profoundly harmful to the fetus.	■ Use of a validated screening tool is recommended. The nurse should refer all screen-positive patients for evaluation and treatment. ■ Nursing care is focused on motivating the patient to abstain from substance use and on supporting the patient through the withdrawal-and-recovery period. ■ For more information, see Module 22, Addiction.
Diabetes mellitus	An endocrine disorder of carbohydrate metabolism resulting from inadequate production or use of insulin. The patient may be diagnosed with diabetes before becoming pregnant or develop gestational diabetes during pregnancy.	■ Patient teaching is important to promote self-care focused on stable glucose levels using a balance of diet, exercise, medications, and frequent monitoring. ■ For more information, see Exemplar 12.A, Type 1 Diabetes Mellitus, in Module 12, Metabolism.
Anemia	Inadequate levels of hemoglobin in the blood, defined as levels of <11 g/dL during pregnancy (ACOG, 2008, reaffirmed 2019), caused by either insufficient hemoglobin production related to nutritional deficiency in iron or folic acid or to hemoglobin destruction in inherited disorders, such as sickle cell disease.	■ Monitor patients for symptoms of anemia (fatigue, pallor, shortness of breath, and alterations in level of consciousness). ■ Promote good nutrition in order to meet the body's metabolic needs. ■ Provide education on iron supplementation, as needed. ■ For more information, see Exemplar 2.B, Anemia, in Module 2, Cellular Regulation.
HIV/AIDS	Viral infection caused by the human immunodeficiency virus (HIV); called AIDS (acquired immunodeficiency syndrome) when symptoms of the disease appear.	■ Reassure the pregnant woman that risk of transmission to the fetus can be reduced by use of antiretroviral medication, that pregnancy is not believed to accelerate progression of the disease, and that most medications used to treat HIV can be safely taken during pregnancy. ■ Cesarean birth and abstaining from breastfeeding are recommended to reduce the risk of transmission to the baby. ■ For more information, see Exemplar 8.A, HIV/AIDS, in Module 8, Immunity.
Heart disease	Pregnancy increases cardiac output, heart rate, and blood volume, which the normal heart can adapt to, but which may put stress on the heart of a patient with decreased cardiac reserve. Women in Class I or II usually experience a normal pregnancy; those in Class III or IV are at risk for more severe complications.	■ Assess the stress of pregnancy on functional capacity of the heart during all antepartum visits. This includes monitoring vital signs and comparing them with pre-pregnancy levels, activity level, and factors that increase strain on the heart, such as anemia, infection, anxiety, lack of a support system, and lifestyle demands (career, home life, and other children to care for). ■ For more information, see Module 16, Perfusion.
Asthma	An obstructive lung condition that can improve symptoms in some pregnant women and worsen symptoms in others. Asthma has also been linked with higher rates of hyperemesis gravidarum, preeclampsia, uterine hemorrhage, and perinatal mortality.	■ Promote oxygenation to prevent hypoxia in both the mother and the fetus. ■ Teach the woman how to recognize signs of preterm labor because the rate of premature birth is higher in patients with asthma. ■ The goal of therapy is to prevent maternal exacerbations because even a mild exacerbation can cause severe hypoxia-related complications in the fetus. If an exacerbation occurs, inhaled albuterol may be recommended by the HCP. ■ For more information, see Exemplar 15.B, Asthma, in Module 15, Oxygenation.

(continued on next page)

Alterations and Therapies *(continued)*

ALTERATION	DESCRIPTION	THERAPY
Epilepsy	Chronic disorder characterized by seizures. Many women have uneventful pregnancies with excellent outcomes. Those with more frequent seizures before pregnancy may have exacerbations during pregnancy. Encourage patients to consult with their neurologists before and during pregnancy.	■ Teach the patient to continue taking recommended antiseizure medication as well as supplementing with folic acid and vitamin K throughout the pregnancy to improve fetal outcome. ■ For more information, see Exemplar 11.B, Seizure Disorders, in Module 11, Intracranial Regulation.
Hyperthyroidism	Enlarged, overactive thyroid gland. This can increase the risk for preeclampsia and postpartum hemorrhage in the mother and for abortion, intrauterine death, and stillbirth in the fetus if not well controlled. Even low doses of antithyroid drug in the mother may produce a mild fetal/neonatal hypothyroidism; higher doses may produce a goiter or mental deficiencies. Fetal loss is not increased in women who are euthyroid.	■ Nursing care is focused on early identification and treatment. ■ For more information, see Exemplar 12.E, Thyroid Disease, in Module 12, Metabolism.
Hypothyroidism	Characterized by inadequate thyroid secretions (decreased thyroxine [T_4]:thyroxine-binding globulin [TBG] ratio), elevated thyroid-stimulating hormone (TSH), lowered basal metabolic rate, and enlarged thyroid gland (goiter). Long-term replacement therapy usually continues during pregnancy at the same dosage as before. If the mother is untreated, the rate of fetal loss is 50%, with a high risk for congenital goiter or congenital hypothyroidism. Therefore, newborns are screened for T_4 level. Mild TSH elevations present little risk because TSH does not cross the placenta.	■ Nursing care is focused on early identification and treatment to prevent potential complications. ■ Teach the patient the importance of taking a thyroid hormone supplement regularly to maintain stable levels. ■ For more information, see Exemplar 12.E, Thyroid Disease, in Module 12, Metabolism.
Multiple sclerosis	Neurologic disorder that destroys the myelin sheath of nerve fibers and affects primarily young women. Pregnancy is associated with remission and slightly increased relapse rates postpartum. Uterine contraction strength is not diminished, but labor may be almost painless because of diminished sensation.	■ Nursing care is focused on promoting rest and nutrition. ■ For more information, see Exemplar 13.D, Multiple Sclerosis, in Module 13, Mobility.
Rheumatoid arthritis	Chronic inflammatory disease believed to have a genetic component. Remission of symptoms is common during the antepartum period, with relapse in the postpartum period. Heavy salicylate use may prolong gestation and lengthen labor. Salicylates may have possible teratogenic effects.	■ Monitor for anemia secondary to blood loss from salicylate therapy. ■ Encourage rest to relieve weight-bearing joints, but the patient needs to continue range-of-motion exercises. ■ The patient in remission may be advised to stop medications during pregnancy. ■ For more information, see Exemplar 8.C, Rheumatoid Arthritis, in Module 8, Immunity.

Alterations and Therapies *(continued)*

ALTERATION	DESCRIPTION	THERAPY
Systemic lupus erythematosus (SLE)	Autoimmune collagen disease characterized by exacerbations and remissions. Women who conceive when the disease is in remission appear to have little risk for adverse outcomes. Those with active disease have less favorable outcomes, as well as increased manifestations of symptoms, which are exacerbated by the physiologic changes associated with pregnancy (American College of Rheumatology, 2020). Increased incidence of spontaneous abortion, preeclampsia, eclampsia, thrombosis, stillbirth, prematurity, and IUGR. Babies born to women with SLE may have a characteristic skin rash, which usually disappears by 12 months. Neonates are at increased risk for complete congenital heart block, a condition that can be diagnosed prenatally (Sonesson, Ambrosi, & Wharen-Herlenius, 2019). When diagnosed, the mother is given corticosteroids that cross the placenta and decrease fetal heart inflammation (Davidson et al., 2020).	▪ Nursing care is focused on providing emotional support throughout the pregnancy and monitoring fetal well-being. Women with SLE have often experienced prenatal loss and may be very fearful about the outcome of pregnancy. ▪ For more information, see Exemplar 8.D, Systemic Lupus Erythematosus, in Module 8, Immunity.
Tuberculosis (TB)	An infection caused by *Mycobacterium tuberculosis*, which often affects the lungs. There has been a significant increase in diagnosis of TB, often associated with HIV infection, living in homeless shelters, and illicit drug use (Cunningham et al., 2018). Eighty percent of new cases are found in developing countries, primarily in Africa and Asia. The relapse rate does not increase if TB is inactive because of prior treatment. Isoniazid crosses the placenta, but most studies show no teratogenic effects. Rifampin also crosses the placenta, and the possibility of harmful effects is still being studied. Rifampin should only be used in patients with isoniazid intolerance or with suspected isoniazid-resistant infection.	▪ When isoniazid is used during pregnancy, the woman should take supplemental pyridoxine (vitamin B_6). ▪ Extra rest and limited contact with others are required until the disease becomes inactive. ▪ If maternal TB is inactive, the mother may breastfeed and care for her baby. If TB is active, the newborn should not have direct contact with the mother until she is noninfectious. ▪ For more information, see Exemplar 9.G, Tuberculosis, in Module 9, Infection.
Gestational Onset		
Vaginal bleeding	Primarily the result of abortion (miscarriage) during the first and second trimesters. Bleeding can also result from complications, such as ectopic pregnancy or gestational trophoblastic disease. In the second half of pregnancy, bleeding is often caused by placenta previa and abruptio placentae.	▪ Monitor blood pressure and pulse frequently. ▪ Observe the woman for behaviors indicative of shock, such as pallor, clammy skin, perspiration, dyspnea, or restlessness. ▪ Count and weigh pads to assess amount of bleeding over a given time period; save any tissue or clots expelled. ▪ If at 12 weeks' gestation or beyond, assess fetal heart tones with a Doppler. ▪ Prepare the woman for intravenous (IV) therapy. There may be standing orders to begin IV therapy on patients who are bleeding. ▪ Prepare equipment for examination. ▪ For more information, see Exemplar 16.L, Shock, in Module 16, Perfusion, and Exemplar 19.C, Menstrual Dysfunction, in Module 19, Sexuality.

(continued on next page)

Alterations and Therapies *(continued)*

ALTERATION	DESCRIPTION	THERAPY
Spontaneous abortion (miscarriage)	Many pregnancies end in the first trimester by spontaneous abortion, often without the woman's awareness that she was even pregnant. Most miscarriages result from chromosomal abnormalities. Other causes include teratogens, faulty implantation because of an abnormal reproductive tract, weakened cervix, placental abnormalities, chronic maternal diseases, endocrine imbalances, trauma, and maternal infections.	■ Miscarriage during the first trimester can rarely be reversed, so nursing care is focused on providing emotional support and preventing complications. ■ Educate the patient to report abdominal pain and vaginal bleeding.
Ectopic pregnancy	Implantation of the fertilized ovum in a site other than the endometrial lining of the uterus. Ectopic pregnancy has many associated risk factors, including tubal damage caused by pelvic inflammatory disease, previous tubal surgery, congenital anomalies of the tube, endometriosis, previous ectopic pregnancy, presence of an IUD, and in utero exposure to diethylstilbestrol.	■ Nursing care is focused on early identification, providing emotional support, and preventing complications secondary to blood loss. ■ Pain management is an important nursing intervention. ■ Assess hCG levels (often lower with ectopic pregnancy and do not increase normally). ■ Prepare the patient for surgery. ■ Provide postoperative reassurance that pregnancy is still possible with one remaining fallopian tube.
Gestational trophoblastic disease (GTD)	Pathologic proliferation of trophoblastic cells (the trophoblast is the outermost layer of embryonic cells). This includes hydatidiform mole, invasive mole (chorioadenoma destruens), and choriocarcinoma.	■ Teach the woman about the need for regular screening for choriocarcinoma. ■ Assess all pregnant women for symptoms of GTD, including vaginal bleeding that is brown with greater uterine enlargement than expected for gestational age. ■ Follow quantitative hCG levels (discussed in greater detail in the Concept section of Module 19, Sexuality).
Hyperemesis gravidarum	Excessive vomiting during pregnancy that progresses to a point at which the woman not only vomits everything she swallows but also retches between meals. Increased hCG levels may play a role.	■ Assess hydration. ■ Administer IV fluids. ■ Assess nutritional status. ■ Total parenteral nutrition may be administered to prevent malnutrition. ■ Keep patient away from food odors that may increase nausea and vomiting. ■ Maintain oral hygiene. ■ For more information on treating dehydration, see Exemplar 6.A, Fluid and Electrolyte Imbalance, in Module 6, Fluids and Electrolytes.
Hypertensive disorders	Preeclampsia, eclampsia, chronic HTN, and gestational HTN.	■ Nursing care focuses on prevention and early detection. ■ For more information, see Exemplar 16.H, Hypertensive Disorders in Pregnancy, in Module 16, Perfusion.
Rh alloimmunization	Destruction of fetal hemoglobin. When the mother is Rh negative and the fetus is Rh positive, alloimmunization may occur in second and successive pregnancies if maternal–fetal blood mixture occurs, whether the pregnancy was carried to term or not. Alloimmunization causes fetal anemia, resulting in marked fetal edema (hydrops fetalis). Congestive heart failure may result. Marked jaundice leading to neurologic damage is also a risk.	■ Administer Rh immunoglobulin at 28 weeks' gestation if the pregnancy continues, or immediately following a spontaneous miscarriage if the mother is Rh negative and the father is Rh positive, or within 72 hours after delivery if the mother is Rh negative and the baby is Rh positive. ■ Assess lab results for positive Coombs test, indicating sensitization, in which case Rh immunoglobulin is not administered.

Alterations and Therapies *(continued)*

ALTERATION	DESCRIPTION	THERAPY
ABO incompatibility	When a woman who has type O blood becomes pregnant with a type A, B, or AB fetus, causing interaction of antibodies present in maternal serum and the antigen sites on the fetal RBCs. ABO incompatibility does not normally cause the severity of hemolysis seen with Rh incompatibility.	■ Assess blood type during prenatal care, and document so that the newborn can be followed after birth for potential hyperbilirubinemia if ABO incompatibility is likely.
Herpes simplex virus	Viral infection causing painful lesions in the genital area; may also occur on the cervix. This infection can profoundly affect the fetus. Primary infection has been associated with spontaneous abortion, low birth weight, and preterm birth. Transmission to the fetus usually occurs with membrane rupture and rarely via transplacental infection. If the fetus is infected, symptoms may include fever or hypothermia, jaundice, seizures, and poor feeding.	■ Educate the patient on the importance of prophylaxis during the last month of pregnancy, to reduce the incidence of active lesions when she goes into labor. ■ Prepare the mother for the need for cesarean delivery if active lesions are present when she goes into labor.
Group B streptococcal (GBS) infection	Bacterial infection is found in the lower GI or urogenital tracts of 10–30% of pregnant women (ACOG, 2020c). Women may transmit GBS infection to their fetus in utero or during childbirth. GBS is one of the major causes of early-onset neonatal infection. Newborns become infected by vertical transmission from the mother during birth or by horizontal transmission from colonized nursing personnel or colonized babies. GBS causes severe, invasive disease in newborns.	■ Nursing care is focused on detection and early intervention during pregnancy in order to resolve the infection before delivery and, through prescribed IV antibiotics, during labor for neonatal prophylaxis.
Urinary tract infection (UTI)	Dysuria, urgency, frequency; low-grade fever and hematuria. If not treated, infection may ascend and lead to acute pyelonephritis, which is associated with increased risk of premature birth and IUGR.	■ Nursing care is focused on teaching the woman the signs to report in order to allow quick intervention and to prevent potential complications. ■ Oral sulfonamides taken in the last few weeks of pregnancy may lead to neonatal hyperbilirubinemia and kernicterus.
Vulvovaginal candidiasis	Fungal infection manifested by thick, white, curdy discharge as well as by severe itching, dysuria, and dyspareunia. If the infection is present at birth and the fetus is born vaginally, the fetus may contract thrush.	■ Nursing care is focused on teaching the woman the signs and symptoms of infection, preventive measures, and rapid recognition so that treatment can be initiated quickly.
Syphilis	Sexually transmitted infection manifested by chancre lasting 3–6 weeks, then often asymptomatic until stage III. Syphilis can be passed transplacentally to the fetus. If untreated, one of the following can occur: second-trimester abortion, stillborn baby at term, congenitally infected baby, or uninfected live newborn. (For more information, see Exemplar 19.E, Sexually Transmitted Infections, in Module 19, Sexuality.)	■ Screening for infections should be part of prenatal care in order to treat and eliminate the infection before delivery.

Source: Adapted from London et al. (2017).

of pregnancy. When the iron needs of pregnancy are not met, maternal hemoglobin falls below 11 g/dL and serum ferritin levels, indicating iron stores, are below 12 mcg/L.

The woman with iron deficiency anemia may be asymptomatic, but she is more susceptible to perinatal infection and has an increased chance of preeclampsia and bleeding. There is evidence of increased risk of low birth weight, prematurity, stillbirth, and neonatal death in babies of women with severe iron deficiency (maternal Hb less than 6 g/dL). The newborn is not iron deficient at birth because of active transport of iron across the placenta, even when maternal iron stores are low. However, these babies do have lower iron stores and are at increased risk for developing iron deficiency during the newborn period and infancy (Means, 2020).

The first goal of healthcare is to prevent iron deficiency anemia. To prevent anemia, the American Academy of Pediatrics (AAP) and ACOG (2017) recommend that pregnant women supplement their diet with at least 30 mg of iron daily. This amount is contained in most prenatal vitamins. In addition, the woman should be encouraged to eat an iron-rich diet. If anemia is diagnosed, the dosage should be increased to 60 to 120 mg/day of iron. Every-other-day dosing has shown to increase absorption and minimize GI side effects (Muñoz et al., 2017). If the woman remains anemic after 1 month of therapy, further evaluation is indicated.

Folic Acid Deficiency Anemia

Folate deficiency is the most common cause of megaloblastic anemia during pregnancy. **Folic acid** is needed for DNA and RNA synthesis and cell duplication. In its absence, immature RBCs fail to divide, become enlarged (megaloblastic), and are fewer in number. Even more significantly, an inadequate intake of folic acid has been associated with neural tube defects (NTDs; spina bifida, anencephaly, myelomeningocele) in the fetus or newborn. With the tremendous cell multiplication that occurs in pregnancy, an adequate amount of folic acid is crucial. However, increased urinary excretion of folic acid and fetal uptake can rapidly result in folic acid deficiency.

Diagnosis of folic acid deficiency anemia may be difficult, and it is usually not detected until late in pregnancy or the early puerperium. This is because serum folate levels normally fall as pregnancy progresses. Even though folate levels are lower with deficiency, they will fluctuate with diet. Measurement of erythrocyte folate status is more reliable but indicates the folate status of several weeks previously. Women with true folic acid deficiency anemia often present with nausea, vomiting, and anorexia. Hemoglobin levels as low as 3 to 5 g/dL may be found. Typically, the blood smear reveals that the newly formed erythrocytes are macrocytic.

Folic acid deficiency during pregnancy is prevented by a daily supplement of 0.4 mg of folate. Treatment of deficiency consists of 1-mg folic acid supplements. Because iron deficiency anemia almost always coexists with folic acid deficiency, the woman also needs iron supplements. The FDA requires the addition of folic acid for all foods labeled "enriched." Even with this addition, the U.S. Public Health Service recommends that all women of childbearing age (15 to 45 years) consume 0.4 mg of folic acid daily. This recommendation is important because half of all U.S. pregnancies are unplanned and NTDs occur very early in pregnancy (3 to 4 weeks after conception), before most women realize they are pregnant (AAP & ACOG, 2017). Nurses can play a crucial role in helping young women become aware of this important recommendation.

Sickle Cell Disease

Sickle cell disease (SCD) is an autosomal recessive disorder in which the normal adult hemoglobin, hemoglobin A (HbA), is abnormally formed. This abnormal hemoglobin is called hemoglobin S. Approximately 1 in 10 African Americans has sickle cell trait and 1 in every 300 African American newborns has some form of SCD (ACOG, 2017b). Diagnosis is confirmed by hemoglobin electrophoresis or a test to induce sickling in a blood sample. Prenatal diagnosis and newborn screening for SCD are important components of perinatal care.

Women with sickle cell trait have a good prognosis for pregnancy if they have adequate nutrition and prenatal care. Maternal mortality due to SCD is rare. Women with SCD may have experienced severe complications by the time they reach childbearing age. Complications include anemia requiring blood transfusion, infections, and emergency cesarean births. Acute chest syndrome, congestive heart failure, or acute renal failure may also occur. Prematurity and IUGR are also associated with SCD. Fetal death is believed to be due to sickling attacks in the placenta.

Because the woman with SCD maintains her hemoglobin levels by intense erythropoiesis, additional folic acid supplements (4 mg/day) are required. Maternal infection should be treated promptly because dehydration and fever can trigger sickling and crisis. Vaso-occlusive crisis is best treated by a perinatal team in a medical center. Proper management requires close observation and evaluation of all symptoms. Women with SCD are at higher risk of developing *sickle cell crisis*, which may increase rates of maternal morbidity and mortality (Alayed, Kezouh, Oddy, & Abenhaim, 2014).

Diabetes During Pregnancy

Carbohydrate metabolism is affected early in pregnancy by a rise in serum levels of estrogen, progesterone, and other hormones. These hormones stimulate maternal insulin production and increase tissue response to insulin; therefore, anabolism (building up) of glycogen stores in the liver and other tissues occurs.

In the second half of pregnancy, the woman demonstrates prolonged hyperglycemia and hyperinsulinemia (increased secretion of insulin) following a meal. Although the mother is producing more insulin, placental secretion of hPL and prolactin (from the decidua) and elevated levels of cortisol (an adrenal hormone) and glycogen cause increased maternal peripheral resistance to insulin. This resistance helps ensure that a sustained supply of glucose is available for the fetus. This glucose is transported across the placenta to the fetus, which uses it as a major source of fuel. Maternal amino acids are also actively transported by the placenta from the mother to her fetus. The fetus uses these amino acids for protein synthesis and as a source of energy. In addition to ensuring that glucose is available to the fetus, the increased maternal resistance to insulin means that the pregnant woman has a lower peripheral uptake of glucose to meet her own needs. This results in a catabolic (destructive) state during fasting periods (e.g., during the night and after meal absorption). Because increasing amounts of circulating maternal glucose are being diverted to the fetus, maternal fat is metabolized (lipolysis) during fasting periods much more readily than in a nonpregnant individual. This process is called *accelerated starvation*. Ketones may be present in the urine as a result of lipolysis.

The delicate system of checks and balances that exists between glucose production and glucose use is stressed by the growing fetus, who derives energy from glucose taken from the mother and by maternal resistance to the insulin her body produces. This stress is referred to as the *diabetogenic effect of pregnancy*. Thus, any preexisting disruption in carbohydrate metabolism is augmented by pregnancy and any diabetic potential may precipitate gestational diabetes mellitus.

Gestational Diabetes Mellitus

Gestational diabetes mellitus (GDM) is defined as a carbohydrate intolerance of variable severity with onset or first recognition during pregnancy. It results from (1) an unidentified preexisting disease, (2) the unmasking of a compensated metabolic abnormality by the added stress of pregnancy, or (3) a direct consequence of the altered maternal metabolism stemming from changing hormonal levels. Diagnosis of GDM is important because even mild diabetes increases the risk of perinatal morbidity and mortality. Many women with GDM progress over time to overt type 2 diabetes mellitus (T2DM).

Influence of Preexisting and Gestational Diabetes During Pregnancy

Pregnancy can affect diabetes significantly. First, the physiologic changes of pregnancy can drastically alter insulin requirements. Second, pregnancy may accelerate the progress of vascular disease secondary to diabetes.

The disease may be more difficult to control during pregnancy because insulin requirements are changeable. Insulin needs frequently decrease early in the first trimester. Levels of hPL, an insulin antagonist, are low; energy demands of the embryo/fetus are minimal; and the woman may be consuming less food because of nausea and vomiting. Nausea and vomiting may also cause dietary fluctuations, which can increase the risk of hypoglycemia or insulin shock. Insulin requirements usually begin to rise late in the first trimester as glucose use and glycogen storage by the woman and fetus increase. As a result of placental maturation and production of hPL and other hormones, insulin requirements may double or quadruple by the end of pregnancy.

Because her energy needs increase during labor, the woman with diabetes may require more insulin at that time to balance IV glucose. After delivery of the placenta, insulin requirements usually decrease abruptly with loss of hPL in the maternal circulation.

Other factors contribute to the difficulty in controlling the disease. As pregnancy progresses, the renal threshold for glucose decreases. There is an increased risk of ketoacidosis, which may occur at lower serum glucose levels in the pregnant woman with diabetes than in the nonpregnant woman with diabetes. The vascular disease that accompanies diabetes may progress during pregnancy. HTN may occur. Nephropathy may result from renal blood vessel impairment, and retinopathy may develop (from occlusion of the microscopic blood vessels of the eye).

Influence of Preexisting Diabetes and Gestational Diabetes on Pregnancy Outcome

The pregnancy of a woman who has diabetes carries a higher risk of complications than a normal pregnancy, especially perinatal mortality and congenital anomalies. The risk has been reduced by the recent recognition of the importance of tight metabolic control (fasting, premeal, and bedtime blood glucose levels of 60 to 95 mg/dL; peak postprandial blood glucose levels of 100 to 129 mg/dL; and glycohemoglobin less than 6%). New techniques for monitoring blood glucose, delivering insulin, and monitoring the fetus have also reduced perinatal mortality (ACOG, 2018c).

Maternal Risks

Maternal health problems in diabetic pregnancy have been greatly reduced by the team approach to preconception planning and early prenatal care and by the increased emphasis on maintaining tight control of blood glucose levels. The prognosis for the pregnant woman with gestational, type 1, or type 2 diabetes that has not resulted in significant vascular damage is positive. However, diabetic pregnancy still carries higher risks for complications than normal pregnancy.

Hydramnios, or an increase in the volume of amniotic fluid, occurs in 10–20% of pregnant women with diabetes. It is thought to be a result of excessive fetal urination because of fetal hyperglycemia (ACOG, 2018c). *Preeclampsia–eclampsia* occurs more often in diabetic pregnancies, especially when diabetes-related vascular changes already exist.

Hyperglycemia due to insufficient amounts of insulin can lead to *ketoacidosis* as a result of the increase in ketone bodies (which are acidic) in the blood released when fatty acids are metabolized. Ketoacidosis usually develops slowly, but it may develop more rapidly in the pregnant woman because of the hyperketonemia associated with accelerated starvation in the fasting state. The tendency for higher postprandial glucose levels because of decreased gastric motility and the contrainsulin effects of hPL also predispose the woman to ketoacidosis. If the ketoacidosis is not treated, it can lead to coma and death of both mother and fetus.

Another risk to the pregnant woman with diabetes is a difficult labor (*dystocia*), caused by fetopelvic disproportion if fetal macrosomia (>4000 g) exists. The pregnant woman with diabetes is also at increased risk for recurrent monilial vaginitis (yeast infection) and UTIs because of increased glycosuria, which contributes to a favorable environment for bacterial growth. If untreated, asymptomatic bacteriuria can lead to pyelonephritis, a serious kidney infection.

Several studies have demonstrated that pregnancy worsens *retinopathy* in women with diabetes. Most investigators agree that during a diabetic pregnancy, good control of blood glucose levels and the use of laser photocoagulation (a treatment used to prevent retinal hemorrhage when the retina shows changes in the blood vessels) when indicated minimize the risk of the negative effects of pregnancy. Hence, women with preexisting diabetes should be referred to an ophthalmologist for evaluation during pregnancy.

Fetal–Neonatal Risks

Many of the problems of the newborn result directly from high maternal plasma glucose levels. The incidence of *congenital anomalies* in diabetic pregnancies is 6–12% and is the major cause of death for babies of mothers with diabetes. Research suggests that this increased incidence of congenital anomalies is related to multiple factors, including high glucose levels in early pregnancy (ACOG, 2018c). The anomalies often involve the heart, CNS, and skeletal system. Septal defects, coarctation of the aorta, and transposition of the great vessels are the most common heart lesions seen. CNS anomalies include hydrocephalus, meningomyelocele, and anencephaly. One anomaly, *sacral agenesis*, appears only in babies of mothers with diabetes. In sacral agenesis, the sacrum and lumbar spine fail to develop and the lower extremities develop incompletely. To reduce the incidence of congenital anomalies, preconception counseling and strict diabetes control before conception and in the early weeks of pregnancy are indicated.

Approximately 18% of newborns of mothers with diabetes are LGA as a result of high levels of fetal insulin production stimulated by the high levels of glucose crossing the placenta from the mother. Sustained fetal hyperinsulinism and hyperglycemia ultimately lead to *macrosomia* and deposition of fat. If born vaginally, the macrosomic newborn is at increased risk for birth trauma such as fractured clavicle or brachial plexus injuries due to shoulder dystocia. Shoulder dystocia occurs when, following birth of the head, the anterior shoulder of the macrosomic fetus does not emerge either spontaneously or with gentle traction (ACOG, 2018c). Macrosomia can be significantly reduced by tight maternal blood glucose control.

After birth, the umbilical cord is severed and, thus, the generous maternal blood glucose supply is eliminated. However, continued islet cell hyperactivity leads to excessive insulin levels and depleted blood glucose (hypoglycemia) within 2 to 4 hours after birth in the neonate. Babies of mothers with diabetes with vascular involvement (see Module 12, Metabolism) may demonstrate IUGR. This occurs because vascular changes in the mother decrease the efficiency of placental perfusion, and the fetus is not as well sustained in utero. *Respiratory distress syndrome* appears to result from inhibition, by high levels of fetal insulin, of some fetal enzymes necessary for surfactant production. Polycythemia in the newborn is due primarily to the diminished ability of glycosylated hemoglobin in the mother's blood to release oxygen. *Hyperbilirubinemia* is a result of the inability of immature liver enzymes to metabolize the increased bilirubin resulting from the polycythemia. Hypocalcemia, characterized by signs of irritability or even tetany, may occur. The cause of these low calcium levels in newborns of mothers with diabetes is not known.

Clinical Therapy

Gestational diabetes is more common than preexisting diabetes. It is estimated to occur in 6–7% of pregnancies, depending on the population studied (ACOG, 2018c). Therefore, screening for its detection is a standard part of prenatal care. If diabetes is suspected, further testing is undertaken for diagnosis.

All pregnant women should have their risk of diabetes assessed at the first prenatal visit (see Exemplar 12.A, Type 1 Diabetes Mellitus, in Module 12, Metabolism). Women at high risk (prior history of GDM or birth of an LGA baby, marked obesity, diagnosis of polycystic ovarian syndrome, presence of glycosuria, or a strong family history of T2DM) should be screened for diabetes as soon as possible. In early pregnancy, the screening criteria for nonpregnant individuals is used: glycoslyated hemoglobin (HbA_{1c}) equal to or greater than 6.5% would be considered diagnostic, as would a fasting plasma glucose level equal to or greater than 126 mg/dL (American Diabetes Association [ADA], 2020).

If there is no preexisting diabetes, screening for GDM is done using one of two approaches performed at 24 to 28 weeks' gestation (ADA, 2020). In the two-step approach, the first step is to give the woman a nonfasting, 50-g, 1-hour oral glucose tolerance test (OGTT). The oral glucose load can be given at any time of the day with no requirement for fasting. One hour later, plasma glucose is measured. If plasma glucose levels are elevated (equal to or greater than 140 mg/dL, depending on the laboratory used), a 100-g, 3-hour glucose test is done. In the second step, a 100-g, 3-hour OGTT is administered. The woman eats an unrestricted diet, consuming at least 150 g of carbohydrates per day for at least 3 days before her scheduled test. She then ingests a 100-g oral glucose solution in the morning after an overnight fast. Plasma glucose is measured fasting and at 1, 2, and 3 hours. A diagnosis of GDM occurs if two or more of the following values are met or exceeded:

Fasting	95 mg/dL
1 hour	180 mg/dL
2 hours	155 mg/dL
3 hours	140 mg/dL

In the one-step approach, the woman ingests a 75-g oral glucose solution in the morning after an overnight fast. Plasma glucose levels are determined fasting and at 1 and 2 hours. A diagnosis of GDM occurs if any one of the following values are equaled or exceeded:

Fasting	92 mg/dL
1 hour	180 mg/dL
2 hours	153 mg/dL

Laboratory Assessment of Long-Term Glucose Control

Glycosylated hemoglobin is a laboratory test that loosely reflects glucose control over the previous 4 to 8 weeks. It measures the percentage of glycohemoglobin in the blood. Glycohemoglobin is the hemoglobin to which a glucose molecule is attached. The test is not reliable for screening for gestational diabetes and is not recommended at this time.

In women with known pregestational diabetes, however, abnormal HbA_{1c} values correlate directly with the frequency of spontaneous abortion and fetal congenital anomalies. Consequently, women with preexisting diabetes who plan to become pregnant should work to achieve HbA_{1c} levels at target levels (less than 6%) without significant hypoglycemia (ADA, 2020). Once pregnant, HbA_{1c} levels should be tested at the initial prenatal visit and monthly if target levels have been achieved (ADA, 2020).

Diet therapy and regular exercise form the cornerstone of intervention for GDM. Insulin therapy is indicated when dietary management is unable to achieve a 1-hour postprandial blood glucose value of less than 130 to 140 mg/dL, a 2-hour postprandial level of less than 120 mg/dL, or a fasting glucose of less than 95 mg/dL. In most instances, the overt diabetic manifestation disappears postpartum, though subtle manifestations of impaired insulin secretory capacity may remain.

Insulin and nutritional therapy are the preferred methods of treatment for gestational diabetes. Oral hypoglycemics can be used during pregnancy, following a discussion regarding the risk of neonatal hypoglycemia and the unknown long-term effects to the infant. If oral hypoglycemics are used, glyburide is the preferred treatment (ADA, 2020).

Evaluation of Fetal Status

Information about the well-being, maturation, and size of the fetus is important for planning the course of the pregnancy and the timing of birth. Because pregnancies complicated by preexisting diabetes are at increased risk of NTDs, an ultrasound to screen for NTDs, in addition to a quadruple screen, which includes testing for maternal serum *α-fetoprotein* (*AFP*), is offered at weeks 16 to 20 of gestation. Daily maternal evaluation of fetal activity, begun at about 28 weeks, is effective and simple to do. The woman is taught a particular method for counting fetal movements.

Nonstress testing should be started at 32 weeks. If evidence of IUGR, preeclampsia, oligohydramnios, or poorly controlled blood glucose exists, testing may begin as early as 26 weeks and may be done more often. If the NST is nonreactive, a fetal biophysical profile is performed. If the woman requires hospitalization (for example, to control glycemia or for complications), NSTs may be done daily.

Ultrasound at 18 weeks confirms gestational age and diagnoses multiple pregnancy or congenital anomalies. It is repeated at 28 weeks to monitor fetal growth for IUGR or macrosomia. Some physicians order *fetal biophysical profiles* (ultrasound evaluation of fetal well-being in which fetal breathing movements, fetal activity, reactivity, muscle tone, and amniotic fluid volume are assessed) as part of an ongoing evaluation of fetal status. Because of the increased risk of macrosomia, an ultrasound at 38 weeks is often performed to estimate fetal weight.

Assessment of Fetal Well-Being

A number of tests are used to obtain accurate and helpful data about the developing fetus. At times, just one test is done; in other circumstances, a combination of testing is necessary. Some of these assessment techniques pose risks to the fetus and, possibly, to the pregnant woman; the risk to both should be considered before deciding to perform the test. The HCP must be certain that the advantages outweigh the potential risks and added expense. In addition, the diagnostic accuracy and applicability of these tests may vary. Although some tests are for *screening* purposes, meaning that they indicate the fetus may be at risk for a certain disorder or anomaly, others are *diagnostic*, meaning that they can diagnose the abnormality. Not all high-risk pregnancies require the same tests.

Before administration of any screening or diagnostic test, the nurse should use the following guide to ensure that the patient knows the reason for performing the procedure:

1. Assess whether the woman knows the reason why the screening or diagnostic test is being recommended:
   - "Has your physician or nurse-midwife told you why this test is necessary?"
   - "Sometimes tests are done for many different reasons. Can you tell me why you are having this test?"
   - "What is your understanding about what the test will show?"
2. Provide an opportunity for questions:
   - "Do you have any questions about the test?"
   - "Is there anything that is not clear to you?"
3. Explain the procedure. For any procedure that requires consent, the HCP, not the nurse, should explain the procedure, paying particular attention to any preparation the woman needs before the test:
   - "The test that has been ordered for you is designed to __________." (*Add specific information about the particular test. Give the explanation in simple language.*)
4. Validate the woman's understanding of the preparation:
   - "Tell me what you will have to do to get ready for this test."
5. Give permission for the woman to continue to ask questions if needed:
   - "I'll be with you during the test. If you have any questions at any time, please don't hesitate to ask."

Selected conditions that indicate a pregnancy is at risk include the following:

- Maternal age less than 16 or more than 35
- Chronic maternal HTN, preeclampsia, diabetes mellitus, or heart disease
- Presence of Rh isoimmunization (immune response to foreign antigen Rh-positive cells)
- Maternal history of fetal demise (stillbirth)
- Suspected IUGR
- Pregnancy prolonged past 42 weeks' gestation
- Multiple gestation
- Prior preterm birth
- Previous pregnancy losses before 20 weeks' gestation or diagnosed cervical insufficiency.

Maternal Assessment of Fetal Activity

Clinicians now generally agree that vigorous fetal activity provides reassurance of fetal well-being and that a marked decrease in activity or cessation of movement may indicate possible fetal compromise (or even death), requiring immediate follow-up (Blackburn, 2018). Maternal assessment is typically used to monitor fetal well-being beginning at approximately 28 weeks of gestation. It provides a low-technology, inexpensive means to evaluate fetal well-being. A reduction of fetal movement has been associated with fetal hypoxia, fetal growth restriction, and fetal death (Malm, Lindgren, Rubertsson, Hildingsson, & Radestad, 2014). A decrease in maternal perception of fetal movement may precede adverse outcomes by several days, thus providing the rationale for educating the woman on the importance of monitoring fetal activity (ACOG, 2014a, reaffirmed 2016).

Although there is no standard definition of how many movements should occur within a specified time, the only evidence-based method is the "count to 10 method." This method was derived from a population-based study and was also evaluated as a screening tool in the same population (Moore & Piacquadio, 1989). The mother should be instructed to rest and focus on fetal movements. She should count the number of fetal movements until she reaches 10. She should be able to count 10 movements in no more than 2 hours. If there are fewer than 10 movements in 2 hours or if the amount of movement is significantly less than normal, the woman should immediately notify her HCP. A maternal perception of decreased movement occurring during a 24-hour period should cause concern and warrant antepartum fetal testing.

Fetuses spend approximately 25% of their time making gross body movements. Fetal movements are directly related to the fetus's sleep–wake cycle and vary from the maternal sleep–wake cycle (Blackburn, 2018). Fetuses may react to maternal hypoglycemia by decreasing their activity level. In women with a multiple gestation, daily fetal movements are significantly higher. After 38 weeks, fetuses spend 75% of their time in a quiet-sleep or active-sleep state. Other factors affecting fetal movement include sound, cigarette smoking, and drugs.

A variety of methods for tracking fetal activity have been developed. These methods focus on having the pregnant woman keep a fetal movement record, such as the Cardiff Count-to-Ten method, the Daily Fetal Movement Record (DFMR), or the Count the Kicks app for smartphones (available at counthekicks.org). A **fetal movement record** is a noninvasive technique that enables the pregnant woman to monitor and record movements easily and without expense. See Patient Teaching: Maternal Assessment of Fetal Activity.

The expectant mother's perception of fetal movements and her commitment to completing a fetal movement record may vary. When a woman understands the purpose of the assessment, how to complete the form, whom to call with questions, and what to report—and has the opportunity for follow-up during each visit—she generally views completing the fetal movement record as an important activity. The nurse should be available to answer questions and clarify areas of concern.

Patient Teaching

Maternal Assessment of Fetal Activity

- Explain that fetal movements are first felt around 18 weeks of gestation. This is called *quickening*. From that time, the fetal movements get stronger and easier to detect. A slowing or stopping of fetal movement may be an indication that the fetus needs some attention and evaluation. The mother's perception of decreased fetal movement is sufficient in most cases. Formal tracking of fetal movement does not lead to improved outcomes in low-risk pregnancies but may have value in high-risk situations.
- Describe the procedures and demonstrate how to assess fetal movement. Sit beside the woman and show her how to place her hand on the fundus to feel fetal movement. Advise the woman to keep a daily record of fetal movements beginning at about 28 weeks of gestation.
- Explain the procedure for the Cardiff Count-to-Ten method:
  a. Beginning at the same time each day, have the woman place an X on the Cardiff card for each fetal movement she perceives during normal everyday activity until she has recorded 10 of them.
  b. Movement varies considerably, but the woman should feel fetal movement at least 10 times in 12 hours, and many women will feel 10 fetal movements in much less time, possibly 2 hours or less.
- Explain the procedure for the DFMR method:
  a. The woman should begin counting at about the same time each day, after taking food.
  b. She should lie quietly in a side-lying position.
  c. The woman should feel at least three fetal movements within 1 hour.
- Explain the procedure for the Count the Kicks smartphone app:
  a. The woman should pick a time to count when the baby is active, preferably about the same time every day, after eating.
  b. Rest in a quiet place and count movements.
  c. She should feel at least 10 movements in 2 hours.
- Instruct the woman to contact her HCP in the following situations:
  a. Using the Cardiff method: If there are fewer than 10 movements in 12 hours.
  b. Using the DFMR method: If there are fewer than three movements in 1 hour.
  c. Using the Count the Kicks method: If there are fewer than 10 movements in 2 hours.
  d. Any method: If overall the fetus's movements are slowing, and it takes much longer each day to note the minimum number of movements in the specified time period, and if there are no movements in the morning.
  e. If there are fewer than three movements in 8 hours.
- Whichever method she is using, encourage the woman to complete her DFMR and to bring it with her during each prenatal visit. Assure her that the record will be discussed at each prenatal visit and that questions may be addressed at that time, if desired.
- Provide the woman with a name and phone number in case she has further questions.

Source: Adapted from Davidson et al. (2020).

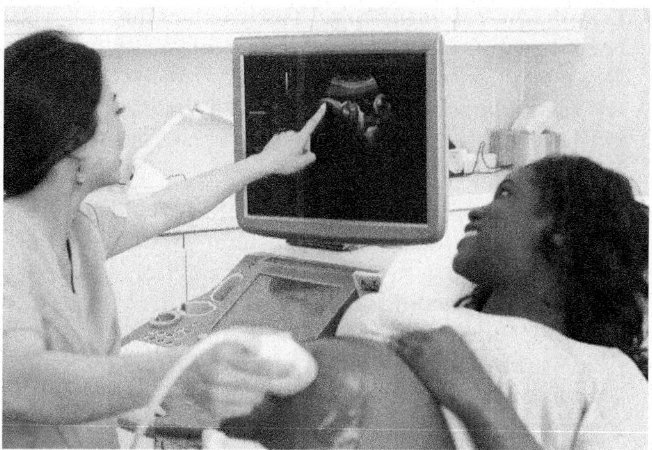

Figure 33.27 » Ultrasound scanning permits visualization of the fetus in utero.
Source: Shutterstock.

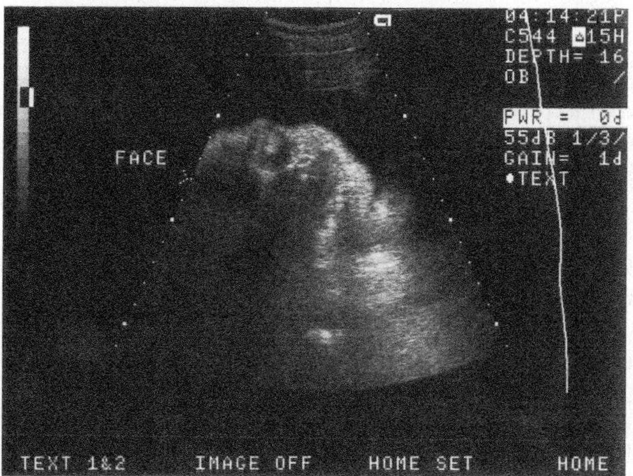

Figure 33.28 » Ultrasound of fetal face.
Source: Pearson Education, Inc.

Ultrasound

Valuable information about the fetus may be obtained from **ultrasound** testing, in which intermittent ultrasonic waves (high-frequency sound waves) are transmitted by an alternating current to a transducer, which is applied to the woman's abdomen. The ultrasonic waves are deflected by tissues within the patient's abdomen, showing structures of varying densities (**Figure 33.27 »** and **Figure 33.28 »**). Ultrasound testing should only be utilized for valid medical testing. The use of nonmedical obstetric ultrasonography is discouraged (ACOG, 2016a, reaffirmed 2020).

Diagnostic ultrasound, when indicated, has several advantages. It is noninvasive, painless, and nonradiating to both the woman and the fetus. Serial studies (several ultrasound tests done over a span of time) may be done for assessment and comparison. Soft-tissue masses (e.g., tumors) can be differentiated, the fetus can be visualized, fetal growth can be followed (especially in the presence of multiple gestation), cervical length and impending cervical insufficiency can be detected, and a number of other potential problems can be averted. In addition, the results are immediately available to the ultrasonographer and physician.

The use of four-dimensional ultrasound may eventually be able to generate future research regarding fetal well-being. Four-dimensional ultrasound combines the components of three-dimensional ultrasound with a fourth dimension, time, because it monitors live action. The technology produces images of photo-like quality, allowing HCPs to better visualize fetal structures and producing better guidance during invasive intrauterine procedures, such as amniocentesis and CVS. Despite these technical advantages, there is insufficient evidence of any clinical advantage of 3D/4D ultrasound. The use of 3D/4D ultrasound should not be a replacement for traditional 2D ultrasound (ACOG, 2016a, reaffirmed 2020).

Although ultrasound is believed to serve as a useful tool in monitoring the fetus throughout pregnancy, it does have limitations. Ultrasound is limited by maternal body habitus, fetal positioning, and technician or physician skill. Another limitation is that ultrasound cannot guarantee that a fetus does not have certain disorders or anomalies. Even though certain fetal problems can be diagnosed via the technology, sometimes abnormalities go unrecognized. A "normal" ultrasound is reassuring for the parents and the healthcare team, but it is important for parents to realize that a normal sonogram is not 100% reliable.

The two most common methods of ultrasound scanning are transabdominal and transvaginal.

Transabdominal Ultrasound

In the transabdominal approach, a transducer is moved across the patient's abdomen. The woman is often scanned with a full bladder because when the bladder is full, the examiner can assess other structures, especially the vagina and cervix, in relation to the bladder. The ability to see the lower portion of the uterus and cervix is particularly important when vaginal bleeding is noted and placenta previa is the suspected cause. The patient is directed to drink 1 to 1.5 quarts of water approximately 2 hours before the examination and to refrain from emptying her bladder. If the bladder is not sufficiently filled, she is asked to drink three to four 8-oz glasses of water and is rescanned 30 to 45 minutes later.

A water-based transmission gel is generously spread over the woman's abdomen, and the sonographer slowly moves a transducer over the abdomen to obtain a picture of the uterine contents and surrounding structures. Ultrasound testing takes 20 to 30 minutes. The patient may feel discomfort caused by pressure applied over a full bladder. In addition, if the woman lies on her back during the test, she may develop shortness of breath. This may be relieved by elevating her upper body during the test.

Transvaginal Ultrasound

The transvaginal approach uses a probe inserted into the vagina. Once inserted, the transvaginal probe is close to the structures being imaged; therefore, it produces a clearer, more defined image. The improved images obtained by transvaginal ultrasound have enabled sonographers to identify structures and fetal characteristics earlier in pregnancy. Internal visualization can also be used as a predictor for preterm birth in high-risk patients (Cunningham et al., 2018). Use of the ultrasound technique to detect shortened cervical length or funneling (a cone-shaped indentation in the cervical os) is helpful in predicting preterm labor, especially in patients who have a history of preterm birth (Cunningham et al., 2018).

After the procedure is fully explained to the woman, she is prepared in the same manner as for a pelvic examination: in the lithotomy position, with appropriate drapes to provide privacy, and a female attendant in the room. It is important that her buttocks be at the end of the table so that, once inserted, the probe can be moved in various directions. A small, lightweight vaginal transducer is covered with a specially fitted sterile sheath, a condom, or one finger of a glove. Ultrasound gel is then applied to both the inside and outside of the covering, making insertion into the vagina easier and providing a medium for enhancing the ultrasound image. The transvaginal procedure can be accomplished with an empty bladder, and most women do not feel discomfort during the exam. The probe is smaller than a speculum, so insertion is usually completed with ease. The woman may feel the movement of the probe during the exam as various structures are imaged. Some patients may want to insert the probe themselves to enhance their comfort, whereas others would feel embarrassed even to be asked. The CNM, physician, or ultrasonographer offers the choice based on personal rapport with the patient.

Benefits of Ultrasound Testing

Ultrasound testing can be of benefit in the following ways:

- ***Early identification of pregnancy.*** Pregnancy may be detected as early as the fifth or sixth week after the LMP by assessing the gestational sac and the presence of a FHR after 6 weeks of gestation.
- ***Observation of fetal heartbeat and fetal breathing movements.*** Fetal breathing movements have been observed as early as 11 weeks of gestation.
- ***Identification of more than one embryo or fetus.***
- ***Comparison of the biparietal diameter of the fetal head, head circumference, abdominal circumference, and femur length to assess growth patterns.*** These measurements help determine the gestational age of the fetus and identify IUGR.
- ***Clinical estimations of birth weight.*** This assessment helps identify macrosomia (newborns > 4000 g at birth) and low-birth-weight newborns (babies < 2500 g at birth). Macrosomia has been identified as a predictor of birth-related trauma and is a risk factor for both maternal and fetal morbidity (ACOG, 2018c). It is used only as a guideline in clinical decision making. Antenatal estimates of fetal weight are poor predictors of both actual fetal weight and outcomes in labor and birth.
- ***Detection of fetal anomalies such as anencephaly and hydrocephalus.***
- ***Examination of nuchal translucency in the first trimester to assess for Down syndrome and other fetal structural anomalies*** (Sahota et al., 2012). Nuchal translucency describes an area in the back of the fetal neck that is measured via ultrasound during the first trimester of pregnancy. *Nuchal translucency testing (NTT),* also known as *nuchal testing* or *nuchal fold testing,* is performed at 11 to 13 weeks of gestation to screen for trisomies 13, 18, and 21 (Miguelez et al., 2012).
- ***Examination of fetal cardiac structures (echocardiography).***
- ***Length of fetal nasal bone.*** The length of the fetal nasal bone during the NTT is used to indicate a risk factor for Down syndrome. Fetuses with a nonvisualized or shortened nasal bone are more likely to have trisomy 21 than are those with a normal-length nasal bone (Sonek, Molina, Hiett, & Glover, 2012).
- ***Identification of amniotic fluid index (AFI).*** Ultrasound can provide a rough measurement of the amount of amniotic fluid, which is an indicator of fetal well-being. There are two methods that can be used to evaluate AFI. Amniotic fluid index is the measurement of the amniotic fluid within four quadrants of the maternal abdomen. The maternal abdomen is divided into quadrants using the umbilicus as the center point. The vertical diameter of the largest amniotic fluid pocket in each quadrant is measured. All measurements are totaled to obtain the AFI in centimeters. Women with an AFI of more than 24 cm are considered to have polyhydramnios (an excessive amount of amniotic fluid in the amniotic sac), and women with an AFI of less than 5 cm at term are considered to have oligohydramnios (not enough amniotic fluid). An AFI of between 5 and 24 cm is considered to be normal. Gestational age has an impact on amniotic fluid volume. After 39 weeks of gestation, the amniotic fluid volume begins to decline (Magann & Ross, 2014). Despite this, gestational age is not considered when evaluating the amniotic fluid index, as the criteria have been established with a focus on adverse outcomes rather than population distribution. The single deepest pocket (SDP) measurement is the vertical measurement of the largest pocket of amniotic fluid that does not contain umbilical cord or fetal extremities (Reddy, Abuhamad, Levine, & Saade, 2014). A depth of < 2 cm is considered oligohydramnios, 2 to < 8 cm is considered normal, and 8 cm or greater is considered polyhydramnios. SDP is the preferred method of amniotic fluid evaluation in twin pregnancies (Ippolito, Bergstrom, Lutgendorf, & Flood-Nichols, 2014). Both polyhydramnios and oligohydramnios are associated with increased risk to the fetus, including nonreassuring fetal status, IUGR, meconium-stained amniotic fluid, and an increase in admissions to the neonatal intensive care unit (NICU).
- ***Location of the placenta.*** The placenta is located before amniocentesis to avoid puncturing it during the procedure. Ultrasound is valuable in identifying and evaluating placenta previa (Cunningham et al., 2018).
- ***Placental grading.*** As the fetus matures, the placenta calcifies. These changes can be detected by ultrasound and graded according to the degree of calcification. Placental grading can be used to identify internal placental vasculature, in which abnormalities can be associated with preeclampsia and chronic HTN.
- ***Detection of fetal death.*** Inability to visualize the fetal heart beating and the separation of the bones in the fetal head are signs of fetal death.
- ***Determination of fetal position and presentation.***
- ***Accompanying procedures.*** Ultrasound guidance is used in a variety of intrauterine procedures, including amniocentesis and CVS.

Nonstress Test

The **nonstress test (NST)**, a widely used method of evaluating fetal status, may be used alone or as part of a more comprehensive diagnostic assessment called a biophysical profile. The NST is based on the knowledge that when the fetus has adequate oxygenation and an intact CNS, accelerations of the FHR occur with fetal movement. An NST requires an external electronic fetal monitor to observe and record these FHR accelerations. A nonreactive NST is fairly consistent in identifying at-risk fetuses (Cunningham et al., 2018).

The advantages of the NST include the following:

- It is quick to perform, permits easy interpretation, and is inexpensive.
- It can be done in an office or clinic setting.
- It is a noninvasive procedure.
- There are no known side effects.

The disadvantages of the NST include the following:

- It is sometimes difficult to obtain a suitable tracing.
- The woman has to remain relatively still for at least 20 minutes.

Procedure for NST

The test can be done with the patient in a reclining chair or in bed with the patient in a left-tilted semi-Fowler or side-lying position. Research has shown that certain maternal positions can help produce more favorable results. Patients in left-tilted semi-Fowler, sitting, and left lateral positions are more likely to have a reactive tracing. Patients should not be placed in a supine position because it decreases cardiac output and uterine perfusion, maternal back pain, and maternal shortness of breath (Cunningham et al., 2018). An electronic fetal monitor is used to obtain a tracing of the FHR and fetal movement. The nurse places the monitor under the woman's clothing. Privacy should be provided. The examiner puts two elastic belts on the patient's abdomen. One belt holds a device that detects uterine or fetal movement; the other belt holds a device that detects the FHR. As the NST is done, each fetal movement is documented so that associated or simultaneous FHR changes can be evaluated.

Interpretation of Test Results

An NST is indicated after 32 weeks at any time fetal well-being needs to be established. It may be used between 26 and 32 weeks with modified criteria for interpretation. The results of the NST are interpreted as follows:

- ***Reactive test.*** A reactive NST shows at least two accelerations of FHR with fetal movements of 15 beats/min, lasting 15 seconds or more, over 20 minutes (**Figure 33.29** »). This is the desired result.
- ***Nonreactive test.*** In a nonreactive test, the reactive criteria are not met. For example, the accelerations do not meet the requirements of 15 beats/min or do not last 15 seconds (**Figure 33.30** »).
- ***Unsatisfactory test.*** An NST is unsatisfactory if the data cannot be interpreted or there was inadequate fetal activity.

It is important that anyone who performs the NST understand the significance of any decelerations of the FHR during testing. If decelerations are noted, the HCP should be notified for further evaluation of fetal status.

Fetal Acoustic and Vibroacoustic Stimulation Tests

Acoustic (sound) and vibroacoustic (vibration and sound) stimulation of the fetus can be used as an adjunct to the NST. A hand-held, battery-operated device is applied to the woman's abdomen over the area of the fetal head. This device generates a low-frequency vibration and a buzzing sound. These are intended to induce movement and associated accelerations of the FHR in fetuses with a nonreactive

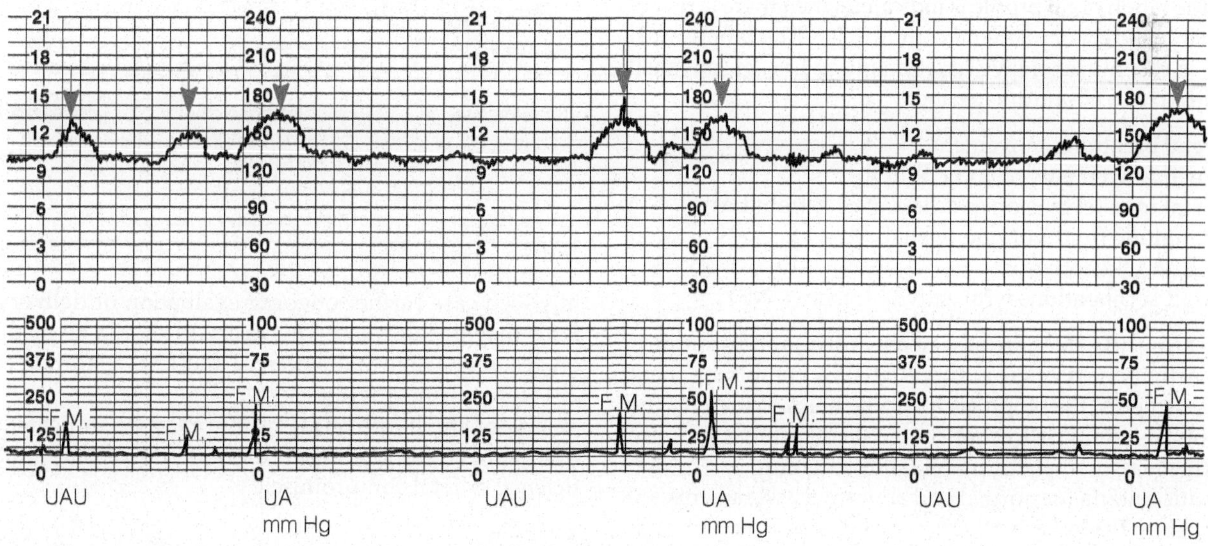

Figure 33.29 » Example of a reactive nonstress test: accelerations of 15 beats/min lasting 15 seconds with each fetal movement. Top of strip shows fetal heart rate; bottom of strip shows uterine activity tracing. Note that FHR increases (above the baseline) at least 15 beats and remains at that rate for at least 15 seconds before returning to the former baseline.

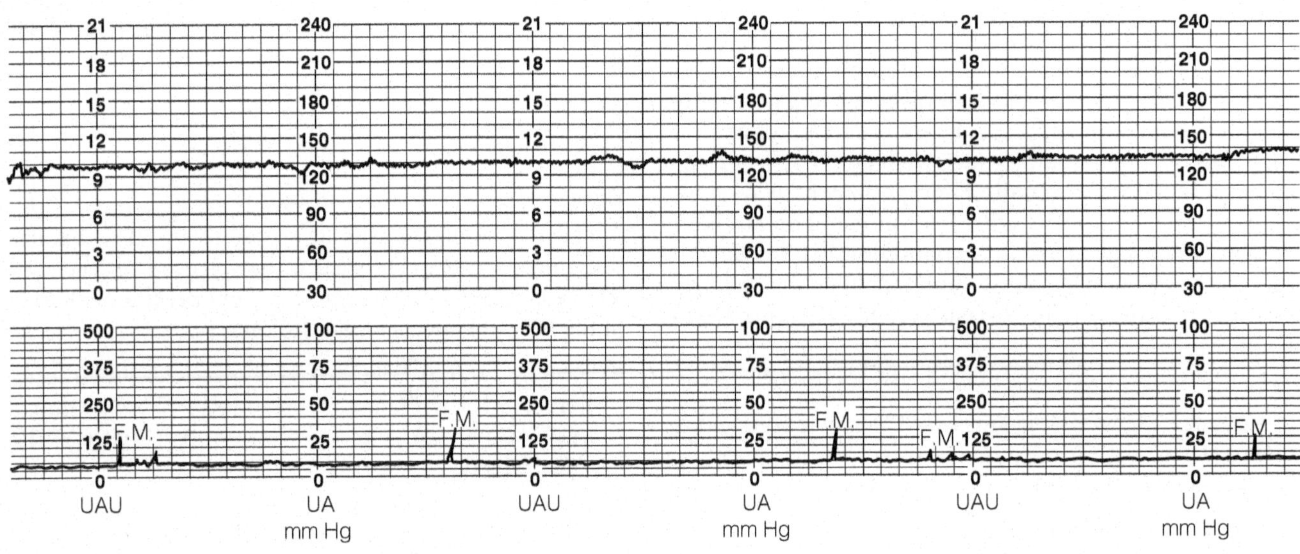

Figure 33.30 ›› Example of a nonreactive nonstress test. There are no accelerations of the FHR with fetal movement. Baseline FHR is 130 beats/min. The tracing of uterine activity is on the bottom of the strip.

NST and in fetuses with decreased variability of the FHR during labor. The sound stimulus persists for 1 second; if no accelerations occur, it is then repeated at 1-minute intervals up to two times and then progresses to 2 seconds waiting 1 minute if no accelerations occur after the stimulus. Whether the fetus responds more to the vibration or to the sound is not known. Two FHR accelerations of 15 beats/min, lasting 15 seconds, in a 20-minute period indicate a reactive test (Cunningham et al., 2018).

Advantages of the fetal acoustic stimulation test and the vibroacoustic stimulation test include the following:

- Both are noninvasive techniques and are easy to perform.
- Results are rapidly available.
- Time for the NST is shortened.

Biophysical Profile

Use of the biophysical profile is indicated when there is risk of placental insufficiency or fetal compromise. The biophysical profile is a comprehensive assessment of five biophysical variables over a 30-minute period:

1. Fetal breathing movement
2. Fetal movements of body or limbs
3. Fetal tone (extension and flexion of extremities)
4. Amniotic fluid volume (visualized as pockets of fluid around the fetus)
5. FHR accelerations with activity (reactive NST).

The first four variables are assessed by ultrasound scanning; FHR reactivity is assessed with the NST. By combining these five assessments, the biophysical profile helps to identify the compromised fetus or to confirm the healthy fetus and also provides an assessment of placental functioning.

Specific criteria for normal and abnormal assessments are presented in **Table 33.3** ››. A score of 2 is assigned to each normal finding, and a score of 0 to each abnormal one, for a maximum score of 10. Scores of 8 and 10 are considered to be normal. Such scores have the least chance of being associated with a compromised fetus unless oligohydramnios is noted, in which case further ongoing evaluation or delivery of the fetus may be indicated. This decision should be made based on gestational age and maternal and fetal condition (ACOG, 2014a, reaffirmed 2016).

TABLE 33.3 Criteria for Biophysical Profile Scoring

Component	Normal (Score = 2)	Abnormal (Score = 0)
Fetal breathing movements	≥1 episode of rhythmic breathing lasting ≥30 seconds within 30 minutes	≤30 seconds of breathing in 30 minutes
Gross body movements	≥3 discrete body or limb movements in 30 minutes (episodes of active continuous movement considered as single movement)	≤2 movements in 30 minutes
Fetal tone	≥1 episode of extension of a fetal extremity with return to flexion or opening or closing of hand	No movements or extension/flexion
Amniotic fluid volume (AFI)	Single vertical pocket > 2 cm AFI > 5 cm	Largest single vertical pocket ≤2 cm AFI < 5 cm
Nonstress test	≥2 accelerations of ≥15 beats/min for ≥15 seconds in 20 minutes	0 or 1 acceleration in 20–40 minutes

Source: From London et al. (2017). Pearson Education, Inc., Hoboken, NJ.

Use of the biophysical profile may be indicated in the following conditions when there is risk of placental insufficiency or fetal compromise:

- IUGR
- Maternal diabetes mellitus
- Maternal heart disease
- Maternal chronic HTN

- Maternal preeclampsia or eclampsia
- Maternal sickle cell disease
- Suspected fetal postmaturity (>42 weeks of gestation)
- History of previous stillbirths
- Rh sensitization
- Abnormal estriol excretion
- Hyperthyroidism
- Renal disease
- Nonreactive NST.

Contraction Stress Test

The **contraction stress test (CST)** is a means of evaluating the respiratory function (oxygen and carbon dioxide exchange) of the placenta. It enables the healthcare team to identify the fetus at risk for intrauterine asphyxia by observing the response of the FHR to the stress of uterine contractions (spontaneous or induced). During contractions, intrauterine pressure increases and blood flow to the intervillous space of the placenta is momentarily reduced, thereby decreasing oxygen transport to the fetus. A healthy fetus usually tolerates this reduction well and maintains moderate variability. If the placental reserve is insufficient, however, then fetal hypoxia, depression of the myocardium, and a decrease in variability to minimal or absent may occur, indicating an altered state in fetal oxygen reserve.

In many areas, the CST has given way to the biophysical profile. The CST is less convenient to perform, can be more time-consuming, and has relative contraindications. It is still used, however, in areas where the availability of other technology is reduced (e.g., during night shifts) or limited (e.g., at small community hospitals or birthing centers). It may also be used as an adjunct to other forms of fetal assessment.

The CST is contraindicated in the patient with third-trimester bleeding from placenta previa, marginal abruptio placentae or unexplained vaginal bleeding, previous cesarean section with classic incision (vertical incision in the fundus of the uterus), premature rupture of the membranes, cervical insufficiency, cerclage in place (gathering stitch around cervix), anomalies of the maternal reproductive organs, history of preterm labor (if being done before term), or multiple gestation.

The critical component of the CST is the presence of uterine contractions. These contractions may occur spontaneously, which is unusual before the onset of labor, or they may be induced (stimulated) with oxytocin (Pitocin) administered IV (also known as an oxytocin challenge test). A natural method of obtaining oxytocin is through the use of breast stimulation (either via nipple self-stimulation or application of an electric breast pump); the posterior pituitary produces oxytocin in response to stimulation of the breasts or nipples.

An electronic fetal monitor is used to provide continuous data about the FHR and uterine contractions. After a 15-minute baseline recording of uterine activity and FHR, the tracing is evaluated for evidence of spontaneous contractions. If three spontaneous contractions of good quality and lasting 40 to 60 seconds occur in a 10-minute window, the results are evaluated and the test is concluded. If no contractions occur, or if the contractions that do occur are insufficient for interpretation, then IV administration of oxytocin, breast self-stimulation, or application of an electric breast pump is done to produce contractions of good quality. The CST should be conducted only in a setting where tocolytic medications are available if a tachysystole pattern occurs or if labor is stimulated from the test.

The CST is classified as follows:

- ***Negative.*** A negative CST shows three contractions of good quality lasting 40 seconds or longer in a 10-minute period without evidence of late decelerations. This is the desired result and implies that the fetus can handle the hypoxic stress of uterine contractions.
- ***Positive.*** A positive CST shows repetitive, persistent, late decelerations, in which the FHR decreases after the onset of a contraction and recovers after the completion of a contraction in more than 50% of the contractions (**Figure 33.31** »). This is not a desired result. The hypoxic stress of the uterine

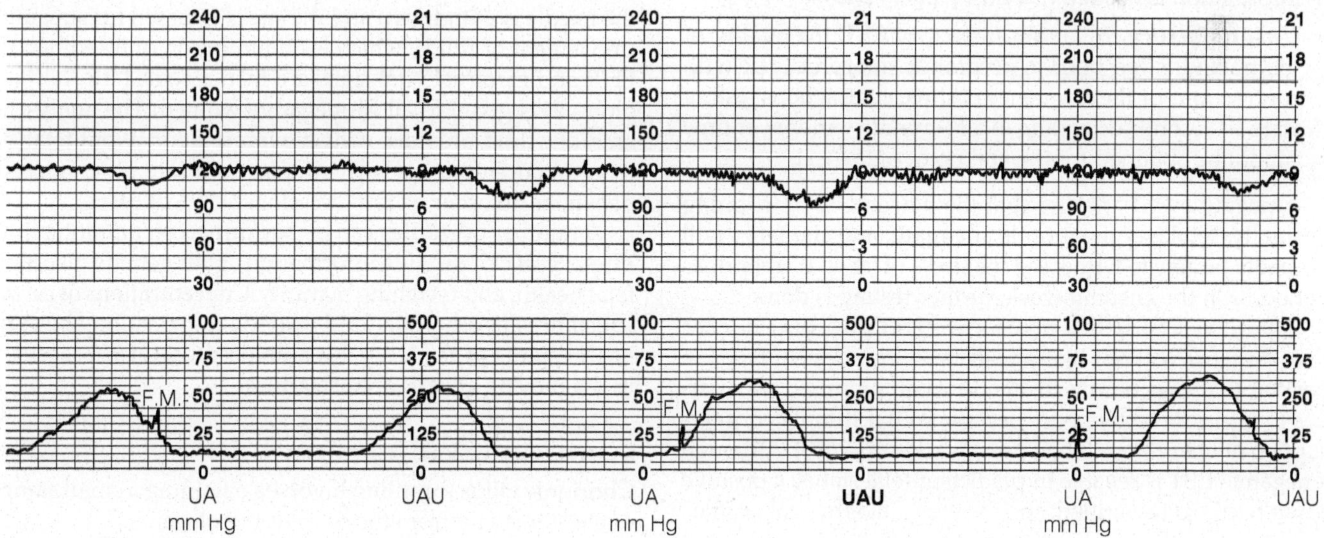

Figure 33.31 » Example of a positive contraction stress test. Repetitive late decelerations occur with each contraction. Note that there are no accelerations of FHR with three fetal movements. The baseline FHR is 120 beats/min. Uterine contractions (bottom half of strip) occurred four times in 12 minutes.

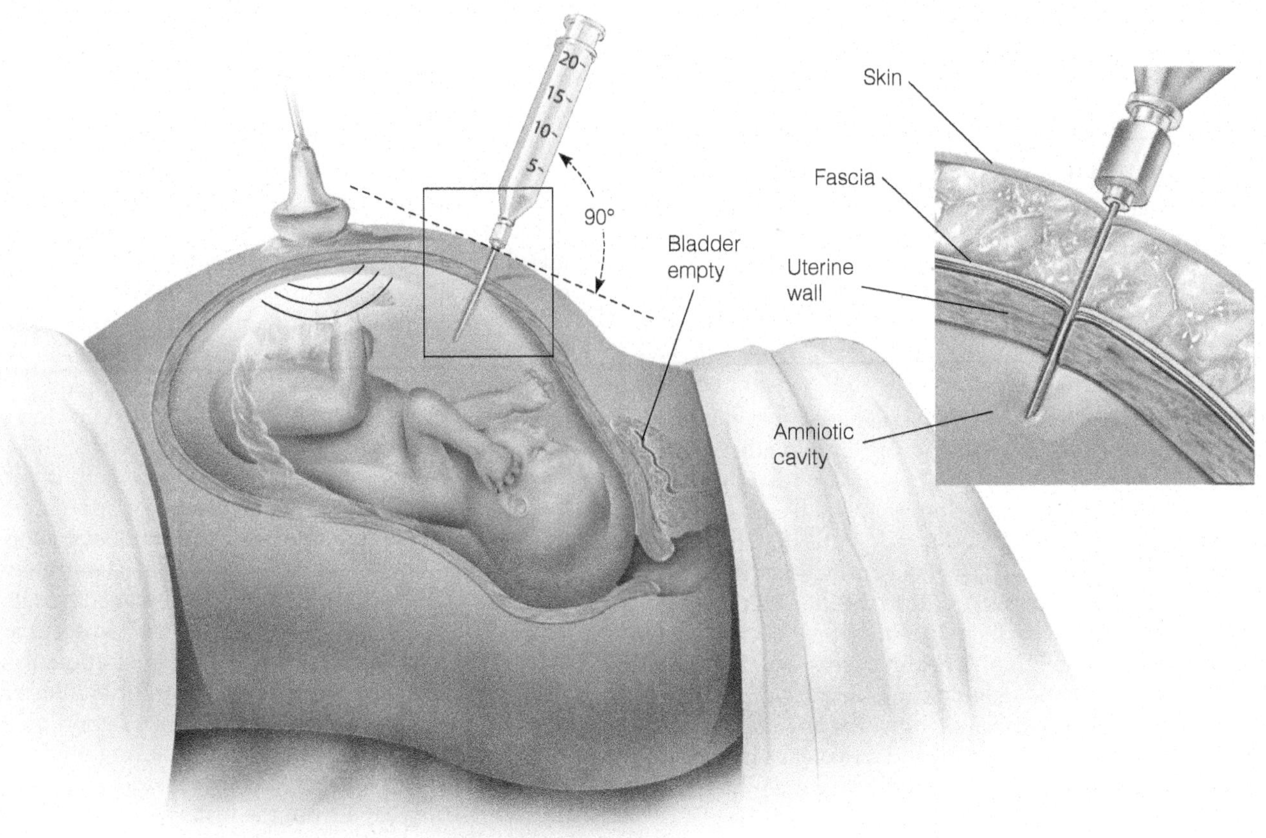

Figure 33.32 ›› Amniocentesis. The woman is scanned by ultrasound to determine the placenta site and to locate a pocket of amniotic fluid. The needle is then inserted into the uterine cavity to withdraw amniotic fluid.

contraction causes a slowing of the FHR. The pattern will not improve and will most likely get worse with additional contractions.

- ***Equivocal.*** An equivocal or suspicious test has nonpersistent late decelerations associated with tachysystole (contraction frequency of every 2 minutes or duration lasting longer than 90 seconds). When this test result occurs, more information is needed (Davidson et al., 2020).
- ***Unsatisfactory.*** In an unsatisfactory CST, the quality of the tracing is too poor to accurately interpret FHR with contractions or the frequency of three contractions lasting 40 to 60 seconds occurring in a 10-minute window of time cannot be obtained for the end point of the test.

A negative CST implies that the placenta is functioning normally, fetal oxygenation is adequate, and the fetus will probably be able to withstand the stress of labor. If labor does not occur in the ensuing week, further testing is done.

A positive CST with a nonreactive NST presents evidence that the fetus will not likely withstand the stress of labor. A positive CST may be able to identify a compromised fetus earlier than a nonreactive NST because of the stimulated interruption of intervillous blood flow (Blackburn, 2018). Although a negative CST is reliable in predicting fetal status, a positive result needs to be verified, such as with a biophysical profile.

Amniotic Fluid Analysis

Amniocentesis is a procedure used to obtain amniotic fluid for genetic testing to determine fetal abnormalities or fetal lung maturity in the third trimester of pregnancy. During an amniocentesis, the physician scans the uterus using ultrasound to identify the fetal and placental positions and to identify adequate pockets of amniotic fluid. The skin is then cleaned with a Betadine solution. The use of a local anesthesia at the needle insertion site is optional. A 22-gauge needle is then inserted into the uterine cavity to withdraw amniotic fluid (**Figure 33.32 ››**). After 15 to 20 mL of fluid has been removed, the needle is withdrawn and the site is assessed for streaming (movement of fluid), which is an indication of bleeding. The FHR and maternal vital signs are then assessed. Rh immune globulin is given to all Rh-negative women. The analysis of amniotic fluid provides valuable information about fetal status. Amniocentesis is a fairly simple procedure, although complications do occur on rare occasions (<1% of cases).

A number of studies can be performed on amniotic fluid. These tests can provide information about genetic disorders, fetal health, and fetal lung maturity. Concentrations of certain substances in amniotic fluid provide information about the health status of the fetus. An amniocentesis is 99% accurate in diagnosing genetic abnormalities.

Chorionic Villus Sampling

Chorionic villus sampling involves obtaining a small sample of chorionic villi from the developing placenta.

The advantages of this procedure are early diagnosis and a short waiting time for results. Whereas amniocentesis is not done until at least 14 weeks of gestation, CVS is typically performed between 10 and 13 weeks of gestation.

Previous studies that evaluated the use of CVS at 9 weeks of gestation found a possible association between limb-reduction anomalies and early CVS. Based on these findings, most practitioners do not recommend early CVS before 10 weeks of gestation (Cunningham et al., 2018). Risks of CVS include failure to obtain tissue, rupture of membranes, leakage of amniotic fluid, bleeding, intrauterine infection, maternal tissue contamination of the specimen, and Rh isoimmunization.

Because CVS testing is performed so early in the pregnancy, it cannot detect NTDs. Patients who desire screening for NTDs would need a quadruple screening or the AFP component of first-trimester integrated screening at 15 to 20 weeks of gestation.

Other Antenatal Screening Tests

The **quadruple screen** is a widely used test to screen for Down syndrome (trisomy 21), trisomy 18, and NTDs. The serum test assesses for appropriate levels of MSAFP, hCG, UE, and dimeric inhibin-A. The newer **penta screen** tests for all that the quadruple screen tests for and also tests for ventral abdominal wall defects. In recent years integrated screening for aneuploidy (chromosome abnormality) has been offered to pregnant women between 11 and 13 weeks' gestation. It consists of an early ultrasound that evaluates markers on the fetus (nasal bone and nuchal fold) and combines these with hCG, estriol, and inhibin A values to generate a more accurate risk profile for trisomy 13, 18, and 21 earlier in the pregnancy. A MSAFP and ultrasound for fetal anatomy are added between 18 and 20 weeks to determine risk or presence of a neural tube defect. Abnormal values on quadruple, penta, and integrated screens are indicators of increased risk only. They must be followed by a diagnostic amniocentesis from which a fetal karyotype is done (Messerlian, Farina, & Palomaki, 2016). Another new development in the diagnosis of fetal aneuploidy is *noninvasive prenatal testing (NIPT)*, also called *cell-free fetal DNA (cffDNA)*. This process detects fetal alleles in maternal serum and can provide accurate information on chromosomal abnormalities without the invasiveness and, albeit small, risk of amniocentesis from 9 weeks gestation onward (Wolfberg, 2016). Aneuploidy detection rates are similar for NIPT, CVS, and amniocentesis (King et al., 2019).

SAFETY ALERT When explaining options for genetic testing to expectant parents, inform them that even if a CVS shows no chromosomal abnormality, it cannot screen for NTDs. Patients who have a normal CVS and an abnormal quadruple screen test are to be offered amniocentesis. Patients with risk factors for NTDs may want to consider amniocentesis instead of CVS because amniocentesis screens for both types of disorders.

The nurse assists the physician during the amniocentesis or CVS and supports the woman undergoing the procedure. Although the physician has explained the procedure in advance so that the patient can give informed consent, the woman is likely to be apprehensive, both about the procedure itself and about the information it may reveal. She may become anxious during the procedure and need additional emotional support. The nurse can provide support by further clarifying the physician's instructions or explanations, by relieving the patient's physical discomfort when possible, and by responding verbally and physically to the woman's need for reassurance.

Factors Affecting Maternal Nutrition

A woman's nutritional status before and during pregnancy can significantly influence her health and that of her fetus. In most prenatal clinics and offices, nurses offer nutritional counseling directly or work closely with a nutritionist to provide nutritional assessment and teaching.

The following factors influence the pregnant woman's ability to achieve good prenatal nutrition:

- ***General nutritional status before pregnancy.*** Nutritional deficits, such as folic acid deficiency, present at the time of conception and during the early prenatal period may influence the outcome of the pregnancy.
- ***Maternal age.*** An expectant adolescent must meet her own growth needs in addition to the nutritional needs of pregnancy.
- ***Maternal parity.*** The mother's nutritional needs and the outcome of the pregnancy are influenced by the number of pregnancies she has had and by the interval between them.

Fetal growth occurs in three overlapping stages:

1. Growth by increase in cell number
2. Growth by increases in cell number and cell size
3. Growth by increase in cell size alone.

Nutritional problems that interfere with cell division may have permanent consequences. If the nutritional insult occurs when cells are mainly enlarging, the changes are usually reversible when normal nutrition resumes.

Growth of fetal and maternal tissues requires increased quantities of essential dietary components. These are listed in the federal government's recommended **Daily Nutritional Goals** for pregnant and lactating women (**Table 33.4** ⟫). Most of the recommended nutrients can be obtained by eating a well-balanced diet each day that includes between four and six 8-ounce glasses of water and a total of between 64 and 80 ounces of total fluid intake daily. The pregnant woman should eat regularly, three meals a day, with nutritious snacks of fruit, low-fat dairy items (such as yogurt or cheese), or other foods between meals, if desired. (More frequent but smaller meals are also recommended.) Between four and six 8-oz glasses of water, and a total of between eight and ten 8-oz cups of total fluid intake, should be consumed daily. Water is an essential nutrient.

It is important to consider the many factors that affect a woman's nutrition. What environmental risks should the woman consider? What are her age, lifestyle, and culture? What food beliefs and habits does she have? What an individual eats is determined by availability, economics, and symbolism. These factors and others influence the expectant mother's acceptance of the nurse's intervention. For more information, see Module 14, Nutrition.

TABLE 33.4 Daily Nutritional Goals for Women Who Are Pregnant and Lactating: Vitamins and Elements

	Age	Vitamin A (mcg/day)	Vitamin C (mg/day)	Vitamin D (IU/day)	Vitamin E (mg/day)
Pregnancy	14–18 yr	750	80	600	15
	19–50 yr	770	85	600	15
Lactation	14–18 yr	1200	115	600	19
	19–50 yr	1300	120	600	19
	Age	**Vitamin K (mcg/day)**	**Thiamine (mg/day)**	**Riboflavin (mg/day)**	**Niacin (mg/day)**
Pregnancy	14–18 yr	75*	1.4	1.4	18
	19–50 yr	90*	1.4	1.4	18
Lactation	14–18 yr	75*	1.4	1.6	17
	19–50 yr	90*	1.4	1.6	17
	Age	**Vitamin B_6 (mg/day)**	**Folate† (mcg/day)**	**Vitamin B_{12} (mg/day)**	**Calcium (mg/day)**
Pregnancy	14–18 yr	1.9	600	2.6	1300*
	19–50 yr	1.9	600	2.6	1000*
Lactation	14–18 yr	2.0	500	2.8	1300*
	19–50 yr	2.0	500	2.8	1000*
	Age	**Iodine (mcg/day)**	**Iron (mg/day)**	**Magnesium (mg/day)**	**Phosphorus (mg/day)**
Pregnancy	≤ 18 yr	220	27	400	1250
	19–30 yr	220	27	350	700
	31–50 yr	220	27	360	700
Lactation	≤ 18 yr	290	10	360	1250
	19–30 yr	290	9	310	700
	31–50 yr	290	9	320	700
	Age	**Potassium (mg/day)**		**Zinc (mg/day)**	
Pregnancy	14–18 yr	2600		11	
	19–50 yr	2900		11	
Lactation	14–18 yr	2500		13	
	19–50 yr	2800		12	

*Values are adequate intakes rather than recommended daily intake.
†In view of evidence linking folate intake with NTDs in the fetus, it is recommended that all women capable of becoming pregnant consume 600 mcg from supplements or fortified foods in addition to intake of food folate from a varied diet.

Sources: Institute of Medicine (IOM; 2006, 2011); National Academies of Sciences, Engineering, and Medicine (2019); U.S. Department of Agriculture and U.S. Department of Health and Human Services (2020).

>> **Stay Current** The U.S. Department of Agriculture provides recommendations regarding nutrition and health for pregnant and breastfeeding women at https://myplate.gov/life-stages/pregnancy-and-breastfeeding.

>> **Stay Current:** The complete *Dietary Guidelines for Americans, 2020–2025* can be found at https://www.dietaryguidelines.gov/.

Socioeconomic Influences

Families living at or near poverty level are not able to afford to make the same food choices that higher-income families can. As a result, many pregnant women are at risk for inadequate nutrition. Disparities in maternal and infant outcomes can be attributed to these factors. These disparities can be reduced by increasing access to resources. Educating pregnant women on access to healthy and affordable food options, including the SNAP and WIC programs, is a priority for the nurse. The Supplemental Nutrition Assistance Program (SNAP) works with state agencies and other organizations to help provide nutrition assistance for families living in poverty. Many pregnant women and children up to 5 years old are eligible for WIC, the Special Supplemental Nutrition Program for Women, Infants, and Children. WIC provides food vouchers and nutrition education to low-income and at-risk pregnant and postpartum women. These programs are primarily federally funded and administered through the states. Applications can be made through local departments of social or children's services.

>> **Stay Current:** More information about the WIC program can be found at the program's website at www.fns.usda.gov/wic.

Cultural, Ethnic, and Religious Influences

Individual food preferences and habits, including cooking methods, may be informed by cultural, ethnic, or religious influences (**Figure 33.33** >>). Availability of foods and methods

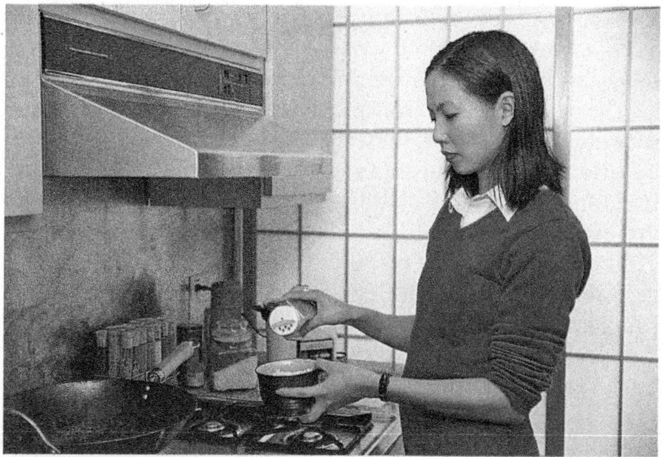

Figure 33.33 ›› Cultural factors affect food preferences and habits.
Source: Pearson Education, Inc.

of preparation also may be based in cultural, religious, or regional factors. For example, many Jewish individuals follow a kosher diet, which forbids the eating of pork products and shellfish. Pregnant Jewish women who observe kosher dietary guidelines may need increased protein, vitamins, and other nutrients. In addition to consuming protein from fish, eggs, legumes, and some meat and poultry, they may benefit from consuming at least one serving of leafy green vegetables and one serving of orange vegetables each day.

In many cultures, certain foods have symbolic significance, often in relation to major life experiences such as birth and death. The extent to which a woman or family follows cultural or religious practices varies widely and often depends on the extent of their exposure to other cultures and on the availability and costs of traditional foods. There are similarities as well: Many cultures recognize the healing properties of chicken soup (Spector, 2017). However, the ingredients and spices used may vary according to ingredients available locally over the course of centuries.

As part of the antepartum assessment, the nurse should identify and understand the extent to which a pregnant woman's cultural and spiritual beliefs affect her eating habits and beliefs about food and pregnancy. The nurse can then provide any nutritional information to help the woman and her family ensure a healthy outcome for the pregnancy.

Psychosocial Influences

The nurse should be aware of the various psychosocial factors that influence a woman's food choices. The sharing of food has long been a symbol of friendliness, warmth, and social acceptance in many cultures. Some foods and food practices are associated with status. Some foods are prepared "just for company"; others are served only on special occasions or holidays.

Knowledge about the basic components of a balanced diet is essential. Often, educational level is related to SES, but even individuals with very limited incomes can prepare well-balanced meals if their knowledge of nutrition is adequate.

The expectant woman's attitudes and feelings about her pregnancy influence her nutritional status. For example, foods may be used as a substitute for expressing emotions, such as anger or frustration, or as a way of expressing feelings of joy. The woman who is depressed or does not wish to be pregnant may manifest these feelings through loss of appetite or overindulgence in certain foods.

Eating Disorders

Two serious eating disorders, anorexia nervosa and bulimia nervosa, develop most commonly in adolescent girls and young women. These conditions are described fully in Exemplar 29.A, Feeding and Eating Disorders, in Module 29, Self.

Women with eating disorders who become pregnant are at risk for a variety of complications. The consequences of the restricting, bingeing, and purging behaviors characteristic of eating disorders can result in a lack of nutrients being available for the fetus. These patients may be at increased risk of miscarriage and postpartum hemorrhage. The babies of these patients are at increased risk for low birth weight, small for gestational age, low Apgar scores (see Exemplar 33.D, Newborn Care, in this module for a discussion of Apgar scores), and intrauterine death (Micali et al., 2012).

Pregnancy can be an especially difficult time for the woman with an eating disorder, even if she has long desired a child. The consumption of additional food and the expectations that she will gain additional weight can result in feelings of fear, anxiety, depression, and guilt. Women with eating disorders also have high rates of postpartum depression (Micali et al., 2012).

When a pregnant woman has an eating disorder, education and individualized meal plans can help the patient increase her dietary intake while maintaining a sense of control. A multidisciplinary approach to treatment, involving medical, nursing, psychiatric, and dietetic practitioners, is indicated. Pregnant women with eating disorders need to be closely monitored and supported throughout their pregnancies.

Pica

Pica is the craving for and persistent eating of nonnutritive substances not ordinarily considered to be edible or nutritionally valuable, such as soil, clay, and soap. Pica appears to occur worldwide but is underreported because women are often embarrassed to discuss it. In the United States, pica is more common among women who are economically disadvantaged, are of Latino or African American descent, live in rural areas, practiced pica before pregnancy, belong to a culture that encourages pica as important for fertility, and have family members who also practice pica (Burke, 2021; Young & Cox, 2019).

Iron deficiency anemia is the most common concern in pica. The connection of ice pica to iron deficiency is well known, but it is unclear if ingestion of large amounts of ice is a sign of iron deficiency or a contributing factor. However, the pica often resolves with iron supplementation (King et al., 2019). The ingestion of laundry starch or certain types of clay may contribute to iron deficiency because they interfere with iron absorption. The ingestion of large quantities of clay could fill the intestine and cause fecal impaction, and the ingestion of starch may be associated with excessive weight gain. Lead poisoning, one of the most serious complications that can result from *geophagia* (eating soil or clay), may affect both the mother and her fetus. Geophagia may produce soilborne parasitic infections, such as toxoplasmosis and toxocariasis. GI tract complications resulting from pica can be mechanical bowel problems, constipation, ulcerations, perforations, and intestinal obstructions. It also can result in impaired cognitive functioning, kidney damage, and encephalopathy. Consequently, blood lead levels should be determined in cases of diagnosed or suspected geophagia.

The nurse should be aware of pica and its implications for the woman and fetus. Assessment for pica is an important part of a nutritional history. However, a patient may be embarrassed about her cravings or reluctant to discuss them for fear of criticism. Using a nonjudgmental approach, the nurse can provide the woman with information that is useful in decreasing or eliminating this practice.

Vegetarianism

Vegetarianism is the dietary choice of many individuals for religious, health, or ethical reasons. There are several types of vegetarians. **Lacto-ovovegetarians** include milk, dairy products, and eggs in their diets. **Lactovegetarians** include dairy products but no eggs in their diets. **Vegans** will not eat any food from animal sources.

The expectant woman who is vegetarian must eat the proper combination of foods to obtain adequate nutrients. If her diet allows, the woman can obtain ample and complete proteins from dairy products and eggs. Plant protein quality can be improved if it is consumed with these animal proteins.

If the woman follows a vegan diet, careful planning is necessary to obtain complete proteins and sufficient calories. An adequate, pure vegan diet contains protein from unrefined grains (brown rice, whole wheat), legumes (beans, split peas, lentils), nuts in large quantities, and a variety of cooked and fresh vegetables and fruits. Adequate dietary protein can be obtained by consuming a varied diet with complementary amino acids, which together provide complete proteins. Complete proteins can be obtained by eating different types of plant-based proteins, such as beans and rice, peanut butter on whole-grain bread, and whole-grain cereal with soy milk, either in the same meal or over a day. Seeds may provide adequate protein in the vegetarian diet if the quantity is large enough. Obtaining sufficient calories to ensure adequate weight gain can be difficult, however, because vegan diets tend to be high in fiber and therefore filling.

Both lacto-ovovegetarians and vegans should eat four servings of vitamin B_{12}–fortified foods (meat substitutes, tofu, cereals, soy milk, and nutritional yeast) daily. A daily supplement of vitamin B_{12} is also recommended during pregnancy and while breastfeeding (London et al., 2017).

The best sources of iron and zinc are animal products; consequently, vegan diets may also be low in these minerals. In addition, a high fiber intake may reduce mineral (calcium, iron, and zinc) bioavailability. Thus, pregnant women who are vegetarians should be advised to have approximately 1200 to 1500 mg/day of calcium, which is higher than the recommended levels for patients who are omnivores. The pregnant woman should also be advised to maintain the recommended daily allowance of 600 IU of vitamin D (ACOG, 2011, reaffirmed 2017).

To achieve optimal nutrition, the nurse should emphasize the use of foods that are nutrient dense and that provide a balanced diet. A vegetarian food group guide appears in **Table 33.5** ».

Special Dietary Considerations

Some foods and food additives require careful consideration during pregnancy. These include folic acid, artificial sweeteners, mercury levels in fish, and lactase/lactose.

Folic Acid

Folic acid, or folate, is required for normal growth, reproduction, and lactation and prevents the macrocytic, megaloblastic anemia of pregnancy. Megaloblastic anemia caused by folate deficiency is rarely found in the United States, but it does occur.

Even more significantly, an inadequate intake of folic acid has been associated with fetal NTDs (spina bifida, meningomyelocele). Although these defects are considered to be multifactorial, research indicates that 50–70% of spina bifida and anencephaly cases could be prevented by adequate intake of folic acid (ACOG, 2017f; CDC, 2019c). Experts recommend that all women of childbearing age (15 to 45 years) consume 400 mcg of folic acid daily because half of all U.S. pregnancies are unplanned and NTDs occur very early in pregnancy (3 to 4 weeks after conception), before most women realize they are pregnant (CDC, 2019c). The best food sources of folate are fresh green leafy vegetables, liver, peanuts, and whole-grain breads and cereals. Folic acid can be made inactive by oxidation, ultraviolet light, and heating. It can easily be lost during improper storage and cooking. To prevent unnecessary loss, foods should be stored covered to protect them from light, cooked with only a small amount of water, and not overcooked.

TABLE 33.5 Vegetarian Food Groups

Food Group	Mixed Diet	Lacto-ovovegetarian	Lactovegetarian	Vegan
Grain	Bread, cereal, rice, pasta	Bread, cereal, rice, pasta	Bread, cereal, rice, pasta	Bread, cereal, rice, pasta
Fruit	Fruit, fruit juices	Fruit, fruit juices	Fruit, fruit juices	Fruit, fruit juices
Vegetable	Vegetables, vegetable juices	Vegetables, vegetable juices	Vegetables, vegetable juices	Vegetables, vegetable juices
Dairy and dairy alternatives	Milk, yogurt, cheese	Milk, yogurt, cheese	Milk, yogurt, cheese	Fortified soy milk, rice milk, almond milk
Meat and meat alternatives	Meat, fish, poultry, eggs, legumes, tofu, nuts, nut butters	Eggs, legumes, tofu, nuts, nut butters	Legumes, tofu, nuts, nut butters	Legumes, tofu, nuts, nut butters

Source: From London et al. (2017). Pearson Education, Inc., Hoboken, NJ.

Artificial Sweeteners

Sweeteners classified as *Generally Recognized as Safe* by the FDA are acceptable for use during pregnancy. As with other foods, moderation should be exercised when using artificial sweeteners, such as saccharin, which can cross the placenta and may remain in fetal tissues. Aspartame also appears to be safe if used within FDA guidelines. Women affected by phenylketonuria should avoid aspartame because it contains phenylalanine. Splenda, or sucralose, is another artificial sweetener that is available to the public. The manufacturers of Splenda and Truvia (stevia) claim that they have no effects on fetal or neonatal development and are therefore safe for use by pregnant or lactating women.

Mercury in Fish

Seafood is an important source of omega-3 fatty acids, which are essential for neural development in the fetus. Of particular interest are the omega-3 fatty acids and their derivative, docosahexaenoic acid (DHA). Maternal dietary intake of DHA during pregnancy may reduce the risk of preterm birth and low birth weight and may enhance fetal and newborn/infant brain development (Julvez et al., 2016). Although the omega-3 in fish is beneficial, pregnant women need to be aware that fish can also contain mercury. Nearly all fish and shellfish contain traces of mercury. Although this is not a concern for most individuals, some fish and shellfish contain higher levels of mercury than others, and mercury can pose a threat to the developing nervous system of a fetus or young child. Mercury exposure also can have a negative effect on cognitive functioning, resulting in deficiencies in language, attention, motor function, memory, and visuospatial abilities (Solan & Lindow, 2014). Consequently, pregnant women need information about the importance of seafood in their diet, but also need to know that they should consume seafood that is low in mercury. The U.S. government has issued the following guidelines for women who are pregnant or may become pregnant, breastfeeding mothers, and young children (U.S. Department of Agriculture, 2015):

- Do not eat swordfish, shark, tilefish, or king mackerel because these fish contain high levels of mercury.
- Eat up to 12 oz/week (two average meals) of a variety of shellfish and fish that are lower in mercury. Commonly eaten fish that are lower in mercury include canned light tuna, shrimp, salmon, catfish, and pollack. Albacore (white) tuna has more mercury than canned light tuna; therefore, only 6 oz/week of albacore tuna is recommended.
- Check local advisories about the mercury content of fish caught by family and friends. If no information is available, limit fish caught in local areas to 6 oz/week and avoid consuming additional fish that week.

Lactase Deficiency (Lactose Intolerance)

Some individuals have difficulty digesting milk and milk products. This condition, known as **lactase deficiency** or **lactose intolerance**, results from an inadequate amount of the enzyme lactase, which breaks down the milk sugar lactose into smaller, digestible substances.

Lactase deficiency is found in many adults of African, Mexican, Native American, Ashkenazi Jewish, and Asian descent and, indeed, in many other adults worldwide. Individuals who are not affected are mainly of northern European heritage. Symptoms include abdominal distention, discomfort, nausea, vomiting, loose stools, and cramps.

When counseling pregnant women who might be intolerant of milk and milk products, the nurse should be aware that even one glass of milk can produce symptoms. Milk in cooked form, such as custards, is sometimes tolerated, as are cultured or fermented dairy products, such as buttermilk, some cheeses, and yogurt. Lactase deficiency need not be a problem for pregnant women because the enzyme is available over the counter in tablets or drops. Lactase-treated milk is also available commercially in most large grocery stores. For more information about lactase deficiency, see Exemplar 4.C, Malabsorption Disorders, in Module 4, Digestion.

Foodborne Illnesses

Foodborne illnesses pose a risk to both fetus and mother. The nurse should provide patient teaching about salmonella, listeriosis, and hepatitis E and reinforce the need for use of proper hand hygiene after food preparation.

Salmonella

Teach pregnant women to avoid eating or tasting foods that contain raw or undercooked eggs, such as cake batter and cookie dough, homemade ice cream made with eggs, and Caesar salad dressing. Reinforce the need to wash and sanitize surfaces that come in contact with raw eggs, poultry, meat, or seafood (FDA, 2018, 2019).

Listeriosis

Listeria moncytogenes is a bacterium that can be found in a number of refrigerated, ready-to-eat foods, including hotdogs and lunch meats, and in unpasteurized milk and milk products. Recommendations for pregnant women include (FDA, 2018):

- Avoid eating lunch meats, hot dogs, and refrigerated patés
- Avoid eating refrigerated smoked seafood (e.g., salmon, mackerel) unless it is in a cooked dish.
- Do not drink raw (unpasteurized) milk or foods made with it
- Refrigerate food and leftovers within 2 hours after eating or preparation
- Keep the refrigerator at 40°F (4°C) or lower and the freezer at 0°F (–18°C). Check the temperature periodically with an appliance thermometer.

Hepatitis E

Hepatitis E is a viral infection found most often in developing countries. This disease is spread through the feces of infected people or animals and is transmitted most often through unclean drinking water, but it can also be contracted by eating contaminated food. Hepatitis E is often more severe in pregnant women, especially during the third trimester, and may lead to maternal death (Gurley et al., 2012; Sherman, 2019).

To prevent hepatitis E, pregnant women should wash their hands thoroughly after using the bathroom, changing diapers, or handling raw foods. When traveling to areas where the quality of the water is uncertain, they should avoid eating raw

TABLE 33.6 Institute of Medicine Weight Gain Recommendations for Pregnancy

Pre-pregnancy Weight Category	Body Mass Index*	Recommended Range of Total Weight (lb)	Recommended Rates of Weight Gain† in the Second and Third Trimesters (lb) (Mean Range [lb/wk])
Underweight	<18.5	28–40	1 (1–1.3)
Normal weight	18.5–24.9	25–35	1 (0.8–1)
Overweight	25–29.9	15–25	0.6 (0.5–0.7)
Obese (includes all classes)	30+	11–20	0.5 (0.4–0.6)

*Body mass index is calculated as weight in kilograms divided by height in meters squared, or as weight in pounds multiplied by 703 divided by square of height in inches.

†Calculations assume a 1.1- to 4.4-lb weight gain in the first trimester.

Note: These guidelines are referenced and used in the U.S. Department of Agriculture and U.S. Department of Health and Human Services' *Dietary Guidelines for Americans, 2020–2025.*

Source: Based on Institute of Medicine (2009). © 2009 National Academy of Sciences.

foods, unpeeled fruit, and uncooked fish. They should also avoid drinking tap water or using ice made with tap water. Rather, they should use bottled or boiled water for drinking, toothbrushing, and formula preparation (Gurley et al., 2012).

Maternal Weight Gain

Maternal weight gain is an important factor in fetal growth and neonatal birth weight. The optimal weight gain depends on the woman's weight for height (BMI) and her pre-pregnant nutritional state. An adequate weight gain indicates an adequate caloric intake. It does not, however, ensure that the woman has a sufficient nutrient intake. The pregnant woman must maintain the nutritional quality of her diet as her weight gain progresses.

The IOM (2009) recommends weight gains in terms of optimal ranges based on pre-pregnant BMI, and ACOG (2015) supports these recommendations. The IOM recommendations are shown in **Table 33.6** ».

The pattern of weight gain is important. The ideal pattern for a normal-weight woman consists of a gain of 0.5 to 2 kg (1.1 to 4.4 lb) during the first trimester, followed by a gain of approximately 0.45 kg (1 lb) per week during the second and third trimesters. The rate of weight gain in the second and third trimesters needs to be slightly higher for underweight women and slightly lower for women who are overweight (ACOG, 2015; IOM, 2009). A normal-weight woman who is expecting twins is advised to gain approximately 0.7 kg (1.5 lb) per week during the second and third trimesters of her pregnancy. Inadequate maternal weight gain has been associated with reduced birth weight of the newborn (ACOG, 2015; IOM, 2009).

Obesity is becoming a major health problem in many developed countries, and more and more women are entering pregnancy already overweight or obese. Pregnant women who are obese are at an increased risk for medical and pregnancy-related complications, such as spontaneous abortion, gestational diabetes, preeclampsia, labor induction, and cesarean birth. They also have a higher incidence of fetal anomalies. They should be considered to be at high risk and counseled accordingly (ACOG, 2015).

Maternal obesity also has implications for children. The children of mothers who are overweight and obese are predisposed to developing obesity and its related health concerns. In fact, the child of an overweight mother is three times more likely to be overweight by the age of 7 than is a child of a normal-weight mother (Voerman et al., 2019).

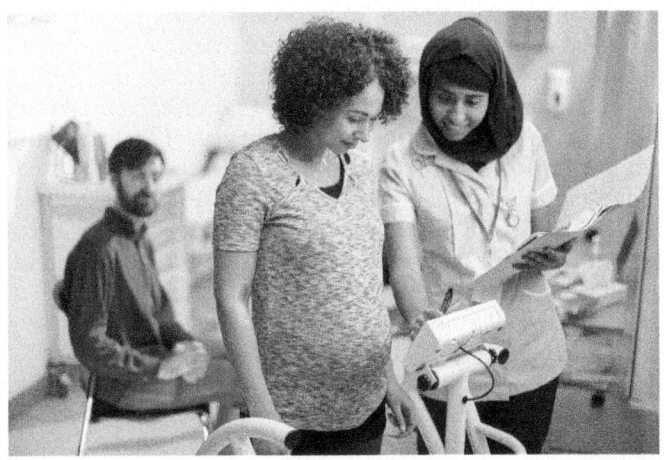

Figure 33.34 » It is important to monitor a pregnant woman's weight over time.

Source: sturti/E+/Getty Images.

Because of the association between maternal weight gain and pregnancy outcome, most HCPs pay close attention to weight gain during pregnancy (**Figure 33.34** »). Weight gain charts can be useful in monitoring the rate and pattern of weight gain over time.

Excessive weight gain during pregnancy also has long-term implications because it is by far the most important predictor of the amount of weight that a woman will retain following childbirth (ACOG, 2015). Counseling the pregnant woman to eat a variety of nutrients from each of the food groups places less emphasis on the amount of her weight gain and more on the quality of her intake. It may also be helpful to encourage the woman to begin a simple exercise program such as walking.

SAFETY ALERT Weight varies with time of day, amount of clothing, inaccurate scale adjustment, or weighing error. Do not overemphasize a single weight; rather, pay attention to the overall pattern of weight gain.

» **Stay Current:** Oregon Health and Science University offers a helpful illustration to assist pregnant women in making healthy food choices. My Pregnancy Plate is available at https://www.ohsu.edu/sites/default/files/2020-10/CWH%203051517%20Pregnancy%20Plate%20FLY%202019.pdf. The American College of Obstetricians and Gynecologists provides FAQ sheets on pregnancy and nutrition at https://www.acog.org/womens-health/faqs/nutrition-during-pregnancy.

Lifespan Considerations

Pregnant adolescents and women over the age of 35 have specific care needs. Some of these considerations are discussed in this section.

Pregnant Adolescents

How adolescents who become pregnant view the pregnancy, and the amount of support they have during the pregnancy, vary greatly. Although specific needs will reveal themselves through assessment and the progression of the therapeutic relationship, nutritional needs and risks associated with adolescence will commonly require the nurse's consideration.

Estimates regarding the nutritional needs of adolescents are generally determined by using the **Dietary Reference Intakes (DRIs)** for nonpregnant teenagers (ages 11 to 14 or 15 to 18) and adding nutrient amounts recommended for all pregnant women (see Table 33.4). If the pregnant adolescent is physiologically mature (> 4 years since menarche), her nutritional needs approach those reported for pregnant adults. However, adolescents who become pregnant less than 4 years after menarche are at risk because of their physiologic and anatomic immaturity. These adolescents are more likely than older adolescents to still be growing, which can affect the fetus's development. Thus, young adolescents (age 14 and younger) need to gain more weight than older adolescents (age 18 and older) to produce babies of equal size.

In determining the optimal weight gain for the pregnant adolescent, the nurse adds the recommended weight gain for an adult pregnancy to that expected during the postmenarchal year in which the pregnancy occurs. If the teenager is underweight, additional weight gain is recommended to bring her to a normal weight for her height.

Specific Nutritional Needs

Caloric needs of pregnant adolescents vary widely. Major factors in determining caloric needs include the physical activity level of the individual and whether her growth is complete. Figures as high as 50 kcal/kg have been suggested for young, pregnant adolescents who are very active physically. A satisfactory weight gain usually confirms an adequate caloric intake.

An inadequate iron intake is a major concern with the adolescent diet. Iron needs are high for the pregnant teen because of the requirement for iron by the enlarging maternal muscle mass and blood volume. Iron supplements—providing between 30 and 60 mg of elemental iron—are definitely indicated.

Calcium is another nutrient that demands special attention from pregnant adolescents. Inadequate intake of calcium is frequently a problem in this age group. Adequate calcium intake is necessary to support the normal growth and development of the fetus and the growth and maintenance of calcium stores in the adolescent. An extra serving of dairy products or other calcium-rich foods is usually suggested for teenagers. Calcium supplementation is indicated for teens who do not consume dairy products or other significant calcium sources in sufficient quantities.

Because folic acid plays a role in cell reproduction, it is also an important nutrient for pregnant teens. As previously indicated, a supplement is usually recommended for all pregnant women, regardless of age.

Other nutrients and vitamins must be considered when evaluating the overall nutritional quality of the teenager's diet. Nutrients that have been found to be deficient in this age group include zinc and vitamins A, D, and B_6. Inclusion of a wide variety of foods—especially fresh and lightly processed foods—is helpful in obtaining adequate amounts of trace minerals, fiber, and vitamins.

Dietary Patterns

Healthy adolescents often have irregular eating patterns. Many skip breakfast and most tend to snack frequently. Teens rarely follow the traditional three-meals-a-day pattern. Their day-to-day intake often varies drastically, and many eat food combinations that may seem bizarre to adults. Despite these practices, adolescents usually achieve a better nutritional balance than most adults would expect.

In assessing the diet of the pregnant adolescent, the nurse should consider the eating pattern over time, not simply a single day's intake. Once the pattern is identified, the nurse can direct counseling toward correcting deficiencies.

Nutrition Education

Counseling about nutrition and healthy eating practices is an important element of care for pregnant teenagers that nurses can provide effectively in a community setting. This counseling may be individualized, involve other teens, or provide a combination of both approaches. If an adolescent's family member does most of the meal preparation, it may be useful to include that individual in the discussion if the adolescent agrees. Involving the expectant father in counseling may also be beneficial. Clinics and schools often offer classes and focused activities designed to address this topic.

The pregnant teenager's understanding of nutrition will influence not only her well-being but also that of her child. However, teens tend to live in the present, and counseling that stresses long-term changes may be less effective than more concrete approaches. In many cases, group classes are effective, especially those that include other teens. In a group atmosphere, adolescents often work together to plan adequate meals, including foods that are special favorites.

Risks to the Adolescent Mother

Risks for the pregnant adolescent may be categorized as physiologic, psychologic, and sociologic.

Physiologic Risks

Adolescents older than 15 years who receive early, thorough prenatal care are at no greater risk during pregnancy than women older than age 20. Unfortunately, adolescents often begin prenatal care later in pregnancy than other age groups. Thus, risks for pregnant adolescents include preterm births, low-birth-weight newborns, cephalopelvic disproportion, iron deficiency anemia, and preeclampsia and its sequelae. In the adolescent age group, prenatal care is the critical factor that most influences pregnancy outcome.

Teenagers age 15 to 19 have a high incidence of STIs, including herpes virus, syphilis, and gonorrhea (U.S. Preventive Services Task Force, 2020). The incidence of chlamydial infection is also increased in this age group. The presence of such infections during a pregnancy greatly increases the risk to the fetus. Other problems seen in adolescents are cigarette smoking and drug use. By the time pregnancy is confirmed, the fetus may already have been harmed by these substances.

SAFETY ALERT Use of nicotine or other substances may have lasting effects on the fetus, even before pregnancy is confirmed. Refer to Module 22, Addiction, for information on the effects of substance use on pregnancy.

Psychologic Risks

Pregnancy interrupts normal developmental tasks of adolescence. This can create an extraordinary amount of psychologic work as the adolescent struggles to complete developmental tasks. Although **Table 33.7** » outlines typical, initial reactions of adolescents to pregnancy, nurses must understand that individual responses may vary based on a number of factors.

Sociologic Risks

Being forced into adult roles before completing adolescent developmental tasks causes a series of events that may result in prolonged dependence on parents, lack of stable relationships, and lack of economic and social stability. Many teenage mothers drop out of school during their pregnancy and then are less likely to complete their schooling. Only 50% of teen mothers receive a high school diploma by age 22, and only 30% have received a GED (general education development) certification (youth.gov, n.d.). Similarly, they are less likely to go to college. In fact, only about 10% of teenagers who give birth before age 18 complete a 2- or 4-year college degree program. In addition, teenage mothers are more likely to have big families and more likely to be single. Certain social determinants of health, such as high unemployment rates, low education, and low income, have been associated with teen pregnancy (CDC, 2019d).

Some pregnant adolescents choose to marry the father of the baby, who may also be a teenager. Unfortunately, most teenage marriages end in divorce. This fact should not be surprising because pregnancy and marriage interrupt the adolescents' childhood and basic education. Lack of maturity in dealing with an intimate relationship also contributes to marital breakdown.

Dating violence is often an issue for teens. When surveyed, 8% of adolescents report some level of physical dating violence, and 6.9% experience some form of sexual dating violence ranging from touching and kidding to forced intercourse. The prevalence of dating violence is highest among white females (Kann et al., 2018). The violence increases in pregnant teens. However, research suggests that this number is significantly lower than the actual number because teens are far less likely to report domestic violence than are adults.

The increased incidence of maternal complications, preterm birth, and low-birth-weight babies among teen mothers also affects society because many of these mothers are dependent on government programs. In the United States, the results of teenage childbearing costs taxpayers $9.5 billion to $11 billion annually, depending on the economic model used (Anthony, Wang, Wani, & Kashani, 2017). Much of this cost comes from

TABLE 33.7 Initial Reaction to Awareness of Pregnancy

Age	Adolescent Behavior	Nursing Implications
Early adolescent (14 years and younger)	Fears rejection by family and peers. Enters healthcare system with an adult, most likely mother (parents still seen as locus of control). Value system closely reflects that of parents, so teen turns to parents for decisions or approval of decisions. Pregnancy probably not a result of intimate relationship. Is self-conscious about normal adolescent changes in body. Self-consciousness and low self-esteem likely to increase with rapid breast enlargement and abdominal enlargement of pregnancy.	Be nonjudgmental in approach to care. Focus on needs and concerns of adolescent, but if parent accompanies daughter, include parent in plan of care. Encourage both to express concerns and feelings regarding pregnancy and options: abortion, maintaining pregnancy, adoption. Be realistic and concrete in discussing implications of each option. During physical exam of adolescent, respect increased sense of modesty. Explain in simple and concrete terms physical changes that are produced by pregnancy versus puberty. Explain each step of physical exam in simple and concrete terms.
Middle adolescent (15–17 years)	Fears rejection by peers and parents. Unsure of whom to confide in. May seek confirmation of pregnancy on own with increased awareness of options and services, such as OTC pregnancy kits and Planned Parenthood. If in an ongoing, caring relationship with partner (peer), may choose him as confidant. Economic dependence on parents may determine if and when parents are told. Future educational plans and perception of parental support or lack of support are significant factors in decision regarding termination or maintenance of the pregnancy. Possible conflict between parental and own developing value system.	Be nonjudgmental in approach to care. Reassure the adolescent that confidentiality will be maintained. Help adolescent identify significant individuals in whom she can confide to help make a decision about the pregnancy. Be aware of state laws regarding requirement of parental notification if abortion intended. Also be aware of state laws regarding requirements for marriage: usually, minimum age for both parties is 18; 16- and 17-year-olds are, in most states, allowed to marry only with consent of parents. Encourage adolescent to be realistic about parental response to pregnancy.
Late adolescent (18–19 years)	Most likely to confirm pregnancy on own and at an earlier date due to increased acceptance and awareness of consequences of behavior. Likely to use pregnancy kit for confirmation. Relationship with father of baby, future educational plans, and personal value system are among significant determinants of decision about pregnancy.	Be nonjudgmental in approach to care. Reassure the adolescent that confidentiality will be maintained. Encourage adolescent to identify significant individuals in whom she can confide. Refer to counseling as appropriate. Encourage adolescent to be realistic about parental response to pregnancy.

Source: Adapted from London et al. (2017).

Medicaid, state health department, maternal care clinics, federal monies for Aid to Families with Dependent Children, the Supplemental Nutritional Assistance Program (SNAP), and direct payments to HCPs. The need for increased financial support for good prenatal care and nutritional programs remains critical.

Early, middle, and late adolescents respond differently to the developmental tasks of pregnancy, reflecting their age and maturity. In addition to her maturational level, the amount of nurturing the pregnant adolescent receives is a critical factor in the way she handles pregnancy and motherhood.

The early-adolescent girl (younger than 15 years) tends to think in a more concrete manner and usually has only a minimal ability to anticipate consequences of her behavior and see herself in the future. In addition, some degree of discomfort with normal body changes and body image may exist. The middle-adolescent girl (15 to 17 years) is prone to experimentation (i.e., drugs, alcohol, and sex), seeks independence, and frequently turns to her peer group for support, information, and advice. Pregnancy at this age can force parental dependency and interfere with attempts at independence. Middle adolescents are capable of abstract thinking but may struggle with anticipating the long-term implications of their behavior. Finally, the late adolescent (17 to 19 years) is developing individuality and can picture herself in control. More sophisticated abstract thinking and an ability to anticipate consequences contributes to the development of problem-solving and decision-making skills (Borca, Bina, Keller, Gilbert, & Begotti, 2015).

*>> Go to **Pearson MyLab Nursing and eText** to see Chart 5: The Early Adolescent's Response to the Developmental Tasks of Pregnancy.*

Pregnant Women over Age 35

Despite advances in maternal care, women over age 35 continue to face medical risks and lifestyle changes that warrant the nurse's attention and understanding.

Medical Risks

Women over the age of 35 face a higher risk of maternal death than younger women who become pregnant. These women are also more likely to have preexisting conditions, such as HTN or diabetes, that can affect maternal health and complicate pregnancy. Pregnant women over the age of 35 face higher rates of miscarriage and stillbirth, preterm birth, cesarean delivery, low birth weight, and perinatal morbidity and mortality. Women over age 35 who become pregnant also have an increased risk for GDM, HTN, placenta previa, difficult labor, and newborn complications (including congenital anomalies) (March of Dimes [MOD], 2016).

Related to congenital anomalies, research has focused on the use of quadruple screening to detect Down syndrome and trisomy 18. First-trimester ultrasound assessment of the thickness of fetal nuchal folds (nuchal translucency) combined with serum screens of free beta-hCG and pregnancy-associated plasma protein A is increasing the detection of Down syndrome, trisomy 18, and trisomy 13. If the screening results are not in the normal range, follow-up testing using ultrasound and amniocentesis is often indicated (ACOG, 2016b).

Amniocentesis or noninvasive prenatal testing through cffDNA are routinely offered to all women over age 35 to permit the early detection of several chromosomal abnormalities, including Down syndrome. Routine genetic testing has not been offered to couples when the only risk is advanced paternal age because there is insufficient evidence to determine a specific paternal age at which to start genetic testing. Advanced paternal age is associated with adverse fetal and neonatal outcomes, including an increased risk of congenital anomalies, childhood cancer, and neurodevelopmental abnormalities (Brandt, Cruz Ithier, Rosen, & Ashkinadze, 2019).

Additional Concerns

The increased medical risks that the pregnant woman over age 35 faces, combined with social, familial, and other health-care concerns, place many of these patients and their families at risk for impaired family processes. In particular, women who are mothers of older children and who provide some level of care for their own older parents may find themselves at their wits' ends trying to find a way to juggle their many responsibilities. The arrival of a new baby in a blended family may cause jealousy among older siblings or strain relationships with in-laws or former partners. The nurse should engage in active listening with these women and their partners, help them prioritize their concerns, and provide referrals to supportive resources as appropriate.

Often, because of their established routines, couples expecting their first child require assistance in understanding how to integrate a newborn into their daily routines. Secondary to increased risk to both the fetus and the pregnant woman, the family is often anxious, and this anxiety can create stress in the household. Encourage the couple to express their fears and concerns and provide support and reassurance. Anxiety may be particularly high when they are waiting for diagnostic test results. Couples may report that they are fighting more than usual. The nurse should help these patients recognize that the role anxiety plays in disrupting their relationships is often an important step to improving the relationship.

If the couple has other children, especially if the siblings are teen or preteen age, they may find their older children are embarrassed by the pregnancy. Older siblings may also fear being asked to contribute to the newborn's care. It is important for the couple to take time to understand their older children's concerns and make it clear to the siblings that the newborn will be the responsibility of the parents, not the responsibility of the older children. Siblings should be welcomed to participate in newborn care but should not be placed in the position of taking on a majority of the responsibility. The nurse can provide a supportive role in this process by encouraging open family communication and trust.

NURSING PROCESS

Most prenatal care is provided in community settings, many of which assign a nurse to coordinate comprehensive care for each family. As some patients may see a different provider at each visit, the nurse may be the only source of continuity for the family. At all stages of the pregnancy, continuity of care and the therapeutic relationship are the foundation for ensuring a healthy pregnancy and delivery.

Assessment

The nurse can complete many areas of prenatal assessment. Advanced practice nurses, such as CNMs and certified women's health nurse practitioners, have the education and skill to perform full and complete antepartum assessments. Areas of assessment may include the following:

- The woman's physical status
- The woman's understanding of pregnancy and the changes that accompany it
- The woman or family's attitudes about the pregnancy and expectations of the impact a baby will have on their lives
- Any health teaching needs
- The degree of support the woman has available to her
- The woman's knowledge of newborn/infant care.

While gathering data, the nurse also has an opportunity to discuss important aspects of nutrition within the context of the family's needs and lifestyle. In addition, the nurse seeks information about psychologic, cultural, and SES factors that may influence food intake.

At subsequent prenatal visits, the nurse continues to gather data about the course of the pregnancy to date and the woman's responses to it (**Box 33.2** »). The nurse also asks about the adjustment of the support person and of other children, if any, in the family. As the pregnancy progresses, the nurse asks about the preparations the family has made for the new baby. The nurse asks specifically whether the woman has experienced any discomfort, especially the kinds of discomfort that are often seen at specific times during a pregnancy. The nurse also inquires about physical changes that relate directly to the pregnancy, such as fetal

Box 33.2
Prenatal Assessment of Parenting Ability

Perception of Complexities of Mothering

A. Desires baby for itself.

Positive:

1. The pregnancy is a planned or desired extension of a stable home life.

Negative:

1. Wants baby to meet own needs, such as someone to love her, someone to get her out of unhappy home, a way to repair faltering relationship.
2. The pregnancy is unwanted.
   - Was the pregnancy planned or a surprise?
   - How do you feel about being a mother?
   - Have you considered terminating the pregnancy or placing the baby for adoption?

B. Expresses consideration of the impact of mothering role on other roles (relationship, career, school).

Positive:

1. Realistic expectations of how baby will affect job, career, school, and personal goals.
2. Interested in learning about child care.

Negative:

1. Lacks insight regarding the physical, emotional, and social demands of parenting.
2. Uninterested in learning about the needs of a baby.

C. Makes lifestyle changes for the baby's benefit.

Positive:

1. Gives up routines not good for baby (quits smoking, adjusts eating habits).
   - What do you think it will be like to take care of a baby?
   - How do you think your life will be different after you have your baby?
   - How do you feel this baby will affect your job, career, school, and personal goals?
   - How will the baby affect your relationship with your significant other?
   - What can you do to help yourself and the baby be as healthy as possible?
   - What can you do to prepare for being a mother?
2. Initiates positive, proactive routines (childbirth classes, prenatal exercise classes, stress reduction).

Negative:

- Rationalizes or denies behavior that places the baby at risk.
- Expresses inability for or lack of interest in proactive behavior.

Attachment

A. Strong feelings regarding sex of baby.

Positive:

1. Verbalizes love and acceptance of either sex.

Negative:

1. Believes baby will be like negative aspects of self and partner.
2. Verbalizes belief that she will be unable to parent a child of a particular gender.
3. Considers a particular gender as conferring more or less status on the family.
   - Why do you prefer a certain gender?
   - How will you feel and what will you do differently if your baby is a boy/girl?

B. Interested in data regarding fetus (e.g., growth and development, heart tones).

Positive:

1. Verbalizes positive thoughts about the baby.
2. Asks questions about the baby's development and status.

Negative:

1. Shows no interest in fetal growth and development, quickening, and fetal heart tones.
2. Expresses negative feelings about fetus.
3. Rejects counseling regarding nutrition, rest, and hygiene.
   - Encourage interest in the fetus. Point out normal development.
   - Explore the mother's reasons for negative feelings and/or rejection of counseling.

C. Fantasizes about baby.

Positive:

1. Prepares for the addition of a baby to her household.
2. Speaks of the baby as her child and her other children's brother and sister.
3. Talks to the baby in utero.

Box 33.2 *(continued)*

4. Makes positive speculations about the baby's appearance and disposition.

Negative:

1. Bonding conditional depending on gender, age of baby, and/or labor and birth experience.
2. Woman considers only own needs when making plans for the baby.
3. Exhibits no attachment behaviors.
4. Failure to prepare.
   - What did you think or feel when you first felt the baby move?
   - Have you started preparing for the baby?
   - What do you think your baby will look like?
   - How would you like your new baby to look?
   - Does this baby have a name?

Acceptance of Child by Significant Others

A. Acknowledges acceptance by significant others of the new responsibility.

Positive:

1. Acknowledges unconditional acceptance of pregnancy and baby by significant others.
2. Partner accepts new responsibility for child.
3. Shares experience of pregnancy with significant others.

Negative:

1. Significant others not supportively involved with pregnancy.
2. Conditional acceptance of pregnancy by significant others depending on sex, ethnicity, and age of baby.
3. Decision making does not take in needs of fetus (e.g., food money spent on new car).
4. Partner and family with no/little responsibility for needs of pregnancy, woman/fetus.
   - How does your partner feel about this pregnancy?
   - How do your parents feel?
   - What do your friends think?
   - Does your partner have a preference regarding the baby's gender? If so, why?
   - How does your partner feel about being a parent?
   - What do you think your partner will be like as a parent?
   - What do you think your partner will do to help you with child care?
   - Have you and your partner talked about how the baby might change your lives?
   - Who have you told about your pregnancy?
   - Do you have family or friends who can help you take care of a new baby?

B. Concrete demonstration of acceptance of pregnancy/baby by significant others (e.g., baby shower, significant other involved in prenatal education).

Positive:

1. Baby shower.
2. Significant other attends prenatal class with woman.
3. Commitment from the mother's community to help take care of the new baby (watch older children when she is in labor and immediately postpartum, meal planning, housework).
   - If partner attends clinic with woman, note partner's degree of interest (e.g., listens to heart tones).
   - Significant other plans to be with woman during labor and birth.
   - Partner is contributing financially.

Ensures Physical Well-Being

A. Concerns about having normal pregnancy, labor and birth, and baby.

Positive:

1. Preparing for labor and birth, attends prenatal classes, interested in labor and birth.
2. Aware of danger signs during pregnancy.
3. Seeks and uses appropriate healthcare (e.g., time of initial visit, keeps appointments, follows through on recommendations).

Negative:

1. Denies signs and symptoms that might suggest complications of pregnancy.
2. Verbalizes extreme fear of labor and birth or refuses to talk about labor and birth.
3. Misses appointments, fails to follow instructions, refuses to attend prenatal classes.
   - Encourage expression of fears so they can be addressed.
   - Ask about reasons for missed appointments in order to assist with obtaining services (medical transportation, social worker, home health nurse).

Note: When "Negative" is not listed in a section, the reader may assume that negative is the absence of positive responses.

Source: Modified and used with permission of the Minneapolis Health Department, Minneapolis, MN.

movement, and asks about the danger signs of pregnancy (**Table 33.8** »).

SAFETY ALERT Pregnancy is a risk factor for intimate partner violence. If a woman presents with suspicious or unexplained injuries, it is essential to assess for intimate partner violence and safety.

Regular physical assessment of pregnant women requires a systematic approach. If the woman's partner is participating in the pregnancy, assessment at each visit should also include the partner. The accompanying Subsequent Prenatal Assessment feature provides a model for assessment and related nursing considerations.

Communicating with Patients and Families

Working Phase

Use compassion and respect when discussing concerns related to the pregnancy with the patient. Provide clear and easy-to-understand education and anticipatory guidance at each visit. Maintain eye contact and use active listening. Use open-ended questions and terminology that the patient will understand.

- Tell me how you have been feeling over the past few weeks.
- I understand that these symptoms are concerning to you. Be assured that the symptoms you are feeling are very normal. I will explain to you why you are experiencing these symptoms.
- You mentioned your partner is concerned about harming the baby during intercourse. Tell me more about that.

TABLE 33.8 Urgent Maternal Warning Signs in Pregnancy

Warning Sign	Possible Cause
Absence of fetal movement	Maternal medication, obesity, fetal death
Temperature above 38°C (100.4°F) and chills	Infection
Dizziness, blurred vision, double vision, spots before eyes	HTN, preeclampsia
Persistent vomiting	Hyperemesis gravidarum
Severe headache	HTN, preeclampsia
Edema of hands, face, legs, and feet	Preeclampsia
Reflex irritability, convulsions	Preeclampsia, eclampsia
Sudden gush of fluid from vagina	Premature rupture of membranes
Vaginal bleeding	Abruptio placentae, placenta previa, lesions of cervix or vagina, "bloody show"
Abdominal pain	Premature labor, abruptio placentae
Epigastric pain	Preeclampsia, ischemia in major abdominal vessel
Chest pain or tachycardia	Worsening cardiac condition, pulmonary embolism, aortic dissection
Trouble breathing	Pulmonary embolism, infection in lungs, worsening cardiac condition
Swelling, redness, or pain in the leg	Deep vein thrombosis
Oliguria	Renal impairment, decreased fluid intake, preeclampsia
Dysuria	UTI
Thoughts of harming herself or the baby	Depression, anxiety
Overwhelming tiredness	Anemia, cardiac disease, diabetes, depression

Sources: Centers for Disease Control and Prevention (2020f); Council on Patient Safety in Women's Health Care (2020); London et al. (2017).

Subsequent Prenatal Assessment

PHYSICAL ASSESSMENT/ NORMAL FINDINGS	ALTERATIONS AND POSSIBLE CAUSES*	NURSING RESPONSES TO DATA†
Vital Signs		
Temperature: 36.2–37.6°C (97–99.6°F)	Elevated temperature (infection)	Evaluate for signs of infection. Refer to HCP.
Pulse: 60–100 beats/min Rate may increase 10 beats/min during pregnancy	Increased pulse rate (anxiety, cardiac disorders)	Note irregularities. Assess for anxiety and stress.
Respiration: 12–20 breaths/min	Marked tachypnea or abnormal patterns (respiratory disease)	Refer to HCP.
Blood pressure: less than 140/90 mmHg (falls in second trimester)	Greater than 140/90 mmHg	Assess for headache, edema, proteinuria, and hyperreflexia. Refer to HCP. Schedule appointments more frequently.
Weight Gain		
First trimester: 1.6–2.3 kg (3.5–5 lb)	Inadequate weight gain (poor nutrition, nausea, SGA)	Discuss appropriate weight gain.
Second trimester: 5.5–6.8 kg (12–15 lb)	Excessive weight gain (excessive caloric intake, edema, preeclampsia)	Provide nutritional counseling. Assess for presence of edema or anemia.
Third trimester: 5.5–6.8 kg (12–15 lb)		

Subsequent Prenatal Assessment *(continued)*

PHYSICAL ASSESSMENT/ NORMAL FINDINGS	ALTERATIONS AND POSSIBLE CAUSES*	NURSING RESPONSES TO DATA†
Edema		
Small amount of dependent edema, especially in last weeks of pregnancy	Edema in hands, face, legs, and feet (preeclampsia)	Identify any correlation between edema and activities, blood pressure, or proteinuria. Refer to HCP, if indicated.
Uterine Size		
See the Initial Prenatal Assessment feature in the Concept section for normal changes during pregnancy	Unusually rapid growth (multiple gestation, hydatidiform mole, hydramnios, miscalculation of EDB)	Evaluate fetal status. Determine height of fundus. Use diagnostic ultrasound.
Fetal Heartbeat		
110–160 beats/min Funic souffle	Absence of fetal heartbeat after 20 weeks of gestation (maternal obesity, fetal demise)	Evaluate fetal status.
Laboratory Evaluation		
Hemoglobin: 12–16 g/dL Pseudoanemia of pregnancy	Less than 11 g/dL (anemia)	Provide nutritional counseling. Hemoglobin check is repeated at 28–36 weeks of gestation. Consider a hemoglobin screen for women of Mediterranean, African, or South Asian descent.
Quad marker screen: blood test performed at 15–22 weeks of gestation. Evaluates four factors—MSAFP, UE, hCG, and inhibin-A: normal levels	Elevated MSAFP (NTD, underestimated gestational age, multiple gestation); lower-than-normal MSAFP (Down syndrome, trisomy 18); higher-than-normal hCG and inhibin-A (Down syndrome); lower-than-normal UE (Down syndrome)	Recommended for all pregnant women; especially indicated for women with any of the following risk factors: age 35 and over, family history of or previous child with a congenital anomaly, insulin-dependent diabetes before pregnancy (Medline Plus, 2021b). If quad screen abnormal, further testing such as ultrasound or amniocentesis may be indicated.
First-trimester integrated screen	Provides the same information as the quad screen in a more accurate and timely fashion as information on trisomy 13, 18, and 21 is available between 11 and 13 weeks' gestation and laboratory tests are combined with ultrasound of the fetal nasal bone and nuchal fold	
NIPT/cffDNA	Allows analysis of fetal alleles in maternal serum; provides information on chromosomal anomalies	
Repeat indirect Coombs test done on Rh-negative women: negative (done at 28 weeks of gestation)	Rh antibodies present (maternal sensitization has occurred)	If Rh negative and unsensitized, Rh immune globulin is given. If Rh antibodies are present, Rh immune globulin is not given; fetus is monitored closely for isoimmune hemolytic disease.
50-g, 1-hour glucose screen (done between 24 and 28 weeks of gestation)	Plasma glucose level greater than 140 mg/dL (GDM) *Note:* Some facilities use a level of greater than 130 mg/dL, which identifies 90% of women with GDM.	Discuss implications of GDM. Refer for a diagnostic 100-g oral glucose tolerance test.
Urinalysis: See the Initial Prenatal Assessment feature in the Concept section for normal findings.	See the Initial Prenatal Assessment feature in the Concept section for deviations.	Repeat urinalysis at 7 months of gestation. Repeat dipstick test at each visit.

(continued on next page)

Subsequent Prenatal Assessment *(continued)*

PHYSICAL ASSESSMENT/ NORMAL FINDINGS	ALTERATIONS AND POSSIBLE CAUSES*	NURSING RESPONSES TO DATA†
Protein: negative	Proteinuria, albuminuria (contamination by vaginal discharge, UTI, preeclampsia)	Obtain dipstick urine sample. Refer to HCP if deviations are present.
Glucose: negative	Persistent glycosuria (diabetes mellitus)	Refer to HCP.
Note: Glycosuria may be present because of physiologic alterations in GFR and renal threshold.		
Screening for GBS: rectal and vaginal swabs obtained at 35–37 weeks' gestation for all pregnant women	Positive culture (maternal colonization)	Explain fetal/neonatal risks and the need for antibiotic prophylaxis in labor. Refer to HCP for therapy.
Determine the mother's (and family's) attitudes about the gender of the unborn child	Some women have no preference about the child's gender, others do; in many cultures, boys are especially valued as firstborn children	Provide opportunities to discuss preferences and expectations; avoid a judgmental attitude to the response.
Ask about the woman's expectations of childbirth. Will she want someone with her for the birth? Whom does she choose? What is the role of her partner?	Some women want their partner present for labor and birth; others prefer a female relative or friend Some women expect to be separated from their partner once cervical dilation has occurred	Provide information on birth options but accept the woman's decision about who will attend.
Ask about preparations for the baby; determine what is customary for the woman	Some women may have a fully prepared nursery; others may not have a separate room for the baby	Explore reasons for not preparing for the baby. Support the mother's preferences and provide information about possible sources of assistance if the decision is related to a lack of resources.
Expectant Mother		
Psychologic status	Increased stress and anxiety	Encourage woman to take an active part in her care.
First trimester: Incorporates idea of pregnancy; may feel ambivalent, especially if she must give up desired role; usually looks for signs of verification of pregnancy, such as increase in abdominal size or fetal movement	Inability to establish communication; inability to accept pregnancy; inappropriate response or actions; denial of pregnancy; inability to cope	Establish lines of communication. Establish a trusting relationship. Counsel as necessary. Refer to appropriate professional as needed.
Second trimester: Baby becomes more real to woman as abdominal size increases and she feels movement; she begins to turn inward, becoming more introspective		
Third trimester: Begins to think of the baby as a separate being; may feel restless and that the time of labor will never come; remains self-centered and concentrates on preparing place for baby		

Subsequent Prenatal Assessment *(continued)*

PHYSICAL ASSESSMENT/ NORMAL FINDINGS	ALTERATIONS AND POSSIBLE CAUSES*	NURSING RESPONSES TO DATA†
Educational needs: Self-care measures and knowledge about the following: Health promotion Breast care Hygiene Rest Exercise Nutrition Relief measures for common discomforts of pregnancy Danger signs in pregnancy (see Table 33.8)	Inadequate information	Provide information and counseling.
Sexual activity: Woman knows how pregnancy affects sexual activity	Lack of information about effects of pregnancy and/or alternative positions during sexual intercourse	Provide counseling.
Preparation for parenting: appropriate preparation	Lack of preparation (denial, failure to adjust to baby, unwanted child)	Counsel. If lack of preparation is caused by inadequacy of information, provide information.
Preparation for childbirth: Patient is aware of the following: 1. Prepared childbirth techniques 2. Normal processes and changes during childbirth 3. Problems that may occur as a result of drug and alcohol use and of smoking	Continued abuse of drugs and alcohol; denial of possible effect on self and baby	If couple chooses a particular technique, refer to childbirth classes. Encourage prenatal class attendance. Educate woman during visits based on current physical status. Provide reading list for more specific information. Refer for thorough evaluation of substance abuse.
Woman has met other physician or nurse-midwife who may be attending her birth in the absence of primary caregiver	Introduction of new individual at birth may increase stress and anxiety for woman and partner	Introduce woman to all members of group practice.
Impending labor: Patient knows signs of impending labor: 1. Uterine contractions that increase in frequency, duration, and intensity 2. Bloody show 3. Expulsion of mucus plug 4. Rupture of membranes	Lack of information	Provide appropriate teaching, stressing importance of seeking appropriate medical assistance.
Expectant Partner		
Psychologic status		
First trimester: May express excitement over confirmation of pregnancy; male partner may be pleased with evidence of his virility; concerns move toward providing for financial needs; energetic, may identify with some discomforts of pregnancy, and may even exhibit symptoms	Increasing stress and anxiety; inability to establish communication; inability to accept pregnancy diagnosis; withdrawal of support; abandonment of the mother	Encourage expectant partner to come to prenatal visits. Establish line of communication. Establish trusting relationship.

(continued on next page)

Subsequent Prenatal Assessment *(continued)*

PHYSICAL ASSESSMENT/ NORMAL FINDINGS	ALTERATIONS AND POSSIBLE CAUSES*	NURSING RESPONSES TO DATA†
Second trimester: May feel more confident and be less concerned with financial matters; may have concerns about expectant mother's changing size and shape, her increasing introspection		Counsel. Let expectant partner know that it is normal to experience these feelings.
Third trimester: May have feelings of rivalry with fetus, especially during sexual activity; may make changes in physical appearance and exhibit more interest in self; may become more energetic; fantasizes about child, but usually imagines older child; fears mutilation and death of woman and child		Include expectant partner in pregnancy activities as the partner desires. Provide education, information, and support. Increasing numbers of expectant partners are demonstrating desire to be involved in many or all aspects of prenatal care, education, and preparation.

*Possible causes of alterations are identified in parentheses.
†This column provides guidelines for further assessment and initial nursing intervention.
Source: From London et al. (2017). Pearson Education, Inc., Hoboken, NJ.

SAFETY ALERT Normal physiologic changes of pregnancy result in a decrease in blood pressure from baseline in the second semester. If this decrease is not noted, further assessment for preeclampsia is necessary.

The woman's individual needs and the assessment of her risks should determine the frequency of subsequent visits. Generally, the recommended frequency of antepartum visits is as follows:

- Every 4 weeks for the first 28 weeks of gestation
- Every 2 weeks until 36 weeks of gestation
- After week 36, every week until childbirth.

During the subsequent antepartum assessments, most women demonstrate ongoing psychologic adjustment to pregnancy. However, some women may exhibit signs of possible psychologic problems, such as the following:

- Increasing anxiety
- Inability to establish communication
- Inappropriate responses or actions
- Denial of pregnancy
- Inability to cope with stress
- Intense preoccupation with the gender of the baby
- Failure to acknowledge quickening
- Failure to plan and prepare for the baby (e.g., living arrangements, clothing, and feeding methods)
- Indications of substance abuse.

If the woman's behavior indicates possible psychologic problems, the nurse can provide ongoing support and counseling and also refer the woman to appropriate professionals.

Diagnosis

Patient needs and priorities for care will vary from one pregnancy to another but may include the following:

- Lack of knowledge of physiologic and psychologic processes of pregnancy
- Learning about self-care needs such as nutrition and fluid requirements
- Potential for fluid volume deficiency if woman experiences vomiting or hyperemesis gravidarum
- Lack of knowledge about how to prepare for the childbirth process
- Ready to learn about parenting and newborn care.

Planning

Together, the nurse and patient will establish the plan of care. Sometimes, priorities of care are based on the most immediate needs or concerns expressed by the woman. For example, during the first trimester, when she is experiencing nausea or is concerned about sexual intimacy with her partner, the woman likely will not want to hear about labor and birth. At other times, priorities may develop from findings during a prenatal examination. For example, a woman who is showing signs of preeclampsia may feel physically well and find it hard to accept the nurse's emphasis on the need for frequent rest periods.

Potential goals of nursing care during pregnancy may include the following:

- The woman will increase her daily intake of calcium to the DRI level.
- The woman will articulate the danger signs during pregnancy and when to call the physician's office or seek emergency care.
- The woman will have the opportunity to express concerns and ask questions.
- The woman will articulate methods of self-care.
- The woman with a chronic condition will consult with her obstetrician and her treating physician during the pregnancy.

Implementation

When providing patient care, the nurse should be sensitive to religious or spiritual, cultural, and socioeconomic factors that may influence a family's response to pregnancy as well as to the woman's expectations of the healthcare system. The nurse can avoid stereotyping patients simply by asking each woman about her expectations for the antepartum period. Although many women's responses may reflect what are thought to be traditional norms, other women may have decidedly different views or expectations that represent a blending of beliefs or cultures.

Promote Knowledge Related to Self-Care

The nurse may see a pregnant woman only once every 4 to 6 weeks during the first several months of her pregnancy, during which time it is important to establish an environment of comfort and open communication with each antepartum visit. The nurse conveys interest in the woman as an individual and discusses her concerns and desires. The nurse can be extremely effective in working with the expectant family by answering questions; providing comprehensive information about pregnancy, prenatal healthcare activities, and community resources; and supporting the healthcare activities of the woman and her family.

Communities often have a wealth of services and educational opportunities available for pregnant women and their families, and the knowledgeable nurse can help expectant families to assess and access these services. A community-based approach supports the family's assumption of equal responsibility with HCPs in working toward their common goal of a positive birth experience.

Home care can be of benefit to any pregnant woman, but it is especially effective in removing barriers for women who have difficulty accessing healthcare. These barriers may include lack of locally available healthcare facilities, problems with transportation to the facility, or schedule conflicts with available appointment times because of employment hours or family responsibilities. A prenatal home care visit or phone contact can also be useful for women who anticipate a short inpatient stay after childbirth. At the prenatal contact, the nurse explains the perinatal program and answers any questions the woman or her family have. Currently, home care is most often used for women with prenatal complications that can be managed without hospitalization if effective nursing assessment and care are provided in the home.

Throughout the prenatal period, the nurse shares information with the family, both verbally and through written materials. This information is designed to help the family carry out self-care and wellness measures as needed and report changes that may indicate a health problem. The nurse also provides anticipatory guidance to help the family plan for changes that will occur after childbirth. The expectant woman and her partner and/or other family members are encouraged to identify and discuss issues that could be sources of postpartum stress. Issues to be addressed before the birth may include sharing of baby and household chores, help during the first few days after childbirth, options for babysitting to allow the mother (and couple) some free time, the mother's return to work after the baby's birth, and sibling rivalry. Families resolve these issues in different ways, but the postpartum adjustment period tends to be easier for those who agree on the issues beforehand than for those who do not confront and resolve them.

Childbirth education classes are important in promoting adaptation to the event of childbirth for expectant couples. Classes for pregnant adolescents and expectant parents over age 35 are now available in many communities.

Important topics for patient teaching include the following:

- Self-care to promote positive outcomes (e.g., nutrition, exercise, avoiding OTC medications, and delegating care of the litter box to other family members)
- Strategies to minimize the discomforts of pregnancy
- Childbirth preparation classes
- Danger signs to report to the provider
- Signs and symptoms of labor.

Exercises to Prepare for Childbirth

Certain exercises help strengthen muscle tone in preparation for birth and promote more rapid restoration of muscle tone after birth. Some physical changes of pregnancy can be minimized by faithfully practicing prescribed body-conditioning exercises. Many body-conditioning exercises for pregnancy are taught; a few of the more common ones are discussed here.

Handouts, videos, and smartphone apps are valuable tools for providing information. When combined, they are especially useful. The nurse can develop a handout that describes the correct way to perform prenatal exercises and include drawings or photos. For exercises that may be new to a woman, such as the pelvic tilt, the nurse can provide a handout for later reference but also demonstrate the exercise and have the woman do a return demonstration. The nurse can also provide a list of recommended smartphone apps or videos that the woman can use to guide her exercise.

Pelvic Tilt

The **pelvic tilt**, or pelvic rocking, is an exercise that helps prevent or reduce back strain as it strengthens abdominal muscles. To do the pelvic tilt in early pregnancy, the woman lies on her back and puts her feet flat on the floor. This flexes the knees and helps prevent strain or discomfort. The woman decreases the curvature in her back by pressing her spine toward the floor. With her back pressed to the floor, the woman then tightens her abdominal muscles as she

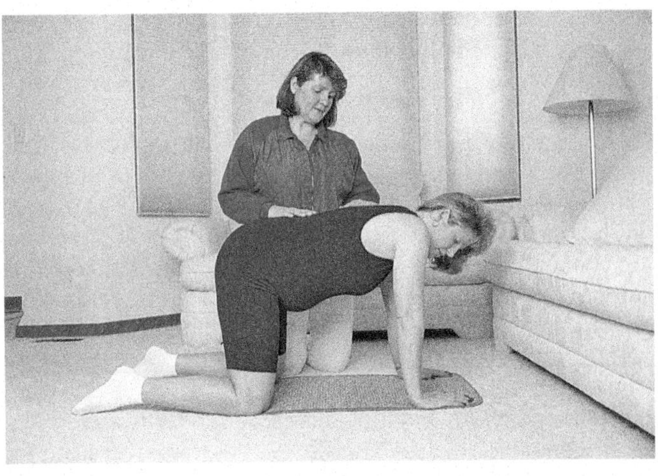

A

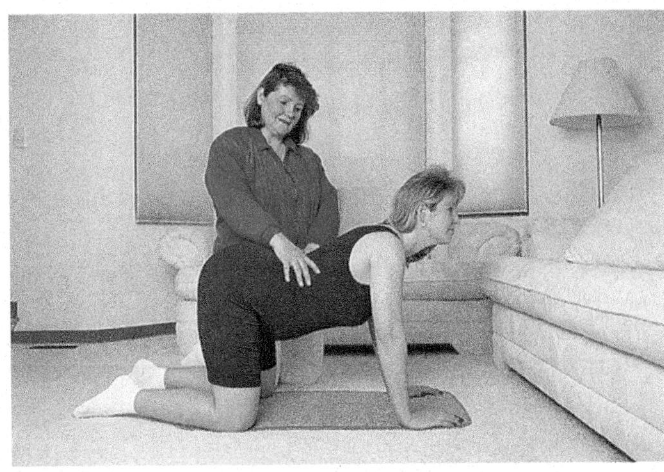

B

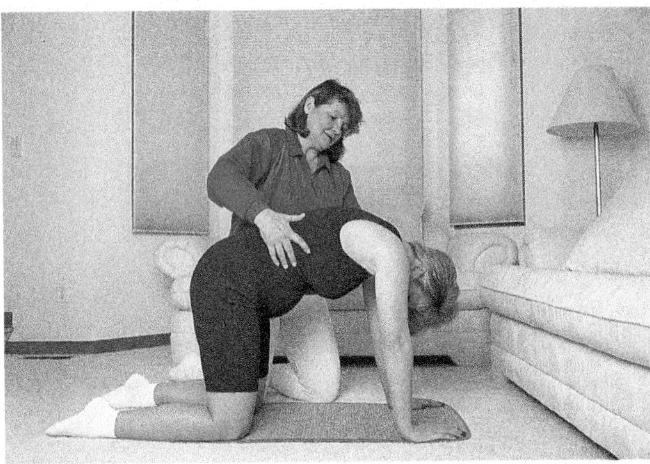

C

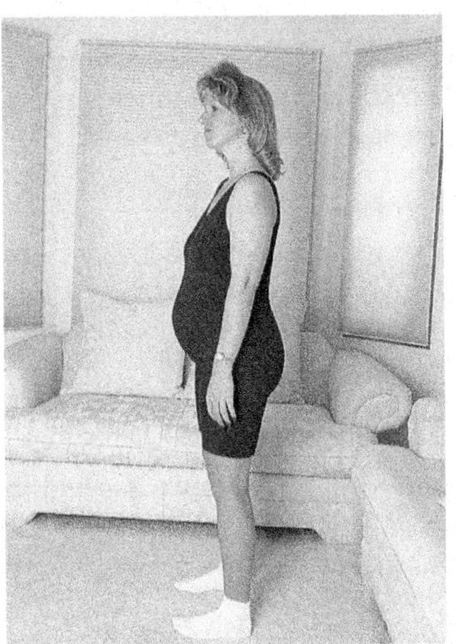

D

Figure 33.35 ›› *A*, Starting position when the pelvic tilt is done on hands and knees. The back is flat and parallel to the floor, the hands are below the head, and the knees are directly below the buttocks. ***B***, A prenatal yoga instructor offers pointers for proper positioning for the first part of the tilt: head up, neck long and separated from the shoulders, buttocks up, and pelvis thrust back, allowing the back to drop and release on an inhaled breath. ***C***, The instructor helps the woman assume the correct position for the next part of the tilt. It is done on a long exhalation, allowing the pregnant woman to arch her back, drop her head loosely, push away from her hands, and draw in the muscles of her abdomen to strengthen them. Note that in this position, the pelvis and buttocks are tucked under and the buttock muscles are tightened. ***D***, Proper posture. The knees are slightly bent but not locked and the pelvis and buttocks are tucked under, thereby lengthening the spine and helping support the weighty abdomen. With her chin tucked in, this woman's neck, shoulders, hips, knees, and feet are all in a straight line perpendicular to the floor. Her feet are parallel. This is also the starting position for doing the pelvic tilt while standing.

Source: ***A***, ***B***, ***C***, ***D***, Pearson Education, Inc.

tightens and tucks in her buttocks. In the second and third trimesters of pregnancy, the woman can also perform the pelvic tilt while on her hands and knees (**Figure 33.35 ››**), sitting in a chair, or standing with her back against a wall. The body alignment that results when the pelvic tilt is done correctly should be maintained as much as possible throughout the day.

SAFETY ALERT Doing the pelvic tilt on hands and knees may aggravate back strain. Teach women with a history of minor back problems to do the pelvic tilt only in the standing position.

Abdominal Exercises

A basic exercise to increase abdominal muscle tone is tightening abdominal muscles with each breath. This exercise can be done in any position, but it is best learned during early pregnancy. The woman lies supine with knees flexed and feet flat on the floor. The woman expands her abdomen and slowly takes a deep breath. Exhaling slowly, she gradually pulls in her abdominal muscles until they are fully contracted. She relaxes for a few seconds and then repeats the exercise. The pregnant woman should avoid the supine position after the first trimester.

Partial sit-ups strengthen abdominal muscle tone and can be done if there is no preexisting diastasis recti. In early pregnancy, partial sit-ups must be done with the knees flexed and the feet flat on the floor to avoid strain on the lower back. The woman stretches her arms toward her knees as she slowly pulls her head and shoulders off the floor to a comfortable level (if she has poor abdominal muscle tone, she may not be able to pull up very far). She then slowly returns to the starting position, takes a deep breath, and repeats the exercise while exhaling. To strengthen the oblique abdominal muscles, the woman repeats the process but stretches the left arm to the side of her right knee, returns to the floor, takes a deep breath, and then, while exhaling, reaches with the right arm to the left knee. During the second and third trimesters, these exercises can be done on a large exercise ball. They can be done approximately five times in a sequence, and the sequence can be repeated at other times during the day as desired. It is important to do the exercises slowly to prevent muscle strain and overtiring. If the pregnant woman does have diastasis recti, isometric abdominal exercises should be done instead.

Perineal Exercises

Perineal muscle tightening, also called **Kegel exercises**, strengthens the pubococcygeus muscle and increases its elasticity (**Figure 33.36** ⟫). The woman can feel the specific muscle group to be exercised by stopping urination midstream. Doing Kegel exercises while urinating is discouraged because this practice has been associated with urinary stasis and UTI.

Childbirth educators sometimes use the following technique to teach Kegel exercises: Tell the woman to think of her perineal muscles as an elevator. When she relaxes, the elevator is on the first floor. To do the exercises, she contracts, bringing the elevator to the second, third, and fourth floors. She keeps the elevator on the fourth floor for a few seconds and then gradually relaxes the area. If the exercise is properly done, the woman does not contract the muscles of the buttocks and thighs.

Kegel exercises can be done at almost any time. Some women use ordinary events—for instance, stopping at a red light—as a cue to remember to do the exercise. Others do Kegel exercises while waiting in a checkout line, talking on the telephone, or watching television.

Inner Thigh Stretch

The nurse can advise the pregnant woman to assume a seated position with the knees bent and the bottoms of the feet together. This "tailor sit" stretches the muscles of the inner thighs in preparation for labor and birth.

Evaluate Patient and Family Well-Being

The problems and concerns of the pregnant woman, the relief of her discomforts, and the maintenance of her physical, psychologic, and spiritual health receive much attention during the antepartum period. However, her well-being is intertwined with the well-being of those to whom she is closest. Thus, the nurse also addresses the needs of the woman's family to help maintain the integrity of the family unit.

Periodic prenatal examinations offer the nurse an opportunity to assess the woman's psychologic needs and emotional status. If the woman's partner attends the antepartum visits, the nurse can also identify the partner's needs and concerns. The interchange between the nurse and the woman or her partner will be facilitated if it takes place in a friendly, trusting environment. The woman should have sufficient time to ask questions and air concerns. If the nurse provides the time and demonstrates genuine interest, the woman will be more at ease bringing up questions that she may believe are silly or has been afraid to verbalize. The nurse who has an accurate understanding of all the changes of pregnancy is most able to answer questions and provide information. For the pregnant woman and her partner who do not speak English, the nurse should ensure that an interpreter is available and provide any written material in the woman's preferred language. The interpreter can be present in person or through a telephone or virtual translation service.

Care of the Partner

While the pregnant woman's partner is present in most cases, the partner's presence cannot be assumed. It is important to assess the woman's support system to determine which significant individuals in her life will play a major role during her childbearing experience.

Anticipatory guidance of the expectant woman's partner, if the partner is involved in the pregnancy, is a necessary part

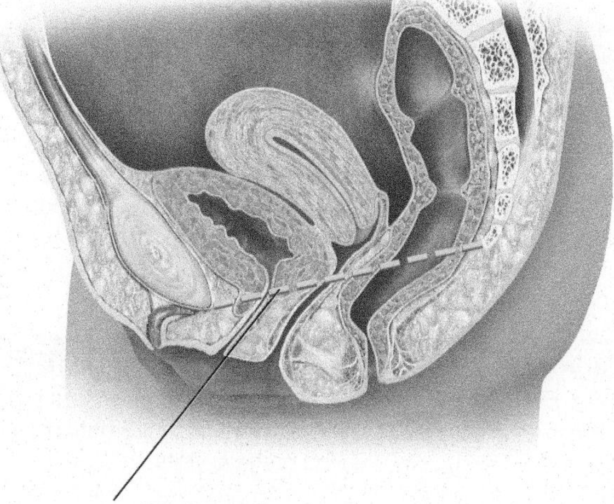

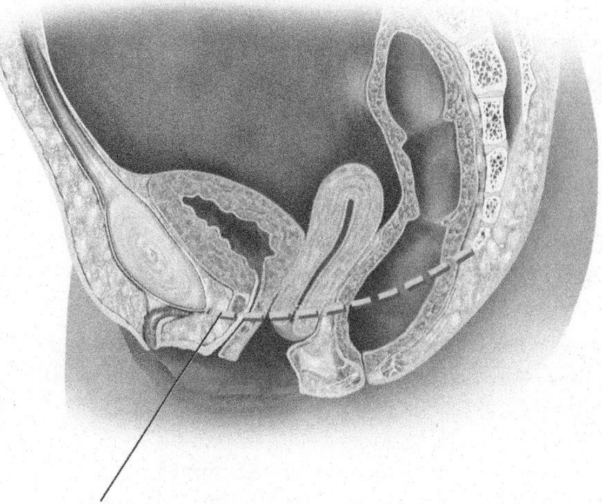

Figure 33.36 ⟫ Kegel exercises. The woman tightens the pubococcygeus muscle to improve support to the pelvic organs.

of any plan of care. The partner may need information about the anatomic, physiologic, and emotional changes that occur during and after pregnancy; the couple's sexuality and sexual response; and the reactions that the partner is experiencing. The partner may wish to express feelings about breastfeeding versus formula feeding, the gender of the child, the partner's own ability to parent, and other topics.

If it is culturally acceptable to the couple and personally acceptable to the partner, the nurse may refer the couple to expectant parents' classes. These classes provide valuable information about pregnancy and childbirth using a variety of teaching strategies, such as discussion, films, demonstrations with educational models, and written handouts. Some classes even give the partner the opportunity to get a "feel" for pregnancy by wearing a pregnancy simulator. Such classes also offer the couple an opportunity to gain support from other couples.

The nurse assesses the partner's intended degree of participation during labor and birth and knowledge of what to expect. If the couple prefers that the partner's participation be minimal or restricted, the nurse must support the decision. With this type of consideration and collaboration, the partner is less apt to develop feelings of alienation, helplessness, and guilt during the pregnancy. As the couple's relationship is strengthened and the partner's self-esteem increases, the partner is better able to provide physical and emotional support to the woman during labor and birth.

At all times, the nurse provides nonjudgmental care of the woman and her partner, regardless of the partner's sex, the relationship status of the couple, or any other factors.

Care of Siblings and Other Family Members

Siblings and other family members may respond in different ways, with feelings ranging from excitement to feelings of insecurity and even anger. The nurse helps facilitate discussions of negative feelings siblings may have and how parents may respond. The nurse encourages open communication between parents and children, providing strategies such as allowing young children to act out feelings with a doll. Open communication with opportunities to share feelings builds trust and promotes the feeling that older children will not be neglected when the new baby arrives. Responses of siblings and other family members are discussed in detail in the Concept section of this module.

Cultural beliefs about parenting practices vary widely, even within a single culture. It is important for the nurse to assess each patient's and each partner's individual beliefs and not make assumptions of the parents' beliefs based on their cultural background.

Identify Concerns and Promote Strengths

To promote a sense of well-being, the nurse treats the pregnancy as normal until or unless specific risks are identified. During the course of the pregnancy, the nurse works with the woman to identify and respond to her specific concerns and promote her strengths as a mother.

The common discomforts of pregnancy—such as nausea and vomiting, urinary frequency, fatigue, breast tenderness, heartburn, ankle edema, and other problems—can contribute to an unpleasant pregnancy for the woman. At each prenatal visit, the nurse can focus teaching on ways to cope with the potential discomforts the woman may experience.

For couples who have amniocentesis or for whom a specific risk to the baby is identified, the nurse helps reduce anxiety by providing information, answering questions, and providing emotional support. When results indicate the possibility of Down syndrome or another genetic abnormality, the nurse provides complete information about the condition, its range of manifestations, and developmental implications.

Evaluation

Anticipated outcomes of nursing care include the following:

- The woman and her partner are knowledgeable about the pregnancy and express confidence in their ability to make appropriate healthcare choices.
- The expectant woman and her partner and their children, if any, are able to cope with the pregnancy and its implications for the future.
- The woman receives effective healthcare throughout her pregnancy as well as during birth and the postpartum period.
- The woman and her partner develop skills in child care and parenting.

Nursing Care Plan

Martina de Herrara and her husband arrived in the United States from Puerto Rico 6 months ago. This is her first prenatal visit since her pregnancy was confirmed 2 days earlier. Mrs. de Herrara's first child is 3 years old and was born in Puerto Rico. Their families live in Puerto Rico, but Mrs. de Herrara's mother has come to visit and help her get settled in their new home. Mrs. de Herrara's husband speaks some English but is unable to attend the prenatal visit, so she has brought her mother to the clinic. Mrs. de Herrara's native language is Spanish. Both women speak very little English and seem uncomfortable as they wait for the provider. The nurse needs to complete a health history, collect some laboratory specimens, and get Mrs. de Herrara scheduled for her next appointment.

ASSESSMENT	DIAGNOSIS	PLANNING
Subjective: Shaking head side to side, no eye contact, anxious Objective: blood pressure 128/82 mmHg, pulse 84 beats/min, respirations 16/min, height 5'4" weight 140 lb, urine negative for protein and glucose	■ Ready to learn about prenatal care related to barriers in communication and sociocultural factors	■ The woman will demonstrate understanding of health information received during prenatal visits.

Nursing Care Plan *(continued)*

IMPLEMENTATION

- Schedule an interpreter during prenatal visits.
- Refer to posters with pictures to explain routine care and procedures during the prenatal exam.
- Use teaching models to demonstrate procedures.
- Provide brochures about prenatal care in the patient's native language.
- Use a professional interpreter to communicate with non-English-speaking parents. If one is not available, use a medical translator smartphone app such as Medibabble, Canopy App, or iTranslate.
- Refer the woman to prenatal classes taught in her native language.
- Involve other members of the healthcare team to assist with prenatal care.

EVALUATION

- The woman responds appropriately to the nurse by using an interpreter.
- The woman demonstrates understanding by pointing to pictures and phrases on posters.
- The woman uses hand gestures to demonstrate understanding.

CRITICAL THINKING

1. Because of the loss of easily understandable tone and correlation with body language in this situation as the patient speaks, how can the nurse assess the woman's anxiety after providing patient teaching?
2. Using an interpreter, how can the nurse determine the woman's understanding of patient teaching?
3. What questions would you ask to assess the patient's cultural beliefs and needs related to her culture?

REVIEW Antepartum Care

RELATE Link the Concepts and Exemplars

Linking the exemplar of antepartum care with the concept of fluids and electrolytes:

1. What recommendations would you make to reduce the risk of dehydration for the pregnant woman who reports vomiting one or two times per day?
2. What electrolyte levels would you want to monitor in the pregnant woman with frequent morning sickness and vomiting?

Linking the exemplar of antepartum care with the concept of stress and coping:

3. You are caring for a woman with four children who had a tubal ligation after delivery of her last baby. During this visit, the woman finds she is pregnant. How can you help her to cope with the discovery and reduce anxiety enough to allow decision making?
4. You are caring for a woman who has been receiving infertility treatments for the past 2 years without success and has just learned she is pregnant. The woman is very anxious about fetal well-being and the possibility of miscarriage. Design a plan of care to promote anxiety reduction.

READY Go to Volume 3: Clinical Nursing Skills

REFER Go to Pearson MyLab Nursing and eText

- Chart 5: The Early Adolescent's Response to the Developmental Tasks of Pregnancy

REFLECT Apply Your Knowledge

Jessica Riley is a single 18-year-old mother with a 1-year-old son, Ryan. Jessica has had no contact with Ryan's father since before Ryan was born. Jessica and Ryan live in a small, one-bedroom apartment with Jessica's boyfriend, Casey. Jessica is now 6 months pregnant with Casey's child. Although Jessica works full time at a restaurant, she has struggled financially. She is glad Casey contributes to paying the bills and is not sure how she could make it financially without him. Her mother, Evelyn, helps by watching Ryan in the evenings. In addition, Jessica has government assistance in the form of WIC coupons and Medicaid. Ryan attends a government-assisted day care program.

Jessica goes to her 24-week prenatal visit. She continues to see the same midwife and likes her a lot because she makes her feel comfortable. Jessica's history indicates she does not exercise and eats mostly fast foods. Jessica smokes about half a pack of cigarettes a day and drinks alcohol socially when she parties.

Jessica tells the nurse who admits her that she tried to stop smoking but hasn't been able to. When asked about alcohol intake, Jessica tells the nurse she is no longer drinking. She shares with the nurse that Casey was giving her a hard time about not drinking, so she has been pretending to drink to keep him happy. While taking Jessica's blood pressure, the nurse notes bruises in the form of fingerprints on her upper arms. While helping Jessica prepare for the examination, the nurse also notes a bruise on her abdomen. When she asks Jessica how it happened, Jessica blushes, stutters, then looks down and mumbles, "I must have bumped into something."

1. Would you assess Jessica further to determine if she has been abused? If so, what specific questions would you ask?
2. What risk factors have you identified related to Jessica's fetus? What nursing strategies can you implement to reduce these risks?
3. What patient teaching would you provide at this prenatal visit?

Exemplar 33.B Intrapartum Care

Exemplar Learning Outcomes

33.B Summarize intrapartum care of the pregnant woman.

- Summarize factors important to labor and birth.
- Describe the physiology of labor.
- Outline the stages of labor and birth.
- Summarize the maternal and fetal response to labor.
- Describe maternal and fetal alterations during the intrapartum period.
- Differentiate considerations related to the assessment and care of pregnant adolescents and women over 35.
- Illustrate the nursing process in providing culturally competent care to the pregnant woman and her family.

Exemplar Key Terms

Overview

In the final weeks of pregnancy, both mother and baby begin to prepare for birth. As the fetus develops and grows in readiness for life outside of the womb, the expectant woman undergoes various physiologic and psychologic changes that prepare her for childbirth. During her prenatal visits, the mother is instructed to call her HCP if any of the following occur:

- Rupture of membranes
- Regular, frequent uterine contractions (nulliparas, 5 minutes apart for 1 hour; multiparas, 6 to 8 minutes apart for 1 hour)
- Any vaginal bleeding
- Decreased fetal movement.

Increasingly, pregnant women and their families are seeking patient- and family-centered care. Patient- and **family-centered care** is a model of care that focuses on the patient, family unit, and the HCPs working as a team to plan and carry out care, with consideration for the physical, sociocultural, spiritual, and economic needs of the mother and family (Kokorelias, Gignac, Naglie, & Cameron, 2019). To reflect the consumer demand for family-centered care, most birthing centers now have *birthing rooms*, single rooms where the woman and her partner or other family members will stay for the labor, birth, recovery, and possibly the postpartum period. These rooms may also be called labor, delivery, recovery, and postpartum rooms, or single-room maternity care.

The atmosphere of a birthing room is more relaxed than that of a traditional hospital room, and families seem to feel more comfortable in birthing rooms. Another benefit is that the woman does not have to be transferred from one area to another for the actual birth. A birthing room setting not only helps the laboring woman create her own space to labor in, but it also enhances the family's comfort and involvement. Birthing rooms usually have beds that can be adapted for birth by removing a small section near the foot. The decor is designed to produce a homelike atmosphere in which families can feel both safe and at ease.

This exemplar discusses in detail the normal progression of labor and culturally appropriate, family-centered care for the laboring mother, fetus, and close family members. A brief discussion of alterations that may occur in the intrapartum period is also provided.

Factors Important to Labor and Birth

Five factors influence the progress of labor: the birth passage, the fetus, the relationship between birth passage and fetus, physiologic forces of labor, and psychologic considerations. Alterations in or abnormalities affecting any one of these can affect the outcome of labor and threaten the health and safety of both mother and baby.

Birth Passage

The true pelvis, which forms the bony canal through which the fetus must pass, is divided into three sections: the inlet, the pelvic cavity (midpelvis), and the outlet. Factors specific to the birth passage are the following:

- Size of the maternal pelvis, including diameters of the pelvic inlet, midpelvis, and outlet
- Type of maternal pelvis (gynecoid, android, anthropoid, platypelloid, or a combination)
- Ability of the cervix to dilate and efface
- Ability of the vaginal canal and external opening of the vagina (the introitus) to distend.

Fetus

The fetal head, attitude, lie, and presentation are critical to the outcome of labor. The size of the fetal head, the largest part of the fetus and the least compressible, is a primary factor in delivery.

Fetal Head

The size of the fetal head is a significant factor in the passage of the fetus during delivery. Once the fetal head has been delivered, the birth of the rest of the body is rarely delayed. The fetal skull (cranium) has three major parts: (1) face, (2) base of the skull, and (3) vault of the cranium (roof).

The bones of the face and cranial base are well fused and essentially fixed. The base of the cranium is composed of the two temporal bones, each with a sphenoid and ethmoid bone. The bones composing the vault are the two frontal bones, the two parietal bones, and the occipital bone (**Figure 33.37 >>**).

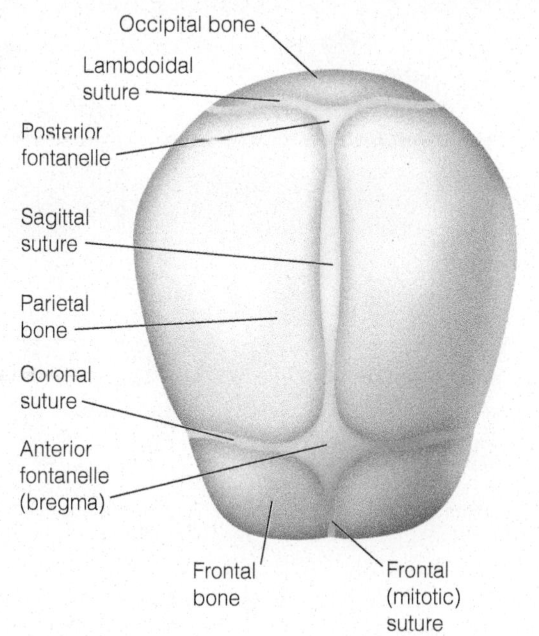

Figure 33.37 >> Superior view of the fetal skull.

These bones are not fused, allowing this portion of the head to adjust in shape as the presenting part passes through the narrow portions of the pelvis. The cranial bones overlap under pressure of the powers of labor and the resistance of the pelvis. This overlapping is called **molding**.

The **sutures** of the fetal skull are membranous spaces between the cranial bones. The intersections of these sutures are called **fontanels**. Cranial sutures allow molding of the fetal head during birth and help the clinician to identify the position of the fetal head during vaginal examination. The important sutures of the cranial vault are as follows (see Figure 33.37):

- ***Frontal (mitotic) suture.*** Located between the two frontal bones, this becomes the anterior continuation of the sagittal suture.
- ***Sagittal suture.*** Located between the parietal bones, this divides the skull into left and right halves; it runs anteroposteriorly, connecting the two fontanels.
- ***Coronal suture.*** Located between the frontal and parietal bones, this extends transversely left and right from the anterior fontanel.
- ***Lambdoidal suture.*** Located between the two parietal bones and the occipital bone, this extends transversely left and right from the posterior fontanel.

The anterior and posterior fontanels (along with the sutures) are clinically useful in identifying the position of the fetal head in the pelvis and in assessing the neurologic and hydration status of the newborn after birth. The anterior fontanel is diamond shaped and measures approximately 2 by 3 cm. It permits growth of the brain by remaining unossified for as long as 18 months. The posterior fontanel is much smaller and closes within 8 to 12 weeks after birth. It is shaped like a small triangle and marks the meeting point of the sagittal suture and the lambdoidal suture.

Following are several important landmarks of the fetal skull (**Figure 33.38 >>**):

- ***Mentum.*** This is the fetal chin.
- ***Sinciput.*** This anterior area is known as the brow.
- ***Bregma.*** This is a large diamond-shaped anterior fontanel.
- ***Vertex.*** This is the area between the anterior and posterior fontanels.
- ***Posterior fontanel.*** This is the intersection between posterior cranial sutures.
- ***Occiput.*** This is the area of the fetal skull occupied by the occipital bone, beneath the posterior fontanel.

The diameters of the fetal skull vary considerably within its normal limits. Some diameters shorten and others lengthen as the head is molded during labor. Fetal head diameters are measured between the various landmarks on the skull. For example, the suboccipitobregmatic diameter is the distance from the undersurface of the occiput to the center of the bregma, or anterior fontanel.

Fetal Attitude

Fetal attitude refers to the relation of the fetal parts to one another, including flexion or extension of the fetal body and extremities. The normal attitude of the fetus is one of

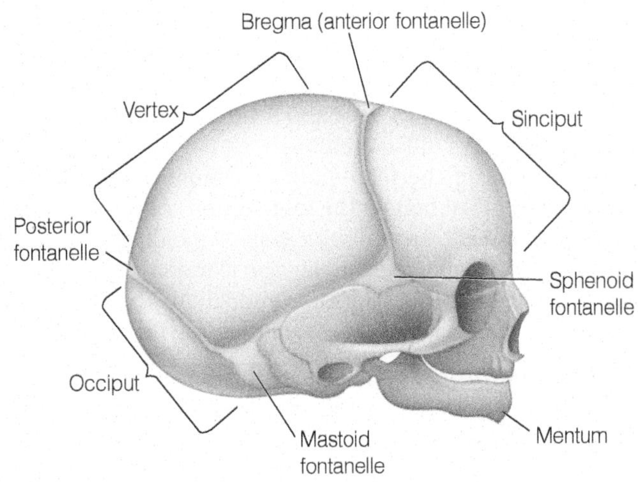

Figure 33.38 » Lateral view of the fetal skull identifying the landmarks that have significance during birth.

moderate flexion of the head, flexion of the arms onto the chest, and flexion of the legs onto the abdomen.

Fetal Lie

Fetal lie refers to the relationship of the cephalocaudal (spinal column) axis of the fetus to the cephalocaudal axis of the woman. The fetus may assume either a longitudinal (vertical) lie or a transverse horizontal lie. A longitudinal lie occurs when the cephalocaudal axis of the fetus is parallel to the woman's spine. A transverse lie occurs when the cephalocaudal axis of the fetus is at a right angle to the woman's spine.

Fetal Presentation

Fetal presentation is determined by fetal lie and by the body part of the fetus that enters the pelvic passage first. This portion of the fetus is referred to as the **presenting part**. Fetal presentation may be cephalic, breech, or shoulder. The most common presentation is cephalic. When this presentation occurs, labor and birth are likely to proceed normally. Breech and shoulder presentations are called **malpresentations** because they are associated with difficulties during labor. With a malpresentation, labor may not proceed as expected.

The fetal head presents itself to the passage in approximately 97% of term births. The cephalic presentation can be further classified according to the degree of flexion or extension of the fetal head (attitude) as follows:

- ***Vertex presentation.*** The fetal head is completely flexed onto the chest, and the smallest diameter of the fetal head (suboccipitobregmatic) presents to the maternal pelvis (**Figure 33.39A »**). The occiput is the presenting part. Vertex is the most common type of presentation.
- ***Military presentation.*** The fetal head is neither flexed nor extended. The occipitofrontal diameter presents to the maternal pelvis (Figure 33.39B). The top of the head is the presenting part.
- ***Brow presentation.*** The fetal head is partially extended. The occipitomental diameter, the largest anteroposterior diameter, is presented to the maternal pelvis (Figure 33.39C). The sinciput is the presenting part (refer to Figure 33.38).
- ***Face presentation.*** The fetal head is hyperextended (complete extension). The submentobregmatic diameter presents to the maternal pelvis (Figure 33.39D). The face is the presenting part.

Breech presentations occur in 3–4% of all births (ACOG, 2020a). In all variations of the breech presentation, the sacrum is the landmark to be noted. These presentations are classified according to the attitude of the fetus's hips and knees:

- ***Complete breech***. The fetal knees and hips are both flexed, the thighs are on the abdomen, and the calves are on the posterior aspect of the thighs. The buttocks and feet of the fetus present to the maternal pelvis.

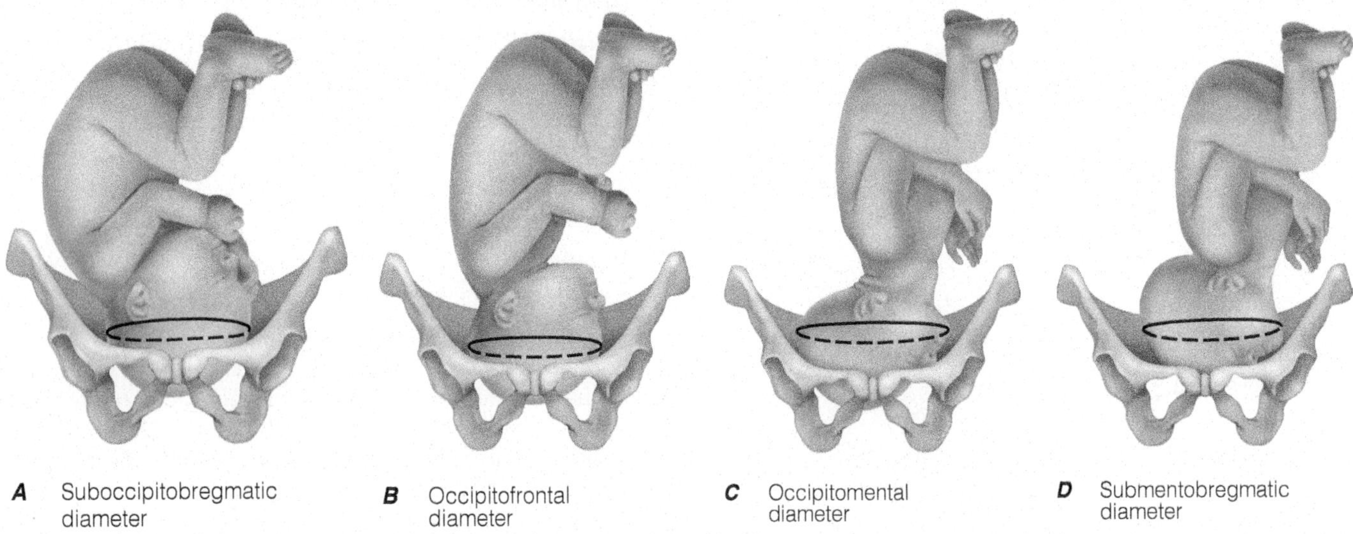

Figure 33.39 » Cephalic presentation. ***A***, Vertex presentation. Complete flexion of the head allows the suboccipitobregmatic diameter to present to the pelvis. ***B***, Military (median vertex) presentation with no flexion or extension. The occipitofrontal diameter presents to the pelvis. ***C***, Brow presentation. The fetal head is in partial (halfway) extension. The occipitomental diameter, which is the largest diameter of the fetal head, presents to the pelvis. ***D***, Face presentation. The fetal head is in complete extension, and the submentobregmatic diameter presents to the pelvis.

- ***Frank breech.*** The fetal hips are flexed, and the knees are extended. The buttocks of the fetus present to the maternal pelvis.
- ***Footling breech.*** The fetal hips and legs are extended, and the feet of the fetus present to the maternal pelvis. In a single footling breech, one foot presents; in a double footling breech, both feet present.

A shoulder presentation is also called a *transverse lie*. Most frequently, the shoulder is the presenting part, and the acromion process of the scapula is the landmark to be noted. However, the fetal arm, back, abdomen, or side may present in a transverse lie.

Relationship Between the Birth Passage and the Fetus

When assessing the relationship between the birth passage and the presenting part of the fetal body, the nurse considers the engagement of the fetus, the location (or station) of the fetal presenting part in the birth passage in relation to the ischial spine, and the fetal position to one of the four quadrants of the maternal pelvis.

Engagement

Engagement of the presenting part occurs when the largest diameter of the presenting part reaches or passes through the pelvic inlet. Whereas engagement confirms the adequacy of the pelvic inlet, it does not indicate whether the midpelvis and outlet are also adequate.

Engagement can be determined by vaginal examinations and Leopold maneuvers. In primigravidas, engagement occurs approximately 2 weeks before term. Multiparas, however, may experience engagement several weeks before the onset of labor or during the process of labor.

Another variable of engagement is the relationship of the fetal sagittal suture to the mother's symphysis pubis and sacrum. The terms *synclitism* and *asynclitism* describe this relationship. **Synclitism** occurs when the sagittal suture is midway between the symphysis pubis and the sacral promontory. Upon vaginal examination, the suture is felt to be midline between these two maternal landmarks and as though it is in alignment. **Asynclitism** occurs when the sagittal suture is directed toward either the symphysis pubis or the sacral promontory and is felt to be misaligned. Upon vaginal examination, the suture feels somewhat turned to one side within the pelvis, making it asymmetrical. Asynclitism can be either anterior or posterior. It is important to identify asynclitism because it can lengthen the time of descent or interfere with the descent process. Sometimes, this can lead to inability of the fetal head to fit through the birth canal and can result in the need for a cesarean delivery.

Station

Station refers to the relationship of the presenting part to an imaginary line drawn between the ischial spines of the maternal pelvis. In a normal pelvis, the ischial spines mark the narrowest diameter through which the fetus must pass. As a landmark, the ischial spines have been designated as zero (0) station (**Figure 33.40** ›››). If the presenting part is higher than the ischial spines, a negative number is assigned, noting the number of centimeters above zero station.

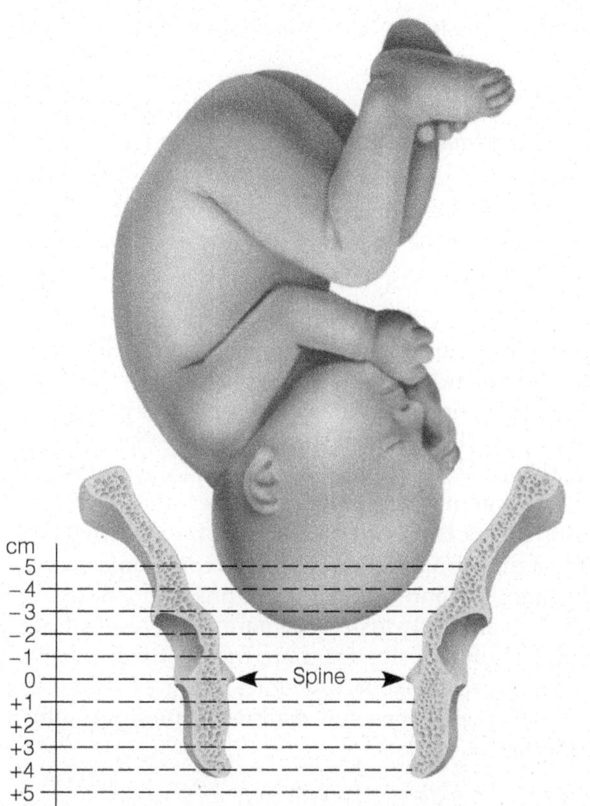

Figure 33.40 ››› Measuring the station of the fetal head while it is descending. In this view, the station is −2/−3.

Engagement is represented when the fetal head reaches zero station. Positive numbers indicate that the presenting part has passed the ischial spines. Station − 5 is at the pelvic inlet, and station +5 is at the outlet.

During labor, the presenting part should move progressively from the negative stations to the midpelvis at zero station and into the positive stations. If the presenting part can be seen at the woman's perineum, birth is imminent. Failure of the presenting part to descend in the presence of strong contractions may be caused by disproportion between the maternal pelvis and the fetal presenting part, malpresentation, asynclitism, or multiple fetuses. Station is assessed by vaginal examination.

Fetal Position

Fetal position refers to the relationship between a designated landmark on the presenting fetal part and the front, sides, or back of the maternal pelvis. The chosen landmarks differ according to presentation as follows:

- The landmark for vertex presentations is the occiput.
- The landmark for face presentations is the mentum.
- The landmark for breech presentations is the sacrum.
- The landmark for shoulder presentations is the acromion process on the scapula.

To determine position, the nurse notes which quadrant of the maternal pelvis the appropriate landmark is directed toward: left anterior, right anterior, left posterior, or right posterior. If the landmark is directed toward the side of the pelvis, fetal position is designated as transverse rather than anterior or posterior. In documentation, the following abbreviations are used:

- Right (R) or left (L) side of the maternal pelvis
- The landmark of the fetal presenting part: occiput (O), mentum (M), sacrum (S), or acromion process (A)
- Anterior (A), posterior (P), or transverse (T), depending on whether the landmark is in the front, back, or side of the pelvis.

These abbreviations help the healthcare team communicate the fetal position. For example, when the fetal occiput is directed toward the back and to the left of the birth passage, the abbreviation used is LOP (left occiput posterior). With a transverse lie, the fetal spine may be either superior (also called back *up*) or inferior (back *down*) (Mayo Clinic, 2017a).

Assessment techniques to determine fetal position include inspection and palpation of the maternal abdomen and vaginal examination. The most common fetal presentation is occiput anterior. When this presentation occurs, labor and birth are likely to proceed normally. Presentations other than occiput anterior are more frequently associated with problems during labor; therefore, they are called *malpresentations*. Presentations and malpresentations are illustrated in **Figure 33.41** ⟫.

Physiologic Forces of Labor

Birth of the fetus, fetal membranes, and placenta occurs through the work of primary and secondary forces. Uterine muscular contractions that occur in the first stage of labor are the primary force. Bearing down, the use of abdominal muscle to push during the second stage of labor, is the secondary force.

Contractions

In labor, uterine contractions are rhythmic but intermittent. Between contractions, there is a period of relaxation. This allows the uterine muscles to rest and provides respite for the laboring woman. It also restores uteroplacental circulation, which is important to fetal oxygenation and adequate circulation in the uterine blood vessels.

Each contraction has three phases:

1. ***Increment:*** the building up of the contraction (the longest phase)
2. ***Acme:*** the peak of the contraction
3. ***Decrement:*** the letting up of the contraction.

When describing uterine contractions during labor, HCPs use the terms *frequency, duration,* and *intensity* (**Figure 33.42** ⟫). **Frequency** refers to the time between the beginning of one contraction and the beginning of the next contraction. **Duration** is measured from the beginning of a contraction to the completion of that same contraction. **Intensity** refers to the strength of the contraction during acme. In most instances, intensity can be estimated by an experienced examiner palpating the uterine fundus during a contraction, but it may be measured directly with an intrauterine catheter. When intensity is measured with an intrauterine catheter, the normal resting pressure in the uterus (between contractions) averages 10 to 12 mmHg. During acme, the intensity ranges from 25 to 40 mmHg in early labor, 50 to 70 mmHg in active labor, 80 to 100 mmHg during transition, and more than 100 mmHg while the woman is pushing in the second stage (Blackburn, 2018).

At the beginning of labor, the contractions are usually mild. As labor progresses, the duration, intensity, and frequency of the contractions increase. Because the contractions are involuntary, the laboring woman cannot control their duration, frequency, or intensity.

Bearing Down

When the cervix is completely dilated and the fetus has descended enough to stimulate the maternal urge to push, the mother's abdominal muscles contract as she bears down. Bearing down assists the expulsion of the fetus and placenta. However, if the cervix is not completely dilated, bearing down can result in cervical edema. This can lead to cervical damage, stalling of dilation, and maternal exhaustion.

Psychosocial Considerations

The final critical factor is the parents' psychosocial readiness, including their fears, anxieties, birth fantasies, excitement level, feelings of joy and anticipation, and level of social support. These psychosocial factors affect both parents. Both are making a transition into a new role, and both have expectations of themselves during the labor and birth experience and as caregivers for their child and their new family. Psychosocial factors that affect labor and birth include the couple's accomplishment of the tasks of pregnancy, usual coping mechanisms in response to stressful life events, support system, preparation for childbirth, and cultural influences. Even pregnant women and partners who attend childbirth preparation classes and have a solid support system can be concerned about what labor will be like. Many couples, even in the intense happiness and excitement of the event, may be concerned about whether they will be able to perform the way they expect, whether the pain will be more than the mother expects or can cope with, and whether the partner can provide helpful support. Although birth is usually a happy and joyful event, it is also a time of physical and emotional stress. Whether that stress is positive or negative, it can affect a couple's responses to the labor itself.

A woman approaching her first labor faces a totally new experience, and the woman who has given birth before knows that this labor might be very different from her previous experience. Most women wonder whether they will live up to their expectations for themselves, whether they will experience a physical injury (e.g., lacerations, episiotomy, or cesarean incision), and whether significant others will be supportive. Many women are excited and happy that labor has begun; however, they may have concerns about the labor process itself.

Expectant women mentally prepare for labor through meaningful action and imaginary rehearsal. The actions frequently consist of "nesting behavior" (housecleaning, decorating the nursery) and a "psyching up" for the labor, which varies depending on the woman's self-confidence, self-esteem, and previous experiences with stress. Specific actions to prepare for labor may focus on becoming better informed and prepared. In addition, just as a woman tries on the maternal role during pregnancy, fantasizing about labor seems to help her understand and become better prepared for it.

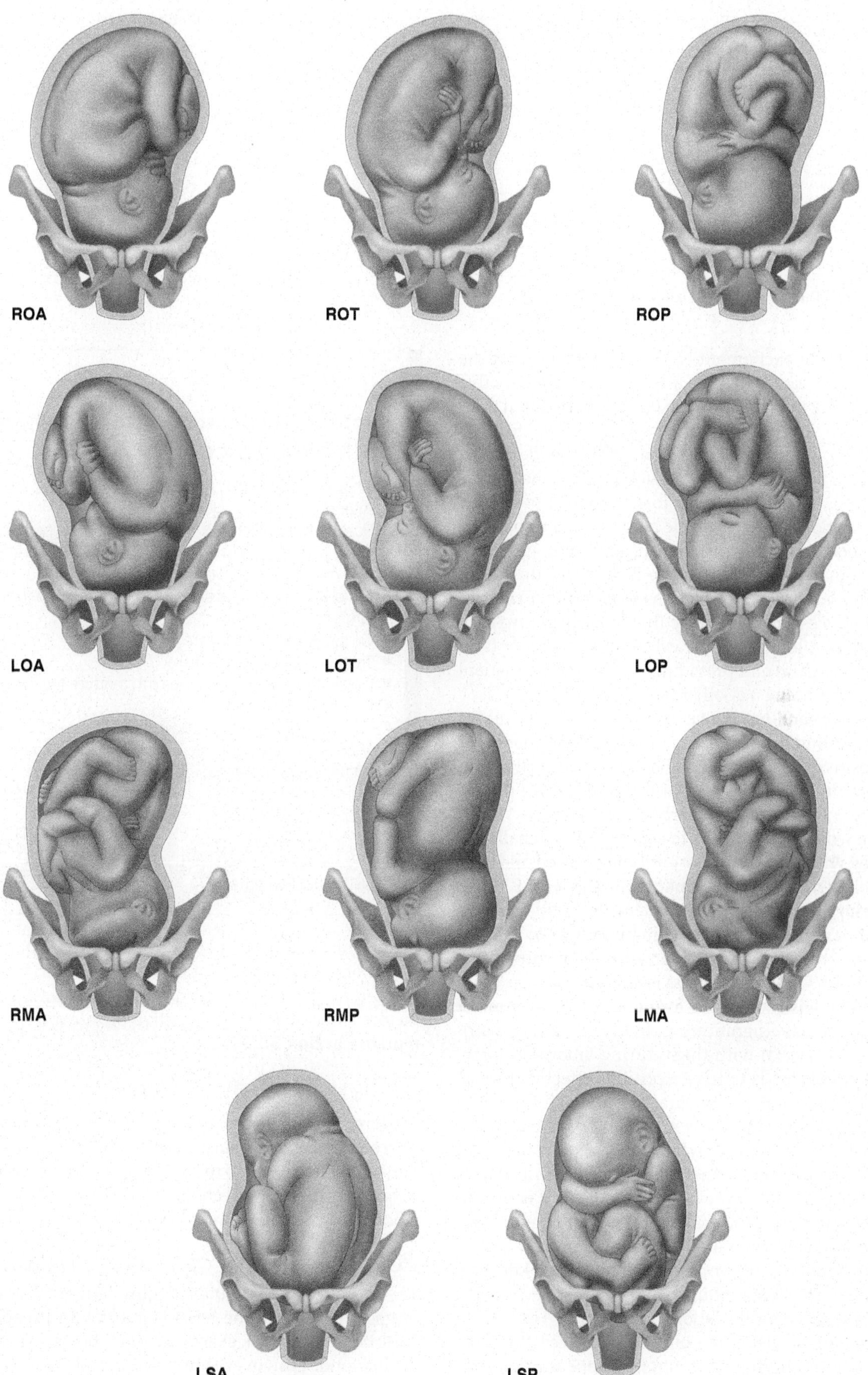

Figure 33.41 ›› Presentations and malpresentations. ***Key:*** FIRST LETTER: R = right, L = left. SECOND LETTER: O = occiput, M = mentum, S = sacrum, A = acromion process. THIRD LETTER: A = anterior, P = posterior, T = transverse.

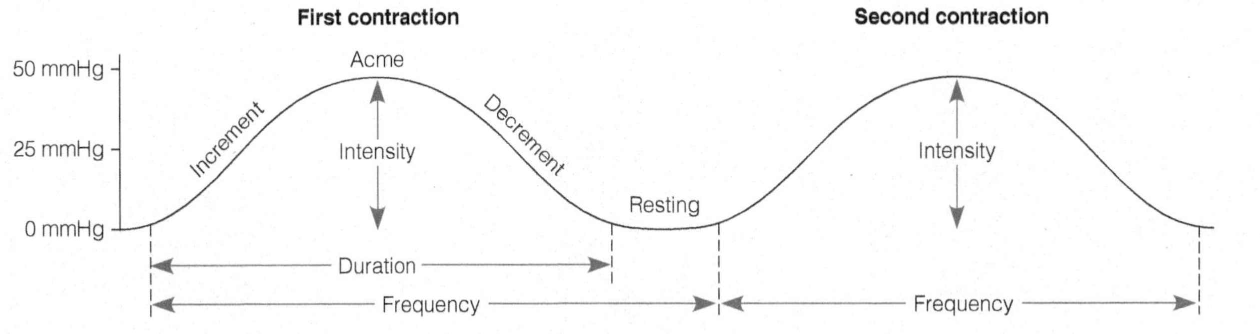

Figure 33.42 ›› Characteristics of uterine contractions.

Fantasies about the excitement of the baby's birth and the sharing of the experience involve the woman in constructive preparation. Many pregnant women have dreams about their baby, labor, birth, and parenting. Some women may fear the pain of contractions, whereas others may welcome the opportunity to feel the birth process. Some women view the pain as threatening and associate it with a loss of control over their bodies and emotions. Others see the pain as a rite of passage into motherhood and a necessary means to an end. It is helpful for the woman to realize that she is safe and that labor pain is not the same sign of danger as pain in other circumstances. Assurances from the nurse that labor is progressing normally can go a long way toward reducing anxiety (and thereby reducing pain) and providing positive reinforcement that the mother is doing a good job.

Empowerment and having control over her body play a key role in determining whether the woman views her labor and birth positively. Mothers who have positive birth experiences are more likely to thrive in the postpartum period and view the transition to motherhood as positive (WHO, 2018a). Some women view the birth experience as a challenge in which they will have the opportunity to succeed and provide their baby with a joyful reception into the world.

The laboring woman's support system also influences the course of labor and birth. Some women prefer not to have a support person or family member with them during the birth process. For some, this process is a private moment that the woman may wish to reserve for herself. However, most women choose to have significant individuals (family members, partner, or friend) with them during labor and birth. This social support tends to have a positive effect. For some families, the birth event is a celebration in which they may want as many significant others present as possible. Some women may want to create a joyful, festive atmosphere that includes the grandparents, friends, and other children. A labor partner's presence at the bedside provides a means to enhance communication and to demonstrate feelings of love. Communication needs may include talking and the use of affectionate and reassuring words from the partner. Affection may also take the form of holding hands, hugging, touching, or gentle reassurance for the laboring woman.

How the woman views the birth experience afterward may affect her mothering behaviors. It appears that any activities by the expectant woman or by HCPs that enhance the birth experience benefit the mother–baby connection. Women who experience traumatic births or have negative feelings about their birth experience are at greater risk for postpartum depression (ACOG, 2018f). The partner's experience of the birth and opportunities for bonding may have important implications for parenting as well. Psychosocial factors associated with a positive birth experience are summarized in **Box 33.3** ››.

Box 33.3
Factors Associated with a Positive Birth Experience

- Choosing or wanting pregnancy
- Attending childbirth classes
- Positive relationship with and support from partner
- Choosing a provider whose philosophy of care is compatible with mother's
- Consistent emotional support from caregivers (professional and family)
- Culturally competent care
- Trust in the healthcare team
- Confidence in ability to give birth, nurture the infant
- Feelings of empowerment
- Use of relaxation strategies (e.g., massage, music)
- Maintaining control during labor, including control of breathing patterns, comfort measures
- Effective, culturally competent communication from nurses, staff about progress, procedures.

Sources: Adapted from London et al. (2017); Nilsson, Thorsell, Wahn, and Ekstrom (2013); Taheri, Takian, Taghizadeh, Jafari, and Sarafraz (2018); World Health Organization (2018c).

Physiology of Labor

Understanding the physiology of normal birth helps the nurse provide information to the mother and her support person, which can help reduce their feelings of anxiety. It also helps alert the nurse to changes from normal that may signal a potential complication of labor.

Possible Causes of Labor Onset

The process of labor usually begins between 37 and 42 weeks of gestation, when the fetus is mature and ready for birth. Despite research, the exact cause of labor onset is not clearly understood. However, some important aspects have been identified: Progesterone relaxes smooth muscle tissue; estrogen stimulates uterine muscle contractions; and connective tissue loosens to permit the softening, thinning, and eventual opening of the cervix (Blackburn, 2018).

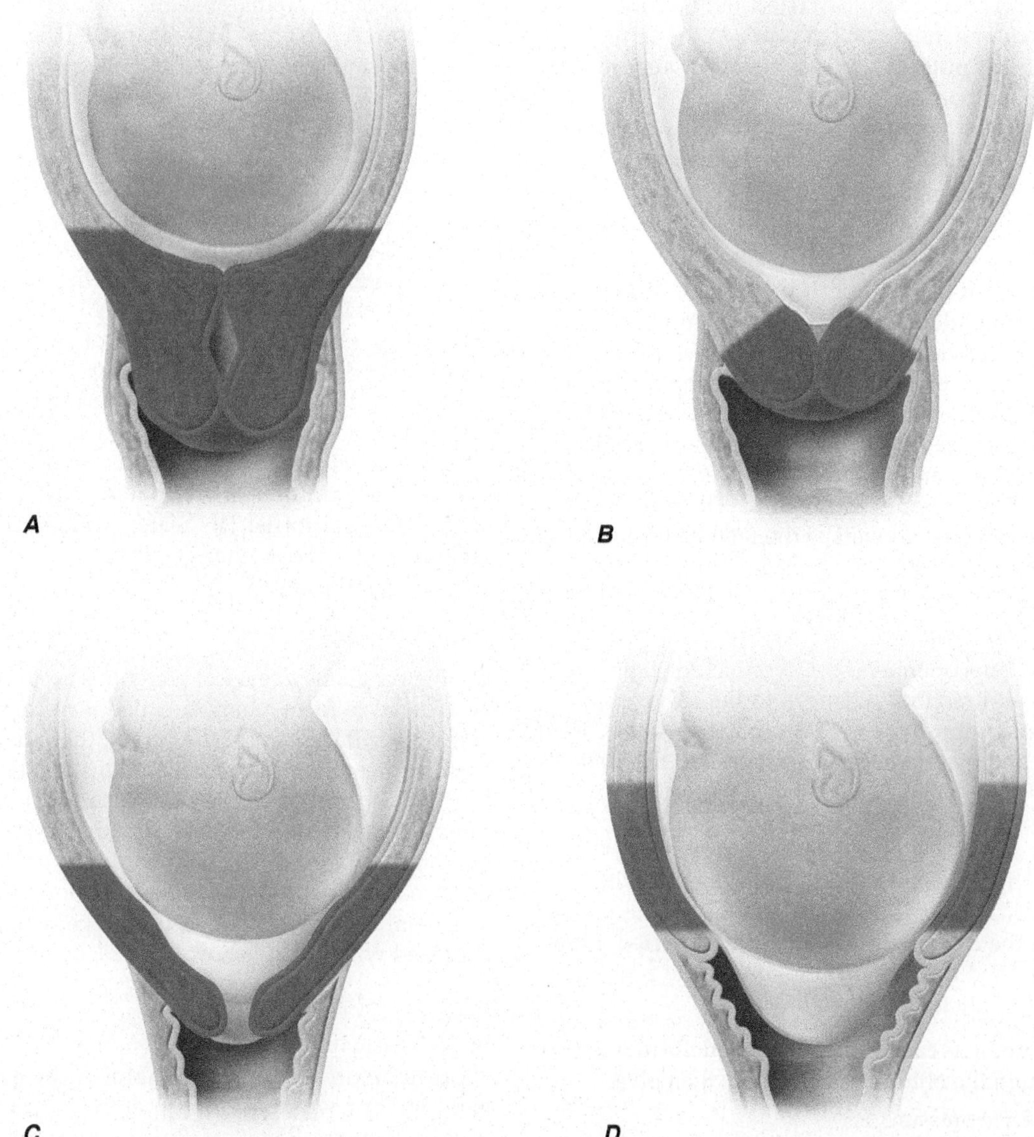

Figure 33.43 ⟫ Effacement of the cervix in the primigravida. ***A***, Beginning of labor. There is no cervical effacement or dilation. The fetal head is cushioned by amniotic fluid. ***B***, Beginning cervical effacement. As the cervix begins to efface, more amniotic fluid collects below the fetal head. ***C***, Cervix is about one-half (50%) effaced and slightly dilated. The increasing amount of amniotic fluid below the fetal head exerts hydrostatic pressure on the cervix. ***D***, Complete effacement and dilation.

Myometrial Activity

In true labor, with each contraction the muscles of the upper uterine segment shorten and exert a longitudinal traction on the cervix, causing effacement. **Effacement** is thinning of the cervix as it is drawn upward into the uterine side walls. The cervix changes progressively from a long, thick structure to a structure that is tissue-paper thin (**Figure 33.43 ⟫**). In primigravidas, effacement usually precedes dilation.

Contractions are stimulated by the hormone oxytocin. Oxytocin is a potent uterine stimulant and is frequently used as an agent to induce or augment labor in term fetuses or when delivery is necessitated. Uterine sensitivity to oxytocin is increased during pregnancy (Blackburn, 2018). Oxytocin is produced in the hypothalamus and secreted into the bloodstream, but it is also produced in uterine tissues during late gestation, with concentrations increasing at the onset of labor. Oxytocin receptors are most likely formed in the gestational tissues, which when stimulated produce myometrial activity (Cunningham et al., 2018).

The uterus shortens with each contraction, which in turn pulls the lower uterine segment upward. This shortening causes flexion of the fetal body, thrusting the presenting part down toward the lower uterine segment and the cervix. The pressure exerted by the fetus is called the fetal axis pressure. As the uterus shortens, the longitudinal muscle fibers elongate, and the lower uterine segment becomes more distensible and removes resistance on the presenting part as the uterus is pulled upward. This action and the hydrostatic pressure of the fetal membranes cause cervical dilation. The cervical os and cervical canal widen from less than 1 cm to approximately 10 cm, allowing birth of the fetus. When the cervix is completely dilated and retracted into the lower uterine segment, it can no longer be palpated. At the same time, the round ligament pulls the fundus forward, aligning the fetus with the bony pelvis.

Note that the metric system is used for measurement in labor and delivery. Dilation of the cervix is measured in centimeters, for example.

Changes in the Pelvic Floor

Direct pressure from the fetal head pushes the rectum and vagina downward and forward with each contraction along the curve of the pelvic floor. As the fetal head descends to the pelvic floor, the pressure of the presenting part causes the perineal structure, which was once approximately 5 cm in thickness, to change to a structure less than 1 cm thick. A normal physiologic anesthesia is produced as a result of the decreased blood supply to the area. The anus everts, exposing the interior rectal wall as the fetal head descends forward (Blackburn, 2018).

Signs of Labor

Signs and symptoms of impending labor include lightening, Braxton Hicks contractions, changes to the cervix, bloody show, membrane rupture, and a sudden burst of energy. Most primigravidas and many multiparas experience these signs.

Lightening

Lightening describes the effects that occur when the fetus begins to settle into the pelvic inlet (engagement). With fetal descent, the uterus moves downward, and the fundus no longer presses on the diaphragm, so breathing is eased. However, with increased downward pressure of the presenting part, the woman may notice the following:

- Leg cramps or pains caused by pressure on the nerves that course through the obturator foramen in the pelvis
- Increased pelvic pressure
- Increased urinary frequency
- Increased venous stasis, leading to edema in the lower extremities
- Increased vaginal secretions resulting from congestion of the vaginal mucous membranes.

Braxton Hicks Contractions

Before the onset of labor, **Braxton Hicks contractions** (irregular, intermittent contractions that occur throughout a pregnancy) may become uncomfortable. The pain seems to be focused in the abdomen and groin but may feel like the "drawing" sensations experienced by some women with dysmenorrhea. Braxton Hicks contractions that are strong enough to disturb the mother without affecting cervical change or fetal descent are sometimes referred to as "false" labor. Prelabor contractions may be exhausting. If the contractions are fairly regular, the woman has no way of knowing whether they are the beginning of active labor, and she may come to the hospital or birthing center for a vaginal examination to determine whether cervical dilation is occurring. These prelabor contractions may be exacerbated by inadequate fluid intake, a full bladder, sexual activity, or a UTI. An episode of regular contractions may resolve or continue, becoming active labor. It is important to remember that women with contractions that occur on a regular basis before 37 completed weeks of gestation should be assessed to determine whether they are experiencing preterm labor.

Cervical Changes

Considerable change occurs in the cervix during the prenatal and intrapartum period. At the beginning of pregnancy, the cervix is rigid and firm, and it must soften so that it can stretch and dilate to allow passage of the fetus. This softening of the cervix is called *ripening*.

As term approaches, the action of enzymes, such as collagenase and elastase, breaks down the collagen fibers of the cervix. As the collagen fibers change, their ability to bind together decreases because of increasing amounts of hyaluronic acid, which loosely binds collagen fibrils, and decreasing amounts of dermatan sulfate, which tightly binds collagen fibrils. The water content of the cervix also increases. All these changes result in a weakening and softening of the cervix.

Bloody Show

During pregnancy, cervical secretions accumulate in the cervical canal to form a barrier called a *mucus plug*. With softening and effacement of the cervix, the mucus plug is often expelled, resulting in a small amount of blood loss from the exposed cervical capillaries. The resulting pink-tinged secretions are called **bloody show**. Bloody show is considered to be a sign that labor will begin within 24 to 48 hours. Vaginal examination that includes manipulation of the cervix may also result in a blood-tinged discharge, which is sometimes confused with bloody show.

Rupture of Membranes

In approximately 10% of women, the amniotic membranes rupture before the onset of labor. After membranes rupture, 90% of women will experience spontaneous labor within 24 hours (Jazayeri, 2018). Membrane rupture prior to the onset of labor is referred to as **premature rupture of membranes (PROM)**. Due to the increased risk for intra-amniotic infection once membranes are ruptured, some clinicians will recommend an induction of labor after PROM, and others may allow the option of awaiting spontaneous labor (Jazayeri, 2018).

At the beginning of labor, the amniotic membranes may bulge through the cervix in the shape of a cone. When the membranes rupture, the amniotic fluid may be expelled in large amounts. **Spontaneous rupture of membranes (SROM)** generally occurs at the height of an intense contraction with a gush of the fluid out of the vagina. If engagement has not occurred, the danger exists that a portion of the umbilical cord may be expelled with the fluid (prolapsed cord). In addition, because of these potential problems, the woman is advised to notify her HCP and proceed to the hospital or birthing center. In some instances, the fluid is expelled in small amounts and may be confused with episodes of urinary incontinence associated with urinary urgency, coughing, or sneezing. The discharge should be checked to ascertain its source and to determine further action. In some instances, the membranes are ruptured by the HCP, using an instrument

TABLE 33.9 Comparison of True and False Labor

True Labor	False Labor
Contractions are at regular intervals.	Contractions are irregular.
Intervals between contractions gradually shorten.	Usually no change.
Contractions increase in duration and intensity.	Usually no change.
Discomfort begins in back and radiates around to abdomen.	Discomfort is usually in abdomen.
Intensity usually increases with change in activity.	Change of activity has no effect on contractions.
Cervical dilation and effacement are progressive.	No change.
Contractions do not decrease with rest or warm tub bath.	Rest and warm tub lessen contractions.

called an *amniohook.* This procedure is called *amniotomy* or **artificial rupture of membranes (AROM)**.

When membrane rupture and leakage of amniotic fluid from the vagina occurs before 37 weeks of gestation, the term **preterm premature rupture of membranes (PPROM)** is used. PPROM occurs in 8–10% of all pregnancies and is the cause of up to one-third of preterm births (Children's Hospital of Philadelphia, 2020). Infection is a common complication of PPROM. When PPROM is suspected, strict sterile technique should be used during any vaginal examination to reduce the risk of infection.

Sudden Burst of Energy

Some women report a sudden burst of energy approximately 24 to 48 hours before labor. This often finds expression in nesting behaviors. The cause of this energy spurt is unknown. In prenatal teaching, warn prospective mothers not to overexert themselves during this energy burst in order to avoid being overtired when labor begins.

Other Signs

Additional signs that labor is imminent include weight loss of 1 to 3 lb and GI symptoms. Weight loss occurs from fluid loss and electrolyte changes due to fluctuations in estrogen and progesterone levels. It is unknown why GI symptoms occur.

Differences Between True and False Labor

The contractions of true labor produce progressive dilation and effacement of the cervix. They occur regularly and increase in frequency, duration, and intensity. The discomfort of true labor contractions usually starts in the back and radiates around to the abdomen. The pain is not relieved by ambulation; in fact, walking may intensify the pain.

The contractions of false labor do not produce progressive cervical effacement and dilation. Classically, they are irregular and do not increase in frequency, duration, and intensity. The contractions may be perceived as a hardening or "balling up" without discomfort, or discomfort may occur mainly in the lower abdomen and groin. The discomfort may be relieved by ambulation, changing positions, drinking a large amount of water, or taking a warm shower or tub bath.

The pregnant woman will find it helpful to know the characteristics of true labor contractions as well as the premonitory signs of ensuing labor. At times, however, the only way to differentiate accurately between true and false labor is to assess dilation. The woman must feel free to come in for accurate assessment of labor and should be counseled not to feel foolish if the labor is false. The nurse must reassure the woman that false labor is common and that it often cannot be distinguished from true labor except by vaginal examination. **Table 33.9** » provides a comparison of true and false labor.

Stages of Labor and Birth

To assist HCPs, common terms have been developed as benchmarks to subdivide the labor process into phases and stages of labor. It is important to note, however, that these represent theoretical separations in the process. A laboring woman will not usually experience distinct differences from one stage to another.

The first stage begins with the onset of true labor and ends when the cervix is completely dilated at 10 cm and the mother has the urge to push. The second stage begins with urge to push in the setting of complete dilation and ends with the birth of the newborn. The third stage begins with the birth of the newborn and ends with the delivery of the placenta.

Some clinicians identify a fourth stage. During this stage, which lasts 1 to 4 hours after delivery of the placenta, the uterus effectively contracts to control bleeding at the placental site (Cunningham et al., 2018).

First Stage

The first stage of labor is divided into the latent, active, and transition phases. Each phase of labor is characterized by physical and psychologic changes and is summarized in **Table 33.10** ».

Latent Phase

The latent (or prodromal) phase starts with the beginning of regular contractions, which are usually mild. The woman feels able to cope with the discomfort. She may be relieved that labor has finally started and that the end of pregnancy has come. Although she may be anxious, she is able to recognize and express those feelings of anxiety. The woman is often smiling and eager to talk about herself and answer questions. Excitement is high, and her partner or other support person is often equally elated.

Uterine contractions become established during the latent phase and increase in frequency, duration, and intensity. They may start as mild contractions lasting 20 seconds with a frequency of 10 to 20 minutes and progress to moderate ones lasting 30 to 40 seconds with a frequency

TABLE 33.10 Characteristics of Labor

	First Stage			
	Latent Phase	**Active Phase**	**Transition Phase**	**Second Stage**
Labor				
Nullipara	<20 hr in most cases	1.1–3.8 hr	1–3.2 hr	≤3 hr, may be longer than 3 hr with epidural anesthesia
Multipara	<14 hr in most cases	0.9–3.2 hr	0.6–2 hr	<1 hr, may be as much as 2 hr with epidural
Cervical dilation	0–6 cm	6–8 cm	8–10 cm	
Contractions				
Note: Contraction patterns may vary considerably. Patterns that do not fit the parameters outlined here are only classified as pathologic in the setting of protraction or arrest of labor.				
Frequency	Every 10–30 min	Every 2–5 min	Every 1.5–2.0 min	Every 1.5–2.0 min
Duration	30–40 sec	40–60 sec	60–90 sec	60–90 sec
Intensity	Begin as mild and progress to moderate; 25–40 mmHg by intrauterine pressure catheter (IUPC)	Begin as moderate and progress to strong; 50–70 mmHg by IUPC	Strong by palpation; 70–90 mmHg by IUPC	Strong by palpation; 70–100 mmHg by IUPC

Source: From London et al. (2017). Pearson Education, Inc., Hoboken, NJ.

5 to 7 minutes. As the cervix begins to dilate, it also effaces, although little or no fetal descent is evident. For a woman in her first labor (nullipara), the latent phase of the first stage of labor generally lasts longer than that for a multipara. Note that specific descriptions of the latent/prodromal phase are guidelines and the actual experiences of women prior to the active phase vary widely. Timing and duration of contractions and time elapsed before the onset of the active phase do not, in themselves, require intervention or influence management. Maternal exhaustion may call for therapeutic rest or in-hospital hydration (King et al., 2019).

Active Phase

When the woman enters the early active phase, her anxiety and her sense of the need for energy and focus tend to increase as she senses the intensification of contractions and pain. She may begin to fear a loss of control or may feel the need to "really work and focus" on the contractions. Women will use a variety of coping mechanisms. Some women exhibit a sense of purpose and the need for regrouping, whereas others may feel a decreased ability to cope or a sense of helplessness. Women who have support persons and family available often experience greater satisfaction and have less anxiety compared to women without support.

During this phase, the cervix dilates from approximately 6 to 8 cm (1.6 to 2.8 in.). Fetal descent is progressive, and the rate of cervical dilation most often increases. During the active phase, contractions become more frequent and longer in duration, and they increase in intensity. By the end of the active phase, contractions may have a frequency of 2 to 5 minutes, a duration of 40 to 60 seconds, and strong intensity.

Transition Phase

The transition phase is the last part of the first stage of labor. When the woman enters the transition phase, she may demonstrate an acute awareness of the need for her energy and attention to be completely focused on the task at hand. She may experience significant anxiety or feel out of control. She becomes acutely aware of the increasing force and intensity of the contractions. Irritability and feelings of self-doubt may occur. She may become restless, frequently changing position in an attempt to get comfortable. The nurse should recognize these behaviors as normal and communicate such to the laboring woman and her support person.

By the time the woman enters the transition phase, she is inner directed and often tired. She may not want to be left alone; at the same time, the support person may be feeling the need for a break. The nurse should reassure the woman that she will not be left alone. It is crucial that the nurse be available as relief support at this time and keep the patient informed about where her labor support people are if they leave the room. Some women have the intuition that the end of labor is occurring and know that birth is near; an instinct to have support people remain often occurs.

During the transition phase, contractions have a frequency of approximately every 1.5 to 2 minutes, a duration of 60 to 90 seconds, and strong intensity. The transition phase does not usually last longer than 3 hours for nulliparas or longer than 1 hour for multiparas (King et al., 2019). The total duration of the first stage may be increased by approximately 1 hour if epidural anesthesia is used.

As dilation approaches 10 cm, there may be increased rectal pressure and an uncontrollable desire to bear down, an increased amount of bloody show, and rupture of membranes (if it has not already occurred). With the peak of a contraction, the woman may experience a sensation of intense pressure. If laboring without anesthesia, she may fear that she will be "torn open" or "split apart." She may also fear that the sensations indicate that something is wrong. The nurse should inform the patient that what she is feeling is normal in this stage of labor. Even with assurance, however, the woman may increasingly doubt her ability to cope with labor and may become apprehensive, irritable, and withdrawn. She may be terrified of being left alone, though she might not want anyone to talk to or touch her. However, with the next contraction, she may ask for verbal and physical support.

Other characteristics of this phase may include the following:

- Increasing bloody show
- Hyperventilation
- Generalized discomfort, including low backache, shaking and cramping in legs, and increased sensitivity to touch
- Increased need for partner's and/or nurse's presence and support
- Restlessness
- Increased apprehension and irritability
- An inner focus on her contractions
- A sense of bewilderment, frustration, and anger at the contractions
- Requests for medication
- Hiccupping, belching, nausea, or vomiting
- Beads of perspiration on the upper lip or brow
- Increasing rectal pressure and feeling the urge to bear down.

The woman in this phase is anxious to "get it over with." She may be amnesic and sleep between her now-frequent contractions. Her support persons may start to feel fatigue and may feel helpless, and they may want more participation from the nurse as their efforts to alleviate the woman's discomfort seem less effective.

Second Stage

The second stage of labor begins with complete cervical dilation and ends with birth of the baby. For primigravidas, the second stage should be completed within 3 to 4 hours after the cervix becomes fully dilated; for multiparas, the second stage should be complete in 2 to 3 hours. Contractions continue with a frequency of about every 15 to 30 minutes, a duration of up to 90 seconds, and strong intensity (Lowdermilk, Perry, Cashion, Alden, & Olshansky, 2020). Descent of the fetal presenting part continues until it reaches the perineal floor.

As the fetal head descends, the woman usually has the urge to push because of pressure from the fetal head on the sacral and obturator nerves. As she pushes, intra-abdominal pressure is exerted from contraction of the maternal abdominal muscles. As the fetal head continues its descent, the perineum begins to bulge, flatten, and move anteriorly. Most women feel acute, increasingly severe pain and a burning sensation as the perineum distends. The amount of bloody show may increase. The labia begin to part with each contraction, and between contractions, the fetal head appears to recede. With succeeding contractions and maternal pushing effort, the fetal head descends farther. **Crowning** occurs when the head no longer recedes and remains visible at the vaginal introitus between contractions; this means that birth is imminent.

The woman may feel some relief that the transition phase of the first stage is over, the birth is near, and she can push. Some women feel a sense of purpose now that they can be actively involved. The woman may be focused and should be encouraged to center all her energy into pushing. The nurse should encourage resting between contractions as well. The support person can offer ice chips, fan her (she is often overheated and fatigued), offer verbal encouragement, and provide support to the legs.

For women without childbirth preparation, this stage can become frightening. The nurse should encourage the woman to work with her contractions and not fight them. A support person who has never seen a labor may also become disconcerted during this time. The nurse can assist the support person in performing activities and offering encouragement that assists the woman during the birth process. The woman may feel she has lost her ability to cope and may become embarrassed, or she may demonstrate extreme irritability toward the staff or her supporters as she attempts to regain control over her body. Some women feel a great sense of purpose and are unrelenting in their efforts to work with each and every contraction, and some women will be very forceful with and directive of staff and support persons. Although not as common, some women may not experience an overwhelming urge to push and will require guidance and encouragement by the nurse to effectively push during contractions. All of these reactions and emotions are normal and should be supported as the woman works toward the birth.

Positional Changes of the Fetus

For the fetus to pass through the birth canal, the fetal head and body must adjust to the passage by certain positional changes. These changes, called **cardinal movements** or *mechanisms of labor*, are described here in the order in which they occur (**Figure 33.44** »):

- ***Descent.*** This occurs because of four forces: (1) pressure of the amniotic fluid, (2) direct pressure of the uterine fundus on the breech, (3) contraction of the abdominal muscles, and (4) extension and straightening of the fetal body. The head enters the inlet in the occiput transverse or oblique position because the pelvic inlet is widest from side to side. The sagittal suture is equidistant from the maternal symphysis pubis and the sacral promontory.
- ***Flexion.*** This occurs as the fetal head descends and meets resistance from the soft tissues of the pelvis, the muscles of the pelvic floor, and the cervix. As a result of the resistance, the fetal chin flexes downward onto the chest.
- ***Internal rotation.*** The fetal head must rotate to fit the diameter of the pelvic cavity, which is widest in the anteroposterior diameter. As the occiput of the fetal head meets resistance from the levator ani muscles and their fascia, the occiput rotates—usually from left to right—and the sagittal suture aligns in the anteroposterior pelvic diameter.
- ***Extension.*** The resistance of the pelvic floor and the mechanical movement of the vulva opening anteriorly and forward assist with extension of the fetal head as it passes under the symphysis pubis. With this positional change, the occiput, and then the brow and face, emerge from the vagina.
- ***Restitution.*** The shoulders of the fetus enter the pelvis inlet obliquely and remain oblique when the head rotates to the anteroposterior diameter through internal rotation. Because of this rotation, the neck becomes twisted. Once the head is born and is free of pelvic resistance, the neck untwists, turning the head to one side (restitution), and aligns with the position of the back in the birth canal.

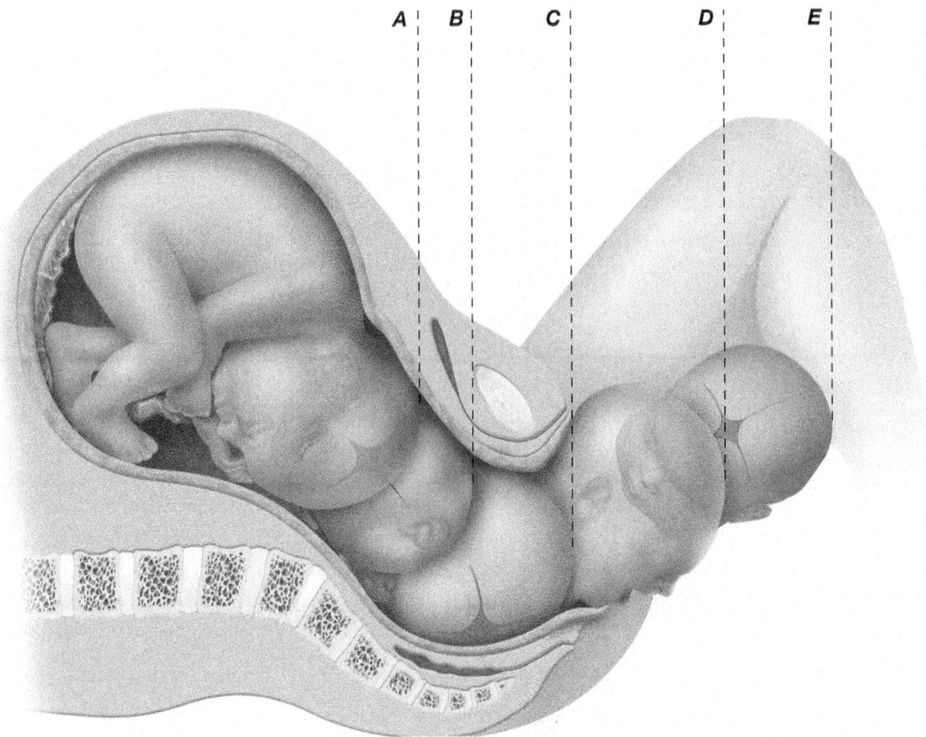

Figure 33.44 ›› Mechanisms of labor. ***A***, Descent. ***B***, Flexion. ***C***, Internal rotation. ***D***, Extension. ***E***, External rotation.

- ***External rotation.*** As the shoulders rotate to the anteroposterior position in the pelvis, the head turns farther to one side (external rotation).
- ***Expulsion.*** After the external rotation, and through the pushing efforts of the laboring woman, the anterior shoulder meets the undersurface of the symphysis pubis and slips under it. As lateral flexion of the shoulder and head occurs, the anterior shoulder is born before the posterior shoulder. The body follows quickly.

Spontaneous Birth (Vertex Presentation)

As the fetal head distends the vulva with each contraction, the perineum becomes extremely thin, and the anus stretches and protrudes. With time, the head extends under the symphysis pubis and is born. When the anterior shoulder meets the underside of the symphysis pubis, a gentle push by the mother aids in the birth of the shoulders. The body then follows. See a birth sequence in **Figure 33.45** ››.

Third Stage

The third stage of labor begins with the birth of the baby and ends with delivery of the placenta, which should be completed within 30 minutes of the birth. Intervention is required if separation of the placenta from the uterine wall has not occurred after 30 minutes (see *Retained placenta* in the Alterations and Therapies feature).

Placental Separation

After the baby is born, the uterus contracts firmly, diminishing its capacity and the surface area of placental attachment. The placenta begins to separate because of this decrease in formation of a hematoma between the placental tissue and the remaining decidua. This hematoma accelerates the separation process. The membranes are the last to separate. They are peeled off the uterine wall as the placenta descends into the vagina. Traditionally, this process was allowed to occur naturally with no intervention. However, newer research has shown that *active management of the third stage of labor* (AMTSL) leads to a shorter third stage, less overall blood loss, and a decreased risk of postpartum hemorrhage. AMTSL includes the administration of oxytocin immediately after birth, gentle traction to the umbilical cord, and mild counterpressure to the uterus until the placenta separates (Lowdermilk et al., 2020).

Signs of placental separation are:

- A globular uterus
- A rise of the fundus in the abdomen
- A sudden gush or trickle of blood
- Further protrusion of the umbilical cord out of the vagina.

Placental Delivery

Once signs of placental separation become apparent, the woman may bear down to assist the process. If this fails and the HCP has determined that the fundus is firm, gentle traction may be applied to the cord while counterpressure is exerted on the lower uterine segment with the provider's opposite hand to guard against uterine inversion (a prolapse of the uterine fundus to or through the cervix). The direction of traction should follow the sacral and symphyseal curves, and care should be taken to avoid allowing the placenta to fall into the collection pan in an uncontrolled fashion. This may snap off adherent membranes, leaving them in the uterus to

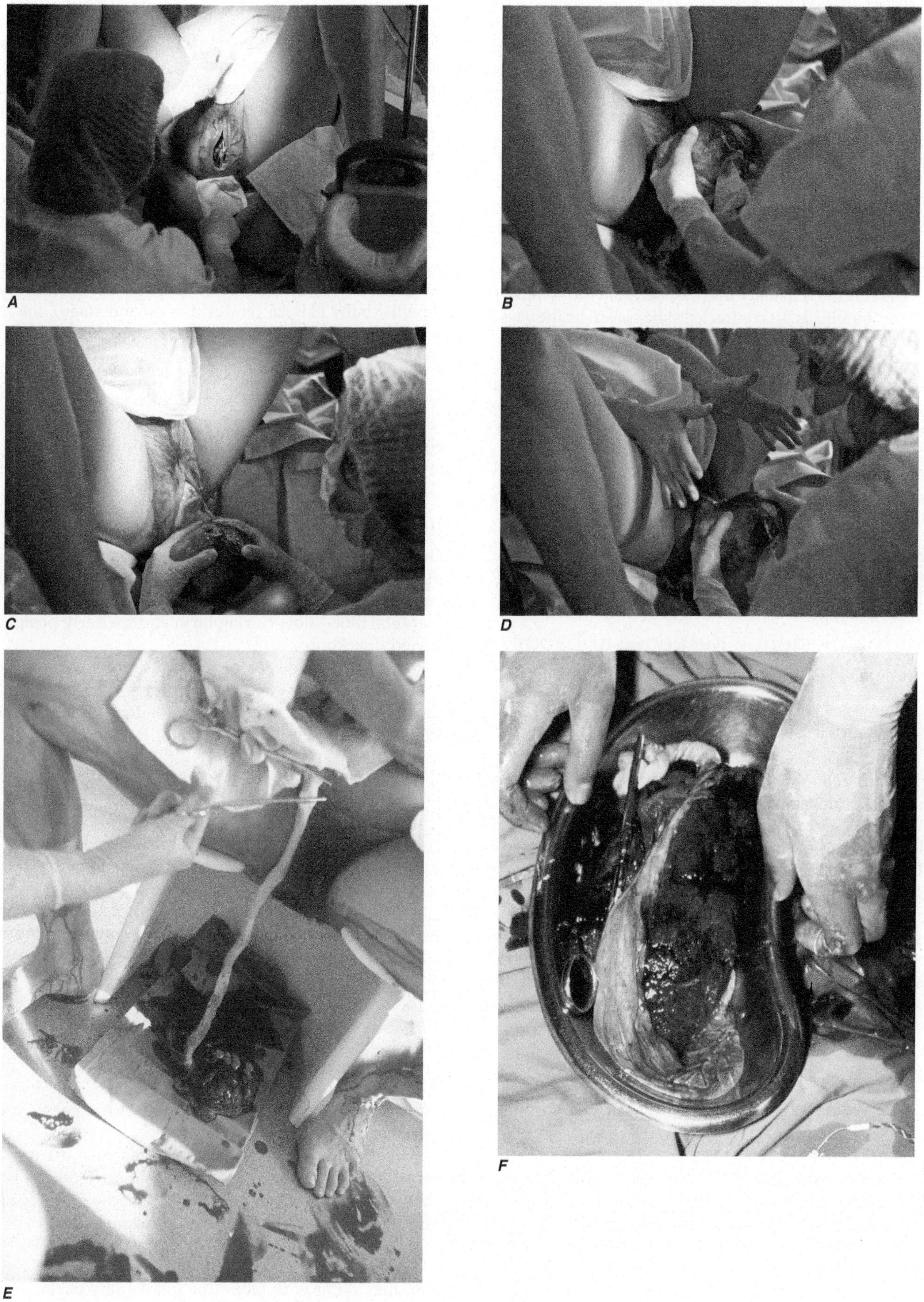

A

B

C

D

E

F

Figure 33.45 ›› A birth sequence.

Source: ***A***, ***B***, ***C***, ***D***, Lionel Souci/BSIP/Science Source. ***E***, EDDIE LAWRENCE/SCIENCE PHOTO LIBRARY/Science Source, ***F***, BIOPHOTO

Fourth Stage

The fourth stage of labor is the time, from 1 to 4 hours after birth, during which physiologic readjustment of the mother's body begins. With the birth, hemodynamic changes occur. Normal blood loss may be as much as 500 mL. With this blood loss and removal of the weight of the pregnant uterus from the surrounding vessels, blood is redistributed into venous beds. This results in a moderate drop in both systolic and diastolic blood pressure, increased pulse pressure, and moderate tachycardia (Cunningham et al., 2018).

The uterus remains contracted in the midline of the abdomen. The fundus is usually midway between the symphysis pubis and umbilicus. Its contracted state constricts the vessels at the site of placental implantation. Immediately after birth of the placenta, the cervix remains open.

Nausea and vomiting usually cease. The woman may be thirsty and hungry. She may experience a shaking chill, which is thought to be associated with the ending of the physical exertion of labor. The bladder may be hypotonic because of trauma during the second stage and/or administration of anesthetics that decrease sensations. Hypotonic bladder can lead to urinary retention.

Maternal and Fetal Response to Labor

Maternal Systemic Response to Labor

Nearly every maternal system is affected by the labor and birth process.

Cardiovascular System

The mother's cardiovascular system is stressed both by the uterine contractions and by the pain, anxiety, and apprehension she experiences. During pregnancy, circulating blood volume increases by 50%. The increase in cardiac output (CO) peaks between the second and third trimester, although during labor there is a significant increase in CO. With each contraction, 300 to 500 mL of blood volume is forced back into the maternal circulation, which results in an increase in CO of as much as 10–15% over the typical third-trimester levels (Blackburn, 2018). Further increases in CO occur as the laboring woman experiences pain with uterine contractions and her anxiety and apprehension increase.

Maternal position also affects CO. In the supine position, CO decreases, heart rate increases, and stroke volume decreases. When the mother turns to a lateral (side-lying) position, CO increases. Women with preexisting heart disease have higher rates of arrhythmias in labor (Blackburn, 2018).

Blood Pressure

As a result of increased CO, blood pressure (both systolic and diastolic) rises during uterine contractions. In the first stage of labor, systolic pressure may increase by 35 mmHg and diastolic pressure may increase by approximately 25 mmHg during a contraction. There may be further increases in the second stage during pushing (Blackburn, 2018). The nurse should ensure that blood pressure measurements are not obtained during uterine contractions because they can result in inaccurate readings.

Respiratory System

Oxygen demand and consumption increase at the onset of labor because of the presence of uterine contractions. As anxiety and pain from contractions increase, hyperventilation frequently occurs. With hyperventilation, the arterial partial pressure of carbon dioxide ($PaCO_2$) falls and respiratory alkalosis results (Sood & Sood, 2020).

By the end of the first stage of labor, most women develop a mild metabolic acidosis that is compensated for by respiratory alkalosis (see Module 1, Acid–Base Balance). As the woman pushes in the second stage of labor, her $PaCO_2$ levels may rise along with her blood lactate levels (because of muscular activity), leading to mild respiratory acidosis. By the time the baby is born (end of the second stage), the metabolic acidosis is uncompensated for by respiratory alkalosis (Blackburn, 2018).

The changes in acid–base status that occur in labor quickly reverse in the fourth stage because of changes in the woman's respiratory rate. Acid–base levels return to pregnancy levels by 24 hours after birth and to nonpregnant levels by a few weeks after birth (Blackburn, 2018; Powrie, Greene, & Camann, 2012).

Renal System

During labor, increases are seen in the maternal renin level, plasma renin activity, and angiotensinogen level. These elevations are thought to be important in the control of uteroplacental blood flow during birth and the early postpartum period (Blackburn, 2018).

Structurally, the base of the bladder is pushed forward and upward when engagement occurs. The pressure from the presenting part may impair blood and lymph drainage from the base of the bladder, leading to edema (Cunningham et al., 2018).

Gastrointestinal System

During labor, gastric motility and absorption of solid food are reduced. Gastric emptying time is prolonged, and gastric volume (amount of contents that remain in the stomach) remains increased, regardless of the time the last meal was taken (Blackburn, 2018). Some narcotics also delay gastric emptying time and add to the risk of aspiration if general anesthesia is used.

Immune System and Other Blood Values

The WBC count increases to 25,000 to 30,000 cells/mm^3 during labor and the early postpartum period. The change in WBCs is mostly because of increased neutrophils resulting from a physiologic response to stress. The increased WBC count makes it difficult to identify the presence of an infection.

Maternal blood glucose levels decrease during labor because glucose is used as an energy source during uterine contractions. The decreased blood glucose levels lead to a decrease in insulin requirements (Blackburn, 2018).

Pain

Pain may occur with labor due to a variety of causes. Each mother experiences and responds to pain differently based on numerous factors. Past experiences of pain may affect how the laboring mother copes with pain.

Causes of Pain During Labor

The pain associated with the first stage of labor is unique in that it accompanies a normal physiologic process. Even though perception of the pain of childbirth varies among women, a physiologic basis exists for discomfort during labor. Pain during the first stage of labor arises from dilation of the cervix, which is the primary source of pain; stretching of the lower uterine segment; pressure on adjacent structures; and hypoxia of the uterine muscle cells during contraction (Blackburn, 2018). The areas of pain include the lower abdominal wall and the areas over the lower lumbar region and the upper sacrum.

During the second stage of labor, pain is caused by hypoxia of the contracting uterine muscle cells, distention of the vagina and perineum, and pressure on adjacent structures. Pain during the third stage of labor results from uterine contractions and cervical dilation as the placenta is expelled. This stage of labor is short, and afterward anesthesia is needed primarily for episiotomy repair.

Factors Affecting Response to Pain

Many factors affect the individual's perception of and response to pain. For example, childbirth preparation classes may reduce the need for analgesia during labor. Preparing for labor and birth through reading, talking with others, or attending a childbirth preparation class frequently has positive effects for the laboring woman and her partner. The woman who knows what to expect and what techniques she may use to increase comfort tends to be less anxious during the labor. A tour of the birthing center and an opportunity to see and feel the environment also help reduce anxiety (especially with the first child) because during admission many new things are happening, and they seem to occur all at once.

In addition, individuals tend to respond to painful stimuli in the way that is acceptable in their culture. In some cultures, it is natural for members to communicate pain, no matter how mild, whereas in other cultures, members stoically accept pain, either out of fear or because it is expected. Nurses need to be aware of cultural norms and demonstrate culturally competent care to women and their families in the intrapartum setting to facilitate satisfying birth experiences.

Response to pain may also be influenced by fatigue and sleep deprivation. The fatigued patient has less energy and ability to use such strategies as distraction or imagination to deal with pain. As a result, she may lose her ability to cope with labor and choose analgesics or other medications to relieve the discomfort.

A woman's previous experience with pain and anxiety also affects her ability to manage current and future pain. Women who have had experience with pain seem to be more sensitive to painful stimuli compared to those who have not. Unfamiliar surroundings and events may increase anxiety, as may separation from family and loved ones. Anticipation of discomfort and questions about whether the mother can cope with the contractions may increase anxiety as well.

Both attention and distraction influence the perception of pain. When the sensation of pain is the focus of attention, the perceived intensity is greater. A sensory stimulus, such as a back rub, can provide distraction and help refocus the woman's attention on the stimulus rather than the pain. Randomized controlled trials have shown that the continuous presence of a support person improves the woman's coping ability and perception of her experience. Furthermore, consistent provision of social support and comfort measures shortens the duration of labor, decreases use of analgesia and anesthesia, and reduces the rate of operative delivery (King et al., 2019).

Pain Management and Nursing Considerations

Many women have anxiety about the pain of labor. It is common for women to create a plan during pregnancy regarding the use of medication to control labor pain. There are many options for pharmacologic pain relief. Some women opt to use intermittent systemic analgesics (opioids). These are given as needed via IV or intramuscular (IM) injections. These medications may offer some mild, temporary relief from pain associated with labor. Systemically administered opioids do cross the placenta and may have a negative effect on the fetus. Another common method of pain relief is epidural anesthesia, which provides regional analgesia or anesthesia. **Epidurals**, a form of regional anesthesia, are considered the most effective form of pain relief for the laboring woman. Medication administered via epidurals has fewer adverse fetal effects compared to IV analgesia or general anesthesia and allows the woman to remain awake to participate in the birth process. The most common complication of epidural anesthesia is maternal hypotension, which can be prevented through IV fluid administration and by positioning the mother on her side. Some women experience a decrease in sensation, which can slow labor progress and fetal descent and affect pushing efforts. Epidurals are contraindicated in the presence of hypovolemic shock, increased intracranial pressure, and maternal coagulopathy.

Any pain management decisions should be made at the request and permission of the patient and information on risks and benefits to the mother and fetus should be provided.

*>> Go to **Pearson MyLab Nursing and eText** for Chart 6, Epidurals.*

Fetal Response to Labor

Physiologic changes associated with normal labor typically have no adverse effects on the healthy fetus. However, some physiologic responses do occur. Nurses should anticipate changes in heart rate, acid–base balance, and fetal sensation, as well as hemodynamic changes.

Heart Rate

Fetal heart rate decelerations (periodic decreases in FHR from the normal baseline) can occur with intracranial pressures of 40 to 55 mmHg as the head pushes against the cervix. The currently accepted explanation of this **early deceleration** is hypoxic depression of the CNS, which is under vagal control. The absence of these head-compression decelerations in some fetuses during labor is explained by the existence of a threshold that is reached more gradually in the presence of intact membranes and lack of maternal resistance. These early decelerations are harmless in a normal fetus.

Acid–Base Balance

Blood flow is decreased to the fetus at the peak of each contraction, leading to a slow decrease in pH status. During the second stage of labor, as uterine contractions become longer and stronger and the woman often holds her breath to push, the fetal pH decreases more rapidly. Although women are encouraged to maintain slow, evenly paced breathing, holding of the breath often occurs. As the base deficit increases, fetal oxygen saturation drops by approximately 10% (Blackburn, 2018).

Fetal Sensation

Beginning at approximately 37 or 38 weeks of gestation (full term), the fetus is able to experience sensations of light, sound, and touch. The full-term fetus is able to hear music and the maternal voice. Even in utero, the fetus is sensitive to light and will move away from a bright light source. In addition, the full-term fetus is aware of pressure sensations during labor, such as the touch of the HCP during a vaginal exam or the pressure on the head as a contraction occurs. Although the fetus may not be able to process this input, it is important to note that as the woman labors, the fetus also experiences the labor.

Hemodynamic Changes

The adequate exchange of nutrients and gases in the fetal capillaries and intervillous spaces depends, in part, on the fetal blood pressure. Fetal blood pressure is a protective mechanism for the normal fetus in the anoxic periods caused by the contracting uterus during labor. The fetal and placental reserves are usually enough to ensure that the fetus comes through these anoxic periods unharmed (Blackburn, 2018).

Alterations During Intrapartum Care

Most women give birth without the need for any procedural interventions to ensure safety. However, sometimes an obstetric procedure is necessary. When the need for additional intervention is unanticipated, some women will feel angry or even guilty that they cannot have a "normal" delivery. Nurses provide support by ensuring that the laboring mother and her partner understand the need for intervention and what the care team is proposing, as well as anticipated benefits, possible risks, and potential alternatives (if any). The most common obstetric procedures are labor induction, episiotomy, cesarean birth, and vaginal birth after cesarean (VBAC).

Cervical Ripening

Induction of labor may be necessary or beneficial in certain clinical situations. When the cervix is unfavorable (usually defined as a Bishop score less than 6; see **Table 33.11** »), the use of cervical ripening agents increases the likelihood of a successful induction of labor. Misoprostol (Cytotec) and formulations of prostaglandin E_2 (PGE_2) gel for **cervical ripening** (softening and effacing of the cervix) are drugs that may be used for the pregnant woman at or near term when there is a medical or obstetric indication for induction of labor. Mechanical methods designed to ripen the cervix include the use of balloon catheters to encourage mechanical dilation.

Use of Misoprostol

Misoprostol (Cytotec) is a synthetic PGE_1 analogue that can be used to soften and ripen the cervix and to induce labor. It is available as a tablet that is inserted into the vagina or it can be taken orally or sublingually. There has been controversy regarding the safety of using Cytotec for cervical ripening and induction of labor. It is not FDA approved for these uses; however, the FDA added special labeling that discusses use in cervical ripening and induction of labor (Vrees, 2018).

Research has shown that the use of Cytotec for ripening the cervix and inducing labor is more effective than the use of oxytocin or prostaglandin agents and is less costly. Women who receive Cytotec to induce labor typically deliver within 24 hours of administration. The use of Cytotec is also associated with lower cesarean birthrates. When compared with women who have been induced using prostaglandin agents or oxytocin, the adverse outcomes do not differ among the three methods (Vrees, 2018). Most adverse maternal and fetal outcomes associated with misoprostol have been associated with the use of doses larger than the recommended 25 mcg. Intravaginal misoprostol has been found to be as efficacious as or superior to dinoprostone gel (Cunningham et al., 2018; Vrees, 2018). Guidelines for misoprostol induction include the following (Goldberg, 2018):

- The initial dosage should be 25 mcg.
- Recurrent administration should not exceed dosing intervals of more than 3 to 6 hours.
- Oxytocin should not be administered less than 4 hours after the last Cytotec dose.
- Cytotec should be administered only where the uterine activity and FHR can be monitored continuously for an initial observation period.

Contraindications for Cytotec include the following:

- Nonreassuring FHR tracing
- Frequent uterine contractions of moderate intensity.

TABLE 33.11 Bishop Scoring System

	Factor				
Score	**Dilation (cm)**	**Position of Cervix**	**Effacement (%)**	**Station (from − 3 to + 3)**	**Cervical Consistency**
0	Closed	Posterior	0–30	−3	Firm
1	1–2	Midposition	40–50	+2	Medium
2	3–4	Anterior	60–70	−1, 0	Soft
3	5–6	—	80	+1, +2	—

Source: Data from Bishop (1964).

Use of Prostaglandin Agents

The two most commonly used types of prostaglandin gel are Prepidil and Cervidil. Prepidil gel contains 0.5 mg dinoprostone (a form of PGE_2 for intracervical application) and is placed intracervically. Cervidil is packaged as an intravaginal mesh insert. It is placed in the posterior vagina and is left in place to provide a slow release of 10 mg dinoprostone over 12 hours.

The advantage of Cervidil is that it can be removed easily if an adverse reaction occurs. Both preparations have been demonstrated to cause cervical ripening, shorter labor, and lower requirements for oxytocin during labor induction (Vrees, 2018). Vaginal birth is achieved within 24 hours for most women. The incidence of cesarean birth is reduced when prostaglandin agents are used before labor induction.

Risks of prostaglandin administration include uterine hyperstimulation, nonreassuring fetal status, higher incidence of postpartum hemorrhage, and uterine rupture. Women with a previous uterine incision should not receive prostaglandin agents because the risk of uterine rupture is greatly increased (Mayo Clinic, 2020b). Prostaglandin should be used with caution in women with compromised cardiovascular, hepatic, or renal function and in women with asthma or glaucoma (Mayo Clinic, 2020a).

Use of Mechanical Methods

Balloon catheters are the safest and most common mechanical method of cervical ripening, although laminaria may still be used in some institutions. Mechanical agents for cervical ripening provide similar efficacy when compared to hormonal agents. Other advantages include lower cost, lower incidence of systemic side effects, and lower incidence of uterine tachysystole (Davidson, 2013; Vrees, 2018).

Balloon catheters have been used for cervical ripening for many years to promote mechanical dilation. A Foley catheter with a 25- to 80-mL balloon is passed through the undilated cervix and then inflated. The weighted balloon applies pressure on the internal os of the cervix and acts to ripen the cervix. This technique can be used alone or in conjunction with pharmacologic or additional mechanical methods. Advantages of the balloon catheter include higher vaginal birth rates and lower rates of tachysystole when combined with PGE_2 gel (Goldberg, 2018).

Nursing Care During Cervical Ripening

Physicians, CNMs, and labor and delivery nurses who have had special education and training may administer agents for cervical ripening. Maternal vital signs are assessed for a baseline, and an electronic fetal monitor is applied for at least 20 minutes to obtain an external tracing of uterine activity, FHR pattern, and a reactive NST. If a nonreactive test is obtained, consultation with the HCP is required. After the gel, intravaginal insert, or tablet has been inserted, the woman is instructed to remain lying down with a rolled blanket or hip wedge under her right hip to tip the uterus slightly to the left for the first 30 to 60 minutes to maintain the cervical ripening agent in place. Gel may leak from the endocervix. The nurse monitors the woman for uterine tachysystole and FHR abnormalities (changes in baseline rate, variability [fluctuations in the FHR], and presence of decelerations) for 30 minutes to 2 hours if a prostaglandin gel agent is used (ACOG, 2013d; Vrees, 2018).

If tachysystole occurs, the woman is positioned on her left side and oxygen is administered to promote fetal perfusion. If uterine tachysystole continues, the administration of a tocolytic agent (such as a subcutaneous injection of 0.25 mg of terbutaline) should be considered. In the presence of severe nausea, vomiting, or tachysystole, the gel may be removed (Vrees, 2018). Treatment with antiemetics, antipyretics, and antidiarrheal agents is usually not indicated. Women who receive Cervidil or Cytotec are admitted for observation so contractions and fetal status can be monitored (ACOG, 2013d; Vrees, 2018).

Women undergoing induction via balloon catheters do not need continuous fetal monitoring. The nurse can perform intermittent monitoring along with the maternal vital signs. The nurse should also assess the location of the catheter to ensure that it has not become displaced. This can be achieved by marking the catheter tubing at the introitus and noting whether movement has occurred. Vaginal examinations should not be performed.

Labor Induction

The ACOG (2017d) defines **labor induction** as the use of medication or other methods to induce (start) labor by stimulating contractions of the uterus to promote vaginal birth. Medical reasons for inducing labor include (MOD, 2019):

- Presence of acute or chronic maternal illness, such as diabetes, preeclampsia/eclampsia, cardiovascular disease, lung disease, or renal disease
- PROM, placental abruption, or infection
- Postterm gestation greater than 42 weeks
- Fetal growth restriction, oligohydramnios (insufficient amniotic fluid)
- Nonreassuring fetal status or fetal demise.

Other indications may include (but are not be limited to) fetal anomalies that require specialized care, previous stillbirth, distance from hospital, psychological health of the mother, and advanced cervical dilation (Cunningham et al., 2018).

Contraindications for spontaneous labor and vaginal birth are also contraindications for inducing labor, which include patient refusal, umbilical cord prolapse, transverse fetal lie, placental previa or vasa previa, previous vertical incision in upper portion of the uterus, and active genital herpes infection (Vrees, 2018).

Assessment prior to induction includes evaluation of fetal maturity and cervical readiness. Evaluation of gestational age may be based on ultrasound prior to 20 weeks' gestation that supports age at delivery above 39 weeks and determination of fetal heart tones for 30 weeks (via Doppler) or 36 weeks since confirmation of pregnancy (Vrees, 2018).

Forceps-Assisted Birth

Forceps are designed to assist the birth of a fetus by providing traction or by providing the means to rotate the fetal head to an occipitoanterior position. In medical literature and practice, **forceps-assisted birth** is also known as *instrumental delivery*, *operative delivery*, or *operative vaginal delivery*. There are many different types of forceps, each with special functions. The type of forceps used is determined by the physician assisting with the birth and the clinical situation.

Indications for Use of Forceps

Indications for the use of forceps include the presence of any condition that threatens the mother or fetus and that can be relieved by birth. Conditions that put the woman at risk include heart disease, acute pulmonary edema or pulmonary compromise, certain neurologic conditions, intrapartum infection, prolonged second stage, or exhaustion. Fetal conditions include premature placental separation, prolapsed umbilical cord, and nonreassuring fetal status. Forceps may be used when the fetal station is very low to shorten the second stage of labor and spare the woman's pushing effort (when exhaustion or heart disease is present) or when regional anesthesia or paralysis has affected the woman's motor innervation and she cannot push effectively (Cunningham et al., 2018).

Risk factors for a forceps- or vacuum-assisted birth (discussion to follow) are as follows (Cunningham et al., 2018):

- Nulliparity
- Maternal age (35 and over)
- Maternal height of less than 150 cm (4 ft 11 in.)
- Pregnancy weight gain of more than 15 kg (33 lb)
- Postdate gestation (41 weeks or more)
- Epidural anesthesia
- Fetal presentation other than occipitoanterior
- Presence of dystocia (labor dysfunction)
- Presence of a midline episiotomy
- Abnormal FHR tracing.

Neonatal and Maternal Risks

Some newborns may develop a small area of ecchymosis or edema, or both, along the sides of the face as a result of forceps application. Cephalohematoma (and subsequent hyperbilirubinemia) may occur as well as transient facial paralysis. Other reported complications include low Apgar scores, retinal hemorrhage, corneal abrasions, ocular trauma, other trauma (Erb palsy, fractured clavicle), elevated neonatal bilirubin levels, and prolonged hospital stay (Cunningham et al., 2018).

Maternal risks may include trauma such as lacerations of the birth canal, periurethral lacerations, and extensions of a median episiotomy into the anus, resulting in increased bleeding, bruising, hematomas, and pelvic floor injuries. Women who give birth with the assistance of forceps are more likely to have a third- or fourth-degree laceration and report more perineal pain and sexual problems in the postpartum period (Cunningham et al., 2018). In addition, an increase in postpartum infections, cervical lacerations, and prolonged hospital stays has been reported (Cunningham et al., 2018). Women who give birth with the assistance of forceps may also experience urinary and rectal incontinence, anal sphincter injury, and postpartum infection (Cunningham et al., 2018).

Vacuum Extraction

Vacuum extraction is an obstetric procedure used by physicians and CNMs to assist the birth of a fetus by applying suction to the fetal head. In 2014, vacuum extraction was used in 3.2% of births in the United States. It is the most commonly used operative method to assist birth, used five times more often than forceps extraction (Cunningham et al., 2018).

The vacuum extractor is composed of a soft suction cup attached to a suction bottle (pump) by tubing. The suction cup, which comes in various sizes, is placed against the occiput of the fetal head, avoiding the fontanels. Care must be taken to ensure that no cervical or vaginal tissue is trapped under the cup. The pump is used to create negative pressure (suction) of approximately 50 to 60 mmHg in a stepwise sequence or rapid application. An artificial caput ("chignon") is formed as the fetal scalp is pulled into the cup.

The longer the duration of suction, the more likely the newborn is to have a scalp injury. While there are no set guidelines, limiting the use of a vacuum to no more than 2 to 33 pop-offs or a maximum of 20 minutes is recommended (Garrison, 2017). Although there are no specifications on the number of attempts, failure to descend with multiple attempts is an indicator that a cesarean birth may be necessary. The most common indication for the use of the vacuum extractor is a prolonged second stage of labor or nonreassuring FHR pattern. Vacuum extraction is also used to relieve the woman of pushing effort, when analgesia or fatigue interferes with her ability to push effectively, or in cases of nonreassuring fetal status when prompt birth is indicated. The vacuum extractor is preferred to forceps in cases of suspected cephalopelvic disproportion (CPD) when successful passage of the fetal head requires all potential space inside the vaginal canal. True CPD is an absolute contraindication to vacuum extraction. Other contraindications include nonvertex presentations, maternal or suspected fetal coagulation problems, known or suspected hydrocephalus, and fetal scalp trauma (Cunningham et al., 2018; Garrison, 2017). Relative contraindications include suspected fetal macrosomia, high fetal station, face or breech presentation, gestation less than 34 weeks, incompletely dilated cervix, and previous fetal scalp blood sampling (Cunningham et al., 2018; Garrison, 2017).

Neonatal complications include scalp lacerations, bruising, subgaleal hematomas, cephalohematomas, intracranial hemorrhages, subconjunctival hemorrhages, neonatal jaundice, fractured clavicle, Erb palsy, damage to the sixth and seventh cranial nerves, retinal hemorrhage, and fetal death. In addition, shoulder dystocia occurs more often (Cunningham et al., 2018; Garrison, 2017). There appear to be more neonatal complications and injuries with use of a metal suction cup device than with soft cup devices. In the presence of a preterm gestation, risk of periventricular–intraventricular hemorrhage has been a concern, and some studies provide conflicting recommendations. Complications to the mother include pain, infection, edema, and trauma to the perineum, including third- and fourth-degree lacerations (Garrison, 2017). Women who give birth with the aid of a vacuum extractor report more sexual difficulties in the postpartum period. Maternal genital tract and anal sphincter injuries occur less frequently with the vacuum extractor than with forceps.

Episiotomy

An **episiotomy** is a surgical incision of the perineal body to enlarge the outlet. The episiotomy has long been thought to minimize the risk of lacerations of the perineum and overstretching of perineal tissues. However, episiotomy may actually increase the risk of fourth-degree perineal lacerations (Blackburn, 2018). Research suggests that (1) rather than protecting the perineum from lacerations, the presence of an episiotomy makes it more likely that the woman will have anal sphincter tears and (2) perineal lacerations heal more quickly than deep perineal tears (Blackburn, 2018). The incidence of major perineal trauma is more likely to happen if a midline episiotomy is done (Mayo Clinic, 2018a). Additional complications associated with episiotomy are blood loss, infection, pain, and perineal discomfort that may continue for days or weeks past birth, including painful intercourse (Lyndon, Lee, Gilbert, Gould, & Lee, 2012; Mayo Clinic, 2018a). Episiotomy is indicated in expediting delivery in the setting of nonreassuring fetal status or enlarging the space in which to apply forceps or disimpact the fetal anterior shoulder. The use of episiotomies has declined greatly over the past several decades.

Overall factors that place a woman at increased risk for episiotomy are primigravid status, large or macrosomic fetus, occipitoposterior position, use of forceps or vacuum extractor, and shoulder dystocia. Other factors that may be mitigated by nurses, physicians, and CNMs include the following:

- Use of lithotomy and other recumbent positions (causes excessive and uneven stretching of the perineum)
- Encouraging or requiring sustained breath holding during second-stage pushing (causes excessive and rapid perineal stretching, can adversely affect blood flow in mother and fetus, and requires woman to be responsive to caregiver directions rather than to her own urges to push spontaneously)
- Arbitrary time limit placed by the physician or CNM on the length of the second stage.

Preventive Measures

General tips to help reduce the incidence of lacerations and episiotomies include the following:

- Perineal massage during pregnancy for nulliparous women
- Natural pushing during labor and avoiding the lithotomy position or pulling back on legs, which tightens the perineum
- Side-lying position for pushing, which helps slow birth and diminish tears
- Warm or hot compresses on the perineum and firm counterpressure
- Encouraging a gradual expulsion of the baby at the time of birth by encouraging the mother to "push, take a breath, push, take a breath," thereby easing the baby out slowly
- Avoiding immediate pushing after epidural placement.

Episiotomy Procedure

The two types of episiotomy are midline and mediolateral, with midline being the most common in current use. Just before birth, when approximately 3 to 4 cm (1.2 to 1.6 in.) of the fetal head is visible during a contraction, the episiotomy is performed by using sharp scissors with rounded points (Cunningham et al., 2018). The midline incision begins at the bottom center of the perineal body and extends straight down the midline to the fibers of the rectal sphincter. The mediolateral incision begins in the midline of the posterior fourchette and extends at a 45-degree angle downward to the right or left.

The episiotomy is usually performed with regional or local anesthesia but may be done without anesthesia in emergency situations. It is generally proposed that as crowning occurs, the distention of the tissues causes numbing. Repair of the episiotomy and any lacerations is completed either during the period between birth of the baby and expulsion of the placenta or after expulsion of the placenta. Adequate anesthesia must be given for the repair.

Cesarean Birth

Cesarean birth (the birth of the baby through an abdominal and uterine incision) is one of the oldest known surgical procedures. Until the 20th century, cesarean procedures were used primarily to save the fetus of a dying woman. As the maternal and perinatal morbidity and mortality rates associated with cesarean birth steadily decreased throughout the 20th century, the proportion of cesarean births increased. The late 1980s saw a temporary decline in cesarean births in an effort to cut healthcare costs. By 2015, the rate of cesarean births performed in the United States reached an all-time high of 32% (ACOG, 2019a).

Cesarean birthrates differ dramatically in other parts of the world. Worldwide, women living in urban areas are four times more likely to have a cesarean compared to women living in rural areas. Countries with low cesarean birthrates (less than 17%) include the Netherlands, Finland, and Norway. The highest rates were found in Italy, Portugal, and the United States, with rates greater than 30%. Overall, the incidence of cesarean birth has continued to increase worldwide (Boerma et al., 2018; WHO, 2015).

The increasing rate of cesarean births in the United States is linked to a rise in repeat cesarean births fueled by concerns about the risk of uterine rupture with a vaginal birth after a previous cesarean birth. There is also an increase in requests from women for cesarean births so that they can avoid the pain of labor and vaginal birth. Statements in some medical literature that vaginal births could result in pelvic floor damage during the birth process have led some women to consider cesarean births (King et al., 2019). While there is little reliable data on the number of cesarean deliveries performed based on maternal requests, estimates are around 2.5% (ACOG, 2019a). Cesarean birth on request is associated with a reduction in maternal hemorrhage risk. However, it is associated with increased complications in subsequent pregnancies, including placenta implantation problems and uterine rupture (Cunningham et al., 2018). Cesarean birth without medical indications should not be recommended for women desiring several children, for women less than 39 weeks of gestation, or when pregnancy dating is unknown or may be inaccurate. ACOG recommendations state that cesarean births at the request of the mother should never be guided by a lack of effective pain management options within the facility (Cunningham et al., 2018).

Many other factors have contributed to the rise in the cesarean birthrate and need to be considered in any discussion about decreasing the rate. These factors include an increased use of epidural anesthesia, maternal age over 35, failed labor inductions, decline in vaginal breech deliveries, decreases in operative vaginal deliveries, increased repeat cesarean rates, reduced VBAC birthrates, increased physician scheduling of cesarean births for personal convenience, political pressure from malpractice insurance carriers who attempt to dictate practice standards, and fear of litigation (ACOG, 2019a).

Indications

Commonly accepted indications for cesarean birth include complete placenta previa, breech presentation, transverse lie, placental abruption accompanied by nonreassuring fetal status, active genital herpes, umbilical cord prolapse, arrest of descent and/or arrest of dilation, nonreassuring fetal status, previous classic incision on the uterus (either previous cesarean birth or myomectomy), more than one previous cesarean birth, benign and malignant tumors that obstruct the birth canal, and cervical cerclage.

Some maternal medical conditions are contraindications to a vaginal birth and warrant a cesarean birth (Cunningham et al., 2018). These medical conditions include some cardiac disorders, disorders that increase intracranial pressure, obstruction of the vaginal canal, and severe mental illness that affects the ability to deliver vaginally. Other indications that are now commonly associated with cesarean birth, although in some circumstances may allow the child to be delivered vaginally, include breech presentation, previous cesarean birth, major congenital anomalies, maternal HIV infection, and severe Rh isoimmunization.

Maternal Mortality and Morbidity

Cesarean births have a higher maternal mortality rate than vaginal births. In the United States, women undergoing a cesarean birth have a twofold risk of most complications associated with delivery compared with women who give birth vaginally (Cunningham et al., 2018). Perinatal morbidity is also considerably higher in women who have had a cesarean. Common postoperative complications include infection, reactions to anesthesia agents, blood clots, and bleeding. Women who have had a cesarean birth are twice as likely to be rehospitalized within 60 days of birth when compared with women who have had a vaginal birth. Other sources of maternal morbidity that are directly associated with cesarean birth include ureteral injury, bladder laceration, and wound infection (Cunningham et al., 2018).

The World Health Organization claims that cesarean births are necessary only in 10–15% of cases and has encouraged countries to maintain levels at or below this. The United States has consistently been well above this goal. The most common complications occurring with cesarean deliveries that lead to the overall increase in maternal morbidity and mortality are hemorrhage, surgical site infection, and venous thromboembolism. All hospitals should create protocols to assess for and prevent these complications (Burke & Allen, 2020).

Evidence-Based Practice

Interprofessional Communication and Maternal Morbidity and Mortality

Effective Communication Among Healthcare Providers Remains Important Evidence-Based Safety Practice to Improve Maternal Morbidity and Mortality Rates

Background

In the United States, the rates of maternal morbidity and mortality related to childbirth are on the rise. Data from the Centers for Disease Control and Prevention (2018) show that pregnancy-related deaths increased from 7.2 (per 100,000 live births) in 1987 to 18.0 in 2014. Data from review boards, which looked at maternal deaths from 2013–2017, showed that 60% of these deaths were preventable. Even greater disparities have been noted for Black women, who are 3.3 times more likely to die due to pregnancy-related complications (ACOG, 2019c). Major maternal morbidity also increased 200% between 1993 and 2014. Some of the common complications seen are hemorrhage, cardiac disorders, infection, and embolisms (CDC, 2020c).

Problem

As the incidence of maternal morbidity and mortality increases, research has focused on ways to improve maternal outcomes in the United States. Because many of the complications are preventable with appropriate care, hospitals have created protocols to address some of the most common issues. ACOG (2014b, reaffirmed 2016) has recognized that the use of interprofessional simulation can improve outcomes in the face of obstetric emergencies. Simulation is considered such an important tool in practice that the American Board of Obstetrics and Gynecology has incorporated it into the certification examination (Deering, 2018).

Implications

Ongoing research continues to show the implications of simulation on practices and maternal outcomes. Some important findings in studies thus far:

- The California Maternal Quality Care Collaborative (CMQCC) created a comprehensive training bundle with protocols, education, and simulation around postpartum hemorrhage and introduced it into 99 hospitals. When compared to hospitals that did not implement the training, the hospitals who utilized the simulation education demonstrated a 20.8% reduction in maternal mortality for patients who experienced a postpartum hemorrhage (Deering, 2018).
- Several studies have shown that practicing maneuvers to deliver babies with shoulder dystocia improve the head-to-body delivery time from 3 minutes to 2 minutes as well as decrease brachial plexus injuries from 10.1 to 4.0% (Deering, 2018).
- Communication and teamwork among HCPs are also improved through simulation. Communication failures have been noted as a cause in up to 70% of maternal deaths in obstetrics. In a three-hospital trial, incorporation of a standardized communication platform (TeamSTEPPS) and simulation proved to decrease maternal mortality rates by 37% (Deering, 2018).

Critical Thinking Application

1. How is simulation being used in the educational setting to help nursing students understand skills and concepts?
2. How can nurses ensure that their voices are heard in simulation scenarios? What are some effective communication measures that nurses can utilize to be an integral part of the team?

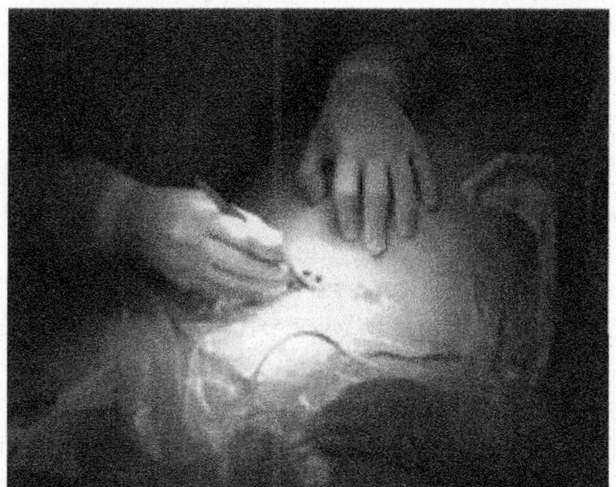

Figure 33.46 ›› Transverse skin incision for a cesarean birth.
Source: Wilson Garcia

Skin Incisions

The skin incision for a cesarean birth is either transverse (Pfannenstiel) or vertical, and it is not indicative of the type of incision made into the uterus (**Figure 33.46** ››). Time factors, patient preference, previous vertical skin incision, or physician preference determines the type of skin incision.

The transverse incision is made across the lowest and narrowest part of the abdomen. Because the incision is made just below the pubic hairline, it is almost invisible after healing. The limitation of this type of skin incision is that it does not allow extension of the incision, if needed. Because it usually requires more time to make and repair, this incision is used when time is not of the essence (e.g., with arrest of descent and/or arrest of dilation and stable fetal and maternal status).

The vertical incision is made between the navel and the symphysis pubis. This type of incision is quicker and, therefore, is preferred in cases of nonreassuring fetal status when rapid birth is indicated, with preterm or macrosomic babies, or when the woman is significantly obese (Cunningham et al., 2018).

Uterine Incisions

The two major locations of uterine incisions are in the lower uterine segment and in the upper segment of the uterine corpus. The type of uterine incision depends on the need for the cesarean. The choice of incision affects the woman's opportunity for a subsequent vaginal birth and her risks of a ruptured uterine scar with a subsequent pregnancy.

The lower uterine segment incision most commonly used is a transverse incision. The lower uterine segment transverse incision is preferred for the following reasons (Cunningham et al., 2018):

- The lower segment is the thinnest portion of the uterus and involves less blood loss.
- It requires only moderate dissection of the bladder from the underlying myometrium.
- It is easier to repair, although repair takes longer.
- The site is less likely to rupture during subsequent pregnancies.
- There is a decreased chance for adherence of bowel or omentum to the incision line.

Disadvantages of this type of segment incision include the following:

- It takes longer to make a transverse incision.
- It is limited in size because of the presence of major vessels on either side of the uterus.
- It has a greater tendency to extend laterally into the uterine vessels.
- The incision may stretch and become a thin window, but it usually does not create problems clinically until subsequent labor ensues.

The lower uterine segment vertical incision is preferred for multiple gestation, abnormal presentation, placenta previa, nonreassuring fetal status, and preterm and macrosomic fetuses. Disadvantages of this type of incision include the following:

- The incision may extend downward into the cervix.
- More extensive dissection of the bladder is needed to keep the incision in the lower uterine segment; hemostasis and closure are more difficult.
- The vertical incision carries a higher risk of rupture with subsequent labor. Consequently, once a vertical incision is performed, future births need to be via cesarean.

One other incision, the classic incision, was the method of choice for many years but is used infrequently today. This vertical incision was made into the upper uterine segment. It resulted in greater blood loss and was more difficult to repair. Most important, it carried an increased risk of uterine rupture with subsequent pregnancy, labor, and birth because the upper uterine segment is the most contractile portion of the uterus.

Analgesia and Anesthesia

All options for analgesia and anesthesia come with advantages, disadvantages, and possible adverse and side effects. Provider and patient preference and patient presentation inform the selection of analgesia and anesthesia, always with the overall goals of safety, comfort, and patient satisfaction.

Preparation for Cesarean Birth

Because cesarean births are common, preparation for this possibility should be an integral part of all prenatal education. The nurse should encourage pregnant women and their partners to discuss the possibility of a cesarean birth, and their specific needs and desires under those circumstances, with their HCP. Their preferences may include the following:

- Participating in the choice of anesthetic
- Partner or significant other being present during the procedures and/or birth
- Partner or significant other being present in the recovery or postpartum room
- Video recording and/or taking pictures of the birth
- Delayed instillation of eyedrops to promote eye contact between parent and newborn in the first hours after birth
- Physical contact or holding the newborn while in the operating and/or recovery room (by the partner if the mother cannot hold the baby)
- Breastfeeding in the recovery area within the first hour after birth.

Information that couples need about cesarean birth includes the following:

- What preparatory procedures to expect
- Description or viewing of the birthing room
- Types of anesthesia for birth and analgesia available postpartum
- Sensations that may be experienced
- Roles of significant others
- Interaction with newborn
- Immediate recovery phase
- Postpartum phase.

Preparing the woman and her family for cesarean birth involves more than the procedures of establishing an IV line, instilling a urinary indwelling catheter, and performing an abdominal prep. Good communication skills are essential in preparing the woman and her support person. The use of therapeutic touch and direct eye contact (if culturally acceptable and possible) assists the woman in maintaining a sense of control and lessens her anxiety.

If the cesarean birth is scheduled and not an emergency procedure, the nurse has ample time for preoperative teaching and to provide an opportunity for the woman and her support person to express their concerns, ask questions, and develop a relationship with the nurse.

In preparation for surgery, the woman is given nothing by mouth. To reduce the likelihood of serious pulmonary damage if gastric contents are aspirated, antacids may be administered within 30 minutes of surgery. If epidural anesthesia is used, the nurse may assist with the procedure, monitor the woman's blood pressure and response, and continue electronic fetal monitoring. An abdominal and perineal prep is done, and an indwelling catheter is inserted to prevent bladder distention. An IV line is started with a large-bore needle to permit rapid administration of blood if that becomes necessary. Preoperative medication may be ordered. The pediatrician should be notified and preparations made to receive the new baby. The nurse ensures that the neonatal radiant warmer is working and that resuscitation equipment is available.

The nurse assists in positioning the woman on the operating table. FHR is assessed before surgery and during preparation because fetal hypoxia can result from the mother lying in the supine position. The operating room table is adjusted so that it slants slightly to one side or a hip wedge (folded blanket or towels) is placed under the right hip to tip the uterus slightly and reduce compression of blood vessels. The uterus should be displaced 15 degrees from the midline. This helps relieve the pressure of the heavy uterus on the vena cava and lessens the incidence of vena cava compression and maternal supine hypotension. The suction device should be in working order, and the urine collection bag should be positioned under the operating table to obtain proper drainage. Auscultation or electronic fetal monitoring of the FHR is continued until immediately before the procedure. If the fetus was monitored internally, a last-minute check is done to ensure that the fetal scalp electrode has been removed.

The nurse continues to provide reassurance and to describe the various procedures being performed (along with their rationales) to ease anxiety and give the woman a sense of control.

Women undergoing elective cesarean birth can be given information about the postoperative experience before their birth experience. Important components of patient education that can be emphasized before birth include dealing with postoperative discomfort, splinting the incision to decrease pain, frequent deep breathing and coughing, and the importance of early ambulation. Patients who receive this information before the birth are more apt to remember it when the information is reviewed in the early postpartum period.

Preparation for Repeat Cesarean Birth

When the parents are anticipating a repeat cesarean birth, they have a general understanding of what will occur, which can help them make informed choices about their birth experience. Those who have had previous negative experiences need an opportunity to describe what they felt. Encourage the parents to identify what they would like to be different and to list options that would make the experience more positive. Those who have already had positive experiences need reassurance that their needs and desires will be met in a similar manner. Provide all families the opportunity to discuss any fears or anxieties. For women who previously labored and then had an unexpected cesarean birth, the experience may be perceived as negative. Emphasize the positive aspects of a repeat cesarean birth. These include participation in selecting the birth date, lack of fatigue related to labor, ability to prepare and make arrangements for other children, and the ability for other family members or friends to be present at the hospital during or immediately after birth if desired by the couple.

Preparation for Emergency Cesarean Birth

When the need for a cesarean birth emerges suddenly, the period preceding surgery must be used to its greatest advantage. It is imperative that the nurse use the most effective communication skills in supporting the parents. The nurse describes what they may anticipate during the next few hours and gives the woman information about (and the rationale for) any procedure before it begins. It is essential for the nurse to explain what is going to happen, why it is being done, and what sensations the woman may experience. This allows the woman to be informed and to consent to the procedure, which gives her a sense of control and reduces her feelings of helplessness.

Supporting the Partner

Every effort should be made to include the partner in the birth experience. When attending a cesarean birth, the partner wears protective coverings similar to those worn by others in the operating suite. A stool can be placed beside the woman's head so that the partner can sit nearby to provide physical touch, visual contact, and verbal reassurance.

To promote the participation of the partner who chooses not to be in the operating suite, the nurse can do the following:

- Allow the partner to be nearby, where they can hear the newborn's first cry.
- Encourage the partner to carry or accompany the newborn to the nursery for the initial assessment.
- Involve the partner in postpartum care in the recovery room.

In some emergency circumstances, a support person may not be permitted in the operating room. Some facilities have policies that prohibit a support person from being in the operating room if the woman requires general anesthesia or if an emergency birth is being performed. In these situations, the support person should receive a thorough explanation of what is happening and why, be advised when the staff will return to provide information, know the expected length of time for the procedure, and be reassured that the mother is receiving the care she and the baby need. Because this exclusion is stressful for family members, the staff needs to provide information as soon as possible after providing emergency care to the mother.

Immediate Postnatal Recovery Period

After birth, the nurse assesses the Apgar score (Apgar scoring is described fully in Exemplar 33.D, Newborn Care, in this module) and completes the same initial assessment and identification procedures used for vaginal births.

Identification bands must be placed on the newborn and the mother (as well as on the support person, if present) before removing the baby from the operating room. The nurse should make every effort to assist the parents in bonding with their baby. If the mother is awake, one of her arms can be freed to enable her to touch and stroke the baby. The newborn may be placed on the mother's chest or held in an *en face* (face-to-face) position. If physical contact is not possible, the nurse should provide a running narrative so that the mother knows what is happening with her baby. The nurse assists the anesthesiologist or nurse anesthetist with raising the mother's head so that she can see her baby immediately after birth. The parents can be encouraged to talk to the baby, and the partner can hold the baby until the family is taken to the recovery room.

The nurse caring for the postpartum woman assesses the mother's vital signs every 5 minutes until they are stable, then every 15 minutes for an hour, and then every 30 minutes until the woman is discharged to the postpartum unit. The nurse remains with the woman until she is stable.

The nurse evaluates the dressing and perineal pad every 15 minutes for at least an hour. Gently palpate the fundus to determine whether it is remaining firm; palpation may be performed by placing a hand to support the incision. IV oxytocin is usually administered to promote the contractility of the uterine musculature. If the mother has been under general anesthesia, she should be positioned on her side to facilitate drainage of secretions, turned, and assisted with coughing and deep breathing every 2 hours for at least 24 hours. If she has received a spinal or epidural anesthetic, the level of anesthesia is checked every 15 minutes for the first 2 hours and then hourly until full sensation has returned. It is important for the nurse to monitor intake and output and to observe the urine for a bloody tinge, which could mean surgical trauma to the bladder. The HCP prescribes medication to relieve the mother's pain and nausea, and that medication is administered as needed.

Bonding can be promoted by encouraging mother and baby skin-to-skin contact for the first hour uninterrupted and performing all assessments and procedures on the newborn at the mother's bedside if both are stable.

Vaginal Birth After Cesarean

In the late 1980s there was an increasing trend to have a *trial of labor after cesarean (TOLAC)* and **vaginal birth after cesarean (VBAC)** in cases of nonrecurring indications for a cesarean (e.g., twins, umbilical cord prolapse, placenta previa, nonreassuring fetal status). This trend was influenced by consumer demand and studies that support VBAC as a viable and safe alternative. VBAC rates peaked in the late 1990s and then the practice came under renewed scrutiny, causing rates to decline into the 2000s. This prompted the National Institutes of Health to review the matter and issue a statement on the safety of TOLAC. Consensus among providers is that all women who meet eligibility criteria should be offered TOLAC (King et al., 2019). The VBAC success rate ranges from 60–80% (ACOG, 2015c; Mayo Clinic, 2018b). The ACOG guidelines have been revised several times over the past decade in an attempt to help improve the rates of TOLAC (Caughey, 2018). Current recommendations state that the following aspects should be met when identifying candidates for a trial of labor:

- No contraindications for vaginal birth
- A woman with one or two previous cesarean births and a low transverse uterine incision
- A clinically adequate pelvis based on clinical pelvimetry or prior vaginal birth
- A woman with one previous cesarean birth with an undocumented uterine scar unless there is a high suspicion there was a classic incision performed previously
- Absence of other uterine scars or history of previous uterine rupture
- A facility that is able to perform emergency cesarean delivery if there is an immediate threat to the life of the mother or fetus.

The incidence of complications with VBACs are low, with uterine rupture occurring in 0.5–1% of all TOLACs (Caughey, 2018). Risks associated with VBAC are listed in **Box 33.4** ».

The nursing care of a woman undergoing VBAC varies according to institutional protocols. Generally, if the woman is at low risk (has had one previous cesarean with a lower uterine segment incision), her blood count, type, and screen are obtained on admission; a heparin lock is inserted for IV access, if needed; continuous electronic fetal monitoring is used; and

Box 33.4

Risks Associated with Vaginal Birth After Cesarean

- Uterine rupture
- Scar dehiscence
- Hysterectomy
- Uterine infection
- Neonatal death
- Intrauterine fetal demise
- Stillbirth
- Transfusion
- Hypoxic ischemic encephalopathy

clear fluids may be consumed. If the woman is at higher risk, NPO status should be maintained and, in addition to the care listed, an intrauterine catheter may be inserted to monitor intrauterine pressures during labor.

Supportive and comfort measures are very important. The woman may be excited about this opportunity to experience labor and vaginal birth but apprehensive if she does not know what to expect from labor. The nurse provides information and encouragement for the laboring woman and her partner.

Intrapartum Risk Factors

A number of other alterations may occur during the intrapartum period. These include precipitous birth, abruptio placentae, placenta previa, premature rupture of membranes, preterm and postterm labor, hypertonic labor, hypotonic labor patterns, fetal malpresentation, fetal macrosomia, nonreassuring fetal status, prolapsed umbilical cord, anaphylactoid syndrome of pregnancy (amniotic fluid embolism), cephalopelvic disproportion, retained placenta, lacerations, placenta accreta, shoulder dystocia, and perinatal loss. These alterations are described in the Alterations and Therapies feature. Perinatal loss is discussed in Module 27, Grief and Loss.

Each of these alterations creates an environment of risk for the woman and/or the fetus. Each requires the immediate attention of the healthcare team. However, the predominant risk factors for maternal morbidity and mortality continue to be cardiovascular disease, prenatal substance exposure, obstetric or postpartum hemorrhage, preeclampsia, venous thromboembolism, and birth equity. **Birth equity** refers to conditions for optimal birth outcomes and the additional risk for morbidity and mortality that Black women face during the peripartum and postpartum periods (CMQCC, 2019). Postpartum hemorrhage is discussed more specifically in Exemplar 33.C, Postpartum Care, in this module. Coverage of the other topics can be found in:

- Cardiovascular disease, preeclampsia, and venous thromboembolism are discussed in Module 16, Perfusion.
- Prenatal substance exposure is covered in Module 22, Addiction.
- Birth equity is discussed in Module 24, Culture and Diversity.

>> *Go to* ***Pearson MyLab Nursing and eText*** *for Chart 7, Intrapartum High-Risk Factors.*

Alterations and Therapies

Intrapartum

ALTERATION	DESCRIPTION	THERAPIES
Precipitous birth	Rapid progression of labor, with birth occurring within 3 hours or less.	▪ The nurse's primary responsibility is to provide a physically and psychologically safe experience for the woman and her baby. ▪ If birth is imminent, do not leave the mother alone, even for a minute. ▪ Provide reassurance and send auxiliary personnel to retrieve the emergency birth pack.
Abruptio placentae	Premature separation of a normally implanted placenta from the uterine wall; may be a catastrophic event depending on the severity of the resulting hemorrhage, which may be vaginal or may be unseen because it collects in the uterus or abdomen.	▪ Monitor uterine resting tone, which is frequently increased with abruptio placentae. ▪ Monitor abdominal girth measurements to determine internal blood collection. ▪ Monitor vital signs, hemoglobin and hematocrit, and urine output.
Placenta previa	Implantation of the placenta in the lower uterine segment rather than the upper portion, resulting in placental separation with dilation of the cervix.	▪ Teach all pregnant women the importance of reporting any bright-red vaginal bleeding, often scant at first. ▪ Avoid vaginal examination if placenta previa is suspected. ▪ Assess blood loss, pain, vital signs, fetal well-being, and uterine contractility. ▪ Provide emotional support for the mother and family.
Premature rupture of membranes	Spontaneous rupture of the membranes before the onset of labor. Preterm PROM is the rupture of membranes occurring before 37 weeks of gestation associated with infection, previous history of PPROM, hydramnios, multiple pregnancy, UTI, amniocentesis, placenta previa, abruptio placentae, trauma, cervical insufficiency, bleeding during pregnancy, and maternal genital tract anomalies.	▪ Assess for duration of rupture, appearance of amniotic fluid, and fetal well-being. ▪ Monitor woman for signs of infection, including WBC count and vital signs. ▪ Assess for potential cord compression if witnessed rupture. ▪ Educate the woman and her partner regarding implications of PROM and all treatments.

Alterations and Therapies *(continued)*

ALTERATION	DESCRIPTION	THERAPIES
Preterm labor	Labor that occurs between 20 and 36 completed weeks of pregnancy. Patients are admitted if at high risk for delivery in the setting of advanced cervical dilation, history of preterm delivery, or positive fetal fibronectin (fFN), a protein in the membranes found in vaginal secretions before 20 weeks and after 37 weeks. Detection of fFN on a vaginal swab between 24 and 34 weeks of gestation increases suspicion of preterm labor (King et al., 2019); if at low risk for imminent delivery, patients are sent home on pelvic rest and normal activity.	▪ Administer IV magnesium sulfate for 12 hours maximum for fetal neuroprotection and IM betamethasone. ▪ Monitor blood pressure every 10–15 minutes, serum magnesium levels, reflexes, respiratory rate, urinary output, and level of sedation and be prepared to administer calcium if toxicity is suspected. ▪ Provide emotional support to the woman, who may be fearful for fetal well-being. ▪ Teach woman to recognize onset of labor, to perform home uterine activity monitoring, to evaluate contraction activity, and symptoms to report.
Postterm labor	A pregnancy that exceeds 42 weeks, occurring most frequently in primigravidas, women with history of postterm pregnancies, or fetal anencephaly.	▪ Conduct ongoing assessment of fetal well-being. ▪ Assess fluid for meconium following rupture of membranes. ▪ Provide patient education. ▪ Provide emotional support, encouragement, and recognition of the woman's anxiety.
Hypertonic labor	Ineffective uterine contractions of poor quality occurring in the latent phase of labor with increased resting tone of the myometrium and frequent contractions.	▪ Provide comfort and support to the laboring woman and her partner. ▪ Provide supportive measures such as change of position, quiet environment, back rubs, or guided imagery. ▪ Consider therapeutic rest.
Hypotonic labor patterns	Usually developing in the active phase of labor, characterized by fewer than two to three contractions in a 10-minute period of low intensity causing minimal discomfort; often the result of overstretching of the uterus, bowel or bladder distention, arrest of descent, or fetal malposition.	▪ Assess contractions, maternal vital signs, and FHR, watching for signs of infection or dehydration. ▪ Promote maternal–fetal well-being. ▪ Monitor for maternal exhaustion. ▪ Assess for meconium if rupture of membranes. ▪ Consider augmentation of labor.
Fetal malpresentation	Any presentation that is not right occiput anterior, occiput anterior, or left occiput anterior, which may prolong labor or require a cesarean section.	▪ Assist with position change to promote fetal repositioning. ▪ Promote rest if labor is prolonged. ▪ Provide patient education. ▪ Prepare for surgery if cesarean section is required.
Fetal macrosomia	A newborn weight of >4000 g at birth, often associated with excessive maternal weight gain, maternal obesity, uncontrolled maternal diabetes, grand multiparity, prolonged gestation, or those with a previous baby with macrosomia >4000 g (Cunningham et al., 2018).	▪ Identify women at risk and assess FHR for nonreassuring fetal status. ▪ Assess for labor dysfunction or lack of fetal descent. ▪ Provide support, encouragement, and education. ▪ Monitor for hemorrhage postpartum. ▪ Assess newborn after delivery for cephalohematoma.
Nonreassuring fetal status	When the oxygen supply is insufficient to meet the physiologic needs of the fetus, a nonreassuring fetal status may result, which may be transient or chronic. Demonstrated by change in FHR, decreased fetal movement, meconium-stained amniotic fluid, or ominous FHR patterns.	▪ Review prenatal history and note any risk factors. ▪ Assess FHR and note characteristics of amniotic fluid with rupture. ▪ Promote maternal positioning to maximize ureteroplacental fetal blood flow.

(continued on next page)

Alterations and Therapies *(continued)*

ALTERATION	DESCRIPTION	THERAPIES
Prolapsed umbilical cord	The umbilical cord precedes the fetal presenting part, placing pressure on the cord and reducing or stopping blood flow to and from the fetus. Of greatest risk when rupture of membranes occurs before engagement of fetal presenting part.	■ Assess FHR and observe for prolapse for a full minute when membranes rupture. If loop of cord is discovered, a gloved hand elevates the fetal presenting part to relieve pressure until the cesarean delivery can be accomplished. ■ Administer oxygen by face mask to increase fetal oxygenation. ■ If the presenting part is well applied to the cervix, then ambulation should be encouraged. If the presenting part is not well applied to the cervix, the woman is at an increased risk of cord prolapse and ambulation should be discouraged; however, the woman can sit with the head of the bed elevated or in a rocking chair to facilitate gravity.
Anaphylactoid syndrome of pregnancy (amniotic fluid embolism)	In the presence of a small tear in the amnion or chorion high in the uterus, an area of separation in the placenta, or cervical tear, a small amount of amniotic fluid may leak into the chorionic plate and enter the maternal circulatory system as an amniotic fluid embolism. The more debris in the amniotic fluid (e.g., meconium), the greater the maternal danger.	■ Administer oxygen under positive pressure and summon emergency assistance. ■ Establish IV access quickly. ■ Perform cardiopulmonary resuscitation if respiratory and cardiac arrest occur. ■ Call anesthesiologist immediately. ■ Provide support to the woman's partner and family members.
Cephalopelvic disproportion (CPD)	Occurs when the fetal head is too large to pass through any part of the birth passage, which can result in prolonged labor, uterine rupture, necrosis of maternal soft tissues, cord prolapse, excessive molding of the fetal head, or damage to the fetal skull and CNS.	■ Assess adequacy of maternal pelvis for a vaginal birth, size of the fetus, and its presentation and position. ■ Suspect CPD when labor is prolonged, cervical dilation and effacement are slow, and engagement of the presenting part is delayed. ■ Provide support to the couple and keep them informed of what is happening and about the procedures being performed. ■ Assess cervical dilation and fetal descent more frequently. ■ Monitor contractions and fetal well-being continuously. ■ Position to optimize pelvic diameters.
Retained placenta	Retention of the placenta beyond 30 minutes after birth, resulting in bleeding that may lead to shock.	■ Assess for excessive bleeding and uterine contraction after delivery. ■ Monitor maternal vital signs.
Lacerations	Tearing of the cervix or vagina, indicated by bright-red vaginal bleeding in the presence of a well-contracted uterus. The highest risk is in young or nulliparous women and during operative vaginal delivery (forceps or vacuum assisted).	■ Monitor for bright-red blood during labor. ■ Promote perineal massage prenatally. ■ If lacerations occur, manage pain and apply ice to the area after delivery to reduce edema. ■ Teach the mother to rinse the perineum after every elimination and use sitz baths to reduce discomfort.
Placenta accreta	The chorionic villi attach directly to the myometrium of the uterus in placenta accreta. Two other types of placental adherence are *placenta increta*, in which the myometrium is invaded, and *placenta percreta*, in which the myometrium is penetrated. The adherence itself may be total, partial, or focal, depending on the amount of placental involvement.	■ Assess for bleeding. ■ Monitor vital signs. ■ Prepare woman for surgical intervention and possible hysterectomy.

Alterations and Therapies *(continued)*

ALTERATION	DESCRIPTION	THERAPIES
Shoulder dystocia	Impaction of the fetal anterior shoulder behind the maternal pubic bone after the birth of the head. Risk factors include macrosomia, history of shoulder dystocia, and rapid labor. However, most shoulder dystocias are not predictable. Pressure from the maternal bone on the fetal brachial plexus can result in paralysis of the arm. Failure to resolve the problem may lead to fetal hypoxia, encephalopathy, and death.	■ The HCP will perform maneuvers to free the shoulder. ■ Call for assistance from the unit and nursery staff. ■ Maintain an orderly atmosphere and clear communication. ■ Emphasize the importance of and helping the mother to cooperate with maneuvers and avoid pushing. ■ Monitor fetal status. ■ Monitor time from birth of the head to fetal expulsion. ■ Reposition the mother to maximize pelvic diameters. ■ Apply suprapubic pressure on provider request to assist in dislodging the shoulder.
Perinatal loss	Death of a fetus or newborn from the time of conception through the end of the newborn period 28 days after delivery.	■ Discussed in detail in Module 27, Grief and Loss.

Source: Adapted from London et al. (2017).

Lifespan Considerations

Nursing care of laboring women who are adolescent and those older than 35 requires some additional considerations.

The Adolescent During Labor and Delivery

As with all women, each adolescent in labor is different. The nurse must assess what each teen brings to the experience as follows:

- Has the young woman received prenatal care?
- What are her attitudes and feelings about the pregnancy?
- Who will attend the birth, and what is each individual's relationship to the woman?
- What preparation has she had for the experience?
- What are her expectations and fears regarding labor and birth?
- What cultural considerations influence her needs and expectations for birth?
- What are her usual coping mechanisms?
- What are her plans for the newborn?

Any adolescent who has not had prenatal care requires close observation during labor. Fetal well-being is established by fetal monitoring. Adolescent women are at risk for pregnancy and labor complications and must be assessed carefully. The nurse must be especially alert for any physiologic complications of labor. The young woman's prenatal record is carefully reviewed for risks, and the adolescent is screened for preeclampsia, cephalopelvic disproportion, anemia, cigarette smoking, alcohol and drugs ingested during pregnancy, STIs (see Exemplar 19.E, Sexually Transmitted Infections in Module 19, Sexuality), and size–date discrepancies.

The support role of the nurse depends on the young woman's support system during labor. The adolescent may not be accompanied by someone who will stay with her during childbirth, or she may have her mother, the father of the baby, or a close friend as her labor partner. Regardless of whether the teen has a support person, the nurse needs to establish a trusting relationship with her. In this way, the nurse can help the teen understand what is happening to her. Establishing a nurturing rapport is essential. Some nurses may view adolescent pregnancy as a negative event; however, it is important to treat the young woman with respect. The adolescent who is given positive reinforcement will leave the experience with increased self-esteem despite the emotional challenges that may accompany her situation.

If a support person accompanies the adolescent, that individual also needs the nurse's encouragement and support. The nurse must explain changes in the young woman's behavior, substantiate her wishes, and describe ways the support person can be of help. The nursing staff needs to reinforce the adolescent's feelings that she is wanted and important.

The adolescent who has taken childbirth education classes is generally better prepared for labor than the adolescent who has not. However, the nurse must keep in mind that the younger the adolescent, the less she may be able to participate actively in the process, even if she has taken prenatal classes.

The very young adolescent (age 14 and younger) has fewer coping mechanisms and less experience to draw on than her older counterparts. Because her cognitive development is incomplete, the younger adolescent may have fewer problem-solving abilities. Her ego integrity may be more threatened by the experience of labor, and she may be more vulnerable to stress and discomfort. She may be more childlike and dependent than older teens. As a result, the very young adolescent needs someone to rely on at all times during labor. The nurse must be sure that instructions and explanations are simple and concrete.

During the transition phase, the adolescent may become withdrawn and unable to express her need to be nurtured. Touch, soothing encouragement, and measures to provide comfort help her maintain control and meet her needs for dependence. During the second stage of labor, the young adolescent may feel as if she is losing control and may reach out to those around her. By remaining calm and giving directions, the nurse helps her cope with feelings of helplessness.

The middle adolescent (age 15 to 17) often attempts to remain calm and unflinching during labor. The experienced nurse realizes that a caring attitude will still help the young woman. Many older adolescents believe that they "know it all," but they may be no more prepared for childbirth than their younger counterparts. The nurse's reinforcement and nonjudgmental manner will help them save face. If the adolescent has not taken childbirth preparation classes, she may require preparation and explanations.

The older teenager (age 18 to 19) responds to the stresses of labor in a manner similar to that of the adult woman.

Adolescents, regardless of their age, need ongoing education throughout labor and in the early postpartum period. Provide clear explanations. Encourage these patients in particular to ask questions and seek information.

Even if the adolescent is planning to relinquish her newborn, she should be given the option of seeing and holding the baby. She may be reluctant to do this at first, but the grieving process is facilitated if the mother sees the baby. However, seeing or holding the newborn should be the young woman's choice.

Adolescents need individualized care for the issues that they face in the postpartum period. They may experience additional psychosocial issues unique to their age group and their developmental level. Adolescents are also at an increased risk for unintended subsequent pregnancies and abortions. Proper discharge teaching for this population should include contraceptive options (CDC, 2019c; Gavin et al., 2013).

Labor and Delivery over Age 35

Generally, women over age 35 respond to the stresses of labor similarly to their younger counterparts.

In the United States and Canada, the risk of death during labor and delivery has declined dramatically during the past 30 years for women of all ages. However, the risk of maternal death is higher for women over age 35 and even higher for women age 40 and older. These women are more likely to have a chronic medical condition that can complicate pregnancy. Preexisting medical conditions such as HTN or diabetes probably play a more significant role than age in maternal well-being and the outcome of pregnancy. For women over the age of 35, the rates of miscarriage, stillbirth, preterm birth, low birth weight, and perinatal morbidity and mortality are increased (Mayo Clinic, 2017b). Nevertheless, while the risk of pregnancy complications is higher in women over age 35 who have a chronic condition such as HTN or diabetes or who are in poor general health, the risks are much lower than previously believed for physically fit women without preexisting medical problems (Cunningham et al., 2018).

NURSING PROCESS

Maternal–newborn nursing offers nurses the opportunity to work with patients and families from diverse backgrounds, each of whom brings their own medical history, personal and cultural preferences and beliefs, anxiety, and desires to the experience of childbirth. Nurses must be prepared for a variety of situations, from emergency cesarean births to families who desire maximum privacy and minimum interaction with the healthcare team. In every case, nurses must be prepared to provide best-practice patient- and family-centered care, whether the mother desires participation of extended family or the mother is alone in her experience of childbirth.

Throughout the process of labor, mother and fetus experience rapid physiologic and psychologic changes. Timely and accurate assessment is critical to ensuring the health and well-being of both mother and baby. Nurses must combine traditional nursing assessment and communication techniques with high-tech electronic monitoring and ultrasound. Regardless of the technology available, it is the nurse's responsibility to monitor the mother and her child.

Maternal Assessment

On admission to the birthing area, the nurse reviews the mother's medical history with her and screens for intrapartum risk factors. Baseline vital signs for both mother and fetus are obtained immediately (**Table 33.12** »). If the vital signs for both patients are within normal limits, the nurse continues the patient interview. One or more abnormal findings from vital signs (for either mother or baby) requires further assessment and prioritization of care.

TABLE 33.12 Nursing Assessments in the First Stage

Phase	Mother	Fetus
Latent	Blood pressure and respirations each hour if in normal range. Temperature every 4 hours unless over 37.5°C (99.6°F) or membranes ruptured, then every 2 hours. Uterine contractions every 30 minutes.	FHR every 60 minutes for low-risk women and every 30 minutes for high-risk women if normal characteristics are present (average variability, baseline in the 110–160 beats/min range, without late or variable decelerations) or assess the heart rate every 30 minutes if the provider orders intermittent auscultation in a low-risk setting. Note fetal activity. If electronic fetal monitor is in place, assess for reactive NST.
Active	Blood pressure, pulse, and respirations every hour if in normal range. Uterine contractions palpated every 15–30 minutes.	FHR every 30 minutes for low-risk women and every 15 minutes for high-risk women if normal characteristics are present.
Transition	Blood pressure, pulse, and respirations every hour. Contractions palpated every 15–30 minutes.	FHR every 15–30 minutes if normal characteristics are present.

Source: From London et al. (2017). Pearson Education, Inc., Hoboken, NJ.

It is common for the HCP to send the prenatal records to the labor and birthing unit before the woman's due date. Review this information to ensure that changes have not occurred since the information was documented. During the initial interview, the nurse is building a trusting relationship. It is often helpful if the nurse sits down and appears unrushed, makes direct eye contact (if culturally appropriate), and begins the interview with a statement such as "I am going to be asking you some very personal and specific questions so that we can provide the best care for both you and your baby." This conveys a nonjudgmental approach, shows respect, and makes the expectant mother feel more at ease. Each agency has its own admission forms, but they usually include the following information:

- Woman's name and age
- Religious preference and spiritual practices
- LMP and estimated date of birth
- Attending physician or CNM
- Personal data: blood type; Rh factor; results of serology testing; pre-pregnant and present weight; allergies to medications, foods, or other substances; prescribed and OTC medications taken during the pregnancy; and history of drug and alcohol use and smoking during the pregnancy
- History of previous illness, such as tuberculosis, heart disease, diabetes, convulsive disorders, and thyroid disorders; asthma; sickle cell, Tay-Sachs, and other inherited disorders; or pregnancy-related complications (e.g., preterm labor, gestational diabetes, preeclampsia, or low platelets)
- Problems in the prenatal period, such as elevated blood pressure, bleeding problems, recurrent UTIs, other infections, abnormal laboratory findings (e.g., abnormal glucose screen indicating gestational diabetes or low hemoglobin or hematocrit indicating anemia), or STIs
- Pregnancy data: gravida, para, abortions, and neonatal deaths
- Method chosen for newborn/infant feeding
- Type of childbirth education or newborn/infant care classes
- Previous newborn/infant care experience
- Woman's preferences regarding labor and birth, such as no episiotomy, no analgesics or anesthetics, or the presence or absence of the partner or others at the birth
- Pediatrician, family practice physician, or nurse practitioner
- Additional data: history of special tests, such as NST, biophysical profile, or ultrasound; history of any preterm labor; onset of labor; amniotic fluid membrane status; and brief description of any previous labor and birth
- Onset of labor, status of amniotic membranes (intact, ruptured, time of rupture, color, and odor).

Because of the prevalence of interpersonal violence in our society (see Exemplar 32.A, Abuse, in Module 32, Trauma), the nurse needs to consider the possibility that the pregnant woman may have experienced abuse at some point in her life. Many victims of interpersonal violence, sexual assault, or childhood abuse may be anxious about the labor process or may experience anxiety during labor. Therefore, it is essential to review the woman's prenatal record and any other available records for information that may indicate abuse or a history of victimization by violence.

Intrapartum High-Risk Screening

Screening for intrapartum high-risk factors is an integral part of assessing the woman in labor. As the history is obtained, the nurse notes the presence of any potential risk factors that may be considered high-risk conditions. For example, the woman who reports a physical symptom such as intermittent bleeding needs further assessment to rule out abruptio placentae or placenta previa before the admission process continues. It is important to determine the difference between vaginal bleeding and bloody show. In addition to identifying the presence of a high-risk condition, the nurse must recognize the implications of the condition for the laboring woman and her fetus. For example, if there is an abnormal fetal position, the nurse understands that the labor may be prolonged and that prolapse of the umbilical cord is more likely, thereby increasing the possibility of a cesarean birth.

Although physical conditions are frequently listed as the major factors that increase risk during the intrapartum period, SES and cultural variables (such as poverty, nutrition, the amount of prenatal care, living conditions, cultural beliefs regarding pregnancy, and communication patterns) may also precipitate a high-risk situation. For patients with mental illness, medications may need to be taken during the pregnancy and prenatal care may be sporadic (Hale & Ngo, 2020). Research indicates that women who experience posttraumatic stress disorder (PTSD) may be at increased risk for pregnancy complications (Lowdermilk et al., 2020). (See Exemplar 32.C, Posttraumatic Stress Disorder, in Module 32, Trauma.) Other risk factors include smoking, drug use, and consumption of alcohol during pregnancy. The nurse can quickly review the prenatal record for number of prenatal visits; weight gain during pregnancy; progression of fundal height; assistance, such as Medicaid and WIC participation; exposure to environmental agents; and history of traumatic life events, including abuse.

A partial list of intrapartum risk factors appears in **Box 33.5** ». Keep these factors in mind during the assessment.

Box 33.5
Selected Intrapartum Risk Factors

- Intermittent bleeding
- Cardiovascular disease
- Abnormal fetal presentation
- Poverty
- Poor nutrition
- Birth equity
- Lack of prenatal care
- Mental illness
- PTSD
- Early elective delivery
- Prenatal/perinatal substance exposure
- Hemorrhage
- HTN/preeclampsia

Intrapartum Assessment

A physical examination is part of the admission procedure and part of the ongoing care of the patient. Although the intrapartum physical assessment is not as complete and thorough as the initial prenatal physical examination (see the Concepts section of this module), it does involve assessment of some body systems and the actual labor process.

The physical assessment portion includes assessments performed immediately on admission as well as ongoing assessments. Nurses conduct ongoing assessments in all clinical situations. For example, when the woman is changing into her gown, the nurse can assess the skin for bruises, needle marks, burns, or other abnormalities. The nurse can also determine whether the woman appears to be undernourished or overnourished. When labor is progressing rapidly, however, the nurse may not have time for a complete assessment. In that case, the critical physical assessments include maternal vital signs, labor status, fetal status, and laboratory findings.

Assessment of psychosocial history is a critical component of intrapartum nursing assessment. An estimated one-third of all pregnant women are exposed to some type of psychotropic medication during their pregnancies. In addition, one in seven women experience depression during pregnancy and an estimated 9% of pregnant women meet the criteria for major depressive disorder (ACOG, 2018f). Perinatal depression is a common complication of pregnancy with potentially devastating consequences if it goes unrecognized and untreated (ACOG, 2018f). Any mental illness can play a role in how the woman copes with the labor and birth experience and should be assessed by the admitting nurse. Women with identified disorders will need ongoing assessment during the labor and birth.

The nurse can begin gathering data about sociocultural factors as the woman enters the birthing area. The nurse observes the communication pattern between the woman and her support person and their responses to admission questions and initial teaching. If the woman and her support person do not speak English and interpreters are not available among the birthing unit staff, the course of labor and the nurse's ability to interact and provide support and education are affected. The couple must receive information in their primary language to make informed decisions (see Nursing Care Plan in Exemplar 33.A, Antepartum Care, in this module). Communication may also be affected by cultural practices, such as beliefs about when to speak, who should ask questions, or whether it is acceptable to let others know about discomfort. People from certain cultures may want to experience birth naturally and may decline pain medications. In some cultures, the partner is not expected to be present in the birthing area. Nurses need to be culturally competent so that this is not interpreted as lack of interest in the birth, the mother, or the baby (Spector, 2017).

Individualized nursing care can best be planned and implemented when nurses know and honor the values and beliefs of the laboring woman (Andrews, Boyle, & Collins, 2020). To avoid stereotyping patients, the nurse always asks the woman and her family about individual beliefs and preferences. Nurses who feel uncertain about what to ask or to consider need to explore the varying cultural values and beliefs of the people residing in their community. Although some communities have a prominent culture that may follow certain rituals, the nurse should still ask each patient about her own individual beliefs and preferences.

The final section of the assessment guide addresses ideas, knowledge, fantasies, and fears about childbearing. The nurse should ask the patient whether she has any special needs. However, because some women may not know what needs may arise, ongoing assessment is imperative. It is important for the nurse to pay specific attention to body language, eye contact, and other nonverbal cues that may indicate the woman is experiencing anxiety or other feelings. By assessing the patient's cultural and psychosocial status, the nurse can better meet the woman's needs for information and support. The nurse can then assist the woman and her partner; in the absence of a partner, the nurse may become the support person.

The Intrapartum Assessment feature provides a framework the nurse can use when examining the laboring woman.

Intrapartum Assessment: First Stage of Labor

PHYSICAL ASSESSMENT/ NORMAL FINDINGS	ALTERATIONS AND POSSIBLE CAUSES*	NURSING RESPONSES TO DATA†
Vital Signs		
Blood pressure (BP): less than 140 systolic and 90 and greater than 90/50 diastolic	High blood pressure (essential HTN, preeclampsia, renal disease, apprehension, anxiety, or pain) Low blood pressure (supine hypotension) Hemorrhage/hypovolemia Shock Drugs Side effect of epidural anesthesia	Evaluate history of preexisting disorders and check for presence of other signs of preeclampsia. Do not assess during contractions; implement measures to decrease anxiety and reassess. Provide quiet environment. Have O_2 available. Notify anesthesiologist.

Intrapartum Assessment: First Stage of Labor *(continued)*

PHYSICAL ASSESSMENT/ NORMAL FINDINGS	ALTERATIONS AND POSSIBLE CAUSES*	NURSING RESPONSES TO DATA†
Pulse: 60–100 beats/min (normal, nonpregnant) Additional 10–20 beats/min during pregnancy	Increased pulse rate (excitement or anxiety, cardiac disorders, early shock, drug use)	Evaluate cause; reassess to see if rate continues; report to HCP.
Respirations: 16–24 breaths/min (or pulse rate divided by 4)	Marked tachypnea (respiratory disease), hyperventilation in transition phase Decreased respirations (narcotics)	Assess between contractions; if marked tachypnea continues, assess for signs of respiratory disease or respiratory distress.
	Hyperventilation (anxiety/pain)	Encourage slow breaths if woman is hyperventilating.
Pulse oximetry 95% or greater	Pulse oximetry less than 90%: hypoxia, hypotension, hemorrhage	Administer O_2; notify HCP.
Temperature: 36.2–37.6°C (97–99.6°F)	Elevated temperature (infection, dehydration, prolonged rupture of membranes, epidural regional block)	Assess for other signs of infection or dehydration.
Weight		
25–35 lb greater than pre-pregnant weight	Weight gain greater than 35 lb (fluid retention, obesity, LGA, diabetes mellitus, preeclampsia) Weight gain less than 15 lb (SGA, substance abuse, psychosocial problems)	Assess for signs of edema. Evaluate dietary patterns from prenatal record.
Lungs		
Normal breath sounds, clear and equal	Rales, rhonchi, friction rub (infection), pulmonary edema, asthma	Reassess; refer to HCP.
Fundus		
At 40 weeks of gestation, located just below the xiphoid process	Uterine size not compatible with estimated date of birth (SGA, LGA, hydramnios, multiple pregnancy, placental/fetal anomalies, malpresentation)	Reevaluate history regarding pregnancy dating. Refer to HCP for additional assessment.
Edema		
Slight amount of dependent edema	Pitting edema of face, hands, legs, abdomen, sacral area (preeclampsia)	Check deep tendon reflexes for hyperactivity; check for clonus; refer to HCP.
Hydration		
Normal skin turgor, elastic	Poor skin turgor (dehydration)	Assess skin turgor; refer to HCP for deviations. Provide fluids per HCP orders.
Perineum		
Tissues smooth, pink color	Varicose veins of vulva, herpes lesions/ genital warts	Note on patient record need for follow-up in postpartum period; reassess after birth, refer to HCP.
Clear mucus that may be blood tinged with earthy or human odor	Profuse, purulent, foul-smelling drainage	Suspected gonorrhea or chorioamnionitis; report to HCP; initiate care to newborn's eyes; notify neonatal nursing staff and pediatrician.
Presence of small amount of bloody show that gradually increases with further cervical dilation	Hemorrhage	Assess BP and pulse, pallor, diaphoresis; report any marked changes. Standard precautions.

(continued on next page)

Intrapartum Assessment: First Stage of Labor *(continued)*

PHYSICAL ASSESSMENT/ NORMAL FINDINGS	ALTERATIONS AND POSSIBLE CAUSES*	NURSING RESPONSES TO DATA†
Labor Status		
Uterine contractions: regular pattern	Failure to establish a regular pattern, prolonged latent phase Hypertonicity Hypotonicity Dehydration	Evaluate whether woman is in true labor. Ambulate if in early labor. Evaluate patient status and contractile pattern. Obtain a 20-minute electronic fetal monitoring strip. Notify HCP. Provide hydration.
Cervical dilation: progressive cervical dilation from size of fingertip to 10 cm (3.9 in.)	Rigidity of cervix (frequent cervical infections, scar tissue, failure of presenting part to descend)	Evaluate contractions, fetal engagement, position, and cervical dilation. Inform patient of progress.
Cervical effacement: progressive thinning of cervix	Failure to efface (rigidity of cervix, failure of presenting part to engage); cervical edema (pushing effort by woman before cervix is fully dilated and effaced, trapped cervix)	Evaluate contractions, fetal engagement, and position. Notify HCP if cervix is becoming edematous; work with woman to prevent pushing until cervix is completely dilated. Keep vaginal exams to a minimum.
Fetal descent: progressive descent of fetal presenting part from station −5 to +4	Arrest of descent (abnormal fetal position or presentation, macrosomic fetus, inadequate pelvic measurements)	Evaluate fetal position, presentation, and size.
Membranes: may rupture before or during labor	Rupture of membranes more than 12–24 hours before onset of labor	Assess for ruptured membranes using Nitrazine test tape before doing vaginal exam. Follow standard precautions. Keep vaginal exams to a minimum to prevent infection. When membranes rupture in the birth setting, immediately assess FHR to detect changes associated with prolapse of umbilical cord (FHR slows).
Findings on Nitrazine test tape: Membranes probably intact: Yellow pH 5.0 Olive pH 5.5 Olive green pH 6.0	False-positive results may be obtained if large amount of bloody show is present, previous vaginal examination has been done using lubricant, or tape is touched by nurse's fingers	Assess fluid for consistency, amount, odor; assess FHR frequently. Assess fluid at regular intervals for presence of meconium staining. Follow standard precautions while assessing amniotic fluid.
Membranes probably ruptured: Blue-green pH 6.5 Blue-gray pH 7.0 Deep blue pH 7.5		Teach woman that amniotic fluid is continually produced (to allay fear of "dry birth"). Teach woman that she may feel amniotic fluid trickle or gush with contractions. Change pads often.
Amniotic fluid clear, with earthy or human odor, no foul-smelling odor	Greenish amniotic fluid (fetal stress) Bloody fluid (vasa previa, abruptio placentae) Strong or foul odor (amnionitis)	Assess FHR; do vaginal exam to evaluate for prolapsed cord; apply fetal monitor for continuous data; report to HCP. Take woman's temperature and report to HCP.
Fetal Status		
FHR: 110–160 beats/min	Less than 110 or greater than 160 beats/min (nonreassuring fetal status); abnormal patterns on fetal monitor: decreased variability, late decelerations, variable decelerations, absence of accelerations with fetal movement	Initiate interventions based on particular FHR pattern.
Presentation: cephalic, 97%; breech, 3%	Face, brow, breech, or shoulder presentation	Report to HCP; after presentation is confirmed as face, brow, breech, or shoulder, woman may be prepared for cesarean birth.

Intrapartum Assessment: First Stage of Labor *(continued)*

PHYSICAL ASSESSMENT/ NORMAL FINDINGS	ALTERATIONS AND POSSIBLE CAUSES*	NURSING RESPONSES TO DATA†
Position: left occiput anterior most common	Persistent occiput posterior position; transverse arrest	Carefully monitor maternal and fetal status. Reposition mother in side-lying or on hands and knees position to promote rotation of fetal head.
Activity: fetal movement	Hyperactivity (may precede fetal hypoxia) Complete lack of movement (nonreassuring fetal status or fetal demise)	Carefully evaluate FHR; apply fetal monitor. Carefully evaluate FHR; apply fetal monitor. Report to HCP.
CULTURAL ASSESSMENT§	**VARIATIONS TO CONSIDER**	**NURSING RESPONSES TO DATA†**
Cultural influences determine customs and practices regarding intrapartum care.	Individual preferences may vary.	
Ask the following questions: ▪ Who would you like to remain with you during your labor and birth?	She may prefer only her partner or other support person to remain or may also want family and/or friends.	Provide support for her wishes by encouraging desired people to stay. Provide information to others (with the woman's permission) who are not in the room.
▪ What would you like to wear during labor?	She may be more comfortable in her own clothes.	Offer supportive materials, such as disposable pads, if needed to protect her clothing. Avoid subtle signals to the woman that she should not have chosen to remain in her own clothes. Have other clothing available if the woman desires. If her clothing becomes contaminated, it will be simple to place it in a plastic bag.
▪ What activity would you like during labor?	She may want to ambulate most of the time, stand in the shower, sit in the Jacuzzi, sit on a chair/stool/birthing ball, remain on the bed, and so forth.	Support the woman's wishes; provide encouragement and complete assessments in a manner so her activity and positional wishes are disturbed as little as possible.
▪ What position would you like for the birth?	She may feel more comfortable in lithotomy position with stirrups and her upper body elevated, side-lying or sitting in a birthing bed, standing, squatting, or on hands and knees.	Collect any supplies and equipment needed to support her in her chosen birthing position. Provide information to the support person regarding any changes that may be needed based on the chosen position.
▪ Is there anything special you would like?	She may want the room darkened or to have curtains and windows open, music playing, her support person to cut the umbilical cord, to save a portion of the umbilical cord, to save the placenta, to videotape the birth, or other particular preferences.	Support requests and communicate requests to any other nursing or medical personnel (so requests can continue to be supported and not questioned). If another nurse or physician does not honor the request, act as advocate for the woman by continuing to support her unless her desire is truly unsafe.
Ask the woman if she would like fluids and what temperature she prefers.	She may prefer clear fluids other than water (tea, clear juice). She may prefer iced, room temperature, or warmed fluids.	Provide fluids as desired.
Observe the woman's response when privacy is difficult to maintain and her body is exposed.	Some women do not seem to mind being exposed during an exam or procedure; others feel acute discomfort.	Maintain privacy and respect the woman's sense of privacy. If the woman is unable to provide specific information, the nurse may draw from general information regarding cultural variation: Southeast Asian women may not want any family member in the room during exam or procedures. The woman's partner may not be involved with coaching activities during labor or birth. Muslim women may need to remain covered during the labor and birth and avoid exposure of any body part. The husband may need to be in the room but remain behind a curtain or screen so he does not view his wife at this time.

Intrapartum Assessment: First Stage of Labor *(continued)*

PHYSICAL ASSESSMENT/ NORMAL FINDINGS	ALTERATIONS AND POSSIBLE CAUSES*	NURSING RESPONSES TO DATA†
If the woman is to breastfeed, ask if she would like to feed her baby immediately after birth.	She may want to feed her baby right away or may want to wait a little while.	
PSYCHOSOCIAL ASSESSMENT	**VARIATIONS TO CONSIDER**	**NURSING RESPONSES TO DATA†**
Preparation for Childbirth		
Does the woman have some information regarding process of normal labor and birth?	Some women do not have any information regarding childbirth.	Add to present information base.
Does the woman have breathing and/or relaxation techniques to use during labor?	Some women do not have any method of relaxation or breathing to use, and some do not desire them.	Support breathing and relaxation techniques that the patient is using; provide information, if needed.
Have the woman and support person done extensive preparation for childbirth?	Some women have strong opinions regarding labor and birth preparation.	Support the woman's wishes to participate in her birth experience; support the woman's birth plan.
Response to Labor		
Latent phase: relaxed, excited, anxious for labor to be well established	May feel unable to cope with contractions because of fear, anxiety, or lack of information.	Provide support and encouragement, establish trusting relationship.
Active phase: becomes more intense, begins to tire	May remain quiet and without any sign of discomfort or anxiety, may insist that she is unable to continue with the birthing process.	Provide support and coaching as needed.
Transitional phase: feels tired, may feel unable to cope, needs frequent coaching to maintain breathing patterns		Provide support and coaching as needed.
Coping mechanisms: ability to cope with labor through use of support system, breathing, relaxation techniques, and comfort measures, including frequent position changes in labor, immersion in warm water, and massage	May feel marked anxiety and apprehension, may not have coping mechanisms that can be brought into this experience, or may be unable to use them at this time. Survivors of sexual abuse may demonstrate fear of IV lines or needles, may recoil when touched, may insist on a female caregiver, may be very sensitive to body fluids and cleanliness, and may be unable to labor lying down.	Support coping mechanisms if they are working for the woman; provide information and support if she exhibits anxiety or needs alternative to present coping methods. Encourage participation of partner or other individual if a supportive relationship seems apparent. Establish rapport and a trusting relationship. Provide information that is true and offer your presence.
Anxiety		
Some anxiety and apprehension is within normal limits.	May show anxiety through rapid breathing, nervous tremors, frowning, grimacing, clenching of teeth, thrashing movements, crying, increased pulse and blood pressure	Provide support, encouragement, and information. Teach relaxation techniques. Support controlled breathing efforts. May need to provide a paper bag to breathe into if woman says her lips are tingling. Note FHR.
Sounds During Labor		
	Some women are very quiet; others moan or make a variety of noises.	Provide a supportive environment. Encourage woman to do what feels right for her.

Intrapartum Assessment: First Stage of Labor *(continued)*

PSYCHOSOCIAL ASSESSMENT	VARIATIONS TO CONSIDER	NURSING RESPONSES TO DATA†
Support System		
Physical intimacy between mother and partner (or mother and support person/doula); caretaking activities, such as soothing conversation and touching	Some women would prefer no contact; others may show clinging behaviors.	Encourage caretaking activities that appear to comfort the woman; encourage support for the woman; if support is limited, the nurse may take a more active role.
Support person stays in proximity	Limited interaction may come from a desire for quiet.	Encourage support person to stay close (if this seems appropriate).
Relationship between mother and partner or support person: involved interaction	The support person may seem to be detached and maintain little support, attention, or conversation.	Support interactions; if interaction is limited, the nurse may provide more information and support. Ensure that the support person has short breaks, especially before transition.

* Possible causes of alterations are identified in parentheses.

† This column provides guidelines for further assessment and initial nursing intervention.

§ These are only a few suggestions that promote cultural competence and are appropriate for assessment of all women regardless of their cultural background. This text does not mean to imply that this is a comprehensive cultural assessment; rather, it is a tool to encourage cultural competence.

Source: From London et al. (2017). Pearson Education, Inc., Hoboken, NJ.

Assessment of Contractions

Once contractions begin, the nurse must assess the nature of the contractions and any accompanying pain. When palpating a woman's uterus during a contraction, compare the consistency to your nose, chin, and forehead to determine the intensity. Many experienced nurses note that the feel during mild contractions is similar in consistency to the tip of the nose, moderate contractions feel more like the chin, and with strong contractions, the uterus feels firm, much like the forehead.

It is also important to assess the laboring woman's perception of pain. How does she describe the pain? What is her affect? Is this contraction more uncomfortable than the last one? Is the nurse's palpation of intensity congruent with the woman's perception? (For instance, the nurse might evaluate a contraction as mild in intensity, whereas the laboring woman evaluates it as very strong.) A nurse's assessment is not complete unless the laboring woman's affect and response to the contractions are also noted and documented.

Electronic monitoring of uterine contractions provides continuous data. Electronic monitoring is routinely used in many birth settings for high-risk patients and those having oxytocin-induced labor. Electronic monitoring may be done externally, with a device that is placed against the maternal abdomen, or internally, with an intrauterine pressure catheter.

External Electronic Monitoring of Contractions

When monitoring contractions by external means, the portion of the monitoring equipment called a tocodynamometer, or "toco," is positioned against the fundus of the uterus and held in place with an elastic belt. The toco contains a flexible disk that responds to pressure. When the uterus contracts, the fundus tightens and the change in pressure against the toco is amplified and transmitted to the electronic fetal monitor. The monitor displays the uterine contraction as a pattern on graph paper.

External monitoring offers several advantages, including a continuous recording of the frequency and duration of uterine contractions, and it is noninvasive. However, it does not accurately record the intensity of the uterine contraction, and it is difficult to obtain an accurate FHR in some women, such as those who are very obese, those who have hydramnios, or those with a very active fetus. In addition, the woman may be bothered by the belt if it requires frequent readjustment when she changes position. Electronic monitoring allows the nurse to continually monitor the fetus if concerns arise based on the FHR. It also enables the nurse and physician or CNM to observe the pattern of the FHR over a period of time by examining the electronic fetal monitoring strip.

Internal Electronic Monitoring of Contractions

Internal intrauterine monitoring provides the same data as external monitoring, as well as accurate measurement of uterine contraction intensity (the strength of the contraction and the actual pressure within the uterus). After membranes have ruptured, the physician or CNM (or the nurse in some facilities) inserts the **intrauterine pressure catheter** into the uterine cavity and connects it by a cable to the electronic fetal monitor. It is important to first assess the fetal position and to review a past ultrasound to determine the location of the placenta because the internal monitor should be placed away from the placenta. If an ultrasound has not been previously obtained, the HCP may wish to obtain one on the unit or have the sonographer perform such an exam.

The pressure within the uterus in the resting state and during each contraction is measured by a small micropressure device located in the tip of the catheter. Internal electronic monitoring is used when it is imperative to have accurate intrauterine pressure readings to evaluate the stress on the uterus or to determine the adequacy of contractions. The advantage of the intrauterine pressure monitor is that it can directly measure the intensity of the contraction. It can be used when the external monitor may not be accurately assessing the contraction strength, such as in cases of maternal obesity. It can also be used when oxytocin is being administered to ensure that uterine contractions are adequate.

During internal electronic monitoring, the nurse should also evaluate the woman's labor status by palpating the intensity and resting tone of the uterine fundus during contractions. Technology is a useful tool if used as an adjunct to good assessment skills, but it is not a replacement for those skills.

Cervical Assessment

Cervical dilation and effacement are evaluated directly by vaginal examination. The vaginal examination can provide information about the adequacy of the maternal pelvis, membrane status, characteristics of amniotic fluid, and fetal position and station.

Fetal Assessment

Thorough intrapartum fetal assessment includes assessment of fetal position, fetal presentation, and fetal status.

Assessment of Fetal Position

Assessment of fetal position combines traditional assessment methods with ultrasound.

Inspection

Inspection includes observation of the shape and size of the mother's abdomen and assessment of fetal lie: longitudinal (whether the uterus projects up or down) or transverse (whether the uterus projects left to right).

Palpation: Leopold Maneuvers

Leopold maneuvers allow the nurse to assess the woman's abdomen and the position and presentation of the fetus (see the Concepts section for information on how to perform Leopold maneuvers). Leopold maneuvers may be difficult to perform if there is excessive amniotic fluid or if the woman is obese. This skill requires that the nurse take care to avoid disturbing the fetus unnecessarily or causing discomfort to the mother.

Vaginal Examination and Ultrasound

Other assessment techniques to determine fetal position and presentation include vaginal examination and the use of ultrasound to visualize the fetus. During the vaginal examination, the examiner can palpate the presenting part if the cervix is dilated. Information about the position of the fetus and the degree of flexion of its head (in cephalic presentations) can also be obtained. Visualization by ultrasound is used when the fetal position cannot be determined by abdominal palpation.

Auscultation of Fetal Heart Rate

The hand-held Doppler ultrasound is used to auscultate the FHR between, during, and immediately after uterine contractions. A fetoscope may also be used. Instead of listening haphazardly over the woman's abdomen for the FHR, the nurse may choose to perform Leopold maneuvers first. Leopold maneuvers not only indicate the probable location of the FHR but also help determine the presence of multiple fetuses, fetal lie, and fetal presentation.

The FHR is heard most clearly at the fetal back (**Figure 33.47** »). In a cephalic presentation, the FHR is best heard in the lower quadrants of the maternal abdomen. In a breech presentation, it is heard at or above the level of the maternal umbilicus. In a transverse lie, the FHR may be heard

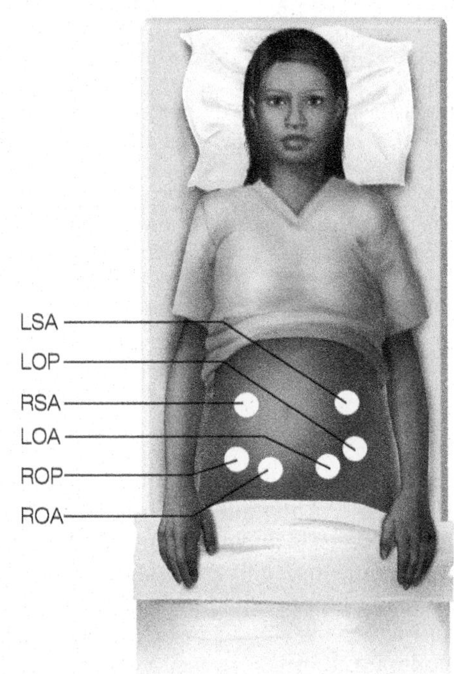

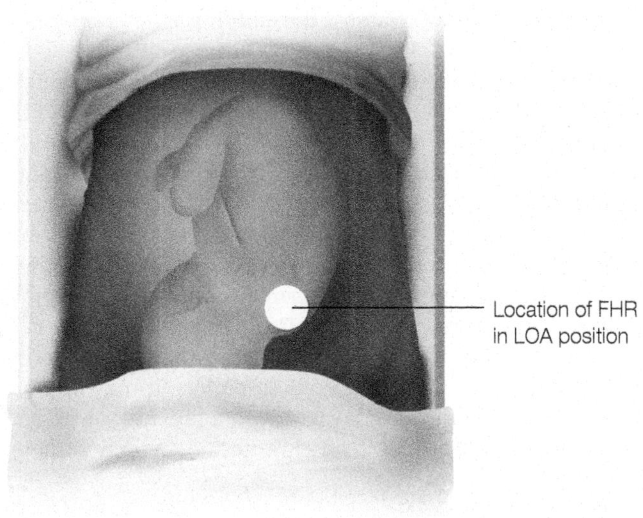

Figure 33.47 » Location of FHR in relation to the more commonly seen fetal positions. The FHR is heard more clearly over the fetal back.

best just above or just below the umbilicus. As the presenting part descends and rotates through the pelvic structure during labor, the location of the FHR tends to descend and move toward the midline.

For many years, the FHR was counted between contractions. However, this technique has been updated, as alterations in the FHR that occurs in relation to contractions can be missed with this method. Current practice is to begin listening at the acme of the contraction and continue listening for 30 to 60 seconds after the contraction has ended. If a deceleration is noted, FHR should be monitored for subsequent contractions for a period of 10 minutes. Electronic monitoring may be more appropriate if decelerations are noted (King et al., 2019). It is important to note that intermittent auscultation has been found to be as effective as the electronic method for fetal surveillance.

Electronic Monitoring of Fetal Heart Rate

Electronic fetal monitoring produces a continuous tracing of the FHR, which allows many characteristics of the FHR to be visually assessed. A growing number of physicians and nurses, however, are beginning to question the widespread use of this technology. Although fetuses who are monitored continuously have a reduction in seizures, there is no reduction in cerebral palsy, newborn/infant mortality, or adverse neonatal outcomes. The incidence of cesarean sections and operative deliveries are higher when continuous fetal monitoring is used (King et al., 2019).

Indications for Electronic Monitoring

If one or more of the following factors are present, the FHR and contractions are monitored electronically:

- Previous history of a stillbirth at 38 or more weeks of gestation
- Presence of a complication of pregnancy (e.g., preeclampsia, placenta previa, abruptio placentae, multiple gestation, and prolonged or premature rupture of membranes)
- Induction of labor (labor that is begun as a result of some type of intervention [e.g., an IV infusion of oxytocin])
- Preterm labor
- Decreased fetal movement
- Nonreassuring fetal status
- Meconium staining of amniotic fluid (meconium has been released into the amniotic fluid by the fetus, which may indicate a problem)
- Trial of labor following a previous cesarean birth (Cunningham et al., 2018)
- Maternal fever
- Placental problems.

Methods of Electronic Monitoring

External monitoring of the fetus is usually accomplished by ultrasound. A transducer, which emits continuous sound waves, is placed on the maternal abdomen. When placed correctly, the sound waves bounce off the fetal heart and are picked up by the electronic monitor. The actual moment-by-moment FHR is displayed graphically on a screen (**Figure 33.48** ›). In some instances, the monitor may track the maternal heart rate instead of the FHR. However, the nurse can avoid this error by comparing the maternal pulse to the FHR.

Recent advances in technology have led to the development of new ambulatory methods of external monitoring. Using a telemetry system, a small, battery-operated transducer transmits signals to a receiver connected to the monitor.

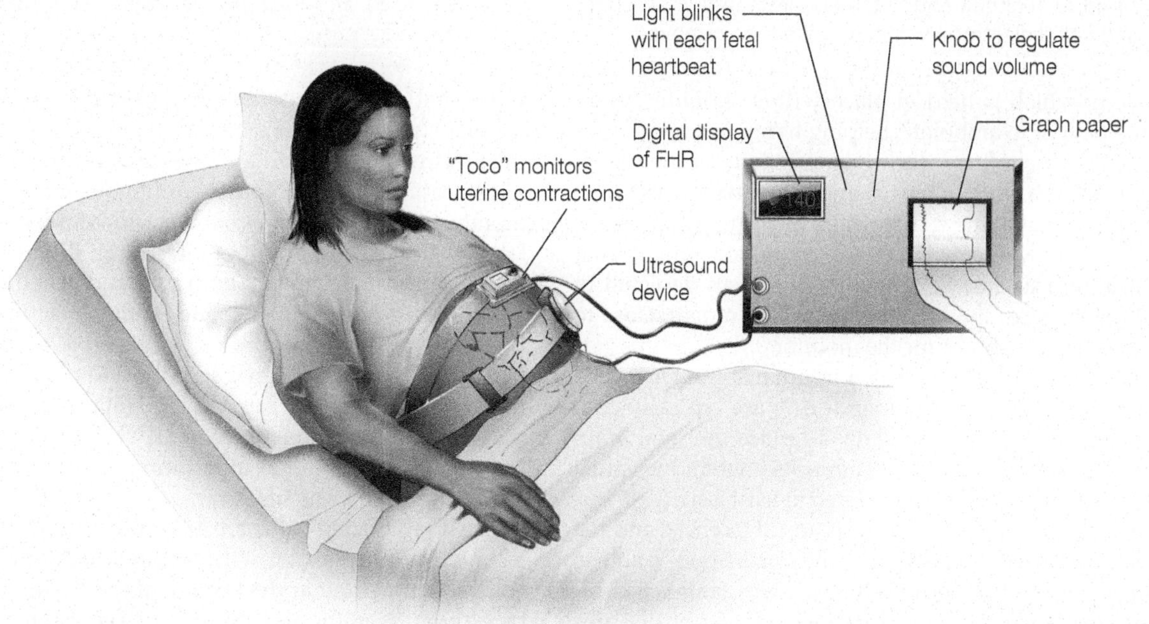

Figure 33.48 › Electronic fetal monitoring by external technique. The ultrasound device, placed over the fetal back, transmits information on the FHR. Information from both the tocodynamometer and ultrasound device is transmitted to the electronic fetal monitor. The FHR is indicated in four ways: on the digital display, as a blinking light, by sound, and on special monitor paper. The uterine contractions are displayed on the graph paper.

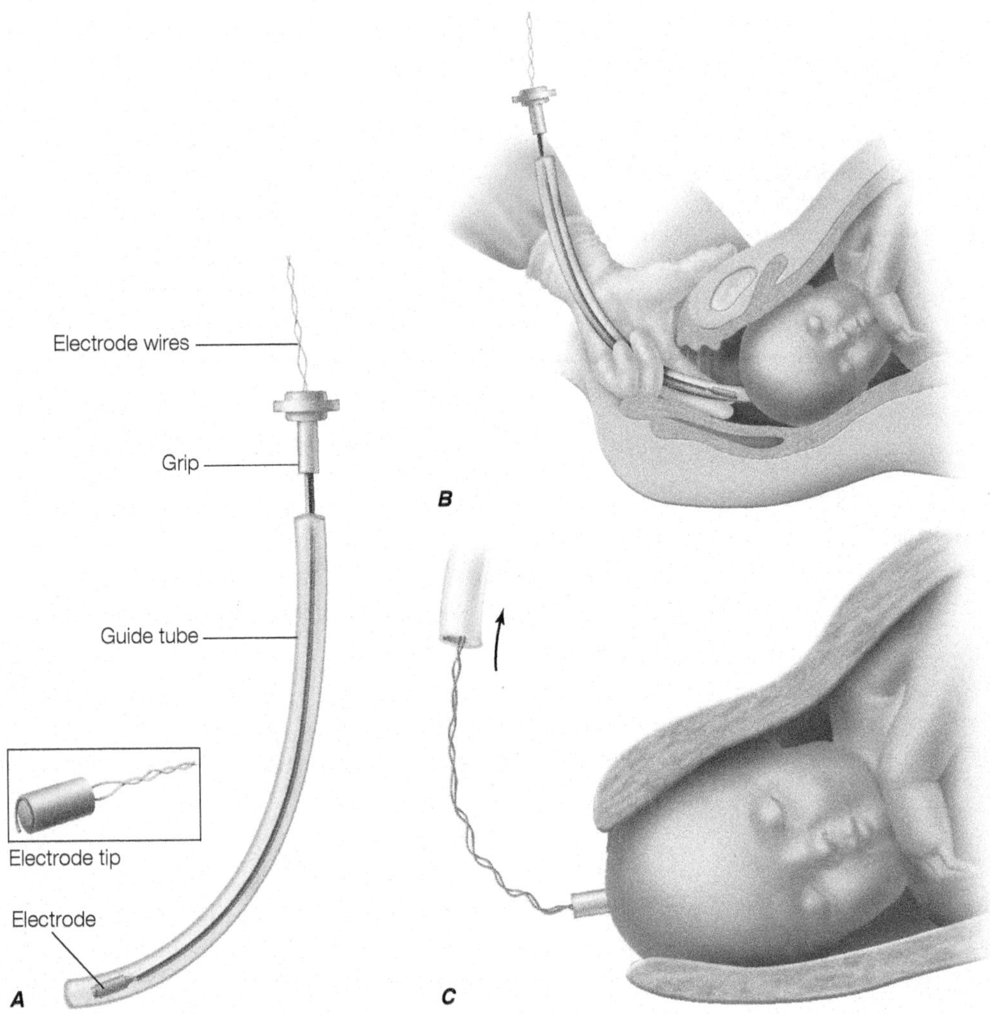

Figure 33.49 ›› Technique for internal, direct fetal monitoring. ***A***, Spiral electrode. ***B***, Attaching the spiral electrode to the scalp. ***C***, Attached spiral electrode with the guide tube removed.

This system, which is held in place with a shoulder strap, allows the patient to ambulate, helping her to feel more comfortable and less confined during labor. Many of the newer models can also be worn in the tub and can be completely submerged in water, making a more natural birthing experience possible even for women who require continuous monitoring for medical indications. In contrast, the system depicted in Figure 33.51 requires the laboring woman to remain close to the electrical power source for the monitor.

Internal monitoring requires an internal spiral electrode. Women who require internal monitoring are typically confined to bed and cannot ambulate. To place the fetal scalp electrode on the fetal occiput, the amniotic membranes must be ruptured, the cervix must be dilated at least 2 cm (0.08 in.), the presenting part must be down against the cervix, and the presenting part must be known (i.e., the nurse must be able to detect the actual part of the fetus that is down against the cervix). If all these factors are present, the labor and birth nurse (if specialty training has been completed), physician, or CNM inserts a sterile internal spiral electrode into the vagina and places it against the fetal head. The spiral electrode is rotated clockwise until it is attached to the scalp. It is essential not to place the electrode over the eye or a fontanel, so the fetal position must be determined before a scalp electrode is applied. Wires that extend from the spiral electrode are attached to a leg plate (placed on the woman's thigh) and then attached to the electronic fetal monitor. This method of monitoring the FHR provides more accurate continuous data than external monitoring because the signal is clearer and movement of the fetus or the woman does not interrupt it (**Figure 33.49 ››**).

Internal monitoring has both risks and benefits. It provides a more accurate fetal tracing and is more effective in monitoring the fetal status. In rare cases, the scalp electrode can be placed on the fetal fontanel or, if the fetus is in a face presentation, on an eye, thus causing fetal injury. Women with certain medical conditions, such as HIV infection, should not be monitored with internal monitoring because it can increase the risk of viral transmission.

The FHR tracing at the top of **Figure 33.50 ››** was obtained by internal monitoring with a spiral electrode; the uterine contraction tracing at the bottom of the figure was obtained by external monitoring with a toco. Note that the FHR is variable (the tracing moves up and down instead of in a straight line). In Figure 33.50, each dark vertical line represents 1 minute; therefore, contractions are occurring about every 2.5 to 3 minutes. The FHR is evaluated by assessing an electronic monitor tracing for baseline rate, baseline variability, and periodic changes.

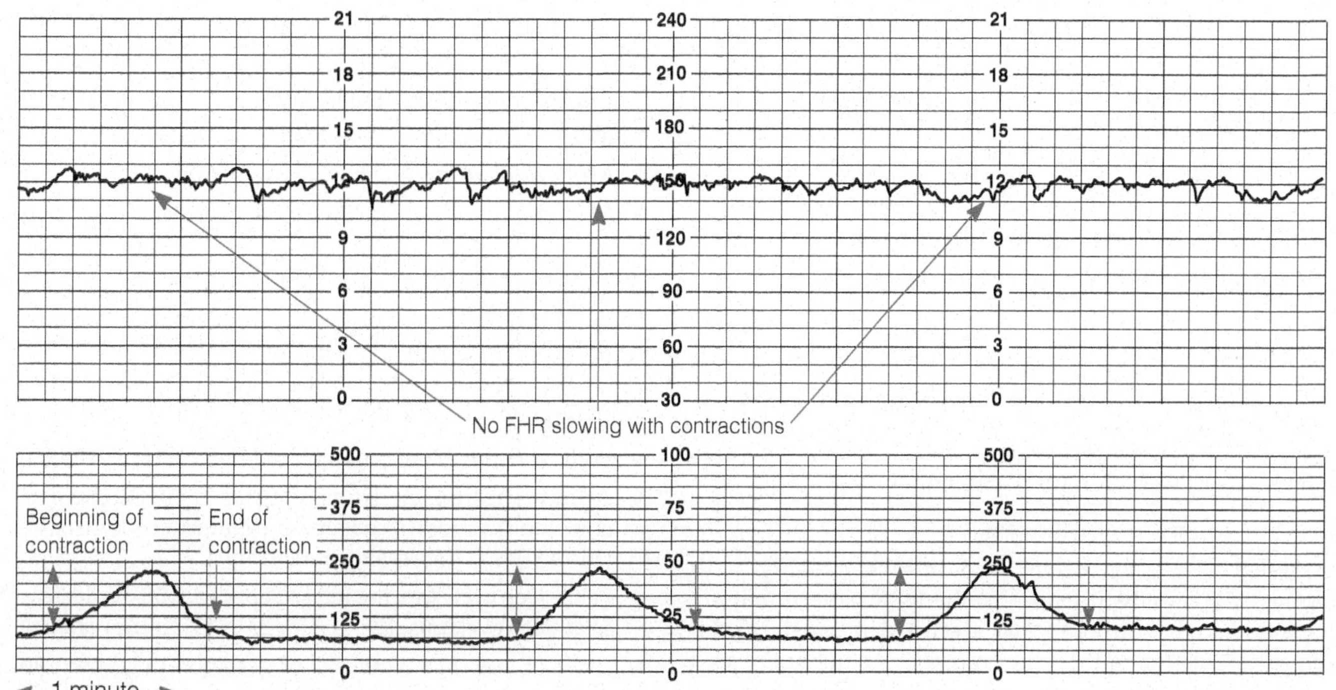

Figure 33.50 » Normal FHR range is from 110 to 160 beats/min. The FHR tracing in the upper portion of the graph indicates an FHR range of 140 to 155 beats/min. The bottom portion depicts uterine contractions. Each dark vertical line marks 1 minute, and each small rectangle represents 10 seconds. The contraction frequency is about every 2.5 minutes, and the duration of the contractions is 50 to 60 seconds.

Baseline Fetal Heart Rate

The **baseline fetal heart rate** refers to the average FHR rounded to increments of 5 beats/min observed during a 10-minute period of monitoring. This excludes periodic or episodic changes, periods of marked variability, and segments of the baseline that differ by more than 25 beats/min. The duration should be at least 2 minutes (King et al., 2019; Menihan & Kopel, 2014). Normal FHR (baseline rate) ranges from 110 to 160 beats/min. There are two abnormal variations of the baseline rate—those above 160 beats/min (tachycardia) and those below 110 beats/min (bradycardia). Another change affecting the baseline is called **baseline fetal heart rate variability**, which is fluctuation in the FHR baseline of two cycles per minute or greater, with irregular amplitude and inconstant frequency (Cunningham et al., 2018; King et al., 2019).

A *wandering baseline* fluctuates between 120 and 160 beats/min in an unsteady wandering pattern and can be associated with neurologic impairment of the fetus or a preterminal event (Cunningham et al., 2018; King et al., 2019). Possible causes for this pattern include congenital anomalies or metabolic acidosis. Immediate interventions are needed to enhance fetal oxygenation and preparation for an emergent operative birth should be made (King et al., 2019).

Fetal tachycardia is a sustained rate of 161 beats/min or above. Marked tachycardia is 180 beats/min or above. Causes of tachycardia include the following (Cunningham et al., 2018):

- Early fetal hypoxia, which leads to stimulation of the sympathetic system as the fetus compensates for reduced blood flow
- Maternal fever, which accelerates the metabolism of the fetus
- Maternal dehydration
- Beta-sympathomimetic drugs, such as ritodrine, terbutaline, atropine, and isoxsuprine, which have a cardiac stimulant effect
- Chorioamnionitis (fetal tachycardia may be the first sign of a developing intrauterine infection)
- Maternal hyperthyroidism (thyroid-stimulating hormones may cross the placenta and stimulate FHR)
- Fetal anemia (the heart rate is increased as a compensatory mechanism to improve tissue perfusion)
- Tachydysrhythmias (fetal dysrhythmias occur in less than 1% of all pregnancies).

Tachycardia is considered to be an ominous sign if it is accompanied by late decelerations, severe variable decelerations, or decreased variability. If tachycardia is associated with maternal fever, treatment may consist of antipyretics and/or antibiotics.

Fetal bradycardia is a rate of less than 110 beats/min during a 10-minute period or longer. Causes of fetal bradycardia include the following (Cunningham et al., 2018):

- Late (profound) fetal hypoxia (depression of myocardial activity)
- Maternal hypotension, which results in decreased blood flow to the fetus
- Prolonged umbilical cord compression (fetal baroreceptors are activated by cord compression, and this produces vagal stimulation, which results in decreased FHR)

- Fetal arrhythmia, which is associated with complete heart block in the fetus
- Uterine tachysystole
- Abruptio placentae
- Uterine rupture
- Vagal stimulation in the second stage (because this does not involve hypoxia, the fetus can recover)
- Congenital heart block
- Maternal hypothermia.

Bradycardia may be a benign or an ominous (preterminal) sign. If there is variability, the bradycardia is considered to be benign. Bradycardia accompanied by decreased variability and late decelerations is considered to be ominous and a sign of nonreassuring fetal status (Cunningham et al., 2018).

Arrhythmias and Dysrhythmias

Arrhythmias, a term often used interchangeably with *dysrhythmias*, are disturbances in the FHR pattern that are not associated with abnormal electrical impulse formation or conduction in the fetal cardiac tissue but are related to a structural abnormality or congenital heart disease. Fetal arrhythmias may be detected when listening to the FHR on a fetal monitor. It is important to rule out artifacts or electrical interference, which may occur. Most true arrhythmias are accompanied by baseline bradycardia, baseline tachycardia, or an abrupt baseline spiking. Most arrythmias are benign, with only about 10% requiring consultation with a cardiologist (King et al., 2019; Miller, Miller, & Cypher, 2017).

Variability

Baseline variability is a measure of the interplay (the push–pull effect) between the sympathetic and parasympathetic nervous systems. Baseline variability is fluctuations in the FHR of two cycles per minute or greater. **Figure 33.51 ››** depicts the different ranges of variability. The amplitudes of the peaks and troughs in beats per minute are defined as follows (King et al., 2019; Papadakis, McPhee, & Rabow, 2014):

- ***Absent:*** amplitude undetectable
- ***Minimal:*** amplitude detectable but less than 5 beats/min
- ***Moderate:*** amplitude 6 to 25 beats/min
- ***Marked:*** amplitude greater than 25 beats/min.

Reduced variability is the best single predictor for determining fetal compromise (Cunningham et al., 2018). Fetal acidosis and subsequent hypoxia are highest in fetuses that have absent or minimal variability.

Causes of decreased variability include the following (Cunningham et al., 2018):

- Hypoxia and acidosis (decreased blood flow to the fetus)
- Administration of drugs such as meperidine hydrochloride (Demerol), diazepam (Valium), or hydroxyzine (Vistaril) that depress the fetal CNS
- Fetal sleep cycle (during fetal sleep, variability is decreased; fetal sleep cycles usually last for 20 to 40 minutes each hour)
- Fetus of less than 32 weeks of gestation (fetal neurologic control of heart rate is immature)
- Fetal dysrhythmias
- Fetal anomalies affecting the heart, CNS, or autonomic nervous system
- Previous neurologic insult
- Tachycardia.

Marked variability is rare and believed to be a result of temporary fetal hypoxia (King et al., 2019). Absent variability that does not appear to be associated with a fetal sleep cycle or the administration of drugs is a warning sign of nonreassuring fetal status. It is especially ominous if absent or minimal variability is accompanied by late decelerations (explained shortly). If decreased variability is noted on

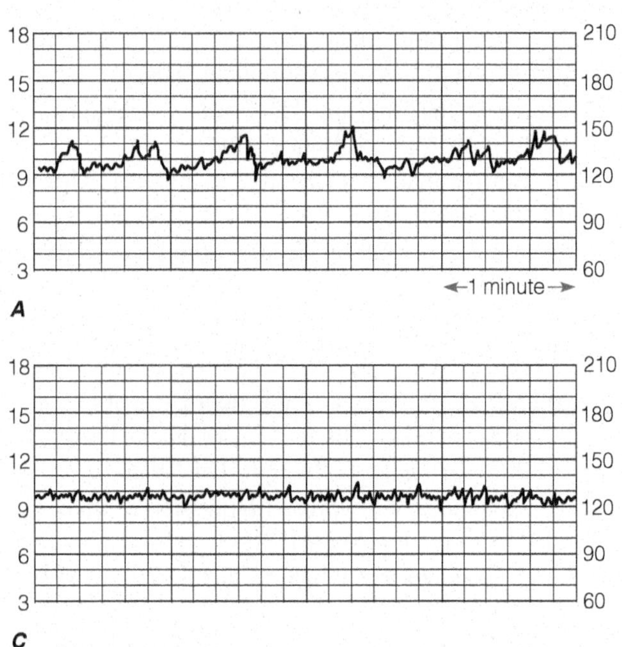

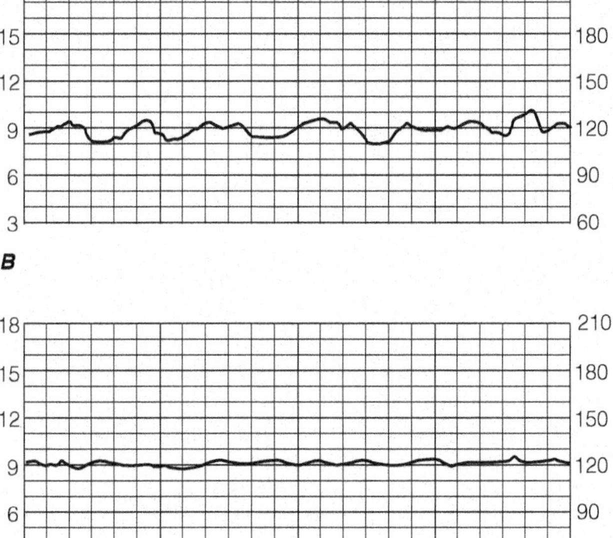

Figure 33.51 ›› Variability. ***A***, Marked variability. ***B***, Moderate variability. ***C***, Minimal variability. ***D***, Absent variability.

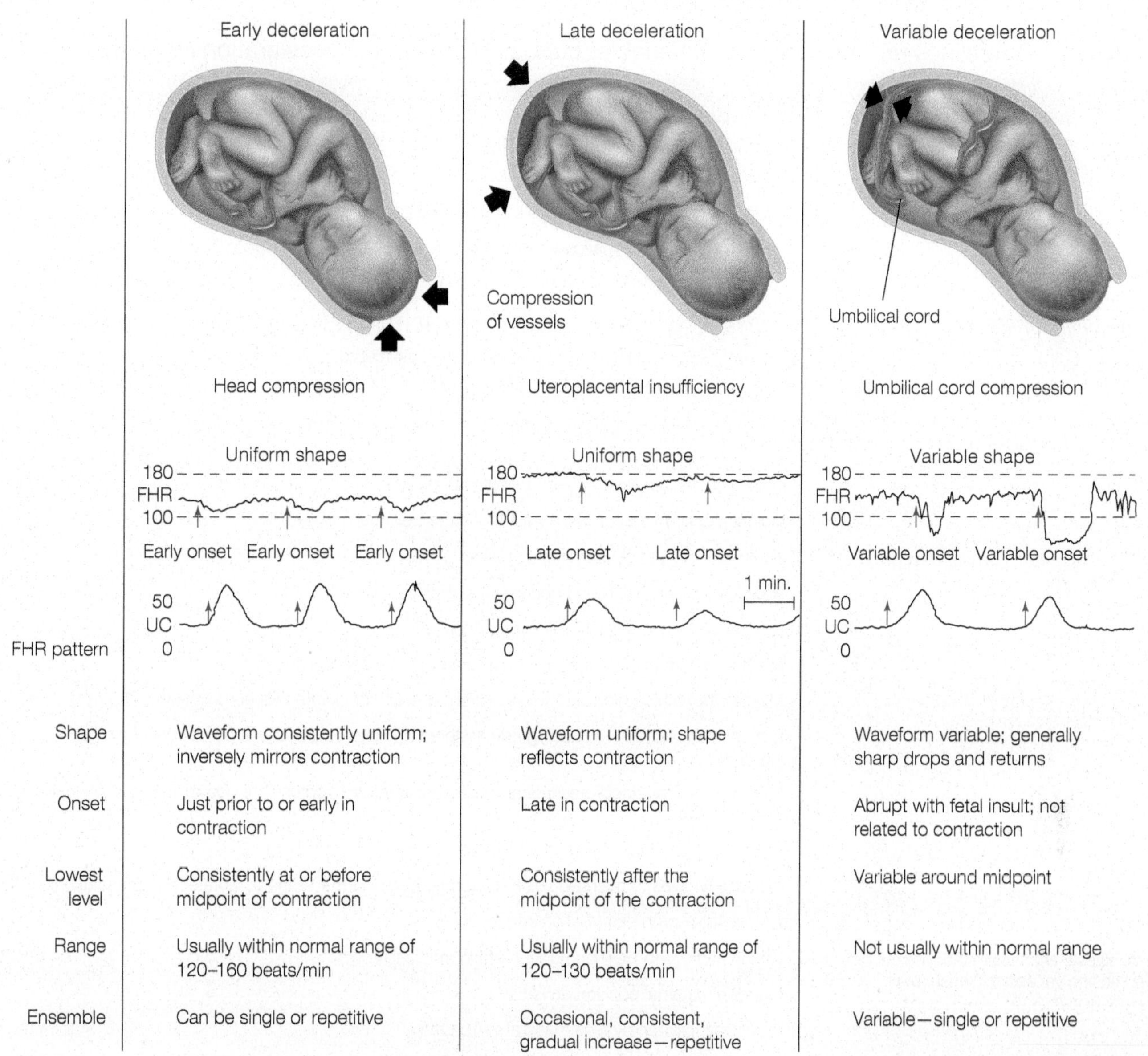

Figure 33.52 ›› Types and characteristics of early, late, and variable decelerations.

monitoring, consider application of a spiral electrode to obtain more accurate information.

Accelerations

Accelerations are transient increases in the FHR normally caused by fetal movement. When the fetus moves, its heart rate increases, just as the heart rates of adults increase during exercise. Often, accelerations accompany uterine contractions, usually because the fetus moves in response to the pressure of the contractions. Accelerations of this type are thought to be a sign of fetal well-being and adequate oxygen reserve. The accelerations with fetal movement are the basis for NSTs.

Decelerations

Decelerations, periodic decreases in FHR from baseline, are categorized as early, late, and variable. This categorization is based on the pattern and timing of the decelerations in the contraction cycle (**Figure 33.52 ››**). See **Table 33.13 ››** for nursing interventions for each deceleration pattern.

When the fetal head is compressed, cerebral blood flow is decreased, which leads to central vagal stimulation and results in early deceleration. The onset of early deceleration is associated with the onset of the uterine contraction. This type of deceleration is of uniform shape, is usually considered to be benign, and does not require intervention.

SAFETY ALERT The presence of repetitive early decelerations may be a sign of advanced dilation or the beginning of the second stage of labor (King et al., 2019). If the monitoring strip shows recurring early decelerations, ask the laboring woman whether she is experiencing any pressure. Pressure that occurs only with the contractions typically indicates advanced dilation. Intense pressure that does not change or ease up when the contractions cease may indicate the beginning of the second stage. A vaginal examination may be performed to establish the amount of dilation.

TABLE 33.13 Guidelines for Management of Variable, Late, and Prolonged Deceleration Patterns

Pattern	Nursing Interventions
Variable decelerations (Cause: umbilical cord compression)	Report findings to HCP and document in medical record. Provide explanation to woman and partner.
Isolated or occasional, moderate	Change maternal position to one in which FHR pattern is most improved. Perform vaginal examination to assess for prolapsed cord or change in labor progress. Monitor FHR continuously to assess current status and for further changes in FHR pattern.
Variable decelerations, severe and uncorrectable (Cause: umbilical cord compression)	Administer oxygen by face mask at 7–10 L/min. Report findings to HCP and document in medical record. Provide explanation to woman and partner. Prepare for probable cesarean birth. Follow interventions listed previously. Prepare for vaginal birth unless baseline variability is decreasing or FHR is progressively rising, in which case cesarean, forceps, or vacuum birth is indicated. Maintain good hydration with IV fluids (normal saline or lactated Ringer solution).
Late decelerations (Cause: uteroplacental insufficiency)	Administer oxygen by face mask at 7–10 L/min. Report findings to HCP and document in medical record. Provide explanation to woman and partner. Monitor for further FHR changes. Maintain maternal position on left side. Maintain good hydration with IV fluids (normal saline or lactated Ringer solution). Discontinue oxytocin if it is being administered and late decelerations persist despite other interventions. Monitor maternal blood pressure and pulse for signs of hypotension; possibly treat with increased flow rate of IV fluids. Follow orders of HCP for treatment for hypotension, if present. Increase IV fluids to maintain volume and hydration (normal saline or lactated Ringer solution). Assess labor progress (dilation and station).
Late decelerations with tachycardia or decreasing variability (Cause: uteroplacental insufficiency)	Report findings to HCP and document in medical record. Maintain maternal position on left side. Administer oxygen by face mask at 7–10 L/min. Discontinue oxytocin if it is being administered. Assess maternal blood pressure and pulse. Increase IV fluids (normal saline or lactated Ringer solution). Assess labor progress (dilation and station). Prepare for immediate cesarean delivery. Explain plan of treatment to woman and partner. Assist HCP with fetal blood sampling, if ordered.
Prolonged decelerations (Cause: multiple issues that result in prolonged impaired perfusion)	Perform vaginal examination to rule out prolapsed cord or to determine progress in labor status. Change maternal position as needed to try to alleviate decelerations. Discontinue oxytocin if it is being administered. Notify HCP of findings/initial interventions and document in medical record. Provide explanation to woman and partner. Increase IV fluids (normal saline or lactated Ringer solution). Administer tocolytic if hypertonus noted and if ordered by HCP. Anticipate normal FHR recovery following deceleration if FHR previously normal. Anticipate intervention if FHR previously abnormal or deceleration lasts > 3 minutes.

Source: From London et al. (2017). Pearson Education, Inc., Hoboken, NJ.

Late deceleration is caused by uteroplacental insufficiency resulting from decreased blood flow and oxygen transfer to the fetus through the intervillous spaces during uterine contractions. The most common causes of late decelerations are maternal hypotension resulting from the administration of epidural anesthesia and uterine tachysystole associated with oxytocin infusion (King et al., 2019). The onset of the deceleration occurs after the onset of a uterine contraction and is of a uniform shape that tends to reflect associated uterine contractions. The late deceleration pattern is considered to be a nonreassuring sign and requires continuous assessment. If late decelerations continue and birth is not imminent, a cesarean delivery may be indicated.

Variable decelerations occur if the umbilical cord becomes compressed, reducing blood flow between the placenta and fetus. The resulting increase in peripheral resistance in the fetal circulation causes fetal HTN. Fetal HTN stimulates the baroreceptors in the aortic arch and carotid sinuses, slowing the FHR. The onset of variable decelerations differs in timing with the onset of the contraction, and the decelerations are variable in shape. This pattern requires further assessment.

A sinusoidal pattern appears similar to a waveform. The characteristics of this pattern include absence of variability and the presence of a smooth, wavelike shape. The pattern resembles a perfect letter "S" lying on its side. These patterns can be pseudosinusoidal (benign) or true sinusoidal. The true pattern is associated with Rh alloimmunization, fetal anemia, severe fetal hypoxia, umbilical cord occlusion, twin-to-twin transfusion, or a chronic fetal bleed. Pseudosinusoidal patterns are associated with medications such as meperidine (Demerol) or butorphanol tartrate (Stadol) (King et al., 2019).

Decelerations are also classified based on the rate in which the FHR leaves the baseline FHR:

- ***Abrupt decelerations*** occur in less than 30 seconds (King et al., 2019)
- ***Variable decelerations*** descend abruptly.
- ***Gradual decelerations*** require 30 seconds or more to descend. Both early and late decelerations descend gradually (King et al., 2019).
- ***Episodic decelerations*** occur independently of the uterine contractions and are frequently the result of external stimulations, such as vaginal exams.
- ***Periodic decelerations*** refer to decelerations that occur with the contractions and are considered to be repetitive if they occur with 50% of the contractions (King et al., 2019).
- ***Prolonged decelerations*** are those that leave the baseline for more than 2 minutes but less than 10 minutes.

Evaluation of Fetal Heart Tracings

Evaluation of the electronic monitor tracing begins by looking at the uterine contraction pattern. To evaluate the contraction pattern, the nurse does the following:

1. Determine the uterine resting tone.
2. Assess the contractions: What is the frequency? What is the duration? What is the intensity?

The next step is to evaluate the FHR tracing as follows:

1. Determine the baseline: Is the baseline within the normal range? Is there evidence of tachycardia? Is there evidence of bradycardia?
2. Determine FHR variability: Is variability absent? Minimal? Moderate? Marked?
3. Determine whether a sinusoidal pattern is present.
4. Determine whether there are periodic changes: Are accelerations present? Do they meet the criteria for a reactive NST? Are decelerations present? Are they uniform in shape? If so, determine whether they are early or late decelerations. Are they nonuniform in shape? If so, determine whether they are variable decelerations.

After evaluating the FHR tracing for the factors just listed, the nurse may further classify the tracing as reassuring (normal) or nonreassuring (worrisome). Reassuring patterns contain normal parameters and do not require additional treatment or intervention. Characteristics of reassuring FHR patterns include the following:

- Baseline rate is 110 to 160 beats/min.
- Variability is moderate.
- Periodic patterns consist of accelerations with fetal movement, and early decelerations may be present.

Nonreassuring patterns may indicate that the fetus is becoming stressed and intervention is needed. Characteristics of nonreassuring patterns include the following:

- Severe variable decelerations (FHR drops below 70 beats/min for longer than 30 to 45 seconds and is accompanied by rising baseline or decreasing variability or slow return to baseline.)
- Late decelerations of any magnitude
- Absence of variability
- Prolonged deceleration (a deceleration that lasts 60–90 seconds or more)
- Severe (marked) bradycardia (FHR baseline of 70 beats/min or less).

Nonreassuring patterns may require continuous monitoring and more involved treatment and intervention (see Table 33.14).

After evaluating the FHR tracing for the factors listed, the nurse may categorize the tracing according to the Three-Tier Fetal Heart Rate Interpretation System shown in **Box 33.6** ». The three-tier system for the categorization of FHR patterns is recommended by ACOG, the Association of Women's Health, Obstetric, and Neonatal Nurses (AWHONN), and the National Institute of Child Health and Human Development (Lowdermilk et al., 2020). Categorization of the FHR tracing evaluates the fetus at that point in time; tracing patterns can and will change. An FHR tracing may move back and forth between categories depending on the clinical situation and management strategies employed.

- ***Category I FHR tracings are normal.*** They are strongly predictive of normal fetal acid–base status at the time of observation. The FHR tracings may be followed in a routine manner, and no specific action is required.

Box 33.6

The Three-Tier Fetal Heart Rate Interpretation System

Category I

Category I FHR tracings include *all* of the following:

- Baseline rate: 110–160 beats/min
- Baseline FHR variability: moderate
- Late or variable decelerations: absent
- Early decelerations: present or absent
- Accelerations: present or absent.

Category II

Category II FHR tracings include all FHR tracings not categorized as Category I or Category III. Category II tracings may represent an appreciable fraction of those encountered in clinical care. Examples of Category II FHR tracings include:

- Baseline rate
  - Bradycardia not accompanied by absent baseline variability
  - Tachycardia
- Baseline FHR variability
  - Minimal baseline variability
  - Absent baseline variability not accompanied by recurrent decelerations
  - Marked baseline variability
- Accelerations
  - Absence of induced accelerations after fetal stimulation
- Periodic or episodic decelerations
  - Recurrent variable decelerations accompanied by minimal or moderate baseline variability
  - Prolonged deceleration of 2 minutes or more but less than 10 minutes
  - Recurrent late decelerations with moderate baseline variability
  - Variable decelerations with other characteristics, such as slow return to baseline, "overshoots," or "shoulders."

Category III

Category III FHR tracings include:

- Absent baseline FHR variability and any of the following:
  - Recurrent late decelerations
  - Recurrent variable decelerations
  - Bradycardia
- Sinusoidal pattern.

Source: Data from American College of Obstetricians and Gynecologists (2009, reaffirmed 2013).

- ***Category II FHR tracings are indeterminate.*** They are not predictive of abnormal fetal acid–base status, yet there is insufficient evidence at present to classify these as Category I or Category III. Category II tracings require evaluation and continued surveillance and reevaluation, taking into account all of the associated clinical circumstances.
- ***Category III FHR tracings are abnormal.*** They are predictive of abnormal fetal acid–base status at the time of observation. They require prompt evaluation. Depending on the clinical situation, efforts to expeditiously resolve the abnormal FHR pattern may include, but are not limited to, provision of maternal oxygen, change in maternal position, discontinuation of labor stimulation, and treatment of maternal hypotension.

It is important to provide information to the laboring woman regarding the FHR pattern and the interventions that will help her fetus. Sharing information with the laboring woman reassures her that a potential or actual problem has been identified and that she is an active participant in the interventions. Occasionally, a problem arises that requires immediate intervention. In that case, the nurse can say something like "It is important for you to turn on your side right now because the baby is having a little difficulty. I'll explain what is happening in just a few moments." This type of response lets the woman know that although an action needs to be accomplished rapidly, information will soon be provided. In the haste to act quickly, the nurse must not forget that it is the woman's body and her baby.

Labor and birth nurses must be skilled and competent in evaluating electronic FHR patterns and responding appropriately (see Table 33.13). Competence can be maintained through frequent in-services, formal courses, and continuing education programs.

Response to Electronic Monitoring

Responses to electronic fetal monitoring can be varied and complex. Many women have little knowledge of monitoring unless they have attended a prenatal class that dealt with this subject. Some women react to electronic monitoring positively, viewing it as a reassurance that "the baby is okay." They may also feel the monitor helps identify problems that develop in labor. Other women may have ambivalent or even negative feelings about the monitor. They may think the monitor is interfering with a natural process and may not want the intrusion. They may resent the time and attention that the monitor requires—time that could otherwise be spent providing nursing care. Some women may find that the equipment, wires, and sounds increase their anxiety. The discomfort of lying in one position and fear of injury to the baby are other objections.

Diagnosis

Priorities for care include labor discomfort (especially pain related to contractions, cervical dilation, the birth process, and/or perineal trauma) and any fears or anxiety the woman and her family may have about the outcome of labor. In addition to fear, anxiety, and pain, nursing diagnoses may address family coping and the need for additional patient information and teaching. At all times, however, the nurse needs to be prepared to prioritize care based on the mother or baby's physiologic state.

Planning

When a plan of care is devised for the intrapartum period, the nurse can develop a general plan that encompasses the total process, from the beginning of labor through the fourth stage, or a plan can be developed for each stage of labor and birth. It is imperative that the nurse assess the couple's understanding of the labor process and provide brief explanations as labor progresses in accordance with the couple's learning needs. The overriding goal is to provide a safe environment for the mother and fetus. Additional goals for care may include:

- Support the mother and family by offering reassurance and information as needed throughout the labor and birth experience
- Promote maternal coping behaviors
- Provide comfort measures to promote pain relief as needed
- Acknowledge and support the mother's desires and choices throughout labor, whenever possible
- Create an environment that is sensitive and supportive of the biophysical, psychosocial, spiritual, and cultural needs of the mother and her family.

Labor can be both an exciting and anxiety-producing time for the mother and her family. Feelings of ambivalence are relatively common as the laboring mother and her partner or support person experience a variety of assessments, care activities, and technologies. Orienting the mother and her family to what to expect can promote feelings of well-being during the labor and birth process (see Patient Teaching: What to Expect During Labor).

Implementation

In most cases, the woman and any support people arrive for admission when the woman is in early labor and there is time for patient education. Some patients, however, will not arrive until birth is imminent. In those instances, the nurse acts to:

- Promote safety of mother and baby
- Provide information about what is happening as it occurs
- Promote maternal and family coping and comfort.

Integrate Cultural Beliefs

Nurses who provide care for pregnant, laboring, and postpartum mothers will have the opportunity to care for women from a variety of cultural and religious backgrounds. Providing culturally competent care is essential to promoting positive outcomes for both mother and baby, to ensuring patient and family satisfaction with the experience, and to reducing any cultural barriers or stigma that might create distrust between the woman or her family and the healthcare team.

Modesty

Regardless of culture, modesty is an important consideration for most women. Many women from a variety of backgrounds find it uncomfortable to be physically examined, so respecting the need for privacy with draping, asking the woman if she would like family members to leave the room, or making other accommodations as needed should be done whenever possible. Some women may be uncomfortable when men are present; others may be uncomfortable with exposure regardless of the sex of the HCPs. It is prudent to assume that embarrassment will occur with exposure and take measures to provide privacy rather than to assume that it will not matter to the woman if she is exposed.

When a woman identifies a cultural or religious preference, it is important to ask questions to gain a specific understanding of what that means to her and how she sees it impacting her care needs. For example, according to the Orthodox Jewish law of *Tznuit*, women should maintain modesty in order

Patient Teaching

What to Expect During Labor

- Provide information on the basic assessment and care activities. Allow time for questions and discussion as the progress of labor permits. Describe aspects of the admission process, including the following:
  - Taking an abbreviated history
  - Physical assessment (maternal vital signs [VS], FHR, contraction status, status of membranes)
  - Assessment of uterine contractions (frequency, duration, intensity)
  - Orientation to surroundings
  - Introductions to other support staff
  - Determination of woman's and any support person's expectations of the nurse.
- Present aspects of ongoing physical care, such as when to expect assessment of maternal VS, FHR, and contractions.
- If an electronic fetal monitor is used, describe how it works and the information it provides. Demonstrate the fetal monitor. Orient the woman to the sights and sounds of the monitor. Explain what "normal" data will look like and what characteristics are being watched for.
- Note that assessments will increase as the labor progresses, especially during the transition phase (usually the time the woman would like to be left alone), to help keep the mother and baby safe by noting deviations from the normal course.
- Describe the vaginal examination and the information it elicits. Use a cervical dilation chart to illustrate the amount of dilation.
- Review comfort techniques that may be used in labor and ascertain what the woman thinks will promote comfort. Focus on open discussion.
- Review the childbirth preparations the woman has learned so that you will be able to support her in their use. Ask the woman to demonstrate the techniques she has learned.
- Review comfort and support measures, such as positioning, back rub, touch, distraction techniques, and ambulation.
- If the woman is in early labor, offer her a tour of the birthing area and explain equipment and routines. Include the woman's partner.

to preserve dignity. For some women, this may be accomplished by providing a long-sleeved gown that covers her elbows and knees, whereas other Orthodox Jewish women may voice no preferences. It is important that the nurse balances knowledge of cultural and religious beliefs with verbal or behavioral cues that support a woman's preferences. The nurse offering to pull the curtain while a woman changes into her patient gown shows understanding that some women prefer not to change in front of their husbands. Women who do not adhere to this belief then have a chance to decline, allowing the nurse to better understand their preferences (Lutwak, Ney, & White, 2020).

Expression and Meaning of Pain

Different cultures also have differing beliefs about the meaning and value of labor pain. As in all cultures, beliefs that were strongly held by one generation may change over time. In the past, many Native American women viewed labor pain as natural and many used meditation, self-control, or indigenous plants or herbs throughout their labor to aid them during birth. Many of these practices go unrecognized by the government-provided Indian Health Services, creating a disconnect between cultural traditions and medical care. Although some Native American women may prefer more modern approaches to pain relief, many seek a return to traditional childbirth practices or to combine them with modern medical care (Gilger, 2019).

Labor and delivery nurses can provide culturally competent care by becoming acquainted with the beliefs and practices of the various subcultures while assessing each woman for her own unique preferences within a cultural context. In the birthing situation, the truly effective nurse supports the family's cultural practices as long as it is safe to do so. See Focus on Diversity and Culture: Childbirth Customs.

Provide Nursing Care on Admission

The manner in which the maternity nurse greets the laboring woman and her partner influences the course of the woman's hospital stay. The arrival at the healthcare setting and the sometimes impersonal and technical aspects of admission can produce profound stress, fear, and anxiety. If women and their families are greeted in a brusque, harried manner, they are less likely to look to the nurse for support. A calm, pleasant manner indicates to the woman that she is important. It helps to instill in the couple a sense of confidence in the staff's ability to provide quality care during this critical time.

Following the initial greeting, the nurse escorts the woman and support person to the birthing room and provides a quick yet thorough orientation to the facility, including the location of the restrooms, waiting area, and nurse-call or emergency-call system. These simple steps can go a long way toward helping the couple feel more at ease. The nurse also explains the monitoring equipment or other unfamiliar technology. Every effort needs to be made to demystify the environment for the laboring woman and her support person. Some women prefer that their partner remain with them during the admission process, although others prefer to have the partner wait outside.

As the nurse helps the woman undress and get into a hospital gown, development of rapport and the assessment process begins. The experienced labor and birth nurse can obtain essential information about the woman and her pregnancy,

Focus on Diversity and Culture

Childbirth Customs

Various cultures have different customs and beliefs surrounding childbearing and childbirth. Generalizations regarding cultural perspectives are discussed with examples designed to provide students with ways to integrate cultural customs into specific individualized labor and birth options for women. Always, the nurse should ask the woman about her own cultural beliefs and obtain specific requests for labor positioning, ambulation in labor, who she would like to provide labor support, preferred birth positions, and temperature of oral fluids. The nurse should advise the laboring woman that a regular diet with her own food preferences can begin immediately following a vaginal birth.

Some Vietnamese women may prefer to walk during labor and to give birth in a squatting position. Like many people from other Asian cultures, some may view labor as a "hot condition" and prefer cold beverages. However, during the postpartum period, which some view as a "cold" condition, they may prefer warm liquids (Kim, 2017). In some cultures, praising a newborn is referred to as the "evil eye" and has negative connotations (Lowdermilk et al., 2020).

Some Latina women desire to have their partners present during labor and birth to show their love and to speak using affectionate words. It is also common for the maternal grandmother to be present in the delivery room (Lowdermilk et. al., 2020). Again, knowledge of traditional cultural norms can help the nurse effectively coordinate care for the woman and her family. Cultural norms should guide, not dictate, the assessment process.

Some Muslim women may have their husband present, whereas others may desire to have a female friend or relative with them during childbirth. Because modesty is of great concern for many Muslim women, care must be taken to cover the woman as much as possible (Spector, 2017). Some women may want to put their *khimar* (head covering) on before a male enters the room. For some Muslim families, it may be important for a female nurse, physician, or CNM to perform examinations when possible. For women who express a preference for female HCPs, it is important to discuss the possibility that a female provider may not always be present and that if a male is required, every effort to provide privacy and advanced notice will be given (Davidson et al., 2020).

Many Orthodox Jewish women observe the law of *niddah*, which requires that couples cease physical contact at the onset of regular uterine contractions or the appearance of bloody show or membrane rupture (Lutwak et al., 2020). The couple may opt for verbal contact and the mother may choose to have another woman present for support (Lutwak et al., 2020). During this time period, the father may provide verbal encouragement and read prayers while in the delivery room or choose not to observe the birth and wait to return to the room until after the woman has completed the third stage of labor and has been assisted in resuming a comfortable position in bed.

initiate any immediate interventions needed, and establish individualized priorities and preferences within a few minutes after admission. Forming realistic objectives for laboring women is a major challenge for nurses because each woman has different coping mechanisms and support systems.

Laboring women often face a number of unfamiliar procedures that may seem routine for HCPs. It is important to remember that all patients have the right to accept or reject care measures. The patient's informed consent is needed before any procedure that involves touching her body. The admission process, therefore, includes signing an informed consent for treatment and providing information regarding advance directives. Typically, an identification bracelet and an allergy band are attached to the expectant woman's wrist.

Laboring families have specific expectations of the labor and birth experience, of themselves, of the nurse, and of the physician or CNM. Sometimes, families have unrealistic expectations, which can increase anxiety, create stress, and end in disappointment if expectations are not met. The nurse should encourage all families to discuss their preferences and special requests. Some families may present to the birthing center with a birth plan. Reviewing the plan provides the nurse with the opportunity to explore the family's wishes. If requests cannot be met, explain the reasons thoroughly. All members of the healthcare team need to be informed of the family's requests.

Some families want the nurse present at all times, whereas others desire privacy and want to spend time alone. Couples may want a great deal of support if they have not attended childbirth education classes or if they are anxious. Others may want to enjoy the experience as a couple, with as few outside interruptions as possible. In this case, the nurse informs the couple of the nurse's availability and of the need to make intermittent assessments.

If indicated, the nurse assists the woman into bed. A side-lying or semi-Fowler position rather than a supine position is most comfortable and prevents supine hypotensive syndrome (vena caval syndrome). After obtaining the essential information from the patient and her records, the nurse begins the intrapartum assessment. Once the assessment is complete, the nurse can make effective nursing decisions about intrapartum care, including the following:

- Should ambulation, bedrest, or a combination of the two be encouraged?
- Is more frequent or continuous electronic fetal monitoring needed?
- What preferences does the woman have for her labor and birth?
- Is a support person available?
- What special needs do this woman and her partner have?

The nurse auscultates the FHR. The nurse assesses the woman's blood pressure, pulse, respirations, oral temperature, and level of pain or discomfort. The nurse also assesses contraction frequency, duration, and intensity (possibly while gathering other data). Before the vaginal examination, the nurse informs the woman about the procedure and its purpose and obtains her consent; afterward, the nurse conveys the findings.

If signs of advanced labor are observed, a vaginal examination must be done immediately upon admission. If the woman shows signs of excessive bleeding or reports episodes of painless bleeding in the last trimester, refrain from performing a vaginal examination and notify the HCP immediately.

Results of the FHR assessment, uterine contraction evaluation, and vaginal examination help determine whether the rest of the admission process can proceed at a leisurely pace or whether additional interventions are required. For example, an FHR of less than 110 beats/min on auscultation indicates that a fetal monitor should be applied immediately to obtain additional data and that continuous fetal monitoring should be performed. The patient's vital signs can be assessed once the monitor is in place.

SAFETY ALERT If the fetal monitor is no longer recording the fetal heart tracing, check for adequate gel under the transducer and reposition it before assuming there is a problem with the fetus. Maternal and fetal movement are the most common causes of an inability to trace the FHR.

The admission process includes collecting a clean, voided, midstream urine specimen. The woman with intact membranes may collect her specimen in the bathroom. Decisions regarding activity level are generally based on physical findings, clinician orders, the patient's desires, agency policy, and safety concerns.

The nurse may test the woman's urine for the presence of protein, ketones, and glucose by using a dipstick before sending the sample to the laboratory. This procedure is especially important if edema or elevated blood pressure is noted on admission. Proteinuria of +1 or more may be a sign of impending preeclampsia. Glycosuria is frequently found in pregnant women because of the increased GFR in the proximal tubules and the inability of these tubules to increase reabsorption of glucose. It may also be associated with gestational diabetes, however, and should not be discounted. While the woman is collecting the urine specimen, the nurse can gather the equipment for any preparation procedures ordered by the HCP.

Laboratory tests are done during early admission. Hemoglobin and hematocrit values help determine the oxygen-carrying capacity of the circulatory system and the woman's ability to withstand blood loss at birth. Elevation of the hematocrit may indicate hemoconcentration of blood, which occurs with edema or dehydration. A low hemoglobin value, in the absence of other evidence of bleeding, suggests anemia. Blood may be typed and crossmatched if the woman is in a high-risk category. Platelets are evaluated as well because low platelets can lead to bleeding problems. Low platelets are also a contraindication for epidural anesthesia. In addition, a type and screen is performed in case an obstetric emergency arises and the woman needs to receive blood products. Additional serologic testing may be performed as indicated, such as HIV testing if the mother was not previously screened (Lowdermilk et al., 2020).

Depending on how rapidly labor is progressing, the nurse notifies the HCP before or after completing the admission procedures. The report includes the following information:

- Parity
- Cervical dilation and effacement

- Station
- Presenting part
- Status of the membranes
- Contraction pattern
- FHR
- Vital signs that are not in the normal range
- Any significant prenatal history
- Woman's birth preferences
- Woman's reaction to labor
- Woman's preferences for pain relief.

The nurse also enters an admission note into the medical record. The admission note should include the reason for admission, the date and time of the woman's arrival and notification of the HCP, the condition of the woman and her baby, and labor and membrane status.

Nursing Care During the First Stage of Labor

The nurse needs to evaluate physical parameters of the woman and her fetus. Maternal temperature is monitored every 2 to 4 hours unless the temperature is over 37.5°C (99.6°F), in which case it is taken every hour. When the amniotic membranes have ruptured, maternal temperature is assessed every 1 to 2 hours, depending on the policy of the institution. Blood pressure, pulse, respirations, and response to pain are monitored as indicated or according to unit policy. If the woman's blood pressure is greater than or equal to 140/90 mmHg or her pulse is more than 100 beats/min, the nurse must notify the HCP and reevaluate the blood pressure and pulse more frequently. Monitor the woman's pain level continually because increased pain can elevate the blood pressure and pulse, especially during contractions.

The nurse palpates uterine contractions for frequency, intensity, and duration every 30 minutes. The nurse also auscultates the FHR every 30 minutes in active labor for low-risk women and every 15 minutes for high-risk women (Miller et al., 2017). Auscultate the FHR throughout one contraction and for approximately 15 seconds after the contraction to ensure there are no decelerations. If the FHR baseline is not in the range of 110 to 160 beats/min or if decelerations are heard, continuous electronic monitoring is recommended (see Table 33.13).

>> *Visit* ***Pearson MyLab Nursing and eText*** *for Chart 8: Psychologic Characteristics and Nursing Support During the First and Second Stages of Labor.*

Latent Phase

The nurse offers food and fluids as desired unless complications exist that may necessitate general anesthesia. Avoiding both liquids and solids during labor, which was once standard practice, is no longer necessary because evidence-based practice research and new guidelines indicate that clear fluids can be consumed throughout labor and up to 2 hours before an elective cesarean birth. Some studies show that consumption of clear fluids 1 hour before cesarean section did not increase the risk of aspiration (Murray, McKinney, Holub, & Jones, 2019). In a low-risk setting, it is not necessary to restrict intake in any way.

Active Phase

During the active phase, the contractions have a frequency of 2 to 5 minutes, a duration of 40 to 60 seconds, and a moderate to strong intensity. As the contractions become more frequent and intense, a woman who has been ambulatory may choose to sit in a chair or lie down. Contractions need to be palpated every 30 minutes.

Vaginal exams may be performed to assess cervical dilation and effacement as well as fetal station and position. Vaginal examinations should be limited, however, because they introduce bacteria, which can lead to maternal infection. During the active phase, the cervix dilates from 6 to 8 cm, and vaginal discharge and bloody show increase; thus, the nurse needs to change the perineal pads more frequently.

During this phase, the FHR is evaluated every 30 minutes for low-risk women and every 15 minutes for high-risk women (Murray et al., 2019). Maternal blood pressure, pulse, and respirations are monitored during the FHR assessment or more frequently, if indicated. The mother's level of pain and coping mechanisms are assessed continuously.

The woman is encouraged to void because a full bladder can interfere with fetal descent. If she is unable to void, catheterization or insertion of an indwelling Foley catheter may be necessary.

If the amniotic membranes have not ruptured previously, they may do so during this phase. When the membranes rupture, the nurse notes the amount, color, odor, and consistency of the amniotic fluid and the time of rupture and immediately auscultates the FHR. The fluid should be clear, with no odor. Nonreassuring fetal status may lead to intestinal and anal sphincter relaxation. This may result in the release of meconium into the amniotic fluid, which turns the fluid greenish brown. When the nurse notes meconium-stained fluid, an electronic monitor is applied to assess the FHR continuously. An additional potential issue during this phase is prolapse of the umbilical cord, which may occur when membranes rupture and the fetal presenting part is not well applied to the cervix. The concern is that the amniotic fluid coming through the cervix will propel the umbilical cord through the cervix (prolapsed cord). The FHR is auscultated because a drop in FHR might indicate an undetected prolapsed cord. Immediate intervention is necessary to remove pressure on a prolapsed umbilical cord.

SAFETY ALERT When rupture of membranes occurs, the priority is assessment of FHR. A drop in FHR may indicate pressure on the umbilical cord, which can become trapped between the maternal pelvis and the fetal head as amniotic fluid releases, resulting in diminished blood flow to the fetus. Diminished FHR may also indicate a prolapsed umbilical cord, which can occur as amniotic fluid moves through the cervix. In either case, immediate intervention is necessary to restore blood flow to the fetus. Fetal demise may result if action is not taken quickly.

>> *Visit* ***Pearson MyLab Nursing and eText*** *for Chart 9: Deviations from Normal Labor Process Requiring Immediate Intervention.*

Transition Phase

During transition, the contraction frequency may be every 1.5 to 2 minutes, duration is 60 to 90 seconds, and intensity is strong. Cervical dilation increases from 8 to 10 cm, effacement is complete (100%), and a heavy amount of bloody show is usually present. Contractions are palpated at least every 30 minutes. Sterile vaginal examinations may be done more frequently because this stage of labor is usually accompanied by rapid change. The FHR is auscultated every 30 minutes for low-risk women and every 15 minutes for high-risk women; maternal blood pressure, pulse, and respirations are monitored when the FHR is assessed or according to unit policy. Note that women may receive more frequent assessments based on individualized needs. The woman's pain level is monitored continuously.

Comfort measures become very important in this phase of labor, but continual assessment is required to ensure appropriate intervention. Women may shake uncontrollably, feel nausea, or vomit during this stage. The woman may rapidly change from wanting a back rub and other hands-on care to wanting to be left completely alone. The support person and the nurse need to follow the woman's cues and change interventions as needed. Because the woman is breathing more rapidly, the nurse can increase the woman's comfort by offering small spoons of ice chips to moisten her mouth or applying an emollient to dry lips. The nurse can encourage the woman to rest between contractions. If analgesics have been administered, a quiet environment enhances the quality of rest between contractions.

Some women have difficulty coping during this time and need help with their breathing. Either the support person or the nurse can breathe along with the woman during each contraction to help her maintain her pattern. A gentle reminder to "slow down your breathing" can help to prevent hyperventilation. It is helpful to encourage the woman and to assure her that she is doing a good job. The woman will begin to feel increased rectal pressure as the fetal presenting part moves down the birth canal. The nurse encourages the woman to refrain from pushing until the cervix is completely dilated. To help the woman avoid involuntary pushing during contractions, the nurse can encourage pant–blow breathing, suggesting that the woman "pant like a puppy" or "blow in short breaths as if you were blowing out a candle." This measure helps prevent cervical edema.

The end of the transition phase and the beginning of the second stage may be indicated by a change in the woman's voice or the sounds that she is making. As the fetus moves down and the woman feels increased pressure and a bearing-down sensation, her voice tends to deepen. If she moans during a contraction, it takes on a more guttural quality. Experienced nurses recognize this sound as a sign of changes in the woman.

Promote Comfort

The nurse identifies factors that may contribute to discomfort for the laboring woman. These factors include uncomfortable positions or infrequent position changes, diaphoresis, continual leaking of amniotic fluid, a full bladder, a dry mouth, anxiety, and fear. The nurse and patient together plan interventions to minimize the effects of these factors.

Women in labor have many types of responses to pain. As the intensity of the contractions increases with the progress of labor, the woman becomes less aware of the environment and may have difficulty hearing and understanding verbal instructions. Some women may become irritable during this time. The pattern of coping with labor contractions varies from the use of highly structured breathing techniques to turning inward. As stated previously, the woman's responses to pain may have a cultural basis. Low moaning that begins deep in the throat, rocking or swaying, counting, facial grimacing, and using loud vocalizations are all effective means of dealing with the discomfort of labor and birth. Some women feel that making sounds helps them cope and do the work of labor, whereas others make loud sounds only as they lose their perception of control.

The most frequent physiologic manifestations of pain are increased pulse and respiratory rates, dilated pupils, increased blood pressure, and muscle tension. During labor, these reactions are transitory because the pain is intermittent. Increased muscle tension is most significant because it may impede the labor process. Women in labor frequently tighten skeletal muscles voluntarily during a contraction and remain motionless. This method of dealing with the contractions may actually increase her discomfort, but the woman may believe it is the only acceptable way to cope with the pain.

A woman generally wants touch, massage, and other forms of physical contact during the first part of labor, but when she moves into the transition phase, she may pull away. Alternatively, the woman may beseech her partner or the nurse to hold her hand or rub her back, or she may even reach out and grasp the support person. Some women are uncomfortable with being touched at all, regardless of the phase of labor; others do not welcome touch from a nonfamily member. It is important to validate the unique strengths and coping techniques of the individual and to meet each family on their own terms, always keeping in mind that this is their experience. Cultural influences can also affect how a woman will react to support and touch in labor. The nurse takes cues from the woman and makes adjustments in her care to meet the patient's specific needs.

- ***General comfort.*** General comfort measures are of great importance during labor. By relieving minor discomforts, the nurse helps the woman optimize her coping abilities to deal with pain. The woman is encouraged to ambulate as long as there are no contraindications, such as vaginal bleeding or rupture of membranes, before the fetus is engaged in the pelvis. Ambulation can increase comfort and aid in fetal descent. Even if the woman prefers not to walk around, upright positions, such as sitting in a rocker or leaning against a wall or bed, can enhance comfort. If the woman stays in bed, the nurse can encourage her to assume positions that she finds comfortable.

  If the woman is more comfortable on her back, the nurse should elevate the head of the bed to relieve the pressure of the uterus on the vena cava. Pillows may be placed under each arm and under the knees to provide support. Because a pregnant woman is at increased risk for thrombophlebitis, it is important to avoid excessive pressure behind the knee and calf. The nurse needs to assess pressure points often. Frequent changes of position contribute to comfort and relaxation. The hands-and-knees posture may be used to relieve persistent back pain during labor.

  Wearing socks or slippers may alleviate cold feet and adjusting the room's thermostat can offset excessive warmth. Attention to such details allows the woman to focus on the more important issues of giving birth. The woman may be offered a warmed or cooled facial cloth, which is placed on her forehead or across or behind her neck. Providing a toothbrush and toothpaste for oral care can also increase comfort.

Diaphoresis and the constant leaking of amniotic fluid can dampen the woman's gown and bed linens. Offering fresh, smooth, dry bed linens promotes comfort. To avoid having to change the bottom sheet following rupture of the membranes, the nurse may replace absorbent underpads at frequent intervals (following standard precautions). To promote comfort and prevent infection, keep the perineal area as clean and dry as possible. A full bladder adds to discomfort during a contraction and may prolong labor by interfering with the descent of the fetus. The bladder should be kept as empty as possible. Even if the woman is voiding, urine may be retained because of the pressure from the fetal presenting part. The nurse can detect a full bladder by palpating directly over the symphysis pubis. Encourage the woman to empty her bladder every 1 to 2 hours. Some of the regional procedures for analgesia and anesthesia during labor contribute to the inability to void, and catheterization may be necessary.

The support person and any family members in attendance also need to be encouraged to maintain their own comfort. Because their attention is directed toward the laboring woman, they may forget their own needs. The nurse may have to encourage them to take breaks, to maintain food and fluid intake, and to rest. Many support persons and family members are reluctant to leave the woman unattended while they meet their own personal needs. Offer to stay with the woman during their absence. This provides reassurance to the support persons or family members that the woman will be well cared for in their absence.

- ***Handling anxiety.*** The anxiety experienced by women in labor is related to a combination of factors inherent to the process. A moderate amount of anxiety about pain enhances the woman's ability to deal with it. However, an excessive degree of anxiety decreases her ability to cope with the pain. Women in the latent phase of labor who are experiencing increased levels of anxiety about their ability to cope and their own personal safety are much more likely to describe their pain as unbearable. Women at risk for greater anxiety during labor include those who are young, poor, and lacking in social support. The incidence of PTSD related to labor and delivery is higher in women who have preexisting mental illness (King et al., 2019). Women with mental illness issues may need additional support to assist them with identifying effective coping mechanisms during the labor and birth process.

  Ways to decrease anxiety not related to pain are to give information, which eases fear of the unknown; to establish rapport with the couple, which helps them preserve their personal integrity; and to express confidence in the couple's ability to work with the labor process. In addition to being a good listener, the nurse must demonstrate genuine concern for the laboring woman. Remaining with the woman as much as possible conveys a caring attitude and dispels fears of abandonment. Praise for breathing, relaxation, and pushing efforts not only encourages repetition of the behavior but also decreases anxiety about the ability to cope with labor.

- ***Patient teaching.*** Providing truthful information about the nature of the discomfort that will occur during labor is important. Stressing the intermittent nature and maximum duration of the contractions can be helpful. The woman can cope with pain better when she knows that a period of relief will follow. Describing the type of discomfort and specific sensations that will occur as labor progresses helps the woman recognize these sensations as normal and expected when she does experience them.

  Advise the woman that although the strength and intensity of contractions are different for each woman, they may feel like a tightening sensation or a menstrual cramp initially. Over time, as the labor progresses, the contractions become more intense and more uncomfortable, with the uterus tightening and becoming very hard and with the pain radiating from the back around to the front. For some women, the pain takes their breath away, or they may feel anxiety and fear. As the contractions become more painful, they also occur closer together. The sensation of having to push occurs as the head progresses into the pelvis and feels like the woman has to have a bowel movement. Once the contraction goes away, this intense feeling of having to have a bowel movement usually lets up somewhat.

  Descriptions of sensations are best accompanied by information on specific comfort measures. As previously noted, some women experience the urge to push during the transition phase, when the cervix is not fully dilated and effaced. This sensation can be controlled by pant–blow breathing (it is difficult to pant or blow and bear down at the same time); the nurse should provide instructions about this technique before it is required.

  Thorough orientation and explanation of surroundings, procedures, and equipment being used also decrease anxiety, thereby reducing pain. Attachment to an electronic monitor may produce fear because the woman may associate equipment of this type with people who are critically ill. It may also limit the woman's ability to move about and comfort herself with position changes and ambulation. If continuous electronic fetal monitoring is needed, the nurse can explain the beeps, clicks, and other strange noises and give a simplified explanation of the monitor strip. The nurse emphasizes that use of the fetal monitor provides a way to assess the well-being of the fetus during the course of labor. If available, a less intrusive telemetry monitor may be applied so that the woman has more freedom to move about. In addition, the nurse can show the woman and her partner or support person how the monitor can help them identify the beginnings of contractions. The nurse should encourage the woman to begin her breathing technique at the onset of each contraction; this may help lessen her perception of pain.

  Labor and childbirth may be a critical time for the woman with a history of childhood physical, emotional, and/or sexual abuse or rape. To develop a competent plan of care, all laboring women should be evaluated on admission for a history of childhood abuse or rape. Depending on their cultural background, women may need specific examples of abuse to determine whether they have had these types of experiences because some behaviors that are considered to be abusive may have been normalized as "ordinary" experiences. Women may or may not be able to address this issue with the nurse because sharing such personal information is difficult and may stir up painful memories. It is therefore especially important for the nurse to be alert for nonverbal cues, such as excessive unexplained anxiety, unrelenting pain, and/or intense fear during vaginal exams, and to be prepared to offer additional teaching to help offset the woman's anxiety.

- ***Supportive relaxation techniques.*** Tense muscles increase resistance to the descent of the fetus and contribute to maternal fatigue. This fatigue increases pain perception and decreases the woman's ability to cope with the pain. Comfort measures, massage, techniques for decreasing anxiety, and patient teaching can contribute to relaxation. Adequate sleep and rest are also important. The laboring woman needs to be encouraged to use the period between contractions for rest and relaxation. A prolonged prodromal phase of labor (also known as false labor or Braxton Hicks contractions) may interfere with sleep. An aura of excitement naturally accompanies the onset of labor, making it difficult for the woman to sleep even though the contractions are mild and infrequent. The nurse may have to act as an advocate for the woman to limit the number of visitors, interruptions, and phone calls.

  Distraction is another method of increasing relaxation and coping with discomfort. During early labor, conversation or activities such as watching television, light reading, or playing cards or other games can serve as distractions. One technique that is effective for relieving moderate pain is to have the woman concentrate on a pleasant experience she has had in the past. Other techniques include the use of a specific visual or mental focal point (e.g., a picture of a loved one), breathing techniques, counting or humming, or visualization.

  Touch is another type of distraction. Although some women regard touching as an invasion of privacy or a threat to their independence, many want to touch and be touched during a painful experience. To determine whether the woman desires touch, the nurse can place a hand on the side of the bed within the woman's reach. The woman who needs touch will reach out for contact, and the nurse can follow through with this behavioral cue.

  Back pain associated with labor may be relieved by firm pressure on the lower back or sacral area. To apply firm pressure, the nurse can place a hand or a rolled, warmed towel or blanket in the small of the woman's back or can instruct the woman's support person to do so.

  In some instances, analgesics or regional anesthetic blocks may be used to enhance comfort and relaxation during labor. The nurse may also enhance the woman's relaxation by providing encouragement and support for her controlled breathing techniques.

- ***Breathing techniques.*** Breathing techniques may help the laboring woman. Used correctly, they raise the woman's pain threshold, permit relaxation, enhance her ability to cope with contractions, provide a sense of control, and allow the uterus to function more efficiently.

  Various types of breathing techniques can be used in labor. Many women learn patterned-paced breathing during prenatal education classes. This type of controlled breathing often has three levels. The woman tends to begin with the first level and then proceed to the next when she feels the need. Regardless of the level of breathing used, a cleansing breath (involving only the chest) begins and ends each pattern. The cleansing breath consists of inhaling slowly through the nose until a sense of fullness in the lungs occurs, and then exhaling slowly through pursed lips. The first pattern may also be called slow, deep breathing or slow-paced breathing. During the breathing movements, only the chest moves. The woman inhales slowly through her nose, moves her chest up and out during the inhalation, and exhales through pursed lips. The breathing rate is six to nine breaths per minute.

  The second pattern may be called shallow or modified-paced breathing. The woman begins with a cleansing breath. At the end of the cleansing breath, she pushes out a short breath. She then inhales and exhales through the mouth at a rate of about four breaths every 5 seconds. This pattern can be altered into a more rapid rate that does not exceed 2 to 2.5 breaths every second.

  The third pattern, introduced earlier, is called pant–blow or patterned-paced breathing. It is similar to modified-paced breathing except that the breathing is punctuated every few breaths by a forceful exhalation through pursed lips. A pattern of four breaths may be used to begin. All breaths are kept equal and rhythmic. As the contraction becomes more intense, the woman may adjust the pattern as needed to 3:1, 2:1, and finally 1:1.

  Abdominal breathing is another technique that can be effective in labor. In abdominal breathing, the woman moves the abdominal wall outward as she inhales and inward as she exhales. This method tends to lift the abdominal wall off the contracting uterus and thus helps to provide pain relief. The breathing is deep and rhythmic and typically relaxing. As transition approaches, the woman using abdominal breathing may feel the urge to breathe more rapidly. The pant–blow pattern discussed earlier can be suggested to slow the breathing and help the woman avoid the urge to bear down.

- ***Hyperventilation.*** **Hyperventilation** is the result of an imbalance of oxygen and carbon dioxide (i.e., too much carbon dioxide is exhaled, and too much oxygen remains in the body). Hyperventilation may occur when a woman breathes very rapidly over a prolonged period. The signs and symptoms of hyperventilation are tingling or numbness in the tip of the nose, lips, fingers, or toes; dizziness; spots before the eyes; or spasms of the hands or feet (carpopedal spasms). If hyperventilation occurs, the nurse encourages the woman to slow her breathing rate and take shallow breaths. With instruction and encouragement, many women are able to change their breathing to correct the problem. Encouraging the woman to relax and counting out loud for her so that she can pace her breathing during contractions are also helpful actions. If the signs and symptoms continue or become more severe, the woman is treated for hyperventilation as appropriate. The nurse remains with the woman to reassure her because hyperventilation can increase anxiety levels.

Communicating with Patients

Introductory Phase

The labor process will be different for each mother. Based on expectations, fears, personal strengths, and supports, the nurse will help the patient find what works for her to manage labor. Getting to know the patient can help the nurse formulate a plan for dealing with the pain and uncertainty they may face. Questions the nurse may ask include:

- Tell me what you have done to prepare for labor, such as classes or learning breathing techniques.
- What are some things you normally do to calm down when you feel stressed or anxious?
- Are there any particular questions about the labor process that you would like answered?
- Do you know if you will want an epidural or would you like to see how labor feels first?
- Are there any important cultural concerns you want the healthcare team to be aware of?

The Role of the Doula

Some women choose to employ a **doula**, a paid caregiver with specialized training or certification in assisting women through labor. Doulas act to enhance comfort and reduce anxiety, and they can be valuable advocates for women in labor and their families. Doulas provide immense benefits by offering presence and continued encouragement throughout the course of labor, and many will remain after delivery to help promote maternal–newborn bonding.

Nursing Care During the Second Stage of Labor

The second stage is reached when the cervix is completely dilated (10 cm [3.9 in.]). The uterine contractions continue as in the transition phase. The mother's blood pressure and pulse should be assessed every 5 minutes, along with the FHR (Lowdermilk et al., 2020). Once the second stage is reached, the nurse remains with the woman continually and generally does not leave the room. Nursing care during the second stage focuses on providing care, promoting comfort, and assisting during the birth.

As the woman pushes during the second stage, she may make a variety of sounds. A low-pitched, grunting sound ("uhhh") usually indicates that the woman is working with the pushing. The nurse who feels comfortable with maternal sounds and stays sensitive to changes in the sounds may be able to detect if the woman is losing her ability to cope. For instance, if the woman feels afraid of the sensations produced by her pushing effort, her sound may change to a high-pitched cry or whimper.

It is not uncommon for the woman to be afraid to push. In these situations, the woman may talk or cry out during the contraction instead of actively pushing. During this time, the nurse provides support, reassurance, and clear directions for the woman to follow. Often, it is helpful to direct the woman to concentrate on a single voice, listen for suggestions, and let her body do the work. Many women find this type of interaction comforting because it allows them to focus on one individual.

When teaching the effective technique for pushing, instruct the woman to bear down and push into her bottom as if she is having a bowel movement. Watch the woman's perineum and rectum while she is pushing and give verbal praise and encouragement when change in the perineum or rectum is seen that indicates she is pushing successfully.

During the second stage, the woman may feel intense rectal pressure. The instinctive response is to resist and to tighten muscles rather than bear down (push). A sensation of "splitting apart" or burning also occurs in the latter part of the second stage when the woman is pushing. The woman who expects these sensations and who understands that bearing down contributes to progress at this stage is more likely to do so.

When the urge to bear down becomes uncontrollable and pushing begins, the nurse can help by encouraging the woman and by supporting her efforts. Most women push spontaneously and effectively in response to messages from their body. Allowing the mother to follow these natural cues has been shown to shorten the pushing phase, lower the risk of perineal tears, and reduce the need for operative delivery (Blackburn, 2018). In some settings, however, sustained, forceful pushing may be useful. In that case, when the contraction begins, the nurse tells the woman to take a cleansing breath or two, then to take a third large breath and hold it while pushing down with her abdominal muscles (called the Valsalva maneuver).

A nullipara is usually prepared for birth when perineal bulging is noted. A multipara usually progresses quickly. As the birth approaches, the woman's partner or support person also prepares.

The nurse monitors the woman's blood pressure and the FHR between contractions, and the nurse assesses the contractions at least every 5 minutes until the birth. The nurse continually assesses the woman's level of pain or her ability to cope with the discomfort of labor. The nurse also continues to assist the woman in her pushing efforts to keep both the woman and the support person informed of procedures and progress and to support them both throughout the birth.

Promoting Comfort

Most of the comfort measures that were used during the first stage remain appropriate during the second stage. Applying cool cloths to the face and forehead may help to cool the woman involved in the intense physical exertion of pushing. The woman may feel hot and want to remove some of her clothing or bed linens. Care still needs to be taken to provide privacy even though covers are removed. The nurse encourages the woman to rest and relax all muscles during the periods between contractions. The nurse and support person can assist the woman into a pushing position with each contraction to further conserve energy. Between contractions, the woman should be assisted into a comfortable position. Sips of fluids or ice chips may be used to provide moisture and relieve dryness of the mouth. Positive reinforcement and encouragement should be continually provided.

For some women, but especially those with epidural anesthesia, the urge to push may not occur spontaneously. The question then becomes whether to encourage passive descent of the fetus versus active pushing.

The natural second stage of labor includes a period of time in which the fetus descends, which the literature refers to as "passive descent." Passive descent allows the woman to delay pushing until she feels the urge to push or until the head is visible. With active pushing, women are directed to push immediately once cervical dilation reaches 10 cm, whether they feel the urge to push or not. The chief concern leading to this practice was that an extended second stage of labor was deleterious for both mother and baby, leading to acidosis, maternal exhaustion, and neonatal morbidity.

Some studies have shown that allowing passive descent to occur results in a decrease in the duration of pushing, fewer operative deliveries, and a higher rate of spontaneous vaginal deliveries. With active pushing, the risk for operative delivery is increased and the second stage of labor has been shown to be longer. The determination to utilize passive descent or active pushing is best made on an individual basis, taking all aspects of labor into account (King et al, 2019).

Assisting During the Birth

In addition to assisting the woman and her partner, the nurse assists the HCP in preparing for the birth. The provider dons a sterile gown and gloves and may place sterile drapes over the woman's abdomen and legs. An episiotomy may be performed just before the actual birth.

Shortly before the birth, the birthing room or delivery room is prepared with the equipment and materials that may be needed. These materials typically come in a prepackaged kit, which contains the instruments and disposable drapes, gowns, and containers that will be used during the birth. The nurse ensures that all supplies and a pair of sterile gloves are placed on the instrument table. This table can be prepared before the birth and covered with a sterile drape. If the birth is to occur in a birthing room, family members do not need to change into other clothing; if the birth is to occur in a delivery room or surgery suite, they don a disposable scrub suit or scrubs provided by the facility. Thorough hand hygiene is required of the nurses and physician or CNM. Nurses who will be in direct contact with the mother at the time of birth need to wear protective clothing, such as an apron or gown with a splash apron, disposable gloves, and eye covering. The physician or CNM also needs to wear a plastic apron or a gown with a splash apron, eye covering, and sterile gloves.

SAFETY ALERT Some physicians and CNMs routinely use other equipment or supplies during the birth. Examples of such equipment include mineral oil, warm water, and clean washcloths for perineal massage. Gathering these supplies early can save time and enable the nurse to stay with the woman during pushing.

If for any reason the laboring woman is to give birth in a location other than the birthing room (e.g., in the case of a forceps-assisted birth where a quick transition to cesarean delivery may be necessary), she is moved on her bed or a gurney shortly before birth. It is important that the woman move from one bed to another between contractions. During the contraction, the woman feels increased discomfort and may be involved in pushing efforts. Perineal bulging may be occurring, which adds to the discomfort and difficulty in moving. Take care to preserve her privacy during the transfer and provide safety by raising the side rails. The bed itself should be placed in a locked position. The labor bed or transfer cart must be carefully braced against the delivery table to ensure the woman's safety during the transfer.

» *See **Pearson MyLab Nursing and eText** for Chart 10: Comparison of Birthing Positions.*

Evidence-based practice research has shown that the squatting position results in a slightly shorter duration of the second stage of labor, reduced instrumental deliveries, fewer episiotomies, and a reduction in abnormal FHR patterns compared to the lithotomy position (King et al., 2019). An upright position, which has been found to be the most effective birthing position, is possible even for women who have received epidural anesthesia.

The woman may be positioned for birth on a bed with use of leg supports in a squatting position, or perhaps on her hands and knees. If a birthing bed is used, the back is elevated 30 to 60 degrees to help the woman bear down. Stirrups, if needed and used, are padded to alleviate pressure. If the nurse is assisting the woman to place her legs in the stirrups, both the woman's legs should be lifted simultaneously to avoid strain on the abdominal, back, and perineal muscles. Stirrups are sometimes needed if the woman is unable to control her legs following epidural anesthesia, if forceps or a vacuum extractor is being used, or if a difficult birth is anticipated. The nurse should adjust the stirrups to fit the woman's legs. The feet are supported in the stirrup holders. The height and angle of the stirrups are adjusted so there is no pressure on the back of the knees or the calves, which might cause discomfort and postpartum vascular problems. Some practitioners may opt to leave the bed assembled and, instead, lower the foot of the bed into a lower position. Many times, women are more comfortable in this position. When stirrups are not used for the birth, the woman's legs may be placed in stirrups after the birth if a repair of the perineum is needed.

- ***Cleansing the perineum.*** After the mother has been positioned for the birth, her vulvar and perineal area are cleansed to increase her comfort, to remove the bloody discharge that is present before the actual birth, and to prevent infection. Perineal cleansing methods range from use of warm, soapy water to aseptic technique, depending on the agency protocol or on physician or CNM orders. Once the cleansing has been completed, the woman returns to the desired birthing position.
- ***Supporting the couple.*** Both the woman's partner or support person and the nurse who has been with the woman during the labor continue to provide support during contractions. They encourage the woman to push with each contraction, and as the fetal head emerges, ask her to take shallow breaths or to pant to prevent pushing. The physician or CNM may instruct the woman to "push and breathe, push and breathe" in an effort to ease the fetal head out to prevent perineal trauma and tearing. While supporting the head, the physician or CNM assesses whether the umbilical

cord is around the fetal neck and removes it if it is, then suctions the mouth and nose with a bulb syringe if there are any obvious obstructions to spontaneous breathing. The mouth is suctioned first to prevent reflex inhalation of mucus when the sensitive nares are touched with the bulb syringe tip. The woman is encouraged to push again as the newborn emerges.

Nursing Care During the Third Stage of Labor

At this stage, nursing care of the mother and newborn focuses on providing initial care of both patients, promoting maternal–newborn bonding, and assisting with the delivery of the placenta. Newborn care is discussed in Exemplar 33.D in this module. This section focuses on care of the mother.

Delivery of the Placenta

After birth, the HCP prepares for the delivery of the placenta. The following signs suggest placental separation:

- The uterus rises upward in the abdomen.
- As the placenta moves downward, the umbilical cord lengthens.
- A sudden trickle or spurt of blood appears.
- The shape of the uterus changes from a disk to a globe.

While waiting for these signs, the nurse palpates the uterus to check for bogginess (soft or mushy feeling) and fullness caused by uterine relaxation and subsequent bleeding into the uterine cavity. After the placenta has separated, the woman may be asked to bear down to aid delivery of the placenta.

Oxytocics are frequently given at the time of the delivery of the placenta so that the uterus will contract and bleeding will be minimized. Oxytocin (Pitocin), 20 units, may be added to an IV infusion, or 10 units may be given IM. In the presence of hemorrhage caused by uterine atony, some HCPs may order up to 40 units of oxytocin in a liter of IV fluid; methylergonovine maleate (Methergine), 0.2 mg, administered IM; or carboprost tromethamine (Hemabate), 250 mcg/mL, administered IM. Cytotec has been commonly used when other pharmacologic interventions have failed. Cytotec is administered rectally in dosages of 600 to 1000 mcg (Lowdermilk et al., 2020). In addition to administering the ordered medications, the nurse assesses and records maternal blood pressure before and after administration of oxytocics and assesses the amount of bleeding.

After delivery of the placenta, the HCP inspects the placenta and membranes to make sure they are intact and that all cotyledons are present. If there is a problem with or a part missing from the placenta, a manual uterine examination or uterine exploration is done. The nurse notes on the birth record the time of delivery of the placenta.

Cord Blood Analysis at Birth

When significant abnormal FHR patterns have been noted, meconium-stained amniotic fluid is present, or the newborn is depressed at birth, umbilical cord blood may be analyzed immediately following the birth to determine whether acidosis is present. ACOG (2017a) recommends performing cord blood analyses when the Apgar score is below 5 at 5 minutes of age (normal Apgar score is 7 to 10) (see Exemplar 33.D, Newborn Care, in this module for an in-depth discussion of the Apgar scoring system).

The cord is clamped before the neonate takes the first breath. Using a Kelly clamp, the HCP clamps a 20- to 25-cm (8- to 10-in.) portion of the umbilical cord. A small amount of blood (1.0 mL is required for a full panel) is aspirated with a syringe from one of the umbilical arteries or from an artery and a vein. If the cord blood will not be analyzed immediately, a heparinized syringe should be used. Normal fetal blood pH should be greater than 7.2 (Lowdermilk et al., 2020). Lower levels indicate acidosis and hypoxia. Many HCPs order cord blood analysis to minimize medicolegal exposure.

Nursing Care During the Fourth Stage of Labor

The HCP inspects the vagina, cervix, and perineum for lacerations and makes any necessary repairs. The episiotomy or laceration may be repaired now if it was not done previously.

The nurse assesses the uterus for firmness by palpating the fundus. The normal position is at the midline and below the umbilicus. A displaced fundus may be caused by a full bladder or by blood collected in the uterus. The clots or blood accumulation in the uterus may be expelled by grasping the uterus transabdominally with one hand anteriorly and posteriorly and then squeezing. The nurse continues to palpate the uterine fundus at frequent intervals for at least 4 hours to ensure that it remains firmly contracted (**Figure 33.53 »**), but it is not massaged unless it is soft (boggy). If the uterine fundus becomes soft (uterine atony) or appears to rise in the

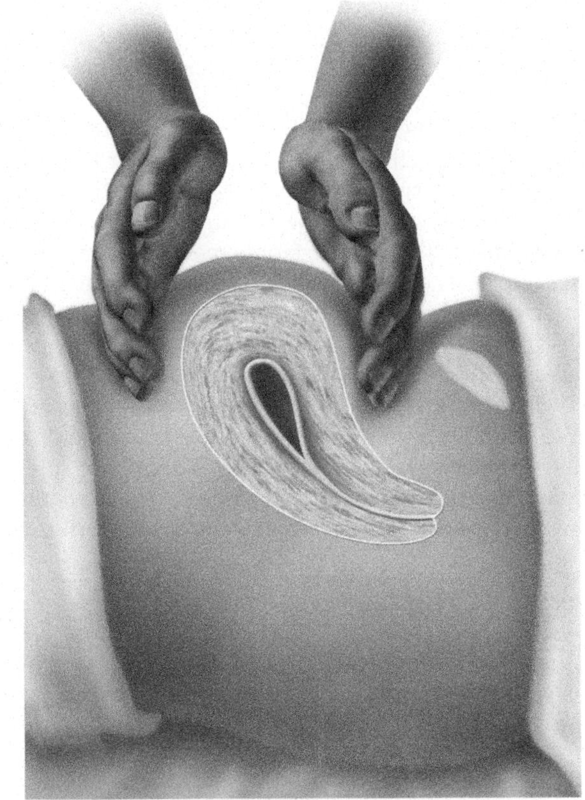

Figure 33.53 » Suggested method of palpating the fundus of the uterus during the fourth stage. The left hand is placed just above the symphysis pubis, and gentle downward pressure is exerted. The right hand is cupped around the uterine fundus.

abdomen, the nurse massages it until firm; then, the nurse exerts firm pressure on the fundus in an attempt to express retained clots. During all aspects of fundal massage, the nurse uses one hand to provide support for the lower portion of the uterus and prevent damage to the round ligaments and uterine eversion. The uterus is very tender at this time; all palpation and massage should be performed as gently as possible.

The nurse washes the woman's perineum with gauze squares and warmed solution and then dries the area well with a towel before placing the sanitary pad. Many times, an ice pack is also placed against the perineum to promote comfort and decrease swelling. If stirrups have been used, both the woman's legs are removed from the stirrups at the same time to avoid muscle strain. The woman is encouraged to move her legs gently up and down in a bicycle motion. The woman remains in the same bed or is transferred to a recovery room bed, and the nurse helps her don a clean gown. Soiled linens are removed, and the woman is typically offered something to drink.

During the recovery period (1 to 4 hours) the nurse monitors the woman closely. The perineum is inspected for edema and hematoma formation, and frequent checking of vital signs for deviations from normal is required. The maternal blood pressure is monitored at 5- to 15-minute intervals to detect any changes. Blood pressure should return to the prelabor level because an increased volume of blood is returning to the maternal circulation from the uteroplacental shunt. Pulse rate should be slightly lower than it was during labor. Baroreceptors cause a vagal response, which slows the pulse. A rise in blood pressure may be a response to oxytocic drugs or may be caused by preeclampsia. Blood loss may be reflected by a lowered blood pressure and a rising pulse rate (**Table 33.14** »).

The nurse also monitors the woman's temperature. Frequently, women have tremors or uncontrollable shaking in the immediate postpartum period that may be caused by a difference in internal and external body temperatures (higher temperature inside the body than outside). Another theory is that the woman is reacting to the fetal cells that have entered the maternal circulation at the placental site. The nurse may place a heated blanket next to the woman's skin to alleviate the problem; this can be replaced as often as the mother desires.

TABLE 33.14 Maternal Adaptations Following Birth

Characteristic	Normal Finding
Blood pressure	Returns to prelabor level
Pulse	Slightly lower than in labor
Uterine fundus	In the midline at the umbilicus, or 1–2 fingerbreadths below the umbilicus
Lochia	Red (rubra), small to moderate amount (from spotting on pads to 1/4–1/2 of pad covered in 15 minutes); does not exceed saturation of one pad in first hour
Bladder	Nonpalpable
Perineum	Without hematomas or open lacerations. Mild to moderate bruising and/or edema is common.
Appetite/thirst	Variations possible. Increased hunger is typical due to the high level of energy expenditure during the labor and birth process. Increased thirst is due to loss of fluids (blood, sweat, urine) and fluid shifts associated with birth process.
Emotional state	Wide variation, including excited, exhilarated, smiling, crying, fatigued, verbal, quiet, pensive, and sleepy

Source: Adapted from London et al. J. (2017).

The nurse assesses the mother's pain level. If the woman is experiencing any type of discomfort, pain medications can be administered as ordered. The nurse also assists with comfort measures, such as position changes, frequent ice pack changes, and administration of topical medications that are often ordered to reduce perineal edema and discomfort.

The nurse inspects the bloody vaginal discharge for amount and documents it as minimal, moderate, or heavy and as with or without clots. This discharge (lochia rubra) should be bright red. A soaked perineal pad contains approximately 100 mL of blood. If the perineal pad becomes soaked in a 15-minute period or if blood pools under the buttocks, continuous observation is necessary. When the fundus is firm, a continuous trickle of blood may signal laceration of the vagina or cervix or an unligated vessel in the episiotomy.

If the fundus rises and displaces to the right, the nurse must be concerned about two factors:

1. As the uterus rises, the uterine contractions become less effective and increased bleeding may occur.
2. The most common cause of uterine displacement is bladder distention.

The nurse palpates the bladder to determine whether it is distended. The bladder fills rapidly with the extra fluid volume returned from the uteroplacental circulation (and with any fluid received IV during labor and birth). The postpartum woman may not realize that her bladder is full because trauma to the bladder and urethra during childbirth and the use of regional anesthesia decrease bladder tone and the urge to void.

All measures should be taken to enable the mother to void. The nurse may place a warm towel across the lower abdomen or pour warm water over the perineum to relax the urinary sphincter and facilitate voiding. The woman may also try running warm water over her hand. If the woman is unable to void, catheterization is necessary.

SAFETY ALERT In the immediate postbirth recovery period, report the following conditions to the HCP:

- Hypotension
- Tachycardia
- Uterine atony
- Excessive bleeding
- Hematoma.

The woman and her partner or support person may be tired, hungry, and thirsty. Some agencies serve them a meal. Most women are very hungry after birth. The tired mother will probably drift off into a welcome sleep. The partner can also be encouraged to rest because the supporting role is physically and mentally tiring. If the mother is not in a birthing room, she is usually transferred from the birthing unit to the postpartum or mother–baby area after 1 hour or more, depending on agency policy and on whether the following criteria are met:

- Stable vital signs
- Stable bleeding
- Undistended bladder
- Firm fundus
- Sensations fully recovered from any anesthetic agent received during birth.

For some women, the childbirth experience has been extremely painful, filled with hours of feeling powerless or out of control. In this circumstance, the woman is at higher risk for developing PTSD. It is estimated that 1–6% of women have symptoms of PTSD in the immediate postpartum period, with 2% continuing to have symptoms at 6 months postpartum (King et al., 2019).

Evaluation

Evaluation provides an opportunity to determine the effectiveness of nursing care. As a result of comprehensive nursing care during the intrapartum period, the following outcomes may be anticipated:

- The mother's physical and psychologic well-being has been maintained and supported.
- The baby's physical and psychologic well-being has been protected and supported.
- The mother and her family members have had input into the birth process and have participated as much as they desired.
- The mother and her baby have had a safe birth.

An additional purpose of care evaluation is to determine if further care is needed based on maternal or neonatal outcomes. If the outcomes are not being met, the nurse may choose to continue or revise the plan of care for optimal outcome attainment. For example, if the mother's or newborn's physical well-being is compromised, transferring them to a more intensive care setting such as an ICU or NICU may be warranted. Likewise, if the mother's psychologic well-being is compromised, a psychologic consult may be needed and safety measures initiated.

Nursing Care Plan

A Patient Requiring Cesarean Section

Lakshmi Pandey is being admitted to labor and childbirth this morning for a scheduled cesarean section due to breech fetal positioning. She is accompanied by her husband, Nitya. Mrs. Pandey is a primigravida at 40 weeks' gestation. She has been experiencing Braxton Hicks contractions during the past week. Mrs. Pandey's membranes are intact, and her vital signs are within normal limits. Her cervix is soft and pliable, 20% effaced, and 1 cm dilated. Fetal station is −3. The nurse confirms breech positioning with bedside ultrasound and admits Mrs. Pandey to the Labor and Delivery unit to prepare for surgery.

ASSESSMENT	DIAGNOSES	PLANNING
Subjective: Braxton Hicks contractions, backache, anxiety. Pain level reported as 2 out of 10. Objective: Cervix is 1 cm dilated, 20% effaced; −3 station; amniotic membranes are intact. Blood pressure 120/84 mmHg, temperature 37.1°C (98.8°F), pulse 94 beats/min, respirations 14/min, fetus in breech position confirmed by ultrasound	▪ Risk for infection related to surgical incision of abdomen and uterus by cesarean section ▪ Anxiety related to fear of surgery	▪ The patient will recover from cesarean section without signs/symptoms of infection. ▪ The patient will experience appropriate healing at the incision site without signs/symptoms of infection. ▪ The patient will be able to understand the implication for cesarean section as a safe delivery option. ▪ The patient will be able to discuss fears and anxieties related to surgery. ▪ The patient will be relaxed and comfortable prior to surgery.

IMPLEMENTATION

- Obtain baseline measurements for maternal blood pressure, pulse, respirations, temperature, and pain level.
- Confirm medical, surgical, obstetric, and prenatal history; confirm any allergies with patient.
- Obtain baseline labs, such as WBCs, to compare postoperative labs with.
- Insert IV line and administer prophylactic antibiotics as ordered.
- Ensure sterile technique is used for operative procedures.
- Monitor incision and drainage post-op for signs of infection, such as redness, warmth, or purulent drainage.
- Monitor maternal vital signs post-op for signs of infection, such as increased temperature.
- Evaluate post-op labs and compare to preoperative baseline to assess for infection.
- Evaluate mother's understanding of the need and benefits of cesarean section.
- Allow mother and support person to ask any questions or express concerns they may have about the procedure.
- Offer mother relaxation techniques to help her remain calm prior to and during surgery.
- Evaluate level of anxiety before, during, and after procedure.
- Ensure that patient and support person are informed throughout the process to help ease anxiety.

(continued on next page)

Nursing Care Plan *(continued)*

EVALUATION

- Vital signs and WBC remain within normal limits during the post-operative period.
- Incision healing appropriately with no signs/symptoms of infection.
- Mother states understanding of procedure and is able to manage anxiety through the use of relaxation techniques.

CRITICAL THINKING

1. Mrs. Pandey is postoperative day 1 on the postpartum floor and has a temperature of 101.2°F with her afternoon vitals. What other assessments should be noted before calling the HCP to report the temperature?
2. Mrs. Pandey has been transferred to the postpartum floor and the nurse is ready to assist her with walking in the halls. She expresses fear about the pain she will feel when getting up for the first time. What actions can the nurse take to ease this fear?.

Source: Adapted from Davidson et al. (2020).

REVIEW Intrapartum Care

RELATE Link the Concepts and Exemplars

Linking the exemplar of intrapartum care with the concept of comfort:

You are caring for a mother in the transition stage of labor when she begins crying and says, "It hurts so much. I don't know if I can take this anymore." As you were admitting her, when contractions were less frequent and intense, the woman told you it was very important to her that she deliver the baby without taking any pain medication and that she would feel like a failure if she gave in and took a narcotic.

1. Will you offer her a narcotic analgesic to reduce her discomfort? Explain your answer.
2. What nonpharmacologic strategies can you implement to help her manage her pain?

Linking the exemplar of intrapartum care with the concept of culture and diversity:

3. When admitting a patient to the labor unit, what cultural assessment will you perform?
4. The woman tells you a cultural belief in her family is that a candle must be burning when the baby is born because they believe the baby will move toward the light, thereby making labor easier and the baby will be born faster. How will you respond to this request?

READY Go to Volume 3: Clinical Nursing Skills

REFER Go to Pearson MyLab Nursing and eText

- Chart 6: Epidurals
- Chart 7: Intrapartum High-Risk Factors
- Chart 8: Psychologic Characteristics and Nursing Support During the First and Second Stages of Labor
- Chart 9: Deviations from Normal Labor Process Requiring Immediate Intervention
- Chart 10: Comparison of Birthing Positions

REFLECT Apply Your Knowledge

Two patients are admitted to the labor and delivery unit at the same time. The first patient is a 24-year-old single woman in labor with her first pregnancy. Her contractions are 8 minutes apart, she is dilated 2 cm (0.8 in.), and is at the +3 station. She rates her pain as 10/10 during contractions and asks how soon the physician can start the epidural. The second patient is 28 years old and in labor with her fourth child. Her contractions are also 8 minutes apart, and she is dilated to 2 cm (0.8 in.) and at the +2 station. She is laughing and joking with her partner between contractions and asks if they are allowed visitors while they wait for labor to progress.

1. What factors may be influencing the different responses of these women to the pain of labor?
2. How would your nursing care differ for these women?
3. Which woman do you anticipate is likely to deliver first? Explain your answer.

Exemplar 33.C Postpartum Care

Exemplar Learning Outcomes

33.C Summarize postpartum care of the mother.

- Summarize physical adaptations of the body systems postpartum.
- Describe the psychologic adaptations of the mother postpartum.
- Outline the nutrition requirements for new mothers.
- Summarize alterations in the postpartum period.
- Differentiate considerations related to the assessment and care of pregnant adolescents and women over age 35.
- Illustrate the nursing process in providing culturally competent care to the new mother and her family.

Exemplar Key Terms

Overview

The **puerperium**, or postpartum period, is a time of physical and psychologic adjustment for the mother. This stage begins immediately after birth and lasts until the woman's body is restored to its (near) pre-pregnant state, which takes about 6 weeks.

Physical Adaptations

As with the many physiologic changes that occurred over the course of the pregnancy, the woman's body goes through many changes as it recovers from pregnancy and birth.

Reproductive System

Postpartum physiologic changes to the woman's reproductive system include (but are not limited to) involution of the uterus; discharge of the lochia; changes to the cervix, vagina, and perineum; return of ovulation and menstruation; changes to the cardiovascular, gastrointestinal, and genitourinary systems; and changes related to the breast and lactation.

Involution

The term **involution** describes the rapid reduction in size of the uterus and the return of the uterus to a nonpregnant state. Following separation of the placenta, the decidua of the uterus is irregular, jagged, and varied in thickness. The spongy layer of the decidua is cast off as lochia (uterine discharge of the debris remaining after birth), and the basal layer of the decidua remains in the uterus to become differentiated into two layers. This occurs within the first 48 to 72 hours after birth. The outermost layer becomes necrotic and is sloughed off in the lochia. The layer closest to the myometrium contains the fundi of the uterine endometrial glands. These glands lay the foundation for the new endometrium. Except at the placenta site, this process is completed in approximately 3 weeks. It takes approximately 6 weeks for the placental site to heal (Cunningham et al., 2018). Bleeding from the larger uterine vessels of the placenta site is controlled by compression of the contracted uterine muscle fibers. The clotted blood is gradually absorbed by the body. Some of these uterine vessels are eventually obliterated and replaced by new vessels with smaller lumens.

The placenta site heals by a process of exfoliation and growth of endometrial tissue. This occurs with upward endometrial growth in the decidua basalis under the placenta site, with simultaneous growth of endometrial tissue from the margins of the site. The infarcted superficial tissue then becomes necrotic and is sloughed off (Blackburn, 2018). Exfoliation is a very important aspect of involution; if healing of the placenta site leaves a fibrous scar, the area available for future implantation is limited, as is the number of possible pregnancies.

With the dramatic decrease in the levels of circulating estrogen and progesterone following placental separation, the uterine cells atrophy and the hyperplasia of pregnancy begins to reverse. Proteolytic enzymes are released, and macrophages migrate to the uterus to promote autolysis (self-digestion), which breaks down and absorbs protein material in the uterine wall. Factors that enhance involution include an uncomplicated labor and birth, complete expulsion of the placenta and membranes, breastfeeding, manual removal of the placenta during a cesarean birth, and early ambulation.

» *Go to **Pearson MyLab Nursing and eText** for Chart 11: Factors That Slow Uterine Involution.*

The **fundus** (top portion of the uterus) is situated in the midline and is palpable below the umbilicus (**Figure 33.54**»).

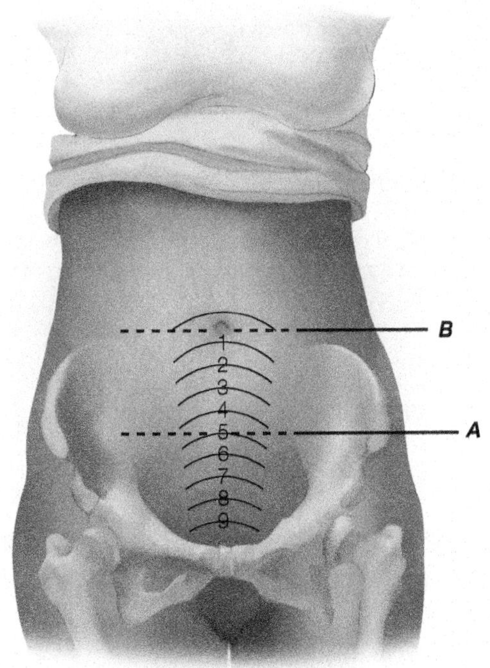

Figure 33.54 » Involution of the uterus. ***A***, Immediately after delivery of the placenta, the top of the fundus is in the midline and approximately halfway between the symphysis pubis and the umbilicus. Approximately 6–12 hours after birth, the fundus is at the level of the umbilicus. ***B***, The height of the fundus then decreases about one fingerbreadth (~1 cm) each day.

Following expulsion of the placenta, the uterus contracts to the size of a large grapefruit. The uterine blood vessels are firmly compressed by the myometrium. Blood and clots that remain within the uterus and changes in support of the uterus by the ligaments cause the fundus of the uterus to rise to the level of the umbilicus within 6 to 12 hours after birth.

A fundus that is above the umbilicus and is boggy (feels soft and spongy rather than firm and well contracted) is associated with excessive uterine bleeding. As blood collects and forms clots within the uterus, the fundus rises, interrupting firm contractions of the uterus and exacerbating **uterine atony** (relaxation of uterine muscle tone).

When the fundus is higher than expected on palpation and is not in the midline (usually deviated to the right), distention of the bladder should be suspected; the bladder should be emptied immediately and the uterus reassessed. If the woman is unable to void, in-and-out catheterization of the bladder may be required. In the immediate postpartum period, many women may not be aware of a full bladder. Because the uterine ligaments are still stretched, a full bladder can move the uterus. By the end of the puerperium, these ligaments regain their nonpregnant length and tension.

After birth, the top of the fundus remains at the level of the umbilicus for about half a day. On the first day postpartum, the top of the fundus is located about 1 cm (0.4 in.) below the umbilicus. The top of the fundus descends approximately one fingerbreadth (width of the index, second, or third finger), or 1 cm (0.4 in.), per day until it descends into the pelvis on about the 10th day.

If the mother is breastfeeding, the release of endogenous oxytocin from the posterior pituitary in response to suckling hastens involution of the uterus. Barring complications, such as infection or retained placental fragments, the uterus approaches its pre-pregnant size and location by 5 to 6 weeks. In women who had an oversized uterus during the pregnancy (because of hydramnios, birth of a LGA baby, or multiple gestation), the time frame for an immediate uterine involution process is lengthened. If intrauterine infection is present, foul-smelling lochia or vaginal discharge results. The infection irritates the uterine muscle, causing the fundus to descend much more slowly. When infection is suspected, other clinical signs, such as fever and tachycardia, and fundal tenderness must be assessed. Any slowing of descent is called **subinvolution**.

Afterpains (cramplike pains caused by intermittent contractions of the uterus that occur after childbirth) are often more severe in multiparas than in primiparas. These afterpains may cause the mother severe discomfort for 2 to 3 days after birth. The administration of uterotonic agents (IV infusion with oxytocin or oral administration of methylergonovine maleate) stimulates uterine contraction and increases the discomfort of the afterpains. A warm water bottle placed against the lower abdomen may reduce this discomfort. In addition, the breastfeeding mother may find it helpful to take a mild analgesic agent approximately 1 hour before feeding her baby. The nurse can assure the mother who is breastfeeding that the prescribed analgesics are not harmful to the newborn and help improve the quality of the breastfeeding experience. If afterpains are interfering with the mother's rest, she may find it helpful to take an analgesic at bedtime.

Lochia

The uterus rids itself of the debris remaining after birth through a discharge called **lochia**, which is classified according to its appearance and contents. These classifications are lochia rubra, lochia serosa, and lochia alba.

Lochia rubra is dark red. It occurs for the first 1–3 days and contains epithelial cells, erythrocytes, leukocytes, shreds of decidua, and occasionally fetal meconium, lanugo, and vernix. Clotting is often the result of blood pooling in the upper portion of the vagina. A few small clots (no larger than a nickel) are common, particularly in the first few days after birth. However, lochia should not contain large (plum-size) clots; if it does, the cause should be investigated without delay.

Lochia serosa is a pinkish color. It occurs from approximately day 3 until day 10. Lochia serosa is composed of serous exudate, erythrocytes, leukocytes, cervical mucus, and numerous microorganisms (Blackburn, 2018; Lowdermilk et al., 2020).

The RBC component decreases gradually, and a creamy or yellowish discharge persists for an additional week or two. This final discharge, termed **lochia alba** (from the Latin word for *white*), is composed primarily of leukocytes, decidual cells, epithelial cells, fat, cervical mucus, cholesterol crystals, and bacteria. Variation in the duration of lochia discharge is not uncommon; however, the trend should be toward a lighter amount of flow and a lighter color of discharge. When the lochia flow stops, the cervix is considered to be closed, and chances of infection ascending from the vagina to the uterus decrease.

Like menstrual discharge, lochia flow has a musty, stale odor that is not offensive. Microorganisms are always present in the vaginal lochia and contaminate the uterus with vaginal bacteria by the second day following birth. It is thought that infection does not develop because the organisms involved are relatively nonvirulent. Any foul smell to the lochia or used peripad suggests infection and the need for prompt additional assessment, such as WBC count and differential and assessment for uterine tenderness and fever.

The total daily volume of lochia gradually decreases over the postpartum period (Blackburn, 2018). Discharge is greater after lying down because of pooling in the vagina and uterus. Temporary increases in lochia may be noted with exertion or breastfeeding. Multiparous women usually have more lochia than first-time mothers. Women who undergo a cesarean birth typically have less lochia than women who give birth vaginally (Blackburn, 2018).

Evaluation of lochia is necessary not only to determine whether hemorrhage is present but also to assess uterine involution. The type, amount, and consistency of lochia determine the stage of healing of the placenta site; a progressive change from bright red at birth to dark red, then to pink, and then to white or clear discharge should be observed over the first 2 weeks. A failure to transition from lochia rubra to lochia serosa within the first week postpartum or a return to lochia rubra may indicate subinvolution or late postpartum hemorrhage. Patients should be instructed to call their doctor if they notice bright red bleeding beyond 4 to 5 days postpartum or a return to bright red bleeding after it had previously ceased.

The nurse should exercise caution in evaluating bleeding immediately after birth. The continuous seepage of blood is more consistent with cervical or vaginal lacerations and may be effectively diagnosed when the bleeding is evaluated in conjunction with uterine consistency. Lacerations should be suspected if the uterus is firm and of expected size and if no clots can be expressed.

Cervical Changes

Following birth, the cervix is flabby, formless, and may appear bruised. The lateral aspects of the external os are occasionally lacerated during the birth process (Cunningham et al., 2018). The external os is markedly irregular and closes slowly. It admits two fingers for a few days following birth, but by the end of the first week, it admits only a fingertip.

The first childbearing permanently changes the shape of the external os. The characteristic dimple-like os of the nullipara changes to the transverse slit (fish-mouth) os of the multipara. After a significant cervical laceration or several lacerations, the cervix may appear lopsided. Because of the slight change in the size of the cervix, changes in maternal weight, muscle tone, and pelvic architecture, a diaphragm or cervical cap will need to be refitted if the woman uses one of these methods of contraception.

Vaginal Changes

The vagina appears edematous and may be bruised following birth. The apparent bruising is caused by pelvic congestion and trauma and quickly disappears. Small, superficial lacerations may be evident, and the rugae are obliterated. The hymen, torn and jagged, heals irregularly, leaving small tags called caruncula myrtiformes.

The size of the vagina decreases, and rugae return within 3 to 4 weeks, although it may never be the same dimensions as prior to delivery (Blackburn, 2018). By 6 weeks, the vagina of a woman who is not breastfeeding usually appears normal. The lactating woman is in a hypoestrogenic state because of ovarian suppression, and her vaginal mucosa may be pale and without rugae. The effects of the lowered estrogen level may lead to dyspareunia (painful intercourse), which may be reduced by the addition of a water-soluble personal lubricant.

Tone and contractility of the vagina may be improved by perineal tightening exercises, such as Kegel exercises (discussed in Exemplar 33.A, Antepartum Care, in this module). The woman may begin these soon after birth. The labia majora and labia minora are more flaccid in the woman who has borne a child than in the nullipara.

Perineal Changes

During the early postpartum period, the soft tissue in and around the perineum may appear edematous, with some bruising. If an episiotomy or a laceration is present, the edges should be approximated. Complete healing of episiotomies or lacerations may take up to 6 months, during which time the woman may experience discomfort (Blackburn, 2018).

Ovulation and Menstruation

The return of ovulation and menstruation varies. Mothers who are not breastfeeding tend to have a return of ovulation and menstruation within 6 weeks (Blackburn, 2018). The return of ovulation is directly associated with a rise in the serum progesterone level.

The length of time for return of ovulation and menstruation in breastfeeding mothers is usually prolonged. It is associated with the length of time the woman breastfeeds and whether formula supplements are used. If a mother breastfeeds for less than 1 month, the return of menstruation and ovulation is similar to that in the woman who is not breastfeeding. Women who exclusively breastfeed usually experience a delay in menstruation. Suckling by the baby typically results in alterations in gonadotropin-releasing hormone production, which is thought to be the cause of amenorrhea (Blackburn, 2018). Although exclusive breastfeeding helps to reduce the risk of pregnancy for the first 6 months after birth, it should be relied on only temporarily and if it meets the criteria for the lactational amenorrhea method. Furthermore, because ovulation precedes menstruation and because women often supplement breastfeeding with bottles and pacifiers, breastfeeding is not considered to be a reliable means of contraception.

Abdomen

The uterine ligaments (notably the round and broad ligaments) are stretched and require the length of the puerperium to recover. Although the stretched abdominal wall appears loose and flabby, it responds to exercise within 2 to 3 months. However, the abdomen may fail to regain good tone and will remain flabby in the grand multipara, in the woman whose abdomen is overdistended, or in the woman with poor muscle tone before pregnancy. **Diastasis recti abdominis** (a separation of the abdominal muscle) may occur with pregnancy. If diastasis occurs, part of the abdominal wall has no muscular support and is formed only by skin, subcutaneous fat, fascia, and peritoneum. This may be especially pronounced in women who have undergone a cesarean section, during which the rectus abdominis muscles are manually separated to access the uterine muscle. Improvement depends on the physical condition of the mother, the total number of pregnancies, pregnancy spacing, and the type and amount of physical exercise. Diastasis may result in a pendulous abdomen and increased maternal backache. Fortunately, diastasis responds well to exercise, and abdominal muscle tone can improve significantly.

The striae (stretch marks), which occur as a result of stretching and rupture of the elastic fibers of the skin, take on different colors based on the mother's skin color. The striae of light-skinned mothers are red to purple at the time of birth, then gradually fade to silver or white. The striae of mothers with darker skin, in contrast, are darker than the surrounding skin and remain darker. Striae gradually fade over time, but they do remain visible.

Breasts and Lactogenesis

During pregnancy, increased levels of estrogen stimulate breast duct proliferation and development, and elevated progesterone levels promote the development of lobules and alveoli in preparation for lactation. Prolactin levels rise from approximately 10 mcg/mL before pregnancy to 200 mcg/mL at term. However, lactation is suppressed during pregnancy by elevated progesterone levels secreted by the placenta. Once the placenta is expelled at birth, progesterone levels fall, and the inhibition is removed, triggering milk production.

This occurs whether the mother has breast stimulation or not. If breast stimulation is not occurring by the third or fourth day, however, prolactin levels begin to drop. By 7 to 14 days postpartum, prolactin levels in nonlactating women will be back to pre-pregnancy levels, and milk production will cease (Blackburn, 2018).

Initially, lactation is under endocrine control. The hormone prolactin is released from the anterior pituitary in response to breast stimulation from suckling or the use of a breast pump. Prolactin stimulates the milk-secreting cells in the alveoli to produce milk, then rapidly drops back to baseline. If more than approximately 3 hours elapse between stimulation, prolactin levels begin to drop below baseline. To reverse the overall decline in prolactin level, the mother can be encouraged to stimulate her breasts more frequently (e.g., every 1.5 to 2.0 hours). Mothers should be strongly encouraged to stimulate their breasts frequently if their babies are not effective feeders or if they are separated from their babies. Prolactin receptors increase quickly after birth with each feeding or breast stimulation (Blackburn, 2018). Inadequate development of prolactin receptors during this time is likely to negatively impact the mother's long-term milk volume.

Colostrum is the initial milk that begins to be secreted during midpregnancy and that is immediately available to the baby at birth. It provides the newborn with all the nutrition required until the mother's milk becomes more abundant in a few days. No routine supplementation of other fluids is necessary unless there is a medical indication. Colostrum is a thick, creamy, yellowish fluid with concentrated amounts of protein, fat-soluble vitamins, and minerals; it has lower amounts of fat and lactose than mature milk. It also contains antioxidants and high levels of lactoferrin and secretory IgA. It promotes the establishment of *Lactobacillus bifidus* flora in the digestive tract, which helps protect the baby from disease and illness. Colostrum also has a laxative effect on the newborn, which helps the baby pass meconium stools, which in turn helps decrease hyperbilirubinemia (Ladewig, London, & Davidson, 2017).

The milk that flows from the breast at the start of a feeding or pumping session is called *foremilk*. The foremilk is watery milk that is high in protein and low in fat (1–2%). This milk has trickled down from the alveoli between feedings to fill the lactiferous ducts, and it is low in fat because the fat globules made in the alveoli stick to each other and to the walls of the alveoli and do not trickle down. In addition to prolactin release, stretching of the nipple and compression of the areola signal the hypothalamus to trigger the posterior pituitary gland to release oxytocin. Oxytocin acts to cause the myoepithelial cells surrounding the alveoli in the breast tissue to contract, ejecting milk (including the fat globules present) into the ducts. This process is called the milk-ejection reflex but is better known in lay terms as the "let-down" reflex (response). The average initial let-down response occurs about 2 minutes after a baby begins to suckle, and between 4 and 10 let-down responses will occur during a feeding session. The milk that flows during "let-down" is called *hindmilk*. Hindmilk is rich in fat (which can exceed 10%) and, therefore, is high in calories. In a sample of expressed breast milk, the average total fat concentration is approximately 4% and the total caloric content is approximately 20 calories/oz.

By 6 months of breastfeeding, prolactin levels are only 5 to 10 mcg/mL, yet milk production continues. A whey protein called feedback inhibitor of lactation (FIL) has been identified as influencing milk production through a negative feedback loop. FIL is present in breast milk and functions to decrease milk production. If there is milk stasis in the breast, FIL levels increase, decreasing overall milk production (Blackburn, 2018). On the other hand, the more often the breasts are emptied, the lower the level of FIL and the faster milk is produced. This mechanism of regulating milk at the local level is called autocrine control.

A number of factors can delay or impair lactogenesis. Maternal factors include the following (Janke, 2014):

- Cesarean birth
- Postpartum hemorrhage
- Type 1 diabetes
- Untreated hypothyroidism
- Obesity
- Polycystic ovary syndrome
- Retained placenta fragments
- Vitamin B_6 deficiency
- History of previous breast surgery
- Insufficient glandular breast tissue
- Significant stress.

Other factors that can interfere with breastfeeding include smoking, use of alcohol, and use of some prescription and OTC medications (e.g., antihistamines, some oral contraceptives).

Stages of Human Milk

During the establishment of lactation, there are three stages of human milk:

1. Colostrum
2. Transitional milk
3. Mature milk.

After 30 to 72 hours of colostrum production, maternal milk production normally becomes noticeably more abundant. The milk "coming in" is called **transitional milk** and has qualities intermediate between those of colostrum and mature milk. It is still light yellow in color, but is more copious than colostrum and contains more fat, lactose, water-soluble vitamins, and calories. By day 5, most mothers are producing approximately 500 mL/day.

Mature milk is white or slightly blue-tinged in color. It is present by 2 weeks postpartum and continues thereafter until lactation ceases. Mature milk contains approximately 13% solids (carbohydrates, proteins, and fats) and 87% water. Mature human milk's appearance, similar to that of skim cow's milk, may cause mothers to question whether their milk is "rich enough." The nurse should reassure the mother that this is the normal appearance of mature human milk and that it provides the baby with all the necessary nutrients. Although gradual changes in composition do occur continuously over periods of weeks to accommodate the needs of the growing newborn, the composition of mature milk in general is fairly consistent with the exception of the fat content as noted previously. Milk production continues to increase slowly during the first month. By 6 months postpartum, a mother produces approximately 800 mL/day (Blackburn, 2018).

Gastrointestinal System

It is common for the mother to be quite thirsty after giving birth due to losing fluids during labor, in urine, and through perspiration. She may also be hungry and need a light meal or snack. While institutional policies may vary, evidence suggests that advancing the diet as desired restores the gastrointestinal system to a normal state more quickly than withholding solids and does not lead to an increased rate of complications, even for women who have undergone a cesarean section (King et al., 2019).

It is normal for bowels to be sluggish immediately after birth due to bowel evacuation during labor and birth, decreased abdominal muscle tone, and continued effects of progesterone. Women who have lacerations or hemorrhoids and those who had an episiotomy may believe that having a bowel movement will tear stitches or increase pain levels. They may try to postpone the first bowel movement to avoid discomfort. However, this can cause increased constipation and more pain when they do finally relieve their bowels.

Women who experience discomfort related to flatulence may find early ambulation, chamomile or peppermint tea, or use of medications to reduce flatulence helpful. Especially if general anesthesia was used, the bowel may take a few days to regain tone. For mothers who had a cesarean or difficult birth, stool softeners may be helpful.

Urinary System

The postpartum woman has increased bladder capacity, swelling and bruising of the tissue around the urethra, decreased sensitivity to fluid pressure, and decreased sensation of bladder filling. Consequently, she is at risk for overdistention, incomplete bladder emptying, and buildup of residual urine. Women who have had anesthesia, such as an epidural or spinal, have inhibited neural functioning of the bladder and are more susceptible to bladder distention, difficulty voiding, and bladder infections. In addition, use of oxytocin to facilitate uterine contractions following expulsion of the placenta has an antidiuretic effect. Following cessation of the oxytocin, the woman will experience rapid bladder filling.

Urinary output increases during the early postpartum period (first 12 to 24 hours) because of postpartum diuresis. The kidneys must eliminate an estimated 2000 to 3000 mL of extracellular fluid with the normal pregnancy, which causes rapid filling of the bladder (Blackburn, 2018). Adequate bladder elimination is an immediate concern. Women with preeclampsia, chronic HTN, and diabetes experience greater fluid retention than do other women, and postpartum diuresis is increased accordingly.

If urinary stasis exists, chances for a UTI increase because of bacteriuria and the presence of dilated ureters and renal pelves, which persist for approximately 6 weeks after birth. A full bladder may also increase the tendency of the uterus to relax by displacing the uterus and interfering with its contractility, leading to hemorrhage. In the absence of infection, the dilated ureters and renal pelves return to pre-pregnant size by the end of the sixth week.

Vital Signs

With the possible exception of the first 24 hours after birth, the woman should be afebrile during the postpartum period. A maternal temperature of up to 38°C (100.4°F) may occur after childbirth as a result of the exertion and dehydration of labor. An increase in temperature to between 37.8 and 39°C (100 and 102.2°F) may also occur during the first 24 hours after the mother's milk comes in (Cunningham et al., 2018). However, in women not meeting these criteria, infection must be considered in the presence of an increased temperature.

Immediately following childbirth, many women experience a transient rise in both systolic and diastolic blood pressures, which spontaneously return to the pre-pregnancy baseline during the next few weeks (Lowdermilk et al., 2020). A decrease may indicate physiologic readjustment to decreased intrapelvic pressure or it may be related to uterine hemorrhage. Orthostatic hypotension, as indicated by feelings of faintness or dizziness immediately after standing up, can develop in the first 48 hours as a result of abdominal engorgement that may occur after birth. A low or decreasing blood pressure may reflect hypovolemia secondary to hemorrhage, but it is a late sign (see discussion of hypovolemia in Module 6, Fluids and Electrolytes). Blood pressure elevations may result from excessive use of oxytocin or vasopressor medications. Because preeclampsia can persist into or occur first in the postpartum period, routine evaluation of blood pressure is needed. If a woman complains of headache, HTN must be ruled out before analgesics are administered.

Puerperal bradycardia with rates of 50 to 70 beats/min commonly occurs during the first 6 to 10 days of the postpartum period. This may be related to decreased cardiac effort, decreased blood volume following placental separation and contraction of the uterus, and increased stroke volume. A pulse rate of greater than 100 beats/min may indicate hypovolemia, infection, fear, or pain and requires further assessment.

Frequently, the mother experiences intense tremors that resemble shivering from a chill immediately after birth. This shivering has been explained as a

- result of the sudden release of pressure on the pelvic nerves after birth,
- response to a fetus-to-mother transfusion that occurred during placental separation,
- reaction to maternal adrenaline production during labor and birth, or
- reaction to epidural anesthesia.

If not followed by fever, this chill is of no clinical concern, but it is uncomfortable for the woman. The nurse can increase the woman's comfort by covering her with a warmed blanket and reassuring her that the shivering is a common, self-limiting situation. If the woman allows herself to go with the shaking, the shivering will last only a short time. Later in the puerperium, chill and fever indicate infection and require further evaluation.

Blood Values

Blood values should return to the pre-pregnant state by the end of the postpartum period. Pregnancy-associated activation of coagulation factors may continue for variable amounts of time after birth. This condition, in conjunction with trauma, immobility, sepsis, obesity, African American ethnicity, diabetes, smoking, and advanced maternal age, predisposes the woman to development of thromboembolism (King et al., 2019). The incidence of thromboembolism is reduced by early ambulation.

Nonpathologic leukocytosis often occurs during labor and in the immediate postpartum period, with WBC counts up to 30,000 cells/mm^3 (Cunningham et al., 2018). These values typically return to normal levels by the end of the first postpartum week. Leukocytosis along with the normal increase in erythrocyte sedimentation rate may make it difficult to determine if acute infection is present (Lowdermilk et al., 2020).

Hemoglobin and hematocrit levels may be difficult to interpret during the first 2 days after birth because of the changing blood volume. Blood loss up to 500 mL for a vaginal delivery and up to 1000 mL for a cesarean delivery is considered normal (King et al., 2019). With larger blood loss, a decrease in hemoglobin and hematocrit will be noted. In addition, the shift in interstitial fluid that occurs after delivery causes hemodilution, further reducing the hemoglobin and hematocrit values. These slowly return to normal levels by 6 weeks postpartum (King et al., 2019).

Platelet levels typically fall as a result of placental separation. They then begin to increase by the third to fourth day postpartum, gradually returning to normal by the sixth week postpartum. Fibrinolytic activity typically returns to normal during the hours following birth. The hemostatic system as a whole reaches its normal pre-pregnant status by 3 to 4 weeks postpartum; however, the diameter of deep veins can take up to 6 weeks to return to pre-pregnant levels (Blackburn, 2018). This explains the prolonged risk of thromboembolism in the first 6 weeks following birth.

Cardiovascular Changes

The mother's cardiovascular system undergoes dramatic changes during the birth that can result in cardiovascular instability because of an increase in CO. The CO typically stabilizes and returns to pre-pregnancy levels within an hour following birth. Maternal hypervolemia acts to protect the mother from excessive blood loss. CO declines by 30% in the first 2 weeks and reaches normal levels by 6 to 12 weeks (Blackburn, 2018).

Diuresis in the first week after birth assists in decreasing the extracellular fluid and results in a weight loss of 3 kg (6.6 lb) (Blackburn, 2018). Failure to have diuresis in the immediate postpartum period can lead to pulmonary edema and subsequent cardiac problems. This is seen more commonly in women with a history of preeclampsia or preexisting cardiac problems (Blackburn, 2018).

Neurologic and Immunologic Changes

Neurologic problems and disorders can predispose women to higher rates of morbidity and mortality during pregnancy and the postpartum period. Headaches are the most common neurologic symptoms encountered by postpartum women. Headaches may have simple causes, such as stress and muscle tension. They may have more complex causes, such as a cerebrospinal fluid leak from an epidural or preeclampsia (Blackburn, 2018). Women with chronic neurologic disorders, such as epilepsy or multiple sclerosis, may find that the hormonal and physiological changes of pregnancy and birth cause changes in their disease processes (Blackburn, 2018).

Psychologic Adaptations

The postpartum period is a time of readjustment and adaptation for the entire childbearing family but especially for the mother. The woman experiences a variety of responses as she adjusts to a new family member, postpartum discomforts, changes in her body image, and the reality that she is no longer pregnant.

The first day or two after birth, the mother may seem passive about the event and may seem more concerned with her own needs. Food and sleep are priority needs, and she begins to process the event. By the second or third day, the new mother is ready to resume control of her mothering and of her body and life in general. At this stage, however, she may experience anxiety and require assurance that she is doing well as a mother. Difficulties with feedings may be a particular source of anxiety.

Maternal Role Attainment

Maternal role attainment (MRA) is the process by which a woman learns mothering behaviors and becomes comfortable with her identity as a mother. Formation of a maternal identity occurs with each child a woman bears. As the mother grows to know this child and forms a relationship, the mother's maternal identity gradually and systematically evolves, and she "binds in" to the newborn (Rubin, 1984).

Maternal role attainment often occurs in four stages (Mercer, 1995):

1. ***The anticipatory stage*** occurs during pregnancy. The woman looks to role models, especially her own mother, for examples of how to mother.
2. ***The formal stage*** begins when the child is born. The woman is still influenced by the guidance of others and tries to act as she believes others expect her to act.
3. ***The informal stage*** begins when the mother starts making her own choices about mothering. The woman begins to develop her own style of mothering and finds ways of functioning that work well for her.
4. ***The personal stage*** is the final stage of maternal role attainment. When the woman reaches this stage, she is comfortable with the notion of herself as "mother."

In most cases, MRA occurs within 3 to 10 months after birth. Social support, the woman's age and personality traits, the marital relationship, the presence of underlying anxiety or depression, the woman's previous child care experiences, the temperament of her infant, and the family's SES all influence the woman's success in attaining the maternal role.

Postpartum women face a number of challenges as they adjust to their new role (Mercer, 1995):

- Finding time for themselves. Mothers must adjust to having less time for self-care.

- Feelings of incompetence because they have not mastered all aspects of the mothering role. Often mothers find themselves unsure of what to do in a given situation.
- Fatigue resulting from sleep deprivation. The demands of nighttime care are tremendously draining, especially when the woman has other children.
- The feeling of responsibility that having a child brings. A woman experiences a sense of lost freedom, an awareness that she will never again be quite as carefree as she was before becoming a mother.
- Finding time for older children following the birth of a new baby. Many women feel guilty because the new baby takes up so much of their time. Sibling rivalry or ill feelings about the baby from other children can put additional stress on the mother.
- The infant's behavior can sometimes be a challenge, especially when the child is about 8 months old. The baby develops stranger anxiety, begins crawling and getting into things, and may be fussy from teething. In addition, the baby's tendency to put things in the mouth requires constant vigilance by the parent.

Mercer (2004) later proposed replacing the term *maternal role attainment* with the term *becoming a mother (BAM)*, which better encompasses the idea that becoming a mother transforms a woman's total persona and is not merely a role to be attained.

A mother's first interaction with her newborn is influenced by many factors, including her involvement with her family of origin, her relationships, the stability of her home environment, the communication patterns she has developed, and the degree of nurturing she received as a child. These factors shaped the person she has become. The following personal characteristics are also important:

- ***Level of trust.*** What level of trust has this mother developed in response to her life experiences? What is her philosophy of childrearing?
- ***Level of self-esteem.*** How much does she value herself as a woman and a mother? Is she generally able to cope with the adjustments of life?
- ***Capacity for enjoying herself.*** Is the mother able to find pleasure in everyday activities and human relationships?
- ***Adequacy of knowledge about childbearing and childrearing.*** What beliefs about the course of pregnancy, the capabilities of newborns, previous experiences with infants or children, and the nature of her emotions may influence her behavior at first contact with her newborn and later?
- ***Prevailing mood or usual feeling tone.*** Is the woman predominantly content, angry, depressed, or anxious? Is she sensitive to her own feelings and those of others?
- ***Reactions to the present pregnancy.*** Was the pregnancy planned? Did it go smoothly? Were there ongoing life events that enhanced her pregnancy or depleted her reserves of energy? How have other life roles changed because of her pregnancy and motherhood?

Initially after birth during the *taking-in* period, the woman tends to be passive and somewhat dependent. She follows suggestions, hesitates to make decisions, and is still rather preoccupied with her needs (Rubin, 1984). She may have a great need to talk about her perceptions of her labor and birth. This helps her work through the process, sort out the reality from her fantasized experience, and clarify anything that she did not understand. Food and sleep are major needs.

By the second or third day after birth, the new mother is often ready to resume control of her body, her mothering, and her life in general. Rubin (1984) labeled this the *taking-hold* period. If she is breastfeeding, she may worry about her technique or the quality of her milk. If her baby spits up after a feeding, she may view it as a personal failure. She may also feel demoralized by the fact that the nurse or an older family member handles her baby proficiently while she feels unsure and tentative. She requires assurance that she is doing well as a mother. Today's mothers seem to be more independent and adjust more rapidly, exhibiting behaviors of "taking-in" and "taking-hold" in shorter periods of time than those previously identified.

Development of Family Attachment

Family assessment that includes long-term stressors affecting family members' adjustments to the arrival of the newborn can help nurses identify issues for anticipatory guidance and patient teaching. Parenting groups—in person or online—may provide opportunities for parents to share problems and seek information and solutions.

Father–Newborn Interactions

Father–child (or partner–child) interactions are influenced by a variety of factors, including cultural and religious expectations and practices, the relationship status of the couple, the father's personal history with his own parents and with other role models, and the father's own perspectives on and ideas about parenting. The attachment that the father and newborn develop after the baby's arrival is called *engrossment*. Engrossment includes both the behaviors and emotions that form between the father and child (Lowdermilk et al., 2020). Early, successful encounters with nurses and other providers can promote confidence and involvement of fathers and partners with their newborns. Nurses can promote their involvement by teaching aspects of newborn care, such as safe holding positions and bathing, and by providing encouragement and positive reinforcement.

LGBTQ Families

It is important for the nurse caring for the new family to be aware of the many types of family variations. Most research regarding the transition to parenthood is linked directly to traditional gender roles and based on heterosexual couples. As legal and social structures within the United States change regarding LGBTQ families, nurses need to provide appropriate care for the mother and her partner, regardless of the partner's gender or the couple's relationship status. Understanding that traditional gender roles may not fit every family, whether they are LGBTQ or not, is an important nursing consideration. Allowing the family to guide care based on their preferences and teaching the patient and family without bias are ways to help them transition to parenthood.

>> **Stay Current:** The National LGBTQIA+ Health Education Center offers educational programs and resources to assist healthcare organizations with optimizing care to this population. For more information, go to lgbtqiahealtheducation.org.

Siblings and Others

Babies are able to form a number of healthy attachments. Many hospitals and birth centers offer extended visiting hours, rooming-in, and other policies that promote opportunities for family members and others to begin the attachment process. Behaviors to encourage in siblings and others to help promote attachment include eye contact, smiling, and cuddling. For siblings who are too young to hold the baby independently, nurses can promote attachment by encouraging the sibling to sit with a parent and cuddle together.

Initial Maternal Attachment Behavior

After labor and birth, a new mother demonstrates a fairly regular pattern of maternal behaviors as she continues to familiarize herself with her newborn. In a progression of touching activities, the mother proceeds from fingertip exploration of the newborn's extremities toward palmar contact with larger body areas and finally to enfolding the newborn with the whole hand and arm. The time she takes to accomplish these steps varies from minutes to days. The mother increases the proportion of time spent in the *en face* position—she arranges herself or the newborn so that she has direct face-to-face and eye-to-eye contact (**Figure 33.55** >>). There is an intense interest in having the newborn's eyes open. When the newborn's eyes are open, the mother characteristically greets and talks to the baby in high-pitched tones.

In most instances, the mother relies heavily on her senses of sight, touch, and hearing in getting to know what her baby is really like. She also tends to respond verbally to any sounds emitted by the newborn, such as cries, coughs, sneezes, and grunts. The sense of smell may be involved as well.

The nurse plays a key role in assessing and assisting the mother–newborn bond. As discussed in detail in Exemplar 33.D in this module, the nurse facilitates a number of activities that help strengthen maternal attachment, including feeding, bathing, and recognizing the baby's specific cues related to sleep and activity. Ongoing assessment of the mother's psychologic adaptation is critical because it allows the nurse to evaluate what patient teaching needs to be provided. Nursing interventions that foster the process of becoming a mother include the following categories:

- Instructing for newborn/infant caregiving
- Building awareness of and responsiveness to newborn/infant interactive capabilities
- Promoting maternal–newborn attachment
- Preparing the woman for maternal social role preparation
- Encouraging interactive therapeutic nurse–patient relationships.

Maternal/social role preparation and interactive therapeutic nurse–patient relationships may have a greater impact on the progress of becoming a mother than formal teaching. A detailed discussion of psychologic assessment of the postpartum mother is included in the Nursing Process section of this exemplar.

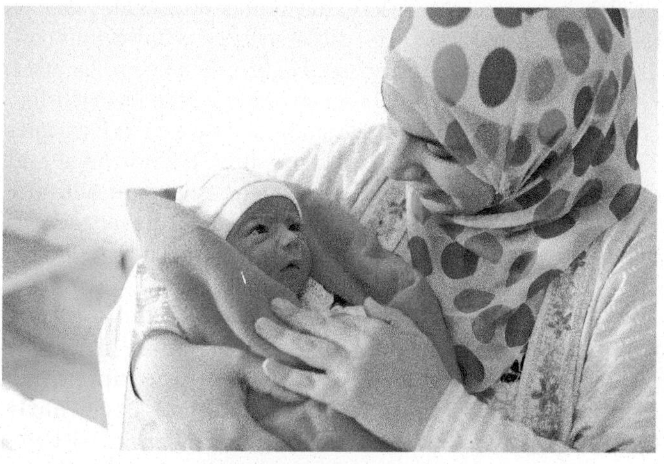

Figure 33.55 >> A mother *en face* with her newborn.
Source: ZouZou/Shutterstock.

Postpartum Weight and Nutrition

An initial weight loss of approximately 4.5 to 5.4 kg (10 to 12 lb) occurs as a result of birth of the baby and expulsion of the placenta and amniotic fluid. Diuresis accounts for the loss of an additional 2.3 kg (5 lb) during the early puerperium. By the sixth to eighth week after birth, many women have returned to approximately their pre-pregnant weight if they had gained the average 11.4 to 13.6 kg (25 to 30 lb) during pregnancy. For others, a return to pre-pregnant weight may take longer. Women often express concern about the slow pace of their postpartum weight loss. Multiparas tend to be more positive than primiparas, probably because a multipara's previous experience has prepared her for the fact that the body does not immediately return to a pre-pregnant state.

Nutritional needs change following childbirth. Nutrient requirements vary depending on whether the mother decides to breastfeed. An assessment of postpartum nutritional status is necessary before giving nutritional guidance. Postpartum nutritional status is determined primarily by assessing the new mother's weight, hemoglobin and hematocrit levels, clinical signs, and dietary history.

Postpartum Nutritional Status

The amount of weight gained during pregnancy is a major determinant of weight loss after childbirth. Generally, women who gain excessive weight during pregnancy are more likely to sustain a weight gain 1 year following childbirth, putting them at increased risk of long-term overweight or obesity. The mother's weight should be considered in terms of ideal weight, pre-pregnancy weight, and weight gain during pregnancy. Women who desire information about weight reduction can be referred to a dietitian or nutritionist for individual counseling or to community-based educational programs.

Hemoglobin and erythrocyte levels should return to normal within 2 to 6 weeks after childbirth. Hematocrit levels gradually rise because of hemoconcentration as extracellular fluid is excreted. Iron supplements are generally continued for 2 to 3 months following childbirth to replenish stores depleted by pregnancy.

The nurse assesses clinical symptoms the new mother may be experiencing. Constipation is a common problem following birth. The nurse can encourage the woman to maintain a high fluid intake to keep the stool soft. Dietary sources of fiber, such as whole grains, fruits, and vegetables, are also helpful in preventing constipation.

The nurse obtains specific information on dietary intake and eating habits directly from the woman. Visiting the mother during mealtimes provides an opportunity for unobtrusive nutritional assessment. Which foods has the woman selected? Is her diet nutritionally sound? A comment focusing on a positive aspect of her meal selection may initiate a discussion of nutrition.

The nurse needs to inform the dietitian if a woman's cultural or religious beliefs require specific foods so that appropriate meals can be prepared for her. The nurse may also refer women with unusual eating habits or numerous questions about good nutrition. In addition, the nurse provides literature on nutrition so that women will have a source of appropriate information at home.

During the childbearing years, the risk for obesity becomes especially problematic for women. Consequently, it is critical to use the postpartum period to change behaviors and help promote effective weight management in women.

Nutritional Care of Formula-Feeding Mothers

After birth, the formula-feeding mother's dietary requirements return to pre-pregnancy levels. If the mother has a good understanding of nutritional principles, it is sufficient to advise her to reduce her daily caloric intake by approximately 300 kcal and to return to pre-pregnancy levels for other nutrients.

If the mother has a limited understanding of nutrition, now is the time to teach her the basic principles and importance of a well-balanced diet. Her eating habits and dietary practices will eventually be reflected in the diet of her child.

If the mother has gained excessive weight during pregnancy (or perhaps was overweight before pregnancy) and wishes to lose weight, the nurse should refer her to a dietitian or a nutritionist. A weight-reduction diet can be designed to meet nutritional needs and food preferences. Weight loss goals of 0.45 to 0.9 kg (1 to 2 lb) per week are usually suggested.

In addition to meeting her own nutritional needs, the new mother is usually interested in learning how to provide for her baby's nutritional needs. A discussion of newborn/infant feeding that includes topics such as selecting newborn/infant formulas, formula preparation, and vitamin and mineral supplementation is appropriate and generally well received.

Nutritional Care of Breastfeeding Mothers

The nutritional needs of the mother are increased during breastfeeding. In Exemplar 33.A in this module, Table 33.4 lists the Dietary Reference Intakes during breastfeeding for specific nutrients. It is especially important for the breastfeeding mother to consume sufficient calories because inadequate caloric intake can reduce milk volume. However, milk quality generally remains unaffected. The breastfeeding mother should increase her calorie intake by approximately 200 kcal over her pregnancy requirement or 500 kcal over her pre-pregnancy requirement. This results in a total of approximately 2500 to 2700 kcal/day for most women.

Because protein is an important ingredient in breast milk, an adequate intake while breastfeeding is essential. An intake of 65 g/day during the first 6 months of breastfeeding, and of 62 g/day during the second 6 months, is recommended. As in pregnancy, it is important for the mother to consume adequate nonprotein calories to prevent the use of protein as an energy source.

Calcium is an important ingredient in milk production, and requirements during lactation remain the same as those during pregnancy—that is, an increase of 1000 mg/day. If the intake of calcium from food sources is not adequate, calcium supplements are recommended.

Liquids are especially important during lactation because inadequate fluid intake may decrease milk volume. Fluid recommendations while breastfeeding are eight to ten 8-oz glasses daily, including water, juice, milk, and soups. In some areas, water quality may be a concern. If this is the case, the mother should be informed that any contaminants in water may be passed through her breast milk to her baby. It may be beneficial for the mother to use filtered water in these situations.

In addition to counseling nursing mothers on how to meet their increased nutrient needs during breastfeeding, it is important to discuss a few issues related to newborn/infant feeding. For example, many breastfeeding mothers are concerned about how specific foods they eat may affect their babies. Generally, the nursing mother need not avoid any foods except those to which she might be allergic. Occasionally, however, some nursing mothers find that certain foods may cause the baby to be colicky or to develop a skin rash. Onions, turnips, cabbage, chocolate, spices, and seasonings are common offenders. The best advice to give the nursing mother is to avoid those foods that she suspects cause distress in her baby. For the most part, however, she should be able to eat any nourishing food she wants without fear that her baby will be affected.

Alterations in the Postpartum Period

Alterations in health occurring at any time during pregnancy and labor may increase risks to the mother during the postpartum period. Table 33.15 lists risks associated with various conditions. Preeclampsia is discussed at length in Exemplar 16.H, Hypertensive Disorders of Pregnancy, in Module 16, Perfusion. Diabetes associated with pregnancy is discussed in Exemplar 33.A, Antepartum Care, in this module. Hemorrhage and **endometritis** (inflammation of the endometrium within 6 weeks after delivery) are two common postpartum alterations that require attention by the nurse. These are discussed here.

Postpartum Hemorrhage

Postpartum hemorrhage is one of the leading causes of maternal mortality and morbidity in the postpartum period. There are two types of postpartum hemorrhage. **Early (primary) postpartum hemorrhage** (PPH) is most common and occurs in the first 24 hours following childbirth. **Late (secondary) postpartum hemorrhage** can occur anywhere from 24 hours to 12 weeks following childbirth.

The traditional definition of PPH was a blood loss greater than 500 mL following a vaginal delivery and 1000 mL following a cesarean birth. In recent years, the American College of Obstetricians and Gynecologists has changed the classification of an early postpartum hemorrhage to a blood loss equal to or greater than 1000 mL along with symptoms of hypovolemia in the first 24 hours after childbirth (Murray et al., 2019).

Uterine atony (relaxation of the uterus) is the leading cause of early PPH. Without proper contraction of the uterine muscle, rapid bleeding from the placental site occurs. Some common causes of uterine atony include overdistention of the uterus, multiple-gestation pregnancies, polyhydramnios and macrosomia. Other causes of postpartum hemorrhage include multiparity, prolonged labor, precipitous delivery, induction of labor, retained uterine segments, uterine rupture, and birth trauma (Murray et al., 2019).

Clinical findings on assessment may include an excessive amount of bright red bleeding, excessive or large clots expelled with fundal massage, a fundus that feels boggy on palpation, a fundus found higher than expected and/or shifted to one side of the abdomen, and a fundus that becomes firm with massage but returns to a boggy state when massage is stopped (Murray et al., 2019). See **Box 33.7** » for an overview of focused assessment parameters.

Box 33.7

Postpartum Hemorrhage: Focused Assessment

Early and accurate identification of obstetric hemorrhage improves outcomes for postpartum mothers and reduces the risk of unnecessary treatments due to overidentification of maternal hemorrhage (Andrikopoulou & D'Alton, 2019). To ensure accurate and timely intervention, a focused nursing assessment that follows facility protocols is essential for each postpartum mother. Nursing actions include:

- Assess lochia every 15 minutes for 1 hour, every 30 minutes for the next 2 hours, every 4 hours for 48 hours, then daily.
- Take vital signs every 5 minutes until stable, then every 15 minutes for 2 hours, then every 30 minutes until discharge to postpartum unit.
- Assess Hgb, Hct, and clotting factors as ordered.
- Weigh saturated perineal pads and dressing every 15 minutes for at least an hour. If the perineal pad becomes soaked in a 15-minute period or if blood pools under the buttocks, continuous observation and weighing of pads and linens is necessary.
- Assess saturated perineal pads and linens (after first hour if bleeding is minimal) visually. If bleeding increases at any time, weighing may be restarted.
- Evaluate fundus height and firmness of uterus.
- Review medical record for history of bleeding problems.
- Assess sensorium and situation of patient.*
- Notify HCP as appropriate.

*As an example, a healthy woman reporting a headache may not be at additional risk. However, a woman with a history of preeclampsia who reports shortness of breath or whose headache does not resolve with comfort measures or medication requires immediate evaluation (CMQCC, 2015). A sudden change from baseline in any patient should prompt further assessment, especially in patients with a history of HTN, venous thrombosis, or bleeding issues. A nurse should remain with the woman until she is stable. Note that facility protocols may vary.

Current recommendations aim to prevent early postpartum hemorrhage with prophylactic administration of oxytocin in the third stage of labor. This is generally administered via IV infusion but can be given by IM injection if IV access is not available (Murray et al., 2019). The nurse will also perform uterine massage frequently in the immediate postpartum period to assess for the size, location, and firmness of the fundus. During these fundal massages, the nurse will note the amount of bleeding on the perineal pads and linens. Ensuring that the mother is effectively and frequently emptying her bladder can also help prevent postpartum hemorrhage.

If a patient is experiencing an early postpartum hemorrhage, nursing care would include the following (Murray et al., 2019):

- Massage the uterus until firm
- Assist the patient to empty her bladder or empty the bladder via catheterization
- Monitor vital signs, watching for signs of hypovolemic shock
- Be prepared to administer medications as prescribed
- Monitor accurate blood loss (via weighing pads, linens, gown, etc.)
- Administer pain medication as needed for procedures (such as bimanual uterine massage)
- Administer fluids or blood products as ordered
- Educate the patient and family on procedures and provide emotional support.

Late postpartum hemorrhages occur anywhere from 24 hours to 12 weeks after birth. Causes for late postpartum hemorrhages are infection, retained placental fragments, and subinvolution of the uterus. Due to shortened hospital stays, many of these will occur at home and not in the hospital setting. Patients should receive education on the signs and symptoms of late postpartum hemorrhage such as prolonged bleeding, excessive bleeding, pelvic pain, and symptoms of infection, such as fever, foul-smelling lochia, or generalized fatigue. Patients should be instructed to notify their HCP if any of these symptoms are present during the first 12 weeks postpartum.

» *Go to* ***Pearson MyLab Nursing and eText*** *for Chart 12: Uterine Stimulants Used to Prevent and Manage Uterine Atony.*

Postpartum Endometritis

Postpartum endometritis (metritis) is an inflammation of the endometrium portion of the uterine lining occurring anytime up to 6 weeks postpartum. It occurs in approximately 1–3% of patients after vaginal delivery and 5–15% of patients after cesarean delivery (Murray et al., 2019). Postpartum infection from vaginal delivery primarily affects the placental implantation site, the decidua, and adjacent myometrium. Bacteria that colonize the cervix and vagina gain access to the amniotic fluid during labor and postpartum and begin to invade devitalized tissue (the lower uterine segment, lacerations, and incisions). The same pathogenesis, polymicrobial proliferation and tissue invasion, is associated with cesarean delivery, but surgical trauma, additional devitalization of tissue, blood and serum accumulation, and foreign bodies (suture, staples) provide additional favorable anaerobic bacterial conditions.

Assessment findings consistent with endometritis are foul-smelling lochia, fever greater than 100.4°F, abdominal pain and cramping, chills, malaise, and anorexia (Murray et al., 2019). Alterations in health during the antepartum and intrapartum period may cause increased risk during the postpartum period. **Table 33.15** >> lists risks associated with various conditions.

TABLE 33.15 Postpartum High-Risk Factors

Risk Factor	Condition
Preeclampsia	↑ Blood pressure ↑ CNS irritability ↑ Need for bedrest → ↑ risk thrombophlebitis ↑ Risk of seizures
Diabetes	Need for insulin regulation Episodes of hypoglycemia or hyperglycemia ↓ Healing
Cardiac disease	↑ Maternal exhaustion ↑ Risk for maternal morbidity and mortality
Cesarean birth	↑ Recovery time ↑ Pain from incision ↑ Risk of infection ↑ Length of hospitalization
Overdistention of uterus (multiple gestation, hydramnios)	↑ Risk of hemorrhage → anemia, hypovolemia ↑ Risk of thrombophlebitis ↑ Risk of anemia ↑ Risk of breastfeeding difficulty (cesarean birth risk) ↑ Stretching of abdominal muscles ↑ Incidence and severity of afterpains
Abruptio placentae, placenta previa	Hemorrhage → anemia, hypovolemia ↑ Uterine contractility after birth → ↑ infection risk
Precipitous labor (< 3 hours)	↑ Risk of trauma to birth canal → hemorrhage
Prolonged labor (> 24 hours)	↑ Exhaustion ↑ Risk of hemorrhage Nutritional and fluid depletion ↑ Bladder atony and/or trauma ↑ Risk for endometritis ↑ Risk for uterine inversion
Extended period of time in stirrups at birth	↑ Risk of thrombophlebitis ↑ Risk of muscle, tendon, ligament, and nerve injury
Trauma due to difficult birth	Exhaustion ↑ Risk for posttraumatic stress disorder ↑ Risk for postpartum depression ↑ Risk of perineal lacerations ↑ Risk of hematomas ↑ Risk of hemorrhage → anemia, hypovolemia
Retained placenta	↑ Risk of hemorrhage → anemia, hypovolemia ↑ Risk of infection
Uterine atony	↑ Risk of hemorrhage → anemia, hypovolemia

Source: Adapted from London et al. (2017).

Lifespan Considerations

Although the nurse considers all new mothers' physical and psychosocial needs, the adolescent mother and the mother over the age of 35 may require specific care and guidance.

Nursing Care of the Postpartum Adolescent

The adolescent mother may have special postpartum needs, depending on her level of maturity and her support system. The nurse needs to assess maternal–newborn interaction, roles of support people, plans for discharge, knowledge of childrearing, and plans for follow-up care. It is imperative that a community health service contact the adolescent shortly after discharge.

Adolescent pregnancies are at higher risks for preterm births, low-birth-weight babies, postpartum depression, PTSD, intimate partner violence, and substance abuse (Lowdermilk et al., 2020). Contraception counseling is an important part of teaching the adolescent mother. The incidence of repeat pregnancies during adolescence is high. Nurses should be aware of the state laws that govern their jurisdiction in order to determine if providing contraception without parental consent is allowed. In states where adolescents can obtain birth control without parental consent, it is often more comfortable for the adolescent to address these issues without others being present. Adolescents also may encounter obstacles when attempting to obtain contraceptives themselves. These may include embarrassment about discussing the topic; concerns about confidentiality, such as not wanting their parents to know or having to give permission; and lack of knowledge regarding available methods. Nurses can play a key role in overcoming these obstacles by providing teaching and referrals that address these barriers. See Exemplar 19.A, Family Planning, in Module 19, Sexuality.

The nurse has many opportunities for teaching the adolescent about her newborn in the postpartum unit. Because the nurse is a role model, the manner in which the nurse handles a newborn greatly influences the young mother. If the father is present, he should be included in as much of the teaching as possible. If the grandparents are going to take an active role in caring for the baby, they should also be included in teaching if this is desired by the new mother.

As with older parents, a newborn examination done at the bedside gives adolescents information about their baby's health and shows possible positions for handling the baby. The nurse can also use this time to provide information about newborn and infant behavior. Parents who have some idea of what to expect from their baby are less frustrated with the baby's behavior.

Providing positive feedback to the adolescent mother about her newborn and her developing maternal responses can increase maternal confidence in this high-risk group. Group classes for adolescent mothers should include information about newborn/infant care skills, such as taking the baby's temperature, clearing the nose and mouth, monitoring growth and development, feeding the baby, providing well-baby care, and identifying danger signals in the ill newborn. These classes can also address unique needs of teen mothers, such as peer relationships, added responsibilities, and goal setting.

Ideally, teenage mothers should visit adolescent clinics for assessments of themselves and their children for several years after birth. Classes in the school system for young mothers are an excellent way of helping adolescents finish school and learn how to parent at the same time. Some public high schools have on-site child care centers to assist adolescent mothers and to provide an opportunity for them to learn important child development principles and child care tasks.

Nursing Care of the Postpartum Mother over Age 35

The mother over age 35 may have special postpartum needs based on her birth experience, personal expectation, and lifestyle choices. Women may delay childbearing for a variety of reasons such as relationship choices, educational opportunities, career options, and financial considerations. In addition, physiologic conditions may impair normal reproductive processes. Because of their greater life experiences, older parents may also be more aware of the realities of having a child and what it means to have a baby at their age (Ladewig et al., 2017).

Although women over 35 experience the same involution process as younger mothers, they may have life experiences and education that better prepare them for parenthood. Despite the potential advantage of more life experiences, older parents must be made aware that the addition of a newborn will alter established routines and practices. In addition to routine postpartum follow-up, some women in this age group with preexisting conditions or complications may need additional follow-up with HCPs other than their obstetrician.

NURSING PROCESS

The Association of Women's Health, Obstetric, and Neonatal Nurses, the American College of Obstetricians and Gynecologists, and *Healthy People 2030* all emphasize health promotion and evidence-based interventions to reduce infant and maternal morbidity and improve outcomes for pregnant and laboring women and their babies, with the overall goal of preventing complications and improving the health of both patients before, during, and after pregnancy. Nurses caring for postpartum women in any setting must be knowledgeable about their needs and recommendations for screenings and evidence-based care.

During the first several weeks postpartum, the woman must accomplish the following physical and developmental tasks:

- Restore physical condition.
- Develop competence in caring for and meeting the needs of her baby.
- Establish a relationship with her new child.
- Adapt to altered lifestyles and family structure resulting from the addition of a new member.

Assessment

Postpartum Physical Examination

Comprehensive care is based on a thorough assessment that identifies individual needs or potential problems. The nurse should remember the following principles in preparing for and completing the assessment of the postpartum woman:

- Use universal precautions, including wearing gloves during this exam.
- Select a time that will provide the most accurate data. Palpating the fundus when the woman has a full bladder, for example, may give false information about the progress of involution. Ask the woman to void before assessment.
- Explain the purpose of regular assessment.
- Ensure that the woman is relaxed before starting. Perform the procedures as gently as possible to avoid unnecessary discomfort.
- Record and report the results as clearly as possible.
- Take appropriate precautions to prevent exposure to body fluids.

While performing the physical assessment, the nurse should also be teaching the woman. The assessment provides an excellent time to provide information about the body's postpartum physical and anatomic changes as well as the danger signs to report. Because the time that new mothers spend in the postpartum unit is limited, nurses need to use every available opportunity for patient education about self-care. To assist nurses in recognizing these opportunities, examples of patient teaching during the assessment are provided throughout the following discussion. See Postpartum Assessment: First 24 Hours After Birth.

Postpartum Psychologic Assessment

The nurse assesses the mother's psychologic adjustment as part of the postpartum evaluation. Psychologic assessment focuses on the mother's attitude toward the baby, ability to engage in maternal–newborn bonding, and caregiving skills; feelings of satisfaction and competence; and support systems and preparations for discharge. The nurse also assesses maternal fatigue level.

Psychologic Assessment Risk Factors

Some new mothers have little or no experience with newborns and may feel totally overwhelmed. They may show these feelings by asking questions and reading all available

Postpartum Assessment: First 24 Hours after Birth

PHYSICAL ASSESSMENT/ NORMAL FINDINGS	ALTERATIONS AND POSSIBLE CAUSES*	NURSING RESPONSES TO DATA†
Vital Signs		
Blood pressure: should remain consistent with baseline BP during pregnancy	High BP (preeclampsia, essential HTN, renal disease, anxiety); drop in BP (may be normal; uterine hemorrhage)	Evaluate history of preexisting disorders and check for other signs of preeclampsia (edema, proteinuria). Assess for other signs of hemorrhage (↑ pulse, cool clammy skin).
Pulse: 60–100 beats/min	Tachycardia (difficult labor and birth, hemorrhage)	Evaluate for other signs of hemorrhage (↓ BP; cool, clammy skin).
Respirations: 12–20 breaths/min	Marked tachypnea (respiratory disease)	Assess for other signs of respiratory disease.
Temperature: 36.6–38.0°C (98–100.4°F)	After first 24 hours, temperature of 38.0°C (100.4°F) or higher suggests infection	Assess for other signs of infection; notify HCP.
Breasts		
General appearance: smooth, even pigmentation; changes of pregnancy still apparent; one may appear larger	Reddened area (mastitis)	Assess further for signs of infection.
Palpation: depending on postpartum day, may be soft, filling, full, or engorged	Palpable mass (caked breast, mastitis); engorgement (venous stasis); tenderness, heat, edema (engorgement, caked breast, mastitis)	Assess for other signs of infection: If blocked duct, consider heat, massage, and position change for breastfeeding. Assess for further signs. Report mastitis to HCP.
Nipples: supple, pigmented, intact; become erect when stimulated	Fissures, cracks, soreness (problems with breastfeeding); not erect with stimulation (inverted nipples)	Reassess technique; recommend appropriate interventions.
Lungs		
Sounds: clear to bases bilaterally	Diminished (fluid overload, asthma, pulmonary embolus, pulmonary edema)	Assess for other signs of respiratory distress.
Abdomen		
Musculature: abdomen may be soft, have a "doughy" texture; rectus muscle intact	Separation in musculature (diastasis recti abdominis)	Evaluate size of diastasis; teach appropriate exercises for decreasing the separation.
Fundus: firm, midline; following expected process of involution	Boggy (full bladder, uterine bleeding, retained products of conception)	Massage until firm. Assess bladder and have woman void, if needed. Attempt to express clots when firm. If bogginess remains or recurs, report to HCP.
May be tender when palpated	Constant tenderness (infection)	Assess for evidence of endometritis.
Cesarean section incision dressing: dry and intact	Moderate to large amount of blood or serosanguineous drainage on dressing	Assess for hemorrhage. Reinforce dressing and notify HCP.
Lochia		
Scant to moderate amount, earthy odor; no clots	Large amount, clots (hemorrhage) Foul-smelling lochia (infection)	Assess for firmness and express additional clots. Begin peripad count. Assess for other signs of infection; report to HCP.

Postpartum Assessment: First 24 Hours after Birth *(continued)*

PHYSICAL ASSESSMENT/ NORMAL FINDINGS	ALTERATIONS AND POSSIBLE CAUSES*	NURSING RESPONSES TO DATA†
Normal progression: first 1–3 days: rubra	Failure to progress normally or return to rubra from serosa (subinvolution)	Report to HCP.
Following rubra: days 3–10: serosa (alba seldom seen in hospital)		
Perineum		
Slight edema and bruising in intact perineum	Marked fullness, bruising, increasing pain (vulvar hematoma)	Assess size. Apply ice glove or ice pack. Report to HCP.
Episiotomy: no redness, edema, ecchymosis, or discharge; edges well approximated	Redness, edema, ecchymosis, discharge, or gaping stitches (infection)	Encourage sitz baths; review perineal care and appropriate wiping techniques.
Hemorrhoids: none present (if present, should be small and nontender)	Full, tender, inflamed hemorrhoids	Encourage sitz baths, side-lying position, Tucks pads, anesthetic ointments, manual replacement of hemorrhoids, stool softeners, and increased fluid intake.
Costovertebral Angle Tenderness		
None	Present (kidney infection)	Assess for other symptoms of UTI; obtain clean-catch urine. Report to HCP.
Lower Extremities		
No pain with palpation; negative calf pain on ambulation	Positive findings (thrombophlebitis)	Report to HCP.
Elimination		
Urinary output: voiding in sufficient quantities at least every 4–6 hours; bladder not palpable	Inability to void (urinary retention); symptoms of urgency, frequency, dysuria (UTI)	Employ nursing interventions to promote voiding; if not successful, obtain order for catheterization. Report symptoms of UTI to HCP.
Bowel elimination: should have normal bowel movement by second or third day after birth	Inability to pass feces (constipation caused by fear of pain from episiotomy, hemorrhoids, perineal trauma)	Encourage fluids, ambulation, roughage in diet, and sitz baths to promote healing of perineum; obtain order for stool softener.
CULTURAL ASSESSMENT§	**VARIATIONS TO CONSIDER**	**NURSING RESPONSES TO DATA†**
Determine customs and practices regarding postpartum care. Ask the mother whether she would like fluids and what temperature she prefers.	Individual preference may include room-temperature or warmed fluids rather than iced drinks.	Provide for specific request, if possible. If woman is unable to provide specific information, the nurse may draw from general information regarding cultural variation.
Ask the mother what foods she would like.	Special foods or fluids to hasten healing after childbirth.	Mexican women may want food and fluids that restore hot–cold balance to the body. Women of European backgrounds may ask for iced fluids.
Ask the mother whether she would prefer to be alone during breastfeeding.	Some women may be hesitant to have someone with them when their breast is exposed.	Provide privacy as desired by the mother.

(continued on next page)

Postpartum Assessment: First 24 Hours after Birth *(continued)*

PSYCHOSOCIAL ASSESSMENT/ NORMAL FINDINGS	VARIATIONS TO CONSIDER*	NURSING RESPONSES TO DATA†
Psychologic Adaptation		
During first 24 hours: passive; preoccupied with own needs; may talk about her labor and birth experience; may be talkative, elated, or very quiet (the taking-in phase)	Very quiet and passive; sleeps frequently (fatigue from long labor; feelings of disappointment about some aspect of the experience; may be following cultural expectation)	Provide opportunities for adequate rest, nutritious meals and snacks that are consistent with what the woman desires to eat and drink, and opportunities to discuss birth experience in nonjudgmental atmosphere if the woman desires to do so.
Usually by 12 hours: beginning to assume responsibility; some women eager to learn; feels overwhelmed easily (the taking-hold phase)	Excessive weepiness, mood swings, pronounced irritability (postpartum blues, feelings of inadequacy, culturally proscribed behavior)	Explain postpartum blues; provide supportive atmosphere. Determine support available for mother. Consider referral for evidence of profound depression.
Attachment		
En face position, holds baby close, cuddles and soothes, calls by name, identifies characteristics of family members in newborn, may be awkward in providing care. Initially may express disappointment over gender or appearance of baby but within 1–2 days demonstrates attachment behaviors.	Continued expressions of disappointment with gender, appearance of baby; refusal to care for baby; derogatory comments; lack of bonding behaviors (difficulty in attachment, following expectations of cultural/ethnic group)	Provide reinforcement and support for newborn caregiving behaviors; maintain nonjudgmental approach and gather more information if caregiving behaviors are not evident.
Patient Education		
Has basic understanding of self-care activities and newborn care needs; can identify signs of complications that should be reported.	Unable to demonstrate basic self-care and newborn care activities (deficient knowledge; postpartum blues; following prescribed cultural behavior; may be cared for by grandmother or other family member)	Identify predominant learning style. Determine whether woman understands English and provide interpreter, if needed. Provide reinforcement of information through conversation and written material (remember that some women and their families may not be able to understand written materials because of language difficulties or inability to read). Provide information regarding newborn/infant care skills that are culturally consistent. Give woman an opportunity to express her feelings. Consider social service home referral for women who have no family or other support, are unable to take in information about self-care and baby care and demonstrate no caregiving activities.

*Possible causes of alterations are identified in parentheses.

†This column provides guidelines for further assessment and initial nursing actions.

§These are only a few suggestions. This text does not mean to imply this is a comprehensive cultural assessment; rather, it is a tool to encourage cultural competence.

Source: From London et al. (2017). Pearson Education, Inc., Hoboken, NJ.

material or by becoming passive and quiet because they simply cannot deal with their feelings of inadequacy. Clues indicating adjustment difficulties include the following:

- Excessive continued fatigue
- Marked depression
- Excessive preoccupation with physical status or discomfort
- Evidence of low self-esteem
- Lack of support systems
- Marital problems
- Inability or unwillingness to care for or nurture the newborn
- Current family crises, such as illness or unemployment.

These characteristics may indicate a potential for maladaptive parenting, which could lead to child abuse or neglect (physical, emotional, or intellectual) and cannot be ignored. A consult for social work to evaluate the patient may be warranted. Referrals to public health nurses or other available community resources may provide greatly needed assistance and alleviate potentially dangerous situations.

Assessment of Early Attachment

A nurse in any postpartum setting can periodically observe and note progress toward attachment. Research shows that fathers experience attachment feelings similar to those experienced by mothers, and the assessment should include both parents when possible. This section, however, focuses primarily on the mother's attachment process.

The following questions can be addressed in the course of nurse–patient interaction:

- Is the mother demonstrating attachment behaviors toward her newborn? To what extent does she seek face-to-face contact and eye contact? Is attachment increasing or decreasing? If the mother does not exhibit increasing attachment, why not? Do the reasons lie primarily within her, the baby, or the environment?
- Is the mother inclined to nurture her baby by feeding every 2 to 3 hours?
- Is she progressing in her interactions with her newborn?
- Does the mother act consistently? If not, is the source of unpredictability within her or her baby?
- Does she seek information and evaluate it objectively? Does she develop solutions based on adequate knowledge of valid data? Does she evaluate the effectiveness of her maternal care and adjust appropriately?
- Is the mother sensitive to the newborn's needs as they arise? How quickly does she interpret her baby's behavior and react to cues? Does she seem happy and satisfied with the baby's responses to her efforts?
- Does the woman state that she is pleased with her baby's appearance and gender? Is she reporting experiencing pleasure during interactions with her newborn? Does she speak to the baby frequently and affectionately? Does she call him or her by name? Does she point out family traits or characteristics she sees in the newborn?
- Are there any cultural factors that might modify the mother's response?

When these questions have been addressed and the facts assembled, the nurse's intuition and knowledge should combine to answer three more questions:

1. Is there a problem in attachment?
2. If so, what is the problem?
3. What is its source?

The nurse can then devise a creative approach to the problem as it presents itself in the context of a unique, developing mother–newborn relationship.

Diagnosis

Nursing diagnoses will vary according to patient needs. Addressing the newborn's need to feed and bond with the mother are among the priorities for care. Common nursing diagnoses for the mother include any of the following:

- Anxiety related to role change
- Readiness to learn about parenting and baby care
- Pain
- Sleep disturbance
- Constipation.

Nursing diagnoses for the family may include those that address the need for information about newborn care, as well as those that address anxiety and family functioning.

Planning

Goals for care may include:

- The mother will demonstrate bonding with newborn as evidenced by using the *en face* position.
- The mother will meet the baby's needs as they arise.
- The mother will demonstrate adequate self-care to meet her needs as they arise.
- The mother will seek assistance as needed to care for self and newborn.
- The mother's physical condition returns to a nonpregnant state.
- The mother will gain competence in caregiving and confidence in herself as a parent.

Implementation

Much of nursing care of the postpartum mother revolves around providing patient teaching and preparation for discharge.

Provide Patient Teaching

An important component of postpartum nursing care is patient teaching, which must be individualized to the learning capability and readiness of the parents. Meeting the educational needs of the new mother and her family can be challenging. Each woman's educational needs will depend on her age, background, educational level, experience, and expectations. However, because the mother spends only a brief period of time in the postpartum area, it can be difficult for the nurse to identify and address individual instructional needs. Effective education provides the childbearing family with sufficient knowledge to meet many of its own health needs and to seek assistance, if necessary. The nurse should have the mother exercise her choices when possible and support those choices, with the help of cultural awareness and a sound knowledge base (see Focus on Diversity and Culture: Postpartum Care).

The nurse first assesses the learning needs of the new mother through observation, sensitivity to nonverbal cues, and tactfully phrased questions. For example, "What plans have you made for handling things when you get home?" may elicit a response of several words and provide the opportunity for some information sharing and guidance. Some agencies also use checklists of common concerns for new mothers. The woman can check the concerns that are of interest to her.

Teaching during the postpartum period is a continuous process in which the nurse takes opportunities during interactions

Focus on Diversity and Culture

Postpartum Care

In many cultures, women and their families may embrace practices involving rest, seclusion, and dietary restraint designed to assist the woman and her baby during the period of postpartum vulnerability. Chou (2017) notes a systematic review of over 50 studies concluded that globally, most cultures identify a specified postpartum period, ranging from 7 to 42 days, in which these practices are common. In some cultures, there is also a period of seclusion that coincides with the period of lochial flow or postpartum bleeding. It should be noted that there are multifaceted variables that formulate a woman's personal beliefs and while cultural traditions will vary, the period of physiological recovery appears to coincide with the need for physical recovery in most cultures (Chou, 2017).

with the new parents to identify learning opportunities and offer teaching interventions. The nurse can also plan and implement teaching in a logical, nonthreatening way based on knowledge of and respect for the family's cultural values and beliefs. Unless the nurse believes a culturally related activity would be harmful, it can be supported and encouraged.

Nurses need to consider the mother's physical and psychosocial needs when conducting postpartum teaching. Initially, the woman may be exhausted from the birth experience and her concentration may be impaired. Later, the new mother may be preoccupied with visitors and phone calls. Information should be delivered a little at a time and repeated to make sure that the parents understand what the nurse has discussed with them. Repetition is a valuable tool in the postpartum environment. Shortened hospital stays also create a barrier to education. When the nurse is performing teaching sessions, she should include the partner or support person. In some cultures, such as the Hispanic culture, female relatives often assist the new mother and baby, so it is important to include any care providers in the teaching session.

Postpartum units use a variety of instructional methods, including handouts, formal classes, videos, and individual interaction. Printed materials are helpful for new mothers to consult if questions arise at home. Some facilities offer a hotline service that new mothers can call with questions or concerns. As the cultural diversity in the United States continues to grow, the need for culturally competent information is imperative. Along with culturally diverse material, teaching aids should be presented in the woman's native language when possible. Written materials should be available, and translators or language lines should be used. Many patients are now accustomed to using the internet and may prefer to visit support groups and access educational materials online. Evaluation of learning may also take several forms, such as return demonstrations, question-and-answer sessions, and even formal evaluation tools. Follow-up phone calls after discharge provide additional evaluative information and continue the helping process for the family.

Teaching content should include information on role changes and psychologic adjustments as well as skills. Risk factors and signs of postpartum depression should be reviewed with every woman. Information is also essential for women with specialized educational needs, such as mothers who have had a cesarean birth, parents of twins, parents of a newborn with congenital anomalies, parents with other young children, parents with a child who will require long-term hospitalization, and so on. More and more women with disabilities are now having children, and they may require additional support and education. Anticipatory guidance can help prepare parents for the many changes they will experience with a new family member.

Following discharge, various services are available in most communities to meet the needs of the postpartum family. These services range from educational, such as classes on nutrition, exercise, newborn/infant care, and parenting, to specific healthcare programs, such as well-baby checks, immunization clinics, family-planning services, new-mother support groups, and more. Some are offered by private caregivers, whereas others are the domain of city, county, state, or federal agencies. In all cases, the goal is to help ensure that all family members have the opportunity to meet healthcare needs, regardless of their resources.

Promote Comfort and Well-Being

The nurse can promote and restore maternal physical well-being by monitoring uterine status, vital signs, cardiovascular status, elimination patterns, nutritional needs, sleep and rest, and learning needs. Some women also require medication to relieve pain, treat anemia, provide immunity to rubella, and prevent development of antibodies in the nonsensitized Rh-negative woman. To promote immunization status, the CDC (2016) recommends that postpartum patients receive the diphtheria, pertussis, and tetanus vaccine and, depending on the time of year, the flu vaccine as indicated. Most postpartum women need nursing interventions to promote their comfort and relieve stress.

» *Go to* ***Pearson MyLab Nursing and eText*** *for Chart 13: Essential Information for Common Postpartum Drugs.*

It is important to ask the mother if she has any special preferences or needs related to her care, including cultural and spiritual needs. For example, Orthodox Jewish families are prohibited from participating in some activities, such as using electrical devices like call bells or light switches, or even opening wrappers on sanitary pads. The nurse should assess the patient's needs related to cultural and spiritual practices before labor begins (Lutwak et al., 2020; Noble et al., 2009).

Many nursing interventions are available for the relief of perineal discomfort. Before selecting a method, the nurse needs to assess the perineum to determine the degree of edema and other problems. Application of ice to an episiotomy can promote comfort. The warmth of the water in the sitz bath provides comfort, decreases pain, and promotes circulation to the tissues, which promotes healing and reduces the incidence of infection. Ice packs and cool sitz baths have been found to be effective in reducing perineal edema and reducing the response of nerve endings that cause perineal discomfort (Lowdermilk et al., 2020).

Complementary health approaches such as the use of lysine may be helpful in decreasing discomfort associated with an episiotomy (see Focus on Integrative Health: Lysine). In addition, patient teaching is imperative to promote healing of the perineum following delivery (see Patient Teaching: Perineal Care).

Focus on Integrative Health
Lysine

Lysine, an essential amino acid, has been identified as a supplement that decreases the incidence of pain following an episiotomy. Lysine is available as a supplement. The recommended adult dosage is 12 mg/kg per day. It is also present in dietary sources, including meat, cheese, fish, eggs, soybeans, and nuts.

Patient Teaching
Perineal Care

Many women do not consider the episiotomy to be a surgical incision. Discussion helps them understand the importance of good wound care.

- Describe the process of wound healing. Discuss the risk of contamination of the episiotomy or laceration repair by bacteria from the anal area.
- Explain techniques that are used to keep the episiotomy clean and promote healing, such as:
  a. Sitz bath
  b. Use of a peribottle following each voiding or defecation. Wash with soap and water at least once every 24 hours. Change peripads at least four times per day.
- Demonstrate correct use of the peribottle or sitz bath, if necessary.
- Describe comfort measures:
  a. Ice pack, glove, or tea pad immediately following birth
  b. Sitz bath
  c. Judicious use of analgesics or topical anesthetics
  d. Tightening buttocks before sitting.
- Identify signs of suture line infection. Advise the woman to contact her HCP if infection develops.
- Encourage discussion and provide printed handouts. Some of this content may also be covered in a postpartum class.

Source: From London et al. (2017). Pearson Education, Inc., Hoboken, NJ.

Some mothers experience hemorrhoidal pain after giving birth. Relief measures include the use of sitz baths, topical anesthetic ointments, rectal suppositories, or witch hazel pads applied directly to the anal area. The woman may be taught to digitally replace external hemorrhoids back into her rectum. Hand washing to prevent contamination to the vagina is essential. The woman may also find it helpful to maintain a side-lying position when possible and to avoid prolonged sitting. The mother is encouraged to maintain an adequate fluid intake, and stool softeners are administered to ensure greater comfort with bowel movements. Mothers should be advised to avoid straining with bowel movements because this can increase the severity and discomfort associated with hemorrhoids. The hemorrhoids usually disappear a few weeks after birth if the woman did not have them before her pregnancy.

To reduce afterpains, the nurse can suggest that the woman lie prone, with a small pillow under her lower abdomen, and explain that the discomfort may feel intensified for approximately 5 minutes but then diminishes greatly, if not completely. The prone position applies pressure to the uterus and, therefore, stimulates contractions. When the uterus maintains a constant contraction, the afterpains cease. Additional nursing interventions include a sitz bath (for warmth), positioning, ambulation, or administration of an analgesic agent. For breastfeeding mothers, an analgesic administered 30 minutes to an hour before nursing helps promote comfort and enhances maternal–newborn interaction.

Discomfort may be caused by immobility. The woman who has been in stirrups or has pulled back on her legs for an extended period of time may experience muscle aches from such extreme positioning. It is not unusual for women to experience joint pain and muscular pain in both arms and legs, depending on the effort exerted during the second stage of labor. Early ambulation is encouraged to help reduce the incidence of complications, such as constipation and thrombophlebitis. It also helps promote a feeling of general well-being. The nurse provides information about ambulation and the importance of monitoring any signs of dizziness or weakness. Despite best efforts by the nurse to teach the mother about postpartum care and anticipated changes following delivery, certain occurrences may cause concern for mothers (see Patient Teaching: Common Postpartum Concerns).

Patient Teaching
Common Postpartum Concerns

Several postpartum occurrences cause special concern for mothers. The nurse will frequently be asked about the following events:

Source of Concern	Explanation
Gush of blood that sometimes occurs upon standing	Result of normal pooling of blood in the vagina when the woman lies down to rest or sleep. Gravity causes blood to flow out when standing.
Passing clots	Blood pools at the top of the vagina and forms clots that are passed upon rising or sitting on the toilet.
Night sweats	Normal physiologic occurrence that results as the body attempts to eliminate excess fluids that were present during pregnancy. May be aggravated by a plastic mattress pad.
Afterpains	More common in multiparas. Caused by contractions and relaxation of uterus. Increased by oxytocin and breastfeeding. Relieved with mild analgesics and time.
"Large stomach" after birth and failure to lose all weight gained during pregnancy	The baby, amniotic fluid, and placenta account for only a portion of the weight gained during pregnancy. The remainder takes approximately 6 weeks to lose. Abdomen also appears large because of decreased muscle tone. Postpartum exercises will help.

Source: From London et al. (2017). Pearson Education, Inc., Hoboken, NJ.

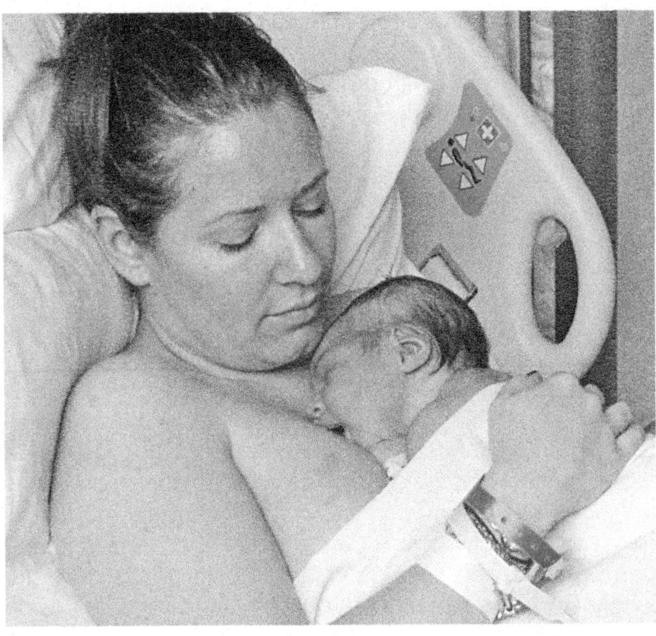

Figure 33.56 ⟫ Mother and newborn skin-to-skin.
Source: Courtesy of Brigitte Hall, RNC, MSN, IBCLC.

Enhance Attachment

The first few hours—and even minutes—after birth are an important period for the attachment of mother and newborn.

If contact can occur during the first hour after birth, the newborn will be in a quiet state and able to interact with parents by looking at them. Newborns also turn their heads in response to a voice. If possible and desired by the mother, the nurse may place the newborn on the woman's chest so that she can see her baby directly (**Figure 33.56** ⟫). This early interaction, particularly skin-to-skin contact between mother and baby, promotes attachment, early breastfeeding, and family interaction.

The first parent–newborn contact may be brief (a few minutes), and it may be followed by more extended contact after the mother completes other uncomfortable procedures (expulsion of the placenta and suturing of the episiotomy or laceration). When the newborn is returned to the mother, the nurse can assist her to begin breastfeeding, if the woman so desires. The baby may seek out the mother's breast, and early contact between mother and newborn can greatly affect breastfeeding success. Even if the newborn does not actively nurse, he or she can lick, taste, and smell the mother's skin. This activity stimulates the maternal release of prolactin, which promotes the onset of lactation. These early interactions are associated with greater breastfeeding success.

Many parents who establish eye contact with the newborn are content to quietly gaze at their baby. Others may show more active involvement by touching or inspecting the newborn. Some mothers talk to their babies in a high-pitched voice, which seems to be soothing to newborns. Some parents verbally express amazement and pride when they see they have produced a beautiful, healthy baby. Their verbalization enhances feelings of accomplishment and ecstasy.

Encourage both parents to do whatever they feel most comfortable doing. Some parents prefer only limited contact with the newborn immediately after birth and, instead, desire private time together in a quiet environment. In spite of the current zeal for providing immediate attachment opportunities, nursing personnel need to be aware of parents' wishes. The desire to delay interaction with the newborn does not necessarily imply a decreased ability of the parents to bond with their newborn.

Communicating with Patients

Working Phase

The role of the nurse after delivery is to provide holistic care for the family. While educating the parents about the benefits of breastfeeding or skin-to-skin contact, the nurse must also respect the parents' wishes regarding newborn care. Asking parents if they are comfortable with skin-to-skin contact or breastfeeding can open discussion about any concerns or questions they may have. This is an excellent time to educate parents on the importance of skin to skin or breastfeeding. The nurse may ask:

- How do you feel about holding your baby in a skin-to-skin position?
- What have you heard about the benefits of skin-to-skin contact for mom and baby?
- What have you heard about breastfeeding? (Ask only if the mother intends to breastfeed.)
- What was your previous breastfeeding experience like?

Discuss Suppression of Lactation

For the woman who chooses not to breastfeed, lactation may be suppressed by mechanical inhibition. Although signs of engorgement do not usually appear until the second or third day postpartum, engorgement is best prevented by beginning mechanical methods of lactation suppression as soon as possible after birth. This involves having the woman wear a well-fitting bra with good support continuously until lactation is suppressed (usually 5 to 7 days), removing it only to shower. The bra provides support and eases the discomfort that can occur with tension on the breasts because of fullness. Ice packs may be applied over the axillary area of each breast for 20 minutes four times daily, to reduce discomfort and inflammation. Cabbage leaves may also be placed inside the bra. The leaves should be chilled prior to use and replaced when they become wilted. The phytoestrogens in the leaves help dry up milk (Lowdermilk et al., 2020).

The nurse should advise the mother to avoid any stimulation of her breasts by her baby, herself, breast pumps, or her sexual partner until the sensation of fullness has passed. Such stimulation increases milk production and delays the suppression process. Heat is avoided for the same reason; therefore, the mother is encouraged to let shower water flow over her back rather than her breasts.

Some mothers may inquire about suppression medications used in the past for non-nursing mothers. The nurse should inform these patients that because of concerns related to side effects, such medications are no longer used. Mechanical, rather than pharmacologic, methods are now employed.

Relieve Emotional Stress

Particularly for the new mother, the birth of a child is a time of stress, bringing role changes and new responsibilities. Early in the postpartum period, it is common for mothers to be tearful and experience mood swings. Sharing the labor and birth experience with family and friends helps the mother integrate her experiences and receive assurances that she is coping well, especially if she believes otherwise or if she is experiencing feelings of inadequacy. In particular, mothers of premature infants often experience feelings of inadequacy and require comfort and reassurance. For the mother whose child is born with a congenital anomaly or is not the desired sex, the postpartum period is a time of grieving the loss of her fantasized child and learning to accept the child that has been born to her.

During the taking-in period (immediately after birth), the mother may be more focused on what is happening with her body and not be ready to learn about newborn and self-care. As the mother begins to take hold, she becomes more concerned about being able to be a good parent, requiring reassurance and becoming more receptive to teaching and demonstration of newborn care and parenting techniques.

Sadness, tearfulness, and feelings of disappointment associated with postpartum blues often come as a surprise to new mothers. Nurses can provide reassurance that these feelings are normal, explain why they occur, and provide a supportive environment that allows mothers to express their feelings without shame or guilt.

The Edinburgh Postnatal Depression Scale (EPDS) is a widely used, validated screening tool that provides the nurse with clear information differentiating normal postpartum adjustment from postpartum depression. It consists of a 10-item questionnaire in which each patient response is given a score from 0 to 3. A total score greater than 12 is strongly associated with depression and indicates a need for intervention (Lowdermilk et al., 2020). See Exemplar 28.C, Peripartum Depression, in Module 28, Mood and Affect, for an in-depth discussion of postpartum depression.

Promote Rest

Energy is needed to make the psychologic adjustments to a new baby and to assume new roles, so it is helpful for the new mother to know that fatigue may persist for several weeks or even months. Although most new mothers feel tired, if they have perceived the pregnancy and birth as a natural process, they tend to view themselves as healthy and well. Mothers who have other children may feel overwhelmed trying to meet the needs of the larger family.

Physical fatigue can affect other adjustments and functions of the new mother as well. For example, fatigue can reduce milk flow, thereby increasing problems with establishing breastfeeding. Persistent fatigue is especially common when mothers attempt to perform activities while the baby is napping instead of resting themselves. The nurse teaches women that failure to get adequate rest can lead to chronic fatigue and should be avoided. Fatigue can be a symptom of postpartum depression and should be discussed with the HCP if symptoms continue or are accompanied by other signs of depression.

Specific groups of mothers at a higher risk for postpartum fatigue include the following:

- Mothers of multiples
- Mothers with babies who are still hospitalized and who engage in multiple trips to the hospital to visit their babies
- Mothers of newborns with congenital anomalies or suspected disabilities
- Mothers who lack social and familial support
- Mothers who return to work before the advised 6-week time period
- Mothers who have been on extended bed rest during the pregnancy.

Discuss Sexual Activity and Contraception

Unless otherwise directed by the HCP, it is safe to resume sexual intercourse once bleeding has ceased and any episiotomy or lacerations are healed (Lowdermilk et al., 2020). Because this usually occurs by the end of the third week, before the 6-week follow-up, it is important that the woman and her partner have information about what to expect. The nurse may inform the couple that because the vaginal vault is "dry" (lacking estrogen), some form of water-soluble lubrication, such as K-Y Jelly or Astroglide, may be necessary during intercourse. The woman-superior and side-lying coital positions may be preferable because they allow the woman to control the depth of penile penetration. Couples should be counseled that intercourse may be uncomfortable for the woman for some time and that patience is imperative.

Breastfeeding couples should be cautioned that during orgasm, milk may spurt from the nipples because of the release of oxytocin. Some couples find this spurt to be pleasurable or amusing, but others choose to have the woman wear a bra during sexual activity.

Other factors may inhibit satisfactory sexual experiences. For example, the baby's crying may be a distraction, the woman's changed body may seem unattractive to her or her partner, maternal sleep deprivation may reduce the woman's desire, or the woman's physiologic response to sexual stimulation may be altered because of hormonal changes. By 3 months postpartum, many couples return to pre-pregnant levels of sexual interest and activity; however, this is highly variable. It is not abnormal for women, especially when breastfeeding, to experience decreased libido for several months. Decreased libido can be associated with hormonal changes, fatigue, stress, and lack of time because of family and work demands.

With anticipatory guidance during the prenatal and postpartum periods, the couple can be forewarned of potential temporary problems. Anticipatory guidance is enhanced if the couple can discuss their feelings and reactions as they experience them.

Information on contraception should be provided as part of discharge teaching if it is permissible within the healthcare agency. The nurse can also be an important resource for the woman and her partner during postpartum follow-up. Couples typically choose to use contraception to control the number of children they will have or to determine the spacing of future children. If the nurse is discussing birth control, it is important to emphasize that in choosing a specific method, consistency of use is essential. The nurse needs to identify the advantages, disadvantages, risks, and contraindications of the various methods to help the couple, or the mother, make an informed choice about the most practical and compatible method. Breastfeeding women are commonly concerned that a contraceptive method will interfere with their ability to breastfeed. Options should be presented to them that are most compatible with maintaining milk production.

» Go to ***Pearson MyLab Nursing and eText*** *for Chart 14: Resuming Sexual Activity After Childbirth.*

Evidence-Based Practice

Optimizing Adherence to the Postpartum Plan of Care

Problem

In the weeks following birth, the plan for postpartum care may become fragmented among HCPs due to inconsistent communication between the inpatient and outpatient settings. As a result, as many as 40% of women do not attend a postpartum visit (ACOG, 2018f).

Evidence

The postpartum visit provides the opportunity for the patient and the HCP to discuss both physical and psychosocial concerns, to establish a plan for contraception, and to determine which HCP will assume primary care. A physical examination and gynecological exam are performed along with a Pap smear and breast exam (Lowdermilk et al., 2020). Women diagnosed with gestational diabetes, hypertensive disorders of pregnancy, or preterm birth should be counseled about these disorders and the associated risks for future pregnancies. The postpartum visit provides an opportunity for women to ask questions about their labor experience, the childbirth process, and any complications that may have occurred (ACOG, 2018f).

Implications

The American College of Obstetricians and Gynecologists (2018f) make the following recommendations regarding optimizing postpartum care:

- Provide anticipatory guidance during antenatal visits to initiate the postpartum plan of care
- Establish a single HCP to assume responsibility for coordinating the woman's postpartum care, including contact information and written instructions
- Discuss pregnancy complications with respect to risks for future pregnancies and recommendations to optimize maternal health
- Emphasize the need for early postpartum follow-up for women with hypertensive disorders and other complications of pregnancy
- Explain the need for a comprehensive postpartum visit within the first 6 weeks after birth, including a full assessment of physical, social, and psychologic well-being
- Establish a system to ensure that women who desire long-acting reversible contraception, or any other form of contraception, receive it during the postpartum visit
- Recommend anticipatory guidance at the postpartum visit that includes newborn/infant feeding, expressing breast milk if returning to work or school, postpartum weight retention, sexuality, physical activity, and nutrition
- Determine who will assume primary responsibility for the woman's ongoing care (ob-gyn or other HCP)

Critical Thinking Application

1. Do you have any biases that may hinder your ability to provide adequate anticipatory guidance for optimization of postpartum care? Think about a variety of situations that may present opportunities for bias, including caring for patients of different cultures and spiritual backgrounds, patients from different age groups, patients of different sexual orientations and marital status, and patients experiencing dysfunctional family dynamics.
2. How will you act as an advocate for a woman who chooses to either breastfeed or bottle feed her baby?
3. How would you approach postpartum teaching about contraceptives for a 17-year-old single mother and a 27-year-old married mother with two children?
4. What are some strategies to improve adherence to the postpartum plan of care? Consider the nurse–patient relationship and how it relates to communication, patient teaching, and collaboration.

Promote Well-Being after Cesarean Birth

The mother who has a cesarean birth usually does extremely well postoperatively. Most women are ambulating by the day after the surgery. By the second postpartum day, the woman usually can shower, which seems to provide a mental as well as physical lift. Most women are discharged by the third day after birth.

The chances of pulmonary infection, however, are increased after a cesarean birth because of immobility after the use of narcotics and sedatives and because of the altered immune response in postoperative patients. Therefore, nurses should encourage the woman to cough and deep-breathe every 2 to 4 hours while awake until she is ambulating frequently.

Nurses should also utilize sequential compression devices or encourage leg exercises every 2 hours until the woman is ambulating. These exercises increase circulation, help prevent thrombophlebitis, and aid intestinal motility by tightening abdominal muscles.

Many of the complications that historically occurred after a cesarean birth were related to postpartum care practices in which mothers were encouraged to stay in bed for prolonged periods of time. Early ambulation, eating a low-roughage diet shortly after birth, and breastfeeding or newborn feeding soon after birth all enhance the recovery of the mother and decrease complications in the postoperative period. Even though a cesarean birth is an operative procedure, most women giving birth are relatively healthy and, therefore, are less likely to experience postoperative complications when compared with other surgical patients.

The nurse monitors and manages the woman's pain experience during the postpartum period. Sources of pain include incisional pain, gas pain, referred shoulder pain, periodic uterine contractions (afterbirth pains), discomfort related to breastfeeding, and pain from voiding, defecation, or constipation. Nursing interventions are oriented toward preventing or alleviating pain or helping the woman cope with pain and include the following:

- Administer analgesics as needed, especially during the first 24 to 72 hours after childbirth. Use of analgesics relieves the woman's pain and enables her to be more mobile and active. Some facilities administer ibuprofen on a continuous basis in the early postpartum period to decrease swelling, reduce pain, and lower the need for narcotic agents.

- Promote comfort through proper positioning, frequent changes of position, massage, back rubs, oral care, and reduction of noxious stimuli, such as noise and unpleasant odors.
- Encourage visits by significant others, including the newborn and older children. These visits distract the woman from the painful sensations and help reduce her fear and anxiety.
- Encourage the use of breathing, relaxation, guided imagery, and distraction techniques taught in childbirth preparation class.

Epidural analgesia administered just after the cesarean birth is an effective method of pain relief for most women in the first 24 hours following birth. Other methods of pain relief that may be ordered by the physician include patient-controlled analgesia and a variety of analgesics. Although the use of general anesthesia continues to decline, women who receive general anesthesia warrant additional assessments in the immediate postpartum period. Vital signs should be monitored continually until the woman has regained consciousness. Cardiopulmonary equipment should be in close range, with cardiac monitoring available as needed. The pulse oximeter should be used to determine the woman's oxygen status.

If a general anesthetic was used, abdominal distention may produce marked discomfort for the woman during the first few postpartum days. Measures to prevent or minimize abdominal distention include leg exercises, abdominal tightening, ambulation, avoiding carbonated or very hot or cold beverages, and avoiding the use of straws. Medical intervention for gas pain includes using rectal suppositories and enemas to stimulate passage of flatus and stool and encouraging the woman to lie on her left side. This position allows the gas to pass from the descending colon to the sigmoid colon so that it can be expelled more readily.

Many physicians also order a nonsteroidal anti-inflammatory drug (NSAID) in addition to the previously mentioned agents once the woman is tolerating oral fluids well. NSAIDs assist with decreasing inflammation and do not have the negative side effects associated with many narcotics, such as sedation and constipation. NSAIDs are often given in combination with narcotic agents during the immediate postpartum period and often result in a decreased intake of narcotic agents.

Sometimes, women who have a cesarean birth have other discomforts that can be relieved with pharmacologic interventions. The nurse assesses the woman for other symptoms, such as nausea, itching (typically related to the morphine used in the epidural), and headache. If the woman is experiencing nausea, an antiemetic can be administered. Itching can also be relieved with pharmacologic interventions. NSAIDs are effective in managing headaches and other body aches.

The nurse can minimize discomfort and promote satisfaction as the mother assumes the activities of her new role. Instruction and assistance in assuming comfortable positions when holding or breastfeeding the baby will do much to increase the mother's sense of competence and comfort. The nurse should teach the woman to splint her incision when she ambulates to decrease pulling on the incision and the discomfort created by contraction of the abdominal muscles.

Other measures are aimed at needs that are unique to the woman who has had an operative birth. These measures include the following:

- Assess for the return of bowel sounds in all four quadrants every 4 hours and assess the consistency of the abdomen. Women with a firm, distended abdomen may have difficulty passing flatus or stool.
- Assess the IV site, flow rate, and patency of the IV tubing.
- Monitor the condition of surgical dressings or the incision site using the REEDA scale (redness, edema, ecchymosis, discharge, and approximation of the suture line) along with skin temperature at and around the incision line.

Provide Care for the Woman Who Places Newborn for Adoption

Women who choose to place their babies for adoption are more likely to be single, white, never-married adolescents than Hispanic or African American women of any age. The majority of women who place their children for adoption have higher education and income levels, higher future educational or career goals, and mothers and fathers who favor adoption. Still others may feel that they are not emotionally ready for the responsibilities of parenthood, or their partner may strongly disapprove of the pregnancy. These and many other reasons may prompt the woman to relinquish her baby.

Increasingly, babies are being placed in foster care because of the mother's illicit drug use, past history of abusing children, or incarceration. The number of babies placed for adoption because of these circumstances is unknown, but several factors must be met, including clear evidence that the parent is unfit and that severing the parental rights is in the best interest of the child (Child Welfare Information Gateway, 2013a). Many of these babies may be placed with relatives or in long-term foster care.

In the 1990s, a number of babies were abandoned and left to die because the mothers did not want them and did not want others to know of their pregnancies. Starting in 1997, Infant Safe Haven Acts were passed that provided a means for a mother to place her baby up for adoption anonymously. The legislation was enacted to protect newborns from death caused by abandonment. Today, all 50 states plus the District of Columbia and Puerto Rico have legislation in place to ensure that relinquished babies are left with safe providers who can care for them and provide medical services. The relinquishing mother is protected from prosecution for neglect or abandonment under the law (Child Welfare Information Gateway, 2013b).

The mother who places her baby for adoption usually experiences intense ambivalence. Several factors contribute to this. First, there are social pressures against giving up one's child. In addition, the woman has usually made considerable adjustments in her lifestyle to carry and give birth to this baby, and she may be unaware of the growing bond between her and her child. Her attachment feelings may peak upon seeing her baby. At the same time, she may not have told friends and relatives about the pregnancy and, therefore, may lack a support system to help her work through her feelings and support her decision making. After childbirth, the mother needs to complete a grieving process to work through her loss and its accompanying grief, loneliness, guilt, and other feelings. The nurse needs to respect any special requests for the birth and encourage the woman to express her emotions. After the birth, the mother should be allowed access to the baby; she is the one who will decide whether she wants to see the newborn. Seeing the newborn often aids in the grieving process and provides an opportunity for the birth mother to say goodbye. When the mother sees her baby, she may feel strong attachment and love. The nurse needs to assure the woman that these feelings do not mean that her decision to relinquish the child is wrong; relinquishment is often a painful act of love.

Postpartum nursing care also includes arranging ongoing care for the relinquishing mother. Some mothers may request an early discharge or a transfer to another medical unit. When possible, the nurse supports these requests.

Evaluation

Anticipated outcomes of comprehensive nursing care of the postpartum family include the following:

- The mother is reasonably comfortable and has learned pain relief measures.
- The mother is rested and understands how to add more activity during the next few days and weeks.
- The mother's physiologic and psychologic well-being have been supported.
- The mother verbalizes her understanding of self-care measures.
- The new parents demonstrate how to care for their baby.
- The new parents have had opportunities to form attachment with their baby.
- The new parents have information and access to community resources. This includes adoptive and relinquishing parents.

An additional purpose of care evaluation is to determine if further care is needed based on the postpartum family's outcomes. If the outcomes are not being met, the nurse may choose to continue or revise the plan of care for optimal outcome attainment (see Nursing Care Plan: A Postpartum Patient).

Nursing Care Plan

A Postpartum Patient

Cathy McGhee delivered Callie, a healthy girl, 4 days ago. At the time of birth, Ms. McGhee was able to put the newborn to breast within the first hour. Callie was very alert at birth, latching on without difficulty. Ms. McGhee was able to breastfeed successfully during the remainder of her hospital stay. Today, she has returned to the clinic complaining of pain and swelling in both breasts and a low-grade fever. She has also had trouble getting Callie to latch on.

ASSESSMENT	DIAGNOSIS	PLANNING
Subjective: Breast pain and tenderness, anxiety Objective: T 38°C (100.4°F). Breast tissue is firm and warm and skin is shiny and taut. Swelling in axillary area and flattened nipples.	Pain related to increased breast fullness secondary to increased blood supply to breast tissue causing swelling of tissue around milk ducts	The patient will remain free of breast fullness and pain. The patient will experience decreased swelling of breast tissue. The patient will exhibit no signs of breast tenderness or firmness.

IMPLEMENTATION

- Instruct woman to breastfeed frequently.
- Instruct woman to breastfeed at least 10 to 15 minutes on each breast per feeding.
- Assist woman to pre-express milk onto nipple or baby's lips.
- Initiate pumping or manually express milk at the beginning of the feeding.
- Instruct woman to pump, hand-express, or massage empty breast when feedings are missed.
- Administer analgesics before breastfeeding.
- Apply warm and/or cold compresses before breastfeeding.
- Apply fresh cabbage leaves to the breast between feedings.

EVALUATION

- No evidence of swelling found in breast tissue.
- Pain has decreased.
- Breast tissue is soft and without tenderness.

CRITICAL THINKING

1. The nurse preparing Ms. McGhee for discharge notices that Callie was breastfed 3 hours ago but for only 3 to 4 minutes on each breast. Ms. McGhee states that the baby is very sleepy and has slept most of the day. She says she will wait to breastfeed again until she is home and more comfortable because her breasts hurt and are swollen. The nurse assesses the woman's breasts, which are firm and tender, with some swelling under the arm. What should the nurse instruct the patient to do before discharge? What can Ms. McGhee do to minimize breast fullness and discomfort?
2. A postpartum nurse is teaching a breastfeeding class to new mothers. During the class, one woman states she had a problem with engorgement after the birth of her first child and wants to know what she can do differently this time in order to avoid the problem again. What strategies can the nurse suggest to help prevent engorgement?

Source: Adapted from Davidson et al. (2020), p. 939.

REVIEW Postpartum Care

RELATE Link the Concepts and Exemplars

Linking the exemplar of postpartum care with the concept of family:

1. What challenges would you anticipate for the new family following the delivery of twins or triplets?
2. How might you assess a family's ability to incorporate a newborn into the family unit?

Linking the exemplar of postpartum care with the concept of stress and coping:

3. What stressors must the mother of a newborn cope with after discharge?
4. How do these stressors impact the risk for child abuse? What nursing implementations and strategies can the nurse offer the new family to reduce this risk?

READY Go to Volume 3: Clinical Nursing Skills

READY Go to Pearson MyLab Nursing and eText

- Chart 11: Factors That Slow Uterine Involution
- Chart 12: Uterine Stimulants Used to Prevent and Manage Uterine Atony
- Chart 13: Essential Information for Common Postpartum Immunizations
- Chart 14: Resuming Sexual Activity After Childbirth

REFLECT Apply Your Knowledge

Jessica Riley is a single, 18-year-old mother with a 1-year-old son, Ryan. Jessica has had no contact with Ryan's father since before he was born. Jessica and Ryan live in a small, one-bedroom apartment with Jessica's boyfriend, Casey. She is currently pregnant with Casey's baby.

Jessica took the evening off from work because she was feeling very tired. She fixes dinner for Casey before he has to go to work. While she is fixing dinner, Ryan begins crying in the other room, and Jessica interrupts making dinner to attend to his needs.

When they all finally sit down to eat, Casey throws his plate against the wall and screams at Jessica for making a "lousy dinner." He then proceeds to yank her out of her chair, hit her in the back, and knock her to the floor. She gets up crying, and Casey hits her in the abdomen and says, "You care more about these damn brats than me and what I want." Jessica falls to the floor, and he kicks her in the abdomen. She screams in pain. She somehow gets off the floor and makes it into the bedroom. The neighbor in the next apartment hears the commotion and calls the police.

When the police arrive, they find Jessica on the bed doubled over and crying, Ryan in his crib crying, and Casey watching TV while smoking a joint. The police note that Jessica is pregnant and call for an ambulance. They ask her whether she was hit, and she denies it. The police tell Jessica they are taking Casey in for drug possession and further questioning. Jessica calls her mother and asks her to come get Ryan and then meet her at the hospital.

When the paramedics arrive, they start an IV line, place Jessica on oxygen, and transport her to the hospital. At the hospital, the obstetrics triage nurse sends her directly to the labor and delivery unit. Jessica delivers a healthy baby girl later in the evening. Because Jessica sustained a small abruption to the placenta, the midwife and physician suspect trauma from abuse.

In the immediate postpartum period, the midwife talks with Jessica privately. She is told that she had a small abruption and that the placenta had an infarct. The midwife tells Jessica that in these situations, trauma is suspected. The midwife also shares with her that sometimes women in abusive relationships get hit or kicked in the abdomen. Jessica cries and admits to the midwife that this is what happened, but she insists that Casey didn't mean to do it and is sure he will never do it again. She tells the midwife she will not press charges.

Social work is called for referral before Jessica goes home. The nurse midwife tells her that a social work referral is required because of the risk of intimate partner violence and the drug charges against Casey. Jessica worries about this, fearing that Casey will be angry. The social worker makes a visit the day after Jessica and the baby are discharged; Jessica is relieved that Casey is not home. She tells the social worker everything is fine and that there are really no problems.

1. As the nurse caring for Jessica, what nursing diagnosis would be appropriate for the plan of care?
2. What risks to parental attachment do you anticipate for Jessica and her new daughter?
3. Create a teaching plan for Jessica before discharge.

Exemplar 33.D Newborn Care

Exemplar Learning Outcomes

33.D Summarize care of newborns.

- Summarize the adaptations of the newborn to extrauterine life.
- Outline alterations found in newborns.
- Summarize collaborative therapies used by interprofessional teams for newborns with alterations.
- Illustrate the nursing process in providing culturally competent care to the newborn.

Exemplar Key Terms

Acrocyanosis, *2393*
Active-acquired immunity, *2384*
Apgar score, *2393*
Barlow maneuver, *2405*
Brazelton Neonatal Assessment Scale, *2410*
Caput succedaneum, *2399*
Cephalohematoma, *2399*
Chemical conjunctivitis, *2400*
Circumcision, *2418*
Congenital dermal melanocytosis, *2398*
Dubowitz tool, *2407*
Epstein pearls, *2401*
Erb-Duchenne paralysis (Erb palsy), *2405*
Erythema toxicum neonatorum, *2397*
Forceps marks, *2398*
Gestational age assessment tools, *2407*
Habituation, *2387*
Harlequin sign, *2397*
Jaundice, *2397*
Lanugo, *2395*
Meconium, *2383*

Milia, *2398*
Molding, *2399*
Mottling, *2397*
Neonatal mortality risk, *2389*
Neonatal transition, *2374*
Neonatology, *2388*
Neutral thermal environment (NTE), *2379*
Nevus flammeus (port-wine stain), *2398*
Nevus vasculosus (strawberry mark), *2398*
New Ballard Score, *2407*
Orientation, *2388*
Ortolani maneuver, *2405*
Passive-acquired immunity, *2384*
Periodic breathing, *2402*
Physiologic anemia of infancy, *2378*
Physiologic jaundice, *2381*
Pseudomenstruation, *2384*
Self-quieting ability, *2387*
Skin turgor, *2398*
Subconjunctival hemorrhage, *2400*
Telangiectatic nevi (stork bites), *2398*
Thrush, *2401*
Vernix caseosa, *2395*

Overview

The newborn (or neonatal) period begins at birth and continues through the baby's 28th day of life, after which the term *infant* may be used until the child's first birthday. The newborn period is a time of complex physiologic adjustment from intrauterine to extrauterine life. Nurses must have a thorough understanding of normal newborn physiologic and behavioral adaptations and be able to identify alterations from normal. Early identification of alterations promotes better outcomes for both newborn and family.

Thorough assessment of the mother and family prior to delivery will have provided important information about cultural considerations, such as beliefs and practices surrounding newborn care and the level of support needed and desired from the nurse. Particularly when working with families whose primary language is not that of the nurse and other HCPs, care must be taken when explaining any changes from normal, even if they are likely to be benign and resolve on their own. Cultural beliefs can affect how mothers and other family members interpret illness, and additional assessment and patient education may be necessary to ensure an environment of trust that promotes maternal satisfaction with the care experience and to promote best outcomes for mother and newborn.

Adaptations to Extrauterine Life

During **neonatal transition**, the first 6 hours of life, the newborn's body begins to adapt to life outside the uterus. Within the first few minutes after birth, the most significant changes occur within the respiratory and cardiac systems.

Respiratory Adaptations

At birth, the newborn must immediately establish gas exchange and changes in circulation to support oxygenation. These changes must occur quickly to ensure the newborn's ability to sustain life outside the womb.

Initiation of Respiration

To maintain life, the lungs must function immediately after birth. Two changes are necessary for this to happen:

1. Pulmonary ventilation must be established through lung expansion.
2. A marked increase in the pulmonary circulation must occur.

The first breath of life—the gasp in response to mechanical and reabsorptive, chemical, thermal, and sensory changes associated with birth—initiates the serial opening of the alveoli. So begins the transition of the newborn from a fluid-filled environment to an air-breathing, independent, extrauterine life. **Figure 33.57** » summarizes the initiation of respiration.

During the latter half of gestation, the fetal lungs continuously produce fluid. This fluid expands the lungs almost completely, filling the air spaces. Production and maintenance of a normal volume of fetal lung fluid are essential for normal lung growth (Cotten, 2017). Through intermittent fetal breathing movements, the fetus practices respiration, develops the chest wall muscles and the diaphragm, and regulates lung fluid volume. Some of the lung fluid moves up into the trachea and into the amniotic fluid; it is then swallowed by the fetus.

During delivery, the fetal chest is compressed, increasing intrathoracic pressure and squeezing a small amount of the fluid out of the lungs. After the birth of the newborn's trunk, the chest wall recoils. This chest recoil creates a negative intrathoracic pressure, which is thought to produce a small, passive inspiration of air that replaces the fluid in the large airways that is squeezed out.

After this first inspiration, the newborn exhales, with crying, against a partially closed glottis, creating positive intrathoracic pressure. The high positive intrathoracic pressure distributes the inspired air throughout the alveoli and begins to establish functional residual capacity (FRC), which is the air left in the lungs at the end of a normal expiration (Blackburn, 2018). The higher intrathoracic pressure also increases absorption of fluid via the capillaries and lymphatic system. The negative intrathoracic pressure created when the diaphragm moves down with inspiration causes lung fluid to flow from the alveoli across the alveolar membranes into the pulmonary interstitial tissue.

At birth, the alveolar epithelium is temporarily more permeable. This permeability, combined with decreased cellular resistance at the onset of breathing, may facilitate passive liquid absorption. With each succeeding breath, the lungs continue to expand, stretching the alveolar walls and increasing the alveolar volume.

Protein molecules are too large to pass through capillary walls. The presence of more protein molecules in the pulmonary capillaries than in the interstitial tissue creates oncotic pressure. This pressure draws the interstitial fluid into the capillaries and lymphatic tissue to balance the concentration of protein.

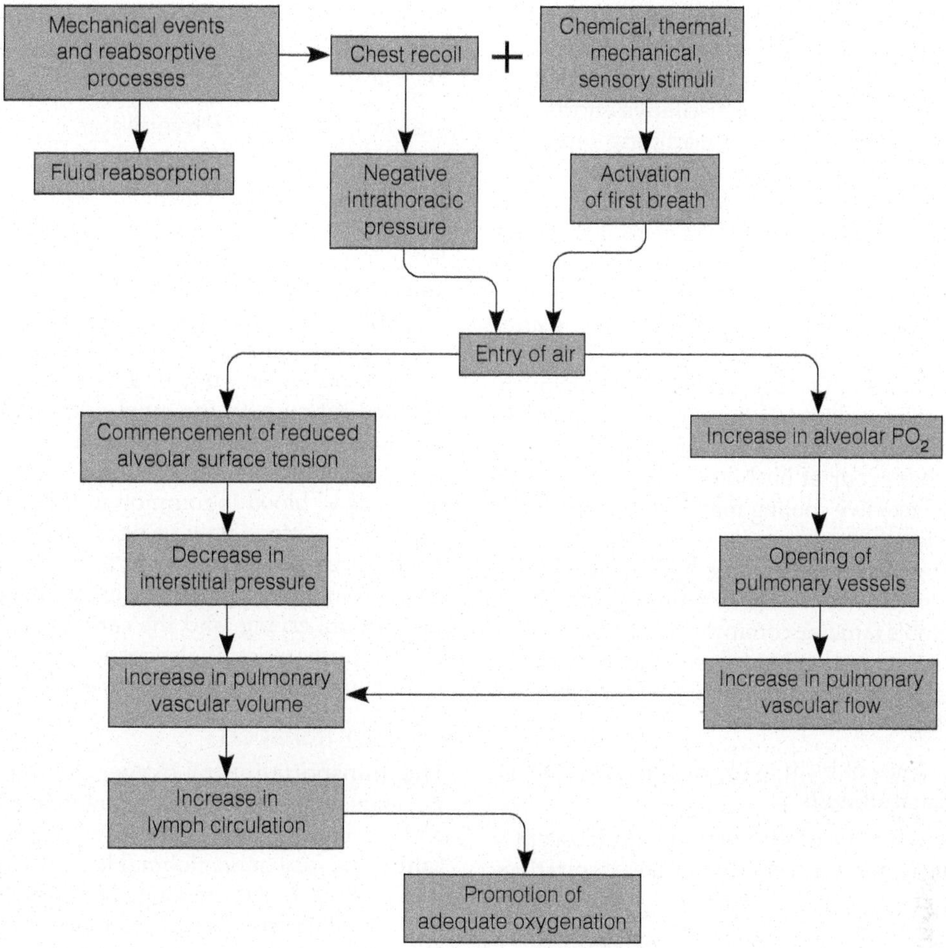

Figure 33.57 ›› Initiation of respiration in the newborn.

Lung expansion helps the remaining lung fluid move into the interstitial tissue. As pulmonary vascular resistance decreases, pulmonary blood flow increases, and more interstitial fluid is absorbed into the bloodstream. In the healthy term newborn, lung fluid moves rapidly into the interstitial tissue, but it may take several hours to move into the lymph and blood vessels (Foglia & Te Pas, 2018). By 30 minutes of age most newborns have a normal FRC with uniform lung expansion. Surfactant is essential for a normal FRC.

Although the initial chest recoil assists in clearing the airways of accumulated fluid and permits further inspiration, most HCPs believe mucus and fluid should be suctioned from the newborn's mouth, nose, and throat. A bulb syringe is used to suction the mouth and nose as soon as the newborn's head and shoulders are delivered and again as the newborn adapts to extrauterine life and stabilizes.

Newborns may have problems clearing the fluid in the lungs and beginning respiration for a variety of reasons:

- The lymphatic system may be underdeveloped, thus decreasing the rate at which the fluid is absorbed from the lungs.
- Complications may occur before or during labor and birth that interfere with adequate lung expansion; thus, the decrease in pulmonary vascular resistance fails to occur, resulting in decreased pulmonary blood flow. These complications include the following:

  a. Inadequate compression of the chest wall in very small newborns (SGA or very low birth weight) because of immature muscular development

  b. The absence of chest wall compression in a neonate born by cesarean delivery, although this compression can be externally applied by skilled HCPs as they deliver the newborn from the uterus

  c. Respiratory depression because of maternal analgesia or anesthesia agents

  d. Aspiration of amniotic fluid, meconium, or blood.

Several chemical factors contribute to the onset of breathing. One of the most important is asphyxia of the fetus and newborn. The first breath is an inspiratory gasp, the result of CNS reaction to sudden pressure, temperature change, and other external stimuli. This first breath is triggered by the slight elevation in partial pressure of carbon dioxide and decrease in pH and PO_2, which are the natural result of a vaginal labor and birth. These changes, which are present in all newborns to some degree, stimulate the aortic and carotid chemoreceptors, initiating impulses that trigger the medulla's respiratory center (Foglia & Te Pas, 2018). Although this brief period of asphyxia is a significant stimulator, prolonged asphyxia is abnormal and depresses respiration. Early cord clamping before the initiation of respirations may result in reflex bradycardia and the need for resuscitative efforts. For term infants, delayed umbilical cord clamping increases hemoglobin levels at birth and improves iron stores for several months, leading to a positive effect on developmental outcomes (Marshall et al., 2019; Nudelman et al., 2020). As a result, it is appropriate for newborns to vigorously cry and be active before the cord is clamped or the placenta separates.

A significant decrease in environmental temperature after birth, from 37°C to between 21 and 23.9°C (98.6 to 70–75°F), results in sudden chilling of the moist newborn (Blackburn, 2018). The cold stimulates skin nerve endings, and the newborn responds with rhythmic respirations. Normal temperature changes that occur at birth are within acceptable physiologic limits. Excessive cooling may result in profound respiratory depression and evidence of cold stress.

Upon birth the newborn experiences light, new sounds, and the full effects of gravity for the first time. As the fetus moves from the womb's familiar, comfortable, and quiet environment to one of sensory abundance, a number of physical and sensory influences help respiration begin. These stimuli include the following:

- The actual experience of birth, with its numerous tactile, auditory, and visual stimuli
- Joint movement, which results in enhanced proprioceptor stimulation to the respiratory center to sustain respirations
- Thorough drying of the newborn and placing the baby on the mother's chest and abdomen for skin-to-skin contact provides ample stimulation in a comforting way and also decreases heat loss.

Factors That Inhibit Respiration

Three major factors may inhibit the initiation of respiratory activity:

- The contracting force between alveoli (alveolar surface tension)
- Viscosity of lung fluid within the respiratory tract, which is influenced by surfactant levels
- The ease with which the lungs are able to fill with air (lung compliance).

Alveolar surface tension is the contracting force between the moist surfaces of the alveoli. This tension, which is necessary for healthy respiratory function, would nevertheless cause the small airways and alveoli to collapse between each inspiration were it not for the presence of surfactant. By reducing the attracting force between alveoli, surfactant prevents the alveoli from completely collapsing with each expiration and thus promotes lung expansion. Similarly, surfactant promotes lung compliance (the ability of the lung to fill with air easily). When surfactant decreases, compliance also decreases. Decreased compliance, combined with the small radii of the newborn's airway, results in an increase in the pressure needed to expand the alveoli with air.

The first breath usually establishes an FRC that is 30–40% of the fully expanded lung volume. This allows alveolar sacs to remain partially expanded on expiration, decreasing the need for continuous high pressures for each of the following breaths. Subsequent breaths require only 6 to 8 cm H_2O of pressure to open alveoli during inspiration. Therefore, the first breath of life is usually the most difficult (Blackburn, 2018).

Cardiopulmonary Physiology

As air enters the lungs, PO_2 rises in the alveoli, which stimulates the relaxation of the pulmonary arteries and triggers a decrease in pulmonary vascular resistance. As pulmonary vascular resistance decreases, the vascular flow in the lungs increases rapidly and achieves 100% normal flow at 24 hours of life. This delivery of greater blood volume to the lungs contributes to the conversion from fetal circulation to newborn circulation.

After pulmonary circulation is established, blood is distributed throughout the lungs, although the alveoli may or may not be fully open. For adequate oxygenation to occur, the heart must deliver sufficient blood to functional, open alveoli. Shunting of blood is common in the early newborn period. Bidirectional blood flow, or right-to-left shunting through the ductus arteriosus, may divert a significant amount of blood away from the lungs, depending on the pressure changes of respiration, crying, and the cardiac cycle. This shunting in the newborn period is also responsible for the unstable transitional period in cardiopulmonary function.

Oxygen Transport

The transportation of oxygen to the peripheral tissues depends on the type of hemoglobin in the RBCs. In the fetus and newborn, a variety of hemoglobins exist, the most significant being fetal hemoglobin (HbF) and adult HbA. Approximately 70–90% of the hemoglobin in the fetus and newborn is of the fetal variety. The greatest difference between HbF and HbA relates to the transport of oxygen.

Because HbF has a greater affinity for oxygen than does HbA, the oxygen saturation in the newborn's blood is greater than that in the adult's, but the amount of oxygen available to the tissues is less. This situation is beneficial prenatally because the fetus must maintain adequate oxygen uptake in the presence of very low oxygen tension (umbilical venous PO_2 cannot exceed uterine venous PO_2). However, this high concentration of oxygen in the blood makes hypoxia in the newborn particularly difficult to recognize. Clinical manifestations of cyanosis (bluish discoloration of skin and mucous membranes) do not appear until low blood levels of oxygen are present. In addition, alkalosis (increased pH) and hypothermia can result in less oxygen being available to the body tissues, whereas acidosis, hypercarbia, and hyperthermia can result in less oxygen being bound to hemoglobin and more oxygen being released to the body tissues. (See Module 1, Acid–Base Balance.)

Maintaining Respiratory Function

Lung compliance is influenced by the elastic recoil of the lung tissue and anatomic differences in the newborn. The newborn has a relatively large heart and mediastinal structures that reduce available lung space. Also, the newborn chest is equipped with weak intercostal muscles and a rigid rib cage, with horizontal ribs and a high diaphragm, which restrict the space available for lung expansion. The large abdomen further encroaches on the high diaphragm to decrease lung space. Another factor that limits ventilation is airway resistance, which depends on the radii, length, and number of airways. Airway resistance is increased in the newborn compared with that in adults.

Characteristics of Newborn Respiration

Initial respirations may be largely diaphragmatic, shallow, and irregular in depth and rhythm. The abdomen's movements are synchronous with chest movements. When the breathing pattern is characterized by pauses lasting 5 to 15 seconds, periodic breathing is occurring. Periodic breathing is rarely associated with skin color or heart rate changes, and it has no prognostic significance. Tactile or other sensory stimulation increases the inspired oxygen and converts periodic breathing to normal breathing patterns during neonatal transition. Cessation of breathing lasting more than 20 seconds is defined as apnea and is abnormal in term newborns. Apnea always needs to be further evaluated.

Newborns tend to be obligatory nose breathers. Although many term newborns can breathe orally, nasal obstructions can cause respiratory distress. Therefore, it is important to keep the nose and throat clear.

Immediately after birth, and for approximately the next 2 hours, respiratory rates of 60 to 70 breaths/min are normal. Acrocyanosis is normal for the first 24 hours. If respirations drop below 30 or exceed 60 breaths/min when the neonate is at rest, or if retractions, cyanosis, or nasal flaring and expiratory grunting occur, notify the healthcare provider.

Cardiovascular Adaptations

During fetal life, blood with higher oxygen content is diverted to the heart and brain. Blood in the descending aorta is less oxygenated and supplies the kidney and intestinal tract before it is returned to the placenta. Limited amounts of blood, pumped from the right ventricle toward the lungs, enter the pulmonary vessels. In the fetus, increased pulmonary resistance forces most of this blood through the ductus arteriosus into the descending aorta.

*» Go to **Pearson MyLab Nursing and eText** to see Chart 15: Fetal and Neonatal Circulation.*

Marked changes occur in the cardiovascular system at birth. Expansion of the lungs with the first breath decreases pulmonary vascular resistance and increases pulmonary blood flow. Pressure in the left atrium increases as blood returns from the pulmonary veins. Pressure in the right atrium drops, and systematic vascular resistance increases as umbilical venous blood flow is halted when the cord is clamped. These physiologic mechanisms mark the transition from fetal to neonatal circulation and show the interplay of the cardiovascular and respiratory systems (**Figure 33.58** »).

Change occurs in five major areas in cardiopulmonary adaptation:

1. ***Increased aortic pressure and decreased venous pressure.*** Clamping of the umbilical cord eliminates the placental vascular bed and reduces the intravascular space. Consequently, aortic (systemic) blood pressure increases. At the same time, blood return via the inferior vena cava decreases, resulting in a decreased right atrial pressure and a small decrease in pressure within the venous circulation.
2. ***Increased systemic pressure and decreased pulmonary artery pressure.*** With loss of the low-resistance placenta, systemic resistance pressure increases, resulting in greater systemic pressure. At the same time, lung expansion increases pulmonary blood flow, and the increased blood PO_2 associated with initiation of respirations dilates pulmonary blood vessels.

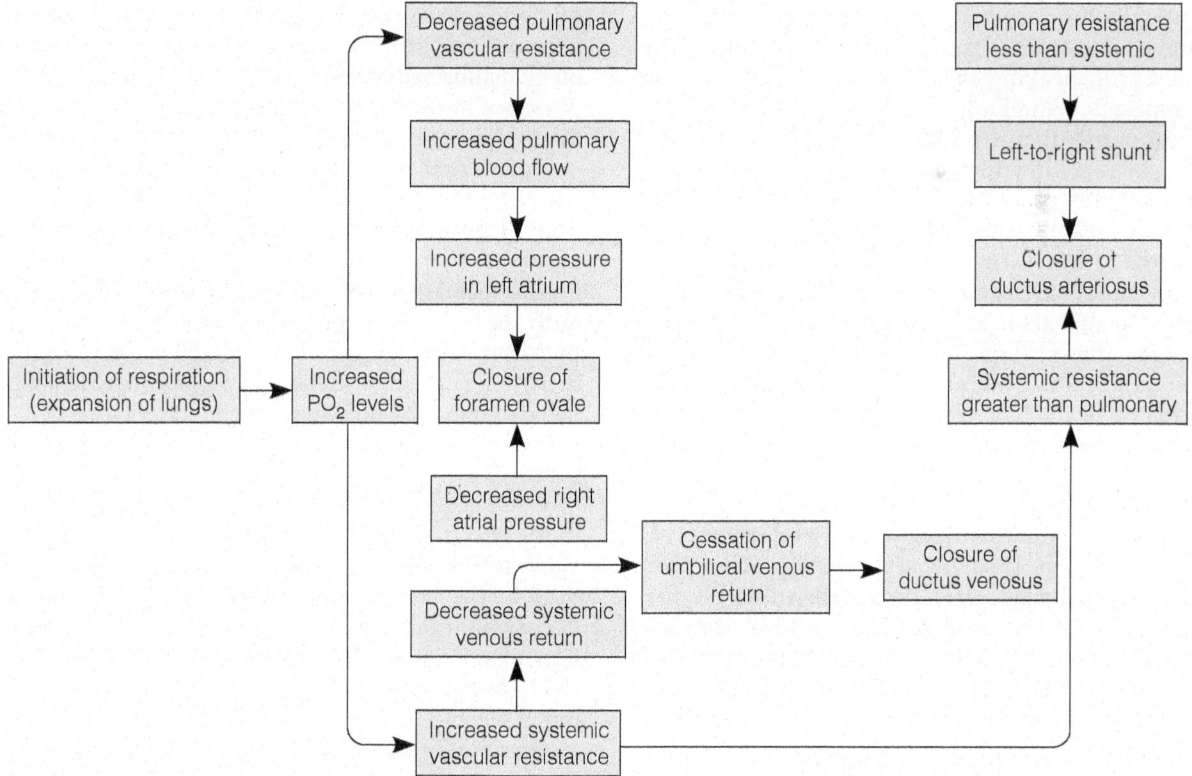

Figure 33.58 » Transitional circulation: conversion from fetal to neonatal circulation.

The combination of vasodilation and increased pulmonary blood flow decreases pulmonary artery resistance. As the pulmonary vascular beds open, the systemic vascular pressure increases, enhancing perfusion of the other body systems.

3. ***Closure of the foramen ovale.*** Closure of the foramen ovale is a function of changing atrial pressures. In utero, pressure is greater in the right atrium, and the foramen ovale is open after birth. Decreased pulmonary resistance and increased pulmonary blood flow increase the pulmonary venous return into the left atrium, thereby increasing left atrial pressure slightly. The decreased pulmonary vascular resistance and the decreased umbilical venous return to the right atrium also decrease right atrial pressure. The pressure gradients across the atria are now reversed, with the left atrial pressure now greater, and the foramen ovale is functionally closed 1 to 2 hours after birth. However, a slight right-to-left shunting may occur in the early newborn period. Any increase in pulmonary resistance or right atrial pressure, such as occurs with crying, acidosis, or cold stress, may cause the foramen ovale to reopen, resulting in a temporary right-to-left shunt. Anatomic closure occurs within 30 months (Blackburn, 2018).
4. ***Closure of the ductus arteriosus.*** Initial elevation of the systemic vascular pressure above the pulmonary vascular pressure increases pulmonary blood flow by reversing the flow through the ductus arteriosus. Blood now flows from the aorta into the pulmonary artery. Furthermore, although the presence of oxygen causes the pulmonary arterioles to dilate, an increase in blood PO_2 triggers the opposite response in the ductus arteriosus—that is, it constricts.

   In utero, the placenta provides PGE_2, which causes ductus vasodilation. With the loss of the placenta and increased pulmonary blood flow, PGE_2 levels drop, leaving the active constriction by PO_2 unopposed. If the lungs fail to expand or if PO_2 levels drop, the ductus remains patent. Functional closure starts within 18 hours after birth, and fibrosis of the ductus occurs within 2 to 3 weeks after birth (Blackburn, 2018; Hooper et al., 2016).
5. ***Closure of the ductus venosus.*** Although the mechanism initiating closure of the ductus venosus is not known, it appears to be related to mechanical pressure changes after severing of the cord, redistribution of blood, and cardiac output. Closure of the bypass forces perfusion of the liver. Fibrosis of the ductus venosus occurs within 2 months.

Assessment of the newborn's heart rate, blood pressure, heart sounds, and cardiac workload provides data for evaluating cardiac function. The newborn's blood pressure tends to be highest immediately after birth and then descends to its lowest level at about 3 hours of age. By days 4 to 6, the blood pressure rises and then plateaus at a level approximately the same as the initial level. Blood pressure is sensitive to the changes in blood volume that occur in the transition to newborn circulation. Peripheral perfusion pressure is a particularly sensitive indicator of the newborn's ability to compensate for alterations in blood volume before changes in blood pressure occur. Capillary refill should be less than 3 seconds when the skin is blanched.

Blood pressure values during the first 12 hours of life vary with the birth weight and gestational age. The average mean blood pressure is 31 to 61 mmHg in the full-term, resting newborn over 3 kg (6.6 lb) during the first 12 hours of life (Hall & Hall, 2020). Crying may cause an elevation of both the systolic and diastolic blood pressure; thus, accuracy is more likely in the quiet newborn. Currently two-point pulse oximetry (right hand and either foot) is recommended to screen for congenital heart disease. Saturation of hemoglobin with oxygen (SpO_2 of $< 95\%$) needs to be referred to a cardiology clinic (Martin et al., 2020).

Shortly after the first cry and the start of changes in cardiopulmonary circulation, the newborn heart rate can accelerate to 180 beats/min. The average resting heart rate in the first week of life is 120 to 160 beats/min in a healthy full-term newborn but may vary significantly during deep sleep or active awake states. In full-term newborns, the heart rate may drop to a low of 80 to 100 beats/min during deep sleep (Blackburn, 2018).

Murmurs are produced by turbulent blood flow. Murmurs may be heard when blood flows across an abnormal valve or across a stenosed valve, when an atrial or ventricular septal defect is present, or when the flow across a normal valve is increased.

In newborns, 90% of all murmurs are transient and not associated with anomalies. These murmurs usually involve incomplete closure of the ductus arteriosus or foramen ovale. Soft murmurs may be heard as the pulmonary branch arteries increase their blood flow from 7 to 50% of the combined ventricular output during transition, causing a physiologic peripheral pulmonary stenosis. Clicks may normally be heard at the lower left sternal border as the great vessels dilate to accommodate systolic blood flow in the first few hours of life. Murmurs are sometimes absent even in seriously malformed hearts.

Before birth, the right ventricle does approximately two-thirds of the cardiac work, resulting in increased size and thickness of the right ventricle at birth. In the first 2 hours after birth, when the ductus arteriosus remains mostly patent, about one-third of the left-ventricular output is returned to the pulmonary circulation. As a result, the left ventricle has a significantly greater increase in volume load than the right ventricle after birth, and it needs to progressively increase in both size and thickness. This may explain why right-sided heart defects are better tolerated than left-sided ones and why left-sided heart defects rapidly become symptomatic after birth.

Hematopoietic Adaptations

In the first days of life, the hematocrit may rise 1 to 2 g/dL above fetal levels as a result of placental transfusion, low oral fluid intake, and diminished extracellular fluid volume. By 1 week after birth, peripheral hemoglobin is comparable to fetal blood counts. The hemoglobin level declines progressively over the first 2 months of life (Blackburn, 2018). This initial decline in hemoglobin creates a phenomenon known as **physiologic anemia of infancy**. One factor that influences the degree of physiologic anemia is the nutritional status of the newborn. Supplies of vitamin E, folic acid, and iron may be inadequate given the amount of growth in the later part of the first year of life. Hemoglobin values fall, mainly from a decrease in red cell mass rather than from the dilutional effect of increasing plasma volume. The facts that red cell survival is lower in newborns than in adults and that red cell production is less also contribute to this anemia. Neonatal RBCs have a lifespan of 60 to 80 days, approximately one-half to two-thirds the lifespan of adult RBCs (Blackburn, 2018). The normal RBC count in a term newborn is in the range of 4.6 million to 5.2 million per milliliter during the first 24 to 48 hours of life (Blackburn, 2018).

Leukocytosis is a normal finding because the stress of birth stimulates increased production of neutrophils during the first few days of life. Neutrophils then decrease to 35% of the total leukocyte count by 2 weeks of age. Lymphocytes play a role in antibody formation and eventually become the predominant type of leukocyte, and the total WBC count falls.

Blood volume is on average 80 to 100 mL/kg for term neonates (Blackburn, 2018). For example, a 3.6-kg (8-lb) newborn has a blood volume of 306 mL. Blood volume varies based on the amount of placental transfusion received during the delivery of the placenta as well as other factors, including the following:

- Delayed cord clamping and the normal shift of plasma to the extravascular spaces
- Gestational age
- Prenatal and/or perinatal hemorrhage
- Site of the blood sample.

SAFETY ALERT Laboratory results may vary between capillary collection and venous collection. Greater variances can be expected if capillary collection was difficult or good blood flow was not obtained and the heel was squeezed excessively, which increases the risk of cellular damage within the specimen, increased serum levels, and micro blood clots.

Temperature Regulation

Newborns are homeothermic: They attempt to stabilize their internal (core) body temperatures within a narrow range in spite of significant temperature variations in their environment. Thermoregulation in the newborn is closely related to the rate of metabolism and oxygen consumption. Within a specific environmental temperature range, called the **neutral thermal environment (NTE)**, the rates of oxygen consumption and metabolism are minimal, and internal body temperature is maintained because of thermal balance (Blackburn, 2018). Thus, the normal newborn requires higher environmental temperatures to maintain a thermoneutral environment.

Several newborn characteristics affect the establishment of thermal stability:

- The newborn has a thinner epidermis and less subcutaneous fat than an adult.
- Blood vessels in the newborn are closer to the skin than the blood vessels of an adult. Therefore, the circulating blood is influenced by changes in environmental temperature and, in turn, influences the hypothalamic temperature-regulating center.
- The flexed posture of the term newborn decreases the surface area exposed to the environment, thereby reducing heat loss.
- Shivering, a form of muscular activity that generates body heat, is common in the cold adult, but is rarely seen in the newborn.

Size and age may also affect the establishment of an NTE. For example, the SGA newborn has less adipose tissue and is hypoflexed and, therefore, requires higher environmental temperatures to achieve an NTE. Larger, well-insulated newborns may be able to cope with lower environmental temperatures. If the environmental temperature falls below the lower limits of the NTE, the newborn responds with increased oxygen consumption and metabolism, which results in greater heat production. As a result, prolonged exposure to the cold may result in depleted glycogen stores and acidosis. Oxygen consumption also increases if the environmental temperature is above the NTE.

A newborn is at a distinct disadvantage in maintaining a normal temperature. With a large body surface in relation to mass and a limited amount of insulating subcutaneous fat, the term newborn loses heat at about four times the rate of an adult. The newborn's poor thermal stability is primarily because of excessive heat loss rather than impaired heat production. Because of the risk of hypothermia and possible cold stress, minimizing heat loss in the newborn after birth is essential (see **Box 33.8** »). This topic is covered in more detail in Module 20, Thermoregulation.

Box 33.8

Thermoregulation and Heat Loss in Newborns

Because of the newborn's large body surface area in relationship to mass and the limited amount of insulating adipose tissue, the newborn loses heat at approximately four times the rate of an adult. Preterm newborns lose heat at an even greater rate. Minimizing heat loss is essential to reduce the risk of hypothermia and cold stress. Systematic reviews have found that skin-to-skin contact of the newborn and its mother is recommended as a mainstay of thermoregulation for most healthy newborns (Feldman-Winter & Goldsmith, 2016; Moore, Anderson, Bergman, & Dowswell, 2016). Skin-to-skin contact promotes conduction of heat directly from mother to baby, and it has been shown to be effective in promoting thermoregulation for babies as small as 1200 g.

For smaller babies, or babies who are too ill to be placed on their mother's skin, resuscitation and other treatments may allow evaporative heat loss. Prewarming the delivery suite to 80°F and placing the newborn in a plastic bag up to the neck during physiologic stabilization prevents heat loss in high-risk babies. Heated mattresses are also effective in preventing hypothermia.

While plastic barriers have been shown to avoid hypothermia in high-risk newborns, no studies have demonstrated that these interventions reduce the long-term risk of death, brain injury, mean duration of oxygen therapy, or hospitalization. Some barrier methods (e.g., occlusive dressings) result in hyperthermia (McCall et al., 2018). Continuous monitoring of the newborn's body temperature should accompany any of the heat loss barrier methods.

Hepatic Adaptations

The newborn liver often is palpable 2 to 3 cm below the right costal margin and occupies about 40% of the abdominal cavity despite having less than 20% of the hepatocytes found in an adult liver. Its essential functions relate to iron storage, metabolism of carbohydrates, conjugation of bilirubin, and coagulation. The newborn liver also plays a role in production of bile, regulation of plasma proteins and glucose, and metabolism of drugs and toxins.

Iron Storage

As RBCs are destroyed after birth, the iron is stored in the liver until needed for new RBC production. Newborn iron stores are determined by total body hemoglobin content and length of gestation. The term newborn has approximately 270 mg of iron at birth, and approximately 140 to 170 mg of this amount is in the hemoglobin. If the mother's iron intake has been adequate, enough iron will be stored to last until the baby is about 5 months of age. After about 6 months of age, the infant requires foods containing iron or iron supplements to prevent anemia.

Carbohydrate Metabolism

At term, the newborn's cord blood glucose level is 15 mg/dL lower than the maternal blood glucose level (Blackburn, 2018). Newborn carbohydrate reserves are relatively low. One-third of this reserve is in the form of liver glycogen. Newborn glycogen stores are twice those of the adult. The newborn enters an energy crunch at the time of birth, with the removal of the maternal glucose supply and the increased energy expenditure associated with the birth process and extrauterine life. The newborn consumes fuel sources at a faster rate because of the work of breathing, loss of heat when exposed to cold, activity, and activation of muscle tone. Glucose is the main source of energy in the first 4 to 6 hours after birth. During the first 2 hours of life, the serum blood glucose level declines, then rises, and finally reaches a steady state by 3 hours after birth (Blackburn, 2018).

The nurse may assess the newborn's glucose level on admission if risk factors are present or per agency protocol. As stores of liver and muscle glycogen and blood glucose decrease, the newborn compensates by changing from a predominantly carbohydrate metabolism to fat metabolism. This allows the newborn to derive energy from fat and protein as well as from carbohydrates. The amount and availability of each of these "fuel substrates" depend on the ability of immature metabolic pathways, which lack specific enzymes or hormones, to function in the first few days of life.

Conjugation of Bilirubin

Conjugation of bilirubin is the conversion of yellow lipid-soluble pigment into water-soluble pigment. Unconjugated (indirect) bilirubin is a breakdown product derived from hemoglobin released primarily from destroyed RBCs. Unconjugated bilirubin is not in an excretable form and is a potential toxin. Total serum bilirubin is the sum of conjugated (direct) and unconjugated (indirect) bilirubin.

Fetal unconjugated bilirubin crosses the placenta to be excreted, so the fetus does not need to conjugate bilirubin. Total bilirubin at birth is usually less than 3 mg/dL unless an abnormal hemolytic process has been present in utero. After birth, the newborn's liver must begin to conjugate bilirubin. This produces a normal rise in serum bilirubin levels in the first few days of life.

The bilirubin formed after RBCs are destroyed is transported in the blood bound to albumin. The bilirubin is transferred into the hepatocytes and bound to intracellular proteins. These proteins determine the amount of bilirubin held in a liver cell for processing and, consequently, the amount of bilirubin uptake into the liver. Direct bilirubin is excreted into the tiny bile ducts, then into the common duct and duodenum. The conjugated (direct) bilirubin then progresses down the intestines, where bacteria transform it into urobilinogen (urine bilirubin) and stercobilinogen. Stercobilinogen is not reabsorbed; rather, it is excreted as a yellow-brown pigment in the stools.

Even after the bilirubin has been conjugated and bound, it can be changed back to unconjugated bilirubin via the enterohepatic circulation. In the intestines, beta-glucuronidase enzyme acts to split off (deconjugate) the bilirubin from glucuronic acid if it has not first been acted on by gut bacteria to produce urobilinogen. The free bilirubin is then reabsorbed through the intestinal wall and brought back to the liver via portal vein circulation. This recycling of the bilirubin and decreased ability to clear bilirubin from the system are prevalent in babies with very high beta-D-glucuronidase activity levels, those who are exclusively breastfed, and those with delayed bacterial colonization of the gut (e.g., because of the use of antibiotics). Very high beta-D-glucuronidase activity levels further increase the newborn's susceptibility to jaundice (yellow pigmentation of body tissues due to high bilirubin levels).

The newborn liver has relatively less glucuronyl transferase activity in the first few weeks of life than an adult liver. This reduction in hepatic activity, along with a relatively large bilirubin load, decreases the liver's ability to conjugate bilirubin and increases susceptibility to jaundice.

Coagulation

The liver plays an important part in blood coagulation during fetal life, and it continues this function following birth. Coagulation factors II, VII, IX, and X (synthesized in the liver) are activated under the influence of vitamin K and, therefore, are considered to be vitamin K dependent. The absence of normal flora needed to synthesize vitamin K in the newborn gut results in low levels of vitamin K, which in turn results in a transient blood coagulation alteration between the second and fifth day of life. From a low point at approximately 2 to 3 days after birth, these coagulation factors rise slowly, but they do not approach adult levels until 9 months of age or later (Stachowiak & Furman, 2020). Other coagulation factors with low umbilical cord blood levels are factors XI, XII, and XIII. Fibrinogen and factors V and VII are near adult levels. Although newborn bleeding problems are rare, an injection of vitamin K (AquaMEPHYTON) is given prophylactically on the day of birth to combat potential clinical bleeding problems.

Platelet counts at birth are in the same range as for older children, but newborns may manifest mild transient difficulty in platelet aggregation functioning. This platelet problem is accentuated by phototherapy. Prenatal maternal therapy with phenytoin sodium (Dilantin) or phenobarbital also causes abnormal clotting and newborn bleeding in the first 24 hours after birth. Neonates born to mothers receiving warfarin (Coumadin) compounds may bleed because these agents cross the placenta and accentuate existing vitamin K–dependent factor deficiencies; therefore, most pregnant women in need of anticoagulant therapy receive heparin, which does not cross the placental barrier (Blackburn, 2018). Transient neonatal thrombocytopenia may occur in newborns born to mothers with severe HTN or HELLP (***h***emolysis, ***e***levated ***l***iver enzymes, and ***l***ow ***p***latelet count) syndrome and in newborns born to mothers who have idiopathic isoimmune thrombocytopenic purpura.

Physiologic Jaundice

Physiologic jaundice (nonpathologic unconjugated hyperbilirubinemia) is caused by accelerated destruction of fetal RBCs, impaired conjugation of bilirubin, and increased bilirubin reabsorption from the intestinal tract. This condition does not have a pathologic basis but is a normal biological response of the newborn.

Muchowski (2014) describes six factors—several of which can also be related to pathologic events—whose interaction may give rise to physiologic jaundice:

1. ***Increased amounts of bilirubin delivered to the liver.*** The increased blood volume because of delayed cord clamping combined with faster RBC destruction in the newborn leads to an increased bilirubin level in the blood. A proportionately larger amount of nonerythrocyte bilirubin forms in the newborn. Therefore, newborns have two to three times greater production or breakdown of bilirubin than adults. The use of forceps or vacuum extraction, which sometimes causes facial bruising or cephalohematoma (entrapped hemorrhage), can increase the amount of bilirubin to be handled by the liver.
2. ***Defective hepatic uptake of bilirubin from the plasma.*** If the newborn does not ingest adequate calories, the formation of hepatic binding proteins diminishes, resulting in higher bilirubin levels.
3. ***Defective conjugation of bilirubin.*** Decreased uridine-diphosphoglucuronosyl activity, as in hypothyroidism or inadequate caloric intake, causes the intracellular binding proteins to remain saturated and results in greater unconjugated bilirubin levels in the blood. The fatty acids in breast milk are thought to compete with bilirubin for albumin-binding sites and, therefore, to impede bilirubin processing.
4. ***Defective excretion of bilirubin.*** A congenital infection may cause impaired excretion of conjugated bilirubin. Delay in introduction of bacterial flora and decreased intestinal motility can also delay excretion and increase enterohepatic circulation of bilirubin.
5. ***Inadequate hepatic circulation.*** Decreased oxygen supplies to the liver associated with neonatal hypoxia or congenital heart disease lead to a rise in the bilirubin level.
6. ***Increased reabsorption of bilirubin from the intestine.*** Reduced bowel motility, intestinal obstruction, or delayed passage of meconium (the first stool) increases the circulation of bilirubin in the enterohepatic pathway, thereby resulting in higher bilirubin values.

Approximately 85% of full-term newborns exhibit physiologic jaundice (Blackburn, 2018). This condition does not have a pathologic basis, but rather is a normal biologic response of the newborn. The characteristic yellow color results from increased levels of unconjugated (indirect) bilirubin, which are a normal product of RBC breakdown and reflect the body's temporary inability to eliminate bilirubin. Bruising, feeding patterns, and GI activity can influence serum bilirubin levels (Pace, Brown, & DeGeorge, 2019). Serum levels of bilirubin reach approximately 4 to 6 mg/dL before the yellow coloration of the skin and sclera appear. The signs of physiologic jaundice appear after the first 24 hours postnatally. This time frame differentiates physiologic jaundice from pathologic jaundice, which is clinically seen at birth or within the first 24 hours of postnatal life. Generally, physiologic jaundice is more prevalent than pathologic jaundice. Sepsis, hypoglycemia, polycythemia, and prematurity contribute to the development of physiologic jaundice (Pace et al., 2019). A major risk factor for developing severe hyperbilirubinemia in term neonates is a total serum or transcutaneous level in the high-risk zone on a bilirubin nomogram. The nomogram created by Bhutani, Johnson, and Sivieri (1999) and approved by the American Academy of Pediatrics (2004) is frequently used, as are bilirubin calculation tools available via the internet.

>> **Stay Current:** Visit www.bilitool.org to see a bilirubin calculation tool based on the nomogram by Bhutani et al. (1999).

There is no consistent definition of neonatal hyperbilirubinemia; what is considered to be in that range varies with population characteristics and age (Blackburn, 2018). Peak bilirubin levels are reached between days 3 and 5 in the full-term newborn. These values are established for European and American white newborns. Chinese, Japanese, Korean, and Native American newborns have considerably higher bilirubin levels that are not as apparent and that persist for longer periods with no apparent ill effects (Blackburn, 2018).

The nursery or postpartum room environment, including lighting, may hinder early detection of the degree and type of jaundice. Pink walls and artificial lights mask the beginning of jaundice in newborns. Daylight assists the observer in early recognition by eliminating distortions caused by artificial light.

If jaundice is suspected, the nurse can quickly assess the newborn's coloring by pressing the skin, generally on the forehead or nose, with a finger. As blanching occurs, the nurse can observe the icterus (yellow coloring).

Several newborn care procedures will decrease the probability of high bilirubin levels:

- Maintain the newborn's skin temperature at 36.5°C (97.8°F) or above because cold stress results in acidosis. Acidosis in turn decreases available serum albumin-binding sites, weakens albumin-binding powers, and causes elevated unconjugated bilirubin levels.
- Monitor stool for amount and characteristics. Bilirubin is eliminated in the feces; inadequate stooling may result in reabsorption and recycling of bilirubin. Encourage early breastfeeding because the laxative effect of colostrum increases the excretion of meconium and transitional stool.
- Encourage early feedings to promote intestinal elimination and bacterial colonization and provide the caloric intake necessary for formation of hepatic binding proteins.

If jaundice becomes apparent, nursing care is directed toward keeping the newborn well hydrated and promoting intestinal elimination.

Physiologic jaundice may be very upsetting to parents; they require emotional support and a thorough explanation of the condition. If the baby is placed under phototherapy, a few additional days of hospitalization may be required; this may also be disturbing to parents. The nurse can encourage parents to provide for the emotional needs of their newborn by continuing to feed, hold, and caress the baby. If the mother is discharged, the parents are encouraged to return for feedings and to telephone or visit when possible. In many instances, the mother, especially if she is breastfeeding, may elect to remain hospitalized with her newborn; the nurse should support this decision. If insurance limitations make this unrealistic, it may be possible to find an empty room for the discharged mother and her family to use while visiting the newborn. As an alternative to continued hospitalization, the newborn may be treated with home phototherapy.

Breastfeeding and Breast Milk Jaundice

Breastfeeding is implicated in prolonged jaundice in some newborns. *Breastfeeding jaundice* occurs during the first days of life in breastfed newborns. It appears to be related to inadequate fluid intake with some element of dehydration and not with any abnormality in milk composition (Pace et al., 2019). Prevention of early breastfeeding jaundice includes encouraging frequent (every 2 to 3 hours) breastfeeding, avoiding supplementation if the newborn is not dehydrated, and accessing maternal lactation counseling. Breastfeeding jaundice is self-limited; it peaks around day 3 as enteral intake increases, then resolves.

In *breast milk jaundice*, the bilirubin level begins to rise after the first week of life, when physiologic jaundice is waning after the mother's milk has come in. The level peaks at 5 to 10 mg/dL at 2 to 3 weeks of age and then declines over the first several months of life.

In contrast to breastfeeding jaundice, breast milk jaundice is related to milk composition. Some women's breast milk contains several times the normal concentration of certain free fatty acids. These free fatty acids may compete with bilirubin for binding sites on albumin and inhibit the conjugation of bilirubin or increase lipase activity, which disrupts the RBC membrane. Increased lipase activity enhances absorption of bile across the GI tract membrane, thereby increasing the enterohepatic circulation of bilirubin. Newborns with breastfeeding jaundice appear well, and at present, development of kernicterus (toxic levels of bilirubin in the brain) has not been documented (Pace et al., 2019). Temporary cessation of breastfeeding may be advised if bilirubin reaches presumed toxic levels of approximately 20 mg/dL or if the interruption is necessary to establish the cause of the hyperbilirubinemia. Most providers believe that breastfeeding may be resumed once other causes of jaundice have been ruled out and as long as serum bilirubin levels remain below 20 mg/dL. In cases of breast milk jaundice, the newborn's serum bilirubin levels begin to fall dramatically within 24 to 36 hours after breastfeeding is discontinued. With resumption of breastfeeding, the bilirubin concentration may have a slight rise of 2 to 3 mg/dL, with a subsequent decline. Breastfeeding mothers need encouragement and support in their desire to breastfeed their babies, assistance and instruction regarding pumping and expressing milk during the interrupted nursing period, and reassurance that they are capable of feeding and nurturing their babies. To diminish misunderstandings by mothers from a variety of cultural backgrounds, careful explanations about newborn jaundice are warranted.

Gastrointestinal Adaptations

The term newborn has sufficient intestinal and pancreatic enzymes to digest most simple carbohydrates, proteins, and fats. The carbohydrates requiring digestion in the newborn are usually disaccharides (lactose, maltose, and sucrose), which are split into monosaccharides (galactose, fructose, and glucose) by the enzymes of the intestinal mucosa. Lactose is the primary carbohydrate in the breastfeeding newborn and generally is easily digested and well absorbed. The only enzyme lacking in the newborn is pancreatic amylase, which remains relatively deficient during the first few months of life. Newborns have trouble digesting starches (changing more complex carbohydrates into maltose), so they should not be fed solid foods until at least 4 to 6 months of age (AAP, 2016; Mayo Clinic, 2016).

Although proteins require more digestion than carbohydrates, they are well digested and absorbed from the newborn intestine. The newborn digests and absorbs fats less efficiently because of the minimal activity of the pancreatic enzyme lipase. The newborn excretes approximately 10–20% of the dietary fat intake, compared with 10% for the adult. The newborn absorbs the fat in breast milk more completely than the fat in cow's milk because breast milk consists of more medium-chain triglycerides and contains lipase.

By birth, the newborn has experienced swallowing, gastric emptying, and intestinal propulsion. In utero, fetal swallowing is accompanied by gastric emptying and peristalsis of the fetal intestinal tract. By the end of gestation, peristalsis becomes much more active in preparation for extrauterine life. Fetal peristalsis is also stimulated by anoxia, causing the expulsion of meconium into the amniotic fluid by more mature fetuses.

Air enters the stomach immediately after birth. The small intestine is filled with air within 2 to 12 hours, and the large bowel is filled within 24 hours. The salivary glands are immature at birth, and the newborn produces little saliva until about 3 months of age. The newborn's stomach has a capacity of approximately 60 to 81 mL by the 10th day of life (Watchmaker, Boyd, & Dugas, 2020). It empties intermittently, starting within a few minutes of the beginning of a feeding and ending 2 to 4 hours after a feeding. Bowel sounds are present within the first 30 to 60 minutes of birth; the newborn can successfully feed during this time. The newborn's gastric pH becomes less acidic about a week after birth and remains less acidic than that of adults for the next 2 to 3 months.

The cardiac sphincter is immature, as is neural control of the stomach. Therefore, some regurgitation may be noted in the newborn period. Regurgitation of the first few feedings during the first day or two of life can usually be lessened by avoiding overfeeding and by burping the newborn well both during and after the feeding.

When no other signs and symptoms are evident, vomiting is limited and ceases within the first few days of life. Continuous vomiting or regurgitation should be observed closely. If the newborn has swallowed bloody or purulent amniotic fluid, lavage of the stomach may be indicated in the term newborn to relieve the problem. Bilious vomiting is abnormal and must be evaluated thoroughly; it may represent a condition that warrants prompt surgical intervention.

Adequate digestion and absorption are essential for newborn growth and development. If optimal nutritional support is available, postnatal growth should parallel intrauterine growth; that is, after 30 weeks of gestation, the fetus gains 30 g per day and adds 1.2 cm (0.5 in.) to body length daily. To gain weight at the intrauterine rate, the term newborn requires 120 calories/kg per day. After birth, caloric intake is often insufficient for weight gain until the newborn is 5 to 10 days old. During this time, the term newborn may experience a weight loss of 5–10%. Because insensible water loss and a shift of intracellular water to extracellular space account for the 5–10% weight loss, failure to lose weight when caloric intake is inadequate may indicate fluid retention.

Term newborns usually pass **meconium** (their first stool) within 8 to 24 hours of life and almost always within 48 hours. Meconium is formed in utero from the amniotic fluid and its constituents, intestinal secretions, and shed mucosal cells. It is recognized by its thick, tarry-black or dark green appearance (**Figure 33.59A** »). Transitional (thin brown to green) stools consisting of part meconium and part fecal material are passed for the next day or two (Figure 33.59B), and then the stools become entirely fecal (Figure 33.59C). Generally, the stools of a breastfed newborn are pale yellow (but may be pasty green); they are more liquid and more frequent than those of formula-fed newborns, whose stools are paler. Frequency of bowel movements varies but ranges from one every 2 to 3 days to as many as 10 a day. Mothers should be counseled that the newborn is not constipated as long as the bowel movement remains soft.

(*A*) Day 1 and Day 2

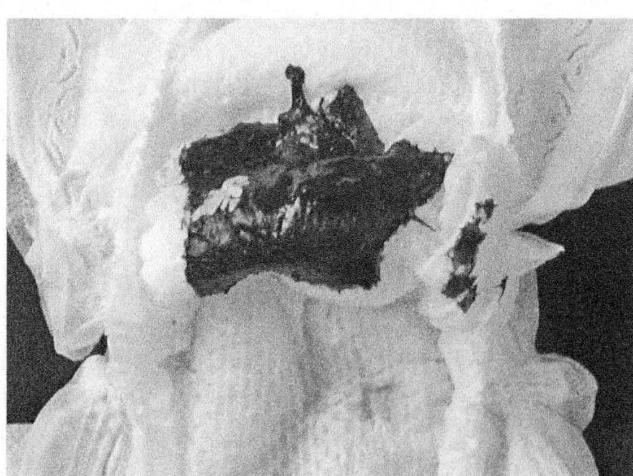

(*B*) Day 3 and Day 4

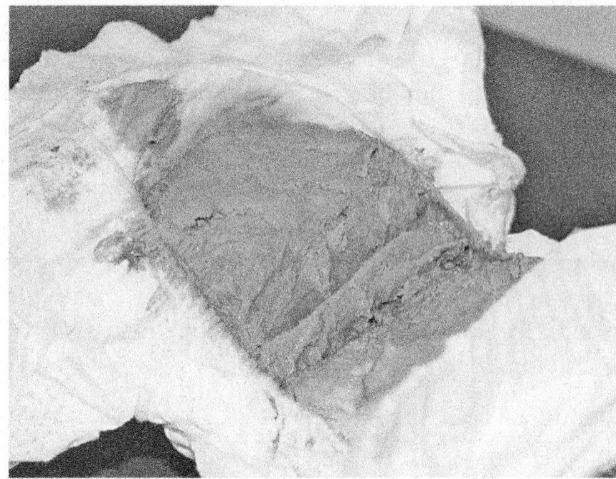

(*C*) Day 5

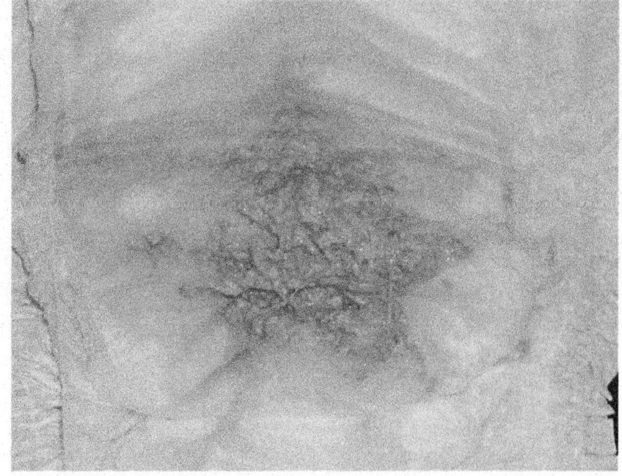

Figure 33.59 » Examples of newborn stools. ***A***, Meconium. ***B***, Transitional stools. ***C***, Fecal stools.

Source: Courtesy of Brigitte Hall, RNC, MSN, IBCLC.

Urinary Tract Adaptations

Certain physiologic features of the newborn's kidneys influence the newborn's ability to handle body fluids and excrete urine:

- The term newborn's kidneys have a full complement of functioning nephrons by 34 to 36 weeks of gestation.
- The GFR of the newborn's kidney is low in comparison with the adult rate. Because of this physiologic decrease in kidney glomerular filtration, the newborn's kidney is unable to dispose of water rapidly when necessary.
- The juxtamedullary portion of the nephron has limited capacity to reabsorb bicarbonate and hydrogen ions and to concentrate urine (reabsorb water back into the blood). The limitation of tubular reabsorption can lead to inappropriate loss of substances present in the glomerular filtrate, such as amino acids, bicarbonate, glucose, and sodium.

Full-term newborns are less able than adults to concentrate urine because their tubules are short and narrow. The limited tubular reabsorption of water and limited excretion of solutes (principally sodium, potassium, chloride, bicarbonate, urea, and phosphate) in growing newborns also reduce their ability to concentrate urine. Although feeding practices may affect the osmolarity of the urine, they have limited effect on the concentration of the urine. The ability to concentrate urine fully is attained by 3 months of age.

The newborn's difficulty concentrating urine makes the effect of excessive insensible water loss or restricted fluid intake unpredictable. The newborn kidney is also limited in its dilutional capabilities. Concentrating and dilutional limitations of renal function are important considerations in monitoring fluid therapy to prevent dehydration or overhydration.

Many newborns void immediately after birth; this voiding frequently goes unnoticed. A newborn who has not voided by 48 hours should be assessed for adequacy of fluid intake, bladder distention, restlessness, and symptoms of pain. The appropriate clinical personnel should be notified, if indicated (Blackburn, 2018).

The initial bladder volume is 6 to 44 mL of urine. Unless edema is present, normal urinary output is often limited, and voidings are scanty until fluid intake increases. (The fluid of edema is eliminated by the kidneys, so newborns with edema have a much higher urinary output.) During the first 2 days after birth, the newborn voids 2 to 6 times daily, with a urine output of 15 mL/kg per day. The newborn subsequently voids 5 to 25 times every 24 hours, with a volume of 25 mL/kg per day.

Following the first voiding, the newborn's urine frequently appears cloudy (because of mucus content) and has a high specific gravity, which decreases as fluid intake increases. Occasionally, pink stains ("brick dust spots") appear on the diaper. These are caused by urates and are innocuous. Blood or whitish discharge may occasionally be observed on the diapers of female newborns; this **pseudomenstruation** is related to the withdrawal of maternal hormones. Males who are circumcised may have bloody spotting following the procedure. In the absence of apparent causes for bleeding, the HCP should be notified. During the early neonatal period, normal urine is straw colored and almost odorless, although odor does occur when certain drugs are given, metabolic disorders exist, or infection is present. Normal urinalysis values for healthy newborns are:

- Protein: <5 to 10 mg/dL
- WBCs: <2 to 3 cells/high power field
- RBCs: 0
- Casts: 0
- Bacteria: 0

Immunologic Adaptations

The newborn's immune system is not fully activated until sometime after birth. Limitations in the newborn's inflammatory response result in failure to recognize, localize, and destroy invasive bacteria. As a result, the signs and symptoms of infection are often subtle and nonspecific in the newborn. The newborn also has a poor hypothalamic response to pyrogens; therefore, fever is not a reliable indicator of infection. In the neonatal period, hypothermia is a more reliable sign of infection.

Of the three major types of immunoglobulins that are primarily involved in immunity—IgG, IgA, and IgM—only IgG crosses the placenta. When the pregnant woman forms antibodies in response to illness or immunization, this process is called **active-acquired immunity**. When IgG antibodies are transferred from the pregnant woman to the fetus in utero, **passive-acquired immunity** results because the fetus does not produce the antibodies. IgG antibodies are very active against bacterial toxins.

Because the maternal IgG is transferred primarily during the third trimester, preterm newborns (especially those born before 34 weeks of gestation) may be more susceptible to infection than term newborns. In general, newborns have immunity to tetanus, diphtheria, smallpox, measles, mumps, poliomyelitis, and a variety of other bacterial and viral diseases. The period of resistance varies: Immunity against common viral infections, such as measles, may last 4 to 8 months; immunity to certain bacteria may disappear within 4 to 8 weeks.

The normal newborn can produce a protective immune response to vaccines, such as hepatitis B immunoglobulin vaccine, when given as early as a few hours after birth. It is customary to begin the majority of routine immunizations at 2 months of age so that the infant can develop active-acquired immunity.

The IgM antibodies are produced in response to blood group antigens, gram-negative enteric organisms, and some viruses in the expectant mother. Because IgM does not normally cross the placenta, most or all of it is produced by the fetus beginning at 10 to 15 weeks of gestation. Elevated levels of IgM at birth may indicate placental leaks or, more commonly, antigenic stimulation in utero. Consequently, elevations of IgM suggest that the newborn was exposed to an intrauterine infection, such as syphilis or TORCH syndrome (***to***xoplasmosis, ***r***ubella, ***c***ytomegalovirus, ***h***erpesvirus hominis type 2 infection). The lack of available maternal IgM in the newborn also accounts for the susceptibility to gram-negative enteric organisms, such as *Escherichia coli*.

The functions of IgA immunoglobulins are not fully understood. IgA appears to provide protection mainly on secreting surfaces, such as the respiratory tract, GI tract, and eyes. Serum IgA does not cross the placenta and is not normally produced by the fetus in utero. Unlike the other immunoglobulins, IgA is not affected by gastric action. Colostrum (the forerunner of breast milk) is very high in the secretory form of IgA. Consequently, it may be of significance in providing some passive immunity to the neonate of a breastfeeding mother. Newborns begin to produce secretory IgA in their intestinal mucosa approximately 4 weeks after birth.

Neurologic and Sensory–Perceptual Function

The postpartum period is considered to be a time of great risk to brain and nervous system development because many of the neurobiochemical changes of the newborn's brain have not yet occurred. The newborn brain is only about one-quarter the size of the adult brain. Myelination of nerve fibers is still progressing. The brain and other nervous system structures must develop in an orderly fashion without insult or interruption to ensure healthy development of neurologic processes, as well as cognition and intellect.

Intrauterine Experience

Newborns respond to and interact with the environment in a predictable pattern of behavior that is somewhat shaped by their intrauterine experience. This intrauterine experience is affected by intrinsic factors, such as maternal nutrition, and by extrinsic factors, such as the mother's physical environment. Depending on the newborn's intrauterine experience and individual temperament, neonatal behavioral responses to different stresses vary. Some newborns react quietly to stimulation, others become overreactive and tense, and still others exhibit a combination of the two.

Factors such as exposure to intense auditory stimuli in utero may eventually manifest in the behavior of the newborn. For example, the FHR initially increases when the pregnant woman is exposed to auditory stimuli, but repetition of the stimuli leads to decreased FHR. Thus, the newborn who was exposed to intense noise during fetal life is significantly less reactive to loud sounds after birth.

Characteristics of Newborn Neurologic Function

Normal newborns are usually in a position of partially flexed extremities, with the legs near the abdomen. When awake, the newborn may exhibit purposeless, uncoordinated bilateral movements of the extremities. The organization and quality of the newborn's motor activity are influenced by a number of factors, including the following (Nugent, 2013):

- Intrauterine growth restriction
- Prenatal stress
- Environmental chemicals
- Obstetric medications
- Acute fetal distress
- Gestational and pregestational diabetes
- Intrauterine drug exposure
- Prematurity and low birth weight.

Eye movements are observable during the first few days of life. An alert newborn is able to fixate on faces and geometric objects or patterns, such as black-and-white stripes. A bright light shining in the newborn's eyes elicits the blinking reflex.

The cry of the newborn should be lusty and vigorous. High-pitched cries, weak cries, and no cries are causes for concern.

The newborn's body growth progresses in a cephalocaudal (head-to-toe), proximal–distal fashion. The newborn is somewhat hypertonic—that is, there is resistance to extending the elbow and knee joints. Muscle tone should be symmetric. Diminished muscle tone and flaccidity may indicate neurologic dysfunction.

Specific symmetric deep tendon reflexes can be elicited in the newborn. The knee-jerk reflex is brisk; a normal ankle clonus may involve three to four beats. Plantar flexion is present. Other reflexes, including the Moro, grasping, Babinski, rooting, and sucking reflexes, are characteristic of neurologic integrity. **Table 33.16** ›› provides a summary of stimulus and response for the common newborn reflexes.

TABLE 33.16 Common Reflexes of the Newborn

Reflex	Stimulus and Response	Visual
Rooting	Elicited when the side of the newborn's mouth or cheek is touched. In response, the newborn turns toward that side and opens the lips to suck (if not fed recently).	*Source:* Pearson Education, Inc.
Sucking	Elicited when an object is placed in the newborn's mouth or anything touches the lips. Newborns suck even while sleeping; this is called *nonnutritive sucking*, and it can have a quieting effect on the baby. Disappears by 12 months.	*Source:* Pearson Education, Inc.
Moro	Elicited when the newborn is startled by a loud noise or lifted slightly above the crib and then suddenly lowered. In response, the newborn straightens arms and hands outward while the knees flex. Slowly the arms return to the chest, as in an embrace. The fingers spread, forming a C, and the newborn may cry. This reflex may persist until about 6 months of age.	*Source:* Pearson Education, Inc.

(continued on next page)

TABLE 33.16 Common Reflexes of the Newborn (*continued*)

Reflex	Stimulus and Response	Visual
Tonic neck (fencer position)	Occurs when the newborn is lying face up and the head is turned to one side. In response, the extremities on the same side extend or straighten, whereas on the opposite side they flex. This reflex may not be seen during the early newborn period, appearing between 1 and 4 months after delivery and resolving within a few months (Arcilla & Vilella, 2020).	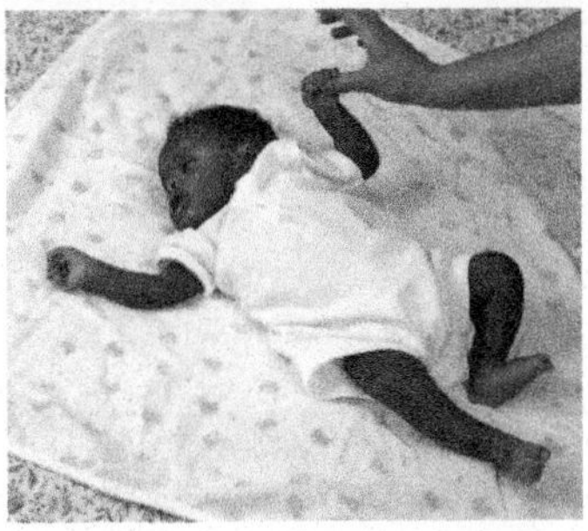 *Source:* Pearson Education, Inc.
Stepping	When held upright with one foot touching a flat surface, the newborn puts one foot in front of the other and "walks" (*stepping reflex*). This reflex is more pronounced at birth and is lost in 4–8 weeks.	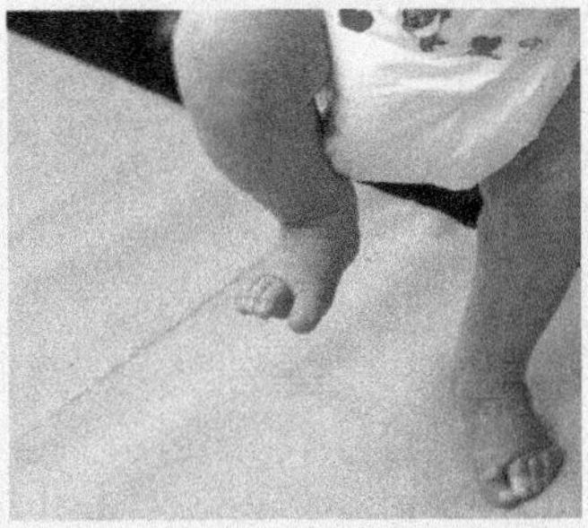 *Source:* Pearson Education, Inc.
Palmar grasping	Elicited by stimulating the newborn's palm with a finger or an object; the newborn grasps and holds the object or finger firmly enough to be lifted momentarily from the crib. This reflex persists until 5–6 months.	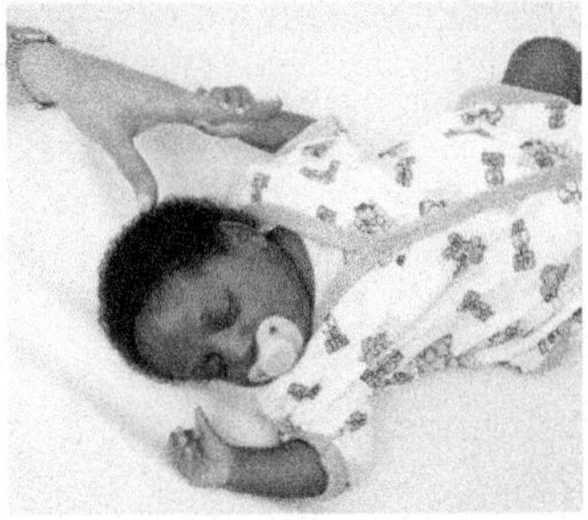 *Source:* Pearson Education, Inc.
Babinski	Fanning and hyperextension of all toes and dorsiflexion of the big toe occurs when the lateral aspect of the sole is stroked from the heel upward across the ball of the foot. In children older than 24 months, an abnormal response is extension or fanning of the toes; this Babinski response indicates upper motor neuron abnormalities.	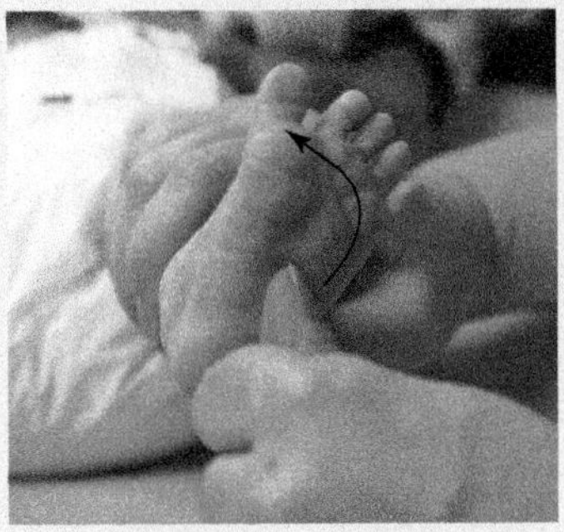 *Source:* Pearson Education, Inc.
Blinking	Flash of light causes eyelids to close.	
Pupillary	Flash of light causes pupils to constrict.	
Startle	Loud noise evokes flexion in arms with fists clenched.	
Abdominal	Tactile stimulation causes abdominal muscles to contract.	
Withdrawal	Slight pinprick to sole of foot causes leg to flex.	
Plantar (toe-grasping) reflex	Pressure applied against the ball of the foot elicits plantar flexion of the toes. Disappears by 12 months.	
Trunk incurvation (Galant reflex)	Stroking the spine of the prone newborn causes the pelvis to turn to the stimulated side.	

Sources: American Academy of Pediatrics (2019); Arcilla and Vilella (2020); Hawes, Bernardo, and Wilson (2020); Ladewig et al. (2017), Table 24-2; MedlinePlus (2019).

Performance of complex behavioral patterns reflects the newborn's neurologic maturation and integration. Newborns who can bring a hand to their mouth may be demonstrating motor coordination as well as a self-quieting technique, thus increasing the complexity of the behavioral response. Newborns also possess complex, organized, defensive motor patterns, as exhibited by the ability to remove an obstruction, such as a cloth across the face.

Periods of Reactivity

Newborns display three behavioral states: the sleep state, the transitional state, and the alert state (McGrath & Vittner, 2018). These are similar to states identified in the fetus during pregnancy. Each state has identified subcategories.

Sleep States

The sleep states are as follows:

- ***Deep or quiet sleep.*** Deep sleep is characterized by closed eyes with no eye movements; regular, even breathing; and jerky motions or startles at regular intervals. Behavioral responses to external stimuli are likely to be delayed. Startles are rapidly suppressed, and changes in state are not likely to occur. Heart rate may range from 100 to 120 beats/min.
- ***Active or light sleep (rapid eye movement [REM] sleep).*** The baby has irregular respirations; eyes closed, with REM; irregular sucking motions; minimal activity; and irregular but smooth movement of the extremities. Environmental and internal stimuli may initiate a startle reaction and a change of state.

Newborn sleep cycles have been recognized and defined according to duration. The length of the sleep cycle depends on the age of the newborn. At term, REM active sleep and quiet sleep occur in intervals of 50 to 60 minutes (Blackburn, 2018). Approximately 45–50% of the newborn's total sleep is active sleep, 35–45% is quiet sleep, and 10% is transitional between these two periods. Growth hormone secretion depends on regular sleep patterns. Any disturbance of the sleep–wake cycle can result in irregular spikes of growth hormone. REM sleep stimulates the highest peaks of growth hormone and the growth of the neural system. Over a period of time, the newborn's sleep–wake patterns become diurnal (the newborn sleeps at night and stays awake during the day).

Transitional State

The transitional state is characterized by *drowsiness*. The behaviors common to the drowsy state are open or closed eyes; fluttering eyelids; semidozing appearance; and slow, regular movements of the extremities. Mild startles may be noted from time to time. Although the reaction to a sensory stimulus is delayed, a change of state often results.

Alert States

In the first 30 to 60 minutes after birth, many newborns display a quiet alert state. After a sleep phase that lasts from a few minutes to between 2 and 4 hours, a second alert state occurs. This second alert period lasts 4 to 6 hours in the normal newborn. The nurse should use these alert states to encourage bonding and breastfeeding.

The newborn's periods of alertness tend to be shorter during the first 2 days after birth; this allows the baby to recover from the birth process. Subsequent alert states are of choice or of necessity. Increasing choice of wakefulness by the newborn indicates a maturing capacity to achieve and maintain consciousness. Heat, cold, and hunger are but a few of the stimuli that can cause wakefulness by necessity. Once the disturbing stimuli have been removed, the baby tends to fall back asleep.

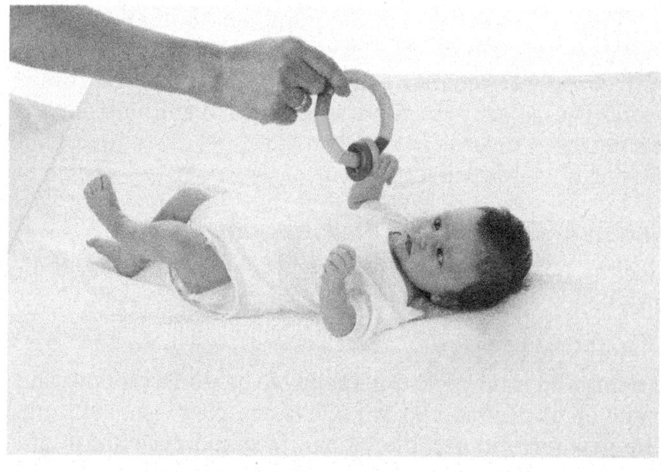

Figure 33.60 » Newborn in active alert state turning his head to follow an object.

Source: Jules Selmes/Pearson Education, Inc.

The following are subcategories of the alert state (McGrath & Vittner, 2018):

- ***Quiet alert.*** In the quiet-alert state, the newborn is alert and follows and fixates on attractive objects, faces, or auditory stimuli. Motor activity is minimal, and the response to external stimuli is delayed.
- ***Active alert.*** In the active-alert state, the newborn's eyes are open and motor activity is quite intense, with thrusting movements of the extremities. Environmental stimuli increase startles or motor activity, but individual reactions are difficult to distinguish because of the generally high activity level (**Figure 33.60 »**).
- ***Crying.*** Intense crying is accompanied by jerky motor movements. Crying serves several purposes for the newborn. It may be a distraction from disturbing stimuli, such as hunger and pain. Fussiness often allows the newborn to discharge energy and reorganize behavior. Most important, crying elicits an appropriate response of help from the parents.

Behavioral Capacities of the Newborn

Newborns have several behavioral capacities that assist them in adapting to extrauterine life. For example, **self-quieting ability** is when newborns use their own resources to quiet and comfort themselves. Their repertoire includes hand-to-mouth movements, sucking on a fist or tongue, and attending to external stimuli. Neurologically impaired newborns are unable to use self-quieting activities and require more frequent comforting from caregivers when stimulated. For example, drug-positive newborns often exhibit abnormal sleep and feeding patterns and irritability.

Habituation is the newborn's ability to process and respond to complex stimulation. For example, when a bright light is flashed into the newborn's eyes, the initial response is blinking, constriction of the pupil, and perhaps a slight startle reaction. However, with repeated stimulation the newborn's response repertoire gradually diminishes and disappears. The capacity to ignore repetitious, disturbing stimuli is a newborn defense mechanism that is readily apparent in the noisy, well-lit nursery.

Sensory Capacities of the Newborn

Healthy, neurologically intact newborns exhibit visual, auditory, olfactory, taste, and tactile capacity.

Visual Capacity

Orientation is the newborn's ability to be alert to, follow, and fixate on appealing and attractive, complex visual stimuli. The newborn prefers the human face and eyes and high-contrast objects and patterns. The newborn is nearsighted and has best vision at a distance of 8 to 15 inches. As the face or object comes into the line of vision, the newborn responds with bright, wide eyes as well as still limbs and a fixed stare. This intense visual involvement may last several minutes. During this time, the newborn is able to follow the stimulus from side to side. The newborn uses this sensory capacity to become familiar with family, friends, and surroundings.

Auditory Capacity

The newborn responds to auditory stimulation with a definite, organized behavioral repertoire. The stimulus used to assess auditory response should be selected to match the state of the newborn. A rattle is appropriate for light sleep, a voice for an awake state, and a clap for deep sleep. As the newborn hears the sound, the cardiac rate rises; a minimal startle reflex may be observed. If the sound is appealing, the newborn will become alert and search for the site of the auditory stimulus. Lack of auditory development is associated with an increased risk of sudden infant death syndrome (SIDS).

Olfactory Capacity

A newborn can differentiate the mother's smell from those of other people (Blackburn, 2018). Olfactory senses help the newborn tell the difference between the mother's breast pad and those of other people, often as soon as 1 week after delivery.

Taste and Sucking

The newborn responds differently to varying tastes. Sugar, for example, increases sucking. Newborns fed with a rubber nipple versus the breast also show sucking pattern variations. When breastfeeding, the newborn sucks in bursts, with frequent regular pauses. The bottle-fed newborn, however, tends to suck at a regular rate, with infrequent pauses.

When awake and hungry, the newborn displays rapid searching motions in response to the rooting reflex. Once feeding begins, the newborn establishes a sucking pattern according to the method of feeding. Finger sucking is seen in utero as well as after birth. The newborn frequently uses nonnutritive sucking as a self-quieting activity, which assists in the development of self-regulation. For bottle-fed babies, there is no reason to discourage nonnutritive sucking with a pacifier. Pacifiers should be offered to breastfed babies only after breastfeeding is well established. If the pacifier is offered too soon, a phenomenon called "nipple confusion" may occur, in which the breastfed baby has difficulty learning to suck from the breast and will nurse less.

Tactile Capacity

Newborns are very sensitive to touch. Supportive touch (such as holding, cuddling, swaddling, or placing a hand on the abdomen) can soothe the newborn and support brain development (Maitre et al., 2017). Touch can also promote alertness and attention to the environment, for example by rousing a sleepy newborn for feeding.

Alterations of the Newborn Period

Neonatology is the field of medicine providing care for sick and premature neonates. Many levels of nursery care have evolved in response to increasing knowledge about at-risk newborns: special care, intensive care, and convalescent or transitional care. Along with the newborn's parents, the nurse is an important caregiver in all these settings. As a member of the multidisciplinary healthcare team, the nurse is a technically competent professional who contributes the high-touch, human care necessary in the high-tech perinatal environment.

Various factors influence the outcome of at-risk neonates, including the following:

- Birth weight
- Gestational age
- Type and length of illness
- Environmental factors
- Maternal factors
- Maternal–newborn separation.

An at-risk newborn is one susceptible to illness (morbidity) or even death (mortality) because of dysmaturity, immaturity, physical disorders, or complications during or after birth. In most cases, the neonate is the product of a pregnancy involving one or more predictable risk factors, including the following:

- Low SES of the mother
- Limited access to healthcare or no prenatal care
- Exposure to environmental dangers, such as toxic chemicals and illicit drugs
- Preexisting maternal conditions, such as heart disease, diabetes, HTN, hyperthyroidism, and renal disease
- Maternal factors, such as age and parity
- Medical conditions related to pregnancy and their associated complications
- Pregnancy complications, such as abruptio placentae, oligohydramnios, preterm labor, premature rupture of membranes, and preeclampsia.

Because these factors and the perinatal risks associated with them are known, the birth of at-risk newborns can often be anticipated. The pregnancy can be closely monitored, treatment can be started as necessary, and arrangements can be made for birth to occur at a facility with appropriate resources to care for both mother and baby.

Whether or not prenatal assessment indicates that the fetus is at risk, the course of labor and birth, as well as the newborn's ability to withstand the stress of labor, cannot be predicted. Thus, the nurse's use of electronic fetal heart monitoring or fetal heart auscultation by Doppler plays a significant role in detecting stress or distress in the fetus. Immediately after birth, the Apgar score may help identify the at-risk newborn, but it is not the only indicator of possible long-term outcome.

The newborn classification and neonatal mortality risk chart is another useful tool for identifying newborns at risk. Before this classification tool was developed, birth weight of less than 2500 g was the sole criterion for determining prematurity. HCPs then recognized that a newborn could weigh more than 2500 g and still be premature. Conversely, a newborn weighing less than 2500 g might be functionally at term or beyond. As a result, birth weight and gestational age together are now the criteria used to assess neonatal maturity, morbidity, and mortality risk.

According to the newborn classification and neonatal mortality risk chart, gestation (postmenstrual age) is divided as follows (ACOG, 2013c, reaffirmed 2017):

- ***Preterm:*** 20 to 36 weeks and 6 days (36 6/7 weeks)
  - Late preterm: 34 to 36 weeks and 6 days (36 6/7 weeks)
- ***Term:*** 37 to 41 6/7 (completed) weeks
  - Early term: 37 to 38 weeks and 6 days (38 6/7 weeks)
  - Full term: 39 to 40 weeks and 6 days (40 6/7 weeks)
  - Late term: 41 to 41 and 6 days (41 6/7 weeks)
- ***Postterm:*** 42 weeks and beyond.

Large-for-gestational-age newborns are those who plot above the 90th percentile curve on an intrauterine growth chart. Appropriate-for-gestational-age newborns are those who plot between the 10th and 90th percentile growth curves. Small-for-gestational-age newborns are those that plot below the 10th percentile growth curve. A newborn is assigned to a category depending on birth weight, length, occipitofrontal head circumference, and gestational age. For example, a newborn classified as Pr SGA is preterm and small for gestational age. The term newborn whose weight is appropriate for gestational age is classified F AGA. It is important to note that intrauterine growth charts are influenced by altitude and by the ethnicity of the newborn population used to create the chart. Also, the assigned newborn classification may vary according to the intrauterine growth curve chart used; therefore, the chart used should correlate with the characteristics of the patient population. Evaluation of gestational age is discussed later in this exemplar in the Assessment section.

Neonatal Mortality Risk

Neonatal mortality risk is a baby's chance of death within the newborn period—that is, within the first 28 days of life. Neonatal mortality risk decreases as both gestational age and birth weight increase. Neonates who are preterm and SGA have the highest mortality risk. The previously high mortality rates for LGA newborns have decreased at most perinatal centers because of both improved management of diabetes in pregnancy and increased recognition of potential complications of these newborns.

Newborn immaturity increases the risk for birth hypoxia or asphyxia and for infections, two frequent causes of neonatal mortality. Worldwide, almost 50% of deaths among children under the age of 5 occur during the newborn period, most within the first week of birth (WHO, 2019b). In the United States, non-Hispanic Black children have the highest infant mortality rates (10.8 per 1000 live births) and Asian American infants have the lowest mortality rate (3.6) (CDC, 2020b). The presence of immaturity (preterm, low birth weight, and SGA) in the newborn indicates a need for careful assessment for distress, hypoglycemia, congenital anomalies, infection, and polycythemia. Exemplar 33.E, Prematurity, in this module discusses care of the premature newborn. Common alterations seen in the newborn are described in Alterations and Therapies: Newborn Care.

COVID-19 and the Newborn

A newborn may be at risk of developing COVID-19 from exposure to respiratory droplets from a parent or caregiver who is infected with the SARS-CoV-2 virus. However, the most recent evidence suggests that this transmission is uncommon (CDC, 2020a). Guidance available as of December 2020 did not include any recommended changes related to skin-to-skin contact but did recommend testing all newborns of mothers with suspected or confirmed COVID-19. Manifestations of COVID-19 observed in newborns include respiratory signs (rhinorrhea, cough, increased work of breathing, tachypnea), as well as fever, poor feeding, vomiting, and diarrhea (CDC, 2020a). For the latest guidance, check the CDC website.

>> *Go to **Pearson MyLab Nursing and eText** to see Chart 16: Potential Birth Injuries and Chart 17: Congenital Anomalies: Identification and Care in the Newborn Period.*

Collaboration

The interprofessional team caring for the newborn often includes a pediatrician or neonatologist, a nurse, a lactation consultant, and an audiologist or audiology technician. Needs of the newborn differ dramatically in the first 4 hours of extrauterine life than in later periods. Assessments and interventions in the first 4 hours involve all organ systems. Because of this, care is divided into initial postpartum care, subsequent care, and discharge preparation. Complications that arise may necessitate involvement by other specialists, such as a pediatric cardiologist or pulmonologist. The nurse's role is described in the following Nursing Process section.

NURSING PROCESS

Thorough and ongoing assessment is necessary to ensure the newborn's safety from delivery to and beyond discharge. The nurse will focus primarily on thermoregulation, oxygenation, and cardiac function, incorporating other needs based on assessment of the newborn and family.

Initial Care of the Newborn

Immediately after birth, the provider places the newborn on the mother's abdomen or under the radiant heat unit. Placing the newborn on the maternal abdomen promotes attachment and bonding and gives the mother the opportunity to immediately interact with her baby. Placing the baby on the mother's chest also promotes early breastfeeding opportunities. Even though the baby may not breastfeed immediately, placement

Alterations and Therapies

Newborn Care

ALTERATION	DESCRIPTION	THERAPIES
Growth		
Small for gestational age (SGA)	Less than the 10th percentile for birth weight; the newborn may be preterm, term, or postterm; often seen in women who smoke, have high blood pressure, or have any condition that reduces blood flow to the fetus. Increased risk of perinatal asphyxia, perinatal mortality, polycythemia, and hypoglycemia.	▪ Care is aimed at promoting growth. ▪ Requires ongoing screening for potential complications related to SGA, including polycythemia, cold stress, asphyxia, hypothermia, and hyperbilirubinemia. ▪ Assess parents and family members because SGA may be an expected finding if short stature runs in the family.
Very small for gestational age (VSGA)	Less than the third percentile for birth weight; the newborn may be preterm, term, or postterm.	▪ Promote weight gain. ▪ Monitor blood sugar levels for hypoglycemia. ▪ Promote smoking cessation or substance abstinence if that is a factor in the newborn's VSGA status.
Large for gestational age (LGA)	Newborn's weight is at or above the 90th percentile; often associated with maternal diabetes, genetic predisposition, multiparous women, erythroblastosis fetalis, Beckwith-Wiedemann syndrome, or transposition of the great vessels.	▪ Accurate estimation of gestational age is important to determining LGA status. ▪ Carefully assess for potential birth trauma, including effects of cephalopelvic disproportion and macrosomia, fractured clavicle or humerus, or damage to the brachial plexus nerves as a result of shoulder dystocia. ▪ Monitor for hypoglycemia, polycythemia, and hyperbilirubinemia.
Intrauterine growth restriction (IUGR)	Pregnancy circumstances of advanced gestation and limited fetal growth most commonly associated with lack of prenatal care, age extremes in the mother, low SES, HTN, multiple-gestation pregnancy, grand multiparity, and primiparity. Environmental factors such as excessive exercise, exposure to toxins, high altitudes, and maternal drug use have also been implicated.	▪ Early identification is important to early intervention. ▪ If IUGR is unexplained, an in utero infection must be ruled out. ▪ Monitor newborn for hypoglycemia. ▪ Provide patient teaching to promote growth after discharge and participation in neonatal stimulation programs to promote neurologic function.
Conditions Present at Birth		
Newborn of a mother with diabetes	Babies born to mothers with diabetes are often LGA, macrosomic, ruddy in color, and have excessive adipose tissue, decreased total body water, edema, cardiomegaly, and often trouble regulating blood sugar levels initially because of higher-than-normal insulin production in utero to cope with the mother's elevated blood sugar levels.	▪ Assess blood sugar levels frequently. ▪ Monitor for signs of hypoglycemia, including tremors, cyanosis, apnea, temperature instability, poor feeding, and hypotonia. ▪ Seizures may occur in severe cases. ▪ Assess lab results for hypocalcemia, hyperbilirubinemia, and polycythemia. ▪ Initial assessment should observe for birth trauma due to large size.
Postterm newborn	Newborn born after 42 weeks of gestation; most often seen in those of Australian, Greek, and Italian heritage. Most are normal size but large because they continued to grow in utero and face higher risk for morbidity, with a two to three times higher mortality rate. Potential complications include hypoglycemia, meconium aspiration, polycythemia, congenital anomalies, seizures, and cold stress.	▪ Many postterm neonates will adapt well to extrauterine life. ▪ Monitor serum blood sugar. ▪ Assess respiratory status, especially in the presence of possible meconium aspiration. ▪ Maintain NTE until newborn demonstrates temperature stability.

Alterations and Therapies *(continued)*

ALTERATION	DESCRIPTION	THERAPIES
Congenital heart defects	Any number of abnormalities can impact the heart during fetal development, increasing the challenge for newborn adaptation to extrauterine life.	▪ One-third of neonates born with congenital heart defects develop life-threatening symptoms in the first few days of life. ▪ Therapies range from palliative care to surgery. ▪ This topic is discussed in more detail in Exemplar 16.B, Congenital Heart Defects, in Module 16, Perfusion.
Newborns with prenatal substance abuse exposure	Substance exposure may include tobacco, marijuana, prescription medications, narcotics, or any number of illegal substances.	▪ Babies are at risk for IUGR, meconium aspiration, reduced birth weight, vomiting, seizures, or irritability depending on the substances the fetus was exposed to. ▪ Sedate newborns to decrease irritability and tremors. ▪ Provide IV fluid therapy for hydration. ▪ Evaluate safety of breastfeeding. ▪ Care of newborns and infants with prenatal substance syndromes is discussed in detail in Module 22, Addiction. Care of children with fetal alcohol syndrome is discussed in Module 25, Development.
Newborns born to mothers with HIV/ AIDS	HIV can be transmitted through the fetal circulation, but the mother who begins antiretroviral medications early in her pregnancy can reduce the risk to the newborn.	▪ Advise mother that taking most HIV medications during pregnancy is safe. ▪ Neonates may be given prophylactic antiretroviral therapy to decrease risk of active infection. ▪ Advise against breastfeeding per CDC recommendations. ▪ This concept is discussed in detail in Exemplar 8.A, HIV/AIDS, in Module 8, Immunity.
Phenylketonuria (PKU)	Amino acid disorders, in which phenylalanine found in dietary protein cannot be converted to tyrosine, result in accumulation of phenylalanine in the blood, which, in turn, results in damage to brain tissue that leads to progressive intellectual disability.	▪ Collect routine screening blood sample before discharge (24–48 hours after first enteral feeding). ▪ Instruct parents that a second screening may be required if initial collection occurs before the initiation of enteral feedings. This follow-up screening often occurs between 7 and 14 days of life.
Maple syrup urine disease	Rapidly progressing and often fatal disease, when untreated, caused by enzymatic defect in the metabolism of the branched-chain amino acids leucine, isoleucine, and alloisoleucine.	▪ Diagnosed by routine newborn screening and confirmed by plasma amino acid assay. ▪ Instruct parents on importance of obtaining second screening exam, as noted for PKU.
Galactosemia	An inborn error of carbohydrate metabolism in which the body is unable to use the sugars galactose and lactose. Enzyme pathways in liver cells normally convert galactose and lactose to glucose. In galactosemia, one step in that conversion pathway is absent because of the lack of either the enzyme galactose 1-phosphate uridyl transferase or the enzyme galactokinase. High levels of unusable galactose circulate in the blood, resulting in cataracts, brain damage, and liver damage.	▪ Instruct parents on importance of routine newborn screening for inborn errors of metabolism.
Homocystinuria	Disorder caused by a deficiency of the enzyme cystathionine beta-synthase, which causes an elevated excretion of homocysteine and methionine.	▪ Screening is included in the Recommended Uniform Screening Panel and is considered an amino acid disorder (U.S. Department of Health and Human Services, 2020). ▪ No symptoms are usually seen in the newborn period.

(continued on next page)

Alterations and Therapies *(continued)*

ALTERATION	DESCRIPTION	THERAPIES
Birth-Related Stressors		
Asphyxia	Asphyxia can occur for a number of reasons, including, but not limited to, abruptio placentae, prolapsed cord, maternal hypoxia or death, difficult or prolonged labor, meconium in the amniotic fluid, intrapartum bleeding, maternal infection, prematurity, multiple births, or narcotic use during labor.	▪ Promote oxygenation, airway clearance, and breathing to reduce newborn hypoxia, which often includes resuscitation. ▪ Monitor blood gas status. ▪ Provide cardiorespiratory monitoring. ▪ Newborn is usually taken to the NICU. ▪ Support parents and family.
Respiratory distress	May result from inadequate production of surfactant, prematurity, excessive airway secretions, narcotic administration to the mother during labor, meconium aspiration, or congenital anomalies, among other factors. Parenchymal damage results in hyaline membrane disease compounded by mechanical ventilation, if required.	▪ Continuous monitoring is conducted with a cardiorespiratory monitor. ▪ Continuous oxygen saturation monitoring is provided. ▪ Determine arterial blood gas levels frequently until stable. ▪ May require assistance with respiration in the form of mechanical ventilation, continuous positive airway pressure (CPAP), bilevel positive airway pressure, and/or oxygen administration. ▪ Parents and family members require emotional support because it can be very frightening to see a small baby that is sick and requires mechanical ventilation.
Transient tachypnea of the newborn	Of particular risk to the LGA and late-preterm neonate because of inadequate clearing of the airways; the newborn will display increased work of breathing 1–6 hours after birth, with rapid respirations, grunting, nasal flaring, and/or mild respiratory and metabolic acidosis. Improvement is usually seen after 24–48 hours.	▪ Monitor newborn's respiratory adaptation to extrauterine life and report any signs of distress immediately to primary HCP. ▪ Administration of oxygen should be in conjunction with oxygen saturation monitoring to prevent complications related to oxygen toxicity. ▪ Promote parental attachment because a newborn requiring oxygen may not be able to feed or spend as much time with parents until breathing improves.
Meconium aspiration syndrome	Meconium is passed in utero secondary to stress and/or hypoxia. This fluid may be aspirated into the tracheobronchial tree in utero or during the first few breaths taken by the newborn. Meconium causes chemical irritation and also forms small balls that become lodged in terminal airways, allowing some air to enter the alveoli but not allowing air to escape. As alveoli continue to expand, they eventually rupture. Complete respiratory collapse may be seen in severe cases.	▪ Avoid positive end-expiratory pressure, which forces more air into the lungs and increases chance that alveoli might rupture. ▪ Mechanical ventilation may be inadequate, and oscillating ventilators that administer 300–400 breaths/minute in small waves of air may be required. ▪ Continuous cardiorespiratory and oxygen saturation monitoring is indicated. ▪ Reduce oxygen demands by keeping the baby quiet; sedation may be required. ▪ Hypoxic newborns should not be fed because oxygen is shunted from the gut; total parenteral nutrition may be administered to meet nutritional demands.
Hypoglycemia	Abnormally low blood sugar (40 mg/dL) can result from a number of conditions, including a mother with diabetes, prematurity, or cold stress.	▪ If possible, feed the baby to raise blood sugar levels. ▪ Provide 40% oral dextrose gel, to attempt reduction in NICU admissions and support exclusive breastfeeding (Watson & Moulsdale, 2020). ▪ If unable to feed, 10% dextrose in water ($D_{10}W$) may be administered IV. ▪ Observe for signs of hypoglycemia, including jitteriness, crying, or in severe cases, seizures.
Cold stress	Results from inadequate temperature regulation; can progress to respiratory distress.	▪ Thermoregulation is discussed in the Nursing Process section that follows and in detail in Module 20.

Alterations and Therapies *(continued)*

ALTERATION	DESCRIPTION	THERAPIES
Polycythemia	Abnormally high hemoglobin levels; can result from placental transfusion caused by delayed cord clamping or cord stripping, fetal asphyxia, or twin-to-twin blood transfusion in utero.	▪ Encourage fluids. ▪ Monitor cardiorespiratory status for tachycardia or congestive heart failure, respiratory distress. ▪ Assess jaundice caused by increased RBC breakdown. ▪ May require patience with feeding because of feeding intolerance, poor feeding, and vomiting.

Source: Adapted from London et al. (2017).

on the mother's chest enables the baby to smell, touch, and lick the mother's nipples. The newborn is maintained in a modified Trendelenburg position, which aids drainage of mucus from the nasopharynx and trachea by gravity. The newborn is dried immediately, and wet blankets are removed. The nurse helps maintain the baby's warmth by placing warmed blankets over the newborn or by placing the newborn in skin-to-skin contact with the mother. If the newborn is under a radiant-heated unit, he or she is dried, placed on a dry blanket, and left uncovered under the radiant heat. Because radiant heat warms the outer surface of objects, a newborn wrapped in blankets will receive no benefit from radiant heat.

The newborn's mouth and nose are suctioned with a bulb syringe as needed. Most immediate care of the newborn can be accomplished while the newborn is in the parent's arms or under the radiant-heated unit. Many women request that their babies be left on their abdomens or chests while initial care is given. Unless a medical complication exists, the nurse should complete assessments in this position to promote parental attachment.

Apgar Scoring System

The Apgar scoring system (**Table 33.17** ›››) is used to evaluate the physical condition of the newborn at birth. The newborn is rated 1 minute after birth and again at 5 minutes and receives a total score (**Apgar score**) ranging from 0 to 10 based on the following assessments:

- ***Heart rate*** is auscultated or palpated at the junction of the umbilical cord and skin. This is the most important assessment. A newborn heart rate of less than 100 beats/min indicates the need for immediate resuscitation.
- ***Respiratory effort*** is the second most important Apgar assessment. Complete absence of respirations is termed *apnea*. A vigorous cry indicates adequate respirations.
- ***Muscle tone*** is determined by evaluating the degree of flexion and resistance to straightening of the extremities. A normal newborn's elbows and hips are flexed, with the knees positioned up toward the abdomen.
- ***Reflex irritability*** is evaluated by stroking the baby's back along the spine or by flicking the soles of the feet. A cry merits a full score of 2. A grimace is given 1 point, and no response is scored as 0.
- ***Skin color*** is inspected for cyanosis and pallor. Generally, newborns have blue extremities with a pink body, which merits a score of 1. This condition is termed **acrocyanosis** and is present in 85% of normal newborns at 1 minute after birth. A completely pink newborn scores a 2, and a totally cyanotic, pale neonate scores a 0. Newborns with darker skin pigmentation will not be pink in color. Their skin color is assessed for pallor and acrocyanosis, and a score is selected on the basis of the assessment.

TABLE 33.17 The Apgar Scoring System

Sign	Score 0	Score 1	Score 2
Heart rate	Absent	Slow—below 100 beats/min	Above 100 beats/min
Respiratory effort	Absent	Slow—irregular	Good crying
Muscle tone	Flaccid	Some flexion of extremities	Active motion
Reflex irritability	None	Grimace	Vigorous cry
Color	Pale blue	Body pink, blue extremities	Completely pink

Source: Data from Apgar (1966).

A score of 7 to 10 indicates a newborn in good condition who requires only nasopharyngeal suctioning and, perhaps, some oxygen near the face (called "blow-by" oxygen). If the Apgar score is less than 7 at 5 minutes, the scoring should be repeated every 5 minutes up to 20 minutes (AAP & ACOG, 2015) and resuscitative measures may need to be instituted. Apgar scores of less than 3 at 5 minutes may correlate with neonatal mortality (Cnattingius, Johansson, & Razaz, 2020).

Clamping the Cord

If the HCP has not placed some type of cord clamp on the newborn's umbilical cord, the nurse must do so. Before applying the cord clamp, the nurse examines the cut end of the cord for the presence of two arteries and one vein. The umbilical vein is the largest vessel; the arteries are seen as smaller vessels. The number of vessels is recorded on the birth and newborn records. The cord is clamped approximately 1.3 to 2.5 cm (0.5 to 1 in.) from the abdomen to allow room between the abdomen and clamp as the cord dries. Abdominal skin must not be clamped because this will cause necrosis of the tissue. The most common type of cord clamp is the plastic Hollister cord clamp (**Figure 33.61** ›››). The Hollister clamp

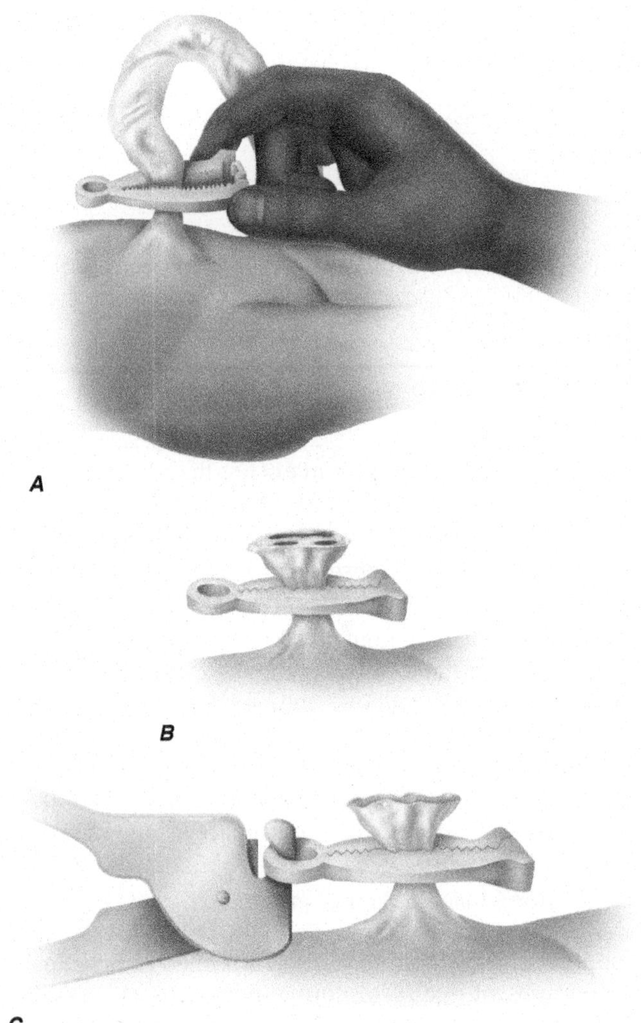

Figure 33.61 ›› Hollister cord clamp. ***A***, Clamp is positioned ½ to 1 in. from the abdomen and then secured. ***B***, Cut cord. The one vein and two arteries can be seen. ***C***, Plastic device for removing the clamp after the cord has dried. After the cord is cut, the nurse grasps the Hollister clamp on either side of the cut area and gently separates it.

is removed in the newborn nursery approximately 24 hours after the cord has dried.

Evidence-based practice suggests that delayed clamping may yield more benefits than immediate cord clamping (ACOG, 2017c). Delaying cord clamping for at least 30 to 60 seconds produces increased blood volume, reduced need for blood transfusions, decreased incidence of intracranial hemorrhage, and a lower frequency of iron deficiency anemia (ACOG, 2017c). One concern with delayed clamping is polycythemia, which is benign. Other concerns include delayed resuscitation of the newborn and interfering with cord blood banking collection (ACOG, 2017c).

Banking Cord Blood

A growing number of parents are arranging for cord blood banking. Parents obtain a special container from the Cord Blood Registry, which they bring with them for the birth. Immediately after the newborn's umbilical cord is clamped and cut, the HCP withdraws blood from the remaining umbilical cord by inserting a large-gauge needle into the umbilical vein. The needle allows the blood to be collected into the container. The nurse labels the specimen immediately and follows the directions required for storage and pickup. The collected cord blood can then be used to treat childhood cancers, rare genetic disorders, and cerebral palsy. There are both public and private cord blood banks. At private banks, the cord blood is stored for possible later use by the donor. Alternatively, cord blood may be donated to public banks for use by anyone in need, much like blood donations. Although cord blood can be donated at some hospital facilities, most hospitals do not have these services available. The main drawback of cord blood banking remains the cost.

Newborn Identification and Security

Identification bands typically come in a set of four, all preprinted with identical numbers. The nurse places two bands on the newborn—one on the wrist and one on the ankle. The newborn bands must fit snugly to prevent their loss. The nurse then gives the mother and her designated significant other each a band. The band number is documented in the maternal and newborn medical records. The bands allow access to the newborn care areas; they must not be removed until the newborn is discharged. In most facilities, as a security measure, only individuals with a band are given unlimited access to the newborn. Some facilities may also include an umbilical clamp with a preprinted number identical to the number printed on the bands.

Hospitals have different safety measures to ensure the safety of newborns. Some institutions rely on an umbilical band system to ensure their safety, whereas others attach an alarm to the ankle band (**Figure 33.62 ››**). The alarm is triggered if the device is tampered with or if the newborn is removed from the perimeters of the security field.

Additional hospital security measures are now commonplace in maternity settings. This includes mandating that all staff wear appropriate identification at all times. Parents are

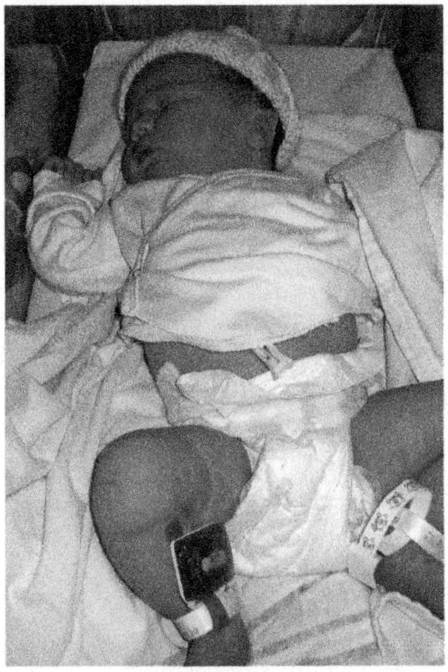

Figure 33.62 ›› Newborn with security device in place on one ankle.

Source: Anne Garcia.

TABLE 33.18 Timing of Newborn Assessments

Time Frame	Assessments
At birth	■ To determine the need for resuscitation or other interventions. ■ The stable newborn can stay with the family after birth in order to initiate early attachment. ■ The newborn with complications is usually taken to the nursery for further evaluation and intervention.
In first 2 hours after birth	■ All newborns in skin-to-skin contact and/or breastfeeding should be continuously monitored by qualified professional personnel. ■ All caregivers should be taught safe positioning of the newborn to ensure airway protection (AWHONN, 2020).
Nursery nurse assessment	■ The nurse conducts a brief physical examination to evaluate the newborn's adaptation to extrauterine life. ■ No later than 2 hours after birth, the admitting nursery nurse should evaluate the newborn's status and any problems that place the newborn at risk (AAP & ACOG, 2017).
Prior to discharge	■ Before discharge, a CNM, physician, or nurse practitioner will carry out a complete physical examination to detect any emerging or potential problems. ■ A general assessment is also performed prior to discharge.

instructed that individuals without appropriate identification should not be allowed to remove their baby under any circumstances. The nurse may also advise the parents to place their baby on the side of the bed away from the window.

Although hospital newborn abductions are rare, they are catastrophic for the family, hospital, and community. Many abductors pose as medical personnel to gain access to the mother and baby. Women should be advised to ask all hospital personnel for proper identification. If the mother or family feels unsure of the individual, they should immediately use the call bell to alert the nurse and ask for other verification. If a woman is reluctant to allow a student nurse to transport her baby, the staff nurse should be asked to assist the student.

Assessment

In addition to clinical signs, such as motion and heart rate, the nurse assesses the newborn's behavior and shares information from the assessment with the parents, so it is incorporated into the plan of care. Assessment in the first 1 to 4 hours is a continuous process to determine how well the newborn is adjusting to extrauterine life (**Table 33.18** ›› outlines the timing of newborn assessments). In addition to careful observation and use of the Apgar score, the nurse also incorporates maternal prenatal history, use of analgesia and anesthesia during delivery, and any complications that occurred during labor or birth into the assessment. Additional assessment considerations include the newborn's gestational age, any treatment provided immediately after birth, and the newborn's physical examination.

It is important that the nurse incorporate parents into the assessment process, either informing them of the assessments as they occur or allowing them to take part in the assessment. Throughout the assessment, the nurse provides nonjudgmental, supportive responses to the parents' questions and encourages them to share their observations. In particular, the Apgar score should be immediately explained to the family. The nurse encourages the newborn's parents to identify behaviors and other characteristics that are unique to the newborn. Providing time for the parents to do this privately with the family is essential.

SAFETY ALERT Sudden, unexpected postnatal collapse is a potentially fatal event in healthy-appearing newborns. It may be related to entrapment or suffocation. Therefore, continuous monitoring by qualified healthcare personnel is necessary for all newborns in skin-to-skin contact and/or breastfeeding (AWHONN, 2020).

Initial Physical Assessment

The nurse performs an abbreviated but systematic physical assessment in the birthing area to detect any abnormalities (**Table 33.19** ››). First, the nurse notes the size of the newborn as well as the contour and size of the head in relationship to the rest of the body. The newborn's posture and movements indicate tone and neurologic functioning.

The nurse inspects the skin for discoloration, presence of vernix caseosa and lanugo, and evidence of trauma and desquamation (peeling of skin). **Vernix caseosa** is a white, cheesy substance normally found on newborns. It is absorbed within 24 hours after birth. Vernix is abundant on preterm babies and absent on postterm newborns. **Lanugo** (fine hair) is seen on preterm newborns, especially on the shoulders, foreheads, backs, and cheeks. Desquamation of the skin is seen in postterm newborns.

In general, expect a scant amount of vernix on the upper back, axilla, and groin. A scant amount of lanugo is found only on the upper back; ears with incurving of upper two-thirds of pinnae and thin cartilage that springs back from folding; male genitals—testes palpated in upper or lower scrotum; and female genitals—labia majora larger, clitoris nearly covered.

In the following situations, the newborn may require stabilization by the nursing staff or the NICU team and may need to be temporarily removed from the birth area.

- Apgar score of less than 8 at 1 minute and less than 9 at 5 minutes or baby requires resuscitation measures
- Respirations below 30 or above 60 breaths/min, with retractions and/or grunting

TABLE 33.19 Initial Newborn Evaluation

Assess	Normal Findings
Respirations	30–60 breaths/min, irregular No retractions, no grunting
Apical pulse	110–160 beats/min, somewhat irregular
Temperature	Skin temp above 36.5°C (97.8°F)
Skin color	Color consistent with genetic background
Umbilical cord	Two arteries and one vein
Gestational age	Should be 37–42 weeks to remain with parents for an extended time
Sole creases	Sole creases that involve the heel

Source: Adapted from London et al. (2017).

- Apical pulse below 110 or above 160 beats/min, with marked irregularities
- Skin temperature below 36.5°C (97.8°F)
- Skin color pale blue or circumoral pallor
- Baby less than 37 weeks or more than 42 weeks of gestation
- SGA or LGA newborns
- Congenital anomalies involving open areas in the skin (meningomyelocele).

The nurse observes the nares for flaring and, as the newborn cries, inspects the palate for cleft palate. The nurse looks for mucus in the mouth and nose and removes it with a bulb syringe as needed. The nurse inspects the chest for respiratory rate and the presence of retractions. If retractions are present, the nurse assesses the newborn for grunting or stridor. A normal respiratory rate is 30 to 60 breaths/min. It is important to note that during the first few hours of life the newborn's respiratory rate may be as high as 80 breaths/min. The nurse auscultates the lungs bilaterally for breath sounds. Absence of breath sounds on one side could indicate a pneumothorax. Because a small amount of fluid may remain in the lungs, rales may be heard immediately after birth; this fluid will be absorbed. Rhonchi indicate aspiration of oral secretions. If there is excessive mucus or respiratory distress, the nurse suctions the newborn with a mucus trap or wall suction. The nurse notes and records elimination of urine or meconium on the newborn record.

Subsequent Physical Assessment

Once the initial assessment process is complete and gestational age has been established, the nurse carries out a thorough, systematic assessment of the newborn. Completing the physical assessment in the presence of the parents provides an opportunity to acquaint them with their unique newborn. The examination is performed in a systematic, head-to-toe manner, and all findings are recorded. When assessing the physical and neurologic status of the newborn, the nurse should first consider general appearance and then proceed to specific areas.

General Appearance

The newborn's head is disproportionately large for its body. The neck looks short because the chin rests on the chest. Newborns have a prominent abdomen, sloping shoulders, narrow hips, and rounded chests. The center of the baby's body is the umbilicus rather than the symphysis pubis, as in the adult. The body appears long and the extremities short.

Newborns tend to stay in a flexed position similar to the one maintained in utero and will offer resistance to straightening of the extremities. This flexed position contributes to the short appearance of the extremities. The hands are tightly clenched. After a breech birth, the feet are usually dorsiflexed, and it may take several weeks for the newborn to assume the typical newborn posture.

Weight and Measurement

The normal, full-term newborn has an average birth weight of 3405 g (7 lb 8 oz) (Martin, Hamilton, Osterman, & Driscoll, 2019). Other factors that influence weight are age and size of the parents, health of the mother (smoking and malnutrition decrease birth weight), and the interval between pregnancies (short intervals, such as every year, result in lower birth weight). After the first week, and for the first 6 months, the baby's weight increases about 198 g (7 oz) weekly.

Approximately 70–75% of the newborn's body weight is water. During the initial newborn period (the first 3 to 4 days), term newborns have a physiologic weight loss of about 5–10% because of fluid shifts. For the term newborn, weight loss that is greater than 10% indicates the need for clinical appraisal. Large babies also tend to lose more weight because of greater fluid loss in proportion to birth weight. Factors contributing to weight loss include insufficient fluid intake resulting from delayed breastfeeding or a slow adjustment to the formula, increased volume of meconium excreted, and urination. Weight loss may be marked in the presence of temperature elevation (because of associated dehydration) or consistent chilling (because of nonshivering thermogenesis).

The length of the average newborn is difficult to measure because the legs are flexed and tensed. To measure length, the nurse should place newborns flat on their backs with their legs extended as much as possible. The average length is 50 cm (20 in.), and the range is 46 to 56 cm (18 to 22 in.). The newborn will grow approximately 2.5 cm (1 in.) a month for the next 6 months. This is the period of most rapid growth.

At birth, the newborn's head is one-third the size of an adult's head. The circumference (biparietal diameter) of the newborn's head is 32 to 37 cm (12.5 to 14.5 in.). For accurate measurement, the nurse places the tape over the most prominent part of the occiput and brings it just above the eyebrows. The circumference of the newborn's head is approximately 2 cm (0.8 in.) greater than the circumference of the newborn's chest at birth and will remain in this proportion for the next few months. It is best to take another head circumference measurement on the second day if the newborn experienced significant head molding or developed a caput from the birth process.

The average circumference of the chest is 32 cm (12.5 in.) and ranges from 30 to 35 cm (12 to 14 in.). Chest measurements are taken with the tape measure placed at the lower edge of the scapulas and brought around anteriorly, directly over the nipple line. The abdominal circumference, or girth, may also be measured at this time by placing the tape around the newborn's abdomen at the level of the umbilicus, with the bottom edge of the tape at the top edge of the umbilicus.

Temperature

Initial assessment of the newborn's temperature is critical; if no heat conservation measures are started, skin temperature decreases markedly within 10 minutes after exposure to room air. The newborn's temperature should stabilize within 8 to 12 hours.

Temperature is monitored when the newborn is admitted to the nursery and at least every 30 minutes until the newborn's status has remained stable for 2 hours. Thereafter, the nurse should assess temperature at least once every 8 hours, or according to institutional policy (AAP & ACOG, 2017; ACOG, 2020c). For neonates who have been exposed to Group B hemolytic streptococcus, more frequent temperature monitoring may be required.

Temperature can be assessed by skin or axillary measurements and through use of manual or servocontrol methods. Although used in the past, rectal temperatures are rarely used today due to the risks of injury, perforation, and potential cross-contamination due to frequent insertions (Blackburn, 2018). If used, normal rectal temperature is 36.6 to 37.2°C (97.8 to 99°F).

Axillary temperatures are the preferred method and are considered to be a close approximation of the core body temperature. Axillary temperature ranges from 36.5 to 37.4°C (97.7 to 99.3°F) (Benitz, 2015). Skin temperature is measured most accurately by means of a continuous skin probe, but this method is generally used only with preterm or high-risk newborns placed under radiant warmers or in isolettes. Normal skin temperature is 36 to 36.5°C (96.8 to 97.7°F).

Temperature instability (a deviation of more than 1°C [2°F] from one reading to the next) or a subnormal temperature may indicate an infection. In contrast to an elevated temperature in older children, an increased temperature in a newborn may indicate a reaction to too many coverings, too hot a room, or dehydration. Dehydration, which tends to increase body temperature, occurs in newborns whose feedings have been delayed for any reason. Newborns may respond to overheating (ambient temperature above 37.0°C (98.6°F) by increased restlessness and, eventually, by perspiration after 35 to 40 minutes of exposure (Blackburn, 2018). The perspiration appears initially on the head and face and then on the chest.

Skin Characteristics

Although the newborn's skin color varies with genetic background, all healthy newborns have a pink tinge to their skin. The ruddy hue results from increased RBC concentrations in the blood vessels and limited subcutaneous fat deposits.

Skin pigmentation is slight in the newborn period, so color changes may be seen even in darker-skinned babies. White newborns have a pinkish-red skin tone a few hours after birth, and Black newborns have a pale pink to reddish-brown skin color. Hispanic and Asian newborns may have an olive skin tone (Eichenwald et al., 2017). Skin pigmentation deepens over time; therefore, variations in skin color indicating illness are more difficult to evaluate in African American and Asian newborns (Eichenwald et al., 2017). A newborn who is cyanotic at rest and pink only with crying may have choanal atresia (congenital blockage of the passageway between the nose and pharynx). If crying increases the cyanosis, heart or lung problems should be suspected. Very pale newborns may be anemic or have hypovolemia (low blood pressure) (see discussion of hypovolemia in Module 6, Fluids and Electrolytes) and should be evaluated for these problems.

Acrocyanosis may be present in the first 24 to 48 hours after birth (**Figure 33.63** ›)). This condition, bluish discoloration of the hands and feet, is caused by poor peripheral circulation, which results in vasomotor instability and capillary stasis, especially when the baby is exposed to cold. Blue hands and nails are a poor indicator of decreased oxygenation in a newborn. If the central circulation is adequate, the blood supply should return quickly (2 to 3 seconds) to the extremity after the skin is blanched with a finger. The nurse should assess the face and mucous membranes for pinkness that reflects adequate oxygenation.

Mottling (lacy pattern of dilated blood vessels under the skin) occurs as a result of general circulation fluctuations. It may last several hours to several weeks, or it may come and go periodically. Mottling may be related to chilling or prolonged apnea, sepsis, or hypothyroidism.

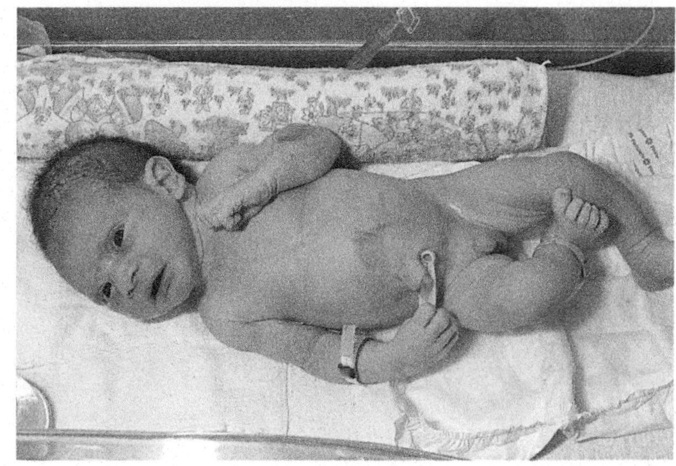

Figure 33.63 ›› Newborn with acrocyanosis.
Source: George Dodson/Pearson Education, Inc.

Harlequin sign color change is occasionally noted: A deep red color develops over one side of the newborn's body while the other side remains pale, so the skin resembles a clown's suit. This color change results from a vasomotor disturbance in which blood vessels on one side dilate while the blood vessels on the other side constrict. It usually lasts from 1 to 20 minutes. Affected newborns may have single or multiple episodes, but they are transient and clinically insignificant. The nurse should document each occurrence.

Jaundice is yellow pigmentation of body tissues caused by the presence of bile pigments. It is first detectable on the face (where skin overlies cartilage) and the mucous membranes of the mouth, and it has a head-to-toe progression (Perry et al., 2017). Jaundice regresses in the opposite direction (from toe to head). It is evaluated by blanching the tip of the nose, the forehead, the sternum, or the gum line. This procedure must be carried out in appropriate lighting. If jaundice is present, the area will appear yellowish immediately after blanching. Another area to assess for jaundice is the sclera. Evaluation and determination of the cause of jaundice must be initiated immediately to prevent possibly serious sequelae. The jaundice may be related to breastfeeding (extremely rare), hematomas, immature liver function, or bruises from forceps, or it may be caused by blood incompatibility, oxytocin (Pitocin) augmentation or induction, or a severe hemolytic process. Any jaundice noted before a newborn is 24 hours of age should be reported to the physician or neonatal nurse practitioner.

Erythema toxicum neonatorum is an eruption of lesions in the area surrounding a hair follicle that are firm, vary in size from 1 to 3 mm, and consist of a white or pale-yellow papule or pustule with an erythematous base. It is often called "newborn rash" or "flea bite" dermatitis. The rash may appear suddenly, usually over the trunk and diaper area, and is frequently widespread (**Figure 33.64** ››). The lesions do not appear on the palms of the hands or the soles of the feet. The peak incidence is at 24 to 48 hours of life. The condition rarely presents at birth or after 5 days of life. The cause is unknown, and no treatment is necessary. Some HCPs believe it may be caused by irritation from clothing. The lesions disappear in a few hours or days. If a maculopapular rash appears, a smear

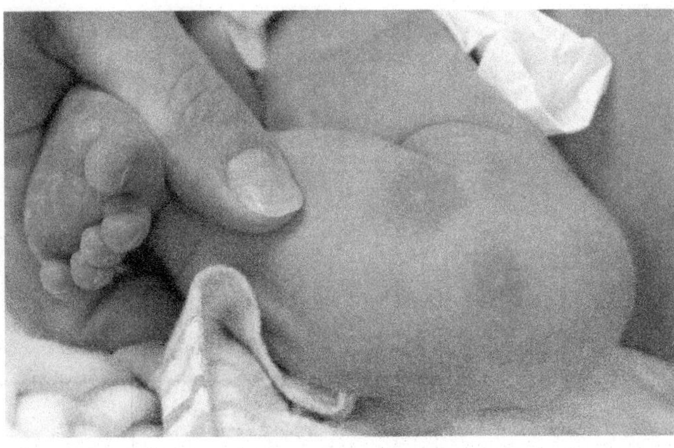

Figure 33.64 » Erythema toxicum on leg.
Source: George Dodson/Pearson Education, Inc.

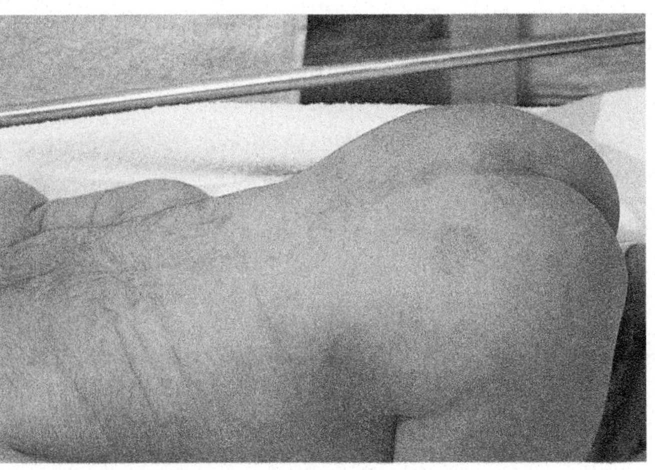

Figure 33.66 » Congenital dermal melanocytosis.
Source: George Dodson/Pearson Education, Inc.

of the aspirated papule will show numerous eosinophils on staining; no bacteria will be cultured.

Milia (exposed sebaceous glands) appear as raised white spots on the face, especially across the nose (**Figure 33.65 »**). No treatment is necessary because they will clear spontaneously within the first month. In dark-skinned infants, a similar condition called *transient neonatal pustular melanosis* can present at birth. These pigmented macules may persist for weeks or months after the pustules have healed (James, Berger, Elston, & Neuhaus, 2019).

Skin turgor (the elasticity of the skin) is assessed to determine hydration status, the need to initiate early feedings, and the presence of any infectious processes. The usual place to assess skin turgor is over the abdomen, forearm, or thigh. Skin should be elastic and return rapidly to its original shape.

Forceps marks may be present after a difficult forceps birth. The newborn may have reddened areas over the cheeks and jaws. It is important to reassure the parents that these marks will disappear, usually within 1 or 2 days. Transient facial paralysis resulting from the forceps pressure is a rare complication.

Vacuum extractor suction marks on the vertex of the scalp are often seen when vacuum extractors are used to assist with the birth. These marks are benign and do not indicate underlying brain lesions.

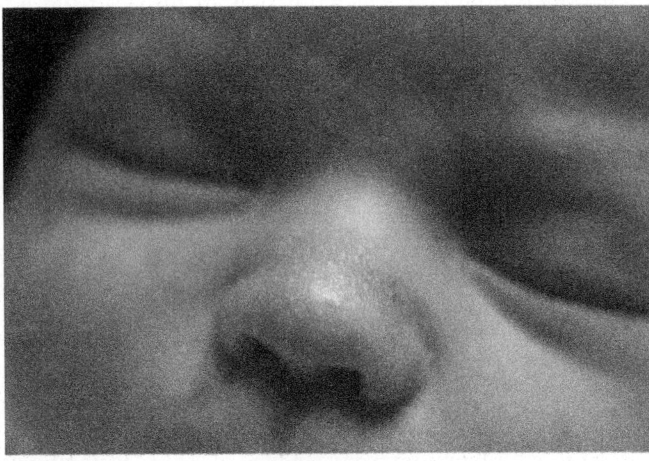

Figure 33.65 » Facial milia.
Source: Jack Sullivan/Alamy Stock Photo.

Birthmarks

Birthmarks are frequently a cause of concern and guilt for parents. The mother may be especially anxious, fearing that she is to blame ("Is my baby 'marked' because of something I did?"). Birthmarks should be identified and explained to the parents. By providing appropriate information about the cause and course of birthmarks, the nurse can relieve the fears and anxieties of the family. The nurse should note any bruises, abrasions, or birthmarks seen on admission to the nursery.

Telangiectatic nevi (stork bites) appear as pale pink or red spots and are frequently found on the eyelids, nose, lower occipital bone, and nape of the neck. These lesions are common in newborns with light complexions and are more noticeable during periods of crying. These areas have no clinical significance and usually fade by the second birthday.

Congenital dermal melanocytosis, sometimes referred to in the literature as Mongolian spots, refers to bluish-black or gray-blue pigmentation on the dorsal area and the buttocks (**Figure 33.66 »**). They are common in newborns of Asian, Hispanic, and African descent and in any newborn with darker skin. They gradually fade during the first or second year of life. They may be mistaken for bruises and should be documented in the newborn's medical record.

Nevus flammeus (port-wine stain) is a capillary angioma directly below the epidermis. It is a nonelevated, sharply demarcated, red-to-purple area of dense capillaries. In newborns of African descent, it may appear as a purple-black stain. The size and shape vary, but it commonly appears on the face. It does not grow in size, does not fade with time, and, as a rule, does not blanch. The birthmark may be concealed by using an opaque cosmetic cream. **Nevus vasculosus (strawberry mark)** is a capillary hemangioma. It consists of newly formed and enlarged capillaries in the dermal and subdermal layers. It is a raised, clearly delineated, dark red, rough-surfaced birthmark commonly found in the head region. Such marks usually grow (often rapidly) starting in the second or third week of life, and they may not reach their full size until about 6 months (Krowchuk et al., 2019). They begin to shrink and start to resolve spontaneously several weeks to months after they reach peak growth. A pale purple or gray spot on the surface of the hemangioma signals the start of resolution. The best cosmetic effect is achieved when the lesions are allowed to resolve spontaneously.

Head

The newborn's head is large (approximately one-fourth of the body size), with soft, pliable skull bones. For most term neonates, the occipitofrontal circumference is 32 to 37 cm (12.6 to 14.6 in.).

The head may appear asymmetric in the newborn of a vertex birth. This asymmetry, called **molding**, is caused by overriding of the cranial bones during labor and birth. The degree of molding varies with the amount and length of pressure exerted on the head. Within a few days after birth, the overriding usually diminishes, and the suture lines become palpable. Because head measurements are affected by molding, a second measurement is indicated a few days after birth.

The heads of breech-born newborns and of those delivered by elective cesarean are characteristically round and well shaped because no pressure was exerted on them during birth. Any extreme differences in head size may indicate microcephaly (abnormally small head) or hydrocephalus (an abnormal buildup of fluid in the brain). Variations in the shape, size, or appearance of the head measurements may be caused by craniosynostosis (premature closure of the cranial sutures), which will need to be corrected through surgery to allow brain growth, and plagiocephaly (asymmetry caused by pressure on the fetal head during gestation) (Hewitt, Kerr, Stanley, & Okely, 2020).

Two fontanels ("soft spots") may be palpated on the newborn's head. Fontanels, which are openings at the juncture of the cranial bones, can be measured with the fingers. Accurate measurement necessitates that the examiner's finger be measured in centimeters. The assessment should be carried out with the newborn in a sitting position and not crying. The diamond-shaped anterior fontanel is approximately 3 to 4 cm (1.2 to 1.6 in.) long by 2 to 3 cm (0.8 to 1.2 in.) wide. It is located at the juncture of the frontal and parietal bones. The posterior fontanel, smaller and triangular, is formed by the parietal bones and the occipital bone and is 0.5 by 1 cm. Because of molding, the fontanels are smaller immediately after birth than they are several days later. The anterior fontanel closes within 18 months, whereas the posterior fontanel closes within 6 to 8 weeks.

The fontanels are a useful indicator of the newborn's condition. The anterior fontanel may swell when the newborn cries or passes a stool or may pulsate with the heartbeat, which is normal. A bulging fontanel usually signifies increased intracranial pressure, and a depressed fontanel indicates dehydration (Lipsett, Reddy, & Steanson, 2020).

The sutures between the cranial bones should be palpated for the amount of overlapping. In newborns whose growth has been restricted, the sutures may be wider than normal, and the fontanels may also be larger because of impaired growth of the cranial bones. In addition to inspecting the newborn's head for degree of molding and size, the nurse should evaluate it for soft-tissue edema and bruising.

Caput succedaneum is a localized, easily identifiable, soft area of the scalp, generally resulting from a long and difficult labor or vacuum extraction. The sustained pressure of the presenting part against the cervix results in compression of local blood vessels, and venous return is slowed. This results in an increase of tissue fluids, edematous swelling, and occasional bleeding under the periosteum. The caput may vary from a small area to a severely elongated head. The fluid in the caput is reabsorbed within 12 hours to a few days after birth. Caputs resulting from vacuum extractors are sharply outlined, circular areas up to 2 cm (0.8 in.) thick. They disappear more slowly than naturally occurring edema. It is possible to distinguish between a cephalohematoma and a caput because the caput overrides suture lines (**Figure 33.67 ››**), whereas the cephalohematoma, because of its location, never crosses a suture line. Also, caput succedaneum is present at birth, whereas cephalohematoma generally is not.

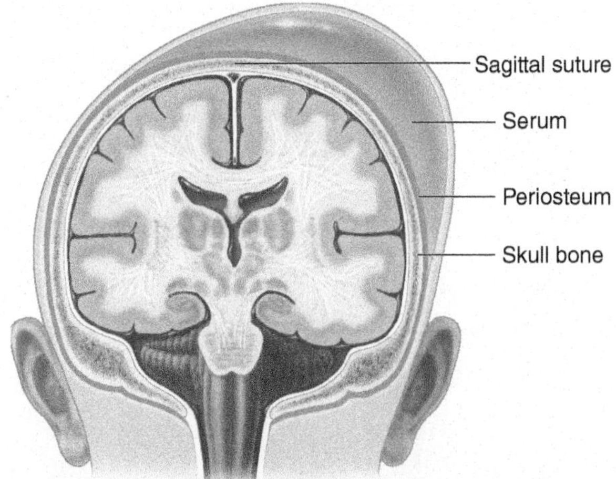

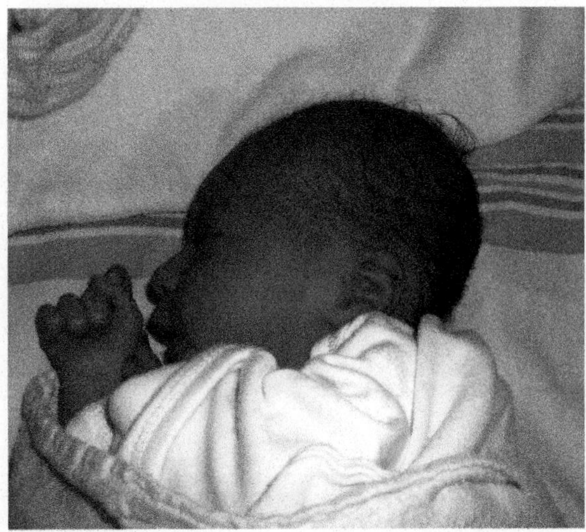

Figure 33.67 ›› Caput succedaneum is a collection of fluid (serum) under the scalp.

Source: George Dodson/Pearson Education, Inc.

Cephalohematoma is a collection of blood resulting from ruptured blood vessels between the surface of a cranial bone (usually parietal) and the periosteal membrane (**Figure 33.68 ››**). The scalp in these areas feels loose and slightly edematous. These areas emerge as defined hematomas between the first and second days. Although external pressure may cause the mass to fluctuate, it does not increase in size when the newborn cries. Cephalohematomas may be unilateral or bilateral and do not cross suture lines. They are relatively common in vertex births and may disappear within 2 weeks to 3 months.

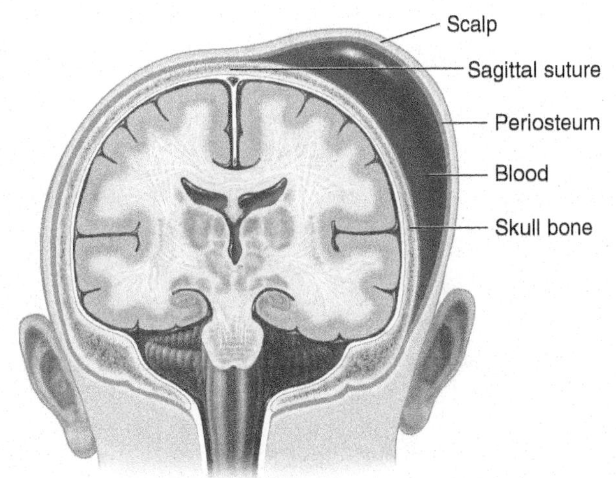

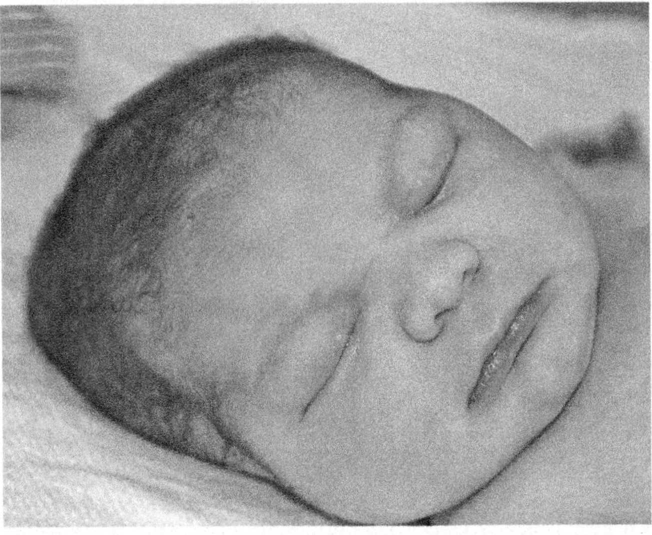

Figure 33.68 ›› Cephalohematoma is a collection of blood between the surface of a cranial bone and the periosteal membrane. This is a cephalohematoma over the left parietal bone.

Source: Courtesy of Jo Engle, RN, MSN, NNP-BC, and Vanessa Howell RN, MSN.

They may be associated with physiologic jaundice because extra RBCs are being destroyed within the cephalohematoma. A large cephalohematoma can lead to anemia and hypotension.

›› *Go to* ***Pearson MyLab Nursing and eText*** *to see Chart 18: Comparison of Caput Succedaneum and Cephalohematoma*

Face

The newborn's face is well designed to help the newborn suckle. Sucking (fat) pads are located in the cheeks, and a labial tubercle (sucking callus) is frequently found in the center of the upper lip. The chin is recessed, and the nose is flattened. The lips are sensitive to touch, and the sucking reflex is easily initiated.

Symmetry of the eyes, nose, and ears is evaluated. Symmetry of facial movement should be assessed to determine the presence of facial palsy.

Facial paralysis appears when the newborn cries: The affected side is immobile, and the palpebral (eyelid) fissure widens. Paralysis may result from forceps-assisted birth or pressure on the facial nerve caused by the maternal pelvis during birth. Facial paralysis usually disappears within a few days to 3 weeks, although in some cases it may be permanent.

Eyes

The eyes of the newborn range from a blue- or slate-gray color to a dark brown color. Scleral color tends to be bluish white in all newborns because of its relative thinness. A blue sclera is associated with osteogenesis imperfecta. The infant's eye color is usually established at approximately 3 months, although it may change any time up to 1 year.

The eyes should be checked for size, equality of pupil size, reaction of pupils to light, blink reflex to light, and edema and inflammation of the eyelids. The eyelids are usually edematous during the first few days of life because of the pressure associated with birth.

Erythromycin is frequently used prophylactically to reduce risk from bacteria to which the neonate may have been exposed during the birth process. Ocular prophylaxis of newborns with 0.5% erythromycin ophthalmic ointment is used most often to prevent gonococcal ophthalmia neonatorum (Curry et al., 2019).

Erythromycin ointment is preferred over the once-popular silver nitrate because erythromycin does not usually cause **chemical conjunctivitis** (irritation of the conjunctiva by chemicals used to treat the eyes, resulting in a purulent greenish-yellow discharge exudate). If infectious conjunctivitis exists, the newborn has the same purulent discharge exudate as in chemical conjunctivitis, but it is caused by gonococcus, *Chlamydia*, staphylococci, or a variety of gram-negative bacteria. It requires treatment with ophthalmic antibiotics. Onset is usually after the second day. Edema of the orbits or eyelids may persist for several days until the newborn's kidneys can eliminate the fluid.

Small **subconjunctival hemorrhages** appear in approximately 10% of newborns and are commonly found on the sclera. These hemorrhages are caused by the changes in vascular tension or ocular pressure during birth. They will remain for a few weeks and are of no pathologic significance. Parents need reassurance that the newborn is not bleeding from within the eye and that the "broken blood vessels" aren't known to cause any vision changes.

The nurse should observe the newborn's pupils for opacities or whiteness and for the absence of a normal red retinal reflex. Red retinal reflex is a red-orange flash of color observed when an ophthalmoscope light reflects off the retina. In a newborn with dark skin color, the retina may appear paler or more grayish. Absence of red reflex occurs with cataracts. Congenital cataracts should be suspected in newborns of mothers with a history of rubella, cytomegalic inclusion disease, or syphilis. Brushfield spots (black or white spots on the periphery of the iris) can be associated with Down syndrome (Salmon, 2020). The newborn may demonstrate transient strabismus caused by poor neuromuscular control of eye muscles (**Figure 33.69** ››). It gradually dissipates in 3 to 4 months.

The cry of the newborn is commonly tearless because the lacrimal structures are immature at birth and are not usually fully functional until the second month of life. However, some babies produce tears during the newborn period.

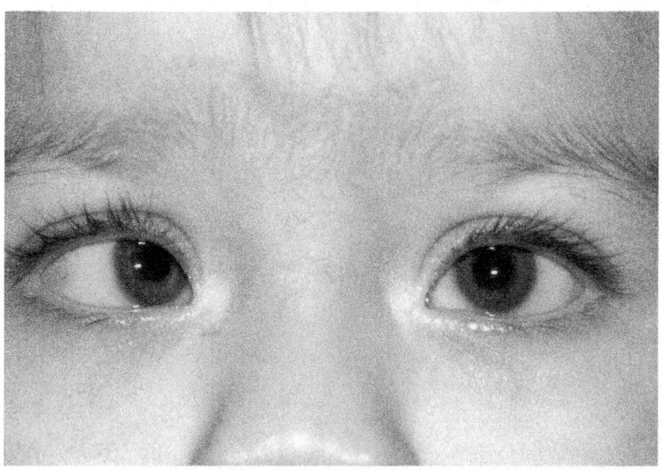

Figure 33.69 ⟫ Transient strabismus may be present in the newborn because of poor neuromuscular control.
Source: Biophoto Associates/Science Source.

Although poor oculomotor coordination and absence of accommodation limit visual abilities, newborns have peripheral vision, can fixate on objects near (20.3 to 38.1 cm [8 to 15 in.]) and in front of their face for short periods, can accommodate to large objects (7.6 cm [3 in.] tall × 7.6 cm [3 in.] wide), and can seek out high-contrast geometric shapes. Newborns can perceive faces, shapes, and colors, and they begin to show visual preferences early. Newborns generally blink in response to bright lights, to a tap on the bridge of the nose (glabellar reflex), or to a light touch on the eyelids. Pupillary light reflex is also present. Examination of the eye is best accomplished by rocking the newborn from an upright position to the horizontal a few times or by other methods, such as dimming overhead lights, which elicit an opened-eye response.

Nose

The newborn's nose is small and narrow. Babies are characteristically nose-breathers for the first few months of life and generally remove obstructions by sneezing. Nasal patency is ensured if the newborn breathes easily with the mouth closed. If respiratory difficulty occurs, the nurse checks for choanal atresia (congenital blockage of the passageway between nose and pharynx). This can be done by observing the newborn feeding or by gently occluding each of the nares (Wegman & McKnight, 2020).

The newborn has the ability to smell after the nasal passages have been cleared of amniotic fluid and mucus. Newborns demonstrate this ability by the search for milk. Newborns turn their heads toward a milk source, whether bottle or breast. Newborns react to strong odors, such as alcohol, by turning their heads away or blinking.

Mouth

The lips of the newborn should be pink. A touch on the lips should produce sucking motions. Saliva is normally scant. The taste buds develop before birth, and the newborn can easily discriminate between sweet and bitter flavors.

The easiest way to examine the mouth completely is to stimulate the baby to cry by gently depressing the tongue, thereby causing the newborn to open the mouth fully. It is extremely important to examine the entire mouth to check for a cleft palate, which can be present even in the absence of a cleft lip. The examiner moves a gloved index finger along the hard and soft palate to feel for any openings.

Occasionally, an examination of the gums will reveal precocious teeth over the area where the lower central incisors will erupt. If they appear loose, they should be removed by the provider to prevent aspiration. Gray-white lesions (inclusion cysts) on the gums may be confused with teeth. On the hard palate and gum margins, **Epstein pearls** (small, glistening, white specks [keratin-containing cysts] that feel hard to the touch) are often present. They usually disappear in a few weeks and are of no significance. **Thrush** may appear as white patches that look like milk curds adhering to the mucous membranes, and bleeding may occur when patches are removed. Thrush is caused by *Candida albicans*, often acquired from an infected vaginal tract during birth, antibiotic use, or poor hand hygiene when the mother handles her newborn. Thrush is treated with an oral preparation of nystatin (Mycostatin).

A newborn who has ankyloglossia (tongue tied) has a ridge of frenulum tissue attached to the underside of the tongue at varying lengths from its base, causing a heart shape at the tip of the tongue. Frenotomy (cutting the ridge of tissue) may be recommended if the newborn has trouble feeding, as the ridge can affect breastfeeding. However, cutting creates an entry for infection. The ridge does not usually affect speech.

Transient nerve paralysis resulting from birth trauma may be manifested by asymmetric mouth movements when the newborn cries or by difficulty with sucking and feeding.

Ears

The ears of the newborn are soft and pliable and should recoil readily when folded and released. In the normal newborn, the top of the ear (pinna) should be parallel to the outer and inner canthus of the eye. The ears should be inspected for shape, size, firmness of cartilage, and position. Low-set ears (**Figure 33.70 ⟫**) are characteristic of many syndromes. Although most often associated with Down syndrome, low-set ears may indicate other chromosomal abnormalities, intellectual disability, and internal organ abnormalities, especially bilateral renal agenesis. Preauricular skin tags may be present just in front of the ear. These skin tags are thought to be embryologic fragments related to either deficient or defective development of the vestigial ear (Rich & Dolgin, 2020). Visualization of the tympanic membrane typically is not done soon after birth because blood and vernix block the ear canal.

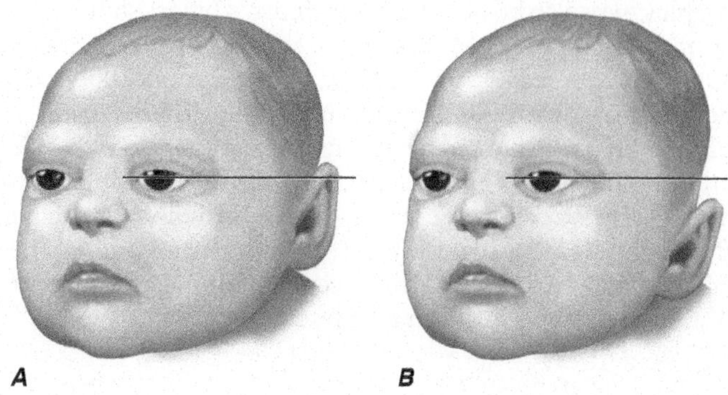

Figure 33.70 ⟫ The position of the external ear may be assessed by drawing a line across the inner and outer canthus of the eye to the insertion of the ear. ***A***, Normal position. ***B***, True low-set position.

The first cry helps initiate hearing improvement as mucus from the middle ear is absorbed, the eustachian tube becomes aerated, and the tympanic membrane becomes visible. Newborns, especially when awake, should startle or respond to loud noise. Although this is not a completely accurate test, absence of this response requires further evaluation.

The newborn can discriminate the individual characteristics of the human voice and is especially sensitive to sound levels within the normal conversational range. The newborn in a noisy nursery may habituate to the sounds and not stir unless the sound is sudden or much louder than usual. An overview of newborn hearing screening is provided later in this exemplar.

Neck

A short neck, creased with skinfolds, is characteristic of the normal newborn. Because muscle tone is not well developed, the neck cannot support the full weight of the head, which rotates freely. The head lags considerably when the newborn is pulled from a supine to a sitting position, but the prone newborn is able to raise the head slightly. The neck is palpated for masses and the presence of lymph nodes and is also inspected for webbing. Adequacy of range of motion and neck muscle function is determined by fully extending the head in all directions. Injury to the sternocleidomastoid muscle (congenital torticollis) must be considered in the presence of neck rigidity.

The nurse evaluates the clavicles for evidence of fractures, which occasionally occur during difficult births or in newborns with broad shoulders. The normal clavicle is straight. If it is fractured, a lump and a grating sensation (crepitus) during movements may be palpated along the course of the side of the break. The nurse also elicits the Moro reflex to evaluate bilateral equal movement of the arms. If the clavicle is fractured, the response will be demonstrated only on the unaffected side.

Chest

The thorax is cylindrical and symmetric at birth, and the ribs are flexible. The general appearance of the chest should be assessed. A protrusion at the lower end of the sternum, called the xiphoid cartilage, is frequently seen. It is under the skin and will become less apparent after several weeks as adipose tissue accumulates.

Enlarged breasts occur frequently in both male and female newborns. This condition, which occurs by the third day, is a result of maternal hormonal influences and may last up to 2 weeks (**Figure 33.71** ››). A whitish secretion from the nipples may also be noted. The newborn's breast should not be massaged or squeezed because this may cause a breast abscess. Extra, or supernumerary, nipples are occasionally noted below and medial to the true nipples. These harmless pink or (in dark-skinned newborns) brown spots vary in size and do not contain glandular tissue. Accessory nipples can be differentiated from a pigmented nevus (mole) by placing the fingertips alongside the accessory nipple and pulling the adjacent tissue laterally. The accessory nipple will appear dimpled. At puberty, this may darken.

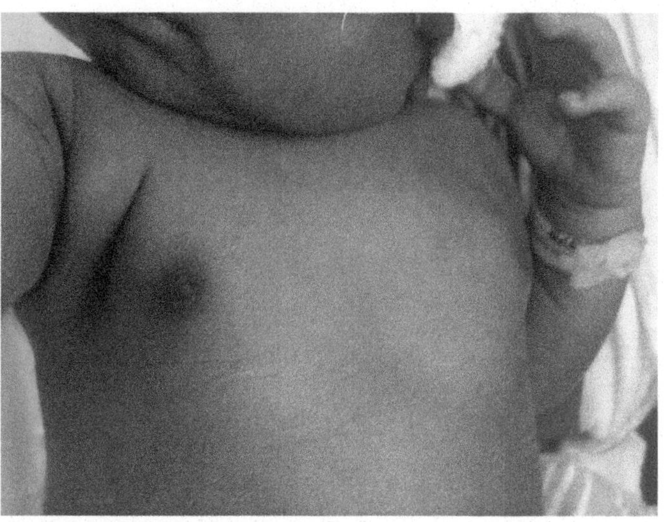

Figure 33.71 ›› Breast hypertrophy.
Source: Pearson Education, Inc.

Cry

The newborn's cry should be strong, lusty, and of medium pitch. A high-pitched, shrill cry is abnormal and may indicate neurologic disorders or hypoglycemia. Periods of crying usually vary in length after consoling measures are used. Babies' cries are an important method of communication; alerting caregivers to changes in a baby's condition and needs.

Respirations

Normal respiration for a term newborn is 30 to 60 breaths/minute and is predominantly diaphragmatic, with associated rising and falling of the abdomen during inspiration and expiration. The nurse notes any signs of respiratory distress, nasal flaring, intercostal or xiphoid retractions, expiratory grunt or sigh, seesaw respirations, or tachypnea (>60 breaths/minute). Hyperextension (chest appears high) or hypoextension (chest appears low) of the anteroposterior diameter of the chest should also be noted. The nurse auscultates both the anterior and posterior chest. Some breath sounds are heard best when the newborn is crying but localizing and identifying breath sounds are difficult in the newborn. Upper airway noises and bowel sounds can be heard over the chest wall, making auscultation difficult. Because sounds may be transmitted from the unaffected lung to the affected lung, the absence of breath sounds may not be diagnosed. Air entry may be noisy in the first couple of hours until lung fluid resolves, especially after cesarean births. Brief periods of apnea (**periodic breathing**) occur, but no color or heart rate changes occur in healthy, term newborns. Sepsis should be suspected in term newborns experiencing apneic episodes.

Heart

The nurse examines the heart for rate and rhythm, position of the apical impulse, and heart sound intensity. The pulse rate is variable and is influenced by physical activity, crying, state of wakefulness, and body temperature. The nurse auscultates the entire chest region (precordium) below the left axilla and below the scapula. Auscultation for a full minute, preferably when the newborn is asleep, allows the nurse to obtain apical pulse rates.

A shift of heart tones in the mediastinal area to either side may indicate pneumothorax, dextrocardia (heart placement on the right side of the chest), or a diaphragmatic hernia. The nurse should auscultate heart sounds using both the bell and the diaphragm of the stethoscope. A slur or slushing sound (usually after the first sound) may indicate a murmur. Although 90% of all murmurs are transient and are considered to be normal, the nurse should document and report them (Blackburn, 2018). Many murmurs are secondary to closing of a patent ductus arteriosus or a patent foramen ovale, which should close 1 to 2 days after birth. A low-pitched, musical murmur just to the right of the apex of the heart is fairly common. Occasionally, significant murmurs are heard, such as the murmur of a patent ductus arteriosus, aortic or pulmonary stenosis, or small ventricular septal defect. Congenital cardiac defects are discussed in Module 16, Perfusion.

The nurse evaluates peripheral pulses (brachial, femoral, and pedal) to detect any lags or unusual characteristics. Brachial pulses are palpated bilaterally for equality and compared with the femoral pulses. Femoral pulses are palpated by applying gentle pressure with the middle finger over the femoral canal (**Figure 33.72** »). Decreased or absent femoral pulses may indicate coarctation of the aorta or hypovolemia and require additional evaluation. A wide difference in blood pressure between the upper and lower extremities also indicates coarctation of the aorta.

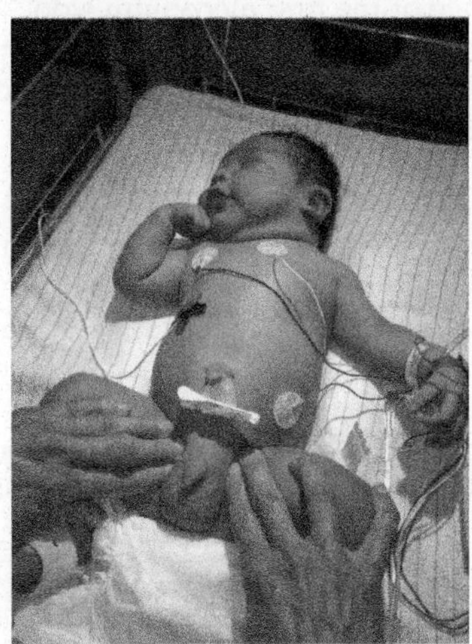

A

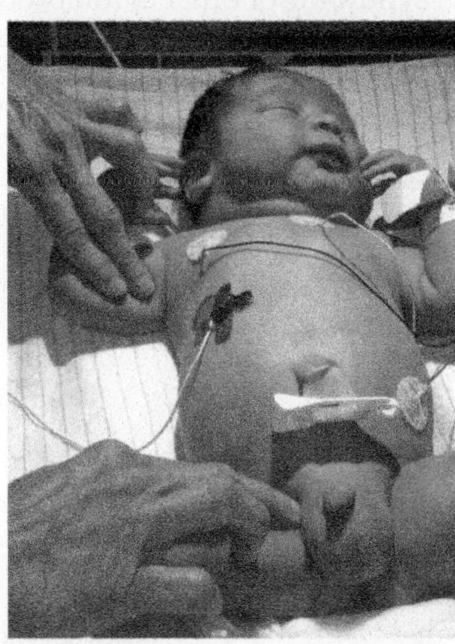

B

Figure 33.72 » ***A***, Bilaterally palpate the femoral arteries for rate and intensity of the pulses. Press fingertip gently at the groin as shown. ***B***, Compare the femoral pulses to the brachial pulses by palpating the pulses simultaneously for comparison of rate and intensity.

Source: Carol Harrigan, RNC, MSN, NNP.

The measurement of blood pressure is best accomplished by using a noninvasive blood pressure device. If a blood pressure cuff is used, the newborn's extremities must be immobilized during the assessment, and the cuff should cover two-thirds of the upper arm or upper leg. Movement, crying, and inappropriate cuff size can give inaccurate measurements of the blood pressure.

SAFETY ALERT If possible, obtain blood pressure measurements during the quiet or sleep state. Place the cuff on the neonate's arm or leg and give the neonate time to quiet. Obtain an average of two to three measurements when making clinical decisions. Follow mean blood pressure to monitor changes because the mean blood pressure is less likely to be erroneous. Noninvasive blood pressure may overestimate blood pressure in very-low-birth-weight neonates.

It is essential to measure blood pressure routinely for newborns who are in distress, premature, or suspected of having a cardiac anomaly (Blackburn, 2018). Neonates who have birth asphyxia and are on ventilators have significantly lower systolic and diastolic blood pressures compared with healthy neonates. If a cardiac anomaly is suspected, blood pressure is measured in all four extremities. At birth, systolic values usually range from 70 to 50 mmHg and diastolic values from 45 to 30 mmHg. By the 10th day of life, blood pressure rises to 90/50 mmHg.

Abdomen

The nurse can learn a great deal about the newborn's abdomen without disturbing the neonate. The abdomen should be cylindrical, protrude slightly, and move with respiration. A certain amount of laxness of the abdominal muscles is normal. A vertical bulge, known as a *diastasis recti*, may be observed down the midline of the abdomen in many newborns. It is caused by a weakness of the fascia between the rectus abdominus muscles but is not pathologic (Stanford Medicine, 2020). A scaphoid (hollow-shaped) appearance suggests the absence of abdominal contents (often seen in diaphragmatic hernias). No cyanosis should be present and few, if any, blood vessels should be apparent to the eye. There should be no gross distention. The more distended the abdomen, the tighter the skin becomes, with engorged vessels appearing. Distention is the first sign of many GI abnormalities.

Before palpating the abdomen, the nurse should auscultate for the presence or absence of bowel sounds in all four quadrants. Bowel sounds may be present by 1 hour after birth. Palpation can cause a transient decrease in the intensity of bowel sounds.

The nurse palpates the abdomen systematically, assessing each of the four abdominal quadrants and moving in a clockwise direction until all four quadrants have been palpated for softness, tenderness, and the presence of masses. The nurse should place one hand under the newborn's back for support during palpation.

Umbilical Cord

The umbilical cord initially appears white and gelatinous, with the two umbilical arteries and one umbilical vein readily apparent. Because a single umbilical artery is frequently associated

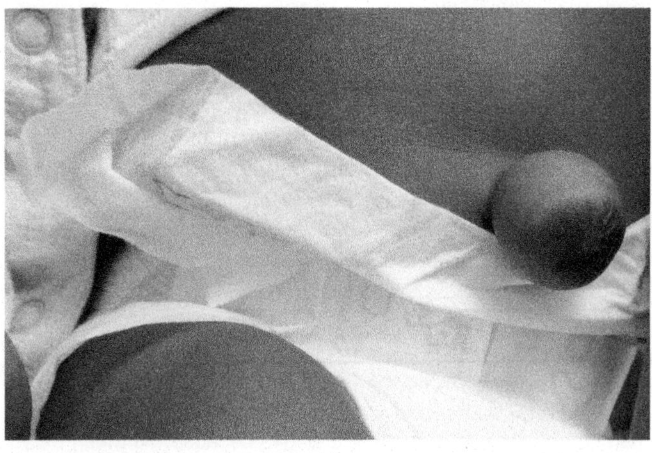

Figure 33.73 ⟫ Umbilical hernia.
Source: George Dodson/Pearson Education, Inc.

with congenital anomalies, the nurse should count the vessels during the newborn assessment. The cord begins drying within 1 or 2 hours of birth and is shriveled and blackened by the second or third day. Within 7 to 10 days, it sloughs off, although a granulating area may remain for a few days longer.

Cord bleeding is abnormal and may result because the cord was pulled inadvertently or the cord clamp was loosened. Foul-smelling drainage is also abnormal and is generally caused by infection, which requires immediate treatment to prevent septicemia. If the newborn has a patent urachus (abnormal connection between the umbilicus and bladder), moistness or draining urine may be apparent at the base of the cord. Another umbilical cord anomaly that can occur is umbilical cord hernia and associated patent omphalomesenteric duct (**Figure 33.73 ⟫**). Umbilical hernias are more common in newborns of African American descent than in white babies (Troullioud Lucas, Jaafar, & Mendez, 2020).

Genitals

For female neonates, the nurse examines the labia majora, labia minora, and clitoris and notes whether the size of each is appropriate for gestational age. A vaginal tag or hymenal tag is often evident and will usually disappear in a few weeks. During the first week of life, the female newborn may have a vaginal discharge composed of thick, whitish mucus. This discharge, which can become tinged with blood, is called pseudomenstruation and is caused by the withdrawal of maternal hormones. Smegma (a white, cheeselike substance) is often present between the labia. Removing it may traumatize tender tissue.

For male neonates, the nurse inspects the penis to determine whether the urinary orifice is positioned correctly. Possible alterations include *hypospadias*, which occurs when the urinary meatus is located on the ventral surface of the penis, and *epispadias*, in which the meatus is located on the dorsal surface of the glans. Hypospadias occurs most commonly among white male newborns. *Phimosis* is a condition in which the opening of the foreskin (prepuce) is so small that the foreskin cannot be pulled back over the glans. This condition may interfere with urination, so the adequacy of the urinary stream should be evaluated.

The nurse then inspects the scrotum for size and symmetry. Scrotal color variations are especially prominent in African American and Hispanic newborns (Vargo, 2014). Palpation allows the nurse to verify the presence of both testes and to rule out cryptorchidism (failure of testes to descend). The nurse palpates the testes separately between the thumb and forefinger, with the thumb and forefinger of the other hand placed together over the inguinal canal. Scrotal edema and discoloration are common in breech births. *Hydrocele* (a collection of fluid surrounding the testes in the scrotum) is common in newborns and should be identified. It usually resolves without intervention. The nurse should report the presence of a discolored or dusky scrotum and solid testis because this may indicate testicular torsion.

Anus

It is essential to inspect the anal area to verify that it is patent and has no fissure. Imperforate anus and rectal atresia may be ruled out by observation. As previously noted, rectal temperatures are rarely used due to the risks of injury and perforation (Blackburn, 2018). Digital examination, if necessary, is done by a physician or nurse practitioner. The nurse also notes the passage of the first meconium stool. Atresia of the GI tract or meconium ileus with resultant obstruction must be considered if the newborn does not pass meconium in the first 24 hours of life.

Extremities

The nurse assesses the newborn's extremities for gross deformities, extra digits or webbing, clubfoot, and range of motion. Normal newborn extremities appear short, are generally flexible, and move symmetrically. Abnormalities should be noted so that a plan of care may be created.

Nails extend beyond the fingertips in term newborns. The nurse should count fingers and toes. Polydactyly is the presence of extra digits on either the hands or the feet. Syndactyly refers to fusion (webbing) of fingers or toes. The hands are inspected for normal palmar creases; a single palmar crease, called a *simian crease* (**Figure 33.74 ⟫**), may be present in children with Down syndrome or other chromosomal anomalies (Wahl, Dupont, & Tubbs, 2019).

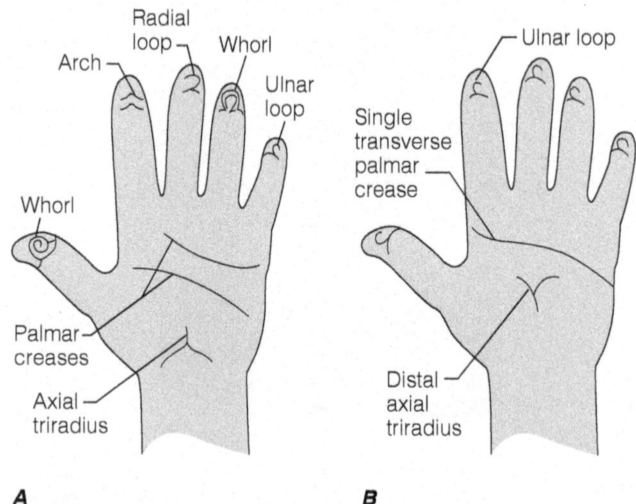

Figure 33.74 ⟫ Dermatoglyphic patterns of the hands in ***A***, a normal individual, and ***B***, a child with Down syndrome. Note the single transverse palmar crease, distally placed axial triradius, and increased number of ulnar loops.

Brachial palsy, paralysis of portions of the arm, results from trauma to the brachial plexus during a difficult birth. It occurs commonly when strong traction is exerted on the head of the newborn in an attempt to deliver a shoulder lodged behind the symphysis pubis in the presence of shoulder dystocia. Brachial palsy may also occur during a breech birth if an arm becomes trapped over the head and traction is exerted.

The portion of the arm affected is determined by the nerves damaged. **Erb-Duchenne paralysis (Erb palsy)** involves damage to the upper arm (fifth and sixth cervical nerves) and is the most common type. Injury to the eighth cervical and first thoracic nerve roots and the lower portion of the plexus produces the relatively rare lower arm injury. The whole-arm type results from damage to the entire plexus.

With Erb-Duchenne paralysis, the newborn's arm lies limply at the side. The elbow is held in extension, with the forearm pronated. The newborn is unable to elevate the arm. Lower arm injury causes paralysis of the hand and wrist; complete paralysis of the limb occurs with the whole-arm type.

Prognosis is related to the degree of nerve damage resulting from trauma and hemorrhage within the nerve sheath. With minimal trauma, complete recovery occurs within a few months. Moderate trauma may result in partial paralysis. With severe trauma, recovery is unlikely, and muscle wasting may develop.

The legs of the newborn should be of equal length, with symmetric skinfolds. However, they may assume a "fetal posture" as a result of the position in utero, and it may take several days for the legs to relax into a normal position. To evaluate for hip dislocation or hip instability, the Ortolani and Barlow maneuvers are performed. The nurse (or, more commonly, the physician or nurse practitioner) performs the **Ortolani maneuver** to rule out the possibility of developmental dysplastic hip, also called congenital hip dysplasia (hip dislocatability). With the newborn relaxed, quiet, and on a firm surface, with hips and knees flexed at a 90-degree angle, the experienced nurse grasps the neonate's thigh with the middle finger over the greater trochanter and then lifts the thigh to bring the femoral head from its posterior position toward the acetabulum. With gentle abduction of the thigh, the femoral head is returned to the acetabulum. Simultaneously, the examiner feels a sense of reduction or a "clunk" as the femoral head returns. This reduction is palpable and may be heard. With the **Barlow maneuver**, the HCP grasps and adducts the neonate's thigh and then applies gentle downward pressure. Dislocation is felt as the femoral head slips out of the acetabulum. The femoral head is then returned to the acetabulum using the Ortolani maneuver, confirming the diagnosis of an unstable or dislocatable hip (**Figure 33.75** »).

The feet are then examined for evidence of a talipes deformity (clubfoot). Intrauterine position frequently causes the feet to appear to turn inward (**Figure 33.76** »); this is termed a "positional" clubfoot. If the feet can easily be returned to the midline by manipulation, no treatment is indicated, and the nurse teaches range-of-motion exercises to the family. Further evaluation is indicated when the foot will not turn to a midline position or align readily. This is considered the most severe type of "true clubfoot," or talipes equinovarus.

Back

With the newborn prone, the nurse examines the back. The spine should appear straight and flat, because the lumbar and sacral curves do not develop until the newborn begins to sit. The base of the spine is examined for a sacral dimple, a hemangioma, a tuft of hair, or a lipoma, findings associated with spina bifida (Blackburn, 2018). A pilonidal dimple should be examined to ascertain that there is no connection to the spinal canal.

Assessing Neurologic Status

The nurse should begin the neurologic examination with a period of observation, noting the general physical characteristics and behaviors of the newborn. Important behaviors to assess are the state of alertness, resting posture, cry, and quality of muscle tone and motor activity.

The usual position of the newborn is with partially flexed extremities, with the legs abducted to the abdomen. When awake, the newborn may exhibit purposeless, uncoordinated bilateral movements of the extremities. If these movements are absent, minimal, or obviously asymmetric, then neurologic dysfunction should be suspected.

Eye movements are observable during the first few days of life. An alert newborn is able to fixate on faces and brightly colored objects. Shining a bright light in the newborn's eyes elicits the blinking response.

The nurse evaluates muscle tone by moving various parts of the body while the head of the newborn is in a neutral position. The newborn is somewhat hypertonic; that is, there should be resistance to extending the elbow and knee joints. Muscle tone should be symmetric. Diminished muscle tone and flaccidity require further evaluation.

Tremors or jitteriness (tremor-like movements) in the term newborn must be evaluated to differentiate the tremors from convulsions. Tremors may also be related to hypoglycemia, hypocalcemia, or substance withdrawal. Environmental stimuli may initiate tremors. Jitteriness may be distinguished from tonic–clonic seizure activity because it usually can be stopped by the baby's sucking on the extremity or by the nurse holding or flexing the involved extremity. A fine jumping of the muscle is likely to be a CNS disorder and requires further evaluation. Newborn seizures may consist of no more than chewing or swallowing movements, deviations of the eyes, rigidity, or flaccidity because of CNS immaturity. In contrast to tremors, seizures are not usually initiated by stimuli, and they cannot be stopped by holding.

Specific deep tendon reflexes can be elicited in the newborn but have limited value unless they are obviously asymmetric. The knee jerk is typically brisk; a normal ankle clonus may involve three or four beats. Plantar flexion is present.

The newborn's immature CNS is characterized by a variety of reflexes. Because the newborn's movements are uncoordinated, methods of communication are limited, and control of bodily functions is restricted, the reflexes serve a variety of purposes. Some are protective (blink, gag, and sneeze), some aid in feeding (rooting and sucking) and may not be very active if the newborn has eaten recently, and some stimulate human interaction (grasping). See Table 33.16 for commonly found reflexes in the normal newborn.

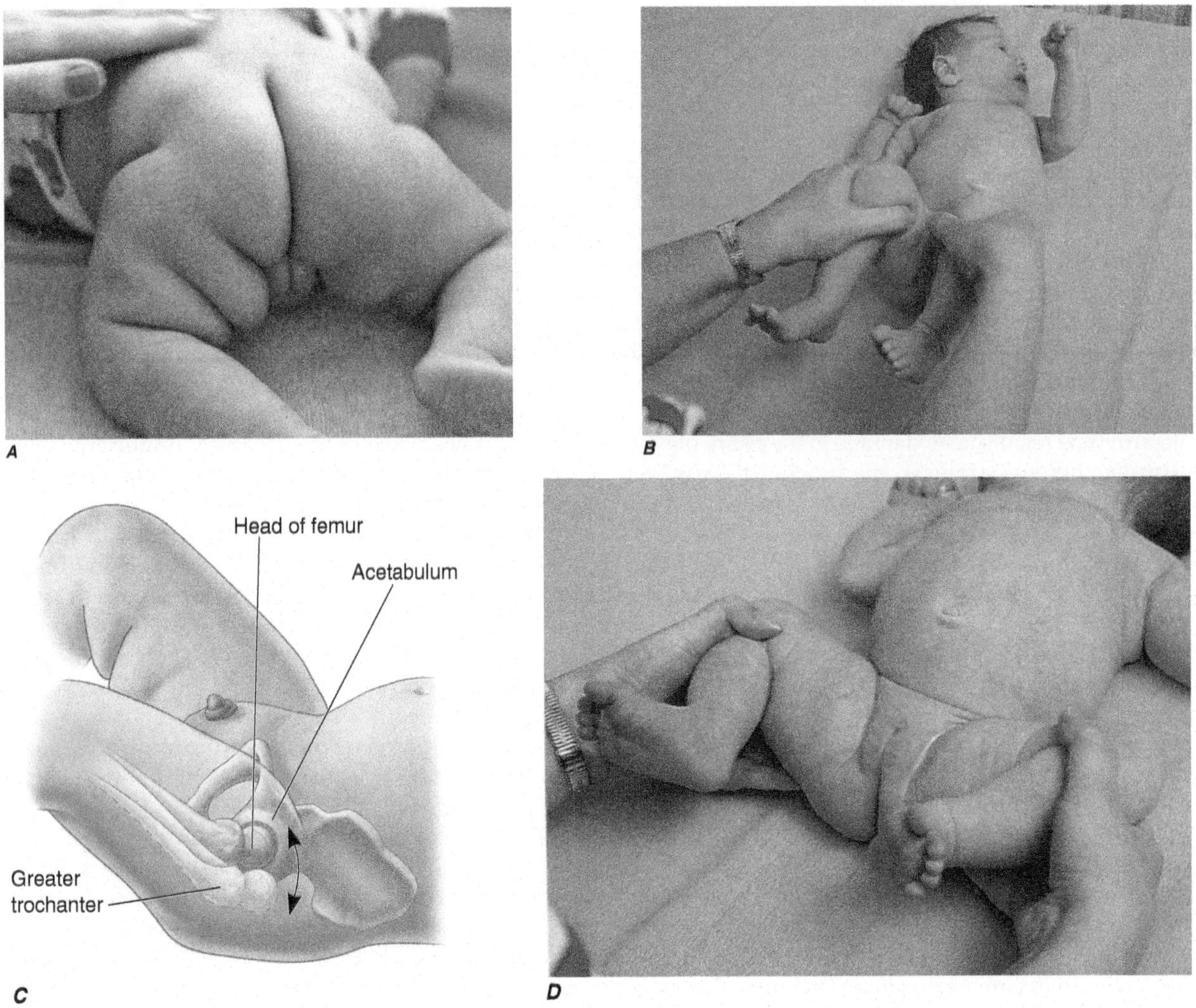

A B

Head of femur
Acetabulum
Greater trochanter

C D

Figure 33.75 ›› ***A***, The asymmetry of gluteal and thigh fat folds seen in a baby with left developmental dysplasia of the hip. ***B***, The Barlow (dislocation) maneuver. The baby's thigh is grasped and adducted (placed together) with gentle downward pressure. ***C***, Dislocation is palpable as the femoral head slips out of the acetabulum. ***D***, The Ortolani maneuver puts downward pressure on the hip and then inward rotation. If the hip is dislocated, this maneuver will force the femoral head back into the acetabular rim with a noticeable "clunk."

Source: (***A***, ***B***, and ***D***) George Dodson/Pearson Education, Inc.

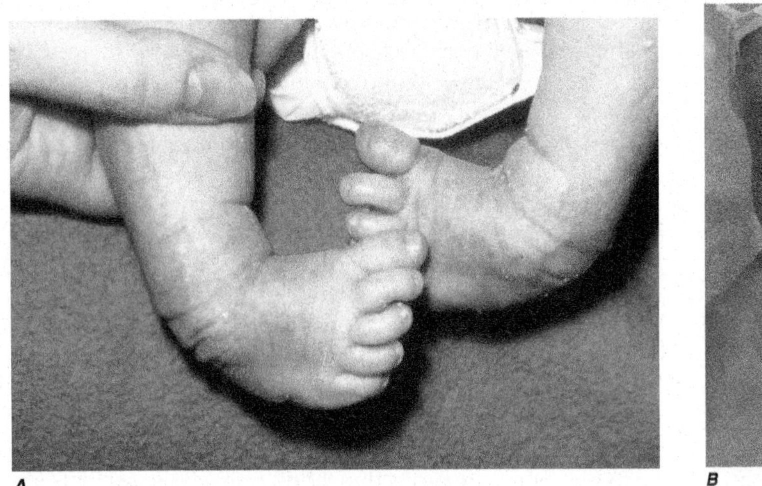

A

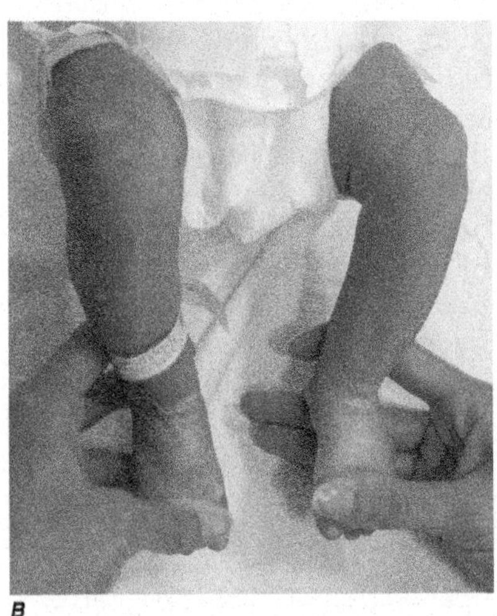

B

Figure 33.76 ›› ***A***, Unilateral talipes equinovarus (clubfoot). ***B***, To determine the presence of clubfoot, the nurse moves the foot to the midline. Resistance indicates true clubfoot.

Source: ***A***, Jim Stevenson/Science Source. ***B***, George Dodson/Pearson Education, Inc.

The nurse assesses CNS integration as follows:

1. The nurse inserts a gloved finger into the newborn's mouth to elicit a sucking reflex.
2. As soon as the newborn is sucking vigorously, the nurse assesses hearing and vision responses by noting changes in sucking in the presence of a light, a rattle, and a voice.
3. The newborn should respond to such stimuli with a brief cessation of sucking, followed by continuous sucking with repeated stimulation.

This CNS integration exam demonstrates auditory and visual integrity as well as the ability to conduct complex behavioral interactions.

As HCPs carry out the newborn physical and neurologic assessment, they are always on the alert to recognize possible alterations and injuries related to the birth process that require further investigation and intervention.

Establishing Gestational Age

In some hospitals, it is standard nursing practice to complete the newborn's gestational age in the first 4 hours after birth so that careful attention can be given to age-related problems (Pickerel, Waldrop, Freeman, Haushalter, & D'Auria, 2020). Once learned, the procedure can be done in a few minutes. Clinical **gestational age assessment tools** have two components: (1) external physical characteristics and (2) neurologic or neuromuscular development.

Physical characteristics generally include sole creases, amount of breast tissue, amount of lanugo, cartilaginous development of the ear, and testicular descent and scrotal rugae or labial development. These objective clinical criteria are not influenced by labor and birth and do not change significantly within the first 12 hours after birth.

Neurologic examination facilitates assessment of functional or physiologic maturation in addition to physical development. However, the newborn's nervous system is unstable during the first 24 hours of life. Therefore, neurologic evaluation findings based on reflexes or assessments that are dependent on the higher brain centers may not be reliable. If the neurologic findings drastically deviate from the gestational age derived by evaluation of external characteristics, a second assessment is done in 24 hours.

The neurologic assessment components (excluding reflexes) can aid in assessing the gestational age of newborns of less than 34 weeks of gestation. Between 26 and 34 weeks, neurologic changes are significant, whereas significant physical changes are less evident. One significant neuromuscular change is that muscle tone progresses from extensor tone to flexor tone in the extremities because the neurologic system matures in a caudocephalad (tail-to-head) progression.

SAFETY ALERT It is essential for the nurse to wear gloves when assessing the newborn in the early hours after birth and before the first bath until amniotic fluid, as well as vaginal and bloody secretions, on the skin are removed.

Ballard et al. (1991) developed the estimation of gestational age by maturity rating, a simplified version of the well-researched **Dubowitz tool**. The Ballard tool omits some of the neuromuscular tone assessments, such as head lag, ventral suspension (difficult to assess in very ill newborns or those on respirators), and leg recoil. In the Ballard tool, each physical and neuromuscular finding is given a value, and the total score is matched to a gestational age. The maximum score on the Ballard tool is 50, which corresponds to a gestational age of 44 weeks.

Postnatal gestational age assessment tools can overestimate preterm gestational age and underestimate postterm gestational age. The tools have been shown to lose accuracy when newborns of less than 28 weeks or more than 43 weeks of gestation are assessed. Ballard et al. (1991), in the **New Ballard Score**, added criteria for more accurate assessment of the gestational age of newborns between 20 and 28 weeks of gestation and less than 1500 g. They suggest that the assessments should be made within 12 hours of birth to optimize accuracy, especially in newborns with a gestational age of less than 26 weeks. Also, the Ballard assessment may be overstimulating to neonates of less than 27 weeks of gestation. Some maternal conditions, such as preeclampsia, diabetes, and maternal analgesia and anesthesia, may affect certain gestational assessment components and warrant further evaluation. Maternal diabetes, although it appears to accelerate fetal physical growth, seems to retard maturation. Maternal HTN states, which retard fetal physical growth, seem to speed maturation.

Newborns of women with preeclampsia have a poor correlation with the criteria involving active muscle tone and edema. Maternal analgesia and anesthesia may cause respiratory depression in the baby. Babies with respiratory distress syndrome tend to be flaccid and edematous and assume a "froglike" posture. These characteristics affect the scoring of the neuromuscular components of the assessment tool used.

Assessing Physical Maturity Characteristics

The nurse first evaluates observable characteristics without disturbing the baby. Selected physical maturity characteristics common to the Dubowitz and Ballard gestational assessment tools are presented in **Figure 33.77** » in the order in which they might be most effectively evaluated.

Other physical characteristics assessed by some gestational age scoring tools include the following:

- ***Vernix*** covers the preterm newborn. The postterm newborn has no vernix. After noting vernix distribution, the birthing area nurse (wearing gloves) dries the newborn to prevent evaporative heat loss, thus disturbing the vernix and potentially altering this gestational age criterion.
- ***Hair*** of the preterm newborn has the consistency of matted wool or fur and lies in bunches rather than in the silky, single strands of the term newborn's hair.
- ***Skull firmness*** increases as the fetus matures. In a term newborn, the bones are hard and the sutures are not easily displaced. The nurse should not attempt to displace the sutures forcibly.
- ***Nails*** appear and cover the nail bed at about 20 weeks of gestation. Nails extending beyond the fingertips may indicate a postterm newborn.

Physical Characteristics of Gestational Age

Skin

Assess for thickness, transparency, and texture.

The preterm newborn's skin appears thin and transparent, and has visible blood vessels.

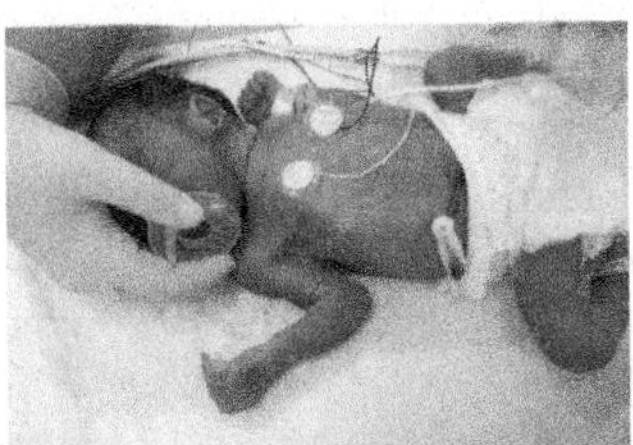

Source: Pearson Education, Inc.

A. Preterm skin

As the newborn approaches term, the skin is thicker and appears opaque because of increased subcutaneous tissue.

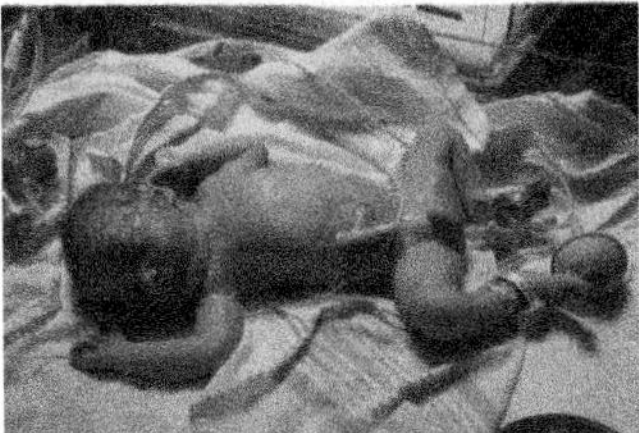

Source: Qwerty/Alamy Stock Photo.

B. Term skin

Disappearance of the protective vernix caseosa promotes skin desquamation; this is commonly seen in postmature neonates and those showing signs of placental insufficiency.

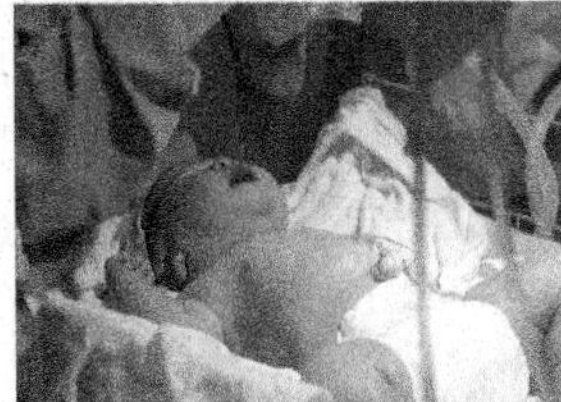

Source: Glenn Kraushar/Alamy Stock Photo.

C. Postterm skin

Lanugo

Assess for the quantity of lanugo, the fine soft hair covering the fetus during intrauterine development.

This hair begins to appear at approximately 19–20 weeks' gestation and is most prominent at 27–28 weeks' gestation.

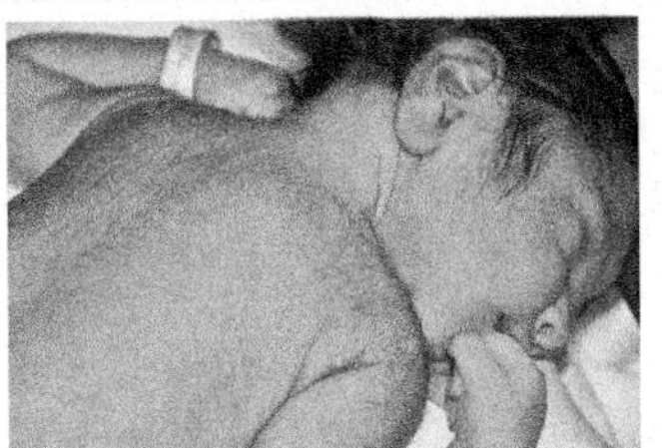

Source: Vanessa Howell, RN, MSN.

D. Lanugo

It is mostly shed by 37 weeks' gestation. It first begins to thin over the lower back and then disappears last from the shoulders.

Plantar surfaces

Assess the number of sole creases over the bottom of the foot. They are reliable indicators of gestational age in the first 12 hours of life.

Plantar creases vary with ethnicity; in Black newborns, sole creases may be less developed at term.

A few creases appear on the anterior portion of the foot and the heel is smooth at approximately 34 weeks' gestation ***(Ballard score 2)***.

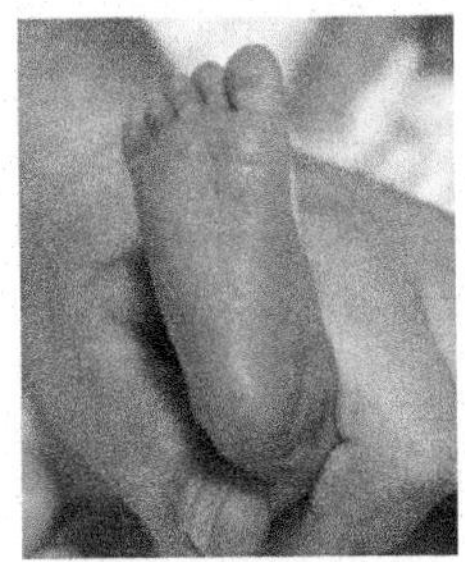

Source: Pearson Education, Inc.

E. Plantar surface, 34 weeks' gestation

By 36 weeks' gestation, a deeper network of creases cover the anterior two thirds of the foot and the heel is smooth ***(Ballard score 3)***.

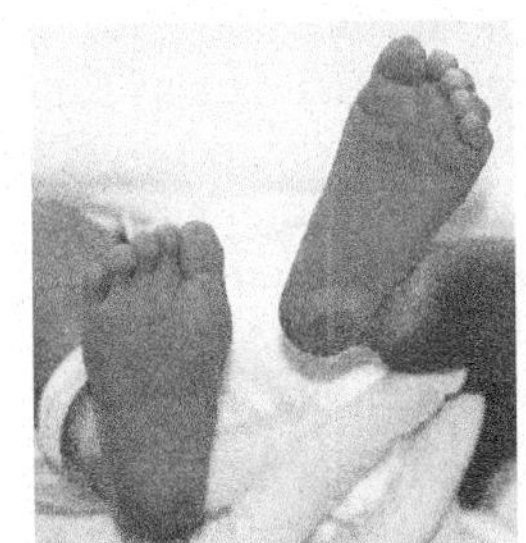

Source: Pearson Education, Inc.

F. Plantar surface, 36 weeks' gestation

At term, deep creases cover the entire foot, including the heel ***(Ballard score 4)***.

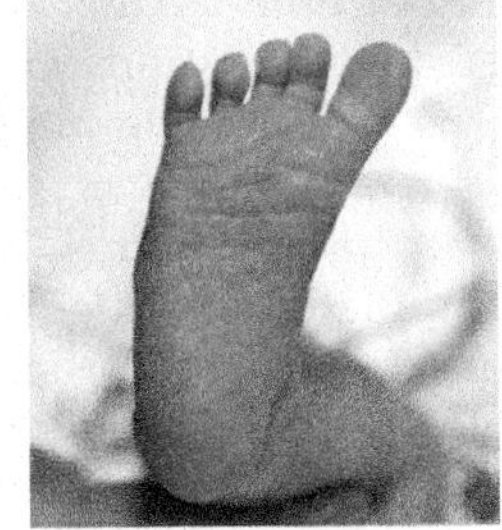

Source: Pearson Education, Inc.

G. Plantar surface, term

Breast

Assess the chest for visibility of the nipple and areola. Then gently palpate the breast bud using the forefinger and middle finger and measure the tissue between them. At term, the tissue will measure between 5 and 10 mm (0.5 cm and 1 cm).

The nurse should not grasp the nipple firmly, because skin and subcutaneous tissue will prevent accurate estimation of size. The nurse must do this procedure gently to avoid causing trauma to the breast tissue.

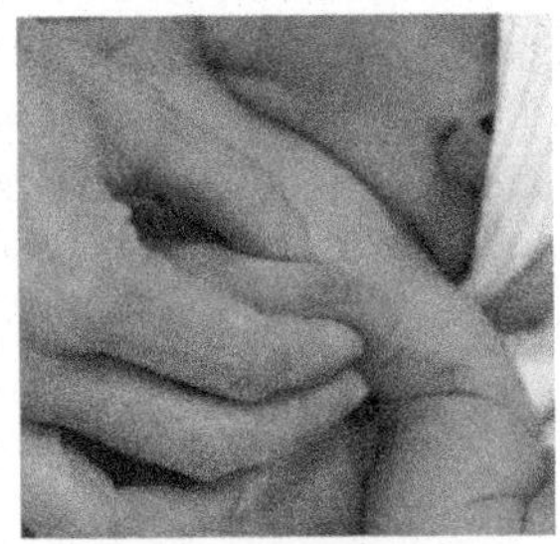

Source: Pearson Education, Inc.

H. At 38 weeks' gestation, this newborn has a visible raised area (breast bud) greater than 0.75 cm in diameter ***(Ballard score 3)***.

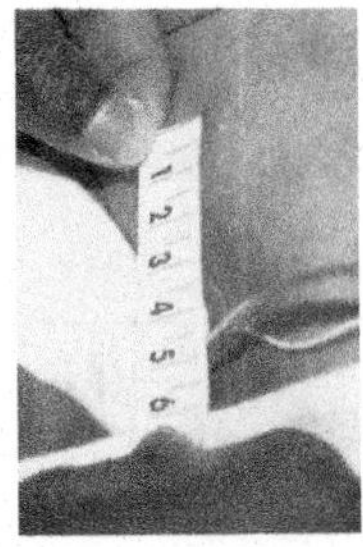

Source: Pearson Education, Inc.

I. Absence of or decreased breast tissue often indicates a premature or SGA newborn.

As gestation progresses, the breast tissue mass and areola enlarge. However, a large breast tissue mass can occur as a result of specific conditions other than advanced gestational age or the effects of maternal hormones on the baby. In the LGA neonate, the accelerated development of breast tissue in a mother with diabetes is a reflection of subcutaneous fat deposits. SGA term or postterm newborns may have used subcutaneous fat, which would have been deposited as breast tissue, to survive in utero; as a result, their lack of breast tissue may indicate a gestational age of 34–35 weeks even though other factors indicate a term or postterm newborn.

Eyes and ears

Assess the eye opening. In extremely preterm neonates, the eyelids are examined with gentle flexion to determine the amount of fusion. Eye opening begins at 22 weeks, and the lids are completely unfused by 28 weeks' gestation.

Assess the formation of the ear cartilage and curving of the pinna. At earlier gestational ages the lack of cartilage allows the ear to fold easily and retain the fold. As gestational age increases, the resistance of the ear to folding increases and recoil is seen. In extremely preterm neonates the pinnae are flat. Incurving proceeds from the top down toward the lobes with advancing gestational age.

The ear of the newborn at approximately 36 weeks' gestation shows incurving of the upper two thirds of the pinna ***(Ballard score 2)***.

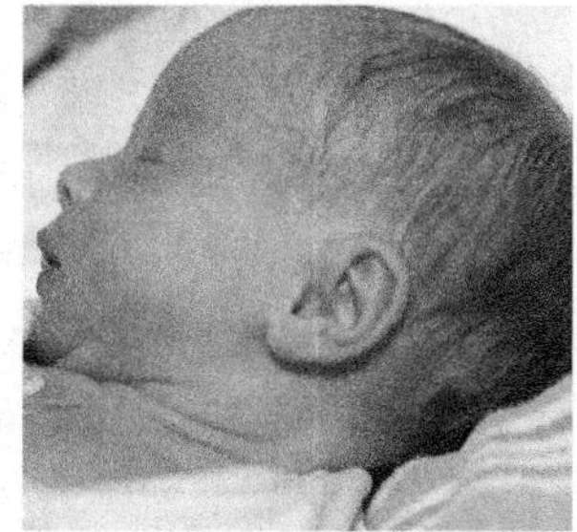

Source: Pearson Educatiotn, Inc.

J. Ear at 36 weeks' gestation

Newborn at term shows well-defined incurving of the entire pinna ***(Ballard score 3)***.

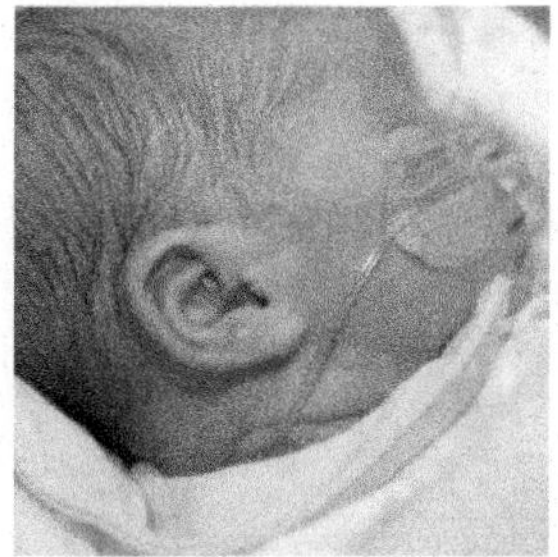

Source: Pearson Education, Inc.

K. Ear at term

The pinna is folded toward the face and released. If the auricle stays in the position in which it is pressed or returns slowly to its original position, it usually means the gestational age is less than 38 weeks.

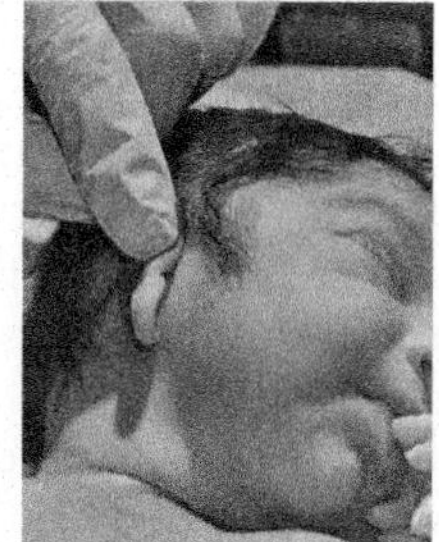

Source: Vanessa Howell, RN, MSN.

L. Assessing the pinna

Male genitals

Assess for size of the scrotal sac, presence of rugae (wrinkles and ridges in the scrotum), and descent of the testes.

Before 36 weeks' of gestation, the scrotum has few rugae, and the testes are palpable in the inguinal canal not within the scrotum ***(Ballard score 2)***.

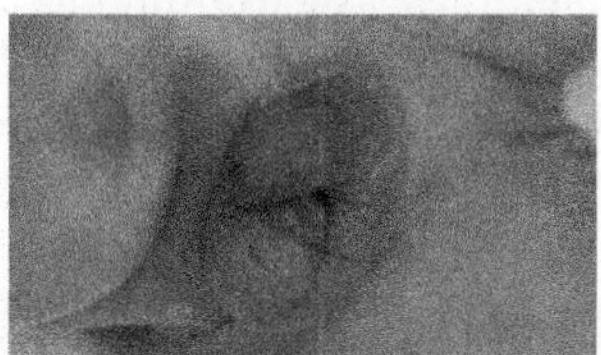

Source: Pearson Education, Inc.

M. Male genitals, preterm

By 36–38 weeks, the testes are in the upper scrotum, and rugae have developed over the anterior portion of the scrotum. By term, the testes are fully descended in the lower scrotum, which is pendulous and covered with rugae ***(Ballard score 3)***.

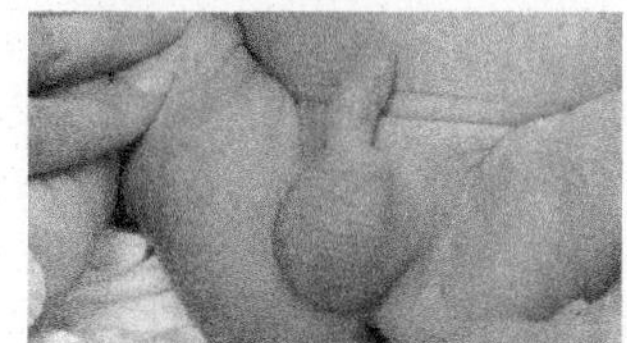

Source: Pearson Education, Inc.

N. Male genitals, term

Female genitals

Assess labial development. Genital appearance depends in part on subcutaneous fat deposition and, therefore, relates to fetal nutritional status. The clitoris varies in size and, occasionally, is so swollen that it is difficult to identify the sex of the newborn. This swelling may be caused by adrenogenital syndrome, which causes the adrenals to secrete excessive amounts of androgen and other hormones.

At 32 weeks' of gestation, the clitoris is prominent and the labia minora are flat ***(Ballard score 1)***.

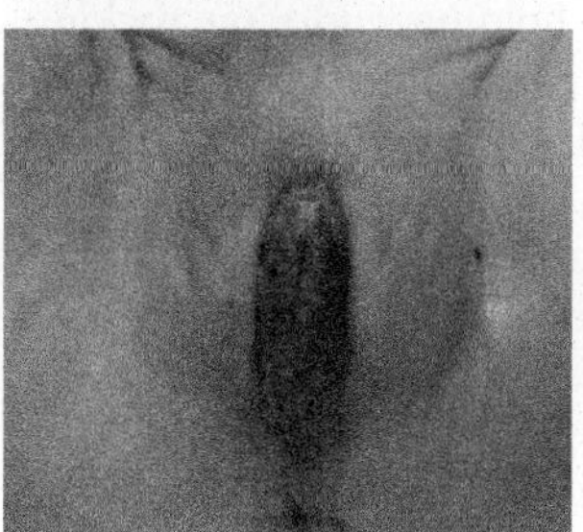

Source: Pearson Education, Inc.

O. Female genitals, 32 weeks' gestation

By 36 weeks' gestation, the labia majora are larger and the clitoris is nearly covered ***(Ballard score 2)***.

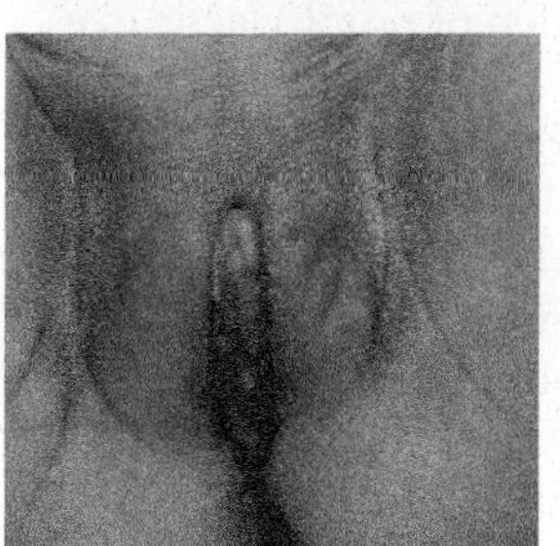

Source: Pearson Education, Inc.

P. Female genitals, 36 weeks' gestation

At term, the labia majora are well developed and cover both the clitoris and labia minora ***(Ballard score 3)***.

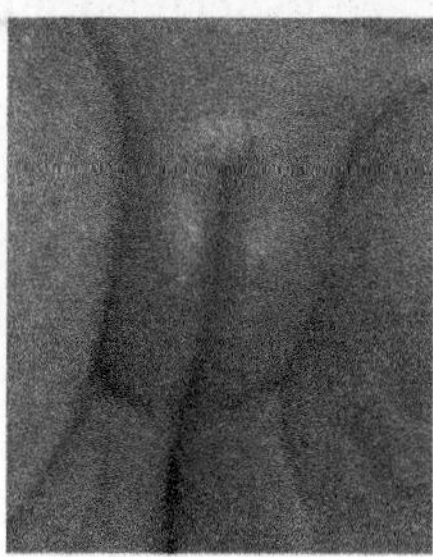

Source: Christine Anderson.

Q. Female genitals, term

Figure 33.77 ›› A–Q Physical characteristics of gestational age. *(continued)*

Assessing Neuromuscular Maturity Characteristics

The CNS of the fetus matures at a fairly constant rate. Tests have been designed to evaluate neurologic status as manifested by development of neuromuscular tone. As noted earlier, neuromuscular tone in the fetus develops in a caudocephalad direction, from the lower to the upper extremities.

The neuromuscular evaluation of the newborn requires more manipulation and disturbances than the physical evaluation. The neuromuscular evaluation is best performed when the newborn has stabilized. Selected neuromuscular maturity characteristics common to the Dubowitz and Ballard gestational assessment tools are presented in **Figure 33.78** ».

Other neuromuscular characteristics assessed by some gestational age scoring tools include the following:

- ***Head lag*** (neck flexor) is measured by pulling the newborn to a sitting position and noting the degree of head lag. Total lag is common in newborns up to 34 weeks of gestation, whereas postterm newborns (> 42 weeks) hold their heads in front of their body lines. Full-term newborns can support their heads momentarily.
- ***Ventral suspension*** (horizontal position) is evaluated by holding the newborn prone on the nurse's hand. The position of the head and back and the degree of flexion in the arms and legs are noted. Some flexion of arms and legs indicates 36 to 38 weeks of gestation; fully flexed extremities, with the head and back even, are characteristic of a term newborn.
- ***Major reflexes***—such as sucking, rooting, grasping, Moro, tonic neck, Babinski, and others—are evaluated during the newborn exam (see Table 33.16).

Additional Methods for Estimating Gestational Age

A supplementary method for estimating gestational age (done by the physician or nurse practitioner) is to view the vascular network of the cornea with an ophthalmoscope. The nurse may need to delay administration of prophylactic eye ointment in preterm neonates until after this vascular eye exam has been done. The amount of vascularity present over the surface of the lens assists in identifying neonates with a gestational age of 27 to 34 weeks (Blackburn, 2018).

When the gestational age determination and birth weight are considered together, the newborn can be identified as one whose growth is classified as SGA (below 10th percentile), AGA (between 10th and 90th percentile), or LGA (above 90th percentile).

This determination enables the nurse to anticipate possible physiologic problems and is used in conjunction with a complete physical examination to establish an appropriate plan of care for the individual newborn. For example, newborns who are SGA or LGA are at risk for hypoglycemia and therefore often require frequent glucose monitoring and early feedings started soon after birth.

The nurse also plots the gestational age against the newborn's length, head circumference, and weight on an appropriate growth chart to determine if these measurements fall within the average range—the 10th to 90th percentile for the corresponding gestational age. These correlations further document the level of maturity and appropriate category for the newborn. The comparison of the newborn's weight–length ratio further facilitates identification of SGA newborns as having symmetric or asymmetric growth restriction. Measuring weight and height often aggravates newborns and may alter their vital signs. For better accuracy, take the newborn's vital signs before weighing and measuring the neonate.

Assessing Newborn Behavior

The **Brazelton Neonatal Behavioral Assessment Scale** provides valuable guidelines for assessing the newborn's state changes, temperament, and individual behavioral patterns (Brazelton, 1984). It provides a way for the nurse, in conjunction with the parents or primary caregivers, to identify and understand the individual newborn's states and capabilities. Families learn which responses, interventions, or activities best meet the special needs of their newborn, and this understanding fosters positive attachment experiences.

The Brazelton assessment tool identifies the newborn's repertoire of behavioral responses to the environment and also documents the newborn's neurologic adequacy and capabilities. The examination usually takes 20 to 30 minutes and involves approximately 30 tests. Some items are scored according to the newborn's response to specific stimuli. Others, such as consolability and alertness, are scored as a result of continuous behavioral observations throughout the assessment. (For a complete discussion of all test items and maneuvers, see Brazelton & Nugent, 1995.)

Because the first few days after birth are a period of behavioral disorganization, the complete assessment should be done on the third day after birth. The nurse should make every effort to elicit the best response. This may be accomplished by repeating tests at different times or by testing during situations that facilitate the best possible response, such as when the parents are holding, cuddling, rocking, and/or singing to their baby.

Assessment of the newborn should be carried out initially in a quiet, dimly lighted room, if possible. The nurse should first determine the newborn's state of consciousness, because scoring and introduction of the test items are correlated with the sleep or waking state (discussed previously). The newborn's state depends on physiologic variables, such as the amount of time from the last feeding, positioning, environmental temperature, and health status; the presence of such external stimuli as noises and bright lights; and the sleep–wake cycle of the neonate. An important characteristic of the newborn period is the pattern of states, as well as the transitions from one state to another. The pattern of states is a predictor of the newborn's receptivity and ability to respond to stimuli in a cognitive manner. Babies learn best in a quiet, alert state and in an environment that is supportive and protective and that provides appropriate stimuli.

Neuromuscular Characteristics of Gestational Age

Resting posture

Assess the posture that the supine newborn assumes at rest. The extremely preterm neonate will lie with arms and legs extended or in any position placed.

At approximately 31 weeks' gestation, the newborn has slightly more flexion in the arms and legs ***(Ballard score 1 or 2)***.

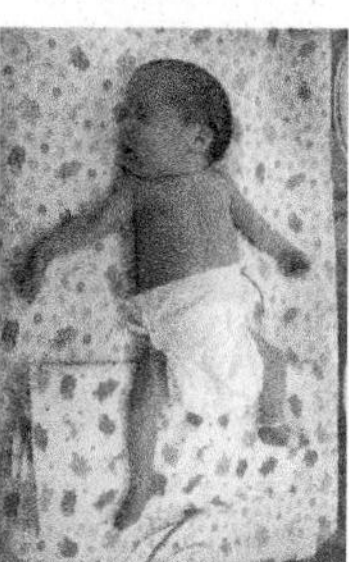

Source: Pearson Education, Inc.

A. Resting posture, 31 weeks' gestation

At approximately 35 weeks' gestation, the newborn exhibits stronger flexion of the arms, hips, and thighs ***(Ballard score 3)***.

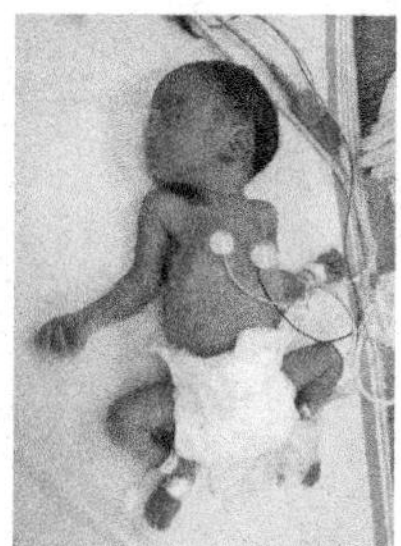

Source: Pearson Education, Inc.

B. Resting posture, 35 weeks' gestation

At term, the newborn exhibits hypertonic flexion of all extremities with arms flexed to the chest, hands fisted, and legs flexed toward the abdomen ***(Ballard score 4)***.

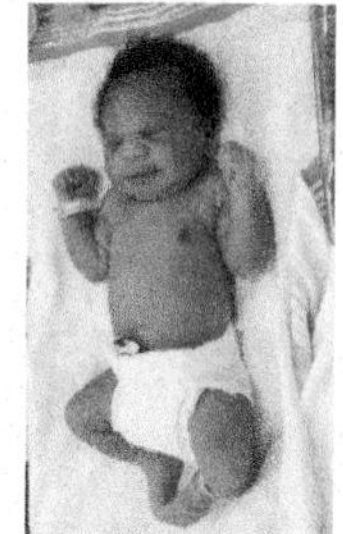

Source: Pearson Education, Inc.

C. Resting posture, term

Square window sign

Assess the angle of the wrist when the palm is flexed toward the forearm until resistance is felt. The angle formed at the wrist is measured. The extremely preterm neonate has no flexor tone and cannot achieve a 90-degree angle. The preterm neonate has poor flexion and is unable to flex the arm at the elbow more than 90 degrees.

At 28–32 weeks' gestation, the angle is 90 degrees ***(Ballard score 0)***.

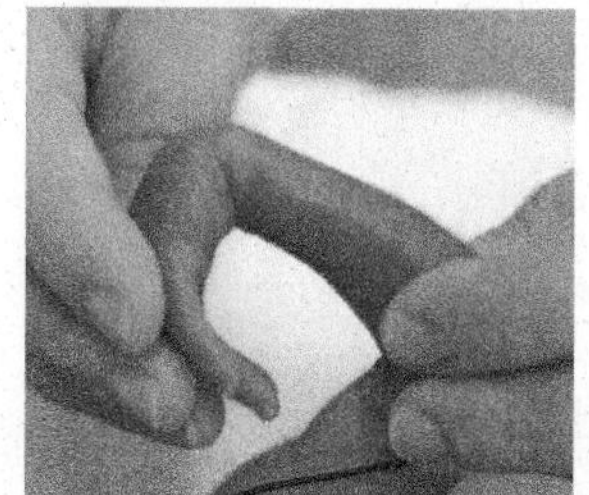

Source: Pearson Education, Inc.

D. Square window sign, 28–32 weeks' gestation

At 38–40 weeks' gestation, the angle is 30 to 40 degrees ***(Ballard score 2 to 3)***.

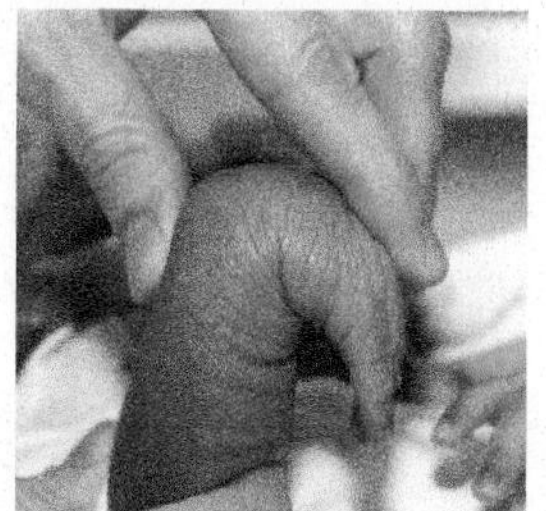

Source: Pearson Education, Inc.

E. Square window sign, 38–40 weeks' gestation

A 0- to 15-degree angle occurs in newborns from 40–42 weeks' gestation ***(Ballard score 4)***.

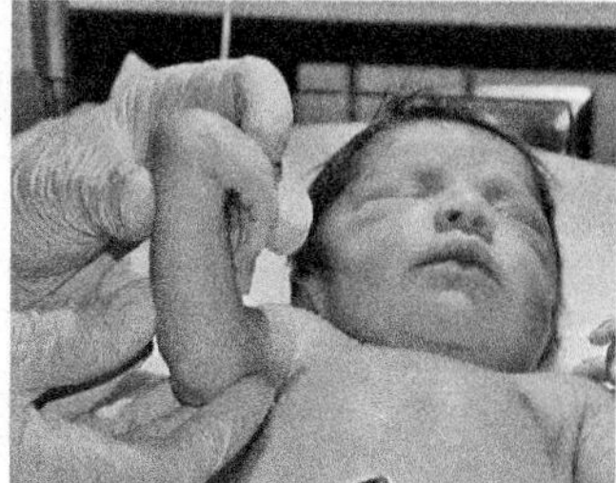

Source: Vanessa Howell, RN, MSN.

F. Square window sign, 40–42 weeks' gestation

Recoil of extremities

Very preterm neonates do not resist extension. They respond with weak and delayed flexion in a small arc. Term newborns resist extension and briskly return their arms to the flexed position.

Arm recoil may be slower in healthy but fatigued newborns after birth; therefore, arm recoil is best elicited after the first hour postbirth, when the baby has had time to recover from the stress of the birth. The deep sleep state also decreases the arm recoil response. Assessment of arm recoil should be bilateral to rule out brachial palsy.

Assess the amount of arm flexion by flexing both arms at the elbows for 5 seconds. Then extend the arms at the elbows

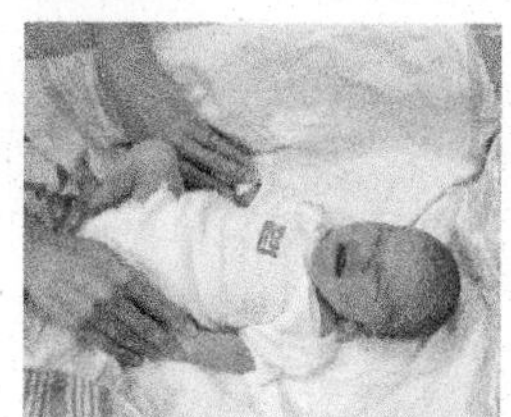

Source: Pearson Education, Inc.

G. Extend arms at elbows

Release the arms to see the amount of recoil

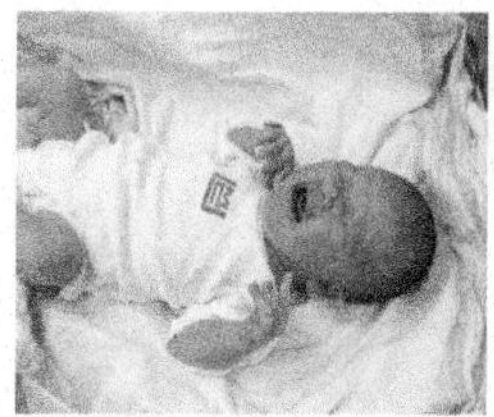

Source: Pearson Education, Inc.

H. Release arms to see recoil

Because flexion first develops in the lower extremities, recoil generally is first tested in the legs. Place the newborn supine on a flat surface. With a hand on the newborn's knees, place the baby's legs in flexion and extend them parallel to each other and flat on the surface. The response to this maneuver is recoil of the newborn's legs. According to gestational age, they may not move or may return slowly or quickly to the flexed position. Preterm neonates have less muscle tone than term neonates, so preterm neonates have less recoil.

Figure 33.78 ›› A–O Neuromuscular characteristics of gestational age.

Popliteal angle

Assess the angle of the knee in the supine newborn. The angle formed is then measured.

Holding the pelvis flat, flex and hold the thigh to the abdomen while extending the leg at the knee until resistance is met

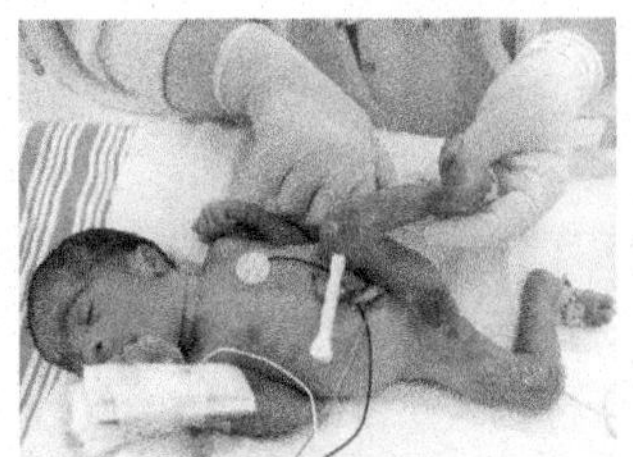

Source: Pearson Education, Inc.

I. Popliteal angle

The newborn with more advanced gestational age has greater flexion. Results vary from no resistance in the very immature newborn to an 80-degree angle in the term newborn.

Scarf sign

Assess the newborn's resistance to pulling the arm across the chest toward the opposite shoulder. The newborn's elbow moves closer to the opposite shoulder with decreasing gestational age.

Until approximately 30 weeks' gestation, the elbow moves past the midline with no resistance ***(Ballard score 1)***.

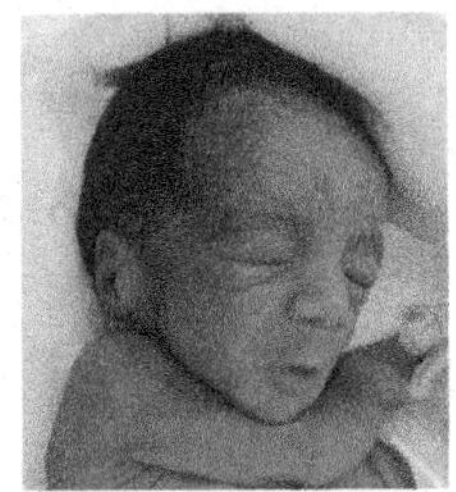

Source: Pearson Education, Inc.

J. Scarf sign, 30 weeks' gestation

At 36–40 weeks' gestation, the elbow is at midline ***(Ballard score 2)***.

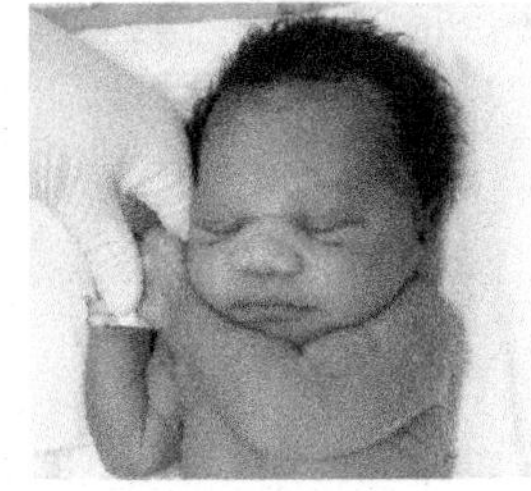

Source: Pearson Education, Inc.

K. Scarf sign, 36–40 weeks' gestation

The term newborn's elbow will not cross the midline of the chest ***(Ballard score 4)***.

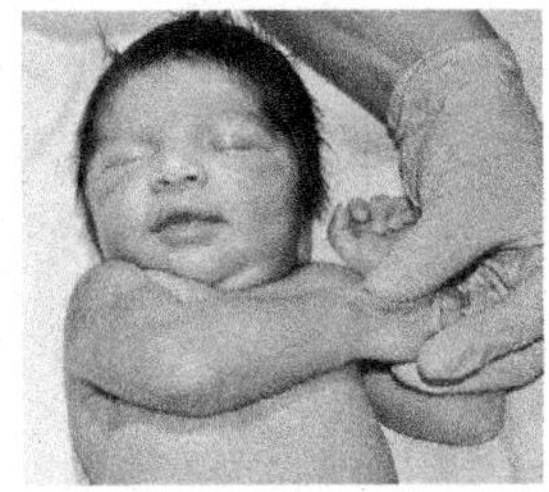

Source: Vanessa Howell, RN, MSN.

L. Scarf sign, term

Heel-to-ear extension

Assess by placing the newborn in a supine position and then gently drawing the foot toward the ear on the same side until resistance is felt. Allow the knee to bend during the test and hold the buttocks down to keep from rolling the baby. Both the proximity of foot to ear and the degree of knee extension are assessed.

A preterm, immature newborn's leg will remain straight, and the foot will go to the ear or beyond ***(Ballard score 0)***.

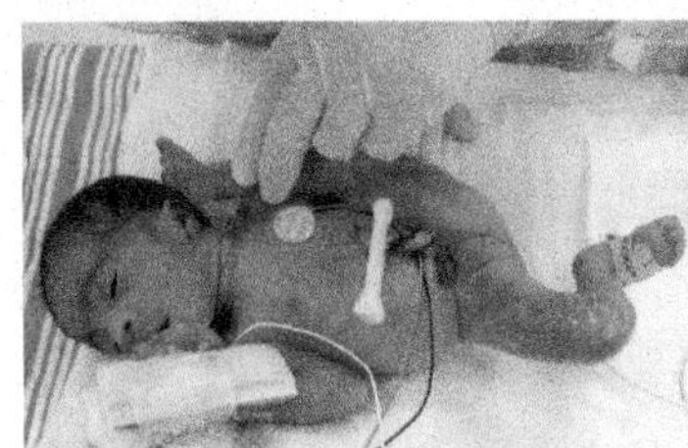

Source: Pearson Education, Inc.

M. Heel-to-ear extension

With advancing gestational age, the newborn demonstrates increasing resistance to this maneuver. Maneuvers involving the lower extremities of newborns who had frank breech presentation should be delayed to allow for resolution of leg positioning.

Ankle dorsiflexion

Assess by flexing the ankle on the shin. Use a thumb to push on the sole of the newborn's foot while the fingers support the back of the leg. Then, measure the angle formed by the foot and the interior leg.

A 45-degree angle indicates 32 to 36 weeks' gestation ***(Ballard score 1)***.

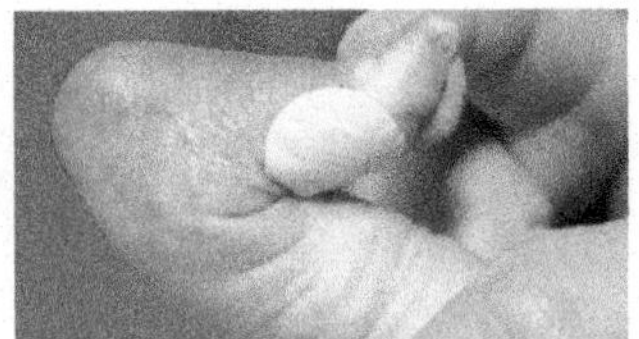

Source: Carol Harrigan, RNC, MSN, NNP.

N. Ankle dorsiflexion, 32–36 weeks' gestation.

A 20-degree angle indicates 36–40 weeks' gestation (Ballard score 2 to 3). A 15- to 0-degree angle is common at 40 weeks or more of gestation ***(Ballard score 4)***.

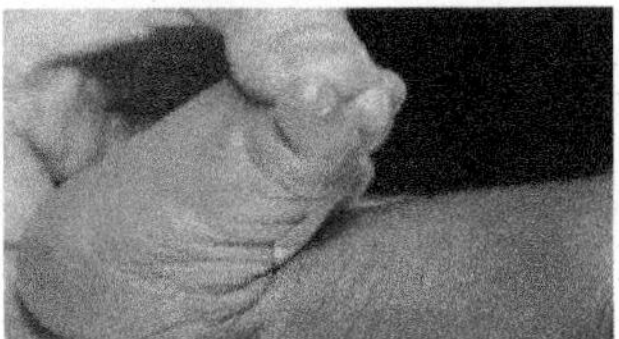

Source: Pearson Education, Inc.

O. Ankle dorsiflexion, 40 or more weeks' gestation

Ankle dorsiflexion findings can be influenced by intrauterine position and congenital deformities.

Figure 33.78 ›› **A–O** Neuromuscular characteristics of gestational age. (*continued*)

The nurse should observe the newborn's sleep–wake patterns, including the rapidity with which the newborn moves from one state to another, the newborn's ability to be consoled, and the newborn's ability to diminish the impact of disturbing stimuli. The following questions may provide the nurse with a framework for assessment:

- Does the newborn's response style and ability to adapt to stimuli indicate a need for parental interventions that will alert the newborn to the environment in order to grow socially and cognitively?
- Are parental interventions necessary to lessen the outside stimuli, as in the case of the baby who responds to sensory input with intensity?
- Can the baby control the amount of sensory input?

The behaviors, and the sleep–wake states in which they are assessed, are categorized as follows:

- ***Habituation.*** The nurse assesses the newborn's ability to diminish or shut down innate responses to specific repeated stimuli, such as a rattle, bell, light, or pinprick to the heel.
- ***Orientation to inanimate and animate visual and auditory assessment stimuli.*** The nurse observes how often and where the newborn attends to auditory and visual stimuli. Orientation to the environment is determined by an ability to respond to clues given by others and by a natural ability to fix on and follow a visual object both horizontally and vertically. This capacity and the parental appreciation of it are important for positive communication between newborn and parents; the parents' visual (*en face*) and auditory (soft, continuous voice) presence stimulates their newborn to orient to them. Inability or a lack of response may indicate visual or auditory problems. It is important for parents to know that their newborn can turn to voices soon after birth or by 3 days of age and can become alert at different times with a varying degree of intensity in response to sounds.
- ***Motor activity.*** Several components are evaluated. Motor tone of the newborn is assessed in the most characteristic state of responsiveness. This summary assessment includes overall use of tone as the newborn responds to being handled—whether during spontaneous activity, prone placement, or horizontal holding—and overall assessment of body tone as the newborn reacts to all stimuli.
- ***Variations.*** Frequency of alert states, state changes, color changes (throughout all states as examination progresses), activity, and peaks of excitement are assessed.
- ***Self-quieting activity.*** This assessment is based on how often, how quickly, and how effectively newborns can use their resources to quiet and console themselves when upset or distressed. Considered in this assessment are such self-consolatory activities as putting a hand to the mouth, sucking on a fist or the tongue, and attuning to an object or sound (**Figure 33.79** »). The newborn's need for outside consolation must also be considered (e.g., seeing a face; being rocked, held, or dressed; using a pacifier; and being swaddled).

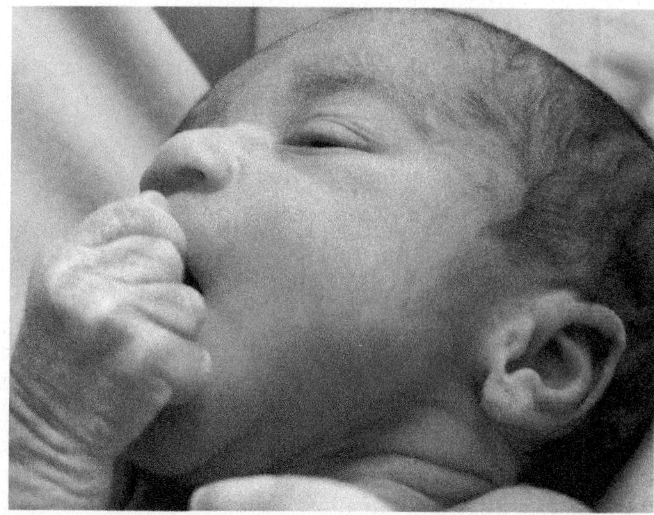

Figure 33.79 » The newborn can bring hand to mouth as a self-soothing activity.

Source: George Dodson/Pearson Education, Inc.

- ***Cuddliness or social behaviors.*** This area encompasses the newborn's need for, and response to, being held. These behaviors influence the couple's self-esteem and feelings of acceptance or rejection. Cuddling also appears to be an indicator of personality. Cuddlers appear to enjoy, accept, and seek physical contact; are easier to placate; sleep more; and form earlier and more intense attachments. Noncuddlers are active, restless, have accelerated motor development, and are intolerant of physical restraint. Smiling, even as a grimace reflex, greatly influences parent–newborn feedback. Parents identify this response as positive.

Once assessment has been completed, the nurse reviews and analyzes the data to determine the newborn's specific needs.

Diagnosis

Analysis of assessment data for salient cues is necessary to determine nursing diagnoses and priorities for care. Physiologic alterations, family processes, and parenting skills necessary to support the healthy newborn as well as the newborn with alterations will be among the priorities for care. Examples of nursing diagnoses commonly appropriate for newborns and their families include:

- Impaired airway clearance if mucus or retained lung fluid is present
- Pain from procedures such as heelsticks for glucose or a vitamin K injection
- Poor thermoregulation if heat loss or immature hypothalamic response are present
- Ineffective breathing pattern related to periodic breathing
- Difficulty breastfeeding
- Undernutrition if the newborn is having difficulty feeding
- Risk for infection at the umbilical cord site, circumcision site, or due to birth trauma or immature immunity
- Impaired family functioning.

Planning

The broad goals of nursing care during this period are the following:

- The newborn will be healthy and well.
- The family unit will function well.

The nurse meets the first goal by providing comprehensive care to the newborn in the mother–baby unit. The nurse meets the second goal by teaching family members how to care for their new baby and by supporting their efforts so that they feel confident and competent. The nurse must be knowledgeable about family adjustments that need to be made as well as about the healthcare needs of the newborn. It is important for the family to return home with the positive feeling that they have the support, information, and skills to care for their newborn. Equally important is the need for each member of the family to begin a unique relationship with the newborn. The cultural and social expectations of individual families and communities affect the way in which normal newborn care is carried out.

Implementation

Nursing care immediately following delivery focuses on ensuring the newborn's successful transition to extrauterine life. Accurate assessment and close observation are essential to planning nursing care that promotes positive outcomes. In addition, the nurse must be familiar with any aspects of the mother's prenatal record that indicate possible risk factors for newborn transition. Relevant maternal data include history of substance use, infection, method of delivery, use of narcotic analgesia, PROM, and any history of psychiatric symptoms or illness.

This section focuses on general care of the newborn, either common or essential interventions that will apply for virtually every newborn until the baby discharged.

Communicating with Families

Introductory Phase

First-time parents may be very nervous about providing care for their newborn. After introducing yourself, share your positive first impressions of their newborn and any bonding behaviors that have been observed. You can:

- Ask if they have picked a name for their newborn.
- Show the parents that by putting a finger in the newborn's hand, the newborn will grasp the finger.
- Explain that the newborn will recognize their voices and that talking to their newborn can be very soothing.

Care of the Newborn During Transition

The nurse responsible for the newborn first checks and confirms the newborn's identification with the mother's identification and then obtains and records all significant information.

Maintaining the Airway

For the neonate with any initial respiratory distress or excessive oral secretions, the nurse should position the newborn on the back (or the side if secretions are copious) and suction the airway using a bulb syringe. When possible, this procedure should be delayed for 10 to 15 minutes after birth to reduce the potential for severe vasovagal reflex apnea. Excessive secretions should be reported to the primary HCP because they may indicate tracheoesophageal fistula.

Taking Vital Signs

In the absence of any newborn distress, the nurse continues to admit the newborn by measuring vital signs. The vital signs for a healthy term newborn should be monitored at least every 30 minutes until the newborn's condition has remained stable for 2 hours (AAP & ACOG, 2017). The newborn's respirations may be irregular yet still be considered normal. Periodic breathing, lasting only 5 to 15 seconds with no color or heart rate changes, is considered to be normal. The normal pulse range is 110 to 160 beats/min (a pulse anywhere from 100 to 205 beats/min may be considered normal), and the normal respiratory range is 30 to 60 breaths/min (during the first several hours after birth it is not uncommon for the newborn to have a respiratory rate as high as 80 breaths/min).

Promoting Thermoregulation

An NTE is best achieved by performing the newborn assessment and interventions with the newborn unclothed and under a radiant warmer. The radiant warmer's thermostat is controlled by the thermal skin sensor taped to the newborn's abdomen, upper thigh, or arm. The sensor indicates when the newborn's temperature exceeds or falls below the acceptable temperature range. The nurse should be aware that leaning over the newborn may block the radiant heat waves from reaching the neonate. In addition to placing the baby under a radiant warmer, it is common practice in some institutions to cover the newborn's head with a cap to prevent further evaporative heat loss (Blackburn, 2018).

When the newborn's temperature is normal and vital signs are stable (2 to 4 hours after birth), the baby may be given a sponge bath. However, the most current evidence supports delaying the first bath until 12 to 24 hours after birth, in order to support breastfeeding success and to decrease the risk for hypothermia and hypoglycemia in healthy newborns (Long, Rondinelli, Yim, Cariou, & Valdez, 2020; Warren, Midodzi, Newhook, Murphy, & Twells, 2020; WHO, 2018a). The baby may be bathed under the radiant warmer or in the parents' room and by the parents. Bathing the newborn offers an excellent opportunity for the nurse to teach and welcome parents' involvement in the care of their baby.

If the baby is bathed under the radiant warmer, the nurse rechecks the baby's temperature after the bath and, if it is stable, dresses and places the newborn in an open crib at room temperature. If the baby's axillary temperature is below that of the hospital's policy, the nurse returns the baby to the radiant warmer. The rewarming process should be gradual to prevent hyperthermia. Once the newborn is rewarmed, the nurse implements measures to prevent further neonatal heat loss, such as keeping the newborn dry, swaddled in one or two blankets with a hat on, and away from cool surfaces or instruments. Newborns are often "double-wrapped" in two or more blankets for temperature maintenance.

Addressing Vitamin K Deficiency

A prophylactic injection of phytonadione (vitamin K) is recommended to prevent hemorrhage, which can occur because of low prothrombin levels in the first few days of life. The potential for hemorrhage is considered to result from the absence of intestinal bacterial flora, which influences the production of vitamin K in the newborn. Newborns should receive a single parenteral dose of 0.5 to 1 mg of phytonadione within 1 hour of birth (Stachowiak & Furman, 2020; Stanford Medicine, 2006). Current recommendations underscore the need for treatment in babies who are exclusively breastfed (Blackburn, 2018).

The phytonadione injection is given IM in the middle third of the vastus lateralis muscle, located in the lateral aspect of the thigh (**Figure 33.80** »). Before injecting, the nurse must thoroughly clean the newborn's skin site for the injection with a small alcohol swab. The nurse uses a 27-gauge, 1/2-in. to 5/8-in. needle for the injection (**Figure 33.81** »).

Preventing Eye Infection

The nurse is responsible for giving the legally required prophylactic eye treatment for *Neisseria gonorrhoeae*, which may have infected the newborn of an infected mother during the birth process. A variety of topical agents appear to be equally effective. Ophthalmic ointments that are used include 0.5% erythromycin (Ilotycin Ophthalmic), 1% tetracycline, or per agency protocol (Curry et al., 2019). All of these ointments are also effective against chlamydia, which has a higher incidence rate than gonorrhea.

Successful eye prophylaxis requires that the medication be instilled into the lower conjunctival sac of each eye (**Figure 33.82** »). The nurse massages the eyelid gently to distribute the ointment. Instillation may be delayed up to 1 hour after birth to allow for the initial breastfeeding in the delivery room as well as eye contact during parent–newborn bonding.

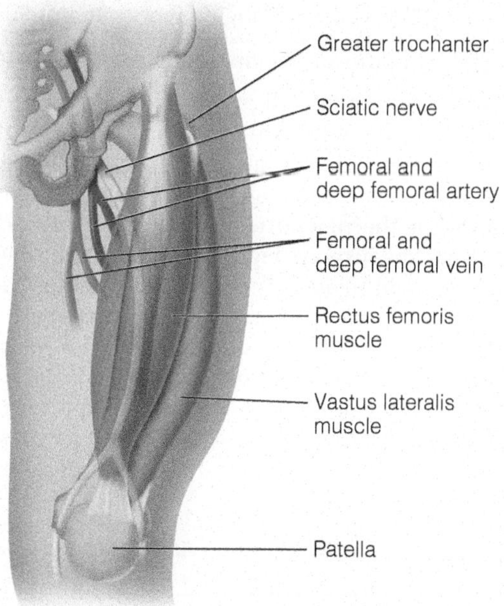

Figure 33.80 » Injection sites. The middle third of the vastus lateralis muscle is the preferred site for intramuscular injection in the newborn.

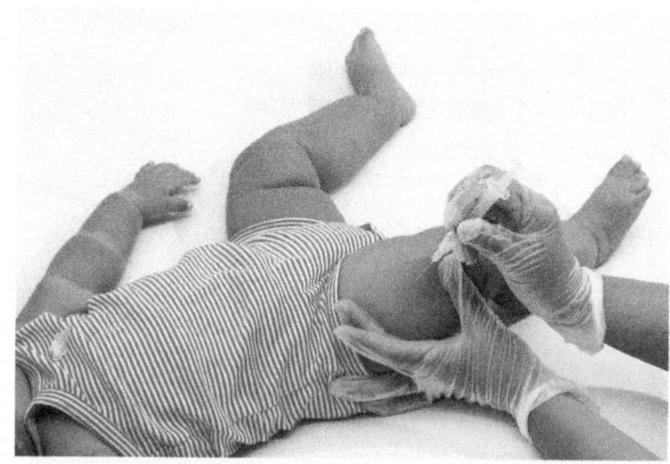

Figure 33.81 » Procedure for vitamin K injection. Cleanse the area thoroughly with an alcohol swab and allow the skin to dry. Hold the tissue of the upper outer thigh (vastus lateralis muscle) taut, and quickly insert a 27-gauge, 1/2-in. to 5/8-in. needle at a 90-degree angle to the thigh. Aspirate, then slowly inject the solution to distribute the medication evenly and minimize the baby's discomfort. Remove the needle and gently massage the site with an alcohol swab.

Source: Marlon Lopez/MMG1 Design/Shutterstock.

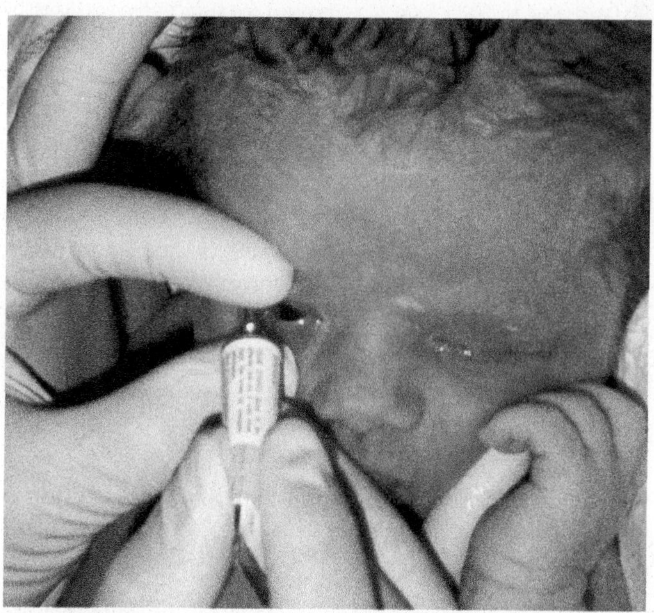

Figure 33.82 » Ophthalmic ointment. Retract the lower eyelid outward to instill a 1-cm-(0.25-in.)-long strand of ointment from a single-dose tube along the lower conjunctival surface. *Make sure that the tip of the tube does not touch the eye.*

Source: Pearson Education, Inc.

Eye prophylaxis medications can cause chemical conjunctivitis, which gives the newborn some discomfort and may interfere with the newborn's ability to focus on the parents' faces. The resulting edema, inflammation, and discharge may cause concern if the parents have not been informed that the side effects will clear in 24 to 48 hours and that this prophylactic eye treatment is necessary for the newborn's well-being.

Box 33.9
Signs of Neonatal Distress

- Respiratory changes
  - Increased respiratory rate (greater than 60/minute) or difficult respirations
  - Sternal, substernal, intercostal retractions
  - Nasal flaring
  - Excessive mucus
- Color change
  - Cyanosis (central: skin, lips, tongue)
  - Pallor
  - Mottling
  - Plethora
  - Jaundice of the skin within 24 hours of birth or because of hemolytic process
- Abdominal distention or mass
- Vomiting bile-stained material
- Absence of meconium elimination within 48 hours after birth
- Absence of urine elimination more than 24 hours after birth (Blackburn, 2018)
- Temperature instability (hypothermia or hyperthermia)
- Jitteriness, irritability, or abdominal movements
- Difficult to wake, lethargy, or hypotonicity
- Weight changes greater than anticipated.

Sources: Data from AAP & ACOG (2017); Blackburn (2018). Reprinted from Davidson et al. (2020), Table 28-1. Reprinted and electronically reproduced by permission of Pearson Education, Inc., Hoboken, NJ.

Assessing Neonatal Distress

During the first 24 hours after birth, assessing and responding to neonatal distress is the nurse's responsibility (**Box 33.9** »). If the newborn remains with the parents during this time, the nurse must provide thorough patient teaching on how to maintain their baby's temperature and to recognize and respond immediately to signs their newborn is in distress. The nurse should teach the parents to observe for:

- Changes in breathing—grunting or sighing sounds with breathing or rapid breathing accompanied by chest retractions
- Facial grimacing
- Changes in skin color
- Changes in activity.

Appropriate interventions to teach the parents include suctioning secretions with a bulb syringe, positioning, and stroking the newborn's spine with a fingertip to stimulate respirations, if needed. The nurse must respond immediately if the parents report signs of distress.

Initiating the First Feeding

The timing of the first feeding varies depending on whether the newborn is to be breastfed or formula-fed and whether there were any complications during pregnancy or birth, such as maternal diabetes or IUGR. The nurse should encourage mothers who choose to breastfeed their newborns to put the baby to the breast during the newborn's first period of reactivity. This practice should be encouraged because successful, long-term breastfeeding during infancy appears to be related to beginning such feedings in the first few hours of life. Sleep–wake states affect feeding behavior and need to be considered when evaluating the newborn's sucking ability.

If the mother decides to formula-feed, the newborn should be offered formula upon exhibiting readiness to feed or per hospital protocol. Signs indicating newborn readiness for the first feeding are licking of the lips, placing a hand in or near the mouth, active bowel sounds, absence of abdominal distention, and a lusty cry that quiets with rooting and sucking behaviors when a stimulus is placed near the lips. Observing the earlier, more subtle cues that the baby is ready to nurse provides an opportunity to teach the parents to recognize these cues and respond before the baby is frustrated and crying.

SAFETY ALERT Newborns with respiratory distress should not be fed orally because of an increased risk of aspiration.

Facilitating Parent–Newborn Attachment

Immediate skin-to-skin care after birth promotes maternal and newborn attachment. The hormonal response to birth sparks behaviors in the newborn that facilitate its transition to postnatal life (Crenshaw, 2019). Eye-to-eye contact between the parents and their newborn can also facilitate parent–newborn attachment and is important during the early hours after birth, when the newborn is in the first period of reactivity. The newborn is alert during this time, the eyes are wide open, and the baby often makes direct eye contact with human faces within optimal range for visual acuity. Parents who cannot be with their newborns in this first period because of maternal or neonatal distress may need reassurance that the bonding process can proceed normally as soon as both mother and baby are stable.

Care of the Newborn after Transition

Following the healthy newborn's successful transition to extrauterine life, continued observations are necessary for the first 6 to 12 hours following delivery and until discharge.

Maintaining Cardiopulmonary Function

The nurse assesses vital signs every 4 to 8 hours or more, depending on the newborn's status. The nurse places the newborn on the back (supine) for sleeping and keeps a bulb syringe within easy reach should the baby need oral–nasal suctioning. If the newborn has respiratory difficulty, the nurse clears the airway. Vigorous fingertip stroking of the baby's spine will frequently stimulate respiratory activity. A cardiorespiratory monitor may be used on newborns who are not being observed at all times and are at risk for decreased respiratory or cardiac function. Indicators of risk are pallor, cyanosis, ruddy color, apnea, and other signs of instability. Changes in skin color may indicate the need for closer assessment of temperature, cardiopulmonary status, hematocrit, glucose, and bilirubin levels.

Promoting Adequate Hydration and Nutrition

The nurse records caloric and fluid intake and enhances adequate hydration by maintaining an NTE and offering early and frequent feedings. Early feedings promote gastric emptying and increase peristalsis, thereby decreasing the potential for hyperbilirubinemia by decreasing the amount of time fecal material is in contact with the enzyme beta-glucuronidase in the small intestine. This enzyme frees the bilirubin from the feces, allowing it to be reabsorbed into the vascular system.

The nurse records voiding and stooling patterns. The first voiding and the first passage of stool should occur within 24 to 48 hours. If they do not occur, the HCP in charge of the newborn needs to be notified. The nurse continues the normal observation routine while assessing for abdominal distention, bowel sounds, hydration, fluid intake, and temperature stability.

The nurse weighs the newborn at the same time each day for accurate comparisons. The newborn must be kept warm during the weighing. A weight loss of up to 10% for term newborns is considered to be within normal limits during the first week of life. This weight loss is the result of limited intake, loss of excess extracellular fluid, and passage of meconium. Parents should be told about the expected weight loss, the reason for it, and the expectations for regaining the birth weight. Birth weight is usually regained by 10 days to 2 weeks if feedings are adequate.

Excessive handling can cause an increase in the newborn's metabolic rate and calorie use and also cause fatigue. The nurse should be alert to the newborn's subtle cues of fatigue, including a decrease in muscle tension and activity in the extremities and neck as well as loss of eye contact, which may be manifested by fluttering or closure of the eyelids. The nurse quickly ceases stimulation when signs of fatigue appear. The nurse demonstrates to parents the need to be aware of newborn cues and to wait for periods of alertness for contact and stimulation.

The nurse also assesses the woman's comfort and latching-on techniques if breastfeeding. If the woman is not breastfeeding, the nurse assesses the mother's bottle-feeding techniques.

Promoting Skin Integrity

Skin care, including bathing, is important for the health and appearance of the individual newborn and for infection control within the nursery. Ongoing skin care involves cleansing the buttock and perianal areas with fresh water and cotton or a mild soap and water during diaper changes. If commercial baby wipes are used, those without alcohol should be selected. Perfume-free and latex-free wipes are also available.

The nurse should assess the umbilical cord for signs of bleeding or infection. Removal of the cord clamp within 24 to 48 hours of birth reduces the chance of tension injury to the area. Keeping the umbilical stump clean and dry can reduce the chance for infection and is best practice for umbilical cord care (Blackburn, 2018). Many types of routine cord care are practiced, including the use of triple dye, an antimicrobial agent (e.g., bacitracin), or application of 70% alcohol to the cord stump, but these are not based on evidence and should not be encouraged. No single method of cord care has proven to be superior in preventing colonization and infection (omphalitis) (AAP & ACOG, 2017). Folding the diaper down to avoid covering the cord stump can prevent contamination of the area and promote drying. The nurse is responsible for cord care per agency policy. It is also the nurse's responsibility to instruct parents in caring for the cord and observing for signs and symptoms of infection after discharge, such as foul smell, redness and drainage, localized heat and tenderness, or bleeding.

Promoting Safety

Safety of the newborn is paramount. Nurses should strictly follow agency policies, which should be based on newborn ID requirements instituted by The Joint Commission (2018), which include:

- Naming systems that use the mother's first and last names and the newborn's sex
- Standardized practices for ID banding systems (such as barcoding and use of two body sites for identification).

The nurse should teach parents the following measures to prevent abduction and provide for safety:

- Parents should check that identification bands are in place as they care for their baby; if the bands are missing, parents should ask that they be replaced immediately.
- Parents should allow only individuals with proper birthing-unit picture identification to bring and/or remove the baby from the room. If parents do not know the staff person, they should call the nurse for assistance.
- Parents should report the presence of any suspicious individuals on the birthing unit.
- Parents should never leave their baby alone in their room. If they walk in the halls or take a shower, parents should have a family member watch the baby or should return the baby to the nursery.
- A parent who is feeling weak, faint, or unsteady should not lift the baby. Instead, the parent should call for assistance.
- Parents should always keep an eye and a hand on the baby when the newborn is out of the crib.
- Parents should ask visitors to leave if they have a cold, diarrhea, discharge from sores, or a contagious disease. Newborns need protection from infection even though they do possess some immunity.

Preventing Complications

Newborns are at continued risk for the complications of hemorrhage, late-onset cardiac symptoms, and infection. Pallor may be an early sign of hemorrhage and must be reported to the HCP. The newborn with pallor is placed on a cardiorespiratory monitor to permit continuous assessment. Several newborn conditions put newborns at risk for hemorrhage. Cyanosis that is not relieved by oxygen administration requires emergency intervention, may indicate a congenital cardiac condition or shock, and requires ongoing assessment.

Hospitals have different safety measures for preventing infection in the nursery and may require that all personnel who have direct contact with newborns scrub for 2 to 3 minutes from the fingertips up to and including the elbows at the beginning of each shift. The use of hand sanitizer before and after contact with every newborn is standard nursing practice. Each caregiver should also clean their hands after touching any soiled surface, such as the floor or their hair or face. Parents are instructed to practice appropriate hand hygiene before touching the baby. They are also instructed that anyone holding the baby should practice good hand hygiene, even after the family returns home.

Jaundice in newborns is caused by the accumulation of the pigment bilirubin in the skin. Jaundice occurs in most newborns.

Most jaundice is benign, but because of the potential toxicity of bilirubin, newborns must be monitored to identify those who might develop severe hyperbilirubinemia and, in rare cases, acute bilirubin encephalopathy or kernicterus (Pace et al., 2019). Current recommendations include obtaining a total serum bilirubin (TSB) level or a transcutaneous bilirubin (TcB) in any neonate who is visibly jaundiced in the first 24 hours of life and obtaining either a TSB or TcB level before discharge (Campbell, 2020). Nomograms for evaluating risk factors based on bilirubin levels and age of the neonate are available.

Circumcision

Circumcision is a surgical procedure in which the prepuce, an epithelial layer covering the penis, is separated from the glans penis and excised. This procedure permits exposure of the glans for easier cleaning. Controversy exists over the need to perform circumcisions.

Originally a religious rite practiced by Jews and Muslims, circumcision has gained widespread cultural acceptance in the United States but is much less common in Europe. Many parents choose circumcision because they want their male child to have a physical appearance similar to that of his father or the majority of other boys; some feel that it is expected by society. Another commonly cited reason for circumcising newborn males is to prevent the need for anesthesia, hospitalization, pain, and trauma if the procedure is needed later in life (Rossi, Buonocore, & Bellieni, 2020). Failure to circumcise is a risk factor related to penile cancer in later life. During the prenatal period, the nurse ensures that parents have clear and current information regarding the risks and benefits of circumcision and supports their decision regarding the choice to circumcise.

As in the past, recommendations regarding circumcision have varied. The 1999 AAP policy statement was reaffirmed in 2012 and does not recommend routine circumcision, but it does acknowledge that medical indications for circumcision still exist (Rossi et al., 2020). The policy recommends that analgesia be used during circumcision to decrease procedural pain (Rossi et al., 2020); the dorsal penile nerve block and subcutaneous ring block are the most effective options (Rossi et al., 2020). If a circumcision is to be performed, it should be done using the least painful method. Studies show that using oral sucrose for painful procedures can be effective in reducing pain for newborns and should be used with other nonpharmacologic measures to enhance its effectiveness (Rossi et al., 2020).

Circumcision should not be performed if the newborn is premature or compromised, has a known bleeding problem, or is born with a genitourinary defect, such as hypospadias or epispadias, which may necessitate use of the foreskin in future surgical repairs.

The nurse plays an essential role in providing parents with current information regarding the medical, social, and psychologic aspects of newborn circumcision. A well-informed nurse can allay parents' anxiety by sharing information and allowing them to express their concerns. In order for parents to make a truly informed decision, they must be knowledgeable about the potential risks and outcomes of circumcision. Hemorrhage, infection, difficulty in voiding, separation of the edges of the circumcision, discomfort, and restlessness are early potential problems. Later, there is a risk that the glans and urethral meatus may become irritated and inflamed from contact with the ammonia from urine. Ulcerations and progressive stenosis may develop. Adhesions, entrapment of the penis, and damage to the urethra are all potential complications of circumcision that could require surgical correction (Rossi et al., 2020).

The parents of a male newborn who will not be circumcised require information from the nurse about good hygiene practices. The nurse should tell the parents that the foreskin and glans are two similar layers of cells that separate from each other. The separation process begins prenatally and is normally completed between 3 and 5 years of age. In the process of separation, sterile sloughed cells build up between the layers. This buildup looks similar to the smegma that is secreted after puberty, and it is harmless. Occasionally during the daily bath, the parent can gently test for retraction. If retraction has occurred, daily gentle washing of the glans with soap and water is sufficient to maintain adequate cleanliness (Campbell, 2020). The parents should later teach the child to incorporate this practice into his daily self-care activities; most uncircumcised males have no difficulty doing so.

If circumcision is desired, the procedure is performed when the newborn is well stabilized and has received his initial physical examination by a HCP. The parents may also choose to have the circumcision done after discharge. However, parents need to be advised that if the baby is older than 1 month, the current practice is to hospitalize him for the procedure.

Before a circumcision, the nurse ensures that the physician has explained the procedure, determines whether the parents have any further questions, and verifies that the circumcision permit is signed. As with any surgical procedure, the neonate's identification band should be checked to verify his identity before the procedure begins. The nurse gathers the equipment and prepares the newborn by removing the diaper and placing him on a padded circumcision board or some other type of restraint, but with only the legs restrained. These restraint measures, along with the application of warm blankets to the upper body, increase the newborn's comfort during the procedure. In Jewish circumcision ceremonies, the newborn is held by the father or godfather and is given wine before the procedure.

Various devices (Gomco clamp, Plastibell, and Mogen clamp) are used for circumcision (**Figure 33.83** ›› and **Figure 33.84** ››), and all produce a small amount of bleeding. Therefore, the nurse should make special note of neonates with a family history of bleeding disorders or with mothers who took anticoagulants, including aspirin, prenatally. During the procedure, the nurse assesses the newborn's response. One important consideration is pain experienced by the newborn. A dorsal penile nerve block or ring block using 1% lidocaine without epinephrine or similar anesthetic significantly minimizes the pain and shifts in behavioral patterns, such as crying, irritability, and erratic sleep cycles, that are associated with circumcision. Studies indicate that a combination of methods is most effective in reducing pain (Rossi et al., 2020). As indicated in Evidence-Based Practice: Breastfeeding to Control Procedural Pain in Newborns, a common method used to control pain associated with circumcision offers an opportunity for the mother

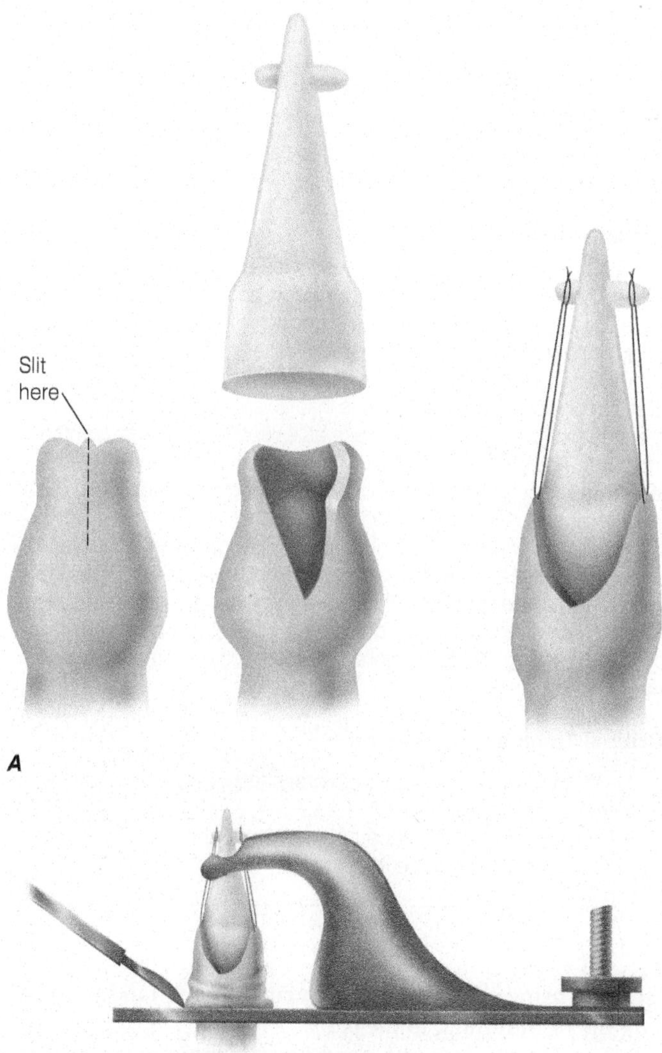

Figure 33.83 ›› Circumcision using a circumcision clamp. *A*, The prepuce is drawn over the cone and *B*, the clamp is applied. Pressure is maintained for 3 to 4 minutes, and then excess prepuce is cut away.

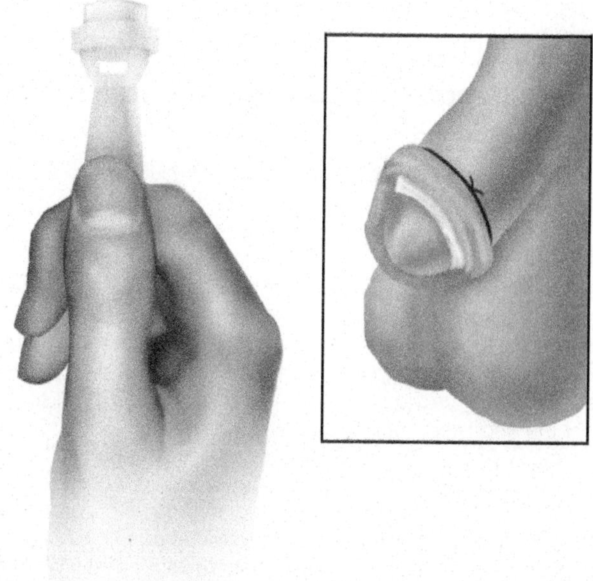

Figure 33.84 ›› Circumcision using the Plastibell. The bell is fitted over the glans. A suture is tied around the bell's rim, and the excess prepuce is cut away. The plastic rim remains in place for 3 to 4 days until healing occurs. The bell may be allowed to fall off; it is removed if still in place after 8 days.

to provide comfort for her newborn while diminishing anxiety related to concern about the procedure.

Following the circumcision, the newborn should be held and comforted by a family member or the nurse. The nurse must be alert to any behavioral cues that these measures are overstimulating the newborn instead of comforting him. Such cues include turning away of the head, increased generalized body movement, skin color changes, hyperalertness, and hiccoughing.

Ideally, the circumcision should be assessed per hospital policy following the procedure. It is important to observe for the first voiding after a circumcision in order to evaluate for urinary obstruction related to penile injury and/or edema. Petroleum ointment and gauze or strictly petroleum ointment may be applied to the site immediately following the procedure to help prevent bleeding and can be used to protect the healing tissue afterward.

The nurse must also teach family members how to assess for unusual bleeding, how to respond if unusual bleeding is present, and how to care for the newly circumcised penis. Parents of babies circumcised with a method other than the Plastibell should receive the following information:

- Clean the site with warm water with each diaper change.
- Apply petroleum ointment for the next few diaper changes to help prevent further bleeding and to prevent the circumcised penis from sticking to the diaper.
- If bleeding does occur, apply light pressure with a sterile gauze pad to stop the bleeding within a short time. If this is not effective, contact the HCP immediately or take the baby to the HCP's office.
- The glans normally has granulation tissue (a yellowish film) on it during healing. Continued application of a petroleum ointment (or ointment suggested by the HCP) can help protect the granulation tissue that forms as the glans heals.
- Report to the HCP any signs or symptoms of infection, such as increasing swelling, pus drainage, and cessation of urination.
- When diapering, ensure that the diaper is not loose enough to cause rubbing with movement and is not tight enough to cause pain.
- If the newborn's HCP recommends oral analgesics, follow instructions for proper measuring and administration.

If the Plastibell is used, parents should receive information about normal appearance and how to observe for infection. Inform parents that the Plastibell should fall off within 8 days. If it remains on after 8 days, they should consult with their HCP. No ointments or creams should be used while the bell remains, but application of petroleum ointment may protect granulation tissue after it falls off.

Evidence-Based Practice

Breastfeeding to Control Procedural Pain in Newborns

Problem

What nonpharmacologic methods can help reduce the pain associated with common neonatal procedures?

Evidence

Assessment and management of pain are important issues in neonatal care. Most newborns will experience a venipuncture or heel lance for blood sampling during their hospital stay. Although HCPs agree that newborns are capable of responding to painful stimuli, most providers do not administer medication to control the short-term pain associated with these common procedures. A Cochrane systematic review investigated the use of breastfeeding—specifically, the oral administration of breast milk—to control the pain associated with common procedures (Harrison et al., 2016). Multiple systematic reviews with this quantity of randomized trials represent the strongest level of evidence for nursing practice.

Newborns who were feeding during heelsticks or venipuncture procedures demonstrated fewer physiologic and behavioral signs of pain. Actual feeding at the breast was associated with a reduction in heart rate change, percentage time crying, duration of crying, and improvement in validated neonatal pain measures. Breastfeeding led to significantly lower increases in heart rate and decreased crying time compared to those who were swaddled. All groups that were fed during the procedure—whether it was breast milk from the mother or expressed breast milk—had better pain control than babies who were swaddled, positioned, or given a pacifier without being held.

Implications

It does not appear that any of these measures completely eliminated the pain of routine procedures. In addition, these studies were focused on healthy newborns undergoing minimally invasive, singular painful procedures. The effectiveness of either breast milk for repeated painful procedures was not studied. With regard to preterm or sick newborns, there is insufficient evidence to support the safety of breast milk or sucrose as a routine, repeated comfort measure. For preterm and sick full-term newborns who are subjected to repeated painful procedures during hospitalization, the ideal analgesic has not yet been identified.

Newborns undergoing single painful procedures, such as venipuncture or heelstick, should be breastfed by the mother during the procedure, if at all possible. If not, the baby can be fed expressed breast milk with a syringe, a bottle, or by dipping a pacifier in the solution. Holding the baby while doing so achieves the best pain control.

Critical Thinking Application

1. What are the challenges with breastfeeding to control procedural pain in newborns?
2. How could the influence of breastfeeding on newborn pain during procedures be measured?

Strengthening Parent–Newborn Attachment

The nurse encourages parent–newborn attachment by involving all family members with the new member of the family. The nurse can discuss waking activities, such as talking with the baby while making eye contact, holding the baby in an upright position (sitting or standing), gently bending the baby back and forth while grasping under the knees and supporting the head and back with the other hand, or gently rubbing the baby's hands and feet. Quieting activities may include swaddling or bundling the baby to increase a sense of security; using slow, calming movements; and talking softly, singing, or humming to the baby.

When fostering parent–newborn attachment, it is important to be sensitive to the cultural beliefs and values of the family. The nurse must also be aware of cultural variations in newborn care (see Focus on Diversity and Culture: Cultural Variations in Newborn Care).

» *Go to **Pearson MyLab Nursing and eText** to see Chart 19: Promoting Attachment.*

Focus on Diversity and Culture

Cultural Variations in Newborn Care

Many cultural variations in the care of newborns exist. Nurses must be sensitive to the needs of the family as they welcome the newborn into their family and culture.

Muslim families may follow one or more of several Islamic practices. Although the mother may choose to have only women attending the birth of the baby, Islam does allow male providers to care for pregnant women and does not prohibit the father from attending the birth. It is common for the father or an elder to speak the first words the newborn hears by whispering into the child's ear. These words are the *Adhan*, or *adhaan*, a call to prayer performed five times a day. By these words, the newborn is welcomed into the Islamic faith and community.

Many Native American (indigenous) women observe different practices depending on their particular tribe. Because many Native American people maintain a close connection to the earth, some maintain the historic practice of touching the newborn's feet to the earth before giving it to the mother.

The best way to learn what aspects of newborn care are culturally informed is to ask the mother and family about their practices and preferences. Then the nurse can provide space and time for families to honor their cultural traditions.

Sources: BBC (2009); Huda (2017); Pember (2018).

Prepare Family for Discharge

The transition from the hospital or birth setting to home presents challenges for any family, as the parents transition to primary caregiver without immediate access to nursing care. Nursing interventions in the period prior to discharge focus on preventing complications and promoting newborn and family health.

Parent Teaching

Nearly every contact with the parents presents an opportunity for sharing information that can facilitate their sense of competence in newborn care. To meet the parents' need for information, the nurse who is responsible for the care of the mother and newborn should assume the primary responsibility for parent education. The nurse should teach the family all necessary caregiving methods before discharge. A checklist may be helpful to determine whether the teaching has been completed and to verify the parents' knowledge on leaving the birthing unit (**Figure 33.85** »). The nurse needs to review all areas for understanding by the mother and father, without rushing, and then take the time to resolve all of their queries. Any concerns of the parents or nurse are noted. Unless their care methods are harmful to the newborn, the parents' methods of giving care should be reinforced rather than contradicted.

Caring for newborns in the hospital setting means that the nurse will have contact with patients from a wide variety of ethnic, religious, and cultural backgrounds. The nurse needs to recognize and respect the many good ways of providing safe care and must be sensitive to the cultural beliefs and values of the family. Although it may not be possible to be conversant with all cultures, the nurse can demonstrate cultural sensitivity with both colleagues and patients as follows (Andrews et al., 2020; Spector, 2017):

- Show respect for the inherent dignity of every human being, whatever the individual's age, gender, or religion.
- Accept the rights of individuals to choose their care provider, participate in care, and refuse care.
- Acknowledge personal biases and prevent them from interfering with the delivery of quality care to individuals of other cultures.
- Recognize cultural issues and interact with patients from other cultures in culturally sensitive ways.
- Incorporate patients' and families' cultural preferences, health beliefs and behaviors, and traditional practices into the plan of care.
- Develop appropriate educational materials that address the language and cultural beliefs of parents and caregivers.
- Access culturally appropriate resources to deliver care to patients from other cultures.

Parents may be familiar with handling and caring for babies or this may be their first time interacting with a newborn. If they are new parents, the sensitive nurse gently teaches them by example and provides instructions geared to their needs and previous knowledge about the various aspects of newborn care.

The length of stay in the birthing unit for mother and baby after birth is often 72 hours or less. The challenge for the nurse is to use every opportunity to teach, guide, and support individual parents, fostering their capabilities and confidence in caring for their newborn. Including mother–baby care and home care instruction on the night shift assists with education needs for early-discharge parents.

Parent Teaching Checklist	
Check off each item once parents understand your instructions	✓
General Baby Care	
Caring for skin	
Caring for cord	
Caring for circumcision and genital area	
What to do if baby is sick	
Using a thermometer	
Using a bulb syringe	
Burping baby	
Comforting baby	
Positioning baby	
Breastfeeding	
Waiting for milk to come in	
Understanding let-down reflex	
Positioning baby for feeding	
Getting baby to latch on	
When to breastfeed	
How long to breastfeed	
Removing baby from nipple	
Understanding supply and demand	
Supplementing	
Comfort measures for sore nipples	
Comfort measures for engorgement	
Using a breast pump	
Breastfeeding after returning to work	
Bottle-feeding	
Choosing formula	
Mixing formula	
Feeding baby from a bottle	
Cleaning bottles	
Safety	
Placing baby to sleep on back	
Preventing shaken baby syndrome	
Using a car seat	
Managing pets	

Figure 33.85 » A parent teaching checklist is completed by the time of discharge.

The nurse observes how parents interact with their newborn during feeding and caregiving activities. Even during a short stay, the nurse will have opportunities to provide information and observe whether the parents are comfortable with changing diapers and with wrapping, handling, and feeding their newborn. Do both parents get involved in the newborn's care? Is the mother depending on someone else to help her at home? Does the mother give reasons (e.g., "I'm too tired," "My stitches hurt," or "I'll learn later") for not wanting to be involved in her baby's care? As the family provides care, the nurse can enhance parental confidence by giving them positive feedback. If the parents encounter problems, the nurse can express confidence in their abilities to master the new skills or information, suggest alternatives, and serve as a role model. All of these factors need to be considered when evaluating the educational needs of the parents. In addition to the learning needs of parents, cultural factors must also be considered when providing patient education. As noted in Focus on Diversity and Culture: Examples of Cultural Beliefs and Practices Regarding Baby Care, parents from different cultures have differing views on subjects such as umbilical cord care, parent–newborn contact, feeding, circumcision, and health and illness.

Several methods may be used to teach families about newborn care. Daily newborn care videos and classes are nonthreatening ways to convey general information. Individual instruction is helpful to answer specific questions or to clarify an item that may have been confusing in class. Currently, many birthing centers have 24-hour educational video channels or videos to be viewed in the mother's room on a variety of postpartum and newborn care issues.

One-to-one teaching while the nurse is in the mother's room is the most effective educational method. Individual instruction is helpful both to answer specific questions and to clarify something that the parents may have found confusing in the educational video. With shorter stays, most teaching unfortunately tends to focus on newborn feeding and immediate physical care needs of the mothers with limited anticipatory guidance provided in other areas.

» *Go to **Pearson MyLab Nursing and eText** to see Chart 20: What to Tell Parents About Newborn Care.*

General Instructions for Newborn Care

Parents who have never picked up and held a baby before may be anxious about doing it correctly. Demonstrate how to slide one hand under the baby's neck and shoulders and place the other hand under the bottom or between the legs and then gently lift the baby up. Talk about the need to support the newborn's head until the baby can do so independently, at about 3 or 4 months of age.

The nurse models and teaches safe care, including putting the newborn to sleep on the back (and not the stomach), never leaving the baby alone anywhere except in the crib, and proper use of a bulb syringe for suctioning secretions.

Focus on Diversity and Culture

Examples of Cultural Beliefs and Practices Regarding Baby Care*

Umbilical Cord

- Individuals from some Latin American cultures and some Filipinos may use an abdominal binder or bellyband to protect against dirt, injury, and umbilical hernia. They may also apply oils to the stump of the cord or tape metal to the umbilicus to ward off evil spirits (Purnell & Fenkl, 2019).
- Individuals of northern European ancestry may expect a sterile cutting of the cord at birth. They may allow the stump to air dry and discard the cord once it falls off.
- Some Latin American parents cauterize the stump with a candle flame, hot coal, or burning stick.

Parent–Newborn Contact

- Individuals of Asian ancestry may pick up the baby as soon as it cries or they may carry the baby at all times.
- Individuals of several native North American nations may use cradle boards so that the baby can be with family even during work to feel secure (Andrews et al., 2020).
- The Muslim father traditionally calls praise to Allah in the newborn's right ear after birth (Purnell & Fenkl, 2019).

Feeding

- Length of time breastfeeding may be culturally influenced. Some Guatemalan women may breastfeed a child for up to 5 years, whereas many Somali women may breastfeed until around the child's second birthday (Purnell & Fenkl, 2019).
- Individuals of Iranian heritage may breastfeed female babies longer than male babies. Many Muslim women will not breastfeed in public.
- Some Asian, Haitian, Hispanic, Eastern European, and American Indian women may delay breastfeeding because they believe colostrum is bad.
- Some Haitian mothers may believe that "strong emotions" spoil breast milk.

Circumcision

- Individuals of Muslim and Jewish ancestry practice circumcision as a religious ritual (Purnell & Fenkl, 2019).
- Many natives of Africa and Australia practice circumcision as a puberty rite.
- Male circumcision is common across diverse cultures and is seen in 37–39% of males worldwide (Morris et al., 2019).

Health and Illness

- Some individuals with Latin American cultural backgrounds may believe that touching the face or head of a baby when admiring it will ward off the "evil eye." They may also neglect to cut the baby's nails to avoid nearsightedness and, instead, put mittens on the baby's hands to prevent scratching. They also may believe that fat babies are healthy (Andrews et al., 2020).
- Some individuals of Asian heritage may not allow anyone to touch the baby's head without asking permission.
- Some Orthodox Jews believe that saying the baby's name before the formal naming ceremony will harm the baby.
- Some Asians and Haitians delay naming their babies until after the confinement month (Purnell & Fenkl, 2019).

**Note:* This information is meant only to provide examples of the behaviors that may be found within certain cultures. Not all members of a culture practice the behaviors described.

In addition to general safety and security reasons, explain that the newborn should not be left alone because newborns spit up frequently during the first day or two and that, when not under direct observation by a parent or caregiver, the newborn is safest in the crib.

Often demonstration with return demonstration is the best way for the nurse to provide parent teaching. Important activities that benefit from demonstration including bathing the newborn, cord care, and taking the newborn's temperature. Regarding cord care, teach parents to contact the HCP if the cord site:

- Develops redness, bright red bleeding, green-yellow drainage, or a bad odor
- Fails to heal within 2 to 3 days after the cord stump sloughs off.

In most settings, dry cord care is preferable to using topical antiseptics.

Nasal and Oral Suctioning

As mentioned, most newborns are obligatory nose-breathers for the first months of life. They generally maintain air passage patency by coughing or sneezing. During the first few days of life, however, the newborn has increased mucus, and gentle suctioning with a bulb syringe may be indicated. The nurse can demonstrate the use of the bulb syringe in the mouth and nose and have the parents do a return demonstration. The parents should repeat this demonstration of suctioning and cleansing the bulb before discharge so that they feel confident in performing the procedure. Care should be taken to apply only gentle suction in order to prevent nasal bleeding.

To suction the newborn, the bulb syringe is compressed before the tip is placed in the nostril. The nurse or parent must take care not to occlude the passageway. The bulb is permitted to reexpand slowly by releasing the compression on the bulb. The bulb syringe is removed from the nostril, and drainage is then compressed out of the bulb and onto a tissue. The bulb syringe may also be used in the mouth if the newborn is spitting up and unable to handle the excess secretions. The bulb is compressed, the tip of the bulb syringe is placed approximately 2.5 cm (1 in.) to one side of the newborn's mouth, and compression is released. This draws up the excess secretions. The procedure is repeated on the other side of the mouth. The roof of the mouth and the back of the throat are avoided because suction in these areas might stimulate the gag reflex. The bulb syringe should be washed in warm, soapy water and rinsed in warm water daily and as needed after use. Rinsing with a half-strength white vinegar solution followed by clear water may help to extend the useful life of the bulb syringe by inhibiting bacterial growth. A bulb syringe should always be kept near the newborn. New parents and nurses who are inexperienced with babies may fear that the baby will choke and are relieved to know how to take action if such an event occurs. They should be advised to turn the newborn's head to the side or hold the newborn with the head down as soon as there is any indication of gagging or vomiting and to use the bulb syringe as needed.

Some newborns may have transient edema of the nasal mucosa following suctioning of the airway after birth. The nurse can demonstrate the use of normal saline to loosen secretions and instruct parents in the gentle and moderate use of the bulb syringe to avoid further irritation of the mucous membranes. If parents will be using humidifiers at home, they should be instructed to follow the manufacturer's cleaning instructions carefully so that molds, spores, and bacteria from a dirty humidifier do not enter the baby's environment.

SAFETY ALERT If parents use humidifiers at home, the nurse should remind them to follow the manufacturer's instructions for cleaning the humidifier. This will prevent molds and bacteria from accumulating in the device and being aerosolized into the newborn's environment.

Sleep and Activity

Current recommendations from the American Academy of Pediatrics are to place healthy term newborns to sleep on their backs (American Academy of Family Physicians, 2017; Task Force on Sudden Infant Death Syndrome, 2016). The nurse provides "Safe to Sleep Guidelines" to reduce the newborn's risk for SIDS. Nurses must model placing newborns to sleep on their backs to help reinforce the behavior for parents. If exceptions are to be made, the nurse should explain the reasons for the exceptions to ensure parents understand them and do not misinterpret exceptions as regular practice. For more information, see Exemplar 15.F, Sudden Unexpected Infant Death, in Module 15, Oxygenation.

Just as infants are placed on their backs to sleep, they should be placed on their stomachs when awake and ready for play. Supervised "tummy time" helps prevent the baby's head from developing a flat spot (plagiocephaly), and it helps promote the development of motor skills such as sitting up and rolling over. Although there are no specific recommendations for how long or how often parents should engage a baby in "tummy time," they can start with just a few minutes at a time and gradually increase the time as the newborn becomes more comfortable (Hoecker, n.d.; Safe to Sleep, n.d.).

In addition to teaching parents about safe sleeping and the importance of tummy time, the nurse assists the parents to begin to recognize their own baby's cues related to sleep and activity.

>> **Stay Current:** Visit the Safe to Sleep website at https://www.nichd.nih.gov/sts/Pages/default.aspx to learn current recommendations for safe sleeping.

Car Safety

Newborns must go home from the hospital or birthing center in an age-appropriate, rear-facing car seat properly secured in the back seat of the car. The back seat is used to prevent injuries from the passenger-side airbag, which may inflate in the front seat in the event of an accident. The nurse can encourage parents to have their car seat checked prior to discharge to make sure it is properly installed. Local fire departments and law enforcement agencies often offer this service free of charge, but detailed instructions and videos are available through the National Highway Transportation Safety Association.

>> **Stay Current:** Visit https://www.nhtsa.gov/parents-and-caregivers to learn how select car seats appropriate to a child's age and how to install car seats properly.

Newborn Screenings and Immunizations

Newborn screenings are completed to identify disorders that can affect life or long-term health prior to them becoming symptomatic. Before the newborn and mother are discharged from the birthing unit, the nurse informs the parents about the newborn screening tests and tells them when to return to their HCP if further tests are needed. Some of the disorders that can be identified from a few drops of blood obtained by a heelstick are cystic fibrosis (see Exemplar 15.D, Cystic Fibrosis, in Module 15, Oxygenation), galactosemia, congenital adrenal hyperplasia, congenital hypothyroidism, maple syrup urine disease, PKU, sickle cell trait (see Exemplar 2.H, Sickle Cell Disease, in Module 2, Cellular Regulation), biotinidase deficiency, and hemoglobinopathies.

Early discharge has affected both the timing of newborn metabolic screening tests and the acquisition of subsequent immunization. Early newborn discharge increases the risk for a delayed or even missed diagnosis of PKU and congenital hypothyroidism because of decreased sensitivity of screening before 24 hours of age. Newborns should be retested by 2 weeks of age if the first test was done before 24 hours of age.

New technology is quickly increasing the number of metabolic and other disorders that can be detected in the newborn period. The Recommended Uniform Screening Panel (RUSP) is a national guideline developed for newborn screening recommendations. The Advisory Committee on Heritable Disorders in Newborn and Children (ACHDNC) makes the decision on which conditions make up the RUSP. The ACHDNC recommends that newborn screening for 35 core disorders and 26 secondary disorders. In most states, newborn screening programs lead to the detection of several conditions before symptoms develop. Each state makes its own decision on what tests are included in the newborn screening (U.S. Department of Health and Human Services, 2020).

Hearing screenings before discharge are now conducted in all 50 states. Hearing loss is found in 1 to 3 per 1000 babies in the normal newborn population (CDC, 2015b). The recommended initial newborn hearing screening should be accomplished before discharge from the birthing unit with appropriate follow-up if the newborn fails to pass the initial screen in all hospitals providing obstetric services (**Figure 33.86** ⟫).

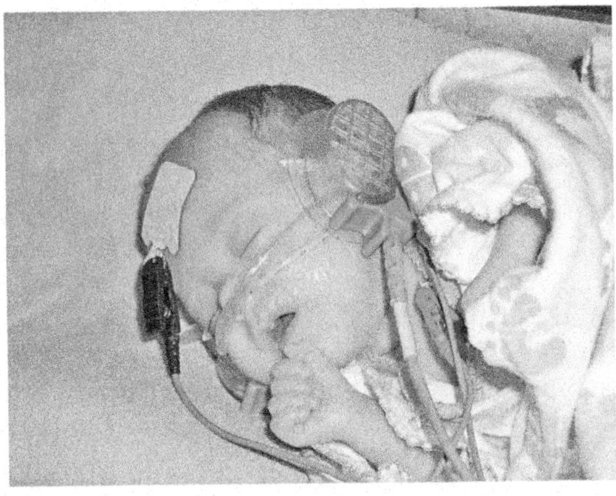

Figure 33.86 ⟫ Newborn hearing screen.
Source: Vanessa Howell, RN, MSN.

Sometimes, newborns fail to pass these tests for reasons other than hearing loss. Amniotic fluid in the ear canals is a frequent cause of suboptimal test results. In these cases, babies are retested in a week or two. The current goal is to screen all babies by 1 month of age, confirm hearing loss with audiologic examination by 3 months of age, and treat with comprehensive early intervention services (CDC, 2020e). Typically, screening programs use a two-stage screening approach (autoacoustic emissions [OAE] repeated twice, OAE followed by auditory brainstem response [ABR], or automated ABR repeated twice). Families need to be educated about appropriate interpretation of screening test results and appropriate steps for follow-up (CDC, 2020e).

The critical congenital heart disease screening is another test completed in the hospital prior to discharge. Pulse oximetry screening is used for early identification of congenital heart disease in the newborn. The screening is typically completed around 24 hours of age and involves obtaining a preductal oxygen saturation (right wrist) and a postductal oxygen saturation (either foot). A passing screen includes an oxygen saturation above 95% in both the right hand and lower extremity, with no more than 3% difference between the hand and foot measurements (Martin et al., 2020).

The most current recommendations state that a passing screen results in providing normal newborn care. A retest is ordered if the obtained oxygen saturation is 90–94% in either the right hand or foot, or a 4% or greater difference exists between the right hand and extremity measurement. The retest should be repeated within an hour of the first measurements. If the rescreen results in the same nonpassing oxygen saturations, the newborn should be referred for immediate assessment. A failed test occurs when an oxygen saturation of 89% or lower is obtained in either the right hand or the lower extremity. A failed screen results in referral for immediate assessment. It is very important to educate families regarding the reason for the screening as well as inform them regarding its results (Martin et al., 2020).

Immunization programs against the hepatitis B virus during the newborn period and infancy are in place in many U.S. states, in at least 20 countries, and in high-incidence areas such as American Samoa. Universal vaccination of newborns and infants is recommended. The most current recommendations are that newborns receive their first dose at birth, the second dose between 1 and 2 months, and the third dose between 6 and 18 months of age. For the newborn who does not receive a birth dose, the hepatitis B series should be started as soon as possible (CDC, 2020d).

⟫ **Stay Current:** Find up-to-date immunization schedules for children from birth to 6 years in English and Spanish at the CDC website at www.cdc.gov/vaccines/schedules/easy-to-read/child.html.

Community-Based Nursing Care

The nurse assists the parents in establishing a relationship with their primary HCP, emphasizing the need to understand how to communicate most efficiently when questions arise and providing patient education related to:

- Recognizing signs of illness and when to call the pediatrician's office

- Contact information for the pediatrician and the nursery unit
- How to reach the pediatrician after hours
- Follow-up care after discharge
- Safe use of OTC medications
- Importance of routine well-baby visits.

In some communities, follow-up postpartum or newborn home visits are available, especially for families discharged within 48 hours after birth. Nursing interventions during home visits include assessing newborn weight, determining how feeding is going, and assessing for hyperbilirubinemia. The nurse also assesses parents' knowledge of newborn care and may assist in helping the family establish follow-up appointments or facilitate referrals (e.g., for a lactation consultant to come to the home). If the nurse notes any signs of maternal depression, the nurse should initiate screening for postpartum depression.

Evaluation

When evaluating the nursing care provided during the period immediately after birth, the nurse may anticipate the following outcomes:

- The newborn's adaptation to extrauterine life is successful, as demonstrated by all vital signs being within acceptable parameters.
- The newborn's physiologic and psychologic integrity is supported.
- Positive interactions between parent and newborn are supported.

When evaluating the nursing care provided during the newborn period, the nurse may anticipate the following outcomes:

- The newborn's physiologic and psychologic integrity is supported by maintaining stable vital signs and interactions based on normal newborn behaviors.
- The newborn feeding pattern has been satisfactorily established.
- The parents express understanding of the bonding process and display attachment behaviors.

When evaluating the nursing care provided in preparation for discharge, the nurse may anticipate the following outcomes:

- The parents demonstrate safe techniques in caring for their newborn.
- The parents verbalize developmentally appropriate behavioral expectations of their newborn and knowledge of community-based newborn follow-up care.

Conducting additional care evaluation determines if further care is needed based on newborn outcomes. If the outcomes are not met, the nurse may choose to continue or revise the plan of care for optimal outcome attainment. Continuation, revision, or discontinuation of a plan of care is decided through the collaboration of all members of the healthcare team.

As noted in the Nursing Care Plan: A Small-for-Gestational-Age Newborn, focused assessments include weight, thermoregulation, perfusion, and metabolism. Because these concepts are closely interrelated, an alteration in one may lead to alterations in others. Accurate assessment and identification of priority diagnoses allow for prompt intervention and improved patient outcomes.

Nursing Care Plan

A Small-for-Gestational-Age Newborn

Ellen, a term baby, was born 8 hours ago weighing 2500 g at 40 weeks of gestation. Two hours after birth, Ellen's temperature was 37.1°C (98.8°F) under the radiant warmer. She was swaddled and placed in an open crib. One hour later, Ellen is returned to the radiant warmer with a falling temperature reading of 36.1°C (97°F). Acrocyanosis has also been detected. The glucose level is 35 mg/dL. The nurse monitors the newborn for signs of hypothermia and hypoglycemia.

ASSESSMENT	DIAGNOSES	PLANNING
Subjective: Alert and active. Objective: 40 weeks of gestation; birth weight, 2500 g; length, 48.3 cm (19 in.); head circumference, 30 cm (11.8 in.); chest circumference, 28 cm (11 in.); temperature, 36.1°C (97°F) axillary; pulse, 140 beats/min; respirations, 45 breaths/min; vigorous cry, alert, and wide-eyed; dry skin; thin, meconium-stained umbilical cord; glucose, 35 mg/dL; and tremors.	■ Hypothermia related to decrease in subcutaneous fat tissue and increased body surface exposure to environment ■ Undernutrition related to increased glucose consumption secondary to metabolic effects of hypothermia and poor hepatic glycogen stores ■ Risk of injury related to hypoglycemia secondary to the metabolic effects of hypothermia and poor hepatic glycogen stores	■ The newborn will maintain stable body temperature within normal range of 36.5–37.4°C (97.7–99.4°F) in an open crib. ■ The newborn will not exhibit signs of acrocyanosis, mottling, or lethargy. ■ The newborn will maintain a glucose level above 40 mg/dL. ■ The newborn's weight will remain stable. ■ The newborn will not exhibit any unusual jitteriness or tremors.

IMPLEMENTATION

- Monitor axillary temperature every 4 hours and prn.
- Monitor pulse and respirations every 4 hours and prn.
- Assess skin color and temperature every 15 to 30 minutes in presence of color change.
- Place newborn skin-to-skin with mother for mild hypothermia if the baby is stable and the parent is willing. If ineffective, place newborn under radiant warmer if temperature falls below 36.5°C (97.7°F).

Nursing Care Plan *(continued)*

- Place newborn in incubator if temperature is unstable.
- Initiate feeding schedule for SGA newborns after screening blood glucose and for symptoms of hypoglycemia (per hospital policy).
- Provide glucose via enteral feeding and/or by IV per HCP order.
- Monitor glucose levels every 4 hours per SGA protocol. Report values below 40 mg/dL or per protocol.
- Monitor for and report signs of hypoglycemia.
- Maintain an NTE.

EVALUATION

- The newborn's temperature remains between 36.5 and 37.4°C (97.7 and 99.5°F) in an open crib.
- The skin is pink in color, with no signs of acrocyanosis or mottling.
- Glucose level remains within acceptable limits per hospital policy.
- The newborn's weight is stabilized.
- No signs of jitteriness or tremors are present.

CRITICAL THINKING

1. What can the nurse do to prevent heat loss through convection when preparing the newborn for the open crib?
2. What measure can the nurse take to reduce heat loss through evaporation and conduction? How many calories can a SGA newborn lose through radiation?
3. Parents of an SGA newborn ask the nurse when they should expect their baby to catch up in weight to normal-growth newborns. What is the nurse's best response?

Source: Adapted from London et al. (2017).

REVIEW Newborn Care

RELATE Link the Concepts and Exemplars

Linking the exemplar of newborn care with the concept of stress and coping:

1. What stressors does a newborn place on the family?
2. What assessment findings might you anticipate in a family that is not coping appropriately with the stress brought on by caring for their newborn? What actions might the nurse take to improve coping strategies?

Linking the exemplar of newborn care with the concept of immunity:

3. What recommendations would you make to the parents during discharge teaching related to their newborn's immune system?
4. While planning for discharge from the hospital, the mother of a newborn asks you, "What vaccinations does my baby need first?" How would you respond to this question?

READY Go to Volume 3: Clinical Nursing Skills

REFER Go to Pearson MyLab Nursing and eText

- Chart 15: Fetal and Neonatal Circulation
- Chart 16: Potential Birth Injuries
- Chart 17: Congenital Anomalies: Identification and Care in the Newborn Period
- Chart 18: Comparison of Cephalohematoma and Caput Succedaneum
- Chart 19: Promoting Attachment
- Chart 20: What to Tell Parents About Newborn Care

REFLECT Apply Your Knowledge

Maria and Carlos Ramirez are preparing to take their newborn daughter home. They have three other daughters, ages 7 years, 3 years, and 2 years. Mrs. Ramirez tells you that the middle child was very jealous when she brought the 2-year-old home from the hospital and is worried about how the children will respond to this new baby.

1. Mrs. Ramirez says she would like to breastfeed the baby but wonders if that will increase the sibling rivalry among her other children. How would you respond to this concern?
2. What strategies might you recommend to Mrs. Ramirez to reduce sibling rivalry when introducing the new baby to the family?
3. Mr. Ramirez shares with you, while Mrs. Ramirez is out of the room, that he had really hoped this new baby would be a boy. What assessment questions might you ask of this father?

» Exemplar 33.E Prematurity

Exemplar Learning Outcomes

33.E Summarize care of premature newborns.

- Describe the physiology and risk factors of the premature newborn.
- Summarize alterations found in premature newborns.
- Describe the nursing process in assessing the premature newborn and implementing culturally competent care to the premature newborn and family.

Exemplar Key Terms

Apnea of prematurity, *2432*
Minimal enteral nutrition, *2430*
Preterm newborn, *2427*

Overview

A **preterm newborn** is a baby born before 37 completed weeks of gestation. The World Health Organization identifies three categories of prematurity: extremely preterm (less than 28 weeks); very preterm (28 to 32 weeks); and moderate to late preterm (32 to 37 weeks). Worldwide, preterm birth complications are the leading cause of death among children under 5 years of age (WHO, 2018b). In the United States, the incidence of preterm births decreased between 2007 and 2014, in part due to declining birthrates among teens and young women. However, after 2014 preterm birthrates rose for the next three years, with preterm birthrates for African American women almost 50% higher than rates for white women (CDC, 2019b). Babies born early are at risk of developing a number of complications, ranging from apnea and respiratory distress to hemorrhage and infection. Preterm babies are at higher risk for disability and even death, with low birth weight associated with about 17% of infant deaths (CDC, 2019b) (**Figure 33.87** »).

The Preterm Newborn

Care of the preterm newborn encompasses the considerations for a healthy term newborn, with additional considerations to the challenges related to the immaturity of the newborn's systems. The degree of severity and variability depends on the length of gestation. The preterm newborn must make the same transitions to extrauterine life as the term newborn but is less prepared physiologically to do so. Specific physiologic parameters provide the focus for care of the preterm newborn (see Exemplar 33.D, Newborn Care, in this module).

Respiratory and Cardiac Physiology

The preterm newborn is at risk for respiratory problems because the lungs are not fully mature and ready to take over the process of oxygen and carbon dioxide exchange without assistance. Critical factors in the development of respiratory distress include the following:

- ***The preterm neonate is unable to produce adequate amounts of surfactant.*** Inadequate surfactant lessens compliance (ability of the lung to fill with air easily), thereby increasing the inspiratory pressure needed to expand the lungs with air. The collapsed (or atelectatic) alveoli will not facilitate an exchange of oxygen and carbon dioxide. As a result, the neonate becomes hypoxic, pulmonary blood flow is inefficient, and the preterm newborn's available energy is depleted. Surfactant may be given during initial resuscitation.
- ***The muscular coat of pulmonary blood vessels is incompletely developed.*** As a result, the pulmonary arterioles do not constrict well in response to decreased oxygen levels. This lowered pulmonary vascular resistance leads to left-to-right shunting of blood through the ductus arteriosus, which increases the blood flow back into the lungs.
- ***The ductus arteriosus of the preterm neonate, who is more susceptible to hypoxia, may respond to increasing oxygen and prostaglandin E levels by remaining open rather than by vasoconstriction, which is how the ductus responds in the term neonate.*** A patent ductus increases the blood volume to the lungs, causing pulmonary congestion, increased respiratory effort, carbon dioxide retention, and bounding femoral pulses.

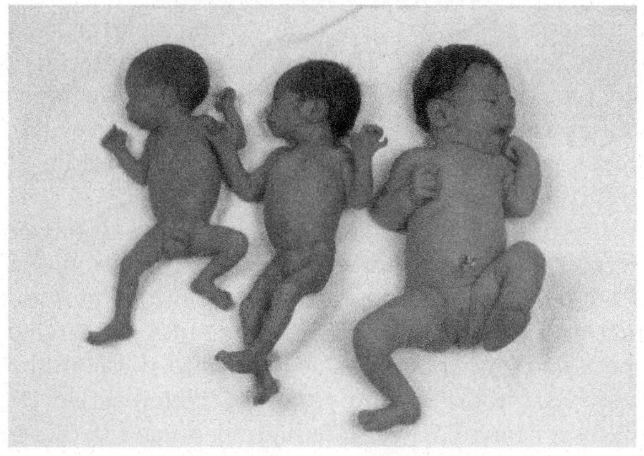

Figure 33.87 » *From left to right:* A 4-week-old neonate who was born 9 weeks prematurely, a 2-week-old neonate who weighed 1200 g at birth, and a full-term neonate, 2 days old, who weighed 3730 g at birth.
Source: Pearson Education, Inc.

Thermoregulation

Heat loss is a major problem in premature newborns. Two factors limiting heat production are the availability of glycogen in the liver and the amount of brown fat available for heat production. Both of these limiting factors appear in the third trimester. In the cold-stressed baby, norepinephrine is released, which in turn stimulates the metabolism of brown fat for heat production. As a complicating factor, the hypoxic newborn cannot increase oxygen consumption in response to cold stress because of the already limited reserves; as a result, the hypoxic newborn becomes progressively colder. Preterm neonates have smaller muscle mass and diminished muscular activity, rendering them unable to shiver and further limiting heat production.

There are five physiologic and anatomic factors that increase heat loss in the preterm neonate.

1. ***The preterm newborn has a higher ratio of body surface to body weight.*** This means that the baby's ability to produce heat (based on body weight) is much less than the potential for losing heat (based on surface area). The loss of heat in a preterm neonate weighing 1500 g is five times greater per unit of body weight than that of an adult.
2. ***The preterm newborn has very little subcutaneous fat, which is the human body's insulation.*** Without adequate insulation, heat is easily conducted from the core of the body (warmer temperature) to the surface of the body (cooler temperature). Heat is lost from the body as the blood vessels, which lie close to the skin surface in the preterm neonate, transport blood from the body core to the subcutaneous tissues.
3. ***The preterm newborn has thinner, more permeable skin than the term neonate.*** This increased permeability contributes to a greater insensible water loss as well as to heat loss.
4. ***The posture of the preterm newborn influences heat loss.*** Flexion of the extremities decreases the amount

of surface area exposed to the environment. Extension increases the surface area exposed to the environment and thus increases heat loss. The gestational age of the neonate influences the amount of flexion, from completely hypotonic and extended at 28 weeks to stronger flexion at 35 weeks and full flexion of all extremities at term.

5. ***The premature newborn has a decreased ability to vasoconstrict superficial blood vessels and conserve heat in the body core.*** This lack of vasoconstriction allows heat to leave the premature neonate's body at a fast rate, thus leading to cold stress.

Thermoregulation is discussed more completely in Module 20. The essential point regarding thermoregulation of the premature neonate is this: Gestational age is directly proportional to the ability to maintain thermoregulation; thus, the more preterm the newborn, the less able the neonate is to maintain heat balance.

The nurse can do much to prevent heat loss by providing an NTE. This is one of the most important considerations in nursing management of the preterm neonate (see Maintain a Neutral Thermal Environment section later in this exemplar). Cold stress, with its accompanying severe complications, can be prevented.

Gastrointestinal Physiology

The basic structure of the GI tract is formed early in gestation. The maturation of the digestive and absorptive process is more variable, however, and occurs later in gestation. As a result of GI immaturity, the preterm newborn has the following ingestion, digestive, and absorption problems:

- A marked danger of aspiration and its associated complications because of the premature neonate's poorly developed gag reflex, incompetent esophageal cardiac sphincter, and poor sucking and swallowing reflexes. The ability to coordinate sucking, swallowing, and breathing is not established until 32 to 34 weeks' gestation.
- Difficulty in meeting high caloric and fluid needs for growth because of small stomach capacity.
- Limited ability to convert certain essential amino acids to nonessential amino acids. Some amino acids, such as histidine, taurine, and cysteine, are essential to the preterm neonate but not to the term neonate.
- Kidney immaturity requires careful consideration regarding increased osmolarity when choosing a formula protein. There are a variety of commercial options specifically designed with this in mind.
- Difficulty absorbing saturated fats because of decreased bile salts and pancreatic lipase. Severe illness of the newborn may also prevent intake of adequate nutrients.
- Initial difficulty with lactose digestion because processes may not be fully functional during the first few days of a preterm neonate's life. The preterm newborn can digest and absorb most simple sugars.
- Deficiency of calcium and phosphorus may exist because two-thirds of these minerals are deposited in the last trimester. This can lead to rickets and significant bone demineralization.
- Activity intolerance—preterm newborns are easily fatigued by simple activities such as sucking.
- Feeding intolerance and necrotizing enterocolitis as a result of diminished blood flow and tissue perfusion to the intestinal tract because of prolonged hypoxia and hypoxemia at birth.

Renal Physiology

The kidneys of the premature neonate are immature compared with those of the full-term neonate, posing clinical problems in the management of fluid and electrolyte balance. Specific renal characteristics of the preterm neonate include the following:

- The GFR is lower because of decreased renal blood flow. The GFR is directly related to lower gestational age, so the more preterm the newborn, the lower the GFR. The GFR is also decreased in the presence of diseases or conditions that decrease renal blood flow and perfusion, such as severe respiratory distress, hypotension, and asphyxia. Anuria and oliguria may also be observed.
- The kidneys of the preterm neonate begin excreting glucose (glycosuria) at a lower serum glucose level than those of the term newborn. Glycosuria with hyperglycemia can lead to osmotic diuresis and polyuria.
- The buffering capacity of the kidney is reduced, predisposing the neonate to metabolic acidosis. Bicarbonate is excreted at a lower serum level, and acid is excreted more slowly. Therefore, after periods of hypoxia or insult, the preterm neonate's kidneys require a longer time to excrete the lactic acid that accumulates. Sodium bicarbonate is frequently required to treat metabolic acidosis in the premature neonate.
- The immaturity of the renal system affects the preterm neonate's ability to excrete drugs. Because excretion time is longer, many drugs are given over longer intervals (i.e., every 24 hours instead of every 12 hours). Urine output must be carefully monitored when the neonate is receiving nephrotoxic drugs, such as gentamicin and vancomycin. If urine output is poor, drugs can become toxic much more quickly in the neonate than in the adult.

Immunologic Physiology

The preterm neonate is at much greater risk for infection than the term neonate. This increased susceptibility may be the result of an infection acquired in utero, which may have precipitated preterm labor and birth. However, all preterm neonates have immature specific and nonspecific immunity.

In utero, the fetus receives passive immunity against a variety of infections from maternal IgG immunoglobulins, which cross the placenta. Because most of this immunity is acquired in the last trimester of pregnancy, the premature neonate has few antibodies at birth, and these antibodies provide less protection and become depleted earlier than in a full-term neonate. The limited number of antibodies in the preterm neonate may be a contributing factor in the higher incidence of recurrent infection during the first year of life as well as in the immediate neonatal period.

As with term newborns, IgA is a significant immunoglobulin. The secretory IgA in breast milk protects the baby from enteric infections such as those caused by *Escherichia coli* and *Shigella*.

Another altered defense against infection in the preterm neonate is the skin surface. In very small neonates, the skin is easily excoriated, and this factor, coupled with many invasive procedures, places the neonate at great risk for healthcare-associated infections. It is vital to use good hand hygiene in the care of these neonates in order to prevent unnecessary infection.

SAFETY ALERT The sudden onset of apnea and bradycardia, coupled with metabolic acidosis or temperature instability in an otherwise healthy, growing premature neonate, may be suggestive of bacterial sepsis, especially if an invasive device, such as a central line or endotracheal tube, is in place.

Neurologic Physiology

The period of most rapid brain growth and development occurs during the third trimester of pregnancy; therefore, the closer to term a neonate is born, the better the neurologic prognosis. A common interruption of neurologic development in the preterm neonate is caused by intraventricular hemorrhage and intracranial hemorrhage. Hydrocephalus may develop as a consequence of an intraventricular hemorrhage caused by the obstruction at the cerebral aqueduct.

Reactivity and Behavioral States

The neonate's response to extrauterine life is characterized by two periods of reactivity. The preterm neonate's periods of reactivity, however, are delayed. In the very ill neonate, these periods of reactivity may not be observed at all because the neonate may be hypotonic and unreactive for several days after birth.

As the preterm newborn grows and the baby's condition stabilizes, identifying behavioral states and traits unique to each baby becomes increasingly possible. In general, stable preterm neonates do not demonstrate the same behavioral states as term neonates. Preterm neonates tend to be more disorganized in their sleep–wake cycles and are unable to attend as well to the human face and objects in the environment. Neurologically, their responses (sucking, muscle tone, and states of arousal) are weaker than those of full-term neonates.

By observing each neonate's patterns of behavior and responses, especially the sleep–wake states, the parents and nurse can plan nursing care around the times when the neonate is alert and best able to attend. In addition, the more knowledge parents have about the meaning of their newborn's responses and behaviors, the better prepared they will be to meet their newborn's needs and to form a positive attachment with their child. (See the Promote Developmentally Supportive Care section later in this exemplar.)

Nutrition and Fluid Requirements

For most newborns, initiating enteral feedings as soon as possible helps maintain normal metabolism and reduces the potential for complications such as hypoglycemia and hyperbilirubinemia. However, the immaturity of the preterm newborn's digestive system creates risk for complications related to feeding. The nurse should confirm that the newborn tolerates enteral feedings before encouraging the mother to feed her newborn. If signs of feeding intolerance or illness develop, feedings should be reassessed.

Nutrition Requirements

Oral (enteral) caloric intake necessary for growth in a healthy preterm newborn is 95 to 130 kcal/kg per day (Blackburn, 2018). In addition to these relatively high caloric needs, the preterm neonate requires more protein than the full-term neonate. To meet these needs, many institutions use breast milk fortifier or special preterm formulas.

Whether breast milk or formula is used, feeding regimens are established on the basis of the neonate's weight and estimated stomach capacity. Initial formula feedings are gradually increased as the neonate tolerates them. It may be necessary to supplement oral feedings with parenteral fluids to maintain adequate hydration and caloric intake until the baby is on full oral feedings. Preterm neonates who cannot tolerate any oral (enteral) feedings are given nutrition by total parenteral nutrition (TPN).

In addition to a higher calorie and protein formula, preterm neonates should receive supplemental multivitamins, including vitamins A, D, and E, as well as iron and trace minerals. A diet high in polyunsaturated fats, which preterm neonates tolerate best, increases the requirement for vitamin E. Preterm neonates who are fed iron-fortified formulas have higher red cell hemolysis and lower vitamin E concentrations and thus require additional vitamin E. Preterm formulas also need to contain medium-chain triglycerides and additional amino acids, such as cysteine, as well as calcium, phosphorus, and vitamin D supplements to increase mineralization of bones. Rickets and significant bone demineralization have been documented in very-low-birth-weight neonates and otherwise healthy preterm neonates.

Whether breast milk or formula is used, feeding protocols are established based on the baby's weight and estimated stomach capacity. Nutritional intake is considered to be adequate when there is consistent weight gain of 20 to 30 g/day, although for smaller premature newborns (24 weeks), it may be as little as 5 g/day (MedlinePlus, 2021a). Initially, no weight gain may be noted for several days, but total weight loss should not exceed 15% of the total birth weight or more than 1–2% per day. Some institutions add the criteria of head circumference growth and increase in body length of 1 cm (0.4 in.) per week once the newborn is stable.

Methods of Feeding

Bottle, breast, and gavage are common methods of feeding the preterm newborn. The newborn's gestational age, neurologic status, and overall health and physical status determine the method of feeding. Some preterm newborns may need TPN, at least in the beginning.

Bottle Feeding

Preterm neonates who have a coordinated and rhythmic suck–swallow–breathing pattern are usually between 32 and 34 weeks of postconceptual age and may be fed by bottle. Oral readiness to feed is best described by the following engagement and hunger cues: bringing hands to mouth, being alert, exhibiting fussiness, sucking on fingers or pacifier, exhibiting rooting behavior, and showing relaxed facial expression and good tone (Lubbe, 2018).

Those premature neonates who root when their cheek is stroked and actively search for the nipple are neurodevelopmentally ready to initiate oral feeding (**Figure 33.88** »).

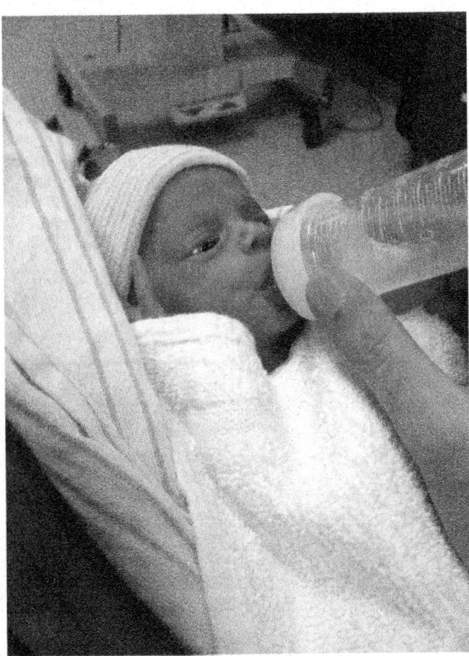

Figure 33.88 » Mother bottle-feeding her premature newborn with expressed breast milk.

Source: Carol Harrigan, RN, MSN, NNP-BC.

To avoid excessive expenditure of energy, a soft, single-hole nipple is generally used (milk flow is less rapid). The neonate is fed in an appropriate position and burped gently after each 0.5 to 1 oz. The feeding should take no longer than 30 minutes (nippling requires more energy than other methods). Premature neonates who are progressing from gavage feedings to bottle feeding should start with one session of bottle feeding a day and have the number of times per day a bottle is given slowly increase until the baby tolerates all feedings from a bottle.

In assessing the premature neonate's readiness for feeding, the nurse assesses the neonate's ability to suck. Sucking may be affected by age, asphyxia, sepsis, intraventricular hemorrhage, or other neurologic insult. Before initiating nipple feeding, the nurse observes for signs of stress, such as tachypnea (>60 respirations/min), respiratory distress, or hypothermia, which may increase the risk of aspiration. During the feeding, the nurse observes the neonate for signs of feeding difficulty (tachypnea, cyanosis, bradycardia, lethargy, or uncoordinated suck and swallow). Difficulty in bottle feeding is often associated with a milk bolus that is too large for the neonate's oral cavity, which can lead to aspiration. Demand feeding protocols, based on the neonate's hunger cues, should be considered for a growing premature neonate only when there is sufficient caloric intake to promote consistent weight gain (Lubbe, 2018; WHO, 2019a).

Breastfeeding

Mothers who wish to breastfeed their preterm neonates are given the opportunity to put the baby to the breast as soon as the baby has demonstrated a coordinated suck-and-swallow reflex. Preterm neonates tolerate breastfeeding with higher oxygen saturation and better maintenance of body temperature than during bottle feeding. Besides breast milk's many benefits for the neonate, breastfeeding allows the mother to contribute actively to the baby's well-being. The nurse should encourage and support mothers to breastfeed if they choose to do so. Even if the neonate cannot be put to the breast, mothers can pump breast milk, which can be given via bottle or gavage. Use of the double-pumping system produces higher levels of prolactin than are obtained using sequential pumping of the breasts.

By initiating skin-to-skin holding of premature neonates in the early intensive care phase, mothers can significantly increase milk volume, thereby overcoming lactation problems (Coşkun & Günay, 2020; Moghadam & Ganji, 2019). The neonate is placed at the mother's breast. It has been suggested that the football hold is a convenient position for breastfeeding preterm babies. Feeding may take up to 30 minutes, and babies should be burped as they alternate breasts. The length of feeding time is monitored so that the preterm neonate does not burn too many calories.

The nurse should coordinate a flexible feeding schedule so that babies can nurse during alert times and be allowed to set their own pace. Feedings should be on demand, but a maximum number of hours between feedings should be set. A similar regimen should be used for the baby who is progressing from gavage feeding to breastfeeding. The mother begins with one feeding at the breast and then gradually increases the number of times during the day that the baby breastfeeds. When breastfeeding is not possible because the neonate is too small or too weak to suck at the breast, an option for the mother may be to express her breast milk into a cup. The milk touches the neonate's lips and is lapped by the protruding motions of the tongue. Include a lactation consultant in such cases, where available.

SAFETY ALERT For an otherwise healthy, growing premature neonate who is receiving enteral intake and who has started to experience apnea and bradycardia, one differential diagnosis to think about is reflux rather than sepsis, although sepsis may need to be ruled out.

Gavage Feeding

The gavage feeding method is used with preterm neonates (32 to 34 weeks of gestation) who lack or have a poorly coordinated suck-and-swallow reflex or who are ill and ventilator dependent. Gavage feeding may be used as an adjunct to nipple feeding if the neonate tires easily. It may also be used as an alternative if a neonate is losing weight because of the energy expenditure required for nippling.

Gavage feedings are administered by either the nasogastric or orogastric route and by intermittent bolus or continuous drip method. Bolus feedings may be preferred because these are thought to be more like natural feedings. In common practice, bolus feedings are usually initiated, but if intolerance occurs, then the feedings are changed to continuous or to infuse on a pump over a set amount of time.

Early initiation of **minimal enteral nutrition** via gavage is now advocated as a supplement to parenteral nutrition. Minimal enteral nutrition refers to small-volume feedings of formula or human milk (usually < 24 mL/kg per day), which are designed to "prime" the premature neonate's intestinal tract, thereby stimulating many of its hormonal and enzymatic functions (Parker, 2021). Benefits of early feeding (as early as within the first 24–72 hours of life) include the following (Kumar et al., 2017):

- No increased incidence of necrotizing enterocolitis
- Fewer days on TPN, thereby decreasing the incidence of cholestatic jaundice

- Increased weight gain
- Shorter time required to reach full-volume enteral feedings
- Increased muscle maturation of the GI function, which can lead to improved feeding tolerance
- Lower risk of osteopenia
- Possible decrease in the total number of hospital days in the NICU.

SAFETY ALERT Orogastric gavage catheter placement is preferable to nasogastric because most neonates are obligatory nose-breathers. If nasogastric is used, the smallest available catheter should be used to minimize airway obstruction.

Total Parenteral Nutrition

When the neonate cannot be fed through the GI tract, TPN is implemented. TPN provides complete nutrition via IV, using hyperalimentation to provide calories and nutrients (including protein), as well as glucose. TPN uses intralipids to ensure provision of essential fatty acids. Use of TPN requires close monitoring via blood and urine tests, as adjustments in nutrient levels may be required to prevent or respond to TPN-related complications.

Fluid Requirements

The calculation of fluid requirements must take into account the neonate's weight and postnatal age. Recommendations for fluid therapy in the preterm neonate are approximately 80 to 100 mL/kg per day for the first day, 100 to 120 mL/kg per day for the second day, and 120 to 150 mL/kg per day by the third day of life. These amounts may be increased up to 200 mL/kg per day if the baby is very small, receiving phototherapy, or under a radiant warmer because of the increased insensible water losses. Fluid losses can be minimized through the use of heat shields and added humidification in the isolette. Daily weights (and, sometimes, twice-a-day weights) are the best indicator of fluid status in the preterm neonate. The expected weight loss during the first 3 to 5 days of life in a preterm neonate is around 10% of birth weight. Premature newborns being treated for complications such as respiratory distress syndrome or patent ductus arteriosus may be on diuretics that can influence their fluid requirements and weight fluctuations.

Long-Term Needs

The care of preterm neonates and their families does not stop on discharge from the nursery. Follow-up care is extremely important: Many developmental problems are not noted until an infant is older and begins to demonstrate delays or disability.

Within the first year of life, low-birth-weight preterm babies face higher mortality rates than term babies. Causes of death include SIDS—which occurs about five times more frequently in the preterm baby than the term baby—respiratory infections, and neurologic issues. (See Exemplar 15.F, Sudden Unexpected Infant Death, in Module 15, Oxygenation.) Morbidity is also much higher among preterm babies, those weighing less than 1500 g being at the highest risk for long-term complications.

The most common long-term needs observed in preterm neonates include the following:

- ***Retinopathy of prematurity (ROP).*** Premature newborns are particularly susceptible to characteristic retinal changes, known as ROP, which can result in visual impairment. The premature newborn's retina does not have all of the blood vessels the term newborn's has. As the blood vessels fill in, they may grow abnormally, with the development of fibrous tissue that can contract and scar, resulting in retinal detachment. The disease is now viewed as multifactorial in origin. Increased survival of very-low-birth-weight babies may be the most important factor in the increased incidence of ROP. The acute stages of ROP may be treated with laser photocoagulation and cryotherapy. Most acute changes with ROP regress spontaneously with no long-term visual impairment. Consultation with an ophthalmologist during the hospital stay and after discharge is recommended.
- ***Bronchopulmonary dysplasia.*** Also known as *chronic lung disease of prematurity*. Long-term lung disease is a result of damage to the alveolar epithelium secondary to positive-pressure ventilator therapy and a high oxygen concentration. These babies have long-term dependence on oxygen therapy and an increased incidence of respiratory infection during their first few years of life.
- ***Speech delays.*** The most frequently observed speech problems involve delayed development of receptive and expressive ability that may persist into the school-age years.
- ***Neurologic deficits.*** Common etiologies of neurologic deficits include cerebral palsy, hydrocephalus, seizure disorders, lower IQ, attention-deficit/hyperactivity disorder, and learning disabilities. (See Exemplar 25.C, Cerebral Palsy, in Module 25, Development.) In the absence of major neurologic disorders, the socioeconomic climate and family support systems are extremely important influences on the child's eventual school performance. Families should be reminded that risk does not equal injury, injury does not equal damage, and description of damage does not allow a precise prediction about recovery or outcome.
- ***Auditory deficits.*** Preterm babies have a 1–4% incidence of moderate to profound hearing loss and should have a formal audiologic exam before discharge and at 3 to 6 months (corrected age). Tests currently used to measure hearing functions of the newborn are the evoked otoacoustic emissions or the automated auditory brain response test. This is especially important for preterm infants who have received ototoxic drugs. Any baby with repeated abnormal results should be referred to speech-language specialists.

When assessing the baby's abilities and disabilities, parents must understand that developmental progress must be evaluated on the basis of chronologic age from the expected date of birth, not from the actual date of birth (corrected age). In addition, the parents need the consistent support of healthcare professionals in the long-term management of their child. Many new and ongoing concerns arise as the former premature neonate grows and develops; the goal is to promote the highest quality of life possible.

Many hospitals and NICUs provide referrals for parents of premature babies to local child health service coordination and early intervention service programs. Early intervention services for newborns, infants, and toddlers are mandated under Part C of the Individuals with Disabilities in Education Act. Nurses working with these families, either in the NICU or hospital setting or in a pediatric setting, should be aware of their agency's referral process or know about services available in their area.

Alterations of Prematurity

The goals of medical and nursing care are to meet the preterm neonate's growth and development needs and to anticipate and manage the complications associated with prematurity. The most common alterations associated with prematurity are as follows:

1. ***Apnea of prematurity.*** **Apnea of prematurity** refers to cessation of breathing for 20 seconds or longer, or for less than 20 seconds when associated with cyanosis, pallor, and bradycardia. Apnea is a common problem in the preterm neonate less than 36 weeks' gestation, presenting between day 2 and day 7 of life. The etiology of apnea is multifactorial, but it is thought to be primarily a result of neuronal immaturity. This factor contributes to the preterm neonate's irregular breathing patterns. Other causes of apnea are obstructive apnea and gastroesophageal reflux. Obstructive apnea can occur when cessation of airflow is associated with blockage of the upper airway (resulting from a small airway diameter, increased pharyngeal secretions, or altered body alignment and positioning). Gastroesophageal reflux is defined as a movement of gastric contents into the lower esophagus caused by poor esophageal sphincter tone, in turn causing laryngospasm, which leads to bradycardia and apnea. Apnea of prematurity is then a diagnosis of exclusion and commonly treated with caffeine citrate.
2. ***Patent ductus arteriosus (PDA).*** The ductus arteriosus fails to close because of decreased pulmonary arteriole musculature and hypoxemia. Symptomatic PDA is often seen around the time when premature neonates are recovering from respiratory distress syndrome. PDA often prolongs the course of illness in a preterm newborn and leads to chronic pulmonary dysfunction.

SAFETY ALERT A growing premature neonate who is showing clinical signs of worsening respiratory status (i.e., increased oxygen needs or increased ventilatory settings), acidosis, and hypotension may be exhibiting signs and symptoms of a PDA.

3. ***Respiratory distress syndrome.*** Respiratory distress results from inadequate surfactant production.
4. ***Intraventricular hemorrhage.*** Intraventricular hemorrhage is the most common type of intracranial hemorrhage in small preterm neonates, especially those weighing less than 1500 g or those born at less than 34 weeks of gestation. Up to 34 weeks, the preterm neonate's brain ventricles are lined by the germinal matrix, which is highly susceptible to hypoxic events, such as respiratory distress, birth trauma, and birth asphyxia. The germinal matrix is highly vascular, and these blood vessels rupture in the presence of hypoxia. Hemorrhage is graded by severity on a scale of I to IV.
5. ***Anemia of prematurity.*** The preterm neonate is at risk for anemia because of the rapid rate of growth required, shorter RBC life, excessive blood sampling, decreased iron stores, and deficiency of vitamin E. The hemoglobin usually reaches its lowest level by 3 to 12 weeks and remains low for 3 to 6 months.

SAFETY ALERT An extremely premature, low-birth-weight neonate who presents with a sudden drop in hemoglobin along with the onset of severe metabolic acidosis, a "waxy" color, and hypotension may have experienced an intracranial hemorrhage.

NURSING PROCESS

Care of the premature newborn is within the scope of practice of the generalist nurse. Onboarding for new nurses and continuing education provided by the employing facility will include facility protocols and use of equipment, among other topics. Families of premature newborns are understandably anxious, making therapeutic communication a key skill when working with this patient population.

Assessment

The nurse needs to assess the physical characteristics and gestational age of the preterm newborn accurately. This allows the healthcare team to anticipate the special needs and problems of the baby.

Determining gestational age in preterm newborns requires knowledge and experience in administering gestational assessment tools. The tool used should be specific, reliable, and valid.

Physical characteristics vary greatly depending on gestational age, but the following characteristics are frequently present:

- ***Color*** is usually pink or ruddy but may show acrocyanosis. (Cyanosis, jaundice, and pallor are abnormal and should be noted.)
- ***Skin*** is reddened and translucent, blood vessels are readily apparent, and there is little subcutaneous fat.
- ***Lanugo*** is plentiful and widely distributed.
- ***Head size*** appears large in relation to the body.
- ***Skull bones*** are pliable; fontanel is smooth and flat.
- ***Ears*** have minimal cartilage and are pliable, folded over.
- ***Nails*** are soft and short.
- ***Testes*** may not be descended and scrotum nonrugated.
- ***Clitoris and labia minora*** are prominent.
- ***Resting position*** is flaccid, froglike.
- ***Cry*** is weak and feeble.
- ***Reflexes*** (sucking, swallowing, and gag) are poor.
- ***Activity*** consists of jerky, generalized movements. (Seizure activity is abnormal.)

Diagnosis

Patient care priorities will depend on a variety of factors, including the newborn's gestational age and parent/caregiver coping skills and resources. Common care issues include:

- Ineffective breathing pattern/inadequate (or imbalanced) gas exchange

- Poor thermoregulation
- Fluid volume disturbance
- Undernutrition/compromised feeding pattern
- Neonatal hyperbilirubinemia
- Potential for injury or infection
- Disturbance in growth and development pattern
- Lack of knowledge by caregiver
- Caregiver conflict or inability/compromised maternal–newborn attachment.

Planning

Important goals of nursing care for the premature neonate often include the following:

- The neonate's oxygenation and normal breathing patterns will be promoted.
- The neonate's weight gain and normal growth will be promoted.
- The neonate's developmental needs will be supported.
- The neonate's parents will be educated to provide care when discharged.
- The neonate will remain free of infection.
- The nurse will support the neonate's parents and suggest strategies to reduce parental anxiety and encourage parent attachment.

Implementation

Premature newborns have many priorities for care, including respiratory function, thermoregulation, fluid and electrolyte balance, and adequate nutrition necessary for healthy growth and development. Preventing and addressing infection and fatigue are essential, as is promoting parent–newborn attachment, providing care that supports best outcomes for growth and development, and preparing parents for care at home (**Figure 33.89** »).

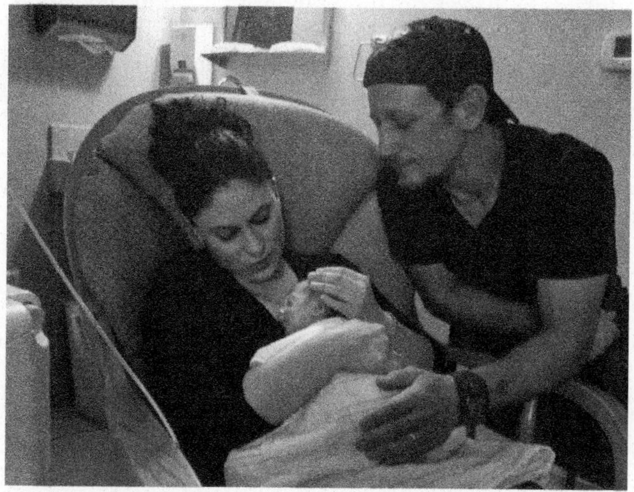

Figure 33.89 » Family bonding occurs when parents have opportunities to spend time with their premature newborn.
Source: Carol Harrigan, RN, MSN, NNP-BC.

Communicating with Parents and Families

It is important for the nurse to foster open communication with the premature newborn's parents or caregiver(s). Language should convey information but not be overly technical. When a parent expresses concern, it is helpful for the nurse to explain the plan of care, expectations for the current stage, and inform the parents about any equipment used on their child. Providing frequent updates and encouraging parent involvement promote parent confidence. Many parents experience some degree of grief and fear when their child is in the NICU environment. Helping parents to have a positive attitude and helping with ways to relate to their child can reduce these feelings. Examples include:

- Take a look at this monitor on Amanda's chest. It's giving us real-time tracking of her heart rate and rhythm, so we'll know right away if there's a problem. These monitors are fancy stickers and do not hurt her one bit.
- I can understand it looks scary seeing Jada hooked up to all these machines. I'll tell you what each of them are doing so you can better understand.
- Brayden's feeding is due in about 10 minutes. Would you like to change his diaper and get him ready?
- (Providing update) Our goal is to wean down the oxygen level, but the last time we tried to turn it down Logan's saturation dropped below his parameters. This is expected during the weaning process, and we will try again in 1 hour. I will call and update you again regarding his progress.

It is important to be encouraging, but realistic. See the sections Parent Support and Prepare for Home Care below.

Promote Respiratory Function

Premature newborns are at increased risk for respiratory obstruction because their bronchi and trachea are so narrow that mucus can obstruct the airway. The nurse must maintain patency through judicious suctioning, but only on an as-needed basis.

Positioning can also affect respiratory function. If the baby is in the supine position, the nurse should elevate the head slightly to maintain the airway, being careful to avoid hyperextension of the neck, which may cause the trachea to collapse. Also, because the newborn has weak neck muscles and cannot control head movement, place a small roll under the newborn's shoulders to maintain this head position. The prone position splints the chest wall and decreases the amount of respiratory effort used to move the chest wall, facilitating chest expansion and improving air entry and oxygenation. Weak or absent cough or gag reflexes increase the chance of aspiration in the premature newborn. The nurse should ensure that the newborn's position facilitates drainage of mucus or regurgitated formula.

SAFETY ALERT Caution must be taken to ensure prone positioning is used only when monitored closely. The nurse should clarify with the parents why prone positioning is being used and not confuse them with recommendations regarding SIDS prevention and the need for the baby to sleep supine at home.

The nurse monitors heart and respiratory rates with cardiorespiratory monitors and observes the newborn to identify alterations in cardiopulmonary status. Signs of respiratory distress include the following:

- Cyanosis (serious sign when generalized) or desaturation
- Tachypnea (sustained respiratory rate >60 breaths/min after first 4 hours of life)
- Retractions, forceful inspirations, or gasping
- Expiratory grunting
- Nasal flaring
- Apneic episodes
- Presence of rales or rhonchi on auscultation
- Diminished air entry.

If respiratory distress occurs, the nurse administers oxygen per provider orders to relieve hypoxemia. If hypoxemia is not treated immediately, it may result in PDA or metabolic acidosis. If oxygen is administered to the newborn, the nurse monitors the oxygen concentration with a pulse oximeter and blood gas analysis. Periodic arterial blood gas sampling to monitor oxygen concentration in the baby's blood is essential because hyperoxemia may lead to ROP and other complications.

The nurse also needs to consider respiratory function before and during feedings. To prevent aspiration and increased energy expenditure and oxygen consumption, the nurse must ensure that the newborn's gag and suck reflexes are intact before starting oral feedings.

Maintain a Neutral Thermal Environment

An NTE minimizes the oxygen consumption required to maintain a normal core temperature; it also prevents cold stress and facilitates growth by decreasing the calories needed to maintain body temperature. The preterm newborn's small brown fat stores and immature CNS provide poor temperature control. A small premature neonate (> 1200 g) can lose 80 kcal/kg per day through radiation of body heat. To minimize heat loss and temperature instability for preterm and low-birth-weight newborns, the nurse should do the following, which addresses all four types of heat loss:

- Monitor ambient temperature of the room where the newborn is kept.
- Allow skin-to-skin contact (*kangaroo care*) between the parents and newborn to maintain warmth and foster security.
- Warm and humidify oxygen to minimize evaporative heat loss and decrease oxygen consumption.
- Place the baby in a double-walled isolette or use a Plexiglas heat shield over small preterm neonates in single-walled isolettes, to avoid radiative heat losses. Some institutions use radiant warmers and plastic wrap over the baby and pipe in humidity (swamping). Do not use Plexiglas shields on radiant warmer beds, however, because they block the infrared heat.
- Avoid placing the baby on cold surfaces, such as metal treatment tables and cold x-ray plates (conductive heat loss). Pad cold surfaces with diapers and use radiant warmers during procedures. Place the preterm newborn on prewarmed mattresses and warm hands before handling the baby to prevent heat transfer via conduction.
- Use warmed ambient humidity. Humidity can decrease insensible and transdermal water loss, especially in very-low-birth-weight newborns.
- Keep the newborn's skin dry (evaporative heat loss) and place a cap on the baby's head. The head makes up 25% of the total body size.
- Keep radiant warmers, isolettes, and cribs away from windows or cold external walls (radiative heat loss) and out of drafts, which cause convection heat loss.
- Open incubator portholes and doors only when necessary and use plastic sleeves on portholes to decrease convective heat loss.
- Use a skin probe to monitor the baby's skin temperature. Correlate ambient temperatures with the skin probe in the isolette using the servocontrol rather than the manual mode. The temperature should be 36–37°C (96.8–98.6°F). Be careful not to place skin temperature probes over bony prominences; areas of brown fat; poorly vasoreactive areas, such as extremities; or excoriated areas.
- Warm formula or stored breast milk before feeding.
- Use a reflector patch over the skin temperature probe when using a radiant warmer bed so that the probe does not sense the higher infrared temperature as the baby's skin temperature and, therefore, decrease the heater output.

Once preterm newborns are medically stable, they can be clothed with a double-thickness cap, cotton shirt, and diaper and, if possible, swaddled in a blanket. The nurse begins the process of weaning to a crib when the premature newborn is medically stable, does not require assisted ventilation, weighs approximately 1500 to 2000 g (depending on facility policy), has had 5 days of consistent weight gain, is taking oral feedings, and when apnea and bradycardia episodes have stabilized. The nurse should be familiar with the individual institution's protocol for weaning preterm babies to a crib.

Maintain Fluid and Electrolyte Status

The nurse maintains hydration by providing adequate fluid intake based on the newborn's weight, gestational age, chronologic age, and volume of sensible and insensible water losses. Adequate fluid intake should compensate for increased insensible losses and the amount needed for renal excretion of metabolic products.

The nurse evaluates the hydration status of the baby by assessing and recording signs of dehydration. Signs of dehydration include the following:

- Sunken fontanel
- Loss of weight
- Poor skin turgor (skin returns to position slowly when squeezed gently)
- Dry oral mucous membranes
- Decreased urine output
- Increased specific gravity (> 1.013).

The nurse must also identify signs of overhydration by observing the newborn for edema or excessive weight gain and by comparing urine output with fluid intake.

A comparison of intake and output measurements over an 8- or 24-hour period provides important information about renal function and fluid balance. Assessment of patterns, and whether they show a net gain or loss over several days, is also essential to fluid management. In addition, the nurse monitors blood serum levels and pH to evaluate for electrolyte imbalances.

Accurate hourly intake calculations are needed when administering IV fluids. Because the preterm newborn is unable to excrete excess fluid, it is essential for the nurse to maintain the correct amount of IV fluid to prevent overload. Accuracy can be ensured by using neonatal or pediatric infusion pumps. To prevent electrolyte imbalance and dehydration, the nurse takes care to give the correct IV solutions as well as the correct volumes and concentrations of formulas. Urinespecific gravity and pH are obtained periodically. Urine osmolality provides an indication of hydration, although this factor must be correlated with other assessments (e.g., serum sodium). Hydration is considered to be adequate when the urine output is 1 to 3 mL/kg per hour.

Provide Adequate Nutrition and Prevent Fatigue During Feeding

The preterm newborn's feeding abilities and health status determine the feeding method. Both nipple and gavage methods are initially supplemented with IV therapy until oral intake is sufficient to support growth. Early, small-volume enteral feedings, called *minimal enteral nutrition via gavage*, have proven to be beneficial for the very-low-birth-weight newborn (see Gavage Feeding earlier in this exemplar). GI priming with these small-volume feedings is not intended to contribute to the total nutritional intake but, rather, to enhance gut metabolism. Trophic feedings may also help encourage earlier advancement to full feedings, thereby decreasing the development of necrotizing enterocolitis and the complications of parenteral nutrition. Formula or breast milk (with or without fortifiers to increase caloric content) is incorporated into the feedings slowly. This is done to avoid overtaxing the digestive capacity of the preterm newborn. The nurse should carefully watch for any signs of feeding intolerance, including the following:

- Increasing gastric residuals
- Abdominal distention (measured routinely before feedings) with visible bowel loops
- Guaiac-positive stools (occult blood in stools)
- Lactose in stools (reducing substance in the stools)
- Vomiting
- Diarrhea
- Water-loss stools.

Before each feeding, the nurse measures abdominal girth and auscultates the abdomen to determine the presence and quality of bowel sounds. Such assessments permit early detection of abdominal distention, visible bowel loops, and decreased peristaltic activity, which may indicate necrotizing enterocolitis or paralytic ileus. The nurse also checks for residual formula in the stomach before feeding when the newborn is fed by gavage. This procedure also can be performed when the nipple-fed newborn presents with abdominal distention. The presence of increasing residual formula is an indication of intolerance to the type or amount of feeding or to the increase in amount of feeding.

SAFETY ALERT Residual feeding may indicate early necrotizing enterocolitis and should be called to the attention of the HCP.

Preterm newborns who are ill or who fatigue easily with nipple feedings are usually fed by gavage. The neonate is essentially passive with these methods, thus conserving energy and calories. As the baby matures, gavage feedings are replaced with nipple (breast or formula) feedings to assist in strengthening the sucking reflex and in meeting the newborn's oral and emotional needs. While their nutrition may come from gavage feedings, nonnutritive sucking is important to the preterm newborn's development and should be encouraged. Signs that indicate readiness for oral feedings include a strong gag reflex, presence of nonnutritive sucking, and rooting behavior. Both low-birth-weight and preterm newborns nipple-feed more effectively in a quiet state. The nurse establishes a gradual nipple-feeding program, such as one nipple feeding per day, then one nipple feeding per shift, and then a nipple feeding every other feeding. The nurse should weigh the baby daily because a small weight loss often occurs when nipple feedings are started. Gastroesophageal reflux is not uncommon in preterm newborns. Long-term gavage feeding may create nipple aversion that will require developmental occupational therapy interventions.

The nurse involves the parents in feeding their preterm baby. This is essential to the development of attachment between parents and baby. In addition, it increases parental knowledge about the care of their baby and helps them cope with the situation.

Prevent Infection

The nurse is responsible for minimizing the preterm newborn's exposure to pathogenic organisms. An immature immune system as well as thin and permeable skin make the preterm newborn susceptible to infection. Invasive procedures, techniques such as umbilical catheterization and mechanical ventilation, and prolonged hospitalization also place the neonate at greater risk for infection.

The practice of strict hand hygiene and use of separate equipment for each neonate help minimize the preterm newborn's exposure to infectious agents. Most nurseries have adopted the Centers for Disease Control and Prevention standard precautions of isolating every baby and The Joint Commission requirement that staff members have short-trimmed nails and no artificial nails. Other specific nursing interventions include limiting visitors, requiring visitors to wash their hands, maintaining strict aseptic practices when changing IV tubing and solutions (which should be changed every 24 hours or per agency protocols), administering parenteral fluids, and assisting with sterile procedures. Isolettes and radiant warmers should be cleaned weekly. The nurse prevents pressure-area breakdown by changing the baby's position regularly, doing range-of-motion exercises, and using water-bed pillows or an air mattress. Chemical skin preps and tape may cause skin trauma and should be avoided as much as possible.

If infection (sepsis) occurs in the preterm newborn, the nurse may be the first to identify its subtle clinical signs, such as lethargy and increased episodes of apnea and bradycardia. The nurse informs the HCP of the findings immediately and implements the treatment plan per clinician orders in the presence of infection.

Promote Attachment

In some cases, preterm newborns are separated from their parents for prolonged periods after illness or complications that are detected in the first few hours or days following birth. This interrupts the bonding process, necessitating intervention to ensure successful attachment.

Nurses need to take measures to promote positive parental feelings toward the preterm newborn. They can give photographs of the baby to parents to take home. Photographs also may be given to the mother if she is in a different hospital or, if in the same hospital, is too ill to come to the nursery and visit. By placing the newborn's first name on the incubator as soon as it is known, nurses help the parents feel that their baby is a unique and special individual. A number of other interventions promote the bonding process, including the following:

- Give parents a weekly card with the baby's footprint, weight, and length.
- Give parents the telephone number of the nursery or intensive care unit and the names of staff members so that they have access to information about their baby at any time of the day or night.
- Encourage visits from siblings and grandparents.
- Use special blanket or clothing from parents as appropriate and encourage them to perform hands-on care whenever able.

Early involvement in the care of and decisions about their newborn provides the parents with realistic expectations for their baby. The individual personality characteristics of the newborn and the parents influence bonding and contribute to the interactive process for the family. By observing each baby's patterns of behavior and responses, especially sleep–wake states, the nurse can teach parents the optimal times for interacting with their babies. The parents and nurse can plan nursing care around the times when the baby is alert and best able to attend.

Parents need education to develop caregiving skills and to understand the premature baby's behavioral characteristics. The more knowledge parents have about the meaning of their baby's responses, behaviors, and cues for interaction, the better they will be able to meet their newborn's needs and form a positive attachment with their child. For parents who cannot stay with their preterm baby, the nurse should encourage their daily participation (if possible) as well as early and frequent visits. The nurse should provide opportunities for parents to touch, hold, talk to, and care for the baby. Skin-to-skin holding (kangaroo care) helps parents feel close to their small newborn (**Figure 33.90 »**). Kangaroo care has been shown to improve outcomes, reduce pain, and increase parents' perception of their caregiving ability (Mu, Lee, Chen, Yang, & Yang, 2020; Sen & Manav, 2020).

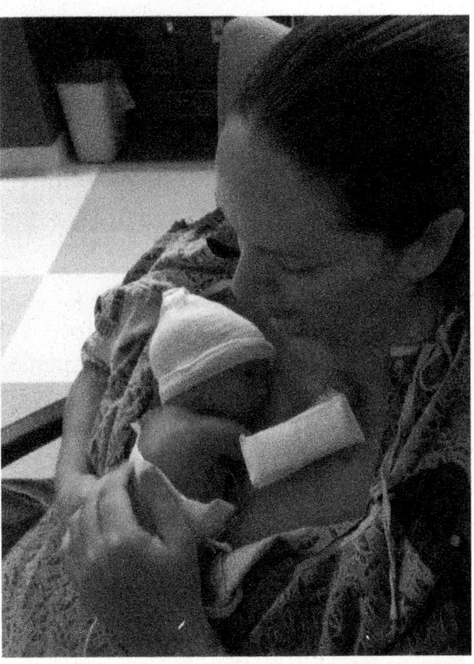

Figure 33.90 » Kangaroo (skin-to-skin) care facilitates closeness and attachment between mother and her premature newborn.

Source: Carol Harrigan, RN, MSN, NNP-BC.

Some parents will progress easily to touching and cuddling their newborn; however, others will not. Parents need to know that their feelings are normal and that the progression of acquaintanceship can be slow. Rooming-in can provide another opportunity for the stable preterm newborn and family to get acquainted; it offers both privacy and readily available help.

Promote Developmentally Supportive Care

Prolonged separation and the NICU environment necessitate individualized baby sensory stimulation programs. The nurse plays a key role in determining the appropriate type and amount of visual, tactile, and auditory stimulation.

Providing developmentally supportive, family-centered care improves the outcomes of the critically ill newborn (Sathish et al., 2019). With this in mind, some hospitals offer specially designed NICUs with the single-room care concept to minimize lighting and noise as well as to provide privacy for the parents of the convalescing newborn.

The NICU environment contains many detrimental stimuli that the nurse can help reduce. Simple actions that nurses can take include the following:

- If possible, replace alarms with lights to lower noise levels.
- Silence alarms quickly.
- Keep conversations away from newborns' bedsides.
- Use dimmer switches to shield newborns' eyes from bright lights.
- Place blankets over the top portion of each isolette.

Nursing care should also be planned to decrease the number of times the baby is disturbed. Signs (e.g., "Quiet Please") can be placed near the bedside to allow the baby some periods of uninterrupted sleep.

Some other suggested developmentally supportive interventions include the following:

- Facilitate handling by using containment measures when turning or moving the neonate or doing procedures such as suctioning. Use the hands to hold the neonate's flexed arms and legs close to the midline of the body. This helps stabilize the newborn's motor and physiologic subsystems during stressful activities, essentially mimicking the environment of the womb.
- Touch the premature newborn gently and avoid sudden postural changes.
- Promote self-consoling and soothing activities, such as placing blanket rolls or approved manufactured devices next to the neonate's sides and against the feet to provide "nesting." Swaddle the premature newborn to maintain extremities in a flexed position while ensuring that the hands can reach the face. This permits the newborn to do hand-to-mouth activities, which can be consoling (**Figure 33.91** »).
- Simulate the kinesthetic advantages of the intrauterine environment by using sheepskin and approved water beds. Positioning aids such as these have been shown to improve sleep and decrease motor activity as well as lead to more mature motor behavior, fewer state changes, and a decreased heart rate (Sathish et al., 2017).
- Provide opportunities for nonnutritive sucking with a pacifier (**Figure 33.92** »). This improves transcutaneous oxygen saturation; decreases body movements; improves sleep, especially after feedings; and increases weight gain.
- Provide objects for the premature newborn to grasp (e.g., a piece of blanket, oxygen tubing, or a finger) during caregiving. Grasping can provide comfort.

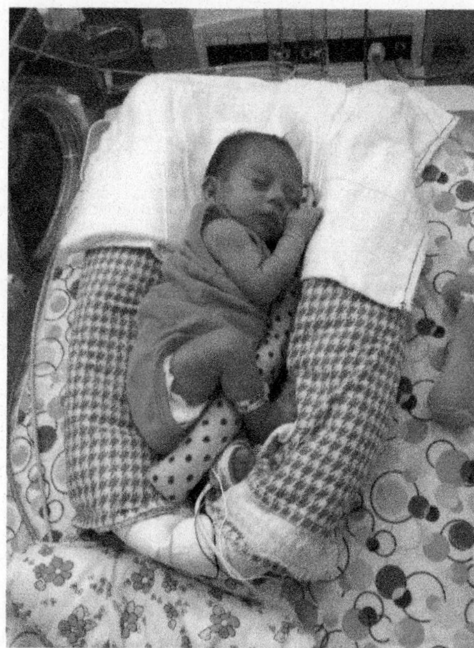

Figure 33.91 » A 3-week-old, 31 weeks' gestational age baby is nested and developmentally positioned. Hand-to-mouth behavior facilitates self-consoling and soothing activities.
Source: Carol Harrigan, RN, MSN, NNP-BC.

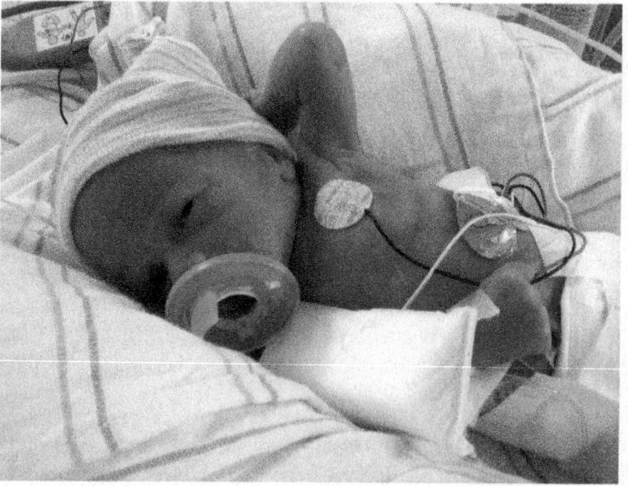

Figure 33.92 » Nonnutritive sucking on a pacifier has a calming effect on the preterm newborn and also facilitates readiness to bottle-feed.
Source: Carol Harrigan, RN, MSN, NNP-BC.

The nurse teaches the parents how to read behavioral cues to help them move at their baby's own pace when providing stimulation. Parents are ideally equipped to meet the baby's need for stimulation. Stroking, rocking, cuddling, quiet singing, and talking to the baby can all be integral parts of the baby's care. Visual stimulation in the form of *en face* interaction with caregivers and mobiles is also important. It is important for the nurse to monitor for overstimulation.

Kangaroo (skin-to-skin) care has become prevalent in NICUs across the United States. Skin-to-skin care is defined as the practice of holding newborns skin-to-skin against their parents. The newborn is usually naked, except for a diaper, and is placed on the parent's bare chest. They are then both covered with a blanket. Benefits of skin-to-skin care as a developmental intervention include the following (Gardner & Goldson, 2021):

- Improved oxygenation, as evidenced by an increase in oxygen saturation levels
- Enhanced temperature regulation
- Decline in the episodes of apnea and bradycardia
- Increased periods of quiet sleep
- Stabilization of vital signs
- Positive interaction between parent and baby, which enhances attachment and bonding
- Increased growth parameters
- Early discharge.

Skin-to-skin care may be limited because of staff uneasiness when moving the neonate while attached to multiple IV lines, monitor leads, and a ventilator. The confines of the nursery may be another limiting factor.

Massage and *gentle touch* have been practiced for many centuries. The types of stimulation include massage with stroking, gentle touch without stroking, and therapeutic touch or "hands-on" containment. Benefits include shorter length of stay, improved weight gain and feeding tolerance, lower pain levels, and improved neurodevelopment

Patient Teaching

Parent Support

For most families, experiencing the birth of a child is an exciting and joyful experience. Unfortunately, parents of babies born prematurely or born with birth anomalies may experience an acute grief response when they realize their newborn is not the "perfect" child they hoped and planned for (Yu, Zhang, & Yuan, 2020). If the baby experiences a life-threatening compromise, the parents may develop anticipatory grieving in advance of the loss of their child. Experiences and expressions of grief are based on numerous factors, including cultural norms and spiritual and religious beliefs. For more information, see Module 27, Grief and Loss.

Evidence suggests that interventions and services that support and empower parents promote feelings of confidence and support the experience of caregiving (Brown, 2016). Many parents who will be taking their premature baby home will not need referrals, but many will need contact information and referrals to appropriate service and support agencies ranging from case management to early childhood intervention services, which can provide nursing and therapy assistance in the home. Support groups and organizations (such as the March of Dimes or United Cerebral Palsy) can assist parents by providing opportunities to share feelings and strategies and provide additional information about resources in the community. Nurses should be careful to instill hope and not make assumptions about the newborn's limitations. With early intervention and other programs, many babies born with congenital anomalies or disabilities can grow into independent, productive adults.

(Pados & McGlothen-Bell, 2019). For premature newborns on ventilators or otherwise confined to the isolette, nurses show and model for parents how to engage with and touch the newborn until they can be held.

For ways to help new parents with a compromised newborn, see Patient Teaching: Parent Support.

Prepare for Home Care

Parents are often anxious when their premature newborn is transferred out of the NICU or is discharged home. Parents of preterm babies should receive the same postpartum teaching as any parent taking a new baby home. In preparing for discharge, the nurse encourages the parents to spend time caring directly for their baby. This process starts on admission. Early education allows parents to digest and begin to understand information in smaller segments, rather than getting everything at once, which can be overwhelming. This familiarizes them with their baby's behavior patterns and helps them establish realistic expectations about the baby. Some hospitals have a special room near the nursery where parents can spend the night with their baby before discharge.

Discharge instruction includes breastfeeding and formula-feeding techniques, formula preparation, and vitamin administration. If the mother wishes to breastfeed, the nurse teaches her to pump her breasts to keep the milk flowing and provide milk even before discharge. The nurse gives information on bathing, diapering, hygiene, and normal elimination patterns and prepares the parents to expect changes in the color of the baby's stool, number of bowel movements, and timing of elimination if feeding methods are changed. This information can prevent unnecessary concern by the parents. The nurse also discusses normal growth and development patterns, reflexes, and activity for preterm newborns. In these discussions, the nurse should emphasize ways to promote bonding behaviors and deal with newborn crying. Caring for the premature newborn with complications, preventing infections, recognizing signs of a sick baby, and the need for continued medical follow-up are other key issues.

Evaluation

Expected outcomes of nursing care include the following:

- The preterm newborn is free of respiratory distress and establishes effective respiratory function.
- The preterm newborn gains weight and shows no signs of fatigue or aspiration during feedings.
- The preterm newborn demonstrates a serial head circumference growth rate of 1 cm (0.4 in.) per week.
- The preterm newborn achieves expected developmental milestones based on corrected age.
- The parent is able to verbalize understanding of infant-specific cares and instructions prior to discharge home.
- The parents are able to verbalize their feelings of anger and guilt about the birth of a preterm baby and show attachment behavior, such as frequent visits and growing confidence in their participatory care activities.

Conducting additional care evaluation determines if further care is needed based on newborn outcomes. If the outcomes are not being met, the nurse may choose to continue or revise the plan of care for optimal outcome attainment. Continuation, revision, or discontinuation of a plan of care is decided through collaboration of all members of the healthcare team.

Nursing Care Plan

A Premature Newborn

Baby Boy Johnson was born 12 weeks early at 28 weeks of gestation to Dennis and Alaina Johnson. He is their first child. The NICU nurse received the baby from the obstetrician after he was delivered vaginally. Apgar scoring was 5 at 1 minute, 5 at 5 minutes, and 4 at 10 minutes. He had a weak cry and was dusky and floppy, with an initial heart rate of greater than 100 beats/min. During resuscitation, the nurse provided blow-by oxygen. When his oxygenation status not only failed to improve but dropped, indicating that resuscitation was not effective, the nurse practitioner inserted an oral endotracheal tube and oxygen was administered by bagging. He was transported to the NICU in a warm isolette, where he was admitted, placed on a ventilator, and had an umbilical artery catheter placed.

His parents come to see him when his mother is moved from the labor area to her room on the postpartum unit. Their first question to the nurse is "Is he okay?" Their next question is "When will he be able to come home?" The nurse encourages his parents to touch him and talk to him before they leave the nursery.

Nursing Care Plan *(continued)*

ASSESSMENT	DIAGNOSES	PLANNING
■ Vital signs T 36°C (96.7°F) axillary; pulse 172 beats/min; respiration 68 breaths/min; BP 42/24 mmHg ■ Endotracheal tube taped in place to ventilator set to deliver 30 breaths/minute, with 4 mmHg of positive end-expiratory pressure ■ Color pink with acrocyanosis ■ Soft murmur audible in left mid-axillary area ■ Hypoactive bowel sounds in all quadrants ■ Has not voided or stooled yet	■ Impaired airway clearance ■ Potential for compromised maternal–newborn attachment secondary to separation ■ Poor thermoregulation secondary to low birth weight ■ Inadequate gas exchange secondary to lung immaturity	■ The newborn will maintain adequate gas exchange to meet tissue requirements. ■ The newborn will maintain a clear airway to promote oxygenation. ■ The parents will bond with the newborn and recognize the characteristics of their baby. ■ The newborn will receive adequate nutrition and fluids to promote growth.

IMPLEMENTATION

- Suction endotracheal tube as needed when secretions are heard in endotracheal tube.
- Monitor arterial blood gas studies to determine adequate gas exchange.
- Assist with surfactant administration as ordered to reduce alveolar collapse on expiration.
- Monitor daily weights.
- Monitor urine output and kidney function by testing urine for pH and specific gravity.
- Encourage parents to visit as often as possible and point out the newborn's characteristics to help parents focus on the baby instead of the medical equipment.
- Assist parents to hold their baby and offer the option of skin-to-skin (kangaroo) care to promote attachment.
- Monitor cardiorespiratory and oxygen saturation on a continuous basis. Change pulse oximeter location frequently (at least every 2 hours) to reduce the risk of altered skin integrity.
- Avoid use of tape to reduce altered skin integrity.
- Promote development by offering a pacifier for the newborn to suck on.
- Provide periods of reduced stimulation to promote rest and comfort.
- Maintain neonate in an NTE, either on a radiant warmer or a heated isolette, until he is able to maintain a normal temperature independently.
- Monitor vital signs at a minimum of every 4 hours.

EVALUATION

After administration of surfactant, Baby Boy Johnson is extubated, placed on CPAP for 2 days, and then weaned to nasal cannula. Feedings are initiated via continuous gavage feedings. Once feedings are tolerated, he is changed to every-3-hour feedings. His murmur is diagnosed as a PDA, and indomethacin is administered, which successfully closes the PDA. He begins to have occasional apneic episodes and is placed on caffeine every 12 hours.

Within 4 weeks, he is showing steady weight gain and is moved to the low-risk NICU. His parents begin participating more in providing care, such as bathing and feeding him, and he is discharged at 12 weeks of age.

CRITICAL THINKING

1. How would you respond to the parents when they ask when the baby is likely to come home?
2. How can you maintain the neonate's temperature while he is being held by his parents?
3. If the neonate weighs 900 g, what are his fluid and caloric needs per day?

REVIEW Prematurity

RELATE Link the Concepts and Exemplars

Linking the exemplar of prematurity to the concept of grief and loss:

1. What factors might induce feelings of loss for the parents of a premature newborn, even if the newborn is doing well?
2. What nursing interventions would you implement to help the parents who are feeling grief and loss over the birth of their premature newborn?

Linking the exemplar of prematurity with the concept of development:

3. What developmental needs does a premature newborn have?
4. What nursing care would you provide the premature newborn in order to promote development?

READY Go to Volume 3: Clinical Nursing Skills

REFER Go to Pearson MyLab Nursing and eText

REFLECT Apply Your Knowledge

Kayla Marshall, 15 years old, delivers a baby girl at 32 weeks of gestation. Kayla sees her baby briefly in the delivery room before the newborn is transported to the NICU. She names the baby Shamika, after her best friend. On the way from the labor and delivery recovery room, the nurse brings Kayla to the nursery to see the baby, who is under an oxygen hood with an IV through her umbilicus and cardiac monitor leads on her chest. When Jessica sees her baby, she begins to cry and says, "She's so small and looks so sick. It's all my fault!" The nurse caring for Shamika points out the baby's beautiful curly hair, long fingers, and aquiline nose. Kayla stops crying and says, "Oh, you're right. Look how beautiful she is—and so perfect." Shamika's nurse takes Jessica to her new room, gives her some information about premature babies to read, and encourages her to come back to visit Shamika as soon as she feels up to it.

1. When assigned to care for Shamika, what nursing diagnoses would you consider to be the greatest priority regarding this family?
2. How would you help Kayla bond with her premature newborn?
3. What risks does this premature newborn face as the result of being born to an adolescent mother?

References

Alayed, N., Kezouh, A., Oddy, L., & Abenhaim, H. A. (2014). Sickle-cell disease and pregnancy outcomes: Population-based study on 8.8 million births. *Journal of Perinatal Medicine, 42*(4), 487–492.

American Academy of Family Physicians. (2017). SIDS and safe sleeping environments for infants: AAP updates recommendations. *American Family Physician, 95*(12), 806–807.

American Academy of Pediatrics (AAP). (2004). AAP Subcommittee on Hyperbilirubinemia. Clinical Practice Guideline: Management of hyperbilirubinemia in the newborn infant 35 or more weeks of gestation. *Pediatrics, 114,* 297.

American Academy of Pediatrics (AAP). (2016). *Infant food and feeding.* https://www.aap.org/en-us/advocacy-and-policy/aap-health-initiatives/HALF-Implementation-Guide/Age-Specific-Content/Pages/Infant-Food-and-Feeding.aspx

American Academy of Pediatrics (AAP). (2019). *Newborn reflexes.* http://www.healthychildren.org/English/ages-stages/baby/pages/Newborn-Reflexes.aspx

American Academy of Pediatrics (AAP) Committee on Fetus and Newborn & American College of Obstetricians and Gynecologists (ACOG) Committee on Obstetric Practice. (2015). The APGAR score. *Pediatrics, 136*(4), 819–822.

American Academy of Pediatrics (AAP) & American College of Obstetricians and Gynecologists (ACOG). (2017). *Guidelines for perinatal care* (8th ed.). Authors.

American College of Obstetricians and Gynecologists (ACOG). (2008, reaffirmed 2019). *Anemia in pregnancy* (ACOG Practice Bulletin No. 95). Author.

American College of Obstetricians and Gynecologists (ACOG). (2009, reaffirmed 2013). *Intrapartum fetal heart rate monitoring: Nomenclature, interpretation, and general management principles* (ACOG Practice Bulletin No. 106). Author.

American College of Obstetricians and Gynecologists (ACOG). (2011, reaffirmed 2017). *Vitamin D: Screening and supplementation during pregnancy* (ACOG Committee Opinion No. 495). Author.

American College of Obstetricians and Gynecologists (ACOG). (2013a, reaffirmed 2016). *Weight gain during pregnancy* (Committee Opinion No. 548). Author.

American College of Obstetricians and Gynecologists (ACOG). (2013b, reaffirmed 2017). *Oral health care during pregnancy and throughout the lifespan* (ACOG Committee Opinion No. 569). Author.

American College of Obstetricians and Gynecologists (ACOG). (2013c, reaffirmed 2017). *Definition of term pregnancy* (ACOG Committee Opinion No. 579). Author.

American College of Obstetricians and Gynecologists (ACOG). (2013d). *Induction of labor* (ACOG Practice Bulletin No. 107). Author.

American College of Obstetricians and Gynecologists (ACOG). (2014a, reaffirmed 2016). *Antepartum fetal surveillance* (ACOG Practice Bulletin No. 145). Author.

American College of Obstetricians and Gynecologists (ACOG). (2014b, reaffirmed 2016). Preparing for clinical emergencies in obstetrics and gynecology (ACOG Committee Opinion No. 590). Author.

American College of Obstetricians and Gynecologists (ACOG). (2015). *Obesity in pregnancy* (ACOG Practice Bulletin No. 156). Author.

American College of Obstetrics and Gynecology (ACOG). (2016a, reaffirmed 2020). *Ultrasound in pregnancy* (ACOG Practice Bulletin No 175). Author.

American College of Obstetricians and Gynecologists (ACOG). (2016b). *Prenatal diagnostic testing for genetic disorders.* (Practice Bulletin No. 162.) Washington, DC: Author.

American College of Obstetricians and Gynecologists (ACOG). (2017a). *The Apgar score.* https://www.acog.org/clinical/clinical-guidance/committee-opinion/articles/2015/10/the-apgar-score

American College of Obstetricians and Gynecologists (ACOG). (2017b). *Carrier screening for genetic conditions* (Committee Opinion No. 691). https://www.acog.org/clinical/clinical-guidance/committee-opinion/articles/2017/03/carrier-screening-for-genetic-conditions

American College of Obstetricians and Gynecologists (ACOG). (2017c). Delayed umbilical cord clamping after birth (Committee Opinion No. 685). *Obstetrics and Gynecology, 129*(1), e5–e10.

American College of Obstetricians and Gynecologists (ACOG). (2017d). *Labor induction.* https://www.acog.org/Patients/FAQs/Labor-Induction

American College of Obstetricians and Gynecologists (ACOG). (2017e). Methods for estimating the due date (Committee Opinion No. 700). *Obstetrics and Gynecology, 129,* e150.

American College of Obstetricians and Gynecologists (ACOG). (2017f). *Neural tube defects* (ACOG Practice Bulletin No. 187). Washington, DC: Author.

American College of Obstetricians and Gynecologists (ACOG). (2018a). *Air travel during pregnancy* (Committee Opinion No. 746). https://www.acog.org/clinical/clinical-guidance/committee-opinion/articles/2018/08/air-travel-during-pregnancy

American College of Obstetricians and Gynecologists (ACOG). (2018b). *Employment considerations during pregnancy and the postpartum period* (ACOG Committee Opinion No. 733). https://www.acog.org/clinical/clinical-guidance/committee-opinion/articles/2018/04/employment-considerations-during-pregnancy-and-the-postpartum-period

American College of Obstetricians & Gynecologists (ACOG). (2018c). *Gestational diabetes mellitus* (ACOG Practice Bulletin No. 190). Author.

American College of Obstetricians and Gynecologists (ACOG). (2018d). *Importance of social determinants of health and cultural awareness in the delivery of reproductive healthcare* (ACOG Committee Opinion No. 729). https://www.acog.org/clinical/clinical-guidance/committee-opinion/articles/2018/01/importance-of-social-determinants-of-health-and-cultural-awareness-in-the-delivery-of-reproductive-health-care

American College of Obstetricians and Gynecologists (ACOG). (2018e). *Nausea and vomiting in pregnancy* (ACOG Practice Bulletin No. 189). Author.

American College of Obstetricians and Gynecologists (ACOG). (2018f). *Screening for perinatal depression* (ACOG Committee Opinion No. 757). https://www.acog.org/clinical/clinical-guidance/committee-opinion/articles/2018/11/screening-for-perinatal-depression

American College of Obstetricians and Gynecologists (ACOG). (2019a). *Cesarean delivery on maternal request* (ACOG Committee Opinion No. 761). https://www.acog.org/clinical/clinical-guidance/committee-opinion/articles/2019/01/cesarean-delivery-on-maternal-request

American College of Obstetricians and Gynecologists (ACOG). (2019b). *Management of patients in the context of Zika virus* (ACOG Committee Opinion No. 784). https://www.acog.org/clinical/clinical-guidance/committee-opinion/articles/2019/09/management-of-patients-in-the-context-of-zika-virus

American College of Obstetricians and Gynecologists (ACOG). (2019c). *Levels of maternal care.* (ACOG Obstetric Care Consensus No. 9). *https://www.acog.org/clinical/clinical-guidance/obstetric-care-consensus/articles/2019/08/levels-of-maternal-care*

American College of Obstetricians and Gynecologists (ACOG). (2020a). *If your baby is breech.* https://www.acog.org/patient-resources/faqs/pregnancy/if-your-baby-is-breech

American College of Obstetricians and Gynecologists (ACOG). (2020b). *Physical activity and exercise during pregnancy and the postpartum period* (ACOG Committee Opinion No. 804). https://www.acog.org/clinical/clinical-guidance/committee-opinion/articles/2020/04/physical-activity-and-exercise-during-pregnancy-and-the-postpartum-period

American College of Obstetricians and Gynecologists (ACOG). (2020c). *Prevention of group B streptococcal early-onset disease in newborns* (ACOG Committee Opinion No. 797). *Obstetrics and Gynecology, 135,* e51–372.

American College of Rheumatology (2020). 2020 American College of Rheumatology guideline for the management of reproductive health in rheumatic and musculoskeletal diseases. *Arthritis and Rheumatology, 72*(4), 529–556.

American Diabetes Association (ADA). (2020). Standards of medical care in diabetes—2020 Abridged for primary care providers. *Clinical Diabetes, 38*(1), 10–38.

American Heart Association. (2019). *Why are black women at such high risk of dying from pregnancy complications?* https://www.heart.org/en/news/2019/02/20/why-are-black-women-at-such-high-risk-of-dying-from-pregnancy-complications

Andrews, M. M., Boyle, J. S., & Collins, J. W. (2020). *Transcultural concepts in nursing care* (8th ed.). Wolters Kluwer.

Andrikopoulou, M., & D'Alton, M. E. (2019). Postpartum hemorrage: Early identification strategies. *Seminars in Perinatology, 43*(1), 11–17. https://doi.org/10.1053/j.semperi.2018.11.003

Anthony, R. S., Wang, H., Wani, R., & Kashani, B. (2017). *The social and economic costs and consequences of teen pregnancy in Nebraska.* Holland Children's Institute. https://hollandinstitute.org/wp-content/uploads/2017/12/HCI_Final_Teen_Pregnancy_Report_FINAL_12_5_16.pdf

Antony, K. M., Racusin, D. A., Aagard, K., & Dildy III, G. A. (2017). Maternal physiology. In S. Gabbe, J. Niebyl, J. Simpson, M. Landon, H. Galan, E. Jauniaux, et al. (Eds.), *Obstetrics: Normal and problem pregnancies* (7th ed., pp. 38–63). Elsevier.

Apgar, V. (1966). The newborn (Apgar) scoring system, reflections and advice. *Pediatric Clinics of North America, 13,* 645.

Association of Women's Health, Obstetrics, and Neonatal Nurses (AWHONN). (2020). Sudden unexpected postnatal collapse in healthy term newborns: AWHONN Practice Brief Number 8. *Nursing for Women's Health, 49*(4), P388–390.

Arcilla, C. K., & Vilella, R. C. (2020). *Tonic neck reflex.* StatPearls. https://www.ncbi.nlm.nih.gov/books/NBK559210/

Babbar, S., & Shyken, J. (2016). Yoga in pregnancy. *Clinical Obstetrics and Gynecology, 59*(3), 600.

Ballard, J. L., Khoury, J. C., Wedig, K., Wang, L., Eilers-Walsmann, B. L., & Lipp, R. (1991). New Ballard Score, expanded to include extremely -premature infants. *Journal of Pediatrics, 119*(3), 417–423.

Barron, M. L. (2020). Antenatal care. In K. R. Simpson & P. A. Creehan (Eds.), *AWHONN's perinatal nursing* (5th ed., pp. 66–98.). Philadelphia, PA: Lippincott Williams & Wilkins.

BBC. (2009). *Muslim birth rites*. http://www.bbc.co.uk/religion/religions/islam/ritesrituals/birth.shtml

Benitz, W. E., & Committee on Fetus and Newborn, American Academy of Pediatrics. (2015). Hospital stay for healthy term newborn infants. *Pediatrics, 135*(5), 948–953.

Bhutani, V. K., Johnson, L., & Sivieri, E. M. (1999). Predictive ability of a predischarge hour-specific serum bilirubin for subsequent significant hyperbilirubinemia in healthy term and near-term -newborns. *Pediatrics, 103*, 6–14.

Bishop, E. H. (1964). Pelvic scoring for elective inductions. *Obstetrics and Gynecology, 24*, 266.

Blackburn, S. T. (2018). *Maternal, fetal, and neonatal physiology: A clinical perspective* (5th ed.). Saunders.

Boerma, T., Ronsmans, C., Melesse, D. Y., Barros, A. J., Barros, F. C., Juan, L., et al. (2018). Global epidemiology of use of and disparities in caesarean sections. *The Lancet, 392*(10155), 1341–1348.

Borca, G., Bina, M., Keller, P. S., Gilbert, L. R., & Begotti, T. (2015). Internet use and developmental tasks: Adolescents' point of view. *Computers in Human Behavior, 52*, 49–58.

Brandt, J. S., Cruz Ithier, M. A., Rosen, T., & Ashkinadze, E. (2019). Advanced paternal age, infertility, and reproductive risks: A review of the literature. *Prenatal Diagnosis, 39*(2), 81–87.

Brazelton, T. B. (1984). *Neonatal behavioral assessment scale* (2nd ed.). Heinemann.

Brazelton, T. B., & Nugent, J. K. (1995). *The neonatal behavioral assessment scale* (3rd ed.). MacKeith.

Brown, J. M. (2016). Recurrent grief in mothering a child with an intellectual ability into adulthood: grieving is the healing. *Child and Family Social Work, 21*(1), 113–122.

Burke, C., & Allen, R. (2020). Complications of Cesarean Birth. *American Journal of Maternal/Child Nursing, 45*(2), 92–99.

Burke, M. (2021). *Pica*. https://emedicine.medscape.com/article/914765-overview

Caldwell, W. E., & Moloy, H. C. (1933). Anatomical variations in the female pelvis and their effect on labor with a suggested classification [Historical article]. *American Journal of Obstetrics and Gynecology, 26*, 479–505.

California Maternal Quality Care Collaborative (CMQCC). (2015). *CMQCC CPMS Early Warning Signs Slideset*. https://www.cmqcc.org/resource/cmqcc-cpms-early-warning-signs-slideset

California Maternal Quality Care Collaborative (CMQCC). (2019). *Birth equity. https://www.cmqcc.org/content/birth-equity*

Campbell, D. E. (2020). *Neonatology for primary care* (2nd ed.). American Academy of Pediatrics.

Cao, C., & O'Brien, K. O. (2013). Pregnancy and iron homeostasis: An update. *Nutrition Reviews, 71*(1), 35–51.

Caudle, P. W. (2019). Reproductive tract structure and function. In R. G. Jordan, C. L. Farley, & K. T. Grace (Eds.), *Prenatal and postnatal care: A woman-centered approach* (2nd ed., pp. 5–18). Wiley.

Caughey, A. B. (2018). *Vaginal birth after cesarean delivery*. Medscape. https://emedicine.medscape.com/article/272187-overview

Centers for Disease Control and Prevention (CDC). (2015b). *Hearing loss in newborn: Screening and diagnosis*. http://www.cdc.gov/ncbddd/hearingloss/screening.html

Centers for Disease Control and Prevention (CDC). (2016). *Guidelines for vaccinating pregnant women*. http://www.cdc.gov/VACCINes/pubs/preg-guide.htm

Centers for Disease Control and Prevention (CDC). (2018). *Pregnancy mortality surveillance System*. https://www.cdc.gov/reproductivehealth/maternalinfanthealth/pregnancy-mortality-surveillance-system.htm

Centers for Disease Control and Prevention. (CDC). (2019a). *About teen pregnancy*. http://www.cdc.gov/-teenpregnancy/about

Centers for Disease Control and Prevention (CDC). (2019b). *Preterm birth*. https://www.cdc.gov/reproductivehealth/maternalinfanthealth/pretermbirth.htm

Centers for Disease Control and Prevention (CDC). (2019c). *Recommendations: Women & folic acid*. https://www.cdc.gov/ncbddd/folicacid/recommendations.html

Centers for Disease Control and Prevention (CDC). (2019d). *Social determinants and eliminating disparities in teen pregnancy*. https://www.cdc.gov/teenpregnancy/about/social-determinants-disparities-teen-pregnancy.htm

Centers for Disease Control and Prevention (CDC). (2020a). *Evaluation and management considerations for neonates at risk for COVID-19*. https://www.cdc.gov/coronavirus/2019-ncov/hcp/caring-for-newborns.html

Centers for Disease Control and Prevention (CDC). (2020b). *Infant mortality*. https://www.cdc.gov/reproductivehealth/maternalinfanthealth/infantmortality.htm

Centers for Disease Control and Prevention (CDC). (2020c). *Pregnancy mortality surveillance system: Trends in pregnancy-related deaths*. https://www.cdc.gov/reproductivehealth/maternal-mortality/pregnancy-mortality-surveillance-system.htm

Centers for Disease Control and Prevention. (CDC). (2020d). *Recommendations for prevention and control of hepatitis C virus (HCV) infection and HCV-related chronic disease*. https://www.cdc.gov/hepatitis/hcv/management.htm

Centers for Disease Control and Prevention (CDC). (2020e). *Screening and diagnosis of hearing loss*. https://www.cdc.gov/ncbddd/hearingloss/screening.html

Centers for Disease Control and Prevention. (2020f). *Urgent maternal warning signs*. https://www.cdc.gov/hearher/maternal-warning-signs/index.html

Centers for Disease Control and Prevention. (2021). *Pregnant and recently pregnant people: At increased risk for severe illness from COVID-19*. https://www.cdc.gov/coronavirus/2019-ncov/need-extra-precautions/pregnant-people.html

Child Welfare Information Gateway. (2013a). *Grounds for involuntary termination of parental rights*. http://www.childwelfare.gov/-systemwide/laws_policies/statutes/-groundtermin.cfm

Child Welfare Information Gateway. (2013b). *Infant safe haven laws*. https://www.childwelfare.gov/pubPDFs/safehaven.pdf

Children's Hospital of Philadelphia. (2020). *Premature rupture of membranes (PROM)/preterm premature rupture of membranes (PPROM)*. https://www.chop.edu/conditions-diseases/premature-rupture-membranes-promPreterm-premature-rupture-membranes-pprom

Chou, C. (2017). Traditional postpartum practices and rituals: A qualitative systematic review. In *The embryo project encyclopedia*. https://embryo.asu.edu/pages/traditional-postpartum-practices-and-rituals-qualitative-systematic-review-2007-cindy-lee

Cnattingius, S., Johansson, S., & Razaz, N. (2020). Apgar score and risk of neonatal death among preterm infants. *New England Journal of Medicine, 383*(1), 49–57.

Coşkun, D., & Günay, U. (2020). The effects of kangaroo care applied by Turkish mothers who have premature babies and cannot breastfeed on their stress levels and amount of milk production. *Journal of Pediatric Nursing, 50*, e26–e32.

Cotten, C. M. (2017). Pulmonary hypoplasia. *Seminars in Fetal and Neonatal Medicine, 22*(4), 250–255.

Council on Patient Safety in Women's Health Care. (2020). *Urgent maternal warning signs*. https://safehealthcareforeverywoman.org/council/patient-safety-tools/urgent-maternal-signs/#link_acc-43-44-d

Crenshaw, J. T. (2019). Healthy birth practice #6: Keep mother and newborn Together—It's best for mother, newborn, and breastfeeding. *Journal of Perinatal Education, 28*(2), 108–115.

Cunningham, F. G., Leveno, K. J., Bloom, S. L., Spong, C. Y., Dashe, G. S., Hoffman, B. L., et al. (2018). *Williams obstetrics* (25th ed.). McGraw-Hill.

Curry, S. J., Krist, A. H., Owens, D. K., Barry, M. J., Caughey, A. B., Davidson, K. W., et al. (2019). Ocular prophylaxis for gonococcal ophthalmia neonatorum: US preventive services task force reaffirmation recommendation statement. *Journal of the American Medical Association, 321*(4), 394–398.

Davidson, M. R. (2013). *Fast facts for the antepartum and postpartum nurse: An orientation in a nutshell*. Springer.

Davidson, M., London, M., & Ladewig, P. (2020). *Olds' maternal–newborn nursing and women's health across the lifespan* (11th ed.). Pearson.

Delprete, H. (2017). Pelvic inlet shape is not as dimorphic as previously suggested. *Anatomical Record, 300*(4), 706–715. https://anatomypubs.onlinelibrary.wiley.com/doi/full/10.1002/ar.23544

Deering, S. (2018). *Using simulation technology to reduce maternal morbidity*. https://www.contemporaryobgyn.net/view/using-simulation-technology-improve-maternal-morbidity

Eichenwald, E. C., Hansen, A. R., Martin, C. R., & Stark, A. R. (2017). *Cloherty and Stark's manual of neonatal care* (8th ed.). Philadelphia, PA: Lippincott Williams & Wilkins.

Feldman-Winter, L., & Goldsmith, J. P. (2016). Safe sleep and skin-to-skin care in the neonatal period for healthy term newborns. *Pediatrics, 138*(3), e1–e10https://doi.org/10.1542/peds.2016-1889

Foglia, E. E., & Te Pas, A. B. (2018). Effective ventilation: The most critical intervention for successful delivery room resuscitation. *Seminars in Fetal and Neonatal Medicine, 23*(5), 340–346. https://doi.org/10.1016/j.siny.2018.04.001

Gabbe, S., Niebyl, J., Simpson, J., Landon, M., Galan, H. Jauniaux, E., et al. (2016). *Obstetrics: Normal and problem pregnancies* (7th ed.). Churchill Livingstone.

Gardner, S. L., & Goldson, E. (2021). The neonate and the environment: Impact on development. In S. L. Gardner, B. S. Carter, M. Enzman Hines, J. A. Hernandez, & S. Niermeyer (Eds.), *Merenstein & Gardner's handbook of neonatal intensive care* (9th ed., pp. 334–406). Mosby.

Garrison, A. (2017). *Vacuum extraction*. Medscape. https://emedicine.medscape.com/article/271175-overview#a6 on 6/10/20.

Gavin, L., Warner, L., O'Neil, M. E., Duong, L. M., Marshall, C., Hastings, P. A., et al. (2013). Vital signs: Repeat births among teens—United States, 2007–2010. *Morbidity and Mortality Weekly Report, 62*(13), 249–255. http://www.cdc.gov/mmwr/preview/mmwrhtml/mm6213a4.htm?s_cid=mm6213a4_w

Gilger, L. (2019, May 31). How one midwife is helping indigenous mothers connect to their childbirth traditions. *America: The Jesuit Review*. https://www.americamagazine.org/politics-society/2019/05/31/how-one-midwife-helping-indigenous-mothers-connect-their-childbirth

Goldberg, A. E. (2018). *Cervical ripening*. Medscape. https://emedicine.medscape.com/article/263311-overview#a6.

Gurley, E. S., Halder, A. K., Streatfield, P. K., Sazzad, H. M., Huda, T. M., Hossain, M. J., & Luby, S. P. (2012). Estimating the burden of maternal and neonatal deaths associated with jaundice in Bangladesh: Possible role of hepatitis E infection. *American Journal of Public Health, 102*(12), 2248–2254.

Hale, T., & Ngo, L. (2020). *Psychiatric conditions surrounding pregnancy*. Infant Risk Center. https://www.infantrisk.com/content/psychiatric-conditions-surrounding-pregnancy

Hall, J. E., & Hall, M. E. (2020). Fetal and neonatal physiology. In *Guyton & Hall textbook of medical physiology* (14th ed., pp. 1061–1070). Elsevier.

Harrison, D., Reszel, J., Bueno, M., Sampson, M., Shah, V., Taddio, A., et al. (2016). Breastfeeding for procedural pain in infants beyond the neonatal period. *Cochrane Database of Systematic Reviews*, Issue 10, Article No. CD011248. https://doi.org/10.1002/14651858.CD011248.pub2

Hawes, J., Bernardo, S., & Wilson, D. (2020). The neonatal neurological examination: Improving understanding and performance. *Neonatal Network, 39*(3), 116–128.

Hewitt, L., Kerr, E., Stanley, R. M., & Okely, A. D. (2020). Tummy time and infant health outcomes: A systematic review. *Pediatrics, 145*(6), e20192168. https://doi.org/10.1542/peds.2019-2168.

Hoecker, J. L. (n.d.). *What's the importance of tummy time for a baby?* https://www.mayoclinic.org/healthy-lifestyle/infant-and-toddler-health/expert-answers/tummy-time/faq-20057755#:~:text=Hoecker%2C%20M.D.,flat%20spots%20(positional%20plagiocephaly).

Hooper, S. B., Te Pas, A. B., & Kitchen, M. J. (2016). Respiratory transition in the newborn: a three-phase process. *Archives of Disease in Childhood (Fetal and Neonatal Edition), 101*(3), F266–F271. https://doi.org/10.1136/archdischild-2013-305704

Huda. (2017). *Common practices of Islamic birth rights*. https://www.thoughtco.com/islamic-birth-rites-2004500

Institute of Medicine (IOM). (2006). *Dietary reference intakes: The essential guide to nutrient requirements*. National Academies Press.

Institute of Medicine. (2009). *Weight gain during pregnancy: Reexamining the guidelines*. National Academies Press. http://www.national-academies.org/hmd/~/media/Files/Report%20Files/2009/Weight-Gain-During-Pregnancy-Reexamining-the-Guidelines/Report%20Brief%20-%20Weight%20Gain%20During%20Pregnancy.pdf

Institute of Medicine (IOM). (2011). *Dietary reference intakes for calcium and vitamin D*. National Academies Press

Ippolito, D. L., Bergstrom, J. E., Lutgendorf, M. A., & Flood-Nichols, S. K. (2014). A systematic review of amniotic fluid assessments in twin pregnancies. *Journal of Ultrasound Medicine, 33*(3), 1353.

James, W. D., Berger, T. G., Elston, D. M., & Neuhaus, I. M. (2019). *Andrews' diseases of the skin: Clinical dermatology* (12th ed., pp. 862–880). Elsevier.

Janke, J. (2014). Newborn nutrition. In K. R. Simpson & P. A. Creehan (Eds.), *Perinatal nursing* (4th ed., pp. 626–661). Lippincott Williams & Wilkins.

Jazayeri, A. (2018). *Premature rupture of membranes*. Medscape. https://emedicine.medscape.com/article/261137-overview#a2

The Joint Commission. (2018). Distinct newborn identification requirement. *Requirement, Rationale, Reference Report, 17.* https://www.jointcommission.org/-/media/tjc/documents/standards/r3-reports/r3_17_newborn_identification_6_22_18_final.pdf?db=web&hash=52948449641735707EDF1CB17A6BDBD9

Julvez, J., Méndez, M., Fernandez-Barres, S., Romaguera, D., Vioque, J., Llop, S., et al. (2016). Maternal consumption of seafood in pregnancy and child neuropsychological development: A longitudinal study based on a population with high consumption levels. *American Journal of Epidemiology, 183*(3), 169–182

Kann, L., McManus, T., Harris, W. A., Shanlin, S. L., Flint, K. H., Queen, B., et al. (2018). Youth risk behavior surveillance–United States, 2017. *Surveillance Summaries, 67*(8), 1–114.

Kim, S. (2017). Sanhujori: Korea's traditional postnatal care culture. *International Journal of Childbirth Education, 32*(3), 13–16.

King, T. K., Brucker, M. C., Kriebs, J. M., Fahey, J. O., Gegor, C. L., & Varney, H. (2019). *Varney's midwifery* (6th ed.). Jones & Bartlett Learning.

Kokorelias, K. M., Gignac, M. A., Naglie, G., & Cameron, J. I. (2019). Towards a universal model of family centered care: A scoping review. *BMC Health Services Research, 19*(1), 564.

Krowchuk, D., P., Frieden, I. J., Mancini, A. J., Darrow, D. H., Blei, F., Greene, A. K., . . . Subcommittee on the Management of Infantile Hemangiomas. (2019). Clinical practice guideline for the management of infantile hemangiomas. Pediatrics, 143(1), e20183475.

Kumar, R.K., Singhal, A., Vaidya, U., Banerjee, S., Anwar, F., & Rao, S. (2017). Optimizing nutrition in pretern low birth weight infants: Consensus summary. *Frontiers in Nutrition*, 4(20). https://doi.org/10.3389/fnut.2017.00020

Ladewig, P. A., London, M. L., & Davidson, M. R. (2017). *Contemporary maternal–newborn nursing care* (9th ed. pp. 528–570). Pearson.

Lipsett, B. J., Reddy, V., & Steanson, K. (2020). *Anatomy, head and neck, fontanelles*. Statpearls. https://www.ncbi.nlm.nih.gov/books/NBK542197/

London, M. L., Ladewig, P. A., Davidson, M. R., Ball, J. W., Bindler, R. C., & Cowen, K. J. (2017). *Maternal and child nursing care* (5th ed.). Pearson.

Long, K., Rondinelli, J., Yim, A., Cariou, C., & Valdez, R. (2020). Delaying the first newborn bath and exclusive breastfeeding. *American Journal of Maternal/Child Nursing, 45*(2), 110–115.

Lowdermilk, D. L., Perry, S. E., Cashion, K., Alden, K. R., & Olshansky, E. F. (2020). *Maternity and women's health care* (12th ed.). Elsevier.

Lubbe, W. (2018). Clinicians guide for cue-based transition to oral feeding in preterm infants: An easy-to-use clinical guide. *Journal of Evaluation in Clinical Practice, 24*(80), 80–88.

Lutwak, R. A., Ney, A. M., & White, J. E. (2020). *Jewish perspectives on the birthing experience*. https://www.mikvah.org/article/jewish_perspectives_on_the_birthing_experience

Lyndon, A., Lee, H. C., Gilbert, W. M., Gould, J. B., & Lee, K. A. (2012). Maternal morbidity during childbirth hospitalization in California. *Journal of Maternal–Fetal and Neonatal Medicine, 12*, 2529–2535.

Magann, E., & Ross, M. G. (2014). *Assessment of amniotic fluid volume*. UpToDate. http://www.uptodate.com/contents/assessment-of-amniotic-fluid-volume

Maitre, N. L., Key, A. P., Chorna, O. D., Slaughter, J. C., Matusz, P. J., Wallace, M. T., & Murray, M. M. (2017). The dual nature of early-life experience on somatosensory processing in the human infant brain. *Current Biology, 27*(7), 1048–1054.

Malm, M. C., Lindgren, H., Rubertsson, C., Hildingsson, I., & Radestad, I. (2014). Development of a tool to evaluate fetal movements in -full-term pregnancy. *Sexual and Reproductive Healthcare, 5*(1), 31–35.

March of Dimes (MOD). (2016). *Pregnancy after age 35*. http://www.marchofdimes.org/pregnancy-after-age-35.aspx

March of Dimes (MOD). (2019). *Medical reasons for inducing labor*. https://www.marchofdimes.org/pregnancy/medical-reasons-for-inducing-labor.aspx

Marshall, S., Lang, A., Perez, M., & Saugstad, O. D. (2019). Delivery room handling of the newborn. *Journal of Perinatal Medicine, 48*(1), 1–10. https://doi.org/10.1515/jpm-2019-0304

Martin, G. R., Ewer, A. K., Gaviglio, A., Hom, L. A., Saarinen, A., Sontag, M., et al. (2020). Updated strategies for pulse oximetry screening for critical congenital heart disease. *Pediatrics, 146*(1), e20191650. https://doi.org/10.1542/peds.2019-1650.

Martin, J. A., Hamilton, B. E., Osterman, M. J., & Driscoll, A. K. (2019). Births: Final data for 2018. *National Vital Statistics Reports, 68*(13), 1–47.

Mayo Clinic. (2016). *Infant and toddler health*. http://www.mayoclinic.org/healthy-lifestyle/infant-and-toddler-health/basics/newborn-health/hlv-20049400

Mayo Clinic. (2017a). *Fetal presentation before birth*. https://www.mayoclinic.org/healthy-lifestyle/pregnancy-week-by-week/multimedia/fetal-positions/sls-20076615?s=6

Mayo Clinic. (2017b). *Pregnancy after 35: Healthy moms, healthy babies*. https://www.mayoclinic.org/healthy-lifestyle/getting-pregnant/in-depth/pregnancy/art-20045756

Mayo Clinic. (2018a). *Episiotomy: When it's needed, when it's not*. https://www.mayoclinic.org/healthy-lifestyle/labor-and-delivery/in-depth/episiotomy/art-20047282

Mayo Clinic. (2018b). *VBAC: Know the pros and cons*. https://www.mayoclinic.org/tests-procedures/vbac/in-depth/vbac/art-20044869

Mayo Clinic. (2020a). *Dinoprostone (vaginal route)*. https://www.mayoclinic.org/drugs-supplements/dinoprostone-vaginal-route/before-using/drg-20063461

Mayo Clinic. (2020b). *Labor induction*. https://www.mayoclinic.org/tests-procedures/labor-induction/about/pac-20385141

McCall, E. M., Alderdice, F., Halliday, H. L., Vohra, S., & Johnston, L. (2018). Interventins to prevent hypothermia at birth in preterm and/or low birth weight infants. *Cochrane Database of Systematic Reviews, 2:* CD004210.

McGrath, J. M., & Vittner, D. (2018). Behavioral assessment. In E. P. Tappero & M. E. Honeyfield (Eds.), *Physical assessment in the newborn* (6th ed., pp. 193–218). Springer.

Means, R. T. (2020). Iron deficiency and iron deficiency anemia: Implications and impact in pregnancy, fetal development, and early childhood parameters. *Nutrients, 12*(2), 447.

MedlinePlus. (2019). *Infant reflexes*. http://www.nlm.nih.gov/medlineplus/ency/article/003292.htm

MedlinePlus. (2021a). *Neonatal weight gain and nutrition*. https://medlineplus.gov/ency/article/007302.htm

MedlinePlus. (2021b). *Quadruple screen test*. http://www.nlm.nih.gov/medlineplus/ency/article/007311.htm

Menihan, C. A., & Kopel, A. (2014). *Point-of-care assessment in pregnancy and women's health: Electronic fetal monitoring and sonography*. Lippincott Williams, & Wilkins.

Mercer, R. T. (1995). *Becoming a mother*. Springer.

Mercer, R. T. (2004). Becoming a mother versus maternal role attainment. *Journal of Nursing Scholarship, 36*(3), 226–232.

Messerlian, G. M., Farina, A., & Palomaki, G. E. (2016). *First trimester combined test and integrated test for screening for Down syndrome and trisomy 18*. UpToDate. http://www.uptodate.com/contents/first-trimester-combined-test-and-integrated-tests-for-screening-for-down-syndrome-and-trisomy-18

Micali, N., Stavola, B. D., Santos-Silva, I., Steenweg-de Graaff, J., Jansen, P. W., Jaddoe, V. W., et al. (2012). Perinatal outcomes and gestational weight gain in women with eating disorders: A population-based cohort study. *British Journal of Obstetrics and Gynecology, 119*(12), 1493–1502.

Miguelez, J., De Lourdes Brizot, M., Liao, A. W., De Carvalho, M. H. B., & Zugaib, M. (2012). Second-trimester soft markers: Relation to first-trimester nuchal translucency and unaffected pregnancies. *Ultrasound in Obstetrics and Gynecology, 39*, 274–278. https://doi.org/10.1002/uog.9024

Miller, C. (2018, April 30). Native's first native birthing facility planned in New Mexico. *Santa Fe New Mexican*. https://www.santafenewmexican.com/news/health_and_science/nation-s-first-native-birthing-facility-planned-in-new-mexico/article_c225ecc6-9e9f-5874-b369-1199e09ac3a7.html

Miller, L., Miller, D., & Cypher, R. (2017). *Mosby's pocket guide to fetal monitoring: A multi-disciplinary approach* (8th ed.). Elsevier.

Moghadam, S. H., & Ganji, J. (2019). The effect of kangaroo care on physical and mental health of infants: A review. *Journal of Pediatrics Review, 7*(5), 12.

Moore, E. R., Anderson, G. C., Bergman, N., & Dowswell, T. (2016). Early skin-to-skin contact for mothers and their healthy newborn infants. *Cochrane Database of Systematic Reviews*, Issue 11, Article No. CD003519. https;//doi.org/10.1002/14651858.CD003519.pub4

Moore, K. L., Persaud, T. V. N., & Torchia, M. G. (2019). *The developing human: Clinically oriented embryology* (11th ed.). Saunders.

Moore, T. R., & Piacquadio, K. (1989). A prospective evaluation of fetal movement screening to reduce the incidence of antepartum fetal death. *American Journal of Obstetrics and Gynecology, 160*(5, Pt. 1), 1075–1080.

Morris, B. J., Hankins, C. A., Lumbers, E. R., Mindel, A., Klausner, J. D., Krieger, J. N., & Cox, G. (2019). Sex and male circumcision: Women's preferences across different cultures and countries: A systematic review. *Sexual Medicine, 7*(2), 145–161.

Mu, P., Lee, M., Chen, Y., Yang, H., & Yang, S. (2020). Experiences of parents providing kangaroo care to a premature infant: A qualitative systematic review. *Nursing and Health Sciences, 22*(2), 149–161.

Muchowski, K. E. (2014). Evaluation and treatment of neonatal hyperbilirubinemia. *American Family Physician, 89(11)*, 873–878.

Muñoz, M., Gómez-Ramírez, S., Besser, M., Pavía, J., Gomollón, F., Liumbruno, G. M., et al. (2017). Current misconceptions in diagnosis and management of iron deficiency. *Blood Transfusion, 15*(5), 422–437.

Murray, S., McKinney, E., Holub, K.S., & Jones, R. (2019). *Foundations of maternal–newborn and women's health nursing* (7th ed.). Elsevier.

National Academies of Sciences, Engineering, and Medicine. (2019). *Dietary reference intakes for sodium and potassium*. National Academies Press.

National Center for Complementary and Integrative Health (NCCIH). (2016). *Ginger*. https://nccih.nih.gov/health/ginger

Niebyl, J. R., Weber, R. J., & Briggs, G. G. (2016). Drugs and environmental agents in pregnancy and lactation: Teratology, epidemiology. In S. Gabbe, J. Niebyl, J. Simpson, M. Landon, H. Galan, E. Jauniaux, et al. (Eds.), *Obstetrics: Normal and problem pregnancies* (7th ed., pp. 136–159). Elsevier Saunders.

Nilsson, L., Thorsell, T., Wahn, E. H., & Ekstrom, A. (2013). Factors influencing positive birth experiences of first-time mothers. *Nursing Research and Practice, 2013*, 349124. https://doi.org/10.1155/2013/349124

Noble, A., Rom, M., Newsome-Wicks, M., Engelhardt, K., & Woloski-Wruble, A. (2009). Jewish laws, customs, and practice in labor, delivery, and postpartum care. *Journal of Transcultural Nursing, 20*(3), 323–333.

Nudelman, M. J., Belogolovsky, E., Jegatheesan, P., Govindaswami, B., & Song, D. (2020). Effect of delayed cord clamping on umbilical blood gas values in term newborns: A systematic review. *Obstetrics and Gynecology, 135*(3), 576–582.

Nugent, J. K. (2013). The competent newborn and the Neonatal Behavioral Assessment Scale: T. Berry Brazelton's legacy. *Journal of Child and Adolescent Psychiatric Nursing, 26*, 173–179.

Pace, E. J., Brown, C. M., & DeGeorge, K. C. (2019). Neonatal hyperbilirubinemia: An evidence-based approach. *Journal of Family Practice, 68*, E4–E11.

Pados, B., F., & McGlothen-Bell, K. (2019). Benefits of infant massage for infants and parents in the NICU. *Nursing for Women's Health, 23*(3), 265–271.

Papadakis, M., McPhee, S., & Rabow, M. W. (2014). *Current medical diagnosis and treatment 2015*. McGraw-Hill.

Parker, L. (2021). Nutritional management. In M. T. Verklan, M. Walden, & S. Forest (Eds.), *Core curriculum for neonatal intensive care nursing* (6th ed., pp. 152–171). Saunders.

Pember, M. A. (2018, January 5). The midwives' resistance: How Native women are reclaiming birth on their terms. *Rewire News*. https://rewire.news/article/2018/01/05/midwives-resistance-native-women-reclaiming-birth-terms/

Perry, S. E., Hockenberry, M. J., Alden, K. R., Lowdermilk, D. L., Cashion, M. C., & Wilson, D. (2017). *Maternal child nursing care*. Mosby.

Pickerel, K. K., Waldrop, J., Freeman, E., Haushalter, J., & D'Auria, J. (2020). Improving the accuracy of newborn weight classification. *Journal of Pediatric Nursing, 50*, 54–58.

Powrie, R., Greene, M., & Camann, V. (2012). *De Swiet's medical disorders in obstetric practice* (5th ed.). Wiley.

Purnell, L. D., & Fenkl, E. A. (2019). *Handbook for culturally competent care*. Springer.

Reddy, U. M., Abuhamad, A. Z., Levine, D., Saade, G. R., & Fetal Imaging Workshop Invited Participants. (2014). Fetal imaging: Executive summary of a joint Eunice Kennedy Shriver National Institute of Child Health and Human Development, Society for Maternal-Fetal Medicine, American Institute of Ultrasound in Medicine, American College of Obstetricians and Gynecologists, American College of Radiology, Society for Pediatric Radiology, and Society of Radiologists in Ultrasound Fetal Imaging workshop. *Obstetrics and Gynecology, 123*(5), 1070.

Rich, B. S., & Dolgin, S. E. (2020). Clarifying misleading lumps and sinuses in the newborn. *Pediatrics in Review, 41*(6), 276–282.

Romm, A. J. (2014). *The natural pregnancy book: Herbs, nutrition, and other holistic choices* (3rd ed.). Crown.

Rossi, S., Buonocore, G., & Bellieni, C. V. (2020). Management of pain in newborn circumcision: A systematic review. *European Journal of Pediatrics, 180*(1), 13–20. https://doi.org/10.1007/s00431-020-03758-6

Rubin, R. (1984). *Maternal identity and the -maternal experience.* Springer.

Sadler, T. W. (2018). *Langman's medical embryology* (14th ed.). Lippincott Williams & Wilkins.

Safe to Sleep. (n.d.). *Babies need tummy time!* https://safetosleep.nichd.nih.gov/safesleepbasics/tummytime

Sahota, D. S., Leung, W. C., To, W. K., Chan, W. P., Lau, T. K., & Leung, T. Y. (2012). Quality assurance of nuchal translucency for prenatal fetal Down syndrome screening. *Journal of Maternal–Fetal and Neonatal Medicine, 25*(7), 1039–1043. https://doi.org/10.3109/14767058.2011.614658

Salmon, J. F. (2020). In *Kanski's clinical ophthalmology: A systematic approach* (pp. 827–880). Elsevier.

Sathish, Y., Lewis, E., Noronha, J. A., George, A., Nayak, B., Pai, M. S., et al. (2017). Clinical outcomes of snuggle up position using positioning aids for preterm (27–32 weeks) infants. *Iranian Journal of Neonatology, 8*(1). https://doi.org/10.22038/ijn.2016.7709

Sathish, Y., Lewis, L. E., Noronha, J. A., Nayak, B. S., Pai, M. S., & Altimier, L. (2019). Promoting developmental supportive care in preterm infants and families in a level III neonatal intensive care unit (NICU) setting in India. *Nurse Education in Practice, 40.* https://doi-org/10.1016/j.nepr.2019.08.006

Sen, E., & Manav, G. (2020). Effect of Kangaroo Care and Oral Sucrose on Pain in Premature Infants: A Randomized Controlled Trial. *Pain Management Nursing, 21*(6), 556–564

Sharifzadeh, F., Kashanian, M., Koohpavehzadeh, J., Rezaiain, F., Sheikhansari, N., & Eshraghi, N. (2018). A comparison between the effects of ginger, pyridoxine (vitamin B6) and placebo for the treatment of the first trimester nausea and vomiting of pregnancy (NVP). *Journal of Maternal-Fetal and Neonatal Medicine, 31*(19), 2509–2514.

Sherman, K. E. (2019). *Hepatitis E virus infection.* UpToDate. https://www.uptodate.com/contents/hepatitis-e-virus-infection

Snijder, C. A., Brand, T., Jaddoe, V., Hofman, A., Mackenbach, J. P., Steegers, E. P., & Burdorf, A. (2012). Physically demanding work, fetal growth and the risk of adverse birth outcomes: The Generation R study. *Occupational Environmental Medicine, 69*, 543–550.

Solan, T. D., & Lindow, S. W. (2014). Mercury -exposure in pregnancy: A review. *Journal of Perinatal Medicine, 42*(6), 725–729.

Sonek, J., Molina, F., Hiett, A. K., & Glover, M. (2012). Prefrontal space ratio: Comparison between trisomy 21 and euploid fetuses in the second trimester. *Ultrasound in Obstetrics and Gynecology, 40*(3), 293–296. https://doi.org/10.1002/uog.11120

Sonesson, S. E., Ambrosi, A., & Wharen-Herlenius, M. (2019). Benefits of fetal echocardiographic surveillance in pregnancies at risk of congenital heart block: Single-center study of 212 anti-Ro52-positive pregnancies. *Ultrasounds Obstetrics and Gynecology, 54*(1), 87–95.

Sood, A., & Sood, N. (2020). Pain relief in labor. In A. Sharma (Ed.), *Labour room emergencies* (pp. 245–256). Springer.

Spector, R. E. (2017). *Cultural diversity in health and -illness* (9th ed.). Pearson Education.

Stachowiak, A., & Furman, L. (2020). Vitamin K is necessary for newborns. *Pediatrics in Review, 41*(6), 305–306.

Stanford Medicine. (2006). *Guidelines for vitamin K prophylaxis.* https://med.stanford.edu/newborns/clinical-guidelines/vitamink.html

Stanford Medicine (2020). *Newborns: Professional education—abdomen.* https://med.stanford.edu/newborns/professional-education/photo-gallery/abdomen.html

Sukumaran, L., McClarthy, N. L., Kharbanda, E. O., Vazquez-Benitez, G., Lipkind, H. S., Jackson, L., et al. (2018). Infant hospitalizations and mortality after maternal vaccination. *Pediatrics, 141*(3), e20173310. https://doi.org/10.1542/peds.2017-3310

Taheri, M., Takian, A., Taghizadeh, Z., Jafari, N., & Sarafraz, N. (2018). Creating a positive perception of childbirth experience: Systematic review and meta-analysis of prenatal and intrapartum interventions. *Reproductive Health, 15*(73). https://doi.org/10.1186/s12978-018-0511-x

Task Force on Sudden Infant Death Syndrome. (2016). SIDS and other sleep-related infant deaths: Updated 2016 recommendations for a safe infant sleeping environment. *Pediatrics, 138*(5), e20162938.

Troullioud Lucas, A. G., Jaafar, S., & Mendez, M. D. (2020). *Pediatric umbilical hernia.* Statpearls. https://www.ncbi.nlm.nih.gov/books/NBK459294/

Udo, I., Lewis, J., Tobin, J., & Ickovics, J. (2016). Intimate partner victimization and health risk behaviors among pregnant adolescents. *American Journal of Public Health, 106*(8), 1457–1459.

U.S. Department of Agriculture. (2015). *Dietary guidelines for Americans 2015–2020* (8th ed.). https://health.gov/our-work/food-nutrition/2015-2020-dietary-guidelines/guidelines/

U.S. Department of Agriculture and U.S. Department of Health and Human Services. (2020). *Dietary guidelines for Americans, 2020–2025* (9th ed). https://www.dietaryguidelines.gov/sites/default/files/2020-12/Dietary_Guidelines_for_Americans_2020-2025.pdf

U.S. Department of Health and Human Services. (2020). *Recommended uniform screening panel.* https://www.hrsa.gov/advisory-committees/heritable-disorders/rusp/index.html

U.S. Food and Drug Administration (FDA). (2014). *Pregnancy and lactation labeling (drugs) final rule.* https://www.fda.gov/drugs/labeling-information-drug-products/pregnancy-and-lactation-labeling-drugs-final-rule

U.S. Food and Drug Administration (FDA). (2018). *Food safety for moms-to-be: At-a-glance.* http://www.fda.gov/Food/FoodborneIllnessContaminants/PeopleAtRisk/ucm081819.htm

U.S. Food and Drug Administration. (FDA). (2019). *Salmonella.* https://www.fda.gov/food/foodborne-pathogens/salmonella-salmonellosis

U.S. Preventive Services Task Force. (2020). *Sexually transmitted Infections: Behavioral counseling.* https://www.uspreventiveservicestaskforce.org/uspstf/recommendation/sexually-transmitted-infections-behavioral-counseling

Vargo, L. (2014). Newborn physical assessment. In K. R. Simpson & P. A. Creehan (Eds.), *Perinatal nursing* (4th ed., pp. 597–625). Lippincott Williams & Wilkins.

Voerman, E., Santos, S., Patro Golab, B., Amiano, P., Ballester, F., Barros, H., et al. (2019). Maternal body mass index, gestational weight gain, and the risk of overweight and obesity across childhood: An individual participant data meta-analysis. *PLoS Medicine, 16*(2), e1002744.

Vrees, R. A. (2018). *Induction of labor.* Medscape. https://reference.medscape.com/drug/cytotec-misoprostol-341995#5 on 6/1/20.

Wahl, L., Dupont, G., & Tubbs, R. S. (2019). The simian crease: Relationship to various genetic disorders. *Clinical Anatomy, 32*(8), 1042–1047.

Waksmonski, C. A., & Foley, M. R. (2020). *Pregnancy in women with congenital heart disease: General principles.* UpToDate. https://www.uptodate.com/contents/pregnancy-in-women-with-congenital-heart-disease-general-principles

Waksmonski, C. A., LaSala, A., & Foley, M. R. (2019). *Acquired heart disease and pregnancy.* UpToDate. https://www.uptodate.com/contents/acquired-heart-disease-and-pregnancy

Warren, S., Midodzi, W. K., Newhook, L. A., Murphy, P., & Twells, L. (2020). Effects of delayed newborn bathing on breastfeeding, hypothermia, and hypoglycemia. *Journal of Obstetric, Gynecologic and Neonatal Nursing, 49*(2), 181–189.

Watchmaker, B., Boyd, B., & Dugas, L. R. (2020). Newborn feeding recommendations and practices increase the risk of development of overweight and obesity. *BMC Pediatrics, 20*(1), 1–6.

Watson, J., & Moulsdale, W. (2020). Translation into practice: Dextrose gel treatment for neonatal hypoglycemia to reduce NICU admissions and increase breastfeeding exclusivity. *Neonatal Network, 39*(2), 57–65.

Wegman, S. J., & McKnight, L. (2020). Case 2: Recurrent respiratory distress in a new born. *Pediatrics in Review, 41*(6), 297–299.

Wolfberg, A. (2016). The evolution of prenatal testing: How NIPT is changing the landscape in fetal aneuploidy screening. *Medical Laboratory Observer, 48*(1), 18.

World Health Organization (WHO). (2015). *The global numbers and costs of additionally needed and unnecessary cesarean sections performed per year: Overuse as a barrier to universal coverage* (World Health Report, Background Paper No. 30). http://www.who.int/healthsystems/topics/financing/healthreport/30C-sectioncosts.pdf

World Health Organization (WHO). (2018a). *Making childbirth a positive experience.* https://www.who.int/reproductivehealth/intrapartum-care/en/

World Health Organization (WHO). (2018b). *Preterm birth: Key facts.* https://www.who.int/news-room/fact-sheets/detail/preterm-birth

World Health Organization (WHO). (2018c). *WHO recommendations: Intrapartum care for a positive birth experience.* https://apps.who.int/iris/bitstream/handle/10665/260178/9789241550215-eng.pdf;jsessionid=569470D12B73D1BD0248954DB3BB0008?sequence=1

World Health Organization (WHO). (2019a). *Demand feeding for low-birth-weight infants.* https://www.who.int/elena/titles/demandfeeding_infants/en/

World Health Organization (WHO). (2019b). *Newborns: improving survival and well-being.* https://www.who.int/news-room/fact-sheets/detail/newborns-reducing-mortality

Young, S., & Cox, J. T. (2019). *Pica in pregnancy.* UpToDate https://www.uptodate.com/contents/pica-in-pregnancy

Youth.gov (n.d.). Adverse effects. https://youth.gov/youth-topics/pregnancy-prevention/adverse-effects-teen-pregnancy

Yu, X., Zhang, J., & Yuan, L. (2020). Chinese parents' lived experiences of having preterm infants in NICU: A qualitative study. *Journal of Pediatric Nursing, 50*, e48–e54.

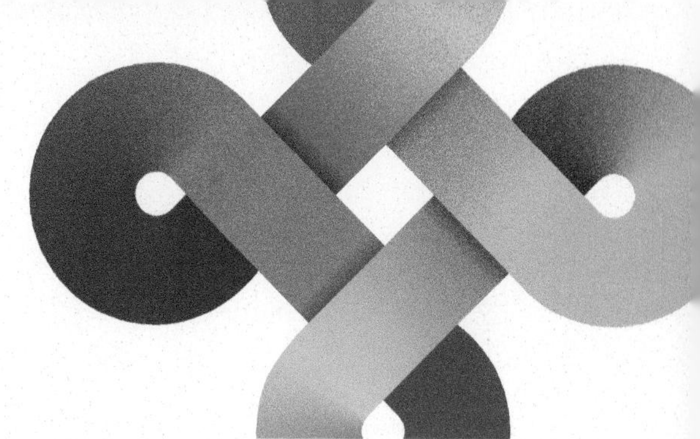

Part IV
Nursing Domain

Part IV consists of modules that define and outline principles of nursing care, including assessment, clinical decision making, and communication. Each module presents a concept that directly relates to professional nursing and its impact on patient health and well-being. Selected principles or topics of that concept are presented as exemplars. In the concept of clinical decision making, for example, the exemplars include the nursing process, the nursing plan of care, and prioritizing care. Each module addresses the impact of that concept and selected exemplars on the care of individuals across the lifespan, inclusive of cultural, gender, and developmental considerations.

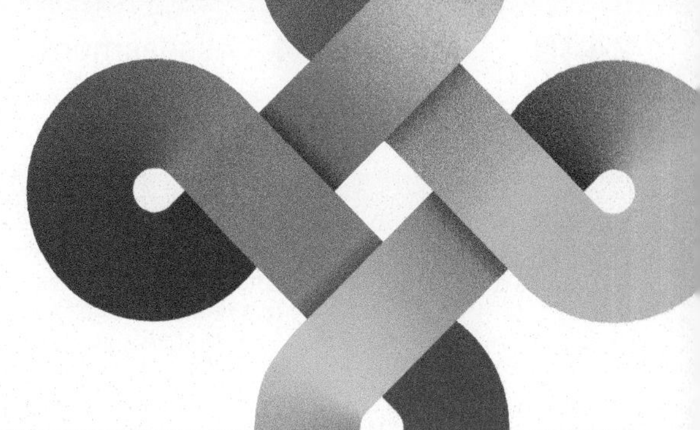

Module 34
Assessment

Module Outline and Learning Outcomes

The Concept of Assessment

Types and Sources of Data

34.1 Analyze the types and sources of data collected during a nursing assessment.

Collecting Data

34.2 Analyze the principal methods used to collect data during a nursing assessment.

Organizing Data

34.3 Analyze various methods of organizing assessment data.

Validating Data

34.4 Analyze the need for validating data collected during the nursing assessment.

Interpreting Data

34.5 Analyze the cues used when interpreting data from a nursing assessment.

Concepts Related to Assessment

34.6 Outline the relationship between assessment and other concepts.

Holistic Health Assessment Across the Lifespan

34.7 Differentiate considerations related to the assessment of patients throughout the lifespan.

›› The Concept of Assessment

Concept Key Terms

Auscultation, **2460**
Benchmark, **2448**
Clinical database, **2448**
Closed questions, **2452**
Communication, **2463**
Crepitation, **2457**
Cues, **2447**
Directive interview, **2450**
Duration, **2460**
Functional status, **2471**
Health assessment, **2447**
Holistic health, **2464**
Hydrocephalus, **2466**
Inspection, **2457**
Intensity, **2460**
Interview, **2449**
Instrumental activities of daily living, **2471**
Leading question, **2453**
Monitoring, **2447**
Neutral question, **2452**
Nondirective interview, **2450**
Objective data, **2448**
Open-ended questions, **2452**
Overnutrition, **2466**
Palpation, **2457**
Percussion, **2459**
Pitch, **2460**
Pleximeter, **2459**
Plexor, **2459**
Quality, **2460**
Rapport, **2450**
Signs, **2448**
Subjective data, **2448**
Symptoms, **2448**
Undernutrition, **2466**
Validation, **2461**

Health assessment is a systematic process through which the nurse collects data about a patient to create a holistic plan of care. The plan of care addresses a patient's current or long-term health status, as well as factors that inform or affect health. The nurse documents an individual's potential for increased risk, current health promotion activities, and relevant physical, psychological, social, cultural, and environmental characteristics. Examples of data gathered about a patient's health include **cues**, signs and symptoms of physical or mental illness or injury, health behaviors, and risk and protective factors. Health assessment includes an interview to determine health history and a patient's current presenting problem and a physical assessment. Accurate recording of findings, both subjective data provided by the patient and objective data collected during the physical examination, is critical to successful interpretation of findings.

When conducting a health assessment, the nurse may use one of four types of assessments depending on the situation: initial (or baseline) assessment, problem-focused (or system-focused) assessment, emergency assessment, and time-lapsed reassessment (**monitoring**) (see **Table 34.1** ››).

Types and Sources of Data

Data collection serves as the foundation for the assessment. The nurse systematically collects information about the patient's health. Significant facts must not be overlooked, and any changes in the patient's health status must be described. Documentation will include both constant data and variable data. Facts, such as birthdate or blood type, are constant and do not change over time. Variable data can change over time. The pace and variability of change can be quick or slow, frequent or rare. Examples of variable data include blood pressure readings and pain levels.

TABLE 34.1 Types of Assessment

Type	Time Performed	Purpose	Example
Initial (or baseline) assessment	Performed within a specified time frame after admission to a healthcare agency (refer to agency policy and procedure)	■ To establish a baseline for problem identification, reference, and future comparison	■ Nursing admission assessment
Problem-focused (or system-specific) assessment	Ongoing process integrated with nursing care	■ To determine the status of a specific problem identified in an earlier assessment	■ Hourly assessment of patient's fluid intake and urinary output in an intensive care unit (ICU) ■ Assessment of patient's ability to perform self-care while assisting a patient to bathe
Emergency assessment	During any physiologic or psychologic crisis	■ To identify life-threatening problems ■ To identify new or overlooked critical problems	■ Rapid assessment of open airway, breathing status, and circulation during a cardiac arrest ■ Assessment of suicidal tendencies or potential for violence
Time-lapsed reassessment (monitoring)	Several months after initial assessment	■ To compare the patient's current status to baseline data previously obtained	■ Reassessment of a patient's functional health patterns in a home care or outpatient setting, or change-of-shift assessments in an acute or long-term care facility

Source: From Berman, Snyder, and Frandsen (2021).

A **clinical database** has components supplied by the entire range of clinicians. Nurses contribute patient health history and physical assessment. Primary care providers document patient history and physical examination. Other health personnel measure the results of laboratory and diagnostic tests and other specialized interventions. For accuracy and completeness, all participants must take an active role in the assessment process.

The nurse compiles data about the patient's past health history, updating the picture to focus on current health problems. For example, evidence of a rash developing from previous penicillin medication is critical to planning care. Other examples of important historical data include previous surgeries, the use of complementary and alternative therapies, and diagnosis of chronic disease. Essential current records describe cues such as pain, nausea, insomnia, and the presence (or absence) of support systems.

Types of Data

It is useful to distinguish between two types of cues: **subjective data (symptoms)** and **objective data (signs)**. Only patients can describe or verify *symptoms*, which are feelings or sensations that the patient experiences but which cannot be objectively measured. Examples of subjective data are sensations of itching, numbness, cold, pain, and feelings of contentment or depression. Important information comes from asking patients about their perceptions of their personal health status and their life situation. Questions can also be asked about patients' values, beliefs, and attitudes that affect their health.

An observer, such as a nurse, can detect, measure, and test objective data against an accepted standard (**benchmark**). *Signs* can be identified by observation or on physical examination by using the senses of sight, hearing, touch, and smell. Examples include temperature, pulse, respirations, and blood pressure. A physical examination can discover visible signs such as pressure sores or swollen joints. The assessment phase of the nursing process is completed when the nurse has obtained sufficient objective data to validate subjective data. For example, if the patient complained of severe throat pain when swallowing (subjective), the nurse might document observation of white patches at the back of the patient's throat and red, swollen tonsils (objective).

Sources of Data

Health data can be collected from primary or secondary (indirect) data sources. The primary source of data is the patient. Interviewing family members, friends, other support people, or other healthcare professionals provides secondary data. Documents such as medical records, laboratory and test reports, and relevant literature also qualify as secondary data sources. Information not supplied directly by the patient is considered as coming from a secondary source, and it should be validated with the patient or during the physical examination, if possible.

Patient

Exceptions to interviewing the patient directly arise in situations of severe illness, mental confusion, or unconsciousness. Fear, embarrassment, lack of trust, or language differences can be barriers to accurate primary assessment. Young age or developmental delay can also present barriers. Otherwise, the best way to gather subjective data is to interview the patient. Some objective data, such as sex and ethnicity, can also be gathered at that time.

Support People

The circle of individuals who support the patient can be valuable resources to supplement or verify patient data. These may include significant others, family members, friends, and caregivers with firsthand knowledge of the patient's health. Members of this circle can often give the nurse a holistic picture about the patient's feelings about and response to illness or injury, as well as information about current stressors and home environment.

Documentation of the assessment data may need to recognize the sensitivity of the information. For example, in cases of physical or emotional abuse, the interviewee might ask to remain anonymous. However, on a routine basis, the nurse should request permission from mentally stable patients to interview support people. The nursing notes should record the fact of the permission and the role of the support person.

The patient is not the only source of subjective information. Significant others, family members, friends, caregivers, and other healthcare professionals can supply their viewpoints. For example, if a nursing assistant said, "The patient is confused," that is secondary subjective data. It is an interpretation of the patient's behavior. However, if the nursing assistant said, "The patient told me, 'I am visiting a zoo right now,'" that statement is secondary objective information. The nursing assistant heard and quoted the patient's words directly.

The nurse should take into account the relationship or lack of connection to support people when asking questions during the patient's assessment interview. Foster parents might have less knowledge of a child's health history than biological parents. An older patient with dementia living alone will require a different interview approach than a healthy patient of the same age enjoying an active lifestyle with a spouse. Adapting assessment tools to personal circumstances customizes the data.

Patient Records

Patient data is present in medical records, documentation of therapies, and laboratory reports. A full range of healthcare professionals contribute to patient data. In many cases, nurses have access to a wide array of information about a patient's current health and health history, illnesses, and injuries. Reviewing medical interviews, physical examinations, surgical and discharge summaries, progress notes, and specialists' consultations could provide valuable information about the patient's allergies, medical crises, health habits, and coping behaviors.

Physical therapists, social workers, nutritionists, and dietitians document their assessments and therapies. In these notes, nurses can find useful information that comes from a different healthcare perspective. For example, a social worker's report about a home visit could shed light on a patient's living situation. A physical therapist's notes could describe the patient's self-care abilities from an objective viewpoint.

Laboratory and diagnostic results can point to areas of the patient's health that might need special attention. For example, the determination of a glycosylated hemoglobin (A1C) level shows the outcome of a diabetic patient's adherence with medications and nutrition over the past 3 months. The nurse should be familiar with agency or industry benchmarks for laboratory results, taking into account the patient's age, sex, and other personal characteristics.

The nurse brings informed awareness of a patient's present health situation to the review of previous patient records. For example, if the last documentation was 10 years ago, the information needs to be updated, as the patient's health and lifestyle habits are likely to be different. Older patients can have a wealth of previous records. If a patient's memory is impaired, their past health history can be summarized and related to findings in the present time.

Healthcare Professionals

Patients' previous or current contacts with other healthcare professionals can provide useful information about their health. Verbal or written sharing of information by nurses, social workers, primary care providers, or physical therapists can ensure continuity of care as patients move from one treatment setting to another.

Literature

Information from professional journals and reference texts can help the nurse develop or interpret an assessment. Available content can include a variety of resources, including:

- Benchmarks (standards or measures against which to compare findings such as height and weight tables or milestones of developmental tasks by age)
- Health practices characteristic of a specific culture or society
- Religious principles or spiritual values
- Additional focused assessment data necessary to plan nursing interventions and evaluate results
- Corresponding medical diagnoses, treatment approaches, and likely prognostic information
- Recent findings from research studies.

Collecting Data

Observation, interview, and examination are the main methods of data collection. The nurse makes observations when meeting with patients or support people. The nurse interviews individuals to produce a nursing health history. The nurse conducts a physical examination to gather objective data about a patient's health status.

The three methods of collecting data are interwoven in practice. When the nurse interviews a patient, the nurse observes the patient's response, listening for cues that need follow-up during the physical examination. Refer to Module 38, Communication, for further details of this process.

Observing

The nurse uses the senses of vision, smell, hearing, and touch to notice, select, organize, and interpret patient data. (See **Table 34.2** >> for types of information found.) For example, when a nurse observes a patient sweating, the nurse will rely on interpretation of the interaction of the patient's vital signs, physical activity, and environmental temperature

To ensure that important signs of illness or injury are not missed, the nurse needs to pay careful attention to detail, focus on potentially useful data (especially with unexpected findings), and not be distracted by the multitude of available data. For example, nurses in the intensive care unit can focus on their assigned patients while ignoring the loud sounds of other patients' monitor alerts. With experience, a nurse learns to continue nursing care activity, such as giving a bed bath or monitoring an intravenous infusion, while simultaneously observing important signs, such as changes in breathing rate or skin color.

Interviewing

An **interview** is defined as a verbal communication that the nurse plans with a definite purpose. The purpose can be to

TABLE 34.2 Using the Senses to Observe Patient Data

Sense	Example of Patient Data
Vision	Overall appearance (e.g., body size, general weight, posture, grooming); signs of distress or discomfort; facial and body gestures; skin color and lesions; abnormalities of movement; nonverbal demeanor (e.g., signs of anger or anxiety); religious or cultural artifacts (e.g., books, icons, candles, beads)
Smell	Body or breath odors
Hearing	Lung and heart sounds; bowel sounds; ability to communicate; language spoken; ability to initiate conversation; ability to respond when spoken to; orientation to time, person, and place; thoughts and feelings about self, others, and health status
Touch	Skin temperature and moisture; muscle strength (e.g., hand grip); pulse rate, rhythm, and volume; palpatory lesions (e.g., lumps, masses, nodules)

Source: From Berman et al. (2021).

get information or give education, identify issues of mutual concern, use criteria to evaluate the healing process, or provide support in the form of counseling or therapy.

The nursing health history is an interview that often forms the starting point for the nursing admission assessment. See **Box 34.1** ›› for the components of a nursing health history.

Nurses can use either a directive or a nondirective approach to interviews. In the **directive interview**, the nurse takes charge of the conversational flow. A template form is often used, as the interview is highly structured, gathering details about specific topics. Both parties understand that the form's completion is their mutual purpose. The discussion pattern is the nurse asking questions and the patient responding with answers. The patient usually has only a limited time for voicing questions or expressing concerns. This approach is useful in emergency situations, for example, when time is limited to identify the clinically appropriate responses. In contrast, a **nondirective interview**, or rapport-building interview, allows the patient to take charge of the conversational flow, its purpose, subject matter, and pacing. **Rapport** is a connection or bond between two or more people.

In most healthcare situations, an interview can combine elements of the directive and nondirective interview methods. As the nurse, using a directive approach, identifies a patient's concerns, the conversation may switch to following that conversational path. For example, if a patient is worried about the possible complications of surgery, the nurse can pause the interview and respond to the patient's fears, giving therapeutic support. Without that response from the nurse, the patient could misunderstand that the nurse does not know about possible complications, does not care about their effects, or dismisses the patient's feelings as unimportant.

Preparing for the Interview

If no standardized interview format is available, most nurses use a guide or notes about topics and subtopics to remember essential information that must be documented. It is not necessary to write out the full narrative. If a standardized interview format is available, such as with electronic health records, the nurse follows that format. Either way, the nurse prepares for the interview by reviewing already-collected relevant information, such as the patient's surgical summary report or current assessment data. The nurse might also want to access current information about the patient diagnosis.

An effective interview depends on balancing several factors to provide comfort for both nurses and patients. The factors are time, place, seating arrangement or distance, and language.

Time

Knowing the patient's clinical condition and the organization's schedule, the nurse plans to interview patients when they are calm and comfortable and when interruptions by other health professional and support people are not expected. In a home interview, the nurse should allow patients to select the interview time, if possible.

Place

Privacy is essential to conducing a comfortable interview—others should not be able to see or overhear the interview. The environment should be well lighted and adequately ventilated. Avoiding excessive noise, movements, and distractions will promote easier communication and comfort.

Seating Arrangement

If the patient is in bed or in a chair, the nurse should avoid conducting the interview while standing, which can intimidate the patient. Instead, the nurse can sit in a chair at a 45-degree angle to the patient's position. Informality helps the conversation and can put the patient at ease, which is less likely to occur if the nurse stands at the foot of the bed or behind a table or desk. Such an arrangement suggests a business meeting of supervisor and subordinate. Before beginning an initial admission interview, the nurse can place the overbed table between interviewer and interviewee to give a sense of personal space. In a clinic environment, a seating arrangement of two chairs at right angles keeps the participants at the same level and adds a sense of informality and being equal partners (see **Figure 34.1** ››). In group interviews, the nurse can arrange the chairs in a horseshoe or circle arrangement to avoid a superior or head-of-the-table position.

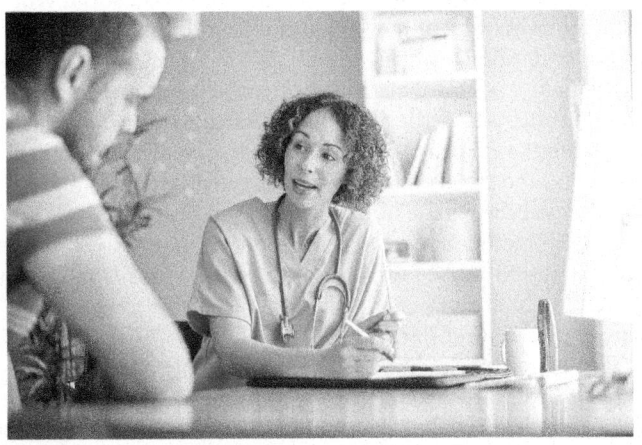

Figure 34.1 ›› A seating arrangement in which the nurse and patient sit on two chairs placed at right angles to a desk puts them on equal terms.

Source: Sturti/E+/Getty Images.

Box 34.1

Components of a Nursing Health History

Biographical Data

The patient's name, address, age, sex, gender, marital status, occupation, religious preference, healthcare financing, and usual source of medical care.

Chief Complaint or Reason for Visit

The chief complaint is the answer given to the question "Can you please tell me the reason you came to the hospital or clinic today?" or "Tell me in your own words why you are here today." It should be recorded in the patient's own words.

History of Present Illness

- When the illness cues started
- Whether the onset of illness cues was sudden or gradual
- How often the problem occurs
- Exact location of the distress
- Character of the complaint (e.g., intensity of pain or quality of sputum, emesis, or discharge)
- Activity in which the patient was involved when the problem occurred
- Cues associated with the chief complaint
- Triggers that aggravate or interventions that alleviate the problem

Past History

- *Childhood illnesses*, such as chickenpox, mumps, measles, rubella (German measles), rubeola (red measles), streptococcal infections, scarlet fever, rheumatic fever, and other significant illnesses
- *Childhood immunizations* and the date of the last tetanus shot
- *Allergies* to drugs, foods, animals, insects, or other environmental agents; the type of reaction that occurs; and how the reaction is treated
- *Accidents and injuries:* how, when, and where the incident occurred, type of injury, treatment received, and any complications
- *Hospitalization for serious illnesses:* reasons for the hospitalization, dates, surgery performed, course of recovery, and any complications
- *Medications and supplements:* all currently used prescription and over-the-counter medications, such as aspirin, nasal spray, vitamins, or laxatives
- *Complementary and integrative health approaches:* use of herbs, chiropractic medicine, acupuncture, or any traditional forms of treatment associated with cultural heritage or spiritual beliefs

Family History of Illness

The nurse needs to ascertain cues that signal increased risk for certain diseases, as well as the ages of siblings, parents, and grandparents and their current state of health or, if they are deceased, the cause of death. Particular attention should be given to disorders such as heart disease, cancer, diabetes, hypertension (HTN), obesity, allergies, arthritis, tuberculosis, bleeding problems, alcoholism, and any mental health disorders.

Lifestyle

- *Personal habits:* the amount, frequency, and duration of use of tobacco, alcohol, coffee, sweetened beverages, tea, and illicit or recreational drugs
- *Diet:* description of a typical diet on a normal day or any special diet, number of meals and snacks per day, who cooks and shops for food, and ethnically distinct food patterns
- *Sleep/rest patterns:* usual daily sleep–wake times, difficulties sleeping, and remedies used for difficulties
- *Activities of daily living (ADLs):* any difficulties experienced in the basic activities of eating, grooming, dressing, elimination, and locomotion
- *Instrumental ADLs (iADLs):* any difficulties experienced in food preparation, shopping, transportation, housekeeping, laundry, and ability to use the telephone, handle finances, and manage medications
- *Recreation/hobbies:* exercise activity and tolerance, hobbies and other interests, and vacations

Social Data

- *Family relationships/friendships:* the patient's support system in times of stress or need, what effect the patient's illness has on the family, and whether any family problems are affecting the patient
- *Ethnic affiliation:* health customs and beliefs, cultural practices that may affect healthcare and recovery
- *Educational history:* data about the patient's highest level of education and past difficulties with learning
- *Occupational history:* current employment status, the number of days missed from work because of illness, any history of accidents on the job, any occupational hazards with a potential for future diseases or accidents, the patient's need to change jobs because of past illness, the employment status of spouses or partners, the way child care is handled, and the patient's overall satisfaction with the work and the workplace environment
- *Economic status:* information about how the patient is paying for medical care (including the kind of medical and hospitalization coverage) and whether the patient's illness presents financial concerns
- *Home and neighborhood conditions:* home safety measures and adjustments in physical facilities required to help the patient manage a physical disability, activity intolerance and difficult ADLs, and the availability of neighborhood and community services to meet the patient's needs

Psychologic Data

- *Major stressors* experienced and the patient's perception of them
- *Usual coping patterns* with a serious problem or a high level of stress
- *Communication style*, or the ability to verbalize appropriate emotions; nonverbal communication—such as eye movements, gestures, use of touch, and posture; interactions with support people; and the congruence of nonverbal behavior and verbal expression

Patterns of Healthcare

Patterns of healthcare are all healthcare resources the patient is currently using and has used in the past. These include the primary care provider, specialists (e.g., ophthalmologist or gynecologist), dentist, traditional healers or folk practitioners (e.g., herbalist or *curandero*), health clinic, or health center; whether the patient considers the care adequate; and whether access to healthcare is a problem.

Source: From Berman et al. (2021).

Distance

The distance between the nurse and patient should be such that both participants can easily see and hear each other without being intrusive. For most people in Western cultures being interviewed, maintaining a separation of 2 to 3 feet feels comfortable. Depending on personal, cultural, or clinical needs, some people will require more or less than that amount of personal space boundaries.

Language

The nurse must communicate in a language that the patient can understand. If the nurse does not speak the patient's language or dialect (a variation spoken in a particular geographic location), the nurse must arrange for an interpreter or translator. If that does not happen, the failure is a form of discrimination.

If the nurse does not speak the patient's language, the person speaking directly to the patient must be able to describe complex medical terms in words that the patient can comprehend. This is a specialized skill. Not everyone who can converse in a foreign language can define anatomic or other health terms. Experienced interpreters make judgments not only about specific words but about subtle meanings of language and ethnicity that need additional explanation or clarification.

When giving written documents to a patient, the nurse must determine whether the patient can read them or if a translator is required. Translators may also be needed to edit the original written source, to ensure the content is comprehensible and culturally appropriate. For in-person interviews, live translation using an experienced interpreter is preferred because the patient can then ask questions for clarification. Services such as LanguageLine Solutions (https://www.languageline.com) are available by telephone or online application 24 hours a day, 7 days a week, in over 200 languages for an hourly fee. Many large agencies have their own on-call interpreters or translation services for the languages or dialects commonly spoken in their area.

SAFETY ALERT Check your healthcare institution's policies about offering interpretive services. Use of family members as interpreters should be avoided as they may insert their own advice or alter information. Using visitors and agency nonprofessional staff should be avoided for reasons of confidentiality. It is important to remember that some patients may be more comfortable with an interpreter who is of the same age and gender as the patient.

Even among patients who speak English, there may be differences in understanding terminology. For example, "cool" may imply something *good* to one patient and something *not warm* to another. For some teenagers and young adults, the term "sick" means something *very good*. The nurse must always confirm accurate understandings.

Telephone and Telehealth Interviews

Increasingly, many intake and preprocedure interviews are being conducted by phone or using a HIPAA-compliant videoconferencing service. In some ways, these types of interviews require even greater attention to detail, looking for changes in patient tone that may signal discomfort in answering questions or attempts to deflect an important question. It is important that nurses use nonjudgmental therapeutic communication to build patient trust and ensure a successful interview. Key strategies for these types of interviews are:

- Beginning with less invasive questions and progressing to more invasive or personal questions as the patient becomes more comfortable with the interview
- Using follow-up questions to clarify important information (such as characteristics of pain) or information that signals a safety issue (such as the patient has not discontinued taking a prescribed blood thinner in advance of a surgical procedure)
- Recognizing cues that indicate patient discomfort or deflection (such as the patient looking away from the camera, talking away from the microphone, asking the nurse to repeat the question several times, or even hanging up).

Types of Interview Questions

Interview questions can be described as closed or open-ended and neutral or leading. The directive interview often uses **closed questions**, which have limited answers of "yes," "no," or a few words of specific facts. Closed questions often start with "when," "where," "who," "what," "do (did, does)," or "is (are, was)." Examples of closed questions include:

- "Are you taking any prescribed medications?"
- "Are you in pain right now? Where?"
- "When did you have your surgery?"

Answers to closed questions are easier than open-ended questions for individuals who are in pain, experiencing high stress, or have difficulty communicating.

The nondirective interview uses **open-ended questions** because it puts patients in charge of the discussion. The conversation gives patients the opportunity to explore, explain, clarify, or describe their thoughts or feelings. The nurse introduces a broad topic that can be answered in the number of words chosen by the patient. Open-ended questions give patients a sense of respect and privacy, as they can share only the information they wish to disclose. That approach is useful at the start of an interview, to change topics, and to understand patients' attitudes.

The first word of an open-ended question is often "what" or "how." Examples of open-ended questions are:

- "What were your first symptoms?"
- "How have you been sleeping recently?"
- "Would you describe more about your relationship with your family members?"
- "What questions do you have for your healthcare provider today?"

It takes flexibility and focused attention to use a combination of closed and open-ended questions during an interview. Nurses need to be open to being flexible to accomplish the objective of the interview, which is to gather all the essential data. See **Box 34.2** » for advantages and disadvantages of open-ended and closed questions.

Nondirective interviews also use open-ended **neutral questions**, questions that can be answered without direction

Box 34.2

Selected Advantages and Disadvantages of Open-Ended and Closed Questions

OPEN-ENDED QUESTIONS

ADVANTAGES	DISADVANTAGES
They develop trust.	They take more time.
They let the patient do the talking.	Patients may give only brief answers.
The nurse is able to listen and observe.	Valuable information may be withheld.
They reveal what the patient thinks is important or what the patient is feeling at the moment.	They can result in more information than necessary.
They may reveal the extent of the patient's knowledge.	Responses may be difficult to document.
They can elicit information the nurse may not ask for.	The nurse requires skill in controlling an open-ended interview.

CLOSED QUESTIONS

ADVANTAGES	DISADVANTAGES
Questions can elicit more targeted information.	They may elicit too little information and require follow-up questions.
They require less effort from the patient.	They may not reveal how the patient feels.
They may be less threatening because they do not require explanations or justifications.	They do not allow the patient to volunteer possibly valuable information.
They take less time.	They may inhibit communication and convey lack of interest by the nurse.
Information can be asked for sooner than it would be volunteered.	The nurse may dominate the interview with questions.
Responses are easily documented.	

Source: Adapted from Berman et al. (2021).

or pressure from the nurse. Examples are "How do you feel about your current living arrangements?" and "Why do you think you chose that line of work?"

A **leading question** is the opposite of the neutral question, usually in the form of a closed question in a directive interview. Examples are "You're stressed about waiting for the biopsy results, aren't you?" and "You will continue to have regular laboratory testing, won't you?" Patients have little time to analyze their responses, since they know what answer is expected of them. This can create problems when patients want to please the interviewer. They can give inaccurate responses, which results in inaccurate data. This can adversely affect nursing care.

Stages of an Interview

Every interview has three stages (Stewart & Cash, 2017):

- Opening (introduction)
- Body
- Closing.

The Opening

The opening stage of an interview is the most important component because its purpose is to establish rapport with patients and orient them to the process of data gathering. The success of the remainder of the interview depends on the nurse's initial words, verbal tone, and body expression.

Creating rapport is the goal of the opening. That connection allows a mutual trust to be established. The script begins with a greeting and introduction ("Hello, Mr. Jones, I'm Pat Perkins, a nursing student"). Nonverbal gestures, such as a smile or a handshake, reinforce a welcoming attitude. This is not a time for superficial talk because that might be construed as unprofessional and make the patient uncomfortable.

In orienting the patient to the process of data gathering, the nurse explains in general terms a description of the needed information, what the data will be used for, the expected duration of the interview, and how the patient can best participate. The nurse usually states that patients' information is treated with confidentiality and they have the right to refuse to provide personal information.

An example of the two-step interview introduction is as follows.

Step 1—Create rapport:

Nurse: Hello, Mr. Jones. I'm Pat Johnson, a senior nursing student. I will be conducting your admission assessment today.

Patient: You're set to graduate this year?

Nurse: Yes, and I hope to continue to work at this hospital. The care team is very supportive of students and new hires.

Patient: It's important to enjoy the people you work with. I've been fortunate that way.

Nurse: I'm glad to hear that.

Step 2—Orientation to the process of data gathering:

Nurse: I can begin your admission assessment right now, if this is a good time for you. May I sit down with you for about half an hour to collect some information that your care team needs? We want to prepare you for before and after your operation.

Patient: Okay. That would be fine.

Nurse: I'm going to ask you questions about your usual daily activities at home and what you expect to be able to do after the operation. I'll take notes on our discussion and share the information with the rest of the care team. If I get to a topic that you don't want to talk about, let me know. All your information is confidential, only shared with those with a legal right to the data.

Patient: I understand. I appreciate your letting me know that.

The Body of the Interview

In the longest part of the interview, the nurse asks the patient a series of questions and notes the patient's responses. The nurse uses communication techniques that expand on the initial comfortable rapport between the participants. To make sure the purpose of the interview is achieved, the nurse should follow these guidelines of "dos" and "don'ts."

Helpful strategies to use during the interview include:

- Do focus your full attention on the patient's responses, with a calm, unhurried, respectful, concerned, and sympathetic attitude.
- Do use all your senses to observe the patient's ongoing reactions, voice characteristics, and body language. Maintain eye contact.
- Do be aware of your own body language and the affect, tone, and inflection of your voice; you need to nonverbally convey interest and acceptance.
- Do speak slowly and clearly. Be ready to repeat or restate your queries if the patient seems confused.
- Do use the spoken language a patient understands or arrange for a translator or interpreter.
- Do follow a logical sequence in asking questions.
- Do acknowledge a patient's right to express personal viewpoints.

Practices or habits to avoid while interviewing patients include:

- Don't ask more than one question at a time. Multiple questions may confuse the patient, and you will not be confident of the accuracy of the response.
- Don't impose your personal value system on the patient's opinions or behavior.
- Don't share your own viewpoint or advice, such as saying, "If I were you . . . "
- Don't position yourself at a different level than the patient or move in too close or too far away.
- Don't interrupt patient-initiated silence; allow the patient to have time to think or organize thoughts.

The Closing of the Interview

The end of the interview usually comes when the nurse has gathered the essential information. However, sometimes patients terminate the data-gathering process. For example, the patient may decline to give further information or be unable to share more details due to a clinical condition, such as fatigue. The closing stage needs to maintain rapport and trust, as well as facilitate future interactions. Several techniques are useful to signal to the patient that the interview process is about to end, including:

1. ***Voice your openness to responding to patient questions.*** "If you have any questions, I'll be glad to answer them." Don't hurry the response. Give the patient time to consider your offer or it will seem insincere.
2. ***Signal the upcoming conclusion, express your support, and thank the patient.*** "Well, I have all the information the care team needs to plan your care. I hope your procedure is successful. Thank you for your time and help." Using the word "well" provides a clue that the interview will be ending. Shaking the patient's hand is another way of smoothly ending the interview.
3. ***Look ahead to the future.*** Let the patient know what comes next, whether it is a follow-up to the interview or another type of meeting. Share as many details as you know at the time. Choices include the day, the time, the place, the topic, and the purpose of the next encounter. "I will see you the afternoon after your operation, to see how you are feeling." Or "Ms. Wong, I am scheduled to take care of you on Monday, Tuesday, and Wednesday mornings between nine o'clock and noon. I can check on your progress those days."
4. ***Summarize your interview information.*** Reviewing the summarized data with the patient verifies its accuracy. Besides helping end the interview, reviewing the information reassures the patient that the nurse has listened carefully and that forward progress has been made in the treatment planning. Introduce the summary by beginning with: "Let me review your information with you." Since this approach is useful for anxious or distractible patients, an offer to gather further data at a later time can be appropriate: "Well, you seem worried about coping with your recovery after your operation. Is that true? I can talk with you tomorrow about what arrangements we can help you make."

Clinical Example A

Rekha Saunders is a 59-year-old recently retired marketing professional who reports continued acute back pain. The findings from the physical assessment are all within normal limits. Ms. Saunders states that the pain started 3 weeks ago and has been getting worse, with only temporary relief with the use of aspirin. The nurse asks about any activities or events associated with the onset of the pain. Ms. Saunders reveals that she took up knitting as a hobby about a month ago. She has been sitting and knitting a blanket for her new grandchild almost every day for an hour or two. In addition, she proudly adds that her garden "has never looked better—not a weed in sight!"

Critical Thinking Questions

1. How does the additional interview information provide cues to assist the nurse in interpretation of Ms. Saunders's back pain?
2. What recommendations could the nurse make to prevent further straining the muscles of Ms. Saunders's back?
3. What timetable should the nurse give Ms. Saunders to expect decreased pain? What is the plan if this target date is not met?

Examining

As part of the assessment process, the nurse conducts a physical examination, systematically collecting data using observation. The nurse uses the senses of sight, hearing, smell, and touch to detect health cues through the techniques of inspection, auscultation, palpation, and percussion. A physical examination satisfies six purposes:

- To gather current data about a patient's functional status
- To add to, verify, or correct data from the nursing history
- To use data as a foundation for nursing diagnoses and plans of care
- To monitor outcomes of healthcare interventions
- To clinically evaluate the patient's health condition
- To discover the patient's health promotion and disease prevention needs.

Nurses conduct three types of physical examinations: (1) the initial admission assessment, (2) the body system–specific assessment (e.g., the neuromuscular system), or (3) an assessment of a body area (e.g., the sacral-lumbar area, when back pain is reported). Physical examinations routinely start by measuring the patient's vital signs. **Table 34.3** » lists normal vital signs across the lifespan.

TABLE 34.3 Normal Vital Sign Ranges Across the Lifespan[a]

	Pulse (per minute)[b]	Respirations (per minute)[b]	Temperature (°C)[c]	Blood Pressure (mmHg)[d]	
				Systolic	Diastolic
Newborn	100–160 (awake) as low as 70 (asleep)	30–60 (over 60 considered tachypnea)	Normal range: (axillary) 36.5–37.4	At birth: 50–70[e] At day 10: 90	At birth: 30–45[e] At day 10: 50
Infant	90–160 (awake) 80–160 (asleep)	30–60	Normal range (axillary): 36.5–37.5	Age 1 Boys: 80–89 Girls: 83–90	Age 1 Boys: 34–39 Girls: 38–42
Toddler	80–140 (awake) 80–120 (asleep)	20–40	Normal range: 36–37.5 Extreme range: 35–40	Age 2 Boys: 84–92 Girls: 85–91	Age 2 Boys: 39–44 Girls: 43–47
Preschooler	80–120 (awake) 80–120 (asleep)	20–35	Normal range: 36–38.5 Extreme range: 35–40	Age 4 Boys: 88–97 Girls: 88–94	Age 4 Boys: 47–52 Girls: 50–54
School age	65–120 (awake) 50–90 (asleep)	16–22	Normal range: 36–38.5 Extreme range: 35–40	Age 9 Boys: 95–104 Girls: 96–103	Age 9 Boys: 57–62 Girls: 58–61
Adolescent	60–100	12–20	Normal range: 36–38.5 Extreme range: 35–40	Age 15 Boys: 109–117 Girls: 107–113	Age 15 Boys: 61–66 Girls: 64–67
Adult	60–100	12–20	Normal range: 36–38.5 Extreme range: 35–40	Less than 120	Less than 80
Older adult	60–100	15–20	Normal range: 36–38.5 Extreme range: 35–40	Less than 120	Less than 80

[a]There is a wide variety of "normal" at each stage of the lifespan, and vital signs are dynamic. While these ranges provide a general sense of the norm, it is important for the nurse to determine what "normal" is for each patient and to base further considerations on those parameters and the context of the patient presentation.
[b]The ranges for pulse and respiration change dramatically from birth through adolescence and then remain fairly stable throughout the rest of life.
[c]The first set of numbers in each cell is the usual range of temperature; the second set shows extremes of normal temperature for when the weather is very cold, when it is early in the morning, or during exercise.
[d]Adult data from American College of Cardiology (2019). Note that blood pressure readings for children are determined using the child's height percentile. The blood pressure values presented here are the 50th percentile for the child's age, sex, and height, which are considered the midpoint of the normal range. A reading above the 95th percentile indicates hypertension. To see the pediatric blood pressure tables, visit https://www.nhlbi.nih.gov/files/docs/guidelines/child_tbl.pdf.
[e]Blood pressure is usually monitored before age 3 only if the patient has cardiac issues. Note that blood pressure readings for children are determined using the child's height percentile. The blood pressure values presented here are the 50th percentile for the child's age, sex, and height, which are considered the midpoint of the normal range. A reading above the 95th percentile indicates hypertension. To see the pediatric blood pressure tables, visit http://www.nhlbi.nih.gov/health-pro/guidelines/current/hypertension-pediatric-jnc-4/blood-pressure-tables.htm.

Alternate Version of Children's BP

	Boys		Girls	
Age, Years	Systolic BP	Diastolic BP	Systolic BP	Diastolic BP
1	Less than 98	Less than 52	Less than 98	Less than 58
2	Less than 100	Less than 55	Less than 101	Less than 58
4	Less than 102	Less than 60	Less than 103	Less than 62
9	Less than 107	Less than 68	Less than 108	Less than 71
More than 13	Less than 120	Less than 80	Less than 120	Less than 80

Source: From Flynn et al. (2017).

Physical examinations typically reveal normal and abnormal findings. The nurse must analyze both types of findings and make critical decisions about their meaning and importance. For example, when a patient is being admitted with a diagnosis of appendicitis, the presence of pain in the right lower quadrant would be an expected initial finding, while a later absence of pain in that same location might be a cue that the appendix has ruptured.

When findings are different than anticipated, the nurse must make decisions about their importance and what to do with the information. If unsure about the significance of a finding or to whom it should be reported, the nurse should consult with a more experienced nurse regarding the best course of action to follow.

A complete physical examination typically follows one of three patterns: (1) head-to-toe process, (2) review of body systems (cardiovascular system, respiratory system, etc.), or (3) a combination of those two formats. See **Box 34.3** ›› for an outline of this combined approach.

Apart from the chosen format, the nurse personalizes the examination according to the patient's age and energy level, illness or injury severity, nurse and patient preferences, examination environment, time constraints, and organizational policies and procedures. In positioning the patient, the nurse has the patient make the fewest movement changes possible.

Often the purpose of the assessment is to check the status of a specific body area, not the entire body. The trigger for these targeted examinations can be the patient's complaints or presenting health problem cues, the nurse's observations or available interventions, or medical therapies. Examples of these situations and assessments are provided in **Table 34.4** ››.

Nurses use national guidelines and evidence-based practice while performing health assessments. For example, when screening for cancer, the nurse should keep in mind the American Cancer Society's (2018) guidelines for early detection. These guidelines include methods for early identification of breast, colorectal, cervical, endometrial, lung, and prostate cancers.

›› **Stay Current:** To see the American Cancer Society's guidelines for early detection of cancer, visit www.cancer.org/healthy/findcancerearly/cancerscreeningguidelines/american-cancer-society-guidelines-for-the-early-detection-of-cancer.

Preparing the Patient

To help the patient feel more comfortable about the physical examination, the nurse briefly explains the entire process. This helps relieve anxiety about unknown findings. A step-by-step explanation provides reassurance and promotes patient relaxation. The details are important: the when, where, why, and what happens. This ensures that the patient gives the necessary informed consent to the examination. The nurse explains that all collected and recorded information is treated with confidentiality, in keeping with the Health Insurance Portability and Accountability Act (HIPAA). The nurse emphasizes that access is restricted to healthcare providers (HCPs) and health insurance companies with legal rights to see the data.

Box 34.3

Outline of Review of Body Systems

- *General survey and health status:* Appearance and mental status, height and weight (including recent changes and duration of time), vital signs, presenting problem or cues suggestive of health problems.

›› **Skills:** For skills related to physical assessment, see Chapter 1, Assessment, in Volume 3.

- *Skin, hair, and nails:* Skin integrity (any cuts, scrapes, burns, moles, lesions, flaking or dry skin), perception of touch, pressure, temperature, pain; evidence of anxiety (hair picking [trichotillomania] or nail biting); overall cleanliness, odor, color; recent changes from normal
- *Head, neck, and related lymphatics:* Color, symmetry, position, movement, tenderness, size, or abnormalities; cues such as headaches, dizziness, or syncope
- *Eyes:* Vision (including any recent changes), function, structure (size, shape, symmetry, movement)
- *Ears, nose, mouth, and throat:* Size, shape, symmetry, color, patency; signs of obstruction, abnormality, or inflammation; hearing (including any recent changes); senses of taste and smell intact, any changes from normal
- *Neurologic system:* Mental status, cranial nerve status (see Module 11, Intracranial Regulation)
- *Lungs and thorax:* Chest symmetry and movement; respiratory rate, rhythm, and effort; presence of any respiratory cues of problems
- *Breasts and axillae:* Skin color and markings; structural symmetry and movement; palpation to assess for tissue abnormalities, tenderness
- *Cardiovascular system:* Heart rate, heart sounds, skin color and temperature (to assess oxygen perfusion), pulses; history of cardiac disease, MI, or chest pain
- *Peripheral vascular system:* Skin color, appearance of superficial vasculature, shape and size of extremities and nails (note any swelling or discoloration), palpation of pulses, auscultation of blood pressure and arteries; sensation (e.g., coldness or numbness)
- *Abdomen:* Skin, shape, abdominal movements; inspection, auscultation, percussion, and palpation in that order
- *Gastrointestinal system:* Appetite; presence of any cues such as indigestion, nausea and/or vomiting; assessment of bowel movements, any changes in stool, or rectal bleeding
- *Genitourinary system:* Urinary frequency and character; changes and cues of problems; genital health; safe sex practices; for women, menstrual history and frequency
- *Musculoskeletal system:* Movement, stability, pain, swelling, deformity, or weakness.

A thorough assessment will also include assessing pain, nutrition and fluid intake and patterns, and psychosocial health (including screening for substance use, depression, and intimate partner violence).

Sources: Adapted from Fenske, Watkins, Saunders, D'Amico, and Barbarito (2019); Jarvis (2019).

TABLE 34.4 Selected Examples of Physical Assessments

Situation (Cue)	Physical Assessment
Patient is admitted with a head injury.	Assess level of consciousness using the Glasgow Coma Scale (discussed in Module 11, Intracranial Regulation); assess pupils for reaction to light and accommodation; assess vital signs. Assess cranial nerve response.
Patient has just had a cast applied to the lower leg.	Assess peripheral perfusion of toes; capillary refill; pedal pulse, if accessible. Take vital signs.
Patient's spouse reports that the patient with limited mobility is "not making sense."	Take vital signs. Check for signs that indicate fall or injury. Assess for signs of infection.
Patient is curled up in a fetal position, holding his head between his hands.	Assess the vital signs, including the possibility of pain or withdrawal. Palpate the forehead to check for elevated temperature.
Patient reports difficulty breathing and is sitting in tripod position.	Take vital signs and conduct focused respiratory assessment.
Patient receiving a blood transfusion reports "itchy skin."	Stop transfusion. Take vital signs and inspect the chest skin for signs of rash.
Parents report their child is unresponsive.	Assess the child's ABCs (airway, breathing, circulation). Intervene as needed.

Before patients are brought into the examination room, they should be given the opportunity to use the restroom. Emptying their bladders helps relaxation and palpation of the lower abdominal area. If a urinalysis is needed, a collection container is provided beforehand. In the examination room, the nurse assists patients as needed to replace their clothes with a gown.

By itself, the physical examination does not usually cause pain. However, the nurse works with the patient to determine if a body position is contraindicated for a particular individual. For example, difficulty breathing might become worse with a supine position or back pain may increase with straight legs on a hard table.

Preparing the Environment

The setting for the physical examination should be well lighted and at a comfortable temperature. Supplies and equipment should be organized and available.

The nurse strives to maintain environmental privacy as much as possible. This prevents the patient's embarrassment at being seen unclothed or fear of being overheard. The culture, age, and gender of both the patient and the nurse should be considered. For example, if the genders of the patient and the nurse are different, the nurse should ask if that difference is acceptable to the patient. If not, special arrangements might be necessary. Unless the patient insists, family and friends should not be in the same room during the examination.

Positioning

The nurse should consider several cues before asking patients to move to different positions during the physical examination. Age, mobility, flexibility, physical condition, and energy level may affect patients' ability to maintain a specific position. Patient embarrassment or discomfort should be minimized as much as possible. Two principles help: not extending the time in any one position and organizing the examination so several body areas can be assessed without the patient moving. **Table 34.5** » summarizes selected positions and areas of assessment.

Methods of Examining

Inspection, palpation, percussion, and auscultation are the four primary techniques of physical examination. Nurses need to practice each method to develop their clinical expertise.

Inspection

Inspection uses the sense of sight to make a visual examination of the patient. Nurses proceed deliberately, purposefully, and systematically either with the naked eye or with a lighted instrument. For example, an otoscope is used to view the inner ear. Simultaneously while looking at the patient, nurses' senses of smell and hearing provide clues to the patient's health status.

Inspection can be used to assess body surfaces for moisture, color, and texture. Examination can reveal if the patient's body has a normal shape, position, size, color, and symmetry. Either natural or artificial light can provide sufficient lighting to see clearly. Similarly, a quiet environment is needed to hear clearly. Nurses can combine observation with other assessment techniques as needed.

Palpation

Palpation is an assessment technique that uses the sense of touch. The fingers pads are highly sensitive due to their high concentration of nerve endings. Palpation can measure the following features, arranged in alphabetical order:

- Amplitude of pulses
- **Crepitation** (cracking or rattling sound)
- Distention (e.g., of the urinary bladder)
- Location, position, size, consistency, and mobility of organs, lumps, or masses
- Moisture
- Pain or tenderness
- Rigidity and spasticity
- Swelling
- Temperature (e.g., of a skin area)
- Texture (e.g., of the hair)
- Vibration (e.g., of a joint).

TABLE 34.5 Patient Positions and Body Areas Assessed

Position	Description	Areas Assessed	Cautions
Dorsal recumbent	Back-lying position with knees flexed and hips externally rotated; small pillow under the head; soles of feet on the surface	Female genitals, rectum, and female reproductive tract	May be contraindicated for patients who have cardiopulmonary problems.
Supine (horizontal recumbent)	Back-lying position with legs extended; with or without pillow under the head	Head, neck, axillae, anterior thorax, lungs, breasts, heart, vital signs, abdomen, extremities, peripheral pulses	Tolerated poorly by patients with cardiovascular and respiratory problems.
Sitting	A seated position, back unsupported and legs hanging freely	Head, neck, posterior and anterior thorax, lungs, breasts, axillae, heart, vital signs, upper and lower extremities, reflexes	Older adults and weak patients may require support.
Lithotomy	Back-lying position with feet supported in stirrups; the hips should be in line with the edge of the table	Female genitals, rectum, and female reproductive tract	May be uncomfortable and tiring for older adults and embarrassing for most patients.
Sims	Side-lying position with lowermost arm behind the body, uppermost leg flexed at hip and knee, upper arm flexed at shoulder and elbow	Rectum, vagina	Difficult for older adults and people with limited joint movement.

Source: Adapted from Berman et al. (2016).

Palpation is either light (superficial) or deep. Light palpation should always be performed before deep palpation. Heavy pressure on the nurse's fingertips can dull the sense of touch. In light palpation, the nurse first places the dominant hand's fingers parallel to the patient's skin surface (see **Figure 34.2** »). Then the nurse moves the hand in a circular motion, while pressing gently, to slightly depress the skin. If the nurse is assessing a mass, the nurse should move and press lightly several times on the skin, rather than holding the pressure in one place. See **Table 34.6** » for the characteristics of masses.

The nurse can perform one- or two-handed (bimanual) deep palpation. In the one-handed technique, the finger pads of the dominant hand move and press over the top of the skin surface. The other hand can be used to support the other side of the mass or organ (see **Figure 34.3** »). For deep bimanual palpation, the nurse uses the dominant hand as the bottom layer on the skin surface. The top layer comes from the finger

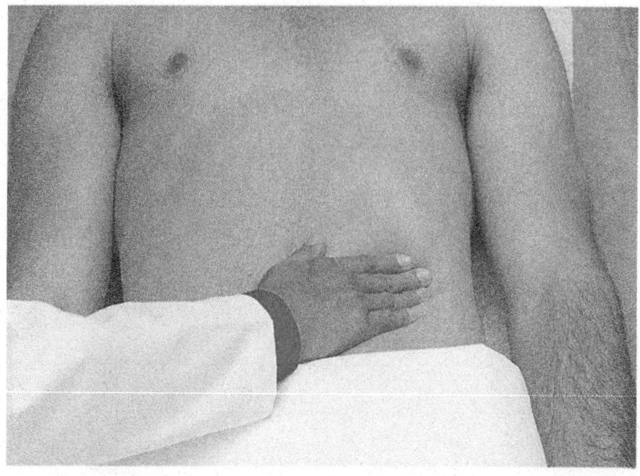

Figure 34.2 ›› The position of the hand for light palpation.
Source: Pearson Education, Inc.

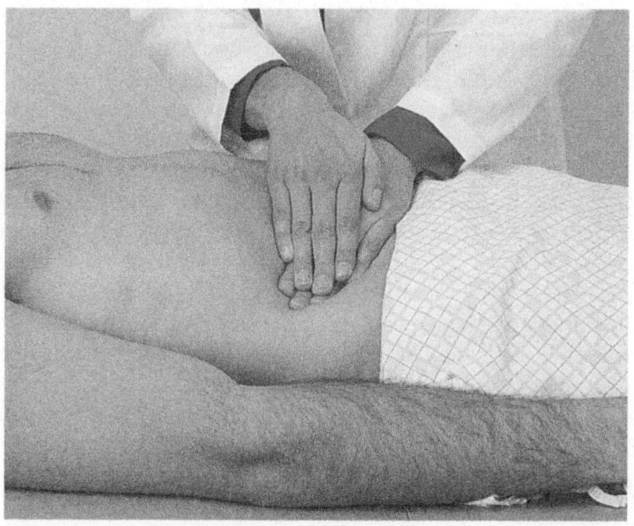

Figure 34.3 ›› The position of the hands for deep bimanual palpation (for a right-handed nurse).
Source: Pearson Education, Inc.

pads of the nondominant hand pushing down upon the surface of the joints of the lower layer's middle three fingers. The top layer provides the pressure, while the bottom layer concentrates on a sensitive touch (see **Figure 34.4** ››).

A routine physical examination does not usually include deep palpation. It needs significant practitioner skill and extreme caution. The applied pressure could damage internal organs. The technique is never used in patients with acute abdominal pain or pain not yet diagnosed.

The patient's level of relaxation and the nurse's correct hand positioning greatly affect the effectiveness of palpation. The nurse uses the dorsal surface (back) of the hand and fingers to test skin temperature. The skin is thinner there than on the palm side. The nurse uses the base of the fingers or palm of the hand to test for vibration. A checklist for palpation includes:

- Appropriate gowning and/or draping of the patient
- Comfortable positioning of the patient
- Clean and warm hands

TABLE 34.6 Characteristics of Masses

Characteristic	Descriptors
Location	Site on the body, dorsal/ventral surface
Size	Length and width in centimeters
Shape	Oval, round, elongated, irregular
Consistency	Soft, firm, hard
Surface	Smooth, nodular
Mobility	Fixed, mobile
Pulsatility	Present or absent
Tenderness	Degree of tenderness to palpation

Source: From Berman et al. (2016).

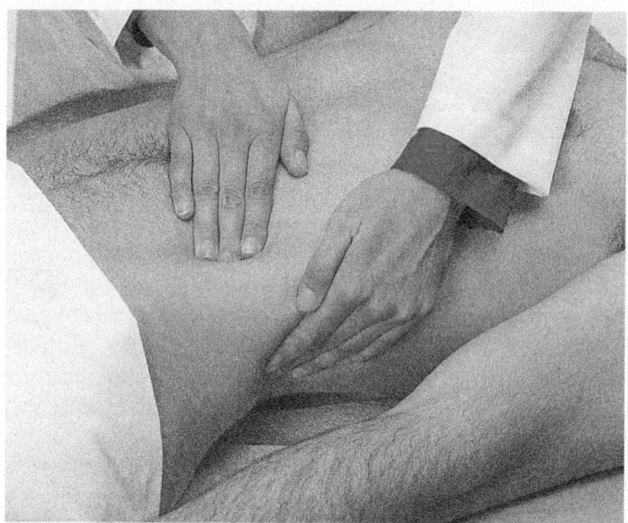

Figure 34.4 ›› Deep palpation using the lower hand to support the body while the upper hand palpates the organ (for a right-handed nurse).
Source: Pearson Education, Inc.

- Short fingernails
- Slow and systematic palpation technique
- Sensitivity to the patient's verbal and nonverbal communications of discomfort
- Tender areas palpated last.

Percussion

Percussion is the assessment technique of striking the surface of a body to hear sounds or feel vibrations. There are two types of percussion: direct and indirect. Direct percussion refers to the nurse striking an area with the pad of the middle finger or with the pads of two, three, or four fingers. The movement uses wrist action with rapid strikes. See **Figure 34.5** ››.

In *indirect percussion*, an object, such as the nurse's distal phalanx and joint of the middle finger of the nondominant hand (**pleximeter**), is held against a body area. The nurse strikes the pleximeter, usually at the distal interphalangeal joint, with the tip of the flexed middle finger of the other hand (**plexor**). Another striking point is between the distal and proximal joints of the nondominant hand (see **Figure 34.6** ››). Just as in direct percussion, indirect

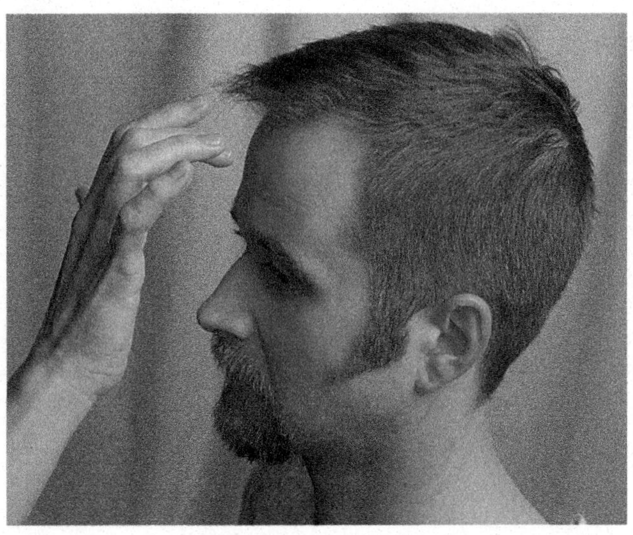

Figure 34.5 » Direct percussion, in which one hand is used to strike the surface of the body.
Source: Pearson Education, Inc.

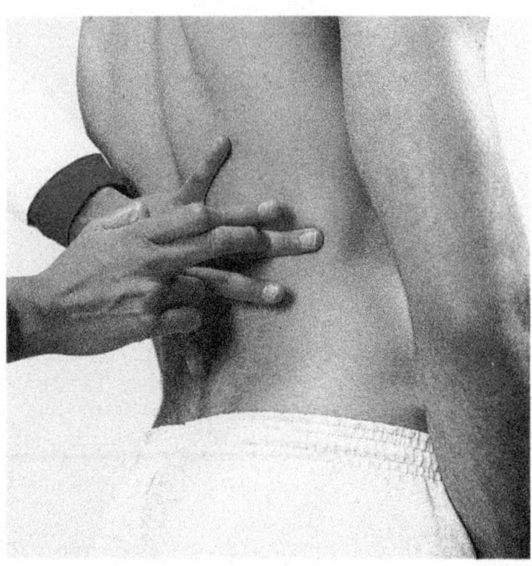

Figure 34.6 » Indirect percussion, in which the finger of one hand taps the finger of the other hand (for a right-handed nurse).
Source: Pearson Education, Inc.

percussion uses wrist action with firm, short, and rapid strikes. A 90-degree angle is maintained between the plexor and the pleximeter. The nurse's forearm does not move.

A percussion technique can define the borders of internal organs, determining their size and shape. The nurse can find out if tissue is fluid filled, air filled, or solid. Characteristics of five types of sound are described in **Table 34.7 »**. On a continuum, a sound of flatness, the top row of the table, comes from percussing the most dense tissue with the least amount of air. A sound of tympany, the lowest row of the table, comes from percussing the least dense tissue with the most amount of air.

Auscultation

Auscultation is an assessment technique that listens to body sounds, either directly or indirectly. The unaided ear uses direct auscultation to listen to a respiratory wheeze or the crackling of a moving joint. A stethoscope provides indirect auscultation to amplify and transmit sounds inside the body to the nurse's ears. For example, it allows bowel sounds or valve sounds of the heart and blood pressure to be clearly heard.

The tubing of a stethoscope should be 30 to 35 cm (12 to 14 inches) long, with an inside diameter of about 0.3 cm (1/8 inch). The nurse should ensure that its earpieces face forward, fitting comfortably. The nurse firmly, but lightly, places the amplifier of the stethoscope against the patient's skin. Dampen excessive body hair with a moist cloth to lie flat against the skin for clear sound transmission.

Auscultated sounds have characteristics of pitch, intensity, duration, and quality. **Pitch** is the vibration frequency, expressed as the number of vibrations per second. Fewer vibrations per second, such as some heart sounds, produce low-pitched sounds. More vibrations per second, such as bronchial sounds, produce high-pitched sounds. **Intensity** (amplitude) describes sounds as loud (e.g., bronchial sounds from the trachea) or soft (e.g., normal lung breathing sounds). **Duration** of a sound measures its length as long or short. **Quality** of sound subjectively describes noises, such as whistling, gurgling, or snapping.

Equipment

Before a physical examination starts, the nurse assembles the required equipment and supplies. Cold equipment that will touch the patient should be warmed up. After each use, equipment should be cleaned according to the manufacturer's or organization's recommendations. Commonly used tools and supplies include:

- *Stethoscope:* For listening to heart, lung, and bowel sounds
- *Sphygmomanometer:* To take blood pressure readings
- *Pulse oximeter:* To assess oxygen saturation

TABLE 34.7 Percussion Sounds and Tones

Sound	Intensity	Pitch	Duration	Quality	Example of Location
Flatness	Soft	High	Short	Extremely dull	Very dense tissue of muscle, bone
Dullness	Medium	Medium	Moderate	Thudlike	Dense tissue of liver, spleen, heart
Resonance	Loud	Low	Long	Hollow	Normal lung filled with air
Hyperresonance	Very loud	Very low	Very long	Booming	Emphysematous lung (not healthy)
Tympany	Loud	High (distinguished mainly by musical or drumlike timbre)	Moderate	Musical	Stomach filled with gas (air)

Source: Adapted from Berman et al. (2021).

- *Ophthalmoscope:* To assess the interior of the eye
- *Otoscope:* To visualize the eardrum and external ear canal
- *Percussion (reflex) hammer:* To test reflexes
- *Tuning fork:* To test hearing acuity and vibratory sense
- *Tongue depressors:* To assess the mouth and pharynx
- *Gloves:* To protect the nurse from patient infections
- *Water-soluble lubricant:* To make the insertion of instruments more comfortable
- *Thermometer:* To take the temperature
- *Clock or watch:* To measure pulse and breathing rate
- *Speculum:* To conduct a pelvic examination
- *Laboratory testing supplies:* As indicated for sending samples out for testing.

Clinical Example B

Clara and Roberto Galvez carry their screaming 7-year-old son Johnnie into the emergency department. They tell the triage nurse that Johnnie woke up before dawn complaining that his stomach hurt. He then vomited and, when touched, he felt very hot and sweaty. Johnnie now holds both hands tightly on his abdomen and cannot be consoled.

The nurse conducts a physical examination that reveals the following: symmetrical abdomen, bowel sounds in all quadrants, tender to palpation in the lower quadrants, guarding. Johnnie has an oral temperature of 101.5°F, pulse of 122 beats/min, and respiratory rate of 24 breaths/min.

Critical Thinking Questions

1. Classify the findings as objective or subjective data.
2. Prepare a narrative nursing note from the data.
3. What cues must be considered in conducting the comprehensive health assessment of Johnnie Galvez? What additional information might prove useful in the assessment? How would you gather that information?

Organizing Data

Collected data must be recorded at the time of collection or shortly thereafter. Data are recorded in written or digital formats that organize assessment data systematically. Most schools of nursing and healthcare agencies have developed their own structured assessment formats for documenting a comprehensive picture of the patient's health. Some ways to organize assessment data are based on selected nursing models or frameworks and other theories. See **Table 34.8** for examples of the foundations of some templates.

See Box 34.3 for an example of an outline based on reviewing body systems.

If the assessment data is less comprehensive and specific to a time frame, a clinical focus, or a patient's physical status, other methods of documentation may be selected. One format for orthopedic patients could focus on musculoskeletal data. Another, more general format uses the mnemonic OLD CART & ICE. For example, for a patient with a cough keeping her awake at night, the findings might look like:

Onset: 10 days ago

Location: Tickle begins in throat

Duration: Daily; coughing fits become worse at night

Characteristics: Painful to cough; can't catch breath; clear mucus coughed up

TABLE 34.8 Selected Frameworks for Assessment Templates

Framework	Topics
Maslow's Hierarchy of Needs for five levels of the pyramid (see Module 31, Stress and Coping)	1. Physiological (survival needs) 2. Safety and security 3. Love and belonging 4. Self-esteem 5. Self-actualization
Gordon's Functional Health Patterns for 11 categories of data	1. Health perception–health management 2. Nutritional-metabolic 3. Elimination 4. Activity-exercise 5. Sleep-rest 6. Cognitive-perceptual 7. Self-perception/self-concept 8. Role-relationship 9. Sexuality-reproductive 10. Coping/stress-tolerance 11. Value-belief
Erikson's Eight Stages of Development by age with primary tasks for that stage (see Table 25.2 in Module 25, Development)	1. Infancy 2. Early childhood 3. Late childhood 4. School age 5. Adolescence 6. Young adulthood 7. Adulthood 8. Maturity
Combination of approaches— often use in gathering complex hospital admission data, both administrative and clinical	See Exemplar 36.A in Module 36 for categories ranging from admission data to education/discharge planning.

Aggravating cues: Worse at night when lying in bed

Relieving cues: Hot liquids, steamy showers

Treatment: Acetaminophen and expectorant

Impact on ADLs: Not had a good night of sleep for over a week; asked other family members to shop and clean

Coping strategies: Afternoon naps

Emotional response: Since the patient has not become better over time, she worries her condition is much more serious than usual cough.

Validating Data

Organized assessment data needs to be validated to confirm completeness and accuracy. The entire nursing process needs to be based on correct facts. **Validation** is the activity of ensuring that data is complete, accurate, and factual. The nurse double-checks that the following statements are true:

- Objective data match subjective data
- Missing information is obtained
- No jumping to conclusions that are unsupported or focusing in the wrong direction.

Factual data collection avoids inference, interpretation, and assumptions. For example, a crying patient is not always experiencing pain or grief. To reduce problems of inaccuracy, nurses need to recognize their own biases, values, and beliefs. A patient ignoring verbal directions might not be noncompliant: The patient might be deaf, preoccupied with fears, or not understanding the language.

Some data can be measured with an accurate scale, be accepted as factual, and not need validation. Examples are height, weight, birthdate, and most laboratory study results. Two situations that need data validation: (1) when the subjective data from the nursing history does not match the objective data from the physical examination and (2) when a patient gives conflicting statements at different times. Validation is needed to ensure patient safety by having a complete and accurate nursing assessment. Guidelines for validating data are shown in **Table 34.9** ».

Interpreting Data

Once data have been collected, organized, and validated, the nurse interprets them to determine priorities for patient care. The nurse analyzes whether the findings are within normal and expected ranges for the patient's age, gender, and race. Then the nurse compares the findings with the patient's health status and immediate and long-range health needs.

Interpretation of findings is influenced by the ability to obtain, recall, and apply knowledge; to communicate effectively; and to take into account family history and dynamics. Other relevant influences include developmental, psychologic, environmental, and cultural/diversity cues.

TABLE 34.9 Validating Assessment Data

Guideline	Example
Compare subjective and objective data to verify the patient's statements with observations made.	Patient's perception of "feeling hot" needs to be compared with measurement of the body temperature.
Clarify any ambiguous or vague statements.	*Patient:* "I've felt sick off and on for 6 weeks." *Nurse:* "Describe what your sickness is like. Tell me what you mean by 'off and on.'"
Be sure assessment data consist of cues and not inferences.	*Observation:* Dry skin and reduced tissue turgor. *Inference:* Dehydration. *Action:* Collect additional data needed to make the inference in the diagnosing phase. For example, determine the patient's fluid intake, amount and appearance of urine, and blood pressure.
Double-check data that are extremely abnormal.	*Observation:* A resting pulse of 30 beats per minute or a blood pressure of 210/95 mmHg. *Action:* Repeat the measurement. Use another piece of equipment to confirm abnormalities or ask someone else to collect the same data.
Determine the presence of factors that may interfere with accurate measurement.	A crying infant will have an abnormal respiratory rate and will need quieting before accurate assessment can be made.
Use references (textbooks, journals, research reports) to explain phenomena.	A nurse considers tiny purple or bluish-black swollen areas under the tongue of an older patient to be abnormal until the nurse reads about physical changes of aging. Such varicosities are common.

Source: From Berman et al. (2021).

Knowledge

A wide variety of resources form the solid foundation necessary for making nursing diagnoses and designing plans of care: research studies; scientific literature; and charts, scales, and graphs. These resources include knowledge from:

- Physical and social sciences
- Nursing theory
- Human anatomy and physiology, with documented ranges of norms and expectations about physical and psychologic development (e.g., mental status examination results)
- Growth and development across the lifespan (e.g., Denver Developmental scores)
- Health-related and healthcare trends in groups and populations, including cues indicative of higher risks for injuries or illnesses (e.g., increasing obesity rates)
- Characteristics specific to age, gender, race, and culture.

Other skills add to interpretive expertise: effective communication, critical thinking, recognition of and response to patient cues, incorporation of a holistic perspective, and determination of data significance. From a combination of knowledge and skills, nurses can immediately recognize emergency situations, initiate essential treatment, and seek additional care support. As nurses gain experience, they learn about how to recognize patterns that predispose patients to illness and injury, how to use health promotion efficiently, and how to provide preventive activities effectively.

Clinical Example C

James Herdman is a 46-year-old man: height 5' 9", weight 230 lb, BP 156/94 mmHg. Both his parents died in their 50s from acute myocardial infarctions. He is worried about his experiencing the same health outcome in the near future.

The nurse shows Mr. Herdman a table of normal vital signs for adults to demonstrate to him that his blood pressure is well above the desired 120/80 mmHg level. The nurse next uses a body mass index table to inform Mr. Herdman that his index measures 34, when the upper limit of normal is 24. This puts him in the obese category. The combination of hypertension, obesity, and a family history of acute myocardial infarctions increase Mr. Herdman's chances of having a heart attack. The nurse combines knowledge of cues about increased risks with his individual data to provide a personalized plan of care. Collaboration with other healthcare professionals and regular monitoring can help Mr. Herdman reduce his weight and lower his blood pressure.

Critical Thinking Questions

1. What are Mr. Herdman's care priorities at this time?
2. What resources are available in your community to assist you with intervening or advocating for patients such as Mr. Herdman?

>> **Stay Current:** A body mass index calculator is available at the National Heart, Lung, and Blood Institute at https://www.nhlbi.nih.gov/health/educational/lose_wt/BMI/bmi_tbl.pdf.

Communication

Communication is the verbal or written purposeful exchange of information, feelings, thoughts, and ideas. That sharing is essential to the assessment process. Techniques, such as open-ended or closed interview questions, statements, clarification, and rephrasing are central to complete and accurate information gathering. Several cues must be acknowledged to personalize the exchange: the patient's age, anxiety level, language differences or difficulties, culture, cognitive ability, affect, appearance, and special needs. That topic is discussed in greater detail in the module on Communication.

Developmental Cues

Developmental cues affect the conduct of the health assessment process. Parents, guardians, or caregivers give the most useful information about young children, patients with developmental disabilities, and those with communication impairments. For patients with developmental disabilities, the nurse considers achievement of milestones of development as the standard, rather than chronological age, when interpreting the data.

The words that nurses use, including medical terminology, are personalized to a patient's situation. For example, the assessment of a pregnant adolescent would be different than for a 36-year-old woman who is having her third child. Differences in assessment approaches are highlighted in Module 25, Development.

Psychologic and Emotional Cues

When interpreting findings from a health assessment, psychologic and emotional cues must be considered as predisposing or contributing cues about the physiologic health status. For example, the autonomic response to anxiety increases pulse rate and blood pressure. Physical problems can affect mental health, such as adolescent obesity contributing to low self-esteem.

Anxiety and depression can block patients' full participation in the health assessment. Grief can limit the ability to recognize health issues or implement healthy habits. See Module 31, Stress and Coping, for more examples of how psychologic and emotional cues affect health status.

SAFETY ALERT Two simple questions—such as "Have you been hit, kicked, punched, or otherwise hurt by someone within the past year? If so, who hurt you?"—can help find out if a patient is at risk at home or in a relationship. The U.S. Preventive Services Task Force (2018) recommends those questions be asked of all women of childbearing age. The same inquiry could be made of older and vulnerable adults to discover situations of abuse. Positive findings might need to be reported to authorities.

Screening for depression is recommended for routine use, but especially for pregnant and postpartum women (Siu et al., 2016). One research study found nearly 10% of women entered their pregnancy with depression, which increased to 16% in the third trimester (Wilcox et al., 2020).

Family History and Dynamics

Because family history for some illnesses results in an increased risk for contracting those diseases, the nurse collects the relevant data in the health assessment. For example, if a female patient's mother, sister, or daughter was diagnosed with breast cancer, she has about double the usual risk of contracting that disease herself (American Cancer Society, 2019).

Also, family dynamics can affect an individual's approach to healthcare decisions. In some families and in some cultures, those decisions are not made independently. Instead, the family leader is the decision maker or, in some families, the final decision is made by group consensus.

Family situations can affect physical and emotional health. For example, a patient with a parent with alcoholism has a higher risk for developing alcoholism. The nurse takes into account the family situation when interpreting unexpected physical or emotional behaviors. Module 26, Family, further explains how the concept of family affects health.

Cultural Cues

Individuals' culture affects their language and expression of feelings, their emotional and physical wellness, and their health habits and practices. Assessment data must be interpreted in light of the cultural norms for the individual patient. For example, some individuals in Asian cultures would not interpret lack of eye contact during a conversation as an inability to interact with the other person or as an indicator of depression or difficulty in paying attention. The nurse must clearly explain abnormal findings, illnesses, and interventions because the patient's culture may influence the patient's views of those issues. Refer to Module 24, Culture and Diversity, for more information on cultural considerations.

Environmental Cues

During the assessment, the nurse gathers data about the patient's internal and external environmental cues. Internal environmental cues are composed of the patient's emotional frame of mind, their response to medications and other treatments, and any individual physiologic or anatomic alterations. External environmental cues are composed of the patient's exposure to the following possible toxins:

- Smoke, chemical substances, and fumes that the patient might have inhaled
- Irritating substances that the patient might have inhaled, ingested, or absorbed topically
- Uncomfortable sensations, such as excessive noise, overly bright lights, or unnerving motions

Allergy triggers, such as animal dander, dust mites, mold or mildew, or perfumes.

For more information about the external environmental cues themselves, consult Module 51, Safety. To become knowledgeable about nurses' exciting roles in making changes in the current environment, refer to Exemplar 43.A, Environmental Quality, in Module 43, Advocacy.

Concepts Related to Assessment

Nursing care always begins with assessment. Nursing care depends on a strong knowledge base and the application of critical thinking. Regardless of the clinical setting, the role of the nurse is multifaceted. Each situation requires the nurse to use the nursing process, starting with strong assessment skills.

In the biophysical realm, thorough nursing assessment (including the fifth vital sign of pain) allows the nurse to identify an individual's problems with acid–base balance, cellular regulation, comfort, digestion, elimination, and fluids and electrolytes. Illness and injury will leave evidence that can be discovered through assessment.

In the psychosocial realm, a similarly thorough nursing assessment can point out a patient's difficulties with trauma, addiction, cognition, grief and loss, mood and affect, and stress and coping. At the same time, an assessment of the patient's strengths in the areas of family and spirituality can be a good foundation on which to build better health and wellness. The Concepts Related to Assessment feature lists some, but not all, of the concepts that are integral to assessment. They are listed in alphabetical order.

Holistic Health Assessment Across the Lifespan

Benchmarks of health status help nurses know normal developmental situations and milestones for children and adults. Monitoring them over time will give nurses evidence-based ideas about how to interpret the complexity of interacting cues, such as genetics and the environment. Patients' responses, especially individual variations, form a picture of current development.

Holistic health describes a clinical approach that includes a broad range of cues that affect patients' biophysical, mental, emotional, and spiritual wellness. The nurse knows that a combination of developmental, psychologic, emotional, family, cultural, and environmental cues influence health status.

In the holistic health approach, the nurse gathers both subjective and objective data to evaluate patients' physical, cognitive, and emotional growth and development. The nurse uses a three-stage process to ensure that the broad range of cues are included in the assessment:

- Obtaining accurate data
- Interpreting findings by using predicted normal milestones and benchmarking personal data against the range of expected outcomes
- Always keeping in mind personal variations in the current health status of individual patients

Module 25, Development, provides an overview of growth and development milestones for each stage of development by age group. Milestones and crises can occur during any stage of development, and they should be documented as part of the complete, holistic assessment.

Along with data about expected milestones, nurses maintain current knowledge related to the leading causes of death by age. This information suggests topics for both assessment and patient teaching. The leading causes of death throughout the lifespan are outlined in **Table 34.10** »». The patient's

Concepts Related to
Assessment

CONCEPT	RELATIONSHIP TO ASSESSMENT	NURSING IMPLICATIONS
Legal Issues	Clinical trial enrollment opportunity → assessment of level of knowledge about risk–benefit ratio → informed consent	■ Nurse offers time and resources to answer questions about research study involvement.
Oxygenation	If assessment shows ↓O_2, prioritize interventions to ↑O_2	■ Decrease oxygen workload by having patient rest; administer O_2 by nasal cannula, if needed.
Perfusion	If assessment shows ↓ blood flow to a limb, prioritize intervention to ↑ blood flow	■ Check for clothes restricting circulation. Use physical movement and exercise to keep fit.
Professional Behaviors	Professional approach ↑ knowledgeable assessment ↑ patient confidence	■ A professional approach helps build confidence and rapport with the patient, making it more likely that the patient will be honest and cooperative during the assessment.
Thermoregulation	If assessment shows ↑ temperature, discover cause of fever	■ Increase fluids and give antipyretic medications.
Safety	If assessment of home environment shows ↑ hazards, intervene to ↓ injury risk	■ Before discharge, scan home environments for obstacles that might cause a patient to slip or fall.
Sensory Perception	If assessment of preschooler shows ↓ visual acuity → assistance device to ↑ vision	■ Refer to optometrist to measure for eyeglasses prescription.
Tissue Integrity and Mobility	If older patient in wheelchair → constant sitting → assess skin → stage 2 pressure ulcer	■ Move patient to positions that do not cause pressure on area of breakdown. Continue to ↑ padding of seat.

TABLE 34.10 Leading Causes of Death Throughout the Lifespan

Age Range	Leading Causes of Death and Number of Deaths in 2018
Birth–age 4 years	■ Conditions originating in the perinatal period (short gestation, maternal pregnancy complications, placenta/cord/membranes): 6198 ■ Congenital anomalies: 4857 ■ Unintentional injuries: 2394 ■ Sudden infant death syndrome (SIDS): 1334 ■ Respiratory distress: 390 ■ Homicide: 353 ■ Cancer: 326
Age 5–9 years	■ Unintentional injuries: 734 ■ Cancer: 393 ■ Congenital abnormalities: 201 ■ Heart and acute/chronic lung diseases: 196 ■ Homicide: 121
Age 10–14 years	■ Unintentional injuries: 692 ■ Suicide: 596 ■ Cancer: 450 ■ Homicide: 168 ■ Heart and acute/chronic lung diseases: 165
Age 15–24 years[a]	■ Unintentional injuries: 12,044 ■ Suicide: 6211 ■ Homicide: 4607 ■ Cancer: 1371 ■ Heart and acute/chronic lung diseases: 1070
Age 25–64 years[b]	■ Cancer: 165,572 ■ Heart and acute/chronic lung diseases: 159,576 ■ Unintentional injuries: 94,030 ■ Suicide: 32,426 ■ Liver disease: 26,218 ■ Diabetes mellitus: 24,474 ■ Cerebrovascular: 20,188 ■ Homicide: 8538
Age 65 and older	■ Heart and acute/chronic lung diseases: 710,957 ■ Cancer: 431,102 ■ Cerebrovascular disease: 127,244 ■ Alzheimer disease: 120,658 ■ Diabetes mellitus: 60,182 ■ Unintentional injuries: 57,213

[a]This is the youngest age group for which diabetes shows up as a leading cause of death, with 246 deaths reported in 2018.
[b]After age 44, homicide was no longer among the 10 leading causes of death; suicide remained a leading cause of death until age 65.
Source: Data from Centers for Disease Control and Prevention (2018).

age; developmental stage; leading causes of illness, injury, and death for the patient's age cohort; and the patient's own health behaviors all inform health promotion and patient teaching. Recommended health promotion activities for different stages of the lifespan are outlined in Module 7, Health, Wellness, Illness, and Injury.

Assessment of Infants, Children, and Adolescents

Assessment findings differ by age group: infants, children, adolescents, and adults vary in physiology, development, and cognition. As a result, the organization of the nursing assessment becomes flexible. For example, the head-to-toe pattern of physical assessment may not be the best choice with young children. Adolescents and young adults will cooperate with examination instructions, but infants and toddlers cannot follow the same complex directions.

Young children are not able to think about and talk about their health problems in detail. Therefore, nurses focus on the parents' voicing of their child's chief complaint and conduct the physical assessment based on those issues and concerns. See **Table 34.11** » for a summary of some interview challenges and strategies for overcoming them. Nurses must overcome many communication and situational obstacles to produce a useful assessment in pediatric patients.

Rapport is necessary when interviewing children and adolescents. Adapting the assessment to begin with comfortable topics, such as asking about nutrition history, can help children feel at ease with a familiar topic. Interviews of infants and younger children will need a caregiver present to answer questions and assist with the physical examination. Caregivers of adolescents might be interviewed separately, so that the teenage patient has privacy during the assessment to supply unpressured answers.

The nurse makes clinical observations and obtains anthropometric measurements using equipment appropriate for the age of the patient. The nurse uses the data to determine if developmental milestones have been achieved. Patterns of eating, sleeping, elimination, exercise, and activity are documented. The nurse also monitors development of speech and language, muscular growth, and strength and coordination. At times, rapid changes might occur between clinical visits. This critical information is part of a complete assessment. Module 25, Development, discusses milestones in more detail.

The length and weight of infants and young children can be measured while lying down. Diapers must be removed. The height and weight of older children can be measured while standing.

The World Health Organization (WHO) recommends weight-for-height as the standard measurement for evaluating children's nutritional health. Other methods, such as skinfold and circumference measurements, are prone to errors in assessing growth and nutritional status. However, at age 3 and younger, head circumference is still measured. That measurement is not useful beyond age 3.

For infants, children, and adolescents under age 20, the Centers for Disease Control and Prevention (CDC) and WHO have age-specific and gender-specific reference charts for height, weight, and body mass index (BMI). For children under 36 months, they give standards for head circumferences. Charts use percentiles to show the distribution of data found in population studies.

Nurses consult these charts to compare their pediatric patients to their age-matched peers. This allows monitoring of individual percentiles within the population, showing individual growth over time. In most cases, children's measurements stay in a narrow percentile range during childhood. For example, a child in the 75th percentile for height (length) for age may have a large frame and parents with large stature. That child may not be at risk for overnutrition. However, a child who drops in height for age from the 75th percentile to the 50th percentile may be at risk for undernutrition. Any significant changes must be investigated.

TABLE 34.11 Strategies for Working Together with Parents or Accompanying Adults

Situation	Possible Causes	Nursing Considerations
Parents unable to recall information or follow complex care instructions given verbally.	Parental distraction and increased stress from interrupted sleep, concern for child, frustration of not knowing reason for child's illness or pain	■ Provide parents with written instructions. ■ Encourage journaling or taking notes about child's illness and treatment. ■ Consider parental stress when designing care plans.
Nannies, babysitters, friends, neighbors, siblings, or stepparents accompany children.	Transportation to healthcare appointments needed Alternate caregiving arrangements in place	■ Verify relationship of adults. Never assume legal or family ties. ■ Know state laws about consent and uphold federal laws about privacy.
Some detailed clinical information missing or not easily understandable to the nurse interviewer.	Child is nonverbal or has limited language ability Previously documented health history is incomplete or not available	■ Listen carefully to parents, especially their report of subtle behavior changes. ■ Use open-ended questions for complete and accurate picture of patient health.

Undernutrition is defined as a BMI for age less than the 5th percentile. Overweight is defined as a BMI for age greater than the 85th percentile. Obesity (overnutrition) is defined as a BMI for age greater than the 95th percentile (CDC, 2018). See Module 14, Nutrition, for more information on overnutrition and undernutrition.

Children and adults are physically different. Specific lifespan variations can be anticipated in assessment findings. Those variations are identified for each concept in the previous individual domains (Modules 1–33). Additional tips for effective assessment of pediatric patients are given in **Box 34.4** ».

Assessment of Newborns

The assessment of newborns is covered in Exemplar 33.D, Newborn Care, in Module 33, Reproduction.

Assessment of Infants

During the first year of life, infants' growth and development should be monitored and compared to norms for their age during frequent assessments. At each assessment, height, weight, and head circumference measurements are plotted on a growth chart. Ideally, each normal measurement should follow the same percentile throughout infancy, keeping the same rate of growth as expected. The nurse can combine information from the patient history, physical assessment, and observation to identify common problems. Early interviews combined with basic parent and caregiver education and support may resolve issues that, if not addressed, could later result in significant health problems or unhealthy parent–child relationships.

For example, infants should feel a sense of attachment with their caregivers. *Attachment* is defined as the bond between the infant and the adults that promotes physical and psychosocial health. Healthy caregiver–infant attachment is seen when an infant is held close, mutual eye contact is encouraged, and smiling and making sounds is exchanged. This position promotes healthy attachment later in life. It also provides support during examinations and procedures.

Signs of interest in the child's development and education also indicate healthy attachment. Regular interaction with the child and timely response to satisfying the child's needs ensure healthy cognitive, psychosocial, and emotional development.

As far as physical development problems, **overnutrition** describes an accelerated rate of weight gain. Caregivers can cause this problem if they assume that all of the infant's cries signal hunger and respond every time by feeding the baby. In other cases, overfeeding results from cultural beliefs that a plump baby is a healthy baby.

Undernutrition describes a diminishing rate of weight gain. Inadequate caloric intake may be caused by a lack of knowledge of normal infant feeding habits, scarce financial resources for baby formula, or not following directions on mixing baby formula. Some parents or caregivers may misinterpret a lack of crying from quiet or passive babies as indicating a lack of hunger. See Exemplar 25.D, Failure to Thrive, in Module 25, Development, for more information about that condition.

Significant change in the percentiles of head growth need to be immediately evaluated. The change may be a sign of **hydrocephalus** (head enlargement caused by inadequate drainage of cerebrospinal fluid). Early diagnosis and interventions for hydrocephalus prevent or lessen serious neurologic problems.

In general, parents and caregivers celebrate infants' achievement of developmental milestones and know their infants' abilities. Especially for first-time parents, nurses may need to provide some education related to developmental milestones. At the first report of an infant not yet meeting an expected milestone, the only intervention needed might be the nurses' suggestion of specific interactive activities. However, further evaluation is required if infants continue to miss meeting normal milestones. **Table 34.12** » describes some instruments to measure aspects of growth and development of infants and children.

Assessment of Toddlers

Toddlerhood spans from 12 to 36 months of age. Toddlers continue to grow, but at a slower rate than infants. Sometimes slight variations are seen, but for the most part, height and weight continue to follow the earlier percentile rate. Feeding patterns can be evaluated by obtaining a 24-hour recall of food intake. Most toddlers feed themselves and interact with family members at mealtimes. Toddlers can change their favorite food from week to week or exercise their autonomy by refusing to eat. When this happens, caregivers can get

Box 34.4

Tips for Effective Assessment of the Pediatric Patient

- Be caring and supportive, yet firm.
- Stay at eye level with smaller patients or keep in eye contact.
- Ask preschoolers and older children directly about their chief complaint and cues indicating problems. Instead of asking "Does your head hurt?" say "Please touch your head where it hurts."
- Give children over age 10 the opportunity to be examined without the accompanying adult. The patient is the child and the individual to whom the nurse has legal and ethical responsibility.
- Encourage children to voice their fears and concerns. Be patient: Excitement and nervousness can cause children to pause between words, repeat themselves, freeze, or become agitated.
- Permit the child to remain in the accompanying adult's lap, if possible (**Figure 34.7** »). However, do not perform painful procedures while the child is sitting in the adult's lap, since the child needs to feel safe and protected there.
- Progress from the least invasive procedures to the most invasive.
- Ensure patient privacy and use standard infection protection precautions.
- Call children by their name and use simple words that children understand to explain examination activities. For example, instead of *abdomen*, use *tummy* or *belly* (**Figure 34.8** »).
- Play should be incorporated into the process. Let children handle equipment or dolls with bandages and syringes (**Figure 34.9** »). Young children can blow bubbles for deep breathing. Use playful language, such as asking about elephants in ears, before using the otoscope. Distract young patients with toys, such as finger puppets.
- Don't let the presence of other children move your focus from the patient. Offer books, crayons, or toys to engage them while you focus on the patient.

Source: Adapted from Fenske et al. (2019).

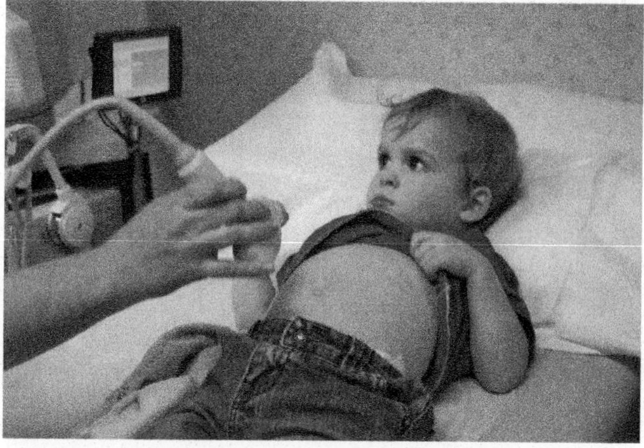

Figure 34.8 » This toddler knows that his belly hurts, but he would not understand if the nurse asked him if his abdomen hurt.

Source: Jessica Lewis/Moment/Getty Images.

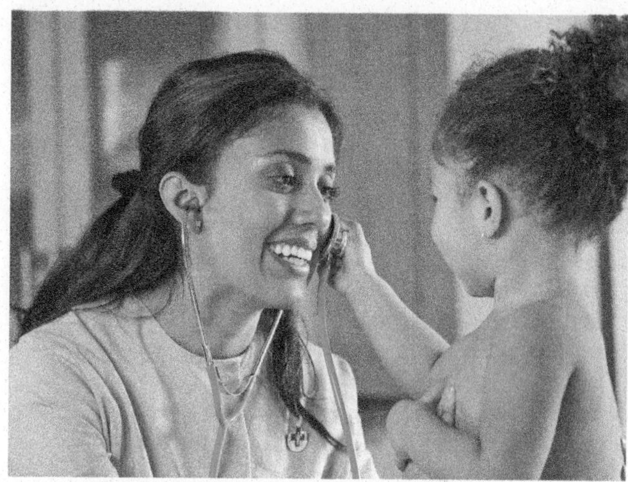

Figure 34.9 » A nurse allows her young patient to play with her stethoscope before using it to assess the child's heart.

Source: Ariel Skelley/Blend Images/Getty Images.

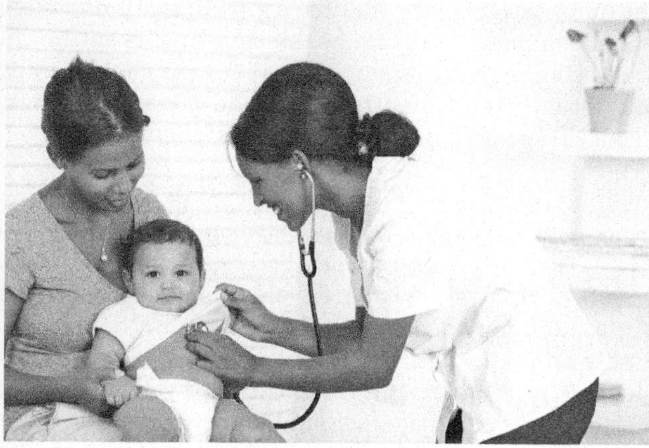

Figure 34.7 » This mother holds her baby while the nurse performs an examination.

Source: Ruslan Dashinsky/iStock/Getty Images.

frustrated and confused. But forced eating can trigger power struggles and cause poor weight gain. On the other hand, if caregivers offer food, especially sweets, to quiet or bribe toddlers, excessive weight gain can occur. Discussion with parents about eating behaviors and weight gain can resolve problems before they get entrenched.

Obtaining the younger toddler's health history from the parent is often the best method of assessing development. Direct observation of older toddlers' development can happen when they are playing with testing materials or being allowed to explore the room with the caregiver present.

TABLE 34.12 Instruments to Assess Growth and Development in Infants and Children

Instrument	Description
ACE Questionnaire for Children and Adolescents	Developed by Dr. Nadine Burke Harris, this questionnaire can help HCPs assess for childhood trauma, which can affect growth and development.
Ages & Stages Questionnaire (ASQ)	Parent questionnaire that covers developmental areas of communication, gross motor, fine motor, problem solving, and personal-social in children. The ASQ:SE assesses social and emotional growth in areas such as self-regulation, adaptive functioning, and interaction with others.
Battelle Developmental Inventory	This inventory assesses adaptive ability; motor, communication, and cognitive skills; and personal-social skills in children from birth through 7 years of age.
Brigance Screens	These screens assess speech–language, motor, readiness, self-help, social-emotional skills, and pre-academics. Used from birth through the end of first grade.
Denver II	Screening test administered to well children between birth and 6 years of age. Assesses four areas: personal-social, fine motor adaptive, language, and gross motor.
Hassles and Uplifts Scale	Scale used to measure adult attitudes about daily situations defined as "hassles" and "uplifts." It focuses on evaluation of positive and negative events in daily life rather than on life events.
Life Experiences Survey	This self-administered questionnaire reviews life-changing events of a given year. Ratings are used to evaluate the level of stress an individual is experiencing.
Pediatric Symptom Checklist	A 35-item parent report questionnaire used to identify conduct behaviors and behaviors associated with depression, anxiety, and adjustment in children ages 4–16 years. Item patterns determine the need for behavioral or mental health referrals.
Stanford-Binet Intelligence Scale: Fourth Edition	Test that measures general intelligence. The areas of verbal reasoning, quantitative reasoning, abstract/visual reasoning, and short-term memory can be tested from age 2 to 23 years.
Wechsler Preschool and Primary Scale of Intelligence—Revised (WPPSI-R)	Standardized test of language and perception for children ages 4½–6 years.

If toddlers perceive the environment as strange or threatening, assessment of language milestones can be difficult. A playroom or waiting room setting can make the child enough at ease to evaluate speech development.

Some challenges arise from normal development. The toddlers' exploration of their environment places them at risk for accidental injury or poisoning. Toddlers have difficulty understanding unwanted limits and little experience dealing positively with frustration. This can lead to frequent temper tantrums. Nurses can discuss how a calm response to outbursts can reduce negative attention-seeking behavior.

The nurse can gather useful information about the relationship of the caregivers and toddlers by observation. What is the toddler's response when seeking comfort? What does the toddler do when confronted by a stranger? What is the adult–child interaction like both verbally and nonverbally?

Some challenges need further evaluation, such as a toddler continuously clinging to a caregiver in a nonthreatening situation. In contrast, the opposite response, not seeking a caregiver's attention for comfort and support, might be a sign of lack of trust. Some caregivers might have unreasonable expectations, such as expecting a toddler to sit quietly in a chair. Inattention to the toddler's activities and not setting appropriate boundaries may hinder the child's development of self-control.

Assessment of Preschoolers

Preschoolers are between 36 and 60 months old. Children of preschool age are generally in a good mood, will cooperate with others, and can communicate verbally. If their caregiver is in sight, they are more relaxed. But they normally do not need that support except in threatening situations.

The nurse can assess language ability, cognitive functioning, and overall development when talking to preschoolers about their favorite activities. The nurse listens for age-appropriate vocabulary and sentence structure. Often the nurse can evaluate the ability to concentrate, magical thinking, and reality imitation. If the preschooler's language ability indicates a lack of environmental stimulation, the nurse should educate caregivers about ways to provide that stimulation. If the nurse observes a clinging, frightened preschooler in a nonthreatening situation, the nurse can recognize a possible lack of trust and communication with caregivers. The nurse should intervene so that the child learns appropriate social interactions and language skills.

Nurses should screen children for parental concerns and health issues and intervene as necessary. For example, if parents are concerned with children's slowed rate of growth, the nurse can show the children's growth charts and discuss nutritional needs. Regular health assessments ensure child well-being, provide an opportunity for parental education, and form the basis to arrange for additional screenings or agency referrals, if needed.

Assessment of School-Age Children

School-age children are those between 5 and 11 years old. They experience a slow, steady body growth with changing proportions. This normal development can make them appear thinner than their parents expect. The nurse can assess children's nutritional intake and review their growth charts to reassure parents about expected weight for height. This relieves parental stress and anxiety, prevents parents from trying to force children to eat, and reinforces healthy food habits to prevent obesity. When children enter the prepubertal growth spurt, their appetites increase. This accompanies a corresponding increase in height and weight, with an increased percentile on the growth chart.

School-age children like to talk about their lives: hobbies, friends, school, and accomplishments. Gross and fine motor control increase with neurologic maturity. This becomes visible in activities such as sports, dancing, music, art, or building structures. School-age children enjoy their newly acquired skills, which can be a source of family pride.

At this age, children may develop lifelong hobbies and are especially interested in collecting items of interest, such as sports or game cards (e.g., Pokemon), dolls and action figures, or Lego sets. School-age children often work hard in school and are proud of their academic progress. Positive feedback and encouragement from families reinforce their children's successes.

School-age children communicate openly with adult family members who set appropriate and necessary boundaries for behavior. The family remains the major influence during most of the school years. As children move toward the teenage years, children find peer relationships becoming increasingly important as they seek greater independence. This can cause strained relationships with family.

Problems can arise when children do not experience these normal milestones. Not having hobbies or visible accomplishments can have negative effects. A disturbed parent–child relationship can result when caregivers speak of children as a burden and do not praise them. Inadequate, ineffective, or negative parent–child relationships can have long-term effects on children's self-esteem and behaviors as they grow into adulthood.

Academic problems may surface, with parents and children in conflict over school attendance, punctuality, grades, homework, and study time. Nurses can encourage parents to establish a consistent time and place for schoolwork and to communicate regularly with their child's teachers. Careful observation of children by teachers, family members, and HCPs may identify learning disabilities or a need for mental health support. Early interventions can be implemented with better opportunities for academic and social success.

SAFETY ALERT Children and adolescents with behavior disorders, low self-esteem, and too little supervision are at increased risk for gang recruitment, regardless of whether they live in an urban, suburban, or rural setting. Information on how to decrease risk for gang membership and identify signs of gang activity is available at https://www.aacap.org/aacap/families_and_youth/facts_for_families/fff-guide/Children-and-Gangs-098.aspx.

Assessment of Adolescents

Nurses should be able to explain the differences between the time frame of adolescence (ages 12 to 18) and the period of puberty. The transition between childhood and adulthood is adolescence. The process of bodily changes by which adolescents become sexually mature is called puberty, with the ability to reproduce as the outcome. In girls, puberty occurs between 10 and 14 years old. It is marked by the beginning of menstruation, development of breasts, growth of axillary and pubic hair, and an increase in height. In boys, puberty occurs between 12 and 16 years old. It is characterized by growth of the penis and testicles; growth of axillary, facial, chest, and pubic hair; and an increase in height. See Module 19, Sexuality, for more information on puberty.

To adults in their environment, adolescents appear to be eating constantly, but never seem satisfied. Adolescents are increasing their calorie intake dramatically to match the needs of their pubertal growth spurt. Even so, adolescents (especially women) are at risk for eating disorders. Information about eating disorders is included in Module 29, Self.

The nurse can assess adolescents together with their parents and then separately with them one-on-one. This gives a more complete picture of the dynamics of the parent–child relationship. It also gives an opportunity for teenagers to express themselves and discuss their concerns, particularly about sensitive issues such as sexual activity, with more freedom. Adolescents are likely to be anxious about their bodies and rapid physical and emotional changes. This anxiety can show up in somatic complaints. The nurse can assure teenagers of the normality of their situations.

Adolescents frequently find it easier to communicate with peers and adults outside their family. They can hold conversations about the important topics in their lives: school, friends, activities, and future plans. As the adolescent asserts increasing independence, adult family members can recognize their decreased influence. Teenage behavior in areas of sexuality, dress, hairstyles, vocabulary, and music can make parents uncomfortable. Lifestyle values may differ greatly, causing difficulties in communication. Some parents respond by severely restricting the activities and freedom of their teenagers. However, this may inhibit progress toward adult independence. Depression can result from a lack of normal social contacts and spending a lot of time alone. In turn, this depressed mood increases the risk for suicide and self-harm. Adolescents' natural inclinations toward exploration and experimentation contribute to an increased risk for injury as well as an increased risk for drug and alcohol use.

Communicating with Patients and Families

Introductory Phase

Respect the confidentiality of information from children. Be aware of state and federal laws about parental notification and mandatory reporting. Both parent and child should be informed about findings that cannot be kept confidential, if they need to be reported to public health de-partments or child protective services. You might say to the young person:

- The things that you and I talk about will always be kept confidential between the two of us, unless you tell me that you are thinking about harming yourself or someone else, or if you tell me that someone is hurting you.

You might say to the child's parents or caregivers:

- I am required by law to report some information to other people. I will let you know if I am going to do that, before I actually talk to them.

Both approaches should aim to maintain rapport at the same time as establishing boundaries in the nurse–child and nurse–parent relationships.

Assessment of Pregnant Women

Prenatal care is important to ensure the health of both the developing fetus and the mother. Briefly, the changes that need to be compared with normal expectations result from hormonal influences, the growing fetus, and the mother's physiologic and psychologic adaptation to pregnancy. She needs regular prenatal checkups to monitor her health and that of her baby (**Figure 34.10** »). Nursing assessment and education activities track the changes over time, comparing them to normal adaptations. For information about how the mother, fetus, and obstetric-gynecologic team ensure a healthy pregnancy, see the four Assessment features in Module 33, Reproduction: Initial Prenatal Assessment, Subsequent

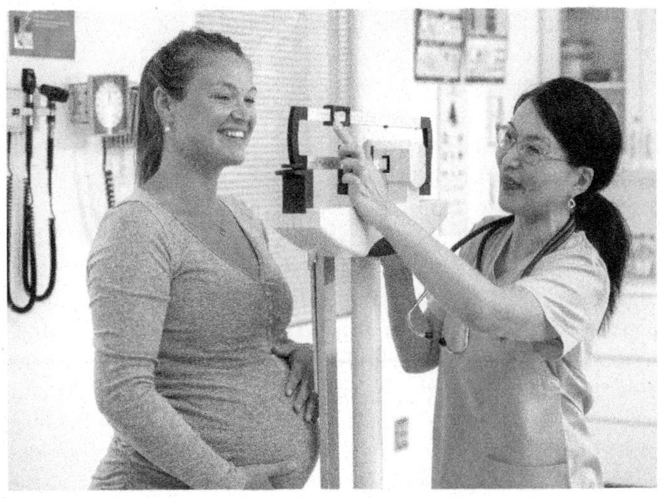

Figure 34.10 » Prenatal checkups include a weigh-in to ensure that the mother is gaining weight appropriately.
Source: Ariel Skelley/Photodisc/Getty Images.

Prenatal Assessment, Intrapartum Assessment during childbirth, and Postpartum Assessment after childbirth. See Module 28, Mood and Affect, for an overview of assessment and nursing considerations related to preventing, identifying, and intervening in peripartum depression.

Assessment of Young Adults

Young adulthood is a busy and productive time of life, occurring from ages 18 to 45. Most young adults are at their maximum physical potential and enjoy good health with sports and physical fitness activities. They enjoy peer activities, and many engage in exploration of creative talents.

Traditionally, young adulthood was a time of forming mature, cooperative friendships and finding a special one-on-one relationship culminating in marriage. Today, a legal union is not the routine expectation. Instead of marriage, informal living-together arrangements are increasingly common. However, the developmental milestone of forming a mature, intimate relationship still should be met.

As far as having children, young adults have a lot of choices:

- Surrogate motherhood
- Artificial insemination
- In vitro fertilization
- Other technological fertility innovations
- Deciding not to have children
- Delaying having children
- Single parenthood
- Adoption.

Other milestones for young adults include choosing an occupation, establishing personal values, and creating a lifestyle. These years are a time for advancing in a career, establishing financial stability, and making an emotional investment. Without these accomplishments, such as a steady job, young adults might lack direction and self-confidence. Feelings of failure and insecurity could develop. These defeats can place the young adult at risk for depression, alcoholism, or substance abuse. Young adults complete their physical and mental structure growth. Their health can be monitored by comparing individual data measures to clinical height and weight growth charts. Eating, sleeping, activity, and exercise patterns can also be compared to their peers.

Assessment of Middle-Aged Adults

Typical middle-aged adults, ages 45 to 65, find satisfaction with previous accomplishments. They are involved in current activities outside of their nuclear family. Many begin to prepare for an active retirement and a healthy adjustment to the physical changes of aging. Financial security is the reward for good financial planning during these years.

The primary and dramatic physical changes in middle-aged adults are related to decreased hormone levels in both men and women. Women begin menopause, which ends the possibility of childbearing. Other decreased functioning applies to the basal metabolic rate, muscle size, nerve conduction, respiratory capacity, kidney excretion, and cardiovascular flow. Adipose tissue deposits increase the weight of middle-aged adults, and skeletal changes decrease their height. Their shorter and heavier bodies experience less sensitivity in the senses of touch, sight, and hearing.

As a member of society, middle age also signals the end of childrearing. Adjustments are made to households without children or children no longer living at home. For couples, their daily lives range from having companions with renewed relationships to marital separation if they find they have little in common at this stage in their lives.

There are some exceptions, for example, women or couples who delayed having children until later in life. These parents are beginning rearing children just as many peers are completing that task.

Assessment of adults includes vital signs and BMI, as well as checking the ability to carry out ADLs and see and hear clearly. These assessments help establish a baseline, assist in determining what is "normal" for the patient, and help identify changes that could be problematic early.

» **Skills:** See Skills 1.5–1.9, Vital Signs, in Volume 3.

Communicating with Patients

Introductory Phase

Give patients an idea of the time frame for their visit. Start by asking about how they are currently feeling, to get a brief summary of their condition. Then inquire about the reason for their visit, so that they are reassured that their clinical issue will be the focus of the visit. If there are delays in their being seen, give an estimate of the amount of time until they can expect to see their HCP.

- Welcome to the clinic. How are you feeling today?
- I am going to take some measurements about your health, and then ask you some questions about it. This should take about 15 to 20 minutes.
- Your healthcare provider is running about 15 minutes behind schedule. Do you have any pain today? Are you comfortable in that chair?

Assessment of Older Adults

Many older adults live healthy, active lives. An annual, comprehensive assessment of older adults, those over 65 years of age, is necessary to help promote maximum health and functioning. The assessment should be repeated after any abrupt change in **functional status** (the ability to safely perform activities of daily living) and **instrumental activities of daily living** (activities that relate to independent living, such as shopping, cooking, managing medications, driving, and using the phone or computer) or any change in functioning in a specific area (such as grasping or gait). A complete assessment is also necessary for any hospitalization, prior to nursing home placement or change in living status, or when a second opinion about a recommended treatment is needed.

Many older adults see multiple providers, making care coordination a challenge. Several strategies can make the assessment process more effective (Kane, Ouslander, Resnick, & Malone, 2018). These include:

- Close communication among members of the interprofessional team with minimal redundancy in the assessments performed
- Use of carefully designed questionnaires that reliable older patients or their caregivers can complete beforehand
- Effective use of assessment forms that are incorporated into computer databases.

The nurse can incorporate a variety of assessment techniques and standardized instruments into routine evaluations (see **Table 34.13** » for a list of instruments used to assess older adults). In addition, the nurse can serve as an advocate for older adults, suggesting appropriate referrals and resources as needed.

» **Stay Current:** Evidence-based protocols, focused on managing over 30 common geriatric cues, are available from the Hartford Institute for Geriatric Nursing (2017), sponsored by the New York University College of Nursing. The general assessment series includes information on the purpose of the clinical measurement, the best tool, the target population, validity and reliability, strengths and limitations, and follow-up suggestions. It is available online at https://consultgeri.org/tools/try-this-series.

Another set of geriatric education resources is available from the Iowa Geriatric Education Center at the University of Iowa. It is one of 48 programs funded by the Health Resources and Services Administration of the U.S. Department of Health and Human Services. The Iowa program targets the "4 Ms of Age-Friendly Health Systems—What Matters, Mentation, Mobility, and Medication." More information is available at https://igec.uiowa.edu/.

Understanding the assessment needs of older adults requires an understanding that the physical, psychological, and sociological domains interact in complex ways to affect the health and functioning of older adults. For example, limited access to transportation for the older adult may result in decreased fluid and nutrition intake if the older adult is unable to shop for groceries as needed. See Exemplar 25.D, Failure to Thrive, in Module 25, Development, for more information about Geriatric Failure to Thrive. Comprehensive health assessment requires asking about psychological and social cues and their impact on functional abilities. Functional status should always be a central focus of the holistic assessment of the older adult (Kane et al., 2018). The nurse is in a unique position to ensure that all aspects of the assessment are addressed and to identify the need for additional resources or referrals.

Arrangements for the Assessment Environment

Ensuring patient safety and comfort when planning the clinical visit will improve the data collection process. A checklist of arrangements to make would include:

- Clear instructions about parking arrangements, including location of handicapped spaces, if appropriate
- Maps showing driving routes and facility entrances; not all adults have smartphones, so this can be particularly important
- Reminders to bring assistive devices, including eyeglasses, hearing aids with full batteries, canes, and walkers. Let patients know if wheelchairs are available for visitor use.
- Written or verbal summary of the steps in the healthcare facility registration process
- Adequate signage and lighting in pathways without hazards for canes and walkers
- Decreased background noise for less competition with clinical conversations
- Comfortable seating, allowing easy sitting down and getting up. Stable chairs with arms to provide an anchor to hold on to.
- Easily accessible elevators and restrooms
- Examination tables that rise or lower to assist patients with disabilities
- Availability of water or juice for patients
- For initial visits, reminder to patient to bring in all prescription and over-the-counter medications. Inclusion of herbal products/vitamins/mineral supplements needs to be specified.
- For initial visits or to update clinical history, request for patient to bring previous medical records, laboratory or x-ray reports, electrocardiograms, reports of vaccination, and other relevant health records

Previsit Review and Recording of Health History by Patient and Family

It is in the best interests of all concerned patients, family members, and HCPs that past health events are recorded accurately and thoroughly. Collecting those details in advance of the clinical visit can make the final medical record much more useful. Many clinics make self-reported history forms available ahead of time either through the mail or online. Completing the past medical history forms at home prepares patients to concentrate on their current clinical situation, confident that the HCPs know the previous medical background. The more complicated the medical history, the greater time savings are achieved. The information that needs to be gathered includes:

- Dates of hospitalization
- Dates of operation and discharge reports
- Dates of more recent procedures such as x-rays or biopsies

TABLE 34.13 Instruments for Evaluation of Older Adults

Instrument	Focus	Measurement	Uses
Tilburg or Groningen Frailty Indicators	Loss of resources causes inability to respond to physical or psychologic stress	Either professional or self-report of functioning in four domains: physical, cognitive, social, psychologic	Vulnerability to future poor health outcomes; to predict disability, healthcare use, and quality of life
World Health Organization Quality of Life questionnaire (WHOQOL-BREF)	Individual's perceptions of culture and value systems and personal goals, standards, and concerns	Brief version is 26 items measuring four domains: physical health, psychologic health, social relationships, and environment	Can be used for people with intact cognitive functioning as well as mild-to-moderate dementia
Short Portable Mental Status	Mental process of knowing and understanding	Ten questions, can adjust for educational level	Assess cognitive functioning; can be repeated to check if decline in cognition
Mini-Mental State Examination (MMSE)	Brief, quantitative measure of cognitive status in adults used to screen for cognitive impairment, to estimate the severity of cognitive impairment at a given point in time, to follow the course of cognitive changes in an individual over time, and to document an individual's response to treatment; used frequently to track cognitive changes in patients with dementia	Eleven questions that assess areas such as orientation, recall, attention, and language	Assess cognitive functioning; can be repeated to check if decline in cognition
Katz's ADL Scale	Ability to independently bathe, dress, toilet, transfer, be continent, feed	Six yes/no questions, one for each functional area	Rate performance of independent activity
Instrumental Activities of Daily Living (iADLs)	Completion of complex activities; need for support services	Measures eight complex activities needed for independent functioning, assessing how much assistance is required, if any	If patient is not able to perform iADLs, assistance will be needed. If caregiver support is inadequate, a change in living situation might be indicated.
Geriatric Depression Scale	Low mood accompanied by low self-esteem and loss of interest or pleasure in normally enjoyable activities	Short form has 15 yes/no questions, completion in 5 minutes; original form had 30 questions	Used to evaluate depression, which can exist alone or accompany dementia, as well as major illnesses: recent stroke, coronary artery bypass graft, or myocardial infarct. Elder abuse can also cause depression.
Barthel Index of Activities of Daily Living	Evaluates if disability is present, estimates its extent, determines when support needed	Can ask information of patient or relatives; can assess improvement over time	Assesses adequate functioning in mobility and daily self-care tasks
Palliative Performance Scale	Progression of disease, symptom management, prognosis, and timing of hospice referral	Scores are given in 10-point increments, ranging from 0 (death) to 100 (full or normal, no disease)	Response to palliative care services. Five categories of function are scored; lower scores indicate greater functional impairment.
Get-Up-and-Go Test	Combination of gait and balance to produce mobility	Patient stands up from seated position in chair, walks short distance, turns around, returns to sitting in chair; can be timed or not	Patient's performance is scored on 5-point scale; higher score indicates greater gait and balance problems as well as an increased risk of falling
Kayser-Jones Brief Oral Health Status Examination (BOHSE)	Rates condition of patient's oral health from 0 (normal) to 2 (problematic)	Ten-item exam identifies oral health problems, using a pen light, tongue depressor, and gauze	Assesses need for referral
Clock Drawing Test (CDT)	Assessment of cognitive decline. If found, medications and management techniques can be used	Patient is asked to draw clock face with a specific time. Score for drawing closed circle, 12 correct numbers in correct positions, with hands pointed accurately	Often given with MMSE. The CDT detects impairments in executive function, while MMSE assesses orientation, memory, and language functions. Useful for detecting dementia in early stages.
Zarit Burden Interview	Patient's care needs effect on daily life of caregiver	Twenty-two items that describe personal strain and role strain on 5-point scale	Used by aging agencies to rate caregiver stress
Braden Scale	Determines an individual's risk for developing pressure ulcers	Level of severity of six indicators: sensory perception, moisture, activity, mobility, nutrition, and friction or shear	Commonly used with older adults who have medical or cognitive impairments, on admission and on regular basis
Berg Balance Test or Single Leg Stance Test	To check for risk of falls; to monitor progress in physical therapy treatment	Choice of 14 tasks range from standing up from a sitting position, to standing on one foot	Clinical balance assessment; rated effective by 70% of physiotherapists
Fullmer SPICES	Conditions that warrant further assessment for fall risk	Checks for six conditions: sleep disorders, problems with eating and feeding, incontinence, confusion, evidence of falls, and skin breakdown	Used on admission to prompt fall risk precautions, if needed
Mini-Nutritional Assessment (MNA)	Malnutrition and risk of developing malnutrition	Six questions on food intake, weight loss, mobility, psychologic stress or acute disease, presence of dementia or depression, and BMI	Suggested use: quarterly for institutionalized older adults and yearly for normally nourished community-dwelling older adults

- Descriptions of injuries or accidents that required immediate medical attention
- Descriptions of medical complications, adverse drug effects, or allergic reactions
- Details about serious illnesses and disabilities
- List of the names and roles of all current HCPs, including primary care providers, specialists, physical therapists, and alternative medicine practitioners such as hypnotists, acupuncturists, massage therapists, and chiropractors.

SAFETY ALERT Polypharmacy is the prescribing of multiple medications. With almost half of individuals over age 65 having three or more chronic diseases, it is a common situation in older adults. The risk comes from the adverse reactions due to drug side effects and interactions and the inability of the older body to efficiently eliminate drug by-products (see Exemplar 51.D, Medication Safety, in Module 51 for more information). Smith and Kautz (2018) offer two recommendations. First, note which medications qualify for the Beers Criteria when recording current medications in the health history. The Beers Criteria, compiled by the American Geriatric Society (www.americangeriatrics.org), lists prescribed medications for older adults to avoid. Second, use the ARMOR approach in polypharmacy situations: Assess, Review, Minimize, Optimize, Reassess.

The health history of an older adult follows the same pattern as for other adults. See Box 34.4 for an example of one approach. **Table 34.14** » lists sample questions to evaluate critical iADLs.

Some potential challenges in completing an accurate health history in older adults, due to age-related issues, are listed in **Table 34.15** ».

Social History

Information about the patient's social support system is a valuable part of the assessment data. Many older adults depend heavily on support and supervision from family members and significant others. That personal assistance allows older adults to compensate for any functional deficits. The components of the social history include personal demographic characteristics, details about relatives, the economic status, and the patient's habits and social activities.

Personal demographic characteristics include current or former marital status, including the quality of the patient's relationships, current living arrangements, and any people with whom the patient lives.

The nurse collects many details about relatives, including the family history. This can be helpful when constructing a family genogram. Names, biological and marital relationships, and place of residence are often documented, concentrating on those individuals with a close involvement in the patient's life. If relevant, family dynamics are categorized as supportive or not, noting the frequency of the interactions. If relevant, family and caregiver expectations are recorded.

TABLE 34.14 Sample Questions for Specific iADLs

Instrumental Activity	Sample Questions
Using transportation	Do you still drive? Do you have an active driver's license?
Managing finances	Do you balance your checkbook yourself? Are you able to afford your prescribed medications?
Shopping	Are you able to buy fresh fruits and vegetables from the grocery store regularly? About how often do you eat fresh fruits and vegetables?
Preparing meals with good nutrition	Do you cook for yourself? What do you usually eat?
Using telephone or other communication devices	Do you use the phone or email to keep up with distant family and friends?
Administering medications	Do you have a method of making sure you take your medicine regularly?
Doing laundry and housework	Are you able to do your own housework?
Maintaining a safe household living environment	How do you keep up with home or equipment repair projects?

TABLE 34.15 Selected Challenges to Assessment of Older Adults

Possible Challenges in Older Adults	Potential Effect on Health History Accuracy
Decreased hearing and vision, decreased cognitive functioning	Pace of communication can be slower. Miscommunication may cause mistakes in understanding on both sides (nurse and patient).
Fears, such as: ■ Being labeled a complainer ■ Being considered for undesired institutionalization ■ Facing a serious illness or death	Fear can lead patients to underreport cues indicating ill health or history of household accidents, such as falls or burns when cooking.
Cognitive impairment due to drug or alcohol use, elder abuse, atypical disease cues	Diagnosis can be difficult without clear knowledge of cues or their etiology.
Undiagnosed depression, multiple chronic illnesses, social isolation	These conditions can make it difficult for healthcare professionals to sort out the clinical priorities from other problems, such as loneliness or suicidal thoughts. Scheduling an appointment with an HCP could be a cry for help.
Need for enough time (at least 1 hour) for appointment	Shorter appointments will result in a hurried interview with missed information (Kane et al., 2018).
Geographical separation from family members, loss of active social support systems due to aging or death	Ask about other social and emotional support methods, such as church, engaged membership in group activities, or spiritual practices.

As far as economic status, the nurse gathers information about current or past occupation and retirement status. The nurse asks about the current financial picture, especially about the adequacy of health insurance coverage.

The nurse asks about the patient's habits, beliefs, and social activities. This includes the patient's transportation options, religion, hobbies, community involvement and support resources used, and spirituality.

As far as religion and spirituality, the nurse should be familiar with the locally available resources or know how to connect individuals and families to them, if needed. Many healthcare facilities and community agencies offer counseling. This can substitute for or enhance a long-term relationship with a chaplain or spiritual counselor. This help is crucial for patients who are depressed or socially isolated, who question the meaning of their existence, or who ask about help with their spiritual concerns. The resources can be a great source of hope in times of despair and crisis.

Some interdisciplinary assessment teams have a social worker on board. The social worker could collaborate with the nurse to identify and address social problems. For example, if the patient has inadequate health insurance coverage, the social worker can serve as a connection to community services, free hospital services, hardship funds for indigent patients, and referrals to community-based free clinics. Patients who might be helped by involving a social worker include those admitted to long-term care facilities, those having severe loneliness or major disabilities, or those not having close relationships with others.

Functional Evaluation

The health history needs to document a systematic evaluation of the patient's functioning level and self-care activities. Regardless of the living environment of the patient—their own home, assisted living, rehabilitation facility, or nursing home—a regular risk assessment for falls and other hazards and measurement of signs of functional decline are important components of ensuring the highest quality of life. Living in an as safe as possible environment promotes the greatest independence and patient satisfaction. Topics to evaluate include cognition, nutrition, continence, mobility, sleep, and skin care. A home visit can be substituted for a comprehensive interview about the patient's home environment. (See Chapter 15, Safety, in Volume 3, especially for Skill 15.2, Fall Prevention, and Skill 15.5, Environmental Safety, for more detail about those assessments.)

Lifestyle and Health Considerations

Older adults can maintain an active lifestyle and satisfying interactions within their community. (**Figure 34.11** »). Activities that promote the older adult's sense of self-worth and usefulness can provide opportunities for developing new friendships. Mental acuity and maximum cognitive functioning can be promoted through pursuing intellectual activities. Some older adults are content with their life review, enjoy their retirement years, and accept death as the inevitable end of a productive life. Other older adults have not successfully resolved developmental crises. They might be depressed and feel that life has been unfair. Declining physical and mental abilities can bring unwanted lifestyle changes. Despair and hopelessness can be the result of a downward spiral of lack of meaningful activity and less ability to take care of oneself.

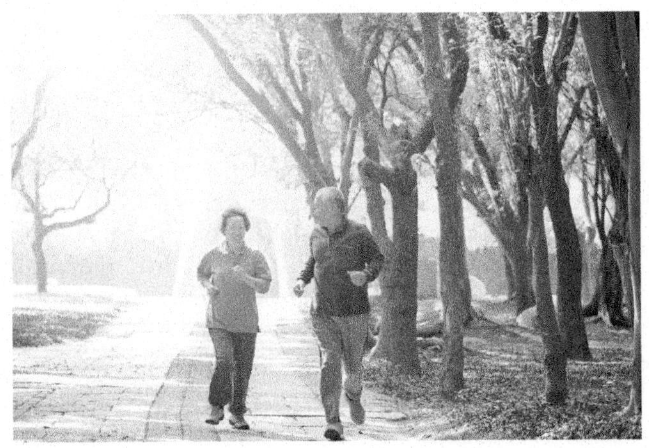

Figure 34.11 » Active older adults continue to enjoy life well into retirement.

Source: Tom Wang/Shutterstock.

Minimum Data Set

Assessment of an older patient for appropriate placement in a nursing home or within a long-term care system is done using the Minimum Data Set (MDS). The MDS is a comprehensive standardized multidisciplinary assessment used throughout the United States. The Omnibus Budget Reconciliation Act of 1987 (OBRA 87) mandated assessment of all residents of facilities funded by Medicare or Medicaid using the MDS. The Department of Veterans Affairs (VA) also collects data for residents of its nursing homes (UCSF Geriatrics, 2018). The MDS is used for validation of the need for long-term care at least every 3 months, reimbursement, ongoing assessment of clinical problems, and assessment of and need to alter the current plan of care due to major changes in health status.

The MDS consists of a core set of screening, clinical, and functional measures:

- *Resident Assessment Protocols (RAPs)* are structured, problem-oriented guidelines that identify unique and relevant information about an older patient. This information is needed for formulating an individualized nursing care plan.
- *Resident Utilization Guidelines (RUGs)* determine the reimbursement the skilled nursing facility will receive for providing care to the older patient. Cues considered include the need for supportive therapy (physical, occupational, and/or speech), self-care ability of the older patient, and the need for special treatments such as feeding tubes or skin care.
- *Resident Assessment Instrument (RAI)* identifies medical problems and describes each older patient's functional ability in a comprehensive and standardized format. This information helps to formulate the plan of care and to evaluate progress toward goals, indicating when changes in the care plan are needed.

Categories of data gathered for the MDS include the following:

- Patient demographics and background
- Cognitive function
- Mobility

- Communication, visual and hearing acuity
- Mood and behavior patterns, including dementia
- Psychosocial well-being, such as resident participation in activities and cues about the presence of depression
- Physical function and ADLs
- Bowel and bladder continence
- Diagnosed diseases
- Health conditions (e.g., pain, shortness of breath, weight loss, pressure ulcers, falls)
- Oral nutritional status
- Oral and dental status
- Skin condition
- Medications (e.g., antipsychotics, sedative–hypnotics)
- Need for special services
- Discharge potential.

Certain information gathered for the MDS, such as data indicating functional decline or a poorly managed chronic disease, may trigger the need for further assessment using the RAPs. For instance, if information gathered for the MDS indicates that the nursing home resident has fallen, a RAP is triggered and indicates the need for direct gait assessment, medication review, and physical/occupational therapy evaluation.

REVIEW The Concept of Assessment

RELATE Link the Concepts

Linking the concept of assessment with the concept of caring interventions:

1. You are assigned to care for a patient who has been receiving tube feedings via a nasogastric tube that has been in place for several days. Prior to administering the first tube feeding of the shift, what assessments would you perform?
2. Would the assessment performed be classified as an initial assessment or a problem-focused assessment? Explain your answer.

Linking the concept of assessment with the concept of clinical decision making:

3. You are assigned care of a 46-year-old man admitted for status asthmaticus. His condition has stabilized and discharge is planned for tomorrow. When you enter his room for the first time, you find that he is short of breath and he requests that you hand him his inhaler, which the physician ordered to be kept at the bedside for self-administration as needed. What will you do first? Which important assessment is needed? How would you handle a possible change in already-set discharge plans?
4. What critical thinking would you apply to the above situation?

Linking the concept of assessment with the concept of communication:

5. When collecting information for a health history, what strategies would you use when communicating with an older adult who is deaf or hard of hearing?
6. You are collecting information from the mother of a 3-year-old for a health history. The mother does not speak any English, but the 3-year-old does speak English. What communication strategies would you employ? What if the child was 9 years old and enrolled in third grade? Would those different characteristics cause you to change your communication strategy?

Linking the concept of assessment with the concept of legal issues:

7. You admit an adolescent to the adolescent unit of a local hospital and begin collecting data when you begin to suspect that the adolescent may be abusing substances. With an understanding of your legal obligation to the adolescent, as well as your knowledge that the parents want to help their child, how would you handle your suspicions if the parents are in the room with the child?
8. You are assessing an older adult and discover bruises that you suspect may be the result of abuse. The patient's son is in the room during the examination. What is the best legally appropriate action for you to take? What will you do if that initial approach does not clarify the situation?

READY Go to Volume 3: Clinical Nursing Skills

REFER Go to Pearson MyLab Nursing and eText

REFLECT Apply Your Knowledge

It was late afternoon in the outpatient clinic, shortly before closing time. The nurse brought Beatriz Clark, a 73-year-old woman, into an examination room to conduct her health history interview before her annual Medicare wellness visit. The following dialogue ensued:

Nurse: "Welcome to our clinic, Beatriz. I have a series of routine, but necessary, questions that I have to ask you before you see your primary care doctor. I apologize for our starting late and your having to sit so long in the waiting room. But if we go fast, we can catch up."

Ms. Clark: "I won't be able to go fast, as I have trouble hearing. If you could speak slower and talk into my good ear, the right one, that would help a lot."

Nurse: "I can do that and make a note of that request for your record, so we can remember that accommodation in the future."

Ms. Clark: "I appreciate that. I keep forgetting to mention that when I come in to see the doctor. I get so worked up when I come into a medical facility. It makes me anxious."

Nurse: "Well now, you just relax. You're in good hands. I see from your last visit that you came in for a urinary tract infection. Did you take your medication as prescribed? Are you still having symptoms 'down there'? Do we need to take a urine specimen today?"

1. How would you change the nurse's introductory remarks to better establish a rapport with the patient?
2. Did the nurse respond appropriately to the patient's sharing her hearing problem? Her anxiety?
3. What are the pros and cons of rescheduling this clinical visit?
4. Critique the nurse's including in the interview questions a reference to the medical concerns prompting the patient's last visit.

References

American Cancer Society. (2018). *American Cancer Society guidelines for early detection of cancer*. https://www.cancer.org/healthy/findcancerearly/cancerscreeningguidelines/american-cancer-society-guidelines-for-the-early-detection-of-cancer

American Cancer Society. (2019). *Breast cancer risk -factors you cannot change*. https://www.cancer.org/cancer/breast-cancer/risk-and-prevention/breast-cancer-risk-factors-you-cannot-change.html

American College of Cardiology. (2019). 2019 *ACC/AHA guideline on the primary prevention of cardiovascular disease*. http://www.onlinejacc.org/sites/default/files/additional_assets/guidelines/Prevention-Guidelines-Made-Simple.pdf

Berman, A., Snyder, S., & Frandsen, G. (2021). *Kozier & Erb's fundamentals of nursing: Concepts, process, and practice* (11th ed.). Pearson.

Centers for Disease Control and Prevention (CDC). (2017). *10 leading causes of death by age group, United States—2017*. https://www.cdc.gov/injury/images/lc-charts/leading_causes_of_death_by_age_group_2017_1100w850h.jpg

Centers for Disease Control and Prevention (CDC). (2018). *Defining childhood obesity*. https://www.cdc.gov/obesity/childhood/defining.html

Fenske, C., Watkins, K., Saunders, T., D'Amico, D., & Barbarito, C. (2019). *Health and physical assessment in nursing* (4th ed.). Pearson.

Flynn, J. T., Kaelber, D. C., Baker-Smith, C. M., Blowey, D., Carroll, A. E., Daniels, S. R., et al. (2017). Clinical practice guideline for screening and management of high blood pressure in children and adolescents. *Pediatrics, 140*(3), e20171904. https://doi.org/10.1542/peds.2017-1904

Hartford Institute for Geriatric Nursing. (2017). *ConsultGeri*. https://consultgeri.org/tools/try-this-series

Jarvis, C. (2019). *Physical examination and health assessment* (8th ed.). Saunders.

Kane, R., Ouslander, J., Resnick, B., & Malone, M. L. (2018). *Essentials of clinical geriatrics* (8th ed.). McGraw-Hill.

Stewart, C., & Cash, W. (2017). *Interviewing: Principles and practices* (15th ed.). McGraw-Hill.

Smith, D. M., & Kautz, D. D. (2018). Protect older adults from polypharmacy hazards. *Nursing 2019*, 48(2), 56–59. https://doi.org/10.1097/01.NURSE.0000527602.17216.6d

Siu, A. L., the U.S. Preventive Services Task (USPSTF), Bibbins-Domingo, K., Grossman, D. C., Baumann, L. C., Davidson, K. W., et al. (2016). Screening for depression in adults: U.S. Preventive Services Task Force Recommendation Statement. *Journal of the American Medical Association, 315*(4), 380–387.

UCSF Geriatrics. (2018). *Minimum Data Set (MDS) data*. https://geriatrics.ucsf.edu/minimum-data-set-mds-data

U.S. Preventive Services Task Force. (2018). *Clinical Summary: Intimate partner violence, elder abuse, and abuse of vulnerable adults: Screening*. https://www.uspreventiveservicestaskforce.org/Page/Document/ClinicalSummaryFinal/intimate-partner-violence-and-abuse-of-elderly-and-vulnerable-adults-screening1

Wilcox, M., McGee, B. A., Ionescu, D. F., Leonte, M., LaCross, L., Reps, J., et al. (2020). Perinatal depression symptoms often start in the prenatal rather than postpartum period: results from a longitudinal study. *Archives of Women's Mental Health*. https://doi.org/10.1007/s00737-020-01017-z

Module 35
Caring Interventions

Module Outline and Learning Outcomes

The Concept of Caring Interventions

Nursing Theories of Caring

35.1 Outline nursing theories that bridge the gap between theory and practice.

Concepts Related to Caring Interventions

35.2 Outline the relationship between caring interventions and other concepts.

Stages of Change

35.3 Discuss application of stage theory as a caring intervention to influence behavior change.

Caring Encounters and Holistic Nursing

35.4 Analyze holistic nursing as it relates to caring interventions.

Lifespan Considerations

35.5 Differentiate caring interventions appropriate for patients at different stages throughout the lifespan.

Caring for the Caregiver: Self-Care in Nursing

35.6 Analyze the importance of nurses caring for themselves.

›› The Concept of Caring Interventions

Concept Key Terms

Caring, **2477**
Compassion, **2483**
Competence, **2483**
Empowerment, **2482**
Motivational interviewing, **2481**
Presencing, **2482**

Caring is generally defined as "feeling or showing concern for others" (Merriam-Webster Dictionary, 2020), but in the context of the nursing profession, caring goes well beyond this simple explanation. Caring has been described as encompassing various intentions and actions. *Caregiving* is a significant role for the practicing nurse (Konuk & Tanyer, 2019). Nurses demonstrate caring behaviors through recognizing and responding to patient status and behaviors, attending to the patient and the family, engaging with the healthcare team, and maintaining a positive attitude (Thompson & McClement, 2019). These are just a few examples of ways in which nurses can exhibit caring to their patients.

Caring is a concept that forms an integral part of nursing theory. That said, the concept of caring is not limited to the realm of academia. Research based on interviews of practicing emergency department nurses revealed that caring is an integral aspect of those called to the nursing profession (Jiménez-Herrera et al., 2020). One nurse participant stated, "helping people makes me feel fulfilled, you are next to them in very serious and critical situations and we are behind the care given at these difficult moments" (p. 6).

Research goes further to describe nursing students who are learning to care as nurses (Young, Godbold, & Wood, 2019). One nursing student stated, "It wasn't just what you were taught to do, everybody has gone that little extra mile of what you can't be taught . . . that feeling you have inside you, it's that empathy" (p. 133). This statement emphasizes the importance of attitude in demonstrating caring behaviors. Nursing students have further described time, personalization, and role modeling as important aspects to developing and learning to care in sometimes challenging healthcare systems (Young et al., 2019). Milton Mayeroff, author of the classic book *On Caring*, argued that at the heart of caring is "helping the other grow" (1971/1990, p. 2). Mayeroff maintained that caring facilitates growth both in the person who exhibits caring and in the recipient, be it a person or thing (such as a concept, cause, or community). Under his framework, caring is not a finite action but rather a process that encourages self-actualization in the caregiver as well as development of the person receiving care. Central to Mayeroff's concept of caring is that the caregiver must respect the individuality and separateness of the other by not inflicting a specific direction in the growth of the other.

Nursing Theories of Caring

Many theories of caring in nursing grew out of humanism, which can be described as the belief in "the potential and dignity of human beings, honoring their freedom and capacity to shape their own destiny from the choices they make throughout their life" (Létourneau, Goudreau, & Cara, 2020, p. 2). Although each caring theory underscores different aspects and perspectives, the sheer number of caring theories highlights the centralization of this concept to nursing practice. Humanism is reflected in many areas of nursing, including respect for patients' autonomy, rights, and cultural and religious preferences.

Bridging the gap between theory and practice has been an ongoing issue in nursing. Roy (2019) noted that it is imperative to incorporate nursing theory into meeting patient healthcare goals and to shape nursing practice. Research of patient experiences supports the work of Roy and other theorists, revealing that patients are clear on what constitutes a good nurse. Patients have identified characteristics and behaviors of a good nurse to include humanistic, supportive, and faithful among essential personality traits, as well as professional traits such as demeanor, competence, patient-centered care, and communication (Lee & Kim, 2019).

Many hospitals around the United States have incorporated caring theories into professional practice models (PPM). For example, at the University of Rochester Medical Center (URMC; 2020), PPM is guided by Watson's theory of human care. Utilizing theory to facilitate professional practice provides both structure and common language to support nursing care (URMC, 2020). By highlighting expectations associated with each of the 10 clinical caritas processes (for example, being authentically present with the patient), this PPM encourages nursing proficiency in interpersonal and technological skills. The culmination of this approach is that patient care is provided holistically to include body, mind, and spirit. Watson's theory is discussed further later in this module.

Although caring theories have been designed with the nurse–patient relationship in mind, the basic tenets of caring can and should be applied to the nurse–nurse relationship. Intense levels of stress caused by staff shortages and high-needs patients underscore the importance of nurses supporting each other. When nurses are supportive of each other, they not only are more satisfied with their roles but patient satisfaction and outcomes also improve (Edmonson & Zelonka, 2019). Inappropriate behaviors, such as bullying, are being scrutinized in healthcare because of the potential negative impact on patient care and safety and worker well-being and satisfaction. These behaviors must not be supported in nursing and should be acknowledged and addressed starting in nursing school (Edmonson & Zelonka, 2019).

Leininger's Theory of Culture Care Diversity and Universality

In the mid-1980s, Madeleine Leininger revolutionized nursing and transformed the concept of caring with the development of a new discipline called transcultural nursing, currently referred to as the theory of culture care diversity and universality (Steefel, 2019). In an early publication, Leininger said that "nurses often labeled, avoided or talked down to the cultural strangers when they did not understand their behavior and needs" (1989, p. 7). Her study of anthropology provided much insight as to how culture played a crucial role in providing nursing care to maintain or encourage health.

For nurses to provide the highest quality of care to culturally diverse patients, Leininger presents three modes of action:

- Culture care preservation and/or maintenance involves nurses and other providers performing actions and making choices that help patients retain their specific cultural values and beliefs.
- Culture care accommodation and/or negotiation refer to nurses' efforts to assist patients in adapting to or working with others to achieve the best possible care.
- Culture care repatterning and/or restructuring is reflected in nursing interventions that support patients in evaluating and changing their approaches to promote improved health outcomes (McFarland & Wehbe-Alamah, 2015).

See Module 24, Culture and Diversity, for more information on culturally competent nursing care.

» **Stay Current:** For additional information on nursing and other cultures, visit the website of the Transcultural Nursing Society at http://www.tcns.org.

Roach's Theory of Caring as the Human Mode of Being

Sister M. Simone Roach's philosophical theory declares caring to be a core element of how humans operate, as well as an expression of interconnectedness: "Caring, as the human mode of being, is caring from the heart; caring from the core of one's being; caring as a response to one's experience of connectedness" (Roach, 1997, p. 16).

Although Roach's theory views humans as caring entities, it also maintains that caring within the context of nursing is distinct in that the specific traits of nurses are all grounded in caring. She has labeled these attributes the six Cs of caring: compassion, competence, confidence, conscience, commitment, and comportment. Refer to **Box 35.1** » for further explanation of each trait.

Boykin and Schoenhofer's Nursing as Caring Theory

In 1993, Anne Boykin and Savina O. Schoenhofer proposed their nursing theory of caring, which maintains that caring is a crucial element of being human, as well as an ongoing

Box 35.1
The Six Cs of Caring in Nursing

Compassion. Awareness of one's relationship to others, sharing their joys, sorrows, pain, and accomplishments. Participation in the experience of another.

Competence. Having the knowledge, judgment, skills, energy, experience, and motivation to respond adequately to others within the demands of professional responsibilities.

Confidence. The quality that fosters trusting relationships. Comfort with self, patient, and family.

Conscience. Morals, ethics, and an informed sense of right and wrong. Awareness of personal responsibility.

Commitment. Convergence between one's desires and obligations and the deliberate choice to act in accordance with them.

Comportment. Appropriate demeanor, dress, and language that are in harmony with a caring presence. Presenting oneself as someone who respects others and in turn demands respect.

Source: From Roach (2002). Adapted with permission.

process rather than a goal to be achieved (Purnell, 2013). They argue that nurses must be willing to accept that caring is never static; it continually changes and evolves throughout the span of their lives. At the heart of it all, nursing is caring. Boykin and Schoenhofer (2001) assume that "people are caring by virtue of their humanness, persons are whole and complete in the moment," and caring is lived moment to moment (p. 1). Self-awareness is also essential to being a caring and effective nurse. Patients respond positively to the nurse's authenticity, which encourages their own growth.

Watson's Theory of Human Care

Jean Watson's (1999) theory of human care (developed in the 1970s) has evolved as a result of her intense interest, varied education, and extensive experience with nursing, philosophy, and metaphysics. At the crux of her theory is the assumption that genuine caring relationships have a positive impact on a patient's health and can facilitate the healing process, putting caring at the core of nursing. The caring moment is thus transpersonal and requires an authentic relationship between the patient and the nurse (Watson Caring Science Institute, 2020).

Furthermore, Watson (1999) maintained that caring involves addressing not just the mind and the body, but also the spirit: "The value of human care and caring involves a higher sense of spirit of self. Caring calls for a philosophy of moral commitment toward protecting human dignity and preserving humanity" (p. 31).

When Watson first developed her theory, she identified what she referred to as the 10 carative factors that needed to exist within a nurse–patient caring relationship. She later updated those characteristics and renamed them the 10 clinical caritas processes. These include the process of practicing loving kindness and equanimity within the context of providing care; being authentically present with the patient; being present to and supportive of patients' expression of feelings—both positive and negative; and creating a healing environment at all levels (Watson Caring Science Institute, 2020).

» **Stay Current:** For an overview of Watson's theory of human caring and the 10 caritas processes, go to https://www.watsoncaringscience.org/jean-bio/caring-science-theory/.

Benner and Wrubel's Theory of Caring

Patricia Benner and Judith Wrubel's contribution to caring theories is grounded in their seminal work *The Primacy of Caring: Stress and Coping in Health and Illness* (1989), which places caring at the heart of providing quality service to patients and their families. They further clarified their perspective as not focusing on nurse caregiving as much as on how care informs stress and coping responses: "Our main goal is to examine the phenomenon of care and caring practices to the experience of health and illness, not the caregiving of nurses" (2001, p. 172). Benner and Wrubel describe a nurse's intent to care as only one factor in how caring is delivered and received. In other words, caring does not happen in a vacuum; it is dependent on other factors, such as the context of the situation, the physical environment, the nurse's training and experience, and the patient's unique capacities and perspectives (Benner & Wrubel, 2001).

Peplau's Theory of Interpersonal Relations

Hildegard Peplau is often referred to as the mother of psychiatric nursing (Haber, 2000; Potter & Moller, 2020). This is largely due to her *Theory of Interpersonal Relations*, first published in the 1950s (Haber, 2000). The theory proposed the importance of the nurse–patient relationship and the therapeutic benefits for the patient (Peplau, 1991). Peplau (1991) identified that the interpersonal relations are unique to the profession of nursing and are a core function to support the professional health team. The interpersonal relationship occurs in phases. The phases are addressed in detail in Exemplar 38.B, Therapeutic Communication, in Module 38, Communication.

Orem's Self-Care Theory

Dorothea Orem (2001) developed her theory of self-care in nursing over several decades, prompted initially by a need to define nursing. Orem hypothesized that nursing was focused on self-care and self-care deficits. Self-care is defined by Orem as the "personal care that individuals required each day to regulate their own functioning and development" (p. 20). Therefore, when an individual experiences a self-care deficit, it means they are unable to provide all of the required personal care. In self-care theory, nurses provide care to meet self-care deficits experienced by patients.

Across the trajectory of illness, it is important to consider how nurses help to address self-care deficits. In acute illness, the nursing role may include completely caring for patients, as patients may be unable to provide any personal care. As patients recover from acute illness, the nurse will need to work with patients to meet their self-care needs, as patients may be able to provide some of their own care. Lastly, as the illness ends, patients are able to complete self-care independently.

Concepts Related to Caring Interventions

Caring interventions are fundamental to the entire nursing process. Caring—both for self and for others—is the essence of nursing. Self-care is also important for nurses and includes recognizing and tending to the nurse's own physiologic and psychosocial needs, as well as seeking out activities that promote professional development. For the nurse, the negative impact of alterations in physical and mental health can extend to patient care, in terms of both the decision-making process and the actual care the nurse provides.

The relationship between caring interventions and professionalism carries important implications for nurses. In work environments where nurse shortages and poor working conditions exist, nurses have reported that quality of care suffers (Halm, 2019). Better work environments are associated with a range of outcomes, including improved job satisfaction, reduced patient mortality, and improved patient satisfaction scores (Lake et al., 2019).

Caring is directly linked to ethics because it "requires nurses who focus on the relationship with the human being by seeing, understanding, and taking responsibility" (Karlsson & Pennbrant, 2020, para. 1). Caring nurses are more inclined to hold high ethical standards, which unfortunately can lead to internal conflict, also referred to as moral distress. Moral distress is a phenomenon that encompasses many issues, such as a nurse knowing the right action to take, but being constrained from taking it; the nurse not sharing an opinion with the healthcare team on an ethical situation; and a lack of preparation to manage ethical conflicts (Morley, Bradbury-Jones, & Ives, 2020).

Cultural influences affect coping styles, which, in turn, affect both care and self-care practices. For example, most Western (North American and western European) cultures are considered to be individualist, placing a high value on facing personal challenges individually and autonomously. In the context of an individualist culture, persons experiencing illness or distress may not seek support out of fear of being perceived as weak by others (Eskin et al., 2020).

Cultural influences also inform the grieving process. Western expectations of autonomy may lead some providers to discount the importance of the family unit during times of grief or illness and may also lead some patients to hesitate to ask family members for help or support. Similarly, individuals from different cultures may observe different rituals during the end of life. Nurses and other healthcare providers (HCPs) assess and facilitate the needs of all patients to observe cultural or traditional practices. Some, but not all, of the concepts integral to caring are shown in the Concepts Related to Caring Interventions feature. They are presented in alphabetical order.

Concepts Related to
Caring Interventions

CONCEPT	RELATIONSHIP TO CARING INTERVENTIONS	NURSING IMPLICATIONS
Culture and Diversity	Western cultural influences → autonomous coping highly valued → sense of weakness associated with seeking social support → tendency to avoid asking for help when needed → ineffective self-care	■ Recognize cultural impact on beliefs about seeking help. ■ Assess personal beliefs regarding the value of social support. ■ Identify trusted sources of support and use resources as needed.
Ethics	Conflict between providing the best possible care for the patient could clash with the family's wishes or the constraining factors of the institution → leads nurse to experience moral distress → ↑ feelings of stress → ↑ risk for burnout	■ Share ethical concerns with supervisor and healthcare team and build supportive networks on the job. ■ Attend workshops on moral distress to increase coping strategies. ■ Identify common causes of moral distress among nursing peers.
Grief and Loss	Western cultural influences assume personal autonomy and involvement in end-of-life decisions and care → disregard for non-Western patient/family preferences regarding end-of-life preferences → impaired patient/family/provider communication → increased grief and unhappiness by patient and family during stressful life event	■ If patients/family from a non-Western culture reject such concepts as palliative care/hospice, advance directives, or organ donation, be respectful of these decisions. ■ Use chaplains and translators (if needed) to ensure that patient/family wishes regarding death and associated practices are fully understood by nurses and assistive personnel. ■ Accommodate patient/family wishes as much as possible to alleviate patient and family stress. ■ Demonstrate respect in all interactions with the patient/family.
Professionalism	Inadequate self-care → decreased level of physical and psychosocial wellness → decreased quality of work performance and weakened affiliation with profession of nursing → decreased level of demonstrated professionalism toward patients, peers, and other members of the healthcare team	■ Assess self-wellness and recognize when limitations are being exceeded. ■ Be aware of warning signs that may signal burnout. ■ Recognize areas of self-care that are unhealthy and identify solutions that promote wellness.
Safety	Lack of knowledge regarding patient culture → incomplete nursing assessment and miscommunication → poor patient outcomes and dissatisfaction with HCPs and facility	■ Use chaplains and translators (if needed) to ensure that information is accurately transmitted to patient and family. ■ Actively seek information about the patient's stated cultural and religious preferences. ■ Ensure that patient teaching is delivered using a culturally sensitive method that enhances understanding and supports decision making. ■ Safeguard against inserting racial or cultural stereotypes, biases, and prejudices that may affect patient care and safety.

Concepts Related to *(continued)*

CONCEPT	RELATIONSHIP TO CARING INTERVENTIONS	NURSING IMPLICATIONS
Stress and Coping	Impaired coping → absence of self-care → stress, anxiety, or mild depression → errors in patient care	■ Identify and acknowledge stressors. ■ Evaluate the efficacy of personal coping methods. ■ Develop healthy, effective coping methods.

Stages of Change

As nurses, one of the most challenging caring interventions is to encourage and facilitate behavior changes in patients. Education alone does not change behavior. A patient's readiness to change affects adherence to the treatment plan (Harrington, 2020). Prochaska and DiClemente (1983) identified a model of change based on five stages, now known as the transtheoretical model of change or *stages of change* model. The stages include precontemplation, contemplation, preparation, action, and maintenance (see **Figure 35.1** »). There is not a smooth transition through these stages for most patients. Often in making behavior changes, patients travel back and forth through the stages of change before reaching the final stage of maintenance (Prochaska, DiClemente, & Norcross, 1992).

During the *precontemplation stage*, patients are unaware a problem needs to be addressed, or they are unable to accept that there is a problem (Prochaska et al., 1992). As the patient becomes aware of the problem and begins to consider making a change, they progress into the contemplation stage. During contemplation, the patient may or may not commit to making changes necessary to resolve the problem. The patient who decides to make changes moves to the third stage, preparation, which is when the patient begins to make plans for behavior change. The action stage begins when the patient starts making changes in one or more behaviors, and the final stage of maintenance is focused on continued preservation of the changed behavior (Prochaska et al., 1992).

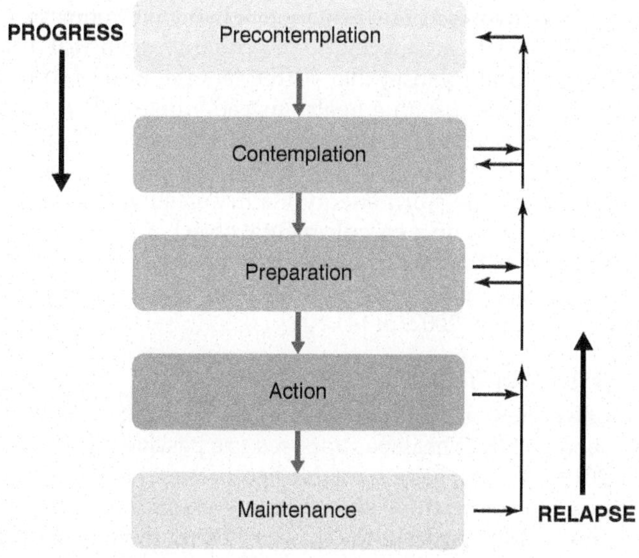

Figure 35.1 » The five stages of change.

While initially developed with addiction behaviors as the key focus for this model, in healthcare today, nurses can utilize this model to approach behavior change of any sort. It can be particularly beneficial when lifestyle changes are needed in response to chronic illness, such as a diagnosis of prediabetes or type 2 diabetes. According to the Centers for Disease Control and Prevention (2020), 60% of American adults have a chronic disease, and 40% have two or more chronic diseases. Lifestyle changes are often required in the areas of diet and exercise to manage these diseases, and the transtheoretical model can help in understanding the patients' willingness to change.

Nurses should work with patients to help encourage behavior changes. One technique that can help to facilitate patient movement through the stages of change model is **motivational interviewing**. Motivational interviewing (MI) is a technique frequently used in addiction counseling. The goal of MI is to explore ambivalence that exists about a behavior change (Li, Yang, Wang, Yang, & Zhang, 2020). There are four key elements in motivational interviewing (Miller & Rollnick, 2013):

- Avoiding the righting reflex (in other words, avoid correcting the patient and telling them what they should do differently)
- Listening with empathy
- Exploring intrinsic motivations
- Encouraging patient self-efficacy.

Nurses work to guide the conversation with the patient to inspire dialogue about the patient's thoughts on change. During the discussion, nurses should be aware of *change talk* and *sustain talk* utilized by the patient. Change talk is any language that expresses a desire to make a change, whereas sustain talk is the patient's language that argues against change (Miller & Rollnick, 2013). For example, the patient who states, "I really need to quit smoking; I know it's making my daughter's asthma worse," is engaging in *change* talk. In contrast, the patient who says, "I just don't have time to go to family therapy; I work two jobs as it is, and besides, I don't have any insurance" is engaging in *sustain* talk. By listening for change talk, the nurse can continue efforts to guide the conversation and explore the ambivalence. The use of OARS is helpful to the nurse in facilitating the discussion. OARS stands for open-ended questions, affirmation, reflection, and summarizing (Motivational Interviewing Network of Trainers, 2020). These techniques set a foundation of collaboration and partnership with the patient that allows the nurse to evoke motivation to make behavior changes and progress through the stages of change.

Clinical Example A

Mr. Bahdoon Osman, a 57-year-old man from Somalia, immigrated to Minnesota 5 years ago with his wife, son, and three daughters. Three days ago, he was rushed to the hospital for breathing and swallowing difficulties, the cause of which was a large tumor. Following emergent surgical resection of the tumor, Mr. Osman was diagnosed with stage IV esophageal cancer. The family is adamant that he not be informed of his terminal diagnosis because Somali culture believes it is cruel to do so. The patient's physician has presented his treatment options.

The charge nurse instructed Mr. Osman's nurse, Joanne Williams, to speak only to the patient's son about Mr. Osman's care and not to his wife, explaining that according to Somali traditions, the father speaks for the family when outside the home. When the father is unable to do so, another adult man in the family, often the son, takes on the responsibility. The nurse finds this instruction challenging, especially seeing the obvious pain the patient's wife is in watching her husband suffer. The son tells Joanne that it is important that they reposition Mr. Osman's bed "so that it faces Mecca." Because Joanne does not understand this request, she asks Mr. Osman's wife for further explanation. His wife avoids Joanne's gaze and does not answer. The son firmly explains to Joanne that his mother does not have a say in the matter and repeats the request. Frustrated and upset at what she feels is a lack of respect for Mr. Osman's wife, Joanne responds by saying it is impossible to move the bed and leaves the room.

Critical Thinking Questions

1. Did Joanne demonstrate caring? If so, how?
2. How could have Joanne dealt with the Osman family differently?
3. What strategies could Joanne have employed to address culturally specific healthcare issues for the family?

Caring Encounters and Holistic Nursing

The healthcare field is moving from its traditional focus on disease management to a more holistic, patient-focused approach to care. The American Holistic Nurses Association (AHNA; 2020a, para. 1) defines holistic nursing as "all nursing practice that has healing the whole person as its goal." Holistic nursing is a philosophy and attitude that facilitates healing by recognizing the intertwined relationships among the "body, mind, emotion, spirit, social/cultural, relationship, context, and environment." Nurses practicing the holistic approach seek to develop a bond with the patient to create a more personal and supportive environment. Complementing traditional treatments with alternative therapies (such as reiki, meditation, biofeedback, and journaling) is also an important part of holistic and integrative nursing (Frisch & Rabinowitsch, 2019). The goal is to go beyond addressing the illness to help patients achieve balance in their lives. In this respect, it places the nurse in the role of health educator and emphasizes the patient's personal responsibility in maintaining health.

This approach to nursing has become more relevant in the face of the nation's changing demographics. Increasingly, the general population is turning to complementary and integrative health practices, formerly known as "alternative" medicine, to address health issues. *Complementary* is a term that refers to a nonmainstream medical therapy or product used in addition to conventional medical practice, whereas the term *integrative* refers to a nonmainstream practice combined with conventional medicine in a seamless approach. The latest figures from the National Health Interview Survey indicate over 30% of adults and almost 12% of children had made use of complementary health approaches in 2012 (National Center for Complementary and Integrative Health, 2018). See Module 7, Health, Wellness, Illness, and Injury, for more information.

Nurses must educate themselves on complementary and integrative health approaches and understand that not all alternative therapies work for all people, and some may even be harmful. Holistic understanding of the patient is required to advise patients on appropriate therapeutic interventions and treatments. Understanding the patient's context is of great importance when deciding on care strategies. For example, recommending costly supplements that can only be found in a few select specialty shops for an older adult who lives alone with limited mobility and income would prove problematic.

Nursing Presence

Presencing is a nursing concept developed by Rosemarie Rizzo Parse that involves the interpersonal arts of perception and communication. Through presencing, the nurse immerses himself in an interaction with the patient that helps the patient define her health choices. It is the patient, then, who has the authority to make decisions about her health. The nurse acts as a guide through use of presence, not in the sense that the nurse tends to the patient, but rather by being open, receptive, and available at all levels without judging or labeling. The nurse's thinking flows with the patient's, and the value systems of the patient direct outcomes, not those of the nurse. Research in this area of nursing resulted in the development of a Presence of Nursing Scale to measure nursing presence, with higher scores indicating enhanced patient–nurse rapport, increased patient coping, and decreased patient anxiety (Hansbrough & Georges, 2019). In this sort of interaction, the nurse lets the patient lead, which could involve dialoguing, simply being there (even if silently), and leaving a lasting memory of the interaction in the patient's mind.

Another important nursing concept in this regard is *intentionality*, which refers to nurses working in conjunction with those involved in the situation at hand as a cooperative force rather than attempting to impose their own will. It is a philosophical mindset that surrenders the idea of directing outcomes and setting goals; instead, nurses allow resistance to dissolve and a course of action to unfold (Watson, 2002). This perspective of "intentionality seeks to access the universal, life-spirit energy via manifesting one's deep intentional focus on a specific mental object of attention and awareness . . . [thus inviting] spirit-energy to enter into one's life and work, and into the caring-healing processes and outcomes" (Watson, 2002, p. 14).

Empowerment

Empowerment is a process whereby patients take a lead role in managing their health as opposed to a passive role (Ison et al., 2019). Nurses, having established personal relationships of mutual respect, trust, and confidence with their patients, are in a unique position to empower them, thus increasing their independence. Nurses can facilitate empowerment by instructing patients on how they should perform certain functions, and in cases where a patient's abilities are hindered, providing only the amount of assistance that is absolutely necessary. In addition, nurses can provide information and resources to patients and their families, explain what they can expect beyond their hospital stay, and give voice to their concerns and desires to administrators and others providing care.

Compassion

When describing the ideal nurse, **compassion** is a must, but debate exists within the nursing community about how to precisely define this quality. It is not uncommon for the terms *compassion* and *compassionate care* to be used interchangeably with other characteristics such as caring and empathy, highlighting the subjective nature of the concept (Su, Masika, Paguio, & Redding, 2020). Compassion is not something a nurse can learn through academic study, but only through the willingness to become intimately involved with the patient's experience. This often involves providing comfort to the patient—anything from validating the patient's experience through attentive listening and eye contact to holding the patient's hand in moments of pain, from adjusting the patient's position in bed to gently providing a warm sponge bath (see **Figure 35.2** »). Another aspect of expressing compassion involves respecting the patient's spiritual beliefs or lack thereof, regardless of the nurse's personal opinions and values. Although nurses frequently cite time constraints as a barrier to compassion, research has shown that patients note a sense of togetherness as evidence of compassion, and togetherness is not the same as time (Durkin, Usher, & Jackson, 2019).

Competence

Similar to Roach's (2002) description of competence, Afshar, Sadeghi-Gandomani, & Alavi (2020) define **competence** as: "Understanding discipline knowledge, mastery of discipline-specific skills, ability to use sound professional judgement, adherence to professional standards and application of skills and knowledge" (para. 1). There are specific attributes inherent in competence, including cognitive ability, participating in professional development, having an awareness of ethical and legal practices, guaranteeing quality and safety in care, and building relationships with patients and fellow nurses. Competence and compassion must coexist, or patient care will inevitably suffer. Competence without compassion can be, at best, off-putting and, at worst, impersonal and insensitive. Compassion in the absence of competence, however, presents real threats to patients' safety and health.

The classic theory regarding the development of nursing competence is Benner's (1982) novice-to-expert research on the lengthy process of nursing skills acquisition. Benner and Wrubel (1989) extended the thesis begun in the novice-to-expert work that caring is central to nursing expertise, to curing, and to healing. One of the unique goals of the latter publication was to distinguish the nursing perspective from purely psychologic, physiologic, or biomedical views.

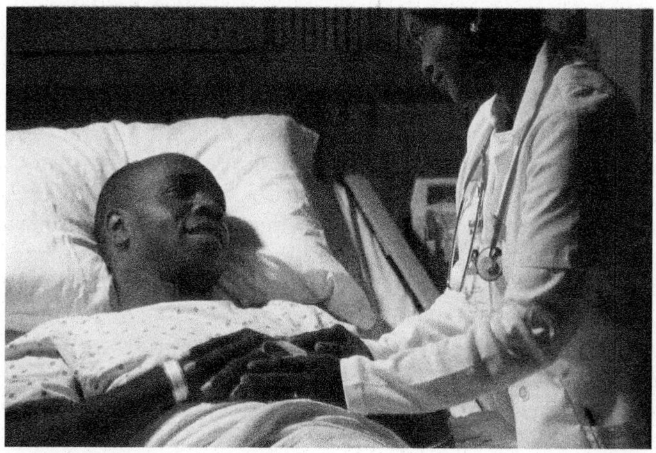

Figure 35.2 » This nurse is using touch and presence to help comfort her patient.

Source: Juan Silva/The Image Bank/Getty Images.

Clinical Example B

Mrs. Julie Briggs is a 29-year-old woman who has undergone a left-breast lumpectomy, which also involved removing cancerous lymph nodes. As a result, she has been admitted to the hospital for a brief recovery period. The first postoperative day, Mrs. Briggs's nurse, Tomas Crespo, overhears an argument between the patient and her father, who is pressuring his daughter to have a double mastectomy as a preventive course of treatment because the patient's mother lost her life to breast cancer at age 36. Mrs. Briggs tells her father that she and her husband hope to conceive a child within the next year and she desperately wants to have the bonding experience of breastfeeding. As he listens, Tomas is reminded of his wife's difficulty in breastfeeding and thinks the patient shouldn't place so much importance on it. After the patient's father leaves, Tomas enters the room and finds Mrs. Briggs crying. He pulls up a chair and asks her if she wants to talk. Mrs. Briggs says she's fine and collects herself. Tomas squeezes her hand and informs her that he is willing to listen, but she shakes her head no. While changing the patient's dressing, he allows a few minutes to pass before providing her with tips on how she can tend to her sutures when she is discharged in a couple of days, adding that he can also instruct her husband when he comes in later that evening. Upon completing Mrs. Briggs's care, Tomas tells her that there are support groups for young breast cancer survivors like her and promises to bring the information to her before the end of his shift.

Critical Thinking Questions

1. Did Tomas demonstrate presencing, empowerment, compassion, and competence in his interactions with Mrs. Briggs? If so, provide specific examples.
2. Could Tomas have approached the patient's dilemma differently? If so, how?

Lifespan Considerations

There are often some overarching themes that influence nurses as they provide caring interventions to patients of all ages. Obviously, one of the most important factors to consider, which is essential to all patient interactions and teaching, is the patient's developmental level. Developmental characteristics across the lifespan are discussed thoroughly in Module 25, Development. The presence of developmental delays and physical impairments will influence interactions with these patients and may require nurses to adjust delivery of caring interventions to achieve optimal outcomes. Many areas can be impacted by developmental factors. Cultural and religious diversity, the presence of pain, the stress of a medical issue or emergency, the unfamiliar environment of the hospital or healthcare facility, and the context of the medical issue (e.g., accidents, chronic illnesses, the possibility of death, and associated psychologic issues such as grief and loss) all influence patient communication.

Furthermore, even though they may be performing caring interventions with only one patient, nurses often find that they are teaching and educating family members and caregivers at the same time. Thus, nurses find themselves accommodating a full range of developmental, psychologic, and sociocultural issues for several people when providing caring interventions. With the addition of family members and caregivers, caregiving becomes increasingly complicated and nuanced.

Caring Interventions for Infants

Nurses interacting with very young infants will likely find that as long as the environment is comfortable and a parent or caregiver is present, infants will not object too much to being handled during caring interventions (see **Figure 35.3 ›››**). Infants are fascinated by faces, and as they age, they prefer faces that are familiar (American Academy of Pediatrics, 2020a). Babies are programmed to inherently provide important information—how they like to be treated, talked to, held, and comforted (American Academy of Pediatrics, 2020a). Aside from assessing developmental milestones and physical issues, nurses caring for infants must consider any pain or discomfort caused by interventions. HCPs now know that infants experience pain and that interventions such as skin-to-skin contact, sucrose, breastfeeding, non-nutritive sucking, swaddling, rocking, and holding are all beneficial in pain management (Hills, Rosenberg, Banfield, & Harding, 2020). Often in these cases, nurses must work with the interprofessional team to advocate for the infant to receive pain-relieving interventions during routine procedures such as heelsticks and circumcision (Hills et al., 2020).

Other areas being assessed with parents and caregivers include whether infants, especially preterm infants, are thriving and gaining weight (American Academy of Pediatrics, 2020a); whether parents have access to adequate community resources consistent with consideration of social determinants of health; whether bonding seems to be taking place between infant and caregiver (American Academy of Pediatrics, 2020b); and the emotional and mental health of the mother and/or caregiver, with special attention given to detection of postpartum (perinatal) depression (Bauman et al., 2020).

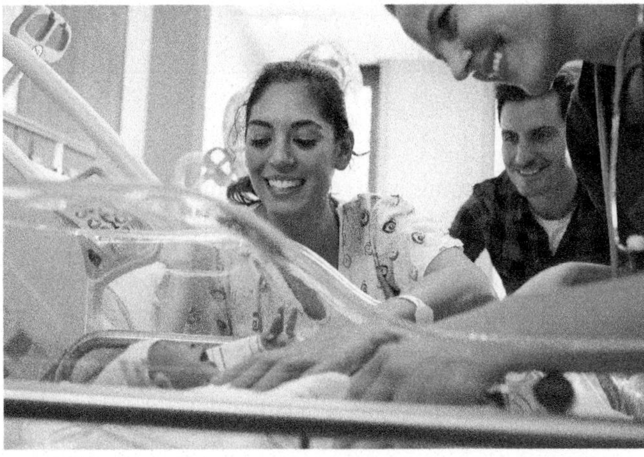

Figure 35.3 ››› Having the parents nearby when providing care for infants is soothing.

Source: iStock/Getty Images.

During the toddler years, physical growth and motor development will slow, but toddlers experience tremendous intellectual, social, and emotional changes. Caring interventions will be affected by the toddlers' self-directed behavior and innate suspicion of strangers. Parents and caregivers will be necessary in providing care during this time.

Caring Interventions for Children

Children during the preschool and school years still need a parent or caregiver present during procedures. If a child has been exposed to uncomfortable medical procedures, they may be leery of or cry during caring interventions. Children at this stage become capable of developing psychic pain that the nurse may have to address. Some of the global issues facing children at this stage are stress, anger, conflict, and bullying; natural and human-caused disasters, such as terrorism and school shootings; poverty and uncertain housing; deployed parents and frequent moves (for children of military personnel); and emotional needs and emerging mental health problems. Nurses should consider the impact of these experiences when providing care.

Caring Interventions for Adolescents

Adolescents may still need parents or caregivers present during times of medical challenge, such as surgery or an accident, but in general, they can handle medical procedures by themselves. They will also prefer privacy when interacting with HCPs. Nurses will find that adolescents will be more forthcoming with sensitive information regarding sexual practices and alcohol or drug use if questioned separately from their parents. Issues of concern with teens and parents include puberty; social development and relationships with peers, especially romantic attachments; family and parent relationships; gender identity; academic pressures; sexual, physical, and emotional abuse; and potential hazardous activities such as drunk driving and contact sports (Allen & Waterman, 2019). The nurse may find that these issues, rather than a procedure or exam, become paramount during patient interactions.

Caring Interventions for Pregnant Women

Regardless of the caring intervention between the provider and pregnant woman, the nurse should keep in mind that they are always dealing with a dyad: the patient and the baby. Obviously, the expectant woman will likely assess every caring intervention in regard to its effect on the baby. Nurses must be sensitive to this concern and include this information in any patient teaching, especially regarding procedures, such as amniocentesis, that can present a genuine risk to the fetus.

Nurses will also assess for signs of maternal alcohol or drug abuse and intimate partner violence (IPV). Some studies have shown IPV to be present in numbers greater than 50% of pregnancies (Udmuangpia, Yu, Laughon, Saywat, & Bloom, 2020). IPV during pregnancy can be associated with negative pregnancy outcomes, including postpartum depression and low infant birth weight. Nurses should be mindful of IPV when caring for pregnant patients.

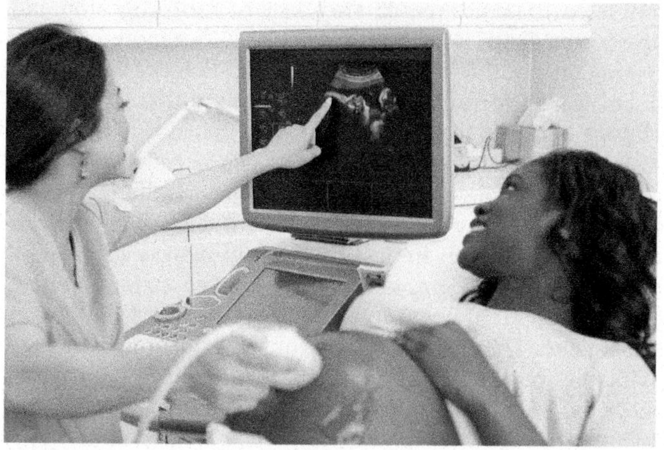

Figure 35.4 ⟫ Having a good rapport with patients is important for nurses in an obstetrics practice.
Source: iStock/Getty Images.

Research has indicated that the quality, rather than quantity, of prenatal care is more important to pregnant women (see **Figure 35.4 ⟫**). Under ideal situations, prenatal care represents an opportunity for health promotion and illness prevention, screening and assessment, information sharing, and person centeredness. Pregnant women, especially those from vulnerable populations, form opinions regarding the quality of care based on access, physical setting, and staff and care provider characteristics. However, they rank as most important interpersonal care processes such as respectful attitude, emotional support, approachable interaction style, and taking time (Wadsworth et al., 2019). Nurses must respect the importance of the patient relationship in all interactions. See Exemplar 33.A, Antepartum Care, in Module 33, Reproduction, for more information.

Caring Interventions for Adults

Perhaps the biggest obstacle nurses and other HCPs face with adults is actually getting them access to healthcare. Lack of time and financial resources are large issues, as well as lack of health insurance coverage and lack of specialty providers in rural and less populated areas. Many young and middle-aged adults use computers regularly, although the abundance of poor-quality health information can complicate nurse–patient interventions and interactions. Nurses are encouraged to become aware of reliable internet sites for healthcare information and steer patients to them (National Institute on Aging, 2018).

Furthermore, many young adults do not connect with the healthcare system for primary care. A large care gap emerges as young adults transition from pediatric care, monitored by parents, into autonomous primary care. The primary concern is that many young adults do not understand the importance of preventive healthcare and require the support of their parents for encouragement (American Academy of Family Physicians, 2020). In all caring interventions and interactions with adults, nurses can emphasize the importance of having a medical home and routinely monitoring and treating chronic conditions.

Caring Interventions for Older Adults

The term *active aging* refers to the fact that many older adults are aging independently or with limited assistance from friends, work associates, neighbors, and family members. Many older adults do not have chronic illnesses or cognitive decline and primarily seek interaction with care providers and other organizations to support quality of life. Healthy active older adults will seek complete and up-to-date information on caring interventions and will be engaged participants in their healthcare. Active older adults also seek opportunities to engage with others and live healthy, purposeful lives. Many communities and organizations have developed extensive volunteer networks through collaborations among local Departments of Aging, Departments of Social Services, hospitals, and other organizations. These volunteer networks may recruit retired and active older adults to participate in meaningful volunteer opportunities in places such as hospitals, airports, libraries, and schools.

In contrast, some older adults will develop physical and functional limitations and need to manage chronic medical conditions and comorbidities as they age. One of the largest issues elders face is securing care from providers who can integrate all the findings from specialists into a comprehensive overview. In the United States, there is a shortage of HCPs who specialize in geriatric care. Reasons for this shortage vary but include insurance reimbursement and low pay (Phillips, Peterson, Fang, Kovar-Gough, & Phillips, 2019) (see **Figure 35.5 ⟫**).

Nurses providing care to older adults should be mindful of negative attitudes that inhibit patient interactions: ageism, which is prejudice or discrimination based on age, and elderspeak, a type of simplified speech, characterized by shorter sentences and words, used when talking to older adults (Zhang, Zhao, & Meng, 2020). Research has shown that the primary factor causing negative nursing attitudes is lack of knowledge about gerontology and the aging process (Rababa, Hammouri, Hweidi, & Ellis, 2020). Nurses can address these factors by continuing their education and by paying careful attention to patient–nurse interactions.

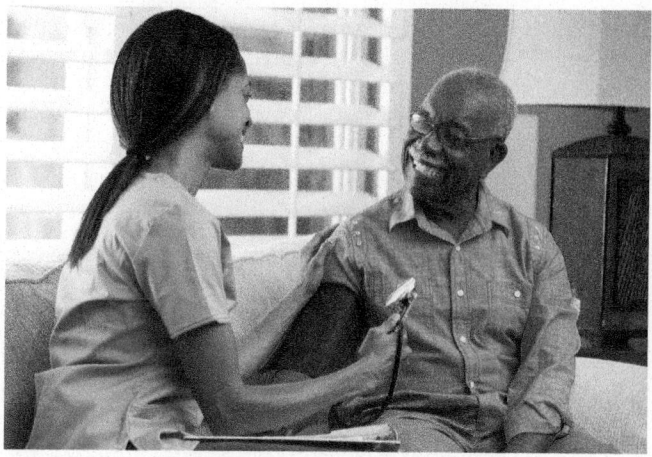

Figure 35.5 ⟫ A home health nurse visits an older adult.
Source: Getty Images.

Caring for the Caregiver: Self-Care in Nursing

Self-care is of vital importance in nursing and should not be treated as peripheral to patient care. Self-care is "engaging in practices that prevent the decline of our health and well-being" (Mahrer, 2019). Examples of such activities include a balanced diet, regular exercise, adequate rest and sleep, recreational activities, and meditation and/or prayer.

Self-care is particularly relevant to the nursing profession because nurses tend to overlook their own well-being while focusing on the health of others. According to the U.S. Bureau of Labor Statistics (2018), registered nurses experience some of the highest rates of illness and injury of any healthcare or related profession. Nurses face a wide range of hazards on the job, including exposure to emerging pathogens, needle-stick injuries, back injuries, latex allergy, violence, and stress.

In addition, the pressures of work, family, school, and community commitments experienced by nurses often lead to exhaustion, burnout, and stress with potentially debilitating effects on the quality of care delivered to patients. One study looking at a multicultural group of nurses noted that absenteeism and job turnover result from the high level of stress and burnout experienced by the profession (Muhawish, Salem, & Baker, 2019). The study concluded that organizational treatment of nurses needs to improve. Additional items that need to be addressed are a lack of team cohesion and heavy workloads (Muhawish et al., 2019). For more information on burnout, see the Evidence-Based Practice feature.

Self-care for nurses encompasses more than just being physically fit and healthy. The practices that lead to increased well-being also build self-esteem, which in turn helps individuals problem-solve critically and face challenges more efficiently. Taking a self-esteem questionnaire helps individuals increase self-awareness by putting them in touch with their feelings and emotions; only through self-awareness can an individual begin to change those aspects that lower self-esteem. There are a number of self-esteem instruments available for use on the internet and at college counseling services. Worthy of note is the connection between self-awareness and self-control. A lack of self-awareness can contribute to decreased self-control (Greater Good in Education, 2019), which could be problematic for nurses and the patients receiving their care.

AHNA (2020b) has maintained that holistic nursing practice requires the integration of self-care and personal development activities into one's life. Holistic nurses engage in self-assessment, self-care, and personal development, aware of being instruments of healing. Holistic nurses value themselves and mobilize the necessary resources to care for themselves, striving to achieve harmony and balance in their own lives and assisting others to do the same.

Evidence-Based Practice

Recognizing and Preventing Burnout in New Nurse Graduates

Problem

Nurses often function in high-pressure, short-staffed situations and are subject to rotating schedules and extended shifts. Despite the challenges associated with functioning in such an intense work environment, nurses tend to ignore feelings of fatigue, exhaustion, depression, and job dissatisfaction, believing that their colleagues must be feeling the same way. Consequently, many push self-care to the bottom of their list of priorities, ignoring even their most basic needs in order to meet job demands. This cycle leads to burnout.

The effects of nursing burnout take not only a personal emotional and physical toll, but they also adversely impact quality of care and patient satisfaction and lead to high turnover rates, contributing to the nursing shortage, which inevitably leads to even more burnout (Bong, 2019). Much research has validated the relationship between poor patient outcomes and nurse burnout, including a systematic review that indicated a correlation with medical errors, neglect of work, inappropriate discharge timing, and decreased patient safety (Tawfik et al., 2019).

Evidence

Most researchers have agreed that burnout consists of three components: emotional exhaustion, depersonalization, and lack of personal achievement, as measured by the Maslach Burnout Inventory questionnaire (Bazmi et al., 2019; Moukarzel et al., 2019). Similar to other helping professions, the prevalence of burnout in nursing is particularly high because of the high emotional and physical demands of the work. Nursing burnout overall has been associated with heavy workloads, inadequate staffing levels, poor work performance, absenteeism, and depression (Dyrbye et al., 2019).

Alarmingly, new-graduate nurses have the highest risk of experiencing burnout and work-related stress, with workload being a significant influencing factor (Feddeh & Darawad, 2020). Almost 30% of pediatric nurses leave the profession after less than a year of practice (Bong, 2019), and this is also seen in other specialty areas. Many factors causing burnout in recent graduates mirrored the concerns of experienced nurses. New-graduate burnout has been significantly related to unmanageable workloads and relationships and conflict with other healthcare professionals (Feddeh & Darawad, 2020).

A significant factor usually considered to be part of the unfavorable working environment is bullying or horizontal violence. Horizontal bullying occurs between colleagues, whereas vertical bullying is between a manager and employee (Cummings, 2020). Furthermore, Cummings (2020) notes that as many as 65% of nurses have observed this type of bullying, and as many as 60% of new nurses who are victims to this leave their jobs in the first 6 months. Education of staff and authentic leadership committed to extinguishing horizontal violence are imperative for creating a zero-tolerance workplace.

Personal and workplace resources can prevent new-graduate burnout. Managers should ensure that empowerment structures are in place to support new-graduate nurses' job satisfaction. Interventions that specifically support nurse graduates include orientation processes and ongoing management supports that decrease turnover, increase stress management, and increased job satisfaction (Perron, Gascoyne, Kallakavumkal, Kelly, & Demagistris, 2020).

Some of the essential components of successful nurse residency programs for transitioning nurse graduates into the workplace have

Evidence-Based Practice *(continued)*

been identified. Formal new-graduate nurse residencies have resulted in good retention and improved competency (Perron et al., 2020). Evidence has suggested that new-graduate education should be at least 10 months in length and should focus on transition to the clinical setting and assimilation into the professional nursing role. A strong preceptor is imperative to this process, so preceptor training must be included in a nurse residency program (Perron et al., 2020).

Implications

Burnout is detrimental to both the nurse and the patient. It is crucial that nurses recognize the signs and symptoms of this phenomenon. The Maslach Burnout Inventory (Maslach & Jackson, 1981) is the most widely used tool for identifying and measuring burnout (Bazmi et al., 2019; Moukarzel et al., 2019). This questionnaire groups symptoms into three categories:

- *Emotional exhaustion.* This is one of the earliest signs of burnout and can cause headaches, insomnia, indigestion, and weight fluctuations. It may manifest itself as feelings of dread about going to work. Examples include uncontrollable crying, queasiness, and/or headaches during the nurse's commute.
- *Personal accomplishment.* Overworked nurses tend to feel that patients, supervisors, and hospital administrators do not appreciate their efforts. This can lead to underperformance, which is an adaptive response to stress.
- *Depersonalization.* When nurses no longer feel compassion for some of their patients, it could cause insensitive behavior when providing care.

New-graduate nurses experiencing any of these symptoms should seek the advice of colleagues and supervisors on how to overcome burnout. Strategies include physical exercise, talking it through, reducing patient load, learning to say "no" to extra assignments and committee appointments, switching shifts, and even changing jobs. Burnout is a sign that something must change. Nurses who choose to ignore it will discover that the symptoms and negative consequences of those symptoms will only worsen.

Critical Thinking Application

1. How can a nurse differentiate between the typical stress experienced by all healthcare professionals and burnout?
2. A nurse is experiencing symptoms of burnout and has approached the supervisor for support and guidance. The supervisor says that it is simply a part of working as a caregiver and to "push through it." What steps can the nurse take to cope and improve her situation?
3. A nurse observes one of his colleagues being brusque with patients (e.g., lack of eye contact, not providing direct answers, cutting off patients when speaking). When he questions his coworker, she says that she doesn't want to get too emotionally involved with her patients and is just maintaining a healthy distance from them. He knows that she is also going through a difficult divorce and custody battle. What should he do?

Maslow's Hierarchy of Needs

Psychologist Abraham Maslow (1943, 1968) identified five levels of needs, the lower of which must be fulfilled before an individual can move to the next level and eventually achieve self-actualization, the highest level. For an illustration of Maslow's human needs hierarchy and a discussion of his work and its implication for the nursing care of patients, refer to Module 31, Stress and Coping.

Physiologic Needs

Physiologic needs are also referred to as survival needs and include the necessities of food, water, air, sleep, and shelter. For example, the extended work hours and rotating shifts common to the nursing profession make it challenging to maintain a regular eating schedule and sleep routine and to participate in regular physical activity. Avoidance of physical activity has been associated with high rates of lower back pain among nurses (Fujii et al., 2019).

Physiologic needs can be satisfied in healthy and unhealthy ways. Nurses practice self-care when they make healthy choices regarding food (e.g., by choosing fruit as a snack between meals), drinks (i.e., by drinking water instead of soft drinks), and sleep. Managing a sleep schedule can be particularly challenging, especially for nurses whose families operate on different schedules than the nurse. Physical recreational activities also help nurses cope with limited sleep while enhancing their fitness level. For more information, see Exemplar 7.A, Physical Fitness and Exercise, and Exemplar 7.C, Normal Sleep–Rest Patterns, in Module 7, Health, Wellness, Illness, and Injury.

>> **Stay Current:** The American Nurses Association launched a challenge for nurses in 2017 called the Healthy Nurse, Healthy Nation Grand Challenge. For more information on this challenge, please visit https://www.healthynursehealthynation.org/en/.

Safety

Needs at this level have both physical and psychologic aspects, including bodily safety, financial security, and personal health. The American Nurses Association's (ANA) *2013–2016 Health Risk Appraisal* (2017) reported workplace stress at significant levels (82%) and musculoskeletal injury (51%) as major health risks. In addition, 25% of nurses reported physical assault by their patients or family members. Moreover, in a study by Gander et al. (2019), 30% of nurses recalled a fatigue-related clinical error in the previous 6 months. The ANA (2020) has endorsed some of the following recommendations:

- Involve nurses in the design of work schedules and use a regular and predictable schedule so nurses can plan for work and personal responsibilities.
- Eliminate the use of mandatory overtime as a "staffing solution."
- Nursing students and precepted students must not be counted into staffing.
- Promote frequent, uninterrupted rest breaks during work shifts.
- Enact official policy that confers RNs the right to accept or reject a work assignment based on preventing risks

from fatigue. The policy should include conditions that a rejected assignment does not constitute patient abandonment and that RNs should not experience adverse consequences in retaliation for such a decision.

Work–family conflict among nurses also has a negative effect on job satisfaction (Galletta et al., 2019). When the quality of a nurse's personal and family life suffers, so does job performance, which directly impacts patient satisfaction and service quality.

Belonging and Love

According to Maslow, when the lower physical needs are met, an individual is in a position to address higher psychologic needs. The sense of love and belonging that comes from relationships with family, friends, and colleagues is particularly important to nurses, who depend on solid support networks to help them talk through and cope with the pressures of work. Venting is a healthy way to unload stress, but it is vital that nurses maintain patient confidentiality at all times, even when venting to other nurses.

Unfortunately, new nurses may find their desire and efforts to fit in at work thwarted by a culture of bullying that is prevalent in the nursing profession. As mentioned in the Evidence-Based Practice feature in this module, newly graduated nurses have significantly higher resignation rates in their first year of practice (Dyrbye et al., 2019). Victims of bullying experience distress, anxiety, feelings of isolation, and depression, and they subsequently show an increased use of sick time. New graduates are particularly vulnerable because they often lack confidence in their skills and thus crave acceptance and positive feedback from their peers. In addition to adversely affecting job performance and satisfaction, bullying leads to increased absenteeism and staff turnover, therefore risking patient safety by interfering with teamwork, collaboration, and communication.

Clinical Example C

Mrs. Oden, the charge nurse on a medical–surgical unit, assigns extra patients to Celia Hammond, a new-graduate nurse, in order to cover for a colleague who left unexpectedly to tend to a family emergency. Mr. Stephen Suskind, a 57-year-old man recovering from knee surgery, is among Celia's patients. In the early afternoon, Mr. Suskind falls while attempting to make his way to the bathroom unassisted. The sound of the fall and his subsequent cry prompt Celia to rush into his room. As Celia helps Mr. Suskind to stand, Mrs. Oden appears in the doorway and criticizes Celia harshly for having neglected her patient, as well as for attempting to move him after his fall. The commotion attracts the attention of other nurses on the floor, who stand behind Mrs. Oden, observing Celia as she is being chastised. Afterward, Celia discusses the incident with an experienced colleague who has worked at the hospital for more than a decade. When Celia complains about having been publicly humiliated, her colleague advises her to "suck it up" and closes the conversation by warning her that "no one likes a whiner."

Critical Thinking Questions

1. What should Celia do next?
2. How have Mrs. Oden, Celia's nurse colleague, and others reinforced a culture of bullying?
3. What actions might the nursing supervisor take to address incidents such as this one?

Self-Esteem

Needs at this particular level include feelings of confidence, independence, competence, respect, and achievement. In nursing, a caregiver's self-esteem is based on how the individual is viewed by others. Nurses strive to be seen as competent and proficient and value the respect of peers. It is important for new nurses to realize that nursing proficiency comes through hands-on practice. Skills are improved and mastered over time; thus, new nurses should not compare themselves to more experienced colleagues by being overly self-critical. Instead, they should maintain a positive mindset and be open to learning. Knowledgeable, sympathetic preceptors can enhance the skills acquisition of new nurses during their orientation to a hospital or other healthcare facility.

A mentor can also play an important role in encouraging a new nurse's self-esteem needs by supporting the new nurse's skill development and sharing experiences. Many healthcare institutions have mentoring programs where new nurses are paired with established colleagues who serve to teach, counsel, aid, and encourage them. Mentoring programs have been shown to positively impact confidence in new nurses (Johnson, Kim, & Punzalan, 2019).

Self-Actualization

After meeting lower-level needs, individuals can then strive to develop their maximum potential and fully realize their abilities and qualities. Part of self-actualization for nurses is the need to make time for themselves. This crucial aspect of self-care includes pursuing activities that bring joy and stimulate creativity. Artistic pursuits—such as writing, playing a musical instrument, and dancing—can serve as important outlets for self-expression. Hobbies are important to personal well-being because they offer a healthy distraction from the pressures of work and encourage personal development. Taking a break to do nothing in particular is also an effective way to relax and reenergize.

Self-Care and COVID-19

The COVID-19 pandemic in 2020 exacerbated the complexity of hospital care environments for a number of reasons, ranging from the physical demands (dehydration, exhaustion) associated with providing long hours of care while wearing protective equipment, to increased risk of infection, to the moral distress associated with watching large numbers of patients struggle for life and die in isolation (U.S. Department of Veterans Affairs [VA], 2020).

In the face of these challenges, the VA (2020) and the American Psychiatric Nurses Association (2020) recommend a multifaceted approach to self-care that includes:

- Self-monitoring and time-outs for hydration, nutrition, and rest
- Regular check-ins with peers, family, and friends
- Focusing on tasks that are achievable
- Fostering a spirit of collaboration and hope
- Engaging in mindfulness activities to activate the parasympathetic nervous system
- Seeking early support for symptoms of moral distress, such as feelings of guilt or self-criticism.

Although these recommendations were issued in response to the overwhelming stress facing nurses and other healthcare workers during the pandemic, they may be applied during any crisis situation that creates high acuity and complexity in a hospital or community.

Choosing Wellness

Wellness is a state of well-being involving sound nutrition, regular physical fitness, stable emotional health, self-responsibility, dynamic personal and professional growth, and preventive healthcare. Just as nurses promote patient wellness, they would do well to avoid unhealthy behaviors and engage in healthy behaviors and activities themselves.

Avoiding Unhealthy Behaviors

In addition to adapting healthy behaviors, self-care is also about avoiding unhealthy ones. Smoking, abusing alcohol and drugs, and misusing medications are all destructive lifestyle choices that impact a nurse's personal and professional life.

An estimated 5–20% of all nurses may be impaired by or in recovery from some form of drug or alcohol addiction (Mumba & Kraemer, 2019). However, the range illustrates a lack of identification of substance use disorders in nurses. Many impaired nurses do enroll in substance abuse monitoring programs, which are often run by state boards of nursing. These programs are often 3 to 5 years in length, correlating well to the risk of relapse that is highest in the first 5 years, particularly in the first year (Mumba, Baxley, Cipher, & Snow, 2019; Smiley & Reneau, 2020). Relapse still occurs, with one study noting 32% of participants experiencing at least one relapse, while 41% completed their program with no relapses (Mumba, Baxley, Snow, & Cipher, 2019). Close monitoring and participation are essential to successful completion.

Another major concern is the alcohol- or substance-impaired student nurse who increases risks to patients by unsafe practices. Nursing students are at risk for alcohol and substance use for various reasons: peer influence and social activities, physical and emotional stress of nursing education and patient care, and exhaustion due to academic rigor, among many other factors (Vorster, Gerber, van der Merwe, & van Zyl, 2019). A recent study demonstrated that of nursing students who consumed alcohol, more than 50% used alcohol in a risky or hazardous manner, with 34% of participants also reporting cannabis use (Tejedor-Cabrera & Cauli, 2019). One identified issue has been a lack of consistency and policies that address impaired nursing students (Nigro, Schwartz, Roche, & Tariman, 2020).

Beyond the harm they do to themselves, nurses who abuse substances may also inadvertently harm patients in their care. Fellow nurses are usually required to report impaired colleagues to management, and it is therefore vital that they recognize the telltale signs of substance abuse. Nurses with a drug or alcohol problem may exhibit one or more of the manifestations described in Module 22, Addiction (e.g., mood swings, tremors, slurred speech, or unsteady gait), as well as any of the following: discrepancies in documentation of controlled substances; volunteering to medicate coworkers' patients; wearing long sleeves in hot weather; committing frequent errors in care, particularly medication errors; arriving to work early or staying late; or coming in when not scheduled to work.

Workplace risk factors for substance use among nurses include the following (Mumba & Kraemer, 2019):

- Easy access to drugs
- High levels of stress in the workplace
- Lack of social support both in and out of the workplace
- Feeling personally invincible
- Self-treating physical pain or stress.

Educating all nurses on signs and symptoms of an impairment is essential to addressing substance use disorder in nurses (Mumba & Kraemer, 2019). Fellow nurses can help by encouraging nurses with substance use disorders to seek assistance options, such as counseling and treatment programs. Before reporting a colleague to management, a nurse may wish to give the fellow nurse the opportunity to self-report.

Addiction is considered to be an illness. Nurses experiencing substance abuse should be referred to treatment, not punished. The majority of states offer alternative-to-discipline programs affiliated with or recognized by their state boards of nursing. Increasingly, professional associations such as state nurses' associations are providing resources to help nurses recover from alcohol and drug addiction.

» **Stay Current:** For more information about nurses and substance abuse, visit https://www.ncsbn.org/substance-use-in-nursing.htm.

Choosing Healthy Behaviors

A healthy lifestyle is particularly important to nurses for two main reasons: (1) They must maintain strong immune systems in order to work with people who are ill and (2) they should act as role models so as to maintain credibility when advising others about healthy choices. Balance and moderation are the keys to a healthy lifestyle, and this is especially true with respect to nutrition and exercise.

Because personal physical, mental, and emotional health is integral to successful nursing practice, the ANA has published a book on the subject, *Self-Care and You: Caring for the Caregiver* (Richards, Sheen, & Mazzer, 2014). Suggestions include the following: Maintain a regular eating schedule; eat balanced, nutritious foods throughout the day; exercise at least three times a week (e.g., take a walk, work out, participate in sports); set aside time for rest and relaxation; seek the company of supportive people; do something enjoyable every day (e.g., play a musical instrument, cook, read, watch TV); avoid tobacco, alcohol, and drugs; maintain an optimistic attitude; set limits with others; and prioritize tasks (Richards et al., 2014).

Maintaining a regular eating schedule is a challenge in a profession where rotating shifts and unexpected events are the norm. Nonetheless, nurses need to make time to address their nutritional needs and not wait until they begin experiencing the effects of hunger and thirst (pangs, dizziness, seeing spots, and so on). Nurses can accomplish this by planning ahead and making sure that healthy snacks and fresh water are on hand to consume at predetermined moments of the work shift. Nurses with physically demanding tasks often make the mistake of thinking they are getting enough physical exercise at work; however, standing for long periods of time, lifting patients, and performing other tasks that require physical exertion are not likely to build muscle tone or contribute to cardiovascular fitness (Richards et al., 2014) (see **Figure 35.6** »).

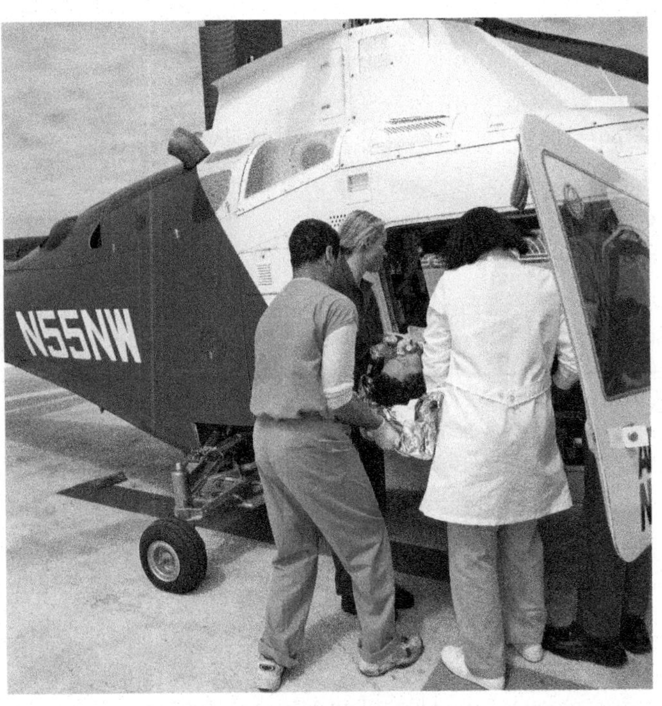

Figure 35.6 » Many nursing tasks are physically demanding. Nurses should incorporate regular exercise into their schedules to build muscle tone and fitness.
Source: Chad Baker/Jason Reed/Ryan McVay/Photodisc/Getty Images.

Self-awareness is the key to effective self-care. It involves self-discovery and leads to personal insights. For instance, a self-aware individual is able to identify personal strengths and weaknesses and is conscious of the assumptions, beliefs, values, and prejudices that can impair judgment. Through self-awareness, a nurse gains greater understanding of others, including patients (Younas, Rasheed, Sundus, & Inayat, 2020). Self-reflection is an important aspect of self-awareness, as it guides personal awareness.

Nurses should take advantage of the support services available to them. At some healthcare facilities, nurses come together for weekly support groups to discuss their cases, providing a venue for them to reflect on their work and receive the benefit of their peers' experiences. Hospital chaplains are also available to listen to and support nurses. For problems such as addiction and depression or health promotion activities such as engaging in a wellness program, nurses may be able to turn to employee assistance programs that are part of their employee benefits or to state nursing boards and nursing associations.

Several professional associations, such as AHNA and state nursing organizations, provide programs and additional resources to help nurses cope with the stressors and pressures of their everyday lives. Online services, such as community forums, offer nurses a safe space where they can vent freely to others who understand the issues they face. Nurses must remember to respect patient privacy and confidentiality during group discussions or in online forums.

REVIEW The Concept of Caring Interventions

RELATE Link the Concepts

Linking the concept of caring interventions with the concept of health, wellness, and illness:

1. Apply theories of caring to discuss how the benefits of self-care (improved physical fitness, overall health, self-esteem, and self-actualization) impact patient care.
2. Explain the relationship between self-care and wellness. Is the absence of illness a requirement for wellness? Why or why not?

Linking the concept of caring interventions with the concept of comfort:

3. In the psychosocial realm, how would an absence of genuine caring impact the nursing care for a patient who is receiving end-of-life care?
4. Describe the application of presencing when caring for the family members of a patient who is receiving end-of-life care.

Linking the concept of caring interventions with the concept of communication:

5. From the patient's perspective, how might inadequate self-care affect facets of the nurse's nonverbal communication, such as personal appearance and facial expression?
6. How does confidence, identified by Roach as a caring trait, impact the quality of communication between the nurse and the patient?

READY Go to Volume 3: Clinical Nursing Skills

REFER Go to Pearson MyLab Nursing and eText

REFLECT Apply Your Knowledge

Ms. Ann Mah, a 26-year-old single woman, was admitted to the hospital following an automobile crash. She lost consciousness at the wheel while driving home from the gym by herself. Since her admission, she has been diagnosed with a neck injury, and a neurologic workup revealed she has epilepsy. Ms. Mah's nurse, Michael Robbins, is monitoring her blood pressure and assessing her for side effects related to her newly prescribed anticonvulsant medication, valproate (Depakote).

When Michael enters the room, he finds Ms. Mah gazing out the window. When he asks how she is doing, she responds with a curt "Fine." As he goes through his list of questions, she answers with just one or two words. He senses that Ms. Mah is a very private person, so he avoids asking her personal questions. Later in the day, Michael asks his mentor for advice on the case, who tells him to be patient and allow the patient time to open up. His mentor also informs him that some patients diagnosed with chronic illness may experience the diagnosis as a loss of their ideal selves and have difficulty accepting the diagnosis at first.

After his next assessment, Michael decides to spend an extra 5 minutes with Ms. Mah. He sits by her bedside quietly, observing her out of the corner of his eye as he pretends to review her file. Suddenly, she blurts out,

"I hate this! My life was perfect. I was promoted to regional director of sales last week. I drove around all over the city and I had a great social life. Now you tell me I'm epileptic. What are they going to say at work?"

Michael responds, "I hear your concern that the diagnosis of epilepsy may interfere with your life and work. And you're right, epilepsy does require adjustments. But you are the same woman you were before the accident. Except that now you know that the woman who was promoted to regional sales director has epilepsy. Tell me what else you're concerned about."

Ms. Mah looks away. "With this stupid medicine, I can't keep any food down!"

"I know that's frustrating, but it is important that we try to prevent another seizure, especially because of your neck injury. The idea is to gradually reduce the dosage to lessen the side effects as much as possible while still controlling the seizures. Does that make sense?"

"Yes, but I really don't want to take medication the rest of my life, especially not this stuff."

Michael nods his head to show that he's listening and answers, "I understand that. Let's do this: I'll email the attending provider who is managing your care and ask her to come around and discuss the medication with you. Would that be all right?"

Ms. Mah turns her head to look at Michael. "Yes. Thank you."

Michael says, "I know you're concerned about work and returning to your social life. How about we come up with a plan for how you might begin to manage your epilepsy after you leave here?"

Ms. Mah replies, "I'd like that. I spoke with my sister yesterday. She told me there are other ways to treat epilepsy. She mentioned acupuncture."

"I've heard that, too. Let's look into it and talk about some more ideas the next time I see you. Deal?"

Michael stretches out his hand and after a few seconds Ms. Mah takes it and they shake on it.

At his next assessment, Michael finds Ms. Mah reading information from an epilepsy website off a tablet.

"How are you today, Ms. Mah?" Michael asks.

"Fine. Today, I'll be asking the questions," Ms. Mah says.

1. Which caring theories are relevant to this case?
2. Which holistic approaches did Michael employ?
3. How did Michael's self-care aid him in caring for Ms. Mah?

References

Afshar, M., Sadeghi-Gandomani, H., & Alavi, N. M. (2020). A study on improving nursing clinical competencies in a surgical department: A participatory action research. *Nursing Open, 7*(4), 1052–1059. https://doi.org/10.1002/nop2.485

Allen, B., & Waterman, H. (2019). *Stages of adolescence.* American Academy of Pediatrics. https://www.healthychildren.org/English/ages-stages/teen/Pages/Stages-of-Adolescence.aspx

American Academy of Family Physicians. (2020). *Adolescent and young adult health.* https://www.aafp.org/family-physician/patient-care/prevention-wellness/emotional-wellbeing/adolescent-and-young-adult-health.html

American Academy of Pediatrics. (2020a). *Ages and stages: Baby.* https://www.healthychildren.org/english/ages-stages/baby/pages/default.aspx

American Academy of Pediatrics. (2020b). *Parenting your infant.* https://www.healthychildren.org/English/ages-stages/baby/Pages/Parenting-Your-Infant.aspx

American Holistic Nurses Association (AHNA). (2020a). *What is holistic nursing?* http://www.ahna.org/About-Us/What-is-Holistic-Nursing

American Holistic Nurses Association (AHNA). (2020b). *What is self care?* https://www.ahna.org/Membership/Member-Advantage/Whatisself-care

American Nurses Association (ANA). (2020). *ANA's principles for nurse staffing* (3rd ed.). Author.

American Nurses Association (ANA). (2017). *2013–2016 health risk appraisal.* https://www.nursingworld.org/~4aeeeb/globalassets/practiceandpolicy/work-environment/health--safety/ana-healthriskappraisalsummary_2013-2016.pdf

American Psychiatric Nurses Association. (2020). *Managing stress & self-care during COVID-19: Information for nurses.* https://www.apna.org/m/pages.cfm?pageID=6685#Moral%20Distress

Bauman, B. L., Ko, J. Y., Cox, S., D'Angelo, D. V., Warner, L., Folger, S., et al. (2020). Vital signs: Postpartum depressive symptoms and provider discussions about perinatal depression - United States, 2018. *Morbidity and Mortality Weekly Report, 69*(19), 575–581. http://dx.doi.org/10.15585/mmwr.mm6919a2

Bazmi, E., Alipour, A., Yasamy, M. T., Kheradmand, A., Salehpour, S., Khodakarim, S., & Soori, H. (2019). Job burnout and related factors among health sector employees. *Iranian Journal of Psychiatry, 14*(4), 309–316. https://ijps.tums.ac.ir/index.php/ijps/article/view/1702

Benner, P. E. (1982). From novice to expert. *American Journal of Nursing, 82*(3), 402–407.

Benner, P. E., & Wrubel, J. (1989). *The primacy of caring: Stress and coping in health and illness.* Addison-Wesley.

Benner, P., & Wrubel, J. (2001). Response to: Edwards, S. D. (2001). Benner and Wrubel on caring in nursing. *Journal of Advanced Nursing, 33*(2), 167–171.

Bong, H. E. (2019). Understanding moral distress: How to decrease turnover rates of new graduate pediatric nurses. *Pediatric Nursing, 45*(3), 109–114. http://www.pediatricnursing.net/issues/19mayjun/abstr1.html

Boykin, A., & Schoenhofer, S. O. (2001). *Nursing as caring: A model for transforming practice.* Jones & Bartlett.

Centers for Disease Control and Prevention. (2020). *About chronic diseases.* https://www.cdc.gov/chronicdisease/about/index.htm

Cummings, R. (2020). Nurse bullying by co-workers. *Journal of Healthcare Protection Management, 36*(1), 40–43.

Durkin, J., Usher, K., & Jackson, D. (2019). Embodying compassion: A systematic review of the views of nurses and patients. *Journal of Clinical Nursing, 28*(9–10). 1380–1392. https://doi.org/10.1111/jocn.14722

Dyrbye, L. N., Shanafelt, T. D., Johnson, P. O., Johnson, L. A., Satele, D., & West, C. P. (2019). A cross-sectional study exploring the relationship between burnout, absenteeism, and job performance among American nurses. *BMC Nursing, 18*, 57. https://doi.org/10.1186/s12912-019-0382-7

Edmonson, C., & Zelonka, C. (2019). Our own worst enemies: The nurse bullying epidemic. *Nursing Administration Quarterly, 43*(3), 274–279. https://doi.org/10.1097/NAQ.0000000000000353

Eskin, M., Tran, U. S., Carta, M. G., Poyrazli, S., Flood, C., Mechri, A., et al. (2020). Is individualism suicidogenic?: Findings from a multinational study of young adults from 12 countries. *Frontiers in Psychiatry, 11*, 259. https://doi.org/10.3389/fpsyt.2020.00259

Feddeh, S. A., & Darawad, M. W. (2020). Correlates to work-related stress of newly-graduated nurses in critical care units. *International Journal of Caring Sciences, 13*(1), 507–516. http://www.internationaljournalofcaringsciences.org/docs/56_darawad_original_13_1.pdf

Frisch, N. C., & Rabinowitsch, D. (2019). What's in a definition?: Holistic nursing, integrative health care, and integrative nursing: Report of an integrated literature review. *Journal of Holistic Nursing, 37*(3), 260–272. https://doi.org/10.1177%2F0898010119860685

Fujii, T., Oka, H., Takano, K., Asada, F., Nomura, T., Kawamata, K., et al. (2019). Association between high fear-avoidance beliefs about physical activity and chronic disabling low back pain in nurses in Japan. *BMC Musculoskeletal Disorders, 20*, 572. https://doi.org/10.1186/s12891-019-2965-6

Galletta, M., Portoghese, I., Melis, P., Gonzalez, C. I. A., Finco, G., D'Aloja, E., et al. (2019). The role of collective affective commitment in the relationship between work–family conflict and emotional exhaustion among nurses: A multilevel modeling approach. *BMC Nursing, 18*, 5. https://doi.org/10.1186/s12912-019-0329-z

Gander, P., O'Keeffe, K., Santos-Fernandez, E., Huntington, A., Walker, L., & Willis, J. (2019). Fatigue and nurses' work patterns: An online questionnaire survey. *International Journal of Nursing Studies, 98*, 67–74. https://doi-org.proxy.sau.edu/10.1016/j.ijnurstu.2019.06.011

Greater Good in Education. (2019). *SEL for students: Self-awareness and self-management.* https://ggie.berkeley.edu/student-well-being/sel-for-students-self-awareness-and-self-management/#tab__2

Haber, J. (2000). Hildegard E. Peplau: The psychiatric nursing legacy of a legend. *Journal of the American Psychiatric Nurses Association, 6*(2), 56–62. https://doi.org/10.1016/S1078-3903(00)90021-1

Halm, M. (2019). The influence of appropriate staging and healthy work environments on patient and nurse outcomes. *American Journal of Critical Care, 28*(2), 152–156. https://doi.org/10.4037/ajcc2019938

Hansbrough, W. B., & Georges, J. M. (2019). Validation of the presence of nursing scale using data triangulation. *Nursing Research, 68*(6), 439–444. https://doi.org/10.1097/nnr.0000000000000381

Harrington, L. (2020). Behavior change techniques in apps: Moving beyond patient education to improve health outcomes. *AACN Advanced Critical Care, 31*(1), 12–15. https://doi.org/10.4037/aacnacc2020244

Hills, E., Rosenberg, J., Banfield, N., & Harding, C. (2020). A multidisciplinary approach to the implementation of non-pharmacological strategies to manage infant pain. *Infant, 16*(2), 78–81. http://www.infantjournal.co.uk/journal_article.html?RecordNumber=7140

Ison, H. E., Ware, S. M., Schwantes, A. T., Freeze, S., Elmore, L., & Spoonamore, K. G. (2019). The impact of cardiovascular genetic counseling on patient empowerment. *Journal of Genetic Counseling, 28*(3), 570–577. https://doi.org/10.1002/jgc4.1050

Jiménez-Herrera, M. F., Llauradó-Serra, M., Acebedo-Urdiales, S., Bazo-Hernández, L., Font-Jiménez, I., & Axelsson, C. (2020). Emotions and feelings in critical and emergency caring situations: A qualitative study. *BMC Nursing, 19*, 60. https://doi.org/10.1186/s12912-020-00438-6

Johnson, J., Kim, J. S., & Punzalan, P. (2019). Mentoring for success: Neurosurgery new hire RN mentorship program. *American Nurse Today, 14*(4), 5. https://www.myamericannurse.com/mentoring-for-success-neurosurgery-new-hire-rn-mentorship-program/

Karlsson, M., & Pennbrant, S. (2020). Ideas of caring in nursing practice. *Nursing Philosophy, 21*(4), e12325. https://doi.org/10.1111/nup.12325

Konuk, T. G., & Tanyer, D. (2019). Investigation of nursing students' perception of caring behaviors. *Journal of Caring Sciences, 8*(4), 191–197. https://dx.doi.org/10.15171%2Fjcs.2019.027

Lake, E. T., Sanders, J., Duan, R., Riman, K. A., Schoenauer, K. M., & Chen, Y. (2019). A meta-analysis of the associations between the nurse work environment in hospitals and 4 sets of outcomes. *Medical Care, 57*(5), 353–361. https://dx.doi.org/10.1097%2FMLR.0000000000001109

Lee, K., & Kim, S. H. (2019). What is a "good nurse"?: An integrative literature review. *Medico Legal Update: An International Journal, 19*(1). https://doi.org/10.37506/mlu.v19i1.1009

Leininger, M. M. (1989). Transcultural nurse specialists and generalists: New practitioners in nursing. *Journal of Transcultural Nursing, 1*(1), 4–16.

Létourneau, D., Goudreau, J., & Cara, C. (2020). Facilitating and hindering experiences to the development of humanistic caring in the academic and clinical settings: An interpretive phenomenological study with nursing students and nurses. *International Journal of Nursing Education Scholarship, 17*(1). https://doi.org/10.1515/ijnes-2019-0036

Li, X., Yang, S., Wang, Y., Yang, B., & Zhang, J. (2020). Effects of a transtheoretical model - based intervention and motivational interviewing on the management of depression in hospitalized patients with coronary heart disease: A randomized controlled trial. *BMC Public Health, 20*(1), 420. https://doi.org/10.1186/s12889-020-08568-x

Mahrer, B. (2019). *Why you struggle with self-care.* National Alliance on Mental Illness. https://www.nami.org/Blogs/NAMI-Blog/December-2019/Why-You-Struggle-with-Self-Care

Maslach, C., & Jackson, S. E. (1981). The measurement of experienced burnout. *Journal of Occupational Behaviour, 2*(2), 99–113.

Maslow, A. (1943). A theory of human motivation. *Psychological Review, 50*(4), 370–396.

Maslow, A. H. (1968). *Toward a psychology of being* (2nd ed.). Van Nostrand Reinhold.

Mayeroff, M. (1990). *On caring.* HarperCollins. (Original work published 1971)

McFarland, M. R., & Wehbe-Alamah, H.B. (2015). *Culture care diversity and universality: A worldwide nursing theory* (3rd ed.). Jones & Bartlett.

Merriam-Webster Dictionary. (2020). *Caring.* https://www.merriam-webster.com/dictionary/caring

Miller, W. R., & Rollnick, S. (2013). *Motivational interviewing: Helping people change* (3rd ed.). Guilford Press.

Morley, G., Bradbury-Jones, C., & Ives, J. (2020). What is "moral distress" in nursing?: A feminist empirical bioethics study. *Nursing Ethics, 27*(5), 1297–1314. https://doi.org/10.1177%2F0969733019874492

Motivational Interviewing Network of Trainers. (2020). *Understanding motivational interviewing.* https://motivationalinterviewing.org/understanding-motivational-interviewing

Moukarzel, A., Michelet, P., Durand, A.-C., Sebbane, M., Bourgeois, S., Markarian, T., et al. (2019). Burnout syndrome among emergency department staff: Prevalence and associated factors. *BioMed Research International, 2019*, Article No. 6462472. https://doi.org/10.1155/2019/6462472

Muhawish, H., Salem, O. A., & Baker, O. G. (2019). Job related stressors and job satisfaction among multicultural nursing workforce. *Middle East Journal of Nursing, 13*(2), 3–16. https://doi.org/10.5742MEJN.2019.93635

Mumba, M. N., Baxley, S. M., Cipher, D. J., & Snow, D. E. (2019). Personal factors as correlates and predictors of relapse in nurses with impaired practice. *Journal of Addictions Nursing, 30*(1), 24–31. https://doi.org/10.1097/jan.0000000000000262

Mumba, M. N., Baxley, S. M., Snow, D. E., & Cipher, D. J. (2019). A retrospective descriptive study of nurses with substance abuse disorders in Texas. *Journal of Addictions Nursing, 30*(2), 78–86. https://doi.org/10.1097/jan.0000000000000273

Mumba, M. N., & Kraemer, K. R. (2019). Substance use disorders among nurses in medical-surgical, long-term care, and outpatient services. *MEDSURG Nursing, 28*(2), 87–118.

National Center for Complementary and Integrative Health. (2018). *Complementary, alternative, or integrative health: What's in a name?* https://www.nccih.nih.gov/health/complementary-alternative-or-integrative-health-whats-in-a-name

National Institute on Aging. (2018). *Online health information: Is it reliable?* https://www.nia.nih.gov/health/online-health-information-it-reliable

Nigro, T. M., Jr., Schwartz, P. S., Roche, B. T., & Tariman, J. D. (2020). Comprehensive reentry policy for student registered nurse anesthetists with substance use disorder. *American Association of Nurse Anesthetists Journal, 88*(4), 319–323. https://www.aana.com/docs/default-source/aana-journal-web-documents-1/nigro-rc4663809bf50486ab502f235d2a7d57c.pdf?sfvrsn=70c8cb2_4

Orem, D. E. (2001). *Nursing: Concepts of practice.* Mosby.

Peplau, H. E. (1991). *Interpersonal relations in nursing.* Springer.

Perron, T., Gascoyne, M., Kallakavumkal, T., Kelly, M., & Demagistris, N. (2020). Effectiveness of nurse residency programs. *Journal of Nursing Practice Applications and Reviews of Research, 10*(1), 48–52. https://doi.org/10.13178/jnparr.2019.09.02.0908

Phillips, J. P., Peterson, L. E., Fang, B., Kovar-Gough, I., & Phillips, R. L., Jr. (2019). Debt and the emerging physician workforce: The relationship between educational debt and family medicine residents' practice and fellowship intentions. *Journal of the Association of American Medical Colleges, 94*(2), 267–273. https://doi.org/10.1097/acm.0000000000002468

Potter, M. L. & Moller, M. D. (2020). *Psychiatric–mental health nursing: From suffering to hope* (2nd ed.). Pearson.

Prochaska, J. O., & DiClemente, C. C. (1983). Stages and processes of self-change of smoking: Toward an integrative model of change. *Journal of Consulting and Clinical Psychology, 51*(3), 390–395. https://doi.org/10.1037/0022-006X.51.3.390

Prochaska, J. O., DiClemente, C. C., & Norcross, J. C. (1992). In search of how people change: Applications to addictive behaviors. *American Psychologist, 47*(9), 1102–1114.

Purnell, M.J. (2013). *Nursing as caring: A model for transforming practice.* Nursing as Caring. https://www.nursingascaring.com/the-theory

Rababa, M., Hammouri, A. M., Hweidi, I. M., & Ellis, J. L. (2020). Association of nurses' level of knowledge and attitudes to ageism toward older adults: Cross-sectional study. *Nursing and Health Sciences,* 22(3), 593–601. https://doi.org/10.1111/nhs.12701

Richards, K., Sheen, E., & Mazzer, M. C. (2014). *Self-care and you: Caring for the caregiver.* American Nurses Association.

Roach, M. S. (Ed.). (1997). *Caring from the heart: The convergence of caring and spirituality.* Paulist Press.

Roach, M. S. (2002). *Caring, the human mode of being: A blueprint for the health professions* (2nd ed.). CHA Press.

Roy, C. (2019). Nursing knowledge in the 21st century: Domain-derived and basic science practice-shaped. *Advances in Nursing Science, 42*(1) 28–42. https://doi.org/10.1097/ANS.0000000000000240

Smiley, R., & Reneau, K. (2020). Outcomes of substance use disorder monitoring programs for nurses. *Journal of Nursing Regulation, 11*(2), 28–35. https://doi.org/10.1016/S2155-8256(20)30107-1

Steefel, L. (2019). *Reflections on Dr. Madeleine M. Leininger.* Transcultural Nursing Society. https://tcns.org/reflections-on-dr-madeleine-m-leininger/

Su, J. J., Masika, G. M., Paguio, J. T., & Redding, S. R. (2020). Defining compassionate nursing care. *Nursing Ethics, 27*(2), 480-493. https://doi.org/10.1177%2F0969733019851546

Tawfik, D. S., Scheid, A., Profit, J., Shanafelt, T., Trockel, M., Adair, K. C., et al. (2019). Evidence relating health care provider burnout and quality of care: A systematic review and meta-analysis. *Annals of Internal Medicine, 171*(8), 555–567. https://doi.org/10.7326/m19-1152

Tejedor-Cabrera, C., & Cauli, O. (2019). Alcohol and cannabis intake in nursing students. *Medicina, 55*(10). https://doi.org/10.3390/medicina55100628

Thompson, G. N., & McClement, S. E. (2019). Critical nursing and healthcare aide behaviors in care of the nursing home resident dying with dementia. *BMC Nursing, 18*, 59. https://doi.org/10.1186/s12912-019-0384-5

Udmuangpia, T., Yu, M., Laughon, K., Saywat, T., & Bloom, T. (2020). Prevalence, risks, and health consequences of intimate partner violence during pregnancy among young women: A systematic review. *Pacific Rim International Journal of Nursing Research, 24*(3), 412–429. https://he02.tci-thaijo.org/index.php/PRIJNR/article/view/217503

University of Rochester Medical Center. (2020). *Nursing professional practice model: Ten steps to delivering unsurpassed patient care.* https://www.urmc.rochester.edu/highland/departments-centers/nursing/nursing-philosophy/professional-practice-model.aspx

U.S. Bureau of Labor Statistics. (2018). *Occupational injuries and illnesses among registered nurses.* https://www.bls.gov/opub/mlr/2018/article/occupational-injuries-and-illnesses-among-registered-nurses.htm

U.S. Department of Veterans Affairs (VA). (2020). *Managing healthcare workers' stress associated with the COVID-19 virus outbreak.* https://www.ptsd.va.gov/covid/COVID_healthcare_workers.asp

Vorster, A., Gerber, A. M., van der Merwe, L. J., & van Zyl, S. (2019). Second and third year medical students' self-reported alcohol and substance use, smoking habits and academic performance at a South African medical school. *Health SA = SA Gesondheid, 24*, 1041. https://doi.org/10.4102/hsag.v24i0.1041

Wadsworth, K. H., Archibald, T. G., Payne, A. E., Cleary, A. K., Haney, B. L., & Hoverman, A. S. (2019). Shared medical appointments and patient-centered experience: a mixed-methods systematic review. *BMC Family Practice, 20*(1), 97. https://doi.org/10.1186/s12875-019-0972-1

Watson, J. (1999). *Nursing: Human science and human care: A theory of nursing.* Jones & Bartlett.

Watson, J. (2002). Intentionality and caring-healing consciousness: A practice of transpersonal nursing. *Holistic Nurse Practitioner, 16*(4), 12–19.

Watson Caring Science Institute. (2020). *Caring science & human caring theory.* https://www.watsoncaringscience.org/jean-bio/caring-science-theory/

Younas, A., Rasheed, S. P., Sundus, A., & Inayat, S. (2020). Nurses' perspectives of self-awareness in nursing practice: A descriptive qualitative study. *Nursing and Health Sciences, 22*(2), 398-405. https://doi.org/10.1111/nhs.12671

Young, K., Godbold, R., & Wood, P. (2019). Nurses' experiences of learning to care in practice environments: A qualitative study. *Nurse Education in Practice, 38*, 132–137. https://doi.org/10.1016/j.nepr.2019.06.012

Zhang, M., Zhao, H., & Meng, F.-P. (2020). Elderspeak to resident dementia patients increases resistiveness to care in health care profession. *Inquiry: The Journal of Health Care Organziation, Provision, and Financing,* 57. https://doi.org/10.1177%2F0046958020948668

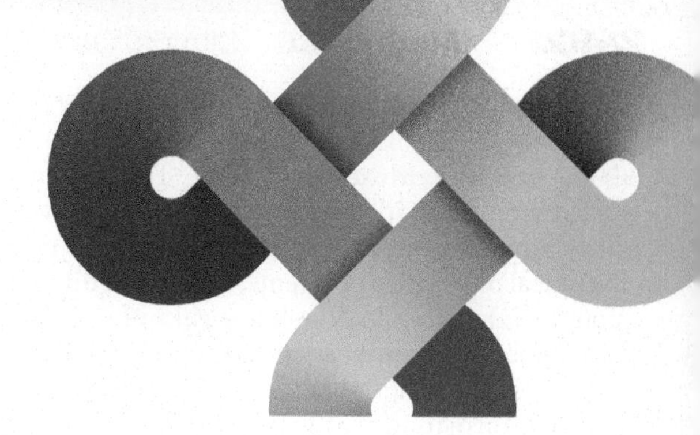

Module 36 Clinical Decision Making

Module Outline and Learning Outcomes

The Concept of Clinical Decision Making

Critical Thinking

36.1 Analyze the use of critical thinking skills in nursing.

Clinical Decision Making

36.2 Analyze the components of clinical decision making.

Clinical Judgment

36.3 Outline the components of clinical judgment.

Lifespan Considerations

36.4 Differentiate considerations related to clinical decision making about patients throughout the lifespan.

Concepts Related to Clinical Decision Making

36.5 Outline the relationship between clinical decision making and other concepts.

Clinical Decision Making Exemplars

Exemplar 36.A The Nursing Process

36.A Analyze the nursing process as it relates to clinical decision making.

Exemplar 36.B The Nursing Plan of Care

36.B Analyze nursing plans of care as they relate to clinical decision making.

Exemplar 36.C Prioritizing Care

36.C Analyze prioritizing care as it relates to clinical decision making.

» The Concept of Clinical Decision Making

Concept Key Terms

Clinical decision making, **2493**
Clinical judgment, **2496**
Clinical reasoning, **2497**
Creativity, **2495**
Critical thinking, **2494**
Deductive reasoning, **2497**
Inductive reasoning, **2497**
Inquiry, **2496**
Intellect, **2494**
Intuition, **2498**
Reflection, **2497**
Salient cue, **2495**

Clinical decision making is a process nurses use in the clinical setting to evaluate and select the best actions to meet desired goals. Nurses use clinical decision making whenever choices are available, even when they evaluate a situation and decide not to act. In some cases, decisions are required in situations that have neither clear answers nor standard procedures and when conflicting forces add to the complexity. At other times, decisions are routine. For example, a nurse is assigned five patients:

- A patient with abdominal surgery postoperative day 1
- A patient who was admitted in sickle cell crisis
- A patient infected with COVID-19 on room air who is in airborne isolation
- A patient who has been crying all night
- A patient who is already up and walking down the hall of the unit.

Clinical decision-making practices affect every aspect of nursing care, from direct client care at the bedside to professional behaviors and accountability inherent in the profession of nursing. The nurse must evaluate each patient's needs and preferences as well as time-constraining activities (such as medication administration) to make appropriate decisions for each patient (see Exemplar 36.C, Prioritizing Care, in this module for further information). To make these decisions, the nurse must use critical thinking to choose among alternatives that support the best patient outcomes for all patients in the nurse's care.

Critical Thinking

Patient outcomes improve when the nurse uses critical thinking. Use of critical thinking skills is also linked to holistic care planning, improved collaboration, and higher nursing job satisfaction (Cooke, Stroup, & Harrington, 2019).

The American Association of Colleges of Nursing's *The Essentials: Core Competencies for Professional Nursing Education* (2021) defines **critical thinking** as "The skill of using logic and reasoning to identify the strengths and weaknesses of alternative healthcare solutions, conclusions, or approaches to clinical or practice problems." The Accreditation Commission for Education in Nursing speaks of critical thinking as "the deliberate nonlinear process of collecting, interpreting, analyzing, drawing conclusions about, presenting, and evaluating information that is both factually and belief based" (Benner, Hughes, & Sutphen, 2008). These statements, and those by other professional nursing organizations, underscore the importance of today's nurses being able to make meaningful observations, solve problems, and decide on a course of action. To do so, nurses must be able to process both previously learned and newly acquired information about their patients, the work environment, and the resources at hand or in the community as well as applicable evidence related to care of the patient; the nurse must then be able to prioritize this information quickly and efficiently.

Nurses use critical thinking skills in a variety of ways. Because nurses manage patient care and human responses holistically, they must draw meaningful information from other disciplines in order to understand the meaning of patient data and plan effective interventions. This can be challenging because nurses work in rapidly changing situations. Routine practice of skill administration does not help the nurse in a situation in which the patient is frightened of the procedure or has altered cognition and is having difficulty understanding why the procedure is necessary. Critical thinking is the process by which the nurse recognizes the need to adapt and respond differently to meet the patient's specific needs. Nurses must use critical thinking, for example, to decide if observations should be reported to the primary care provider immediately or if those observations can wait to be reported after morning rounds. The skills and abilities necessary to develop critical thinking include intellect, creativity, inquiry, reasoning, reflection, and intuition (**Figure 36.1** >>). Critical thinking also requires maintaining an attitude that promotes critical thinking and working in an environment that encourages this skill (**Table 36.1** >>).

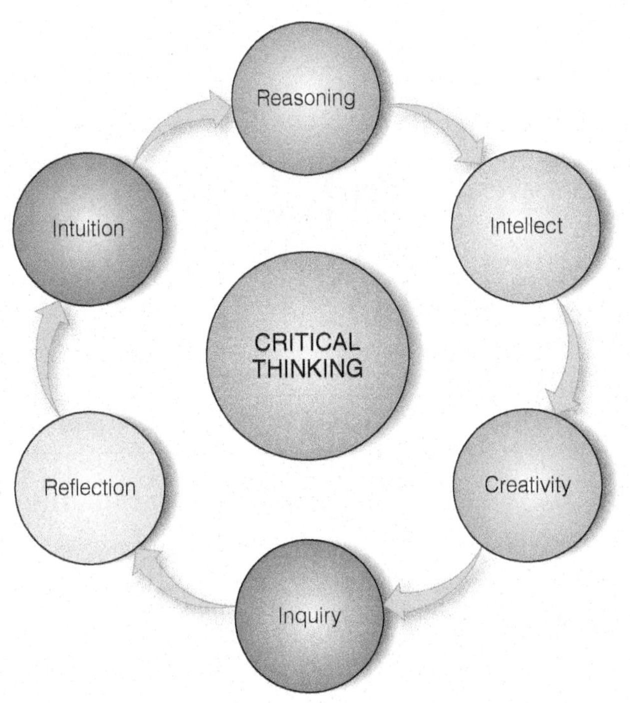

Figure 36.1 >> Critical thinking skills are essential for making clinical decisions.

TABLE 36.1 Common Attitudes of Critical Thinkers

Attitudes	Examples
Independence	▪ Does own thinking, objectively and honestly. ▪ Is open minded about different methods used to reach same goal. ▪ Looks for the facts; not easily swayed by opinions.
Fair-mindedness	▪ Has neutral judgments without bias. ▪ Considers opposing views to understand all aspects before making decisions. ▪ Is open to new ideas and ways of doing things.
Aware of self-limits	▪ Knows limits of intellect and experience. ▪ Seeks new knowledge or skills in current evidence. ▪ Expresses a willingness to self-reflect on own beliefs and ideas.
Integrity	▪ Challenges own ideas and methods of doing nursing care. ▪ Evaluates inconsistencies within own nursing practice. ▪ Chooses the right thing to do over the popular thing to do.
Perseverance	▪ Has stick-with-it motivation to find the best solution for quality patient outcomes. ▪ Is patient with processes.
Confidence	▪ Knows both the extent and limitations of existing knowledge base. ▪ Trusts the skills and abilities of intellect, creativity, inquiry, reasoning, reflection, and intuition.

SAFETY ALERT A cross-sectional review of 2699 patient medical records from hospitals found that 76.8% of patient-related adverse events were attributable to nursing. Patients had an average 15.3% risk of experiencing an adverse event. Of those patients who experienced adverse events attributed to nursing, 30% experienced at least two adverse events (D'Amour, Dubois, Tchouaket, Clarke, & Blais, 2014). In a time of economic restraint with healthcare reimbursement linked to patient satisfaction, adverse healthcare events are costly for institutions, pose a risk to patient safety, and diminish patient confidence in healthcare institutions and in nursing (D'Amour et al., 2014).

Intellect

Intellect is defined as the ability to think, understand, and reason. Building on clinical knowledge and skills expands the knowledge base nurses use for reasoning, analyzing, and predicting patient outcomes. Intellect helps to differentiate facts from opinions, approach situations objectively, and clarify concepts. Thinking becomes an intentional action to identify **salient cues** within a clinical situation. *Salient*, or significant, means the leading, most noticeable, or most important, and *cue* refers to significant data that informs and influences conclusions about the patient's health status. Salient cues can cluster to form a pattern that can be translated into a nursing diagnosis for the patient. A salient cue does one of the following:

- ***Points to a change in the patient's condition with positive or negative implications.*** For example, the patient states, "I have suddenly lost more than 20 pounds without dieting."
- ***Differs from expected findings in the general population.*** For example, a 7-year-old patient who is 60 inches tall, but the nurse knows that the typical 7-year-old is closer to 48 or 50 inches tall.
- ***Suggests delayed development.*** For example, by 6 months of age an infant should be rolling over in both directions (Centers for Disease Control and Prevention, 2019). The nurse who is aware of developmental milestones knows that a 7-month-old who cannot roll over has not achieved an important milestone, indicating a possible developmental delay.

Once salient cues are recognized, they can be clustered to determine whether any patterns are present. The nurse can then interpret the pattern and take appropriate action. Awareness of cues and their significance can be valuable in making clinical decisions essential to nursing care for ever-changing conditions and reordering of priorities to meet patient needs (Dickson, Haerling, & Lasater, 2019). This dynamic method of thinking evolves over time, very much in the way that nurses advance through the stages of skill acquisition as they gain experience in clinical care. New nurses need to write down the assessment data and search the data for abnormal cues to help cluster significant cues that can be translated into a nursing diagnosis. See **Figure 36.2** » for an example of cues and clustering of data.

Continuous learning is necessary for nurses to remain current with the best evidence for quality patient outcomes (see the feature on Evidence-Based Practice for further information). Many states now require that for licensure renewal, nurses complete continuing education credits to demonstrate up-to-date and current knowledge in patient care.

Creativity

Creativity is an outlet for the imagination that allows a nurse to take what can be seen in the mind and make it tangible. **Creativity** means finding unique solutions to unique problems when traditional interventions are not effective; for example, finding just the right way to connect with a patient who does not want to talk about her diabetes or finding interventions that best help a patient meet a goal so he can be discharged from the hospital.

A modification to the old adage "One size does not fit all" describes the importance of individualizing nursing care

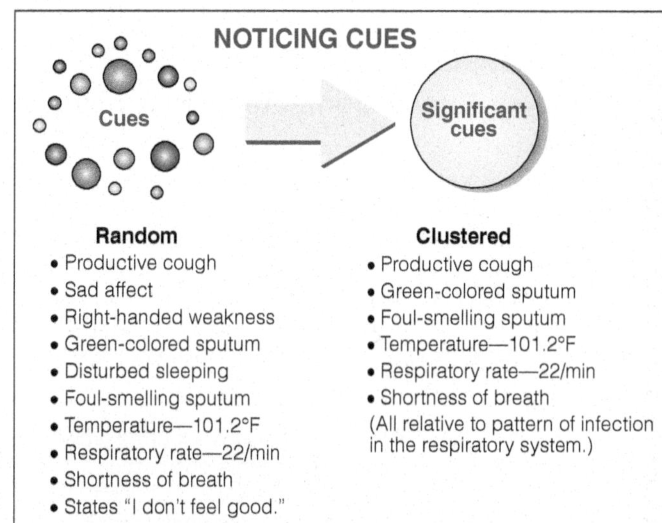

Figure 36.2 » Random cues are not similar to each other, whereas significant cues that relate to each other can be clustered to form a pattern.

for each patient. When an attempt to help a patient is not successful, the nurse changes tactics and asks the question, "What other approach might help this patient to succeed?" The ability to look for alternatives by "thinking outside the box" is necessary because the need for creative problem solving occurs every day. Some examples of opportunities for nurse creativity are:

- Helping a patient who is dehydrated to drink more liquids by mouth
- Helping a patient newly diagnosed with diabetes learn appropriate foods for controlling blood glucose levels
- Finding alternatives for an IV tubing label when a traditional label is not available
- Finding something to write vital signs on when paper, laptop, or computer are not at hand
- Using tape and tongue blades to make a toy house for a young child.

Sometimes the best way to find a good alternative is to increase the number of options available. This is where creativity and reality meet in much the same way creativity is used to figure out how many words can be spelled using the letters in "nursing care." Initially, you may have minimal success, but after more thought, you will begin to "see" more possibilities and spell more words from these few letters. Nurses can promote creative problem solving if they begin with asking, "What if we . . . ?"

Thinking creatively requires a deep understanding of the issue at hand. Nurses first assess problems and then apply their understanding to creatively solve a problem. In Clinical Example A, the nurse has a working knowledge of the concepts of mobility and development of pediatric patients. Creative thinking enables the nurse to process that knowledge into an appropriate plan of care for the client.

Evidence-Based Practice

Evidence-Based Competencies for Nurses

Problem

Evidence-based practice (the integration of research into practice), **clinical judgment** (the nurse's determination and provision of appropriate care to the patient), and patient preferences together ensure the use of scientific rigor when providing high-quality healthcare to patients. Although the benefits of evidence-based practice (EBP) have been well established, a lack of consistency exists in its use among healthcare providers (HCPs), including nurses (Melnyk et al., 2018; Valdez, 2018).

Evidence

Clinicians fail to use EBP for several reasons, including provider lack of knowledge and understanding and the misperception that implementing EBP is time-consuming. These clinicians often follow traditional practices rather than evidence-based practices because that's the way it's always been done, even when traditional practices can harm patients (Upvall, 2019). Furthermore, many healthcare organizations fail to support EBP, and academic institutions continue to teach only traditional nursing methods. To begin implementing EBP, nurses must become proficient in critiquing current evidence, evaluating current practices, developing strategies to implement practice changes, and evaluating the outcomes related to changes in practice. Well-informed nurses become champions for safe, current EBP (Upvall, 2019).

Implications

Evidence-based practice has been an integral part of healthcare for at least a generation. Professional nursing and medicine strive to use this patient-centered practice methodology because it relies on the clinician's appraisal of the best evidence appropriate for the population the clinician serves. Furthermore, the added dimension of patient preference empowers patients in healthcare decision making and allows individuals to be active participants in their care as opposed to being recipients of the traditional paternalistic physicians' orders or nursing interventions.

The National League of Nursing (NLN), American Association of Critical-Care Nurses, and Quality and Safety Education for Nurses (QSEN) have undertaken efforts to advance implementation of EBP among nurses at both the national and international levels (Melnyk et al., 2018). Research by Melnyk et al. (2018) supports both organizational and individual strategies for integrating EBP competencies into nursing practice, nursing research, organizational policies, management, and education.

Critical Thinking Application

1. How well do you understand EBP? Are you familiar with a healthcare institution or a HCP that uses this practice? How does their use of EBP affect patient satisfaction and outcomes?
2. In your own words, describe how EBP affects the care patients receive.
3. How will you integrate evidence-based care into clinical decision making in your professional nursing practice?

Clinical Example A

A home health nurse is caring for Tyesha, a 9-year-old girl who has limited mobility of her left arm following a severe shoulder injury sustained during a playground accident. The provider has ordered active range-of-motion (ROM) exercises. Tyesha becomes anxious during the exercises. With her parents' permission, the nurse offers to bring in a trained therapy support dog. Tyesha is excited about playing with the canine. The nurse knows that the movements Tyesha uses while playing with the dog will promote active range of motion. After seeing how well she responds to the dog, the nurse suggests that future caregivers collaborate with trained therapy dog handlers to make Tyesha's active ROM exercises less intimidating and more productive.

Critical Thinking Questions

1. What questions might the nurse ask of Tyesha to isolate the reasons the active ROM exercises cause her to be anxious?
2. How might the nurse explain the purpose of the exercises to Tyesha in a way that would decrease her fear?
3. Why is playing with a professionally trained therapy animal an effective part of the treatment plan for Tyesha? How much does it depend on her understanding the therapeutic component of what she is doing?
4. If Tyesha didn't want to engage with the therapy dog, what might an effective alternative be that could fulfill the same purpose?
5. If an older, teenage child didn't want to actively participate in ROM exercises, what might be an effective alternative?
6. How might the nurse measure the positive effect of Tyesha's activity time with the dog?

Inquiry

Inquiry, a form of research, is defined as a search for knowledge or facts. When nurses use inquiry, they examine objective information to gain clarification and find solutions to problems. Inquiry differs from query in that a query is simply a question that requires an answer. Critical thinking requires nurses to use inquiry to examine both the situation at hand and their own nursing practice: "Why do we always need to apply the dressing this way?" "How can I help a patient who is on a salt-free diet avoid problems with her serum potassium levels?" "What would happen if we helped the patient exercise more than twice a day?" "Is there something else we can try when a patient is having trouble swallowing?" Nurses continuously use inquiry in the clinical setting. Nurses are inquisitive decision makers who ask questions about physician orders they do not understand, seek more information about an alternative therapy, or wonder if there is a better way of accomplishing an outcome for a patient. Nurses make changes in their practice based on new information, evidence, or innovative ways of doing things better. Clinical inquiry can resolve clinical problems and issues to promote improved patient outcomes.

Reasoning

To be able to walk into a patient's room and immediately observe significant data, come to a conclusion about the patient, and begin appropriate actions takes clinical reasoning by an experienced nurse. To be objective, the nurse needs to focus on salient cues and not be influenced by personal beliefs, biases, or assumptions that can result in errors, as illustrated by this statement made by a nurse: "The patient's a man, so I didn't think he was really in enough pain for an injection of morphine."

To help determine if decisions are reasonable, nurses use one of two forms of logical reasoning: deductive and inductive. In **deductive reasoning**, the nurse works from the "top down" by starting with general ideas, observations, or principles and analyzing them to develop specific predictions (Polit & Beck, 2017). For example, based on prior knowledge, the nurse knows that older adults have increased susceptibility to infection (general). Using deduction, the nurse can predict that when an 88-year-old man arrives at the emergency department (ED) with a 2-day complaint of increased sputum production, decreased appetite, productive cough, low energy, and complaints of chest pain when coughing, he has pneumonia (specific). Ask these questions: "What is the general idea?" and "What cues observed support it?" and, finally, "Do the significant cues make sense? Are they logical?"

Inductive reasoning involves working from the "bottom up." The nurse observes specific behaviors or symptoms and develops a general conclusion by putting significant, specific cues together (Polit & Beck, 2017). For example, the nurse has observed the following specific symptoms in patients diagnosed with pneumonia: increased sputum production, poor appetite and fluid intake, productive cough, little energy, and complaints of chest pain with coughing. Using inductive reasoning, the nurse concludes that the presence of these same signs and symptoms in other patients strongly indicates they may also have pneumonia. Ask these questions: "What are the significant cues observed?" and "What is the conclusion from the cues (the end result)?" And again, "Does the conclusion make sense? Is it logical?"

When engaging the reasoning process, the nurse listens intently to a patient to determine if information shared is based on fact, an inference, a judgment, or an opinion (see **Table 36.2** »). The nurse cannot accept every statement heard as factual. The same approach applies to communication with colleagues. It is crucial to evaluate statements based on accuracy. The most effective way to accomplish this is through a literature search or review, a medical record documentation search, or through conversations with experts in the subject matter (e.g., nurse manager or nurse educator).

Clinical reasoning, the use of careful reasoning in the clinical setting to improve patient care, is a learned skill that novice nurses must practice. Clinical reasoning requires critical thinking and the ability to reflect on previous situations and decisions and evaluate their effectiveness. With effort and time, new nurses learn critical thinking and integrate it into daily routines. Here are a few actions new nurses can take to improve their clinical reasoning:

1. On entering a patient's room, look around and observe the patient, any other people in the room, where they are positioned in the room, and what they are doing. Observe what items, smells, and sounds are present and what actions are taking place. This is similar to doing a 60-second safety check, a 3-minute brief assessment, or a 5-minute general survey of the patient. Careful use of the senses can help the nurse collect important cues.
2. Common cues nurses learn to recognize include facial expressions, patient activity, degree of respiratory effort, smell of cigarette smoke, complaints made by the patient, bed safety (e.g., rails up or down, bed low and locked, call bell within reach), patient affect, and colors (e.g., red indicating bleeding, yellow indicating infection). These common cues can provide meaningful information quickly and help the nurse determine which cues are salient and if they form a pattern. Clusters of information may bring attention to a problem or issue the patient is having (e.g., presence of infection) or that is in the patient's immediate environment (e.g., visitors preventing appropriate rest). The nurse can then determine the best course of action and intervene as appropriate (Georg, Welin, Jirwe, Karlgren, & Ulfvarson, 2019; Tedesco-Schneck, 2019).
3. Nurses can evaluate previous actions and turn those actions into experiences that can be drawn upon in the future. New nurses may ask themselves questions about a situation in order to analyze and learn from the experience. For example, "How well did that work?" "How did the patient respond?" "What could be done better next time?"
4. Build awareness of faulty reasoning, an occurrence that may cause new nurses to make mistakes in reasoning. Types of faulty reasoning are outlined in **Table 36.3** ».

TABLE 36.2 Differentiating Types of Statements

Statement	Description	Example
Facts	Can be verified through investigation	Blood pressure is affected by blood volume.
Inferences	Conclusions drawn from facts; going beyond facts to make a statement about something not currently known	If blood volume is decreased (e.g., in hemorrhagic shock), the blood pressure will drop.
Judgments	Evaluation of facts or information that reflect values or other criteria; a type of opinion	It is harmful to the patient's health if the blood pressure drops too low.
Opinions	Beliefs formed over time; may include judgments that may fit facts or be in error	Nursing intervention can assist in maintaining the patient's blood pressure within normal limits.

Source: From Berman, Snyder, and Frandsen (2021). Pearson Education, Hoboken, NJ.

Reflection

Reflection is the action of retrospectively making sense of occurrences, experiences, situations, or decisions and consequently learning from them. It is the process of questioning what worked or did not work in a situation, what could have been done differently to achieve better outcomes, which actions contributed to the situation, and what was done well

TABLE 36.3 Types of Faulty Reasoning

Type of Faulty Reasoning	Action	Example
Bandwagon	Doing something because everyone else is doing it	Changing a patient's dressing without indicating date and time new dressing is applied because the dressing removed did not have this information.
Cause-and-effect fallacy	Linking something that happens to something that occurs before it happens	Thinking that the patient's nasogastric (NG) tube was draining fine until the nurse cleaned up the patient's bedside table; therefore, the nurse interfered with the NG tube drainage setup when cleaning up.
Circular reasoning	Supporting an opinion by restating it using different words	Saying that a new dressing is very popular to use because a lot of nurses like using it. (The terms *popular* and *a lot of nurses like using it* are saying the same thing.)
Either–or fallacy	Assuming that a problem has only two solutions	Thinking that the only way to help a patient with a headache is either with medication or a cold cloth on the head. (This ignores other interventions that may be helpful such as dimming the lights, decreasing noise, or giving the patient something to eat.)
Overgeneralizations	Coming to a conclusion when there is not enough evidence to do so	Concluding that a postoperative patient eats all of his meals based on the observation that he ate 100% of his last meal.
Using emotions instead of words	Reporting feelings about a situation rather than the facts	Saying the patient is an angry old man instead of saying that the older patient is anxious about being in the hospital.

(Parissopoulos, 2019). To reflect on an experience, nurses need to learn to observe the significant factors of an experience that need to be included in reflective thinking. See **Box 36.1** ›› for an example of guided reflection.

Reflection requires continuous and open-minded consideration of strengths, weaknesses, behaviors, and opportunities to improve practices. Evidence shows that taking the time to reflect on simulated learning experiences helps learners apply information from simulation to real clinical situations (Grant et al., 2018). Reflective thinking can change a situation that is obscure, uncertain, and disturbing into one that is clear, understandable, and settled. For example, a nurse might be assigned to a patient who is anxious about going for surgery. The nurse can use guided reflection to help the patient "see" the surgical experience with better clarity, which may result in less anxiety for the patient.

Intuition

At times, nurses may experience what they call a "gut reaction" or a "feeling that something is wrong" when working with patients. Even though this awareness seems abstract and mysterious, it may be part of the nurse's reasoning and analysis of the constant data the nurse receives through the senses below a level of conscious awareness. In their article "How Expert Nurses Use Intuition," Benner and Tanner (1987) conclude that **intuition** is the use of nursing knowledge, experience, and expertise for understanding without the conscious use of reasoning. Many argue that intuition is a valuable cognitive skill in clinical decision making among professional expert nurses (Chilcote, 2017; Melin-Johansson, Palmqvist, & Rönnberg, 2017).

Intuition is a process. The data that are continuously received through the senses are not always recognized consciously. Patterns and similarities of patterns are clustered and analyzed. Comparisons are made between a current patient's significant patterns and past patients' patterns in response to similar situations. If the mind recognizes that a new pattern is similar to an old pattern, this recognition may bring the information to a level of cognitive awareness, making it available for the nurse to use in determining a course of action. Although the intuitive method of problem solving is gaining recognition as part of nursing practice, it is not recommended for new nurses or nursing students because they usually lack the knowledge base and clinical experience on which to make a valid judgment.

Critical thinking remains the cornerstone of nursing care and patient intervention. As nursing continues to evolve, so too do the methods of thinking that influence those interventions that directly affect patient care. Benner (2015) emphasizes shifting from critical thinking alone to multiple thinking methods that expand the nurse's understanding and include understanding the patient's experience, the family's experience, and also the nurse's experience. Benner reasons that the complexity of the illness and its effect on the patient and all elements of his being beyond that of being a patient are too broad and far-reaching to be explained by a single theory. Benner recommends multiple methods of thinking in addition to critical thinking, including practical reasoning, in which decisions for actions are determined in part by the actions that provide the best outcome for the patient.

Clinical Decision Making

Nurses make many decisions every day:

- "Which patient should I see first?"
- "When can I teach my patient with congestive heart failure about a low-salt diet?"
- "How long should I wait before doing a bladder scan on my patient who hasn't voided since the indwelling catheter was removed?"

Box 36.1

Guided Reflection

This activity illustrates how one new nurse reflected on a situation he encountered during a day at work that caused him to think about what happened and how he responded. Learning to organize thinking about patient care and professional nursing practice is an acquired skill. Reflecting on thinking processes supports recognizing the "lessons learned" for personal improvement in clinical judgment.

TASK	GUIDED REFLECTION	NEW NURSE RESPONSE
Understanding the background of situation	**1.** Briefly describe what happened and what emotions you experienced during the situation.	**1.** "I was so busy giving my patient his bath that I forgot to give him a scheduled medication."
	2. What previous personal experience with a similar situation helped guide you through the situation?	**2.** "I have worked as a UAP [unlicensed assistive personnel] in the past; I know that baths have to be given around other interventions that the patient has scheduled during the day."
Observing	**3.** What did you initially notice about the situation?	**3.** "I started bathing the patient about 0850. I thought I had enough time to finish it, change his dressing, and then give him his medication that was scheduled to be given at 0930."
	4. As time passed, what did you then notice?	**4.** "The patient needed more time than I thought to bathe. When I checked my watch, it was already 1003, and the medication was late."
Interpreting	**5.** What further information about the situation did you decide you needed, and how did you get it?	**5.** "I should have remembered that some patients, particularly older adults, need more time to do things. I could have started the bath earlier, or I could have given the patient his medication first and then helped him with his bath."
Responding	**6.** What was your nursing response to the situation? What interventions did you do?	**6.** "I had to tell the charge nurse what had happened. I then had to give the medication late."
	7. Describe stresses you experienced as you responded to the situation.	**7.** "It stressed me out that I made a medication error. I felt stupid and was so embarrassed."
Reflecting	**8.** How did the situation end, and what emotion did you feel when the situation was over?	**8.** "The patient received the medication 37 minutes late, so my actions didn't negatively impact the patient, but I could have kicked myself for this."
	9. What might you do differently if this situation happens again?	**9.** "I need to plan my work around medication administration times when I help a patient with morning care—or any intervention."
	10. What was your "take-away" from the experience?	**10.** "Keep an eye on the clock and give priority to interventions and activities I need to do at specific times—work the other interventions around the timed ones."

Source: Based on Tanner (2006).

- "When's the best time for me to watch the video on that new dressing?"
- "Where can I find more linens for the UAP to finish patient morning care?"

Wouldn't it be nice if there was a book to show nurses how to guarantee all clinical decisions they make would be 100% "successful"?

Sound clinical decisions require the ability to weigh the evidence and consider various options for interventions while considering the consequences of each action. Decision making includes many factors such as the needs and desires of the patient, the nurse's experience with similar situations, knowledge, related skill, critical thinking, reasoning, and clinical judgment. Nursing actions are the result of clinical decision making.

Examples of types of decisions are:

- *Ethical and value based.* Decisions in which the action and/or its consequences could compromise the beliefs, privacy, dignity, identity, or other moral or value-based aspect of the patient's being.
- *Prioritization.* Decisions in which the nurse must decide quickly what is most important in a given situation, what must be done personally, what can be delegated, and what can wait (e.g., seeing a patient with a new onset of symptoms first while delegating a vital sign check in a stable patient's room).
- *Time management.* Decisions in which the nurse considers the most efficient use of time for each patient based on factors such as anticipated duration and complexity of tasks and delegation availability of staff (e.g., performing

a physical assessment and mediation administration during the same round).

- *Scheduling.* Decisions that are bound by set time parameters (e.g., medications to be given at a prescribed time, treatments that are time-driven, dialysis, therapy).
- *Personal and professional.* Nurses make decisions surrounding where to work, certifications to obtain, and what career path to take.

It is also important for the nurse to advocate for the patient's right to make decisions regarding healthcare (American Medical Association, 1995–2020). In the role of patient advocate, the nurse can provide resources and age-appropriate information (see the Lifespan Considerations section) to facilitate autonomy and patient-centered care.

The constantly changing healthcare environment requires strong clinical decision-making skills. New technology, expanding roles for nurses in healthcare systems, the complexity of patients entering the healthcare system, and the expanding body of knowledge and skills all add to the complexity of clinical decision making.

When nurses do not have enough clinical experience or nursing knowledge, skills, or imagination to make decisions, they can turn to available guidelines for help. Decision trees and protocols can assist in decision making for many aspects of nursing and nursing subspecialties. For example, many facilities have an emergency protocol for starting a patient on low-flow oxygen when the patient meets listed criteria. Sometimes when cycling through the alternatives, one alternative will just be exactly what is needed and may be chosen for use without further consideration of other alternatives. Many models for decision making are available, each suggesting steps in how to use cognitive processes to choose among alternatives. The following common steps are used in making decisions:

1. Recognize the situation or problem: What decision needs to be made?
2. Analyze the information (e.g., pros and cons of each alternative or solution).
3. Prioritize options and alternatives to try in a given environment.
4. List or make a mental inventory of solutions.
5. Put the best solution into action.
6. Evaluate the success of the action taken by considering alternative solutions or no action (Brenton & Petersen, 2019).

As nurses apply critical thinking to challenges in the workplace, they typically must choose among possible alternatives, engage in problem solving, use the nursing process, employ the scientific method, and sometimes engage in trial and error.

SAFETY ALERT The Texas Board of Nursing (n.d.-b) recommends the following six questions as part of a decision-making model and a tool for clinical judgment in order to ensure patient safety:

1. Is the activity consistent with your state's nurse practice act?
2. Is the activity appropriately authorized by a valid order or protocol, and is it in accordance with established policies and procedures?
3. Is the act supported by either research reported in nursing- and health-related literature or in scope-of-practice statements by national nursing organizations?
4. Do you possess the required knowledge and have you demonstrated the competency required to carry out this activity safely?
5. Would a reasonable and prudent nurse perform this activity in this setting?
6. Are you prepared to assume accountability for the provision of safe care and the outcome of care rendered?

Choosing Among Alternatives

Many clinical situations present possible alternatives that must be considered prior to taking action. In clinical situations, alternatives may be selected from a range of nursing interventions or patient care strategies. Often priorities for care suggest or even determine the alternative chosen, but not always. For example, pain may be treated with oral or injectable medications as needed (prn) or on a schedule or without any pharmacologic intervention by using nursing measures to support the patient's comfort. In all cases, the nurse analyzes the alternatives to ensure that there is an objective rationale for choosing one alternative over another. For example, for the patient with kidney stone pain, common nursing measures may not provide strong enough relief, and oral medication may take effect too slowly, so an intravenous narcotic might be the best choice. The nurse must consider the possibilities of adverse consequences due to a decision. This is also part of the decision-making process. If the intravenous narcotic is selected, should safety measures such as a narcotic antidote and supplemental oxygen be in place? Think about the following questions when choosing between alternatives in decision making:

1. Is there always just "one best" alternative?	Finding the "one best" alternative is very time-consuming and may result in unnecessary delay.
2. Can consideration always be given to every alternative?	The list of alternatives could be quite lengthy, so limit the list to the top five options for serious consideration.
3. Is there always time to gather all the information about alternatives and consequences and then to think about them one at a time?	Is there ever enough time?

The nurse recognizes significant cues that form patterns and then uses intellect, intuition, and reasoning to quickly make decisions and choose a plan of action based on past experiences. Experienced nurses will recognize more patterns and possess a greater wealth of knowledge, enabling them to come to decisions quickly. Regardless of experience, all nurses cycle through alternatives until they find an appropriate choice based on their past experience, knowledge, and skills. At this point, the nurse mentally rehearses the choice and, if the alternative looks like it will work, selects a course of action. Every decision-making process helps nurses improve their decision-making skills and adds to their clinical experience.

Problem Solving

Problem solving is the norm rather than the exception for routine nursing responsibilities today. Nurses become skilled problem solvers in order to manage obstacles and maintain an unencumbered flow of care as they manage their workday. Sometimes patients are scheduled to be in two places at one time for various diagnostic tests, or perhaps a patient received the wrong diet tray and needs a different diet meal, or a patient needs a medication that has yet to arrive from the pharmacy department. Sometimes the problem itself is the number of problems that must be addressed in a short amount of time. Because some patients have complex health issues, their care is equally complex and involve problems that are not always easy to "fix." Some problems may occur repeatedly—for example, the nurse may realize that the pharmacy has been late delivering medications for several days. Nurses must be alert to recurrent problems and new problems and find the time to step in and correct the cycle (see Module 50, Quality Improvement, for more information).

When problems arise, nurses use decision making as part of the problem-solving process. In problem solving, the nurse obtains information that clarifies the nature of the problem and identifies possible solutions. The nurse then carefully evaluates the possible solutions and chooses the best one to implement. After implementing the solution, the nurse monitors the situation over time to ensure the initial and continued effectiveness of the solution. The other possible solutions are held in reserve in the event that the first solution is not effective. The nurse may also encounter a similar problem in a different patient situation where another solution is found to be the most effective. Therefore, problem solving for one situation contributes to the nurse's body of knowledge for problem solving in similar situations. Commonly used approaches to problem solving include the nursing process, trial and error, intuition, and the scientific method.

The Nursing Process

The nursing process includes five phases that organize the problem-solving process (see Exemplar 36.A in this module for more information). Nurses make clinical decisions using critical thinking during every phase of the nursing process. Experienced nurses also use their experiences, knowledge, skills, and current nursing research evidence to make decisions. As nursing students' knowledge, skills, and attitudes progress, they will be able to make better decisions faster using the nursing process as a decision-making tool. Clinical Example B outlines the five phases of the nursing process as they relate to problem solving:

Clinical Example B

1. ***Assessment:*** *Gathering information to determine the problem*
   The nurse admits a 4-year-old patient, Austin Gates, who is suspected of having asthma. The patient has a history of frequent colds and has an allergy to grasses. His dad smokes three packs of cigarettes a day. Austin's mother tells the nurse that Austin has been playing with the neighbor's cats for the past few days. The nurse determines it is important to assess Austin for shortness of breath, respiratory effort, use of accessory muscles, lung sounds, vital signs, oxygen saturation, and the results of lab studies, including a complete blood count (CBC) and chest x-ray. With the help of Austin's mother, the nurse collects other data that may be relevant, such as the patient's past medical history, developmental behaviors, and activity level.
2. ***Nursing diagnosis:*** *Stating the specific problem to solve*
   Based on the assessment data obtained, the nurse caring for Austin determines that his main complaint is difficulty in breathing secondary to airway obstruction. The obstruction is caused by both narrowing of airways and increased mucus production, evidenced by audible wheezing and adventitious lung sounds. The patient is anxious secondary to his shortness of breath and being in a strange environment. The patient has an elevated WBC and an increased respiratory rate. The nurse must decide which of these symptoms are top priorities for nursing care.
3. ***Planning:*** *Stating how to know when the problem is resolved*
   During the planning phase, the nurse caring for Austin decides that an important priority would be to monitor his wheezing, which indicates patency of airways. The goal might be "Austin's lung sounds will be clear bilaterally."
4. ***Implementation:*** *Giving solutions to resolve the problem*
   - Interventions to help Austin meet his goal might be:
     - Assess lung sounds every 4 hours.
     - Maintain supplemental oxygen via nasal cannula as ordered by physician.
     - Administer medication prescribed by provider.
     - Encourage oral (PO) fluids.
5. ***Evaluation:*** *Evaluating if the problem has been resolved*
   Nursing staff has documented, "For the past 12 hours, Austin's lung sounds have been free from wheezes and are now clear."

Critical Thinking Questions

1. What interventions must the nurse address immediately in caring for Austin?
2. What interventions can be delayed?
3. What actions should the nurse anticipate related to Austin's presentation?

Trial and Error

One way to solve problems is through trial and error—trying out a solution, seeing if it works, and, if it does not, reflecting on why and making another, different attempt. Trial and error is an option only when time and safety allow multiple opportunities to select the correct solution. This problem-solving process is not an option when an error may result in harm to the patient. Trial and error may be more useful in situations related to patient comfort or preference. Two trial-and-error examples are when determining how far to raise the head of the bed for the patient to be comfortable enough to eat, or trying different methods to communicate with a patient who has a hearing impairment. The trial-and-error process is primarily used to solve problems; it may not result in the best solution, but it may reveal a workable solution. The use of trial and error requires creativity and patience, two qualities essential to nursing.

Intuition

Intuition is an immediate unconscious awareness of a potentially compromising or dangerous situation. It is known as the "gut feeling." Intuition is an aspect of critical thinking. It is also relevant to problem solving. With practice, solving problems using rules and anticipatory thinking transforms into the ability to use thinking processes, knowledge, and intuition almost unconsciously.

The Scientific Method

The scientific method is a systematic, analytical approach to solving problems. The step-by-step method includes the formulation of a question, data gathering or research, formation of a hypothesis, experimenting with variables, observing and analyzing differences or changes, and drawing conclusions. The scientific method requires a controlled environment, or one in which control of variables is possible. This method is not ideal for nursing practice. Patients, their support systems, and environments, conditions, and contributing factors are too widely varied. While this may not be the ideal approach for problem solving in direct patient care, it is a reliable method for research to discover, appraise, and establish evidence-based practices.

Many aspects of nursing practice involve clinical decision making. Any time a patient's condition changes, those caring for the patient must decide how to respond. Decisions are usually made by problem solving or by choosing among alternatives. Some actions are performed routinely, such as measuring vital signs at the beginning of the shift or introducing oneself when meeting a new patient. Other actions require careful consideration, critical thinking, problem solving, and decision making in order to provide the highest quality nursing care and ensure the safety of patients and staff. See Clinical Example C for an example of clinical decision making.

Clinical Example C

Anna Nadine, 64 years old, is admitted to the medical unit at a local healthcare facility with a medical diagnosis of pulmonary edema secondary to left-sided heart failure. Ms. Nadine has a history of type 2 diabetes requiring insulin injections, hypertension, and early-stage chronic renal failure. She is married, has no children, and lives with her husband in a high-rise apartment building that has a functioning elevator. Initial vital signs are T 99.2°F, P 90 bpm, R 24/min, and BP 136/86 mmHg. Oxygen saturation (O_2 Sat) is 91% on room air. Ms. Nadine is 5′2″ and weighs 168 pounds. She has the following physician orders:

- Vital signs, including O_2 Sat every 1 hour × 3, then every 2 hours × 3, then every 4 hours
- Give oxygen at 2 LPM via nasal cannula titrate to maintain $PaO_2 \geq 94\%$
- Chest x-ray
- Electrocardiogram
- Lab work: CBC with differential, electrolytes, urinalysis (voided)
- Arterial blood gases (ABGs) on oxygen
- Daily weights
- No-added-salt regular diet
- Accu-Chek before meals and at bedtime, with sliding scale—cover with regular insulin

  200 or less = 0 coverage
  201–250 = 2 units subcutaneous injection
  251–300 = 4 units subcutaneous injection
  301–350 = 6 units subcutaneous injection
  351–400 = 8 units subcutaneous injection
  401 and higher = 10 units subcutaneous injection and call physician

- Activity—out of bed to chair with assistance
- Intake and output every 12 hours
- D_5 ½ NS with 10 mEq potassium chloride (KCl) at 50 mL/hr
- Lasix 40 mg IV STAT, then Lasix 20 mg PO daily (am)
- Digoxin 0.125 mg PO daily (am)
- Clonidine 0.1 mg PO BID.

Within 12 hours of admission, Ms. Nadine's weight is 160 pounds and she is breathing more comfortably with breath sounds mostly clear with some fine crackles in the bases. Vital signs are T 99.2°F, P 78 bpm, R 18/min, BP 118/80 mmHg, and O_2 Sat 97% on 2 LPM via nasal cannula.

The next day when you return to the unit and are again assigned to Ms. Nadine's care, you receive a report from the previous shift that she has been confused and disoriented for the past 2 hours. Her blood sugar when last checked 30 minutes ago was within normal limits. Her husband has been notified and plans to come in and sit with her today, but he has not yet arrived.

Critical Thinking Questions

1. What assessment information do you need to obtain?
2. What are the top three priority nursing actions for Ms. Nadine at this time?
3. What factors could be contributing to this patient's confusion?
4. How important is it to gather additional assessment data prior to implementing any interventions for Ms. Nadine?
5. What discussion might you want to have with Mr. Nadine when he arrives?
6. Use critical thinking to determine what physician orders you would anticipate receiving for Ms. Nadine.

Clinical Judgment

Clinical judgment is a highly complex cognitive process through which nurses solve problems by applying clinical reasoning, critical thinking, and decision-making skills. Ultimately, it is through clinical judgment that the nurse determines which actions to take to provide appropriate care to the patient (Martin, Greenawalt, Palmer, & Edwards, 2020). Clinical judgment can be used in emergency situations and also for long-term planning of care.

This dynamic cognitive process brings all the elements of critical thinking and clinical decision making together in making clinical judgments about patient care through the application of nursing knowledge, skills, and attitudes. New nurses may find this skill difficult and slow to use, whereas experienced nurses will be faster and will be able to use their intuition for clinical judgment. Clinical judgment is a competency for graduates of nursing programs. The National Council of State Boards of Nursing (NCSBN; 2020) has models available for states to use in revising their scopes of nursing practice that relate to the accountability for clinical judgments. According to NANDA International (NANDA-I; 2018), a nursing diagnosis is a clinical judgment about an individual or family's situation or their response to a health concern or life process. Three nurse researchers have given the nursing profession important clinical research evidence related to clinical judgment: Patricia Benner, whose skill acquisition model describes five levels of clinical competence; Christine Tanner, whose clinical judgment model supports "thinking like a nurse;" and Kathie Lasater, who promotes the use of a clinical judgment rubric. Based on the work of these and other nurse researchers, the NCSBN has proposed a new framework for measuring clinical judgment and critical thinking ability.

Benner's Skill Acquisition Model

The ability to make clinical judgments improves as nurses gain experience and build on their critical thinking and decision-making skills. A study in the late 1970s compared the performance of senior nursing students, new nurses, and experienced nurses over a 3-year period of time. The results of this study demonstrated distinct differences in clinical performance at these varying levels of nursing education and nursing experience (Benner, Tanner, & Chesla, 2009). Benner adapted these findings to the Dreyfus Model of Skill Acquisition and organized the evidence from the study into five levels of proficiency nurses progress through as they gain additional clinical experience (Benner, 2020). These levels are novice, advanced beginner, competent, proficient, and expert (see **Figure 36.3** »).

The different levels of competence reflect four progressive changes in thinking processes:

1. Moving from not having nursing experiences on which to relate to having concrete clinical experiences to relate to new situations that require critical thinking
2. Progressing from following steps in a specific sequential order to customizing and adapting actions using nursing experience and intuition
3. Moving from taking in many significant cues and trying to make sense of all of them to identifying significant cues and clustering them to form patterns
4. Progressing from being an observant bystander to being an active participant.

Each level builds on the previous level as critical thinking skills are mastered and decision making becomes routine for nurses. Experience further expands this process as nurses gain confidence in their nursing skills.

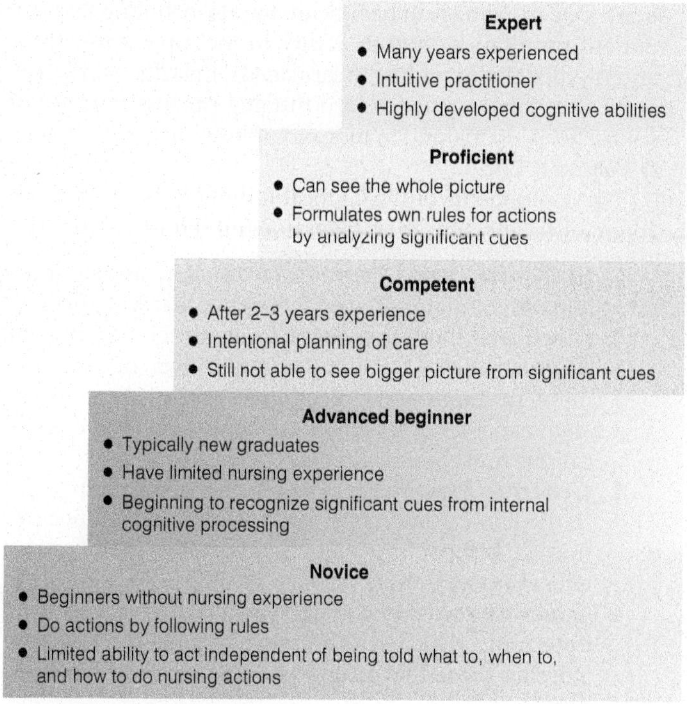

Expert
- Many years experienced
- Intuitive practitioner
- Highly developed cognitive abilities

Proficient
- Can see the whole picture
- Formulates own rules for actions by analyzing significant cues

Competent
- After 2–3 years experience
- Intentional planning of care
- Still not able to see bigger picture from significant cues

Advanced beginner
- Typically new graduates
- Have limited nursing experience
- Beginning to recognize significant cues from internal cognitive processing

Novice
- Beginners without nursing experience
- Do actions by following rules
- Limited ability to act independent of being told what to, when to, and how to do nursing actions

Figure 36.3 » Benner's five levels of clinical competence from nursing student to graduate to professional.

Source: Data from Benner (2011).

TABLE 36.4 Features of the Tanner Clinical Judgment Model

Feature	Description
Noticing	■ Having a sense of what is happening in the patient situation ■ May include recognition of or absence of expected significant cues from the patient's response to illness or a medical condition ■ Includes influences of the nurse's own health beliefs about patient situations and expectations of the work culture for patient care
Interpreting	■ Using logical reasoning to gain understanding about a situation and determine appropriate actions
Responding	■ Includes analyzing a situation and choosing the best course of action ■ Includes intuitive "knowing" from past similar experiences ■ Includes using past similar experiences to "make sense" of a present clinical situation ■ Includes responsive actions by the nurse
Reflecting	■ Using cognitive processes to review a clinical situation ■ Considering appropriateness of assessment data obtained in the situation, actions taken, and positive and negative outcomes for the patient ■ Making mental response adjustments for similar future situations ■ Learning from actions (done or not done)

Sources: Based on Alfaro-Lefevre (2017); Alfayoumi (2019); Tanner (2006).

Tanner's Clinical Judgment Model

Clinical judgment does not always include standard decision making or require all the skills of critical thinking. Tanner's (2006) "thinking like a nurse" approach in her clinical judgment model emphasizes the importance of elements the nurse uses in cognitive processing: different types of knowledge (e.g., textbook, transferred, on-the-job, abstract), length of nursing experience, values, morals, intuition, and knowing the patient (i.e., being familiar with expected patterns of responses to a medical condition or knowing the individual patient). Another element that influences clinical judgment is the culture of the work environment, including group norms and expectations of work routines. The Tanner model includes four features: noticing, interpreting, responding, and reflecting (**Table 36.4** »).

Nursing education teaches fundamental nursing knowledge, skills, and attitudes that lay the foundation for expected high-level performance from students. Nursing education, both didactic and clinical, promotes safe and quality nursing performance. Nursing programs teach students to develop knowledge of their patients in order to care for them responsibly and to develop a sense of their patients' situations in which they will need to intervene. Reflecting on clinical situations and learning from them help students build experiences they can use for future reference. In other words, "thinking like a nurse" begins with learning as a nursing student (Tanner, 2006). See **Figure 36.4** » for a diagram of these sequential cognitive steps.

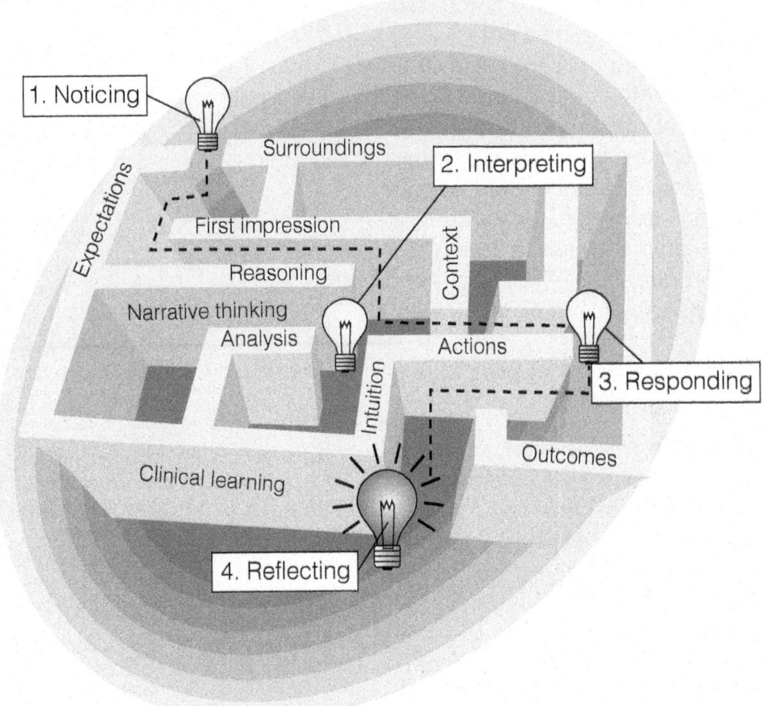

Figure 36.4 ››› Tanner's clinical judgment model includes four major sequential cognitive steps: (1) noticing, (2) interpreting, (3) responding, and (4) reflecting.
Source: Based on Tanner (2006).

Lasater's Clinical Judgment Rubric

Lasater developed the clinical judgment rubric to measure and evaluate clinical judgment using simulation (Bussard, 2018). Tanner's clinical judgment model served as the foundation for the rubric (see Figure 36.4). The rubric serves as a guide for learners to know the specific characteristics needed to reach quality levels of clinical judgment performance (**Figure 36.5** ›››). The rubric has been used successfully while observing learners in a simulation environment.

The rubric uses the four aspects of the Tanner model: noticing, interpreting, responding, and reflecting. Lasater developed additional dimensions for each of these aspects to describe associated behaviors and actions for each (see Figure 36.5, the vertical axis): for example, prioritizing data is an essential behavior of *interpreting* information. Lasater proposes measuring the four aspects of Tanner's model in a progressive developmental order: beginning, developing, accomplished, and exemplary (see Figure 36.5, the horizontal axis). The table provides descriptors and behavioral dimensions for each performance level. Students can use the rubric to measure their progress in using clinical judgment. The rubric clearly defines characteristics for clinical judgment levels and dimensions (Bussard, 2018).

NCSBN Clinical Judgment Model

Reliable clinical judgment is considered integral to safe and effective nursing practice (Dickson et al., 2019). The NCSBN developed the Clinical Judgment Model (CJM), or Clinical Judgment *Measurement* Model, to establish a standardized method of measuring clinical judgment and clinical decision making. The NCSBN is responsible for the creation and regulation of the national licensure exam, the NCLEX-RN, among other nursing licensure exams. The CJM aligns with the steps of the long-accepted nursing process (i.e., assessment, diagnosis, planning, implementation, evaluation). Due to changes in healthcare trends including an older patient population, higher acuity in the inpatient setting, and rapidly changing healthcare needs, the CJM was developed to augment the standard nursing process to facilitate sound decision making in more complex situations (Brenton & Peterson, 2019).

The components of the Clinical Judgment Model include (Brenton & Peterson, 2019; Hensel, 2020) (**Figure 36.6** ›››):

1. ***Recognize cues.*** Determine factors that are important and differentiate between those cues that will affect the patient and those that distract from the clinical picture.
2. ***Analyze cues.*** Consider the implications of all assessment findings and "recognized cues." As cues are analyzed, pathophysiology, patient needs, and complications must be considered.
3. ***Generate hypotheses.*** Prioritizing is key in this step in the clinical judgment cycle. Decide which need or finding is most important and consider the cues that affect the client most.
4. ***Generate solutions.*** Weigh various interventions and determine which will be most beneficial while considering those that would not help or could harm the patient.
5. ***Take action.*** Determining which intervention is the priority and understand why the specific action will best meet the need of the patient based on personal factors and resources. Nursing interventions, delegation,

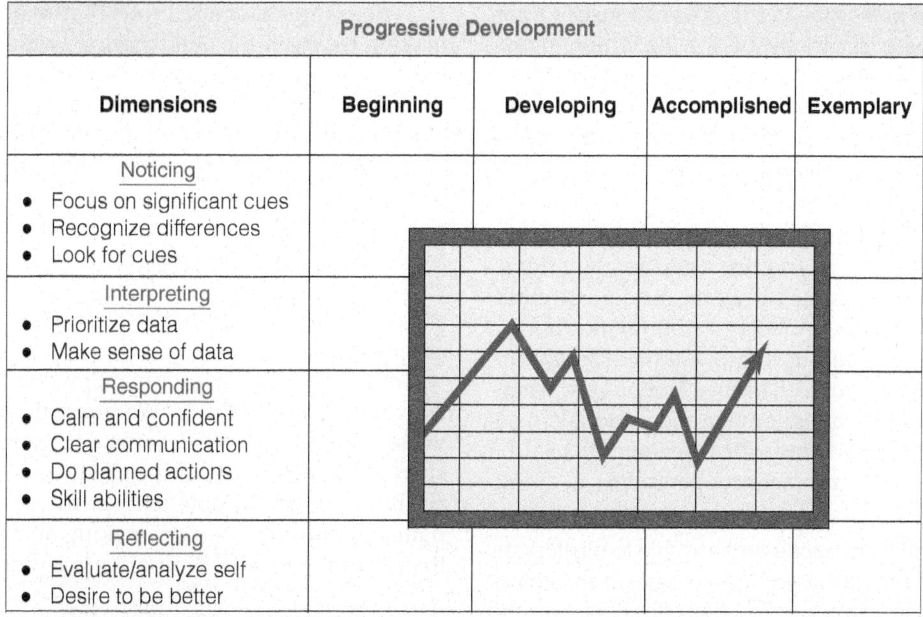

Progressive Development
Dimensions
Beginning
Developing
Accomplished
Exemplary
Noticing
Focus on significant cues
Recognize differences
Look for cues
Interpreting
Prioritize data
Make sense of data
Responding
Calm and confident
Clear communication
Do planned actions
Skill abilities
Reflecting
Evaluate/analyze self
Desire to be better

Figure 36.5 » Lasater used the dimensions from Tanner's clinical judgment model and created developmental levels of clinical judgment for her rubric.
Source: From Bussard (2015).

time management, and professional communication are also considered in this step.

6. ***Evaluate outcomes.*** Consider which outcomes are anticipated and assess the actual outcomes of actions that were taken

The goal of the NCSBN in creating the Clinical Judgment Model is to facilitate a higher level of clinical judgment among new nurses to reduce medical errors linked to poor clinical decision-making skills (Hensel, 2020).

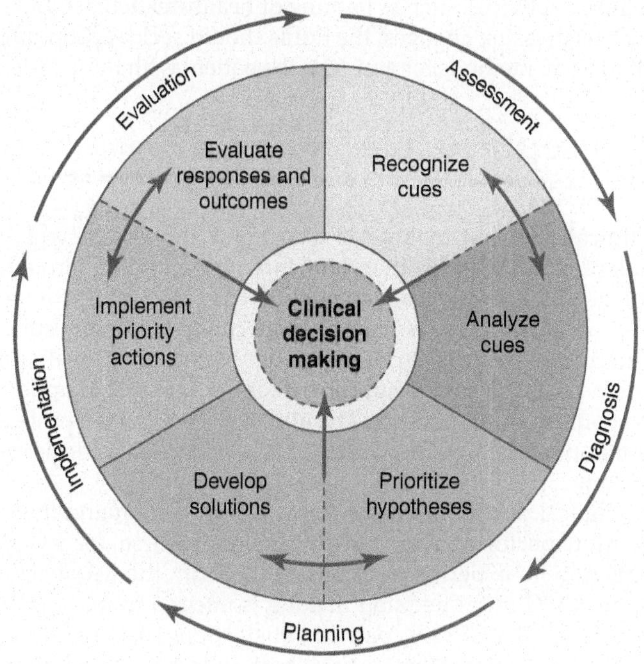

Figure 36.6 » Interrelatedness and overview of the nursing process and the NCSBN Clinical Judgment Model. Adapted from Brenton and Petersen (2019).

Lifespan Considerations

Clinical Decision Making Involving Children

Parents often make decisions about the healthcare of their children. Growing children can participate in those decisions in developmentally appropriate ways. As children mature and develop, they gain decision-making ability and an understanding of the consequences of their decisions. They can contribute to decisions about their health; however, HCPs must carefully evaluate and follow an established process if the child or adolescent is involved in making healthcare decisions (Sawyer & Rosenberg, 2020). Children's ability to reason and think critically about themselves and their situation develops gradually. At each stage, nurses should be aware of the way children think and should be sensitive to how the child can be involved in healthcare decisions at each developmental stage:

- At birth, infant behavior is reflex-driven and completely dependent on others. From birth to approximately one year of age, the infant begins to mimic and repeat actions and behaviors. Through playing games such as peek-a-boo and discovery (e.g., dropping items), infants discover basic principles of object permanence and cause and effect (Cherry, 2019). Infants clearly cannot make healthcare decisions. They require the protection, security, and support of adults during the healthcare experience.
- Toddlers and preschoolers engage their imaginations in self-centered thought processes. Children in these age groups have varying abilities to understand age-appropriate instructions and explanations related to healthcare. Nurses and other HCPs may incorporate toys and games into treatments and instructions. Toddlers and

preschoolers can express whether they are interested in or willing to participate in care by answering simple questions, such as *Do you want to eat your jello?* They have limited decision-making capability but are capable of making choices when presented with alternatives; for example, *Would you like to practice breathing with this tube [incentive spirometer] before or after lunch?*

- School-age children think in concrete terms and require straightforward, simple instructions and explanations. When safe and appropriate to do so, the school-age child may benefit from hands-on teaching opportunities by touching, holding, or even trying to use medical equipment (e.g., stethoscope, reflex hammer, incentive spirometer). Experimenting with equipment and materials may give children at this age a sense of involvement in healthcare, reduce anxiety, and promote cooperation.
- Adolescents begin to develop the ability to control emotions, are able to think abstractly, and are able to participate in healthcare decisions. Adolescent involvement in clinical decision making is complex and, when possible, should involve the patient's assent to a procedure, though parental consent is still required. In some instances, an adolescent may provide assent as well as possess autonomous decision-making ability for clinical care. In such cases, the adolescent is also afforded both confidentiality and the ability to provide consent for procedures (Sawyer & Rosenberg, 2020). HCPs and ethics committees or attorneys (if required) must evaluate the situation and the adolescent and determine competence and capability of making informed decisions.

Clinical Decision Making Involving Pregnant Women

Three decision-making models prevail in the health of the pregnant woman: paternalism, consumerism, and mutualism (Health Care, 2020; Newnham & Kirkham, 2019; Yuill, McCourt, Cheyne, & Leister, 2020). Paternalism assumes that the HCP, because of education and experience, knows best and will make the best decisions for the woman and the fetus. This assumption is based on the further assumption that the HCP will make the best decision because of the need for a positive reputation among present and future patients.

The consumerism model takes a hands-off approach to decision making on the part of the clinician. In this model, the woman or her insurance provider pays for a service. The HCP gives the woman what is believed to be the best information based on science and research. There is a transfer of essential information, enabling the woman to make an informed decision, but there is little engagement.

Mutualism is the most complex of the three models and involves shared decision making between the woman and her HCP. In the mutualism model, the HCP gives the woman information regarding any decision that must be made. The woman informs the HCP of her preferences, values, expectations, previous knowledge, and other factors that may influence her decision making. In turn, the HCP molds the information from the general to the specific as it relates to the unique individual woman and her pregnancy. Together, the patient and the provider discuss scenarios and options, deliberate, and arrive at a mutual decision.

Two examples of situations that require mutual decision making between the childbearing woman and her HCP are women who have previously undergone cesarean birth but wish to consider a trial of labor after cesarean (Kuppermann et al., 2020), and women who prefer intermittent fetal monitoring during labor in contrast to constant fetal monitoring. In these cases, as in others, women should be informed of risks, benefits, evidence, possible occurrences, and support measures (Chuey, De Vries, Dal Cin, & Low, 2020). Mutualism and shared decision making provide the best model for managing these and other issues related to pregnancy, labor, and delivery.

For the childbearing woman, pregnancy, labor, and delivery can be intense times. Women value the input of HCPs, yet some women have described them as inadequate, insensitive, and coercive. Childbearing women expect HCPs who are both knowledgeable and sensitive and who value their patients' input in decision making about their bodies, their lives, and the lives of their unborn children.

Clinical Decision Making Involving Older Adults

All adult patients should be involved in clinical decision making and planning their nursing care; however, older adults with impaired cognition related to disease processes such as Alzheimer disease present a challenge. The nurse should allow these patients as much control and input as possible, keeping discussions simple, direct, and easy to understand. Older adults with impairments may be unable to perform multiple tasks or to think of more than one step at a time. The nurse must be willing to calmly repeat instructions as necessary. Presenting and discussing issues in basic terms helps maintain the older adult's respect and dignity and allows older adults to participate in their care for as long and as much as possible. If the older adult is unable to perform self-care activities such as bathing or health-related activities such as dressing changes, the nurse should seek appropriate alternative methods for assisting the patient with these tasks.

Concepts Related to Clinical Decision Making

Clinical decision making is a complex process in which nurses observe and gather data, interpret that data through the use of salient cues, and identify patterns that provide critical information. Nurses analyze cues and patterns and determine patients' priority needs. Nurses also evaluate alternatives to provide appropriate interventions to support best outcomes for patients. The nursing process is the professional process by which nurses engage in clinical decision making.

Clinical decision making impacts every action and intervention performed by the professional nurse for every patient who experiences an alteration from the usual state of health. Clinical decision making is integral to nursing: it affects quality of care, patient satisfaction, cost, and care-related outcomes. Nurses make critical decisions and intervene to maintain the essential states necessary for life: airway, breathing, and circulation (ABC). Rapid clinical decisions and interventions maintain a patient's airway, ventilation, and perfusion, as well as the patient's oxygen supply to meet the body's demands. The nurse's clinical decision to initiate cardiopulmonary resuscitation (CPR) immediately can help restore circulation to major organs, including the brain and the heart. Nurses' critical decision making addresses the patient's actual or potential risk for compromised airway that may lead to respiratory arrest and alteration in the body's acid–base balance.

The nurse uses a vast body of knowledge in deciding appropriate interventions to resolve dehydration for the patient with fever in order to restore the patient to a state of normal hydration and to minimize the patient's electrolyte imbalance. However, the nurse's decisions and interventions must also reflect caution to avoid causing fluid overload that may exacerbate heart failure, compromise circulatory perfusion, and lead to respiratory failure.

The nurse caring for patients with neurologic deficits makes clinical decisions that reduce environmental stimuli with the potential to increase the patient's intracranial pressure. The nurse makes clinical decisions that avoid overwhelming the patient's sensory perceptions.

Nursing clinical decision making is integral to the postoperative patient, as the nurse's decision-making capability leads to interventions that assist patients who required surgical intervention for an inflammatory process, who undergo an orthopedic procedure related to mobility or orthopedic function, or have alteration in cellular regulation such as breast or colorectal cancer. The nurse uses knowledge and clinical decision making to perform interventions to decrease pain and promote patient comfort while continually assessing the patient and noting any postoperative alterations, including fever, a possible sign of infection; urinary retention after removal of an indwelling urinary catheter; or gastric alterations, a possible sign of digestive system complications that may compromise the patient's nutritional status. All hospitalized patients have increased risk of infection. Nurses' clinical decisions about a patient's already compromised immunity or recent surgery can alter the patient's risk of exposure to infection. Nurses' clinical decisions and interventions in the postoperative patient include interventions to promote tissue integrity and wound healing at the surgical site.

Almost every patient–nurse encounter requires a clinical decision that draws on the nurse's academic knowledge and work experience. Patients who benefit from nurses' sound decision-making ability experience satisfaction with quality nursing care. Sound decision making often calls for shared decision making, in which the nurse engages the patient and advocates for the patient's participation in all aspects of care planning (see the Focus on Diversity feature). The Concepts Related to Clinical Decision Making feature links some, but not all, of the concepts integral to clinical decision making. They are presented in alphabetical order.

Concepts Related to Clinical Decision Making

CONCEPT	RELATIONSHIP TO CLINICAL DECISION MAKING	NURSING IMPLICATIONS
Accountability	Standards of care set benchmarks for nursing performance expectations, including evidence of competent and effective clinical decision making that reflects professional behavior.	■ Nurses are responsible for the clinical decisions and judgments they make to support desired patient outcomes.
Cognition	The nurse assesses the cognitive ability of the patient and determines the severity of cognitive impairment. Based on this assessment, the nurse decides on the most effective way to communicate and to teach the patient.	■ Nurses are knowledgeable about the progression of cognitive impairment. Based on the patient's history and the nurse's assessment, the nurse decides on those interventions that have been found to be effective means of communicating and teaching patients who are cognitively impaired. The nurse creatively employs those methods.
Collaboration	The nurse's assessment determines the patient's postdischarge needs, which may include the need for subacute care; visiting nurse services for wound care, vital sign monitoring, teaching, and safety assessment; and the need for home physical therapy.	■ Nurses participate in a collaborative team approach when caring for patients. ■ Nurses refer patients to social services and case management to provide services outside of the hospital while continuing certain interventions for goal attainment.
Communication	Priorities of patient care need to be communicated to achieve continuity of care. Passing on correct information about patient status helps nurses on the next shift make competent decisions about patient care.	■ Nurses use the patient's plan of care, written or electronic, to communicate priority goals of the patient; document treatments, interventions and outcomes, and teaching; and record their work.

(continued on next pag

Concepts Related to *(continued)*

CONCEPT	RELATIONSHIP TO CLINICAL DECISION MAKING	NURSING IMPLICATIONS
Safety	All clinical decisions, actions, and interventions on the part of the nurse must protect patients from harm. Clinical decision making and nursing actions and interventions must protect the nurse and nursing colleagues from harm.	■ Protecting patients from harm, or nonmaleficence, is one of the ethical foundations of nursing care. ■ Behaviors that endanger the nurse, nursing colleagues, and staff increase the risk of serious injury, loss of staff members due to injury, and possible health repercussions such as needlesticks and back injuries.
Thermoregulation	Patients with thermoregulatory dysfunction require immediate interventions to begin cooling and minimize organ and brain injury in cases of hyperthermia and immediate warming for patients with hypothermia to minimize tissue injury, loss of limb, or in cases of extreme exposure, death.	■ The nurse is knowledgeable about the need for immediate interventions and the necessary precautions in treating patients with exposure and thermoregulatory disorders. This knowledge, in combination with patient assessment, helps the nurse make appropriate decisions about the independent actions the nurse will take.

Focus on Diversity and Culture

Shared Decision Making and Patient–Provider Relationships

Shared or inclusive clinical decision making (the combination of clinical expertise and patient values and preferences) is an important part of the patient–provider relationship. Shared decision making can help break down barriers between providers and patients to help increase trust and improve clinical outcomes.

Patients who belong to more than one marginalized group (e.g., patients who are lesbian, gay, bisexual, or transgender and also identify with an ethnic or cultural minority) are at risk for suboptimal shared decision making (Howard et al., 2019; Tan, Arshiya, Baig, & Marshall, 2017). This often results in poor clinical outcomes (Margolies & Brown, 2019). Patients describe healthcare providers' lack of knowledge regarding gender identity, cultural barriers, and distrust as factors that contribute to stigmatization and discrimination in the healthcare system (Margolies & Brown, 2019). Tan et al. (2017) provide an extensive list of components for both patients and providers to assist in overcoming barriers to shared or inclusive decision making. These range from recognizing that patients of color may have experiences that are different from white patients, even when patients share other characteristics (such as being transgender or living in poverty), to creating more inclusive environments by making sure that signage and symbols represent diverse populations, among other recommendations.

REVIEW The Concept of Clinical Decision Making

RELATE Link the Concepts

Linking the concept of clinical decision making with the concept of legal issues:

1. What legal actions may occur if the nurse fails to make prudent clinical decisions? Explain your answer.
2. What role regarding sound clinical decision making in patient care is expected of the licensed registered nurse?
3. What role regarding sound clinical decision making in the workplace does the employer expect of the nurse?

Linking the concept of clinical decision making with the concept of evidence-based practice:

4. How does the nurse with strong critical thinking maintain an evidenced-based practice?
5. A nurse reads a peer-reviewed article that recommends changing currently accepted practice. What critical thinking will the nurse perform before accepting the article's recommendations?

Linking the concept of clinical decision making with the concept of ethics:

6. What ethical obligation does the nurse hold toward the patient related to clinical decision making?
7. What ethical obligation does the nurse hold toward the hiring facility related to clinical decision making?

REFER Go to Pearson MyLab Nursing and eText

REFLECT Apply Your Knowledge

The nurse is caring for a patient who was admitted 3 days ago with acute abdominal pain. Following extensive diagnostic testing, the patient has received a medical diagnosis of stomach cancer, with suspected metastasis to the liver and pancreas. The oncologist has informed the patient that there are several options related to treatment. Option 1 is to surgically remove as much of the tumor as possible, followed by chemotherapy and radiation therapy. This is the most aggressive approach with the best odds for survival, but the oncologist tells the patient that with the amount of metastasis that has already occurred, the odds for survival are still not very good (less than 10%). The second option is to do nothing, allowing the patient to remain as comfortable as possible (palliative care) until death, which will likely occur in 3 to 6 months. The third option is the moderate option and involves chemotherapy to slow cancer growth, which may prolong the patient's life but will result in side effects (e.g., hair loss, vomiting, weakness) that will likely impact the patient's quality of life. After the oncologist leaves the room, the patient looks to the nurse and asks, "What do you think I should do? What would you do if you were me?"

1. What actions by the nurse would be most appropriate for this patient?
2. What ethical, legal, and moral duties guide the nurse when responding to this patient's questions?
3. How would you respond to each of the patient's questions?

» Exemplar 36.A The Nursing Process

Exemplar Learning Outcomes

36.A Analyze the nursing process as it relates to clinical decision making.

- Describe the assessment phase of the nursing process.
- Describe the diagnosis phase of the nursing process.
- Describe the planning phase of the nursing process.
- Describe the implementation phase of the nursing process.
- Describe the evaluation phase of the nursing process.
- Differentiate the use of the nursing process in caring for patients across the lifespan.

Exemplar Key Terms

Assessment, *2510*
Cognitive skills, *2526*
Collaborative interventions, *2523*
Defining characteristics, *2514*
Dependent interventions, *2523*
Diagnostic label, *2514*
Etiology, *2514*
Evaluation, *2521*
Evaluation statement, *2528*
Goal, *2519*
Health promotion diagnosis, *2513*
Implementation, *2522*
Independent interventions, *2523*
Interpersonal skills, *2526*
Modifiers, *2514*
NANDA-I, *2512*
Nursing diagnosis, *2512*
Nursing process, *2509*
Outcome, *2519*
Planning, *2519*
Problem-focused diagnosis, *2513*
Risk factors, *2513*
Risk nursing diagnosis, *2514*
SMART, *2521*
Syndrome diagnosis, *2514*
Technical skills, *2526*

Overview

The **nursing process** is a systematic, scientific method nurses use to make decisions and determine the effectiveness of patient (individual, family, community, group) care. The nursing process includes the assessment of the patient, diagnosis of problems or potential problems, planning nursing interventions and anticipated medical or interprofessional actions, implementing the planned actions, and evaluating the effectiveness or outcomes of interventions or treatments (**Figure 36.7 »**).

The term *nursing process* was first coined in the 1950s by nursing theorist Ida Orlando (1972). The five steps of the nursing process include assessment, diagnosis, planning, implementation, and evaluation (sometimes referred to by the mnemonic *ADPIE*). In the early 1970s, the nursing process became a standard of nursing practice that remains in use. It has long been the framework for the Nursing Scope and Standards of Practice, national licensure exams, and for nurse practice acts in most of the United States (American Nurses Association [ANA], 2015). Although the NCSBN's Clinical Judgment Model is becoming the standard for national licensure exams, it was developed around and remains anchored by the scientific methodological steps of the nursing process (Brenton & Peterson, 2019; Dickson et al., 2019).

A few general characteristics of the nursing process complement its ease to organize the flow of nursing care and produce an individualized plan of care for all patients across the lifespan. The nursing process is *dynamic* and *cyclical* rather than static so that it can adapt to changes in the patient's status. While it is called the *nursing* process, the *patient* is the focus. Nurses utilize the process to provide individualized, patient-centered care.

For the purposes of nursing practice, *health* is considered to be an optimal state of overall wellness and not just the absence of disease processes. Nurses cannot strictly think of a disease while providing care. Nurses recognize that patients are biological, spiritual, psychological, and social beings. Additionally, nurses are cognizant of environmental and social determinants of wellness, including education level and accessibility, shelter, relationships, and other external factors when providing holistic care to individuals, families, or groups of people (Petiprin, 2020).

Problem-solving processes are used in many professions. Physicians employ the medical model to evaluate pathophysiological processes. Scientists use the scientific method. However, the medical model and scientific method are examples of very focused, problem-centered processes. The nursing process is focused holistically on the patient and not exclusively the patient's presenting problem. This means that the nurse is considering the person and all internal and external influences. The nursing process helps the nurse evaluate responses to any disruptions in wellness as well as

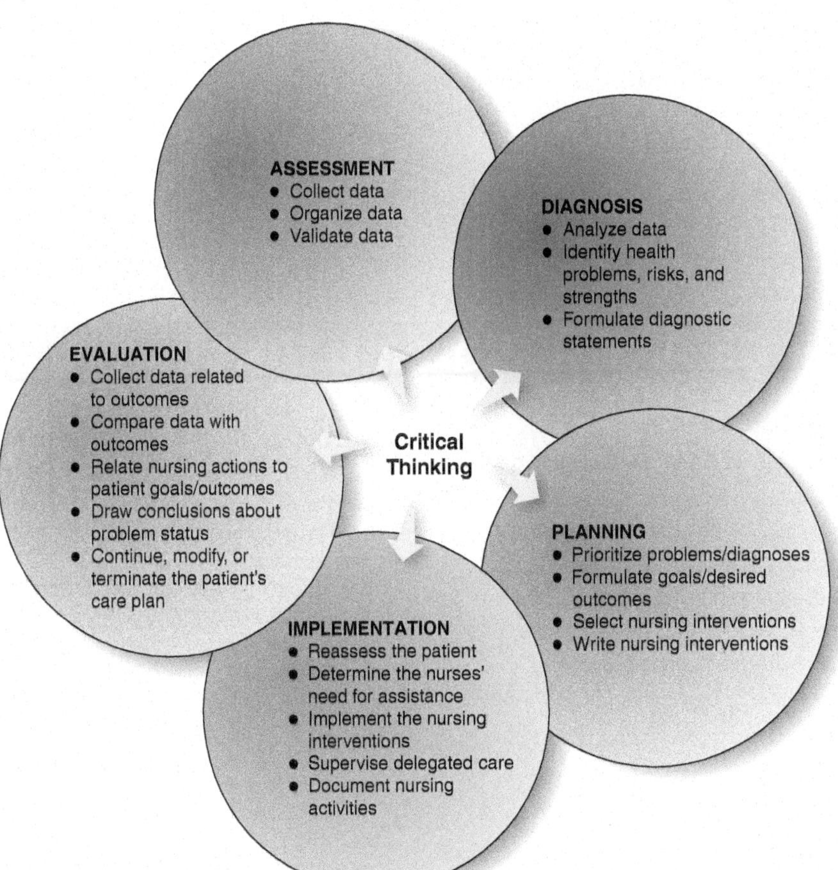

Figure 36.7 » The nursing process in action.

interventions implemented during care. Ultimately, the nurse is concerned with helping the patient return to an optimal state of being, or health.

Nurses must make decisions in each step of the nursing process. For example, the nurse must decide which assessment is most important (e.g., head-to-toe or focused assessment, or which assessment equipment to utilize). Decisions made within the structure of the nursing process can include techniques and lessons that have been memorized or learned, checklists and protocols, or creative, intuitive decisions that come with experience. Many of the decisions made include the necessity of both intraprofessional (nurses) and interprofessional (e.g., physicians and other non-nursing professionals) team members. While there are few one-size-fits-all systems in healthcare, the adaptable elements of the nursing process provide the foundation and structure for patient-centered care in all settings and for all people (e.g., all beliefs, sexual identities and orientations, genders, cultures, ages, and religions).

An overview of the five phases of the nursing process is given in **Table 36.5** ». The phases of the nursing process are not separate entities—they are interrelated and they overlap and cycle. For example, assessment, which may be considered the first phase of the nursing process, is also carried out during the implementation and evaluation phases. For instance, while administering medications (implementation), the nurse assesses the patient to determine the patient's continued need for the medication, response to the medication, and potential side effects of the medication.

The nursing process lends organization and structure to clinical decision-making practices. The phases of the process do not exist in vacuums. Each one impacts the others. Without expert assessment, an accurate diagnosis cannot be made, resulting in the implementation of subpar interventions and the evaluation of insufficient outcomes. Even though the phases may be repeated and the nurse may move back and forth across some of the steps, the first and most important block on which the nursing process is built is *assessment*. Sound clinical decision making is not possible without collecting the appropriate information (data) through patient/situation assessment.

Assessment

Assessment is the systematic collection of data and recognition of cues related to the patient's state of being (Brenton & Peterson, 2019; Mousavinasab, Rostam, Zarifsanaiey, Rakhshan, & Ghazisaeedi, 2020). It is the foundation of all phases in the nursing process, and all other components of patient care are built on the accurate collection of assessed data. Assessment is continuous throughout the nursing process and is especially important during the implementation and evaluation phases. Evaluation is sometimes referred to as *reassessment*. It is not possible to determine patient needs, diagnose, plan, implement treatments, or evaluate without skillful and accurate data collection through assessment.

A nursing assessment focuses both on an actual or potential problem and on a patient's responses to a health

TABLE 36.5 The Phases of the Nursing Process

Phase and Description	Purpose	Activities
Assessment		
Collecting, organizing, validating, and documenting patient's assessment data Begin noting significant cues and how they may be clustering.	To establish a database about the patient's response to health concerns or illness and the ability to manage healthcare needs.	■ Establish a database: —Obtain a nursing health history. —Conduct a physical assessment. —Review patient records. —Speak with family members and significant support persons. —Speak with appropriate health professionals. ■ Update data to keep it current.
Look for significant cue clusters and patterns.		■ Organize data.
Seek more assessment data to clarify cue clusters and patterns.		■ Validate data. ■ Communicate/document data.
Diagnosis/Nursing Diagnosis		
Analyzing and synthesizing data	To identify patient strengths and health problems that can be prevented or resolved by collaborative and nursing interventions. To develop a list of nursing and collaborative problems.	■ Interpret and analyze data: —Compare data against standards. —Cluster or group data (generate tentative hypotheses). —Identify gaps and inconsistencies. ■ Determine patient's strengths, risks, diagnoses, and problems. ■ Formulate diagnostic statements. ■ Document priority nursing diagnoses on the nursing plan of care.
Planning		
Determining how to prevent, reduce, or resolve the identified priority patient problems; how to support patient strengths; and how to implement nursing interventions in an organized, individualized, and goal-directed manner; anticipating interprofessional care and patient responses to interventions	To develop an individualized plan of care that specifies patient goals/desired outcomes and related priority nursing interventions.	■ Set priorities and goals/outcomes in collaboration with patient. ■ Write goals/desired outcomes. ■ Select nursing strategies/interventions. ■ Consult other healthcare professionals. ■ Write nursing interventions and nursing plan of care. ■ Communicate plan of care to relevant HCPs.
Implementation		
Carrying out (or delegating) and then documenting the planned nursing interventions	To assist the patient to meet desired goals/outcomes; promote wellness; prevent illness and disease; restore health; and facilitate coping with altered functioning.	■ Reassess the patient to update the database to keep it current. ■ Determine the nurse's need for assistance. ■ Perform planned priority nursing interventions. ■ Communicate what nursing actions were implemented: —Document care and patient responses to care. —Give organized reports as necessary.
Evaluation		
Measuring the degree to which goals have been achieved and identifying factors that positively or negatively influence goal achievement. Identifying outcomes.	To determine whether to continue, modify, or terminate the plan of care.	■ Collaborate with patient and collect data related to desired outcomes. ■ Judge whether goals/outcomes have been achieved. ■ Relate nursing actions to patient outcomes. ■ Make decisions about problem status. ■ Review and modify the plan of care as indicated or terminate it. ■ Document achievement of outcomes and modification of the plan of care.

problem or change in health status. Nursing assessment includes subjective data obtained from the patient or family about the patient's needs, health condition, health practices, values, health history, and lifestyle. It also includes objective data obtained through assessment and physical examination of the patient. Available sources, including the patient's medical record or office visit records, are used to assist the nurse in developing a database that includes the patient's past medical history and previous current health status (see Module 34, Assessment, for further information).

The data collected through assessment can be organized using various models. Nursing curricula worldwide have adopted a concept-based model for learning and for organizing nursing information, including assessment data. Conceptual areas can be divided into biophysical, psychosocial, and professional nursing domains. Health assessment data can be organized using broad based, conceptual labels to define not only the problem area but also the effect a disturbance may have on the patient to help guide decision making. A few examples include:

1. Oxygenation
2. Perfusion
3. Intracranial regulation
4. Sensory perception
5. Cognition
6. Mood and affect.

See Module 34, Assessment, for an overview of other frameworks of assessment, including a review of body systems (Box 34.3) and Gordon's Functional Health Patterns (Table 34.8).

Nurses collect and validate assessment data before analyzing the information for salient cues. Analyzing assessment data requires that the nurse compare data against standards or norms to identify cues; cluster cues to begin to form an understanding of what is happening with the patient; and identify gaps and inconsistencies in data to determine what additional information is needed.

As nurses gain experience, they develop the ability to perform the phases of the nursing process in an ongoing cycle while constantly analyzing assessment data. It can appear to happen without conscious thought. That kind of *intuitive processing* comes with years of experience. New nurses tend to think in sequences, following checklists, guides, and worksheets to collect and analyze data. Evidence-based written cues promote safe practice and should be utilized while the new nurse gains experience. All nurses need to critically think about assessment, prioritize clustered data, and focus on the most important information (cues) that require intervention.

When gathering and clustering assessment data for children, the nurse will need to include the parents or guardians as a major source of subjective data as well as asking the child about feelings. Assessment of the family's needs related to the child's illness (e.g., Does lack of insurance present a barrier to accessing services or paying for prescriptions?) is also necessary. See the Lifespan Considerations section for more detail on using the nursing process with children.

Case Study » Part 1

Aarti Kher, a 28-year-old married professional with three children, was admitted to the medical unit of the local hospital with a medical diagnosis of pneumonia throughout her right lung. She has been assigned to Nurse Maya Park, RN. After Mrs. Kher is oriented to her room by the UAP, Nurse Park does her admission assessment.

During the interview, Nurse Park learns that Mrs. Kher has had a "chest cold" for 2 weeks and has been experiencing shortness of breath when she tries to cook dinner or clean the house. Even putting her child to bed makes her short of breath. Mrs. Kher reports that for the past few days, she has not felt like eating very much and is only drinking a couple of glasses of tea every day. She states she has had a productive cough with a medium amount of thick, foul-smelling, pink sputum. Mrs. Kher tells Nurse Park that she hasn't felt like going to work; she just feels tired all the time. She states she doesn't smoke and only drinks a glass of beer or wine occasionally. Mrs. Kher jogs every morning and walks the family dog in the evenings after work, but lately she has not had the energy to exercise. She currently takes levothyroxine 0.1 mg daily, and her last hospitalization was for the delivery of her youngest child 3 years ago. Mrs. Kher states she is allergic to penicillin but not to foods, latex, or iodine.

On physical examination, Mrs. Kher is 62 in. (157 cm) tall and weighs 125 lb (56.7 kg). Vital signs are T 103°F (39.4°C), P 92 bpm, R 28/min, BP 122/80 mmHg, and oxygen saturation (O_2 Sat) 95% on room air. Nurse Park observes that Mrs. Kher's skin is dry, her cheeks are flushed, and she is experiencing chills. Auscultation reveals inspiratory rhonchi with diminished breath sounds in the right lung. Respirations are shallow. Mrs. Kher's oral mucous membranes are pale and dry and her skin turgor when tented is > 3 seconds. She speaks in short sentences. Peripheral pulses are weak and equal bilateral in all four extremities.

Clinical Reasoning Questions Level I

1. Which assessment data are salient cues?
2. Do these cues form any clusters? If so, what are they?

Clinical Reasoning Questions Level II

3. Are there any other questions you would ask Mrs. Kher to further clarify her health status?
4. Which cluster of significant cues would be the priority? Why?

Diagnosis

In the diagnosis phase of the nursing process, nurses use critical thinking and reasoning to analyze the cues from the assessment and identify priority problems. Diagnosis is the phase in which data comes together to determine the first steps that need to be taken to support the patient. Cues that the nurse recognizes and analyzes inform the diagnoses that will lead to the nursing plan of care.

NANDA-I (formerly the North American Nursing Diagnosis Association) has developed, established, and periodically updates the NANDA-I nursing diagnoses and taxonomy. In 1990, NANDA-I adopted an official working definition of **nursing diagnosis**, "a clinical judgment concerning a human response to health conditions/life processes, or a vulnerability for that response, by an individual, family, group or community. A nursing diagnosis provides the basis for selection of nursing interventions to achieve outcomes for which the nurse has accountability" (2018, p. 38). This definition implies the following:

- Registered nurses are responsible for making nursing diagnoses, even though other nursing personnel may contribute data to the process of diagnosing and may implement specified nursing care. In *Nursing: Scope and Standards of Practice*, Standard 2 addresses the fact that registered nurses determine the diagnoses or issues from analysis of the assessment data (ANA, 2015). The Joint Commission embraces the ANA's standards and therefore requires evidence of nursing diagnoses in patients' medical records.
- The domains of nursing diagnoses include only those health states that nurses are educated and licensed to treat within their scope of practice (see Module 49, Legal Issues, for further information about scope of practice). For example, nurses can diagnose and treat *confusion*, *dehydration*, and *inadequate gas exchange*, all of which are human responses that may occur with a medical diagnosis of pneumonia.
- A nursing diagnosis is a judgment made only after thorough, systematic assessment and data collection.
- Nursing diagnoses describe a continuum of health states: deviations from health, presence of risk factors, and areas of enhanced personal growth.

The current organization of NANDA-I nursing diagnoses is called Taxonomy II (NANDA-I, 2018). Taxonomy II has three levels: domains, classes, and nursing diagnoses. The diagnoses are coded according to seven axes that reflect elements of a patient's response addressed in the diagnosis: diagnostic focus, subject, judgment, location, age, time, and status.

>> **Stay Current:** For more information about NANDA-I-approved nursing diagnoses, refer to the NANDA-I website at www.nanda.org.

To identify nursing diagnoses effectively and then create and complete a nursing plan of care, the nurse must be familiar with:

- Common terms used with nursing diagnoses
- Difference between a nursing diagnosis and a medical diagnosis
- Types of nursing diagnoses
- Components of a nursing diagnosis.

Common Terms

A diagnosis is the identification of a condition, situation, or occurrence after assessment and analysis are performed. Many electronic documentation systems have made moves toward the use of *plain-language diagnoses* rather than NANDA-I-specific nursing diagnosis wording. In the examples used in this text, NANDA-I nursing diagnosis labels are capitalized, whereas plain-language diagnoses are not. A nursing diagnosis includes the problem area, causation, and related factors and is crafted into a statement intended to address the issue and potential patient responses. Potential problems are identified as risks. **Risk factors** identify vulnerabilities in the patient's current state that could threaten wellness. The nursing plan of care is based on prioritized diagnoses formulated after analyzing assessment data.

Nursing diagnoses are developed using a multiaxial system. Axes are categories that address components of the diagnostic process. There are seven axes: the focus of the diagnosis, the subject of the diagnosis (patient, family, etc.), nursing judgment (impaired, inefficient, ineffective, etc.), locations (cardiac, pulmonary, leg, etc.), age (infant, child, adolescent, adult, etc.), time (chronic, acute, intermittent, constant, etc.), and status of the diagnosis (problem focused, risk, or health promotion) (NANDA-I, 2018).

- Axis 1, the focus of the diagnosis, is the fundamental basis of traditional nursing diagnosis (NANDA-I, 2018). In the NANDA-I diagnosis *Compromised Family Coping*, coping is the principal element.
- Axis 2, the subject, may be explicit or implicit. For example, in the nursing diagnosis *Compromised Family Coping*, the subject, "family," comes from Axis 2. In the plain-language nursing diagnosis, *impaired airway clearance ability*, the subject, "patient," is implied.
- Axis 3 consists of modifiers that give meaning to the focus of the diagnosis. In the diagnosis *Compromised Family Coping*, the judgment is compromised (Axis 3). Other judgments in nursing diagnoses include complicated, decreased, delayed, ineffective, insufficient, inadequate, impaired, and several other modifiers and descriptors.
- Axis 4 provides a description, location, system, or function affected by the focus. In some cases, the location may not be a part of the body—for example, bed, wheelchair, or crutches. In the diagnosis *impaired airway clearance ability*, "airway" reflects Axis 4: airway is the location of the focus.
- Axis 5, age, represents the categorical age of the subject. Ages are categorized as fetus, neonate, infant, child, adolescent, and adult. For example, a nursing diagnosis that categorizes the age of the subject could be *Ineffective Infant Feeding Pattern*.
- Axis 6 describes time as it relates to the nursing diagnosis. Time may be episodic, for example, perioperative, the time before and after surgery; it may be situational and relate to a set of circumstances, for example labor and delivery; or it may be periodic (e.g., daily). Time can also be acute, lasting less than 3 months, or chronic, lasting more than 3 months. In the diagnosis *Ineffective Coping Related to Chronic Back Pain*, the subject has endured back pain for at least 3 months. Other time-related terms include *continuous* and *intermittent*.
- Axis 7, the status of a diagnosis, determines an actual or current health problem (a problem-focused diagnosis), a future problem (a risk diagnosis), or a desire to improve health and well-being (a **health promotion diagnosis**).

Nurses develop diagnoses by determining the focus (Axis 1) and adding a judgment (Axis 3). There are times when Axes 1 and 3 are combined—for example, *nausea* or *fatigue*. After determining the focus and the judgment, the subject is added. However, this is not necessary if the subject is an individual. Additional axes are then used to provide further detail and clarity.

Nursing Diagnosis versus Medical Diagnosis

Nursing diagnoses are statements formulated by nurses that describe holistic patient conditions, responses, and risks that are within the nursing scope of practice, training, and expertise to treat. Unlike medical diagnoses that are focused on pathophysiological changes, nursing diagnoses describe the patient's responses to physical, sociocultural, psychologic, and spiritual changes in wellness. Nursing diagnoses change as the patient's responses change. Medical diagnoses are made by licensed physicians, nurse practitioners, and physician assistants to label standardized disease processes and conditions rather than the patient's response to the pathophysiological process.

Types of Nursing Diagnoses

The current types of nursing diagnoses are problem-focused diagnoses (also referred to as actual diagnoses), risk diagnoses, health promotion diagnoses, and syndrome diagnoses (NANDA-I, 2018). Additionally, plain-language diagnoses may be used in some clinical settings following similar axes and patterns:

1. **Problem-focused diagnosis** involves a prioritized diagnosis made when recognizing and analyzing cues during patient assessment. An example of a NANDA problem-focused diagnosis would *Deficient Fluid Volume*. A plain-language version of that diagnosis would be *fluid volume deficiency*. Regardless of the formatting, problem-focused nursing diagnoses are based on cues that are recognized, analyzed, and prioritize during patient assessment.

2. **Risk nursing diagnosis** requires anticipation of a problem that has not yet occurred or a condition that has not yet been diagnosed but is within the realm of probability for a patient. Nurses apply clinical judgment to discern potential issues based on existing clinical cues assessed. It is within the nurse's scope of practice to intervene to prevent diagnoses based on risks. For example, it is possible for any patient to develop an allergy to latex while hospitalized. The nurse knows that patients with allergies to bananas and mangos are at significantly higher risk of latex allergy. Therefore, a nursing diagnosis of *potential for allergic reaction to latex* would be appropriate. The risk diagnosis documents a patient's health status vulnerability for a single diagnosis or the risk for a syndrome diagnosis.
3. A **health promotion diagnosis** reflects a patient's readiness to improve an aspect of health. For example, if a patient expresses the desire to improve eating habits, an appropriate diagnosis would be that the patient is *ready to learn about and receive improved nutrition*. Similarly, if a woman expresses the desire to improve her health in order to prepare for pregnancy, the nurse may note that the woman is *prepared to learn about improving pregnancy and childbirth outcomes*. Health promotion diagnoses reflect patient awareness of well-being and the desire to maintain or enhance this state.
4. A **syndrome diagnosis** recognizes a cluster of individual nursing diagnoses that occur simultaneously and may result in the best patient outcomes if addressed concurrently (NANDA-I, 2018). Syndrome diagnoses may be problem-focused or risk diagnoses. For example, a diagnosis of *potential for disuse syndrome* may be assigned to patients who are bedridden. The cluster of nursing diagnoses associated with disuse syndrome include *compromised physical mobility, potential for impaired tissue integrity, inability to tolerate activity, risk of infection, risk of injury, potential for constipation, inadequate gas exchange*, and *risk for feelings of powerlessness*.

Components of a Nursing Diagnosis

A nursing diagnosis has three components, and each component serves a specific purpose:

1. The **diagnostic label** ("What is the focus or subject of the problem?")
2. The **etiology** ("Where did it come from?" "What is it related to?")
3. The **defining characteristics** ("What does it look like?").

Diagnostic Label

A *diagnostic label* is a clear and concise description of the patient's response to a specific condition or situation, sometimes referred to as the *problem statement*. To be clinically useful, the diagnostic labels must be specific. It is customary to use as few words as possible to describe what the patient is experiencing (e.g., *constipation, dry mouth*, or *confusion*). Regardless of whether plain language or a specific model such as NANDA-I (2018) is used, the diagnostic label indicates the focus of any planning and goals setting, interventions, and evaluations of patient care.

Modifier words are used in Axis 3 to indicate the direction, intensity, or severity of the problem. Establishing a modifier in the diagnosis process requires the analysis of assessment cues and application of clinical judgment to form a hypothesis or prediction or identify trends in data.

- *Deficient:* too little to be sustainable, inadequate amount or quality, not complete
- *Impaired:* diminished, reduced, worsened or worsening, hindered, injured
- *Decreased:* declining, lessened amount, quality, or measurement
- *Ineffective:* unproductive, inadequate
- *Compromised:* threatened integrity, vulnerable

Each diagnostic label approved by NANDA-I carries a definition that clarifies its meaning. For example, the definition of the diagnostic label *Activity Intolerance* is given in **Table 36.6** ».

Etiology (Related Factors and Risk Factors)

Nursing diagnosis includes the *etiology*, or likely causes of the problem facing the patient. Causation guides the actions taken by the nurse when selecting individualized, patient-centered interventions. Table 36.6 demonstrates the etiologies of *Activity Intolerance*. It is important to identify different likely causes when formulating a nursing diagnosis because each etiology may require specific and different actions. For example, **Table 36.7** » illustrates how the diagnosis of constipation can have many different causes and each etiology requires specific interventions.

TABLE 36.6 Example of the Components of a Nursing Diagnosis

Diagnostic Label and Definition	Related Factors	Defining Characteristics
Activity Intolerance: Insufficient physiologic or psychologic energy to endure or complete required or desired daily activities	Bedrest or immobility Generalized weakness Imbalance between oxygen supply/demand Sedentary lifestyle	Verbal report of fatigue or weakness Abnormal heart rate or blood pressure response to activity Electrocardiographic changes reflecting arrhythmias or ischemia Exertional discomfort or dyspnea

Source: From NANDA-I. (2018). NANDA International, Inc. nursing diagnoses: Definitions and classification 2018–2020 (11th ed.). [e-book]. Chichester, UK: Wiley-BlackwellThieme.

TABLE 36.7 Example of a Nursing Diagnosis with Different Etiologies

Diagnostic Label (Problem)	Patient	Etiology
Constipation	Al Martinez	Long-term laxative use
	Jerry Wong	Inactivity and insufficient fluid intake
	Tanya Brown	Depression
	Caitlin Shea	Change in eating pattern

Defining Characteristics

Defining characteristics refer to the cluster of signs and symptoms that indicate the presence of a particular diagnostic label. For actual nursing diagnoses, the defining characteristics are the patient's signs and symptoms. For risk nursing diagnoses, subjective and objective signs are not present. Thus, the factors that cause the patient to be more vulnerable to the problem are the etiology of a risk nursing diagnosis. Characteristics can be listed separately according to whether they are subjective or objective in nature. For example, the problem-focused diagnostic label *fear* includes the following defining characteristics:

- Report of apprehension, being scared, having increased tension
- Diminished learning ability, unable to solve problems
- Diarrhea, vomiting, dry mouth, increase in pulse rate.

The risk diagnostic label *Risk for Falls* includes the following defining characteristics:

- Having a history of falling, using a cane to walk
- Lack of gate on the stairs, lack of parental supervision
- Tranquilizer use, anemia, visual difficulties.

Developing a Nursing Diagnosis

The nurse uses critical thinking skills, discussed earlier in this module, to analyze clinical cues and apply clinical reasoning to make nursing diagnoses. Data gathered during assessment of the patient and from the patient's medical record are analyzed based on accepted norms within the population and trends found in the patients' past and current history. The nurse reviews standardized ranges for lab results, age-appropriate values for vital signs, and established norms for height and weight through the lifespan. The nurse also compares the patient's current values to the medical history. See **Table 36.8** ›› for examples of analyzing cues by comparing to norms.

Experienced nurses demonstrate the ability to rapidly assess and recognize important cues when entering a patient's environment. This rapid assessment leads to immediate analysis, identification of priorities, instant planning, and appropriate actions. Expert nurses perform this process intuitively at times, as if an expert level of clinical judgment becomes automatic. The expert level of clinical decision making comes with years of experience, education, and practice. In contrast, new nurses require tools such as checklists and specific guidelines to recognize and analyze cues and formulate an appropriate plan of action or make a clinical decision (see the Critical Thinking section at the beginning of this module for more information).

Skilled and accurate nursing assessment reduces the risk of misread cues leading incorrect or incomplete diagnoses, goals, and interventions. The nurse should ask, Did the data from any assessment match the patient's clinical picture? Do the cues make sense to the nurse? Is the present situation congruent with the history? Are the findings consistent? For example, a patient may report not touching alcohol for 2 years, but the blood alcohol level on admission was elevated. Without criticism or bias, the nurse must clarify all such inconsistencies before drawing conclusions about patterns and behaviors. See **Table 36.9** ›› for examples of nursing diagnoses based on immediate and gathered assessment cues.

After clustering the cues and data, the nurse works with the patient to identify problems that support the various types of nursing diagnoses (e.g., problem focused, risk, or health promotion). The steps of determining the appropriate type of diagnosis is a decision-making process. The nurse must also decide if the problem is something within the nursing scope of practice, experience, and skill to treat; if the issue requires a medical diagnosis; or if the problem presents a collaborative opportunity for the interprofessional team. **Figure 36.8** ›› is a diagram designed to aid in the process of determining the most appropriate type of diagnosis for a given scenario.

During the assessment, the nurse identifies the patient's physical strength, supportive resources, and coping skills. While providing holistic care, nurses know that most people are more aware of their strengths and abilities than they may realize. Through history taking, chart review, psychosocial assessment, and skillful therapeutic communication, the nurse is able to inventory the assets a patient brings into the care setting and transform the patient from simply being a consumer or recipient of care into a collaborator in care. Empowering the patient to participate is not only important

TABLE 36.8 Examples of Patient Cues Compared to Standards/Norms

Cues from Patient	Standard/Norm	Interpretation of Cues
Height is 5 ft., 2 in. Woman with small frame Weighs 240 lb	Height and weight tables indicate that the healthy weight for a woman 5 ft., 2 in. with a small frame is 108–121 lb.	Deviation from population norms
Child is 17 months old. Parents state child has not yet attempted to speak. Child laughs aloud and makes cooing sounds.	Children usually speak their first word by 10–12 months of age.	Developmental delay
States, "I'm just not hungry these days." Ate only 15% of food on breakfast tray. Has lost 30 lb in past 3 months.	Patient usually eats three balanced meals per day. Adults typically maintain stable weight.	Changes in patient's usual health status
Mrs. Stuart reports that lately her husband angers easily. "Yesterday he even yelled at the dog." "He just seems so tense."	Mr. Stuart is usually relaxed and easygoing. He is friendly and kind to animals.	Changes in patient's usual behavior

TABLE 36.9 Nursing Diagnoses Derived from Patient Cues

Patient Cues	Potential Problems	Diagnostic Statements
Restlessness; tossing and turning, pulling at bed sheets Unable to answer basic questions Not orientated to time, place, situation; only oriented to person	Confusion	*Acute confusion related to medications for pain, changes in oxygenation, and current disease process*
Tachypneic; Respiratory rate >30 Unable to speak in full sentences Shallow breathing Worsening over past 12 hours States "I . . . can't . . . breathe."	Irregular or insufficient breathing pattern	*Ineffective breathing pattern related to physical compensation to maintain adequate oxygenation; infectious process*
Skin pale-to-bluish around the mouth, dark nails Oxygenation saturation of 86% Diminished breath sounds bilaterally	Inadequate gas exchange	*Impaired gas exchange related to inability to meet physical oxygenation demands*
Febrile temp of 39.6°C (103°F) Pallor Dry, hot skin	Poor thermoregulation	*Impaired thermoregulation related to increased cellular metabolism triggered by infectious process*
Tachycardia >115 beats per minute Pallor Sluggish capillary refill >3 seconds Decreased oxygen saturation Mild cyanosis	Potential for impaired tissue perfusion	*Risk for ineffective peripheral tissue perfusion related to decreased oxygen reaching tissues secondary to tachypnea, shallow breathing*

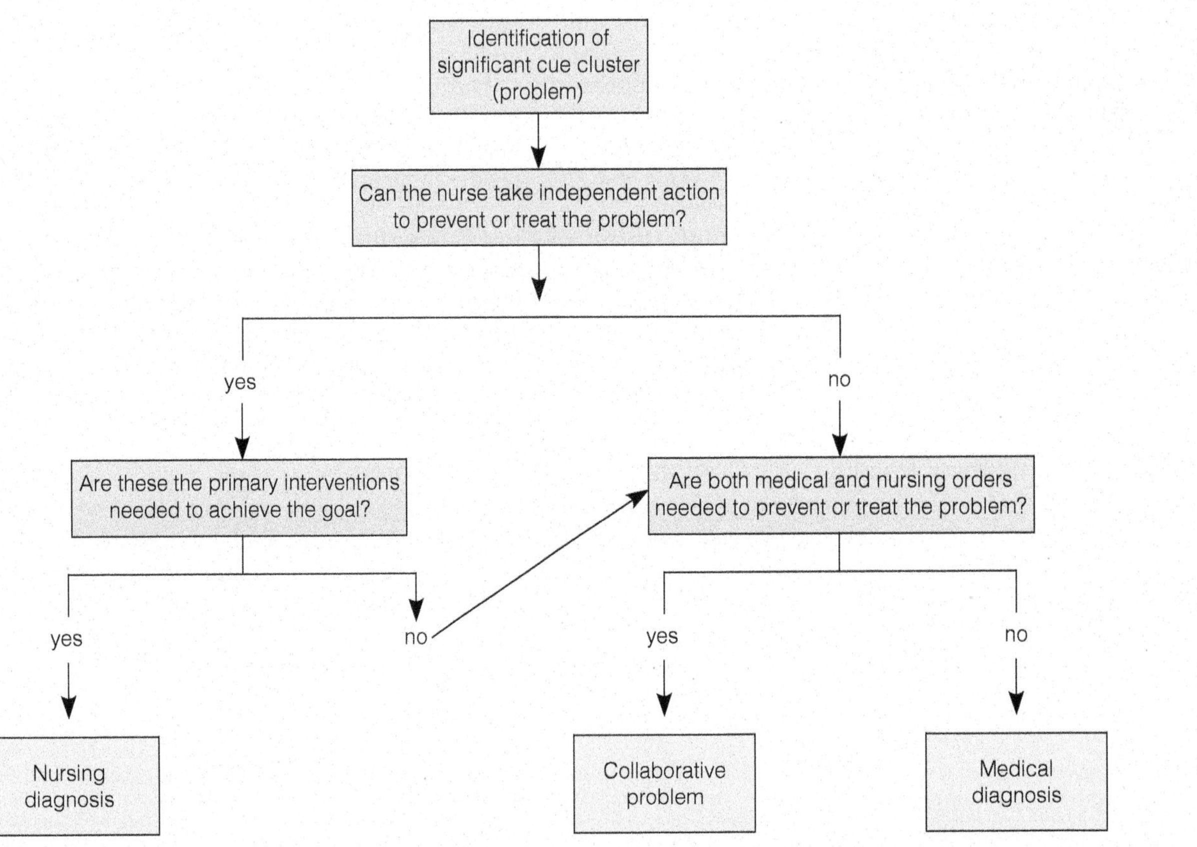

Figure 36.8 » Decision tree for differentiating among nursing diagnoses, collaborative problems, and medical diagnoses.

TABLE 36.10 Examples of Two-Part Nursing Diagnosis Statements

Problem	Related to	Etiology
Nausea	related to	early pregnancy
Anxiety	related to	threat to safety: loss of home

in providing patient-centered care, but it can also serve as a great motivator to achieving goals and sustaining progress. The experienced nurse also knows that patients possess physiological strengths, such as a healthy weight, absence of drug allergies, and a history of no substance abuse. Each of these strengths can help to improve outcomes and can drastically influence or change the direction of a plan of care.

Writing a Nursing Diagnosis Statement

Nursing diagnoses are typically written as two-part (identifying actual or potential problems) or three-part (for actual problems only) statements.

Basic Two-Part Statement

The basic two-part nursing diagnosis statement (*PE format*) may be used for the diagnosis of risks or for actual or potential problems.

1. *Problem (P):* NANDA-I or other diagnostic label to identify the type of diagnosis is needed (e.g., problem-focused, risk, health promotion, or syndrome)
2. *Etiology (E):* Identify the probable cause of the problem.

The two parts are joined by the words *related to* or *due to* because of the causal relationship. Some examples of two-part nursing diagnoses are shown in **Table 36.10** ».

Basic Three-Part Statement

The basic three-part nursing diagnosis statement (*PES format*) is used for the diagnosis of actual problems. The three-part nursing statement includes the following:

1. *Problem (P):* NANDA-I or other diagnostic label to identify the type of diagnosis is needed (e.g., problem focused, risk, health promotion, or syndrome)
2. *Etiology (E):* Identify the probable cause of the problem.
3. *Signs and symptoms (S):* State the signs and symptoms that support the diagnosis. Think of this as the evidence or manifestations of the issue.

Actual problems can be documented by using a three-part statement (see **Table 36.11** ») because the signs and symptoms or manifestations of the condition are recognized and can be documented. Signs and symptoms or manifestations are not a part of risk or potential diagnoses because there are no physical manifestations of a risk. The risk diagnosis is in place to prevent the problem from occurring. The PE/PES formatting is highly useful for novice nurses who need more structure when making decisions. The listing of signs and symptoms validate the diagnosis and help guide actions.

Basic One-Part Statement

There are some exceptions to the two-part/three-part nursing diagnosis guidelines. Diagnostic statements, especially syndrome and health promotion–based statements, may stand alone as labels. If nursing actions can be determined based solely on the label, no further etiology or manifestations need to be defined. Examples of this type of syndrome nursing diagnostic label are *posttrauma syndrome* and *rape-trauma syndrome*. Etiologies and manifestations do add clarity to those labels.

Health promotion diagnoses include descriptions of how the patient or group is prepared to improve, grow, or learn about a certain health-related concern. Health promotion nursing diagnoses begin with the words *Readiness for Enhanced* or *prepared to learn more or improve* followed by the health-related area in need of growth (e.g., *Readiness for Enhanced Parenting* or *ready to improve parenting*). Examples of NANDA-I health promotion nursing diagnoses are *Readiness for Enhanced Spiritual Well-Being*, *Communication*, *Coping*, and *Sleep*. Health promotion diagnoses stand alone as one-part statements or they may be clarified by adding a descriptor, for example, *Readiness for Enhanced Breastfeeding* (lactation consultant session). See **Table 36.12** » for guidance on writing each type of nursing diagnostic statement.

Common Variations

Some variations in creating the one-, two-, and three-part diagnostic statements include:

1. The condition has an *etiology* that is unknown. Situations in which the defining characteristics are present but the nurse cannot identify the causes lead to the development of *unknown etiology* statements. For example, *anxiety* related to *unknown etiology*.
2. Nursing diagnoses are intended to be succinct. It may become necessary to define the etiology of a diagnostic statement as involving complex factors. Using the term *complex factors* ensures that nursing diagnoses remain brief. For example, the etiology of a chronic disrupted body image, for instance, extremely complex and long lasting, as in the following nursing diagnosis: *chronic disrupted body image related to complex factors.*
3. The phrase *secondary to* clarifies and further describes the etiology of a nursing diagnosis by dividing it into two parts. The words following *secondary to* are often pathophysiologic processes or medical diagnoses, as in *reduced cardiac output related to reduced myocardial contractility secondary to heart failure manifested by ejection fraction of <40%, edema, crackles in the lungs, and other manifestations as appropriate.*

TABLE 36.11 Example of a Three-Part Nursing Diagnosis Statement

Problem	Related to	Etiology	As Manifested by	Signs and Symptoms
Chronic pain	related to (r/t)	Back injury	as manifested by (amb)	Rates pain as 7 on a 0–10 scale and as 10 during exacerbations; difficulty sleeping due to pain; difficulty engaging in typical activities due to pain

TABLE 36.12 Guidelines for Writing a Nursing Diagnostic Statement

Guideline	Correct Statement	Incorrect or Ambiguous Statement
1. State in terms of a problem, not a need.	Inadequate fluid volume (problem) related to fever	Fluid replacement (need) related to fever
2. Word the statement so that it is legally advisable.	Altered skin integrity related to immobility (legally acceptable)	Altered skin integrity related to improper positioning (implies legal liability)
3. Use nonjudgmental statements.	Impaired spirituality related to inability to attend church services secondary to immobility (nonjudgmental)	Impaired spirituality related to strict rules necessitating church attendance (judgmental)
4. Make sure that both elements of the statement do not say the same thing.	Potential for altered skin integrity related to immobility	Altered skin integrity related to ulceration of sacral area (response and probable cause are the same)
5. Be sure that cause and effect are correctly stated (i.e., the etiology causes the problem or puts the patient at risk for the problem).	Pain: Severe headache related to fear of addiction to narcotics	Pain related to severe headache
6. Word the diagnosis specifically and precisely to provide direction for planning nursing interventions.	Alteration in mucous membrane integrity related to decreased salivation secondary to radiation of neck (specific)	Alteration in mucous membrane integrity related to noxious agent (vague)
7. Use nursing terminology rather than medical terminology to describe the patient's response.	Potential for altered respiratory status related to accumulation of secretions in lungs (nursing terminology)	Potential for pneumonia (medical terminology)
8. Use nursing terminology rather than medical terminology to describe the probable cause of the patient's response.	Potential for altered respiratory status related to accumulation of secretions in lungs (nursing terminology)	Potential for altered respiratory status related to emphysema (medical terminology)

Source: From Berman et al. (2021). Pearson Education, Hoboken, NJ.

4. Statements can be added to the nursing diagnosis to specify the location. For example, *impaired tissue perfusion* is a very general statement that could apply to generalized perfusion issues. However, if the patient has experienced a traumatic brain injury, the impaired perfusion will be limited to the brain. Adding the word *cerebral* to the diagnosis clarifies where the issue is. *Impaired cerebral tissue perfusion* is specific and labels the real problem.

Avoiding Errors in Diagnostic Statements

Accuracy is imperative when formulating nursing diagnoses. Nursing diagnosis, whether written in NANDA-I, plain language, or from customized databanks provided by electronic health records, must be deliberately formulated using critical thinking and clinical reasoning. The nursing diagnosis establishes the plan of care for the patient. To avoid making diagnostic mistakes while collecting, interpreting, and clustering relative data cues, nurses can perform the following steps:

- ***Verify*** the information by communicating with the patient and patient's support system. Ensure that the cues the nurse recognized and analyzed match the clinical picture, personal history, and medical or psychosocial diagnosis of the patient. It is also a good idea to ask the patient and family members if they agree with the nurse's interpretation of the data and the diagnosis.
- ***Gain experience and practice knowledge building.*** Be intentional about building a database of knowledge while increasing experience in a clinical area. It is not possible to properly diagnose a patient issue without recognizing cues during an assessment. Recognition occurs when the nurse recalls prior experiences, knowledge, and skills practice in similar situations.
- ***Know what is normal so you can recognize what is not.*** Wherever nurses practice, they need to know the expected ranges for laboratory values, vital signs, growth and development, physical assessment findings, cognition, and other areas for that population. Some *normal* values vary greatly depending on the patient's age. For example, neonatal patients have vastly different vital signs from young adults. What is normal in a pediatric patient could be life-threatening for a geriatric patient. Additionally, a firm grasp of normal assessment findings helps the nurse cue into changes from normal. Upon an initial assessment, the nurse compares assessment findings to learned cues and established milestones or ranges of normal. Subsequent assessments and evaluations of medical data should compare the updated findings to the initial, baseline assessments.
- ***Search the evidence and consult expert resources.*** No matter what stage of career the nurse is in, the astute professional seeks out evidence-based literature and expert resources for diagnostic support. Research, experienced colleagues, and respected members of the interprofessional team are valuable resources. Current nursing texts and nursing diagnosis books can help the nurse determine if the appropriate diagnosis has been selected based on whether manifestations meet defined criteria.
- ***Nursing diagnoses are based on trends and patterns, not on isolated occurrences.*** A young adult may be greatly concerned about caring for a 55-year-old parent after an uncomplicated outpatient cholecystectomy. It is

likely that the recovery from the procedure will be very brief and there will be no lasting limitations from the procedure. Therefore, a nursing diagnosis of *caregiver burden* would not be appropriate in that instance.

- ***Strengthen critical thinking skills.*** Strong critical thinking skills help to prevent the nurse from committing the mistakes of forming assumptions, stereotyping, or making sweeping generalizations about patients. While medical diagnoses are similar, patients are unique and the critically thinking nurse becomes more aware of individual patient problems and experiences.

Case Study » Part 2

Nurse Park wants to use the assessment data she obtained during the admission assessment of Mrs. Kher to identify the priority nursing diagnosis. First, she makes a list of all of the assessment data and then separates the significant cues that form clusters. Some of the significant cues Nurse Park identifies include:

- "Chest cold" for 2 weeks
- Shortness of breath with activity
- Lung sounds—inspiratory crackles with diminished breath sounds in right lung
- Insufficient fluid intake
- Feels tired all the time; no energy to do home activities or go to work
- Does not smoke
- T 103°F (34.4°C), P 92 bpm, R 28/min, BP 122/80 mmHg, and O_2 Sat 95% on room air
- Productive cough with thick, foul-smelling green sputum
- Speaks in short sentences.

Based on the above assessment cluster and the fact that Mrs. Kher has a medical diagnosis of pneumonia, Nurse Park feels confident that the priority nursing diagnosis would involve Mrs. Kher's response to the infection in her right lung. There are many potential nursing diagnoses related to the respiratory system. Nurse Park decides that *inadequate airway clearing ability* best fits Mrs. Kher's signs and symptoms. So the diagnostic statement for the top-priority nursing diagnosis for Mrs. Kher is *inadequate airway clearing ability* related to accumulated mucus obstructing airways (secondary to pneumonia).

Clinical Reasoning Questions Level I

1. How do the assessment data support the nursing diagnosis made by Nurse Park?
2. Can you identify the different components in this two-part diagnostic statement?

Clinical Reasoning Questions Level II

3. What might be the second- and third-priority nursing diagnoses for this patient?
4. What other assessment data could you hypothesize might be a potential problem for Mrs. Kher because of her medical diagnosis of pneumonia?

Planning

The **planning** phase is a deliberate, systematic phase of the nursing process during which the nurse refers to the patient's assessment data and nursing diagnoses for direction in formulating patient goals. Goals are different from outcomes, although many times these words are used to mean the same thing; the difference is outlined in **Box 36.2** ». The goals become the basis for the nursing interventions that are developed to prevent, reduce, eliminate, or improve the situation identified by the nursing diagnosis. For the plan of care to be effective, it is important for the patient and support persons (if applicable) to participate in the development of the plan: Nurses plan care *with* the patient, encouraging the patient to participate actively to the extent possible (**Figure 36.9** »). In a home setting, the patient's family members and caregivers are the ones who implement the plan of care; thus, its effectiveness depends largely on them.

Box 36.2

The Difference Between a Goal and an Outcome

Goals are observable patient responses—what the nurse hopes to achieve through nursing actions. Goals are developed in the planning phase of the nursing process. They are broad statements about something the patient strives to achieve and indicate progress toward desired patient behaviors or actions. Goals are what nurses and patients want to happen. They are individualized and specific for each patient. Goals are the responses to nursing interventions.

Outcomes are used to evaluate the patient's response to the plan of care. Desired outcomes are specific, observable criteria used to evaluate whether goals have been met. Desired outcomes are identified during the planning phase; during the evaluation phase, the nurse determines if outcomes have or have not been met. Outcomes are the end results of nursing actions—both desirable and undesirable. Outcomes indicate the effectiveness of nursing actions. For example, for the patient experiencing impaired airway clearing ability related to poor cough effort:

Goal: Patient will demonstrate an effective cough by 1400 this afternoon.

Desired outcome: Patient maintains a clear airway during the postoperative period.

The terms *goal* and *desired outcome* are often used interchangeably. Sometimes the word *or* is used between them ("goals or outcomes") and sometimes they are written "goals/outcomes." In this text, goals are developed in the planning phase of the nursing process and desired outcomes are used to evaluate the patient's response to the plan of care.

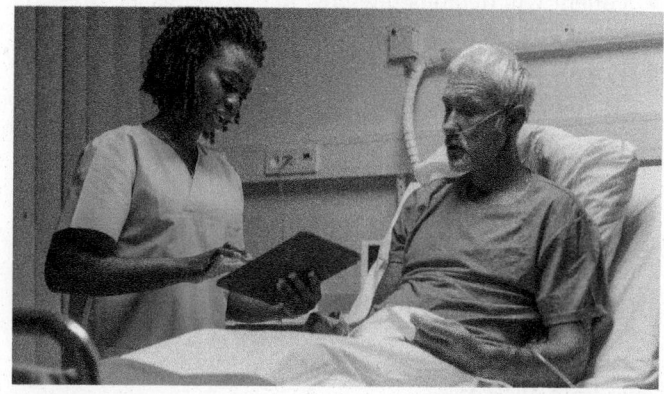

Figure 36.9 » Nurses plan care collaboratively with the patient.
Source: Gorodenkoff/Shutterstock

When the nurse and patient identify a goal for every nursing diagnosis together, it helps support the nurse–patient relationship. This partnership achieves these other purposes as well:

1. Provides direction for selecting nursing interventions. Ideas for interventions come more easily if the goal clearly and specifically states what the patient is to achieve.
2. Serves as criteria for evaluating patient progress. Although developed in the planning phase of the nursing process, goals serve as the criteria for determining the effectiveness of nursing interventions and patient progress for desired outcomes in the evaluation phase.
3. Enables closure of the nursing diagnosis situation when the patient and nurse determine the goal has been achieved.
4. Helps motivate the patient and nurse by providing a sense of achievement. As goals are met, both patient and nurse can see that their efforts have been worthwhile. This provides motivation to continue following the plan, especially when difficult lifestyle changes need to be made by the patient.
5. Supports a therapeutic nurse–patient relationship. Anytime the nurse and patient are able to move forward together in the patient's plan of care, the patient gains trust in the nurse, further increasing the likelihood of the plan's success.

Long-Term and Short-Term Goals

Goals are customized to individual patients, which means they take varying amounts of time to achieve. Because of differences in time, goals are categorized as either short term or long term, depending on the time frames necessary to achieve them.

Short-term goals are useful for patients who require healthcare for a short time. In an acute care setting, much of the nurse's time is spent on the patient's immediate needs, so most goals are short term and can be achieved by the patient in a range of a few hours to a few days. Examples of short-term goals are:

- Patient will raise her right arm to shoulder height 4 days from today, January 23.
- Patient will identify five salty foods to avoid while on a low-sodium diet by tomorrow, May 7.
- Patient will demonstrate how to change his leg dressing before discharge.
- Patient will use a cane to walk 20 feet down the hallway by April 22.

Long-term goals are often used for patients who live at home and have chronic health problems and for patients in nursing homes, extended care facilities, and rehabilitation centers. However, patients in acute care settings also need long-term goals to guide planning for their discharge to long-term care agencies or home care, especially in a managed-care environment. Long-term goals can be achieved by the patient in a range of 1 week to several months. Examples of long-term goals are:

- Patient will regain full use of her right arm 6 weeks from today, June 6.
- Patient will be able to discuss five effective coping strategies for dealing with stressful situations that he has used over a 6-month period of time from today, September 25.
- Patient will eat at least 60% of all meals by the end of 3 weeks from today, June 1.
- Patient will participate in two weekly group activities by sitting quietly and listening attentively by 3 months from today, May 13.

Developing a Goal

Goals are derived from the patient's nursing diagnoses—primarily from the diagnostic label. Each nursing diagnosis has one goal for the patient to achieve. When developing goals, the nurse should ask the following questions:

1. What about the nursing diagnosis needs to be changed for or by the patient?
2. Is there a healthy response to correct a problem stated in the nursing diagnosis that the patient can achieve as a goal?
3. How will the patient look or behave if the healthy response as a goal is achieved? (What will be seen, heard, measured, palpated, smelled, or otherwise observed through the senses?)
4. What action must the patient do and how well must the patient do it to demonstrate problem resolution or achievement of the goal?

For example, the nursing diagnosis is:

Fluid volume deficiency related to diarrhea and inadequate intake secondary to nausea

The *diagnostic label* is "*fluid volume deficiency*."	This is the problem.
Related to is "diarrhea and inadequate intake."	This is the source of the problem.
Secondary to "nausea"	This is the origin of the "related to" factors.

The goal for this nursing diagnosis might be "Patient's intake and output of fluids will be balanced during his hospitalization." The patient's goal reflects maintaining a fluid balance during the time interval he is losing fluids through diarrhea.

Writing a Goal

Goals have specific characteristics that should be included when writing them to fulfill their purpose in the planning phase of the nursing process. Setting a goal helps to identify desired change in a patient's situation and define the focus of nursing interventions. Common characteristics of goals include being:

- Patient centered (not about nurse activities)
- Specific and concise single action
- A single goal for each nursing diagnosis
- Directional for nursing interventions
- Measurable
- Quantifiable

- Attainable for an individual patient
- Realistic to an individual patient
- Relevant to an individual patient
- Time limited.

All goals are patient centered in that the patient is always the subject, as indicated by beginning the goal with the words "The patient will" much of the time. Sometimes these three words are omitted in goals because it is assumed that the subject is the patient unless indicated otherwise. A quick and user-friendly format to follow to write a goal statement is the acronym SMART (Stonehouse, 2018), which stands for:

Specific single action
Measurable
Attainable (achievable)
Relevant
Time limited.

Specific Single Action

The goal includes a clearly stated, single action for the patient to do that can be observed directly or indirectly. Any additional information defining how the action is to be done is included in this part of the statement. These are sometimes called *qualifiers* of the action. Information provided about the action is detailed so that other nurses following the nursing plan of care will be able to understand what the patient is to achieve to reach the goal.

Here are some examples of specific single actions for goals. The patient will:

- Walk 20 feet down the hall using a walker.
- Demonstrate giving herself an insulin injection using aseptic technique.
- Identify six foods to avoid that are high in salt content.
- State the purpose of his new medication, nitroglycerin, and when and how to take it.

Measurable

The goal includes a specific, measurable observation or result that is quantifiable. Any nurse observing the patient attempting the single action of the goal will be able to recognize when the patient reaches the goal. In the following examples, the first column does not provide specific measurements or quantities that all nurses would define the same, whereas the second column does. The patient will:

Poorly Written Quantified Measure	Correctly Written Quantified Measure
Go for a walk (need to know distance for goal to be reached).	Walk 20 feet down the hall using a walker.
Understand how to give insulin (understanding doesn't mean being able to do it).	Demonstrate giving herself an insulin injection using aseptic technique.
State foods not to eat (quantify how many and what kind so the understanding is consistent).	Identify six foods to avoid that are high in salt content.
Know about nitroglycerin (need to be specific about what to know).	State the purpose of his new medication, nitroglycerin, and when and how to take it.

Nurses must be aware that some phrases can lead to disagreements about whether the outcome was met. Avoid statements that start with *enable, facilitate, allow, let, permit,* or similar verbs followed by the word *patient*. These verbs indicate what the nurse hopes to accomplish, not what the patient will do.

Attainable (Achievable)

The goal is appropriate for the individual patient. The single action to be measured is realistic and one that the patient can complete based on the patient's physical, emotional, and psychologic capabilities and limitations (e.g., finances, equipment, family support, and social services). For example:

- Walking a mile would not be achievable for an end-stage COPD patient (20 feet might be more realistic).
- A 2-year-old would not be able to give her own insulin.
- A 24-year-old could identify foods high in salt content.
- A 68-year-old could discuss nitroglycerin.

Relevant

The goal is applicable to the individual patient. The attainable single action to be measured has a purpose that has been customized for the patient based on the needs of the individual. For example, typically:

- A patient on bedrest would not need a goal about walking.
- A nondiabetic patient does not need to know about insulin injections.
- An ordinary teenager does not need to watch his salt intake.
- A 22-year-old patient without angina does not need to know about nitroglycerin.

Time Limited

The goal has a specific time frame and deadline for the goal to be achieved. During this time period, the nurse evaluates the patient's progress in achieving the goal. **Evaluation** is a planned activity in which patients and HCPs examine the patient's progress. Evaluation may serve as motivation for the patient to continue working to achieve the goal. The time frame is specific to date and hours, days, weeks, or months. For example:

- 3/2 at 0800
- In two months, starting 6/2
- Four hours from 1330
- 6/24 in the morning.

Putting all the SMART components together in the previous examples results in the following appropriate goals:

- The patient will walk 20 feet down the hall using a walker by 3/3 at 0800.
- The patient will demonstrate giving herself an insulin injection using aseptic technique by discharge.
- The patient will identify six foods to avoid that are high in salt content in 4 hours from 1330.
- The patient will state the purpose of his new medication, nitroglycerin, and when and how to take it by discharge.

See **Table 36.13** >> for examples of goals written in SMART format.

TABLE 36.13 SMART Format

Specific, Single Action	Measurable (Quantifiable, Determines How Often)	Appropriate for Patient	Realistic and Attainable for Patient	Time Frame for Patient to Reach Goal
Patient will drink	2500 mL of fluids daily	Ask yourself "Is this goal appropriate for this specific patient?"	Ask yourself "Is this goal realistic and attainable for this specific patient?"	by ________ (time, date)
Patient will administer	correct insulin dose using aseptic technique			by day of discharge
Patient will list	three hazards of smoking			by ________ (time, date)
Patient will walk	30 feet down the hall with his cane			by day of discharge
Patient's right ankle will measure	less than 10 inches in circumference			in 48 hours from ________ (time, date)
Patient will identify	five foods that are allowed on a low-salt diet			by ________ (time, date)

The nurse writes the goal statement in the format of subject, verb, goal, and time limit. The *subject* in the goal statement is the patient. The *verb* is the specific action the patient is to perform that can be observed. The *goal* is the patient and nurse's intended achievement, and the *time limit* determines by when the goal should be accomplished. Examples of action verbs include:

apply	discuss	select
change	drink	sit
demonstrate	explain	state
describe	inject	verbalize
differentiate	prepare	walk

Make sure the patient considers the goals important and valuable. Patients are motivated if goals are associated with personal meaning. The nurse should assess the patient's motivation to achieve goals or make behavioral changes. Some patients may know what they wish to accomplish with regard to their health problem; others may not be aware of their possible health goals. The nurse must actively listen to the patient to determine the individual's personal values and goals in relation to current health concerns. Patients are usually motivated and expend the necessary energy to reach goals they consider important.

Case Study » Part 3

Nurse Park has formulated this diagnostic statement to be the top priority for Mrs. Kher based on the assessment cluster of significant cues: *inadequate airway clearing ability* related to accumulated mucus obstructing airways (secondary to pneumonia). She is now ready to collaborate with Mrs. Kher to establish a goal. The following reasoning is part of this discussion:

- Mrs. Kher hasn't been drinking much lately, so her mucus is thick and hard to expel.
- She has inspiratory rhonchi with diminished breath sounds in the right lung, which indicate partial obstructions from the thickened mucus in her airways.
- Because Mrs. Kher has increased mucus production from the infection in her lungs, she is experiencing impairment in gas exchange, which results in her intolerance to activities and shortness of breath.
- Because she is breathing faster, she is using more energy to breathe.
- Mrs. Kher is experiencing general fatigue as her body fights the lung infection.

Nurse Park helps Mrs. Kher understand that many of her problems are a result of the amount and type of mucus in her airways from the lung infection. Nurse Park further explains the importance of liquefying the mucus so she can cough more effectively and help clear her airways. Together, they decide on a goal: "The patient will drink 3000 mL of fluids daily by 8/12." Both are satisfied that Mrs. Kher can reach this goal within the time frame. Now that the goal has been identified, they begin thinking about interventions that can help her reach her goal.

Clinical Reasoning Questions Level I

1. What role did the critical thinking skill of reasoning play in the discussion between Nurse Park and Mrs. Kher?
2. Identify the different components of the SMART format in the goal they created together.

Clinical Reasoning Questions Level II

3. Why does Nurse Park include Mrs. Kher in deciding what the goal will be instead of just letting her know she needs to drink more every day?
4. If Mrs. Kher did not feel she could drink 3000 mL of fluids daily, what other goal would you suggest based on the information provided in the case study?

Implementation

Implementation is the action phase of the nursing process. In this phase, nurses take all the data acquired in the first three phases of the nursing process and determine interventions that would be most appropriate to help the patient reach the goal stated in the planning phase. Interventions provide data that will be used during the evaluation phase to determine patient outcomes. Implementation is a two-step process. The first step is identifying the best priority interventions for an individual patient, and the second step is the implementation of these interventions.

Nursing Interventions

Interventions include nursing actions, delegation of tasks, and documentation completed to help the patient achieve the goal based on the nursing diagnosis. These actions are listed in priority order (see Exemplar 36.C, Prioritizing Care, in this module for further information). Nursing interventions focus on:

- Assessing for changes in the patient's status
- Preventing complications

- Reducing risk factors
- Treating through teaching and providing physical care
- Improving health through health promotion and achieving higher levels of wellness.

Correct identification of the etiology during the assessment and nursing diagnosis phases provides the framework for choosing successful nursing interventions. For example, the diagnostic label *Activity intolerance* may have several etiologies: pain, weakness, sedentary lifestyle, anxiety, or cardiac arrhythmias. Interventions will vary according to the cause of the problem. Sometimes nursing actions treat the patient's response to a disease, illness, or medical condition. Interventions for risk nursing diagnoses focus on measures to reduce the patient's risk factors found in the etiology of the risk nursing diagnosis. **Table 36.14** ›› shows examples of typical nursing interventions based on the nursing diagnosis and its etiology.

Types of Nursing Interventions

Nursing interventions include both direct and indirect care. Direct care is an intervention performed through interaction with the patient. Indirect care is an intervention performed away from, but on behalf of, the patient. Attending an interprofessional meeting and managing the care environment are two examples of indirect care. Nursing interventions are classified as independent, or nurse initiated; dependent, or physician initiated; and collaborative, or involving other providers (e.g., physical therapist) involved in the patient's treatments.

Independent interventions are those activities that nurses are licensed to do within their scope of practice; in other words, areas of healthcare that are unique to nursing and separate and distinct from medical management. These interventions include physical care, ongoing assessment, emotional support and comfort, teaching, counseling, environmental management, and making referrals to other healthcare professionals. For example, most patients with a nursing diagnosis of pain have medical orders for analgesics, but many independent nursing interventions also can alleviate pain (e.g., guided imagery, teaching a patient to "splint" an incision using a pillow). Recall that many nursing diagnoses are patient problems that can be treated primarily by independent nursing interventions. In performing an autonomous activity, the nurse determines that the patient requires certain nursing interventions. The nurse either carries these out or delegates them to other nursing personnel and is accountable or responsible for the decision and the actions (see Module 42, Accountability, for further information). An example of an independent action is planning and providing special mouth care for a patient after diagnosing impaired oral mucous membranes.

Collaborative interventions encompass **dependent interventions** employed by the nurse under a physician's orders, under supervision, or according to specified routines and protocols, as well as actions the nurse carries out in collaboration with other healthcare team members, such as physical therapists, social workers, dietitians, and physicians. Collaborative nursing activities reflect the overlapping responsibilities of, and cooperative relationships among, healthcare personnel and demonstrate the benefits of multidisciplinary patient care. For example, the physician might order physical therapy to teach the patient crutch-walking. The nurse would be responsible for informing the physical therapy department and for coordinating the patient's care to include the physical therapy sessions. When the patient returns to the nursing unit, the nurse would assist with crutch-walking and collaborate with the physical therapist to evaluate the patient's progress.

Healthcare providers' prescriptions commonly direct nurses to provide medications, IV therapy, diagnostic tests, diet, and activity for patients. The nurse is responsible for assessing the need for, explaining, and administering medical orders. Nursing interventions should be written to customize the medical order based on the individual patient. For example, instead of writing "Administer NSAID as ordered" as an intervention, the nurse can write "Give ketorolac 15 mg IV every 6 hours prn pain × 5 days as prescribed by physician."

The amount of time the nurse spends in an independent versus a collaborative or dependent role varies according to the clinical area, type of facility, and specific position of the nurse.

Considerations When Selecting Interventions

Usually several potential interventions can be identified for each nursing goal. The nurse's task is to select those that are most likely to achieve the desired patient outcomes. There is also a need to prioritize potential interventions and include the patient's input. Weighing the pros and cons of each intervention can help the nurse make these decisions. For example, "Provide accurate information about diabetes" as an intervention could result in any one of the following patient responses:

- Increased anxiety
- Decreased anxiety
- Wish to talk with the primary care provider
- Desire to leave the hospital
- Relaxation.

TABLE 36.14 Examples of Typical Nursing Interventions Based on Nursing Diagnosis and Etiology

Type of Nursing Diagnosis	Etiology	Nursing Interventions
Problem focused	*Acute pain* related to surgical site	■ Assess pain level using a pain rating scale of 0–10 at frequent intervals. ■ Give ketorolac 15 mg IV every 6 hours prn pain × 5 days.
Risk	*Potential for falling* related to use of walker	■ Assess ability to move when using the walker. ■ Keep area from bed to bathroom free from clutter.
Health promotion	*Ready to improve parenting* related to newborn in the home	■ Assess parents' feelings of impact of having a newborn in the home. ■ Discuss infant stimulation techniques with both parents.

TABLE 36.15 Examples of Priority Nursing Interventions

Nursing Interventions	Rationale
Nursing Diagnosis: *Inadequate airway clearing ability* related to viscous secretions and shallow chest expansion secondary to pneumonia	
Monitor respiratory status q4h: rate, depth, effort, skin color, mucous membranes, lung sounds, amount and color of sputum, and sensorium.	To identify progress toward or away from goal (i.e., pallor, cyanosis, lethargy, and drowsiness).
Monitor vital signs q4h: temperature, pulse, respiratory rate, blood pressure, and oxygen saturation.	To identify changes in vital signs, which may indicate changes in the patient's condition.
Administer oxygen at 2 L/min via nasal cannula as prescribed by physician.	Supplemental oxygen makes more oxygen available to the cells, which reduces the work of breathing.
Maintain in Fowler or semi-Fowler position.	Gravity allows for fuller lung expansion by decreasing pressure of abdomen on diaphragm.
Administer prescribed antibiotic to maintain therapeutic blood level.	Resolves infection by bactericidal effect.
Administer prescribed expectorant.	Helps loosen secretions so they can be coughed up and expelled.
Administer prescribed analgesic.	Controls pleuritic pain, enabling patient to increase thoracic expansion.
Encourage fluids by mouth (except when contraindicated by medical conditions such as cardiovascular or renal problems).	Helps liquefy the mucus, making it easier to cough up and expel.
Instruct in breathing and coughing techniques. Remind patient to perform, and assist as needed q2–3h.	To enable patient to cough up secretions.

Determining the pros and cons of each intervention requires nursing knowledge and experience. For example, the nurse's experience may suggest that providing information the night before the patient's surgery may increase the patient's worry and tension, whereas maintaining the usual rituals before sleep is more effective. The nurse might then consider providing the information several days before surgery. See examples of priority nursing interventions for the patient in **Table 36.15** ».

The following guidelines can help the nurse choose the most appropriate priority nursing interventions to support patients in reaching their goal. Interventions need to be:

- Safe and appropriate for the individual patient's age, health, and condition (see the Lifespan Considerations feature).
- Achievable with the resources available. For example, a home care nurse might wish to include an intervention for an older adult patient to "check blood glucose daily," but in order for that to occur the patient must have intact sight, cognition, and memory to carry this out independently, or daily visits from a home care nurse must be available and affordable.
- Congruent with the patient's values, beliefs, and culture (see Module 24, Culture and Diversity).
- Congruent with other therapies (e.g., if the patient is not permitted food, the strategy of an evening snack must be deferred until health permits).
- Based on current best nursing research evidence.
- Within established standards of care as determined by state laws, professional associations (e.g., ANA), and the policies of the facility. Many agencies have policies to guide the activities of health professionals and to safeguard patients. For example, there may be policies for visiting hours and procedures to follow for the patient who has had a cardiac arrest.

Writing a Nursing Intervention

After choosing the best priority nursing interventions, the nurse writes them in the patient's nursing plan of care. Interventions are dated when they are written and then reviewed regularly. Common characteristics of nursing interventions include that they:

- Are patient centered
- Have a specific and concise single action
- Include detailed information about the action (i.e., when, how, time, and where)
- Are realistic for the individual patient
- Are relevant to helping the patient reach goal set in planning phase.

Only the top three to five priority interventions are usually listed for each nursing diagnosis (instead of the six to ten that could be listed). Nursing students often include a rationale for each selected intervention as they are learning about nursing actions expected with patient conditions and diseases. The table below shows examples of poorly and correctly written interventions:

Poorly Written Intervention	Correctly Written Intervention
Tell the patient about insulin.	Explain to the patient the actions of insulin.
Assess edema of left ankle daily.	Measure and record patient's left ankle circumference daily at 0800.
Apply dressing to left leg.	Change spiral dressing to left leg every shift as needed.
Give pain medication as needed.	Give acetaminophen 325 mg/oxycodone 5 mg 1 tablet PO 30 minutes prior to going to physical therapy and every 6 hours prn per physician order.

The Process of Implementation

Implementation refers to doing the actions in the interventions. The process of implementation commonly includes the following:

- Preassessment of the patient
- Determining the nurse's need for assistance
- Implementing the nursing interventions
- Supervising any delegated care
- Documenting nursing actions.

Preassessment of the Patient

Just before implementing an intervention, the nurse must reassess the patient to make sure the intervention is still needed and appropriate because the patient's condition may have changed. For example, a patient experiences sleep disturbance related to anxiety and unfamiliar surroundings. During rounds, the nurse discovers that the patient is sleeping; the nurse decides to defer the back massage intervention that had been planned as a relaxation strategy.

New data may indicate a need to change the priorities of care or the nursing activities. For example, a nurse begins to teach a patient who has diabetes how to give himself insulin injections. Shortly after beginning the teaching, the nurse realizes that the patient is not concentrating on the lesson. Subsequent discussion reveals that he is worried about his eyesight and fears he is going blind. Realizing that the patient's level of stress is interfering with his learning, the nurse ends the lesson and arranges for a primary care provider to examine the patient's eyes. The nurse also provides supportive communication to help alleviate the patient's stress.

Determining the Nurse's Need for Assistance

When implementing some nursing interventions, the nurse may require assistance for one or more of the following reasons:

- The nurse is unable to implement the nursing activity safely or efficiently alone (e.g., ambulating a patient who is obese and needs assistance).
- Assistance would reduce stress on the patient (e.g., turning an individual who experiences acute pain when moved).
- The nurse lacks the knowledge or skills to implement a particular nursing activity (e.g., a nurse who is not familiar with a particular type of orthopedic traction equipment needs assistance the first time turning the patient).

Implementing Nursing Interventions

Before beginning implementation, explain to the patient what interventions will be done, what sensations to expect, what the patient is expected to do, and the purpose of the intervention. For many nursing activities, it is important to ensure the patient's privacy by closing doors, pulling curtains, or draping the patient. The number and types of direct nursing interventions are almost unlimited and include coordination of patient care. Interventions involve scheduling patient contacts with other HCPs (e.g., laboratory and x-ray technicians, physical and respiratory therapists) and serving as a liaison among the members of the healthcare team.

When implementing interventions, nurses should follow these guidelines:

- ***Support nursing interventions with scientific evidence, the body of nursing literature, research, and professional standards.*** The nurse is responsible for understanding the rationale for interventions. A patient admitted with a peptic ulcer wants to chew an enteric-coated medication. The nurse knows that the enteric coating is present to protect the stomach lining from erosion and chewing removes that protective barrier. It is necessary for the nurse to provide the scientific reason for the enteric coating to explain to the patient why the practice of chewing that medication is not acceptable.
- ***Understand how and why to implement an intervention, its possible consequences, and to clarify or question anything that is not clear prior to implementing the intervention.*** The nurse cannot blindly follow orders and protocols. The nurse must fully understand interventions ordered by physicians and those indicated by protocols or order sets. The rationale or indications for interventions must be clear to the nurse, as should any contraindications that would affect the implementation of an order. It is the nurse's responsibility to question interventions that may be inappropriate as well as those that are unfamiliar.
- ***Customize interventions to suit the individual patient's needs.*** The patient's health status is directly affected by environmental factors, belief systems, and personal characteristics. Age, developmental stage, cognitive and physical ability, relationships, and resources are a few examples of factors that can influence the patient's health. The nurse understands the medical diagnosis of a patient but focuses holistically on the individual when carrying out interventions.
- ***Keep safety as the primary focus of all nursing interventions.*** Safe practice involves preventing complications, adverse events, or injuries while providing care. The Joint Commission (2020) provides a list of National Patient Safety Goals each year to focus on safety issues in healthcare and help improve safety. Examples of practices that can improve patient care and nursing interventions include excellent communication among patient care staff, safe medication administration, consistent patient identification, infection prevention, and the safe use of alarms in the clinical setting.
- ***Teach, support, and comfort the patient before, during, and after interventions.*** Patient consent and participation are integral to the effective implementation of interventions. The nurse provides intervention-specific teaching to support the autonomy of the patient and gives support and comfort throughout interventions.
- ***Respect the sociocultural experiences, ethnicity, and religious beliefs of the patient.*** Nursing care is holistic. Patients are more than physical beings and the nurse should always be mindful of all factors that make every human unique. Caring for the whole person means paying attention to preferences, beliefs, practices, and other aspects of life that are valuable to the patient. One example of holistic care involves observing the religious practices of a patient and planning rounds and treatments around designated prayer times.

- ***Protect the patient's dignity and build self-confidence and autonomy.*** Patients have a right to privacy and to be treated with dignity. Nurses advocate for patients' rights to be partners in their healthcare by empowering them to participate in decision making in developmentally appropriate ways.
- ***Empower the patient with opportunities to participate in implementing care.*** Patients who actively take part in healthcare are more likely to gain the ability to care for themselves. The nurse provides teaching and demonstrations and allows the patient to demonstrate both the willingness to be involved in care and the ability to take part. It is important for the nurse to perform appropriate learning assessments, identifying physical, cognitive, and developmental barriers to care and provide education on the appropriate level. Nurses must also understand that degrees of pain, severity of the problem, and cultural and psychosocial issues such as fear may affect the patient's ability to actively participate in care.

Delegation

Delegating patient care and assigning tasks are important responsibilities for registered nurses (RNs) because healthcare facilities use licensed practical nurses (LPNs) and many UAPs. To delegate appropriately, the nurse must match the needs of the patient and family with the scope of practice of the available caregivers. The RN remains responsible for making sure delegated tasks are carried out properly. Many states clearly outline the rules of delegation within various nurse practice acts.

The nurse is not expected to perform all patient care alone. The RN must learn to work interprofessionally with members of the healthcare team. That includes delegating tasks to the appropriate personnel. Delegation is a skill that requires practice and competence. The nurse must determine if the skill or task is within the scope of practice of the team member (e.g., UAP, tech, licensed vocational nurse). If the task does not require a registered nurse license or licensed HCP, the nurse selects the correct person for the task. Clear communication is key to delegating tasks and the RN must assess to ensure that the task was carried out correctly, providing feedback as needed (Texas Board of Nursing, n.d.-a). Registered nurses cannot delegate nursing assessment, the analysis of patient data, establishing or changing the plan of care, or the evaluation of patient responses to treatments (see Module 39, Managing Care, for further information).

Documentation

Nursing interventions must be accurately documented after completion. The documentation must include the procedure, timing, technique, teaching, and patient responses. The medical record serves as a resource for patient assessment and history, a database of critical patient information, a communication tool between nurses and others on the healthcare collaborative team, and legal record of nursing and interprofessional patient care. Even verbal communication needs to be documented and acknowledged.

Critical Implementation Skills

Successful implementation of nursing interventions requires knowledge, skills (technical), and attitudes (KSAs) to meet the task. Knowledge is a cognitive skill involving learned facts and evidence to support interventions. Technical skills are gained through the demonstration of hands-on competency and deliberate practice of properly performed interventions. Attitudes are the interpersonal abilities needed to perform patient teaching and effective communication and to provide comfort and protect the privacy and dignity of the patient. Consider the intervention of changing the dressing on a central line. The nurse has knowledge of the requirement of maintaining a sterile field, demonstrates competency in the steps of the actual procedure, and provides reassurance and teaching to the patient while protecting patient safety and privacy by asking visitors to exit during the intervention.

Cognitive skills include the processes involved in decision making, including the ability to critically think and creatively solve problems. Cognitive skills require knowledge, memory, reasoning, and attentiveness.

Interpersonal skills are critical to nursing communication and include both verbal and nonverbal cues. The most technically skilled nurse must expertly communicate or risk creating distress and mistrust among patients and family members. Interpersonal skills require emotional intelligence and are required for building both patient and professional relationships. The nurse who is competent in the domain of interpersonal skills is self-aware, reflective, respectful, and genuinely interested in the lifestyles, beliefs, values, and cultural and ethnic differences among fellow healthcare professionals and patient populations.

Technical skills are also known as procedural or psychomotor skills and include the practice-oriented, tactile skills performed in patient care. These skills include but are not limited to dressing changes, equipment use, venous access initiation, sterile procedures, and other direct patient-care interventions. Procedural interventions require knowledge of steps and safeguards in addition to the actual physical coordination and dexterity needed to competently perform the tasks. Technical skills must be properly taught, demonstrated, and correctly practiced to gain precision and reduce the likelihood of patient injury or nursing error. The number of technical skills the nurse is responsible for performing depends on the policies and procedures at each facility.

Relationship to Other Nursing Process Phases

To determine which intervention to implement, the nurse must first perform an assessment by recognizing specific patient cues, determine an appropriate diagnosis through analysis of the assessment cues, and prioritize a plan for the patient. The implementation phase involves the generation of solutions and actions taken to solve the problems faced by the patient. Patient responses to nursing actions are examined in the last phase of the nursing process, evaluation.

Case Study » Part 4

The goal for Mrs. Kher is "The patient will drink 3000 mL of fluids daily by 8/12." Nurse Park and Mrs. Kher are now discussing interventions that will help her reach her goal. Here is the list of potential interventions they have come up with:

- Measure and document intake and output every shift.
- Perform postural drainage daily.
- Record daily weights.

- Encourage Mrs. Kher to drink a variety of beverages so she does not get bored with water.
- Have Mrs. Kher's favorite beverages available so she can drink them frequently.
- Do coughing and deep-breathing exercises every 2 hours.
- Have Mrs. Kher's favorite snacks readily available.
- Assess sputum for consistency, color, amount, and odor.

Nurse Park explains to Mrs. Kher that they need to select the top four priorities from this list to add to her plan of care. She further explains the importance of assessment to measure progress toward reaching the goal. Together, they decide these are the top four priorities:

- Measure and document intake and output every shift.
- Perform postural drainage daily.
- Have Mrs. Kher's favorite beverages available so she can drink them frequently.
- Do coughing and deep-breathing exercises every 2 hours.

Clinical Reasoning Questions Level I

1. What is the importance of conducting an assessment before performing any interventions?
2. Would you have selected other interventions for Mrs. Kher? If so, what are they and why would you have selected them?

Clinical Reasoning Questions Level II

3. Which of the interventions listed are independent interventions nurses can do without physician orders?
4. Why do you think assessment of the sputum for consistency, color, amount, and odor was not selected as an intervention specific to helping Mrs. Kher reach her goal?

Evaluation

Every nursing intervention requires appropriate evaluation to determine the effectiveness or need for further actions. Evaluation is the planned, continuous, intentional reassessment of cues to accomplish two primary purposes. First, the nurse evaluates to determine whether the intervention helped the patient make progress toward goals. Second, the nurse evaluates the effectiveness of the action taken as it relates to the plan of care. The evaluation phase allows the nurse to determine if the plan of care is appropriate and whether it needs to be advanced, changed, or maintained. Patients and their support persons are integral to the evaluation of care as their feedback and participation are key indicators of the quality and effectiveness of interventions.

Evaluation is ongoing until the patient achieves goals of care or has reached an optimal state of well-being within realistic limitations and is released from nursing care. Evaluation is a planned and deliberate activity that occurs during, immediately after, or at time intervals after an intervention takes place. For example, a home health nurse may evaluate a patient's ability to ambulate on a weekly basis to determine progress made in therapy. In the acute care setting, the nurse administering an intravenous medication to lower blood pressure evaluates the patient's blood pressure during the administration, immediately after administration, and at regular intervals for a period time. As a patient is discharged from nursing care, a discharge nurse completes a broad evaluation and considers cues that indicate whether the patient achieved goals within the plan of care. The nurse must also evaluate to determine the patient's ability to perform self-care and participate in a follow-up plan for HCP office visits and therapy. The outcomes of each of these evaluations are documented in the patient's medical record as it is noted that the patient *met*, *partially met*, or *did not meet goals*.

Evaluation is the phase in which the nurse closes the loop on decisions made while providing patient care. The nurse knows that it is important to take ownership of interventions, even when the evaluation determines that the outcome was not what was intended or desired. Nurses who perform competent evaluations demonstrate accountability and take responsibility for the outcomes of their actions. An intervention is a single factor in the scope of patient care. Therefore, professionals should not assume that a positive evaluation is an indicator of an action being the sole factor in a patient's progress.

Clinical Example D

Ruth Horowitz, a patient with obesity, needed to lose 14 kg (30 lb). When the nurse and Mrs. Horowitz drew up a plan of care, one goal was "Lose 1.4 kg (3 lb) in 4 weeks." A nursing intervention listed in the plan of care was "Explain how to plan and prepare a 1200-calorie diet." Four weeks later, Mrs. Horowitz weighed herself and had lost 1.8 kg (4 lb). The goal had been met—in fact, exceeded. It is easy to assume that the nursing intervention was highly effective. However, it is important to collect more data before drawing that conclusion. On questioning Mrs. Horowitz, the nurse might find any of the following: (a) She planned a 1200-calorie diet and prepared and ate the food; (b) she planned a 1200-calorie diet but did not prepare the correct food; or (c) she did not understand how to plan a 1200-calorie diet so she did not bother with it.

If the first possibility is found to be true, the nurse can safely judge that the nursing intervention "Explain how to plan and prepare a 1200-calorie diet" was effective in helping Mrs. Horowitz lose weight. However, if the nurse learns that either the second or third possibility actually happened, then it must be assumed that the nursing strategy did not affect the outcome. The next step for the nurse is to collect data about what Mrs. Horowitz actually did to lose weight. It is important to establish the relationship (or lack thereof) of the nursing actions to the patient responses.

Critical Thinking Questions

1. How might a nurse explain how to plan and prepare a 1200-calorie diet?
2. If a SMART goal is specific, measurable, attainable, realistic, and time limited, then how do these criteria apply to the statement that "Ruth Horowitz, a patient with obesity, needs to lose 14 kg (30 lb)"?
3. If Ruth did not prepare the correct food, should the goal be explained more practically, revised, or abandoned?
4. What questions should the nurse ask to determine how Ruth lost weight if she did not follow her diet plan?
5. If Ruth did not understand how to plan and prepare the 1200-calorie diet, what should the nurse do first to determine how to better explain the practical steps involved?
6. What are potential indications that the problem might be Ruth's attitude and not her intellectual understanding of the practical issues involved in the 1200-calorie diet?

Source: Adapted from Berman et al. (2021).

Drawing Conclusions

Clinical judgment helps the nurse determine if the plan of care was an effective approach to treat, lessen, or prevent the development of various nursing diagnoses. While evaluating the overall plan of care, the nurse draws one of the following conclusions:

- The patient's actual problem as stated in the nursing diagnosis has been resolved, or the risks for a problem have been eliminated. Upon resolution of the problem or elimination of the risk factors, the nurse notes that the goals of care have been met. Once the goals are met, the nurse no longer focuses care on that nursing diagnosis or problem.
- The patient still has risk factors for a potential problem. The actual nursing diagnosis is prevented, but a risk diagnosis is still needed. In this situation, the nurse continues to document on this problem and the risk diagnosis remains in the plan of care.
- The problem at the focus of the patient's actual nursing diagnosis persists, although some progress is made. For example, in a patient with impaired airway clearance ability, a goal in the plan of care is "Oxygen saturation will remain above 95% on room air." The patient's oxygen saturation may be 96% on room air, but wheezing and coughing can still be heard. Therefore, the patient is still showing signs of impaired airway clearance. Therefore, the nurse must continue to implement care related to the airway. This evaluation of the nursing diagnosis would be documented as a goal that is in progress or partially met.

When goals of care are not met or partially met, the nurse draws one of two conclusions:

- The nurse may need to revise the plan of care. In this case, the process of decision making starts back at square one, with assessment. During the analysis of cues from the assessment, a new diagnosis may be formulated and a new plan and implementations are determined.

OR

- The nurse may recognize that the patient simply needs time and further intervention to achieve goals. At this time, the nurse will need to evaluate patient cues to determine if the partially met goals are moving the patient in the desired direction. It could be that the evaluation was completed too early for measurable progress to be made. The nurse needs to apply clinical reasoning and judgment to determine why the goal was only partially met. It could be that progress is expected to be slow or that the patient is having difficulty adhering to the treatment.

Developing an Evaluation

Objective and subjective data help the nurse draw conclusions. Objective data is verifiable, measurable, fact-based information (e.g., urine output is 42 mL per hour, respiratory rate is 18 breaths/min, blood pressure 135/90 mmHg). Subjective data is qualitative and subject to opinion or experience (e.g., the patient states, "I feel better," "This food is terrible," or "My pain is worse"). Assessment cues, or data, whether objective or subjective, are important and need to be accurately documented in the medical record.

When evaluating whether a patient has achieved the goals within a plan of care or if the goal of an action was achieved, the nurse simply needs to ask if the patient's response to an intervention aligns with the purpose of the action.

1. A goal was met if the response to an intervention matched or fulfilled the goal.
2. A goal was partially met if the response did not achieve the purpose of the goal but only more time was needed to make more progress.
3. The goal was not met if the patient did not achieve the desired outcome within the desired time.

Writing an Evaluation

An **evaluation statement** must be written to document if goals were met, partially met, or not met. The evaluation may be documented in the plan of care, in narrative notes within the patient assessment, or in another designated area in the medical record and should contain these elements:

- Date and time of the evaluation
- Whether the goal was met, partially met, or not met
- Evidence to support the conclusion (e.g., subjective and objective assessment data).

The table below outlines sample statements of evaluation:

Date and Time of Evaluation	Conclusion Statement	Supporting Statement
12/3, 1345	Goal met.	Patient walked with cane 20 feet down hallway.
9/22, 0900	Goal partially met.	Patient is able to identify three foods instead of five foods high in sugar content.
5/14, 1030	Goal not met.	Patient did not change the dressing on his right arm using aseptic technique.

Continuing, Modifying, or Terminating the Nursing Plan of Care

The nursing plan of care is updated once a goal is met. Updates or changes to the plan of care will look different depending on the facility's documentation system. The important point is to realize that a goal that has been met no longer requires nursing care. When a goal is met, the nurse must make a decision about refocusing on a new problem area or continuing to work on other goals in the care plan. Regardless of the status of the goals (met, partially met, not met), the nurse makes decisions to continue, modify, or terminate care for each diagnosis. See **Table 36.16** » to guide care plan review. The list uses closed-ended questions to help the nurse recognize cues that require further actions.

It is possible that a plan of care was not appropriate for a patient. A situation like this requires a complete review of the existing plan, which is accomplished through a step-by-step application of the nursing process, beginning with assessment. Once the nurse has a current set of data and analyzes the salient cues, the nurse updates the priority nursing diagnoses and begins revising patient goals.

Revising Patient Goals

During reassessment of the patient, the nurse confirms if the initial assessment data and the nursing care priorities

TABLE 36.16 Evaluation Checklist

Phase of Nursing Process	Checklist
Assessment	_______ Are data complete, accurate, and validated?
	_______ Do new data require changes in the care plan?
Diagnosis	_______ Are nursing diagnoses relevant and accurate?
	_______ Are nursing diagnoses supported by the data?
	_______ Has problem status changed (i.e., potential, actual, risk)?
	_______ Are the diagnoses stated clearly and in the correct format?
	_______ Have any nursing diagnoses been resolved?
Planning	***Desired Outcomes***
	_______ Do new nursing diagnoses require new goals?
	_______ Are goals realistic?
	_______ Was enough time allowed for goal achievement?
	_______ Do the goals address all aspects of the problem?
	_______ Does the patient still concur with the goals?
	_______ Have patient priorities changed?
	Nursing Interventions
	_______ Do nursing interventions need to be written for new nursing diagnoses or new goals?
	_______ Do the nursing interventions seem to be related to the stated goals?
	_______ Is there a rationale to justify each nursing diagnosis?
	_______ Are the nursing interventions clear, specific, and detailed?
	_______ Are new resources available?
	_______ Do the nursing interventions address all aspects of the patient's goals?
	_______ Were the nursing interventions actually carried out?
Implementation	_______ Was patient input obtained at each step of the nursing process?
	_______ Were goals and nursing interventions acceptable to the patient?
	_______ Did the caregivers have the knowledge and skill to perform the interventions correctly?
	_______ Were explanations given to the patient prior to implementing?

that were based on the assessment were accurate. If the data were accurate and the patient is not meeting goals, the nurse should determine whether they need revision or if patient priorities have changed. Another important consideration is whether the patient is in agreement with the plan. While revising the plan of care, the nurse establishes new goals for all new diagnoses.

Selecting New Nursing Interventions

Perhaps the reason for a patient not achieving goals of care was due to the interventions that were implemented. Poorly prioritized or inappropriate interventions will not yield desired outcomes and can actually hinder patient progress. Or perhaps the patient has improved in another area, changing the needs and reprioritizing interventions. The nurse must select and implement new interventions in response to patient status changes.

Method of Implementation

While analyzing the plan of care using the nursing process to frame the investigation, the nurse may find that all aspects of the plan are appropriate. In this case, the nurse considers the methods for implementing interventions and whether all interventions were actually completed. Medications given at wrong times, the lack of staffing or resources to carry out orders, or errors could lead to missed interventions. Before modifying the plan of care, the nurse must ensure that the necessary interventions were carried out appropriately and if interventions were not realistic for the patient, facility, or caregivers due to issues involving resources, staffing, and time.

Using the nursing process to modify the plan of care results in the implementation of the new plan and the systematic evaluation of nursing care continues. Refer to **Table 36.17** » for examples of a systematic evaluation of the plan of care. Revisions to the care plan are italicized. In this example, the nurse is not only evaluating the patient's responses but also evaluating the nursing care given (see Module 50, Quality Improvement, for further information).

Relationship to Other Nursing Process Phases

Successful evaluation depends on the effectiveness of the phases that precede it. Assessment data must be accurate and complete so that the nurse can formulate appropriate nursing diagnoses and desired goals. The goals must be stated concretely to be useful for evaluating patient responses. And finally, without the implementing phase in which the plan is put into action, there would be nothing to evaluate.

The evaluation phase includes assessment. As previously stated, assessment (data collection) is ongoing and continuous at every patient contact. However, data are collected for different purposes at different points in the nursing process. During the assessment phase, the nurse collects data for the purpose of making diagnoses. During the evaluation phase,

TABLE 36.17 Example of Plan of Care Evaluation

Planned Outcomes	Goals with Judgment Statements	Nursing Interventions	Nursing Interventions with Notes
Nursing Diagnosis: ***Impaired airway clearance ability*** **related to nonproductive cough with thick mucus and poor respiratory effort secondary to decreased fluid volume, pain, and fatigue**			
Oxygenation–pulmonary status: effective gas exchange as evidenced by:			*Continue nursing interventions and assess for progress. Problem remains unresolved.*
■ Skin and mucous membrane free from pallor and cyanosis	Goal partially met. Absence of cyanosis. Skin remains pale.	Assess respiratory status every 2 hours: Skin and mucous membrane color, respiratory rate, effort, depth, sputum (amount, quality, and color).	
■ Improved respiratory effort with use of incentive spirometer and flutter valve breathing device as instructed	Partially met. Demonstrates appropriate flutter valve use but only uses incentive spirometer when pain is well controlled.	Continue to analyze ABG results, chest imaging, continuous pulse oximetry, volume of incentive spirometry, and frequency flutter valve breathing device with quality of cough.	
■ Productive cough	Met. Use of flutter valve breathing device yields productive cough with copious amounts of thick, greenish mucus.	Continue to encourage use of flutter valve breathing device, assess pain, administer mucolytics as ordered with appropriate amounts of water	
■ Lung sounds clear to auscultation within 72 hours of admission	Not met. Scattered rhonchi and wheezes auscultated throughout all lung fields.	Continue to assess vital signs every 4 hours, reassess lung sounds every 8 hours and PRN, encourage deep breathing	
■ Respiration rate 16–24/min; pulse rate <100 bpm	Met. Respirations 24/min, pulse 90 bpm.	Support and encourage progress in continued breathing and coughing techniques. Remind to continue to perform I/S at least every 3 hours. *(11/22/2020, RW)*	*Goal was met. Issue resolved. Patient still needs support due to adventitious lung sounds, intermittent pain, and fatigue.*
■ Incentive spirometer use reaching established volume of 600mL	Not met. Tidal volume 400 mL. *(Evaluated 2/22/2020 RW)*	Continue to encourage I/S use. Maintain semi- to high-Fowler position to encourage chest expansion and teach the importance of positioning at home. Administer mucolytic as ordered. Administer pain medications needed to encourage deep breathing. Administer antibiotic therapy and provide teaching for antibiotic timing and use at home. Administer oxygen, if needed, to maintain $PaO_2 > 94\%$. If needed, ensure portable O_2 is available for transporting.	*Patient is making some progress on I/S use. Will be ready to discharge home after pain, fever, and hydration status are controlled.*

Revisions to the care plan are *italicized*.

the nurse collects data for the purpose of comparing it to the goal developed in the planning phase and making decisions about the effectiveness of the nursing care.

Case Study » Part 5

It is 8/12 and time for Nurse Park and Mrs. Kher to evaluate whether she has reached her goal. The first day her intake was 3100 mL and output was 2600 mL; the second day her intake was 3050 mL and output was 2825 mL. Mrs. Kher is pleased that she was able to increase her intake of fluids to at least 3000 mL daily. Nurse Park was happy that she has reached her goal that supports the outcome "to restore an effective breathing pattern." The goal statement was "Goal met. Patient has consumed at least 3000 mL of liquids daily by 8/12."

Clinical Reasoning Questions Level I

1. Can you identify the different components in the goal statement?
2. How important is it for Nurse Park to give Mrs. Kher positive feedback on reaching her goal?

Clinical Reasoning Questions Level II

3. If Mrs. Kher was not able to reach her goal, what would be Nurse Park's next action?
4. Once a goal has been met successfully by the patient, what happens to this nursing diagnosis in the plan of care?

Lifespan Considerations

Applying the Nursing Process to Children

Assessment of a child is complex and can vary significantly depending on the child's chronologic age and developmental stage. Neonates and infants are not able to verbalize their complaints; therefore, collecting "subjective" data relies heavily on parents and caregivers; objective data are based on nursing observations, child–caregiver interactions, and physical assessment. Nevertheless, assessment of the child is a continuous process of collecting and developing a database of information. The nurse analyzes the data and develops accurate nursing diagnoses.

Data analysis supports a nursing diagnosis or diagnoses addressing the child's health-focused problem. Nursing diagnoses may also address risk problems that require interventions in order to decrease the risk of the child or family developing an actual problem. Furthermore, nurses must become familiar with the defining characteristics of diagnoses that address parenting, role conflict, and family processes and observe for cues that accurately support these diagnoses.

After developing nursing diagnoses, the nurse identifies a priority outcome that will be used to evaluate the pediatric patient's plan of care. A priority outcome states that (1) a healthcare problem does not exist and therefore health promotion is stressed; (2) a risk for health dysfunction is present that requires intervention to decrease or eliminate development of an actual problem; (3) an actual health-focused problem is present that requires interventions; or (4) the nurse identifies an outcome that addresses the child and the family's healthcare goals.

In addition to identifying an outcome to evaluate the plan of care, the nurse, the patient, and, when applicable, the patient's family develop a plan with patient goals that will evaluate the patient's response to nursing interventions. Once the nurse develops patient- or family-focused goals, the next step is to develop and implement planned interventions and assess feedback by observation or by communication with the patient, family, and other HCPs in order to determine the effectiveness of the interventions. The nurse ensures the child's physical and emotional safety and comfort while nurses or other HCPs perform interventions.

In the final step of the nursing process, the nurse evaluates data to determine that previously established goals and outcomes have been met and that nursing interventions were appropriate to the child's needs. If the goals have not been met, have been partially met, or have been met because of interventions not included in the plan of care, the nurse considers altering the plan of care, its goals, and its interventions.

Expected outcomes are not reviewed only during the child's hospitalization and at discharge but also at follow-up appointments with the child's pediatrician to evaluate for complete resolution of the actual health problem and, if applicable, the risk problem. School nurses and providers in daycare centers should also review expected outcomes for children with chronic diseases such as asthma, cystic fibrosis, diabetes, and other chronic diseases.

Clinical Example E

A 4-year-old girl is admitted following emergency surgery for a ruptured appendix. She is awake and alert but refuses to talk. Her parents have had little sleep for over 24 hours and are extremely anxious.

- Gathering assessment data in this situation requires the nurse to be sensitive to the parents' needs for rest and assurance; at the same time, the nurse must collect information to compile an adequate database that can be used to make appropriate nursing care decisions. Assessment will be problem focused, monitoring the condition of the child as she recovers from surgery and being alert to potential problems.
- Objective data collected include vital signs; level of and response to pain (often called the fifth vital sign); bleeding or discharge from the incision; mobility; integrity of dressings, intravenous lines, catheters, nasogastric tubes, or other medical devices; and affect.
- Because most children are a part of families, assessment will include observation of family dynamics and questions that could lead to care of the family system.

Critical Thinking Questions

1. What are the nursing priorities for the 4-year-old child?
2. What are the patient-centered outcomes for the child?
3. What might be an effective method of getting the patient to talk?
4. List three strategies that you would use to allay the parents' anxiety.
5. What objective data about the patient's parents is important for you to assess in relation to her care?

Source: From Berman et al. (2021). Pearson Education, Hoboken, NJ.

Applying the Nursing Process to Older Adults

Older adults make up the greater proportion of all hospital admissions. As the older adult population increases, so does the cultural diversity of this segment of the population (Administration for Community Living, 2019). Nurses are challenged to provide culturally sensitive care to the older population without cultural or age-related bias and assumptions.

In addition to acute care facilities, older adults function and seek care in various community settings. Nurses are involved in the care of older adults in patients' homes, nursing homes, adult daycare facilities, assisted-living communities, and various categories of subacute care facilities.

Assessment of the older adult in the acute care or community setting may be complex because of factors related to physical health, cognition, and functionality. However, the nurse should not assume that all older adults have poor memory or impaired functionality; that they all experience depression, social isolation, or financial hardship; or that all older adults are dependent individuals.

The older adult has the potential for a complex and lengthy assessment database as the nurse attempts to organize information that spans a lifetime. For the older adult who may have visual and auditory impairment, assistive devices such as glasses and hearing aids should be used in order to engage in conversation with the nurse and to respond to questions appropriately. Some older adults may respond to questions with slower but accurate answers. The nurse allows the patient time to respond and does not rush the patient or fill in answers based on assumptions about older adults. Some older adult patients may have less than adequate recall due to cognitive dysfunction, medication, or illness. Patients with previous admissions to an institution should have an established database of health-related information that is supplemented and updated with each new admission. Assessment of the older adult should include up-to-date assessment of each patient's strengths, limitations, and means of social support and factors that may change over short periods of time due to illness, change in functionality, and death of spouse or friends.

The nurse must be aware that changes in an older adult's mental status, often reported by family members or caregivers, may indicate an underlying illness. In many cases, older adults do not present with typical signs and symptoms associated with infections or other healthcare problems. An acute change in mental status of the older adult is a cue for a high level of suspicion for a focused health problem and the need for thorough assessment.

The nurse determines the patient's diagnosis or diagnoses based on subjective data and observations from family members and caregivers and from objective data, including observations, physical and cognitive exams, and test results. The nurse then identifies a priority outcome related to the patient's diagnosis and identifies short- and long-term goals that will be used to evaluate nursing interventions. Outcomes and goals for the older adult must be realistic, individualized, and within the realm of the patient's capability. As much as possible, older adult patients should be included when determining goals and interventions related to their care. Although care for every patient is individualized, common goals in caring for older adults revolve around learning needs related to chronic illnesses and medication regimens, safety concerns related to mobility and polypharmacy, and in some cases issues of physical and emotional safety related to caregiver mistreatment or socioeconomic well-being.

Once the nurse develops patient goals, the next step is to develop and implement planned interventions and assess feedback by observation or by communication in order to determine the effectiveness of the interventions. The nurse must take into consideration certain factors that prove challenging when developing interventions for some older adults, including the need for additional time, the patient's level of education and health literacy, the need to interact or teach the patient during the most energetic time of day, and the need to use everyday language. The nurse may consider using multiple teaching modes and creativity when educating older adults.

In the final step of the nursing process, the nurse evaluates data to determine that previously established outcomes have been met and that nursing interventions were appropriate to the patient's goals. If the goals have not been met, have been partially met, or have been met because of interventions not included in the plan, the nurse considers altering the plan of care.

Expected outcomes are reviewed during the patient's hospitalization and at discharge. Outcomes should also be evaluated as patients return to the community because health maintenance minimizes patient readmission. Although many older adults have chronic illnesses and actual health problems, nurses should not focus on these alone. Risk diagnoses are significant to the health of older adults, some of whom are vulnerable to additional healthcare, social, and socioeconomic problems.

Healthcare providers often associate health promotion with children and young adults; however, many older adults at various functional levels express the desire to maintain their level of health, improve their health status and functionality, and prevent disease. For older adults who express interest in improving their health status and in preventive care, health promotion diagnoses and interventions should be included in each patient's plan of care.

REVIEW The Nursing Process

RELATE Link the Concepts and Exemplars

Linking the exemplar of the nursing process with the concept of communication:

1. How does the nurse communicate the use of the nursing process when documenting?
2. The nurse is caring for a patient with postoperative pain and administers an analgesic 10 minutes before the end of the shift. How does the nurse communicate the need for evaluation of effectiveness of pain management to the oncoming shift?

Linking the exemplar of the nursing process with the concept of legal issues:

3. How does use of the nursing process in providing and documenting care reduce the nurse's risk of malpractice claims?
4. What legal obligations does the nurse have related to use of the nursing process?

REFER Go to Pearson MyLab Nursing and eText

REFLECT Apply Your Knowledge

Dr. Danilo Ocampo is a 74-year-old retired pathologist. He lives in his home with Lydia, his wife of 51 years. Their only child, a son, was killed at age 22 in an automobile crash. Dr. Ocampo was born and raised in the Philippines and came to the United States when he was 23. He is the last living member of his immediate family. He has a few nephews and nieces in the Philippines, but no relatives live nearby.

Dr. Ocampo's health has been declining for the past few years. He has a medical history that includes hypertension, myocardial infarction, angina, and heart failure. Because of these cardiovascular disorders, he takes multiple medications, including metoprolol, lisinopril, furosemide, clopidogrel, atorvastatin, aspirin, and nitroglycerin. Dr. Ocampo understands the pharmaceutical properties of the medications. At times, he is doubtful of the quality of healthcare he receives because of all the medications he has been prescribed. He often does not believe the medications are helpful because he experiences many side effects, and he has been readmitted to the hospital multiple times. Dr. Ocampo usually feels better after a few days in the hospital but typically checks himself out of the hospital before his physicians are ready to discharge him.

Because Lydia has dementia, most of Dr. Ocampo's time and energy are spent managing their household and taking care of her. He has been resistant to outside help, believing he can care for her better than anyone else. Dr. Ocampo maintains a consistent schedule, and he and his wife get along quite well. Although at one time in their lives they were very socially active, at this point, they rarely go out.

Dr. Ocampo has become increasingly short of breath and is very fatigued. He notices his legs have become edematous. He goes to the neighborhood drugstore to use the "self-serve" blood pressure machine and finds his blood pressure to be 152/106 mmHg. Dr. Ocampo is resistant to the idea of seeing his physician or going to the ED for fear of being admitted. Instead, he increases the dose of furosemide and lisinopril by one tablet per day and tries to get a bit more rest. A week later when his symptoms fail to improve and seem to worsen slightly, Dr. Ocampo visits his HCP's office and reports his symptoms and increase in medication dosages.

1. What are the priorities of care for this patient?
2. What data would you collect from Dr. Ocampo on initial examination?
3. Develop a nursing plan of care for this patient.

Exemplar 36.B The Nursing Plan of Care

Exemplar Learning Outcomes

36.B Analyze nursing plans of care as they relate to clinical decision making.

- Define the nursing plan of care.
- Describe the column plan type of nursing care plan.
- Describe the concept map type of nursing care plan.
- Describe the standardized plan type of nursing care plan.
- Describe the clinical pathway type of nursing care plan.

Exemplar Key Terms

Clinical pathway, *2538*
Column plan, *2535*
Concept map, *2535*
Nursing plan of care, *2533*
Standardized plan, *2536*

Overview

A **nursing plan of care** is a written or electronic guideline that organizes information about an individual patient or family's care. One plan may include several nursing diagnoses for a single patient. It is important to prioritize nursing diagnoses and to list only three to five nursing diagnoses; this helps the nurse focus on nursing care that provides the best patient outcomes. The RN initiates the plan when the patient is admitted to the facility. The plan of care is then constantly updated throughout the patient's stay in response to changes in the patient's condition and evaluations of goal achievement. Keeping the plan of care current is necessary to ensure appropriate, individualized care for the patient. When the patient is discharged from the facility, the plan is included as part of a patient's permanent record of the care received and care the patient should have received (see Module 38, Communication, for further information).

Although formats differ from facility to facility, the plan of care is often organized using the five phases of the nursing process (see **Figure 36.10** »). Whether written or electronic, plans have the following purposes:

- Provide individualized patient-centered care to meet the unique needs of each patient.
- Provide for continuity of care through communication with nursing staff and other HCPs involved with the care of the patient.
- Inform the nurse about which specific observations or actions need to be documented in the nurse's progress notes about the patient's care.
- Provide health insurance companies documented proof for reimbursement amount to pay for services rendered to the patient.
- Provide the nurse with a guide when assigning nursing staff to care for each patient.

Accessibility

Nursing plans of care need to be readily accessible to all healthcare team members involved with the care of the patient. Availability of the plan supports communication with others for better continuity of care. The plan of care may be kept at the bedside but is more commonly kept within the medical record. In most institutions, the nursing plan of care is part of the electronic medical record (EMR), which requires specific information about the patient's plan of care. The EMR is accessible to all staff with appropriate access to the patient's record on all units and departments to which the patient may be transferred. The EMR provides the healthcare team with information about the patient, such as demographic data, routines of daily care (i.e., bathing, nutrition), diagnostic studies, social history, oxygen therapy, monitoring needs, medications and IV fluids, and surgical drains.

Guidelines

The nurse should follow the guidelines in **Table 36.18** » when writing nursing plans of care. Note that the guidelines include specificity and customization.

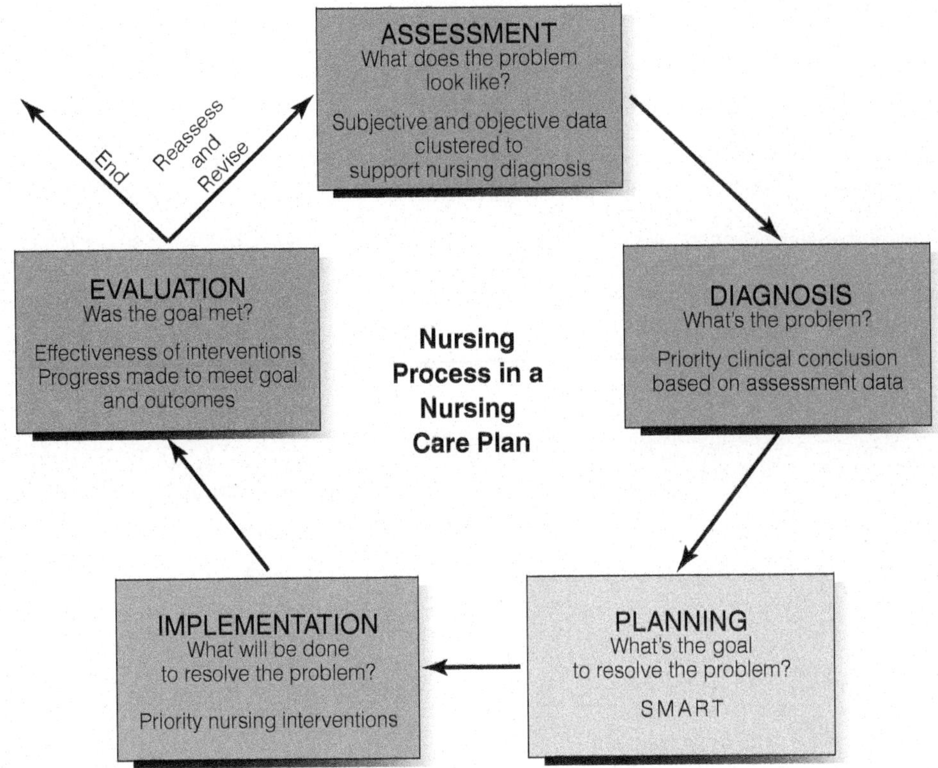

Figure 36.10 » Using the nursing process in a nursing plan of care.

TABLE 36.18 Guidelines for Writing a Nursing Plan of Care

Guideline	Description
Date and sign the plan.	The date the plan is written is essential for evaluation, review, and future planning. The nurse's signature or login demonstrates accountability since the effectiveness of nursing actions can be evaluated.
Use category headings "Assessment," "Nursing Diagnoses," "Goals/Desired Outcomes," "Nursing Interventions," and "Evaluation."	Headings may vary slightly with different facilities but are relative to the nursing process phases.
Use approved abbreviations and key words rather than complete sentences to communicate ideas unless facility policy dictates otherwise.	For example, write "Turn/reposition q2h" rather than "Turn and reposition the patient every two hours." Or, write "Clean wound c̄ H_2O_2 bid" rather than "Clean the patient's wound with hydrogen peroxide twice a day, morning and evening." (See Module 38, Communication, for more information.)
Be specific, short, and concise.	Because nurses are now working shifts of different lengths (e.g., 12- or 8-hour shifts), the nurse must be specific about the timing of an intervention. An intervention reading "Change incisional dressing q shift" could mean either twice in 24 hours or three times in 24 hours, depending on the length of the facility's shifts.
Refer to facility resources, such as procedure books, rather than including all of the steps on a written plan.	For example, write "See unit procedure book for tracheostomy care" or attach a standard nursing plan about such procedures as preoperative or postoperative care.
Customize the plan to include patient's choices, such as preferences about the times of care and the methods used.	This reinforces the patient's individuality and sense of control. For example, the written nursing intervention might read "Provide partial bath in the evening per patient's preference."
Ensure that the nursing plan incorporates preventive and health maintenance aspects as well as restorative ones.	For example, carrying out the intervention "Provide active assistance ROM exercises to affected limbs q2h" prevents joint contractures and maintains muscle strength and joint mobility.
Ensure that the plan contains interventions for ongoing assessment of the patient.	For example, "Inspect incision q8h."
Include collaborative activities in the plan.	For example, the nurse may write interventions to ask a nutritionist or physical therapist about specific aspects of the patient's care.
Include plans for the patient's discharge and health teaching needs.	The nurse begins discharge planning as soon as the patient has been admitted, often consulting and making arrangements with a community health nurse, social worker, and other community agencies to supply patient services, needed equipment, and supplies.

Clinical Example F

Marlene Fisher is a 52-year-old woman whose husband of 35 years died 5 weeks ago after a long battle with lung cancer. She says that she has come to the clinic today because she does not sleep more than 3 hours at night and feels tired all the time. She tells the nurse that she has lost about 15 pounds since her husband died because she is too tired to fix anything to eat.

Mrs. Fisher has two sons, both of whom attended the funeral, but they have not contacted Mrs. Fisher since then. One lives on the other side of town, and the other lives out of state.

For more than 40 years, Mrs. Fisher attended her place of worship every time the doors were opened for an activity. She also enjoyed singing in the choir. For the past couple of weeks, she has not been able to attend any activities because she doesn't understand why her husband had to die, and she feels disconnected from her place of worship. She stopped singing at home because she says she "doesn't feel the music anymore." Mrs. Fisher says she stays at home every night now to avoid seeing people that are "smiling and happy" when she feels so lost and alone.

Clinical Reasoning Questions Level I

1. What are the significant assessment data for Mrs. Fisher?
2. What related clusters do the significant assessment data form?

Clinical Reasoning Questions Level II

3. What are the top three nursing priorities based on the clustered assessment data?
4. What goal would be appropriate for each of the three nursing care priorities?
5. What are the top three priority nursing interventions to support Mrs. Fisher reaching her goals?

Written nursing plans of care are used in facilities that do not have EMRs. Plans can be kept in a separate notebook or with the patient's medical record. Similar to the EMR, written plans of care support communication and continuity of care when patients are transferred from one unit to another or from one facility to another. The plan of care becomes a part of the patient's permanent record upon the patient's discharge from the facility. Each facility decides the format used for the plan of care. Facilities customize the following common types of plans of care for their patients: column plan, concept map, standardized plan, and clinical pathway.

Column Plan

Nursing students learn to develop patient plans of care and to organize the patient data from working with patients assigned to them for learning activities. As a result, care plans developed by students are usually lengthier and more detailed than plans of care used by experienced nurses. Students may be required to give a rationale, or reason, for selecting a particular nursing intervention as a priority. Students may also be required to cite research evidence from literature to support their stated rationale and to develop evidence-based practice habits.

The **column plan** of care uses columns to categorize data for each phase of the nursing process. This type of care plan may include four columns: (1) nursing diagnoses, (2) goals/desired outcomes, (3) nursing interventions, and (4) evaluation. Some agencies use a three-column plan in which evaluation is done in the goals column or in the nurses' notes; other agencies use a five-column plan that adds a column for assessment data preceding the nursing diagnosis column. **Figure 36.11 ››** shows a five-column framework for a nursing care plan for the patient in Clinical Example F, Mrs. Fisher.

Concept Map

A **concept map** is a visual representation of a nursing plan of care in a patterned diagram with data and ideas. Various shapes and colors are used to show relationships and connections in combination with lines or arrows. Concept maps are creative, conceptual images of concrete critical thinking. The visual image enhances clinical reasoning by "showing" how nursing diagnoses, goals, interventions, and evaluations relate to each other in a logical pattern. Concept maps can take many different forms and encompass various categories of data according to the creator's interpretation of the patient or health condition. They are an offshoot of mind maps or cognitive maps. A concept map can be a visual guide for analyzing relationships among clinical data to help prioritize meeting patient needs.

Assessment	Nursing Diagnosis	Plan	Implementation	Evaluation
■ Doesn't understand why her husband died ■ Stopped attending place of worship because feels disconnected from it ■ Stopped singing in the choir	Spiritual crisis	Patient will meet with religious adviser by 4/12.	■ Establish therapeutic relationship with patient. ■ Assist patient to cope with lifestyle changes. ■ Assist patient in finding a reason for living. ■ Discuss visit with religious adviser. ■ Encourage patient to talk about her feelings.	4/12 Goal ongoing; patient has appointment with religious adviser on 4/13.
■ Not sleeping well ■ States she "feels so lost" ■ Lost 15 pounds ■ Not eating well	Inadequate coping skills	Patient will eat three meals a day by 4/8.	■ Assess for risk of hurting self or others. ■ Refer patient to counseling. ■ Discuss sleep promotion behaviors. ■ Have dietitian discuss cooking for one with patient.	4/8 Goal met—patient has eaten three meals a day ×4 days.
■ No contact with sons since husband's death ■ Husband died 5 weeks ago ■ Avoids people ■ Stays at home every night	Social isolation	Patient will phone each son by 4/10.	■ Discuss promotion of social contacts. ■ Assist patient in developing a support system. ■ Support patient in reconnecting with sons. ■ Encourage outside activity, like walking.	4/10 Goal not met—patient has spoken with only one of her sons.

Figure 36.11 ›› Five-column nursing plan of care for situational distress.

The concept map is another way of depicting the nursing plan of care. Concept maps can help nursing students view patients and their problems holistically rather than as a single problem or medical diagnosis. Students are often asked to complete concept maps as a method of learning and demonstrating the links among disease processes, laboratory data, medications, signs and symptoms, risk factors, and other relevant data.

There are many different ways to make a concept map. Sticky notes are useful because they already come in a variety of colors and shapes; they also make it easy to move data around until the concept map is finished. Colored pencils or markers and paper cut into various shapes can be used as well. Software programs are available for creating electronic concept maps, and many websites offer free concept-mapping programs.

Hints when making a concept map:

- Follow the sequence of the nursing process phases; always begin with assessment data collection and cluster significant related data to determine nursing diagnoses (see Exemplar 36.A, The Nursing Process, in this module for further information).
- Keep it simple. The more lines cross each other, the more difficult it is to follow the connections among data.
- Many nursing programs have developed a concept map format for nursing students to follow, but the nurse can still use creativity to individualize patient concept maps.
- Avoid becoming caught up in the artistic expression. Do not spend hours matching colors and shapes and coordinating patterns while developing a concept map: it is a visual representation of important concepts focused on nursing care for best patient outcomes.

Many approaches can be used to build a concept map. Here is an example that is basic and can be expanded if more data are being used:

1. Develop a legend for the concept map by assigning shapes and colors for each nursing process phase and one for other categories of patient information: demographics, outcomes, lab results, risk factors, or medications.
2. Put the shape with the patient's initials, age, gender, and priority medical diagnosis in the middle of the paper to illustrate the patient-centered nature of nursing care.
3. Look at the assessment data, subjective and objective, and then gather and sort the significant clusters. Each piece of significant data goes on one assessment shape. Place the clustered groups around the patient shape.
4. Determine the priority nursing diagnoses that are relative to each of the clusters and place one nursing diagnosis with each of them. Draw connecting lines from each shape with assessment data to the nursing diagnosis for which it is relative.
5. Determine one appropriate goal for each nursing diagnosis cluster and add its shape to the side of the nursing diagnosis cluster. Select priority nursing interventions for each goal. Write separate interventions on their designated shape. Draw connecting lines from each shape with an intervention to the goal or patient outcome to which it is related. As needed, identify specific activities related to the nursing intervention.
6. Evaluate whether the goal was met, partially met, or not met and place the evaluation shape on the side of the nursing diagnosis cluster. It can be located under the goal shape or on the opposite side.
7. The concept map is now complete. See **Figure 36.12 »** for an example of a concept map for a patient at risk for declining health.

Standardized Plan

A **standardized plan** of care specifies the nursing care for groups of patients with common needs (e.g., all patients with myocardial infarction). These plans can be developed by a standardized care committee composed of facility staff that use both medical and nursing research evidence. Facilities may also purchase standardized plans to complement their policies and procedures. Once the nursing assessment is completed, the standardized plan of care that is appropriate for the patient is selected, and the nurse adds or deletes information to individualize it to the unique needs of a particular patient.

A standardized plan of care frequently includes checklists, drop-down menus, blank lines, or empty spaces to allow the nurse to individualize goals and nursing interventions. Standardized plans of care should not be confused with standards of care. Although the two have some similarities, they have important differences.

SAFETY ALERT Standards of care are nursing actions for patients that describe achievable nursing care. They define the interventions for which nurses are held accountable. Standards of care are developed by individual healthcare facilities for nurses working in the facility. National organizations and agencies, such as the ANA, The Joint Commission, and state boards of nursing, also set standards of nursing practice for nurse accountability (see Module 42, Accountability, for further information). A standardized plan of care provides general nursing care for specific medical diseases or conditions. If the nurse determines that following any part of a standardized plan of care would jeopardize a patient's safety or health outcomes, the nurse is responsible for taking appropriate action to ensure the health and safety of the patient by altering or deleting that section of the plan of care.

Standardized care plans are usually categorized according to specific age groups, patient problems, and specialty categories. Standardized plans follow the nursing process phases so nurses are familiar with their format. Regardless of whether plans of care are handwritten, computerized, or standardized, nursing care must be individualized to fit the unique needs of each patient (see the Focus on Diversity and Culture feature). In practice, a plan of care usually consists of both computer-generated and nurse-created sections. The nurse uses standardized care plans for predictable, commonly occurring problems and creates an individual plan for unusual circumstances or problems that require special attention and are unique to the individual patient's needs.

For example, a standardized care plan for "patients with a medical diagnosis of pneumonia" would probably include a nursing diagnosis of *fluid volume deficiency* and direct the nurse to assess the patient's hydration status. On a respiratory or medical unit, this would be a common

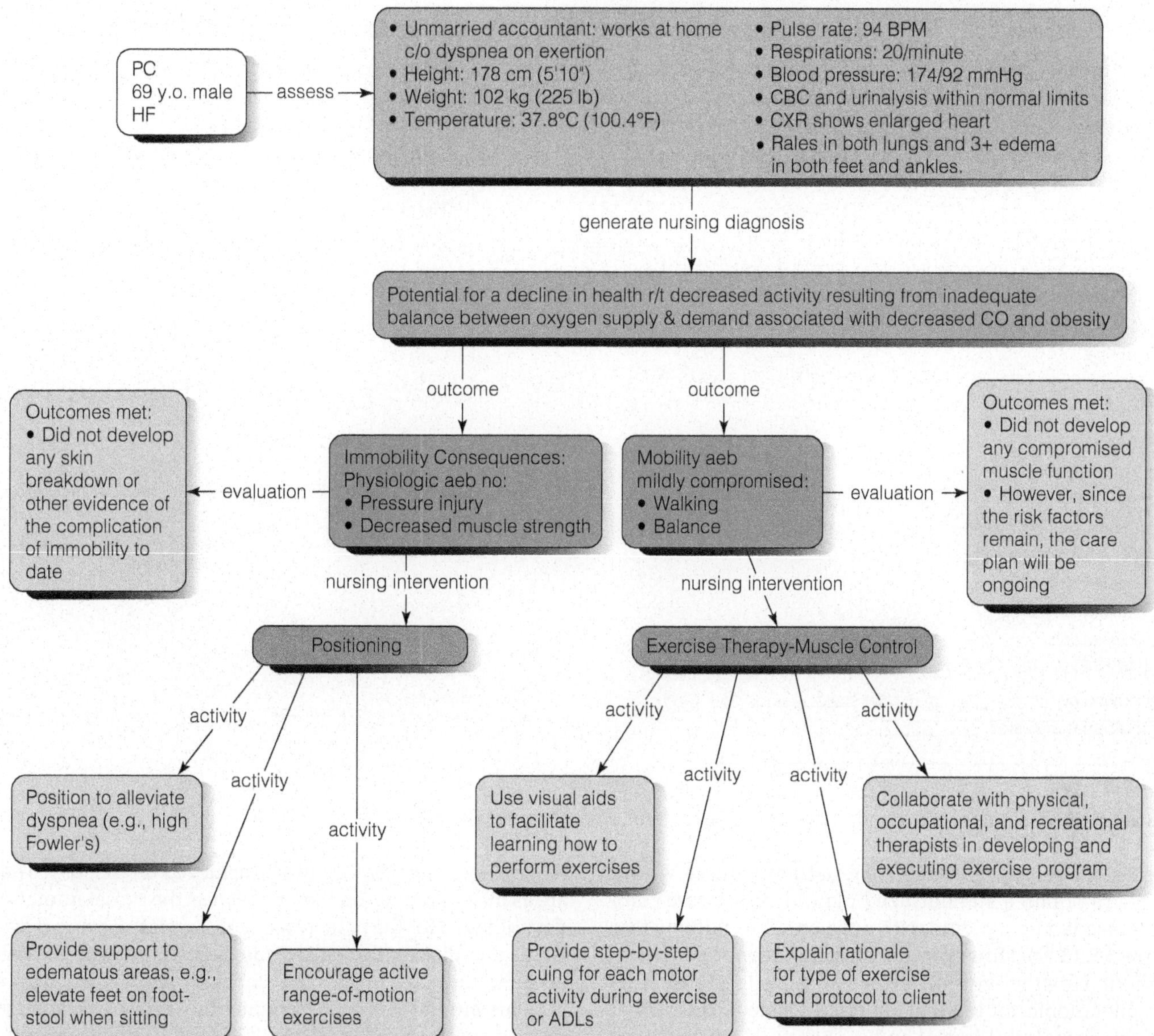

Figure 36.12 >> Concept map for potential for decline in health.
Source: Berman et al. (2021).

Focus on Diversity and Culture

Planning Culturally Competent Care

The nurse develops the patient's plan of care with respect to the patient and family's sociocultural background, including the family's structure and organization, religious values, cultural beliefs, and the way in which culture and ethnicity relate to roles within the family. A patient's plan of care must address the role of family and family function within a specific culture because after discharge, the family will be involved in the daily care of the patient. Nurses should employ effective communication, a holistic patient perspective, and respectful cultural care when caring for patients of varied cultures. Both in the hospital and at home, dietary recommendations should, as much as possible, fall within the patient's cultural dietary habits; it may be necessary to consult a dietitian for assistance with regard to dietary changes and recommendations. The nurse should note the patient's religious observances that may require fasting and the manner in which this practice can affect the patient's medication regimen and health. Religious practices may also influence the gender of the nurse who is able to care for the patient during hospitalization. This should also be taken into consideration if the patient is discharged to home with an order for visiting nurse services. In addition, patients who receive skilled nursing and other health-related therapies at home may benefit from having healthcare personnel who speak the same language or who share or have superior understanding of the patient's culture.

Sources: Based on Agency for Healthcare Research and Quality (2013); Giger (2017); Lopes et al. (2018).

Etiology	Desired Outcomes	Nursing Interventions (Identify Frequency)
___ Decreased oral intake	___ Urinary output >30 mL/hr	___ Monitor I&O q___ hr
___ Nausea	___ Urine specific gravity 1.005–1.025	___ Weigh daily
___ Depression	___ Serum Na^+ within normal limits	___ Monitor serum electrolyte levels × ___________
___ Fatigue, weakness	___ Mucous membranes moist	___ Assess skin turgor and mucous membranes q ___
___ Difficulty swallowing	___ Skin turgor elastic	___ Administer prescribed IV therapy ___________
___ Other: ________	___ No weight loss	___ Offer oral liquids frequently
___ Excess fluid loss	___ 8-hour intake = ________	___ Mouth care as needed
___ Fever or increased metabolic rate	___ Other: ________	___ Teach patient about importance of fluid intake
___ Diaphoresis		___ Other: ___________
___ Vomiting		
___ Diarrhea		
___ Burns		
___ Other: ________		
Defining Characteristics		
___ Insufficient intake		
___ Negative balance of I&O		
___ Dry mucous membranes		
___ Poor skin turgor		
___ Concentrated urine		
___ Rapid, weak pulse		
___ Lowered BP		
___ Weight loss		

Plan initiated by: ____________ Date: ________

Plan/outcomes evaluated: ____________ Date: ________

Patient: ______________________

Figure 36.13 ›› Example of a standardized plan of care for fluid volume deficiency.

nursing diagnosis; therefore, the patient's nurse would be able to obtain a standardized plan directing care commonly needed by patients with deficient fluid volume (see **Figure 36.13 ››**). However, the nursing diagnosis *impaired family functioning* would not be common to all patients with pneumonia, although it would be needed for a mother with three small children at home. Therefore, the goals and nursing interventions for that diagnosis for that patient would need to be created by the nurse.

Clinical Pathway

A **clinical pathway** is a standardized, evidence-based, interprofessional plan that outlines the expected care required for patients with common, predictable health conditions. To initiate a clinical pathway, the HCP writes an order for one that is appropriate for the patient. The clinical pathway documents are part of the patient's permanent record and are integrated into the clinical documentation.

Sometimes clinical pathways are referred to as *collaborative plans* or *case management plans*, and they sequence the care that must be given on each day during the projected length of stay for the specific type of condition. They include clinical interventions, time frames for completion, usual expectations of response, and expected outcomes. They are also sometimes called *multidisciplinary* or *interprofessional plans* because they include medical treatments to be performed by different types of HCPs.

The plan is usually organized with a section for each day, listing the interventions that should be carried out and the patient outcomes that should be achieved on that day. There are as many sections on the care plan as the preset number of days allowed for the patient's diagnosis-related group (DRG). Clinical pathways do not include detailed nursing activities because they are interprofessional in nature. Because all patients are unique, each patient's care will be customized to meet specific needs while keeping the guidelines in mind. Clinical pathways minimize variance in treatment plans in order to reduce cost, increase efficiency, and improve patient care outcomes.

Patient-specific clinical pathways are given to patients to help them understand what to expect in terms of time frames, actions, and results as related to DRGs. For example, a clinical pathway for a vaginal birth will include information about activity, nutrition, medications, treatments, patient teaching, tests, and discharge planning for specific times from delivery time of the baby (see **Figure 36.14 ››**).

Clinical pathways may be developed as an algorithm or path, as shown in the example in **Figure 36.15 ››**. This clinical pathway is for pediatric patients with asthma and is directed toward the interprofessional team. It includes separate assessment and treatment progressive guidelines for the pediatric patient with mild, moderate, severe, and near-death signs and symptoms of asthma. Medications, treatments, and teaching instructions are listed. The pathway includes information about the assessment, pretreatment, and treatment of these patients and steps to be taken if the patient has not improved. Pathways like this one are designed to improve the quality of care and outcomes as well as to standardize care provided across clinical disciplines.

	MOTHER		NEWBORN	
	24 HOURS	**48 HOURS**	**24 HOURS**	**48 HOURS**
Activity	■ Up with assistance as needed, progress to up by self ■ Shower ■ Self-care with assistance ■ Baby care with assistance	■ Total self-care ■ Baby care by self with assistance as needed ■ Vaginal exercises	(To be done by nursing staff; continuous monitoring for first 2 hours)	(To be done by nursing staff)
Nutrition	■ Regular diet as tolerated	● Regular diet	■ Encourage mothers to put newborn to breast during first period of reactivity; thereafter breastfeed on cue to meet a minimum 6 feeds in 24 hours ■ Initiate bottle feeding on signs of readiness to feed or per protocol; minimum 6 feedings in 24 hours (each 15–30 mL) ■ SGA and LGA newborns often require early initiation of feedings and frequent glucose monitoring	■ Breastfeeding on cue; minimum 8 feeds in 24 hours ■ Scheduled bottle feeding; minimum 6 feedings in 24 hours (each 30–60 mL)
Medications	■ Pain medications as needed ■ Routine medications	■ Laxative as needed ■ Routine medications	■ Sucrose orally prior to procedures	● Sucrose orally prior to procedures
Interventions/ Treatments	■ Routine vital signs and assessment ■ Comfort measures for perineum/episiotomy/ hemorrhoids ■ Monitoring for signs of complications (e.g., excessive bleeding, difficulty urinating, constipation) ■ Promote attachment ■ Assess for depression, anxiety	■ Routine vital signs and assessments ■ Sitz bath as needed ■ Comfort measures continued as needed ■ Monitoring for signs of complications continued ■ Continued assessment for depression and anxiety.	■ Routine vital signs and assessment related to transition to extrauterine life ■ Vitamin K injection and erythromycin ointment to eyes at birth ■ Examination by physician ■ Newborn care, height, weight ■ Circumcision if requested	■ Routine vital signs and assessment ■ Continued newborn care, weight ■ Infant hearing screening ■ Circumcision care as needed
Patient Teaching	■ Discussion about self-care and newborn care, including safe positioning of newborn to protect head, airway and instruction on safe sleep practices for newborn. ■ Review s/sx of late postpartum hemorrhage and to notify provider if any symptoms occur within first 12 weeks ■ Review perineal care ■ Review learning materials provided and address concerns ■ Discussion about breastfeeding or bottle feeding. ■ Discussion about newborn safety, cord site care, comfort, bathing, sleeping, activity ■ Discussion about signs and symptoms of postpartum depression.	■ Continue learning about at-home care for self and newborn ■ Continue learning about at-home newborn feeding needs	None	None
Tests	■ Procedures and diagnostic tests as needed	● Procedures and diagnostic tests as needed	● Newborn screening as needed before discharge	● Newborn screening as needed before discharge
Discharge Planning	■ At-home care of self and newborn ■ Discussion about community resources available ■ Discussion about birth certificate, newborn's name, and health coverage	■ Continue at-home care of self and newborn discussions ■ Follow-up appointments for mother, newborn scheduled	■ Appointment for newborn screening if needed	● Follow-up appointment for newborn scheduled before discharge

Figure 36.14 ›› Sample clinical pathway for mother and newborn post vaginal delivery.

EMERGENCY DEPARTMENT: PROTOCOL FOR ASSESSMENT AND TREATMENT OF PEDIATRIC ASTHMA

	ASSESSMENT	SYMPTOMS PRIOR TO TREATMENT	INTERVENTIONS AND THERAPIES	NEXT STEPS IF NOT IMPROVED
MILD ASTHMA	■ May be agitated ■ Can lie down ■ Nocturnal cough ■ Exertional dyspnea ■ Plays quietly ■ Can talk ■ Increased use of β-agonist ■ Good response to β-agonist	■ O_2 saturation >95% ■ Increased respiratory rate ■ Moderate wheeze-end expiratory Respiratory rates: *Age* — *Normal rate* <2 months — <60/min 2–12 months — <50/min 1–5 years — <40/min 6–8 years — <30/min	■ O_2 to achieve $SaO_2 \geq 95\%$ ■ β-agonist—nebulizer, up to 3 doses in first hour ■ Oral systemic corticosteroids	
MODERATE ASTHMA	■ Agitated ■ Prefers sitting ■ Shorter cry ■ Difficulty feeding ■ Increased work of breathing ■ Some difficulty talking ■ Partial relief with β-agonist ■ β-agonist needed >q4h	■ SaO_2 92–95% room air ■ Increased respiratory rate ■ Increased heart rate ■ Wheezing throughout exhalation Pulse rates *Age* — *Normal rate* 2–12 months — <160 bpm 1–2 years — <120 bpm 2–8 years — <110 bpm	■ O_2 to achieve $SaO_2 \geq 95\%$ ■ β-agonist and anticholinergic—nebulizer, up to 3 doses in first hour or continuous treatment for 1 hour ■ Systemic corticosteroids	**ADMIT**
SEVERE ASTHMA	■ Very agitated ■ Sits upright ■ Stops feeding ■ Marked limitation in talking ■ Dyspnea at rest ■ Grunting	■ $SaO_2 < 92\%$ ■ Labored respirations ■ Persistent tachycardia ■ Breath sounds are decreased ■ Unusually loud wheezing throughout inhalation and exhalation	■ 100% O_2 ■ Continuous β-agonist and anticholinergics ■ Systemic corticosteroids ■ Systemic magnesium sulfate	**ADMIT TO ICU or TERTIARY CARE**
NEAR DEATH	■ Exhausted ■ Drowsy or confused ■ Diaphoretic ■ Cyanotic ■ Apnea ■ Unable to talk ■ Use of accessory muscles to breathe ■ Suprasternal retractions	■ $SaO_2 < 80\%$ ■ Decreased respiratory effort ■ Falling heart rate ■ Paradoxical thoracoabdominal movement ■ Silent chest	■ Cardiac monitoring ■ Oximetry, ABGs ■ Chest x-ray ■ Frequent reassessment ■ Medical supervision until clear signs of improvement ■ Consider alternative drugs: IV β-agonist Inhalation anesthetics Aminophylline Epinephrine	**RAPID-SEQUENCE INTUBATION**

Figure 36.15 ›› Sample clinical pathway for pediatric asthma for interprofessional team.

REVIEW The Nursing Plan of Care

RELATE Link the Concepts and Exemplars

Linking the exemplar of the nursing plan of care with the concept of communication:

1. What information in the nursing plan of care is communicated to members of other disciplines who are taking care of the same patient?

Linking the exemplar of the nursing plan of care with the concept of managing care:

2. How can using a standardized plan of care influence the cost of patient care?

Linking the exemplar of the nursing plan of care with the concept of professional behaviors:

3. Why is use of a nursing plan of care considered a professional behavior?

REFER Go to Pearson MyLab Nursing and eText

REFLECT Apply Your Knowledge

Devon Bynum, an 11-year-old, is admitted to the hospital in sickle cell crisis. This is the first time he has been admitted to a hospital. He states he hurts all over and rates his pain as 7 out of 10. Devon has been in the ED all night and last received morphine 2 mg IV at 0400 for his pain. He is receiving oxygen at 2 liters per minute (LPM) via nasal cannula. He has an IV of D5 ½NS running at 83 mL/hr. Devon's mom, who has been with him throughout the night, is anxious for her son to feel better. His latest vital signs are T 99.3° F; P 122 bpm; R 22/min; BP 100/64 mmHg; and oxygen saturation 93% on oxygen at 2 LPM. He says he is tired and just wants to go to sleep. Devon's mom tells the nurse that she doesn't know how she will be able to pay the hospital bills. She shares that she is a single parent with two other children at home.

1. What type of nursing plan of care would you use for Devon? Why?
2. Would you include his mom's concern about finances in his plan of care? How?
3. What other healthcare discipline(s) would you expect to include in Devon's plan of care?

» Exemplar 36.C Prioritizing Care

Exemplar Learning Outcomes

36.C Analyze prioritizing care as it relates to clinical decision making.

- Describe the need for nurses to prioritize care.
- Describe methods for identifying what to prioritize.
- Describe various processes of categorizing priorities.
- Outline factors to consider when prioritizing care.
- Summarize pitfalls of prioritization.

Exemplar Key Terms

ABC, *2543*
ABCD, *2543*
Effectiveness, *2542*
Efficiency, *2542*
Pitfall, *2548*
Pop-ups, *2547*
Prioritizing care, *2541*
Priority, *2541*
Resources, *2546*
Time constraints, *2544*
Time priority, *2544*
Triage, *2545*
Urgency factor, *2544*

Overview

The term **priority** refers to using judgment to discern which among competing problems should be addressed immediately. **Prioritizing care** is a process that helps nurses manage time and establish an order for completing responsibilities and care interventions for a single patient or for a group of patients. The ability to set priorities is a critical thinking skill that can optimize a nurse's time and productivity by categorizing responsibilities and care interventions in an order based on significance and urgency. Time is a constant factor in prioritizing care: Nurses have only a limited amount of time to make clinical judgments about which interventions to perform and when to do them, whether for one patient or for several patients. Without some forethought and planning, a nurse may work for hours and yet accomplish very little. Nurses must learn to use time and energy wisely in today's busy healthcare settings.

A nurse's workload includes many objectives that need to be completed during each shift. Time management is an important skill that helps the nurse ensure that necessary activities are completed. Nurses can use a variety of approaches to accomplish nursing responsibilities and interventions. Unfortunately, some of these approaches may result in interventions being done poorly, incompletely, late, or not at all.

For example, some nurses simply plow through their work. They complete tasks as they go from patient to patient in no particular order, keeping busy by doing activities to meet patients' needs. They may start at one room and simply work their way down the hallway doing things for their patients. This strategy raises a number of questions. What about the nursing interventions with time constraints, such as medication administration? Are all nursing interventions equally important? Do all nursing interventions impact patients equally?

Sometimes nurses choose to work on the easiest tasks first, postponing the more challenging, complex tasks for a later time, but then find themselves rushing to finish the complex tasks during that inevitable "crunch" time. Nurses may decide they do not have time to perform an important intervention and leave it undone. A nurse working at a hurried pace experiences an increased stress level, which interferes with clear thinking, clinical judgment, and decision making. As time to complete actions decreases, this can negatively impact both the quality of professional performance and the quality of patient care.

Due in part to struggles with assessment skills, many new nurses have difficulty prioritizing patient care. New nurses benefit from adequate orientation and preceptorship (or residency programs) that include discussions about delegation, but they also benefit from having a mentor to address issues such as critical thinking, time management, and prioritization of patient care. As new nurses learn from preceptors, they can gain skill, confidence, experience, and competency. They develop the ability to distinguish tasks that can be delegated from nursing care and they develop time management skills built on improved critical thinking and prioritizing patient care (Shaw, Abbott, & Spalla King, 2018).

In contrast to less productive methods of completing activities, nurses can learn to prioritize their actions according to the importance of tasks and interventions and the appropriate timing for accomplishing them. As a result, interventions that have a high priority will be completed early. Just like learning any new skill, learning to prioritize care will take practice. When developing this skill, nurses have the advantage of being able to transfer other skills they have learned in nursing: assessment, critical thinking, clinical judgment, decision making, planning, implementation, and ongoing evaluation (see the Critical Thinking section earlier in this module for more information).

Identifying What to Prioritize

Three factors can influence patient satisfaction with nursing care: availability of nursing staff to care for patients, the amount of time it takes nursing staff to meet patients' needs, and the quality of the care provided. **Effectiveness** (doing the right things) and **efficiency** (doing things right) are two qualities that impact patient perception of nursing care. Nurses employ effectiveness and efficiency by using the strategies of setting priorities, managing time, and delegating to staff. To support these qualities, nurses need to limit distractions and interruptions. Patients may perceive the nurses' distractions and interruptions as signs of inefficiency and conclude that the actions nurses perform are simply tasks instead of individualized personal care. When providing patient-centered care, nurses treat all patients with respect, dignity, and necessary attention.

Assessment

"Look before you leap" reflects the need to have accurate information prior to taking action. Setting priorities for nursing care always begins with assessment. Assessment includes observing and asking questions to gather the information necessary for decision making. Helpful assessment data include the following:

- Observing for cues about pace and emotions of staff already working on the unit (e.g., are they relaxed or stressed?).
- After receiving information from the previous nurse in shift report, conducting one's own assessment by making a quick safety check of patients.
- Becoming aware of any patients who have an unstable status, a risk of change in their condition, or who require closer observation.
- Asking if there are any complexities to patient problems.
- Asking about any special safety concerns for the patients (e.g., high risk for falls).
- Making note of routine responsibilities and interventions that have time constraints (e.g., physician rounds at 0900, medication administration at 1000 and 1200, nursing meeting at 1330).
- Knowing how many and what level of nursing staff are available for delegation of tasks to help with patient care. Delegation is the transfer of responsibility and authority for completing an activity to a qualified individual (see Module 39, Managing Care, for additional information), although accountability for the task remains with the nurse.
- Noting the presence (and absence) of necessary resources on the unit (e.g., linens, supplies, and nourishments).
- Asking about patient preferences to take into consideration when providing care.

Airway, breathing, and circulation are vital for life. If a safety risk or physiologic deterioration threatens any one of these functions, the situation may quickly become life-threatening without prompt assessment and intervention. Nurses must be able to assess and prioritize threats to these functions as they arise (see **Box 36.3** »).

The Nursing Process

Since the 1950s, the nursing process has been used as a method of organizing nursing care of patients, and this process was made mandatory when it was codified by the ANA in 1973. The steps in the nursing process provide the framework nurses use to determine priorities when working with a single patient or a group of patients (see Exemplar 36.A in this module for further information).

The National Council of State Boards of Nursing provides models for states to use when revising their nurse practice acts and nursing administrative rules. The sections covering the scope and standards of nursing practice list the steps of the nursing process that develop a nursing plan of care. These sections also support accountability for clinical judgments, decision making, critical thinking, and competence of interventions in the course of nursing practice (prioritizing care and performing interventions). The NCSBN (2020) also provides easy access to each state's nurse practice act. See **Box 36.4** » for an example of state rules about prioritization of care.

Maslow's Hierarchy of Needs

Maslow's hierarchy of needs is a well-known method of assessing and organizing patients' needs. This hierarchy is typically displayed as a five-level triangle or set of steps (see Module 31, Stress and Coping, for further information). Beginning at the bottom, the levels of need progress from the most basic physiologic needs to more complex psychologic and social needs at the top. The most basic needs include food, air, water, shelter, elimination, and sleep (McLeod, 2020).

According to Maslow, these needs motivate behavior. The first four needs—physiologic, safety, social, and esteem—are sometimes called "deficiency needs" and indicate the patient is experiencing deprivation of one or more of those four needs. Needs on the lower levels must be met before an individual can move to higher levels. The last need, self-actualization, is called a "being need" and does not result from a deficiency but rather indicates a desire for growth as an individual (McLeod, 2020).

Maslow ranked his hierarchy of needs with essential needs on the first (bottom) level and lowest needs on the last (top) level. Nurses can use Maslow's hierarchy as they establish priorities of patient care. For example, ineffective breathing pattern, a physiologic need, takes priority over body image disturbance, a self-esteem need.

The nursing process and Maslow's hierarchy of needs can be used to guide the nurse in thinking critically about the order in which patient needs should be addressed. Nurses can then use their clinical judgment to make decisions about ranking patient needs as low, medium, and high priorities.

Box 36.3

Priority Assessment of Safety Risks and Physiologic Deterioration

A nurse walks into a patient's room and finds the patient pulling out his tracheostomy tube. Another nurse walking down the hallway passes the visitors' waiting room and finds a pediatric patient climbing up a high metal file cabinet. A third nurse finds her patient unresponsive, not breathing, and without a pulse. These situations involve safety and physiologic deterioration; all require prompt assessment for the potential to become life-threatening. Removal of the tracheostomy tube could leave the patient without a patent airway; the pediatric patient could cause the file cabinet to fall and possibly crush his head; and the patient who is unresponsive with no respirations or pulse could die within minutes. Nurses continuously assess patients in their environments to recognize harmful situations. If the patient is in danger, intervention becomes a priority.

The mnemonic **ABC** represents the essential functions of airway, breathing, and circulation. It provides a guideline for use when assessing a patient. An initial assessment of basic body functions necessary to sustain life precludes a more definitive assessment or any patient intervention (discussed in Module 16, Perfusion). The initial ABC assessment includes:

Airway: A patent airway so oxygen will have a pathway into the lungs for gas exchange and for carbon dioxide to be expelled from the body

Breathing: An effective breathing pattern and respiratory effort to take in enough oxygen to meet cellular demands for oxygen throughout the body

Circulation: An effective circulatory system to deliver oxygen throughout the body and exchange carbon dioxide and oxygen through the pulmonary circulatory network.

Nurses working in a variety of settings follow priority emergency protocols developed by the American Heart Association (2020) to standardize CPR. Since its development, the ABCs of CPR have been enhanced and altered by various specialty groups and professional organizations, adding more letters or changing the meaning of the letters; however, ABC is the universally accepted priority in managing life-threatening emergencies.

Another popular enhancement to the basic ABCs mnemonic is to add a *D* at the end, creating **ABCD** to help define other priority emergency assessments to complete. The meaning of D varies from one organization to another, but *D* may stand for:

- Defibrillation (use an automated external defibrillator for an absent pulse)
- Deficiency (assess for sensory or neurologic changes)
- Deadly bleeding (assess for massive hemorrhaging and shock)
- Disability (assess for spinal cord trauma and injury with movement or sensory deficits) (American College of Surgeons Committee on Trauma, 2017; Katsaphourou, 2019).

The few seconds taken by the nurse to assess for a patent airway, an effective breathing pattern, and an effective circulation system are essential. If life-threatening problems are found on assessment, the nurse intervenes with appropriate nursing actions. When initiated immediately, these interventions can positively affect patient outcomes by preventing complications, resolving a deteriorating condition, or saving a life.

Assessment of airway, breathing, and circulation can be done very quickly by observing the patient. Is the patient awake? Moving? Talking? Responding? If there is no problem with airway, breathing, or circulation, a nurse can move on to a more holistic assessment to identify other patient needs. Assessment may include lung sounds, heart sounds, sensorium, emotional status, and psychologic status.

Box 36.4

Example of Board of Nursing Rules Addressing Prioritization of Care

Tennessee Board of Nursing

1000-01-.14 Standards of Nursing Competence

(1) (a). 2. Establish critical paths and teaching plans based on individual patient's plans of care after prioritizing need upon completion of a comprehensive assessment.

Source: From Tennessee Board of Nursing (2019). Published by the Department of Health Services.

Low Priority

Problems that typically can be resolved easily with minimal interventions and do not cause significant dysfunction are included in the low-priority category. For example, responding to a patient's request for a midafternoon snack could be delegated to UAP.

Medium Priority

These are problems that may result in unhealthy physical or emotional consequences but that are not life-threatening. For example, the nurse could ask a patient who exhibits spiritual distress by saying, "God has forgotten about me" if she would like to have a hospital chaplain come visit.

High Priority

This category includes life-threatening problems of airway, breathing, circulation, deteriorations in vital signs, or other conditions that have a potential to become life-threatening within a short amount of time (Allen, 2020). An example of a high-priority intervention is frequent monitoring for unexpected changes in the vital signs and drainage for a patient who has just had a chest tube inserted.

SAFETY ALERT A survey of perioperative nurses indicated that priority safety issues exist for surgical patients despite increased efforts to reduce surgery-related errors. Researchers identified wrong site/wrong side and wrong procedures to be the most common surgical errors (Geraghty, Ferguson, McIlhenny, & Bowie, 2020). Other possible errors that can occur in surgery include medication errors, pressure injuries from poor positioning, and surgical site contamination, among other serious surgical patient safety concerns. Patient safety is the responsibility of the entire healthcare team. As advocates for patients, nurses should voice their concerns and question and clarify any situation that may compromise patient safety.

Categorizing Priorities

Nurses must set priorities for nursing activities and interventions using assessment data with consideration of the category of the intervention: low, medium, or high priority. In addition, nurses must consider other priorities, including time constraints and the significance of the activities and interventions on patient outcomes. The urgency factor model will help nurses learn how to rank priorities based on time imperatives and severity of patient needs.

Time Constraints

When setting priorities, it is important to remember that some nursing interventions have **time constraints**, or deadlines, for completion. One common intervention bound by time constraints is the administration of scheduled medications. Setting priorities for patient care includes planning the day in advance and determining which direct- and indirect-care activities must be completed at expected times (Antinaho, Kivinen, Turunen, & Partanen, 2017). Essential activities not performed by the nurse may result in negative consequences for patients.

The Urgency Factor

Organizing times to provide nursing care is influenced by the urgency factor. The word *urgency* reflects the need to act. **Time priority** means a time constraint is present when completing actions. The **urgency factor** is a way to illustrate how much time can safely lapse before a patient's health status is compromised. Do all nursing interventions require an immediate action? Can some actions be performed within a short amount of time and others be delayed for a longer period without negative consequences for the patient?

Changes in the patient's condition, deterioration of status, or the complexities of a patient's condition can impact the urgency of performing interventions and the order in which the nurse performs those interventions. The urgency factor comprises four levels. These levels progress from not urgent (a low time priority) to high urgency (the highest time priority). The nurse can use the levels of the urgency factor to assist in setting patient-care priorities. By using the levels of urgency, the nurse can identify interventions that need to be completed and the order in which they should be accomplished. See **Figure 36.16** ≫ and the following sections for a diagram and discussion of the urgency levels when setting time priorities.

Nonacute

Interventions with a low urgency factor may be termed *nonacute*. A delay in providing these interventions would not negatively impact patient outcomes. Interventions at this level do not take priority. For example, at the beginning of a shift, the nurse could discuss with a patient scheduling a later time to teach him about changing a dressing.

Acute

Acute interventions are often considered medium priority: There is a low potential for the patient's condition to become life-threatening if these interventions are not accomplished within a short amount of time. Typically, these are actions that nurses are expected to complete to meet identified patient needs. Interventions at this level can be scheduled during the shift when time constraints of higher-priority interventions allow. For example, a nurse can schedule with UAP to turn and reposition a patient with impaired bed mobility every 2 hours to prevent skin breakdown.

Critical

This level is considered medium-high urgency: There is an urgent need for the nurse to respond quickly to high-priority physical or psychologic problems within a short amount of time because the potential exists for a patient's condition to become more serious and even life-threatening if interventions are delayed. Quick recognition and a rapid response time are necessary to prevent further exacerbation of the patient's problem. For example, a patient develops shortness of breath and air hunger. If the patient does not receive high-flow supplemental oxygen, the patient may develop impaired gas exchange problems that may progress to severe hypoxemia and become life-threatening.

Imminent Death

The highest urgency factor is *imminent death*. The time to take action to prevent threat to life takes priority over everything else. When the patient's airway is obstructed, the patient stops breathing, or the patient's heart becomes ineffective in pumping blood through the circulatory system, immediate intervention is necessary to try to save the patient's life. The nurse must act now, STAT, to prevent further deterioration and threat to life.

Of course, there are countless possible life-threatening situations. For example, a patient on suicide precautions is holding a knife against his neck and is threatening to kill himself.

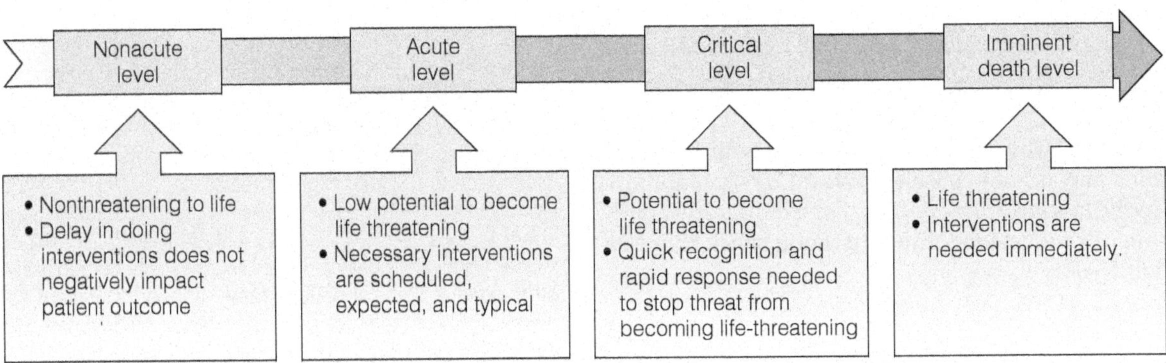

Figure 36.16 ≫ Urgency factor levels for setting time priorities.

Immediate actions must be taken to try and prevent him from harming, and possibly killing, himself. Nurses are always on alert for situations that could result in death for patients. Many of the more common situations, including medication errors, patient identification errors, and other safety issues, are identified in the National Patient Safety Goals (see Module 51, Safety, for additional information).

Ranking Activities

Learning to set priorities is the key to organizing patient care and using time efficiently to provide valued care. Setting priorities leads to providing efficient and effective patient care and can increase patient satisfaction, but it is important to understand that prioritizing does not mean it is acceptable to omit or unnecessarily delay nonurgent interventions (Papastavrou et al., 2020). Nurses can set priorities by thinking in terms of these categories: "must (or *need* to) do," "should do," and "*nice* to do."

Priority 1 or Must Do

These activities carry the highest priority for completion, take priority over other interventions, and must be done. For example, suctioning secretions from a tracheostomy tube to keep a patient's airway patent is a *must-do* priority.

Priority 2 or Should Do

These activities should be done, but are not essential. These interventions can be accomplished once *must-do* activities have been completed or covered. For example, restocking dressing supplies in the room of a patient who needs frequent dressing changes is a *should-do* priority.

Priority 3 or Nice to Do

These activities are important to complete, but only after priority 1 and 2 actions have been completed. These actions can be done when time is available, but they are not essential. Nurses should also use their judgment to determine which "should-do" and "nice-to-do" actions may be delegated to UAP.

Other category names for level of urgency can be used to rank priorities. See **Table 36.19** » for examples of category names.

Triage

In EDs, emergency situations, and prehospital care, the process of identifying priorities for implementing care is called **triage**. Triage allows nurses and other healthcare staff to set priorities based on the severity and urgency of a patient's illness, injury, and condition (see Module 46, Healthcare Systems, for additional information). Common categories used to set priorities are discussed next.

Emergent (or Immediate)

This category is for life-threatening issues that require prompt treatment and care. Stabilization of the patient's condition is critical. For example, a trauma patient with a blood pressure of 88/56 mmHg and a pulse of 108 bpm is emergent.

Urgent (or Delayed)

This category is for serious health conditions in which a delay of treatment and care would not result in life-threatening situations. For example, a patient who complains about having a productive cough for the past 4 days is urgent.

Nonurgent (or Minor)

Patients in this category have minor issues that do not require prompt care. Many of these patients can ambulate and are stable in their conditions. For example, a patient with a splinter in his foot that needs to be removed is nonurgent. Some EDs use satellite divisions for patients with nonurgent issues. This allows the main ED to manage patients with emergent and urgent health problems with immediacy while decreasing wait times for nonurgent patients.

See **Figure 36.17** » for a diagram of the prioritization of care process.

TABLE 36.19 Examples of Common Names for Priority Categories

Priority 1	Priority 2	Priority 3
Need to do	Try to do	May not do
Vital to do	Important to do	If time permits
Must do	Should do	Nice to do
High priority	Medium priority	Low priority
Most important	Less important	Least important

Factors to Consider When Prioritizing Care

Prioritization means more than just making decisions about which interventions to do first, second, third, and so forth. The assumption that nurses accomplish all of the things they want or need to do for all of their patients regardless of what order they do them in is no longer true. In some situations, nurses cannot get everything done within an allotted period of time. When nurses experience demands on their services that exceed the time available, they must be able to set priorities of care. Because of this, prioritization sometimes means the most important interventions get done, activities of lesser priority *may* get done, and the least important actions *may not get done at all* because there is insufficient time to complete them.

Prioritizing care in and of itself does not result in nurses being more productive in a given time period. Interventions take the same amount of time to complete regardless of the order in which they are done. Multitasking and learning to perform certain actions faster may improve effectiveness and efficiency but should never compromise patient safety.

Ethics

A holistic approach to nursing means caring for the physical, psychologic, spiritual, cultural, emotional, and developmental needs of patients. Often, patients have many more needs than nurses are able to meet. The principle of *justice* guides nurses in making decisions about setting priorities (see Module 44, Ethics). Nurses show *fairness* in treating individuals as equals. The difference among patients is the urgency of their needs; for example, a life-threatening situation will take

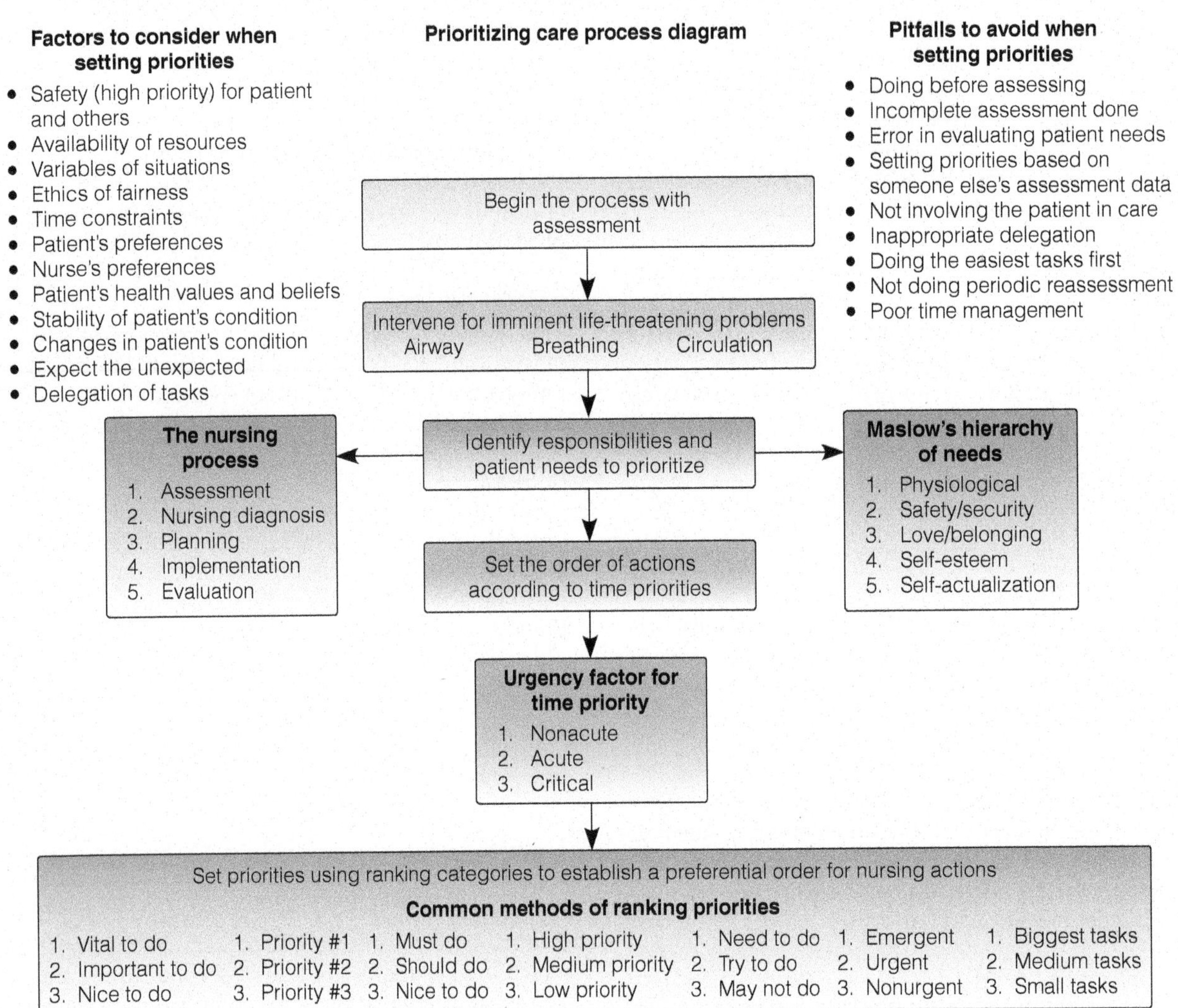
Factors to consider when setting priorities
Safety (high priority) for patient and others
Availability of resources
Variables of situations
Ethics of fairness
Time constraints
Patient's preferences
Nurse's preferences
Patient's health values and beliefs
Stability of patient's condition
Changes in patient's condition
Expect the unexpected
Delegation of tasks
Prioritizing care process diagram
Pitfalls to avoid when setting priorities
Doing before assessing
Incomplete assessment done
Error in evaluating patient needs
Setting priorities based on someone else's assessment data
Not involving the patient in care
Inappropriate delegation
Doing the easiest tasks first
Not doing periodic reassessment
Poor time management
Begin the process with assessment
Intervene for imminent life-threatening problems
Airway Breathing Circulation
Identify responsibilities and patient needs to prioritize
The nursing process
1. Assessment
2. Nursing diagnosis
3. Planning
4. Implementation
5. Evaluation
Maslow's hierarchy of needs
1. Physiological
2. Safety/security
3. Love/belonging
4. Self-esteem
5. Self-actualization
Set the order of actions according to time priorities
Urgency factor for time priority
1. Nonacute
2. Acute
3. Critical
Set priorities using ranking categories to establish a preferential order for nursing actions
Common methods of ranking priorities
1. Vital to do 2. Important to do 3. Nice to do
1. Priority #1 2. Priority #2 3. Priority #3
1. Must do 2. Should do 3. Nice to do
1. High priority 2. Medium priority 3. Low priority
1. Need to do 2. Try to do 3. May not do
1. Emergent 2. Urgent 3. Nonurgent
1. Biggest tasks 2. Medium tasks 3. Small tasks

Figure 36.17 ›› Prioritizing care process diagram.

priority over a psychosocial problem. Decisions are sometimes based on consideration of which actions will result in the best outcomes for the patient (Zahednezhad, Hosseini, Ebadi, Dalvandi, & Tabrizi, 2018).

Safety

Protecting patients and providing them with a safe environment is another aspect of justice. Safety in doing no harm to patients is a professional behavior (see Module 40, Professionalism, for further information). The Institute of Medicine (IOM; 2011) published a document that emphasized the need to improve safety for patients that led to the National Patient Safety Goals developed by The Joint Commission. For example, safely administering medications to patients is a high priority (see Module 51, Safety, for additional information). The IOM, now the National Academy of Medicine (2020), updated the document related to the future of nursing to reflect the profession of nursing during the coronavirus pandemic response and beyond.

Nurses can be fair in their allocation of time, attention, and skills to ensure patient safety. Unrealistic demands on nurses' physical and emotional abilities may result in nurses minimizing what they can do for their patients and may lead to feelings of dissatisfaction and exhaustion. Nurses' desire to help patients requires an environment that supports the delivery of quality care.

Availability of Resources

Resources are assets that help nurses meet patient needs. Problems arise when necessary resources are not available in the required quantity. Rationing or making decisions about which patients will receive the available resources may require prioritization. For example, a linens cart that has not been replenished leaves everyone without enough towels, washcloths, and gowns for patients. A nurse's creativity and resourcefulness can be valuable in finding solutions, such as borrowing the needed linens from another nursing unit and replenishing it when new linens arrive on the unit.

Nurses should use their time and resources efficiently and minimize activities that detract from patient care. Nurse managers should be made aware of situations that potentially compromise patient care, such as lack of sufficient resources. For example, in the previous scenario, the nurse may suggest borrowing linens from another unit to the nurse manager, who then facilitates that arrangement and delegates assistive or supportive personnel to deliver the linens.

Time Management

Time priorities are determined by the urgency of completing interventions for patients. As nurses become proficient, they develop a sense of how long it takes to complete certain interventions for patients, a skill that helps nurses better manage their time. Part of developing good time management is taking into account specific considerations, such as patient health preferences, changes in patient's condition, unexpected occurrences, and appropriate delegation of tasks.

Multiple Patients

Nurses generally take care of more than one patient at a time. Nurses can identify and plan interventions for all patients based on assessments of assigned individual patient needs, changes in patient status, and complexity of patient problems. Setting priorities is determined by the significance of the interventions for each of the individual patients. Time constraints such as medication administration for multiple patients requires more organization and focus from the nurse in order to complete medication administration within an allotted time frame. The pathophysiology of the individual patients would also require consideration when setting priorities among the assigned patients.

Patient Preferences

Patients are unique individuals who grow and develop as a result of genetic and environmental factors. Although patients share many similarities, such as the need for oxygen, they differ in terms of cultural rituals, spiritual practices, and routines of daily living. Some of these practices have time constraints, such as praying at specific times of day.

Health practices and beliefs of patients may conflict with some physicians' orders. Helping a patient maintain cultural or religious practices without compromising the patient's treatment plan sometimes requires extra effort on the part of the nursing staff. The goal is to strive for a win–win situation by honoring the patient's wishes as much as possible and completing nursing interventions as needed. Working together for a mutually beneficial solution strengthens the patient–nurse relationship.

Prioritizing activities for the day can be done with most patients. The patient's individual preferences and expectations of care can help set time priorities. For example, some patients may prefer to have a shower in the evening instead of the morning. The patient can plan individual activities around nursing actions that are scheduled at certain times. For example, if the patient knows he needs to get medications at 1000 and 1400, he could schedule his walk down the hall at 1100. Activities the patient considers as priorities may differ from those ranked as priorities by the nurse. By assessing for patient preferences, nurses can help strengthen patient participation in and support for the plan of care. Such actions may result in improved patient outcomes, a positive experience for the patient, and greater patient satisfaction.

Change in Patient Condition

Patients need to be monitored continuously for changing circumstances. Assessing patients at 1200 and reporting on them at 1900 without reassessing them means 7 hours have elapsed in which one or more patients have likely experienced a change of status without reassessment by the nurse. Such infrequent assessments may result in the nurse receiving the shift report getting inaccurate or incomplete data about the patient.

Nurses depend on other nurses to let them know of problems and changes in their patients. Assessment is an ongoing process to recognize changes and provide appropriate interventions early. When a patient's condition changes or becomes unstable, the earlier it is discovered and addressed, the more quickly nurses and the healthcare team can intervene and prevent further deterioration. A change in patient status may require reevaluating priorities and changing the planned order of interventions. Revising priorities is especially important when planning care for multiple patients.

The Unexpected

Things do not always go as planned. Nurses could plan their workday more efficiently if they could depend on the initial schedule set at the beginning of the shift and follow that plan throughout the day. However, on most days, nurses encounter unexpected events, or **pop-ups**, that require their time and attention and take them away from their plan for the day. For example, a new admission to the unit, a patient whose blood pressure is dropping, or a patient complaining of shortness of breath all take precedence over interventions such as teaching a patient about food choices for a low-salt diet, changing a dressing for a surgical patient, or any number of other nursing interventions. Pop-ups can challenge the time management and organizational skills of the most experienced nurses.

Nurse Self-Care

A nurse's plan for a quick 15-minute break and a 30-minute meal break at the beginning of a shift may sound simple. However, when it is time for nurses to take a break, they often are busy with their patients or other responsibilities; because breaks are not considered a priority, they do not always happen. "I'll go when I finish this" may be a never-ending refrain.

A short time away for self-care can provide quality time to refresh, reenergize, and take care of body functions (drink some water, eat some food, go to the restroom, or do some stretching). A few quiet minutes can help break up the intensity of the work environment and relieve stress for nurses (American Holistic Nurses Association, n.d.).

Delegation

Delegating tasks to other nursing staff, such as LPNs and UAP, can improve time management. Registered nurses must be aware of the legal responsibilities involved in delegating a task. The task must be within the scope of practice for the nursing staff member to whom the task has been delegated. The nurse who delegates the task must evaluate the task upon its completion (Campbell, Layne, Scott, & Wei, 2020; Wagner, 2018). See Exemplar 39.C, Delegation, in Module 39, Managing Care, for more information.

Delegation between the RN and UAP requires mutual trust and demonstrates the RN's confidence in staff members' abilities to assist in patient care. New RNs often do not delegate tasks because they are not sure of their role or they fear taking responsibility for the work of another person. Also, they are often unsure of which tasks may be delegated to UAP, and they have yet to develop the skills to determine trustworthiness of

UAP (Campbell et al., 2020; Wagner, 2018). Furthermore, novice nurses often fail to see themselves as leaders and fear being perceived as assertive by UAP (Wagner, 2018). Role-playing during orientation and preceptorship and discussions with a mentor may help the new nurse recognize when it is appropriate to delegate lower-level priorities to UAP and that leadership is an inherent role of RNs.

Pitfalls of Prioritization

Nurses should learn to avoid pitfalls when prioritizing care. A **pitfall** is an unforeseen situation that often harbors consequences for nurses and can result in patient harm. Although nurses may not know all of the possible pitfalls, there are some they can learn to recognize and avoid. When nurses follow ethical practices, use available resources, know the health concerns of their patients, have a sense about patient priorities, prioritize care appropriately, and use questions from clinical decision-making models, they can avoid many pitfalls. Common pitfalls are described in the following sections.

Prioritizing Without Assessment

Nurses need as much information as they can gather about their assigned patients, especially when they are assigned more than one patient. When providing care to multiple patients, nurses must consider interventions for all patients separately and set priorities. Without assessment, the first step in the prioritization process, nurses may forget important interventions or provide interventions based on old data. Patients may sustain severe consequences as a result.

Incomplete Assessment

Part of knowing how to do an assessment is learning what information is required to set priorities for patient care. Accurate and timely information about patient status, resources, available nursing staff, time constraints, and complexity of interventions is needed to prioritize care. If any of these are not assessed first, nurses will fail to include important and necessary information when setting priorities.

Relying Solely on Another's Assessment

Obtaining assessment data from another nurse, such as during shift report, can provide insight and give a picture of a patient's status during the previous shift. However, using only this information to set priorities, without also performing one's own assessment, may negatively affect patient outcomes.

Failing to Do Periodic Reassessments

Reassessment allows the nurse to adjust the time and order of actions to support completing interventions and activities on time and in order of importance. Sometimes the unexpected happens, taking the nurse in another direction and interrupting planned activities. Examples of these situations include a change in a patient's condition, arrival of a new patient who needs to be admitted to the unit, and a request from a relative or visitor to speak with the nurse. Periodic reassessments give the nurse a sense of the time available to perform actions, determine which actions still need to be done, and when to perform these actions throughout the shift.

Poor Time Management

Time management can be difficult for nurses to master, especially for those who do not check the clock every couple of hours to sense where they are in terms of accomplishing patient-care activities. Nurses may find that some actions have taken longer than expected to complete, while others have taken less time. Some actions have time constraints that may not be altered. Proficient time management ensures that priority tasks are accomplished in a timely manner and that the nurse remains productive during the shift. See **Box 36.5** >> for suggestions on managing time.

Box 36.5

Time Management Suggestions

At home, the night before your shift:

1. Make a list of scheduled medication administration times (i.e., 0730, 0800, 1000, 1200, 1400, and 1600).
2. Under each time, list expected patient interventions that will happen close to the times (i.e., meals, safety checks, IV checks, pain management checks, physician rounds, morning care, and documentation). This is the blueprint to follow for managing your time.
3. If you know of any procedures you may need to do the next day, review and visualize how to do them so you will be prepared and not use time the next day to refresh how to perform the procedure (e.g., giving an IV piggyback medication, inserting an indwelling urinary catheter).

At the beginning of your shift:

1. Arrive early to put your things away. Eat prior to arrival.
2. Set priorities as you attentively listen to change of shift report. Remember to include the urgency factor for time priorities.
3. Consider unexpected events that could occur and allow some time for them.
4. Stay focused. Remember to perform actions you've designated as priorities or difficult actions early and check them off of your to-do list. Learn to say no.
5. Make safety check rounds on your patients to assess for additional information. This will make your practice efficient and ensure that you are taking the correct actions.
6. Learn how to delegate.
7. Take notes and keep them in a designated area. This will help you remember important points and will also keep your workspace neat and reduce frustration.
8. Exercise flexibility by reprioritizing your time as needed when pop-ups or unplanned events occur.
9. Stay organized.
10. Celebrate your success as you complete priority interventions. Do not waste time agonizing over time management mistakes. This will only lead to becoming overwhelmed. Be kind to yourself. You will develop time management skills as you gain experience (Dragon, 2019).

Patient care is individualized even when addressing routine tasks. When working with children and with older adults, more time may be needed for discussions, answering questions, and teaching, based on the patient's developmental stage and cognitive ability. In addition, during the course of the work shift, the nurse can expect to encounter family members and caregivers, in person and by phone, who will also require time as they present questions about the state of the patient's health. Nurses often forget to include these occurrences when considering their plan for the day. By recognizing that interactions with patients and families will take time away from tasks, the nurse is able to plan the workday with consideration for such encounters. Patients and families must perceive that the nurse is fully engaged in responding to their needs: they should not feel rushed or hurried. Both patients and families recognize meaningful encounters and nursing attention as signs of quality care.

SAFETY ALERT Nurses are aware of healthcare organizations' policies and procedures related to quality nursing care, patient safety, and general institutional safety guidelines—three essential factors in prioritizing patient care. However, a recent study concluded that nursing leaders need to advocate for nurses, provide professional development opportunities, and build a culture of safety where nurses are free to question decisions and actions as needed without fear of being penalized. Factors such as nurse-to-patient ratio, improving interprofessional communication through simulation experiences, and forming professional relationships with HCPs are among other recommendations that may help improve the quality and safety of patient care (Clark & Lake, 2020). These factors may also help nurses avoid pitfalls that occur because of short staffing or, in some cases, lack of participation in nursing governance.

Not Involving Patients in Their Care

Nurses assess and determine patient needs when setting priorities. Nurses are also accountable for planning and carrying out interventions, but it is a mistake not to include patients in planning their care. Patients have preferences in how they do things, when they want things to happen, and what they want to do. Preferences may be a result of culture, family influences, spirituality, or heritage. Asking patients about their needs is a way to recognize their individuality and deliver patient-centered nursing care. Observing patient behaviors can also provide the nurse with cues about time and order of patients' preferences.

Inappropriate Delegation

Nurses must follow certain rules when delegating tasks to others (see Module 39, Managing Care, for further information). Other nursing staff, LPNs, and UAP can assist in completing tasks for patients if the tasks are within the scope of practice found in their state's nurse practice act. Transferring responsibility for a task to an LPN or UAP does not remove accountability for the outcome from the RN. Inappropriate delegation may result in the RN having to repeat an intervention or may even result in harm to the patient. Inappropriate delegation can have immediate ramifications for patient care.

Completing the Easiest Tasks First

Setting priorities means determining those actions that are more important than others and ordering actions based on their priority. Nurses become competent in the process of prioritizing through practice. Completing important, necessary, and sometimes complicated nursing tasks and interventions before easier, less complicated ones makes good, professional common sense. Positive patient outcomes occur when nurses provide intentionally planned care services to meet patients' needs.

REVIEW Prioritizing Care

RELATE Link the Concepts and Exemplars

Linking the exemplar of prioritizing care with the concept of clinical decision making:

1. What are some commonalities between these two processes?

Linking the exemplar of prioritizing care with the concept of safety:

2. Why is safety a high priority for patients who have *potential for* or *risk for . . .* nursing diagnoses?

Linking the exemplar of prioritizing care with the concept of professionalism:

3. What aspects of setting priorities for care are professional behaviors for nurses?

Linking the exemplar of prioritizing care with the concept of managing care:

4. Name some ways setting priorities for care contributes to improved management of care.

REFER Go to Pearson MyLab Nursing and eText

REFLECT Apply Your Knowledge

You have been assigned to take care of Mr. J. Rodriguez, a 48-year-old male patient, during clinical from 0645 to 1300. This patient was admitted to the medical unit yesterday with bilateral pneumonia. He has a history of shortness of breath and exertional dyspnea for the past week. Mr. Rodriguez states he has had a productive cough for the past 4 days, with thick, green, foul-smelling sputum. He complains of chest pain when he has to cough. His appetite is diminished and he is not drinking very much because he says he is too tired. He also states he was not able to go to work the 2 days before he was admitted to the hospital. Mr. Rodriguez lives with his wife and four children. His wife speaks very little English. His last set of vital signs were temperature 102.2°F (39°C), pulse 98 bpm, respirations 22/min; blood pressure 134/86 mmHg. He is friendly, quiet, and wants to get better. He is in no distress at this time.

Physician orders include:

- IV D_5 1/2NS with 20 mEq KCl at 100 mL/hr
- Rocephin 1 gram IV piggyback every 12 hours
- Intake and output every shift
- Vital signs every 4 hours, including pulse oximetry
- Out of bed to chair with assistance

(continued on next page)

- Regular diet, encourage fluids
- Use an incentive spirometer 10 times every hour while awake
- Oxygen via nasal cannula at 2 LPM oxygen.

Nursing interventions include:

- Assisting with bath and morning care as needed
- Changing bed linens on patient's bed
- Administering medications at 0800, 1000, and 1200
- Assisting with breakfast as needed at 0800
- Assisting with lunch as needed at 1230
- Doing a 60-second patient safety check every 2 hours
- Doing a complete assessment on the patient early morning
- Reassessing the patient's condition every 4 hours
- Doing vital signs at 0800 and 1200
- Assisting the patient with incentive spirometry during morning hours
- Encouraging the patient to drink fluids
- Checking for new physician orders
- Checking for diagnostic test results
- Listening to report from previous shift nurse
- Assisting patient in menu selection for tomorrow's meals
- Teaching the patient how to splint his chest with a pillow when he needs to cough to prevent chest muscles from hurting with coughing
- Documenting in patient's electronic medical record throughout the day
- Checking the patient's IV every 4 hours
- Providing fresh ice water in the patient's water pitcher
- Measuring and tallying the intake and output for the patient during the shift
- Assisting the patient to get up to the chair in the morning and again in the afternoon.

List any additional interventions you would want to do with this patient:

1.

2.

3.

Decide the priority of each of the above nursing interventions, both those listed and your own. Indicate your priority choice beside each one by writing a "1" for a high priority, a "2" for a medium priority, and a "3" for a low priority. Now decide which actions can be delegated to UAP to assist in completing them all. Write a "D" beside the interventions that can be appropriately delegated to UAP.

References

Agency for Healthcare Quality and Research. (2013). *Re-engineered discharge to diverse populations*. http://www.ahrq.gov/professionals/systems/hospital/red/toolkit/redtool4.html

Alfaro-Lefevre, R. (2017). *Critical thinking, clinical reasoning, and clinical judgment*. Elsevier.

Alfayoumi, I. (2019) The impact of combining concept-based learning and concept-mapping pedagogies on nursing students' clinical reasoning abilities. *Nurse Education Today, 72*, 40–46. https://doi.org/10.1016/j.nedt.2018.10.009

Allen, G. (2020). Barriers to non-critical care nurses identifying and responding to early signs of clinical deterioration in acute care facilities. *MEDSURG Nursing, 29*(1), 43–52.

American Association of Colleges of Nursing. (2021). *The essentials: Core competencies for professional nursing education*. https://www.aacnnursing.org/Portals/42/AcademicNursing/pdf/Essentials-Final-Draft-2-18-21.pdf?ver=hNeCl7OjgamIA9sHgDi_Yw%3d%3d×tamp=1613742420447

American College of Surgeons Committee on Trauma. (2017). *Advanced trauma life support* (10th ed.). Author.

American Heart Association. (2020). *2020 American Heart Association guidelines for CPR and ECC*. https://cpr.heart.org/en/resuscitation-science/cpr-and-ecc-guidelines

American Holistic Nurses Association. (n.d.). *Holistic stress management for nurses*. http://www.ahna.org/Resources/Stress-Management

American Medical Association (AMA). (1995-2020). *Ethics: Patient rights*. https://www.ama-assn.org/delivering-care/ethics/patient-rights

American Nurses Association (ANA). (2010). *Principles for nursing documentation*. http://www.nursingworld.org/MainMenuCategories/ThePracticeofProfessionalNursing/NursingStandards/ANAPrinciples/PrinciplesforDocumentation.pdf

American Nurses Association (ANA). (2015). *Nursing: Scope and standards of practice* (3rd ed.). https://www.lindsey.edu/academics/majors-and-programs/Nursing/img/ANA-2015-Scope-Standards.pdf

Antinaho, T., Kivinen, T., Turunen, H., & Partanen, P. (2017). Increasing value-adding patient care by applying a modified TCAB program. *Leadership in Health Services, 30*(4), 411–427.

Benner, P. (2015). Curricular and pedagogical implications for the Carnegie Study, educating nurses: A call for radical transformation. *Asian Nursing Research, 9*(1), 1–6. https://doi.org/10.1016/j.anr.2015.02.001

Benner, P. (2020). From novice to expert. *Current Nursing*. http://currentnursing.com/nursing_theory/Patricia_Benner_From_Novice_to_Expert.html

Benner, P., Hughes, R. G., & Sutphen, M. (2008). Clinical reasoning, decision making, and action: Thinking critically and clinically. In R. G. Hughes (Ed.), *Patient safety and quality: An evidence-based handbook for nurses*. Agency for Healthcare Research and Quality. http://www.ncbi.nlm.nih.gov/books/NBK2643

Benner, P., & Tanner, C. (1987). How expert nurses use intuition. *American Journal of Nursing, 87*(1), 23–31.

Benner, P., Tanner, C., & Chesla, C. (2009). *Expertise in nursing practice: Caring, clinical judgment and ethics* (2nd ed.). Springer.

Berman, A., Snyder, S., & Frandsen, G. (2021). *Kozier & Erb's fundamentals of nursing: Concepts, process, and practice* (11th ed.). Pearson.

Brenton, A. & Petersen, E. (2019). *Next Generation NCLEX (NGN) Educator Webinar Part 1* [Presentation slides]. National Council of State Boards of Nursing. https://www.ncsbn.org/NGN-Educator-Webinar.pdf

Bussard, M. (2015). The nature of clinical judgment development in reflective journals. *Journal of Nursing Education, 54*(8), 451–454. https://doi.org/10.3928/01484834-20150717-05.

Bussard, M. (2018). Evaluation of clinical judgment in prelicensure nursing students. *Nurse Educator, 43*, 106–108. https://doi.org/10.1097/NNE.0000000000000432

Campbell, A., Layne, D., Scott, E., & Wei, H. (2020). Interventions to promote teamwork, delegation, and communication among registered nurses and nursing assistants: An integrative review. *Journal of Nursing Management, 28*(7), 1465–1472. https://doi.org/10.1111/jonm.13083

Centers for Disease Control and Prevention (CDC). (2019, December 5). *CDC's developmental milestones*. https://www.cdc.gov/ncbddd/actearly/milestones/index.html

Cherry, K. (2019). *Object permanence and Piaget's theory of development*. Verywellmind. https://www.verywellmind.com/what-is-object-permanence-2795405

Chilcote, D. R. (2017). Intuition: A concept analysis. *Nursing Forum, 52*(1), 62–67. https://doi.org/10.1111/nuf.12162

Chuey, M., De Vries, R., Dal Cin, S., & Low, L. K. (2020). Maternity providers' perspectives on barriers to utilization of intermittent fetal monitoring: A qualitative study. *Journal of Perinatal and Neonatal Nursing, 34*(1), 46–55. https://doi.org/10.1097/JPN.0000000000000453

Clark, R. R. S., & Lake, E. T. (2020). Association of clinical nursing work environment with quality and safety in maternity care in the United States. *American Journal of Maternal Child Nursing, 45*(5), 265–270. https://doi.org/10.1097/NMC.0000000000000653

Cooke, L., Stroup, C., & Harrington, C. (2019). Operationalizing the concept of critical thinking for student learning outcome development. *Journal of Nursing Education, 58*(4), 214–220. https://doi.org/10.3928/01484834-20190321-05

D'Amour, D., Dubois, C. A., Tchouaket, E., Clarke, S., & Blais, R. (2014). The occurrence of adverse events potentially attributable to nursing care in medical units: Cross sectional record review. *International Journal of Nursing Studies, 51*(6), 882–891. https://doi.org/10.1016/j.ijnurstu.2013.10.017

Dickson, P., Haerling, K. A., & Lasater, K. (2019). Integrating the National Council of State Boards of Nursing Clinical Judgment Model into nursing educational frameworks. *Journal of Nursing Education, 58*(2), 72–78. https://doi.org/10.3928/01484834-20190122-03

Dragon, N. (2019). 10 time management tips for nurses and midwives. *Australian Nursing and Midwifery Journal*. https://anmj.org.au/10-time-management-tips/

Freysteinson, W. M. (2018). A synopsis of Ricoeur's phenomenology of the will: Implications for nursing practice, research, and education. *Journal of Holistic Nursing, 37*(1), 87–93. https://doi.org/10.1177/0898010118778904

Georg, C., Welin, E., Jirwe, M., Karlgren, K., & Ulfvarson, J. (2019). Psychometric properties of the virtual patient version of the Lasater Clinical Judgment Rubric. *Nurse Education in Practice, 38*, 14–20. https://doi.org/10.1016/j.nepr.2019.05.016

Geraghty, A., Ferguson, L., McIlhenny, C., & Bowie, P. (2020). Incidence of wrong-site surgery list errors for a 2-year period in a single national health service board. *Journal of Patient Safety, 16*(1), 79–83. https://doi.org/10.1097/PTS.0000000000000426

Giger, J. N. (2017). *Transcultural nursing: Assessment and intervention* (7th ed.). Mosby.

Grant, V. J., Robinson, T., Catena, H., Eppich, W., & Cheng, A. (2018). Difficult debriefing situations: A toolbox for simulation educators. *Medical Teacher, 40*(7), 703–712.

Health Care 2020 Part 2: Consumerism. (2017). *Healthcare Financial Management, 71*(1), 50–53.

Hensel, D. (2020). Strategies to teach the National Council of State Boards of Nursing Clinical Judgment Model. *Nurse Educator, 45*(3), 128–132.

Howard, S. D., Lee, K. L., Nathan, A. G., Wenger, H. C., Chin, M. H., & Cook, S. C. (2019). Healthcare experiences of transgender people of color. *Journal of General Internal Medicine, 34*(10), 2068–2074. https://doi.org/10.1007/s11606-019-05179-0

Institute of Medicine (IOM). (2011, January 26). *The future of nursing: Focus on education*. http://www.iom.edu/Reports/2010/The-Future-of-Nursing-Leading-Change-Advancing-Health/Report-Brief-Education.aspx

The Joint Commission. (2020). *2021 Hospital national patient safety goals*. https://www.jointcommission.org/-/media/tjc/

documents/standards/national-patient-safety-goals/2021/simplified-2021-hap-npsg-goals-final-11420.pdf

Katsaphourou, P. (2019). Initial assessment of the trauma patient: A nursing approach. *Journal of Research and Practice on the Musculoskeletal System, 3*(4), 139–142. https://doi.org/10.22540/JRPMS-03-139

Kuppermann, M., Kaimal, A., Blat, C., Gonzalez, J., Thiet, M., Bermingham, Y., et al. (2020). Effect of a patient-centered decision support tool on rates of trial of labor after previous cesarean delivery: The PROCEED randomized clinical trial. *Journal of the American Medical Association, 323*(21), 2151–2159. https://doi.org/10.1001/jama.2020.5952

Lopes C., Alves de Sousa, S., Carvalho Silva, L. D., Dias, R. S., Ribeiro Azevedo, P., Oliveira Nunes, F. D., & de Souza Paiva, S. (2018). Patient safety culture and the cultural nursing care. *Journal of Nursing UFPE/Revista de Enfermagem UFPE, 12*(9), 2500–2506. https://doi.org/10.5205/1981-8963-v12i9a235048p2500-2506-2018

Margolies, L., & Brown, C. (2019). Increasing cultural competence with LGBTQ patients. *Nursing, 49*(6), 34–40. https://doi.org/10.1097/01.NURSE.0000558088.77604.24

Martin, B., Greenawalt, J. A., Palmer, E., & Edwards, T. (2020). Teaching circle to improve nursing clinical judgment in an undergraduate nursing program. *Journal of Nursing Education, 59*(4), 218–221. https://doi.org/10.3928/01484834-20200323-08

McLeod, S. (2020, March 3). *Maslow's hierarchy of needs*. Simply Psychology. https://www.simplypsychology.org/maslow.html

Melin-Johansson. C., Palmqvist, R., & Rönnberg, L. (2017). Clinical intuition in the nursing process and decision-making: A mixed-studies review. *Journal of Clinical Nursing*, 26(23–24), 3936–3949. https://doi.org/10.1111/jocn.13814

Melnyk, B. M., Gallagher, F. L., Zellefrow, C., Tucker, S., Thomas, B., Sinnott, L. T., & Tan, A. (2018). The first U.S. study on nurses' evidence-based practice competencies indicates major deficits that threaten healthcare quality, safety, and patient outcomes. *Worldviews on Evidence-Based Nursing, 15*(1), 16–25. https://doi.org/10.1111/wvn.12269

Mousavinasab, E. S., Rostam, S., Zarifsanaiey, N., Rakhshan, M., & Ghazisaeedi, M. (2020). Nursing process education: A review of methods and characteristics. *Nurse Education in Practice, 48*, 102886–102886. https://doi.org/10.1016/j.nepr.2020.102886

NANDA International (NANDA-I). (2018). *NANDA International, Inc. nursing diagnoses: Definitions and classifications* (11th ed.) (T. H. Herdman & S. Kamitsuru, Eds.). Thieme.

National Academy of Medicine. (2020). *A consensus study from the National Academy of Medicine*. https://nam.edu/publications/the-future-of-nursing-2020-2030/

National Council of State Boards of Nursing (NCSBN). (2020). *Find your nurse practice act*. https://www.ncsbn.org/npa.htm

Newnham, E., & Kirkham, M. (2019). Beyond autonomy: Care ethics for midwifery and the humanization of birth. *Nursing Ethics, 26*(7/8), 2147–2157. https://doi.org/10.1177/0969733018819119

Orlando, I. J. (1972). *The discipline and teaching of the nursing process: An evaluative study*. Putnam.

Papastavrou, E. (2020). The ethics of nursing care rationing in the context of COVID-19 Pandemic. *Rostrum of Asclepius/Vima Tou Asklipiou, 19*(4), 252–255.

Parissopoulos, S. (2019). Reflection and reflective practice: a cornerstone value for the future of nursing. *Rostrum of Asclepius/Vima Tou Asklipiou, 18*(3), 200–203.

Petiprin, A. (2020). *Roy's adaptation model of nursing*. Nursing Theory. https://nursing-theory.org/theories-and-models/roy-adaptation-model.php

Polit, D. F., & Beck, C. T. (2017). *Nursing research: Generating and assessing evidence for nursing practice* (10th ed.). Wolters Kluwer.

Roy, C. (2009). *The Roy adaptation model* (3rd ed.). Prentice Hall.

Sawyer, K., & Rosenberg, A. R. (2020). How should adolescent health decision-making authority be shared? *AMA Journal of Ethics, 22*(5), E372–E379. https://doi.org/10.1001/amajethics.2020.372

Shaw, P., Abbott, M., & Spalla King, T. (2018). Preparation for practice in newly licensed registered nurses: a mixed-methods descriptive survey of preceptors. *Journal for Nurses in Professional Development, 34*, 325–331. https://doi.org/10.1097/NND.0000000000000487

Stonehouse, D. (2018). How SMART are your patient goals? *British Journal of Healthcare Assistants, 12*(5), 233–235. 10.12968/bjha.2018.12.5.233

Tan, J.Y., Arshiya, A, Baig, M., & Marshall, H. (2017). High stakes for the health of sexual and gender minority patients of color. *Journal of General Internal Medicine, 32*, 1390–1395. https://doi.org/10.1007/s11606-017-4138-3

Tanner, C. (2006). Thinking like a nurse: A research-based model of clinical judgment in nursing. *Journal of Nursing Education, 45*(6), 204–210. http://www.mccc.edu/nursing/documents/Thinking_Like_A_Nurse_Tanner.pdf

Tedesco-Schneck, M. (2019). Use of script concordance activity with the think-aloud approach to foster clinical reasoning in nursing students. *Nurse Educator, 44*, 275–277. https://doi.org/10.1097/NNE.0000000000000626

Tennessee Board of Nursing. (2019). *Rules of the Tennessee Board of Nursing*. https://publications.tnsosfiles.com/rules/1000/1000-01.20190805.pdf

Texas Board of Nursing. (n.d.-a) *Delegation principles*. https://www.bon.texas.gov/pdfs/delegation_pdfs/Delegation-Principles.pdf

Texas Board of Nursing. (n.d.-b). *Six-step decision-making model for determining nursing scope of practice*. https://www.bon.texas.gov/pdfs/publication_pdfs/dectree.pdf

University of Iowa, College of Nursing. (2018). *Overview: Nursing outcomes classification (NOC)*. https://nursing.uiowa.edu/cncce/nursing-outcomes-classification-overview

Upvall, M. J. (2019). Exemplars illustrating de-implementation of tradition-based practices. *Critical Care Nurse, 39*(6), 64–69. https://doi.org/10.4037/ccn2019534

Administration for Community Living. (2019). *Diversity and cultural competency*. U.S. Department of Health and Human Services. *https://acl.gov/programs/strengthening-aging-and-disability-networks/diversity-and-cultural-competency*

Valdez, A. (2018). What guides your practice? *Journal of Emergency Nursing, 44*(1), 3–4. 10.1016/j.jen.2017.11.010

Wagner, E. (2018). Improving patient care outcomes through better delegation-communication between nurses and assistive personnel. *Journal of Nursing Care Quality, 33*, 187–193. https://doi.org/10.1097/NCQ.0000000000000282

Yuill, C., McCourt, C., Cheyne, H., & Leister, N. (2020). Women's experiences of decision-making and informed choice about pregnancy and birth care: A systematic review and meta-synthesis of qualitative research. *BMC Pregnancy Childbirth, 20*, 343. https://doi.org/10.1186/s12884-020-03023-6

Zahednezhad, H., Hosseini, M., Ebadi, A., Dalvandi, A., & Tabrizi, K. N. (2018). Exploring fair decision-making rules in nursing: A qualitative study. *Nursing Ethics*. https://doi.org/10.1177/0969733018791313

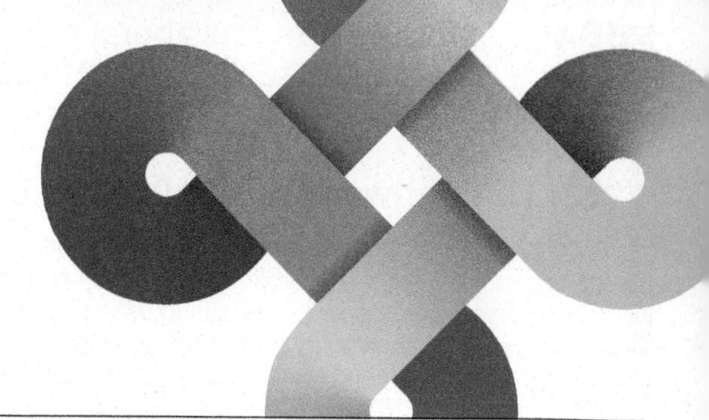

Module 37
Collaboration

Module Outline and Learning Outcomes

The Concept of Collaboration

The Nurse as Collaborator

37.1 Describe the nurse's role as a collaborative member of the healthcare team.

Concepts Related to Collaboration

37.2 Describe the relationship between collaboration and selected other concepts and implications for nursing care.

Competencies Basic to Collaboration

37.3 Identify competencies necessary for successful collaboration.

Interprofessional Collaborative Practice

37.4 Summarize the benefits and nature of interprofessional collaborative practice.

Conflict Prevention and Management

37.5 Analyze aspects of conflict prevention and management.

Incivility in the Workplace

37.6 Describe the effects of incivility in the workplace.

›› The Concept of Collaboration

Concept Key Terms

Call-out, 2557
Collaboration, 2553
Conflict, 2559
Conflict competence, 2562
Covert conflict, 2560
Handoff, 2557
Horizontal violence, 2563
Incivility, 2563
Interdisciplinary, 2553
Intergroup conflict, 2560
Interorganizational conflict, 2560
Interpersonal conflict, 2560
Interprofessional, 2553
Intrapersonal conflict, 2560
Mutual respect, 2556
Overt conflict, 2560
Verbal abuse, 2563
Workplace bullying, 2563

The nature of healthcare today is so complex that it is impossible for any single professional to provide high-quality patient care without working with other members of the healthcare team. The best care is delivered in a collaborative environment with all members of the healthcare team working together to improve patient health outcomes. **Collaboration** among members of an interprofessional team occurs when two or more individuals work together toward a common goal by combining their skills, knowledge, and resources to deliver high-quality care while avoiding duplication of effort (World Health Organization [WHO], 2010). Ideally, collaboration is a dynamic process in which patients (individuals, groups, or communities) work together with physicians, nurses, and other healthcare providers (HCPs) to meet their health objectives. There is growing support to provide interprofessional education to students in healthcare fields to prepare them for interprofessional practice.

Collaborative care is fundamental to nursing practice. Virginia Henderson (1991), one of the pioneers of professional nursing, defined collaborative care as "a partnership relationship between doctors, nurses, and other healthcare providers with patients and their families" (p. 44).

To prepare nurses with the knowledge, skills, and attitudes needed to improve the quality and safety of the patient care environment, QSEN (Quality and Safety Education for Nurses) identified teamwork and collaboration as two necessary competencies, along with patient-centered-care, evidence-based practice, quality improvement, safety, and informatics (Cronenwett et al., 2007) (**Box 37.1** ››). The American Nurses Association (ANA) *Standards of Professional Nursing Practice* has also recognized collaboration as a key component of nursing practice. Standard 10 outlines specific competencies related to the nurse's role in collaboration (ANA, 2015b). Additionally, the National League for Nurses (NLN; 2015), whose mission is to promote excellence in nursing education, has called for schools of nursing to work with other professions to establish interprofessional education.

The term **interprofessional** usually refers to professionals from various disciplines, whereas the term **interdisciplinary** is often used to denote that paraprofessionals are also included. For this module and throughout this text, the term *interprofessional* refers to professionals from various disciplines along with support staff, the patient, and family members—anyone who is working together for the benefit of the patient.

Successful collaboration requires that nurses develop skills in communication and teamwork, value the roles and responsibilities of other team members, and work to establish

Box 37.1
QSEN: Teamwork and Collaboration

According to QSEN, nurses should function effectively within nursing and interprofessional teams, fostering open communication, mutual respect, and shared decision making to achieve quality patient care. The knowledge (K), skills (S), and attitudes (A) necessary to do this include:

- (K) Describe one's personal strengths, limitations, and values in functioning as a member of a team. (S) Demonstrate an awareness of personal strengths and limitations; initiate a plan for self-development as a team member and act with integrity, consistency, and respect for differing views. (A) Acknowledge your potential to be a contributing team member while appreciating the importance of collaboration.
- (K) Describe the scope of practice and roles of other health team members the strategies for identifying and managing overlaps in team member roles and recognize the contributions of other team members in helping patients and families to achieve goals. This can be achieved by (S) functioning within your scope of practice, assuming the role of team member or leader as appropriate, requesting help when needed, clarifying roles, and integrating the contributions of others in a (A) respectful manner.
- (K) Analyze differences in communication style and understand the impact of your own communication style on others by (S) communicating with and soliciting input from team members and initiating actions to resolve conflict by (A) actively participating in the resolution process.
- (K) Describe the impact of team functioning on patient safety and quality care and explain how levels of authority have the potential to affect teamwork. (S) Follow best practice to minimize risks associated with handoffs and (A) acknowledge that care transition is risky.
- (K) Identify system barriers and facilitators of effective team functioning and examine strategies for improving systems to support team performance by (S) participating in designing systems that support teamwork and (A) valuing the influence of system solutions in achieving effective team functioning.

Source: Based on Cronenwett et al. (2007).

a climate of mutual respect. Successful interprofessional education and practice depend on healthcare professionals working in teams to provide safe, quality care (NLN, 2015).

The Nurse as Collaborator

Collaboration may occur between nurses, between HCPs and patients, and between HCPs from different professional backgrounds (**Figure 37.1** »). Collaborative interprofessional teams recognize each individual profession's value and contributions in an atmosphere of mutual trust and respect through open discussion and shared decision making (ANA, 2015b). Nurses may also be involved in collaborating to develop community initiatives, write or revise legislation, or conduct health-related research. **Table 37.1** » lists professionals who may serve as members of an interprofessional healthcare team and their respective roles.

To fulfill a collaborative role, nurses need accountability and increased authority in their practice areas. Continuing education in role exploration, communication, group work, and other areas helps members of the healthcare team understand the collaborative nature of their roles, specific contributions of each professional member, and the importance of working together. Each professional needs to understand how an integrated delivery system centers on the patient's healthcare needs rather than on the care given by any one group. **Box 37.2** » describes selected aspects of the nurse's role as a collaborator.

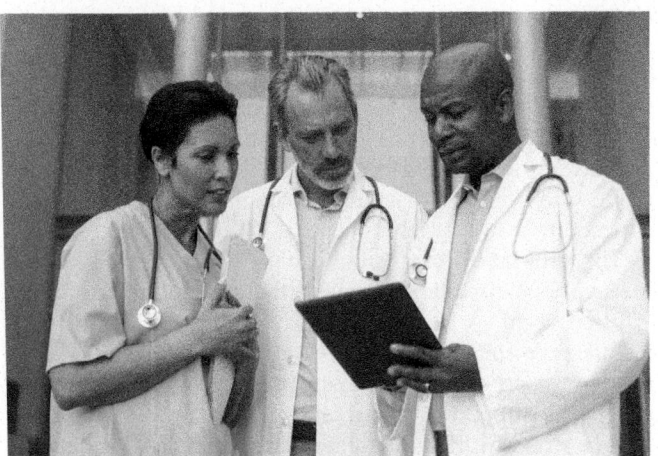

Figure 37.1 » The healthcare team works together to communicate concerns and mutually problem solve.
Source: Wavebreak Media Ltd/123RF.

Concepts Related to Collaboration

Effective collaboration influences healthcare on every level. At the organizational level, collaboration leads to increased efficiency, staff retention, and cost effectiveness. For patients, collaboration promotes safety, decreasing morbidity and mortality rates. Patients who are involved in the collaborative process report an increased sense of autonomy, which leads to greater overall satisfaction with care. Nurses who participate in collaboration report an increased sense of perceived autonomy and professionalism, along with greater job satisfaction. Some of the concepts integral to collaboration are shown in the Concepts Related to Collaboration feature. They are presented in alphabetical order.

Competencies Basic to Collaboration

Core competencies to improve patient outcomes and improve quality of care through interprofessional collaboration include values and ethics, roles and responsibilities, communication, and teams and teamwork (Interprofessional Education Collaborative [IPEC], 2016).

Values and Ethics

Members of the interprofessional team have a duty to work with other professionals and the patient in a mutually respectful manner that promotes trust and supports the shared goals

TABLE 37.1 Potential Members of Interprofessional Healthcare Teams

Healthcare Professional	Role
Nurse	The nurse's role is to meet the unique healthcare needs of a patient, community, or population. A registered nurse (RN) uses the nursing process to assess health, identify health concerns, and develop, implement, and direct a plan of care. A licensed practical nurse (LPN) or licensed vocational nurse (LVN) assists in the delivery of patient care under the supervision of a RN, physician, or other licensed practitioner. The advanced practice registered nurse (APRN) diagnoses and treats healthcare problems, holds a graduate or doctoral degree, and includes the roles of nurse practitioner, clinical nurse specialist, nurse anesthetist, and nurse midwife.
Unlicensed assistive personnel	Unlicensed assistive personnel (UAP) are not licensed to perform nursing care but work in a supportive role to nurses by carrying out delegated patient care activities, such as assisting with personal hygiene, feeding, and ambulating. UAPs may include certified nursing assistants (CNAs), home health aides, and nursing and patient care technicians. UAPs are not licensed but some, such as CNAs, may hold a certification to perform certain tasks. Each state board of nursing delineates the process of delegation by the RN to the UAP in their nurse practice acts.
Complementary healthcare providers	Nonmainstream practice used along with conventional medicine is considered complementary. Examples of complementary practitioners include chiropractors, herbalists, acupuncturists, massage therapists, reflexologists, and holistic health healers. These professionals, when used in conjunction with providers of allopathic or Western medicine, are considered to be complementary providers.
Case manager	The case manager works collaboratively with HCPs to coordinate quality care and resources for the patient across all settings to ensure quality, timely, and fiscally sound outcomes. Case managers are often nurses but may also be social workers and other healthcare team members.
Dentist	Dentists promote oral health and diagnose and treat problems of the teeth and oral cavity. Many hospitals, especially long-term care facilities, have dentists on staff.
Dietitian or nutritionist	A registered dietitian (RD) or registered dietitian nutritionist (RDN) is board-certified and has passed a registration exam after completing a bachelor's or master's program. RDs manage medical nutrition therapy to prevent and manage acute and chronic medical conditions. The RD/RDN assesses nutritional status of individuals, diagnoses nutritional problems, and develops and evaluates a nutritional plan of care. A nutritionist is knowledgeable about food and nutrition but may not have an academic degree in the field of nutrition. Nutritionists teach about healthy diets to promote or prevent disease but do not diagnose and treat disease. A nutritionist may, for example, teach parents about a balanced diet to promote health for all members of the family.
Information technologist	The information technologist (IT) works with the healthcare team to manage patient health information. The IT expert supports electronic health records, personal health records, telehealth, and electronic prescribing, while ensuring the privacy and security of patient data. The IT expert also supports and educates healthcare staff in the use of healthcare information systems.
Occupational therapist	The occupational therapist (OT) provides rehabilitation to individuals with mental, physical, or developmental needs due to injury, illness, or disability. The OT helps individuals perform daily activities needed for school, work, home, and recreation. The OT may use exercises, interventions, assistive devices, and technology to improve an individual's functioning.
Medical technologist	Medical technologists, such as laboratory, radiological, and nuclear medicine technologists, assist the healthcare team by providing data used to diagnose and treat medical conditions and illnesses. A paramedical laboratory technologist, for example, uses specialized instruments and automated equipment to analyze blood, body fluids, and other tissues (such as wound drainage or feces) to provide information used in making therapeutic decisions.
Pharmacist	In addition to preparing and dispensing medications, pharmacists perform medication reconciliation and patient education and work with the healthcare team to develop and evaluate the pharmacologic plan of care for patients.
Physical therapist	A physical therapist (PT) assesses, diagnoses, and develops a plan of care to help patients with musculoskeletal problems improve mobility, manage pain, restore function, and prevent disability. The goal of physical therapy is to maintain or restore function through physical interventions such as exercise, massage, electrical stimulation, hydrotherapy, heat and cold therapy, and ultrasound. A PT also educates patients about their conditions, such as caring for an artificial limb or using a cane or walker.
Physician	A physician diagnoses and treats diseases and injuries and works with patients to promote health and prevent or delay the onset of disease. A physician may be a general practitioner in internal medicine, primary care, or family health or a specialist in areas such as pediatrics, psychiatry, obstetrics and gynecology, neurology, dermatology, ophthalmology, or surgery.
Physician assistant	Physician assistants (PAs), under the direction of a physician, diagnose and treat medical problems and assist in surgery. PAs work in all medical and surgical settings, such as hospitals, offices, health centers, long-term care, and the workplace. Nurses should check the Nurse Practice Act in the state where they work and their workplace policies before following orders written by a PA.
Respiratory therapist	Respiratory therapists (RTs) provide care to patients with conditions affecting breathing and the airways, such as asthma, pneumonia, emphysema, trauma, cystic fibrosis, and muscular dystrophy. Care provided by an RT may include oxygen therapy, mechanical ventilation, breathing treatments, pulmonary function testing, chest physiotherapy, and patient education.
Social worker	A social worker helps patients and their families to cope, problem solve, adjust to illness or life events, and may provide counseling or psychotherapy. Social workers protect vulnerable populations, such as children and older adults, but they also work with others who need assistance due to, for example, finances, lifestyle, substance abuse, relationships, or psychologic issues.
Speech–language pathologist (SLP)	Also referred to as speech therapists, SLPs work with individuals who have communication problems, speech disorders, and difficulties with eating, drinking, or swallowing.

Box 37.2
The Nurse as a Collaborator

With Patients

- Acknowledges, supports, and encourages patients' active involvement in healthcare decisions.
- Encourages patient autonomy and equal position with other members of the healthcare team.
- Helps patients set mutually agreed-on goals and objectives for healthcare.
- Provides patients with consultation in a collaborative fashion.

With Peers

- Shares personal expertise with other nurses and elicits the expertise of others to ensure high-quality patient care.
- Develops a sense of trust and mutual respect with peers who value each member's unique contributions.

With Other Healthcare Professionals

- Recognizes the contribution by members of the interprofessional team by virtue of their expertise.
- Listens to each individual's viewpoints.
- Shares responsibilities with other members of the team to explore care options, set realistic goals, and make decisions about the plan of care with patients and their families.
- Participates in collaborative interprofessional research to increase knowledge of a clinical problem or situation.

With Professional Nursing Organizations

- Seeks opportunities to collaborate with and within professional organizations.
- Serves on committees in state (or provincial), national, and international nursing organizations or specialty groups.
- Supports professional organizations in political action to create solutions for professional and healthcare concerns.

With Legislators

- Offers expert opinions on legislative initiatives related to healthcare.
- Collaborates with other HCPs and consumers on healthcare legislation in order to best serve the needs of the public.

of quality care and safety (IPEC, 2016). **Mutual respect** occurs when team members value the contributions and knowledge of each team member and treat all members as equals (Emich, 2018). Respect also includes acknowledging the uniqueness and differing views that each member and profession brings to the team (Cronenwett et al., 2007). Trust occurs when a team member is confident in the actions of another individual. The healthcare team must also acknowledge the diversity, values, and preferences of each patient and of each other. Mutual respect and trust do not just happen, rather, they are shared processes that are nurtured and developed over time (Karam, Brault, Van Durme, & Macq, 2018).

The healthcare system itself has not always created an environment that promotes respect or trust of the various HCPs.

Concepts Related to
Collaboration

CONCEPT	RELATIONSHIP TO COLLABORATION	NURSING IMPLICATIONS
Health Policy	↑ Job satisfaction	■ Support by leadership to endorse new approaches in workforce development and innovations that improve work environments and increase job satisfaction.
Healthcare Systems	↑ Collaboration among healthcare team members → ↓ duplication of patient services and ↓ healthcare costs	■ Support and promote collaboration among healthcare team members. ■ Apply principles of effective collaboration, including principles that facilitate clear communication. ■ Participate in interprofessional committees to build collaboration on a systemwide level.
Professionalism	↑ Nurse–physician collaboration → ↑ perceived professional autonomy → ↑ nursing professionalism	■ Recognize the impact of collaboration on job satisfaction in nursing. ■ Apply principles of collaboration to promote collaborative nurse–physician relationships. ■ Educate members of the team about nursing roles and responsibilities.
Quality Improvement	↑ Situational awareness ↑ Teamwork among healthcare team members	■ Identify threats to patient safety through open communication, identification of purpose and skill, and established plan of action.
Safety	↑ Collaboration among healthcare team members → ↓ patient morbidity and ↓ patient mortality rates	■ Support and promote collaboration among healthcare team members. ■ Participate in interprofessional team meetings and discuss concerns with team members. ■ Educate healthcare team members about the safety-related benefits of collaboration.

Although progress has been made toward creating more trusting relationships, past attitudes may continue to impede efforts toward collaborative practice (see the Evidence-Based Practice feature).

Roles and Responsibilities

Each member of the interprofessional team should be committed to understanding and appreciating the role and scope of practice of other members of the team. Moreover, the team should work toward using the skills of each team member to enhance patient care. Each team member is also responsible for continuing education and professional development to develop their interprofessional skills. Each role should also be clearly communicated to the patient (IPEC, 2016).

Communication Skills

Communication is crucial to developing mutual respect and trust. It is the basic method through which interprofessional collaboration occurs and is essential to ensuring patient safety (Karam et al., 2018). Communication failures among providers have been identified as a major cause of adverse events (Umberfield, Ghaferi, Krein, & Manojlovich, 2019). The typical patient environment is fraught with interruptions, distractions, conflicting goals, anxieties, and stressors that often hamper the best intentions. Even the most well-intended comment or instruction can be misinterpreted or misunderstood and can compound the problem (Burgener, 2020).

Members of the healthcare team should be sensitive to differences in communication styles and the effects that their own style has on successful collaboration (IPEC, 2016) (see Module 38, Communication, for information about communication styles). For example, in a study of team communication patterns, Walter and colleagues (2019) found that physicians on a pediatric cardiac intensive care unit team spoke an average of 89.9% more than other team members in family case planning meetings. Style of communication also differs among healthcare professionals. In an integrated review of the literature, Tan and colleagues (2017) noted that physicians communicate more concisely than nurses, who tend to use a descriptive communication style.

Team-centered communication, as opposed to status-based communication, demonstrates appreciation for each member's contributions and can flatten perceived hierarchies, such as those that have historically existed between physicians and nurses (Armstrong, 2019). Status-based communication is a hierarchical model that can be intimidating, keeping team members from speaking up and increasing the risk of errors. Team-centered approaches focus on the "we"—the work "we will do for this patient"—versus one-sided commands such as "give this, do that" statements that do not invite dialogue and do not promote collaboration. Acknowledging alternative perspectives, articulating one's own viewpoint, and engaging in mutual give-and-take are necessary qualities for effective collaboration. Using an attentive style of communication that encompasses active listening (instead of a dominant, take-charge, or argumentative style) helps to remove the barriers that impede effective communication and collaboration (Harper & Kracun, 2019; IPEC, 2016).

Communication among team members should reduce risks that may occur during patient handoffs or transitions in care and communicate in a manner that reduces poor communication associated with hierarchies among team members (Cronenwett et al., 2007). Standardized communication strategies have been developed to facilitate interprofessional communication and reduce errors. To improve team collaboration and communication skills, the Department of Defense's Patient Safety Program and the Agency for Healthcare Research and Quality (AHRQ; 2019) developed *TeamSTEPPS* (Team Strategies and Tools to Enhance Performance and Patient Safety). These strategies and tools include the following:

SBAR (Situation, Background, Assessment, Recommendation/Request) is a tool to communicate critical information about a patient that requires attention, especially during a patient **handoff** (the transfer and acceptance of patient care responsibility from one nurse to another, such as at the end of a shift (The Joint Commission, 2017). See Exemplar 38.D, Reporting, in Module 38, Communication, for more detailed information on SBAR. Table 38.10 gives an overview of critical information to include in an SBAR report.

Call-out is used to report critical information to all members of the team at the same time. For example, at the bedside of a patient with chest pain, the physician might ask, "Electrocardiogram findings?" The medical resident might respond, "ST segment elevation in anterior leads." The physician then asks, "Blood pressure?" to which the nurse responds "86/60."

Checkback is a technique of repeating back information to check that critical information by the speaker is understood by the receiver. For example, in a code, a physician might order, "Atropine 0.5 mg IV push." The nurse would respond, "Atropine 0.5 mg IV push." The physician then confirms the order, saying "You are right, atropine 0.5 mg push."

CUS (I am Concerned, I am Uncomfortable, this is a Safety issue/I don't feel this is Safe) is a technique to let the team know your concerns. For instance, a nurse might say, "I am *concerned* about Mrs. Abbott's blood pressure. I am *uncomfortable* with how low it is. I don't think it is *safe* to give this medication right now."

Two-challenge rule gives team members the right to voice safety concerns twice to ensure that they have been heard. The challenged team member then needs to acknowledge that the concern was heard. If the safety issue is not addressed, the concerned team member should take additional actions and go up the chain of command, if required.

I PASS THE BATON is a structured method of handing off a patient to another team member using the following steps:

Introduce self and patient

Patient's name, identifiers, and basic information

Assessment, including chief complaint, symptoms, diagnosis, and vital signs

Situation: Current status of patient

Safety issues: Critical lab values, allergies, falls, infection, social issues

THE

Background: Health and family history, medications

Action: Interventions carried out or needed, with reasoning

Timing: Degree of urgency, clear timing, prioritizing actions

Ownership: Assign responsibility for actions

Next: What are next steps?

>> **Stay Current:** Visit the TeamSTEPPS 2.0 website at https://www.ahrq.gov/teamstepps/instructor/fundamentals/index.html.

Teams and Teamwork

Teams depend on each member to interact with other members toward the goal of patient care and to put team goals before individual goals (AHRQ, 2019). Patients and families should be included as members of the team and given the opportunity to voice concerns, ask questions, have access to information, and participate in care. Members should understand the role and scope of practice of each team member as well as their own scope of practice. When addressing patient care or concerns, all team members should provide discipline-specific input, followed by discussion and shared decision making. Team members should also acknowledge each other and work together to resolve areas of conflict and disagreement.

Clinical Example A

Bill Hainsley, 67 years old, is ready for discharge following a knee replacement. His surgeon recommends discharge to a rehabilitation facility to gain strength in his leg and to learn to navigate his home safely. Although Mr. Hainsley believes that he can manage his rehabilitation at home, his wife is concerned about her ability to help him navigate their two-story house, which has only a small half-bath on the first floor. Mr. Hainsley is worried about the cost of going to a rehabilitation facility. A team meeting takes place to plan for Mr. Hainsley's discharge. In attendance are Mr. and Mrs. Hainsley and a primary care nurse, RN case manager, physical therapist, social worker, and surgical resident.

The team discusses what is needed for Mr. Hainsley to be safely discharged to his home and makes key decisions for his home care.

Evidence-Based Practice

Overcoming Barriers: The Benefits of Nurse–Physician Collaboration

Problem

Despite research-based evidence that supports the benefits of effective collaboration between nurses and physicians, barriers to this process—several of which relate to the relationship between the nurse and the physician—remain intact.

Evidence

While nurse–physician communication is at the core of interprofessional collaboration, a systematic review of the literature indicates that barriers, such as power struggles and hierarchical relationships, can deter collaboration (Karam et al., 2018). Although the nurse–physician relationship is shifting from subservient–superior to collegial, differences still exist in how nurses and physicians communicate and think about collaboration (Tan, Zhou, & Kelly, 2017).

Understanding the roles of each discipline is important to the collaboration process. In a study of shared mental models and mutual respect between nurses and physicians on a medical–surgical unit, researchers found that physicians and nurses viewed role responsibilities and mutual trust differently, creating potential barriers to nurse–physician collaboration (McComb, Lemater, Hennneman, & Hinchey, 2017). They recommend that healthcare professionals learn about the roles of each profession represented on the team so that there is a shared understanding of each member's responsibilities.

In another systematic review, House and Havens (2017) found that nurses and physicians perceived interprofessional collaborative relationships differently. Nurses wanted to be part of the decision-making process, participate in developing the plan of care, have a reciprocal sharing of expertise, have their feedback about patients considered, share concerns, and offer suggestions. Furthermore, nurses wanted physicians to actively listen and to communicate in an open and clear manner. Alternatively, physicians saw themselves as the key decision maker and the person in control of patient care. Some felt that collaboration meant that nurses were easily accessible to assist or answer questions about patients. Other physicians felt that information from nurses was critical in their care of patients.

Tan and colleagues (2017), in an integrated review on factors impacting interprofessional communication, concluded that segregated professional education promotes differing views on communication by nurses and physicians. Interestingly, in evaluations of communication by physicians and nurses, physicians were more likely to rate the communication as effective than nurses. Similarly, Collette and colleagues (2017), in a study of hospital nurses and physicians, also found that physicians viewed collaboration more positively than nurses did.

Implications

Overcoming barriers to collaboration is essential to providing quality patient care.

Interprofessional education can improve the way nurses and physicians regard other healthcare disciplines, collaborative behaviors, and the benefits of an interprofessional approach to patient care (Spaulding et al., 2019). To improve interdisciplinary collaboration, Collette et al. (2017) recommend emphasis on interdisciplinary rounding, understanding the roles of team members, respecting team members, and improving communication. Support from administration is important in creating a culture that supports positive interdisciplinary relationships.

Critical Thinking Application

Development of a collaborative relationship requires mutual trust and respect, an understanding of the roles and responsibilities of each team member, clear methods of communication, and professionalism. The common goal of providing the best care possible for the patient should be the starting point of all discussions and remain as the focal point throughout patient care. The expertise of each team member needs to be shared and appreciated: the physician or advanced practice nurse for the diagnostic information, the nurse for the patient- and family-specific knowledge, and other health team members (e.g., PT, OT, social work) for their skill and capability in condition-specific treatment and follow-up.

Mr. Hainsley expresses his desire to go home, and his wife discusses her concerns about her ability to provide care for him. The nurse and physical therapist convey their concerns about the ability of the couple to manager safe transfers and ambulation. The social worker discusses financial resources available to Mr. Hainsley, while the case manager will coordinate care to ensure a timely and safe discharge for him. The surgical resident describes activity restrictions that Mr. Hainsley needs to follow until his follow-up appointment with the surgeon.

The RN case manager contacts the home care department and arranges for the home care nurse to see Mr. and Mrs. Hainsley on the day of discharge. The primary care nurse explains Mr. Hainsley's medications, activity restrictions, and signs and symptoms to report to the surgeon. The hospital's physical therapist teaches safe transfer and ambulation techniques using a walker to Mr. Hainsley and his wife and then makes a call to the physical therapist working on the home care team to relay Mr. Hainsley's progress and needs. The social worker reviews costs and financial issues and recommends places that loan medical equipment. In addition, the primary nurse documents in the chart that the meeting occurred, who was involved, and the final decision by the patient and team about discharge.

Critical Thinking Questions

1. What collaborative skills were used by Mr. Hainsley's team to ensure a safe and timely discharge?
2. What other skills and team competencies could the team have used during the collaborative meeting?
3. Describe the role of Mr. and Mrs. Hainsley during the team meeting.

Interprofessional Collaborative Practice

Interprofessional collaboration is essential in an increasingly specialized and fragmented healthcare system. An interprofessional collaborative framework can improve the delivery of care, manage costs, enhance quality, and increase patient satisfaction with care. Interprofessional collaborative practice models attempt to achieve the following objectives:

- Provide patient-directed and patient-centered care using a participative framework.
- Enhance continuity of care across the continuum of health, from wellness and prevention through acute illness to recovery or rehabilitation.
- Improve patient and family satisfaction with care.
- Provide high-quality, cost-effective, evidence-based care that improves patient outcomes.
- Promote mutual respect, communication, and understanding between the patient and the healthcare team.
- Provide opportunities to address and resolve system-related issues and problems.
- Develop interdependent relationships and understanding among providers and patients.

Benefits of Interprofessional Collaboration

Because collaborative care is patient-centered and patient-directed, collaborative care empowers patients to be informed consumers and actively work in partnership with the healthcare team in the decision-making process. When patients are empowered to participate and professionals share mutually set goals with patients, quality of care improves and everyone—including the organization and healthcare system—ultimately benefits. When quality improves, adherence to therapeutic regimens increases, lengths of stay decrease, and overall costs to the system decline. Sound application of collaborative strategies leads to decreased patient morbidity and mortality rates (Goldsberry, 2018) and reduced complications, error rates, and patient length of stay (WHO, 2010). When team members collaborate, evidence-based care, decision-making skills, and creativity improve among team members. Because collaborative teams tend to have less of a hierarchical structure, team members may report greater feelings of empowerment, respect, and appreciation. Other benefits include higher staff satisfaction and retention rates (Morley & Cashell, 2017), as well as improved coordination of care, use of specialists through referrals, and access to healthcare (WHO, 2010).

Interprofessional Settings

Interprofessional collaboration can occur in any setting in which healthcare is provided, not just within a hospital. Examples of interprofessional settings outside the hospital environment include:

- ***Skilled nursing, rehabilitation, and long-term care facilities:*** Patients admitted to these facilities require care from multiple disciplines, including nursing; medical (physician, nurse practitioner, specialist); physical, occupational, speech–language, or respiratory therapy; social services; and mental health or psychiatric services.
- ***Schools and educational settings:*** Children with disabilities, who are medically fragile, or who have acute or chronic conditions may require interprofessional care from nurses, teachers, school administrators, counselors, mental health specialists, physical therapists, occupational therapists, speech–language therapists, physicians, and others.
- ***Assertive community treatment (ACT):*** ACT provides mental health and support services for individuals with serious mental illness (such as schizophrenia or bipolar disorder) to promote optimal functioning at home and within the community. Professionals participating in a patient's care team may include psychiatrists, psychologists, social workers, pharmacists, advanced practice nurses, employment counselors, and peer support specialists.
- ***Elder care services:*** Options such as Programs of All-Inclusive Care for the Elderly (PACE) offer services for older adults to meet their healthcare needs in the community. Services may include medical care, respite care for caregivers, transportation to medical and social services appointment, and mental healthcare. Collaborative team members may include physicians, nurses, therapists, social workers, and mental health professionals.

Conflict Prevention and Management

Conflict occurs when there is disagreement or discord among individuals, groups, or organizations that prevents problem solving and interferes with effective communication (McKibben, 2017). Conflict is a normal part of the work environment. Responses to conflict depend on the nurse's leadership communication skills for achieving positive outcomes within the work environment. Conflict can never be eliminated; however, it can be managed, and it takes both skill and competence to handle it successfully.

Types of Conflict

Conflict can take place between nurses, between nurses and patients or family members, between nurses and other members of the healthcare team, or within a unit or a department, or it can affect the entire organization. Conflict may also occur between units and departments, between organizations, and between an organization and the community.

Levels of Conflict

Levels of conflict may be categorized in a variety of ways. This section approaches conflict as existing on four levels:

- **Intrapersonal conflict**, which occurs within an individual, is stress or tension that results from real or perceived pressure generated by incompatible expectations. This may occur when an individual has role conflict or confusion (Barr & Dowding, 2019). For example, intrapersonal conflict may occur when a nurse must choose between accepting a day-shift position that interferes with fulfilling family-related responsibilities or staying on the night shift and always feeling sluggish and fatigued.
- **Interpersonal conflict** occurs between two or more individuals (Barr & Dowding, 2019). It can arise from differences in goals or personalities, competition, or concern about territory, control, or loss. Interpersonal conflict may occur when one staff member misunderstands the roles or responsibilities of another or when one member of the team belittles or bullies another.
- **Intergroup conflict** occurs between teams that are in competition or opposition to one another. In some cases, the groups are competing for rewards or scarce resources (Barr & Dowding, 2019). An example of this type of conflict is the debate occurring between physicians who want to bring nurse practitioners under the control of the medical board and nurse practitioners who feel strongly that they should remain under the control of the board of nursing.
- **Interorganizational conflict** commonly involves competition between two organizations that exist within one market (Black, Gardner, Pierce, & Steers, 2019). For example, hospitals within the same community may demonstrate interorganizational conflict, with different institutions advertising superior care for a subset of patients, or colleges of nursing may compete for qualified applicants for program admission.

Covert and Overt Conflict

At any level, conflict may be overt or covert. **Overt conflict** occurs when people or groups openly disagree. Since this type of conflict is apparent, it can be more easily addressed and plans for resolution can be made. **Covert conflict** is not obvious or may be underlying, expressed in reactive or avoidant behaviors. Examples of reactive behaviors include complaining, gossiping, and using passive-aggressive behaviors. Covert conflict may also be at play if repressive behaviors, such as absenteeism and tardiness, occur.

Although sustained avoidance may be associated with negative outcomes, avoidance may be an effective method of temporarily managing conflict. For instance, avoidance may be appropriate when emotions are flaring and the individuals involved would benefit from taking time to regain composure before discussing the issues at the foundation of the conflict (Schermerhorn & Bachrach, 2018). However, sustained tactics of covert conflict result in increased stress, distress, and confusion about how to address the conflict. Acknowledging covert conflict is not easy, and everyone involved may have different perceptions of the conflict because it operates below the surface.

Causes of Conflict

To resolve conflict effectively, nurses must understand its cause. Kim and colleagues (2017) identified sources of individual, interpersonal, and organizational conflict in healthcare. Sources of individual conflict included personal characteristics, communication styles, and conflict management methods. Factors that influenced interpersonal conflict included various forms of incivility, degree of support, communication, differences in education, and generational characteristics. Organizational conflict arose from professional role ambiguity, scope of practice, organizational structure and workflow, work environment, and resource constraints.

The Nurse–Physician Relationship

The nurse–physician relationship should be the strongest collaboration that nurses have in order to meet the needs of their patients. Unfortunately, this is not always the case. Factors that can undermine the nurse–patient relationship include lack of confidence on the part of the nurse, a need to save face when mistakes are made (by either the nurse or the physician), or an attempt or need to preserve a patriarchal nurse–physician relationship (Goldsberry, 2018; Zuzelo, 2019). Both nurses and physicians can contribute to inadequacies in this relationship. When conflict does occur, it often becomes a barrier to effective patient care. Cooperation and collaboration are integral to the success of this relationship.

The Nurse–Patient Relationship

Although the nurse–patient relationship is fundamental to nursing, conflict with patients or their family members or caregivers can arise. Causes of conflict in this relationship include lack of knowledge on the part of the patient or family member, poor coping skills by the patient or family member, fear or anxiety resulting in the patient or family member expressing frustration, and failure of the nurse to assess or meet patient needs or promote the therapeutic relationship. If not resolved in a timely and satisfactory manner, conflict between the nurse and patient or family member can become a barrier to effective care.

The Nurse–Nurse Relationship

Nurse–nurse and nurse–coworker conflicts can also occur. When not managed properly, these may rise to the level of workplace bullying or incivility. Strategies for preventing and managing conflict (including workplace bullying and incivility) are outlined in the sections that follow.

Clinical Example B

Josiah Elliot, 72 years old, is admitted to the hospital with diagnoses of congestive heart failure, chronic renal failure, hypertension, and benign prostatic hypertrophy. The nurse develops his plan of nursing care and identifies the problems of fluid volume excess, urinary retention, inadequate gas exchange, and anxiety. Three days later, Mr. Elliot has lost 9 pounds and is breathing more easily. He also denies feeling anxious and reports, "I'm relaxed now that I can breathe!" The patient's problems of fluid volume excess, inadequate gas exchange, and anxiety are all marked as resolved. During morning rounds with Mr. Elliot's healthcare team, the nurse gives an update on the patient's condition and questions the need to continue administering the large doses of diuretics that were ordered when the patient was admitted. The team addresses the nurse's concerns, and the physician reduces the dosage of the diuretics. The physician asks about Mr. Elliot's nutritional status and suitability for discharge to home. The dietitian notes that Mr. Elliot has been educated about the need to limit his sodium intake and understands the importance of following this diet. After a discussion that includes Mr. Elliot and his wife, there is agreement that he is ready for discharge with home care follow-up. The RN case manager will work with the patient to arrange home care.

Critical Thinking Questions

1. Describe the impact of the collaborative approach by the healthcare team on Mr. Elliot's outcomes.
2. How might this patient's care have differed if the healthcare team had not collaborated?
3. What further collaboration is indicated in providing care for Mr. Elliot?

Preventing Conflict

Workplace conflict is inevitable as long as there are differences between people. While these differences add to the diversity and vigor of an organization, they can also lead to conflict.

Preventing conflict involves being aware of personal and situational cues that indicate a rise in tension and negative behaviors (Weberg, Mangold, Porter-O'Grady, & Malloch, 2019). Addressing these cues promptly can prevent escalation to higher levels that can be more difficult to resolve. Moreover, teams that promote learning, member accountability, and continued development experience less conflict (Ellis & Abbott, 2020).

Nurses and other members of the healthcare team should recognize their feelings of increased tension and anxiety. They should also be alert for situations that suggest a rise in tensions in others, such as:

- Arguments
- Excluding a coworker
- Acting out
- Snide remarks.

Developing unit procedures that address workplace conflict and engagement in discussions that address sources of conflict can help keep conflict from escalating to a point that is difficult to control. Healthcare teams need to know that conflict can be handled through open communication. Teams that do not have confidence and trust in their workplace are less likely to recognize potential conflict or unsafe conditions (Weberg et al., 2019).

The hierarchical nature of healthcare can cause some team members to feel subordinate to other team members, lacking a voice and feeling unimportant or appreciated (McKibben, 2017). Creating a shared understanding about roles and responsibilities in team members increases respect and trust (McComb et al., 2017). The move toward interprofessional education has increased this understanding of the roles and responsibilities, leading to improved communication and collaboration and reducing the hierarchy among team members (Armstrong, 2018).

Taking steps to decrease or manage stress levels helps to reduce the likelihood of initiating conflict (see Focus on Integrative Health: Stress Reduction). Other strategies that help prevent conflict include the following (Choudhary, 2018; Weberg et al., 2019):

- Address issues as they arise.
- Avoid destructive criticism, including harsh words, threats, and generalized condemnation of behaviors or performance.
- Address team members in a respectful manner.
- Avoid arguing and maintain a calm demeanor.
- Discuss the situation in a private place, away from patient care areas.
- Practice active listening.
- View the situation from the perspective of the other individual.

Strategies to promote conflict prevention for nursing leaders include the following (Weberg et al., 2019):

- Allocate resources fairly, including fair distribution of workload balance and intensity when assigning patient care.
- Define role expectations for all team members.
- Encourage staff to provide feedback and identify potential concerns without the threat of punitive action.
- Acknowledge team members' accomplishments and achievements, as well as significant life events.

Focus on Integrative Health

Stress Reduction

Integrative health approaches can have a positive impact on stress reduction. Knowing oneself and what is likely to trigger a reaction or a response to stress can be tempered by using integrative approaches, such as meditation, guided imagery, and progressive relaxation. In a study of mindfulness meditation and self-compassion training on perceived stress and compassion in nurses, researchers found that perceived stress scores decreased and compassion scores increased after 6 weeks of mindfulness practice and compassion training. These two integrative approaches can be used by nurses to improve their own well-being. Moreover, the researchers suggest that mindfulness meditation and compassion training by nurses can increase the quality of care they deliver to their patients (Mahon, Mee, Brett, & Dowling, 2017).

Conflict Management Styles

Not everyone responds to conflict in the same way, and individuals vary in how they respond to conflict in different circumstances. While an individual may prefer to use a certain mode of response, sometimes other modes may be more effective, depending on the situation. Five modes for responding to conflict have been identified and can be assessed in individuals using the Thomas–Kilmann Conflict Mode Instrument (TKI; Yoder-Wise, 2019). Those styles include:

1. ***Competing:*** An assertive, power-oriented approach; competing can be seen as self-centered or as defending one's position on behalf of the patient.
2. ***Collaborating:*** A cooperative approach; gaining insight to the perspectives of others can lead to creative problem solving.
3. ***Compromising:*** An approach in which both parties are partially satisfied; compromising, at the very least, addresses rather than avoids the issue.
4. ***Avoiding:*** Seen as uncooperative or a preference to avoid addressing the conflict; however, avoidance can be a helpful approach when more information is needed or when the issue is not worth risking further conflict or a loss of opportunity or consideration.
5. ***Accommodating:*** An attempt to satisfy the concerns of others while neglecting the self; accommodation works best when one individual or group is less interested in the issue than the other.

The ability manage conflict differently depending on the situation is sometimes referred to as **conflict competence**. It is a skill that requires practice and self-awareness to develop (Thomas & Kilmann, 1974).

Responding to Conflict

Not everyone responds to conflict in the same way, and individuals vary in how they respond in different circumstances. Often, interactions and their accompanying behaviors may be unpredictable. In turn, how a person responds to another's behaviors can trigger an unreasonable or inappropriate retort. For example, a coworker's argumentative response when being asked for assistance can trigger an inappropriate retort by the nurse who asked for assistance. Unpredictable and inappropriate responses can create barriers and prevent successful engagement and problem solving.

When conflict occurs, each individual involved has a personal perspective of the conflict. The nurse who can recognize the types of responses to conflict will be better equipped to predict and manage it. To respond effectively to conflict, the nurse should apply the following guidelines:

- Demonstrate honesty, trustworthiness, and respect.
- State the issue objectively and provide a factual basis for the concern.
- Avoid emotion-based discussions.
- Hear all individuals' viewpoints and avoid passing judgment.
- Allow all individuals to express their concerns without interruption.
- Apply active listening techniques.
- Focus on identifying solutions as opposed to exacerbating the problem.
- Recognize that the delivery of safe, effective patient care is the central concern.

As stated earlier, communication, an essential component of conflict resolution, can be status-based or team-centered. Team-centered communication emphasizes shared problem solving, which in turn can prevent conflict. Rather than "I want" or "You need to do x" with the status-based approach, the team-centered approach uses "How can we solve x" as a common strategy. Team-centered communication focuses on "we" statements such as "Mr. X is concerned about. . . . What are your thoughts on this?" or "How can we work together to help him?" Statements such as these reflect shared responsibility and encourage open discussions. Team-centered communication focuses on respect, being self-aware, maintaining boundaries within the professional team, being empathetic, accepting individuality, and promoting equality among team members.

Managing Conflict within the Healthcare Team

Although it is often viewed as negative, conflict can be an impetus for better communication, stronger team relationships, and healthy changes. When effectively managed, conflict can bring to light issues that need to be addressed and result in beneficial outcomes for individuals, groups, and organizations (Bochatay et al., 2017).

When faced with conflict, some individuals may resort to positions of avoidance, compromise, or accommodation rather than address an issue or deal with the conflict. Such approaches, over time, can lead to resentment, which can lead to feelings of ambivalence. Nurses should anticipate that conflict will occur and be prepared to manage conflict constructively. Learning to manage and resolve conflict successfully is essential for professional growth. Nurses need to learn to address difficult situations in a constructive and confident manner and in a safe space where all parties feel that they can have conversations about perceptions or misperceptions without fear of retribution.

Successfully addressing conflict requires self-awareness: Nurses who understand how they respond in times of conflict will be better able to change their behaviors in times of conflict from reactionary to more reflective, allowing them to better see all sides of the conflict and respond appropriately rather than merely reacting to conflict. Self-inventory tools can help nurses better understand how they respond to situations that trigger conflict. Two such tools are the Thomas–Kilmann Conflict Mode Instrument (Thomas & Kilmann, 1974) and Emotional Intelligence Inventory (Stein & Book, 2000).

At an organizational level, leaders need to promote programs that go beyond assertiveness training, conflict management, and collaborative processes. Agencies must engage employees in institution-wide programs that emphasize respect, use communication to improve patient safety, use nondisciplinary approaches to resolve issues, and model language and tactics that reduce tension and remove the barriers that impede resolution, such as TeamSTEPPS and Crew Resource Management (AHRQ, 2019).

Managing Conflict with Patients and Families

Recognize that patients who are sick or injured may be scared and often feel a lack of control (Ilse & Neilipovitz, 2019).

As a result, they may respond in atypical ways, such as yelling or using abusive language. Anger and inappropriate behavior may also be due to pain, medications, anxiety, dementia, and dysfunctional communication. Cultural differences and language barriers can lead to misunderstandings that are displayed as anger.

When conflict arises with a patient or family member, utilize the basic nonverbal and verbal communication skills presented in Module 38, Communication. Try to determine what triggered the patient's or family member's behavior by acknowledging that they seem upset, and then address the trigger. See the Communicating with Patients feature. As appropriate, use available resources to help defuse the situation and offer support, such as the hospital chaplain or social worker. While managing the situation, the nurse should also set limits on negative behaviors. If a patient is using foul language and yelling, the nurse should acknowledge that the patient is upset and set boundaries, such as "I know the delay in surgery is upsetting. I will call the operating room to see what is happening, but I will not tolerate foul language." Any escalation in behavior should be reported immediately to the nurse manager and actions should focus on nurse, visitor, and patient safety. See The Concept of Trauma in Module 32 and Module 51, Safety, for information on handling workplace violence.

Communicating with Patients

Working Phase

When patients are upset or angry, it is important for the nurse to remain calm and understand that the attack is not personal. The nurse should engage the patient in conversation and try to determine the cause of the patient's emotions but avoid arguing. The nurse should show empathy and treat the patient respectfully, For example:

- I can see that you are upset—let's talk. Tell me what is bothering you.
- I know you normally have lunch and take your medications at home around 11:00, but the cafeteria here delivers meal trays around 12:30. What if I bring you a snack and your medications around 11:00?

Incivility in the Workplace

Incivility in the workplace is described as rude and disruptive behaviors that can progress to aggression, bullying, and violence (Schoville & Aebersold, 2020). These behaviors not only intimidate and undermine the victim, but they also negatively impact patient outcomes and the healthcare team, workplace, and nursing profession.

The problem is more widespread than reports indicate, partly because individuals may not report incivility and bullying behaviors out of fear of retribution, lack of knowledge of the reporting process, or an assumption that the behavior is acceptable. Other factors that discourage reporting of incivility in the workplace include the failure of administration to support or respond to previous reports and the overall lack of awareness on the part of the individual or the staff as a result of the normalization of the activity.

Incivility and disruptive behaviors violate professional nursing practice. The ANA (2015a) *Code of Ethics for Nurses* provision 1.5 speaks to collegial relationships with others and the nurse's obligation to create a culture of civility and kindness. Provision 6 addresses the nurse's responsibility for creating a culture of excellence. Despite these ethical expectations, incivility and bullying by nurses is a problem. As a result of bullying behaviors in the workplace, the ANA (2015c) issued a position statement, *Incivility, Bullying, and Workplace Violence*, to promote safe and healthy work environments for nurses, employers, interprofessional team members, and patients. Interprofessional groups have also taken a stance against incivility, bullying, and workplace confidence. For example, within the *Core Competencies for Interprofessional Collaborative Practice* is the values/ethics competency stipulating that healthcare team members must place the interests of patients and populations at the center of care (IPEC, 2016). Other organizations that are working to create healthy work environments include the American Association of Critical Care Nurses, American Nurses Credentialing Center (Magnet recognition), Institute for Safe Medication Practices, and The Joint Commission (Gosselin & Ireland, 2020).

Workplace Bullying

Workplace bullying consists of verbal attacks, refusal to help others, speaking negatively, or taunting. The ANA (2015c) defines bullying as "repeated, unwanted harmful actions intended to humiliate, offend, and cause distress in the recipient" (p. 3). Workplace bullying can cause physical and psychological stress to the victim, adversely affect patient safety and outcomes, and create a negative work environment.

Bullies use power to make victims feel defenseless and demoralized. When not effectively managed or controlled, workplace bullying can escalate to physical threats. The term **horizontal violence** is used to describe aggressive acts committed against a nurse by a nursing colleague. *Vertical violence* occurs when one person has power over another person, such as in a chain of command (Caristo & Clements, 2019). **Verbal abuse** in professional settings is defined as malicious, repeated, harmful mistreatment of an individual with whom one works, regardless of whether that individual is an equal, a superior, or a subordinate. Verbal abuse occurs in healthcare settings between patients and staff, nurses and other nurses, physicians and nurses, and all other staff relationships.

Manifestations of Bullying

Bullying behaviors can be overt or covert. Overt or blatant bullying behaviors are easier to recognize and include gossiping, withholding or hiding information, condescending or patronizing behavior, sabotaging or preventing the nurse from performing duties, intimidating or belittling speech, name-calling, calling out shortcomings, blaming, and forming cliques. Covert bullying behaviors are indirect and may include unkind or even antagonistic interactions, divisive behavior, inequitable patient assignments, failing to act when asked for help, making faces, and eye rolling (Caristo & Clements, 2019).

Impact of Bullying

Workplace bullying produces serious negative consequences to the patient, the nurse being bullied, and the workplace.

Adverse Patient Outcomes

Incivility and bullying prevent team members speaking out against conditions that can cause a patient harm.

When team communication and collaboration are negatively impacted, patient safety and quality of care are affected (Schoville & Aebersold, 2020). Bullying and disrespectful behavior can, for instance, pressure a caregiver to perform an action despite safety concerns (Gosselin & Ireland, 2020). Bullying has also been linked to increased patient falls, medication errors, treatment errors, delayed care, and mortality (Clark, 2019; Houck & Colbert, 2017; Rehber et al., 2020).

Adverse Nurse Outcomes

The nurse who has been bullied often does not report the bullying and bears the brunt of negative behaviors alone, which can affect decision making and performance (Wallace & Gipson, 2017). Victims of bullying experience adverse psychologic effects, including depression, anxiety, isolation, irritability, and posttraumatic stress disorder (Caristo & Clements, 2019). Other psychologic consequences include anger, anxiety, poor self-confidence, exhaustion, helplessness, powerlessness, and sadness (Gosselin & Ireland, 2020). Being bullied can also negatively impact a nurse's ability to think critically and make sound clinical judgements (Clark, 2019). Physical effects that a bullied nurse may experience include weight gain or loss, hypertension, palpitations, headache, insomnia, and irritable bowel syndrome (Houck & Colbert, 2017). Those who witness bullying or who work in a negative environment are also affected by such harmful behaviors, making it difficult to deliver quality care and to maintain a culture of excellence (Schoville & Aebersold, 2020). Moreover, the destructive effects of bullying are cumulative, with the harmful effects becoming worse over time (ANA, 2015c).

Adverse Organizational Outcomes

In healthcare organizations, bullying is linked to nurse burnout, poor staff retention rates, decreased job satisfaction, increased absenteeism, work-related injuries, and decreased productivity (Schoville & Aebersold, 2020). Bullying also places a significant financial burden on the institution due to absenteeism, overtime pay, nurse turnover, and recruiting and orienting new nurse hires. Nurses who are bullied are more likely to change work units or place of employment (Gosselin & Ireland, 2020). In a study of nurse bullying and intent to leave, Sauer and McCoy (2018) found that 40% of nurse participants were bullied in the past 6 months and 68% witnessed bullying. Nurses who were bullied were more likely to leave the employer than to transfer to another unit. The financial burden of nurse turnover for a hospital is estimated to be between $5.2 million and $8.1 million annually (University of New Mexico, 2016).

Responding to Bullying

The first step when encountering bullying is to ensure the safety of staff, patients, and visitors. See Exemplar 51.C, Nurse Safety, in Module 51 for tips on protecting against workplace violence. If there is no threat to safety, respond to the disruptive behavior using assertive and nonthreatening language. A lack of response to negative behaviors sends a message that such actions are acceptable (Wallace & Gipson, 2017). If the disruptive behaviors are taking place in a public or patient area, try to calmly move the bully to a private space. If the bully refuses to move, walk away to show that the behavior is not appropriate. This gives the people involved time to calm down and reflect.

Professional communication skills can diffuse a tense situation and help move toward conciliation when confronting disruptive or bullying behaviors. *Cognitive rehearsal* is a behavioral technique that can help nurses develop and practice responses, under nonstressful conditions, allowing them to respond confidently and professionally to incivility or bullying when it occurs (Armstrong, 2018). The rehearsed response allows the nurse to communicate calmly, acknowledge the situation, and convey expectations (Longo, 2017). (See Clinical Example C). The use of "I" messages is also a useful technique because "you" messages may be construed as accusatory, putting the other person on the defensive (Clark, 2019). The CUS communication technique discussed earlier can also be used by the nurse to express concern about a potentially harmful situation. See Techniques for Assertive Communication in Module 38, Communication.

Clinical Example C

Nevaeh Hasbrough, who has been a registered nurse for more than 5 years but has recently transferred to the medical–surgical unit at a large hospital, is trying to start an IV on a patient with congestive heart failure in order to administer parenteral diuretics. After several unsuccessful attempts, Nevaeh asks Callie Waddell, another nurse on the unit who's worked there "forever," for help. Callie, with a roll of the eyes, responds, "Don't you know anything?" Since Callie has engaged in this type of behavior before, Nevaeh is prepared through cognitive rehearsal and decides to use the "I" message approach. Nevaeh takes a few deep breaths and calmly responds: "I have inserted many IVs successfully, but this patient is very edematous. I am concerned that she is not receiving her diuretics on time. It would be helpful if you could come in with me and give me some pointers. If you are busy, who do you suggest I ask?"

Critical Thinking Questions

1. What is the benefit to Nevaeh's approach?
2. What might have happened if Nevaeh had ignored Callie's comment, "Don't you know anything?"

Nurses need to report each incident of bullying and incivility to the nurse manager. Ignoring and not responding to bullying may be interpreted as the behavior being acceptable (Longo, 2017). Reports of bullying should include details such as the date, time, and description of events, as well as identification of any witnesses. See **Box 37.3** », Recommendations Following a Bullying Incident.

At the organizational level, each workplace should have a zero-tolerance policy and be committed to making positive changes in the work environment. All employees should know the policies regarding expected behaviors and the consequences of violating bullying policies. Nurses should trust that they can report bullying, their report will be acted upon, and no retaliation will take place (Caristo & Clements, 2019). Fear of conflict often keeps nurses from addressing unprofessional behavior (Martinez et al., 2017).

Disruptive behaviors, by even one person, can affect a workplace, prompting others to engage in disruptive behaviors and creating an unsafe environment. Disruptive behaviors destroy the trust that healthcare teams need to communicate and collaborate to provide high-quality patient care. Failure to address disruptive and bullying behaviors also leads to an erosion of trust in leadership (Rehber et al., 2020).

Box 37.3

Recommendations Following a Bullying Incident

If you are the subject of a bullying event:

- Promptly report the event to the appropriate person, following organization policy.
- Document the event, including date, time, name of bully, names of witnesses, the words and actions of the bully, and your responses.
- Seek support through peers, employee assistance programs, psychologic counseling, or healthcare practitioner.

If you witness bullying:

- Support your peers and let them know that bullying behavior is not tolerated.
- Refer your peer to the policies for documenting and reporting bullying.

If you have engaged in bullying:

- Take responsibility for your actions.
- Apologize to the person you bullied and take measures to correct your action.
- Reflect on own behavior and how you can improve interactions with others.

Source: Adapted from American Nurses Association (2015c).

Box 37.4

Strategies for Preventing Workplace Bullying Among Nurses

- Educate team members about bullying behaviors and their adverse effects.
- Develop codes of conduct that clearly outline unacceptable behaviors.
- Promote a "zero-tolerance" attitude toward bullying.
- Encourage nurses to report bullying without fear of punishment or negative consequences.
- Offer the option of reporting bullying behaviors or recommendations for improvement of antibullying policies through use of comment or suggestion boxes.
- Assure nurses that reports of bullying will be taken seriously and thoroughly addressed, including through mandatory investigations of all allegations of bullying.
- Train leadership and management personnel to work collaboratively to prevent, identify, and address bullying behaviors.
- Create an environment in which courtesy and respect are valued.

Education programs should address the issues of incivility and bullying, including associated behaviors; impact on the patient, victim, workplace, and profession; available resources to support the victim; communication skills; and consequences to the bully. The program may include time for role playing to develop communication skills, such as cognitive rehearsal (Gosselin & Ireland, 2020). See **Box 37.4** » for an overview of guidelines for prevention of bullying among nurses in the workplace.

Maintaining a Culture of Excellence

Nurses have a responsibility to create and maintain a culture of excellence, and within that is the obligation to report bullying. When bullying is allowed to persist, bullying behaviors become the norm (Caristo & Clements, 2019). Nurses should recognize workplace bullying, be aware of its effects, and follow organizational policies and procedures for reporting the behavior. Ideally, individuals in leadership positions within the organization will address the issue in such a manner that the bullying stops. Empowered nurses have access to information, support, and resources and work in environments whose leaders are committed to providing opportunities to learn and grow, all in an effort to minimize or greatly reduce workplace incivility. **Box 37.5** » outlines the standards set by the American Association of Critical Care Nurses

Box 37.5

AACN Standards for Healthy Work Environments

The American Association of Critical Care Nurses has worked diligently to promote healthcare environments that focus on meeting the needs of patients, families, nurses, and other healthcare professionals. As part of this work, the AACN has identified six essential standards based on evidence-based principles of professional performance. The six standards with sample critical elements include:

1. *Skilled communication*, with the expectation that individuals advance collaborative relationships, improve communication styles, establish zero-tolerance policies to protect against disrespectful behavior in the workplace, maintain accountability for words and actions, and encourage a focus on finding solutions and achievable outcomes.
2. *True collaboration*, wherein team members have access to interprofessional education opportunities, have high levels of integrity, and demonstrate competence in their roles.
3. *Effective decision making*, which ensures that nurses participate in all levels of decision making within their organizations, that team members share fact-based information, and that effective processes are in place to objectively evaluate the results of decisions.
4. *Appropriate staffing* based on the professional obligation for nurses to provide high-level quality care and that organizations adopt technologies that increase the effectiveness of care.
5. *Meaningful recognition*, which acknowledges that team members should be recognized for the value they bring to the organization.
6. *Authentic leadership*, whereby leaders fully embrace and sustain a healthy work environment that promotes professional advancement.

Source: Based on American Association of Critical Care Nurses (2016).

for establishing a healthy workplace. The *Code of Ethics for Nurses with Interpretive Statements* by the ANA (2015a) states that nurses must "create an ethical environment and culture of civility and kindness, treating colleagues, coworkers, employees, students, and others with dignity and respect." Thus, both bullying as well as not taking action against bullying violate the Code of Ethics (ANA, 2015c). By following these standards, nurses and healthcare agencies can work to establish a culture of excellence.

Clinical Example D

Dee Johnston has worked in pediatric intensive care at General Hospital for the past year. She decides to leave her current position because she feels that her coworkers do not value the knowledge and skill that she has gained since she graduated from nursing school. Coworkers still make remarks such as "She's just the newbie on the block" or "Wait until she has a really sick baby to deal with." Dee begins to feel nervous at the thought of going to work and is afraid she is going to make a mistake. She decides to accept a position as a staff nurse in the pediatric ICU at University Hospital. Within 3 weeks of orientation, her preceptor quickly recognizes her expertise and feels that additional orientation is unnecessary. Dee begins to gain more self-confidence and enjoys going to her job once again.

Critical Thinking Questions

1. How is Dee interpreting her coworkers' behavior at General Hospital?
2. Why might Dee's coworkers be making such comments about Dee?
3. Do you think that leaving was the right thing for Dee to do? Why or why not?

REVIEW The Concept of Collaboration

RELATE Link the Concepts

Linking the concept of collaboration with the concept of communication:

1. How do communication skills affect a nurse's ability to collaborate?
2. How does communication style affect the process of collaboration? Give some examples.

Linking the concept of collaboration with the concept of oxygenation:

3. How would the care of a patient with chronic obstructive pulmonary disease (COPD) benefit from a collaborative healthcare team?
4. In caring for the patient with COPD, what aspects of care would require collaboration?

Linking the concept of collaboration with the concept of stress and coping:

5. How do different levels of stress affect both the occurrence of conflict and the management of conflict that arises?
6. How can an understanding of different individuals' coping mechanisms improve the ability to manage conflict?

REFER Go to Pearson MyLab Nursing and eText

REFLECT Apply Your Knowledge

Abigail Lessarian, a 32-year-old patient, delivered her first baby prematurely at 32 weeks' gestation. Her infant son, Garrett, was apneic at birth and required a brief period of tracheal intubation and mechanical ventilation. Immediately after his delivery, Garrett was admitted to the neonatal intensive care unit (NICU) for treatment of neonatal respiratory distress syndrome (RDS). By day 3, Garrett had made excellent progress; he was extubated and oxygen administration was implemented via nasal cannula with continuous positive airway pressure (CPAP). By day 14 in the NICU, Garrett was breathing effectively enough to maintain his oxygen saturation at >98% on room air with CPAP via nasal cannula; however, he experienced intermittent apneic spells with bradycardia until day 22. Garrett also was diagnosed with an atrial septal defect (ASD), for which his surgeon recommended monitoring because ASD often resolves without requiring surgical treatment. Garrett received gavage feedings via a nasogastric tube.

By day 30 in the NICU, Garrett had experienced no apneic spells for 7 days. On day 32, Garrett's gavage tube was removed, and he successfully transitioned to bottle feeding over a period of several days. On day 43, Garrett began transitioning to breastfeeding; despite having difficulty with sucking, his progress was slow but steady. By day 46, Garrett's neonatologist (pediatrician specializing in neonatal care) cleared him for discharge to home.

Prior to Garrett's discharge, his mother and father are scheduled to complete an infant CPR course. They also will receive teaching about the use of a home apnea monitor. During discussion of the numerous topics about which Garrett's parents will receive instruction, Garrett's mother states, "I don't know if I can handle much more. I feel so overwhelmed." When she becomes tearful, her husband puts his arm around her and says, "We'll do whatever it takes to help him get healthy. I can't believe I was concerned about whether or not he'd like playing baseball or football. Now, that seems so silly. I just want him to survive."

1. Identify three nursing priorities that are appropriate for inclusion in Garrett's nursing plan of care.
2. Identify three nursing priorities that are appropriate for inclusion in the nursing plan of care for Garrett's parents.
3. During preliminary discharge planning, Garrett's interprofessional team's recommendations include home visits by a nurse, occupational therapist, and social worker. What roles might each of these professionals serve in the care of Garrett and his family?
4. What other professionals might be beneficial to the care of Garrett and his parents in the home setting?

References

Agency for Healthcare Research and Quality (AHRQ). (2019). *TeamSTEPPS 2.0 fundamentals*. https://www.ahrq.gov/teamstepps/instructor/fundamentals/index.html

American Association of Critical Care Nurses (2016). *AACN Standards for Establishing and Sustaining Healthy Work Environments*. https://www.aacn.org/nursing-excellence/standards/aacn-standards-for-establishing-and-sustaining-healthy-work-environments

American Nurses Association. (2015a). *Code of ethics for nurses with interpretive statements*. Author.

American Nurses Association (ANA). (2015b). *Nursing: Scope and standards of practice*. Author.

American Nurses Association. (2015c). *Position statement: Incivility, bullying, and workplace violence*. https://www.nursingworld.org/~49d6e3/globalassets/practiceandpolicy/

nursing-excellence/incivility-bullying-and-workplace-violence-ana-position-statement.pdf

Armstrong, G. (2019). Quality and safety education for nurses teamwork and collaboration competency: Empowering nurses. *Journal of Continuing Education in Nursing, 60*(96), 252–255.

Armstrong, N. (2018). Management of nursing workplace incivility in the healthcare settings. *Workplace Health & Safety, 66*(8), 403–410.

Barr, J., & Dowding, L. (2019). *Leadership in healthcare*. Sage.

Black, S., Gardner, D. G., Pierce, J. L., & Steers, R. (2019). *Organizational behavior*. Openstax. https://opentextbc.ca/organizationalbehavioropenstax/front-matter/preface/

Bochatay, N., Bajwa, N. M., Cullati, S., Muller-Juge, V., Blondon, K. S., Junod Perron, N., et al. (2017). A multilevel analysis of professional conflicts in health care teams: Insights for future training. *Academic Medicine, 92*(11), S84–S91.

Burgener, A. M. (2020). Enhancing communication to improve patient safety and to increase patient satisfaction. *The Health Care Manager, 39*(3), 128–132.

Caristo, J. M., & Clements, P. Y. (2019). Let's stop "eating our young": Zero-tolerance policies for bullying in nursing. *Nursing 2019 Critical Care, 15*(4), 45–48.

Choudhary, L. (2018). Educational strategies for conflict management. *Nursing2018, 48*(12), 14–15.

Clark, C. M. (2019). Combining cognitive rehearsal, simulation, and evidence-based scripting to address incivility. *Nurse Educator, 44*(2), 64–68.

Collette, A. E., Wann, K., Nevin, M. L., Rique, K., Tarrant, G., Hickey, L. A., et al. (2017). An exploration of nurse–physician perceptions of collaborative behavior. *Journal of Interprofessional Care, 31*(4), 470–478.

Cronenwett, L., Sherwood, G., Barnsteiner, J., Disch, J., Johnson, J., Mitchell, P., et al. (2007). Quality and safety education for nurses. *Nursing Outlook, 55*(3), 122–131.

Ellis, P., & Abbott, J. (2020). Managing conflict in the workplace: Reducing and managing it. *Journal of Kidney Care, 5*(3), 140–143.

Emich, C. (2018). Conceptualizing collaboration in nursing. *Nursing Forum, 53*, 567–573.

Goldsberry, J. W. (2018). Advanced practice nurses leading the way: Interprofessional collaboration. *Nurse Education Today, 65*, 1–3.

Gosselin, T. K., & Ireland, A. M. (2020). Addressing incivility and bullying in the practice environment. *Seminars in Oncology Nursing, 36*, 1–6.

Harper, J. C., & Kracun, M. D. (2019). Interprofessional communication: How do we do it? *Journal of Nursing Education and Practice, 9*(4), 48–58.

Henderson, V. A. (1991). *The nature of nursing: Reflections after 25 years*. National League for Nursing.

Houck, N., & Colbert, A. (2017). Patient safety and workplace bullying: An integrative review. *Journal of Nursing Care Quality, 32*, 165–171.

House, S., & Havens, D. (2017). Nurses' and physicians' perceptions of nurse–physician collaboration: A systematic review. *Journal of Nursing Administration, 47*(3), 165–171.

Ilse, R., & Neilipovitz, D. (2019). Addressing bullying behavior by patients and families. *Healthcare Management Forum, 32*(4), 224–227.

Interprofessional Education Collaborative (IPEC). (2016). *Core competencies for interprofessional collaborative practice: 2016 update*. https://nebula.wsimg.com/2f68a39520b03336b41038c370497473?AccessKeyId=DC06780E69ED19E2B3A5&disposition=0&alloworigin=1

Karam, M., Brault, I., Van Durme, T., & Macq, J. (2018). Comparing interprofessional and interorganizational collaboration in healthcare: A systematic review of the qualitative research. *International Journal of Nursing Studies, 79*, 70–83.

Kim, S., Bochatay, N., Relyea-Chew, A., Buttrick, E., Amdahl, C., Kim, L., et al. (2017). Individual, interpersonal, and organisational factors of healthcare conflict: A scoping review. *Journal of interprofessional Care, 31*(3), 282–290.

Longo, J. (2017). Cognitive rehearsal. *American Nurse Today, 12*(4), 41–42, 51.

Mahon, M. A., Mee, L., Brett, D., & Dowling, M. (2017). Nurses' perceived stress and compassion following mindfulness meditation and self compassion training. *Journal of Research in Nursing, 22*(8), 572–583.

Martinez, W., Lehman, L.S., Thomas, E. J., Etchegaray, J. M., Shelburne, J. T., Hickson, G. B., et al. (2017). Speaking up about traditional and professionalism-related patient safety threats: a national survey of interns and residents. *BMJ Quality & Safety, 26*(11), 869–880.

McComb, S. A., Lemaster, M., Henneman, E. A., & Hinchey, K. T. (2017). An evaluation of shared mental models and mutual trust on general medical units: Implications for collaboration, teamwork, and patient safety. *Journal of Patient Safety, 13*(4), 237–242.

McKibben, L. (2017). Conflict management: importance and implications. *British Journal of Nursing, 26*(2), 2–5.

Morley, L., & Cashell, A. (2017). Collaboration in health care. *Journal of Medical Imaging and Radiation Sciences, 48*, 207–216.

National League for Nursing (NLN). (2015). *NLN Vision Series: Transforming nursing education; leading the call to reform. Interprofessional Collaboration in Education and Practice: A living document from the National League for Nursing*. http://www.nln.org/docs/default-source/default-document-library/ipe-ipp-vision.pdf?sfvrsn=14

Rehber, K. J., Adair, K. C., Hadley, A., McKittrick, K., Frankel, A., Leonard, M., et al. (2020). Associations between a new disruptive behaviors scale and teamwork, patient safety, work–life balance, burnout, and depression. *The Joint Commission Journal on Quality and Patient Safety, 46*, 18–26.

Sauer, P. A., & McCoy, T. P. (2018). Nurse bullying and intent to leave. *Nursing Economic$, 36*(5), 219–224, 245.

Schermerhorn, J. R., & Bachrach, D. G. (2018). *Exploring management*. Wiley.

Schoville, R., & Aebersold, M. (2020). How workplace bullying and incivility impacts patient safety: A qualitative simulation study using BSN students. *Clinical Simulation in Nursing, 45*, 16–23.

Spaulding, E. M., Marvel, F. A., Jacob, E., Rahman, A., Hansen, B. R., Hanyok, L. A., et al. (2019). Interprofessional education and collaboration among healthcare students and professionals: A systematic review and call for action. *Journal of Interprofessional Care*. https://doi.org/10.1080/13561820.2019.1697214

Stein, S. J., & Book, H. E. (2000). *The EQ edge: Emotional intelligence and your success*. Stoddart.

Tan, T.-C., Zhou, H., & Kelly, M. (2017). Nurse–physician communication: An integrated review. *Journal of Clinical Nursing, 26*, 3974–3989.

The Joint Commission. (2017). *Sentinel alert event: Inadequate hand-ff communication*. https://www.jointcommission.org/-/media/tjc/documents/resources/patient-safety-topics/sentinel-event/sea_58_hand_off_comms_9_6_17_final_(1).pdf?db=web&hash=5642D63C1A5017BD214701514DA00139

Thomas, K. W., & Kilmann, R. H. (1974). *Thomas-Kilmann Conflict Mode Instrument*. Consulting Psychologists Press.

Umberfield, E., Ghaferi, A. A., Krein, S. L., & Manojlovich, M. (2019). Using incident reports to assess communication failures and patient outcomes. *The Joint Commission Journal on Quality and Patient Safety, 45*(6), 406–413.

University of New Mexico. (2016). *The high cost of nurse turnover*. https://rnbsnonline.unm.edu/articles/high-cost-of-nurse-turnover.aspx

Wallace, S., & Gipson, K. (2017). Bullying in healthcare: A disruptive force linked to compromised patient safety. *PA Patient Safety Advisory, 14*(2), 64–70.

Walter, J. K., Schall, T. E., DeWitt, A. G., Faerber, J., Griffis, H., Galligan, M., et al. (2019). Interprofessional team member communication patterns, teamwork, and collaboration in pre-family meeting huddles in a pediatric cardiac intensive care unit. *Journal of Pain and Symptom Management, 58*(1), 11–18.

Weberg, D. Mangold, K., Porter-O'Grady, T., & Malloch, K. (2019). *Leadership in nursing practice: Changing the landscape of health care*. Jones & Bartlett.

World Health Organization (WHO). (2010). *Framework for action on interprofessional education & collaborative practice*. https://apps.who.int/iris/bitstream/handle/10665/70185/WHO_HRH_HPN_10.3_eng.pdf;jsessionid=EBD24EE341C71F6B1D3147950C6666BA?sequence=1.

Yoder-Wise, P. S. (2019). *Leading and managing in nursing*. Elsevier.

Zuzelo, P. R. (2019). Partnering for holistic and safe care. *Holistic Nursing Practice, 33*(5), 316–318.

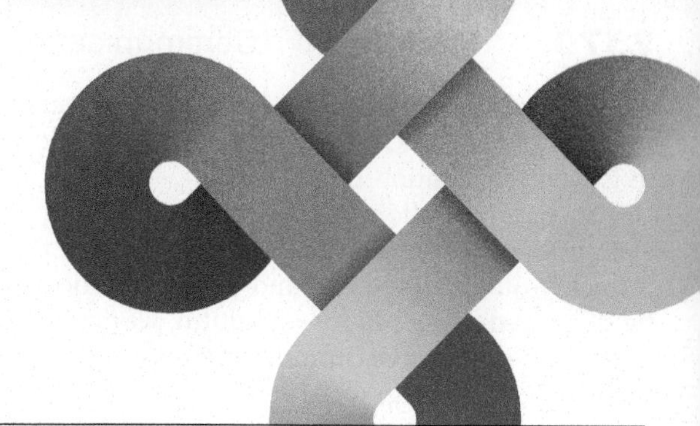

Module 38
Communication

Module Outline and Learning Outcomes

The Concept of Communication

Modes of Communication

38.1 Differentiate the various forms of communication.

Concepts Related to Communication

38.2 Outline the relationship between communication and other concepts.

Factors Influencing the Communication Process

38.3 Analyze the factors that influence the communication process.

Barriers to Communication

38.4 Analyze barriers to effective communication.

Types of Communicators

38.5 Analyze the various types of communicators.

Assertive Communication

38.6 Summarize the attributes of a nurse who uses assertive communication.

Lifespan Considerations

38.7 Differentiate considerations related to communication throughout the lifespan.

Nursing Process

38.8 Analyze the nursing process as it relates to a patient with impaired verbal communication.

Communication Exemplars

Exemplar 38.A Groups and Group Communication

38.A Analyze groups and group communication.

Exemplar 38.B Therapeutic Communication

38.B Analyze the interactive process of therapeutic communication.

Exemplar 38.C Documentation

38.C Analyze documentation as it relates to communication.

Exemplar 38.D Reporting

38.D Analyze reporting as it relates to communication.

›› The Concept of Communication

Concept Key Terms

Active listening, **2577**
Aggressive communicators, **2579**
Assertive communicators, **2579**
Communication, **2569**
Congruent communication, **2570**
Credibility, **2571**
Elderspeak, **2579**
Electronic communication, **2570**
Intimate distance, **2578**
Nonverbal communication, **2570**
Passive communicators, **2579**
Perceptions, **2577**
Personal distance, **2578**
Personal space, **2578**
Proxemics, **2578**
Public distance, **2578**
Social distance, **2578**
Territoriality, **2578**
Values, **2577**
Verbal communication, **2570**

Nursing involves interactions between nurses and patients, nurses and other health professionals, and nurses and the community. The process of human interaction occurs through communication: verbal and nonverbal, written and unwritten, planned and unplanned. Communication between individuals conveys thoughts, ideas, feelings, and information. To be effective in their interactions, nurses must be proficient in their verbal and written communication skills. They must be aware of what their words and body language say to others. Nurses also must demonstrate competency in computer and electronic communication skills.

The term *communication* has various meanings, depending on the context in which it is used. For example, communication can be the interchange of information, thoughts, or ideas between two or more individuals. This kind of communication uses methods such as talking and listening or writing and reading. However, thoughts and ideas can be conveyed to others not only through spoken or written words but also through gestures or body actions.

Poor communication between a healthcare professional and a patient can result in poor health outcomes for the patient and can even lead to distrust of healthcare professionals in general. This section on the concept of communication provides nurses with essential information necessary to communicate successfully with patients, family members, peers, and other healthcare professionals. For the purposes of this text, **communication** is any means of exchanging information or feelings between two or more individuals. The sender gives or shares a message with the person or persons receiving the message, who may or may not understand or respond to the communication.

All communication has the *intent* of eliciting a response. The process of communication has two main purposes: to influence others to respond and to obtain information. It can be described as helpful or unhelpful. Communication that is positive or effective promotes the sharing of information, thoughts, or feelings between individuals. Ineffective or negative communication can hinder or block the successful sharing of information, thoughts, or feelings. In nursing, any type of breakdown in communication can lead to negative patient outcomes.

Four specific types of communication are explored in the exemplars of this module. Each of these is essential to successful nursing practice. Group communication is becoming ever more important in the process of making decisions in the current healthcare system. Therapeutic communication is an essential tool for developing the nurse–patient helping relationship and promoting best patient outcomes. Documentation is the primary form of written communication used by nurses in all aspects of healthcare. Finally, reporting through handoff communication is the process of nurse-to-nurse communication that ensures continuity of care for the patient from one shift change or visit to another.

Modes of Communication

Communication typically occurs through either verbal or nonverbal methods. **Verbal communication** involves the use of written or spoken words. In contrast, gestures, facial expressions, and touch are forms of **nonverbal communication**. Both forms of communication occur simultaneously; however, most communication is nonverbal. Nurses can develop effective communication patterns and relationships with patients by being knowledgeable about nonverbal communication.

Electronic communication is a mode of communication that evolves with technology. One of the most common forms of electronic communication used in the workplace is email, whereas social networking and text messaging are more frequently used for social purposes. Nurses should be aware of the appropriateness of email and other forms of electronic communication when communicating with patients, families, and other healthcare professionals.

Verbal Communication

Verbal communication is primarily a conscious and purposeful activity because individuals choose the words they use. The words and type of phrasing used differ among individuals according to culture, age, education, and socioeconomic background. An abundance of words can be used to form messages and a wide variety of feelings can be expressed when people talk. This results in countless possible ways for ideas and information to be exchanged.

When selecting what words to say or write, nurses should consider pace and intonation, simplicity, clarity and brevity, timing and relevance, adaptability, credibility, and humor.

Pace and Intonation

The feeling and impact of a person's message can be influenced by the pace or rhythm and intonation in which it is delivered. Intonation or inflection can express excitement, joy, anger, sadness, or amusement. The pace or tempo of speech may indicate interest, boredom, anxiety, or fear. Speaking slowly and softly, for example, may help to calm an anxious or excited patient.

Simplicity

Simplicity of speech refers to using commonly understood words in a way that promotes understanding for the person receiving the information. Words that are meaningful to the nurse and that may be easy for the nurse to use, such as *hysterectomy* or *vasodilation*, are not meaningful to patients with no background in healthcare. Nurses need to select terms patients are likely to understand and that are appropriate based on the patient's developmental age, knowledge, educational level, and culture of the patient. For example, if an order is received for nasogastric (NG) tube insertion, instead of saying to the patient, "Another nurse and I will need to put an NG tube in your nose," it might be better to say, "In an hour, we need to place a small, thin tube called a nasogastric, or NG, tube through your nose and into your stomach to make it easier for you to take your medications." The second statement is more simply worded, making it easier to understand. It also expresses to the patient why the procedure is necessary.

Clarity and Brevity

A message that is direct and simple is the most effective type of message. The use of *clarity*, saying exactly what is meant, and *brevity*, using the fewest words needed to convey the message, results in a clear and simple message. Essential to clarity is **congruent communication**, in which the behavior or nonverbal communication of the nurse is congruent (consistent) with the words being spoken. If a nurse says to a patient, "I am interested in hearing what you are feeling," the nonverbal behavior of the nurse should include facing the patient, making eye contact (if culturally appropriate), and leaning slightly forward. The goal is to facilitate clear communication so that all parts of the situation or incident are understood. The nurse should also speak slowly and pronounce words carefully to ensure clarity in communication. Careful pronunciation, however, does not necessitate speaking louder. Speaking loudly can be interpreted by the patient as being patronizing or aggressive, even if the patient is hard of hearing, and can damage the nurse–patient relationship.

Timing and Relevance

Words can be stated or written clearly and simply, but the timing needs to be appropriate to guarantee that the words are heard and understood. Furthermore, the message being delivered should relate to the person or interests of the person receiving it and requires nurses to be sensitive to a patient's needs and concerns. For example, a patient who has just received a possible terminal diagnosis may not hear the nurse's explanation of an upcoming CT scan. Similarly, patients experiencing acute anxiety have trouble taking in new information.

To promote timing and relevance of communications, nurses can encourage patients to share their concerns and then discuss with them how to address those concerns before imparting new or important information. Explanations related to the diagnostic procedure can be provided to the patient after the patient's concerns or anxieties have been addressed, or later when the patient is able to listen.

Adaptability

Nurses must alter spoken messages in response to behavioral cues from the patient. This adjustment is referred to as *adaptability*. Nurses carefully consider and individualize what they say and how they say it. This requires both astute assessment and sensitivity. For example, suppose that a nurse who usually smiles, appears cheerful, and greets a patient with an enthusiastic "Hi, Mrs. Brown!" notices that the patient is not smiling and appears distressed. In this situation, the nurse should modify her tone of speech and express concern via facial expressions while moving toward the patient.

Credibility

Credibility is the quality of being trustworthy, truthful, and reliable. Nurses promote credibility in themselves and their profession by being honest, consistent, and dependable. This includes being knowledgeable about any topic being discussed, providing accurate information to the patient, and being willing to admit uncertainty by saying, "I don't know, but I will find out for you."

Humor

Humor can be used to help patients find a brief emotional release during difficult or painful situations. When used appropriately, humor can reduce tension and promote well-being. However, not everyone finds humor in the same situations. Humor also depends on both relevance and timing. Although humor and laughter can help reduce stress and anxiety, the nurse should assess the situation and allow the feelings of the patient to guide the use of humor by the nurse (Sousa et al., 2019).

Nonverbal Communication

Nonverbal communication (also called *body language*) includes gestures, facial expressions, use of touch, body position and movement, and physical appearance (including hairstyle, clothing, and accessories). Nonverbal communication can express more about an individual's feelings than what the person actually says, because nonverbal behaviors are less consciously controlled than verbal behavior (**Figure 38.1** »).

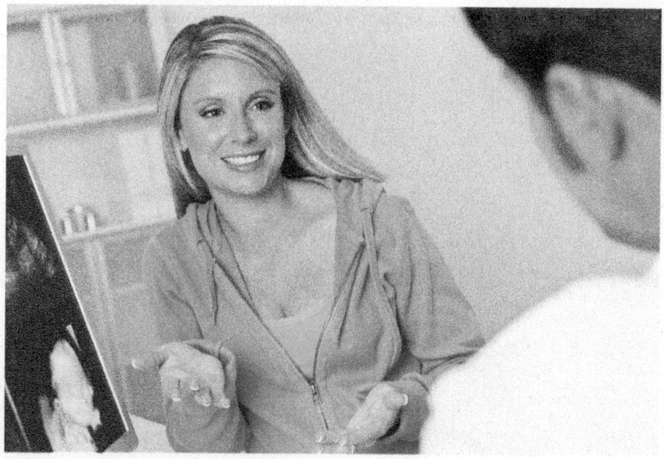

Figure 38.1 » Nonverbal communication sometimes conveys meaning more effectively than words. This patient is clearly receptive to the HCP's message.

Source: SDI Productions/E+/Getty Images.

Nonverbal communication has the ability to either support (congruence) or contradict (incongruence) what is expressed verbally. The nurse who says to a patient, for example, "I would be happy to stay and answer your questions," yet glances at the clock every few minutes is contradicting her verbal statement with her nonverbal behaviors. The patient is most likely to interpret this nonverbal behavior as indicating the nurse's disinterest. In contrast, if the nurse enters the patient's room and observes that the patient is gazing out the window and crying, and then pulls a chair up to the bed and asks softly, "You appear to be upset, can you tell me what is bothering you?" conveys the message that the nurse cares and is willing to allow time to listen to the patient.

Every nurse must develop the ability to observe and interpret a patient's nonverbal behaviors. Efficient observation of nonverbal behaviors by the nurse requires a systematic assessment that includes the patient's overall appearance and mental status, gestures and facial expressions, and posture and gait.

Patients with alterations in cognition, patients with autism or intellectual disability, and others may have difficulty expressing themselves clearly or understanding nonverbal communication. See **Box 38.1** » for information about communicating with patients with limited communication skills.

Box 38.1

Nonverbal Communication in Patients with Altered Thought Processes

Patients who have altered thought processes (e.g., schizophrenia or dementia) may have moments when it is difficult or impossible for them to express themselves clearly. Their nonverbal communication may or may not be congruent with what they are trying to express. For example, a patient with psychosis who is experiencing a hallucination will have difficulty perceiving nonverbal communication or understanding directions from others. Similarly, a patient with dementia may not be able to form words necessary to communicate intent or feeling. Yet both may be communicating important information that the nurse will need to interpret.

Patients with autism spectrum disorder can have difficulty understanding nonverbal communication and may avoid or have difficulty making eye contact, which can cause them to seem uninterested or inattentive. They may not be able to interpret nonverbal communication.

Strategies to use when communicating with a patient with altered cognition, dementia, or autism depends on accurate interpretation of the individual assessment. When available, caregivers may be able to help the nurse interpret a patient's message and suggest strategies for the nurse to use that work with that individual. Without this helpful information, the nurse should be alert for nonverbal expressions of anxiety and pain, such as:

- Guarding an affected area or a change in posture or gait
- Withdrawal or combativeness
- Sudden change in mental status
- Crying, inconsolability
- Repeated groaning or calling out in distress.

Nurses who are attentive, calm, and clarify observations convey a message of caring and acceptance to the patient. In doing so they promote the development of a trusting nurse–patient relationship, even for patients who have difficulty with appropriate communication.

Nonverbal communication, even for behaviors such as smiling and shaking hands, can vary widely among cultures. Many individuals feel that smiling and shaking hands are integral parts of an interaction and crucial to establishing trust. However, other individuals may perceive these actions as disrespectful or purposeless. Additional information related to cultural differences in communication can be found in Module 24, Culture and Diversity.

It can be difficult to know if the nurse has interpreted nonverbal communication accurately. The same feeling can be expressed nonverbally in multiple ways, even within the same cultural group. For instance, anger may be communicated through aggressive or excessive body movement or through silence or stillness. When the nurse is uncertain of her interpretation of a patient's nonverbal communication, the nurse can validate the interpretation directly with the patient by saying something like, "I see you frowning. Is there something upsetting you?"

Personal Appearance

As stated earlier, personal appearance (hairstyle, clothing, and accessories) can convey information about an individual. For example, clothing may indicate social and financial status, self-concept, and/or religious or cultural affiliation (**Figure 38.2** »). Some people wear jewelry as a fashion statement; others may wear amulets or charms for health protection. If a patient is wearing an object or piece of clothing whose symbolic meaning is unfamiliar to the nurse, the nurse can ask about its significance and use that as an opportunity to learn more about the patient and the individual's customs or beliefs.

Personal grooming and dress can be affected by either financial status or illness. Patients who have infrequent access to a washer and dryer may not be able to keep clothes clean. Patients with acute or chronic illness may not have the energy or desire to engage in regular self-care and personal hygiene. Disinterest in grooming and hygiene may also indicate the development of depression. Nurses observing a sudden change in personal appearance can validate their observations by asking the patient or caregiver directly about the changes.

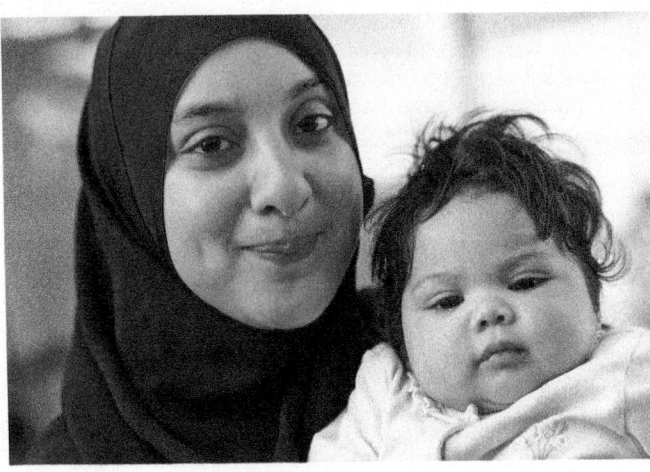

Figure 38.2 » Women who are Muslims may wear a headscarf (or hijab) or another form of head covering as a sign of modesty, to reflect their devotion to God, or as a means to express their Muslim identity. Not all Muslim women wear headscarves; many choose not to veil. In many American families who practice Islam, it is the woman's choice whether to wear a hijab (The Conversation, 2019).

Source: Yuri Arcurs/E+/Getty Images.

Posture and Gait

Self-concept, current mood, and health are often indicated by the way individuals walk or carry themselves. Erect posture and a stable, purposeful gait suggest well-being, whereas slouching and a slow, shuffling gate may indicate discomfort or depression. In contrast, tense, quick movements may indicate anxiety or anger. The nurse can clarify the interpretation of observations by saying something like, "I see you're hunching your shoulders and holding your arm. I'm wondering if you're in pain and if you need something to help you be more comfortable."

Facial Expression

The face is the most expressive part of the body (see **Figure 38.3** »). Facial expressions can convey feelings of happiness, sadness, fear, anger, surprise, or disgust. Often a person's face expresses genuine emotions, but most people are able to control their facial muscles to hide their emotions from others. When a patient's facial expression is unclear or is inconsistent with the individual's stated emotions, it is important for the nurse to investigate further to clarify the meaning of the expression. Accurate interpretation of a single expression cannot occur without considering other reinforcing physical cues (including the expressions of others in the immediate area), the setting in which the expression occurs, and the cultural background of the patient.

Because most patients will quickly note the facial expressions of the nurse, it is important for nurses to be aware of their own facial expressions and what they are communicating to others. A patient who is questioning the nurse about an anxiety-producing procedure or lab result will notice whether the nurse maintains eye contact or looks away when answering. A patient who has had a disfiguring accident will

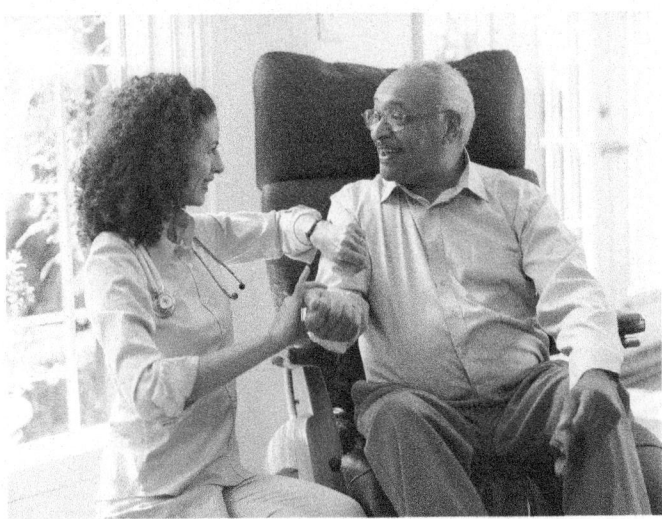

Figure 38.3 » The nurse's facial expression communicates warmth and caring.

Source: Fuse/Corbis/Getty Images.

analyze the nurse's face for evidence of disgust. Although it is impossible to control all facial expressions, nurses need to be able to maintain professional facial expressions that are appropriate to the situation and supportive of the patient and the situation.

One essential element of facial communication is eye contact. Many cultures use mutual eye contact to acknowledge another person and to express a willingness to maintain communication. Other cultures, however, consider direct eye contact to be impolite (see Module 24, Culture and Diversity). A patient who averts the eyes may be signaling embarrassment or view the nature of the contact as threatening.

Gestures

Gestures of the hands and body may be used for emphasis or clarification of a verbal message or to communicate without words. For example, a spouse who is worried about his partner in surgery may pace back and forth or wring his hands. A patient who is despondent over being in a hospital or long-term care facility might simply shrug the shoulders when asked if they want something to eat. Some gestures, such as waving hello or goodbye, may have universal meanings. Others may be culturally specific. For example, "thumbs-up," which indicates approval in the United States, is considered an insult in some countries. See the Focus on Diversity and Culture feature for more information.

The hands are central to communication for individuals with special communication problems such as hearing impairments. Many individuals with a hearing impairment learn and use sign language to communicate. The hands, along with facial expressions and other body language, are used with signing to form expressions with accepted meanings. As with spoken language and dialects, signs used in sign language will vary; a patient from another country who is deaf and fluent in that country's sign language may not be able to communicate in American Sign Language. Similarly, individuals who are unable to reply verbally may be able to communicate using their hands. For example, the patient who is intubated may be able to raise an index finger once for "yes" and twice for "no." Other signals for communication can often be created by the patient and nurse to indicate various meanings.

Focus on Diversity and Culture

Nonverbal Communication

Language barriers and differing cultural values create the most evident communication issues when working with patients from backgrounds different from that of the nurse. Nonverbal communication, however, presents an equally complicated set of issues. Just as languages and accents vary across the world, nonverbal communication patterns vary across cultures. Standards for personal space also vary widely by culture (Ao, 2019; International Institute of Minnesota, 2020).

Every culture interprets gestures and other modes of nonverbal communication differently, so exercise caution when working with patients from cultures with which you are unfamiliar. This is particularly true when it comes to the use of therapeutic touch. Many cultures have specific rules or practices regarding the use of touch, especially between individuals of different sexes (International Institute of Minnesota, 2020). When working with a patient from another culture, always follow the patient's lead and do not be afraid to ask, clarify, and validate the meaning of a gesture or nonverbal response. Use hand and arm gestures with great caution, be careful in interpreting facial expressions, and do not force a patient to make eye contact (EveryNurse.org, 2019; U.S. Department of State, n.d.).

Electronic Communication

Today's nurses increasingly use electronic communication methods such as email, text messaging, and online portals to communicate with patients, other nurses, other departments in their employment setting, and resources outside the facility. It is important for nurses to follow their agency's guidelines for the use of electronic communication and to understand the associated advantages and disadvantages.

Advantages

Electronic communication using patient portals has many advantages. As Dendere and colleagues (2019) note, patient portals can provide secure access to patient health information, including scheduled appointments, laboratory results, discharge information, and medication lists. Patient portals also allow for secure patient–provider communication, appointment and payment management, as well as prescription refill requests (Dendere et al., 2019). Any email communication to or from a patient using a patient portal automatically becomes part of that patient's record.

The use of email communication between healthcare providers (HCPs) and patients and nurses and patients has become increasingly popular due to the numerous advantages, ranging from email's instantaneous nature to the fact that email addresses tend to change less frequently than residential addresses. Additional benefits of email include increased efficiency, strengthened patient–provider communications, and informed decision making. Some healthcare facilities provide information to their patients on how to reach specific staff members by email. This improves communication and continuity of patient care.

Social networks such as Facebook and Instagram are less commonly used in healthcare, but they represent an important opportunity for the distribution of general information, such as operating hours and after-hours contact information. Nurses can use social networking to connect with colleagues worldwide for continuous learning through organizations such as the American Nurses Association. Posts on hospital Facebook and Instagram pages can provide followers with helpful information about community events such as health fairs or reminders about influenza vaccinations. During natural disasters, emergency management personnel and healthcare facilities may use social media as an additional method for sharing critically important information (such as evacuation orders and the location of shelters or medical care facilities).

Text messaging is another form of electronic communication for HCPs, and it offers the benefits of convenience, ubiquity, immediacy, monitoring of symptoms, dissemination of emergency alerts, and multimedia capability.

In communicating with patients, text messaging has been useful for disseminating public service announcements. Between nurses and other HCPs, text messaging can provide a convenient and low-cost means of electronic communication.

Disadvantages

The main disadvantage of electronic communications methods is the heightened risk to patient confidentiality. Healthcare organizations are required by the Health Insurance Portability and Accountability Act (HIPAA) to apply "reasonable and appropriate safeguards" when emailing protected health information (PHI). Every healthcare agency should have an email encryption system to ensure PHI security.

Another disadvantage is one of socioeconomics. Not everyone has a computer or a cell phone capable of accessing the internet. Even if internet access is possible, not everyone has the necessary computer skills. Email, patient portals, and social media may enhance communication with some patients, but others may not have access to it at all. Alternative forms of communication will be needed for patients who have limited access to or limited abilities with using the internet. Similarly, patients who do not use cell phones with text-messaging capability will not be able to receive appointment reminders or patient intake surveys using this method.

The major drawbacks of text messaging in a healthcare context are related to its strengths of ubiquity and instantaneousness. Nurses who constantly receive work-related text messages may check their messages at inappropriate times or even use their devices for personal messages while at work. This can prove to be a barrier to effective communications with patients.

When Not to Use Electronic Communications Media

Nurses and other healthcare staff should avoid using electronic communications when:

- ***Information must be communicated urgently.*** There is no guarantee when a patient (or another HCP) may read an email or receive a text message.
- ***Diagnostic findings are abnormal.*** Abnormal test findings can cause anxiety. Patients need the opportunity to ask questions at the time the results are shared and to schedule any follow-up appointments promptly.
- ***Information to be relayed is highly confidential.*** There is no guarantee that information relayed electronically can be accessed by only the patient. Highly confidential information should be shared directly with the patient.

Other Guidelines

Nurses are responsible for following their facility's guidelines for using electronic communications with patients as well as with other members of the healthcare team. Patients are generally asked to complete a form indicating they would like to receive email or text-based communication and confirming the patient's preferred means of communication and email address. The website of the National Council of State Boards of Nursing also provides guidance to nurses on the use of social and electronic media in healthcare.

When using email, nurses should identify the email as confidential in the subject line. Healthcare-related email typically includes a disclaimer in the body of the message stating that the message is to be read only by the person to whom it is addressed and that if the email is mistakenly sent to an individual other than the intended person, the recipient should contact the sender.

Email communication, like other documentation in the patient's record, may be used as evidence in court. Email communication must also comply with the rules for written communication (see the next section).

Email communication can enhance effective communication with patients; however, it is not a substitute for effective in-person communication. Nurses should use their professional judgment when determining which form(s) of communication will best meet the patient's health needs.

Written Communication

Written communication can be considered a form of verbal communication. Examples of forms of written communication include notes, letters, email messages, and text messages. Written communication has some limitations. For example, it lacks the nonverbal cues that accompany verbal communication. For example, you may receive a text message from a friend that says, "GET OUT OF HERE!!" Without an understanding of context, this message could be interpreted as shock and disbelief at something you told your friend, anger and the wish for you to vacate the friend's life, or a request to be left alone. Only by hearing tone of voice and seeing body language can context be relayed. As a result, rules for written communication differ from rules for other forms of communicating.

The most common form of written communication used by nurses are the nursing notes documented in the medical record related to a patient's status and assessments or interventions performed (see Exemplar 38.C, Documentation, later in this module). Nurses also use written communication when providing discharge instructions and patient education information to patients and their families and in messages to nursing colleagues and other healthcare professionals. Employee evaluations, policies and procedures, and other communications to administrators, colleagues, and nursing staff are ways that nurse managers use written communication. One important consideration in written communication is that receipt and interpretation of written communication does not always happen immediately. In some cases, it may be days before the intended recipient reads the information. This makes it essential to use clarity in written communication because it may not be possible for the recipient to ask questions or clarify areas of confusion.

Characteristics of Effective Written Communication

In addition to the characteristics of effective oral communication (simplicity, brevity, clarity, relevance, credibility, and humor), written communication must contain the following:

- ***Appropriate language and terminology.*** Language and terminology must be appropriate for the patient's developmental age, education and reading level, and culture. If English is not the primary language of an individual, it may be more effective to have a professional translator translate the written materials into the patient's primary language. In addition, written materials should use lay terminology instead of or alongside medical terminology.

Box 38.2

National Standards for Culturally and Linguistically Appropriate Services (CLAS) in Health and Health Care

Standard 1: Provide effective, equitable, understandable, and respectful quality care and services that are responsive to diverse cultural health beliefs and practices, preferred languages, health literacy, and other communication needs.

Standard 2: Advance and sustain organizational governance and leadership that promotes CLAS and health equity through policy, practices, and allocated resources.

Standard 3: Recruit, promote, and support a culturally and linguistically diverse governance, leadership, and workforce that are responsive to the population in the service area.

Standard 4: Educate and train governance, leadership, and workforce in culturally and linguistically appropriate policies and practices on an ongoing basis.

Standard 5: Offer language assistance to individuals who have limited English proficiency and/or other communication needs, at no cost to them, to facilitate timely access to all healthcare and services.

Standard 6: Inform all individuals of the availability of language assistance services clearly and in their preferred language, verbally and in writing.

Standard 7: Ensure the competence of individuals providing language assistance, recognizing that the use of untrained individuals and/or minors as interpreters should be avoided.

Standard 8: Provide easy-to-understand print and multimedia materials and signage in the languages commonly used by the populations in the service area.

Standard 9: Establish culturally and linguistically appropriate goals, policies, and management accountability, and infuse them throughout the organization's planning and operations.

Standard 10: Conduct ongoing assessments of the organization's CLAS-related activities and integrate CLAS-related measures into measurement and continuous quality improvement activities.

Standard 11: Collect and maintain accurate and reliable demographic data to monitor and evaluate the impact of CLAS on health equity and outcomes and to inform service delivery.

Standard 12: Conduct regular assessments of community health assets and needs and use the results to plan and implement services that respond to the cultural and linguistic diversity of populations in the service area.

Standard 13: Partner with the community to design, implement, and evaluate policies, practices, and services to ensure cultural and linguistic appropriateness.

Standard 14: Create conflict and grievance resolution processes that are culturally and linguistically appropriate to identify, prevent, and resolve conflicts or complaints.

Standard 15: Communicate the organization's progress in implementing and sustaining CLAS to all stakeholders, constituents, and the general public.

Source: Based on Office of Minority Health (2018); Think Cultural Health (n.d.); Thompson (2018).

For example, *stroke* may be used instead of *cerebrovascular accident*. National standards for culturally and linguistically appropriate services (CLAS) in health and healthcare are listed in **Box 38.2** ».

- ***Correct grammar, spelling, and punctuation.*** Use of correct grammar, spelling, and punctuation helps promote clarity of the message being communicated. Incorrect grammar, errors in punctuation, and misspelled words can change the intended meaning, create confusion, and undermine the reader's confidence in the sender.
- ***Logical organization.*** When written materials are well organized, they are easier to read. For example, a logical order for providing information is to begin with basic, foundational information before introducing more complex information.
- ***Appropriate use and citation of resources.*** If borrowing information from other sources, credit must be given to the original source. For example, a patient information pamphlet that includes information from the Centers for Disease Control and Prevention (CDC) should cite that organization and provide a full reference where the reader may find the information. Failure to reference information borrowed from another writer is called plagiarism; it is considered unethical and may violate copyright laws. Nurses and other healthcare professionals often follow either the American Psychological Association or American Medical Association style guidelines when using citations and references.

» **Stay Current:** For more information regarding the CLAS standards, go to https://www.thinkculturalhealth.hhs.gov/clas/standards.

Concepts Related to Communication

Communication is a concept that relates to every healthcare concept and is used in every healthcare setting. Communication is the cornerstone of patient care, and nurses, along with all HCPs, must be mindful of their communication techniques when providing care, regardless of setting. Communication binds healthcare workers, patients, and institutions together and is the means through which nurses provide both hospital-based and community-based care. Nurses should keep in mind the patient's needs and limitations and always take care to use simple, understandable phrases and not technical terms and medical terminology during communication (Sibiya, 2018). Listening is an essential component in nursing communication, and it is the foundation of responsible nursing practice. When listening, nurses should assess both the verbal and nonverbal statements of the patient. By being attentive to unspoken needs, nurses can enhance nursing diagnoses and the quality of care.

One of the most important components of providing effective communication in real-world nursing practice is tailoring communication efforts to the particular situation of the patient. Patients will vary dramatically in their ability to communicate and listen effectively at the time of treatment.

Physiologic illness, cognitive impairment, substance abuse, mental illness, the emotional context of the healthcare encounter, and linguistic and cultural differences are all factors that can affect a patient's ability to communicate with the healthcare team. In all cases, the nurse is responsible for ensuring successful communication and for advocating for patients who are unable to advocate for themselves. The Concepts Related to Communication feature provides examples of some of the many concepts integral to communication. They are presented in alphabetical order.

Concepts Related to **Communication**

CONCEPT	RELATIONSHIP TO COMMUNICATION	NURSING IMPLICATIONS
Advocacy	Communication among nurses, patients, and physicians is a key component of effective healthcare. In addition to communication with patients, nurses directly or indirectly influence physician–patient communications.	■ Assess what the HCP has told the patient regarding the patient's condition. ■ Encourage the patient to clarify understanding with the HCP. ■ Help the patient identify and access high-quality sources of healthcare information. ■ Always advocate for the best interests of the patient and the patient's expressed wishes.
Comfort	Pain → communication ability. Impaired communication may ↓ ability to report pain.	■ Take patient's report of pain levels seriously. ■ Assess for nonverbal signs of pain such as wincing and guarding. ■ Communicate equally with patients across the lifespan. ■ Use a pain management scale such as a numeric rating scale or the FACES pain rating scale that is appropriate for the patient's age and ability to communicate. ■ Investigate palliative care options for patients at the end of life.
Grief and Loss	Grief or loss can adversely affect the way in which an individual communicates. Not only does the person experiencing the loss have trouble communicating needs to others, but others often do not know how to communicate their condolences to those who have experienced a loss. Cultural differences can exacerbate communication issues.	■ Determine the effects of the loss on the patient. If the patient is grieving the loss of a primary caregiver or a spouse who provided financially for the patient, the individual may have a number of immediate needs. ■ Consider the stages of grief when communicating with patients. ■ Consider the cultural background of the patient and family related to expressions of grief and loss.
Intracranial Regulation	Impaired intracranial regulation → impaired communication. Traumatic brain injury → difficulty with word finding, sentence formation, and expression. Patients with severe increased intracranial pressure may enter a coma state.	■ Recognize the communication difficulties caused by traumatic brain injuries early and respond appropriately. ■ Help the patient with cognitive and/or physical limitations find an appropriate therapist to help the patient regain lost abilities. ■ If patients have difficulty expressing their thoughts, calmly help them find ways of communicating.
Mood and Affect	A diagnosis of mental illness ↑ likelihood patient will experience discrimination/stigma and may ↑ reluctance to trust healthcare personnel. In addition, HCPs may miss signs that these patients are experiencing these disorders.	■ Be aware that people of all ages can experience from mental and psychiatric disorders. ■ Do not assume that someone does not have one of these conditions because of their physical appearance. ■ Screen patients for depression or other psychiatric illness by asking open-ended questions with empathy. ■ Research medical records for histories of mental illness and cognitive issues and shape communication appropriately. ■ Be consistent and predictable in your nursing practice and communication.
Oxygenation	Decreased O_2 → hypoxemia → decreased level of consciousness (LOC) → decreased ability to communicate verbally (due to shortness of breath and LOC) and nonverbally (due to decreased LOC).	■ Position patient in Fowler or semi-Fowler position as indicated to promote ease of breathing. ■ Administer medications and supplemental oxygen as ordered. ■ Consider other methods of communication for the patient (e.g., a tablet, a family member).

Concepts Related to *(continued)*

CONCEPT	RELATIONSHIP TO COMMUNICATION	NURSING IMPLICATIONS
Safety	Impaired communication ↑ risk for illness and injury.	■ Create a supportive environment that promotes communication and safety. ■ Introduce opportunities for the patient to communicate needs and concerns. ■ Be tactful and avoid abrupt, offensive, and accusatory statements. ■ Maintain a nonthreatening approach and validate cooperation. ■ Listen to the concerns of other members of the healthcare team. ■ Apologize when needed. ■ Agree when possible. ■ Encourage the team to follow national standards.

Factors Influencing the Communication Process

Many factors influence the communication process. Some of these are development, gender, values and perceptions, personal space, territoriality, roles and relationships, environment, congruence, and attitudes. Some sociocultural factors, such as cultural aspects and language, have already been discussed.

Development

A patient's stage of development affects the ability to communicate with and understand the communication of others. For example, when communicating with infants and toddlers who do not have well-developed language skills, the nurse may rely more on the child's nonverbal communications when assessing comfort and pain levels. The nurse may hold the child and use touch to demonstrate caring and provide comfort. In contrast, the nurse working with older children may use pictures or dolls to enhance communication. As children reach adolescence, they are better able to understand and participate in verbal communication. Hearing or visual impairments may affect communication with patients of any age but are more common in older adulthood. For these patients, it may be helpful to use visual or audio communication methods to enhance communication. Further information related to aspects of communicating with children can be found in the Lifespan Considerations section.

Gender

From an early age, girls and boys may exhibit differences in language development and communication tendencies that can persist into adulthood. Examples often cited include the tendency of women to make requests and men to make demands, of men to address issues more directly and women to be more active listeners, often using statements that encourage a response. **Active listening**, also known as *attentive* or *mindful listening*, involves fully concentrating on both the content and emotion of a person's message, rather than just passively hearing the words a person says. (For more information on this topic, see Exemplar 38.B, Therapeutic Communication, later in this module.) Although it has long been believed that these perceived differences result from psychosocial development, more recent research indicates that language development proceeds differently in girls than in boys, indicating that neuronal factors, psychosocial factors, and hormonal differences may influence language and communication discrepancies (Wilder, 2020).

When working with patients or colleagues, nurses should be aware that men and women might interpret the same communication differently. Thus, nurses should always work to assess the ways in which a patient's or colleague's communication is gendered. Maintaining an understanding of the ways in which people communicate differently because of their socialization allows the nurse to respond accordingly.

An area of awareness that continues to develop in healthcare communities is communicating with transgender individuals and individuals who are nonbinary or gender nonconforming (identifying as neither male nor female). In everyone, gender identity (how one sees oneself), gender expression (the outward expression of an individual's sense of maleness or femaleness), biological sex (one's anatomy), and sexual attraction (to whom one is sexually attracted) are distinct, and each element of identity can be well defined or ambiguous. Transgender individuals who have not had sex reassignment surgery have a gender identity that may not align with their biological sex characteristics, and therefore, their name or appearance may not "match" their stated (or legal) sex. The nurse should always use a patient's stated name and pronoun (whether *he*, *she*, *them*, or something else) and guard the patient's privacy. By protecting the privacy and personal expression of transgender and nonbinary individuals and treating them with respect, nurses can reduce undue stress, promote the therapeutic relationship, and help these individuals feel safe in healthcare contexts (Centers for Disease Control and Prevention, 2020).

Values and Perceptions

Values, standards that influence behavior, and **perceptions** (a person's interpretation of issues or events) are unique to each individual and can influence how they receive and interpret verbal, nonverbal, and electronic communication. Values and perceptions also influence personal preferences. For example, one patient may want the curtain around the bed drawn in an effort to maintain privacy, whereas another patient may fear staff will forget if the curtain is drawn. The nurse needs to be aware of a patient's values and perceptions in order to promote trust in the nurse–patient relationship.

Personal Space

Personal space is the distance individuals prefer to keep between themselves and others during social, family, or work-related interactions. **Proxemics** refers to the amount of space individuals are comfortable putting between themselves and others when interacting. Most people who live in North America use definitive distances in a variety of interpersonal relationships, in addition to specific voice tones and body language altered, changing their communication in accordance with four ranges of physical distance in this culture, each with a near and a far phase (Oxford Reference, 2020):

1. ***Intimate:*** touching to 1½ feet
2. ***Personal:*** 1½ to 4 feet
3. ***Social:*** 4 to 12 feet
4. ***Public:*** 12 feet or more

Intimate distance is used for confidential communication and is characterized by body contact, increased awareness of body heat and smell, and lowered voices. Nurses use intimate distance when performing actions such as cuddling a baby, positioning a patient, observing a wound, or auscultating the lungs.

Individuals have a natural protective instinct to maintain a certain amount of space immediately around them. This amount varies among individuals and cultures. When a person who wants to communicate moves too close, most people automatically take a step or two backward to maintain their personal space. Nurses are often required to violate this personal space when performing therapeutic nursing interventions and should know when this will occur so they can inform the patient in advance.

Personal distance typically refers to the physical distance between two individuals in a social, family, or work setting. Within this zone, voice tones are moderate, physical contact is possible (e.g., a handshake or touching a shoulder), and body odor is less noticeable. The majority of communication between nurses and patients occurs at a personal distance. For example, the nurse is observing personal distancing while sitting with a patient, giving medications, or establishing an intravenous infusion. Although communication at a close personal distance can facilitate the sharing of personal information and feelings, it can also create tension if it invades the other person's personal space (**Figure 38.4 ⟫**).

Social distance provides a clear view of the whole person. At this distance conversations are loud enough to be overhead by others, body odor is imperceptible, and eye contact is increased. Social distance is often associated with more formal communication. It is also convenient for communicating with several individuals at the same time or within a short period of time. Individuals may use social distance out of convenience, or intentionally if they want to remain beyond the potential for sharing thoughts or feelings. Examples include when the nurse waves to a colleague when walking by the nurse's station or when someone chooses to sit at a distance from others during lunch.

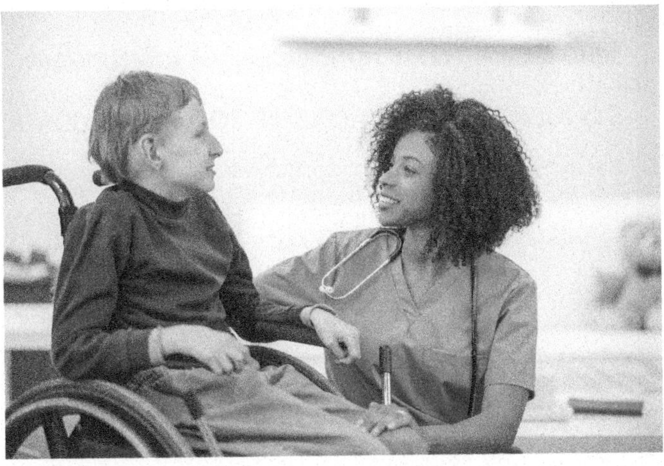

Figure 38.4 ⟫ Personal space influences communication in social and professional interactions. Encroachment into another individual's personal space may create tension.

Source: Fat Camera/E+/Getty Images.

Social distance can be misused in situations when personal distance would be more appropriate. For example, the nurse who stands in the doorway and asks a patient, "How are you today?" is not likely to elicit as meaningful a response from a patient as the nurse who takes time to come into the room and speak with the patient from within the boundaries of personal distance.

Public distance requires loud, clear vocalizations with careful articulation. With public distance, the perception is of the group or community and, although the faces and forms of people are visible, individuality is lost.

Territoriality

Territoriality is a term that refers to the use of space to establish or convey ownership and belonging. Territories may or may not be visible. Examples of visible territories include the walls of a private room, the curtains around the bed unit, and even the bed itself. Patients often feel the need to defend their territory when it is invaded by others, such when a nurse removes a chair for use in another room. Because claiming territory is a natural human tendency, the nurse should recognize the boundaries of the patient's territory and obtain permission from the patient to remove, rearrange, or borrow objects in the patient's hospital area.

Roles and Relationships

Role relationships (such as nursing student and instructor, parent and child, nurse and patient) can affect the communication process, as can other factors already discussed, such as clarity and nonverbal communication. The length of the relationship can also affect communication. For example, the nurse who has cared for a patient previously and developed a relationship with that individual will communicate differently from the nurse who is meeting with that patient for the first time. The nurse may choose a more formal stance when communicating with HCPs or administrators and a more informal or comfortable stance when communicating with patients or colleagues.

Environment

A comfortable environment is usually most conducive to effective communication. Distractions in the environment such as temperature extremes, excessive noise, and poor ventilation can result in impaired or distorted communication. Lack of privacy may also interfere with a patient's communication about issues the patient considers to be private or personal. For example, a patient who is concerned about sexual dysfunction may not wish to discuss this concern with a nurse within hearing distance of others.

Congruence

Congruent communication—in which the nurse's verbal expression and nonverbal behaviors match others—promotes the patient's trust in the nurse and helps prevent miscommunication. If there is any discrepancy between verbal and nonverbal communication, the real meaning is usually conveyed in the sender's body language. For example, when teaching a patient how to perform wound care for a surgical site after an operation, the nurse may say, "It's easy, you won't have any problem doing this." However, if the nurse looks concerned or makes a disgusted face while saying this, the patient is less likely to trust what the nurse is saying.

Nurses must strive to improve their nonverbal communication skills. One strategy is to refrain from indiscriminate use of nonverbal gestures, such as the overuse of smiling or nodding the head, which can cause the patient to doubt the nurse's sincerity. Another strategy is to convey a calm, relaxed attitude, rather than a distressed attitude. Being relaxed makes it easier for patients to feel at ease around the nurse.

Interpersonal Attitudes

Most individuals communicate their thoughts and feelings about others or about their current situation through their attitude. In turn, attitude can affect how others perceive that communication. A caring, respectful attitude facilitates communication with and acceptance of others. In contrast, a condescending or judgmental attitude can inhibit communication and acceptance.

Lotfi and colleagues (2019) found that effective nursing communication is significantly related to patient satisfaction. When nurses communicate (both verbally and nonverbally) warmth, positivity, energy, and capability, patients express greater satisfaction with both competence and interpersonal care. Caring involves giving feelings, thoughts, skill, and knowledge. It requires psychologic energy and poses the risk of gaining little in return; yet by caring, both nurses and patients usually reap the benefits of greater communication and understanding.

Respect and civility are two qualities that promote effective communication. *Respect* is an attitude that emphasizes the other person's worth and individuality while conveying that the person's hopes and feelings matter. *Civility* (politeness or courtesy in speech or behavior) communicates respect for others and facilitates successful communication.

Healthcare providers may unknowingly show disrespect or incivility by using speech that they believe shows caring but that the patient perceives as demeaning or patronizing. This can happen in settings that provide healthcare to older adults and/or individuals with obvious physical or mental disabilities. **Elderspeak** is a style of speech similar to baby talk that sends the message to patients, especially older adults, that they are dependent and incompetent. It does not communicate respect. Many HCPs are not aware that they use elderspeak or that it can have negative meanings to the patient. The characteristics of elderspeak include use of inappropriate terms of endearment (such as "honey" or "dear"), plural pronouns (e.g., "Are we having a good day?"), tag questions, and slow, loud speech. Tag questions are short statements followed by a mini-question, such as "You feel better now, don't you?" Tag questions and other types of elderspeak should not be used with any age group. Alternative strategies to elderspeak include:

- Refer to and call patients by their full name (e.g., Ms. Lakewood) or preferred name instead of using diminutives or terms of endearment.
- Always speak to patients by using "you" instead of using inappropriate plural pronouns such as "we."
- Ask questions directly. Avoid using phrases or tags that make patients think that you are leading them to answer in a certain way.
- Always address patients as the adults that they are and avoid the use of baby talk, which is demeaning to patients.

In all cases, the nurse conveys *acceptance* rather than approval or disapproval when communicating with patients. The nurse willingly accepts or receives patients' honest expressions of feelings, allowing them to be themselves. Acceptance, however, does not mean there are no limits to patient behavior. Nurses may set limits or boundaries when a patient's behavior is inappropriate or aggressive. When that happens, the nurse can also give the patient examples of what comments or behaviors are appropriate.

Barriers to Communication

Just as there are characteristics of effective communication, there are barriers to effective communication. Nurses need to be aware of these barriers and avoid them. Major barriers to communication include not listening, improperly interpreting the person's intended message, and placing the nurse's needs above those of the patient. **Table 38.1** » outlines other barriers to communication.

Types of Communicators

Individuals tend to express themselves in various ways. **Aggressive communicators** are those who tend to focus on their own needs and become impatient when their needs are not met. **Passive communicators** are those who focus on the needs of others. They often deny that their own needs are important, which causes them to become frustrated. **Assertive communicators** are those who declare and affirm their needs or opinions. In doing this, however, they respect the rights of others to communicate in the same fashion. Assertive communicators have the most productive communication with others. **Table 38.2** » compares and contrasts the three styles of communicating.

Assertive communicators stand up for themselves while remaining open to ideas and respecting the rights of others (Mayo Clinic, 2020). By communicating directly, honestly, and appropriately, assertive communicators minimize the risk for miscommunication with others. By using assertive communication, nurses promote patient safety.

TABLE 38.1 Barriers to Communication

Technique	Description	Examples
Stereotyping	Offering generalized and oversimplified beliefs about groups of individuals that are based on experiences too limited to be valid. These responses categorize patients and negate their uniqueness as individuals.	"Two-year-olds are brats." "Women are complainers." "Men don't cry." "Most people don't have any pain after this type of surgery."
Agreeing and disagreeing	Similar to judgmental responses, agreeing and disagreeing imply that the patient is either right or wrong and that the nurse is in a position to judge this. These responses deter patients from thinking through their position and may cause a patient to become defensive.	*Patient:* "I don't think Dr. Broad is a very good doctor. He doesn't seem interested in his patients." *Nurse:* "Dr. Broad is head of the department of surgery and is an excellent surgeon."
Being defensive	Attempting to protect an individual or healthcare service from negative comments. These responses prevent the patient from expressing true concerns. The nurse is saying, "You have no right to complain." Defensive responses protect the nurse from admitting weaknesses in the healthcare services, including personal weaknesses.	*Patient:* "Those night nurses must just sit around and talk all night. They didn't answer my light for over an hour." *Nurse:* "I'll have you know we literally run around on nights. You're not the only patient, you know."
Challenging	Giving a response that makes patients prove their statement or point of view. These responses indicate that the nurse is failing to consider the patient's feelings, making the patient feel it necessary to defend a position.	*Patient:* "I felt nauseated after that red pill." *Nurse:* "Surely you don't think I gave you the wrong pill?" *Patient:* "I feel as if I am dying." *Nurse:* "How can you feel that way when your pulse is 60?" *Patient:* "I believe my husband doesn't love me." *Nurse:* "You can't say that. Why, he visits you every day."
Probing	Asking for information chiefly out of curiosity rather than with the intent to assist the patient. These responses are considered prying and violate the patient's privacy. Asking "why" is often probing and places the patient in a defensive position.	*Nurse:* "Tell me about how you were sexually abused when you were a teenager." *Patient:* "I didn't ask the doctor about that when he was here." *Nurse:* "Why didn't you?"
Testing	Asking questions that make the patient admit to something. These responses permit the patient only limited answers and often meet the nurse's need rather than the patient's.	"Who do you think you are?" (forces the individual to admit to a lower status) "Do you think I am not busy?" (forces the patient to admit that the nurse really is busy)
Rejecting	Refusing to discuss certain topics with the patient. These responses often make patients feel that the nurse is rejecting not only their communication but also the patients themselves.	"I don't want to discuss that. Let's talk about. . . . " "Let's discuss other areas of interest to you rather than the two problems you keep mentioning." "I can't talk now. I'm on my way for a coffee break."
Changing topics and subjects	Directing the communication into areas of self-interest rather than considering the patient's concerns is often a self-protective response to a topic that causes the nurse anxiety. These responses imply that what the nurse considers important will be discussed and that patients should not discuss certain topics.	*Patient:* "I'm separated from my wife. Do you think I can start sleeping with other women?" *Nurse:* "I see that you're 36 and that you like gardening. I bet you're looking forward to summer."
Unwarranted or false reassurance	Using clichés or comforting statements of advice as a means to reassure the patient. These responses block the fears, feelings, and other thoughts of the patient.	"You'll feel better soon." "I'm sure everything will turn out all right." "Don't worry."
Passing judgment	Giving opinions and approving or disapproving responses, moralizing, or imposing one's own values. These responses imply that the patient must think as the nurse thinks, fostering patient dependence.	"That's good (bad)." "You shouldn't do that." "That's not good enough." "What you did was wrong (right)."
Giving common advice	Telling the patient what to do. These responses deny the patient's right to be an equal partner. Note that giving expert advice that is appropriate for the patient's individual situation rather than common advice is therapeutic.	*Patient:* "Should I move from my home to a nursing home?" *Nurse:* "If I were you, I'd go to a nursing home where you'll get your meals cooked for you."

Source: From Berman, Snyder, and Frandsen (2021). Pearson Education, Inc., Hoboken, NJ.

TABLE 38.2 Aggressive, Passive, and Assertive Styles

Aggressive Individuals	Passive Individuals	Assertive Individuals
■ Engage in heated arguments, often using insults ■ May resort to violence ■ Refuse to accept blame or responsibility ■ Walk out in the middle of arguments	■ Hide or deny their feelings ■ Avoid arguments ■ Are noncommittal	■ Express their feelings honestly and appropriately ■ Acknowledge feelings of others ■ Are open to discussion ■ Use "I" statements to express concerns or reduce conflict

Assertive communication uses "I" statements rather than "you" statements. "You" statements imply blame and can put the listener on the defensive. In contrast, "I" statements foster communication. For example, when a nurse states "I am concerned about . . . " to another colleague, the nurse will be more likely to gain that person's attention and convey the importance of working together for the benefit of the patient. Once the nurse has the other person's attention, the nurse uses principles of effective communication (such as clarity and brevity) to explain the concern.

Individuals who are passive communicators often try to meet the needs and requests of others without regard to their own, believing their needs are not as important. In some cases, passive communicators may lack self-esteem and communicate passively in an attempt to avoid negative criticism or conflict from others. They often prioritize and meet the demands and requests of others without regard to their own feelings and needs. They believe their own thoughts and feelings are not as important. It is believed by some experts that individuals who use submissive behaviors or communication styles are insecure and avoid conflict such as negative criticism or disagreement from others to try to maintain their self-esteem.

Individuals who use aggressive communication assert their rights without consideration for the needs or feelings of others. Aggressive communication undercuts trust and is often perceived as a personal attack by the recipient because it usually seeks to embarrass, humiliate, control, or bully the recipient. The person using aggressive communication may appear self-righteous or feel superior, which helps to increase their self-esteem while lowering others'. Aggressive communicators may fail to understand that the very nature of their communication causes others to resent or avoid them. Screaming, sarcasm, belittling jokes, bullying, and personal insults are examples of aggressive communication.

A nurse's approach to communication can have far-reaching impact on the quality of patient care delivered. See clinical example A.

Clinical Example A

You are a nurse who is caring for Shannon Collins, a 41-year-old woman. She has a standing order for vital signs every 2 hours because her temperature was elevated on admission to the facility. Since admission, Mrs. Collins's temperature has normalized, and her vital signs have consistently been within normal limits. She tells you that she isn't sleeping well because the nurses keep coming in and waking her every 2 hours and it takes her almost an hour to fall back to sleep. As a result, Mrs. Collins is sleeping in 1-hour intervals and feels extremely sleep deprived. You approach the HCP and request that the order be changed to every 4 hours during the day with 6 hours of uninterrupted sleep from midnight to 6:00 a.m. The HCP responds by saying, "If she wants to sleep, she'll have to wait until she goes home. I want vital signs every 2 hours as ordered."

Critical Thinking Questions

1. Which type of communication style will best serve the needs of the patient? Provide a rationale for your response.
2. What type of response will the nurse have using an aggressive communication style?
3. What type of response will the nurse have using a passive communication style?
4. What type of response will the nurse have using an assertive communication style?

Assertive Communication

The goal of all healthcare professionals is to promote the best outcome for everyone involved. Assertive communication allows the nurse to express all ideas in a direct and nonconfrontational manner that promotes the rights of the nurse or the patient while respecting the rights of others to have a different outlook. Assertive communication does not use name-calling, is not judgmental, and does not blame others. It increases the likelihood of creating a win–win result in which both parties walk away feeling that their point of view was heard and understood while reaching a conclusion satisfactory to them both.

Characteristics of assertive communicators include freedom to express themselves, awareness of their own rights, and self-control over strong emotions such as anger, fear, or frustration. Assertive communicators are professional and serve as the best advocate for the patient. They express their opinions but are open to listening to others' points of view. They do not use sarcasm, biting comebacks, or passive-aggressive sniping to promote their superiority. Assertive communicators use body language that is relaxed and open to the words of others. They use a tone of voice that is well modulated with appropriate inflection and avoid raising their voice, whispering, or using aggressive overtones.

An assertive individual receives feedback from others with a willingness to consider both the positive and negative perspectives of the evaluator. Although assertive individuals may not believe everything that is said, they will listen to another individual's opinion without becoming defensive or angry and without attacking the speaker. Seeking clarification is appropriate to be sure that the perception of the message is the same as what the sender intended.

Some individuals may have more trouble accepting positive feedback and will dismiss it or negate it when offered. The assertive individual simply says, "Thank you" and considers the value of the positive feedback for later application to similar situations.

Benefits of Assertive Communication

Assertiveness is an effective and professional communication style because it is based on mutual respect. An assertive style improves communication and reduces stress by deescalating conflict, improving outcomes, and reducing the likelihood of angry encounters.

Techniques for Assertive Communication

Because no one technique works in every situation, the nurse must have an arsenal of strategies to use when faced with a situation requiring assertive communication. These techniques include the following:

- ***"I" statements.*** Assertive communicators voice their own feelings and wishes based on sound evidence without placing blame or raising the defenses of the individual to whom they are speaking. For example, "I have assessed that Patient A is . . . ."
- ***Fogging.*** Finding some area, no matter how small, on which both parties agree and building from there is a technique that assertive communicators use. In the example of the sleep-deprived patient described previously, both the nurse and the HCP can agree that they want to maintain patient

safety through careful monitoring of the patient's condition. This gives them a starting point from which to reach consensus where both can feel patient care has been optimized.

- ***Negative assertion.*** An assertive communicator can agree with criticism without becoming upset or angry, thus moving the focus of the communication toward the desired goal. This can be particularly important to the nurse when receiving feedback related to the quality of the care the nurse delivers. For example, when the evaluator says, "Although you are very caring, I would like to see you improve your decision-making ability," the nurse may respond, "I could stand to improve my decision-making ability, but I believe the quality of the care I deliver is excellent." This prevents an ongoing debate about something that both parties agree on and allows the communication to move forward regarding the more important topic.
- ***Repetition.*** When being met with resistance to a request, repeating the request can be useful. However, each time the request is repeated, the power of the words is diminished. This strategy is effective only if the nurse has power within the relationship. For example, suppose the nurse calls the pharmacy to request a newly ordered medication that is to be given within the hour. The pharmacist explains that the pharmacy is very busy, cannot fill the prescription right now, and will not be able to deliver it to the unit for 3 to 4 hours. The nurse repeats, "I must give this medication within the hour" or "The patient needs the medication within the hour." The effectiveness of this approach may improve if the nurse attempts to find a compromise. The nurse might say, "I need to administer this medication within the hour," to which the pharmacy responds, "I'm sorry, I can't have it to the floor that quickly." The nurse then responds, "The patient needs that medication within the hour. What if I come to the pharmacy so you don't have to deliver it?" This allows for the nurse and the pharmacy to collaborate to reach a mutually effective solution to the problem through compromise.
- ***Confidence.*** Confidence is essential to assertive communication. A choppy or weak tone of voice implies uncertainty. The nurse should maintain an air of confidence in order to help others see their needs and wants as having merit.
- ***Managing nonverbal communication.*** Getting too close to the other individual, wagging a finger in someone's face, or glaring at the other person can all counteract assertive words. By maintaining open, assertive body language and keeping a neutral voice, the nurse promotes shared decision making and compromise.
- ***Thinking before speaking.*** Consider both the choice of words and the tone of voice before speaking. This helps the nurse avoid saying something they will later regret or that will reduce the effectiveness of the nurse's communication style.
- ***Avoiding apologizing whenever possible.*** This is particularly important for women, who have a tendency to say "I'm sorry" even when there is no call for an apology. A woman may say, "I'm sorry, I didn't hear you," or "I'm sorry to bother you, but . . . ." An unnecessary apology immediately places the communicator in a somewhat submissive position. Apologies should be given only when warranted.
- ***Performing a postconversation evaluation.*** Assertive communicators can continue to improve their skills by reviewing what was said and how the communication might have been handled differently to improve the final outcome. This should be done even when the communication interaction was successful because evaluation of what went well, in contrast to what did not, helps the nurse improve assertive communication skills.

Although some individuals may not prefer or feel comfortable with assertive communication, it is possible for all nurses to become assertive communicators and reach more positive outcomes through practice, self-evaluation, and ongoing efforts to improve their communication approach.

Lifespan Considerations

Developmental level, cognitive ability, sensory and motor systems, and previous experiences communicating all affect the ability to communicate. Communication abilities change significantly as individuals grow and mature.

Communicating with Infants

Infants communicate nonverbally, often in response to bodily sensations rather than in a conscious effort to be expressive. Infants' perceptions are related to sensory stimuli. For example, a gentle voice is soothing, whereas tension and anger displayed around an infant create distress. Infant body language can provide important cues about their needs and feelings. Infants use two types of nonverbal cues: engagement and disengagement cues. Each type of cue may be expressed in a subtle or direct manner. Disengagement cues include crawling away, crying, or lip compression. Engagement cues include smiling, babbling, and opening hands (Raising Children Network Australia, 2020). Nurses can familiarize themselves with the expressive but nonverbal messages of infants to better communicate with their youngest patients.

Communicating with Toddlers and Preschoolers

As they grow and develop, toddlers and young children gain skills in both expressive (i.e., telling others what they feel, think, want, and care about) and receptive (hearing and understanding what others are communicating to them) language. Toddlers need time to complete verbalizing their thoughts without interruption. Adults should provide simple responses to questions and straightforward, one-step directions because toddlers have short attention spans. Around the age of 4, children begin to follow two- and three-step directions and become more able to express feelings and sensations. For children at this age, drawing pictures or using pictures and photos to communicate can be helpful in a variety of settings.

Communicating with School-Age Children

In interactions with school-age children, it is important to give them opportunities to be expressive, listen openly, and respond honestly, using words and concepts they understand. Talk to children at their eye level to help decrease any feelings of intimidation. Children have the ability to express themselves and take part in their healthcare, so if the child is present, include the child in the conversation. Several techniques are helpful when communicating with children. Play, the universal language, allows children to use other symbols, not just words, to express themselves. Drawing, painting, and other art forms can be used even by nonverbal children. Storytelling, in which the nurse and child take turns adding to a story or putting words to pictures, can help the child safely express emotions and feelings. Word games that pose hypothetical situations or put the child in control, such as "What if . . . ?" "If you could . . . ," or "If a genie came and gave you a wish . . . " can help a child feel more powerful or explore ideas about how to manage an illness. Reading books with a theme similar to the child's condition or problem and then discussing the meaning, characters, and feelings generated by the book can help the nurse communicate with the child about the condition and the child's experiences with it. Movies or videos can also be used in this way. Older children can use writing to reflect on their situation, develop meaning, and gain a sense of control.

Communicating with Adolescents

Adolescents have the ability to think abstractly and make decisions about their own healthcare. Adolescents are focused on the development of effective communication skills and feel a strong need to share thoughts, facts, and feelings with others (Koutoukidis & Stainton, 2020). It takes time to build rapport with adolescents. Nurses working with this age group should use active listening and project a nonjudgmental attitude and nonreactive behaviors, even when an adolescent makes disturbing comments. Adolescents are very sensitive to feelings of judgment, so it is essential to remain open minded when communicating with them. Adolescents prefer expectations to be clearly explained, and they appreciate when praise is given.

Communicating with Adults

Young adults and middle-aged adults are at the peak of their communication abilities. They are fully grown/developed, and many have either completed their education or are earning advanced degrees. However, there is a wide range of communication abilities among adults based on cognitive ability, education levels, socioeconomic levels, exposure to professional and work environments, and health literacy. Young adults may still display some adolescent patterns of communication. At the upper end of middle age, some adults may begin to have some of the physical and cognitive problems usually seen in older adults. Nurses should identify any barriers to communication with adults and plan accordingly.

Communicating with Pregnant Women

Optimal pregnancy outcomes depend on clear communication, effective decision making, and teamwork (Chang, Coxon, Portela, Furuta, & Bick, 2018). Effective therapeutic communication is essential to patient safety, creates a climate of confidence, and strongly affects the patient's comfort with the process of pregnancy and birth. Nurses can promote the patient's self-expression by establishing a therapeutic relationship, making the family feel welcome, and being nonjudgmental. Keys to communication during pregnancy include determining the cultural values of the family about birth, engaging in shared decision making, and listening to the patient as well as providing support. Refer to Module 33, Reproduction, for more information on communicating with pregnant women.

Communicating with Older Adults

Older adults may have physical or cognitive problems that necessitate nursing interventions to improve communication. Some of the common problems include sensory deficits; cognitive impairment; neurologic deficits from stroke or other neurologic conditions; and psychosocial problems, such as depression. Recognizing specific needs and obtaining appropriate resources for patients can greatly increase their socialization and quality of life. Nurses can use a number of different interventions to improve communication with patients who need assistance. For example, nurses can ensure that the patient is using assistive devices, glasses, and hearing aids, and that these are in good working order. Nurses can also use communications aids, such as paper and pencil, communication boards, tablets or computers, or pictures, when possible. Referral to appropriate services and resources, such as speech therapy, may provide further support for the older adult who experiences communication difficulties.

To communicate effectively with older adults, the nurse should keep environmental distractions to a minimum. The nurse should seek to speak in short, simple sentences, one subject at a time, and reinforce or repeat what is said when necessary. In communicating effectively with older adults, the nurse must avoid elderspeak and should always face the patient when speaking; coming up behind someone may be frightening. Include family and friends in conversation. When verbal expression and nonverbal expression are incongruent, believe the nonverbal; clarification of this and careful attention to the patient's feelings will help promote a feeling of caring and acceptance. Find out what has been important and what has meaning to the patient and try to maintain these things as much as possible. Simple things such as bedtime rituals become more important, especially in a hospital or extended-care setting.

NURSING PROCESS

Communication is essential to assessing, monitoring, and evaluating patients; planning care in collaboration with patients and other members of the healthcare team; and providing direct patient care and education.

Assessment

Assessment strategies related to communication include evaluating the patient's communication style and appraising any language or communication barriers. Remember that cultural values and practices may influence when and how a patient speaks. Obviously, language varies according to age and development. For example, with children, the nurse observes sounds, gestures, facial expressions, and vocabulary.

Throughout the process of collecting data, the nurse uses communication skills to increase nurse–patient rapport, put the patient at ease when discussing personal matters, and interpret the patient's nonverbal communication, and assess for and overcome barriers to communication as outlined below. Exemplar 38.B in this module discusses the role of therapeutic communication in creating a helping relationship with the patient.

Language Deficits

The nurse needs to assess the ability of the patient to communicate both verbally (with or without assistive devices) and nonverbally. Assessment of communication ability includes determining if the patient speaks another language or has any kind of cognitive, speech, or hearing impairment that affects communication. Patients who use English as a second language may not be able to speak or understand English well enough to meet their needs in a healthcare environment.

Sensory Deficits

All of the senses assist in the process of communication. A hearing impairment can significantly alter the message a patient receives. Vision impairment may affect a patient's ability to observe nonverbal behavior, such as a smile or a gesture. Sensing danger, such as smoke from a fire or heat from a stove, depend on the ability to feel and smell.

Strategies for working with patients who have hearing impairment include the following:

- Note the presence of a hearing aid, medical alert bracelet, necklace, or tag indicating hearing loss.
- For patients who use hearing aids, confirm that the hearing aid is turned on and functioning.
- Observe if the patient is trying to see your face to read lips.
- Observe if the patient is trying to use the hands to communicate with sign language.
- Evaluate feedback to validate that effective communication is taking place.

Refer to Box 18.2, Communicating with Patients Who Have a Visual or Hearing Deficit, in Module 18, Sensory Perception, for more information.

Cognitive Impairments

Disorders that impair cognitive functioning, such as stroke, traumatic brain injury, brain tumors, or dementia, may affect a patient's ability to use and understand language. Some patients may lose the ability to find or name words, may experience impaired articulation, or may completely lose their ability to speak. They may also experience difficulty understanding others or following conversations, which may manifest through withdrawal, frustration, or changing the subject. Some medications (including some sedatives, neuroleptics, and antidepressants) can impair speech, causing patients to slur their words or use incomplete sentences.

Assessment of patients' ability to respond to verbal communication includes:

- Does the patient speak fluently or hesitate when speaking?
- Does the patient use words in the correct manner, putting words in the right order and using them appropriately to their meaning?
- Can the patient understand instructions, as evidenced by following directions?
- Can the patient repeat words or phrases when instructed to do so?

In addition, the nurse should assess the patient's ability to comprehend and follow written directions. Asking the patient to read a selected sentence or sentences out loud or asking patients to identify specific words are strategies for assessing a patient's ability to understand written directions. Nurses should use large, clearly written words when assessing patients in this area.

SAFETY ALERT When the patient is unconscious, the nurse looks for any indication that suggests the patient has some ability to comprehend and communicate, such as attempting to arouse the patient verbally and through touch. The nurse may also ask a closed question such as "Can you hear me?" or "Squeeze my hand if you can hear me," and observe for a nonverbal response. Attempts to determine comprehension must be individualized to the specific needs of the patient.

Other Impairments

Extreme shortness of breath, airway obstruction, or structural defects of the oral and nasal cavities (e.g., cleft palate, artificial airways, laryngectomy) can impair speaking ability and speech patterns. Verbal impairment combined with paralysis of the upper extremities (affecting ability to write) requires assessment of the patient's ability to blink, nod, point, or squeeze a hand. A simple and effective communication system can be created using any of these actions.

Style of Communication

Nurses should consider both verbal and nonverbal communication when assessing communication style. In addition to physical barriers, the patient's ability to communicate can be influenced by cognitive impairment, psychosis, delirium, or severe depression. Altered thought processes that may present as a result of these illnesses include (but are not limited to) repeated verbalization of the same words or phrases, talking about people or things that are not present, and flight of ideas (a continuous, rapid flow of speech that quickly changes from one topic to the next).

Verbal Communication

The content and themes of a patient's message as well as the patient's verbalized emotions are the focus of the nurse's assessment of verbal communication. Other indicators to consider include:

- The pattern of communication: Is the patient's speech slow, rapid, spontaneous or hesitant, quiet or overly loud or aggressive, or evasive?
- Vocabulary and any deviations from normal vocabulary. For example, acute illness or extreme distress may cause patients to use language they may not normally use, such as curse words, or may cause them to rely more on nonverbal communication to reduce the work of breathing.
- Changes in articulation of words, such as slurring or stuttering, inability to pronounce a specific sound, lack of clarity in enunciation, inability to speak in sentences, loose association of ideas, flight of ideas, or the inability to find or name words or identify objects.
- The refusal or lack of ability to speak.

SAFETY ALERT Neurologic impairment may be indicated by changes in the patient's ability to put words together into sentences, to properly name an item, or a struggle to find the right word for common objects. Assessment of communication ability is especially important following any type of head injury and in cases of suspected cerebrovascular accident (stroke).

Diagnosis

A nursing diagnosis related to communication may be made if the patient has difficulty with communication, including *receptive* communication (difficulty hearing or understanding words) or *expressive* communication (difficulty speaking).

Planning

Once the nurse determines that a communication impairment exists, the nurse works with the patient to plan strategies to ensure successful communication between the healthcare team. Whiteboards, tablets, and smartphones are among the devices patients and healthcare teams can use to establish communication. For example, smartphone apps are available that use symbols and pictures to help people communicate with others.

Specific goals for patients with a communication impairment will vary depending on the stated etiology and may include the following:

- The patient will have an effective method for communicating needs.
- The patient will maximize the ability to understand and be understood by others.

Once a successful method of communicating has been established, the nurse should facilitate access to any assistive communication devices or other strategies to assist the patient. For example, if the patient hears better in the left ear, that information should be noted in the patient's electronic health record and made available to all members of the patient's healthcare team.

Implementation

Appropriate nursing interventions to facilitate communication include manipulating the environment, providing support to patients and caregivers, using tools to enhance communication, and avoiding or reducing any cultural barriers to communication.

Manipulate the Environment

A quiet environment with limited distractions provides the best setting for, and increases the possibility of, effective communication. Adequate light is beneficial for reducing anxiety and conveying nonverbal messages, which are especially important if the patient has visual or auditory impairment. Impairments in communication can contribute to patient anxiety and feelings of isolation. Successful nurse–patient communication reduces feelings of anxiety and loneliness. To further reduce patient feelings of isolation, the nurse should acknowledge and praise the patient's attempts at communication and assist family members to learn to communicate with the patient regardless of the nature of the impairment.

Provide Support

Providing encouragement and nonverbal reassurance are essential to supporting patients with altered communication. If the nurse has difficulty understanding a patient's communication, the nurse must make the patient aware so that the individual can provide clarification by using other words or through alternative forms of communication. When speaking with a patient who has difficulty understanding, stop frequently during the conversation to determine that the patient has heard and understood what has been communicated. Asking open-ended questions will assist the nurse to obtain more accurate information about the effectiveness of communication.

Clinical Example B

You are providing care to Maria Perez, a 52-year-old Latina patient who has limited English skills. As part of the discharge teaching for this patient, you are teaching her about dietary changes that are necessary for managing Crohn disease. You ask Ms. Perez, "Do you understand what to eat?" She nods her head yes. You realize that the question did not elicit an answer that sufficiently confirms that Ms. Perez understood. You ask a follow-up question: "What do you think will be good for you to eat when you go home?" At the same time, your body language (e.g., gestures, posture, facial expression, and eye contact) conveys acceptance and approval. When Ms. Perez begins to explain what foods she should avoid, you are confident that you communicated the information to Ms. Perez successfully.

Critical Thinking Questions

1. What resources are available for teaching patients whose primary language is not English?
2. How does culture affect communication?
3. How does body language affect the communication process?

Source: Adapted from Berman et al. (2021).

Employ Measures to Enhance Communication

To facilitate communication, the nurse first needs to assess how the patient best receives information: by listening, looking, or reading; through touch; or through using an interpreter. The use of augmentative and alternative communication strategies, such as word boards, pictures, paper and pencil, or smartphone, laptop, or tablet may be helpful (see the Evidence-Based Practice feature). Whether using alternative communication strategies or normal verbal or nonverbal communication, the nurse should use words with simple and concrete meanings and stay on the topic at hand before moving on to another topic.

Avoid Potential Cultural Barriers to Communication

The nurse should remember several strategies when communicating with a patient whose primary language is not English:

- Avoid the use of slang, buzzwords, and medical terminology when possible. Show the patient respect by speaking clearly, directly, and at a normal pace.
- Avoid words that may impede the communication process, such as words that are slurred and those that have several syllables.
- Speak at a speed that does not overload the patient and allows the patient to follow the conversation. However, avoid speaking too slowly because this may cause the nurse to lose the patient's attention.
- Use open-ended questions and rephrase them as necessary to obtain accurate information.

When using nonverbal communication with these patients, select gestures with care. This form of nonverbal communication underscores both words and actions and can be used to clarify meaning; however, gestures may have different meanings for different cultures. Therefore, the nurse must validate words and gestures with each patient on an individual basis.

Evidence-Based Practice

The Role of Alternative Communication Strategies and Time in Caring for the Patient with Complex Communication Needs

Problem

Effective nurse–patient communication is an essential aspect of healthcare. As Sibiya (2018) notes, "The quality of communication in interactions between nurses and patients has a major influence on patient outcomes." Unfortunately, time to communicate is often limited and subject to the workload demands of the nurse. Especially in the current era of healthcare institutions cutting costs and staff to stretch their limited resources, nurses are faced with more time pressure, a development that has been shown to undercut the quality of care for all patients (Perez-Francisco et al., 2020). There are also difficulties with using appropriate communication strategies and inexperience using augmentative and alternative communication (AAC) (Stans, Dalemans, Roentgen, Smeets, & Beurskens, 2018). Little research has been conducted related to the way nurses manage the "lack of time" or use AAC strategies when caring for patients with developmental disabilities and those with complex communication needs. These groups tend to communicate at slower rates and at a more concrete level, which can further undermine the communication process.

Evidence

Stans and colleagues (2018) investigated "communication-vulnerable" patients residing in a long-term care facility for individuals with acquired brain injury and physical limitations and their experiences in communicating with healthcare professionals. They conducted 11 interaction observations between pairs of healthcare professionals and patients and conducted 22 interviews.

Seven key themes were identified during this study; three were related to adaptation of the communication process and one identified time as a barrier to successful communication. Improvement was noted when communication took place in calm, quiet, distraction-free environments that allowed patients to concentrate on what was being discussed. Tailoring the communication to the patient was also identified as important. Healthcare professionals should speak slowly, use simple words, ask one question at a time, and repeat information as necessary to facilitate the communication process. Inexperience using AAC in both patients and healthcare professionals and allowing patients adequate time to communicate were identified as barriers to successful communication.

Implications

To improve communication between "communication-vulnerable" patients and healthcare professionals, time must be used efficiently, using appropriate alternative communication strategies tailored to the patient. These changes will support effective communication and promote better patient involvement with the healthcare process.

Critical Thinking Application

1. What resources can the nurse use to communicate with patients with complex communication needs in the hospital setting?
2. What resources might the nurse use to communicate with patients with complex communication needs once they are discharged into the community?

If language is a barrier, the use of an interpreter may be necessary. In 2000, the federal Office for Civil Rights (OCR) of the Department of Health and Human Services mandated that any HCPs and agencies that receive federal funds must communicate effectively with patients, family members, and visitors who are deaf or hard-of-hearing and must take steps to provide meaningful access to their programs for persons who have limited English proficiency (LEP). Failure to do so is considered discrimination. The OCR provides information, tools, and resources that allow healthcare organizations to assist people who are not proficient in English and people who are deaf or hard of hearing.

Because the use of family members as interpreters can raise confidentiality and privacy issues, the nurse should enlist the aid of bilingual staff members or a professional interpreter to communicate information effectively. Most healthcare institutions have a list of bilingual staff members who can be used as personal interpreters, medical interpreters, or both. When working with an interpreter, the nurse must remember to always speak directly to the patient and not to the interpreter.

The nurse who is culturally competent will be appreciated by the patient. The following strategies can be used when caring for patients from a different culture:

1. Use the proper form of address for the patient's culture.
2. Know how individuals in the patient's culture greet one another. This may include the use of handshake, embraces, or kissing the cheeks. In some cultures, physical contact is prohibited.
3. Be aware of what a smile means in the patient's culture. A smile may indicate friendliness or be considered taboo. Also be aware of what eye contact means; in some cultures, it indicates respect, whereas in others, it may indicate aggression or be considered impolite.
4. Remember that not all gestures have a universal meaning.

While similarities may enhance the therapeutic relationship, differences can serve as topics for open discussion. Having an open and ongoing conversation between all parties will promote understanding.

Evaluation

To determine whether patient outcomes have been met as they relate to communication, the nurse should listen actively and observe nonverbal cues. The overall patient outcome for individuals who have impaired verbal communication is reduction or resolution of the factors impairing the communication. Examples of statements indicating outcome achievement include, "Patient used the whiteboard to state absence of pain."

Examples of outcomes of care for the patient who has impaired communication may include the following:

- The patient communicates effectively that needs are being met.
- The patient demonstrated appropriate use of the inhaler.
- The patient communicates effectively, using ________ (insert method of communication here).
- The patient is expressing reduced frustration, fear, or anxiety.
- The patient uses available resources appropriately.

REVIEW The Concept of Communication

RELATE Link the Concepts

Linking the concept of communication with the concept of culture and diversity:

1. How can misunderstanding the patient's culture act as a barrier to communication when the nurse's culture differs from that of the patient?
2. The nurse is studying a culture different from the one in which the nurse was raised. What aspects of the culture would the nurse wish to learn about in order to understand how that culture's communication style may differ?

Linking the concept of communication with the concept of professional behaviors:

3. How do the nurse's communication skills affect the perceptions of others (both patients and other members of the healthcare team) regarding the nurse's professionalism?
4. A patient asks the nurse a question. Although the nurse is very knowledgeable about the subject, the nurse stumbles over words while answering the patient, repeatedly starts sentences over again, uses "ahh" and "umm" a number of times, and gives the impression of weighing each word carefully. What impact will this delivery have on the patient's perception of the nurse's professionalism and knowledge of the subject matter being explained?

Linking the concept of communication with the concept of immunity:

5. How can a nurse's communication skills produce positive and negative patient teaching outcomes for patients with a chronic illness such as systemic lupus erythematosus?
6. Discuss some of the difficulties in communicating about a condition such as HIV/AIDS, which carries a social stigma. How can a nurse most effectively provide communication and allow patients to express themselves?

REFER Go to Pearson MyLab Nursing and eText

REFLECT Apply Your Knowledge

Madeline McCormick, 24 years old, is an RN who has worked in the local acute care hospital on the medical floor for the past 3 years. Last night her boyfriend proposed. She accepted and is so thrilled she can't wait to show her new diamond ring to all of her coworkers and tell them the good news. Ms. McCormick arrives at work early to share the news and they all congratulate her and shower her with questions about her ideas for the wedding.

You are a student nurse assigned to Ms. McCormick's floor today. As you walk by one of the patients' rooms you hear Ms. McCormick, who is providing morning care to a patient, talking to the patient and telling her all about how her boyfriend proposed, her wedding plans, and how happy she is.

1. Is it appropriate for Ms. McCormick to share her good news with her coworkers? Why or why not?
2. Is it appropriate for her to share her news with a patient? Why or why not?
3. How does Ms. McCormick's excitement over her engagement affect the nurse–patient communication process?

Exemplar 38.A Groups and Group Communication

Exemplar Learning Outcomes

38.A Analyze groups and group communication.

- Describe the types, functions, levels of formality, and characteristics of effective groups.
- Outline the aspects of group dynamics.
- List group problems that nurses should recognize and avoid.
- Describe types and functions of healthcare groups.

Exemplar Key Terms

Apathy, *2591*
Cohesiveness, *2591*
Creativity techniques, *2590*
Decision trees, *2590*
Formal groups, *2588*
Group, *2588*
Groupthink, *2591*
Informal groups, *2588*
Monopolizing, *2591*
Pilot projects, *2590*
Primary group, *2588*
Scapegoat, *2591*
Scenario planning, *2590*
Secondary group, *2588*
Self-help group, *2592*
Semiformal groups, *2588*
Transference, *2591*
Trial and error, *2590*
Worst-case scenario, *2590*

Overview

A **group** is defined as three or more people who interact with each other, often with a shared purpose, or who are classified or considered together because they have something in common. Nurses regularly participate in groups and, depending on their qualifications and nature of the group, may function as either group leader or participant. The way a group functions is determined by group processes or *group dynamics.* Group dynamics must be effective in order for the work of the group to be successful.

In healthcare, decisions related to policy and practice are made by groups of individuals ranging from research groups and think tanks, advocacy groups, professional groups, and institutional groups (such as an ethics committee) to politicians at local, regional, state, national, and international levels. Nurses in all settings participate as active members of one or more decision-making groups, making it essential that all nurses be knowledgeable about the dynamics of group interaction so they can be effective group participants and leaders.

Groups

The primary purpose of any group is to achieve goals that would be unattainable through individual effort alone. Successful groups combine the ideas and expert knowledge of the various group members, disseminate information among the group quickly and consistently, and often take greater risks than the individual members might do alone. For example, in 2020, the American Association of Critical Care Nurses invited a team to submit a review about how to protect nurses and others during aerosol-generating procedures performed on tracheostomy patients not on ventilators. Pandian et al. (2020), a team of content experts in clinical and research settings, conducted a study of existing research and submitted a guideline for using a T-piece with a heat and moist exchanger (HME) with expiratory filter to maintain a closed system.

In healthcare settings, nurses work in groups whenever they collaborate with other nurses, other healthcare professionals, patients, and family members when planning and providing care. In professional, specialty, civic, and community organizations, groups of nurses work together to promote the goals of nursing on a number of levels. Therefore, it is important for nurses to be able to function successfully in different types of groups regardless of setting.

Types of Groups

Groups are classified as either primary or secondary. A **primary group** is a close, personal, and inclusive group, with members seeing the group as cooperative and inclusive. These types of groups include informal work groups and friendship groups. A family may also be a primary group, often with membership including extended family members or long-time friends considered to be family. Communication between members of a primary group generally takes place in face-to-face interactions, and members develop a strong sense of unity, although group texting and use of group apps are becoming increasingly popular. In primary groups, one person's accomplishments are often viewed as a success for the group as a whole. Similarly, a challenge experienced by one member may be viewed as a challenge for the group as a whole to help solve. For example, when one member falls seriously ill or becomes injured, the other members will pitch in to assist with transportation to healthcare appointments, pick up children from school, or organize additional resources as necessary.

A **secondary group** is usually larger and less interconnected than a primary group. Professional associations, committees, task groups, and political parties and their affiliated groups are all examples of secondary groups. In most cases, members view secondary groups as a way to accomplish goals without a lot of personal interaction. Secondary groups often have a set of bylaws or rules that defines the purpose of the group and the nature of the working relationship.

Functions of Groups

Primary groups tend to function around the needs of group members, providing a source for shared experiences and support at different times. Secondary groups, however, generally function relative to their stated purpose. For example, a therapy group functions to provide a safe environment in which group members can build the skills necessary to help them function better either as a member of a family or as a member of society. In contrast, a political party functions to try to get members who represent its interest elected to government.

Levels of Group Formality

Groups may be **formal**, **semiformal**, and **informal**. Typical features of each type of group are shown in **Box 38.3** ».

Characteristics of Effective Groups

In order for a group to be effective, the group must develop and retain some level of cohesiveness, modify its structure as necessary to ensure effectiveness, and accomplish its goals.

The ability of a group to achieve these functions can be promoted or inhibited by many factors, including the cohesion, communication, and creativity of its members (**Figure 38.5** »). These and other factors are compared in **Table 38.3** ».

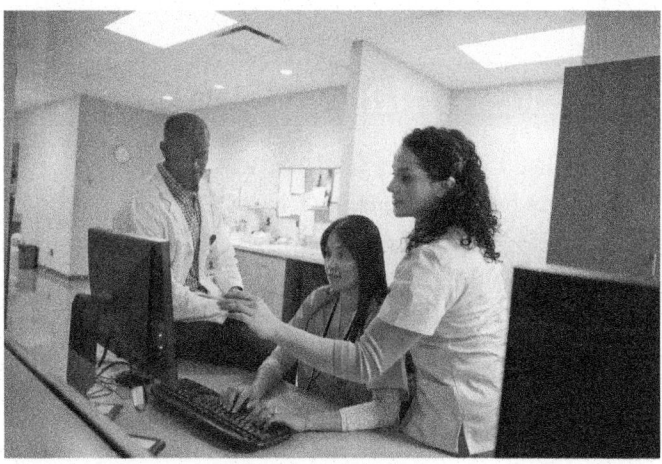

Figure 38.5 » A healthcare team gathers to discuss issues affecting a patient's care.

Source: Hero Images/Getty Images.

Box 38.3

Characteristics of Formal, Semiformal, and Informal Groups

FORMAL GROUPS	SEMIFORMAL GROUPS	INFORMAL GROUPS
▪ Authority is imposed from above. ▪ Leadership selection is assigned from above and made by an authoritative and often arbitrary order or decree. ▪ Managers are symbols of power and authority. ▪ The goals of the formal group are normally imposed at a much higher level than the direct leadership of the group. ▪ Management is endangered by its aloofness from the members of the work group. ▪ Behavioral norms (expected standards of behavior), regulations, and rules are usually superimposed. The larger the turnover rate of members, the greater the structuring of rules. ▪ Membership in the group is only partly voluntary. ▪ Rigidity of purpose is often a necessity for protection of the formal group in the pursuit of its objectives. ▪ Interactions within the group as a whole are limited, but informal subgroups often are formed.	▪ The structure is formal. ▪ The hierarchy is carefully delineated. ▪ Membership is voluntary but selective. ▪ Prestige and status are often accrued from membership. ▪ Structured, deliberate activities absorb a large part of the group's meeting time. ▪ Objectives and goals are rigid; change is not recognized as desirable. ▪ In many cases, the leader has direct control over the choice of a successor. ▪ The day-to-day operating standards and methods (group norms) are negotiable. Because most people become bored at quibbling about norms, someone can often "railroad" acceptance of a list of norms that person desires.	▪ The group is not bound by any set of written rules or regulations. ▪ Usually governed by a set of unwritten laws and a strong code of ethics. ▪ The group is purely functional and has easily recognized basic objectives. ▪ Rotational leadership is common. The group recognizes that only rarely are all leadership characteristics found in one person. ▪ The group assigns duties to the members best qualified for certain functions. For example, the person who is recognized as outgoing and sociable will be assigned responsibilities for planning parties. ▪ Judgments about the group's leader are made quickly and surely. Leaders are replaced when they make one or more mistakes or do not get the job done. ▪ The group is an ideal testing ground for new leadership techniques, but there is no guarantee that such techniques can be transferred effectively to a large, formal organization. ▪ Behavioral norms are developed either by group effort or by the leader and adopted by the group. ▪ Deviance by one member from the group's behavioral norms is more threatening to the perpetuation of small, informal groups than to large, formal, heterogeneous groups. Conformity and group solidarity are important for the protection and preservation of small groups. ▪ Group norms are enforced by sanctions (punishments) imposed by the group on those who violate a norm. Different values are placed on norms in accordance with the values of the leader. One leader may regard the action as a gross violation, whereas another leader may find it quite acceptable. ▪ Interpersonal interactions are spontaneous.

Group Communications

Group Dynamics

Group dynamics, also referred to as group processes, are the way the group communicates, functions, and sets and achieves goals. Five characteristics of group dynamics are commitment, decision-making ability, member behavior, cohesiveness, and power.

Commitment

Groups are effective when the members are committed to the goals and success of the group. Commitment requires that individual members give up some of their own autonomy to put the goals of the group before their own interests. Commitment also requires that individual members manage conflicts that arise appropriately and work together to find resolution. Committed group members:

- Share a strong sense of belonging
- Act truthfully and provide support to the group as a whole
- Value the contributions of other members
- Are motivated by working in the group and desire to perform their roles well
- Identify and amplify the positive contributions of other members
- View the goals of the group as achievable and important.

Decision-Making Ability

Another characteristic essential to effective group functioning is the ability to make sound decisions. Effective decisions are

TABLE 38.3 Features of Effective and Ineffective Groups

Factor	Effective Groups	Ineffective Groups
Atmosphere	Informal, comfortable, and relaxed. It is a working atmosphere in which individuals demonstrate their interest and involvement.	Obviously tense. Signs of boredom may appear.
Goal setting	Goals, tasks, and objectives are clarified, understood, and modified so that members of the group can commit themselves to cooperatively structured goals.	Unclear, misunderstood, or imposed goals may be accepted by members. The goals are competitively structured.
Leadership and member participation	Shift from time to time, depending on the circumstances. Different members assume leadership at various times because of their knowledge or experience.	Delegated and based on authority. The chairperson may dominate the group or the members may defer unduly. Members' participation is unequal, with high-authority members dominating.
Goal emphasis	All three functions of groups are emphasized: goal accomplishment, internal maintenance, and developmental change.	One or more functions may not be emphasized.
Communication	Open and two-way. Ideas and feelings are encouraged, both about the problem and about the group's operation.	Closed or one-way. Only the production of ideas is encouraged. Feelings are ignored or taboo. Members may be tentative or reluctant to be open and may have "hidden agendas" (personal goals at cross purposes with group goals).
Decision making	By consensus, although various decision-making procedures appropriate to the situation may be instituted.	By the higher authority in the group, with minimal involvement by members; an inflexible style may be imposed.
Cohesion	Facilitated through high levels of inclusion, trust, liking, and support.	Either ignored or used as a means of controlling members, thus promoting rigid conformity.
Conflict tolerance	High. The reasons for disagreements or conflicts are carefully examined, and the group seeks to resolve them. The group accepts unresolvable basic disagreements.	Low. Attempts may be made to ignore, deny, avoid, suppress, or override controversy by premature group action. The group may choose to live with conflict rather than attempt to resolve it.
Power	Determined by the members' abilities and the information they possess. Power is shared. The issue is how to get the job done.	Determined by position in the group. Obedience to authority is strong. The issue is who controls.
Problem solving	High. Constructive criticism is frequent, frank, relatively comfortable, and oriented toward removing an obstacle to problem solving.	Low. Criticism may be destructive, taking the form of either overt or covert personal attacks. It prevents the group from getting the job done.
Self-evaluation of the group	Frequent. All members participate in evaluation and decisions about how to improve the group's functioning.	Minimal. What little evaluation there is may be done by the highest authority in the group rather than by the membership as a whole.
Creativity	Encouraged. There is room within the group for members to become self-actualized and interpersonally effective.	Discouraged. People are afraid of appearing foolish if they put forth a creative thought.

Sources: Data from Arnold and Boggs (2019); Eventus (2020); Lukic (2020).

made when members of the group listen to each other's ideas and feel engaged in the decision-making process; maintain a positive atmosphere; use time efficiently by focusing on the matters at hand; and feel responsible for the outcomes of any decisions made by the group.

Huber (2017) describes several techniques groups can use when making decisions: trial and error, pilot projects, creativity techniques, decision trees, scenario planning, and worst-case scenario. **Trial-and-error** techniques are the most haphazard: in these situations, a solution that seems viable is simply attempted. Managers and groups who use these techniques are typically seen as poor problem solvers, especially in a healthcare context. Evidence-based practice protocols have replaced trial and error as the standard in the nursing profession.

Pilot projects make use of limited trials to determine problems with problem-solving alternatives. Pilot project strategies may resemble research projects and may be linked to quality improvement initiatives. **Creativity techniques** such as brainstorming sessions use the creative potential of the group to generate a large number of possible options quickly. A **decision tree** is a graphic model that visually represents the choices, outcomes, and risks to be anticipated. A decision tree helps groups visualize the results of a series of branching options and helps streamline decision making by clearly spelling out alternative options as decisions lead to subsequent options.

Scenario planning is a group process strategy that encourages members of a group to create a hypothetical or "possible future" situation. Scenario planning is most applicable to fluid and changing environments. Participants are encouraged to ask themselves, "What if?" Group members imagine pathways, forces in play, turning points, and deep behavioral undercurrents. Scenario planning helps illuminate early warning signs, create opportunities, and ensure against risks.

Worst-case scenario is a technique designed to help groups make decisions that involve risk. The worst-case outcome is outlined for each alternative, and then the scenario with the comparatively best outcome is selected as the preferred outcome. This technique helps ensure that the "least of all evils" is selected.

Member Behavior

Members of a group are responsible for their own behavior and participation. Group structure and leadership style can influence the amount of input by members and how the group functions as a whole. Individuals may perform one or more different roles depending on the needs of the group at the time. These roles include:

- ***Information givers***, who offer facts relevant to the work of the group.
- ***Information seekers***, who seek facts in order to make informed decisions.
- ***Opinion givers***, who offer beliefs and alternate suggestions.
- ***Facilitators***, who clarify relationships among ideas and keep discussions focused on the topic at hand.

Cohesiveness

Cohesiveness is defined as the attachment that members feel toward each other, the group, or the group's purpose. Cohesive groups possess specific characteristics, such as a sense of common purpose. There is a greater level of satisfaction within groups that have a high level of cohesiveness. Groups lacking cohesiveness tend to be unstable and are more prone to member disengagement, making it less likely that the group will achieve its goals.

SAFETY ALERT Effective group communication is essential for the patient's safety because the patient's care is overseen by an interdependent healthcare team. Team members must coordinate their efforts to ensure that medications are given in the correct dose at the correct time, that necessary education is provided, and that all interventions are implemented correctly. Poor group atmosphere, goal setting, leadership, goal emphasis, and all the other elements of group cohesion have a direct and cumulative impact on patient outcomes and safety.

Power

Power can greatly affect the patterns of behavior within groups. In group settings, power can be defined as the ability of one member to act individually to influence the group's dynamic or decisions.

Many individuals have a negative perception of power, comparing it to the control or intimidation of others. However, the overall purpose of power within a group is to encourage cooperation and collaboration in achieving a task or goal of the group.

Group Problems

A variety of problems can occur and prevent a group from accomplishing its goals. Beyond general conflict, other problems include monopolizing, group think, scapegoating, silence and apathy, and transference or countertransference.

Monopolizing

Domination of a discussion by one member of a group is referred to as **monopolizing**. Monopolizing threatens the group by taking up time, depriving others of the opportunity to participate, and increasing frustration levels of all members.

Monopolizing behavior may result from a need for attention or approval. Many times, individuals who monopolize conversations are unaware of how their behavior affects others.

Strategies for dealing with monopolizing include the following:

- ***Interrupt simply, directly, and supportively.*** This strategy is an initial attempt to get the individual to hear others.
- ***Reflect the member's behavior.*** This strategy is an attempt to help the individual become aware of the monopolizing behavior.
- ***Reflect the group's feelings.*** This strategy is an attempt to help the individual member become aware of the effects of the behavior on others.
- ***Confront the person and/or the group.*** This strategy can be directed toward the individual or toward the group to help members realize their own responsibility for the problem.

Groupthink

Groupthink is a type of decision making characterized by a group's failure to critically examine its own processes and practices. Groupthink may also occur when members of a group fail to recognize and respond to change. It may occur in highly cohesive groups when group members do not want to disagree or criticize the majority of the group's thinking for fear of being considered disloyal. For example, the administrators of a local urgent care center, failing to recognize that the staff is struggling to communicate with their many Latino patients, refuse to hire Spanish-speaking staff or engage the services of a full-time interpreter. Symptoms of groupthink include the group overestimating its power and morality, the group becoming closed minded, and group members experiencing pressure to conform.

Scapegoating

A **scapegoat** is someone who has been targeted to take blame for a failure or problem. Individuals and groups who participate in scapegoating deflect their own errors or failures onto others. Scapegoating is grossly unprofessional behavior that has no place within the profession of nursing, which emphasizes responsibility and accountability, or in the larger healthcare setting.

Silence and Apathy

Apathy, or lack of interest or enthusiasm, of one or more group members can destroy a group. Lack of enthusiasm can result when a group member doesn't have a real interest in the group; if a group member expresses ideas or suggestions that are never considered; or if a group member otherwise feels disengaged from the group. When there are multiple group members who disengage, the group risks becoming dysfunctional and unable to achieve its goals.

Transference and Countertransference

When a group member transfers feelings they have toward someone in their personal life to a member of the group, it is called **transference**. An example is a group member who acts toward another as the member would act toward a sibling o a parent. Members can unwittingly transfer any number of personal feelings toward others in the group. *Countertransference* occurs when leaders transfer emotions based on outside interactions onto group members. When working in groups, it is important for both members and leaders to try to recognize times at which they may be overacting because they are transferring emotions from previous relationships onto someone else in the group.

Healthcare Groups

Nurses spend a great deal of time working in groups, where they may be required to take on different roles as member or leader, teacher or learner, adviser or advisee. Committees or teams, task forces, teaching groups, self-help groups, therapy groups, and work-related social support groups are some of the common types of healthcare groups in which nurses may participate. There are various similarities and differences between the groups as well as the roles of nurses participating in them. Cultural competence is equally necessary when working in groups as it is when working with a patient and family (see the Focus on Diversity and Culture feature).

Committees or Teams

Committees are the most common type of work-related group. Committees typically have a specific purpose that, in part, determines their organizational structure, and they generally meet at specified intervals. Examples include policy committees, quality improvement committees, ethics committees, and governmental affairs committees. Committees may also be referred to as teams, which are smaller groups of individuals who share a common purpose such as a rapid response team or a wound care team. Team members share a common approach to their work, have complementary and overlapping skills, and performance goals that may vary depending on their role on the team.

> ## Focus on Diversity and Culture
> ### Cross-Cultural Group Communication
>
> Group communication is difficult under any circumstances, but it can be especially hard when members of the group have different cultural standards. Brenner (2018) provides some ideas for managing cross-cultural concerns in group communication. When communicating with members of the group who speak a different language or dialect, nurses should slow their rate of speech, attempt to communicate clearly and concisely, and keep statements simple. When group members come from different cultures, nurses should maintain respect and courtesy and avoid slang. Nurses should avoid humor, as humor does not necessarily translate across cultures, and nurses should adopt a formal communication approach until a group rapport is established. Nurses should ask for feedback to determine whether or not they are being understood and adjust accordingly. No matter the patient or colleague's culture, the nurse should honor the differences in cultures by using neutral tones, categorizations, and behaviors that are respectful of the person's culture and avoiding those that could be interpreted as offensive (Arnold & Boggs, 2019).

Every team or committee selects or is designated a leader. Successful leaders are experienced in the committee's focus area and are acknowledged as an appropriate leader by the other members. The leader has the responsibility of identifying tasks that will move the group toward its goals and clarifying communication among members. Within a single organization, members of a committee or team are generally selected based on their individual functional roles and employment status. If a committee or team is made up of members from multiple organizations, the member organizations typically designate who will serve on the committee, although in some cases membership designation may be determined by rule or law. For example, membership in county child fatality review teams is normally designated by law and includes representatives of local hospitals, emergency medical systems, law enforcement, community health nurses, the district medical examiner's office, and so forth. "At-large" positions may be designated to allow local committees to add additional members from community organizations who would be helpful to achieving the goals of the group but that are not recognized as being required by rule or law.

Task Forces

Task forces (sometimes called *ad hoc committees*) are work groups that may be designated to come together to perform a specific activity, such as preparation for an accreditation visit or preparing for an upcoming health fair. Once the activity has been completed, the task force is dissolved. Task forces function in the same manner as other committees or work teams, but with a designated duration of work.

Teaching Groups

A *teaching group* has the main purpose of imparting information to the participants. Teaching groups can include continuing education and patient healthcare groups. Teaching groups may be formed to address any number of topics ranging from childbirth techniques and preoperative information sessions to instructions to family members about follow-up care for discharged patients. A nurse must be skilled in the teaching–learning process when leading a group in which the primary purpose is to teach or learn. See Module 41, Teaching and Learning, for further discussion.

Self-Help Groups

A **self-help group** is comprised of individuals who come together to share and discuss a common problem or issue. These groups are centered around the helper-therapy principle: Those who help someone who is also struggling are helped most. The self-help movement has a central belief that individuals who experience a specific social or health problem have a better understanding of the condition than those who have no experience with it. Alcoholics Anonymous (AA), Narcotics Anonymous (NA), and cancer survivor groups are examples of self-help groups.

Therapy Groups

Therapy groups offer group psychotherapy to individuals to help them work together toward better communication with others, more satisfactory ways of relating or handling stress, and changing patterns of behavior around health. Members are selected by health professionals based on the approach to psychotherapy (i.e., cognitive-behavioral therapy or dialectical behavioral therapy), personalities, behaviors, needs, and identification of group therapy as the treatment of choice. The number of sessions or the termination date is usually mutually determined by the therapist and members.

Work-Related Social Support Groups

Many nurses, especially those working in specialty areas such as hospice, emergency, and critical care and psychiatric nursing, experience high levels of work-related stress. To reduce vocational stress, nurses can participate in *work-related social groups*, where members who are knowledgeable about the work they do can offer encouragement and provide enthusiasm as well as resources and ideas for solving problems or resolving conflicts.

REVIEW Groups and Group Communication

RELATE Link the Concepts and Exemplars

Linking the exemplar of groups and group communication with the concept of addiction:

1. How do individuals work in groups and use group communication when dealing with addiction?
2. What are some group communication types that may be useful when working with addicts in a group setting?

Linking the exemplar of groups and group communication with the concept of family:

3. How can families use group communication techniques to increase communication?
4. How might communication within a family be affected as a result of health alterations?

REFER Go to Pearson MyLab Nursing and eText

REFLECT Apply Your Knowledge

As a substance abuse nurse, you are responsible for leading daily meetings for a group of people who have addiction challenges. You have been asked to lead your first meeting now that you have finished your 6-week preceptorship and are now taking your own patient assignments on the unit. You are nervous about running a group independently. You begin to plan your session and want your mentor's input on whether you are planning a session that will be effective for the participants.

1. What type of meeting should you plan for this group?
2. What type of group problems might occur during the session?
3. After the session you feel that the group is ineffective. What characteristics would lead you to believe this?

» Exemplar 38.B Therapeutic Communication

Exemplar Learning Outcomes

38.B Analyze the interactive process of therapeutic communication.

- Summarize the various techniques used by nurses to support patients.
- Outline the phases of the therapeutic relationship.
- Explain ways that nurses can develop therapeutic relationships with patients.
- Differentiate considerations related to therapeutic communication throughout the lifespan.

Exemplar Key Terms

Physical attending, *2595*
Therapeutic communication, *2593*
Therapeutic relationship, *2593*

Overview

Therapeutic communication is an interactive process between the nurse and the patient. It is an integral part of the **therapeutic relationship**, which is the caring relationship between a nurse and a patient that is based on mutual trust and respect, sensitivity, and nurturing. Therapeutic communication helps the patient overcome temporary stress, get along with other people, adjust to situations that cannot be changed, and overcome any psychologic blocks that may stand in the way of self-realizations. Therapeutic communication promotes understanding and can help establish a constructive relationship between the nurse and the patient. Unlike the social relationship, which might not have a specific purpose or direction, the nurse establishes a therapeutic relationship with the purpose of helping the patient achieve health goals.

In therapeutic communication, the nurse responds not only to the content (words and thoughts) of a patient's verbal message but also to feelings the patient expresses and to nonverbal cues. It is important for the nurse to understand how the patient perceives a situation and feels about it before responding. Sometimes the words someone speaks will be incongruent with their feelings. For example, a patient might say, "I'm glad she's gone. She was so mean to me these last few years." However, the nurse observes the patient holding back tears. By responding to the patient's nonverbal expression of emotion by saying something like, "You seem sad that your spouse has died," instead of responding only to the patient's words, the nurse helps the patient focus on their feelings.

Many times, patients need time to process emotions before they can participate in healthcare interventions, including care planning. This can be especially true when patients receive a serious or terminal diagnosis. How patients respond in these situations will vary. Some may need days or weeks to process it and make decisions, whereas others may be ready to move forward more quickly. Some will want to begin processing the information alone, others will want someone to listen to them and help them identify and verbalize emotions, and some will want more information in order to plan next steps. Although it is appropriate for nurses to help patients explore alternatives, nurses should not participate in the decision-making process with patients or their families.

Therapeutic Communication Techniques

Therapeutic communication is intended to help patients reach an understanding about their condition or treatment while encouraging them to express feelings and ideas. Therapeutic communication is rooted in acceptance of the patient's point of view. Nontherapeutic communication, on the other hand, interferes with the nurse–patient relationship by putting barriers in the way of open communication (Evesham, 2017).

Therapeutic communication relies on active listening and continuous confirmation that both the nurse and the patient are being understood. In therapeutic communication, nurses take time to answer questions and encourage patients to satisfy their curiosity. In therapeutic communication, the nurse focuses on the most important issues and summarizes important points of communication to ensure that the patient understands the nurse and that the nurse understands the patient. Nontherapeutic communication detracts from patient care and includes behaviors such as asking irrelevant personal questions, sharing unnecessary personal information of your own, or showing disapproval. False reassurance and sympathy are also aspects of nontherapeutic communication.

The nurse can employ a number of different communication techniques to support patients as they deal with their feelings related to their health and healthcare. The nurse must embrace these techniques and adapt them to each situation to improve communication with patients. However, no one technique will guarantee a successful encounter with all patients. Each situation is unique. The nurse should use a holistic approach to communicating with patients in each situation that is presented.

Empathizing

Active listening (described in the next section) is a skill that nursing students are taught throughout their education. Merely listening, however, is not enough. The nurse must have an empathetic understanding of the situation and offer appropriate feedback to the patient. *Empathy* is best described as a process in which individuals are able to put themselves in someone else's situation. By using empathy, the nurse is able to embrace the attitudes of each patient in each encounter.

To be able to empathize with patients, the nurse must be able to understand and acknowledge the ideas that the patient is expressing or that the patient feels are important to the situation. The nurse must also accept and respect the patient's feelings as valid for the individual, whatever those feelings may be, even if the nurse would not feel the same way in similar circumstances. Using empathy allows the nurse to connect with patients, and it also validates the importance of the patient's message to the nurse.

The term *empathy* is often mistakenly used to mean *sympathy*. Empathy, however, contains no elements of condolence, agreement, or pity. Empathy focuses on the patient's feelings, not the nurse's feelings. Nurses who sympathize rather than empathize assume that there is a parallel between their own feelings and the patient's feelings. This perceived similarity can make professional judgment and objectivity difficult. Nurses who empathize can interpret patients' feelings and do not insert their own feelings into the current situation. The process of establishing empathetic understanding has four phases:

1. ***Identification.*** This phase involves the relaxation of conscious control. In this phase, the nurse is able to envision the patient and the patient's experiences.
2. ***Incorporation.*** In this phase, the nurse considers the patient's experiences and feelings rather than the nurse's own experiences.
3. ***Reverberation.*** This phase involves an interplay of the patient's internalized feeling with the nurse's own experiences or fantasies. The nurse is fully absorbed in the patient's identity but is able to experience it separately.
4. ***Detachment.*** In this phase, the nurse withdraws from subjective involvement with the patient and resumes the nurse's own identity. The nurse uses the insight that was gained from the reverberation phase, along with reason and objectivity, to offer meaningful and useful responses to the patient.

Empathizing with patients who are troubled can have some stressful consequences for nurses. Problems can arise at any phase of the process, and when a nurse fails to cope with one of the four phases of achieving empathy, obstacles occur in terms of the nurse–patient relationship. The nurse should not identify too closely with the patient because this can lead to sympathy rather than empathy.

Active Listening

Active listening is perhaps the most important technique in therapeutic communication and is the basis of all other techniques. Also called *attentive* or *mindful listening*, it involves listening with multiple senses, in contrast to listening only with the ear. Active listening is more than just being quiet while the other individual talks. It involves paying attention to the patient's verbal and nonverbal messages and noting congruency between them. Active listening means that the nurse does not select or listen solely to what the nurse wants to hear. While listening to the patient the nurse maintains the focus on the patient's needs while exhibiting an attitude of caring and interest in order to encourage the patient to talk (**Figure 38.6** »).

Active listening requires that the nurse be careful not to interrupt or react too quickly to the message while looking for key themes in the patient's message. At appropriate times, the nurse should ask questions to obtain additional information or clarify information to ensure the nurse fully understands what the patient is trying to convey.

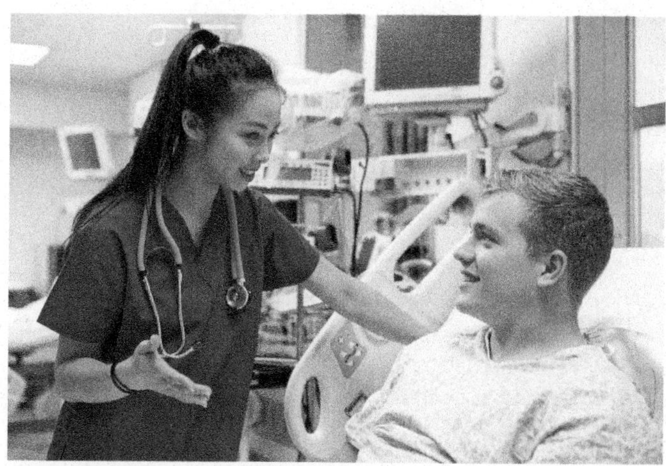

Figure 38.6 » The nurse conveys active listening through a posture of involvement.

Source: Cathy Yeulet/123RF.

Active listening requires that nurses be aware of their own biases. A message that reflects values or beliefs that differ from the nurse's should not be discredited for that reason. The patient, who is the sender, should decide when to close the conversation, and the nurse should listen for the signal that the patient is ready to do so. When the nurse closes the conversation, the patient may assume that the nurse considers the message unimportant.

There are some specific blocks to listening that may prevent the nurse from actually hearing what the patient says. This may convey a message to patients that what they have to say is not important (**Box 38.4 »**).

Active listening is an advanced skill that can be learned with practice. A nurse can listen actively and attentively to patients in various ways. Common responses that indicate active listening include nodding the head, uttering "uh huh" or "mmm," repeating the words that the patient has used, or saying "I see what you mean." Nurses have individual ways of responding and must be cautious not to sound insincere or condescending.

Box 38.4

Blocks to Active Listening

- ***Rehearsing:*** When the nurse is busy planning what to say next in the conversation
- ***Being concerned with oneself:*** When the nurse focuses on the nurse's own intelligence, competence, feelings, or accomplishments instead of focusing on the patient
- ***Assuming:*** When the nurse makes assumptions about what the patient is really trying to convey in the conversation
- ***Judging:*** When the nurse frames messages in the context of the nurse's own judgment about whether what the patient is saying is right or wrong, mature or immature, calm or anxious, sensible or paranoid, or depressed or simply quiet
- ***Identifying:*** When the nurse focuses on the nurse's own experiences, beliefs, or feelings; this may occur when what the patient communicates triggers memories or concerns from the nurse's own personal experiences
- ***Getting off track:*** When the nurse changes the subject or makes light of what the patient is expressing because the nurse is uncomfortable, bored, or tired
- ***Filtering:*** When the nurse tunes out certain topics in the conversation or hears only certain items that the patient is saying; this may occur because of anxiety on the part of the nurse.

Physical Attending

Physical attending describes nonverbal language that expresses attention to another person. Nonverbal communication that indicates the nurse is present and attending to a patient includes looking at the patient when speaking, maintaining an open posture, and leaning toward the person.

Maintaining an open posture means that the nurse maintains a relaxed posture with natural gestures rather than crossing the arms or acting in any way that might convey judgment or make it seem as though the nurse's interest in the patient is forced. Leaning toward a person conveys interest, as does moving closer to the patient. Speaking to a patient from the door rather than moving to the bedside conveys disinterest.

Maintaining good eye contact, preferably at the patient's level, is another method of physically attending to the patient, provided the patient is not from a culture that views eye contact as intrusive or inappropriate.

Therapeutic communication techniques facilitate communication and focus on the patient's concerns. **Table 38.4 »** lists some common therapeutic communication techniques with their descriptions and examples of use. Touch can also be used as a part of therapeutic communication, but nurses are advised to use it with caution and intention (Vera, 2020). As stated earlier, people from different cultures may view the use of touch differently. In addition, patients with a history of physical or sexual abuse and trauma and patients with certain mental illnesses, such as some personality disorders, may misinterpret the use of touch (Potter & Moller, 2019).

Using Silence

Nurses often feel that they must respond to each statement that is made by a patient. This, however, is not necessary. The use of *silence* can be therapeutic and goes beyond active listening. The nurse who uses silence may sit or walk quietly with the patient. The goal is to provide a therapeutic purpose, such as:

- Encouraging the patient to communicate with the nurse
- Allowing the patient time to think about what has been said or to make connections
- Allowing the patient the necessary time to collect personal thoughts
- Allowing the patient time to consider possible alternatives.

The nurse who uses silence while remaining interested in what the patient is communicating maintains an open posture or a questioning look, which will encourage the patient to use the time effectively.

Silence is an effective communication technique only when it is used appropriately and purposefully for therapeutic communication. When an uncomfortable silence occurs, the nurse should break the silence and then analyze it. It is important not to allow the patient to become anxious or resistive.

TABLE 38.4 Therapeutic Communication Techniques

Technique	Description	Examples
Using silence	Accepting pauses or silences that may extend for several seconds or minutes without interjecting any verbal response.	Sitting quietly (or walking with the patient) and waiting attentively until the patient is able to put thoughts and feelings into words.
Providing general leads	Using statements or questions that (1) encourage the patient to verbalize, (2) choose a topic of conversation, and (3) facilitate continued verbalization.	"Tell me how it is for you." "Perhaps you would like to talk about . . . ." "How might it help to discuss your feelings?" "Where would you like to begin?" "And then what?"
Being specific and tentative	Making statements that are specific rather than general and tentative rather than absolute.	"Rate your pain on a scale of 0 to 10" (specific statement) versus "Are you in pain?" (general statement) "You seem unconcerned about your diabetes" (tentative statement) versus "You don't care about your diabetes and you never will" (absolute statement)
Using open-ended questions	Asking broad questions that lead or invite the patient to explore (elaborate, clarify, describe, compare, or illustrate) thoughts or feelings. Open-ended questions specify only the topic to be discussed and invite answers that are longer than one or two words.	"I'd like to hear more about that." "Tell me about . . . " "How have you been feeling lately?" "What brought you to the hospital?" "What is your opinion?" "You said you were frightened yesterday. How do you feel now?"
Sharing observations	The nurse openly informs the patient of the assessment and observations, especially those involving unconscious patient behavior.	"You are shaking." "You are biting your nails."
Restating or paraphrasing	Actively listening for the patient's basic message and then repeating those thoughts and/or feelings in similar words. This conveys that the nurse has listened and understood the patient's basic message and also offers the patient a clearer idea of what it said.	*Patient:* "I couldn't manage to eat any dinner last night—not even the dessert." *Nurse:* "You had difficulty eating yesterday?" *Patient:* "Yes, I was very upset after my family left." *Patient:* "I have trouble talking to strangers." *Nurse:* "You find it difficult talking to people you do not know?"
Seeking clarification	A method of making the patient's broad overall meaning of the message more understandable. It is used when paraphrasing is difficult or when the communication is rambling or garbled. To clarify the message, the nurse can restate the basic message or confess confusion and ask the patient to repeat or restate the message. Nurses can also clarify their own message with statements.	"I'm puzzled." "I'm not sure I understand that." "Would you please say that again?" "Would you tell me more?" "I meant this rather than that." "I'm sorry that wasn't very clear. Let me try to explain another way."
Perception checking	A method similar to clarifying that verifies how the patient is experiencing a situation.	*Patient:* "My mother yelled at me." *Nurse:* "Tell me how you felt when your mother yelled at you."
Offering self	Suggesting one's presence, interest, or wish to understand the patient without making any demands or attaching conditions that the patient must comply with to receive the nurse's attention.	"I'll stay with you until your daughter arrives." "We can sit here quietly for a while. We don't need to talk unless you would like to." "I'll help you dress to go home if you'd like."
Giving information	Providing, in a simple and direct manner, specific factual information the patient may or may not request. When information is not known, the nurse states this and indicates who has it or when the nurse will obtain it.	"Your surgery is scheduled for 11:00 a.m. tomorrow." "You will feel a pulling sensation when the tube is removed from your abdomen." "I do not know the answer to that, but I will find out from Ms. King, the nurse in charge."
Acknowledging	Giving recognition, in a nonjudgmental way, of a change in behavior, an effort the patient has made, or a contribution to a communication. Acknowledgment may be with or without understanding, verbal or nonverbal.	"You trimmed your beard and mustache and washed your hair." "I notice you keep squinting your eyes." "You walked twice as far today with your walker."
Clarifying time or sequence	Helping the patient clarify an event, situation, or happening in relationship to time.	*Patient:* "I vomited this morning." *Nurse:* "Was that before or after breakfast?" *Patient:* "I feel like I have been asleep for weeks." *Nurse:* "You had your operation Monday, and today is Tuesday."
Presenting reality	Helping the patient differentiate the real from the unreal.	"The doorbell sound came from the program on television." "Your hairbrush is right here in the drawer. It has not been stolen."

TABLE 38.4 Therapeutic Communication Techniques (*continued*)

Technique	Description	Examples
Focusing	Helping the patient expand on and develop a topic of importance. It is important for the nurse to wait until the patient finishes stating the main concerns before attempting to focus. The focus may be an idea or a feeling; however, the nurse often emphasizes a feeling to help the patient recognize an emotion disguised behind words.	*Patient:* "My wife says she will look after me, but I don't think she can, what with the children to take care of. They're still little, and they need a lot of attention." *Nurse:* "Sounds like you are worried about how well she can manage."
Reflecting	Directing ideas, feelings, questions, or content back to patients to enable them to explore their own ideas and feelings about a situation.	*Patient:* "What can I do?" *Nurse:* "What do you think would be helpful?" *Patient:* "Do you think I should tell my husband?" *Nurse:* "You seem unsure about telling your husband."
Summarizing and planning	Stating the main points of a discussion to clarify the relevant points discussed. This technique is useful at the end of an interview or to review a health teaching session. It often acts as an introduction to future care planning.	"During the past half hour we have talked about . . . " "Tomorrow afternoon we may explore this further." "In a few days I'll review with you what you have learned about the actions and effects of your insulin." "Tomorrow I will look at your feeling journal."
Exploring	Investigating a patient's feeling related to a subject or idea.	"Would you describe your experience with that in more depth?" "Tell me more about your childhood."

Source: Adapted from Berman et al. (2021).

The nurse who is silent out of discomfort or a lack of knowledge or skill on how to communicate effectively should seek guidance from someone more experienced in order to analyze the personal and professional areas that are in need of growth.

Reflecting

There are a number of other patient teaching techniques that can augment general therapeutic communication skills. One therapeutic teaching skill is the ability to assess a patient for individualized teaching. This requires the nurse to assess the patient's education and developmental level and also to determine what motivates the specific patient. Nurses can optimize the learning environment by turning off distractions and shutting the door, as well as sitting with the patient to create "space" for learning. Nurses should use effective teaching strategies such as demonstrating, involving the learner in the education process, and using videos for educational purposes (PracticalNursing.org, 2020). Nurses should confirm that their teaching efforts are understood. Nurses should ask themselves "Does my teaching reach the patient?" to help determine whether the patient is able to put the teaching into practice.

When nurses use reflection in the communication process, they are actively acknowledging what they have heard or seen from patients. *Reflecting* is what takes place when the nurse repeats the patient's verbal or nonverbal messages for the patient's benefit.

Reflecting Content

By reflecting the content of the message that the nurse receives from the patient, the nurse is essentially repeating the patient's statement. This allows the patient the opportunity to both hear and reflect on what is told to the nurse in the course of the conversation.

The technique of content reflecting is often misused or overused in the mental health environment. Overuse of this technique causes it to lose effectiveness. The nurse should use this technique judiciously.

Clinical Example C

Jason Smith is a 48-year-old man who has been admitted to the hospital with the diagnosis of acute inferior myocardial infarction (MI). He says to the nurse, "I can't believe I had a heart attack. Those are for old people! I still feel young, but I guess I have to slow down." The nurse, using reflection, asks Mr. Smith, "Do you feel that you can no longer lead an active life because you have had a heart attack?" The nurse's statement will encourage Mr. Smith to continue sharing thoughts and explain why he believes this to be true. This will allow the nurse to correct any misunderstanding that he has about the recovery process after an MI.

Critical Thinking Questions

1. What physical attending communication techniques could be used in this interaction, and how might they impact the patient's communication?
2. How might the nurse use acknowledging in this encounter? What impact do you think it would have on this interaction?
3. What other communication techniques could the nurse use, and how might those impact the interaction with Mr. Smith?

Reflecting Feelings

In using the technique of *reflecting feelings*, the nurse verbalizes the feelings that are implied in the patient's comment. The nurse should respect that patients have the right to their own opinions and feelings even when the nurse personally disagrees with them. Some examples of reflecting feelings are as follows:

- "Sounds like you're really angry at your sister."
- "You're feeling anxious about being discharged from the hospital later today."

By reflecting feelings, the nurse attempts to identify any latent or connotative meanings that can either clarify or distort the content that is communicated. Reflection of feelings is useful because it will encourage the patient to make additional, clarifying comments in the conversation.

Imparting Information

In *imparting information*, the nurse is helping the patient by supplying additional data for consideration. This encourages further clarification because it is based on new or additional input. Some examples of statements that impart information are as follows:

- "Group therapy will be held on Wednesday afternoon from 3:30 until 5:00."
- "I am a mental health nursing student."

Note that it is inappropriate to withhold information from a patient when the patient asks an information-seeking question. The nurse must be mindful not to cross the line between giving information and giving the patient advice. Also, the nurse should not give information as a way of avoiding conflict. Nurses who give patients personal or social information are moving outside of the realm of therapeutic communication. Information that the nurse must share with the patient includes the nurse's name, title, and position. New nurses must be cautioned to resist the temptation to divulge inappropriate information to patients.

Patients' participation in the decision-making process begins with patients taking in and understanding information regarding their own condition. The ultimate goal of sharing essential information with patients is to provide effective education that empowers them. Empowered patients are more likely to achieve a positive mental health and physical health outcome. They are also less likely to be admitted for inpatient therapy or be readmitted after discharge.

Additional examples of therapeutic techniques, annotated with the techniques used by the nurse, are provided in **Box 38.5** ».

Avoiding Self-Disclosure

Patients have been known to ask personal questions of nurses who are caring for them. This may include inquiring about the nurse's marital status, where the nurse lives, what religion the nurse practices, or information about personal issues. The best methods for deflecting requests for self-disclosure, outlined by Auvil and Silver in their classic 1984 study, include the following:

- ***Using honesty:*** "I don't feel comfortable sharing my address with you."
- ***Using benign curiosity:*** "Why are you asking me this today?"
- ***Using refocusing:*** "You were talking about how your mother treats you. Why are you changing the topic? You were saying . . . ."
- ***Using interpretation:*** "I notice that every time you talk about your sister, you change the subject and ask me a question." (pause)
- ***Seeking clarification:*** "You keep asking me where I live. I wonder, do you have any concerns about me today?"
- ***Responding with feedback and limit setting:*** "I'm uncomfortable when you ask me who pays my tuition for school. Talking about my finances isn't part of our agreement to work together." Adding something like "The last time we met, you were deciding whether you were going to call your sister on the phone . . . " helps restructure the situation.

These communication techniques should be used within the context of the therapeutic relationship.

Therapeutic communication revolves around the needs of the patient. It is not appropriate for nurses to talk to patients about their own experiences, such as what they did last night or their thoughts on a given subject. This wastes time that could be spent on learning about the patient's needs, thoughts, concerns, or problems. Nurses should always maintain a patient focus during communication.

Clarifying

Even when the nurse has listened carefully and thoughtfully to the patient, there may be a need to clarify information. *Clarifying* is an attempt to understand the basic nature of a patient's statement.

- "I'm confused about what is upsetting you. Could you go over that again, please?"
- "You say you're feeling anxious now. What's that like for you?"

Asking the patient to give an example allows the patient to clarify the meaning of the communication and helps the nurse understand the intended message. Clarification may be needed because of the language that the patient employs, such as slang used by adolescent patients, or when the nurse is not certain of adequate interpretation of what the patient is trying to convey.

Clinical Example D

The nurse is caring for Sara Kim, a 36-year-old woman who was recently diagnosed with breast cancer. The HCP has informed Ms. Kim that her chance of full recovery is excellent and has recommended a course of treatment to include removal of the involved breast followed by chemotherapy. While the nurse is providing preoperative instructions, Ms. Kim says, "I'll sign the consent form, but I'll be dead before the surgery date." The nurse is not sure whether Ms. Kim is fearful of dying from cancer or whether this may be a statement of suicidal ideation. The nurse seeks clarification by asking, "Why do you think you'll be dead before the date for surgery arrives?"

Critical Thinking Questions

1. What would be an appropriate next step if Ms. Kim clarifies that she is considering suicide?
2. What would be an appropriate next step if Ms. Kim clarifies that she believes she will die from the cancer before the surgery can take place?
3. What is another therapeutic communication tactic that the nurse could have used instead of clarifying? How might the outcome have been changed with the use of a different technique?

Box 38.5

Additional Examples of Therapeutic Communication

Example 1

Jeff Mastin, a 49-year-old man, is at the dermatologist's office having a basal cell carcinoma removed from his temple. He teaches history and coaches baseball at the local high school. The procedure requires only a local anesthetic. Mr. Mastin's wife sits in a chair in the corner during the procedure. Dr. Keisha Thompson, the dermatologist, is conducting the procedure, assisted by two nurses, Sheila Webber and Karl Kline. Ms. Webber's son is on the baseball team, and much of the conversation during the procedure revolves around baseball.

As Dr. Thompson finishes the procedure, Mr. Kline begins giving discharge instructions.

"You need to keep the bandage dry and intact for 48 hours. It's also important to minimize movement for 48 hours." **<giving information>**

"His baseball bag is in the trunk of the car, and he's planning on dropping me off at the house and going on to practice this afternoon." Ms. Mastin says.

"I understand you don't want to miss practice," Ms. Webber says, **<acknowledging>** "but the reason for limiting movement for 48 hours is because strenuous activity increases the risk of bleeding." **<being specific>**

Example 2

Junot Martinez, a 62-year-old man, is a professor of anthropology at the local college, and he was admitted to the hospital yesterday to have a noncancerous astrocytic brain tumor removed. Mr. Martinez just regained consciousness after being under anesthesia for many hours, and he is disoriented, asking disjointed questions of family, friends, and members of the healthcare team. Clark Karabell, the nurse on duty, checks on Mr. Martinez during the period of his greatest confusion. He has been mumbling for quite a few hours but eventually he poses a question to Mr. Karabell, "I feel like I've been asleep forever. How long have I been here?"

"You were admitted to the hospital yesterday morning, Mr. Martinez," Karabell responds. "That was Thursday morning, and now it is 4:00 p.m. on Friday." **<clarifying time>**

"Which one of you people stole my wallet?" Martinez asks, agitated.

"No one stole your wallet, Mr. Martinez," Mr. Karabell responds. "Your wife has your wallet, and she is downstairs at the food court right now." **<presenting reality>**

"Well, I guess nobody is looking out for me, then," Mr. Martinez says, looking downcast.

"Would you like me to stay with you until she returns?" Mr. Karabell asks. **<offering self>**

Example 3

Shuka Mansoori, a 50-year-old woman, is being released from the hospital following a heart attack. She is in a room with her husband, Blake, and seems withdrawn and moody despite being described normally as a sociable person. Francine Muhly, the nurse on duty, provides patient teaching on post–heart attack lifestyle changes when Ms. Mansoori unexpectedly asks, "Am I going to be okay?"

Ms. Muhly responds, "What specifically are you worried about, Ms. Mansoori?" **<seeking clarification, using open-ended questions>**

"I'm worried that I won't be able to play with the grandkids. I'm worried that I'm going to die," she says.

"So you're worried that you won't be able to do the things you enjoy and that you might have another heart attack?" Ms. Muhly summarizes. **<restating>**

"Yes," Ms. Mansoori says.

"I understand your concerns. However, if we work together to make a few simple changes to your diet, exercise routine, and smoking habit," Ms. Muhly says, "your overall health will improve. This will help reduce your risk of additional cardiovascular problems." **<planning>**

Example 4

Shen Liao, an 8-year-old boy, is admitted to the emergency department with significant bruising on his body. He is accompanied by his mother, Anya, and his 3-year-old sister, Laura. When asked how he received the bruises, Shen is silent, but his mother provides the explanation that he fell down a flight of stairs while playing with his younger sister.

Dave Musharraf, the nurse, is suspicious that the patient may have received the injuries through abuse because most of the bruises are concentrated on the patient's back and forearms. He asks Shen and his mother, "Could you tell me more about the accident?" **<using open-ended questions, exploring>**

"Well," Mrs. Liao says, "he was at the top of the stairs and . . . tripped over a playground ball."

Musharraf turns to Shen and says "Shen, I'd like to hear your explanation. Could you tell me how the accident happened?" Musharraf then sits quietly while waiting for Shen to respond. **<using silence>**

"My dad hit me," Shen says quietly, looking away as his mother recoils.

"Thank you for telling me that, Shen," **<acknowledging>** responds Musharraf. "Can you tell me exactly what happened?" **<exploring>**

Paraphrasing

By *paraphrasing*, nurses restate in their own words what the patient has said. Some examples of paraphrasing statements are as follows:

- "In other words, you're tired of being treated like a child."
- "I hear you saying that when people compliment you, you feel embarrassed and if they knew the real you, they would not provide such praise."

The nurse is able to test understanding of what the patient is trying to communicate through paraphrasing. Paraphrasing is reflective in nature, as it lets the patient know what the nurse heard and how the nurse understands what is being discussed. It is also an opportunity for the patient to clarify the content of the message or the feelings behind it.

Checking Perceptions

Nurses can *check perceptions* by sharing how they perceived and heard the information. Once the nurse's perceptions have been shared, it is important to ask the patient to verify the perception by using statements such as the following:

- "Let me know if this is how you see it, too."
- "I get the feeling that you're uncomfortable when we're silent. Does that seem right?"

The effective use of perception checking conveys that the nurse wants to understand what the patient is communicating. It gives the patient the opportunity to correct inaccurate perceptions that the nurse may have. Essentially, *checking perceptions* allows the nurse to avoid actions that are based on false assumptions about the patient.

Questioning

Questioning is a very direct way of speaking that the nurse can use when communicating with a patient. This technique is quite useful when the nurse is seeking specific information. If the nurse is trying to engage in meaningful dialogue with a patient, questions should be limited because they can affect the nature and the ranges of responses from the patient.

Open-ended questions can be used to elicit more information than closed questions. An *open-ended question* allows the nurse to focus the topic while allowing the patient freedom with responses. Examples of this include the following:

- "How did you feel when your brother said that to you?"
- "What's your opinion about . . . ?"

Closed questions should be used sparingly because they typically limit the patient's responses to "yes" or "no." Closed questions also limit therapeutic exploration. This type of question can be useful, however, to guide the patient who may have disorganized thinking.

Questions that ask "why" are typically less helpful than open-ended questions. These questions tend to be hard to answer, in part because they require a higher level of insight on the part of the patient, and they rarely lead to the nurse having a clearer understanding of the current situation. Other types of closed questions, such as "who," "what," "when," and "how," can be useful if the nurse uses them wisely.

Nurses must be careful when questioning not to steer the patient to answer questions in a certain way. For example, "You don't exercise in excess, do you?" may suggest that the patient answer this question with a "no." Refer to Module 34, Assessment, for more information on using open-ended and closed questions.

Structuring

The nurse can use a technique known as *structuring* in an attempt to create order or establish guidelines for patients. This helps patients become aware of their problems and the order in which they should deal with them. Examples of structuring statements are as follows:

- "You've mentioned that you want to improve your relationships with your husband, your son, and your boss. Let's put them in order of importance."
- "No, I won't be giving you advice, but we can discuss some solutions to these issues together."

The nurse can use structuring when a patient introduces a number of issues in a brief period and doesn't know where to begin. This technique can also be used to define the parameters of the nurse–patient relationship in terms of how the nurse will participate with the patient to facilitate the problem-solving process.

Pinpointing

The nurse can use a technique known as *pinpointing* to call attention to specific statements and relationships. For example, when the nurse points out inconsistencies among statements or similarities and differences in points of view, feelings, or actions, the nurse is engaging in pinpointing. This can also be used to determine differences between what an individual says and what one does. Examples of pinpointing statements include the following:

- "So, you and your husband aren't in agreement about how many children you want."
- "You say you're happy, but you're frowning."

Linking

When using the technique known as *linking*, the nurse responds to the patient in a way that ties together events, experiences, feelings, or people. Nurses often use linking to connect past experience with current behaviors that the patient is exhibiting. The nurse can also use linking when there is tension between two individuals during times of stress. Examples of statements that use linking include the following:

- "You felt depressed after the death of both of your parents."
- "So, the arguments didn't really begin until after you lost your job."

Giving Feedback

In using *feedback*, the nurse shares reactions to the patient's statements or behaviors. This technique can help patients become aware of how their own actions and behaviors can affect others. The nurse who responds with feedback may engage in therapeutic self-disclosure because it allows the nurse to offer constructive information regarding how the patient's words or actions have affected the nurse as a communication partner. Total self-disclosure, however, is inappropriate in the nurse–patient relationship and should be avoided. This can place a burden of interdependence on the patient and may limit the time and energy the nurse has available to work on the patient's concerns. The use of reciprocal self-disclosure is more appropriate in friend and colleague relationships than in nurse–patient relationships.

Effective feedback should have three distinct qualities. It should be *immediate*, meaning that it is given as soon as possible; it should be *honest*, meaning that it provides a true reaction; and it should be *supportive*, meaning that it is provided in a way that is tolerable to comprehend and never hurtful or disrespectful to the patient. Examples of effective feedback statements include the following:

- "When you cross your arms while speaking, I feel your apprehension."
- "Sometimes when you look down while we are talking, I think you're angry."

Feedback should always be provided to the patient in a nonthreatening manner. Threatening feedback may increase the patient's defensiveness. The more defensive the patient is when engaging in therapeutic communication, the less able

TABLE 38.5 Giving Helpful, Nonthreatening Feedback

Strategy	Rationale
Focus the feedback on behavior.	Feedback should relate to what the patient actually does rather than how the nurse imagines the patient to be.
Focus the feedback on observations.	Feedback should relate to what the nurse actually sees or hears the patient do. When inferences are used rather than observations, the nurse is drawing conclusions or making assumptions.
Focus the feedback on description.	Description reports what actually occurred rather than evaluating it in terms of good or bad, right or wrong.
Focus feedback on "more or less" rather than "either/or" descriptions of behaviors.	"More or less" descriptions stress quantity rather than quality (which may be value laden).
Focus feedback on here-and-now behavior rather than on there-and-then behavior.	The most meaningful feedback from the nurse is given as soon as it is appropriate to do so.
Focus feedback on sharing of information and ideas.	Sharing of ideas and information helps the patient make decisions about the individual's own well-being. In contrast, by giving advice, the nurse takes away the patient's freedom to be self-determining.
Focus feedback on exploration of alternatives.	Focusing on a variety of alternatives for accomplishing a particular goal for the patient prevents premature acceptance of answers or solutions that may not be appropriate.
Focus feedback on its value to the patient.	Feedback should serve the patient's needs, not the needs of the nurse.
Limit feedback to the appropriate amount of information.	Overload of information will decrease the effectiveness of feedback for the patient.
Limit feedback to the appropriate time and place.	For feedback to be effective, it must be presented at the appropriate time.
Focus feedback on what is said rather than why it is said.	Focusing on why the patient has said something or done something moves away from observations and toward patient motive or intent. Motive or intent can only be assumed and, unless verified, such an assumption is counterproductive.

the patient is to hear and understand the feedback that the nurse is providing. Patients often feel offended if they perceive the nurse to be rejecting them. Feedback that is nontherapeutic, meaning that it is harsh, hurtful, cruel, or rejecting of the patient, will create an unnecessary boundary between the patient and the nurse. The nurse should take great care to prevent the patient from feeling personally rejected as a result of feedback from the nurse. **Table 38.5** » lists strategies and rationales that the nurse can use for giving helpful, nonthreatening feedback.

Feedback goes both ways. Patients usually want to accomplish several items during their interactions with the nurse. They want to express themselves and they want to express information about their perception of the nurse. The nurse should be open and receptive when receiving cues from the patient, either solicited or unsolicited, because these can be useful in a more meaningful working relationship. **Box 38.6** » provides strategies to help nurses reflect on feedback from patients.

Box 38.6

Reflecting on Feedback from Patients

Input can be both positive and negative. Input can be received from a wide variety of individuals, including classmates, instructors, and patients. Input can allow the nurse to become more aware of "blind spots," that is, those characteristics about the self that are ignored, denied, or defended. Self-deception can interfere with the nurse's ability to relate and to communicate. Strategies to increase self-awareness include:

- Think about recent interactions with patients and how those patients responded to you.
- Identify the positive/negative elements in these interactions.
- Try to determine what the patients were telling you about yourself in the interactions. Ask these questions: What characteristics do you possess that enable patients to openly express their thoughts and feelings? What characteristics do you possess that prevent patients from openly expressing their thoughts and feelings?
- Discuss the interactions and your interpretations of them with an instructor, mentor, or preceptor.
- Ask for feedback on your behavior from others.

Confronting

Used in a constructive way, confrontation can lead to productive change. *Confronting* is defined as the deliberate invitation to examine some aspect of personal behavior. Typically, confronting is used when there is a discrepancy or incongruence between what an individual says and what that individual does. It can also be used when expected behavior differs from actual behavior, such as when a patient who is prescribed a liquid diet asks family members to sneak in food from a restaurant. Confrontation requires careful attention to nonverbal communication and to both verbal and nonverbal discrepancies between messages.

The two basic types of confrontation are informational and interpretive. Each type can be directed toward the patient's resources and limitations. An *informational confrontation* describes the visible behavior of another individual (e.g., "You look sad and say you're 'not as smart as your brother and sister,' yet you are the only one who made the honor roll in school"). *Interpretive confirmation* expresses thoughts and feelings about behavior and draws inferences (e.g., "Ever since Emily and Frank criticized the way you conducted the assembly, you haven't spoken to them. It looks like you're feeling angry").

Six skills can be used in incorporating constructive confrontations:

1. Use personal statements with the words *I*, *my*, and *me*.
2. Use relationship statements that express thoughts and feelings about the patient in the present.
3. Use statements that describe visible patient behaviors. This is known as behavior descriptions.
4. Use the description of personal feelings in which you specify the feeling by name.
5. Use responses that are aimed at understanding. Examples of these include paraphrasing and perception checking.
6. Use constructive feedback skills.

Summarizing

Summarizing is a technique that the nurse can use to highlight the main ideas that are expressed during interactions. It is used to convey the nurse's understanding to the patient and it allows both nurse and patient to benefit from a review of the main ideas of a conversation. Summarizing can also be useful when the nurse wants to focus the patient's thinking and to aid in conscious learning.

In certain instances, summarizing is particularly appropriate. The nurse may want to use this technique in the first few minutes of patient interaction because it is useful to review what occurred during previous interactions. This helps the patient recall items that were discussed and gives the patient an opportunity to see how the nurse synthesized the information from previous encounters. Summarizing also keeps all participants directed toward a common goal.

Processing

The nurse can also use a technique known as processing. *Processing* is a complex and sophisticated technique used to direct attention to the interpersonal dynamics of the nurse–patient relationship in terms of content, feelings, and behaviors that have been expressed. This is an advanced skill. Processing is most useful and meaningful when therapeutic intimacy has been achieved.

Clinical Example E

The nurse is preparing to conduct a home visit to Emily Bardinovich, an 86-year-old woman who has lived in an assisted living apartment for the past 5 years. Mrs. Bardinovich was recently discharged back to her apartment following an exacerbation of chronic obstructive pulmonary disease. The nurse has cared for Mrs. Bardinovich for many years and knows her as a friendly, outgoing woman with a great sense of humor who loves to tease people. Today, the nurse finds her very quiet and reserved with little to say. The nurse comments, "You're very quiet today; you haven't teased me at all," to which Mrs. Bardinovich responds, "I'm just not in a teasing mood." The nurse has used processing to help the patient begin to talk about how she feels. This will allow the nurse to perform a more in-depth assessment of the patient's mood and thoughts.

Critical Thinking Questions

1. What therapeutic communication strategies could the nurse use to respond to the patient's statement, "I'm just not in a teasing mood"?
2. What are some potential outcomes if the nurse does not ask Mrs. Bardinovich why she is being so quiet?
3. Describe how the outcome might differ if the nurse uses linking instead of processing in this situation.

Common Mistakes

Nurses often make mistakes when it comes to therapeutic communication. It can be difficult for the nurse to both empathize and communicate with patients when the nurse is feeling uncomfortable with the situation. In addition to the barriers to communication discussed earlier and outlined in Table 38.1, some common mistakes the nurse should take care to avoid include the following:

- ***Giving advice.*** This carries the message that the patient is not capable of solving problems.
- ***Minimizing or discounting feelings.*** Attempts at reassurance often minimize and discount what the patient is feeling.
- ***Deflecting.*** Changing the subject or making jokes in an attempt to move the conversation to something that is less painful is not considered a positive shift because it gives the patient the message that the nurse does not know how to cope with the patient's experience.
- ***Interrogating.*** Asking a series of questions implies that the nurse is more interested in gaining information than in listening to what the patient has to say.
- ***Sparring.*** Debating or disagreeing with the patient sets up an adversarial dynamic and prevents the nurse from listening to what the patient is trying to communicate.

Clinical Example F

Anita Alvarez, a nurse, is providing care to Mark Walton, a 27-year-old man who has just been diagnosed with irritable bowel syndrome. She is teaching him about the dietary changes that he will need to make to manage his condition. Anita asks a series of questions quickly, changing the subject rapidly and not allowing Mr. Walton to provide answers or ask clarifying questions. During the session, she reads directly off a computer screen. When he does get a chance to ask questions, Anita takes several seconds to respond because she is busy looking at her phone. She focuses on herself for several minutes when Mr. Walton asks a question about her work. When he leaves, Anita says, "Everything's going to be all right" as she slams the door.

Critical Thinking Questions

1. Which mistakes or barriers to communication did Anita engage in?
2. What could Anita have done better or differently to ensure that Mr. Walton retained the information and to promote the therapeutic relationship?

The Therapeutic Relationship

The therapeutic nurse–patient relationship is one of helping the patient achieve maximum physical and emotional health.

By maintaining the focus on the patient, the nurse promotes trust and helps patients (Egan & Reese, 2018):

1. Manage their health challenges more effectively and find and use opportunities and resources more effectively
2. Become better at managing their own needs and resources
3. Develop the tools to prevent health problems and recurrences.

To develop a therapeutic relationship with a patient requires time and attention to promote the patient's trust in the nurse and acceptance of the nurse's role in providing care. Good communication skills and a sincere interest in the patient's well-being can help the nurse overcome factors that can affect the development of the relationship, including gender, age, or cultural differences; differences in values and backgrounds; and differences in expectations between the nurse and the patient.

At all times, the therapeutic relationship:

- Is patient-focused, seeking a bond of trust between the nurse and the patient
- Respects the patient as an individual by:
    a. Providing opportunities for the patient to participate in decision making and care provision
    b. Being considerate of the patient's ethnic background and cultural practices
    c. Understanding family relationships and values.
- Respects patient modesty, privacy, and confidentiality.
- Centers on the patient's well-being.
- Fosters mutual trust, respect, and acceptance.

Phases of the Therapeutic Relationship

The process of developing a therapeutic relationship can be described in terms of four phases:

- Preinteraction
- Introductory
- Working (maintaining)
- Termination.

Each phase of the therapeutic relationship necessitates specific tasks and builds upon the phase that precedes it.

Preinteraction Phase

The preinteraction phase takes place before the nurse actually meets the patient, when the nurse receives initial information about the patient. This may be information gathered during intake, information relayed during a change-of-shift report, or information relayed by emergency medical services either en route to the facility or during a handoff report. Sometimes processing information and planning for the initial interview with the patient can cause the nurse to feel some anxiety. By recognizing and processing any anxious feelings, the nurse can address them and better focus on the patient.

Introductory Phase

The introductory phase, also called the orientation or pretherapeutic phase, sets the tone for the nurse–patient relationship. It is during the initial interaction with the patient that first impressions are formed as each sizes up the other. The nurse's goal during this phase is to promote the patient's trust and help the patient feel safe and confident in the nurse (Wofford, 2019).

Patients who have difficulty acknowledging they need help may display resistive behaviors that inhibit cooperation and communication. Patients may fear exposing their feelings, may be uncomfortable confronting and changing their own problem-causing behaviors, or may reject the nurse's approach to the situation.

Nurses who convey a nonjudgmental attitude of caring can overcome patient resistance and begin to establish trust. *Trust* can be described as the knowledge that the other person is reliable in times of illness, injury, or distress. Patients often come to the nurse at times when they are at their most vulnerable and feel exposed. By trusting the nurse, patients become able to share their problems and feelings more openly, which is essential to accurate assessment, care plan development, and adherence to the treatment regimen.

By the end of the introductory phase, patients should begin to:

- Develop trust in the nurse.
- View the nurse as an honest, open, and competent professional who is concerned about their welfare and capable of helping.
- Believe the nurse will attempt to recognize and respect their cultural values and beliefs.
- Trust that the nurse will respect their privacy and confidentiality.
- Feel comfortable discussing sensitive issues and emotions with the nurse.
- Feel comfortable in engaging in the plan of care.

Clinical Example G

While working in an ambulatory care setting, the nurse is asked by the primary HCP to talk with a 24-year-old female patient named Raissa Kunin to explain the need for phlebotomy secondary to her diagnosis of polycythemia. Her hemoglobin is 17.4 mg/dL; it has been steadily increasing for the past year , when it was 16.2 mg/dL. The nurse enters the room and says, "Hello, Ms. Kunin, my name is Mikela Mathews. I'm a registered nurse working for Dr. Shah. He asked me to speak with you about the need to remove blood to lower your hemoglobin." Ms. Kunin says, "I'm just not sure I want to do that, but I'll call you after I have time to think about it." The nurse responds by stating, "You have every right to make a decision in your own best interest. What if I just give you some information while you're here so you can make your decision based on all the details. I can explain the risks of polycythemia, the process of removing blood, and answer any questions you may have." The nurse attempts to overcome resistance behavior by allowing the patient to maintain control. This also promotes a trusting relationship with the patient.

Critical Thinking Questions

1. How would you respond if the patient answered, "No, thank you. That's not necessary. I can look it up on the internet"?
2. If the patient agrees to listen to the nurse, what phase of the relationship will they be in once the nurse begins teaching?
3. What other types of resistive behaviors might you encounter, and how would you attempt to overcome them?

Working Phase

The working or middle phase of the nurse–patient relationship has two major stages: *identification* of problems and plans to address the problems and *exploitation*, in which the nurse assists the patient to participate in health services. During the exploitation stage, the nurse and patient work together to help the patient meet the goals set during the identification stage.

Nursing skills essential to this phase include:

- ***Empathy.*** Nurses must listen attentively and respond with empathy, validating their understanding of the patient's needs and progress while acknowledging the patient's expressed concerns and feelings.
- ***Respect.*** Nurses exhibit a nonjudgmental attitude while respecting the patient's willingness to be available and participate and exhibiting a desire to work with the patient. Nurses take the patient's point of view into consideration while promoting the importance of the patient adhering to the treatment plan.
- ***Genuineness.*** Nurses display genuine care for patients by showing unconditional positive regard for them and maintaining professional behaviors that promote the therapeutic helping relationship. Professional behaviors that convey genuineness include being consistent and reliable, keeping the focus on the patient, not being defensive, suspending judgment, and being spontaneous (Egan & Reese, 2018; Potter & Moller, 2020).
- ***Reflecting, paraphrasing, clarifying, and confronting.*** Nurses use these skills (described earlier) to make sure they understand the patient's point of view and to assist the nurse in helping the patient explore new areas of understanding.

Patients may express feelings such as anxiety, anger, or even shame during this first stage of the working phase as the intensity of the interaction increases. Nurses assist patients to address and resolve these feelings in the pursuit of a better understanding of how these feelings may affect their health status.

Patients often have difficulty moving between the phases of the nurse–patient relationship, especially if they have dementia, cognitive impairment, or severe anxiety. Nurses working with these patients may find they need to reintroduce themselves and reorient the patient to the need for interventions.

Termination Phase

The termination phase, in which the nurse concludes the relationship, can be challenging, especially for patients who don't have a positive outlook or are unable to handle problems independently. Some patients may be ambivalent about ending the relationship, but some may feel a sense of loss, especially if they have been working with the nurse over a period of days or longer. Because each therapeutic relationship is specific to that nurse and that patient, strategies for terminating the relationship will vary.

In some cases, nurses will summarize what occurred during the relationship, sharing recollections of how things were at the beginning of the relationship and comparing them to the present. Both the nurse and the patient may find it helpful to openly and honestly express their feelings about termination. Therefore, termination discussions need to start prior to the termination interview to allow time for the patient to adjust to the idea that the nurse will no longer be a supportive presence.

Some patients will require a termination process that looks more like a transition, with the nurse offering telephone or email support for a specified period for follow-up. In other situations, the nurse may transition the patient to another service (such as home health) or simply affirm the patient's improvement and efforts as the nurse says goodbye at the end of shift or at discharge.

Developing Therapeutic Relationships

Regardless of setting, the purpose of the therapeutic relationship is to establish mutual goals (outcomes) with the patient or with support people if the patient is unable to participate. Although it is advantageous to have special training in counseling techniques, it is not required to be able to help patients. In addition to listening attentively, the nurse can:

- ***Help identify what the person is feeling.*** Patients who are distressed often have difficulties identifying or labeling their feelings and may have problems talking about them. Responses from the nurse such as "You look as if you have been crying since the HCP talked to you about your diagnosis" or "You sound as if you've been lonely since your husband died" can help patients acknowledge their feelings and talk about them.
- ***Be honest.*** Honesty is necessary to an effective therapeutic relationship. Nurses maintain honesty when they acknowledge their limitations (for example, by saying "I don't know the answer to that right now, but I'll do my best to find out) and by setting limits, such as by saying, "This discussion is making me uncomfortable."
- ***Be genuine and credible.*** Nurses who are consistent, reliable, and genuine promote their patients' trust in the therapeutic relationship.
- ***Use your ingenuity.*** Consider all the possible ways to help patients meet their goals while ensuring that interventions are congruent with patients' value systems and likely to promote success.
- ***Be aware of cultural differences that may affect meaning and understanding.*** Recognize the language(s) and/or dialect(s) that the patient uses to promote understanding. Provide interpreters as needed for patients with limited English proficiency. This helps promote the therapeutic relationship and patients' overall trust in the healthcare system.
- ***Maintain patient confidentiality.*** Share patient information only as necessary with other members of that patient's healthcare team in order to provide effective care and treatment and maintain the patient's right to privacy.
- ***Know your role and your limitations.*** Roles and functions should be clarified, specifically what the expectations are of the patient, the nurse, and the primary care provider. Strengths and problems are unique to each individual. If the nurse feels unable to handle some of the patient's problems, the nurse should notify the patient of this and provide a referral to the appropriate healthcare professional.

Lifespan Considerations

Communicating with Children and Families

In caring for pediatric patients, the nurse should implement interventions that will establish an effective nurse–child–family relationship. The nurse must provide an appropriate environment that will foster nurse–child–family communication and ensure confidentiality while doing so. The techniques the nurse uses to develop this relationship are similar to the techniques that the nurse uses with an individual patient, tailoring communication techniques to the needs of both the child and the family (**Figure 38.7** »).

The nurse can use any of several communication techniques with children. These include accepting, active listening, broad openings, clarifying, collaborating, exploring, focusing, giving recognition, observation, offering self, placing an event in time or sequence, reflection, restating or paraphrasing, summarizing, and validating perceptions. The nursing implications for each technique are explored in **Table 38.6** ».

Establishing Rapport with Children

First and foremost, the nurse must establish rapport with the child to set the stage for a productive therapeutic relationship. All patients, including children, will be more responsive to the nurse who makes an effort to help them feel that they are important in an interaction.

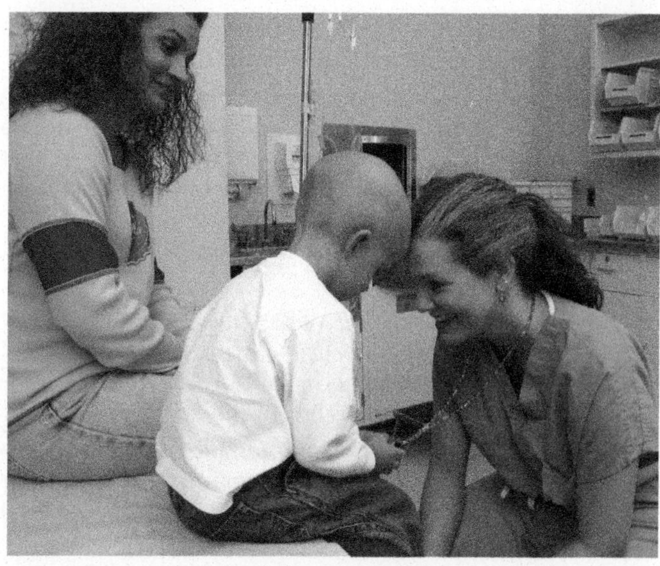

Figure 38.7 » Taking time to listen to the child and family members is important for establishing trust and developing rapport.
Source: Pearson Education, Inc.

The following guidelines can be used by the nurse to establish rapport with a child and encourage the sharing of information and feelings:

- ***Position yourself on the same eye level as the child.*** This suggests that the nurse cares about and respects the child.

TABLE 38.6 Nursing Implications of Using Therapeutic Communication Techniques with Children

Communication Technique	Nursing Implications
Accepting	By conveying acceptance, the nurse respects the child's emotions and allows the child to cry when in pain or lets the child know that crying is okay.
Active listening	The nurse involves the child in the discussion and encourages communication of the child's point of view. It is important to face the child and parents when speaking. This conveys to the family that the nurse is listening and understands what is being said.
Broad openings	This includes using open-ended questions that allow the child to choose the topic for discussion.
Clarifying	By asking the child to clarify or elaborate on what is being expressed, the nurse communicates understanding.
Collaborating	The nurse suggests collaboration with the child and family and then assists them through the problem-solving process.
Exploring	This helps the child to organize their thoughts and focus on the current issue. It will also encourage the child to discuss the issue in more detail.
Focusing	This guides the direction of the conversation. It is useful with small children who may wish to discuss a variety of topics.
Giving recognition	This identifies observed behaviors and indicates an interest in the child.
Observation	This is particularly important with the behavioral aspect of communication. The nurse acknowledges behaviors that indicate the child's thoughts and feelings.
Offering self	This indicates that the nurse is available and willing to listen to the child.
Placing the event in time or sequence	The goal of this technique is to help the child and the nurse understand the order of events.
Reflection	This indicates that the nurse is interested in the discussion and also validates the child's concerns.
Restating or paraphrasing	This acknowledges to the child that the nurse is listening. It also validates appropriate interpretation of what the child is communicating.
Summarizing	This highlights the key facts of the conversation and also provides an opportunity to consider the direction for future discussions. It can also provide closure. Summarizing can occur at varying points in the communication process.
Validating perceptions	This is when the nurse shares conclusions that have been drawn as a result of the discussions with the child. It provides an opportunity for the child to confirm or deny interpretations that the nurse has made throughout the process.

- ***Show interest in what the child is doing.*** This displays that the nurse is interested and encourages security.
- ***Agree with the child when it is appropriate.*** It may be appropriate for the nurse to share feelings. An example of this is telling the child, "I don't like the taste of that medicine either, but sometimes I have to take it when I am sick—but then afterward I drink something that I like." Sharing experiences with the child offers encouragement to the child and family.
- ***Compliment the child.*** Examples include "You are really strong" or "You picked really nice colors for that picture." Complimentary statements by the nurse may reduce anxiety while conferring status on the child.
- ***Use a calm tone of voice and language that is developmentally appropriate.*** It is important to talk and share information with children that is on an appropriate level of comprehension.
- ***Pace the discussion or procedure so that the child does not feel rushed.*** Feeling rushed will increase the child's anxiety.
- ***Explain concepts in terms the child can understand.*** This is especially important for preschool-age children, who have a limited concept of time. For example, stating "Your mother will be back after lunch" is appropriate for this age level because it provides a concrete time frame that the child can understand.
- ***Include the child in the discussion of care if developmentally appropriate.*** This is particularly important for adolescents because they have the cognitive ability to participate in abstract conversation and to comprehend some medical terminology.
- ***Listen more than you talk and avoid distractions.*** This shows the child that the nurse is interested in what the child has to say.

Establishing Trust with Children and Families

Trust is critical to an effective nurse–child–family relationship. Strategies to establish trust with children and families include following through on promises made to the child and family, respecting confidentiality, and being truthful, even when the truth is not what they want to hear.

If a child asks whether a procedure is painful, answer truthfully, but follow with positive words. For example, if a child asks if a "shot" is going to hurt, you might reply, "Yes, some people say that a shot hurts, but it will hurt only for a moment, and then it will be over. Your mother can hold your hand while I give you the shot if that will make you feel better." By following difficult information with a positive rationale or comforting statement, the nurse can maintain credibility while still providing compassionate care.

Communicating with Pregnant Women

Whether a pregnancy is planned or unplanned, the patient is likely to experience stress and emotional distress. Therapeutic communication with pregnant women is especially important because the woman's emotional and physical health—as well as the health of the child—is at stake during pregnancy (Goodtherapy.org, 2019). Sources of emotional distress during pregnancy include worries about the health of the child, independent mental health issues such as anxiety and depression, strained romantic partnerships, financial issues, and physical challenges. Physical health issues include fetal development, physical strain on the mother, proper nutrition, and many others outlined in Module 33, Reproduction.

Keys to communicating with pregnant women are relating medical information clearly and listening for their questions and concerns. Nurses should use active listening techniques to be attentive to the patient's verbal and nonverbal communication. Silence can be a powerful tool to allow the patient to express herself fully so the nurse can address her concern. Making observations fills a similar role in that it allows the patient to communicate without the need for lengthy questioning. For example, the nurse can make observations such as "You look tired" to solicit communication by the patient. Using therapeutic communication techniques can help clarify patient concerns and protect the health of both mother and child.

Communicating with Older Adults and Their Families

Most older adults respond well to the therapeutic communication strategies outlined previously. However, many older adults have conditions that make communication difficult and require the nurse to adjust the therapeutic communication strategy. Approximately half of older adults have hearing loss, and many experience vision loss. These sensory impairments require the nurse to select communication techniques specifically tailored to the needs of the individual older adult (National Institute on Aging, 2017). For example, a nurse can change the environmental conditions of the individual with hearing loss to promote effective communication. Many of the difficulties in communicating effectively with older adults arise when the nurse and patient fail to establish a reliable nurse–patient communication system. The nurse can overcome communication impairments of all kinds by researching assistive communication devices and involving the patient's family in the communication process.

Establishing a reliable communication system with an older adult requires the nurse to continuously reevaluate the patient's communication needs. For instance, for a patient with a cognitive impairment such as dementia, the nurse can use simple, concrete sentences, ask one question at a time, allow time for the patient to reflect, be an active listener, and include family in conversations to ease the burden on the patient. For patients who are visually impaired, nurses can check for use of glasses, identify themselves when coming into contact with the patient, speak in a normal tone of voice, use gestures sparingly, and employ fonts of readable size in printed materials. If the patient seems to not understand the nurse's questions or teaching, the nurse can reevaluate whether they can take any specific steps to change the communication pattern, such as moving to a different room or involving another member of the healthcare team. To communicate most effectively with the older patient, nurses should acquaint themselves with the patient's family and friends to learn about relevant health concerns and favorite conversational topics.

Conclusion

Effective communication is essential to the nurse's ability to provide high-quality care to patients throughout each stage of care: assessment, planning, implementation, and evaluation. It is important that nurses be understood and understand the messages they receive when communicating with patients, other members of the healthcare team, family members, or peers.

REVIEW Therapeutic Communication

RELATE Link the Concepts and Exemplars

Linking the exemplar of therapeutic communication with the concept of advocacy:

1. How do strong therapeutic communication skills contribute to the nurse's role as a patient advocate?
2. How do strong therapeutic communication skills contribute to the nurse's ability to work within groups to advocate for patients?

Linking the exemplar of therapeutic communication with the concept of teaching and learning:

3. The nurse is preparing to teach a patient who is newly diagnosed with diabetes about self-care. Describe the four phases of the therapeutic relationship as it applies to the patient-teaching plan.
4. While teaching the patient with diabetes, the nurse accidentally creates a barrier to the therapeutic relationship by misspeaking. What should the nurse do next?

REFER Go to Pearson MyLab Nursing and eText

REFLECT Apply Your Knowledge

Zainah Kattan is a newly licensed nurse working at the Neighborhood Hospital. She is assigned the care of Lydia Ocampo, a 70-year-old woman who was born and raised in the Philippines who has been diagnosed with Alzheimer disease. She was admitted with a fractured hip following a fall at home. Mrs. Ocampo experienced some delirium during the night and pulled out her IV. The night nurse calmed her down, replaced the IV, and bandaged it in a bulky bandage to prevent her from pulling it out again. This has distressed Mr. Ocampo, who is now afraid to leave his wife's side. Ms. Kattan is happy to act as her primary nurse. She develops rapport with Mr. Ocampo and gets satisfaction from caring for his wife by helping her to feel more comfortable.

1. When communicating with a patient diagnosed with later-stage Alzheimer disease, what strategies will the nurse employ?
2. Why does the development of rapport with Mr. Ocampo improve the patient's ability to meet expected outcomes?

›› Exemplar 38.C Documentation

Exemplar Learning Outcomes

38.C Analyze documentation as it relates to communication.

- Outline the legal and ethical considerations of documentation.
- Summarize the purposes of patient records.
- Outline various types of documentation systems.
- Summarize the documentation of nursing activities.
- Describe facility-specific documentation.
- Outline general guidelines for recording documentation.

Exemplar Key Terms

Assessment, *2609*
Charting, *2607*
Charting by exception (CBE), *2610*
Discussion, *2607*
Documenting, *2607*
Evaluation, *2609*
Flow sheet, *2610*
Focus charting, *2610*
Intervention, *2609*
Objective data, *2609*
Patient record, *2608*
PIE documentation model, *2610*
Plan of care, *2609*
Planning, *2609*
Problem-oriented medical record (POMR), *2609*
Problem-oriented record (POR), *2609*
Record, *2607*
Recording, *2607*
Report, *2607*
Revision, *2609*
SOAP, *2609*
SOAPIER, *2609*
Subjective data, *2609*
Variance, *2612*

Overview

The quality of care patients receive depends on clear, effective communication among HCPs. Healthcare personnel normally communicate through a variety of methods, including verbal communication, medical records, and reports. A **discussion** is an informal verbal communication by a group of two or more people for the purpose of identifying and solving a problem. A **report** is communication intended to convey information to others (such as an end-of-shift report between nurses) and can be presented in oral, written, or electronic form. Until 2014, when the Patient Protection and Affordable Care Act took effect, a **record** could be handwritten or electronic. Currently, all patient records are required to be electronic (USF Health, 2020). **Recording**, **charting**, and **documenting** are terms used to describe the process of making an entry into a patient record.

Each **patient record** is a formal, legal document that provides evidence of the patient's health status and care provided. Regardless of the healthcare organization or records system used, all patient records include similar information, including patient demographic information, health history, nurse or provider notes, and medication administration records.

The Joint Commission and other accrediting agencies require patient record documentation to be performed in a timely, complete, accurate, and confidential manner and be specific to the patient. Nurses are responsible for following the requirements of their employing organization's accrediting agency, as well as the organization's specific policies for documenting and reporting patient information.

The need for documentation to be specific to the patient goes beyond simply ensuring that the individual patient's information is entered correctly in the healthcare record. Complete, accurate, and specific patient information includes entering relevant, objective information about cultural and other considerations that will help other members of the healthcare team who work with the patient to provide culturally appropriate, respectful care.

Ethical and Legal Considerations

As stated in the American Nurses Association's *Code of Ethics* (2015), "[T]he nurse has a duty to maintain confidentiality of all patient information" (p. 9). In practice, the nurse follows agency policies to maintain the privacy of the patient's record, which is legally protected as official documentation of care provided to the patient. Only those healthcare professionals involved in assessing or providing care to a patient may access the patient's record. Although patient medical records are legally owned by the healthcare agency, patients have the right to request digital or paper copies of their medical records.

The Health Insurance Portability and Accountability Act (HIPAA) includes regulations about maintaining the privacy, confidentiality, and security of *protected health information*, or PHI. PHI is identified as any health information about a patient that is recorded or maintained in any format (electronically, digitally, or on paper) or that is transmitted about a patient (for example, during a handoff report or a telephone report to the patient's HCP).

In most clinical settings, student healthcare professionals (such as nursing, medical, and physician assistant students) may access patient records for the purposes of education and research and for use in patient studies and conferences and in clinical rotations or rounds. As with other healthcare professionals, students are bound by strict ethical codes and have a legal obligation to maintain the privacy and confidentiality of the patients with whom they interact and whose records they access. Part of that legal responsibility includes not writing or noting patients' names on any paperwork or notes that could potentially leave the facility's premises—including not making notes on their personal cell phones.

With the use of electronic records came the need for policies and procedures to ensure the security and confidentiality of patient information stored electronically. The Security Rule of HIPAA governs the protection of electronic forms of health information and establishes sanctions and fines for healthcare organizations and providers who violate the privacy of electronic patient records. To protect electronic patient information, each member of the healthcare team should:

- Have a personal login and password for accessing patient records that is not to be shared with anyone else, including other members of the healthcare team.
- Log off a computer when not actually using it to prevent unintended access to patient information.
- Make sure patient information is not displayed for anyone else to see while in use.
- Know the agency's policy for correcting an entry error.
- Follow agency policies for documenting sensitive material (such as diagnosis of a sexually transmitted infection or evidence of assault or abuse).

Purposes of Patient Records

Patient records are kept for a variety of reasons:

- ***Communication.*** Patient records allow for members of the healthcare team assigned to that patient to review each other's findings and care provided, reducing the possibility of duplication of interventions.
- ***Planning patient care.*** Every member of the healthcare team working with a patient has access to the same data to inform and plan care. For example, a physical therapist can review the orthopedist's orders and the nurse's notes prior to making an initial assessment of the patient who is recovering from hip replacement surgery.
- ***Research.*** Patient data may be used for research, normally with the provision that personally identifying information such as names, birthdates, and patient identification numbers be excluded from the information culled for research. Age, sex, and some socioeconomic data may be reported under certain circumstances. In most cases, information about multiple patients is culled and reviewed to look for trends. For example, the year 2020 saw a number of high-quality randomized controlled trial (RCT) studies of the use of corticosteroids in the treatment of patients with severe COVID-19, with the research groups agreeing to share data. The results of using corticosteroids in this patient population were reported and shared without breaching patient confidentiality (Prescott & Rice, 2020).
- ***Education.*** Patient records may be used as a teaching tool for students from a variety of healthcare disciplines to provide a comprehensive view of the patient, the illness, effective treatment strategies, and any factors that affect the outcome of the illness.
- ***Reimbursement.*** Healthcare facilities use diagnosis-related group (DRG) codes associated with patient records to indicate provision of appropriate care and to bill health insurance policies for payment. Codable diagnoses, such as DRGs, are supported by thorough and accurate documentation of a patient's care by nurses. If a patient requires additional care, treatment, or length of stay in a facility, thorough documentation will help justify these needs.
- ***Auditing health agencies.*** Accrediting agencies, such as The Joint Commission, and oversight agencies, such as the Centers for Medicare and Medicaid Services or state

health departments, may audit patient records for quality assurance purposes. For more information, see Module 50, Quality Improvement.

- ***Legal documentation.*** The patient's record is a legal document and is typically admissible as evidence in court. In some jurisdictions, however, if the patient objects because the record contains confidential information, the record is considered inadmissible as evidence.
- ***Healthcare analysis.*** Information from patient records can be used to analyze different aspects of service provision in order to make improvements or adjustments at the unit or agency level. For example, analyzing the number of nights in the hospital required to recover from a specific type of surgery can help determine recovery costs associated with that type of surgery.

Documentation Systems

The most common documentation systems used by healthcare agencies are the problem-oriented medical record (problem, intervention, evaluation [PIE] model); focus charting (data, action, response [DAR] format); charting by exception (CBE); and electronic documentation (Lockwood, 2019). In the American Recovery and Reinvestment Act of 2009, the federal government mandated that all healthcare facilities move to electronic medical records from paper records.

Problem-Oriented Medical Record

In a **problem-oriented medical record (POMR)**, or **problem-oriented record (POR)**, the data are arranged according to the problems the patient has rather than the source of the information. Each member of the healthcare team contributes information to the problem list, plan of care, and progress notes. Plans for each active or potential problem are developed, and progress notes are written for each problem.

The advantages of POMRs are that they encourage collaboration, allow for rapid identification of current patient needs, and make it less difficult to track the status of each problem. The disadvantages of a POMR are that caregivers vary in their ability to use the required charting format. It is challenging and inefficient to maintain a current problem list because assessments and interventions that apply to more than one problem must be repeated, causing documentation to be extremely time-consuming.

The POMR is comprised of four basic components:

- ***Database.*** The database of a POMR contains all the data gathered on admission, including the results of initial assessments and baseline diagnostic tests. As additional assessments and care is provided, that information is updated in the database.
- ***Problem list.*** From the data available, a problem list is generated. Problems are listed in the order in which they are identified. All members of the healthcare team may contribute to a patient's identified problem list, with primary HCPs entering medical diagnoses and orders. Problems may be redefined as the patient's condition changes.
- ***Plan of care.*** In the POMR method, the member of the healthcare team who identifies the problem is the one who generates the care plan for addressing that problem. The written **plan of care** is listed in progress notes associated with the problem and not isolated in a separate list of orders or interventions.
- ***Progress notes*** may be made by any member of the healthcare team who is providing care to the patient. Progress notes correlate to the identified problem on the problem list. Progress notes often use the **SOAP** or **SOAPIER** format:

Subjective data: obtained from statements made by the patient

Objective data: information that can be measured or observed

Assessment: interpretations or evaluations about data collected

Planning: goals and outcomes developed to resolve identified problems

Intervention: identification of specific measures to achieve expected outcomes

Evaluation: analysis of patient response to interventions or treatments

Revision: modifications to initial desired outcomes or interventions.

Figure 38.8 » illustrates a nursing progress note using the SOAPIER format.

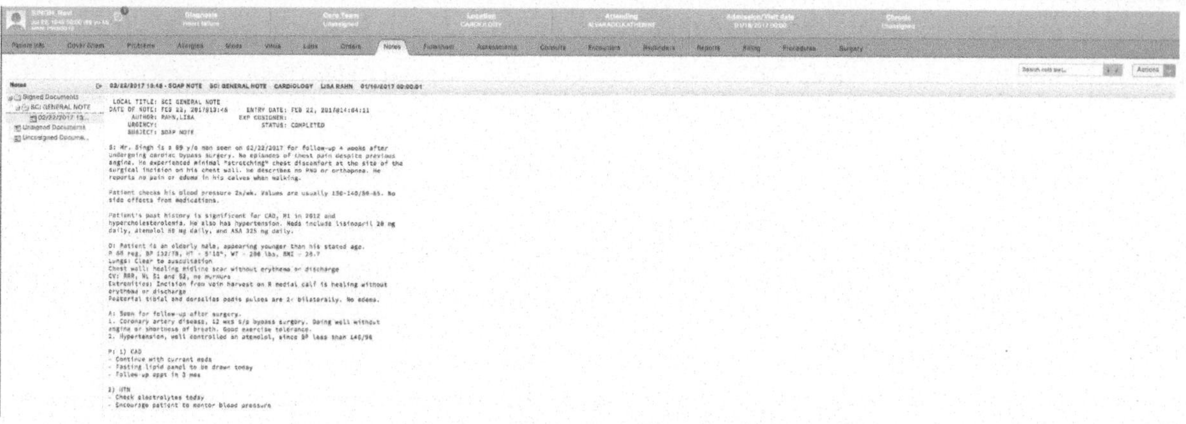

Figure 38.8 » An example of a nursing progress note using SOAPIER in an EHR.

PIE Model

The **PIE documentation model** is a simplified approach to problem-oriented documentation that focuses on the nursing process and is an acronym for:

Problems

Interventions

Evaluation of nursing care.

This system, based on the nursing process, consists only of a patient care assessment flow sheet and progress notes. The **flow sheet** follows a specific format, such as basic human needs or functional health patterns (e.g., nutrition, elimination, activity). The parameters for a flow sheet differ based on the setting. For example, a postpartum patient's vital signs may be monitored by the quarter hour for the first few hours after labor and delivery, whereas in an outpatient clinic a patient's warfarin level may be recorded monthly.

After the assessment is completed, the nurse establishes and records identified problems on the progress notes, frequently using nursing diagnoses following a three-part format: the problem, contributing or probable causes of the problem, and signs and symptoms manifested by the patient.

- The *problem statement*, which is labeled "P" and identified by a number (e.g., P #3).
- The *interventions* planned to address the problem are labeled "I" and are numbered to match the problem (e.g., I #3).
- The *evaluation* of the patient's response to interventions is labeled "E" and is also numbered to match the problem (e.g., E #5).

Focus Charting

Focus charting is a systematic approach to documentation that is intended to make the patient's strengths and needs the focus of care. This format uses three columns for recording: date and time, focus, and progress notes. The *focus* identifies the content of the entry and may be a sign or symptom, nursing or medical diagnosis, or a change in the patient's condition. The progress notes are organized into (D) data, (A) action, and (R) response categories, referred to as DAR. The *data* are information gathered during assessment and consist of both objective and subjective information that describe the focus. This information may include observations of patient status and behaviors or data from laboratory diagnostics or assessment information from other members of the health-care team.

The *action* category reflects the planning and implementation phase and includes immediate and future nursing interventions, including changes to the plan of care based on ongoing monitoring of the patient. The *response* category reflects the nurse's evaluation of patient outcomes or response to any nursing or medical care.

The focus charting system provides a holistic view of the patient's strengths and needs and responses to nursing and medical interventions This format also provides a nursing process framework for the progress notes (DAR). The three categories do not need to be recorded in order, and each note does not need to contain all three categories; they should only be used as they are relevant. Checklists and drop-down menus are often used on the patient's chart to record routine nursing tasks and assessment data.

Charting by Exception

In **charting by exception (CBE)**, only significant or unexpected findings or exceptions to defined norms are recorded. CBE incorporates flow sheets, standards of nursing care, and bedside access to the patient's record (Guido, 2019):

1. ***Flow sheets***. Examples of flow sheets include a graphic record (**Figure 38.9** ››) and daily nursing assessments record (**Figure 38.10** ››), but flow sheets may be used to record other information, such as patient teaching and focused assessments.
2. ***Standards of nursing care***. Standards of nursing care allow for consistent quality of care and documentation. Agencies using CBE must develop

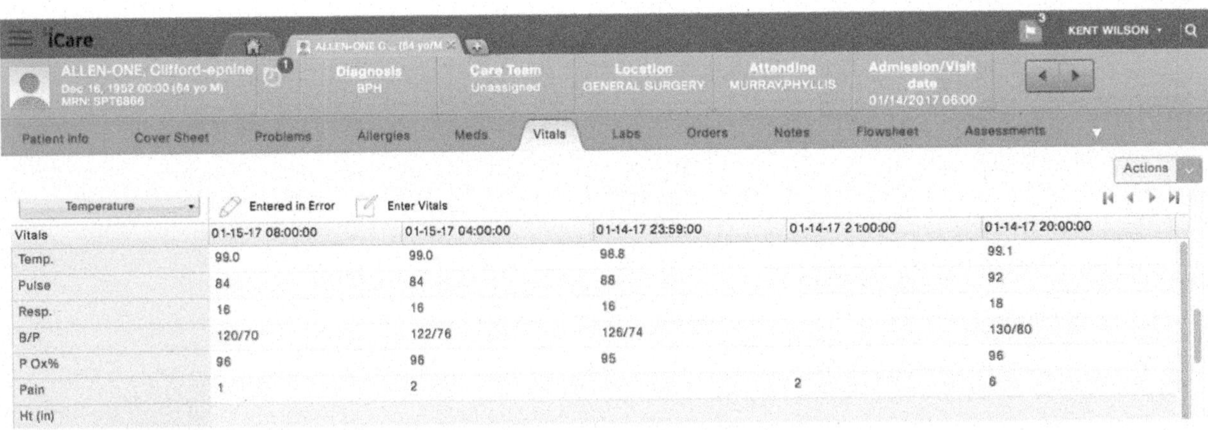

Vitals	01-15-17 08:00:00	01-15-17 04:00:00	01-14-17 23:59:00	01-14-17 21:00:00	01-14-17 20:00:00
Temp.	99.0	99.0	98.8		99.1
Pulse	84	84	88		92
Resp.	16	16	16		18
B/P	120/70	122/76	126/74		130/80
P Ox%	96	96	95		96
Pain	1	2		2	6
Ht (in)					

Figure 38.9 ›› A sample vital signs graphic record in an EHR.

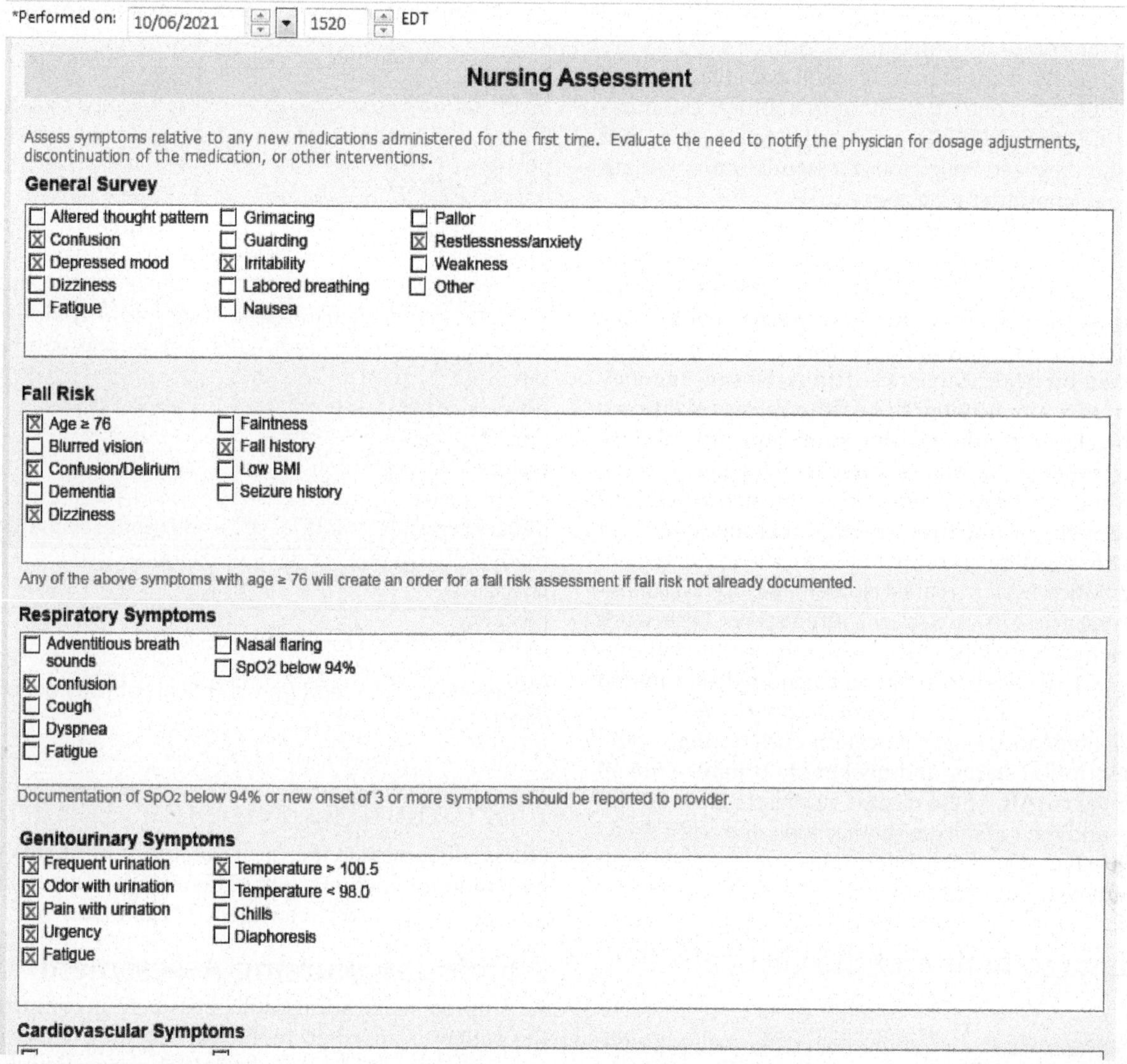

*Performed on: 10/06/2021 1520 EDT

Nursing Assessment

Assess symptoms relative to any new medications administered for the first time. Evaluate the need to notify the physician for dosage adjustments, discontinuation of the medication, or other interventions.

General Survey

- [ ] Altered thought pattern
- [x] Confusion
- [x] Depressed mood
- [ ] Dizziness
- [ ] Fatigue
- [ ] Grimacing
- [ ] Guarding
- [x] Irritability
- [ ] Labored breathing
- [ ] Nausea
- [ ] Pallor
- [x] Restlessness/anxiety
- [ ] Weakness
- [ ] Other

Fall Risk

- [x] Age ≥ 76
- [ ] Blurred vision
- [x] Confusion/Delirium
- [ ] Dementia
- [x] Dizziness
- [ ] Faintness
- [x] Fall history
- [ ] Low BMI
- [ ] Seizure history

Any of the above symptoms with age ≥ 76 will create an order for a fall risk assessment if fall risk not already documented.

Respiratory Symptoms

- [ ] Adventitious breath sounds
- [x] Confusion
- [ ] Cough
- [ ] Dyspnea
- [ ] Fatigue
- [ ] Nasal flaring
- [ ] SpO2 below 94%

Documentation of SpO2 below 94% or new onset of 3 or more symptoms should be reported to provider.

Genitourinary Symptoms

- [x] Frequent urination
- [x] Odor with urination
- [x] Pain with urination
- [x] Urgency
- [x] Fatigue
- [x] Temperature > 100.5
- [ ] Temperature < 98.0
- [ ] Chills
- [ ] Diaphoresis

Cardiovascular Symptoms

Figure 38.10 » Sample of a portion of a daily nursing CBE assessment form in an EHR.
Source: Pearson Education, Inc.

their own specific standards of nursing care that establish minimum criteria of patient care. Examples include standards for frequency of oral care for unconscious or debilitated patients or frequency of assessments of postpartum patients for complications. Documentation of care according to these specified standards may be indicated by checking a box next to the standard met. If a standard is not implemented, the nurse enters an asterisk on the flow sheet and describes any exceptions to the standards in narrative form in the nurses' notes.

3. ***Bedside access to records***. In the CBE system, all information is recorded and available at the bedside.

Electronic Documentation

Computerized clinical record systems have been the fastest-growing sector in the field of documentation. Electronic health record (EHR) or electronic medical record (EMR) systems provide an efficient way to manage the huge volume of information required in contemporary healthcare. Nurses use computer databases to store the patient data, add new data, create and revise care plans, and document patient progress. Some institutions provide a computer terminal at each patient's bedside or a laptop or tablet for the nurse to carry; these technologies enable the nurse to document care immediately after providing it.

EHRs and EMRs use standardized lists, drop-down menus, and narrative information entered by the nurse or other HCP to document and record patient assessment and care information. Some information systems allow nurses and other providers to enter information verbally through dictation. A role that has expanded in healthcare is that of the "medical scribe or documentation assistant" who is a paraprofessional trained to enter physician assessment data and medical orders directly into the EMR on behalf of the provider and accordingly free the physician to focus more attention on the patient than the computer (Robeznieks, 2018).

Electronic health records have made it possible to transmit information from one care setting to another. The nursing Minimum Data Set (MDS) is a classification system that allows for standardized collection of essential nursing data for inclusion in computer databases.

Electronic medical records contain the standard medical and clinical data gathered in one provider's office. EHRs go beyond data collected at the individual HCP's office and over time compile a comprehensive patient history (HealthIT.gov, 2019). EHR data can be created, managed, and consulted by healthcare staff within the same agency as well as across any number of healthcare organizations. EMRs and EHRs are more useful than paper records by most measures. Specifically, electronic records can track data over time, identify patients who are due for certain procedures, monitor patients' vaccination schedules, and improve patient safety.

Documentation systems called *electronic medication administration records (eMARs)* are specifically used to keep track of patient medication information (InSynch Healthcare Solutions, 2020). eMARs use barcodes and a hand-held scanner to send and fill prescriptions. Medication dosages, number of refills, types of medications, medication classifications, refill history, prescription status, and tracking information are all included in the eMAR. These records accelerate the prescribing process, and their quality assurance tools and audit tracking features enhance available information and severely limit the possibility of a medication error.

Case Management and the Critical Pathway

The case management model emphasizes high-quality, timely, complete, and cost-effective care provided within an established length of stay. This model uses an interprofessional approach to planning and documenting patient care using *critical pathways* (**Figure 38.11** ››). Critical pathways identify the outcomes that certain groups of patients are expected to achieve during care, along with anticipated interventions (Vikrant, 2019). For example, the critical pathway for patients with a hip replacement might include that the patient's lungs are clear to auscultation and the patient expresses comfort with pain control measures.

Case management models incorporate the use of graphics, flow sheets, and critical pathways. Nurses can enter progress or narrative notes to chart by exception if goals on a critical pathway are not met or the patient experiences an unexpected response that affects that plan of care, called a **variance** (deviation from the plan). When a variance occurs, the nurse writes a narrative note documenting the unexpected event (such as an adverse reaction to a medication), the cause, and interventions used in response to the variance.

The case management model promotes collaboration among members of the healthcare team and reduces length of stay. Critical pathways generally work best, however, for patients with only one or two diagnoses and few individualized needs. Patients with multiple high-acuity diagnoses or an unpredictable course are difficult to document using critical pathways.

CRITICAL PATHWAY: TOTAL HIP REPLACEMENT

	DOS/Day 1	Days 2–3
Pain Management	Outcome: • Verbalizes comfort or tolerance of pain Circle: V NV Variance:	Outcome: • Verbalizes comfort with pain control measures Circle: V NV Variance:
Respiratory	Outcomes: • Breath sounds clear to auscultation • Achieves 50% of volume goal on incentive spirometer Circle: V NV Variance:	Outcomes: • Breath sounds clear to auscultation • Achieves 100% of volume goal on incentive spirometer Circle: V NV Variance:
Key: V = Variance	NV = No Variance	
Signature:	Initials:	
Signature:	Initials:	

Figure 38.11 ›› Excerpt from a critical pathway documentation form.

Documenting Nursing Activities

Nurses document evidence of nursing assessments, interventions, and interactions with patients regardless of the type of records system used in an agency (**Table 38.7** ››).

Admission Nursing Assessment

A comprehensive admission assessment is completed when the patient is admitted to the nursing unit. This assessment may also be referred to as an initial assessment, health history, or nursing assessment. The purpose of the assessment is to evaluate the patient's health status, identify functional health problems, and establish a comprehensive database for comparison with future assessments and for evaluation of changes in patient health status. The admission assessment may be organized according to the type of healthcare setting (e.g., intensive care unit, labor and delivery, or pediatric clinic) or according to body systems, functional health patterns or abilities, or nursing or medical diagnoses. Ongoing assessments are entered as part of the critical pathway or through nursing progress notes.

TABLE 38.7 Documentation for the Nursing Process

Step	Documentation Forms
Assessment	Initial assessment form, various flow sheets
Nursing diagnosis	Nursing care plan, critical pathway, progress notes, problem list
Planning	Nursing care plan, critical pathway
Implementation	Progress notes, flow sheets
Evaluation	Progress notes

Note: All steps are recorded on discharge/referral summaries.
Source: From Berman et al. (2021).

Nursing Care Plans

The Joint Commission and other accrediting agencies require that each patient's medical record include documentation of assessments, nursing diagnoses or patient care priorities, nursing interventions, patient outcomes, and evidence of a current nursing plan of care. See Module 36, Clinical Decision Making, for information on types of nursing care plans and approaches to their development and use.

Flow Sheets

A flow sheet allows the nurse to record nursing data in a concise and rapid manner and provides an easy-to-read record of the patient's condition over time.

- ***Graphic record***. The graphic record usually captures essential clinical data such as vital signs and oxygen saturation. It may also capture clinical data relevant to the setting, such as bowel movements, pain levels, or activity.
- ***Intake and output (I&O) record***. The I&O record documents all fluid intake and fluid loss and the routes for each type of fluid measured. Daily weights and percentage of meal consumption may also be included.
- ***Medication administration record***. The MAR is a chart or flow sheet for recording all information related to prescribed medications:
    a. The initial order, including the date of entry, date/time of expiration, and the name of the medication with the route, dose, and frequency of administration.
    b. Confirmation of any assessments prior to medication administration (such as checking for allergies)
    c. Documentation of the administration of the medication, including the time, dose, and route and the nurse's signature or initials. If the medication order is based on a sliding scale (such as an insulin sliding scale) or a scoring system (such as the Richmond Agitation Scoring Scale), or is PRN, the nurse enters all data that supports the determination of the dose administered (e.g., the patient's blood glucose level for an insulin sliding scale).
- ***Skin assessment record***. A skin or wound assessment documents the stage of injury or wound appearance, color and amount of drainage, odor, wound culture results, and interventions and treatments.

Progress Notes

Nurses enter progress notes to document the patient's progression toward expected or desired outcomes, any problems or exceptions, nursing interventions, and evaluations of patient responses to interventions.

Nursing Discharge Plan and Referral

A discharge plan and referral summary are completed when the patient is being discharged and transferred to another facility or to home with follow-up home health care. Forms for these summaries are developed and provided by the healthcare facility and usually include the discharge plan with instructions for care, as well as medication administration, and the final progress note.

If the discharge plan is given directly to the patient and family, it is imperative that information be provided in the language the patient understands. The nurse reviews the plan with the patient and family and offers the opportunity for them to ask questions and seek clarification.

If a patient is to be transferred to another unit or to another facility, it is essential that a report accompany the patient to ensure continuity of care. This report should include all components of the discharge instructions as well as a description of the patient's condition prior to transfer and documentation of any teaching or patient instruction that has been given, as well as the last dose of all medications and the next time prescribed medications are to be administered.

For patients discharged home with follow-up home health services, the discharge plan becomes part of the referral made to the home health service. Information included in the referral will include the following:

- Description of the patient's physical, cognitive, and mental health status at discharge
- Continuing health problems and current care needs
- Treatments that are to be continued (e.g., wound care, oxygen therapy)
- Current medications list
- Any restrictions regarding moving, diet, or bathing
- Patient functional ability and ability to manage activities of daily living (ADLs) with help or assistance
- Patient education/instruction provided prior to discharge.

The home health agency will require a provider's order to initiate the first home health assessment and follow-up care. The home health nurse can request additional orders following the first nursing assessment in the patient's home. For patients with multiple high acuity or chronic conditions (such as Parkinson disease), a PRN order, which allows the nurse to visit on an as-needed basis in consultation with the family until the patient is discharged from home health services, can be helpful to patients and their family members in the first few days following discharge from a hospital or rehabilitation facility.

Facility-Specific Documentation

Documentation systems and requirements vary by facility. The documentation required in an acute care setting, as discussed in the early part of this exemplar, is different from the documentation required by long-term care, home care, or other care delivery sites such as outpatient clinics.

Long-Term Care Documentation

Long-term facilities provide intermediate care for patients who need rehabilitation and assistance with ADLs following discharge from the hospital but who will be able to return home safely within 3 to 4 weeks. Some provide comprehensive and specialized nursing care for patients with medical conditions that have progressed to the point they can no longer be cared for safely at home.

A number of laws provided standards for documentation systems in long-term care settings. For example, the Omnibus Budget Reconciliation Act of 1987 requires that long-term care facilities conduct a comprehensive patient assessment (called the Minimum Data Set for Resident Assessment and Care Screening) within 4 days after admission and formulate a plan of care within 7 days after admission. Every 3 months thereafter, the patient plan of care must be reviewed by the healthcare team providing care to the patient. Documentation in long-term care facilities must also fulfill the requirements set by Medicare and Medicaid, which reimburses facilities for skilled nursing care, such as tube feedings and chemotherapy administration. For patients receiving skilled nursing care, the nurse must provide daily documentation to verify the need for service and reimbursement.

Nurses typically complete a weekly nursing care *summary* for patients requiring skilled care and every 2 weeks for patients who require intermediate care. Nursing care summaries document patient mental status, ADLs, safety measures needed, medications administered and other treatments, nutrition and fluid status, and any assistive devices the patient requires.

Home Care Documentation

Home health services follow documentation requirements for Medicare, Medicaid, and other third-party reimbursement plans. The home health nurse assigned to the patient is responsible for completing a home health certification and plan of treatment, which is signed by the nurse and authorized by the patient's HCP. The home health nurse documents in the patient's medical record each interaction with the patient. Information in a home care medical record often includes reports to third-party payers, a list of medications, an interprofessional plan of care, referral and intake forms, and patient assessments.

General Guidelines for Recording

In addition to maintaining confidentiality of records, nurses and other healthcare personnel are charged with meeting legal standards of documenting information because the patient's medical record is a legal document that can be used as evidence in court.

Date and Time

Although many electronic records systems automatically document the date and time, the nurse is responsible for making sure that the date and time of each entry are recorded. Some systems use conventional time (e.g., 8:00 a.m. or 2:15 p.m.), but many use the 24-hour clock (e.g., 0800 or 1415).

Timing

Documentation should follow agency policies. As a rule, nurses should document an assessment finding, a patient statement, or a nursing action as soon as possible after it occurs. Documentation should not be recorded *before* the event.

Accepted Terminology

Documentation should contain only abbreviations, symbols, and terms approved by the healthcare facility. A large number of healthcare facilities are moving away from the use of any abbreviations. When there is doubt about using an abbreviation, write the term out completely. **Table 38.8** » lists some common abbreviations used in healthcare.

To reduce errors in healthcare settings, accrediting agencies require all organizations requesting accreditation to develop a "Do Not Use" list of abbreviations, acronyms, and symbols, which must include those abbreviations banned by the accrediting agency.

» **Stay Current:** Keep up with The Joint Commission's "Do Not Use" list by visiting its website at http://www.jointcommission.org/-/media/tjc/documents/fact-sheets/do-not-use-list-8-3-20.pdf.

Correct Spelling

To reduce the potential for errors, it is essential that nurses use correct spelling and that they look up any words they do not know how to spell. This is particularly important when documenting medications, many of which have similar spellings.

Signature

Nurses must sign or otherwise confirm their name in any nursing notes or other documentations using both name and title; for example, "Mary K. Green, RN" or "M. K. Green, RN." If the nurse has been assigned a personal identification code for use in EMRs, the nurse should include the assigned ID number.

Accuracy

Before making an entry, nurses should ensure they are in the correct chart or electronic record. Documentation in patient records must be accurate and correct. Accurate documentation requires that the nurse document objective observations or facts and not personal opinions. For example, it is more accurate to write that the patient "refused medication" than to document that the patient "was uncooperative," which is an opinion. Similarly, the nurse should quote patient statements in documentation, such as "I don't like that medication, it makes me dizzy," rather than recording the nurse's interpretation that "The patient doesn't like the medication." Similarly, it is necessary to document observations specifically, such as "2 cm of swelling around the injection site, red and warm to touch" rather than "swollen, warm area around the injection site."

Sequence

Events should be documented in the order in which they occur, for example, assessments should be recorded first, then the nursing interventions, and then the patient's responses. Update as needed or according to agency protocols.

Appropriateness

Document only information that is relevant to the patient's health status and care. It is inappropriate to document personal information the patient shares with the nurse that is not relevant to care, as doing so can be considered an invasion of patient privacy.

Completeness

Nurses should document all care provided and any care omitted or refused by the patient. Documenting care provided should reflect the nursing process, including all assessments and findings, dependent and independent nursing interventions, patient comments and responses to interventions, patient progress and variances toward goals, and nurse communications with other members of the healthcare team.

TABLE 38.8 Commonly Used Abbreviations

Abbreviation	Term	Abbreviation	Term
Abd	Abdomen	(L)	Left
ABO	The main blood group system	LMP	Last menstrual period
ac	Before meals	meds	Medications
ad lib	As desired	mL	Milliliter
ADL	Activities of daily living	mod	Moderate
Adm	Admitted or admission	neg	Negative
a.m.	Morning	Ø	None
amb	Ambulatory	#	Number or pounds
amt	Amount	NPO, NBM	Nothing by mouth
approx	Approximately	NS, N/S	Normal saline
bid, BID	Twice daily	OOB	Out of bed
bm, BM	Bowel movement	pc	After meals
BP	Blood pressure	PE, PX	Physical examination
BRP	Bathroom privileges	per	By or through
c̄	With	p.m.	Afternoon
C	Celsius (centigrade)	PO	By mouth
CBC	Complete blood count	postop	Postoperatively
c/o	Complains of	preop	Preoperatively
DAT	Diet as tolerated	prep	Preparation
drsg	Dressing	prn, PRN	When necessary
Dx	Diagnosis	qid, QID	Four times a day
ECG	Electrocardiogram	(R)	Right
F	Fahrenheit	s̄	Without
fld	Fluid	stat	At once, immediately
GI	Gastrointestinal	tid, TID	Three times a day
gtt	Drops	TPR	Temperature, pulse, respirations
hr	Hour	VO	Verbal order
H_2O	Water	VS	Vital signs
I&O	Intake and output	WNL	Within normal limits
IV	Intravenous	wt	Weight

Note: Institutions may elect to include some of these abbreviations on their "Do Not Use" list. Check the agency's policy.

Care that is omitted due to the patient's condition or refusal must also be documented. For example, if the patient's ordered antibiotic is changed after a culture and sensitivity test, the nurse should document the test results, that the nurse discontinued the antibiotic and administered the new antibiotic following updated orders from the HCP.

Conciseness

Brevity is important. The patient's name and the word *patient* can be omitted. For example, the nurse may write "Reports pain as 2 on a 1 to 10 scale."

Legal Prudence

The clinical record provides proof of the assessments and interventions and the overall quality of care provided to a patient. It is admissible in court as a legal document. By adhering to professional standards of nursing care as well as facility policies and procedures for intervention and documentation, nurses ensure the best possible care is provided to the patient while protecting themselves, other members of the healthcare team, and the healthcare facility from issues of liability (**Box 38.7** »).

Provider–Patient Communications

The use of electronic records has expanded to *patient portals,* secure email services used by many primary and specialty providers to communication information between the patient and the provider and the nurse who works most closely with that provider. Any email messages to or from a patient become part of that patient's record. Nurses communicating with patients through patient portals should follow their organization's policies for communication and all the best practice recommendations reflected in this exemplar.

Box 38.7
Dos and Don'ts of Documentation

DO

- Document a change in a patient's condition *and* show that follow-up actions were taken.
- Read the nurses' notes prior to care to determine whether there has been a change in the patient's condition.
- Be timely. A late entry is better than no entry; however, the longer the period of time between actual care and charting, the greater the risk for recording inaccurate information or omitting necessary information.
- Use objective, specific, and factual descriptions.
- Correct documentation errors in the manner specified by agency policy.
- Document all teaching.
- Record the patient's actual words by putting quotation marks around the words.
- Document the patient's response to interventions.
- Review your notes. Are they clear? Do they reflect what you want to say?

DON'T

- Document in advance of the event (e.g., procedure, medication).
- Use vague terms (e.g., "appears to be comfortable," "had a good night").
- Document for someone else.
- Use "patient" instead of the patient's name.
- Alter a record even if requested by a superior or a physician.
- Record assumptions or words reflecting bias (e.g., "complainer," "disagreeable").

REVIEW Documentation

RELATE Link the Concepts and Exemplars

Linking the exemplar of documentation with the concept of legal issues:

1. How does proper documentation reduce the risk of lawsuits?
2. What components of nursing care must be included in the nurse's documentation to meet legal requirements?

Linking the exemplar of documentation with the concept of quality improvement:

3. How is nursing documentation used to assess the quality of nursing care delivered?
4. How can incomplete documentation result in a negative evaluation of the quality of nursing care delivered?

REFER Go to Pearson MyLab Nursing and eText

REFLECT Apply Your Knowledge

Kelly Riley is a 23-year-old nurse from a small, rural community. Kelly graduated from nursing school a few months ago and took a job working on a general medical–surgical inpatient unit at the local hospital. Her goal is to eventually work in an adult intensive care unit. She recently received a sign-on bonus and looks forward to buying her first new car.

Kelly has a busy week because of increased patient loads. She has seven to eight patients of her own, and she has trouble managing her charting with all the patient care she has to do. She ends up staying up to 2 hours after each shift to get the charting done. Kelly's manager, Pat, talks with her about this and reviews the importance of point-of-care charting. The feedback he gives Kelly is generally positive.

1. Why is Kelly's manager trying to improve her point-of-care charting?
2. What are the potential drawbacks of waiting until the end of the shift to document care?
3. What strategies might you suggest to Kelly to help her improve point-of-care charting during a busy shift?

Exemplar 38.D Reporting

Exemplar Learning Outcomes

38.D Analyze reporting as it relates to communication.

- Explain the purposes of reporting.
- Describe the handoff report.
- Outline the SBAR technique of communication.
- Describe the process of telephone communication.
- Summarize the care plan conference.

Exemplar Key Terms

Change-of-shift report, *2617*
Handoff, *2617*
Handoff communication, *2617*
Reporting, *2616*
SBAR, *2617*
SHARE, *2617*

Overview

Reporting is the communication of specific information to a designated individual or group. Oral or written reports, such as change-of-shift or telephone reports, should be concise and include only pertinent information. Reporting can also occur in settings such as nursing rounds and care team meetings, when nurses and other members of the healthcare team share information about the patient's care.

The national CLAS standards (Office of Minority Health, 2018) have established a framework for agencies to follow to ensure that reporting mechanisms within agencies consider culturally and linguistically appropriate services at all levels of communication throughout the agency. For example, consider a healthcare agency located in an urban area serving English-speaking, Spanish-speaking, and Arabic-speaking patients. As the agency employs more native Spanish and Arabic speakers to meet the needs of its patients, the agency must have policies and procedures in place to ensure that nurses and other HCPs who engage in reporting both in person (e.g., handoff reports) or through electronic means are able to communicate successfully with each other. Agencies must also ensure that communication and reporting mechanisms include opportunities for nurses and other providers to report pertinent cultural information about patients' healthcare and cultural needs.

Handoff Communication

Ineffective communication is the primary cause of sentinel events, which are serious, unexpected events (The Joint Commission, 2020). As a result, hospitals are required to implement a standardized approach to "handing off" communication. **Handoff** is defined as "the transfer of information (along with authority and responsibility) during transitions in care across the continuum. It includes an opportunity to ask questions, clarify, and confirm" (Agency for Healthcare Research and Quality [AHRQ], 2020). Hospital handoffs occur at many times, including but not limited to when a patient is transferred between units, at the change of shift, and at discharge (AHRQ, 2019). The **handoff communication** is a verbal or written exchange of information that encompasses the nursing care that has been provided along with all members of the healthcare team who have cared for the patient during the relevant time period (AHRQ, 2020).

The handoff process involves two groups, the senders and the receivers. The senders are the caregivers who are transmitting patient information and releasing care; the receivers are the caregivers who are accepting the patient and the patient's information.

The SHARE method can be used to accomplish a successful handoff:

Standardize critical content.

Hardwire within your system.

Allow opportunity to ask questions.

Reinforce quality and measurement.

Educate and coach.

The Joint Commission Center for Transforming Healthcare (2020) provides several items that can be helpful in the handoff communication process. The goal of the Hand-off Communications Targeted Solutions Tool (TST) is "to assist health care organizations with the process of passing necessary and critical information about a patient from one caregiver to the next, or from one team of caregivers to another, to prevent miscommunication-related errors" (The Joint Commission Center for Transforming Healthcare, 2020).

>> **Stay Current:** For more information regarding the handoff communication process, visit https://www.aorn.org/about-aorn/aorn-newsroom/or-exec-newsletter/2017/2017-articles/hand-off-communication-5-areas-of-focus-for-safer-care.

Change-of-Shift Report

Nurses use a type of handoff communication known as a **change-of-shift report** to provide nurses on the next shift with a concise summary of patient needs and details of care to be given. Change-of-shift reports are essential to ensure continuity of care and safety for patients.

Change-of-shift reports occur in person at the bedside, elsewhere on the unit, in writing, or by audio or video recording. Face-to-face reporting, whether at the bedside or elsewhere on the unit, allows the nurse who is coming on shift to ask questions during report. A thorough change-of-shift report:

- Follows a specific order (such as by room number on the unit or, if at the bedside, by following the SBAR format).
- Provides essential identifying information for each patient (e.g., name, room number, bed designation).
- For patients new to the nurse, provides the reason for admission diagnosis (or diagnoses) the patient's current status, and any diagnostic tests or interventions that occurred in the past 24 hours.
- Includes significant changes in the patient's condition and presents the information in a specific order (i.e., assessment, nursing diagnoses, interventions, outcomes, and evaluation). For example, "Mr. James Kelly said he had burning pain, rated at 7, at his abdominal incision site at 1300 hours. Inspection revealed an intact incision with no signs of inflammation or drainage. Incisional pain is related to the surgical procedure. Administration of morphine 2 mg IV at 1310 provided relief."
- Provides exact information, such as "Ms. Sara Jenkins received ondansetron 2 mg IV at 1600 hours," not "Ms. Jenkins received some ondansetron during the evening."
- Reports patients' need for holistic care. For example, a patient who has just learned that a recommended treatment carries some substantial risks needs time to talk about his feelings before discussing the next stages of care, and another patient requires care to be planned around specific prayer times.
- Includes newly initiated HCP orders.
- Provides a summary of newly admitted patients, their diagnosis, age, general health status, status of prescribed orders and independent interventions, and information about family members or other support persons.
- Reports on patients who were transferred or discharged from the unit prior to shift change.
- Clearly states priorities of care and care that will be needed immediately after the shift begins. For example, in an 0700 report, the nurse might say, "Carl Sullivan's vital signs are due at 0730, and his IV bag will need to be replaced by 0815."
- Is concise. Do not elaborate on background data, routine care, or unit standards (such as vital signs taken per protocol).

SBAR

The SBAR technique, which was developed by the U.S. Navy, provides a framework for safe, efficient communication between members of the healthcare team. SBAR stands for:

Situation

Background

Assessment

Recommendation.

The tool provides an easy way to develop team cohesion and create a culture of patient safety (Institute for Healthcare Improvement, 2020). In the Situation step, the nurse provides a concise statement of the problem. In the Background step, the nurse relates information relevant to the situation. In the Assessment step, the nurse provides an analysis and consideration of options. And in the Recommendation step, the nurse provides a recommendation based on the relevant evidence. Using the SBAR technique during handoffs, transfers, and shift changes will reduce miscommunications that have the potential to cause patient harm, including those surrounding cultural considerations in patient care, as seen in the clinical example below. Improving communication skills among team members overall, and specifically in critical clinical situations, will help the nurse manager and the team improve patient safety and, in turn, team satisfaction.

Clinical Example H

Thomas Fullerton is a nurse in the postoperative recovery wing of a hospital. He is monitoring the vital signs of Mrs. Hussein, a 41-year-old woman who is recovering from a percutaneous endoscopic gastrostomy (PEG) placement earlier today. Thomas notices that Mrs. Hussein is having increasing dyspnea and complaining of chest pain, so he decides to alert the patient's HCP. Thomas provides the information in SBAR format. He calls the physician and states the situation: "Mrs. Hussein is experiencing dyspnea and complaining of chest pain." Then, he provides background: "Mrs. Hussein had a PEG placement today, and a few hours ago she started complaining of chest pain. Her pulse is 122 and her blood pressure is 129 over 53. She is short of breath and restless." Then, Thomas provides his assessment: "I think she may be having a cardiac event or a pulmonary embolism." And finally, his recommendation: "I recommend that you see the patient as soon as possible and that we start her on O_2 stat." See a condensed version of Thomas's SBAR report in **Table 38.9** ».

Critical Thinking Questions

1. Would you have provided any information that Thomas did not? Why or why not?
2. Is the SBAR an appropriate format in which to convey this information? Can you think of any mistakes that Thomas avoided by using SBAR?
3. Explain why this phone call between Thomas and the HCP is a type of handoff event.

TABLE 38.9 Example of an SBAR Report

Phase	Action
Situation	Provide description of the patient's dyspnea and chest pain.
Background	Provide an explanation that the patient had a PEG placement this morning and that relatively recently she began complaining of chest pain.
Assessment	Provide an assessment that the patient is most likely having a cardiac event or pulmonary embolism.
Recommendation	Provide a recommendation that the physician see the patient immediately and that the patient be started on an O_2 stat.

Sources: Based on Missouri Department of Health and Senior Services (2017); Shahid and Thomas (2018).

» **Stay Current:** Learn more about the SBAR technique by reading the article titled "SBAR Tool: Situation–Background–Assessment–Recommendation" at http://www.ihi.org/resources/Pages/Tools/SBARToolkit.aspx.

SAFETY ALERT Employing effective communication techniques is essential throughout the nursing process, but communication may be most critical during reporting situations. If nurses do not receive adequate information from patients, provide the healthcare team with relevant details, and communicate effectively in groups, the patient's health may be jeopardized. Reporting techniques such as SBAR and handoff protocols are standardized techniques that streamline reporting safety.

Telephone Communication

Telephone Reports

Nurses and other members of the healthcare team frequently provide reports of patient issues by telephone when the patient experiences a change in status or a significant diagnostic finding is returned that indicates the need to consult quickly with the HCP or another member of the healthcare team.

When receiving a telephone report, the nurse should document the date and time and note the name of the individual providing the information and subject of the information received. The nurse should repeat the information back to the caller to confirm understanding before either ends the call.

When delivering a telephone report to a patient's HCP or another member of the care team (such as the wound or ostomy nurse), the nurse making report must be concise and accurate. Telephone reports generally include the patient's name and medical diagnosis, significant changes in nursing assessment, current vital signs, pertinent laboratory data, and related nursing interventions. The nurse should make the report while the patient's healthcare record is open and accessible in case there any additional questions. After reporting is complete, the nurse should document the date, time, and content of the call.

Telephone Orders

Healthcare providers may order treatments or therapies for a patient by telephone. Facilities have specific policies about receiving and documenting telephone orders, and most allow only registered nurses to receive telephone orders. The increased use of EHRs has reduced the use of telephone orders, as electronic transmission of orders allows for greater accuracy.

When receiving a telephone order, the nurse must *write* down or enter the complete order following facility policy and *read* it back to the primary care provider to ensure accuracy. The nurse should question any order that is ambiguous, outside of the normal parameters (e.g., an abnormally high dosage of a medication), or contraindicated by the patient's condition or other treatments. When the nurse enters the order into the patient's EHR, the nurse indicates how the order was prescribed (e.g., by using TO for telephone order) following facility policy. Once transcribed into the EHR, the primary care provider countersigns the order within the time period described by facility policy. Many facilities require that this be done within 24 hours, however, this may vary by state and agency. Guidelines for telephone and verbal orders include:

1. Know the position of the state's nursing board related to who can give and accept verbal and phone orders.
2. Follow the facility's policy and procedure regarding phone orders.
3. Ask the HCP to spell the name of the medication if you are not familiar with it.
4. Question the drug, dosage, or changes if they do not seem appropriate for the patient.
5. Write down the order or enter it into the EHR per facility policy.
6. Read the order back to the HCP. Use words instead of abbreviations.
7. Have the HCP confirm the read-back.
8. Transcribe the order onto the provider's order form, recording the date and time the order was received, and indicate it was a telephone order.
9. Sign your name and credentials as required by facility policy and the EHR database.
10. Follow agency protocol to have the HCP sign or verify the order within the required time.

Also:

- Follow facility protocols and best-practice recommendations for entering dosages (e.g., by writing out units, i.e., 15 units rather than 15 U).
- Do not accept orders made in a voice mail message. Call the HCP and follow facility protocol for accepting telephone orders.

Care Plan Conference

Care plan conferences allow the members of a healthcare team working with a specific patient to be able to share information and discuss the patient's care together in real time. They are often used for patients with high acuity and complex care needs. The patient (or family members for patients who are unable to participate) is invited. Attendance at the care plan meeting may include a social worker, pharmacist, or other professionals involved in the patient's care.

Care plan conferences that engage in respectful, nonjudgmental acceptance of all team members are more effective than meetings in which there is conflict or a lack of concern for others' contributions. See Module 37, Collaboration, for more information.

REVIEW Reporting

RELATE Link the Concepts and Exemplars

Linking the exemplar of reporting with the concept of legal issues:

1. What are the legal obligations of a nurse who is providing change-of-shift reporting to the oncoming nurse?
2. How can the nurse ensure that all legal obligations have been met when accepting telephone orders from the primary provider?

Linking the exemplar of reporting with the concept of safety:

3. How does handoff communication contribute to patient safety?
4. In providing a telephone report to a primary care provider because of a patient's sudden change in condition, what information should be included to maintain the safe care of the patient?

REFER Go to Pearson MyLab Nursing and eText

REFLECT Apply Your Knowledge

Marjorie Newman, a 64-year-old woman, was admitted to the coronary care unit (CCU) with a diagnosis of acute anterior myocardial infarction. Her condition has remained stable, and she is to be transferred to the telemetry unit tomorrow or sooner if the CCU bed is required for an acutely ill patient. The nurse assigned to her care is called to the monitors by the monitor technician because Ms. Newman has suddenly begun having frequent premature ventricular contractions (PVCs). When the nurse enters Ms. Newman's room, she assesses the patient and finds her to be short of breath, experiencing severe left-sided chest pain radiating to the left arm, and very diaphoretic. Vital signs are T 98.6°F; P 108 beats/min and irregular; R 28/min; and BP 92/44 mmHg. The nurse analyzes Ms. Newman's rhythm strip and finds elevated ST segments, tachycardia, with 10–14 PVCs per minute. A coworker agrees to stay with Ms. Newman and monitor her condition while the nurse assigned to her care calls the primary care provider.

1. What information would the nurse report to the primary care provider when calling to notify of the change in the patient's condition?
2. Why did the nurse have a coworker stay with the patient while calling the primary care provider?
3. How should the nurse report Ms. Newman's condition in the SBAR portion of the handoff report?

References

Agency for Healthcare Research and Quality (AHRQ). (2019). *Handoffs and signouts*. https://psnet.ahrq.gov/primer/handoffs-and-signouts

Agency for Healthcare Research and Quality (AHRQ). (2020). *Pocket Guide: TeamSTEPPS*. https://www.ahrq.gov/teamstepps/instructor/essentials/pocketguide.html

American Nurses Association (ANA). (2015). *Code of ethics for nurses with interpretive statements*. Author.

Ao, W. (2019, May 15). Nonverbal communication in different cultures. *Freely Magazine*. https://www.freelymagazine.com/2019/05/15/nonverbal-communication-different-cultures

Arnold, E. C., & Boggs, K. U. (2019). *Interpersonal relationships: Professional communication skills for nurses* (8th ed.). Elsevier Saunders.

Auvil, C. A., & Silver, B. W. (1984). Therapist self-disclosure: When is it appropriate? *Perspectives in Psychiatric Care*, *22*(2), 57–61.

Berman, A., Snyder, S. J., & Frandsen, G. (2021). *Kozier and Erb's fundamentals of nursing: Concepts, processes, and practice* (11th ed.). Pearson

Brenner, L. (2018). *How to use good communication skills for cross-cultural diversity*. Chron. https://work.chron.com/use-good-communication-skills-crosscultural-diversity-8317.html

Centers for Disease Control and Prevention (CDC). (2020). *Patient-centered care for transgendered people: Recommended practices for health care settings*. https://www.cdc.gov/hiv/clinicians/transforming-health/health-care-providers/affirmative-care.html#

The Conversation. (2019). *Why do Muslim women wear a hijab?* https://theconversation.com/why-do-muslim-women-wear-a-hijab-109717?gclid=CjwKCAjwgOGCBhAlEiwA7FUXkrcHR7-op0eZP2fRx3vyArETMPKDFUZ8NsB516-l4-EdruWdNbgkxyxoC-zEQAvD_BwE

Chang, Y. S., Coxon, K., Portela, A. G., Furuta, M, & Bick, D. (2018). Interventions to support effective communication between maternity care staff and women in labour: A mixed-methods systematic review. *Midwifery*, 59, 4–16. https://doi.org/10.1016.j.midw.2017.12.014

Dendere, R., Slade, C., Burton-Jones, A., Sullivan, C., Staib, A., & Janda, M. (2019). Patient portals facilitating engagement with inpatient electronic medical records: A systematic review. *Journal of Medical Internet Research*, *21*(4), e12779. https://doi.org/10.2196/12779

Egan, G., & Reese, R. J. (2018). *The skilled helper: A problem-management and opportunity-development approach to helping* (11th ed.). Cengage Learning

Eventus. (2020). *Effective vs. ineffective teams*. https://www.eventus.co.uk/effective-vs-ineffective-teams/

EveryNurse.org. (2019, June 4). Seven steps to becoming a more culturally sensitive nurse. EveryNurse. https://everynurse.org/blog/7-steps-culturally-sensitive-nurse/

Evesham, F. (2017). Therapeutic and non therapeutic communication. *Healthfully*. https://healthfully.com/188795-therapeutic-and-non-therapeutic-communication.html

Goodtherapy.org. (2019). *Pregnancy and childbirth*. GoodTherapy. https://www.goodtherapy.org/learn-about-therapy/issues/pregnancy-and-birthing

Guido, G. W. (2019). *Legal and ethical issues in nursing* (7th ed.). Pearson.

HealthIT.gov. (2019). *What are the differences between electronic medical records, electronic health records, and personal health records*. Office of the National Coordinator for Health Information Technology. https://www.healthit.gov/faq/what-are-differences-between-electronic-medical-records-electronic-health-records-and-personal

Huber, D. (2017). *Leadership and nursing care management* (6th ed.). Elsevier Saunders.

Institute for Healthcare Improvement. (2020). *SBAR tool: Situation-background-assessment-recommendation*. https://www.ihi.org/resources/Pages/Tools/SBARToolkit.aspx

InSync Healthcare Solutions. (2020, Mar. 25). *What is EMAR?* https://www.insynchcs.com/blog/emar

International Institute of Minnesota. (2020). *Body language and personal space*. https://iimn.org/publication/finding-common-ground/culture-at-work/body-language-and-personal-space/

The Joint Commission. (2020). *Sentinel event alert 58: Inadequate hand-off communication*. https://www.jointcommission.org/resources/patient-safety-topics/sentinel-event/sentinel-event-alert-newsletters/sentinel-event-alert-58-inadequate-hand-off-commuication/

The Joint Commission Center for Transforming Healthcare. (2020). *Hand-off communication*. https://www.centerfortransforminghealthcare.org/improvement-topics/hand-off-communications/

Koutoukidis, G., & Stainton, K. (2020). *Tabbner's nursing care* (8th ed.). Elsevier.

Lockwood, W. (2019). *Documentation: Accurate and legal*. RN.org. https://www.rn.org/courses/coursematerial-66.pdf

Lotfi, M., Zamanzadeh, V., Valizadeh, L., & Khajehgoodari, M. (2019). Assessment of nurse-patient communication and patient satisfaction from nursing care. *Nursing Open*, 6(3), 1189–1196. https://doi.org/10.1002/nop2.316

Lukic, M. (2020, August 6). *Top 10 characteristics of effective teamwork*. Active Collab. https://activecollab.com/blog/collaboration/top-10-characteristics-of-effective-teamwork

Mayo Clinic. (2020). *Being assertive: Reduce stress, communicate better*. https://www.mayoclinic.com/healthy-lifestyle/stress-management/assertive/art-20044644

Missouri Department of Health and Senior Services. (2017). *Best practice: Physician relationships*. https://health.mo.gov/seniors/hcbs/pdf/physiciannursetrack.pdf

National Institute on Aging (NIA). (2017). *Tips for improving communication with older patients*. https://www.nia.nih.gov/health/tips-improving-communication-older-patients

Office of Minority Health. (2018). *The national CLAS standards*. https://www.minorityhealth.hhs.gov/omh/browse.aspx?lvl=2&lvlid=53

Oxford Reference. (2020). *Overview: Interpersonal zones*. https://www.oxfordreference.com/view/10.1093/oi/authority.20110803100008289

Pandian, V., Morris, L. L., Brodsky, M. B., Lynch, J., Walsh, B., Rushton, C., . . . & Lami, L. (2020). Critical care guidance for tracheostomy care during the COVID-19 pandemic: A global, multidisciplinary approach. *American Journal of Critical Care*, 29(6), e116–e117.

Perez-Francisco, D. H., Duarte-Climents, G., del Rosario-Melian, J. M., Gomez-Salgado, J., Romero-Martin, M., & Sanchez-Gomez, M. B. (2020). Influence of workload on primary care nurses' health and burnout, patients' safety, and quality of care: Integrative review. *Healthcare*, *8*(1), 12. https://doi.org/10.3390/healthcare8010012

Potter, M. L., & Moller, M. D. (2019). *Psychiatric-mental health nursing: From suffering to hope* (2nd ed.) Pearson Education.

Practical Nursing.org. (2020). *Five tips for providing effective patient education*. https://www.practicalnursing.org/five-tips-providing-effective-patient-education

Prescott, H. C., & Rice, T. W. (2020). Corticosteroids in COVID-19 ARDS. Evidence and hope during the pandemic. *JAMA Network*, 324(13), 1292–1295. https://doi.org/10.1001/jama.2020.16747

Raising Children Network Australia. (2020). *Baby cues and baby body language: A guide*. https://raisingchildren.net.au/babies/connecting-communicating/communicating/baby-cues

Robeznieks, A. (2018). *The overlooked benefits of medical scribes*. American Medical Association. https://www.ama-assn.org/practice-management/sustainability/overlooked-benefits-medical-scribes

Shahid, S., & Thomas, S. (2018). Situation, background, assessment, recommendation (SBAR) communication tool for handoff in health care – A narrative review. *Safety in Health*, 4(7). https://doi.org/10.1186/s40886-018-0073-1

Sibiya, M. N. (2018). *Effective communication in nursing*. Intechopen. https://doi.org/10.5772/intechopen.74995

Sousa, L. M. M., Marques-Vieira, C. A. M., Antunes, A. V., Frade, M. G., Severino, S. P. S., & Valentim, O. S. (2019). Humor intervention in the nurse–patient interaction. *Revista Brasileria de Enfermagem*, 72(4), 1078–1085. https://doi.org/10.1509/0034-7167-2018-0609

Stans, S. E., Dalemans, R. J. P., Roentgen, U. R., Smeets, H. W. H., & Beurskens, A. J. H. M. (2018). Who said dialogue conversations are easy?: The communication between communication vulnerable people and health-care professionals: A qualitative study. *Health Expectations: An International Journal of Public Participation in Health Care and Health Policy*, *21*(5), 848–857. https://doi.org/10.1111/hex.12679

Think Cultural Health. (n.d.). *National standards for culturally and linguistically appropriate services (CLAS) in health and health care*. U. S. Department of Health and Human Services. https://thinkculturalhealth.hhs.gov/assets/pdfs/EnhancedNationalCLASStandards.pdf

Thompson, V. S. (2018, March 27). *Cultural and linguistically appropriate services in health care (CLAS standards)*. Gateway Region YMCA. https://gwrymca.org/blog/cultural-and-linguistically-appropriate-services-health-care-clas-standards

U.S. Department of State. (n.d.). *So you're an American? A guide to answering difficult questions abroad*. https://www.state.gov/courses/answeringdifficultquestions/htm/app.htm?p=module3_p2.htm

USF Health. (2020). *Federal mandates for healthcare: Digital record-keeping requirements for public and private healthcare providers*. https://www.usfhealthonline.com/resources/healthcare/electronic-medical-records-mandate

Vera, M. (2020). *Communication in nursing: Documenting and reporting*. Nurseslabs. https://nurseslabs.com/communication-in-nursing

Vikrant, K. (2019). *Seminar on critical pathway* [PowerPoint slides]. https://www.slideshare.net/kulthevikrantcritical-pathway-for-nursing-administration

Wilder, A. (2020). *Gender differences in language development and disorder*. DLD and Me. https://dldandme.org/gender-differences-in -language-development-and-disorder

Wofford, P. (2019). *4 essential skills that will make you the best nurse*. Nurse.org. https://nurse.org/articles/4-best-nursing-soft-skills

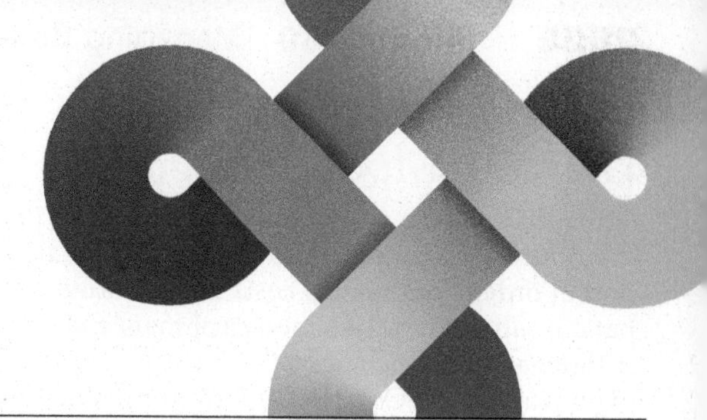

Module 39
Managing Care

Module Outline and Learning Outcomes

The Concept of Managing Care

Managed Care and Care Delivery Models

39.1 Analyze frameworks for delivering care.

Concepts Related to Managing Care

39.2 Outline the relationship between managing care and other concepts.

Managing Care Exemplars

Exemplar 39.A Case Management

39.A Analyze case management as it relates to managing care.

Exemplar 39.B Cost-Effective Care

39.B Analyze cost-effective care as it relates to managing care.

Exemplar 39.C Delegation

39.C Analyze delegation as it relates to managing care.

Exemplar 39.D Leadership and Management

39.D Analyze leadership and management as they relate to managing care.

» The Concept of Managing Care

Concept Key Terms

Case management, **2622**
Case method, **2623**
Differentiated practice, **2623**
Functional method, **2623**
Licensed practical nurses (LPNs), **2623**
Managed care, **2621**
Patient-focused care, **2622**
Primary nursing, **2624**
Registered nurses (RNs), **2623**
Shared governance, **2623**
Team nursing, **2623**
Unlicensed assistive personnel (UAP), **2623**

Managed care is a healthcare delivery system that focuses on decreasing costs and improving outcomes for groups of patients. In this type of system, care is carefully planned from the initial contact with the patient through the conclusion of the patient's specific health problem. Although exact methods used to manage care differ depending on the delivery model used, the overarching goals of lower costs and better outcomes remain constant.

Managed care is an important topic in nursing practice because it shapes numerous aspects of the healthcare system. As payers search for ways to better contain rising costs, they continue to develop new incentives and standards, which in turn create trends in healthcare. Some of these trends have positive consequences, such as an increased focus on preventive care. Others have the potential to create negative consequences, such as increases in hospital readmission following early release.

Within the managed care system, nurses may be involved in a variety of processes aimed at promoting high-quality care for patients while maintaining cost effectiveness. Delegation is one such process; by distributing routine tasks to other staff members, nurses are able to devote more time to skills unique to or required of the registered nurse role. Care coordination and case management are other examples. Care coordination is a collaborative effort in which an interprofessional team provides cohesive care as a patient proceeds from hospitalization to recovery and health maintenance. The case manager coordinates and facilitates patient use of healthcare services in the long term. These processes eliminate redundancy and promote consistency, therefore lowering costs and improving quality. Successful delegation, care coordination, and case management depend on the ability of nursing leaders and managers to inspire staff, monitor patients, and adhere to organizational requirements. As a result, nurses' interpersonal skills are at the heart of good managed care.

Understanding the basics behind managed care is important for nurses as they move through their careers, no matter their level of leadership or managerial responsibility. Each healthcare organization uses a specific model and understanding of managed care, and each organization layers its own goals, ethical standards, and legal requirements into its model of choice. Therefore, as nurses move from one organization or setting to another, they must have knowledge of these models in order to successfully care for patients and mature in their profession. With this requirement in mind, this module and its exemplars introduce the many facets of managed care.

Managed Care and Care Delivery Models

Managed care is a system of healthcare used to coordinate distribution of resources to a subscribed patient population in order to minimize costs and increase efficiency and patient satisfaction. Two models of managed care are health maintenance organizations (HMOs) and preferred provider organizations (PPOs). HMOs incorporate the use of a gatekeeper to track provided services and act as a referral agent for the patient population. PPOs allow patients to select from a larger network of physicians without having to use direct referrals to specialists.

Nurses incorporate the nursing process in providing evidence-based care as they work within the managed care system. The nurse's work has important implications for direct patient care, coordination of care, and cost containment. For example, the nurse knows that the patient has an order for physical therapy and swallowing evaluations but also knows the patient tires easily. By scheduling the swallowing test and the physical therapist at different times, the nurse can make sure that neither professional wastes time waiting on the other and that the patient has time to rest in between evaluations.

Effective managed care requires the abilities to prioritize, identify clinical pathways, and create concept maps and care plans (see Module 36, Clinical Decision Making). The nurse must also understand patients' rights (Module 44, Ethics) and advance directives (Module 49, Legal Issues) and must be committed to quality improvement (Module 50, Quality Improvement).

From an organizational perspective, managed care has been embraced as a model for healthcare reform, but some people question the application of a business approach to something as personal and important as healthcare. Despite these concerns, many organizations have effectively combined managed care principles with a number of delivery models. As described in the following sections, each of these models requires nurses to draw upon their skills in different ways as they seek to promote patient well-being while controlling the costs of care.

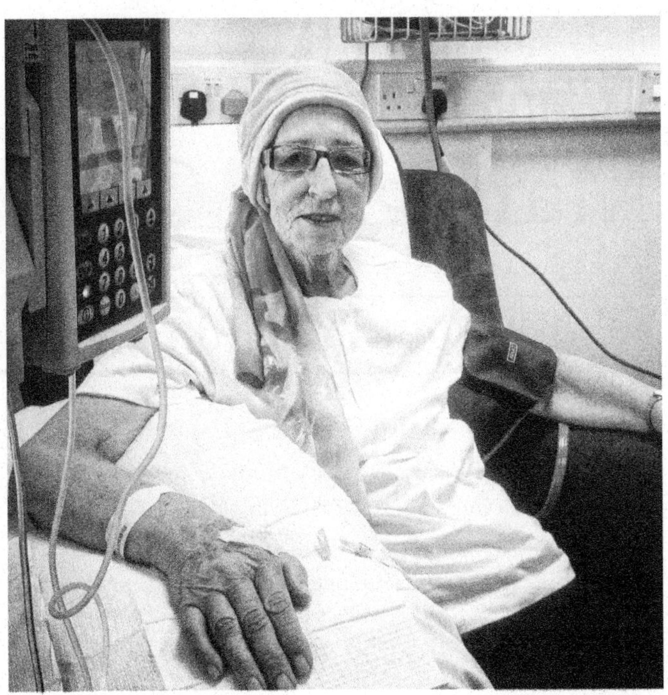

Figure 39.1 » Case management usually focuses on ongoing care of patients with chronic conditions or long-lasting problems, such as this patient who is receiving chemotherapy for cancer.

Source: CaroleGomez/E+/Getty Images.

Case Management

Case management is the coordination of patient care over time using the combination of health and social services necessary to meet the individual patient's needs. Case management is a fundamental element of many managed care systems. Case management offers intensive services, so it is most effectively and efficiently used for patients with multiple or complex chronic health problems (**Figure 39.1 »**). For example, a patient with chronic obstructive pulmonary disease (COPD) who has just had hip replacement surgery would benefit from case management beginning at admission and continuing at the rehabilitation center or the skilled nursing facility to which the patient is discharged from the hospital.

Generally, case management involves interprofessional teams that collectively assume responsibility for planning and assessing the needs of groups of patients. These teams are also responsible for coordinating, implementing, and evaluating patient care from preadmission through discharge or transfer and recuperation. Each team is led by a case manager who is a nurse, social worker, or other appropriate professional. In some areas of the United States, case managers are referred to as discharge planners. These individuals may work for a patient's healthcare provider (HCP) (e.g., clinic, hospital, or long-term care facility), insurance company, or perhaps even the patient's employer.

Patient-Focused Care

Patient-focused care organizes the framework of healthcare services with the patient at the center. Patient-focused or patient-centered care ensures that patients (and their families or caregivers) are integral to planning and making decisions about care.

In patient-focused care, the nurse takes time to learn about the patient's lifestyle, habits, and family. This includes being sensitive to diverse religious or cultural preferences. These preferences can impact diet, activity, and health practices, thus affecting patient adherence to the care regimen. After gathering the necessary information about the patient's way of life, the nurse works with the patient to develop a plan of care that addresses both health and personal needs. As part of this plan, the nurse helps the patient acquire the knowledge and skills necessary to manage the health condition and make informed choices. The patient-focused model recognizes it is critical for patients to retain autonomy and dignity while healthcare decisions are being made to improve health outcomes (Burton, 2018).

SAFETY ALERT With patient-focused care, the nurse should seek to honor the patient's preferences to the greatest degree possible. Still, the nurse has a duty to "do no harm." At no point should the nurse agree to a request that will potentially jeopardize the patient's well-being. Instead, the nurse should carefully and nonjudgmentally inform the patient of the risks associated with the requested practice or intervention.

Differentiated Practice

Differentiated practice is a system that uses academic credentialing, clinical training, and expertise to differentiate how roles are assigned. This practice model organizes the various roles/job descriptions (licensed vocational nurse/licensed practical nurse, registered nurse, and nurse practitioner) in nursing practice to facilitate improved patient outcomes. Determination of best practice includes the identification of skill sets attributable to each level of nursing. The ability to delegate care is specified based on established nursing competencies at the organizational level. By differentiating practice in this manner, healthcare organizations ensure that nurses are delivering high-quality, top-of-license care and not spending time on tasks (such as changing the bed linens or assisting the patient to the toilet) that may be assigned to staff who are unlicensed or at a lower level of licensure. Differentiation helps maximize the quality and affordability of care.

Shared Governance

The **shared governance** model focuses on the key element of "sharing" as being the driving framework between bedside nurses and nursing leaders to affect clinical decision making and allocation of resources to improve patient outcomes (McKnight & Moore, 2020). By using a shared approach, nurses become more invested at the organizational level. Shared decision making results in increased nursing satisfaction, which in turn leads to improved patient outcomes (McKnight & Moore, 2020).

Case Method

The **case method** focuses on the assignment of a single nurse to provide all aspects of patient care and care coordination during the designated shift. This model assumes that the nurse utilizes nursing process (assessment, nursing diagnoses, implementation, planning, and evaluation) in the coordination of care for all assigned patients. Primary care nursing was derived from the case method and further defines elements of patient complexity to establish nursing assignments with the goal of minimizing the number of patients assigned to a nurse to promote best practice (Sharafi, Chamanzari, Pouresmail, Rajabpour, & Bazzi, 2018). The case method is often used in high acuity settings, such as emergency departments and intensive care units (**Figure 39.2** »).

SAFETY ALERT Information gaps often develop when patients are transferred from one facility to another, such as when a patient moves from the hospital to a rehabilitation facility. They may also occur during nursing shift changes. Communication breakdown during the transfer or shift-change process can result in life-threatening situations for the patient. To help prevent such situations, be sure to carefully and completely document all care provided to the patient, as well as to verbally communicate with a patient's new nursing staff whenever possible.

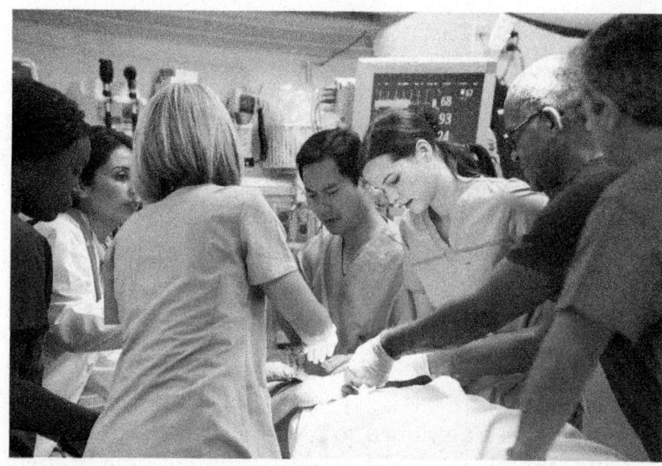

Figure 39.2 » The case method is often used in emergency departments.

Source: Shutterstock.

Functional Method

The **functional method** focuses on tasks as the primary factor in delivery of care by nurses to patients. Efficiency is the core element, with staff members who have less professional education than the nurse providing care with less complex requirements. Although this approach is economical and efficient, it can easily result in fragmented care (with multiple staff members providing patient care on a single shift) and may not capture tasks that are more difficult to qualify and assign, such as responding to patient anxiety or promoting culturally competent care.

Team Nursing

Team nursing focuses on the delivery of care to a group of patients by a professional nursing team that is typically led by a registered nurse. Depending on the type of available nurse staffing at an institution, a nursing team may include:

- **Registered nurses (RNs)**, who are specially licensed and trained to deliver direct patient care, including patient assessment, identification of health problems, and development and coordination of care
- **Licensed practical nurses (LPNs)** or licensed vocational nurses (LVNs), who provide direct patient care under the direction of an RN, physician, or other licensed practitioner
- **Unlicensed assistive personnel (UAP)**, sometimes called *assistive personnel* or *healthcare staff*, who assume delegated aspects of basic patient care such as bathing, assisting with feeding, and collecting specimens. UAP include certified nurse assistants, hospital attendants, nurse technicians, and orderlies.

In team nursing, the assigned team leader (the RN) is responsible for the overall care of the group of patients and uses delegation principles as needed to coordinate care between members of the team. Depending on the acuity of the patient group and adequate staffing, team nursing can be an efficient approach in the delivery of care to patients.

Primary Nursing

In the **primary nursing** model, the RN oversees the comprehensive care for the assigned patient(s) (**Figure 39.3 ›››**). Primary nursing focuses on best practice and patient acuity to coordinate and implement consistency of care across the length of stay for a patient. The primary nurse coordinates the patient's care and is responsible for coordinating information and facilitating care with the other members of the interprofessional care team.

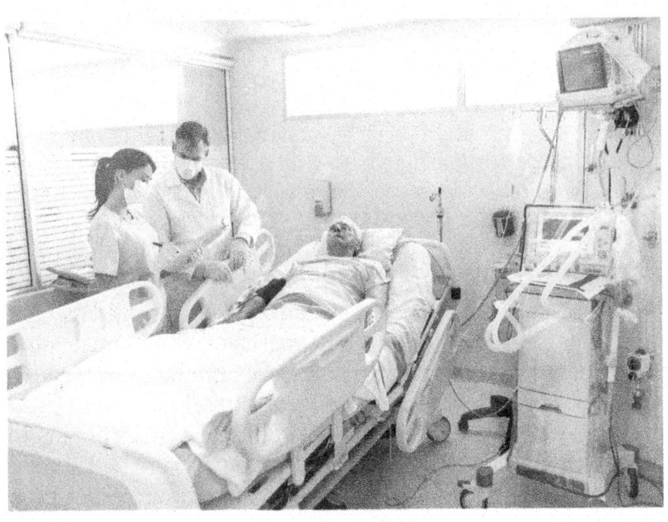

Figure 39.3 ››› The primary nursing model is often used in intensive care units.
Source: Andresr/E+/Getty Images.

Concepts Related to Managing Care

Managed care is designed to provide cost-effective, high-quality care for groups of patients from the time of their initial contact with the healthcare system through the conclusion of their health problem. Managed care relies on collaboration among the patient, the patient's family, and HCPs. Care coordination and case management are significant components of managed care.

Communication is a key concept in managed care, and it encompasses both communication within the healthcare team and communication between the care team and the patient. Clear communication among nurses, doctors, and other care providers ensures continuity in patient care, improving the patient's perception and experience of care and eliminating costly duplications. Communication among team members and patients creates a relationship based in trust and helps patients be informed and active participants in the care they receive.

Evidence-Based Practice

Nursing Ratio, Patient Outcomes, and Cost Effectiveness

Problem

The nursing ratio (i.e., the number of patients assigned to one nurse) in inpatient settings has long been thought to impact patient outcomes. Seminal research provided by the Institute of Medicine in 2010, now known as the National Academy of Medicine, determined that it is not only the *number* of nurses but their academic *qualifications* and *experience* that can impact care (Paulson, 2018). Addressing issues associated with the nursing ratio has the potential to influence the cost of care, which is a concern for organizations that adhere to the principles of managed care.

Evidence

Using objective measures such as the number of patients per nurse or the number of nursing hours per patient day, researchers have attempted to measure the impact of nursing ratios on patient outcomes. Relevant factors examined include patient acuity/complexity, designated levels of care facilities, and academic/clinical training of nursing staff as having an impact on patient morbidity and mortality (Aiken, Clarke, Cheung, Sloane, & Silber, 2003; Driscoll et al., 2017; Lee et al., 2017; Livanos, 2018). Two additional factors are the nursing shortage and the number of nurses who may be nearing retirement. Research indicates that there are more nurses are nearing the age of retirement while demand for nurses is increasing, both at the bedside as well as in different types of specialty nursing (e.g., psychiatric, geriatric, and pediatric nursing). The nursing shortage has only been exacerbated by the COVID-19 pandemic in 2020 (Avant Healthcare, 2020; Juraschek, Zhang, Ranganathan, & Lin, 2019). In the face of the pandemic, current research has shown that nursing shortages have contributed to further stress and burnout as nurses deliver frontline care under harrowing conditions (Lasater et al., 2020).

Although 14 states have regulations that address nurse staffing, only California mandates nurse–patient ratios in hospital settings (Advanced Medical Reviews, 2019). This is despite the fact that research has clearly shown that improved outcomes are consistent with adequate nurse–patient ratio (Heath, 2018). Clearly, it is important that legislative proposals include required elements of nurse–patient ratios such as minimum/maximum numbers of nurses, correlation with patient acuity levels, regulation of unlicensed staff to perform activities based on competencies and standards, recognition of appropriate training for nurses, and enforcement of prescribed ratios at all times (National Nurses United, 2020).

Finding the right ratio of nurses to patients and the right mix of licensed and unlicensed staff has important implications for both patient care and healthcare costs. The ideal blend will vary from organization to organization, and it is affected by the care delivery model used. Organizations committed to managed care models that emphasize best patient outcomes stand to benefit from determining their ideal balance in both areas.

Critical Thinking Application

1. Evaluate how the loss of three licensed staff members from your unit might affect patient outcomes.
2. If these staff members cannot be replaced, how would you, as the unit's director, prepare the remaining licensed and unlicensed personnel to prevent the most common adverse events that result from reductions in nursing staff?
3. If these staff members cannot be replaced, what case management approach would you use to ensure that patients on your unit are adequately cared for and that their health is not jeopardized?

To provide high-quality, effective care, the nurse must have a clear understanding of the best ways to manage personal time and patient time, as well as the best ways to work with the schedules of other professionals on the care team. Flexibility and patience are key to effective time management, as is a clear understanding of a patient's care priorities. These skills are learned through practice and lead to more efficient clinical decision making. They are discussed in more detail in Module 36, Clinical Decision Making. In addition, when making clinical decisions, nurses must be aware of the types of care that will be most beneficial for patients and advocate for that care when necessary.

Nurses maintain high ethical standards as they work with other members of the healthcare team to ensure that the care provided is cost effective yet meets the patient's needs and does no harm. The nurse must also assume the role of teacher in managed care in order to educate the patient and family about the patient's acute and ongoing healthcare needs after discharge. This teaching role is especially important because it helps the patient maintain health and reduce or avoid the costs associated with an acute exacerbation or recurrence of disease or injury.

Some, but not all, of the concepts integral to managing care are shown in the Concepts Related to Managing Care chart. They are presented in alphabetical order.

Concepts Related to
Managing Care

CONCEPT	RELATIONSHIP TO MANAGING CARE	NURSING IMPLICATIONS
Advocacy	Nurses advocate to protect the rights of patients and defend patients from harm. Vulnerable populations depend on nurses to speak up for them as decisions about availability of healthcare services and resources are made.	■ Nurses work in a variety of healthcare settings with heterogeneous populations that need advocates to protect their rights. Nurse advocates empower and educate patients while managing their care.
Clinical Decision Making	Making decisions about patient care begins with analyzing assessment data to identify priorities of actions for best patient outcomes. Having a plan of care helps the nurse manage care by preventing duplication of services and communicating patient goals to other healthcare professionals.	■ Prioritizing care is a process nurses use to manage time and to establish an order for completing responsibilities and care interventions for a patient or group of patients. Competing priorities for care may mean initiating some interventions at a later time.
Communication	Communication among members of the collaborative team of HCPs is essential to ensure continuity of patient care. It also eliminates redundancy in testing and procedures. Therapeutic communication helps patients learn about their condition and the care process.	■ Nurses direct communication within the collaborative team. They facilitate patient interactions with team members and coordinate care activities. In addition, they familiarize patients with their conditions and any necessary procedures. They also listen to patient concerns and answer patient questions.
Ethics	The ethical principles of altruism, autonomy, human dignity, integrity, and social justice influence decisions made in dispersing services and resources throughout healthcare systems.	■ Nurses need to provide patient-centered care to all patients in accordance with the common ethical nursing values of being truthful, promoting good, maintaining fairness, and doing no harm.
Healthcare Systems	Delivering and managing healthcare includes coordinating services and allocating resources as a means of meeting multiple patient needs and keeping costs in check. There is a need to close the gap between financial reimbursement and advances in medical interventions.	■ Nurses work with federal, state, and local guidelines in private and public healthcare settings to provide preventive, acute, chronic, and palliative care to patients. Adaptability, flexibility, and creativity are attributes nurses use to achieve good patient outcomes.
Teaching and Learning	Educating patients about their condition and health management is essential for enabling them to maintain health and avoid future complications. Mentoring staff members with less experience and familiarizing them with the components of managed care helps improve care delivery.	■ Nurses are primarily responsible for patient teaching; as such, they lay groundwork essential for keeping patients healthy and reducing the costs of care. Nurses also play an important role in helping other staff members develop their skills, particularly when tasks are delegated to less experienced staff members.

REVIEW The Concept of Managing Care

RELATE Link the Concepts

Linking the concept of managing care with the concept of communication:

1. How does the nurse's ability to communicate effectively contribute to managing the patient's care?
2. Describe a situation in which conflict management may be necessary when managing care for a patient who requires the services of several departments within a hospital.

Linking the concept of managing care with the concept of collaboration:

Mr. Montoya, a 54-year-old man, is to be discharged from an acute care facility after removal of a metastatic brain tumor. He will receive chemotherapy intrathecally as well as intravenously. The unit clerk has scheduled follow-up appointments with Mr. Montoya's surgeon, family provider, oncologist, and neurologist as well as with the infusion therapy department. The physician has provided referrals for consultation with a dietitian, social services, and home nursing care.

3. How can the nurse prioritize care to meet Mr. Montoya's needs while also ensuring that all of the services provided (e.g., predischarge nutritional screening, social services interview, and home nursing assessment to determine home-care needs) fulfill the nurse's responsibilities to prepare him for discharge?
4. What is the nurse's role in managing Mr. Montoya's care and collaborating with the other members of the healthcare team?

REFER Go to Pearson MyLab Nursing and eText

REFLECT Apply Your Knowledge

John Seitz is the nursing director at a skilled nursing facility (SNF). He has received multiple complaints from patients and their families that care provided in one of the facility's units is inconsistent. For example, sometimes residents' trays are brought to the room, but no one helps the residents eat. Similarly, beds often go unchanged, and baths are not always provided as requested by the residents.

1. Evaluate what type of nursing model may work best in an SNF.
2. Plan how you, as the nursing director, would ensure that the appropriate model is implemented by the facility's team members.
3. What tools would you design and apply to evaluate the effectiveness of the new plan?

» Exemplar 39.A Case Management

Exemplar Learning Outcome

39.A Analyze case management as it relates to managing care.

- Describe the purpose of case management and the role of the case manager.
- Identify key elements of case management.
- Explain the need for critical pathways in the case management process.

Exemplar Key Terms

Case management, *2626*
Critical pathway, *2626*
Patient-centered medical home (PCMH), *2626*

Overview

Case management is the integration of care across various disciplines through an interconnected interprofessional approach. The goals of case management are to improve patient-care experiences, decrease costs, provide options for patient decision making, and improve the overall health of the population (Armold, 2019).

Case managers are nurses, social workers, or other healthcare professionals who coordinate care for patients across disciplines. Responsibilities of case managers generally include:

- Assessment of patient strengths and needs, including home life and family members or caregivers who help meet the needs of the patient
- Coordination of patient care
- Collaboration with other healthcare professionals to meet the patient's needs to provide cost-effective care
- Monitoring and evaluating patient progress toward mutually determined goals.

Case management models often use **critical pathways,** standardized plans of care developed for groups of patients with similar, predictable medical conditions. For example, the care team may follow a critical pathway in providing care for a patient receiving a complete knee replacement but may make adjustments to the pathway if the patient has a comorbidity such as COPD or dementia.

The Nurse as Case Manager

As mentioned previously, case management takes a variety of forms within the U.S. healthcare system. For instance, with the **patient-centered medical home (PCMH)** model, a patient's primary care provider works with the patient and family to develop a personalized plan that addresses the patient's physical and mental health needs across the lifespan. In this model, the provider's office serves as a "home base" from which the patient can access comprehensive preventive, acute, and chronic care services in a manner specific to needs, values, and cultural and linguistic preferences (Patient-Centered Primary Care Collaborative, 2020). Of course, provider-based case management also occurs in other settings. For example, hospital-based case managers plan and coordinate pre- and postdischarge care for patients with chronic or complex conditions, whereas community-based case managers work with patients in their homes to ensure they receive adequate ongoing care. In addition, many insurance companies and even some large employers have case managers on staff to control costs while obtaining better health outcomes.

Regardless of the exact setting, approximately 89% of case manager positions are filled by RNs (Armold, 2019). In order to become certified as a case manager, nurses must meet a combination of criteria including academic preparation (BS or MS degree in a health or human services area) and experiential clinical work (case manager with supervision of experience criteria) (Armold, 2019).

Nurse case managers help to coordinate all aspects of care, advocate for patients at each stage of care, and plan an overall strategy to address each patient's problems. The caseload varies depending on the clinical facility and clinical unit, with the case manager facilitating patient care, coordinating with the interprofessional team, and monitoring and evaluating patient outcomes.

Clinical decision making and critical thinking skills are crucial to the development and execution of a well-coordinated care plan. The nurse case manager assesses the patient's needs holistically to ensure that those needs are met and that the patient's independence and quality of life are maximized. The nurse case manager also explores available resources to assist the patient with achieving or maintaining homeostasis and independence, including determining what materials or equipment (such as oxygen or assistive devices) the patient may need.

Actual and potential problems should be identified during care plan development. The nurse case manager is responsible for identifying potential coordination challenges and ensuring that those challenges are addressed during the development phase. For example, challenges may arise related to a patient's religious practices, cultural beliefs and practices, or use of complementary approaches. The nurse case manager assesses for any potential conflicts and works with the patient and the healthcare team to resolve them to ensure the provision of safe, appropriate care and the best possible outcomes for the patient.

Case managers must also ensure that planned care follows standard protocols or critical pathways and evidence-based guidelines. After evaluating the patient's care needs, the nurse case manager organizes the required components of care and develops the nursing care plan in consultation with the patient and any caregivers. The care plan then serves as the nurse's framework for care coordination.

The nurse case manager initiates consultation with the interprofessional care team, recognizes the needs for referral, and obtains necessary orders. As consultations and referrals are implemented, the case manager updates the critical pathway and informs the other members of the interprofessional team. On an ongoing basis, the nurse case manager communicates with patients, family members, and members of the healthcare team to ensure that the plan is executed and continues to meet the patient's needs. It is critical that the nurse coordinator monitor the plan execution and follow up with the patient, family, and team members when adjustments are needed. When necessary, the nurse case manager revises the care plan. Changes in a patient's condition and plans to discharge or transfer the patient are automatic flags that the plan must be updated. The nurse case manager is responsible for documenting the original care plan and any modifications.

Key Elements of Case Management

Nursing case management organizes patient care by major diagnoses or *diagnosis-related groups (DRGs)*. DRGs standardize clinical diagnoses as they relate to care provision and cost reimbursement for patients with identified clinical conditions. Working within this framework, nurse case managers identify expected patient outcomes that should occur within a defined time frame and coordinate the interprofessional care necessary for patients to achieve the expected outcomes. Nurse case managers also ensure that care provided meets the legal and ethical standards of professional practice, promotes best practices alongside cost effectiveness, and uses principles of continuous quality improvement.

Research suggests that case managers should be actively involved from the time of admission to facilitate patient outcomes regardless of the setting or point of access (inpatient, outpatient, or home) (Geld, 2020).

In many cases, the need for case management is identified based on the patient being identified with one or more of several high-volume or high-risk diagnoses, such as total hip replacements on an orthopedic unit or traumatic brain injury in the emergency department. High-risk cases include those patients with multiple comorbidities, admission to an acute care unit of 3 days or more, or the need for ventilatory support or home healthcare. For example, a patient with Parkinson disease is admitted for suspected infection and deterioration of mental function likely brought on by the infection. Over the course of the 4 days it takes to identify and begin to treat the infection, he loses some functional capacity, although his cognition improves with treatment for the infection. The case manager works with the patient, his spouse, and the care team to determine whether he can be discharged home with home health and some physical and occupational therapy or if he should be discharged to a rehabilitation facility.

In summary, successful case management requires several elements:

- A qualified case manager
- A dedicated interprofessional team
- Organizational support at every level (administration, medical, and support staff)
- A quality management system (see Module 50, Quality Improvement)
- Critical pathways for patient care (see the next section).

Clinical Example A

Tanya Calder, RN, is a board-certified (NARON) case manager at an orthopedic hospital. She is currently managing 10 patients on the unit: two adults with multiple fractures due to motor-vehicle crashes; one 55-year-old with hip replacement surgery who is expected to be discharged later that evening; one older adult who just came up from the postanesthesia care unit and is recovering from knee replacement surgery; two older adults, each with a fractured hip; and four adolescent patients who required placement of pins and traction to stabilize fractures. Ms. Calder compares each patient's progress to the critical pathway for that patient and makes recommendations to the physician managing their care related to meeting specific needs.

One of the patients involved in a motor-vehicle crash sustained a traumatic brain injury as well as multiple fractures. Ms. Calder collaborates with the neurologist and the physical therapy team to optimize the patient's status in preparation for rehabilitation. She has been in discussion with the admissions coordinator for the rehabilitation facility to which the patient will be discharged. For the other patients, Ms. Calder is collaborating with physical therapy and the floor nurse to ensure their recovery is going according to plan.

Critical Thinking Questions

1. Identify the different individuals and organizations with whom Ms. Calder is collaborating. Explain why collaboration is essential to meeting a patient's needs.
2. What is the purpose of a critical pathway? What are some other names for a critical pathway?
3. In the care of patients with orthopedic injuries, explain how case management for the older adult patient might differ from that needed for the younger adult patient.

Critical Pathways

Critical pathways (also known as *care maps*, *critical paths*, *clinical pathways*, or *action plans*) provide a therapeutic plan of care based on evidence-based practice methods to help direct clinical decision making. These pathways are used in managed care systems to track patients' progress, maintain interprofessional communication, and help improve patient outcomes (Aspland, Gartner, & Harper, 2019).

Critical pathways organize standardized treatment plans into time frames and the expectation is that the patient will meet outcomes as prescribed in the critical pathway. Even though the pathway is standardized, there is room for individual variations and/or complications that may affect the ability of the patient to meet these outcomes in the specified time frame (for example, if the patient develops delirium during the inpatient stay). Variances are noted for both time frame issues and/or interventions provided to address either patient complications and/or a patient's ability to respond. All members of the interprofessional team share a vested interest in caring for the patient. Ongoing data analysis of patients receiving care using a critical pathway can contribute to the body of knowledge and help foster improvement where needed.

For the unit or floor nurse working directly with the patient, the critical pathway serves as an outline for providing care during each day or time frame. For example, the critical pathway might specify a time frame in which the postsurgical patient should be up and walking once the anesthesia wears off. If the patient is unable to meet the expected outcomes within the time frame, the nurse outlines in the critical pathway whom the nurse should notify (in this example, either the surgeon or the case manager) and next steps to take in patient care. As mentioned earlier, the case manager tracks variances for patients assigned to case management. At some point, the care team may analyze variances, especially variances that occur regularly across the group. In the same example, if multiple postoperative patients are taking longer than expected to come out of anesthesia or to begin walking following anesthesia, that issue will need to be examined and possible modifications made to the critical pathway. Typically, critical pathways identify:

- A medical diagnosis (or diagnoses)
- Anticipated interventions across disciplines (e.g., nursing care, pharmacology needs, physical or other therapy needs)
- Time frames for care (in days, hours, minutes, or visits)
- Expected patient outcomes.

All critical pathways should include the ability to identify and document variances and adjustments to the pathway based on variances.

>> **Stay Current:** Clinical pathways vary according to patient needs, agency protocols, and current best practices for care. Examples of research information related to the concept of clinical pathways can be found at the homepage of the *Journal of Clinical Pathways* (https://www.journalofclinicalpathways.com/interviews).

Case Management Across the Lifespan

Case management can yield positive results for patients of all ages and with any number of health concerns. However, some patients are more likely to benefit from case management than others. Prominent examples of such patients include at-risk pregnant women; children with congenital conditions or disabilities; children, adolescents, and adults with behavioral, intellectual, or mental health disorders or disabilities; and older adults who have chronic conditions or are approaching the end of life.

At-Risk Pregnant Women

Maternity case managers specialize in working with women who have one or more health-related, social, or economic factors in their lives that place them at increased risk for problems during pregnancy or childbirth. For example, a woman might benefit from maternity case management if she has a chronic disease, uses drugs or alcohol, is experiencing mental illness, lives in extreme poverty, and/or is involved in an abusive relationship. In such cases, the maternity case manager can help promote the health of mother and infant alike by ensuring receipt of adequate prenatal care and referring the patient to various community and government services as appropriate. The case manager also plays a critical role in educating the woman about such topics as obtaining proper nutrition and exercise during pregnancy; recognizing perinatal mood disorders; avoiding fetal exposure to alcohol, tobacco, and drugs; understanding the benefits of breastfeeding; and reducing the risk of maternal–fetal disease transmission at birth.

Children with Disabilities

Many children sustain physical and/or mental disability as a result of premature delivery, congenital disease, birth injury, childhood illness, or some other cause. Case managers are a valuable resource for these children and their families, not only at the time of the initial diagnosis or injury but for months and sometimes years afterward.

For those children whose conditions can be remedied by surgical and other means (e.g., those with correctable heart or musculoskeletal defects), case managers help plan and coordinate the medical procedures required to correct the problem. They also arrange for the child and family to receive other services necessary to support their well-being throughout the entire treatment period, such as physical and occupational therapy, psychologic counseling, pharmacotherapy, and in-home nursing care.

For children whose conditions will persist for the rest of their lives, case managers perform a similar set of actions. However, in addition to coordinating medical care and connecting patients and their families with available support services, they also work to ensure that the child receives adequate educational and other accommodations throughout childhood. Frequently, this requires the case manager to engage in advocacy efforts on behalf of these patients.

Patients with Behavioral, Intellectual, or Mental Health Disorders or Disabilities

Patients of all ages may be affected by behavioral, intellectual, or mental health disorders or disabilities that limit their ability to participate in school, obtain or retain a job, engage in self-care, live independently in the community, or engage in any number of other activities of daily living. After working with these individuals to determine their unique limitations, case managers can help each patient formulate a set of realistic goals and expectations, then connect the patient with any number of resources necessary for meeting these goals. Examples include (but are not limited to) individual and/or group counseling; vocational training and structured workshops; nutritional services; disability advocacy organizations; group homes; housekeeping services; home care aides; transportation services; assistive technology; and resources for ensuring adherence with pharmacologic and other therapeutic regimens.

Older Adults

Case management is often a critical component of care for older adult patients. One reason is that many older adults experience multiple and/or chronic health conditions that require ongoing care and coordination. For patients like these, case management helps promote continuity of care, prevents duplication of services, and ensures that patients are not receiving therapies that counteract or otherwise work against one another. In this way, case management helps promote better patient outcomes while simultaneously fostering more efficient, cost-effective use of healthcare resources.

Case management is also an increasingly common aspect of end-of-life care for many older adults (as well as patients of any age who are affected by terminal illness). By working closely with these individuals and their families, case managers help ensure that their patients are able to achieve death with dignity. This means that patients are empowered to choose which treatments they wish to receive without feeling pressured to undergo potentially painful and/or expensive treatments that may only minimally extend their lifespan, yet they are not automatically precluded from receiving these treatments if they so choose. It also means that patients are able to die in the place of their choosing and/or in the presence of loved ones. Often, the case manager's first step in ensuring patients' wishes are met is to simply speak honestly with patients about their health and impending mortality—something that many HCPs and family members are reluctant to do. From this foundation of honesty and understanding, the case manager and patient together can explore options for many end-of-life decisions, including choices related to hospice, palliative care, financial affairs, advance directives, power of attorney, and other medical and legal concerns.

REVIEW Case Management

RELATE Link the Concepts and Exemplars

Linking the exemplar of case management with the concept of perfusion:

1. A neonate born with a severe congenital heart defect will require numerous open-heart surgeries and regular follow-up with cardiology and pediatrics. The parents, who carry comprehensive medical insurance, will require assistance paying for medical bills because the cost of care is expected to exceed the child's lifetime maximum coverage within a few years. How might this family benefit from case management? What specifically would the case manager do for this family?

Linking the exemplar of case management with the concept of oxygenation:

2. The nurse is caring for two patients. One patient has pneumonia that is resolving with IV antibiotics; the other patient has had asthma for many years. Which patient would benefit most from case management? Explain your answer.
3. The nurse is caring for a patient with a chronic alteration in oxygenation requiring many different medications, frequent physician visits, and a history of two to three hospital admissions per year. How might case management help this patient?

REFER Go to Pearson MyLab Nursing and eText

REFLECT Apply Your Knowledge

Curt Ranier is a 42-year-old man who sustained a right femur fracture during a motor-vehicle crash. Following surgical repair of his femur fracture, he is admitted to the orthopedic unit. Mr. Ranier's surgery and anesthesia were uneventful, and he is stable and alert. His medical history includes type 2 diabetes, which he manages through his diet. He also has a prior history of deep vein thrombosis in his left leg. During his admission to the orthopedic unit, Mr. Ranier expressed his motivation to heal and go home; however, he states that he is concerned about caring for himself outside the hospital setting, as he lives alone and has no relatives nearby.

1. Considering Mr. Ranier's current condition and medical history, which nursing diagnoses (both actual and risk) should be included in his nursing plan of care?
2. How would Mr. Ranier benefit from case management? In addition to nursing, describe several other professional disciplines that should collaborate in this patient's care.
3. Describe the benefits of using a critical pathway to guide Mr. Ranier's care. In addition to his medical diagnosis and patient identification data, identify three categories that would be included in Mr. Ranier's critical pathway.

Exemplar 39.B Cost-Effective Care

Exemplar Learning Outcomes

39.B Analyze cost-effective care as it relates to managing care.

- Summarize payment sources in the United States.
- Describe the international perspective of healthcare.
- Outline factors influencing the provision of healthcare.
- Describe cost-containment strategies.
- Summarize the economics of nursing.

Exemplar Key Terms

Diagnosis-related groups (DRGs), *2632*
Mandatory health insurance, *2631*
Private insurance, *2630*
Prospective payment system (PPS), *2632*
Public insurance, *2630*
Socialized insurance, *2630*
Socialized medicine, *2630*
Voluntary insurance, *2631*

Overview

The healthcare system has increasingly become involved in and affected by aspects of commercial (entrepreneurial) and government (state and federal) marketplaces (Vogenberg & Santilli, 2019). As healthcare costs rise, a greater share of these costs is passed on to the consumer (patient) in the form of out-of-pocket (OOP) expenses. Aspects impacting the delivery of care include costs, access to care, quality of care, and adaptations to improve efficiency. Related to increased costs, efforts are directed to reduce risks that result in increased costs to healthcare organizations (Vogenberg & Santilli, 2019). Access to and quality of care remain issues in the search for cost-effectiveness. To improve access to care, efforts are aimed at increasing distribution of services to those in need either geographically or via telehealth modalities. To improve quality of care, attention is focused on maintaining a consistent process by continued monitoring and increased transparency.

Healthcare expenditures in the United States are at a staggering level. The Commonwealth Fund (Tikkanen & Abrams, 2020) notes that the United States spends more on healthcare than any other country, yet has:

- The highest obesity rate
- The highest chronic disease burden
- The highest suicide rate
- The lowest life expectancy.

Reasons for high healthcare costs in the United States range from administrative waste, the high cost of pharmaceutical drugs (medications typically cost more in the United States than in other developed countries), and other factors. The COVID-19 pandemic is expected to cost the United States more than $16 trillion across all areas of the economy, not just healthcare (Cutler & Summers, 2020).

Prior to the pandemic, recommendations for controlling healthcare costs included increasing opportunities for small businesses to be able to afford to provide health insurance for employees, permitting short-term insurance plans to come into the marketplace, and erasing state borders by allowing patients to shop for health insurance plans in other states (Council of Economic Advisors, 2019). Some groups and congresspeople increased or renewed their calls for a Medicare for All program or public insurance option to ensure more people have access to affordable healthcare. This exemplar looks at some of the issues in providing cost-effective care, including payment options.

Payment Sources in the United States

Payment for healthcare services in the United States is made through **public insurance** (government funded), **private insurance** (private or publicly owned companies), or directly from the patient (personal OOP expense). Examples of public insurance in the United States are Medicare or Medicaid, for which individuals must meet selected criteria to enroll. Examples of private insurance in the United States are Blue Cross Blue Shield, Kaiser Permanente, and Aetna.

Insurance plans (regardless of type) typically have a yearly deductible requirement, may require a co-payment for selected services or prescriptions, and may define criteria for treatment and reimbursement. Individuals may have to incur OOP expenses based on care that is needed but does not meet specified criteria or if they receive care from an out-of-network or nonparticipating provider.

The International Perspective

How a society views the role of government in people's lives influences the development of its healthcare systems and policies. In contrast to other developed countries such as Canada and the United Kingdom, the United States has not adopted a nationalized or socialized form of medicine as the mode of healthcare delivery. As mentioned earlier, comparisons between the United States and other countries reveal declining health outcomes and a higher overall burden of disease. For example, in 2017, the U.S. disability-adjusted life years (DALY) rate was an average of 31% higher than that of other developed countries. **Table 39.1** » examines health outcomes between the U.S. in relation to healthcare in other countries.

Each country has its own unique healthcare system, but these systems can be broadly divided into four categories based on the organization and financing of healthcare:

- The first category is **socialized medicine**, in which the state owns and controls healthcare services. Examples of socialized medicine are seen in the United Kingdom, Sweden, and Denmark, where physicians derive virtually all their income from the government and have employment contracts with the state.
- The second category is **socialized insurance**, in which all medically necessary services are covered by the government (including physician care, hospital services, and, to some

TABLE 39.1 Health Outcomes in the United States Compared to Other Developed Countries

Outcome	United States (rate per 100,000 population)	Other Developed Countries (rate per 100,000 population)
All-cause mortality	840.2	690.63
Respiratory disease mortality	83.4	59.16
Circulatory system mortality	254.8	210.07
Cancer mortality	183.1	197.73
Maternal mortality	16.9	4.44

Source: Data from Kurani, McDermott, and Shanosky (2020).

extent, prescription drugs), but these services are delivered by a blend of private and public providers. Canada, France, and Australia have this form of healthcare system.

- **Mandatory health insurance** is the third category and is found in Germany and Japan. These nations have large, nonprofit health insurance organizations called "sickness funds." Sickness funds are usually organized around large employers or work-based associations. Government-sponsored programs cover citizens who are not part of a sickness fund. Everyone belongs to one of these two types of plans, thus ensuring universality of coverage.
- Finally, **voluntary insurance** provides no guarantee of universality because coverage may be expensive and difficult to purchase. The United States currently has this type of system, under which millions of Americans lack coverage due to financial and other constraints (see Focus on Diversity and Culture: Health Insurance and Socioeconomic Status). A major goal of the Patient Protection and Affordable Care Act, signed into law in March 2010 and often referred to as the ACA or "Obamacare," was to reduce the difficulties associated with securing voluntary insurance in the United States. Initially under the ACA, most individuals who did not have health insurance through their employer or a government program were required to purchase coverage or pay a financial penalty. To make such coverage more accessible and affordable, the ACA established subsidies for some Americans and called for the establishment of health insurance exchanges in all 50 states. Subsequently, the financial penalty for individuals was removed. Presently, the ACA is undergoing discussion for transformation by legislative action.

Factors Influencing the Provision of Healthcare

Several factors influence provision of and access to healthcare, regardless of the types of coverage available. Within the United States, economic factors including but not limited to supply and demand and the inability to account for the actual costs of critical services (e.g., nursing services) are important influences on the provision of healthcare, but there are other economic variables that should be considered for their relative impact on the rising costs of healthcare.

Healthcare costs are increasing dramatically in the United States and can no longer be explained simply by the concept of supply and demand. Nunn, Parson, and Shambaugh (2020) identified several key findings:

- Healthcare spending quadrupled from 1980 to 2018
- U.S. healthcare expenditures are 50% higher, on average, than other developing countries
- The majority of healthcare expenditures focus on hospital/professional services
- Individuals with the poorest health spend more on healthcare services
- Variations in private insurance occur throughout the country
- Variations in costs of services occur throughout the country
- Physician provider services are not well dispersed based on demographics and geographical locations
- Surprise costs to patients can occur.

These findings illustrate the complexity of the economic marketplace in healthcare and how merely looking at supply and demand does not afford an explanation of why healthcare costs have increased.

Access and Affordability

In the mid- to late 20th century, it was common for many employers to provide employer-subsidized health insurance. However, with the 2008 economic downturn, many employers reduced the benefits they offered, passed increasing costs of health insurance premiums onto employees, or stopped providing health insurance altogether. This resulted in large numbers of Americans no longer having health insurance, reducing their access to healthcare, especially preventive care (see the Focus on Diversity and Culture feature).

Kerns and Willis (2020) identified a variety of factors affecting access to primary care providers:

- Unequal distribution of providers across different geographical areas
- Inability of individuals (uninsured) to afford payment for provided services.
- Hours of clinical practice not available for some patient populations
- Care models may not provide reimbursement benefits for other professionals outside of the defined "physician model" and/or patients may not be aware that they can receive quality services from nonphysician practitioners (such as nurse practitioners or physical therapists).
- Increased requirements of documentation (electronic charting) to meet established criteria for reimbursement, which takes away from clinical practice hours.

SAFETY ALERT Under federal law, patients who are experiencing a true medical emergency cannot be denied treatment, regardless of their ability to pay. Specifically, the Emergency Medical Treatment and Labor Act (EMTALA) of 1986 requires all Medicare-participating hospitals that offer emergency services to examine and stabilize any patient who presents for an emergency medical condition, even if that patient cannot pay for services. Once the patient is stabilized, however, EMTALA protections no longer apply, and the patient may be transferred or discharged at the hospital's discretion.

Focus on Diversity and Culture

Health Insurance and Socioeconomic Status

Health insurance is a major determinant of access to care—and in the United States, health insurance coverage is strongly tied to socioeconomic status.

According to the Kaiser Family Foundation (Tolbert, Orgera, & Damico, 2020), in 2019:

- 28.9 million nonelderly people in the United States did not have health insurance.
- Most uninsured Americans came from families in which at least one member worked.
- 73.7% reported that the high cost of insurance as being the primary reason for no coverage.
- Individuals at highest risk (82.6%) of being uninsured lived at or below 200% of the federal poverty level.
- People of color accounted for over half of the nation's uninsured, even though they made up only 43.1% of the overall U.S. population. Uninsured rates were especially high among American Indians/Alaskan Natives (51.5%), Hispanics (21.7%), and non-Hispanic Blacks (20.0%) as compared to whites, who had an uninsured rate of 7.8%.

These statistics also underline the importance of finding solutions to the current healthcare crisis in the United States. Making care more affordable for patients with low socioeconomic status will improve health and reduce suffering. It will also save money in the long run by eliminating costly complications associated with conditions that are preventable or more easily treated in the early stages.

Separate Billing for Nursing Services

Within the United States, bills for hospital and other inpatient care services continue to bundle nursing services with flat daily charges (e.g., the cost of the room and housekeeping). Aiken and Lasater (2017) commented on the ability of the professional nurse to function as an integral part of the medical division of labor, but there is no specific metric value as it relates to professional nursing care. There is still much work to be done in this area to define the inherent monetary value for reimbursement of care delivered by a licensed nurse (registered or licensed vocational/practical) within a clinical facility environment.

Cost-Containment Strategies

Over the past few decades, a number of cost-containment strategies have been implemented, including competition, price controls, managed care, health promotion and illness prevention, and vertically integrated healthcare services. Various measures aimed at controlling the costs of care are discussed in the sections that follow.

Competition

Competition can be an effective strategy to contain costs, but it is subject to government regulations that decrease the ability of individual markets to compete. With restrictions and regulations in place, healthcare practices have transitioned from private practice to multiprovider conglomerate practices in order to align with regulations and help defray costs. Although competition can sometimes increase care options for patients, evidence linking competition to reduced costs in the healthcare system is often lacking or unclear. Some private and public insurers have assumed the task of providing information to patients to help them make choices for healthcare based on costs, and this may, in turn, promote competition in the marketplace and drive down costs. For example, Blue Cross Blue Shield of North Carolina offers an online tool to help patients find a provider and estimate costs for a variety of services. However, whether or not these tools result in competition that creates change has yet to be determined.

Price Controls

Changes in government policies have been instituted to provide increased transparency related to costs and removal/modification of paperwork processes that are considered obsolete, repetitive, or burdensome ("Patients over Paperwork"; Verma, 2019). However, despite these changes, healthcare costs were showing no signs of stabilization even before the COVID-19 pandemic.

Price controls for healthcare services have been established in various ways. Some organizations have established a "case fee" that provides a coordinated treatment plan to a patient for a prescribed fee within a specific time period (90 days). Most insurers, including Medicaid and Medicare, limit reimbursement for services provided using a **prospective payment system (PPS)** whereby billing is predetermined based on the defined diagnosis/procedure. Factored into this are the **diagnosis-related groups (DRGs)** that correlate reimbursement with length of stay (LOS). Reimbursement to the facility is based on the typical standard of care for the DRG and LOS. For example, a hospital that admits a patient with a diagnosis of myocardial infarction is reimbursed for a specific dollar amount, regardless of the cost of services, the length of stay, or the acuity or complexity of the patient's illness. DRG rates are set in advance of the year during which they apply and are fixed unless major, uncontrollable events occur.

Group insurance plans can help reduce costs for affiliated members. Unions, employers, and professional organizations are among those that offer group insurance plans. Group plans are essentially a "buy in bulk" model—members can access health insurance and healthcare at lower rates than if they participated as individuals.

Cost-containment strategies such as PPS and group self-insurance plans have driven several trends in healthcare delivery. These include increased emphasis on preventive care to reduce the incidence of illnesses, provision of treatment in noninstitutional settings such as clinics or patients' homes and use of best practices as documented in protocols and guidelines. These strategies focus on avoiding hospital and institutional placement unless necessary and ensuring that all care provided is scientifically based.

Vertically Integrated Health Services Organizations

Yet another cost-containment practice is the use of *vertically integrated health services organizations*, or networks of hospitals, clinics, and individual providers that offer a broad range of care and support services to patients across the entire wellness spectrum. By integrating the provision of hospital care, ambulatory care, outpatient surgery, and home health services, these systems allow patients to receive the precise level of care they need in the most cost-effective way possible.

With the establishment of the ACA, attention was focused on *integration* as a mechanism for distributing services. Advances in technology accompanied the focus on integration, resulting in best practice delivery of care and redistribution of where and how services are offered. LOS decreased for surgical care procedures and alternative sites (outpatient vs. inpatient) were used to provide and deliver care.

The goal of vertical integration is to create a seamless system of coordinated care to reduce duplication of care, improve patient outcomes, and control costs through the efficient use of resources. For example, the patient's primary care provider can see results of labs and diagnostics ordered by a specialty care provider in the same system, as well as order medications and make care decisions in a timely manner without having to request records or wait for a call to be returned.

Cost Containment in the Context of Federal Laws

The ACA legally compelled healthcare organizations to adopt various cost-containment measures aimed at improving the quality of care provided, redesigning healthcare delivery systems, determining appropriate payment for services provided, modernizing the financial systems used to pay for services, and eliminating fraud and abuse. For example, the law established payment penalties as an incentive to prevent hospital readmissions and healthcare-associated conditions such as pressure injuries and infections. The ACA also called for provision of coordinated care by healthcare teams rather than individual providers and mandated reduction of medically unnecessary services that may be detrimental to a patient's health. Despite the unpopularity of the ACA among some critics, these measures have largely been welcomed and become the standard.

Nursing Economics

As discussed earlier, placing a value on nursing care is a major challenge. How many nursing care hours are required for each DRG? What is the best skill mix—that is, ratio of RNs to LPNs to UAP—for an intensive care unit in comparison to a medical–surgical unit? These questions persist despite decades of attempts to determine the actual costs and cost-effectiveness of nursing care.

To a certain extent, the cost of advanced practice care has been quantified. Advanced practice nurses receive reimbursement for their services but often at a lower rate than their medical counterparts and/or physician assistants. Consumer confidence in the quality of care that NPs can provide at lower costs is increasing. However, the economic value of the bedside nurse still remains unquantifiable.

Nursing Shortages

Current data obtained from the 2021 Nursing Solutions Incorporated (NSI) National Health Care Retention & RN Staffing Report, focuses on factors that contribute to nurse turnover, which in turns leads to increased economic costs for the healthcare industry. Two factors that influence nurse turnover are the *nurse vacancy rate* (percentage of unfilled positions) and the *RN Recruitment Difficulty Index* (average days needed to replace an experienced nurse). According to the 2021 NSI report, in 2019 the nurse vacancy rate was 9.9%, with the RN Recruitment Difficulty Index indicating approximately 3 months to find a replacement. High nurse vacancy rates and lengthy recruitment times often result in facilities using contract or travel nurses to maintain nurse–patient ratios.

An overall vacancy rate of 9.9% may seem low, but in reality that means 10 of 100 nurse positions are vacant. And that is an across-the-board average. In some communities and at some facilities vacancy rates are much higher. By 2030, the shortage of registered nurses is expected to be over 500,000 across the country (Zhang, Tai, Pforsich, & Lin, 2018).

A number of factors affect staffing (American Association of Colleges of Nursing [AACN], 2020; NSI, 2021):

- The expansion of the profession has led to more and more options for advanced certification, education, and specialization, giving registered nurses many more options than working in a hospital or other inpatient setting
- The high number of nurses leaving the profession, with universities and colleges unable to enroll enough students to meet current needs
- Salaries for services in some areas are not competitive enough
- Staffing shortages combined with high patient acuity increase nurse stress levels and impact job satisfaction, increasing the number of nurses leaving the profession before they reach retirement age.

Ending the cycle of nurse shortages will require significant changes at the state and national levels. Currently nursing schools are forming strategic partnerships and trying to find private support to help expand the number of students they can enroll. AACN, the American Nurses Association, and other professional organizations are working to expand awareness and bring public and private resources to bear. These and other strategies will be necessary to combat the problem of nursing shortages and ensure patients receive high-quality care across settings (AACN, 2020).

Cost-Conscious Nursing Practice

All nurses must understand the costs associated with healthcare and the ways in which these costs impact nursing practice. Because the nursing staff is the largest professional group in a hospital, it is the most expensive. However, the nursing staff does not produce revenue because nursing services are included as part of patients' room and board charges. Research has demonstrated that both academic (BSN preparation) and clinical experience of registered nurses help to improve patient outcomes but that recognition at the facility level is often not connected with financial recognition (Paulson, 2018). It is therefore important for additional research to be done to examine the correlation between perceived value and engagement of nursing staff by hospital facilities to lead to better nurse retention and more cost-conscious nursing practice.

Nursing practice based on use of evidence-based measures and resources will help to support cost containment within the clinical practice setting. Safe nursing practice and simple measures such as hand hygiene help reduce the risks for injuries and illnesses in the workplace, thereby reducing costs. Effective coordination of care, as discussed in Exemplar 39.A, Case Management, can also help reduce costs. Diligent documentation reduces the risk for errors and inadvertent delay in or duplication of services. These and other best-practice nursing strategies help to reduce costs and improve outcomes for patients across settings.

REVIEW Cost-Effective Care

RELATE Link the Concepts and Exemplars

Linking the exemplar of cost-effective care with the concept of health, wellness, and illness:

1. Explain how health promotion activities reduce the cost of care.
2. You are caring for an adolescent patient who admits to smoking "a couple" of cigarettes per week. What impact would helping this patient quit smoking have on the lifetime cost of his healthcare?

Linking the exemplar of cost-effective care with the concept of infection:

3. How does the cost of a healthcare-associated infection impact the cost of a patient's admission?
4. How does the cost of reducing the risk of healthcare-acquired infections compare to the cost of treating a patient who contracts a healthcare-acquired infection?

REFER Go to Pearson MyLab Nursing and eText

REFLECT Apply Your Knowledge

A group of nurses works on an oncology unit with 30 beds, including a six-bed bone marrow transplant unit. Each nurse is usually assigned four or five patients, depending on acuity levels. Only nurses with advanced training can administer chemotherapy, so it is not uncommon to have one nurse assigned to be a medication nurse when many others on the same shift have not yet attended or completed the chemotherapy certification course.

1. What actions could you, as a staff nurse on this unit, take to reduce the cost of providing care to these patients?
2. The hospital is considering replacing its 10-year-old x-ray machine with a newer model that uses less radiation and is completely digital, thereby eliminating the need for film cartridges and making it easier for radiologists to read x-rays from computers in their offices or homes. However, the cost of the machine is very high. You are asked to join the committee that will make the decision about whether to purchase this equipment. What are the pros and cons of buying this new radiology equipment?

» Exemplar 39.C Delegation

Exemplar Learning Outcomes

39.C Analyze delegation as it relates to managing care.

- Summarize principles of delegation.
- Describe benefits of delegation.
- Outline the delegation process.
- Outline factors affecting delegation.
- Describe how liability affects delegation.

Exemplar Key Terms

Assignment, *2634*
Delegate, *2634*
Delegation, *2634*
Delegator, *2634*

Overview

Nurses play a major role in healthcare, and the United States continues to experience a nursing shortage secondary to increases in lifespan, the number of older adults requiring medical care, and the need for nursing care in nonhospital environments. As a result, registered nurses must dedicate increasingly larger portions of their time to the performance of highly skilled tasks. This often leaves them with little time to complete the less complex interventions required for attainment of successful patient outcomes. For such tasks to be accomplished, RNs frequently rely on the process of delegation.

In general terms, **delegation** is a process in which one individual transfers the responsibility and authority of completing an activity to another individual. The individual who transfers the activity or assignment to another is known as the **delegator**. The individual who accepts responsibility for completing the task is the **delegate**. Delegation in the setting of nursing care allows for increased efficiency and coordination of efforts at the individual and/or group level. Delegation of care relies on the five rights of delegation : the "*right*" time, task, person, communication/instructions, and supervision/evaluation (National Council of State Boards of Nursing [NCSBN] & American Nurses Association [ANA], 2019).

Delegation is often confused with work allocation or assignment. Although the two concepts are related, they are not the same. **Assignment** refers to a skill or task that is a fundamental part of an individual's job that is expected to be accomplished on a regular basis (NCSBN & ANA, 2019). Asking an individual to perform a task that is a part of their regular responsibilities and job description is not delegating. In *delegation*, the nurse asks another individual to perform a task or skill that is not part of the individual's regular assigned work. In delegating, the nurse transfers the *responsibility* for completing the task to the delegate, but not the *accountability* for the task. Accountability remains with the nurse (NCSBN & ANA, 2019). Delegation is not easy. Complications may arise due to several factors, including variations in titles and terminology, lack of training, issues of accountability and responsibility, and the nurse's discomfort with the delegation process. Still, today's emphasis on "doing more with less" means it is more critical than ever before that nurses master the skill of delegation. Once nurses learn how to delegate, they extend their ability to accomplish more by using others' help. Guidelines for successful delegation are listed in **Box 39.1** ⟫ and are described in detail throughout this exemplar.

Principles of Delegation

The principles of delegation can be applied at multiple levels that follow the hierarchy of nursing practice: advanced practice nurses, who in turn can delegate to registered nurses, licensed vocational/practical nurses, or unlicensed assistive personnel. Aspects of delegation are also defined by state practice acts and specified by healthcare organizations in terms of policy and procedure. The key issue with delegation is that the individual who delegates still assumes accountability and responsibility for the action.

Delegating to Other Nurses

Registered nurses frequently delegate tasks to other RNs. For example, a charge nurse is engaging in delegation when she makes assignments for a shift. A nurse may also opt to delegate certain care activities for a patient to another nurse, if the second nurse is free and can accept the additional responsibility. For instance, an RN may assign a float RN to an unstable patient with a high temperature and high blood pressure. Caring for an unstable patient is within the RN scope of practice, so the RN who accepts the assignment will be responsible for completing the patient's care safely, ethically, and completely. In addition, it may be appropriate for an RN to delegate specific interventions to an LPN or LVN. In these cases, the RN remains responsible for ensuring that the LPN or LVN completes the interventions both correctly and appropriately.

Box 39.1

Guidelines for Successful Delegation

1. Follow your state's nurse practice act and your facility's policies and procedures when delegating.
2. Delegate only tasks for which you have both accountability and responsibility.
3. Follow state regulations, job descriptions, and agency policies when delegating.
4. Follow the delegation process and key behaviors for delegating.
5. Only accept delegation when you have a clear understanding of the task, time frame, reporting requirements, and other expectations.
6. Confront your fears about delegation; recognize which fears are realistic and which are not.

When delegating to other nurses of any type, the RN must use critical thinking and professional judgment. RNs must also follow the widely accepted *Five Rights of Delegation*:

1. ***Right task:*** The delegator must ensure that the task is one that can be delegated according to the agency's policies and procedures and is appropriate for the specific patient.
2. ***Right circumstance:*** The delegator must determine that the task addresses the patient's needs and contributes to a desired outcome and that adequate supervision is available.
3. ***Right person:*** The delegator must assign the task to a delegate who has the necessary skills and experience. Moreover, the task must be within that delegate's job description.
4. ***Right directions and communication:*** The delegator must provide a clear, concise description of the task, along with its objectives, limits, and expectations. This material may be communicated orally or in written format. The delegator must also verify that the delegate understands the information that has been communicated.
5. ***Right supervision and evaluation:*** The delegator must monitor and evaluate the delegate's performance. This includes providing feedback and intervening if necessary (NCSBN & ANA, 2019).

Delegating to Unlicensed Assistive Personnel

Unlicensed assistive personnel, who provide care to patients but are not professionally licensed as a nurse, are identified by a variety of titles, including certified nursing aides/assistants (CNAs), home health aides (HHAs), medical technicians, orderlies, assistive personnel (AP), and surgical technicians. Each category and the individuals within it have diverse levels of training and experience. Even though UAP lack licensure, nurses may delegate to them as appropriate because they are employees of the HCP. (Conversely, nurses may not delegate to family members or friends of patients even if these individuals provide personal care to the patients because these individuals do not work for the HCP.)

It is not possible to generate an exhaustive list of exactly which actions are acceptable for delegation to UAP. Remember, each state's nurse practice act defines what acts may or may not be delegated to UAP within that state. Still, some general examples of tasks that may and may not be delegated are provided in **Box 39.2** ⟫.

SAFETY ALERT Care of unstable patients should *never* be delegated to an LPN, LVN, or UAP. If an RN must delegate all or part of the care of an unstable patient, these tasks must be delegated to another RN as appropriate.

Principles guiding the nurse's decision to delegate help ensure the safety and quality of outcomes. These principles include the Five Rights of Delegation, along with those listed in **Box 39.3** ⟫. Note that even if a task is one that may be delegated legally, the individual nurse must still determine whether the task can be delegated to a particular UAP for a

Box 39.2

Examples of Tasks That May and May Not Be Delegated to Unlicensed Assistive Personnel

TASKS THAT MAY BE DELEGATED TO UAP

- Taking vital signs
- Measuring and recording intake and output
- Patient transfers and ambulation
- Postmortem care
- Bathing
- Feeding
- Gastrostomy feedings in established systems
- Attending to safety
- Weighing
- Suctioning chronic tracheostomies

TASKS THAT MAY NOT BE DELEGATED TO UAP

- Assessment
- Interpreting data
- Making a nursing diagnosis or a problem list
- Creating a nursing care plan
- Evaluating care effectiveness
- Care of invasive lines
- Administering parenteral medications
- Inserting nasogastric (NG) tubes
- Patient education
- Performing triage
- Giving telephone advice

specific patient. Note also that UAP may not delegate tasks to another person.

Once a nurse has made the decision to delegate, the nurse must communicate clear instructions to the UAP, confirm the UAP understands the instructions, and then validate that the action has been completed. The delegator must provide information about the specific task as it relates to the patient(s), timing for task completion, whether additional resources may be needed, expected outcomes for the task, communication of findings, and how the documentation for task completion will be noted.

Certain tasks should never be delegated by the RN. For example, discipline of other employees, highly technical tasks, and complex patient care tasks that require specific levels of licensure, certification, or training should not be delegated. Also, any situation that involves confidentiality or controversy should not be delegated to others.

SAFETY ALERT Each HCP, licensed or unlicensed, is responsible for their own actions. Anyone who feels unqualified to perform a delegated task must decline to perform it until receiving appropriate training and assessed for competency.

Delegation versus Dumping

Nurses should delegate because it allows them to make better use of their time. They should not delegate in order to dump an undesirable task on someone else or to reward a

Box 39.3

Principles Used by the Nurse to Determine Delegation to Unlicensed Assistive Personnel

1. The nurse must assess the individual patient before delegating tasks.
2. The patient must be medically stable or in a chronic condition and not fragile.
3. The task must be considered routine for this patient.
4. The task must not require a substantial amount of scientific knowledge or technical skill.
5. The task must be considered safe for this patient.
6. The task must have a predictable outcome.
7. The nurse must know and understand the agency's procedures and policies about delegation.
8. The nurse must know the scope of practice and the customary knowledge, skills, and job description for each discipline represented on the healthcare team.
9. The nurse must be aware of individual variations in work abilities and training. Each individual UAP has different experiences and may or may not be capable of performing the task to be delegated.
10. The nurse, when unsure about a UAP's ability to perform a task, must observe while the UAP performs the task or must demonstrate the task to the UAP and get a return demonstration before allowing the UAP to perform it independently.
11. The nurse must clarify reporting expectations to ensure the task is accomplished.
12. The nurse must create an atmosphere that fosters communication, teaching, and learning. For example, the nurse should encourage the UAP to ask questions, listen carefully to concerns, and make use of every opportunity to teach.

Source: Adapted from Sullivan (2019).

productive employee with more work. Sometimes, a nurse may fear that he is "dumping" on another staff member by delegating routine care; in such cases, however, the nurse needs to maintain perspective on what tasks he can complete in a timely fashion and what tasks could be performed effectively by the delegate. Delegation should always be practiced in a way that provides the greatest benefit to the patient, makes the best use of the time of all staff members, and provides delegates with opportunities for growth.

Benefits of Delegation

The proper delegation of duties can benefit the nurse, the delegate, the manager, and the organization.

Benefits to the Nurse

By delegating some tasks to UAP, nurses can devote more time to those tasks that cannot be delegated, such as complex patient care. For example, a nurse has three central line dressing changes and two patients who require daily weights to be completed before the shift ends in 1 hour. The nurse may delegate the task of obtaining the patients' daily weights to a UAP and complete the central line dressing changes herself. In this example, delegation improves patient care in that all the necessary tasks are done but the nurse is not rushed to complete more complex tasks. By alleviating task overload, delegation also increases nurses' job satisfaction and improves an organization's employee retention rate.

Benefits to the Delegate

Delegates benefit from the process of delegation as it promotes confidence, builds on communication skills, allows for more transparency of delivery of care, and fosters a renewed commitment to the patient(s) who are placed in their care. Delegation allows the delegate to form collaborative partnerships, problem-solve potential delivery of care issues, and achieve a consensus whereby the patient, not the individual task, becomes the central focus. Delegation, when done effectively and efficiently, helps to build a cohesive team. Most delegates also feel a strong sense of internal satisfaction from knowing that their contributions assisted in the achievement of desired patient outcomes.

Benefits to the Manager

Delegation benefits the manager as it allows for more efficient use of time in the clinical environment. Management can thereby focus on additional responsibilities such as clinical decision making and policy development at the unit level. Effective delegation will lead to a more efficient nursing unit, which, in turn, will benefit nursing management.

Benefits to the Organization

Delegation benefits the organization due to increased efficiency of task(s) completion and accountability and responsibility for actions, which in turn lead to improved patient outcomes. As team and patient satisfaction increase, the organization benefits from goals being met. As team satisfaction increases, employee absences and turnover decrease and productivity increases, improving the organization's overall financial position as well as perception of care provided.

The Delegation Process

Nurses may delegate only those tasks for which they have responsibility and authority. These include tasks that are routine, tasks for which the nurse does not have time, and tasks that have moved down in priority. Whenever a nurse opts to transfer authority for one or more of these tasks, the nurse must engage in the delegation process. According to the NCSBN and ANA (2019), this process begins at the administrative level and consists of interrelated responsibilities whereby each participant (employer/nurse leader, licensed nurse, and delegate) understands their role and responsibilities and operates with transparency in the environment. The roles and responsibilities of each of these participants are described in detail in the following sections.

Employer/Nurse Leader

At the organizational level, direction is aimed at the development of policies and procedures that support delegation by outlining what tasks can be delegated in what circumstances. Monitoring and evaluation of stated delegation policies should be ongoing, and the organization should assume the responsibility of promoting a positive work environment based on evidence-based practice and safety (NCSBN & ANA, 2019).

Licensed Nurse

The licensed nurse assumes the responsibility and accountability for selection of tasks to be delegated for the patient(s) assigned to her care. As the delegator, the licensed nurse must select the appropriate delegate based on competency requirements. The licensed nurse must remain available to the delegate in case questions or problems arise and must follow up with both the delegate and the patient to ensure the task was completed correctly and to evaluate any issues the delegate discovered in the process of completing the tasks (for example, if the patient reports pain to the UAP) (NCSBN & ANA, 2019).

Appropriate communication goes both ways: from the delegator to the delegate and from the delegate to the delegator. Specifically, the delegator must allow enough time to clearly describe the task and expectations for completing it, answer the delegate's questions, address any situations that must be reported to the delegate, and inform the delegate of the nurse's own availability in the event the delegate has further questions or needs assistance. Some behaviors that can assist in the accomplishment of these tasks are described in **Box 39.4** ». The delegator must also consider any cultural factors that might affect the delegation process.

Box 39.4

Key Behaviors When Delegating Tasks

When delegating a task to another staff member, the nurse should:

- Describe the task using "I" statements (e.g., "I would like . . . ") and appropriate nonverbal behaviors (e.g., open body language, face-to-face positioning, and eye contact). The delegate needs to know what is expected and when, where, and how the task should be completed. More experienced delegates may be able to define for themselves the where and how. The nurse must decide whether written reports are necessary or if brief oral reports are enough. If written reports are required, the nurse should indicate whether tables, charts, or other graphics are necessary. The nurse should be specific about reporting times. In patient care tasks, it is also important to determine who has responsibility and authority to chart certain tasks: UAP can enter vital signs, but if they observe changes in patient status, RNs must investigate and chart their assessment.
- Describe the importance of the task to the organization, the delegator, the patient, and the delegate.
- Clearly describe the expected outcome and the timeline for completion. Here, the nurse must also establish how closely the assignment will be supervised.
- Identify any constraints on completing the task or any conditions that could change. For example, the nurse may ask an assistant to feed a patient as long as the patient is not having difficulty swallowing; should the patient begin to demonstrate dysphagia, then the nurse will take over feeding activities.
- Have the delegate repeat back the task and specific directions. The nurse should further validate the delegate's understanding of the task and its expectations by eliciting questions and providing feedback.

Source: Adapted from Sullivan (2019).

Delegate

The delegate also has certain responsibilities. In particular, the delegate needs to communicate understanding of the task, have competency in the performance of the task, and describe what communication and action should be undertaken in an emergency. For delegation to be effective, delegates should not accept a task they are unqualified to perform. Additional instruction/resources may be required in order to facilitate task completion, but the act of delegation carries shared responsibility on the part of both the delegator and the delegate. Both the delegator and the delegate should also have a clear understanding of how the delegated task will be documented in the nursing record (NCSBN & ANA, 2019).

Supervision and Evaluation

Supervision and evaluation are the final elements of the delegation process, for they combine the critical elements of accountability, responsibility, and communication. When engaging in evaluation, the delegator must compare the delegate's performance against appropriate policies, procedures, and standards of practice. The delegator must also determine whether the delegate's actions contributed to achievement of the agreed-upon objectives. Specific questions that can help the nurse evaluate the effectiveness of delegation include the following:

- Was the delegated task performed appropriately and successfully?
- Was the desired outcome achieved in a satisfactory manner?
- Was communication between the delegator and delegate both timely and effective?
- Which aspects of the task and/or the delegation process went well? Which aspects did not proceed so smoothly?
- Did any problems arise? If so, how were they addressed?
- Could the patient's need(s) be met in a more effective way?
- Should any adjustments be made to the patient's overall plan of care considering the delegated task or activity?

If a problem arises, the nurse should investigate the problem and explain any concerns to the delegate. It is equally important for the nurse to provide positive feedback, to validate what the delegate did correctly in order to promote correct completion of tasks in the future, and to help the delegate achieve satisfaction in a job well done.

An often-overlooked consideration related to the practice of delegation is how new (novice) nurses receive training in the clinical environment. Delegation is a complex process in which individual nurses should have training and adequate resources to perform. Strategies that may prove to be helpful for the new nurse who is delegating include adhering to the scope of practice, being aware of the level of competency of potential delegates, maintaining clear communication pathways, and knowing not only when to delegate but when not to delegate (Anderson, 2018).

The following Clinical Example explores how a school nurse would use this overall process when delegating the task of medication administration.

Clinical Example B

Colleen Key is a school nurse for a large school district. She has responsibility for two elementary schools, one of which serves several children whose native language is other than English, a preschool that serves children age 3 to 5 with moderate and severe disabilities, and two middle schools. Colleen's management responsibilities include providing health services for 1825 students, coordinating with staff members at the various schools including members of the exceptional children's services department, and supervising three unlicensed school health aides. The logistics of managing multiple school sites means that Colleen must delegate many daily tasks, including medication administration, to the school-based health aides. The nurse practice act in this state allows for delegation of medication administration in the school setting. Colleen is responsible for training the school health aides to safely administer medication to students, documenting the training, evaluating the aides' performance, and providing ongoing supervision.

To delegate medication administration to a health aide, Colleen must do all the following:

- Understand the state nurse practice act and its applicability to the school setting.
- Implement school district policies related to health services and medication administration.
- Develop and implement an appropriate training program.
- Limit opportunities for error and decrease liability by ensuring that unlicensed health aides are appropriately trained to handle delegated tasks.
- Maintain documentation related to training and observation of medication administration by unlicensed staff.
- Audit medication administration records to ensure accuracy and completeness.
- Conduct several "drop-in" visits during the school year in order to track the competency of health aides.
- If necessary, report any medication errors to administration and follow up with focused training and closer supervision.
- Provide constructive feedback and address any concerns.
- Acknowledge the effectiveness of the unlicensed health aide's efforts.

Critical Thinking Questions

1. If you were a school nurse, what would you include in your training of unlicensed health aides for medication administration?
2. Other than medication administration, what duties typically needed at a school could be delegated to the unlicensed personnel? What duties could not be delegated?
3. How would you respond if a task that you delegated to an unlicensed health aide was completed incorrectly and resulted in harm to a child?

Source: Adapted from Sullivan (2019).

Factors Affecting Delegation

Several factors may affect delegation, including organizational culture, assignment patterns, and the personal qualities of the participants. Resource availability, such as having enough staff to whom the nurse may delegate tasks, also impacts delegation.

Assignment Patterns

Three assignment patterns affect delegation: unit-based assignment, pairing, and partnering. The unit-based approach assigns assistive personnel such as UAP to serve everyone on the unit by working from a task list. Limited planning between the RNs and support staff is a feature of unit-based assignment patterns; consequently, there is no sense of teamwork. With this type of assignment, RNs frequently ask for assistance as needed. Their requests are made in a vacuum; that is, none of the nurses are aware of the demands being placed on the UAP by others, thus placing the UAP in the position of managing conflicting requests. Not surprisingly, this approach does not lend itself to effective delegation and causes dissatisfaction among both RNs and support staff.

A more effective means of delegation is pairing, or the assignment of an RN, LPN, and/or UAP to work together as a team for a shift. Pairs are not scheduled to work together consistently; therefore, the team's composition varies from day to day. Pairs are able to plan care; team members identify priorities and plan each patient's individual outcomes for the shift. Pairing increases satisfaction among team members and facilitates delegation.

Partnering is the best assignment pattern. It is the consistent scheduling of a set team, such as an RN, LPN, and/or nursing assistant, who always work together. This consistency creates healthy interpersonal relationships and increases trust. Each partner is able to anticipate the others' needs and expectations. Inclusion of annual competency-based training in the clinical environment can also assist the nursing team to stay current on best-practice methods of delegation (Potter, Perry, Stockert, & Hall, 2021; Wagner, 2018).

Delegate Understanding, Acceptance, and Communication

Delegates are responsible for making sure they fully understand a task before accepting it. Before accepting the task, a determination must be made whether the delegate has the skills and abilities to complete it. If the delegate does not possess the necessary skills and abilities, the individual must inform the delegator. The delegate must also discuss with the delegator whether or not there is sufficient time to complete the task.

If the delegate does not have the necessary skills or abilities but the delegator is willing to train the delegate to complete the task, the delegate may accept the task provided there is time for sufficient training and questions before the task must be completed.

By accepting delegation, the delegate accepts full responsibility for the outcome of the task. Note that the delegate has the option to negotiate to perform only those parts of the task for which the individual has been trained.

Once the delegate and delegator have agreed on the nature of the assignment and their roles and responsibilities, they should clarify the time frame and other expectations of the task as well as how the delegate is to report the outcome of the task and what kind of assistance and feedback the delegate can expect from the delegator. The delegate should keep the delegator informed of progress and report any concerns or unexpected events. Finally, the delegate should complete the assignment as agreed and report the task as completed in a timely manner. This fosters trust between delegator and delegate and builds the delegate's reputation for dependability and credibility.

Obstacles to Delegation

Delegation can yield many benefits, but it also has barriers that can potentially endanger patients and/or lead to unsuccessful outcomes. For example, when a patient does not receive ambulation because nursing staff fails to follow through on this important activity, the patient may be at increased risk for falls, pneumonia, and development of deep vein thromboses and pressure ulcers.

Some barriers to delegation are environmental, whereas others are the result of the delegator's or delegate's experience or behaviors, as described in the sections that follow.

Environmental Barriers to Delegation

- *Nonsupportive Environment.* Depending on the organization and the type of leadership hierarchy, delegation may be limited and/or not even allowed (autocratic leadership).
- *Lack of resources.* Inadequate staffing and limited physical resources can impact the ability to delegate.
- *Limited training.* There must be enough training of staff/personnel in order to maintain competency related to delegated tasks and adherence to policy and procedures.
- *Time.* There must be enough time for preparation for procedural aspects related to delegation.

Staff Experience and Behavior

Delegation depends on the delegator transferring full authority for the tasks to the delegate and providing the delegate with the necessary instructions and information, the delegate accepting the authority for the task and completing it appropriately, and the delegator taking back responsibility and evaluating the completion of the task. In delegating the task, the nurse retains accountability for it while the delegate has the responsibility for completing it. The delegated task must be (1) within the nurse's scope to delegate the task and (2) within the delegate's competency to complete it. Failure to follow the five rights of delegation, assigning tasks that are outside the scope of practice for the nurse or outside the competency of the delegate, and any failures in communication or documentation can adversely impact patient outcomes, patient trust in the healthcare team, and the working relationship of both the delegator and the delegate.

Clinical Example C

After completing training for the health aides (see the prior Clinical Example), Colleen gives them the authority to begin administering medications to the students in their schools. During the first week of classes, one of the health aides decides to set the students' medications out in individual cups for ease of administration but fails to label the individual containers. Colleen is called back to the school to administer the correct medications, which makes the students late to class.

Critical Thinking Questions

1. Which of the four steps of the delegation process did Colleen fail to follow?
2. Which step or steps did the aide fail to follow?
3. What should Colleen do to prevent this situation from happening again?

Source: Adapted from Sullivan (2019).

Legal Aspects of Delegation

Nurse practice acts define the scope of practice based on professional licensure, which is utilized to establish safe practice by nurses to the community/population that is under their care. NCSBN has also identified the responsibilities and accountabilities of the clinical triad (employer/nurse leadership, licensed nurse, and delegatee) as being the foundation for delegation practice (Miller, 2018). State practice acts outline parameters for practice and organizational policies determine how delegation may occur in the specific workplace. Adherence to these rules should protect nurses from liability, but several additional guidelines can provide extra peace of mind when delegating. Perhaps the most useful guidelines for nurses to remember are the five rights of delegation described earlier in this exemplar. Another helpful guide is a decision tree based on the NCBSN and ANA guidelines (see **Figure 39.4** »)

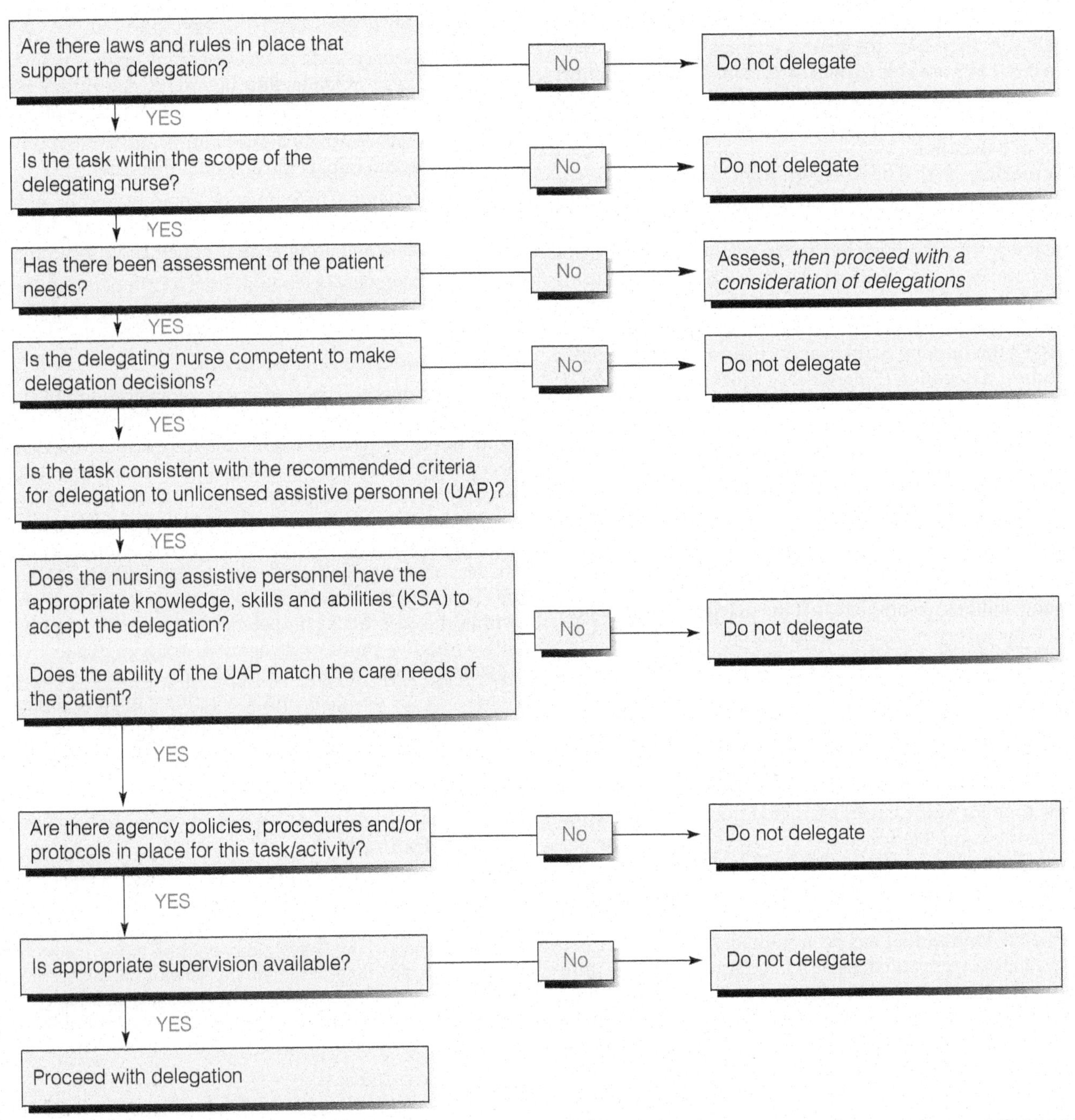

Figure 39.4 » Decision tree for delegation to unlicensed assistive personnel.

Source: Adapted from "Appendix B NCSBN, Decision Tree for Delegation to Nursing Assistive Personnel" from Joint Statement on Delegation by the American Nurses Association and the National Council of State Boards of Nursing. Used by permission of the National Council of State Boards of Nursing.

REVIEW Delegation

RELATE Link the Concepts and Exemplars

You are an RN working on a medical unit with two other RNs, an LPN, and two UAP. You receive a call informing you that two patients (both of whom are assigned to your care) must be transferred to another unit in order to make room for two patients who are to be admitted as soon as the rooms are ready.

Linking the exemplar of delegation with the concept of collaboration:

1. You delegate collection of one patient's possessions in preparation for transfer to one of the UAP, who says, "Why are you dumping this work on me? You do it." How would you manage this conflict?
2. The LPN working on the unit is newly licensed and has been employed for only 4 weeks. How would you collaborate with this nurse when delegating tasks for completion?

Linking the exemplar of delegation with the concept of teaching and learning:

3. How can you facilitate the new LPN's education in performing tasks that are commonly delegated?
4. How would you evaluate the LPN's learning related to delegated tasks?

REFER Go to Pearson MyLab Nursing and eText

REFLECT Apply Your Knowledge

You are working the night shift on a medical unit and have been assigned charge nurse responsibilities. You are working with four RNs, one LPN, and two UAP. A patient becomes pulseless and is not breathing, and the nurse assigned to the patient's care calls a code. The nurse is occupied at this patient's bedside for 1.5 hours until the resuscitation effort is completed, and the patient is transferred to the intensive care unit. This nurse also has four other assigned patients. In addition to the nurse assigned to care for the patient requiring resuscitation, two of the other nurses working on your unit are assisting in the code.

1. What tasks could you delegate to the UAP?
2. How will you maintain the safety of the other patients on your unit while the three nurses are occupied with the patient who requires resuscitation?
3. How might effective delegation to other team members contribute to care of the patients on the unit?

» Exemplar 39.D Leadership and Management

Exemplar Learning Outcomes

39.D Analyze leadership and management as they relate to managing care.

- Differentiate managers from leaders.
- Outline classic and contemporary leadership theories.
- Outline the four functions of management.
- Describe selected principles of management.

Exemplar Key Terms

Accountability, *2644*
Authoritarian leader, *2642*
Autocratic leader, *2642*
Bureaucratic leader, *2642*
Charismatic leader, *2642*
Commanding, *2644*
Contingency plan, *2643*
Controlling (monitoring), *2644*
Coordinating (directing), *2644*
Democratic leader, *2642*
Effectiveness, *2645*
Efficiency, *2645*
Formal leader, *2641*
Informal leader, *2641*
Laissez-faire leader, *2642*
Leader, *2641*
Manager, *2641*
Organizing, *2644*
Planning, *2643*
Productivity, *2645*
Quantum leadership, *2643*
Responsibility, *2644*
Servant leadership, *2643*
Shared leadership, *2643*
Situational leader, *2642*
Strategic plan, *2643*
Transactional leader, *2642*
Transformational leader, *2642*

Overview

Although leadership and management are important concepts in nursing, some nurses struggle to understand the difference between leaders and managers. In broad terms, **leaders** are individuals who use interpersonal skills to influence others to accomplish specific goals. Leaders tend to be productive and persuasive and exhibit initiative and confidence, and they play a significant role in organizational success. Leadership may be formal or informal. A **formal leader** is one who is given official authority to make decisions and to act in that capacity within an organization. An **informal leader** is one who by virtue of selected factors (talent, ability, seniority, or age) assumes a leadership position but is not officially appointed to direct the activities of others. Each type of leader (formal or informal) helps to contribute to the healthcare environment.

In contrast to leadership, management is always formal. **Managers** are individuals who hold an official position within an organization and are essential to the organization's success. Managers go by a variety of titles, including (but not limited to) *manager*, *director*, *supervisor*, and *administrator*. Nurse managers may manage units, departments, or entire facilities. On any given day, they must balance the needs of patients, professional staff, nonprofessional staff, contractors, the organization, and themselves. In order to meet the needs of these groups, nurse managers require a body of knowledge and skills distinct from those used in general nursing practice. Unfortunately, a gap often exists between what managers know and what managers need to know. New managers tend to apply skills learned through experiences with former supervisors rather than through formal management training. Increasing the number of nurses who hold BSN and MSN degrees could help close this gap.

All nurses manage and lead—at least in a practical sense. Whether through example, delegation, or the authority of their position, they formally and informally direct the work of professional and nonprofessional staff in order to achieve desired outcomes in patient care. As a result, all nurses should seek to build their leadership and management skills, no matter their current position or career aspirations.

Leadership Theories

Because leadership is a learned process, being an effective leader requires an understanding of the needs, goals, and rewards that motivate people. It also requires knowledge of leadership skills and of the group's activities as well as possession of the interpersonal skills necessary to influence others.

When learning leadership skills, it is helpful to be familiar with leadership theories. These theories describe the traits, behaviors, motivations, and choices leaders use to influence others. Classic leadership theories focus on what leaders are (trait theories), what leaders do (behavioral theories), and how leaders adapt their style according to the situation (contingency theories). Contemporary theories look at the emotions and relationships involved in leadership, as well as the importance of empowerment and shared responsibility. In practice, good leaders combine components of classical and contemporary theories into their daily interactions with others, and no single theory or type of theory adequately describes all the components of leadership.

Classic Leadership Theories

Most classic leadership theories are classified as trait based or behavior based. Trait theories hold that successful leaders have certain traits or characteristics such as knowledge, judgment, decision making, integrity, and self-confidence associated with leadership. These theories have traditionally posited that leader traits and abilities are something an individual is born with, not something that is learned or acquired. In contrast, behavioral theorists believe that leadership characteristics are learned through life experience and training. According to this point of view, an individual's leadership style can be described as autocratic, democratic, laissez-faire, or bureaucratic.

An **autocratic leader**, also called an **authoritarian leader**, assumes the decision-making process for a group and directs all activities based on a prescribed protocol. Depending on the task or process designed, this type of leadership style can be effective as it promotes efficiency when urgent decisions must be made (e.g., in the case of a cardiac arrest, unit fire, or terrorist attack), when one individual must assume responsibility without being challenged by other team members. The task or goal is the focus rather than the needs of the group members.

In contrast, a **democratic leader** (also called a *participative or consultative leader*) encourages group engagement, discussion, and decision making, which in turn promote productivity related to the task or goal at hand. This type of leadership requires a coordinated effort between the leader and group members and places value on all members of the group to contribute toward goal completion.

A **laissez-faire leader** allows for the group to make decisions based on their expertise and internal motivation to achieve goals. This type of leadership assumes that the group will work collaboratively rather than at cross purposes. The laissez-faire leader takes a hands-off approach. This type of leadership can be effective when the group is composed of committed members who have the experience to accomplish the task or project at hand without much help or direction from the leader.

A **bureaucratic leader** works within the confines of the organization's values as they relate to policy and procedures to serve as the framework for group process. Similar to the group members, the bureaucratic leader often focuses leadership on the organization's rules and procedures, allowing for little flexibility. This can lead to dissatisfaction among group members, especially if they may have more experience than the leader.

In addition to trait and behavioral theories, contingency theories account for a third category of classic leadership theories. These theories propose yet another type of leader: the **situational leader**, who adapts the leadership style to the situation. Flexibility is a key component of the situational leader. This type of leader focuses on being not only aware of tasks and/or relationship but utilizes encouragement and selects activities that help promote participation of group members.

Contemporary Leadership Theories

Contemporary leadership theories are categorized as charismatic leaders, transactional leaders, and transformational leaders. Embedded in these categories are shared leadership, shared governance, and servant leadership.

A **charismatic leader** engages group members with personality and enlists them to follow the leader's cause and beliefs. The connection between the charismatic leader and the group is strong and fosters commitment, faith, and perseverance in completing tasks.

The **transactional leader** forms a transactional relationship between the leader and group members that helps to promote loyalty and engagement. The connection between the transactional leader and the group is based on the perceived value of the exchange. Tasks are performed as needed and completed efficiently.

In contrast, a **transformational leader** focuses on using adaptation and change to encourage and motivate group members to participate in a shared vision to complete tasks. The connection between the transformational leader and group members focuses on creativity and inspiration to help achieve independence, individual growth and change.

The National Academy of Medicine (NAM) and researchers are beginning to focus on how nursing leadership is affected by transitioning roles, technology, and the social environment (Miceli, 2019). The NAM's *The Future of Nursing 2020–2030* (2020) consensus report provides information related to emerging challenges to nursing in view of the current health pandemic.

For more information on the traits required by transformational nursing leaders, see **Box 39.5** ».

Shared leadership focuses on the commonality of the experience and collective action serves as the motivating factor for group action rather than any action by a single leader. By working collaboratively, group actions allow for a broader decision-making process in this type of leadership.

Quantum leadership examines the context of leader, the group, and the task to be accomplished or problem to be solved. Quantum leaders focus on connections within the group, are flexible rather than controlling, and are able to view the big picture while still anticipating and planning how to respond to problems or barriers.

Finally, **servant leadership** focuses on the belief that the most effective leaders are those who are motivated primarily by a desire to serve, rather than a desire to lead. According to this theory, by placing others' needs before their own, servant leaders inspire their followers to grow and become more self-directed. As a result of this personal growth, the followers themselves feel more empowered to act in the best interests of both the organization and the people around them. Servant leadership's emphasis on service, caring, and compassion make it an especially good fit for the healthcare environment and nursing. Use of this leadership model cultivates not only stronger staff relationships but also stronger nurse–patient relationships. Characteristics of the servant leader include strong communication skills (listens and is empathic), the ability to resolve issues (by being aware, healing, and persuasive) and think ahead (conceptualizing, visionary, and being an effective steward of resources), and commitment to the process at the individual group level, organizational level, and community level (Sherman, 2019).

Regardless of which type of leadership model is in effect in the healthcare environment, the focus remains on the ability of the model to translate theory into reality. Working toward achievement of a goal requires determination, perseverance, and buying into the perceived value. Combine that with respect, integrity, recognition, and inclusion of how diversity can be incorporated into a realistic approach, leadership in nursing practice will evolve and continue to lead to improved health outcomes.

Box 39.5

Transformational Leadership in Nursing

Transformational leadership in nursing looks to inspire and motivate others and is considered an intentional action on the part of the leader. The transformational leader focuses on open communication, creative engagement, and fostering a sense of commitment and empowerment regarding decision making.

Transformational leaders:

- Model healthy professional behaviors and decision making
- Inspire a shared vision among team members
- Enable others to act based on that vision
- Maximize team capacity
- Offer solutions when challenging processes
- Provide support and recognition.

With the concept of transformational leadership as the core, the model allows for a circular pathway whereby motivations and actions are encouraged and realized through group effort.

Sources: Based on Clavelle and Prado-Inzerillo (2018); Morales (2020).

Clinical Example D

Lauren Chavoen works in a hospital where senior management believes it is essential to engage nursing staff in planning, implementing, and evaluating patient care policies. She realizes that she is not yet ready to assume a management position, but she understands that senior management's beliefs offer her a chance to develop some leadership and management skills through participation in policy development.

Critical Thinking Questions

1. How should Lauren convince her manager that her participation would benefit not only herself but also her unit?
2. Evaluate what skills Lauren will need to be successful on the committee she joins.

Management Functions

Management and leadership are closely tied to each other, although the functions associated with management tend to be more clearly defined than those associated with leadership. These functions were first described by French industrialist Henri Fayol in 1916 as *planning, organizing, commanding, coordinating (directing)*, and *controlling (monitoring)*. Though a century has passed, the fundamental functions identified by Fayol remain relevant for nurse managers today (Acob, 2018).

Planning

Planning is a multistage process whereby goals are established based on assessment data and a course of action is developed to help realize and achieve the intended goals. Planning may occur at the individual, group (unit or department), or organizational level. The number of individuals involved in the decision-making and problem-solving process is reflective of the defined planning level. At higher levels of planning that involve more people or groups, planning becomes more comprehensive and should be aligned with the mission and goals of the organization. Nurse managers would be involved and accountable for goals developed at the unit level.

Planning is either strategic or contingent. A **strategic plan** focuses on organizational outcomes and results to be achieved and typically involves a committee working over several months, engaging with various stakeholders to gather and analyze data to inform the strategic plan. The strategic plan outlines the desired results of the organization and describes the actions that will be taken to achieve those results. For example, to hire a more diverse staff, the organization will take specific steps outlined in the strategic plan for recruitment.

In contrast, a **contingency plan** focuses on preparation for occurrences based on the probability that an event might occur. For example, many organizations have contingency plans for weather events or a fire occurring inside the facility. Contingency plans help to provide a framework for intervention and planning should an event occur so that a response can be initiated quickly.

Consider this example of strategic planning at the unit level: A nurse manager might be charged with developing a plan to add a time-saving device to commonly used equipment. The manager must present the plan persuasively and develop operational strategies for implementation, such as acquiring the device and training staff in its use.

At the unit level, the nurse manager may have a contingency plan for a number of possibilities, ranging from staffing shortages to bed shortages. Contingency plans will vary based on the potential problem identified. For example, a contingency plan for unintentional exposure of a patient to an infection will be different than a contingency plan for staffing if two nurses call in sick for the same shift on the same unit.

Organizing

Organizing is the process of identifying and assigning assets and resources—everything from staff to equipment and supplies. An organization that has inherent systematic reviews of assets (personnel, equipment, and finances) is more efficient and better able to succeed. Identification of participants within the organization structure in terms of leadership and chain of command should align with the stated mission values of the organization.

Commanding

Commanding is the supervision of work to communicate and achieve goals. Commanding or supervising employees should be done in line with the standards and values of the organization.

Coordinating (Directing)

Coordinating (directing) is the process of using communication to motivate individuals in a group process. Inherent in this process is the act of delegation. When group function is supported by management, the process will be more efficient in working toward achieving outcomes.

Controlling (Monitoring)

Controlling (monitoring) uses metrics to monitor and evaluate processes and resources leading to goal achievement. Inherent in this process are establishing performance standards, a metric for evaluation of standards, comparison between a real and actualized process with feedback, and ways of identifying and tracking use of resources and supplies. Based on reported comparisons and feedback, if needed, subsequent action can be undertaken to help achieve goals.

While Fayol's functions of management may reflect historical insight, they are still in use today as a key framework to establish effective management. Fayol's work is also seen in nursing research. Acob (2018) utilized Fayol's work in a research study that focused on nursing management in the Philippines. Results indicated that out of the five functions of management, nurse managers used "commanding" the most and "planning" the least in their roles. Supervision and authority in the clinical environment were the main management focus.

SAFETY ALERT Improving patient safety is an important function of the nurse manager. In doing so, the nurse manager must identify errors in patient care and help staff learn from those errors. When using errors as a teaching tool, it is essential that the manager do so without singling out the staff member or members who committed the error or attaching blame to those individuals.

Principles of Management

In addition to understanding managerial functions, nurse managers must have knowledge of the basic principles of management, including authority, accountability, and responsibility. *Authority* is the right to direct others along with their activities in order to achieve outcomes. Authority to supervise or direct is realized through various leadership models. Implied within the context of authority is that individuals having authority will be accountable and take responsibility for their own actions.

Accountability and **responsibility** are terms that are applied in nursing and in management. Smith and Karakashian (2018) clarify that the nurse is *accountable* to something as in adhering to the scope of practice, whereas the nurse is *responsible* for performing professional roles and duties, such as administering a medication. Taken together, the professional nurse is both accountable and responsible for the delivery of care as defined by the standards of care and scope of practice. In management, the manager has accountability for the outcomes of the organization and a responsibility to the organization for achieving those outcomes. Depending on the values of the organization, the manager may also have a responsibility to employees and consumers (patients), but the manager is employed by and accountable to the organization.

Managing Resources

The ability to manage resources (personnel and fiscal) is a critical element in any type of organization. Nurse managers must be aware of how budgets impact delivery of care and how to incorporate best-practice methods to determine and adapt as needed between projected and actual expenses. For more information about the allocation of resources, see Module 46, Healthcare Systems.

Enhancing Employee Performance

Nurse managers should focus on best-practice methods to foster engagement and participation for their staff in order to improve outcome measures. Lifelong learning is an integral core of nursing practice, and nurse managers should promote educational opportunities as well as achievement of advanced certification for their staff. Nurse managers who lead by example, offer support and guidance, and foster a commitment to the institution will help promote staff confidence.

Building and Managing Teams

The manager is responsible for building and managing the work team by utilizing the group process. The term *group process* focuses on the ability of each member of the team to understand not only the group's purpose but what specific role each individual member fulfills as part of that team. An effective manager recognizes contributions at the individual or group level, thereby fostering engagement and confidence. The interprofessional team is an example of a group that follows a group process.

Yet another way that nurse managers can promote more effective group processes is through recognition and appreciation of the differences among staff members, as described in the Focus on Diversity and Culture.

Communication is a critical element used in working with healthcare teams. Healthcare teams come together to deliver care and improve outcomes for patient populations. It is therefore important that communication is effective, transparent, and understood within group interactions. The nurse manager is in an excellent position to facilitate communication and make sure that documentation is aligned with the management of care.

Evaluating the group's work is another responsibility of the manager. Effectiveness, efficiency, and productivity are three frequently used outcome measures. **Effectiveness** refers to the ability to provide the best care based on evidence-based practice methods. **Efficiency** refers to providing timely, cost-effective care without any unnecessary waste or expense. **Productivity** refers to best-practice methods where the outcome measurement of performance is evaluated in terms of effectiveness and efficiency. To be productive, nurses must use effective methods to deliver nursing care in an efficient manner.

Managing Conflict

In the healthcare setting, nurse managers often are asked to resolve conflicts related to individual, groups, or teams to help maintain and improve outcomes. Areas of conflict include but are not limited to differences in personal or interpersonal matters such as values or philosophical beliefs or fiscal issues such as competition for resources and/or distribution of services.

A nurse can use any of the available methods for managing conflict, each of which has its advantages and disadvantages (see Module 37, Collaboration). New nurse managers may require training to become proficient in the use of these methods.

Managing Time

Effective time management is an essential quality of nurse managers. Leading by example, nurse managers should remain focused on the task(s) at hand while being able to adjust for unanticipated events. Strategies that the nurse manager (and all nurses) can rely on in order to use time efficiently include the use of prioritized actions based on best-practice methods, knowing when to ask for assistance, and establishing a routine (protocol) that helps promote consistency and at the same time can be adaptable to patient care situations as needed.

Focus on Diversity and Culture

Research on Cultural Competence Training

Today's nursing workforce is increasingly diverse, not only in terms of culture and ethnicity but also in terms of age, experience, education, gender, religion, and many other factors. Increased diversity is beneficial because it means America's nurses are better equipped than ever before to address the needs of a rapidly changing population. However, if not properly addressed and embraced, diversity among staff members can also serve as a potential impediment to communication, teamwork, and effective group processes. There is strong support for cultural competence training based on federal and state organizations that mandate delivery of healthcare. However, it is equally important to assess and evaluate the training that is being used to promote and satisfy the ability to be culturally aware.

Research by Kaihlanen et al. (2019) examined the perception of nurses regarding cultural competence training by looking at the parameters of content, utility, and implementation. Results revealed that when nurses first understood their own "self-bias," they were better apt to adapt and/or understand cultural aspects of other populations. Research has demonstrated that with cultural competence training not only do healthcare workers collaborate more effectively but patient satisfaction improves, leading to better outcomes (University of Wisconsin Public Health Institute, 2021). Guyton (2019) stresses the fact that it is not only important to understand the levels of cultural competence (be knowledgeable, be aware, be sensitive, and be competent [operationalize the process]) but to be more self-aware so as to move to a multicultural mindset.

REVIEW Leadership and Management

RELATE Link the Concepts and Exemplars

Linking the exemplar of leadership and management with the concept of quality improvement:

1. What effects might shared leadership and shared governance have on the quality improvement process?

Linking the exemplar of leadership and management with the concept of communication:

2. What is the nurse manager's role in improving communication at the time of patient hand-offs to promote patient safety?
3. Can an individual with poor communication skills act as a competent leader? Why or why not?

REFER Go to Pearson MyLab Nursing and eText

REFLECT Apply Your Knowledge

Taylor Bradakis graduated 2 years ago and worked in labor and delivery after graduation. He recently was transferred to the neonatal intensive care unit (NICU). Martha Rivaldo is a staff nurse on Taylor's new unit; she has been in the NICU for 13 years and has a reputation for being an exceptionally skilled and competent nurse. She also has a reputation for being critical and unkind to new nurses on the unit. Taylor has yet to have an unpleasant encounter with Martha, but he has overheard her complaining to her friends about younger staff members and about the way the unit is managed. Several nurses confide in Taylor that they have complained about Martha to the nurse manager, but the nurse manager never does anything about her behavior. Instead, the nurse manager simply says, "How do you suggest correcting this issue?"

1. Is Martha a leader? Explain your answer.
2. Why might the nurse manager ask for staff nurses' input when they report problems with Martha?
3. If you were the NICU nurse manager and you had received several complaints about Martha's behavior, how would you respond?
4. What is Taylor's best course of action when he overhears complaints from both Martha and the other nurses on the unit?

References

Acob, J. R. (2018). Nurse managers' utilization of Fayol's theory in nursing. *Journal of Health Science and Prevention, 2*(2), 62–66. https://pdfs.semanticscholar.org/a079/0607df5371d81d201b5315dbb75fe68ece0e.pdf

Advanced Medical Reviews. (2019). *Mandated nurse-to-patient staffing ratios: Benefits at the bedside and beyond.* https://www.admere.com/amr-blog/mandated-nurse-to-patient-staffing-ratios-benefits-at-the-bedside-and-beyond

Aiken, L. H., Clarke, S. P., Cheung, R. B., **Sloane, D. M., & Silber, J. H.** (2003). Educational levels of hospital nurses and surgical patient mortality. *Journal of the American Medical Association, 290,* 1617–1623.

Aiken, L. H., & Lasater, K. B. (2017). Commentary on "The changing medical division of labor." *Journal of Ambulatory Care Management, 40*(3), 176–178.

American Association of Colleges of Nursing (AACN). (2020) *Nursing shortage.* https://www.aacnnursing.org/News-Information/Fact-Sheets/Nursing-Shortage

Anderson, A. (2018). Delegating as a new nurse. *American Journal of Nursing, 118*(12), 51–55.

Armold, S. (2019). Case management: An overview for nurses. *Nursing, 49*(9), 43–45. https://journals.lww.com/nursing/Fulltext/2019/09000/Case_management__An_overview_for_nurses.11.aspx

Aspland, E., Gartner, D., & Harper, P. (2019). Clinical pathway modelling: A literature review. *Health Systems.* https://www.tandfonline.com/doi/full/10.1080/20476965.2019.1652547

Avant Healthcare. (2020). *2020 Trends in nurse staffing. A national survey on the state of nurse staffing in 2020.* https://avanthealthcare.com/pdf/2020-Trends-in-Nurse-Staffing.pdf

Burton, L. (2018). *What is person-centered care and why is it important?* https://www.highspeedtraining.co.uk/hub/what-is-person-centred-care/

Clavelle, J. T., & Prado-Inzerillo, M. (2018). Inspire others through transformational leadership. *American Nurse Today, 13*(11), 39–41. https://www.myamericannurse.com/inspire-transformational-leadership/

Council of Economic Advisers. (2019). *Deregulating health insurance markets. Value to market participants.* https://www.whitehouse.gov/wp-content/uploads/2019/02/Deregulating-Health-Insurance-Markets-FINAL.pdf

Cutler, D. M., & Summers, L. H. (2020). The COVID-19 pandemic and the $16 trillion virus. *Journal of the American Medical Association, 324*(15), 1495–1496.

Driscoll, A., Grant, M. J., Carroll, D., Dalton, S., Deaton, C., Jones, I., et al. (2017). The effect of nurse-to-patient ratios on nurse-sensitive patient outcomes in acute specialist units: A systematic review and meta-analysis. *European Journal of Cardiovascular Nursing, 17*(1), 6–22.

Geld, B. (2020). *Case management managing access protecting hospital resources and patient's benefits.* https://www.cfcm.com/wp-content/uploads/2020/03/Case-Management-Managing-Access-The-Center-for-Case-Management.pdf

Guyton, G. (2019). *Promoting cultural competence in the workplace: Understanding the difference between cultural competence and awareness.* https://www.glenguyton.com/2019/09/11/promoting-cultural-competence-in-the-workplace-understanding-the-difference-between-cultural-competence-and-awareness/

Heath, S. (2018). *How nurse staffing ratios impact patient safety, access to care.* https://patientengagementhit.com/news/how-nurse-staffing-ratios-impact-patient-safety-access-to-care

Institute of Medicine (IOM). (2010). *The future of nursing: Leading change and advancing health.* Washington, DC: National Academies Press.

Juraschek, S. P., Zhang, X., Ranganathan, V., & Lin, V. W. (2019). United States registered nurse workforce report card and shortage forecast. *American Journal of Medical Quality, 34*(5), 241–249.

Kaihlanen, A.M., Hietapakka, L. & Heponiemi, T. (2019). Increasing cultural awareness: Qualitative study of nurses' perceptions about cultural competence training. *BMC Nursing, 18*(38), 1–9. https://bmcnurs.biomedcentral.com/articles/10.1186/s12912-019-0363-x

Kerns, C., & Willis, D. (2020, March 16). The problem with U.S. health care isn't a shortage of doctors. *Harvard Business Review.* https://hbr.org/2020/03/the-problem-with-u-s-health-care-isnt-a-shortage-of-doctors

Kurani, N., McDermott, D., & Shanosky, N. (2020). *How does the quality of the U.S. healthcare system compare to other countries?* https://www.healthsystemtracker.org/chart-collection/quality-u-s-healthcare-system-compare-countries/#item-start

Lasater, K. B., Aiken, L. H., Sloane, D. M., French, R., Martin, B., Reneau, K., et al. (2020). Chronic hospital nurse understaffing meets COVID-19: An observational study. *BMJ Quality & Safety.* https://qualitysafety.bmj.com/content/qhc/early/2020/08/13/bmjqs-2020-011512.full.pdf

Lee, A., Cheung, Y. S. L., Joynt, G. M., Leung, C. C. H., Wong, W.-T., & Gomersall, D. (2017). Are high nurse workload staffing ratios associated with decreased survival in critically ill patients?: A cohort study. *Annals of Intensive Care, 7*(46). https://doi.org/10.1186/s13613-017-0269-2

Livanos, N. (2018). A Broadening coalition: Patient safety enters the nurse-to-patient ratio debate. *Journal of Nursing Regulation, 9*(1), 68–70.

McKnight, H., & Moore, S. M. (2020). *Nursing shared governance.* StatPearls. https://www.ncbi.nlm.nih.gov/books/NBK549862/

Micelli, S. (2019). *The next decade of nursing. NAM town halls explore how new roles, new tech, and social needs are transforming the field.* https://www8.nationalacademies.org/onpinews/newsitem.aspx?RecordID=8262019&_ga=2.67085102.1060025698.1566825267-978273653.1546549226

Miller, L. A. (2018). Delegation. Legal issues for clinicians. *Journal of Perinatology and Neonatal Nursing, 32*(2), 104–106.

Morales, M. (2020). *Characteristics and examples of transformational leadership in nursing.* https://www.relias.com/blog/transformational-leadership-in-nursing

National Academy of Medicine. (2020). *The future of nursing 2020–2030.* https://nam.edu/publications/the-future-of-nursing-2020-2030/

National Council of State Boards of Nursing (NCSBN) & American Nurses Association (ANA). (2019). *National guidelines for delegation.* https://www.ncsbn.org/NGND-PosPaper_06.pdf

National Nurses United. (2020). *RN staffing ratios: A necessary solution to the patient safety crisis in U.S. hospitals.* https://www.nationalnursesunited.org/ratios

Nunn, R., Parson, J., & Shambugh, J. (2020). *A dozen facts about the economics of the US health-care system.* Brookings Institution. https://www.brookings.edu/research/a-dozen-facts-about-the-economics-of-the-u-s-health-care-system/

Nursing Solutions Inc. (NSI). (2021). *2021 NSI National health care retention & RN staffing report.* https://www.nsinursingsolutions.com/Documents/Library/NSI_National_Health_Care_Retention_Report.pdf

Patient-Centered Primary Care Collaborative. (2020). *Defining the medical home: A patient-centered philosophy that drives primary care excellence.* https://www.pcpcc.org/about/medical-home

Paulson, R. A. (2018). Taking nurse staffing research to the unit level. *Nursing Management, 49*(7), 42–48. https://www.ncbi.nlm.nih.gov/pmc/articles/PMC6039374/

Potter, P. A., Perry, A. G., Stockert, P. A., & Hall, A. M. (2021). *Fundamentals of nursing* (10th ed.). Elsevier.

Sharafi, S., Chamanzari, H., Pouresmail, Z., Rajabpour, M., & Bazzi, A. (2018). The effect of case method and primary nursing method on the social dimension in quality of patient care. *Journal of Holistic Nursing and Midwifery, 28*(4), 252–258.

Sherman, R. O. (2019). The case for servant leadership. *Nurse Leader, 17*(2). 86–87. https://www.nurseleader.com/article/S1541-4612(18)30397-5/fulltext

Smith, N., & Karakashian, A.L. (2018). *Accountability in nursing practice. Evidence-based care sheet.* CINHAL. https://www.ebscohost.com/assets-sample-content/NRCP_EBCS_Accountability-in-NursingPractice.pdf

Sullivan, E. J. (2019). *Effective leadership and management in nursing* (9th ed.). Pearson.

Tikkanen, R., & Abrams, M. K. (2020). *U.S. health care from a global perspective, 2019: Higher spending, worse outcomes?* The Commonwealth Fund. https://www.commonwealthfund.org/publications/issue-briefs/2020/jan/us-health-care-global-perspective-2019

Tolbert, J., Orgera, K., & Damico, A. (2020). *Key facts about the uninsured population.* Kaiser Family Foundation. https://www.kff.org/uninsured/issue-brief/key-facts-about-the-uninsured-population/

University of Wisconsin Public Health Institute. (2021). *Cultural competence training for healthcare professionals.* https://www.countyhealthrankings.org/take-action-to-improve-health/what-works-for-health/strategies/cultural-competence-training-for-health-care-professionals

Verma, S. (2019). *Competition as the engine for lowering healthcare costs.* Centers for Medicare and Medicaid Services. https://www.cms.gov/blog/competition-engine-lowering-healthcare-costs

Vogenberg, F. R., & Santilli, J. (2019). Key trends in healthcare for 2020 and beyond. *American Health & Drug Benefits, 12*(7). https://www.ncbi.nlm.nih.gov/pmc/articles/PMC6996619/pdf/ahdb-12-348.pdf

Wagner, E. A. (2018). Improving patient care outcomes through better delegation-communication between nurses and assistive personnel. *Journal of Nursing Care Quality, 33*(2), 187–193.

Zhang, X., Tai, D., Pforsich, H., & Lin V. W. (2018). United States registered nurse workforce report card and shortage forecast: A revisit. *American Journal of Medical Quality, 33*(3), 229–236.

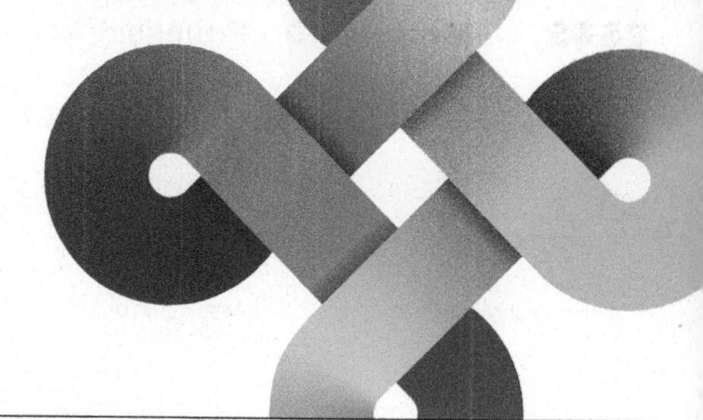

Module 40
Professionalism

Module Outline and Learning Outcomes

The Concept of Professionalism

Components of Professionalism in Nursing

40.1 Analyze the components of professionalism within the practice of nursing.

Concepts Related to Professionalism

40.2 Outline the relationship between professionalism and other concepts.

Unprofessional Behaviors

40.3 Analyze the components of unprofessional behaviors.

Professionalism Exemplars

Exemplar 40.A Commitment to Profession

40.A Analyze commitment to profession as it relates to professionalism.

Exemplar 40.B Professional Development

40.B Analyze professional development as it relates to professionalism.

Exemplar 40.C Work Ethic

40.C Analyze work ethic as it relates to professionalism.

>> The Concept of Professionalism

Concept Key Terms

Abuse of power, **2652** Compassion, **2650** Formation, **2649** Integrity, **2650** Profession, **2647**

Nursing has taken great strides to be viewed and accepted as a profession. **Profession** can be defined as work that requires specialized training and/or skills. A profession is differentiated from other occupations by knowledge and skills acquired in a particular area (Berman, Snyder, & Frandsen, 2021). To be viewed as a professional, a person possesses the characteristics, traits, behaviors, and training that align with a particular occupation (Byars, Camacho, Earley, & Harrington, 2017).

Nurses hold the public's trust. In Gallup's annual survey of professions published on January 6, 2020, 85% of Americans called nurses' honesty and ethical standards either high or very high (Reinhart, 2020). This rating has remained consistent for the last 18 years, with nurses ranking the highest among all professionals for honesty and ethics.

Nurses are visible and present across the continuum of healthcare services, advocating for and caring for patients through the many facets of health promotion, education, maintenance, and restoration. Nurses may be found in diverse healthcare settings, including acute hospital settings, clinics, public health departments, private practice, hospice centers, birthing centers, schools, pharmacies, and doctors' offices. Nursing care extends beyond the confines of institutions and facilities. It is given in parish ministries, on military bases and in mobile field hospitals, at children's camps, at community health fairs, at motor-vehicle crashes by emergency flight nurses, at places of employment in corporate health clinics, and in patients' homes. Nurse educators and researchers practice in colleges and universities and in clinical settings, and there are school nurses in schools and colleges. Nurses are accessible 24 hours a day in the acute care setting and may also be available via telehealth lines. Given that they interact so often with the community in health and wellness, in sickness, at work, at school, or at recreation sites, is it any wonder that nurses have secured trust in the community?

The first step in fostering trust is to be present and engaged in a professional manner. How then does the nursing profession, with such a large and varied practice arena, define professional behaviors for nurses?

Components of Professionalism in Nursing

Upon receiving their licenses, members of the nursing profession commit to a fundamental social contract that sets rules to guide the professional conduct of licensed registered nurses (American Nurses Association [ANA], n.d.). Nurses, however, do not become professionals just by receiving a license. The complexities of professionalism are learned by nurses over years of engagement with comprehensive educational programs, competent role models, and field experiences (Bimray, Jooste, & Julie, 2019). Through learning, interaction, development, and adaptation, nurses gradually

TABLE 40.1 Characteristics Exhibited by Professional Nurses

Characteristic	Description
Professional Behaviors	Nurses convey professionalism by maintaining calm demeanors, refraining from inappropriate electronic media use, demonstrating a strong work ethic, and dressing appropriately.
Teaching and Learning	Nurses attain an expert level of nursing practice by actively engaging with both on-the-job learning opportunities and formal education programs.
Competence	Nurses demonstrate competence through rigorous application of universally accepted standards of care and evidence-based practice.
Collaboration	By working respectfully and communicating fluently with other members of the healthcare team, nurses display professional collaboration skills.
Advocacy	Nurses are accountable for advocating for patient safety and needs at all times and in all settings. Nurses act to reduce risk and improve patient outcomes.
Caring Interventions	By exemplifying a positive attitude and demonstrating compassion and cultural awareness for patients' needs, nurses provide a crucial aspect of patient care.
Ethics	By adhering to accepted nursing standards and considering the ethical implications of their actions, nurses protect patients and the healthcare team and demonstrate integrity.

learn to respond to novel situations with independent and creative applications of their nursing training. A brief overview of the characteristics of professionalism in nursing is presented in **Table 40.1** ».

As the nursing profession expands to include the dynamic roles of case managers, nurse educators, and clinical nurse specialists, it is essential for nurses to educate the public to keep the image of nursing professionalism current (Gunawan, Aungsuroch, Sukarna, Nazliansyah, & Efendi, 2018). As the public and the healthcare team arrive at a coherent understanding of nursing as a healthcare profession in its own right, nurses gain incentive to perform to the best of their professional ability.

Professional Behaviors

One key component of professionalism is the nurse's commitment to behaving professionally by looking and acting like a professional, acting autonomously, and demonstrating a commitment to nursing. As a member of the profession of nursing, the individual nurse is always being observed and judged as a representative of that profession, even when off duty. How a nurse dresses, behaves, and communicates sets the stage for the development of trust or mistrust. Most healthcare employers provide employees with guidance and expectations for proper attire and conduct. Although most facilities have specific policies, those of one healthcare facility might not be relevant in another facility, and best practices are constantly being revised in light of new findings on patient safety, public perception, and shifting cultural attitudes. However, there are commonly accepted guidelines about dress, professional demeanor, and electronic media use (see **Table 40.2** »).

Appearance also affects how others within the medical community see the nurse (**Figure 40.1** »). Appearance is a form of nonverbal communication that evokes a response from others. Imagine a nurse talking on a cell phone while approaching a physician or other healthcare provider (HCP) to question the validity of an order. Will the colleague have enough confidence in the nurse to accept the expressed concern and change the decision regarding the patient's plan of care?

Behavioral factors also play a large role in the nurse's self-identification and public presentation as a professional. In the past, nurses have been seen as accessories to doctors, but as nursing knowledge and practices have developed, nurses increasingly act autonomously in delivering care and prescribing nursing treatments (Oshodi et al., 2019). As nursing continues to be increasingly recognized as an independent profession, patients and other members of the healthcare team alike will prize nurses' commitment to their profession and autonomy in performing their work.

An essential quality in acting with professionalism is demonstrating a strong work ethic. Nurses who go above and beyond to provide exemplary care, resolve conflicts, and collaborate respectfully with patients and the healthcare team will inevitably be seen as professionals.

Teaching and Learning

For generations, the on-the-job work of becoming a nurse has been considered a process of socialization. The old model of socialization carries with it a long history of subservient,

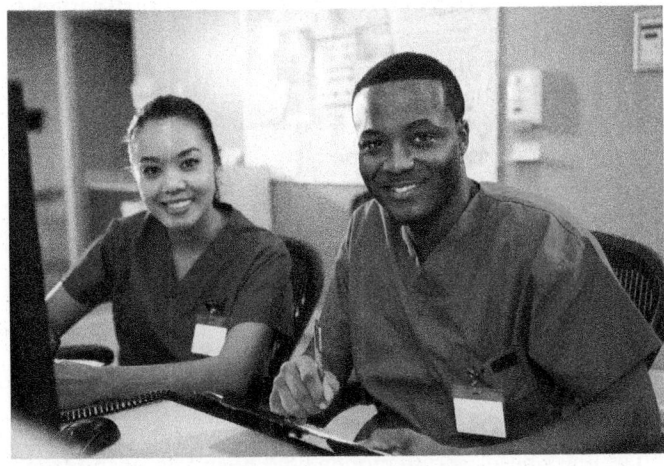

Figure 40.1 » A professional appearance supports the nurse's credibility.
Source: Shutterstock.

TABLE 40.2 Common Guidelines for Professional Attire, Demeanor, and Electronic Media Use

Guidelines	Rationale
Professional Dress	
No excessive jewelry, long fingernails or artificial nails, or chewing gum	Avoidance of items that may harbor pathogens and threaten patient safety
Hair secured away from contact with the individual receiving care	Prevents contamination of sterile fields and spread of bacteria
Personal cleanliness, avoiding strong odors and perfumes	Prevents patient discomfort and annoyance Instills patient confidence and trust Shows respect for needs of allergic or nauseated patients
Clean uniform or clothing	Promotes good sanitation Builds patient trust
Follow facility policy regarding piercings, tattoos, and other body modifications	Piercings can create a safety issue if they fall out or are pulled out by patients. Visible body modifications and tattoos may cause patient discomfort.
Professional Demeanor	
Avoid loud talking	Respect patients' need for rest
Maintain a positive attitude and instill hope	Encourages and shows respect for patients and families
Maintain a clean, uncluttered workstation	Shows respect for peers
Avoid taking personal calls at work	Keeps focus on patient care
Do not discuss personal problems with patients	Maintains professional boundaries
Never breach patient confidentiality	Avoids violation of HIPAA
Avoid gossiping with and bullying coworkers	Maintains and promotes civility and patient safety
Do not complain to patients or family members	Maintains professional boundaries
Do not use illegal substances	Shows respect for self and patient safety
Electronic Media Use	
Do not use personal cell phones to document patient information	Prevents the sharing of photos, videos, and sound recordings that may violate HIPAA
Do not share patient information over social media	Avoids the violation of HIPAA Ensures that patient information cannot be shared or retrieved from servers later, even after the nurse removes the offending content from social media

dependent roles for women, the acceptance of dominant behaviors for men, and a hierarchical structure in healthcare organizations. As an alternative to the socialization model of becoming a nurse, the concept of **formation**, a process that facilitates the transformation of an individual from a layperson to a professional nurse, can be used. Formation is an evolutionary process that requires the acquisition of lifelong learning, experience, technical expertise, and interdependent professional collaboration (Haugland, Lassen, & Giske, 2017). The resulting integration of the nurse's thoughts, feelings, education, experience, and ethical behavior contributes to the formation of a professional nurse from novice to expert (see Box 42.3, Benner's Stages of Nursing Expertise, for more information). Transformation can occur only with personal commitment to self, individuals, the community, organizations, society, lifelong learning, and the profession.

Continuously gaining knowledge is central to providing high-quality care and maintaining patient safety. Nursing students are required to learn the information the entry-level practicing nurse needs, but learning does not stop at graduation. Once licensed, nurses are expected to maintain and update their knowledge base throughout their career by engaging in continuing education programs and maintaining their licensure. Healthcare is changing constantly as new drugs enter the market, new treatments and technology are introduced, and ongoing research confirms or calls into question the effectiveness of past information. If nurses do not participate in continuing education, their knowledge base quickly becomes obsolete, and their practice may even endanger patients. Each state's board of nursing outlines requirements for nurses to participate in classes designed to help maintain and improve their knowledge (ANA, 2015). Many nurses also choose to pursue advanced degrees in nursing and other healthcare fields. See Module 41, Teaching and Learning, for more information on the nurse as a student.

Accountability

A key component in nursing professionalism is accountability to expected standards of care. Organizations such as The Joint Commission, the ANA, and the National League for Nursing (NLN) define standards of care against which nurses' performance is measured (Guido, 2020). A nurse's competence, or ability to perform the job correctly, is the practical measure of accountability. The expectation of competence begins when the student enrolls in a nursing program and continues throughout nursing practice, whether the nurse is caring for patients, managing a department, or acting in an advanced practice role. The nurse must learn how to operate new equipment before it is put into general use; maintain an evidence-based practice that is current on the latest findings; and seek help from peers, mentors, and instructors to learn new skills and techniques. Each nurse is responsible for pinpointing personal areas of strength and weakness. Once an area of weakness has been identified, the nurse should seek opportunities to gain competence in that area. This self-examination is a necessary ingredient in the formation of a truly professional nurse.

Nursing is defined as a profession in part because nurses are guided and assisted by professional organizations. In addition to the state boards of nursing and the National Council of State Boards of Nursing (NCSBN), which license nurses and define the standards of safe conduct, nurses can join a large number of professional organizations that promote information sharing, community building, and problem solving within the nursing profession. Nurses can join these organizations as a way of continuing their education and keeping up-to-date on the most recent developments in nursing practice. Module 47, Health Policy, fully describes the professional organizations that govern and differentiate the profession of nursing.

Collaboration

How to work as a member of the team is discussed in detail in Module 37, Collaboration. Skill in working as a team member contributes to others' opinions of the nurse as a professional and improves the quality of care delivered to the patient.

Clinical Example A

Caroline Nava is a 28-year-old nursing student who is enrolled in her final clinical rotation and due to graduate in 2 months. She is working on a surgical unit managing care for five individuals. After completing her documentation, she leaves the nursing unit 2 hours late. Caroline returns home, exhausted from a particularly busy clinical day. Just as she sits down to enjoy some relaxation time, she remembers that she failed to obtain information from the chart of a new postoperative patient. Earlier today, her instructor asked Caroline to report back to her about this individual's laboratory results by the end of the day. The patient returned to the unit late from postanesthesia care, as Caroline was about to leave.

Caroline begins to panic and is uncertain what to do. Suddenly, she remembers that her friend Joan McIntyre, another student, is in clinical on the same unit until late that evening. Caroline calls Joan and asks her for a favor. She explains to Joan that she is in a bind and has to call her nursing instructor with the information as soon as possible. Caroline asks Joan to take a picture with her cell phone of the laboratory results in the patient's chart and send her the picture. Joan is glad to be able to help her friend and successfully sends the information to Caroline. Caroline is able to contact her instructor with the necessary information about her patient.

Critical Thinking Questions

1. Do you think Caroline handled the situation ethically? Support your answer.
2. If you were Joan, what would you have done in this situation?

Advocacy

Advocacy, the practice of expressing and defending patients' needs, is an essential component of professional nursing practice. The ANA Code of Ethics for Nurses emphasizes patient advocacy as a key concern (see Module 44, Ethics, for more information). A nurse may be a patient advocate by conveying patients' wishes to members of the healthcare team, by communicating with patients' families, or simply by encouraging patients to express their wishes. Patient advocacy is essential for patients in vulnerable populations, such as those with disabilities or mental health diagnoses. Promotion of an organizational culture that is conducive to patient advocacy is of central importance to the development of professionalism rooted in advocacy (Gerber, 2018). See Module 43, Advocacy, for more information.

Caring Interventions

The caring interventions of attitude and compassion are key to nursing professionalism. *Attitude* is a mental state involving values, beliefs, feelings, and mood. Each individual's attitude affects the individual and all others who are nearby. Professional behavior for the nurse includes maintaining a positive attitude while working with patients, their family members, and other healthcare professionals. A nurse with a positive attitude refrains from complaining and expresses an optimistic outlook. Attitude is discussed in more detail in Exemplar 40.C, Work Ethic, in this module.

Compassion is an awareness of and concern about other individuals' suffering. Nurses demonstrate compassion when they recognize a patient's need and respond appropriately to meet that need. In showing compassion, the nurse treats the patient as a unique and special individual and not as a number or a diagnosis. The nurse further demonstrates compassion by advocating in the community and communicating with politicians to develop laws that protect and promote the health of individuals and families. See Module 35, Caring Interventions, for more information on compassion and attitude.

Ethics

As professionals, nurses adhere to the ANA Code of Ethics for Nurses, as well as evaluate the potential for any ethical conflicts between their personal ethical codes and their work as nurses. Nurses who successfully engage in consistently ethical behavior demonstrate **integrity**, or adherence to a strict moral or ethical code. For nurses, integrity involves consistent behaviors based on the internalization of the values, ethics, and best practices of the profession of nursing. Nurses demonstrate integrity by accepting feedback (positive or negative) as a tool for improving their delivery of patient care, by maintaining accountability for their actions and freely admitting when they make mistakes, and by following their state's nurse practice act and never working outside their scope of practice.

Concepts Related to Professionalism

Professionalism is a central component of all effective nursing actions. Being professionally engaged enables nurses to make accurate assessments, perform caring interventions, collaborate, make clinical decisions expediently, and teach with compassion and care. How the concepts of accountability, collaboration, advocacy, and ethics relate to professionalism are outlined elsewhere in this module. Communication and application of culturally respectful, caring interventions through the nursing process are key elements valued by nursing students and nurses (Brooks, Manias, & Bloomer, 2019). The profession of nursing is based on teamwork and respectful communication with patients as well as colleagues, and nurses must be fluent communicators to attain expert status.

Nurses' success within the discipline is predicated on a careful adherence to codes of ethics in all healthcare settings for all patients. The role of professional nurses is to incorporate ethical values of patient safety into decision making for nurses at every level of a healthcare organization or system, so that nurses in all roles consider ethical values when administering care (Haddad & Geiger, 2020).

Professional nurses are above all accountable to deliver the highest standard of care. Nursing programs should prepare students for the necessity of delivering safe, culturally competent, and compassionate care despite busy schedules, an intervention that can be aided in practice by nurses' membership in nursing organizations and ongoing education programs (Su, Masika, Paguio, & Redding, 2020). Some, but not all, of the concepts integral to Professionalism are outlined in the Concepts Related to Professionalism feature. The concepts are in alphabetical order.

Concepts Related to **Professionalism**

CONCEPT	RELATIONSHIP TO PROFESSIONALISM	NURSING IMPLICATIONS
Caring Interventions	Professional behaviors help nurses provide caring interventions to patients and themselves.	■ Practice theories of caring to ensure comprehensive patient care. ■ Emphasize caring to facilitate patients' empowerment. ■ Engage in self-care to promote holistic personal and professional wellness.
Clinical Decision Making	Nurses who engage in professional behaviors are better able to provide high-quality, evidence-based nursing care at all stages of the nursing process.	■ Use careful reasoning to ensure accurate and timely assessment while providing maximum comfort to the patient. ■ Use clinical decision making to determine priorities for care to ensure the best outcomes for the patient. ■ Use clinical decision making to determine the timing and order of interventions to promote patient trust and comfort.
Communication	Professional behaviors promote reliability and accountability for information and the methods by which it is conveyed.	■ Establish trust and rapport with patients and team members. ■ Ensure accurate and complete documentation and reporting, decreasing risks to patient safety.
Culture and Diversity	Professional standards of nursing require the nurse to work toward cultural competency and refrain from imposing the nurse's own values on the patient.	■ Assess patient and family cultural needs and practices. ■ Ensure that care provided incorporates patient and family cultural needs and practices whenever doing so will not cause injury to the patient. ■ Support the patient and family in maintaining cultural practices and rituals in outpatient, inpatient, and home care settings.
Healthcare Systems	Professional behaviors assist nurses in promoting patient trust and in advocating for patients with other members of the healthcare team.	■ By participating in primary prevention using evidence-based standards and professional guidelines, the nurse can help promote the health of the individual and the larger community. ■ By assessing the patient's insurance status and ability to access healthcare, the nurse can assist the patient in finding affordable and practical ways to meet healthcare needs.
Safety	Professional behaviors ensure that nurses follow safety guidelines and the principles of evidence-based practice.	■ Maintain current knowledge of evidence-based practices to promote patient safety. ■ Administer interventions according to knowledge of best practices across the lifespan to facilitate optimal health outcomes. ■ Maintain a sense of one's own physical limits and boundaries to promote nurse and healthcare team safety.

Unprofessional Behaviors

Unprofessional behaviors undermine an individual nurse's credibility and negatively affect group morale, and they may affect patient outcomes.

Types of Unprofessional Behaviors

Unprofessional behaviors come in many forms, but they all make members of the healthcare team and patients feel uncomfortable, hurt, intimidated, threatened, or targeted in ways that interfere with the provision of high-quality patient care (Sauer & McCoy, 2018). Some examples of unprofessional behaviors include the following:

- Belittling someone's opinion or using patronizing language
- Delivering negative or disparaging nonverbal messages
- Engaging in constant criticism, scapegoating, and fault-finding
- Engaging in elitism about experience, education, or practice area
- Undermining someone's activities or causing unnecessary disruptions
- Having emotional outbursts
- Being reluctant to answer questions
- Pitting staff members against one another and propagating rumors.

Unprofessional behaviors such as breach of confidentiality, as defined by state nurse practice acts, are discussed in Module 49, Legal Issues. Other unprofessional behaviors, such as substance abuse and discrimination, are discussed in other modules. Excessive absenteeism and tardiness, two other unprofessional behaviors, are discussed in Exemplar 40.C, Work Ethic, in this module.

It is important to recognize that the work environment sometimes carries over to social events, such as unit parties, company picnics, and informal gatherings. The rules of professionalism and the pitfalls of unprofessional behavior extend to these types of situations as well.

Abuses of Power

Any discussion of unprofessional behavior must include a discussion about abuses of power. An **abuse of power** is any attempt to use one's position or authority to shame, control, demean, humiliate, or denigrate another individual in order to gain emotional, psychologic, or physical advantage over that individual. In any professional environment, including the nursing profession, abuses of power such as sexual harassment, improper use of authority, bullying, and intimidation must be addressed immediately and appropriately.

SAFETY ALERT Acting with professionalism is not merely a matter of ensuring group cohesion and mutual respect. Behaving professionally is essential to healthcare workers' ability to ensure patient safety. According to the Agency for Healthcare Research and Quality (2019), 77% of healthcare staff report witnessing physicians engaging in disruptive behavior, and 65% report nurses engaging in these communication patterns. Most healthcare staff also believe that disruptive actions increase the potential for medical error and preventable deaths. Disruptive behaviors have been tied to nurses' workplace dissatisfaction in addition to sentinel events in the operating room. There is no standard healthcare definition of disruptive behavior, but it is commonly defined as any behavior that shows disrespect for others or impedes the delivery of patient care.

Bullying

Evidence of bullying, lateral violence (violence directed toward peers), and incivility in the healthcare environment has been well documented in nursing research for over three decades. These behaviors are commonplace because of widespread tolerance within the healthcare arena. Furthermore, the long history of a hierarchical or tiered power structure perpetuates the dominance and empowerment of unprofessional individuals. The Joint Commission has identified "behaviors that undermine a culture of safety" in healthcare (such as bullying and incivility) as being among the leading causes of sentinel events (The Joint Commission, 2018). The Joint Commission calls for zero tolerance of intimidation and bullying in the workplace and recommends that healthcare facilities implement policies to stop such bullying. See the Evidence-Based Practice feature for more information.

Sexual Harassment

According to the Equal Employment Opportunity Commission (EEOC), the definition of *sexual harassment* is "unwelcome sexual advances, requests for sexual favors, and other verbal or physical conduct of a sexual nature" (Code of Federal Regulations, 2009). Because *sexual harassment* violates the harassed person's rights, it is a form of discrimination and is prohibited by federal law. According to the Code of Federal Relations, sexual harassment occurs in any of the following circumstances:

- An individual's employment is conditional on compliance with sexual requests or tolerance of sexual behavior, regardless of whether that condition is explicitly stated or simply implied.
- Employment decisions that affect the individual, such as promotion, are based on whether that individual can be coerced into accepting a sexual request or tolerating sexual behavior. (Whether the individual rejects or is coerced into accepting the sexual request or behavior is irrelevant; it is sexual harassment in either event.)
- Sexual conduct interferes with an individual's performance on the job or creates an "intimidating, hostile, or offensive working environment."

The victim or violator may be male, female, or nonbinary in any of these cases, and it is not necessary for the victim and violator to be of a different gender.

To address any sexual harassment encountered in the workplace, nurses must develop their assertiveness skills to be able to say no when necessary. They must also familiarize themselves with the sexual harassment policy and procedures at the institution that employs them. They must know the procedure for reporting sexual harassment (including to whom they should report incidents), the investigative process, and how their confidentiality will be protected and to what extent.

Evidence-Based Practice

Bullying and Disruptive Behavior in the Workplace

Problem

Bullying and disruptive behaviors in the healthcare environment can have adverse effects on quality of care and patient safety (Omar, Salam, & Al-Surimi, 2019).

Evidence

Over the past several decades, the phenomenon of disruptive behavior in the healthcare environment has been referred to as *lateral violence*, *incivility*, and *workplace bullying (WPB)*. According to the World Health Organization (WHO), WPB is caused by psychosocial, cultural, or individual factors (Omar et al., 2019). Behaviors that indicate WPB include eye rolling, making faces, snide and rude comments, hiding supplies, and setting others up for failure (Butler, 2018). Covert and overt actions are defined as verbal outbursts and physical threats as well as passive reluctance or refusal to answer questions, failure to return phone calls or pages, use of condescending language or voice intonation, and impatience with questions. A study published by WHO found that healthcare professionals in various countries around the world experienced WPB; however, the ability to tolerate such behavior depends on the country's culture and the morals and values of the healthcare professional (Omar et al., 2019). A recent study conducted with nurses on the prevalence of bullying found that patients and visitors taking out frustrations on the nurse was the highest source of bullying. However, other studies identify supervisors and managers as the most common source of these offensive behaviors. Being exposed consistently to WPB can lead to low self-esteem and low job satisfaction and productivity, which can cause high absenteeism and staff turnover (Butler, Prentiss, & Benamor, 2018).

Implications

The National Academy of Medicine (n.d.) is currently working on the future challenges for nursing during the years 2020–2030. One of the challenges being considered is the importance of nurse well-being and resilience in ensuring the delivery of high-quality care. Although a specific challenge does not address WPB, nurses must possess and use good communication and conflict resolution skills to address bullying in the workplace and transform the healthcare environment in which they practice. The continued training of point-of-care nurses in assertiveness and leadership skill is necessary to effect a change.

Critical Thinking Application

Bullying is a threat to patient safety and the emotional well-being of nurses. What cues might a student or novice nurse use to address bullying by more experienced nurses in the healthcare setting? Describe a situation in which you may have observed or experienced incivility. Write down practical comments you would feel comfortable making to address the behavior in real time.

When providing patient care, nurses must use caution to avoid having patients misinterpret nursing behaviors as sexual harassment. For example, in lifting a patient's breast to bathe the chest or to place leads when performing an electrocardiogram, it is best to use the back of the hand rather than the palm of the hand. It is also important to explain the procedure and seek the patient's permission. In this way, the nurse can reduce the possibility that the action will be misinterpreted as sexual harassment and can avoid responses by the patient that might tend toward sexual harassment of the nurse.

Improper Use of Authority

Improper use of authority is widespread and has no place in the practice of nursing. A nursing manager may use intimidation to show favoritism and to foster subordinate compliance, bias, and group pressure to exclude employees toward whom the manager has a less favorable attitude or who challenge the manager. Nurses in authority who emphasize principles over personality and who focus on patient safety can extinguish these negative behaviors and encourage nurses at the point of care. Nurses can facilitate effective leadership by becoming active in nursing leadership organizations such as the American Organization of Nurse Executives (AONE) and the ANA Leadership Institute following licensure and by lifelong learning within the discipline to promote professionalism and support the larger nursing community. Transformational leadership, which is discussed in the exemplar on Management and Leadership Principles in Module 39, Managing Care, is recommended as the leadership style for facilitating progress and innovation in nursing.

Clinical Example B

Mary Reynolds, who is a nurse of the baby-boomer generation, disagrees with Ashley Maloney, a newly licensed nurse, about how Ms. Maloney handled a situation with a patient's family. You overhear Ms. Reynolds telling a friend of hers that she hopes that Ms. Maloney never takes care of her or her family. Later, while you are on break, Ms. Reynolds repeats to you her story about Ms. Maloney. She informs you that Ms. Maloney "ignored the family" sitting at the bedside and that the family complained to Ms. Reynolds. She apologized for Ms. Maloney and told the family, "She is a problem. Thanks for telling me. I will take care of it for you." The family rewards Ms. Reynolds by writing a supportive note to the nurse manager about her and also detailing their perception of how Ms. Maloney dealt with their family.

Critical Thinking Questions

1. Using your knowledge of formation of professional behavior and bullying, how might you respond to Ms. Reynolds?
2. Using what you have learned about communication, frame a respectful response to Ms. Reynolds.
3. If you were the nurse manager, how would you handle this situation while applying a provision of the ANA Code of Ethics?

Intimidation

Intimidation is bullying, threatening, or forcing someone who is physically or emotionally weaker to do something (or refrain from doing something) in order to avoid retribution. It is never appropriate for a nurse to threaten someone, whether a coworker, a patient, a patient's family member, or anyone else. Intimidation can be subtle, such as standing close to another individual with a hostile look on one's face, or it can be overt, such as telling someone to do something or that person will be "sorry." Even nurses with the best of intentions may not realize that they are using intimidation when they say things like "If you don't take your medicine [or go to physical therapy, or follow the treatment plan], you're only going to get worse." Even though what the nurse says may be true, this approach is intimidating and lacks professionalism.

REVIEW The Concept of Professionalism

RELATE Link the Concepts

Linking the concept of professionalism with the concept of addiction:

1. What impact does a nurse's use of addictive substances (legal or illegal) have on the practice of nursing?
2. What is your professional responsibility when a nurse on your unit appears to be under the influence of a substance?

Linking the concept of professionalism with the concept of clinical decision making:

3. How do professional behaviors result from effective clinical decision making? How do competent clinical decisions stem from professional behaviors?
4. What conclusions would you draw, or have you drawn, about a nurse's ability to make clinical decisions on the basis of the nurse's professional or nonprofessional behaviors?

REFER Go to Pearson MyLab Nursing and eText

REFLECT Apply Your Knowledge

Cheryl Goodwin is a nurse executive who is widely respected for her rapport with nurse educators. She is the dean of a nursing college and is a doctoral-prepared nurse who maintains a small private practice. She is active in state organizations and willing to help both faculty and students. A hospital administrator calls Ms. Goodwin in for a private meeting. In the course of the meeting, Ms. Goodwin is told that a faculty member in the nursing college has committed an act of abuse and neglect toward a patient in the hospital. The Chief Nurse Executive (CNE) of the hospital, who is also at the meeting, informs Ms. Goodwin that the faculty member is no longer permitted to practice at that hospital.

Upon questioning the faculty member involved, Ms. Goodwin discovers that the individual did in fact commit the offenses willfully, as reported by the CNE. Ms. Goodwin informs this faculty member that his actions created dire consequences for the patient involved and that his position at the college is terminated. He had been on probation for bullying and maltreatment of students before this incident.

The college administration permits the nursing faculty member to resign his position. He then begins a campaign to attack Ms. Goodwin, accusing her of making a number of false accusations. Friends rally around the dismissed employee, who has taught at the college for a number of years. He has been known for covering for and doing favors for other faculty members for extra cash, such as picking up an extra clinical day, and for granting favors to the faculty members who reported to him. As a senior faculty member, he also coordinated clinical rotations and scheduling.

Ms. Goodwin is not at liberty to discuss the incident that led to this faculty member's resignation. The other faculty members at the college are not aware of the consequences suffered by the hospital patient and family. The hospital has requested that the situation remain confidential, as the family has not been notified of the abuse. Faculty members who have known Ms. Goodwin for many years begin questioning her motives and labeling her as "sick." They talk behind her back and do not invite her to nursing functions that she has always attended. They bully any faculty member who associates with her. Ms. Goodwin acquires another position and leaves a position that she loved.

1. How would you describe the behaviors and actions of the faculty members in the scenario?
2. What recourse does Ms. Goodwin have?
3. Why do you suppose the faculty members who had a prior satisfactory relationship with Ms. Goodwin did not support her? Do you believe they did the right thing? How and why might they have handled the situation differently?

» Exemplar 40.A Commitment to Profession

Exemplar Learning Outcomes

40.A Analyze commitment to profession as it relates to professionalism.

- Describe factors associated with professional commitment.
- Describe types of commitment.
- Outline the stages of the commitment process.
- Discuss ways to manage stress associated with commitment to a profession.

Exemplar Key Terms

Affective commitment, *2655*
Burnout, *2656*
Commitment, *2655*
Continuance commitment, *2656*
Normative commitment, *2656*
Organizational commitment, *2655*

Overview

Many experienced nurses view nursing as a vocation or calling. It is not a job or what they *do*; it is a part of who they *are*. They have made a commitment to their profession, incorporating the ethics and expectations of nursing into every aspect of their lives, whether at home, work, or play. This commitment is in essence a duty to the individual who is at the center of nursing care. Over time, some nurses may confuse professional commitment with organizational or corporate commitment.

Commitment can be defined as an agreement or promise to do something, to act. To understand the term *commitment* as it is applied to the profession of nursing, one must first look at the concept of organizational commitment. The most widely accepted definition of **organizational commitment** is that it is the relative strength of an individual's relationship to and sense of belonging to an organization. Although organizational commitment and professional commitment may intersect, it is important for nurses to distinguish between the two. Experienced nurses can cite many instances in which nursing ethics and corporate goals collide. The business of healthcare and the provision of care to the patient are not always the same issue. The nursing profession holds the trust of the community and individuals in our society. With this trust comes the moral responsibility of nurses to address the needs of patients and to advocate for safe care within the business of healthcare.

Factors of Professional Commitment

Factors associated with professional commitment include the following:

1. A strong belief in and acceptance of the profession's code, role, goals, values, and morals.
2. A willingness to exert considerable personal effort on behalf of the profession.
3. A strong desire to maintain membership in the profession.
4. A pattern of behaviors congruent with the nurses' professional code of ethics.

As discussed earlier, nursing education concerns not only teaching students how to think like nurses and perform nursing tasks but also is charged with the acculturation and formation of professional behaviors in students and novice nurses. This process begins when the student enters the first nursing class. Many of the policies and rules associated with a nursing program are intended to prepare the student for entry into the profession of nursing. The student who violates or ignores school policy is in danger of becoming the nurse who ignores practice and agency policy. For example, tardiness in coming to clinicals may result in significant consequences for the offender. Time and attendance are critical in nursing, as patients depend on the nurse for their safety. Especially during a nursing shortage, the nurse who is chronically late for work or excessively absent is subject to disciplinary action that could include suspension and termination. With frequent staff shortages, it is even more important for managers to be able to rely on staff members to be on the job when scheduled. Chronic lateness and frequent absenteeism place a greater burden on colleagues, compromise patient care, and lead to conflict among staff.

The values and goals of professional nursing are clearly delineated by standards of nursing practice, codes of ethics, nurse practice acts, national patient safety goals, accrediting agencies, and many other such resources. Entering the nursing profession is not just taking a job. It is assuming the obligation to protect, advance, and promote the health of self, individuals, and groups in the community, and it involves many role expectations not inherent in occupations that are just "jobs."

Most students can easily identify with the willingness to exert considerable effort on behalf of the profession. Nursing programs have high standards of admission, and many programs receive far more applications than they have openings available. In times of economic recession, this imbalance is even more evident as displaced workers seek job security in the healthcare professions that have staff shortages. Nursing education is a rigorous program of study requiring considerable time and effort to prepare for entry into a demanding yet rewarding profession. The applicants who are accepted into nursing programs tend to be those who have demonstrated the ability to expend such time and effort to achieve their goals.

Students also can identify with the strong desire to maintain membership in the profession. Most students have already made sacrifices while taking related general education and science courses in preparation for the nursing major. The sacrifices required during nursing courses are even greater, as the number of hours required per credit earned increases when hours spent in lab and clinical are added. Most students who are accepted into a nursing program have a strong desire to complete it, especially as their time in the program increases.

After graduation, the commitment to maintain membership in the nursing profession is demonstrated by membership in professional organizations and on various committees and by contributing to community organizations seeking input on laws related to healthcare and health promotion. Nurses must always maintain current knowledge related to changes in healthcare and the profession of nursing to keep their nursing practice up to date and keep their patients safe. Commitment to the profession of nursing is an obligation to behave in accordance with accepted codes of nursing professional practice.

Types of Commitment

Three types of commitment describe the psychologic link between an individual and the decision to continue in a profession: affective, normative, and continuance. **Affective commitment** is an attachment to a profession and includes identification with and involvement in the profession. Affective commitment develops when involvement in a profession produces a satisfying experience. The student or nurse who has a strong desire to continue in the profession, who is involved in keeping up with current information, and who becomes involved with profession-specific organizations and service activities demonstrates affective commitment (**Figure 40.2** »). This individual is in nursing school or working as a nurse because of the desire to do so.

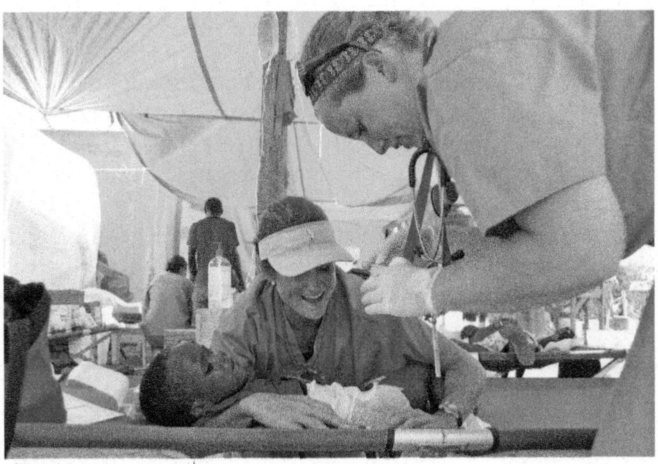

Figure 40.2 ›› Affective commitment leads nurses and other healthcare professionals to volunteer their services to help in disasters, such as the January 2010 earthquake in Haiti. Here, Tiffany Young, a pediatric nurse from North Carolina (center), holds a child with cholera who is receiving treatment.

Source: Roseann Dennery/Samaritan's Purse/Charlotte Observer/Tribune News Service/Getty Images.

Normative commitment is a feeling of obligation to continue in the profession. Normative commitment develops as a result of having received benefits or having had positive experiences through engagement in the profession. The nurse who enters the field or remains in it because personal or family experiences with illness have created a desire to work in the healthcare field exemplifies normative commitment.

Continuance commitment, or the awareness of costs associated with leaving the profession, develops when negative consequences of leaving, such as loss of income, are seen as reasons to remain. Individuals who experience this type of commitment do not manifest the same ties to the profession as do those who are motivated by affective or normative commitment. In general, such individuals are not inclined to promote their profession. These students and nurses are in the field for the money and job security.

Stages of Commitment Development

The commitment to a profession develops in stages. The first stage is the *exploratory stage*, in which individuals explore the positive aspects of the profession. An example of this stage is the excitement of nursing students during the first weeks of their program as they model their new uniforms and ransack their lab kits. Commitment that begins as exploration leads to a positive orientation toward the profession.

The second stage is the *testing stage*, during which individuals discover negative elements of the profession. In this stage, individuals start to assess their willingness and ability to deal with those negative elements. Some nursing students never get beyond this stage and drop out of school or change majors, deciding that the sacrifices are not worth the effort or that they are not suited to the nursing profession.

The third stage is the *passionate stage* of commitment, which begins as the individual synthesizes the positive and negative elements from the first two stages. Students in this stage are not only willing to commit to the profession, but they are also willing to contribute to its well-being. These students are the ones who become involved in student nursing associations, serve as class officers, or volunteer for activities not associated with a grade.

The fourth stage is the *quiet-and-bored stage* of commitment, in which students settle into the humdrum routines of the nursing program. This stage often occurs during the middle or late middle of the program, as students begin to become more comfortable in their role and feel less anxiety about their performance.

The *integrated stage* is the final stage of commitment. Individuals who reach this stage have integrated both positive and negative elements of the profession into a more flexible, complex, and enduring form of commitment. They act out their commitment as a matter of habit. These students are in the final stages of their nursing program and are beginning to see themselves as nurses, eager to take the NCLEX-RN® exam and begin employment. As new graduates, they will once again proceed through the stages of commitment while transitioning from being nursing students to being registered nurses.

Managing Stress

Part of a commitment to any profession is learning how to manage the stress associated with that profession. Although most nurses find healthy ways to cope with the physical and emotional demands of the profession, these demands do create stress that can be difficult to manage. Nurses in some situations are overcome and develop **burnout**, which is similar to the exhaustion stage of the general adaptation syndrome (see Module 31, Stress and Coping) and should be understood as a complex syndrome of behaviors. In extreme cases, burnout may cause affected nurses to abandon the nursing profession altogether. The signs that a nurse is experiencing burnout include feelings of helplessness and hopelessness, a negative attitude and self-concept, and physical and emotional exhaustion.

The use of healthy stress management techniques can help nurses prevent burnout. The first step is to recognize their stress and how they respond to stress. Some common responses to stress are angry outbursts, fatigue, feelings of being overwhelmed, physical illness, and increases in coffee drinking, smoking, or using alcohol or other mood-enhancing substances. After nurses learn to recognize their stress and how they personally react to it, they must identify the trigger situations that tend to provoke the most pronounced stress reactions in them. Going through this recognition process will help nurses choose the stress reduction techniques that are best for them, which include the following:

- To reduce tension, engage in quiet activities that are personally meaningful (such as reading, listening to music, soaking in a tub, or meditating) for daily relaxation.
- To direct energy outward, establish and follow a regular exercise regimen.

- To overcome a feeling of powerlessness in relationships with others, learn techniques to increase assertiveness and develop the ability to say no.
- Turn errors and failures into constructive learning experiences by learning to accept such missteps as a part of life. By recognizing that most people do the best they can but do not always succeed, nurses learn to open up about their feelings with colleagues, ask for help, and reciprocate by supporting colleagues in their times of need.
- By recognizing that no situation is perfect and that certain limitations always exist, nurses learn to accept what cannot be changed; acceptance can decrease negative responses to stress.
- To improve organizational policies and procedures that may generate stress, nurses may get involved in efforts toward constructive change.
- To constructively handle the feelings and anxieties of working in a high-stress setting, nurses may develop collegial support groups.
- To address workplace issues, nurses may participate in professional organizations.
- To help clarify their problems and reactions to those problems, nurses may seek counseling.

Few professions are as demanding as nursing, which imposes unusual work schedule requirements, heavy demands on time and energy, and great responsibility. The work that nurses do often involves life and death, and nurses must face that possibility every day. Although the work of nursing can be highly satisfying and meaningful for many nurses as they help patients survive trauma and cope with problems to improve their lives, sustained professional commitment is necessary to avoid potential burnout.

REVIEW Commitment to Profession

RELATE Link the Concepts and Exemplars

Linking the exemplar of commitment to profession with the concept of development:

1. How might nurses in different life stages commit themselves to the profession of nursing in different ways?
2. Describe the impact of the nurse's moral development, according to Kohlberg's theory, on commitment to the profession of nursing.

Linking the exemplar of commitment to profession with the concept of collaboration:

3. How is nurses' commitment to profession demonstrated by their ability and willingness to collaborate with others?
4. A nurse working on a medical unit is approached by a newly graduated licensed practical nurse who asks for help in improving her skill in initiating an IV catheter. How would nurses with different levels of commitment to the profession respond to this request?

REFER Go to Pearson MyLab Nursing and eText

REFLECT Apply Your Knowledge

Andrea Kamara is a nurse working on a very busy and often understaffed oncology unit. Two patients have died within the past week. They were both well known to the staff because each had been admitted several times with complications of their disease and treatment. The staff members who were working all cried, first for one patient and then, a few days later, for the other. Today, one of Ms. Kamara's assigned patients required cardiopulmonary resuscitation and was sent to the ICU, another developed septicemia and required many diagnostic tests and procedures, and a third was given bad news about her prognosis and was tearful and frightened. At the end of the day, Ms. Kamara felt that she had not done her best job because she was so busy. She wished she could have spent more time with each of her assigned patients, caring more for their emotional needs.

1. How will Ms. Kamara's commitment to the profession of nursing affect how she responds to her feelings of inadequacy and grief?
2. If Ms. Kamara is fully committed to nursing, how will she resolve her feelings about the quality of the care she delivers?
3. If Ms. Kamara has a continuance commitment to nursing, how will she respond to the shift she just worked and her feelings?

Exemplar 40.B Professional Development

Exemplar Learning Outcomes

40.B Analyze professional development as it relates to accountability.

- Analyze the history of nursing.
- Explain the effects of women's status, religion, war, and societal attitudes on nursing.
- List nursing leaders who made notable contributions to the profession.
- Differentiate the components of contemporary nursing practice.
- Differentiate expanded careers for nurses.

Exemplar Key Terms

Authority, *2660*
Chain of command, *2660*
Line authority, *2660*
Organizational chart, *2661*
Responsibility, *2660*
Staff authority, *2660*

Overview

Professional development or *professional growth* is an expectation of all professional nursing practice. Being an accountable practitioner means being knowledgeable, able, and up-to-date with the current trends influencing one's area of practice. Continuous personal and professional growth is one of the provisions of the *Code of Ethics for Nurses* (ANA, 2015). Provision 5.5 speaks to the importance of continually seeking competence and of developing, maintaining, and evaluating criteria for which competence is evaluated. It also speaks to the importance of providing holistic care to patients. Provision 5.6 addresses the need for nurses to participate in activities that broaden their growth and ultimately lead to a better understanding of patients, particularly in increasingly diverse environments.

Influence of Nurse Leaders

Traditional historical overviews often speak to the factors that influenced nurses' struggle for autonomy. Recurring themes include the status of women in society, religion, and war. Of these, large-scale events such as war were catalysts for change in both the perception and role of the nurse. With the perspective of time, the COVID-19 pandemic in 2020 may bring about additional changes in the perception and role of the nurse and other HCPs.

Contributions of Past Nurse Leaders

Leaders such as Florence Nightingale, Clara Barton, Lillian Wald, Lavinia Dock, Margaret Sanger, and Mary Breckinridge made notable contributions to both nursing's history and women's history, and their skills at influencing others and bringing about change make them potent models for political nurse activists today. Contemporary nursing leaders have also played important roles in the profession. For example, Virginia Henderson created a modern worldwide definition of nursing, and Martha Rogers made important theoretical contributions.

Florence Nightingale (1820–1910)

Florence Nightingale's contributions to nursing are well documented. During the Crimean War, she made such great strides in improving standards of care for war casualties that her efforts earned her the title "Lady with the Lamp." She also became an accomplished political nurse—the first nurse, in fact, to exert political pressure on government—in her zeal to reform hospitals and produce and implement public health policies. Her greatest achievements, however, were her contributions to nursing education and her pioneering work *Notes on Nursing: What It Is, and What It Is Not* (1859/1969), which established Nightingale as nursing's first scientist–theorist.

Clara Barton (1812–1912)

A schoolteacher who volunteered as a nurse during the American Civil War, Clara Barton was given the responsibility of organizing the nursing services. She established the American Red Cross and in 1882 persuaded Congress to ratify the Treaty of Geneva (the first Geneva Convention), which linked the American Red Cross with the International Red Cross to perform humanitarian efforts in times of peace.

Linda Richards (1841–1930)

Linda Richards graduated from the New England Hospital for Women and Children in 1873, thereby becoming America's first trained nurse. Richards did pioneering work in psychiatric and industrial nursing, and the practices of nurse's notes, doctor's orders, and nurses wearing uniforms all originated with her (ANA, 2016a).

Mary Mahoney (1845–1926)

In 1879, Mary Mahoney graduated from the New England Hospital for Women and Children to become the first African American professional nurse. Mahoney promoted equal opportunities and worked tirelessly for African Americans to be accepted in nursing (Donahue, 1996, p. 271). The ANA (2016b) gives the Mary Mahoney Award biennially to recognize significant contributions, whether by individual nurses or groups of nurses, to the advancement of racial integration in nursing.

Lillian Wald (1867–1940)

Lillian Wald is considered the founder of public health nursing. Wald and Mary Brewster provided nursing and social services as well as organized educational and cultural activities to economically disadvantaged people in New York City. Wald pushed for school nursing as an adjunct to visiting nursing soon after founding the Henry Street Settlement.

Lavinia Dock (1858–1956)

A friend of Lillian Wald and a feminist, prolific writer, political activist, and suffragist, Lavinia L. Dock campaigned both for the passage of the 19th Amendment securing women's right to vote, but also for legislation to make the profession of nursing autonomous by allowing nurses, not physicians, to control it. Dock, assisted by Mary Adelaide Nutting and Isabel Hampton Robb, founded the American Society of Superintendents of Training Schools for Nurses of the United States and Canada in 1893; this was a precursor to the current National League for Nursing.

Margaret Sanger (1879–1966)

A public health nurse in New York, Margaret Higgins Sanger had a lasting impact on women's healthcare and reproductive rights. She was imprisoned for opening America's first birth control information clinic and is considered the founder of Planned Parenthood. Sanger brought attention to the large number of unwanted pregnancies among the working poor and pushed for this issue to be addressed.

Mary Breckinridge (1881–1965)

In 1918, immediately following the end of World War I, Mary Breckinridge worked with the American Committee for Devastated France to distribute food, clothing, and supplies to rural villages and care for sick children. After returning to the United States in 1921, Breckenridge acted on her plans to provide healthcare to the people of rural America, establishing the Frontier Nursing Service (FNS) in 1925 with two other nurses in Leslie County, Kentucky. Within the FNS, Breckinridge started one of the first midwifery training schools in the United States.

Contemporary Nurse Leaders

Nurses today usually do not think of themselves as leaders unless they have been given a title or are in a position of management. Often, textbooks focus on contemporary nurse thought leaders such as Patricia Benner and Hildegarde Peplau (considered the founder of modern psychiatric nursing) or nurses such as Ernest Grant, the first male president of the American Nurses Association (and also the first African American man to serve as its vice-president).

However, accountable behavior and safe practice are the qualities of clinical leaders. Clinical leaders are frontline providers who contribute to quality patient care by identifying inefficiencies in workflow and procedures and policies that impinge on safe patient care. Clinical leaders motivate others to do well, to be leaders of change in correcting problems or intervening in situations of potential harm. The behaviors of clinical leaders contribute to job satisfaction and retention of workers and higher patient satisfaction (Mianda & Voce, 2018).

The clinical environment plays a large role in nurses' ability to be clinical leaders. Nurses have an obligation to put patient safety in the forefront. A supportive environment is one that supports open communication and collaborative problem solving and believes that patient safety is a shared responsibility (Yoo & Kim, 2017). Sufficient resources are needed so that each nurse is empowered to continue to grow and learn and ultimately provide the best care possible for their patients and excel as clinical leaders (Raymond, Toloiy, & Bergman, 2020). A culture of high performance is one where everyone is important and everyone is accountable regardless of whether the task is as simple and routine as communicating one to one with a patient or as complex as a multidisciplinary approach for problem solving (Cochrane, 2017).

Contemporary Nursing Practice

Examining the definitions of nursing, who receives nursing services, the settings for nursing practice, nurse practice acts, and current standards for clinical nursing can help cultivate a deeper understanding of contemporary nursing practice.

Definitions of Nursing

More than 150 years ago, Florence Nightingale (1859/1969) highlighted the importance of environment in *Notes on Nursing*, her seminal work defining nursing. She considered a clean, well-ventilated, and quiet environment to be essential for patient recovery. Nightingale raised the status of nursing through education and is often considered the first nurse theorist. Thanks to her efforts, nurses were no longer untrained housekeepers, but professional individuals formally educated in the care of the sick.

Virginia Henderson helped define nursing. In her words, "The unique function of the nurse is to assist the individual, sick or well, in the performance of those activities contributing to health or its recovery (or to peaceful death) that he would perform unaided if he had the necessary strength, will, or knowledge, and to do this in such a way as to help him gain independence as rapidly as possible" (1966, p. 3). Henderson described nursing in relation to the patient and the patient's environment, just as Nightingale did. However, unlike Nightingale, Henderson saw the nurse as concerned with both healthy and ill individuals. She acknowledged that nurses interact with patients even when it might not be possible for them to recover and promoted the role of the nurse as both teacher and advocate.

In 1952, Hildegard Peplau published her landmark *Interpersonal Relations in Nursing*, which described and emphasized the importance of the nurse–patient relationship as a therapeutic process. Her pioneering work on nurse–patient relations and on anxiety led to her being widely considered as the founder of modern psychiatric nursing.

In the late 20th century, a number of nurse theorists worked to describe not only what nursing is, but also the interrelationship among nurses, nursing, the patient, the environment, and the intended patient outcome. Certain themes are common to many of these definitions; for example, most theoretical definitions view nursing as:

- Caring
- An art
- A science
- Patient centered
- Holistic
- Adaptive
- Concerned with health promotion, health maintenance, and health restoration
- A helping profession.

Professional nursing associations have also scrutinized the nursing profession and contributed their own definitions of nursing. In 1973, the ANA described nursing practice as "direct, goal oriented, and adaptable to the needs of the individual, the family, and community during health and illness" (p. 2), but the organization changed its definition of nursing in 1980 to this: "Nursing is the diagnosis and treatment of human responses to actual or potential health problems" (p. 9). Later, in 1995, the ANA recognized the contribution that the science of caring had made to nursing philosophy and practice. Its current definition of professional nursing is therefore much broader than earlier definitions: "Nursing is the protection, promotion, and optimization of health and abilities, preventions of illness and injury, alleviation of suffering through the diagnosis and treatment of human response, and advocacy in the care of individuals, families, communities, and populations" (ANA, 2003, p. 6).

Settings for Nursing

The many and varied settings for nursing practice include acute care hospitals, community agencies, ambulatory clinics, long-term care facilities, health maintenance organizations, nursing practice centers, and patients' homes (see **Figure 40.3** »).

Depending on the setting, nurses may have different degrees of autonomy and responsibility. They may provide direct care or they may teach patients and support individuals. They may also serve as advocates and agents of change, helping determine the health policies that affect consumers in hospitals and in the community.

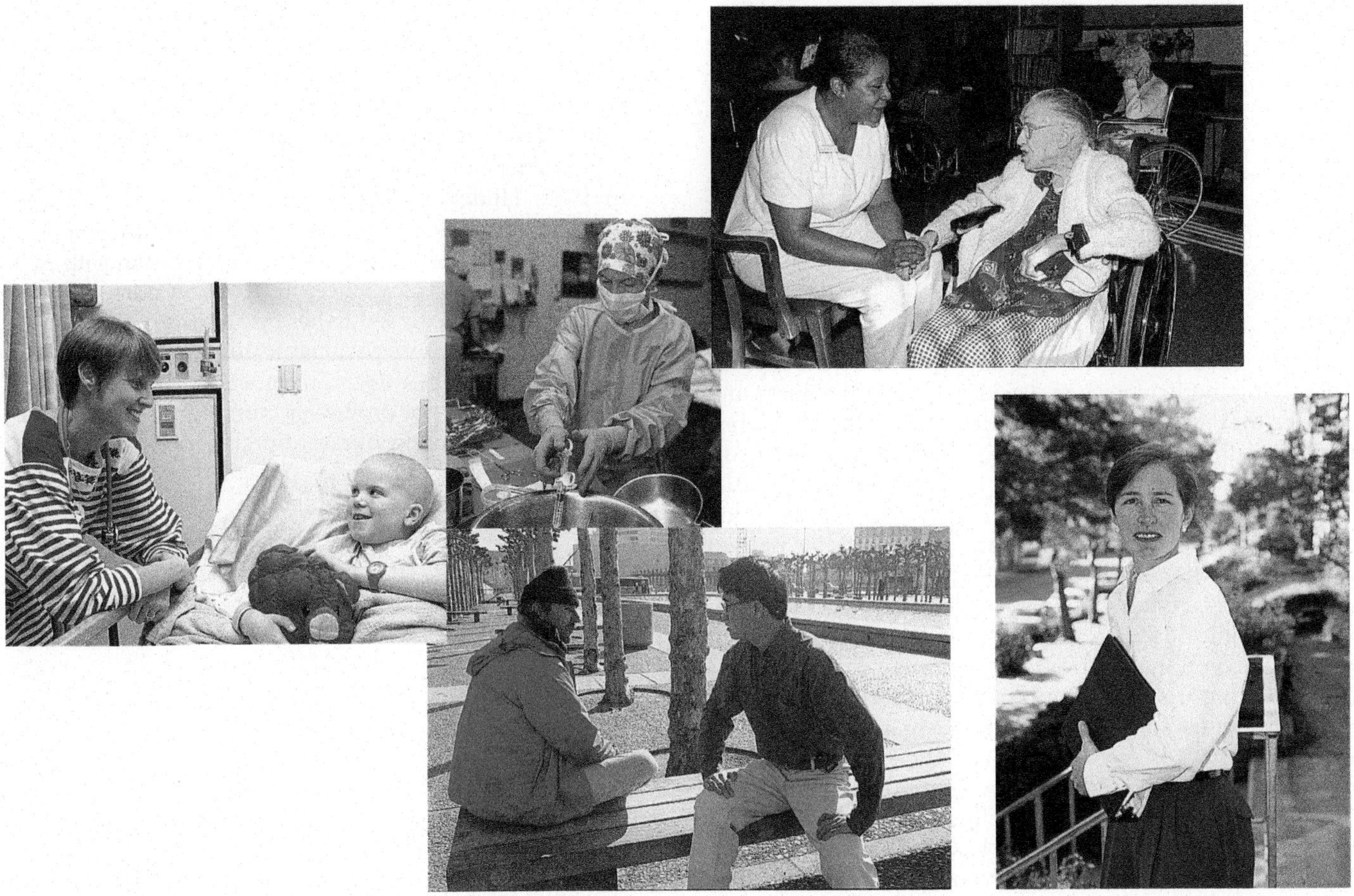

Figure 40.3 ›› Nurses practice in a variety of settings. Clockwise from left: pediatric nursing, perioperative nursing, geriatric nursing, home nursing, and community nursing.

Source: Pearson Education, Inc.

Chain of Command

The **chain of command** is the hierarchy within an organization. The authority and responsibility of the individuals in the organization depend on their position in the chain of command. **Authority** is the power to command other individuals and direct their activities; **responsibility** is being accountable for meeting personal or organizational objectives and performing required tasks.

Line authority is the power to direct the activities of subordinates within the organization. In **Figure 40.4** ››, examples of line authority include the relationships among the chief nurse executive, the nurse manager, and the staff nurse. **Staff authority** is the power to provide advice and support to employees or departments but not to assign tasks. In Figure 42.2, staff authority is illustrated by the relationship between the acute care nurse practitioner and the nurse manager. Neither is responsible for the work of the other; rather, they collaborate to optimize care in the unit for which the nurse manager is responsible.

A chain of command provides structure, so employees understand how to perform their tasks and how to manage supervisory relationships within the organization. It also provides a structure for reporting issues that need management's

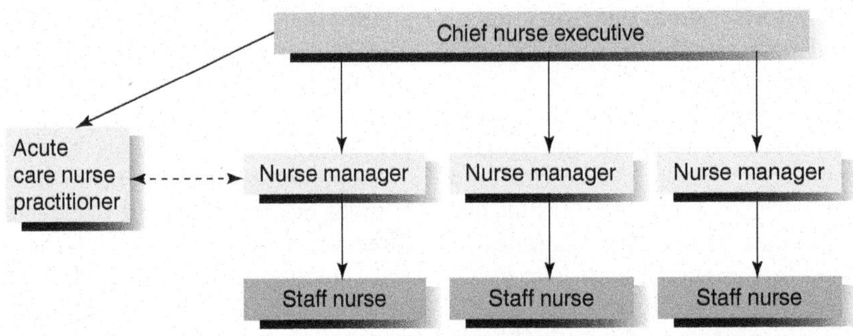

Figure 40.4 ›› Organizational chart showing chain of command in a nursing unit.

attention. Any nurse who identifies such an issue should follow the organization's chain of command. For example, in a hospital, a problem is usually first reported to the charge nurse, then to the unit manager. If the problem is still not resolved, the nurse may approach someone in middle or upper management.

The student nurse should always follow the chain of command, and the nursing instructor acts as the first link in that chain. When a problem arises in the clinical area, the student should discuss the problem with the instructor first and then with the nurse manager. Failure to follow the chain of command is considered unprofessional and slows the resolution process. In some organizations, failure to follow the chain of command may result in disciplinary action.

In traditional organizations, an **organizational chart** shows the formal hierarchical structure and related responsibilities of individuals or positions. However, organizations also have informal structures that are not reflected in a chart. For instance, nurses who function as leaders but do not have a formal title in the hierarchy would not appear in the organizational chart. Similarly, managers who have strong personalities or other characteristics may have more actual power than other managers with the same formal level of authority, but these differences are not shown in the chart.

The traditional hierarchical structure is not the only model used in healthcare settings. Many organizations have moved toward a shared governance model. Shared governance incorporates the principles of "partnership, equity, accountability, and ownership" and, as such, empowers nurses to have an impact on their work environments (Kroning & Hopkins, 2019, p.13).

Roles and Functions of the Nurse

Nurses perform a number of roles, often simultaneously. The nurse, for example, may not only provide physical care, but also act as an educator to teach the patient aspects of that care. The needs of the patient and the aspects of the patient's environment at a particular time determine which roles a nurse will be required to fulfill. These roles, briefly outlined in **Table 40.3** », are discussed throughout this text.

As the nursing profession has grown in autonomy through professional organizations, nursing leaders and managers have seen a need for a number of expanded roles

TABLE 40.3 Roles and Functions of the Nurse

Nursing Role	Functions
Caregiver	The nurse engages in activities that assist the patient physically, psychologically, spiritually, and emotionally in a culturally competent manner.
Communicator	The nurse identifies patient problems, advocates on their behalf, shares information, and functions as an active member of an interprofessional healthcare team. (See Module 38, Communication.)
Teacher	Nurses help patients learn about their health and health-promoting behaviors that help to restore or maintain their health, and they encourage patients and families to seek information from reliable resources. Nurses also mentor unlicensed assistive personnel (UAP) to whom they delegate care and share expertise with other nurses and healthcare professionals. (See Module 41, Teaching and Learning.)
Patient advocate	The nurse may represent the patient's needs and wishes to other health professionals, such as relaying the patient's requests for information to the physician or speaking out in situations of potential harm. The nurse also assists patients in exercising their rights and helps them advocate for themselves.
Counselor	Nurses counsel and/or seek professional help for individuals needing support adjusting to a new normal following hospitalization or treatment. Nurses encourage individuals to look at alternative behaviors and identify support systems to foster a sense of personal control. Nurses counsel ill patients in how to develop healthy and self-protective behaviors and recognize and respond to triggers, signs, and symptoms indicative of a problem or a potential problem in a timely manner.
Change agent	Nurses assist patients to make modifications in their behavior. Nurses act as change agents by voicing concerns about policies and procedures that impact patient care.
Leader	A leader influences others to work together to accomplish specific goals. The leader role can be employed at different levels: individual patient, family, groups of patients, colleagues, or the community. Effective leadership is a learned skill requiring an understanding of the needs and goals that motivate individuals, the knowledge to apply the leadership skills, and the interpersonal skills to influence others. (Leadership is discussed further in Module 39, Managing Care.)
Manager	The nurse manages the nursing care of individuals, families, and communities. The nurse manager also delegates nursing activities to ancillary workers and other nurses in addition to supervising and evaluating their performance. Managing requires knowledge about organizational structure and dynamics, authority and accountability, leadership, change theory, advocacy, delegation, and supervision and evaluation. Managers also serve as mentors and role models to staff personnel.
Case manager	Nurse case managers work with the interprofessional healthcare team to measure the effectiveness of the case management plan and to monitor outcomes. Each agency or unit specifies the role of the nurse case manager. In some institutions, the case manager works with primary or staff nurses to oversee the care of a specific caseload. In other agencies, the case manager is the primary nurse or provider of direct care to the patient and family. Insurance companies have also developed a number of roles for nurse case managers, and responsibilities may vary from managing acute hospitalizations to managing high-cost patients or case types. Regardless of the setting, case managers help ensure that care is oriented to the patient while also controlling costs. (See Module X39, Managing Care, for more information.)
Research consumer	Nursing practice should be evidence based. Whenever possible, nurses should use research to improve patient care. Nurses need to have knowledge of the process and language of research, be protective of the rights of patients as human subjects, participate in the identification of significant researchable problems, and be a discriminate consumer of research findings.

in the nursing profession. Some of these roles, such as that of the nurse-midwife, have come about partly as a response to needs expressed by patients. Others, such as that of the nurse educator, have resulted primarily from the profession's desire to continue to improve, educate, and renew its own members.

Expanded Career Roles for Nurses

Expanded career roles that allow greater independence and autonomy are available to many nurses. Such roles include nurse practitioner, clinical nurse specialist, nurse-midwife, nurse educator, and nurse anesthetist. Although exact requirements for these roles are defined in each state's nurse practice act, they almost universally reflect the standards below.

Nurse Practitioner

The basic requirements for becoming a nurse practitioner are advanced education (master's degree or higher), graduation from a nurse practitioner program, and American Nurses Credentialing Center (ANCC) certification in a particular area. These areas include adult nurse practitioner, family nurse practitioner, school nurse practitioner, pediatric nurse practitioner, and gerontology nurse practitioner. Nurse practitioners must hold both an RN license and a nurse practitioner license in order to practice. Nurse practitioners usually provide primary ambulatory care as well as care for patients with nonemergency acute or chronic illness, and they are employed in healthcare agencies or in community-based settings.

Clinical Nurse Specialist

A clinical nurse specialist is a nurse who possesses an advanced degree (master's or higher) with emphasis on a specialized area of practice, such as gerontology or oncology. To become a clinical nurse specialist, the nurse must hold RN licensure and pass a certification exam administered by the ANCC. Most states then require the nurse to obtain separate licensure as a clinical nurse specialist. Depending on their specialty and job setting, clinical nurse specialists provide direct patient care, educate others, consult, conduct research, and manage care.

Nurse Anesthetist

Nurse anesthetists administer general anesthetics for surgery under the supervision of a physician prepared in anesthesiology, as well as carry out preoperative and postoperative patient assessments. A nurse may qualify to be a nurse anesthetist after completing advanced education (master's degree or higher) in an accredited program in anesthesiology. Nurses who obtain this degree and already hold RN licensure may then sit for a certification examination offered by the National Board on Certification and Recertification of Nurse Anesthetists (NBCRNA). Nurses who pass this exam earn the title of Certified Registered Nurse Anesthetist (CRNA). Maintenance of the CRNA credential requires nurses to meet certain continuing education requirements set by the NBCRNA. Some states also require that CRNAs obtain separate licensure beyond that of a registered nurse.

Nurse-Midwife

Nurse-midwives provide prenatal and postnatal care and manage deliveries in normal pregnancies. They practice in association with a healthcare agency, which enables them to quickly obtain medical services should complications occur. Nurse-midwives may also conduct routine Papanicolaou tests, family planning counseling, and routine breast examinations. To become a nurse-midwife, a registered nurse must complete an accredited graduate program in midwifery, earning a master's degree or higher. The nurse must then pass a certification exam offered by the American College of Nurse-Midwives. In many states, specialized licensure is also required.

Nurse Researcher

The role of the nurse researcher is to investigate problems in nursing and to discover solutions that may improve nursing care and refine and expand nursing knowledge. Academic institutions, teaching hospitals, and research centers, such as the National Institute for Nursing Research in Bethesda, Maryland, all employ nurse researchers. Nurse researchers typically have advanced education at the doctoral level.

Nurse Administrator

A nurse administrator manages patient care, including delivery of nursing services. He or she may have a middle management position, such as head nurse or supervisor, or a more senior management position, such as director of nursing services. The nurse administrator's functions include budgeting, staffing, and planning programs. To prepare for their role, nurse administrators complete at least a baccalaureate degree in nursing and frequently a master's or doctoral degree as well.

Nurse Educator

The nurse educator usually has a baccalaureate degree or more advanced preparation and frequently has expertise in a particular area of practice. Nurse educators work in nursing programs, at educational institutions, or in hospital staff education programs. They are responsible for classroom, skills laboratory, and often clinical teaching.

Nurse Entrepreneur

A nurse entrepreneur is someone who manages a health-related business and typically has an advanced degree. The nurse entrepreneur's business may involve education, consultation, or research.

Clinical Nurse Leader

The American Association of Colleges of Nursing (2020) developed the role of clinical nurse leader to address the challenges of providing high-quality healthcare in the current environment. Quality improvement and use of evidence-based solutions are hallmarks of this role. Clinical nurse leaders must hold a master's degree and have completed specialized coursework in areas such as pathophysiology, clinical assessment, finance management, epidemiology, and pharmacology. They must also pass a certification examination offered by the Commission on Nurse Certification.

REVIEW Professional Development

RELATE Link the Concepts and Exemplars

Linking the exemplar on professional development with the concept of legal issues:

1. What role does the nurse's continued professional development play in meeting the legal requirements for the profession?
2. What nursing regulations require continued professional development?

Linking the exemplar on professional development with the concept of ethics:

3. Can the nurse meet the ethical responsibilities of the profession without belonging to a professional organization? Explain.
4. How does the nursing code of ethics address the issue of professional development?

REFER Go to Pearson MyLab Nursing and eText

REFLECT Apply Your Knowledge

Francois Guardiene graduated from nursing school 4 years ago and accepted a position working in the coronary care unit (CCU) of a large metropolitan hospital. He was required to attend 6 weeks of hospital orientation and a 3-month class for CCU nurses. He worked under the supervision of a preceptor for an additional 3 months. During his first year of practice, Francois checked with more experienced nurses frequently, but with time, he began to have more confidence in his competence and established a more autonomous practice. Over the past 2 years, he has noticed that some individuals seek to collaborate with him, and he considers himself a good CCU nurse.

1. Has Mr. Guardiene satisfied the need for professional development? Explain your answer.
2. What obligations does Mr. Guardiene have to continue developing his professional practice?
3. How would a nurse's hospital orientation differ if the position involved an area less specialized than the CCU?

Exemplar 40.C Work Ethic

Exemplar Learning Outcomes

40.C Analyze work ethic as it relates to professionalism.

- Describe the relationship of attendance and punctuality to work ethic.
- Outline the importance of reliability and accountability for the professional nurse.
- Describe the influence of attitude and enthusiasm on the work environment.
- Summarize generational differences in work ethic.

Exemplar Key Terms

Arrogance, *2664*
Corrective action, *2664*
Dismissal, *2664*
Generational cohort, *2665*
Insubordination, *2664*
Optimism, *2664*
Pessimism, *2664*
Punctual, *2663*
Work ethic, *2663*

Overview

A majority of employers identify a "strong work ethic" as the most important characteristic of a good employee. A belief in the importance and moral worth of work constitutes a **work ethic**. Because they place a high value on hard work and diligence, people with strong work ethics tend to stay focused on the job and leave their personal problems at home. Because they value doing the work right the first time, they take a thorough approach to tasks and apply themselves fully to what they do. People with strong work ethics assume responsibility for any mistakes they do make, fixing the mistakes if they can, and willingly accepting the consequences of their actions. They know what management expects of them, and they exercise self-discipline and self-control to meet these expectations. They are proactive, taking the initiative, and approaching work tasks positively and enthusiastically.

Nursing students may develop a better grasp of the expectations of the nursing profession by examining the components of a strong work ethic and, through developing a strong work ethic themselves, demonstrating a commitment to their job and to their employer.

Attendance and Punctuality

Attendance is a fundamental requirement to demonstrate commitment to a job. To perform the duties of a job requires showing up for work every day. A key component of attendance is being on time, or **punctual**.

Other employees are required to take on more than their usual workloads to cover for employees who do not come to work. An employee may have a legitimate reason for being absent, but even so, frequent absences increase stress for other employees and decrease productivity. Funding shortages force many healthcare agencies to employ no more employees than are absolutely required. Accordingly, all employees have full workloads that, even under the best of circumstances, require their full commitment and the best of their ability. If employees have to take on some or all of an absent employee's work, this increases the burden for everyone. Accordingly, every nurse (and nursing student) has the responsibility to be at work and to arrive on time.

Employees who arrive late for work create delays and other inconveniences for their coworkers. A nurse's failure to be punctual might force the rescheduling of a patient's procedure and could delay that patient's (or another's) diagnosis, treatment, surgery, or discharge from the hospital. That nurse might be late in delivering needed supplies and filing paperwork by its appointed deadline, forcing other people to work overtime to compensate for the delays. Nurses must report to work on time because of the interconnected nature of professional healthcare roles. Being "on time" does not mean arriving at the parking lot at the time work is scheduled to begin; "on time" means that at the start of a nurse's shift, that nurse is already at work and in place, ready to begin.

It is inevitable for almost everyone to occasionally miss work or arrive late. However, habitual poor attendance and lack of punctuality are performance issues and may be grounds for steps to overcome the problem (**corrective action**) or even terminate employment (**dismissal**).

Professional commitment, then, dictates that nursing students must arrive on time for work every day and be ready to work immediately when the shift starts. To assist with this, nursing students should anticipate potential emergencies, such as a child being sick or a car being in the shop, and set up contingency plans to prepare for them.

For nurses, one component of forming a good work ethic is taking steps to protect their own health and safety, such as by getting enough rest, avoiding unnecessary risks, and taking preventive measures such as receiving flu shots.

Another part of maintaining a good work ethic is avoiding excessively long or unscheduled breaks. This includes nurses trying to allow some extra time at the end of every shift in case they are held over. Above all, nurses must never rush out the door the minute the shift ends if that might mean leaving a patient, coworker, visitor, or guest hanging. Staying long enough to complete work or to hand it off properly to the individual who follows is every nurse's (and nursing student's) responsibility. Doing so facilitates a smooth transition between shifts and ensures that work in progress is not left for other people to finish.

Reliability and Accountability

Professionalism involves the essential factors of reliability and accountability. From a systems perspective, each nurse must complete the duties of the job appropriately so that others who depend on the nurse can complete their own work. Part of reliability and accountability is following through on commitments—for example, honoring agreements to trade shifts or taking on additional work when someone is absent. Honoring commitments helps the team function properly and builds trust and team cohesion (**Figure 40.5** ›››). It is also important to take responsibility for the consequences of one's actions. Professionals do not blame others for their mistakes but instead hold themselves personally accountable.

The professional nurse refuses work assignments only when the nurse is not qualified or is not prepared to perform the assignment. In either case, the nurse should discuss the situation immediately with the supervisor. Otherwise, the nurse should be ready to complete all assigned tasks, especially because refusal to do so may be regarded as **insubordination** (defiance of authority) and grounds for dismissal.

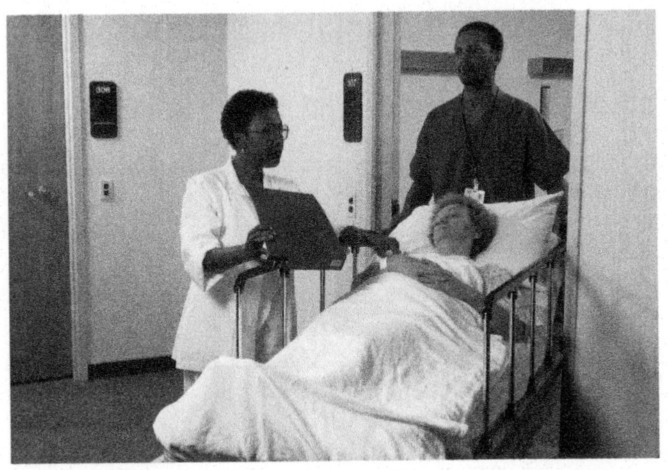

Figure 40.5 ››› Nurses are responsible for completing their duties so that other people can complete their own work.
Source: Pearson Education, Inc.

Nurses act professionally when they avoid judging patients or forcing their own personal beliefs onto patients. When a nurse feels a conflict between an assigned task and the nurse's religious beliefs, morals, or values, it is the nurse's responsibility to bring this conflict to the supervisor's attention and discuss it reasonably. Many employers will allow a nurse to opt out of participation in activities to which the nurse has moral objections, but the nurse should anticipate such conflicts and report them to the employer at the earliest opportunity. For more information, refer to Module 42, Accountability.

Attitude and Enthusiasm

A positive attitude—an essential professional characteristic for nurses—involves a sense of **optimism**, or a feeling that things will turn out for the best. Professional nurses are typically optimistic, but unfortunately, a negative attitude is a way of life for some people. This negativity expresses itself as **pessimism**, or the belief that the current situation is always bad and may become worse. Pessimists complain about everything and tend to be dissatisfied with what they have. Pessimists do not convey enthusiasm about their work. They rarely smile and often appear unhappy, which, whether the pessimist consciously intends it or not, may spread negativity to their coworkers, undermining morale, teamwork, and cooperative spirit. Pessimism is a dangerous attitude that nurses must guard against because it erodes trust and confidence. Instead, nurses should convey optimism and enthusiasm about their work, especially to patients and their families. A commitment to positivity contributes to a more pleasant, collegial, and productive work environment.

Arrogance is another negative attitude that can damage a nurse's professionalism. **Arrogance**, or excessive pride and a feeling of superiority, can be an extremely dangerous characteristic in the nurse, as it can lead to a false belief that the nurse is always right and does not need input from others. For example, when the unit begins using a new IV infusion pump, the arrogant nurse does not bother attending the in-service, believing that it is possible to "figure things out" independently. Accurate self-assessment of strengths and weaknesses, as well as acceptance of feedback from others, promotes both safety and growth and is therefore an essential ability for the nurse.

Generational Differences in Work Ethic

Discussions about cultural diversity often focus on differing ethnic, national, or religious perspectives. But in the United States, a major cultural divide impacting nurses' work ethic is the generation gap.

Throughout America, multiple generations of people are working shoulder to shoulder. Different generations hold different ideals, values, traits, goals, and characteristics, which play a significant role in how employees of one generation relate to those of other generations. These differences can be seen in communication styles, expectations, work styles, values and norms, attitudes about work and life, comfort with technology, views regarding loyalty and authority, and acceptance of change.

The term **generational cohort** refers to people born in the same general time span who share key life experiences, including historical events, public heroes, pastimes, and early work experiences. These common life experiences create cohesiveness in perspectives and attitudes and lead generational cohorts to develop distinct values and workforce patterns. Differences between generations (sometimes called a *generation gap*) can have negative effects in the workplace, causing conflicts and interpersonal tension. Learning to create collegial relationships with people from different generations is a critical skill for nurses who work in multigenerational teams.

While the literature sometimes disagrees on specific years or generational names, there is consistent agreement on the characteristics of each generational cohort. An understanding of the historical influences on each generation, their common life experiences, and the workforce the members entered when first employed is necessary to understand their attitudes and values related to work (see **Table 40.4** »).

Different generational styles can lead to workplace conflict. Older nurses may experience considerable conflict over younger nurses' behaviors and may describe younger nurses as arrogant, lacking in commitment, and having a "slacker" attitude. Younger nurses may see themselves as self-reliant rather than arrogant. Older nurses may be dismayed and struggle with a perceived lack of professionalism among their younger colleagues, evidenced by younger nurses' dress, hairstyles, piercings, and tattoos. Younger nurses may be disillusioned by older nurses' perceived unwillingness to become technologically competent.

While differences between generations are not new, two significant changes over the past 60 years have forced the current generations in the workforce into more intense interaction. First, the nature of the work itself has shifted. In traditional bureaucratic structures, interactions between generations followed hierarchical lines. People from younger generations traditionally held entry-level positions and reported to people of the older generation in more senior positions. As a result, younger employees took direction from and followed the rules of people who were older. With the advent of continuous quality improvement and shared governance structures, individuals from various "levels" of the organization are now equal members of a team. This arrangement has increased the interaction of employees from different generations.

Second, the transformation from the industrial age to the information age has altered the interactions between people of differing generations. Historically, the most senior members of an organization offered the most reliable information and knowledge. Young nurses relied on their more senior colleagues for instruction and advice when confronted with an unusual diagnosis or a complex patient situation. With the advent of the information age, young nurses are not as reliant on their older peers, since they can easily access information from around the world on their computers and smartphones. Computerization has not only broken the dependence of younger generations on more senior generations for information, it has also resulted in the unprecedented situation in which the youngest individuals in the workforce are the most expert at a critical skill. Instead of younger nurses turning to their older colleagues for advice, older nurses often depend on their younger peers for guidance in using new technologies.

Note: Generational trends exist and everyone is, to some extent, shaped by things that happened in their particular generation; however, nurses should approach each colleague as an individual and should not stereotype based on generation.

Members of each generation typically operate as if their own values and expectations are universal. For example, baby-boomer nurses who entered the workforce during a flourishing economy embrace professionalism and love to work and assume that those of younger generations have the same values. These nurses may see younger colleagues' frequent job changes or working as independent agents as unreliability or a lack of commitment. Younger nurses may assume that their older peers who are workaholics focus on having money, when in reality older nurses love the work and want to share experiences and expertise with the younger nurses. Also, having grown up in a world in which their voice and contributions are expected, millennial nurses are often misunderstood when they advise their more senior colleagues who were raised as the "me" generation. A baby-boomer nurse may see the voiced criticisms of a novice millennial nurse at a staff meeting as arrogant and question the younger nurse's work ethic. From the younger nurse's perspective, speaking up even with limited experience is contributing to the unit.

Learning to develop collegial relationships with people from different generations is a critical skill for all nurses. Working with nurses from different generations offers the opportunity to explore new and different ways of thinking. Rather than focusing on what is "wrong" with another generation, nurses should look for ways to capitalize on each generation's strengths. Nurses of the baby-boomer generation value teamwork, Generation X nurses value self-reliance, millennial nurses value achievement, and Generation Z nurses learn by doing. In the workplace, a baby-boomer nurse might say, "Let's get together and reach a consensus about how to

TABLE 40.4 Description of Four Generations in the American Workforce

Generational Cohort and Their Historical Influences	Life Experiences	Workforce Entered	Work Ethic
Baby Boomers: Born 1945–1960			
Introduction of television Humans landed on the moon Assassination of President Kennedy Assassination of Dr. Martin Luther King, Jr. Civil rights movement Summer of Love Vietnam War Woodstock Watergate	Grew up in a healthy, flourishing economy Watched variety shows, movies, and sitcoms in their own home News became more visual and dramatic Raised in two-parent households in which father worked and mother was home caretaker Were members of smaller families	Emphasis was on freedom to be yourself—the "me" generation Heroes were those who questioned the status quo People in positions of power were not to be trusted Raised to be independent, critical thinkers Many female college graduates went on to become secretaries, nurses, or teachers because of the perception that these were primarily female professions	Are workaholics. Embrace sense of professionalism. Self-worth closely tied to work ethic Question authority Status quo can be transformed by working together Desire financial prosperity but long to make a significant contribution with their experience and expertise
Generation X: Born 1961–1980			
Rising divorce rates Microwave ovens Video games Computers Space shuttle *Challenger* disaster Numerous scandals involving high-profile public figures Operation Desert Storm	Lived in two-career households Many raised in single-parent homes "Latch key" generation; learned to manage on their own, becoming adept, clever, and resourceful Allowed to be equal participants in family discussions	Dramatic downsizing, reengineering, and layoffs seen Hierarchical structures had begun to flatten, eliminating promotion opportunities for younger workers Large cohort of baby boomers remained in workforce, filling limited managerial positions Keep themselves employable by constantly updating their skills	Seek challenges Are self-directed Expect instant access to information Desire employment in which they can create balance in work and personal life Prefer managers to be mentors and coaches Desire more control over their own schedule
Millennials (Generation Y): Born 1981–1996			
Established infrastructure (child care, preschool, after-school care) to assist dual-career parents Global generation Internet School shootings Terrorist attack of September 11, 2001 Wars in Afghanistan and Iraq Obama presidency	Life highly structured and scheduled Parents heavily involved in their upbringing, often chaperoning or coaching extracurricular activities Accept multiculturalism Raised enmeshed in digital technology Mass consumption of pop culture but via the internet	Economic downturn Drying-up of job opportunities in many industries Belief that education is the key to success Resurgence of heroism and patriotism Diversity a given Renewed sense of interest in contributing to collective good Volunteering for community service Joining organizations in record numbers	Collaborative, open-minded, achievement oriented Expectation of daily feedback, high maintenance Potential to become the highest-producing workforce in history Personal smart devices a necessity for daily life
Generation Z (GenTech, iGen) Born 1997–2012*			
Has never known a time without internet Less interested in identifying with a political party Aware and concerned about an economy shaped by income inequality Grew up in the era of school shootings Forced to embrace distance learning due to the coronavirus pandemic	More supervised and protected growing up Greater need for immediate gratification Greater distrust in government and religious authority figures Desire to help others and contribute to society Less likely to take risks Greater fear of personal interactions	Growth of the gig economy Increase in use of teleconferencing, telemedicine Opportunities available may not always provide the diverse, inclusive, collaborative environments attractive to Gen Zers	More individualistic, less developed social skills Capable of multitasking Respond to supportive feedback Willing to work hard, but need reward for efforts

* *Sources:* Chicca and Shellenbarger (2019); Patel (2017).

do it." The Generation X staff nurses might say they will do it themselves, whereas the millennial nurses might not care who does it as long as the work gets done. The Generation Z staff nurse might say "let me figure it out."

Baby boomers should be valued for their clinical and organizational experience and should be used to coach and mentor younger nurses. Generation X nurses should be valued for their innovative ideas and creative approaches to unit issues and problems. They can be important in helping organizations design new approaches to nursing care delivery. Millennial nurses should be valued for their understanding of technology and insights into how it can be used in practice. They can also serve as technology coaches for members of older generational cohorts. Generation Z nurses should be encouraged to participate and be given permission to learn and make mistakes.

Appreciation of the unique strengths of each generation can decrease interpersonal tension and facilitate personal growth. Nurses who learn to acknowledge and appreciate their colleagues from different backgrounds, including generational backgrounds, have a distinct advantage. Successful teamwork is increasingly required for job satisfaction and the ability to positively affect patient outcomes. This teamwork requirement is reflected in the recent introduction of relationship-based nursing care delivery systems, as discussed in Module 46, Healthcare Systems. All too frequently, intergenerational interactions lead to conflicts due to lack of appreciation or understanding or simply to misinterpretation of other perspectives.

Particular attention should be paid to engaging the perspective of younger nurses, as the youngest generation is always at a distinct disadvantage. Existing organizational structures are often based on strategies that were used successfully in the past rather than having been designed for the future. Because of their longevity, older generations often dominate in the powerful leadership positions and are more influential when changes are made. These nurses update processes and rewards in a way that makes sense from their generational perspective, often not recognizing that younger nurses might not hold the same perspective and might have a valuable perspective of their own. Incorporating younger nurses' values of participation, access to information, and balance into nursing operations is important. Older nurses need to learn to welcome input from their younger colleagues, encouraging them to use their fresh viewpoints to identify where opportunities exist. Younger nurses need to be taught and learn to value the experience and expertise of more senior nurses who have a wealth of lived experiences to share.

The best teams use the contributions of each generation's skill set and strengths. The idealist, passionate baby boomers; the techno-literate, adaptable Generation Xers; the young, optimistic millennials; and the quiet, multitasking Generation Zers can come together in a powerful network of nurses with a remarkable ability to support each other and maximize each nurse's contribution to patient care (**Figure 40.6 »**).

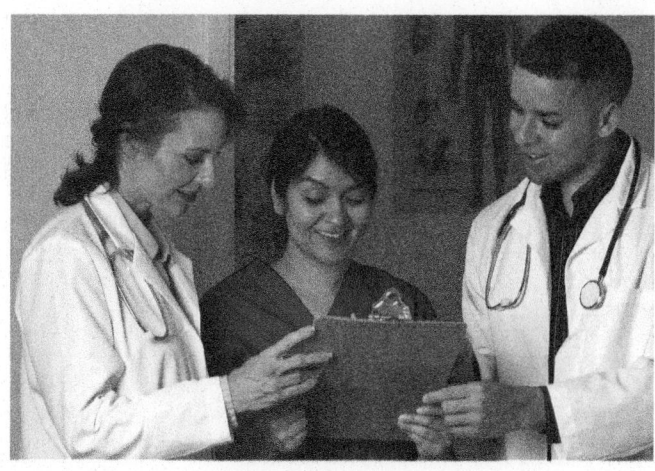

Figure 40.6 » The best nursing teams use the contributions of each generation's strengths.
Source: JHDT Productions/Shutterstock.

REVIEW Work Ethic

RELATE Link the Concepts and Exemplars

Linking the exemplar of work ethic with the concept of collaboration:

1. How does the work ethic of the individual nurse affect collaboration?
2. How might nurses from different generations respond to a rude and confrontational coworker?

Linking the exemplar of work ethic with the concept of teaching and learning:

3. How does the nurse's generational work ethic affect how the nurse teaches patients?
4. How does the nurse's generational work ethic affect learning style?

REFER Go to Pearson MyLab Nursing and eText

REFLECT Apply Your Knowledge

How would you respond in each of the following situations?

1. You were out with friends until very late last night and were scheduled to report for work this morning at 7:00. You arrive on time, but you know that your coworkers won't get there for another half hour. You have just enough time for a quick run to the corner coffee shop before your coworkers arrive.
2. You promised your coworkers that you would work the day shift on Thanksgiving so they could be home with their families. Two days before the holiday, an old friend from out of town calls to say that he would like you to be his guest for lunch on Thanksgiving Day.
3. You have an appointment with your supervisor next week to review the results of your annual performance evaluation. You overhear one of your teammates telling another individual that they gave you a low score on your 360-degree feedback evaluation because you refused to trade shifts over the Easter weekend.

4. Your shift ends in 30 minutes, and you have about 30 minutes of work left to do, but you have not been able to take your afternoon break yet.
5. One of your neighbors is admitted to the unit where you work. A member of your family calls to tell you that he has heard a rumor that the neighbor has a communicable disease. Because you work on the unit and have access to patient records, your family member asks you to find out whether the rumor is true.
6. A new piece of equipment has been installed in your department, but you missed the in-service session in which everyone was trained in how to operate it. Today a procedure is to be done using this equipment and it is your responsibility to use it.
7. A coworker invites you to a party. When you arrive, you notice three other people you work with complaining about low wages and telling a group of strangers that one of the surgeons at your hospital made a mistake in surgery last week and lied to the patient's family to try to cover it up.

References

Agency for Healthcare Research and Quality. (2019). *Disruptive and unprofessional behavior*. https://psnet.ahrq.gov/primer/disruptive-and-unprofessional-behavior

American Association of Colleges of Nursing. (AACN). (2020). *Clinical nurse leader (CNL)*. https://www.aacnnursing.org/CNL

American Nurses Association (ANA). (n.d.). *Bill of Rights FAQs*. https://www.nursingworld.org/practice-policy/work-environment/health-safety/bill-of-rights-faqs/

American Nurses Association (ANA). (2015). *Standards of nursing practice* (3rd ed.). Author.

American Nurses Association (ANA). (2016a). *ANA hall of fame*. https://www.nursingworld.org/ana/about-ana/history/hall-of-fame/inductees-listed-alphabetically/American Nurses Association (ANA). (2016b). *ANA hall of fame*. https://www.nursingworld.org/ana/about-ana/history/hall-of-fame/inductees-listed-alphabetically/American Nurses Association. (2003). *Nursing's social policy statement*. Washington, DC: Author.

Berman, A., Snyder, S., & Frandsen, G. (2021). *Kozier & Erb's fundamentals of nursing: Concepts, process, and practice* (11th ed.). Pearson.

Bimray, P., Jooste, K., & Julie, H. (2019). Professionalism experiences of undergraduate learner nurses during their 4-year training programme at a higher education institution in the western cape, South Africa. *Curationis*, 42(1). https://doi.org/10.4102/curationis.v42i1.2030

Brooks, L. A., Manias, E., & Bloomer, M. J. (2019) Culturally sensitive communication in healthcare: A concept analysis. *Collegian*, 26(3), 383–391. https://doi.org/10.1016/j.colegn.2018.09.007

Butler, E., Prentiss, A., & Benamor, F. (2018). Exploring perceptions of workplace bullying in nursing. *Nursing & Health Sciences Research Journal*, 1(1), 19–25. https://scholarlycommons.baptisthealth.net/cgi/viewcontent.cgi?article=1015&context=nhsrj

Byars, M., Camacho, M., Earley, D., & Harrington, L. (2017). Professionalism in the critical care setting: A concept analysis. *Nursing 2017 Critical Care*, 12(3), 5–8. https://doi.org/10.1097/01.CCN.0000515987.70483.8d

Chicca, J., & Shellenbarger, T. (2019). A new generation of nurses is here: Strategies for working with generation Z. *American Nurse Today*, 14(2), 48–50. https://www.myamericannurse.com/wp-content/uploads/2019/02/ant2-GenZ-117.pdf

Cochrane, B. S. (2017). Leaders go first: Creating and sustaining a culture of high performance. *Health Management Forum*, 30(5), 229–232.

Code of Federal Regulations. (2009). *Title 29—Labor: Section 1604-11—Sexual harassment*. U.S. Government Publishing Office. https://www.gpo.gov/fdsys/pkg/CFR-2009-title29-vol4/pdf/CFR-2009-title29-vol4-sec1604-11.pdf

Donahue, M. P. (1996). *Nursing: The finest art. An illustrated history* (2nd ed.). Mosby.

Gerber, L. (2018). Understanding the nurse's role as a patient advocate. *Nursing 2019*, 48(4), 55–58. https://doi.org/10.1097/01.NURSE.0000531007.02224.65

Guido, G. W. (2020). *Legal and ethical issues in nursing* (7th ed.). Pearson.

Gunawan, J., Aungsuroch, Y., Sukarna, A., Nazliansyah, A. S., & Efendi, F. (2018). The image of nursing as perceived by nurses: A phenomenological study. *Nursing and Midwifery Studies*, 7(4), 180–185. https://doi.org/10.4103/nms.nms_24_18

Haddad, L. M., & Geiger, R. A. (2020). *Nursing ethical considerations*. StatPearls. https://www.ncbi.nlm.nih.gov/books/NBK526054/

Haugland, B. O., Lassen, R. M., & Giske, T. (2017). Professional formation through personal involvement and value integration. *Nurse Education in Practice*, 29, 64–69. https://doi.org/10.1016/j.nepr.2017.11.013

Henderson, V. (1966). *The nature of nursing: A definition and its implications for practice, research, and education*. Macmillan.

Kroning, M., & Hopkins, K. (2019). Healthcare organizations thrive with shared governance. *Nursing Management (Springhouse)*, 50(5), 13–15.

Mianda, S., & Voce, A. (2018). Developing and evaluating clinical leadership interventions for frontline healthcare providers: A review of the literature. *BMC Health Services Research*, 18. https://doi.org/10.1186/s12913-018-3561-4

National Academy of Medicine. (n.d.). *The future of nursing 2020–2030*. https://nam.edu/publications/the-future-of-nursing-2020-2030/

Nightingale, F. (1969). *Notes on nursing: What it is, and what it is not*. Dover. (Original work published 1859)

Omar, M. A., Salam, M., & Al-Surimi, K. (2019). Workplace bullying and its impact on the quality of healthcare and patient safety. *Human Resources Health*, 17, 89. https://doi.org/10.1186/s12960-019-0433-x

Oshodi, T. O., Bruneau, B., Crockett, R., Kinchington, F., Nayar, S., & West, E. (2019). Registered nurses' perceptions and experiences of autonomy: A descriptive phenomenological study. *BioMed Central Nursing*, 18, 51. https://doi.org/10.1186/s12912-019-0378-3

Patel, D. (2017, September 21). 8 ways generation Z will differ from millennials in the workplace. *Forbes*. https://www.forbes.com/sites/deeppatel/2017/09/21/8-ways-generation-z-will-differ-from-millennials-in-the-workplace/#68b7f00a76e5

Peplau, H. (1952). *Interpersonal relations in nursing: A conceptual frame of reference for psychodynamic nursing*. Putnam.

Raymond, C., Toloiy, R., & Bergman, J. (2020). Exploring the professional responsibility concern process. *Journal of Nursing Care Quality* 35(2), E20–E26.

Reinhart, R. J. (2020). *Nurses continue to rate highest in honest, ethics*. Gallup. https://news.gallup.com/poll/274673/nurses-continue-rate-highest-honesty-ethics.aspx

Sauer, P., & McCoy, T. (2018). Nurse bullying and intent to leave. *Nursing Economic$*, 36(5), 219–224, 245. https://insights.ovid.com/nursing-economic/nrsec/2018/09/000/nurse-bullying-intent-leave/6/00006073

Su, J. J., Masika, G. M., Paguio, J. T., & Redding, S. R. (2020). Defining compassionate nursing care. *Nursing Ethics*, 27(2), 480–493. https://doi.org/10.1177/0969733019851546

The Joint Commission. (2018). *Sentinel event: Physical and verbal violence against health care workers*. https://www.jointcommission.org/-/media/tjc/documents/resources/patient-safety-topics/sentinel-event/sea_59_workplace_violence_4_13_18_final.pdf

Yoo, M. S., & Kim, K. J. (2017). Exploring the influence of nurse work environment and patient safety culture on attitudes toward incident reporting. *Journal of Nursing Administration* 47(9), 434–440.

Module 41
Teaching and Learning

Module Outline and Learning Outcomes

The Concept of Teaching and Learning

Nurses as Teachers and Learners

41.1 Analyze the nurse's role in teaching and learning.

Concepts Related to Teaching and Learning

41.2 Outline the relationship between teaching and learning and other concepts.

The Art of Teaching

41.3 Summarize the art of teaching.

Aspects of Learning

41.4 Analyze aspects of learning.

Lifespan Considerations

41.5 Differentiate considerations related to teaching and learning throughout the lifespan.

Technology, Health Information, and Patient Teaching

41.6 Analyze the impact of the internet on teaching and learning.

Teaching and Learning Exemplar

Exemplar 41.A Patient/Consumer Education

41.A Analyze patient/consumer education as it relates to teaching and learning.

» The Concept of Teaching and Learning

Concept Key Terms

Adherence, **2672**
Adult learning theory, **2673**
Behaviorist theory, **2673**
Cognitive theory, **2673**
Compliance, **2672**
Constructivist theory, **2673**
E-health, **2680**
Emotional intelligence, **2674**
Feedback, **2674**
Learning, **2669**
Learning need, **2672**
Mentors, **2670**
Modeling, **2673**
Observational learning, **2673**
Positive reinforcement, **2673**
Social learning theory, **2673**
Teaching, **2669**
Theory of multiple intelligences, **2673**

Teaching is a process that uses planned strategies and approaches with the goal of changing behavior. **Learning** is an outcome that occurs after being exposed to information that adds to knowledge and skill. Evidence of learning is a change in behavior that can be observed and measured and becomes a part of routine activities.

Some additional attributes of learning are described in **Box 41.1**».

> **Box 41.1**
>
> **Attributes of Learning**
>
> **Learning is:**
>
> - An experience that occurs within the learner
> - The discovery of the personal meaning and relevance of ideas
> - A consequence of experience
> - A collaborative and cooperative process
> - An evolutionary process that builds on past learning and experiences
> - A process that is both intellectual and emotional
>
> *Source:* Berman, Snyder, and Frandsen (2021). Pearson Education, Inc., Hoboken, NJ.

The teaching–learning process is a unique exchange that occurs between the person imparting information, or the teacher, and the one who is receiving the information, or the learner. Actions that occur within this process include sharing information and skills to influence or change attitudes, perceptions, values, and/or behaviors. Because nurses constantly gather information from and provide information to patients and other individuals, they require a clear understanding of the roles of teacher and learner alike.

This concept takes an in-depth look at the teaching–learning process and the nurse's responsibility as a patient and family educator. In doing so, it examines major domains and theories of learning as well as factors that affect an individual's ability to learn. The concept concludes with a discussion of ways in which nurses can use their knowledge of the teaching–learning process to design more successful patient and family education activities.

Nurses as Teachers and Learners

Nurses as Teachers

In the most recent publication of the American Nurses Association (ANA) *Scope and Standards of Practice* (2015), teaching is an expectation of the nurse when providing care.

Even though nurses teach a variety of topics to different populations, the main population of focus for teaching is the patient and family. Topics vary according to the individual patient's or family's needs and may include everything from instructions on administering medication to a family member to teaching which symptoms should prompt the parent to call a healthcare provider (HCP). Teaching may also be focused on therapies or treatments such as performing chest physiotherapy for a child with cystic fibrosis or changing a lower-extremity dressing for an older patient with a stasis ulcer caused by peripheral vascular disease.

Nurses also teach other nurses and staff in healthcare settings. Many teach students in traditional academic settings as well as in online education and certification programs offered through colleges and universities. Opportunities for nurses to teach may also occur when precepting new staff, mentoring, and while working with nursing students during clinical practicums. **Box 41.2** » describes the mentoring relationship among nurses.

The teaching of patients, families, and other healthcare professionals is monitored by different agencies. Federal and state regulatory organizations have specific expectations that must be documented and demonstrated by schools of nursing to achieve and maintain accreditation. Agencies that employ and train nurses and other healthcare professionals must meet specific requirements in order to gain certification. Because the nurse may be teaching a variety of populations, there is a need to be aware of changes in treatments, therapies, and medications. The nurse must be equipped to research current information and be aware of various approaches to facilitate learning. Since the individuals requiring instruction are diverse, the nurse needs to be prepared to address the learning needs of different learners in a variety of situations.

Nurses as Learners

A science-based education is the foundation for the profession of nursing. Today there are several avenues for individuals to become a nurse. Formal educational tracks range from diploma to university programs. However, nursing education does not end at graduation. The professional nurse needs to remain current with treatments and approaches to care by participating in continuing education programs, which are mandatory to maintain licensure for many states. This is supported by the ANA (2015) *Scope and Standards of Practice*, which states that nurses "seek knowledge and competence that reflects current nursing practice and promotes futuristic thinking."

Continuing education for nurses is supported by healthcare organizations and facilities through the use of impromptu and formal continuing education programs. Nurses also have opportunities to attend educational programs designed and accredited through regulatory agencies. The continuing education opportunities for nurses range from earning advance degrees to proving competency and becoming credentialed. Continuing education programs are also offered to provide information on changes in regulations and requirements, evidence-based protocols, and other changes relevant to maintaining a current and safe nursing practice.

Concepts Related to Teaching and Learning

The concepts of development, communication, health, wellness, and illness are directly related to the concepts of teaching and learning. Nurses must understand various theories of psychosocial development and basic principles of communication to create effective teaching plans and

Box 41.2

Mentoring

Mentoring is an important career development tool for nurses in any setting or specialty. **Mentors** are experienced nurses who coach, advise, and support the personal and professional growth of a less-experienced or novice mentee or protégé in a professional relationship by discussing mutual goals and providing accountability (Erikson, 2018). Fortunately, modern technology provides more opportunities for mentoring via the internet and other rapid communication methods when the protégé is not physically in the same location as the mentor.

Often, the mentor relationship is one of teacher–learner. The mentor instructs the protégé in the expected role, introduces the protégé to individuals important to the achievement of goals, helps the protégé evaluate new ideas, and challenges the protégé to advance in the practice of nursing. Mentor programs are important for both student nurses and newly licensed nurses when transitioning from the role of a student into the role of a professional nurse. Mentoring is also important for professional development in nursing administration, nursing education, and when nurses enter a new position (Erikson, 2018; Goodyear & Goodyear, 2018a, 2018b).

Nurse mentor programs also benefit the nursing profession as a whole. Transitioning to practice can affect a new nurse's job satisfaction, job retention, and stress levels, as well as patient safety (Welch, Strickland, & Sartain, 2019). Hospitals with an evidence-based, structured transition-to-practice program have higher job satisfaction, retention, and competency levels. They also have decreased stress and patient care errors among newly licensed nurses compared to hospitals without transition-to-practice programs (Welch et al., 2019).

The mentoring relationship requires work and time from both the mentor and protégé. Some mentoring relationships have negative effects, including power struggles, intimidation, and loyalty issues. Nurses should recognize their individual strengths and encourage excellence in one another rather than feeling intimidated by each other. Employees must feel safe in their workplace, and a commitment to improving intrapersonal and interpersonal communication among nurses should provide a safe learning environment and encourage growth. Mindful creation of collaborative work environments is an essential task of nurse leaders (Klaber, 2018). Such environments help nurses unite and support each other, which helps ensure safety and excellence in nursing practice.

transmit information appropriate to each patient's level of understanding. Combining psychologic theories such as Erik Erikson's stages of psychosocial development, Jean Piaget's phases of cognitive development, and John B. Watson's behaviorism theory will provide direction and explanations for a fundamental understanding of mental, emotional, and social development during the lifespan. Similarly, cultural competency has become increasingly relevant for nurses providing teaching and therapeutic communication to diverse populations and in diverse settings. Educational materials and care plans must be patient specific and written after all aspects of a patient's cultural, mental, and physical status are assessed.

Knowledge of basic principles of teaching and learning is crucial because nurses empower individuals to lead healthier lives. Teaching and promoting general health principles such as good nutrition practices, illness and infection prevention, and safety measures are among the primary roles and responsibilities of nurses as patient advocates and, in some cases, professional educators of colleagues. Education empowers individuals to be active participants in their healthcare and promotes individual recovery, self-care, and personal responsibility for health and well-being. Some, but not all, of the concepts that are integral to teaching and learning are outlined in the Concepts Related to Teaching and Learning feature. They are presented in alphabetical order.

Concepts Related to
Teaching and Learning

CONCEPT	RELATIONSHIP TO TEACHING AND LEARNING	NURSING IMPLICATIONS
Communication	Teaching and learning processes require nurses and patients alike to engage in verbal, nonverbal, and written communication.	■ Use various elements of verbal communication—including pace, intonation, clarity, credibility, timing, relevance, and humor—in ways that are appropriate and help promote desired learning outcomes. ■ Effectively employ different elements of nonverbal communication, including posture, appearance, facial expressions, and gestures. ■ Create, distribute, and recommend written communication items (e.g., handouts, computer programs, mobile device apps) that are reflective of patients' literacy levels.
Culture and Diversity	Understanding and appreciating cultural diversity will encourage and promote trusting, interactive communication in patient care and interprofessional relationships.	■ Evaluate personal attitudes and beliefs regarding cultural diversity. ■ Recognize and consider patients' cultural background when planning care. ■ Coordinate interprofessional participation for resources such as interpreters or social and faith-based services to meet patients' culture-specific needs.
Development	As children develop, their learning abilities become more complex. As adults age, their vision, hearing, and motor function may become impaired. They may also experience declines in cognitive functioning.	■ Assess patient's age and developmental stage. ■ Use teaching methods appropriate to the patient's age and level of development. ■ Be aware that age does not always indicate specific developmental characteristics.
Health, Wellness, Illness, and Injury	Knowledge empowers individuals to make lifestyle choices that promote health and may prevent illness and injury.	■ Educate patients to be effective healthcare consumers. ■ Reinforce healthy patient behaviors. ■ Guide patients to problem-solve health-related issues.
Nutrition	Understanding basic nutritional requirements and food preparation guidelines can help individuals promote health, prevent illness, and manage existing disease processes.	■ Promote the importance of a balanced diet for disease prevention. ■ Provide information and teaching on specific diets related to disease management. ■ Provide referrals to a nutritionist or dietitian.
Safety	Knowledge of safe practices can help both patients and healthcare personnel avoid accidents and injury.	■ Assess patient's level of safety and risk for injury related to the environment. ■ Evaluate safety risks related to patient's cognitive and/or physical development. ■ Provide information about and teach basic safety precautions.

The Art of Teaching

Some may believe that teaching is simply a process by which the teacher speaks or imparts knowledge to another. In reality, teaching is much more than talking to someone about a particular subject or topic. Effective teaching follows a series of planned steps with the goal of changing a behavior, learning a skill, or gaining an understanding about a particular topic or activity. When the art of teaching takes place, the teacher uses creativity, strategies, and environmental changes to engage the learner.

Effective teaching begins with a thorough assessment of the learner's needs and particular style, which are then incorporated into an individualized teaching plan. The ability to capture the learner's attention exemplifies the art of teaching.

When teaching, the nurse should continually assess the patient's comprehension to limit or prevent misunderstanding. The nurse should support and encourage the learner to participate in the process through asking questions and seeking clarification.

Nurses should have a firm understanding of their personal strengths and confidence when planning and providing patient teaching. They should also be aware of their personal limitations on knowledge of a particular topic or skill. Additional information about the characteristics of effective teaching is located in **Box 41.3** ».

SAFETY ALERT It is essential that the nurse be knowledgeable about the subject matter to prevent the patient receiving any incorrect information that may compromise the patient's safety.

Box 41.3
Characteristics of Effective Teaching

Effective Teaching

- Identifies the learner's preferred learning styles (e.g., visual, auditory, verbal, written) and language.
- Uses several methods of teaching to accommodate a variety of learning styles, and provides learning opportunities through hearing, seeing, and doing.
- Asks the learner to identify areas of major interest as a strategy to enhance engagement.
- Involves the learner in the learning process, keeping the individual engaged and building a partnership between the learner and the teacher.
- Is appropriate for the learner's age, condition, and abilities.
- Sets realistic goals directed at helping the learner meet objectives.
- Uses accurate and current evidence-based information from reliable sources.
- Helps the learner believe that learning is possible and likely.
- Supports the learner with optimistic, positive reinforcement and feedback.
- Uses a variety of age-appropriate methods to evaluate learning.
- Is cost-effective (i.e., the cost of the nurse's time spent teaching is less than the cost of treating health problems that occur when patients do not follow recommended treatments, fail to take medications correctly, or do not adapt their lifestyle to changing health needs).

Source: Adapted from Blais and Hayes (2016).

When engaging in the teaching–learning process, the relationship between the nurse and patient transcends to being one of teacher and learner. However, the steps of the nursing process are still followed and serve as a guide during the process. Through careful assessment and thorough planning, the nurse as teacher creates a plan of instruction with the intention of achieving the patient's goals. The nurse then evaluates the effectiveness of strategies used to determine if outcomes (successful learning that will promote patient change) are met.

The teaching–learning process is grounded on specific theories that address the way people learn and the best strategies to facilitate a change in behavior. Understanding learning theories better equips the nurse to prepare individualized teaching plans for patients, families, and other populations of learners.

Aspects of Learning

To understand the process of learning, it is essential to identify the learner's needs. A **learning need** is an identified deficit in knowledge, information, or skills needed to achieve a particular goal. Goals may be focused on basic content (such as when to take a rescue inhaler), learning a new skill (such as how to use a rescue inhaler), or actions to change a specific behavior (such as avoiding asthma triggers).

One important aspect of learning is compliance, or the individual's desire to learn and to act on that learning. In the healthcare context, **compliance** refers to the extent to which an individual's behavior follows medical or health advice. Compliance is best illustrated when the individual accepts the need to learn, then follows through with appropriate actions that reflect the learning. For example, a patient who is diagnosed with diabetes would be compliant if he willingly learned about the recommended special diet and then followed that diet. However, many people view the term *compliance* negatively because it implies learners are passive participants, without the right to make their own healthcare decisions, or external factors that might affect the learners' participation in the treatment plan. At the same time, some professionals are too quick to label a patient as noncompliant. It is important to determine why a patient is not following a recommended course of action before applying this label. For example, a patient may have intended to comply with a prescription regimen but was unable to do so because of not affording the cost of the medications.

Many nurses and other healthcare professionals today prefer the term **adherence**, or attachment to a prescribed regimen. Modern healthcare promotes and encourages patients to be committed, active participants in maintaining personal health and wellness. Adherence identifies the level of a patient's behavioral patterns in response to mutually agreed-upon HCPs' teaching and treatment recommendations (Kim, Combs, Downs, & Tillman, 2018).

Mutual agreement does not always imply shared decision making, in which the patient plays an active role in determining the course of treatment. Studies indicate that shared decision making between provider and patient increases patient adherence with treatment recommendations, resulting in improved outcomes (De las Cuevas, de Leon, Peñate, & Betancourt, 2017; Lofland et al., 2017). Shared decision making ensures that the provider considers the individual patient's preferences and other factors that affect adherence, such as cultural practices, work schedules, and ability to afford treatment.

When evaluating responses and results of treatment plans, nurses may use the terms *adherence* and *compliance* interchangeably. Although both terms convey the same general concept, adherence has more positive connotations and emphasizes the collaborative nature of the patient–provider relationship (Ross, 2018). The terms *adherence* and *nonadherence* recognize that factors other than patient willingness to comply (e.g., financial considerations) may affect the treatment process.

Learning Theories

A number of different theories can help nurses understand the ways in which people learn. Adult learning theory, behaviorist theory, cognitive theory, social learning theory, and humanistic learning theory are among the theories most commonly used by nurses when teaching individuals and groups of learners. Additional concepts that the nurse should keep in mind when formulating teaching plans include the theories of categorization and constructivism. **Table 41.1** » provides a brief description of these theories and highlights some ways nurses can apply each theory in the teaching process.

In addition to the learning theories discussed in the table, nurses should understand the **theory of multiple intelligences**. This theory was presented by researcher Howard Gardner and is based on observations of the ways in which stroke damage can impact one area of the brain while leaving other areas of mental functioning intact. Initially, Gardner (1983; see also Marenus, 2020) cited seven intelligences:

1. Linguistic
2. Musical/rhythmic (music)
3. Logical/mathematical
4. Spatial (visual)
5. Kinesthetic/movement (body)
6. Personal
7. Symbols as intellectual strengths or ways of knowing.

Gardner has since added an eighth intelligence, naturalist intelligence, which is associated with recognition of environmental elements and patterns (Marenus, 2020).

TABLE 41.1 Major Learning Theories and Their Implications for the Teaching Process

Learning Theory	Summary	Implications for Teaching
Adult learning theory	Adult learners differ from child learners in fundamental ways. In particular, adults: ■ Need to know why they should learn something. ■ Prefer that others treat them as capable of self-direction. ■ Have accumulated life experiences that can enhance their current learning. ■ Are often ready to learn what they must know in order to take care of themselves.	When providing teaching to adult patients or caregivers, communicate how and/or why information is important and useful. Respect the learner as an independent, competent adult. Identify previous experiences and help the learner scaffold or incorporate new information with previous experiences.
Behaviorist theory	Learning occurs when an individual's response to a stimulus is either positively or negatively reinforced. It is possible to change an individual's behavior by either altering the stimulus condition or altering what happens after the individual responds to the stimulus. Providing **positive reinforcement**, or a pleasant experience such as praise and encouragement, is especially useful in fostering repetition of an action.	Provide praise or encouragement with each attempt or at each phase of the learning process. Allow sufficient time for the learner to practice new skills (e.g., return demonstrations). Consider environmental influences that affect the learning process.
Cognitive theory	Learning involves three mental processes that can occur sequentially or simultaneously: (1) acquiring information, (2) processing the information, and (3) using the information. Individuals' capacity to learn is shaped by their developmental level as well as by the social, emotional, and physical contexts in which learning takes place. Learning occurs across three primary domains: the cognitive (or "thinking") domain, the affective (or "feeling") domain, and the psychomotor (or "skill") domain.	Develop appropriate strategies to meet each learner's unique learning style and preferences. Assess each learner's developmental stage and emotional readiness to learn, then adapt teaching strategies to the learner's level. Select behavioral objectives and teaching strategies that encompass the cognitive, affective, and psychomotor domains of learning.
Constructivist theory	Learning is a developmental process constructed from individual experiences. Knowledge acquisition is the ongoing assimilation and accommodation of new experiences and interpretations. Cooperative learning and problem solving in collaboration with others promote learning.	Acknowledge the importance of and build on the learner's prior learning experiences. Encourage the learner to engage with the nurse and others during the learning process.
Social learning theory	Learning primarily results from instruction and **observational learning**, or the process of acquiring new skills or altering old behaviors by watching other people. This process focuses on imitation and **modeling**. The cognitive aspect of social learning theory suggests that an individual's beliefs, perceptions, and cognitive competencies influence the way in which the individual interacts with the environment.	By modeling how to perform skills (such as changing a wound dressing) and asking for repeat demonstrations until the patient can perform the skill satisfactorily, the nurse provides an opportunity for imitation and modeling.

Sources: Data from Bloom (1956); Bruner (1966); Candela (2012); Knowles, Holton, and Swanson (2005).

Gardner's work is one of several theories that challenge the notion that intelligence is static and is solely based on the learner's intelligence quotient, or IQ, which is a score derived from standardized tests. Another important theory that disputes the concept of IQ was put forth by researcher Daniel Goleman (1995) and later reinforced by Brandon Goleman (2019). They propose that **emotional intelligence**—or EQ—is as relevant to learning and success as IQ, or even more so. EQ measures individuals' abilities to differentiate between their own thoughts and feelings, recognize the thoughts and feelings of others, and show discernment when using emotions to influence decisions.

It is important for nurses to understand the focus and limitations of the various learning theories, as well as Gardner's and Goleman's theories. Intelligence levels are unique and specific to every person, and individuals can exhibit one or more intelligences at higher operant levels than the others. By knowing the various theories, the nurse can select the most appropriate theory or theories when developing a teaching plan for a specific patient.

Clinical Example A

Patrick Johnson is a 60-year-old man who owns a small business. He underwent coronary bypass surgery 3 days ago after experiencing a myocardial infarction at his retail store. He is scheduled for hospital discharge within the next 48 hours. The nurse responsible for Mr. Johnson's care and discharge planning notes that the HCP has ordered several new medications, as well as dietary restrictions and follow-up appointments.

Mr. Johnson is used to working 7 days per week. He lives with his 56-year-old wife, who occasionally helps at the store but also works as a part-time substitute teacher. The Johnsons have two grown children who are married and reside out of state. Mr. Johnson states that he is very worried that his business (and therefore his income) will decline due to his recent health problems and potential lifestyle changes.

Critical Thinking Questions

1. Discuss the impact of Mr. Johnson's recent health impairment and stated concerns on his ability to "learn," and apply information based on the cognitive and psychomotor domains of learning. What factors might hinder Mr. Johnson's ability to learn? Do any real and/or potential factors exist to promote his learning?
2. Is teaching a priority of care for Mr. Johnson at this time? Why or why not?

Factors Affecting Learning

Numerous factors can facilitate or impede learning. Factors that can facilitate learning include motivation, readiness, and feedback. Factors that can impede learning include illness status, stress and anxiety, medication side effects, pain, and fatigue. Nurses should keep these in mind because they impact the patient's response to teaching.

Factors That Facilitate Learning

There are specific conditions that positively impact learning. These conditions may be present in people at different times and influence the outcome of instruction. What motivates one individual to learn, for example, may not motivate another individual at all.

- ***Motivation.*** Motivation to learn is personal and affects how much an individual learns. It can also influence the rate of learning. Motivation must be identified and experienced by patients—the nurse's recognition of a need is not sufficient to motivate patients, although the nurse can help individuals identify and embrace the need. Furthermore, the nurse can help persuade support people that a need exists by providing information and/or reminding patients how their behaviors affect the people around them. For example, a man who has smoked for 20 years may not embrace the need to quit for the benefit of his own health. However, if the nurse provides patient education that includes the dangers of secondhand smoke, especially to young children, the man may recognize the need to quit smoking for the benefit of a child or grandchild.
- ***Readiness.*** Readiness to learn is a concept that is not always easy to recognize in another. It is characterized by curiosity, attention, and willingness to accept new or different information about a particular situation. Readiness is not something that can be planned; however, it can be facilitated when caring for patients. Since every nurse–patient encounter is an opportunity to teach, the nurse needs to implement strategies that enhance the situation and transform usual patient care activities into an active learning session. This is done by anticipating patients' basic needs and creating an environment that facilitates learning. Nurses can assess patient motivation and inspire patient readiness to learn through a process called *motivational interviewing* (see Module 35, Caring Interventions).
- ***Active involvement.*** Active involvement means the learner is engaged in the process and focused on the content being taught. When caring for adult patients, nurses promote active involvement by focusing on problems or situations that they find troubling or for which they are seeking a particular solution. This type of focused instruction increases the likelihood that the teaching will be effective. For example, an adult with a condition that limits hand mobility may be reluctant or fearful to participate in learning about self-injection of medications. With careful planning, the nurse can offer suggestions to reduce the patient's hesitancy and support learning a new skill despite the physical limitation. Active participation facilitates learning better than passive learning, in which the patient is merely an observer and not an active participant.
- ***Relevance.*** For teaching to be effective, it needs to be relevant to the learner. Prior to any teaching, inquire if there is any particular aspect of their health or treatment that patients want to learn more about. With this information, the nurse can tailor the instruction to meet patients' identified needs. During the teaching, the nurse should periodically stop and reassess patients to determine if the content continues to meet their learning needs.
- ***Feedback.*** The purpose of **feedback** is to determine if the information met the patient's goals or to evaluate the effectiveness of the instruction provided. Ask the patient if the content fills the identified knowledge gap. Evaluate the effectiveness of the instruction based on the content provided and any tasks or skills addressed during the instruction. Evaluating the effectiveness of teaching a particular skill can be done by observing the patient perform the skill or asking the patient to "teach back" the activity. The nurse can then gently reinforce any teaching the patient misunderstood or provide recommendations on how to improve skill performance. The nurse should find opportunities to offer praise when providing feedback as this will encourage the patient to continue with the learning process.

- ***Nonjudgmental support.*** Not all adults will admit the need to learning something. It may take creativity to determine if patients require specific instruction to address an identified health need, change a behavior, or learn a skill. The nurse is in the unique position to provide instruction without making patients feel like they need special help. Encouraging patients to watch while changing a dressing or filling a medication syringe at the bedside while they observe are beginning steps in the teaching process. After a while, asking if patients could "help" with the process encourages them to participate and limits resistance to performing the skill.
- ***Information that proceeds from simple to complex.*** Although teaching cannot always be planned in advance, regardless of the situation, the best approach is to begin with simple information and then proceed to the more complex topics. The simple information serves as a foundation on which more complicated concepts can be applied. This approach helps patients assimilate previous information with the new and encourages understanding. Keep in mind, however, that what one person finds simple may be complex for another.
- ***Repetition.*** It is unrealistic to expect patients to master new information after one exposure. The role of repetition in teaching is essential. Repeating instructions helps patients understand new unfamiliar terms and concepts and offers them an opportunity to practice a new skill under the supervision of the nurse.
- ***Timing.*** Timing is a challenging issue when providing patient teaching. Patients' health status may limit the amount and type of teaching to provide at any given time. Often teaching is not "scheduled in advance," but rather occurs when the ideal time presents itself. Patients' comfort plays a role in learning. Teaching episodes should be of short duration so as not to unnecessarily fatigue patients. Teaching sessions should be adequately spaced so that patients do not forget what was instructed during the previous session. During the session, patients should be given adequate time to demonstrate a skill, ask questions, and receive feedback to reinforce learning.
- ***Environment.*** It may be challenging to create an ideal environment for learning in the healthcare setting. Patients may be surrounded with machinery; a person in the next bedspace might have the television on; or visitors may be in the room. Every effort should be made to create an environment that is conducive to learning. This includes providing for patients' comfort, having all of the required supplies and materials prepared in advance, and reducing the noise or interruptions during the teaching session.

Depending on the type of instruction, patients might need to have a support person in attendance. For example, a family member may need to be instructed on filling syringes for insulin injections in the event the patient becomes unable to do so at home. The patient may also have a wound that is difficult to change independently. In these situations, teaching should be planned so that the support person is in attendance.

Clinical Example B

Angela Simpson, a 22-year-old woman, recently gave birth to her first child, and she is eager to learn how to safely care for her newborn. Angela believes that babies should sleep on their stomachs (prone position), and she has grown up observing family members, including her own mother, use this position with her younger siblings at naps and bedtime. As Angela's nurse, you know that evidence-based research discourages this tradition because stomach sleeping is linked to an increased risk for sudden infant death syndrome. You also note that Angela is currently staying with her mother (the baby's grandmother), who is actively involved in caring for her grandchildren.

Critical Thinking Questions

When developing a plan for teaching infant care to this mother:

1. What essential information would you want Ms. Simpson to learn?
2. How could you assess this patient's motivation to apply this information?
3. In what setting would Ms. Simpson be most likely to learn and retain the information?

Factors That Inhibit Learning

Many factors can inhibit patient learning. Some of the most common barriers to learning are described in **Table 41.2** ». Several of these barriers are described below:

- ***Emotions.*** Emotions such as fear, anger, and depression can impede learning. Similarly, high levels of anxiety can result in agitation and an inability to focus or concentrate, thereby also inhibiting learning. Patients or families who are experiencing extreme emotional states may not hear spoken words or may retain only part of the communication. However, emotional responses such as fear and anxiety decrease with information that relieves uncertainty. By providing information at appropriate times and repeating teaching sessions as needed, the nurse can help reduce anxiety and promote learning for patients and families in distress.
- ***Physiologic status.*** The patient's physical status should be the priority before providing any teaching. If the patient is experiencing pain or fatigue, learning will not be effective. Nursing care should focus on ensuring the patient's comfort and well-being before initiating any teaching plan. Encourage patients to rest before any planned teaching session as the actual time spent in learning may produce fatigue.
- ***Cultural considerations.*** Nurses should consider cultural factors before initiating any teaching. As with all aspects of care, patients should be provided with information in their native language. This includes the provision of verbal information as well as written teaching materials. Another consideration is the patient's health beliefs and practices. Health teaching should be congruent with the patient's cultural and religious practices, otherwise the patient is likely to ignore the teaching or perceive bias on the part of the instructor. The nurse should practice cultural competence when instructing patients from different cultures. Cultural competence begins with assessment. A holistic nursing assessment will assist the nurse in determining when the recommendations for the patient complement the patient's cultural and religious preferences and when they collide. When they collide, the nurse and healthcare team should take the time to consult with the patient to develop treatment and educational plans together. Engaging in shared decision making will increase patient adherence and facilitate patient learning.

TABLE 41.2 Common Barriers to Learning

Barrier	Explanation	Nursing Implications
Acute illness	Patient requires all resources and energy to cope with illness.	Defer teaching until patient's health status has improved.
Anxiety level	Severe and panic anxiety levels interfere with the ability to focus and pay attention.	Provide interventions to reduce anxiety. Plan teaching when anxiety is reduced. Defer any teaching if the patient's anxiety level is severe as teaching will be ineffective.
Biorhythms	Mental and physical performances have a circadian rhythm.	Adapt time of teaching to suit patient's circadian rhythms. For example, plan a teaching session during the part of the day when the patient is most alert.
Cognitive impairment or intellectual disability	Impaired cognitive ability may affect a patient's capacity for learning.	Assess patient's capacity for learning. Plan teaching activities to complement the patient's ability while also planning more complex learning for the patient's caregivers.
Culture/religion	Specific cultural or religious practices may impact healthcare beliefs and preferences.	Assess the patient's cultural and/or religious needs when planning learning activities.
Developmental level and age-related changes	Children have a shorter attention span and different vocabulary than adult patients. Older adults are more likely to have sensory or motor impairments that impede learning.	Adapt duration of teaching sessions, vocabulary, materials used, and other methods to meet the needs of the individual learner.
Emotions (e.g., denial, depression, grief)	Emotions require energy and distract from learning.	Deal with emotions and possible misinformation prior to providing patient teaching. Defer teaching if emotions are interfering with the patient's ability to focus.
Language	Patient may not be fluent in the nurse's language.	Obtain the services of an interpreter or nurse with appropriate language skills.
Pain	Pain decreases the ability to concentrate.	Conduct pain assessment before teaching. Engage in nonpharmacologic pain measures or allow ordered pain medication to take effect before providing teaching for patients reporting pain.
Physical disability	Visual, hearing, sensory, or motor impairments may affect a patient's ability to learn or perform certain tasks.	Plan teaching activities appropriate to the learner's physical abilities. For example, provide audio learning tools for a patient who is blind or work with occupational or physical therapists to adapt skills for patients with paralysis or prosthetics.
Prognosis	Patient can be preoccupied with illness and unable to concentrate on new information.	Defer teaching to a better time.

Source: Adapted from Berman et al. (2021).

- ***Psychomotor ability***. When determining a patient's learning needs, the nurse needs to consider the patient's ability to perform psychomotor skills. These skills can be altered by a health problem or side effect of a medication. Alterations in hand mobility can impact a patient's ability to fill a syringe, provide an injection, instill eyedrops, or open a container for an oral medication. Specific physical attributes that need to be considered before instructing a psychomotor skill include:
  - ***Muscle strength***. Muscle strength can be affected by an acute illness or chronic health problem. Assess the patient's strength before teaching a new skill. For example, a patient who has limited arm strength might not be able to safely walk with crutches.
  - ***Motor coordination***. There are two types of motor coordination: gross and fine. Gross motor coordination is that used to walk or throw an object, while fine motor coordination is that used to fill a syringe or write with a pen. The type of coordination required should be determined before teaching a new skill.
  - ***Energy***. Energy is needed to learn a new psychomotor skill. A patient who is acutely ill will have limited energy reserves, which will interfere with the ability to learn new information or perform a new skill or task. Older patients may have even greater energy needs to learn and perform a new skill. The nurse needs to assess the patient's energy level before initiating instruction so as not to create unnecessary fatigue.
  - ***Sensory acuity***. The patient's sensory status needs to be considered before teaching. Vision will be required to observe a skill and hearing will be required to understand verbal instructions. The patient with a sensory impairment may need to have a support person in attendance during teaching sessions to ensure the patient's safety.

Clinical Example C

Margaret Kim, a 36-year-old woman, is being transferred from the hospital to a long-term care facility to recover following a motor-vehicle crash. She sustained multiple fractures resulting in partial paralysis on her right side. She and the nurse planned a learning session at 1:00 p.m. to discuss wound care and medications for post-hospitalization treatment and care. At 1:00 p.m., the nurse comes to Ms. Kim's room with supplies and handouts to help her learn. The nurse finds Ms. Kim crying.

Critical Thinking Questions

1. What actions should the nurse take at this time?
2. Can learning take place? Why or why not?
3. Discuss strategies that the nurse could use to enhance Ms. Kim's readiness to learn.

Lifespan Considerations

As individuals progress from infancy to older adulthood, their capacity to learn changes in many different ways. To ensure that efforts to educate patients are as successful as possible, nurses must carefully assess each patient's level of development before creating a teaching plan. Generally speaking, patients within certain age groups tend to be at similar levels of development, and they often face similar physical, cognitive, and psychosocial factors that impact learning (see Module 25, Development). The following sections highlight some of the most important points to keep in mind when planning and delivering teaching to patients at various stages throughout the lifespan.

Teaching Children

Children are constantly developing new cognitive and motor skills and becoming increasingly purposeful when interacting with their environment. When developing a teaching plan for a pediatric patient, the nurse must first assess the child's level of development. Teaching plans for patients in this age group typically focus on primary healthcare, health promotion, and illness/injury prevention. In most cases, the teaching plan should be directed toward the parent or primary caregiver; however, the nurse must include the child in the teaching and provide basic instructions at the child's level of understanding.

To ensure successful outcomes, seek to establish trust by addressing the child by name. Be sure all teaching interventions are implemented in a safe environment using a calm approach and take care to address any concerns or fears of the child or parent/caregiver. Allow time for questions and practice if the teaching involves patient or caregiver performance of a skill or task. When appropriate, use props to demonstrate treatment procedures (**Figure 41.1** »). Always provide feedback, praise, and encouragement; evaluate the effectiveness of the teaching–learning experience; reinforce teaching as needed; and document the intervention (Ball, Bindler, Cowen, & Shaw, 2022). See the Patient Teaching feature for tools to use when teaching children.

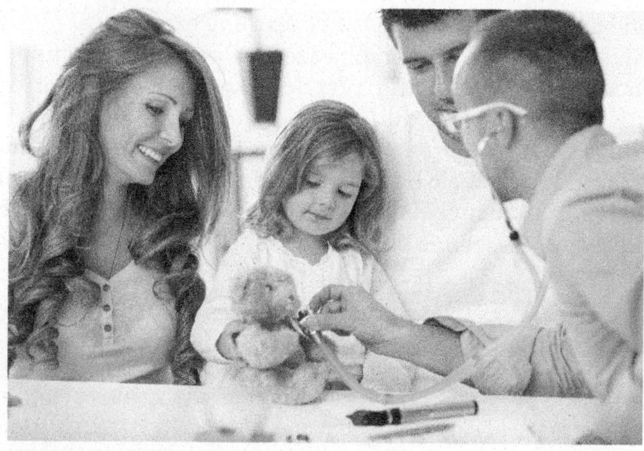

Figure 41.1 » This preschooler is holding a teddy bear that the nurse "examined" first to show the child what to expect.
Source: Vgajic/iStock/Getty Images.

Patient Teaching

Tools for Teaching Children Prior to Procedures and Hospitalizations

- Teaching should be age-appropriate.
- ***Toddlers:*** Use simple terminology and short explanations. Have the child visit the hospital in advance to reduce fear. Have the child play dress-up with a hospital gown (**Figure 41.2** »).
- ***Preschool age:*** Provide coloring books to show the child the types of rooms, people, and equipment that may be used. Use storybooks to describe what the child will be experiencing. Puppets may also be used to role-play situations.
- ***School-age:*** Dolls or stuffed animals can be used to show the site for a procedure. Some facilities have custom dolls available to help with teaching about tubes and injections.
- ***Preadolescent:*** Provide oral instructions and samples of the equipment that may be used. Encourage the child to handle the equipment and answer any questions. Ensure the child's privacy.
- ***Adolescent:*** Provide oral instructions and use of other strategies such as video. Stay with the adolescent during the video to answer any questions and allay any anxiety. Encourage adolescent friends to visit and participate in the teaching if the patient desires.

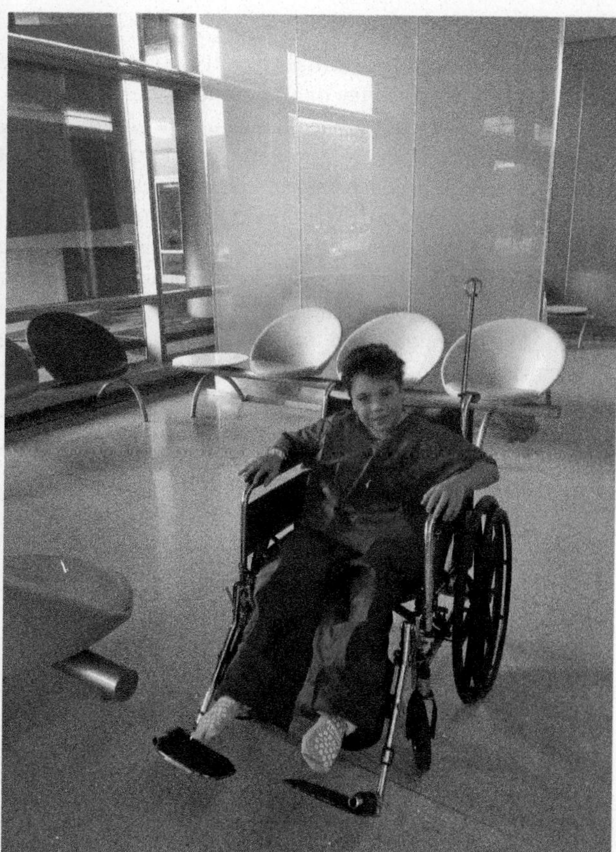

Figure 41.2 » Aiden, age 11, visited the hospital in preparation for upcoming surgery. While there, he got to have a wrist band, try on a hospital gown, and use a wheelchair.
Source: Courtesy of Kelly Block.

Teaching Adolescents

Adolescents experience many cognitive, moral, and physical changes as part of the transition from childhood to adulthood. Interpersonal communication, development of trusting relationships, and increased independence are of primary importance to patients in this age group. Health alterations can deeply affect personal identity, including feelings of well-being and perceptions of body image, and may carry long-term effects.

Before constructing a teaching plan for an adolescent patient, assess the patient's level of development and independence from parents and caregivers. During the teaching session, acknowledge and show respect for the patient's fears and feelings, and strive to provide a calm environment. Involving adolescents in the teaching effort facilitates a trusting relationship between the nurse and the patient and is essential for successful teaching. Teaching and health promotion for adolescent patients should focus on safety, consequences, and personal responsibility due to environmental influences that may involve peer pressure and risk-taking behavior. As with younger patients, allow time for questions and practice if teaching involves performance of a skill or task; provide feedback, praise, and encouragement. Always evaluate the effectiveness of the learning and teaching, reinforce teaching as needed, and document the intervention (**Figure 41.3** »).

Teaching Adults

An individual's critical thinking skills, cognitive development, and learning styles or preferences are influenced by personal experience and may change over a lifetime. Accordingly, before teaching, the nurse must seek to determine the adult patient's unique learning preferences, even if the nurse has worked with the individual in the past. In addition, gathering subjective and objective data regarding the patient's personal demands, responsibilities, educational level, cultural influences, and motivation to learn is essential to setting realistic teaching goals and preparing the patient for success.

Because teaching is one of the most critical nursing interventions, nurses' self-awareness of their personal learning style may be helpful when developing individualized patient teaching plans. Adult learners have a "need to know," so it is important for the nurse to allow time for questions and practice if teaching involves return demonstrations of skills or tasks (**Figure 41.4** »). Providing feedback, reassurance, and support promotes a positive learning experience.

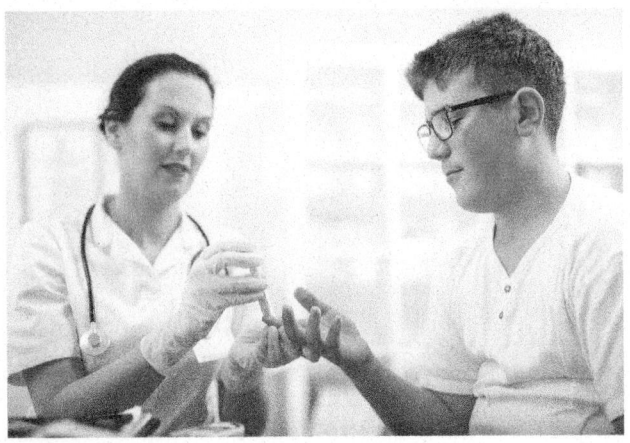

Figure 41.3 » An adolescent with diabetes is learning how to check his blood sugar. The nurse will next provide an opportunity for the patient to try it on his own.

Source: Jovanmandic/iStock/Getty Images.

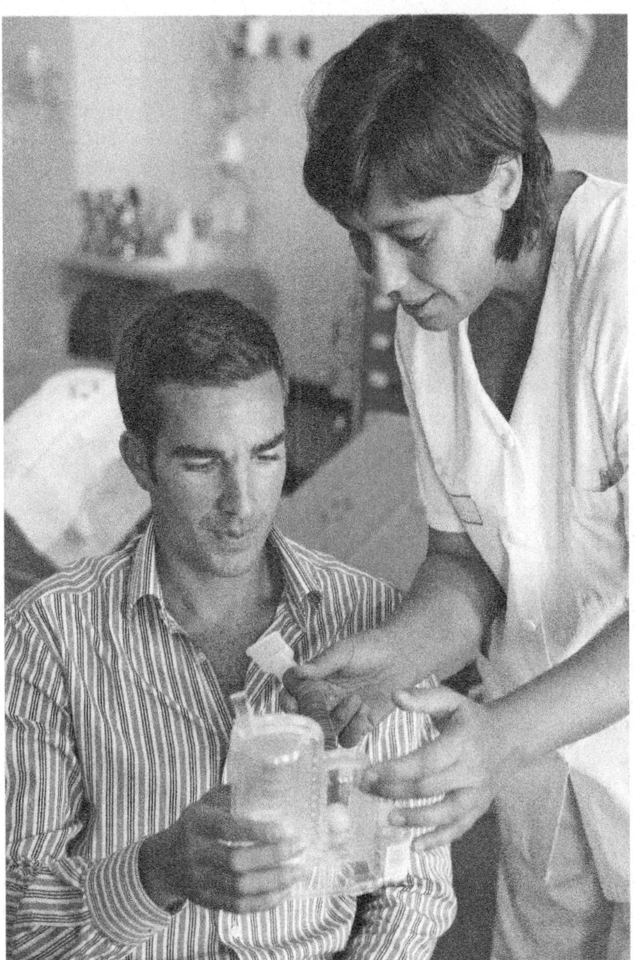

Figure 41.4 » When teaching adult patients, make sure to answer all their questions so that they understand the need for and benefit from the treatment.

Source: Javier Larrea/age fotostock/Alamy Stock Photo.

Nurses should also emphasize and promote the importance of positive health practices and actively involve patients in their care during patient teaching. However, it is imperative for nurses to remember that adult patients are responsible for their behaviors, and nurses cannot control responses or change patients' habits. Providing knowledge and awareness are the primary goals.

SAFETY ALERT According to The Joint Commission, patient education material should be written at the fifth-grade level; assessment of these materials is a part of the facility's accreditation. There are online websites available to analyze written material to ensure that it is prepared at the appropriate reading level (Readability Formulas, n.d.).

Teaching Older Adults

Many older adults have chronic illnesses that require various medications and therapies, so teaching with regard to these

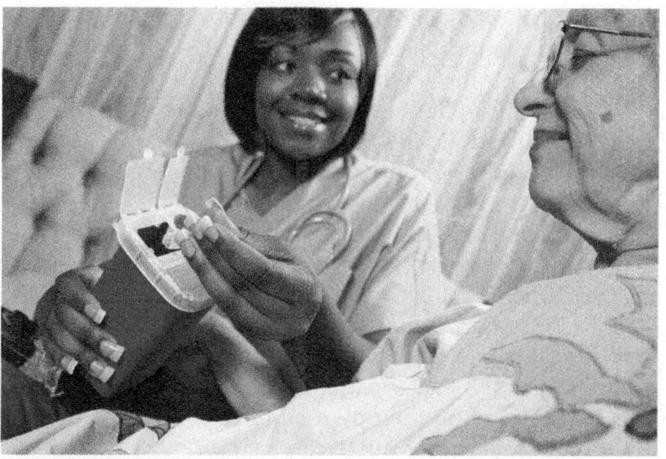

Figure 41.5 » A home healthcare nurse demonstrates for an older patient how to properly dispose of unused medication.
Source: Fstop123/E+/Getty Images.

treatments is essential for symptom control and prevention (**Figure 41.5 »**). Teaching plans for older adults commonly center on nutrition, physical activity, personal safety, medications, and the need for follow-up healthcare appointments (Bastable, 2020).

When teaching older adults, nurses must address aging factors that influence comprehension and develop teaching plans that ensure maximal learning can take place. Sensory alterations (especially hearing, vision, and touch), energy level, physical abilities, cultural influences, memory, response time, and stress can all affect an older adult's ability to learn and/or retain information, and they may be significant factors in nonadherence with treatment regimens. Older adults also have past experiences, insight, and knowledge that affect their current attitudes toward healthcare teaching. The nurse should respect older patients and use these past experiences, knowledge, and skills to help them learn.

To maximize learning and establish trust, the nurse must include older adults when developing a teaching plan and setting goals. Moreover, to achieve outcomes specific to older adults, the nurse should allow adequate time for processing information, provide repetition, and include significant others or primary caregivers as necessary. Teaching handouts that are written at a fifth- to sixth-grade reading level and use of large (e.g., at least 14-point font) black print on matte paper are practical and effective tools. As with all age groups, the nurse should use a calm approach, create a peaceful environment, allow time for questions and practice if teaching a skill or task, and provide feedback and encouragement. The nurse must also evaluate the effectiveness of the teaching and learning, reinforce teaching as needed, and document the intervention (Berman et al., 2021).

Teaching to Patients' Individual Needs

Each patient's individual needs should inform the teaching plan. One patient may have an impairment of mobility or cognition, whereas another may have an illness affected by environmental issues. When planning individual teaching, the nurse should perform a complete assessment of the individual's home environment, support systems, and unique level of development prior to any teaching efforts. Later, during teaching, the nurse may need to stress the importance of interprofessional interventions from therapists or medical social workers to ensure that all of the patient's health and wellness needs are met.

Clinical Example D

Lily is an active 5-year-old girl who fell off a swing at the playground, fracturing her left clavicle for the second time in 18 months. The physician tells Lily's mother that CT scans reveal the need for minor surgical correction that will require an overnight hospital stay. As the nurse prepares to teach both Lily and her mother about the upcoming procedure, Lily begins tearfully asking for her favorite doll "so my boo-boo can feel better." Lily's mother also verbalizes concern about what her daughter's postsurgical care may require. She is a single working mother with minimal support and another daughter who is 11 years old and too young to stay home alone. She further explains that she cannot afford to take much time off from work.

Critical Thinking Questions

1. What priority actions should the nurse take at this time?
2. Can learning take place? Why or why not?
3. What strategies could the nurse use to enhance Lily's learning and calm her fears?
4. Discuss strategies that the nurse could use to teach and provide reassurance to Lily's mother and address her concerns.

Technology, Health Information, and Patient Teaching

Technology has dramatically transformed many aspects of healthcare, including the ways in which patients and HCPs obtain and use health information.

Patients and Online Health Information

Increased use of the internet has changed the way people locate and access health-related information (Katzby, 2021). Many published articles, clinical studies, and scholarly journal publications are available online and through health-related applications. Unfortunately, there are also many websites that contain unreliable, questionable, and biased information. HCPs must review online sources carefully to identify those that are reliable. They must also teach patients how to discern trustworthy information from false or potentially dangerous health advice. The following points may be helpful for both nurses and patients who are searching for health information on the internet:

- Consider the author's credentials and whether the information is on a personal website or a site sponsored by an organization.
- Review any "About Us," "Philosophy," or "Background" links on the page.
- Look for citations or references documented with footnotes and working links to other sources of information.
- Check the publication or posting date on the page.

Authors with credentials from known and respected universities or organizations are preferable to authors with unknown or questionable credentials. However, information provided on a blog or personal website should be questioned, even if the author appears credible.

Organizational websites should be carefully vetted as well. In general, websites associated with reputable organizations such as the Mayo Clinic, the Cleveland Clinic, or the American Heart Association are reliable, whereas sites associated with private companies promoting medical products should be viewed cautiously. Reputable sites will often acknowledge that the information they provide is not a substitute for professional advice and will encourage individuals to follow up with their HCPs. In addition, *.gov* and *.edu* domains are generally reliable sources of health information. The domain *.org* is generally reserved for nonprofit organizations. The information from nonprofit professional organizations, such as the American Academy of Allergy, Asthma, and Immunology, and nonprofit advocacy organizations, such as the Alzheimer's Association and the National Parkinson Foundation, is usually helpful and reliable, but caution patients to vet information from sites that are less well known.

Citations and references should be reliable and of high quality. Journal articles, research studies, and documents from the National Institutes of Health and the Centers for Disease Control and Prevention (CDC) are examples of quality references; popular nonscientific or "wiki" websites are not. References should be current unless they are classic or foundational studies in a particular field or area of medicine (National Institute on Aging, 2018). The publication or posting date on the page itself should also be current.

» **Stay Current:** The Health on the Net Code of Conduct (HONcode) was established by the Health on the Net Foundation (n.d.) to accredit health-related websites for reliability. It has become an important resource for validating ethical, internet-based information. Any health or medical website intended for patients, health professionals, or the general public can request a review in order to receive the HONcode certification of reliability. Once approved, the HONcode logo can be publicly displayed on the website to indicate its credibility. For further information, see Health on the Net Foundation at https://www.hon.ch/en/.

Incorporating Technology in Patient Teaching

Technology-based tools offer nurses new and innovative methods for working with patients. These tools are part of the **e-health** movement, which focuses on making healthcare resources more accessible to patients by transferring them to electronic media (Phaneuf, 2020). Incorporating technology into patient teaching will depend on the particular health topic; the resources available; and patients' comfort with, preferences about, and willingness to use technology.

Some hospitals and clinics have e-health portals that enable nurses and providers to print educational information personalized for each patient based on condition and age. These resources may be particularly useful for patients who are not tech-savvy or who prefer to keep printed information on hand. If patients show interest in accessing this information on their own and the portal is structured for patient access, the nurse can also provide information to patients about logging on to the portal from a home computer.

Some facilities also have smart TVs that enable patients to watch videos and use health learning applications. Some of these applications may be downloadable to patients' tablets or mobile phones, enabling them to work through them at their own pace or revisit them at a later time. The applications may also include tutorials and quizzes that can help reinforce patient learning.

More individualized uses of technology may also be used in patient teaching, such as HIPAA-compliant video conferencing when working with patients who are homebound. It can also be effective for observing patients performing self-care tasks in the home.

Use of e-health interventions may be especially helpful with the adolescent population, which is acclimated to obtaining and sharing information online. Döğer et al. (2019) examined the effect of telehealth interventions on the control of type 1 diabetes in children and adolescents. After 6 months, the results showed that increased frequency of counseling by the diabetes team through the use of an instant chat application improved blood glucose control and promoted better self-care.

REVIEW The Concept of Teaching and Learning

RELATE Link the Concepts

Linking the concept of teaching and learning with the concept of communication:

1. How does the quality of a nurse's communication skills impact the ability to teach?
2. How does the ability to communicate with people who speak a different language impact the teaching process?

Linking the concept of teaching and learning with the concept of advocacy:

3. How does the role of the nurse as teacher combine with the role of the nurse as advocate?
4. A nurse teaches a patient newly diagnosed with diabetes how to provide self-care to reduce the risk of complications. How does teaching this patient serve the nurse's advocacy role?

REFER Go to Pearson MyLab Nursing and eText

REFLECT Apply Your Knowledge

Samuel Jordan is a 33-year-old man who has worked as a nurse on the medical unit of a local acute care facility for the past 4 years. He has 9 years of nursing experience, having worked at another facility for 5 years before accepting this position. The unit is usually staffed with registered nurses, nursing assistants, and licensed practical nurses, along with a clinical secretary who transcribes orders, answers the phone, and obtains supplies. Throughout the course of an average day, Samuel interacts with many different members of the healthcare team.

1. What teaching opportunities is Samuel likely to encounter on a normal workday?
2. What teaching opportunities might Samuel encounter on his days off?
3. How does teaching impact Samuel's self-evaluation of his work performance?

» Exemplar 41.A Patient/Consumer Education

Exemplar Learning Outcomes

41.A Analyze patient/consumer education as it relates to teaching and learning.

- Differentiate environments where nurses teach.
- Outline the steps of developing a teaching plan.
- Summarize the aspects of identifying learning needs.
- List special teaching strategies.

Exemplar Key Terms

Anticipatory guidance, *2691*
Anticipatory problem solving, *2692*
Health literacy, *2685*
Return demonstration, *2682*
Teach-back method, *2693*

Overview

The American Nurses Association, The Joint Commission, the American Hospital Association, and many other professional and accrediting organizations identify patient education as a standard of practice for nurses, providers, and healthcare organizations. In particular, The Joint Commission requires accredited agencies to provide education to patients in a language and manner that supports patients' communication level (Bastable, 2020). In addition, state nurse practice acts include teaching as a function of nursing and a legal and professional responsibility.

Although nurses play a key role in educating patients, patients are not passive recipients of information. In fact, many patients are taking an increasingly active role in all aspects of their health.

Good patient education efforts recognize the patient's role as consumer. Accordingly, education should help patients take a more active role in their health by providing them with information about methods for reducing health risk factors, increasing their level of wellness, and taking protective measures. **Box 41.4** » lists specific areas of health teaching that address these areas.

This exemplar takes a closer look at the steps nurses can take to provide teaching that promotes patient health and empowers patients as consumers. It begins with a discussion of the different environments in which nurses may engage in teaching. It also discusses methods for developing specific, individualized patient teaching plans. In addition, it looks at methods for identifying patient learning needs and implementing teaching plans. Finally, the exemplar explores methods for evaluating teaching and learning.

Teaching Environments

Patient teaching can occur in a variety of settings, including acute care hospitals, physician practices and clinics, urgent care centers, the patients' homes, and extended-care facilities. Teaching may also occur in community settings such as schools, libraries, community health centers, and child or adult day care centers.

Box 41.4

Common Topics for Patient Education

Health Promotion

- Human growth and development
- Exercise
- Family planning
- Hygiene
- Nutrition
- Safe sex
- Smoking cessation
- Substance use
- Stress management
- Resources within the community
- Weight management

Illness/Injury Prevention

- Health screening (e.g., blood glucose levels, blood pressure, blood cholesterol, Pap tests, mammograms, vision and hearing tests, routine physical examinations)
- Reducing health risk factors (e.g., lowering cholesterol levels, weight management)
- Specific protective health measures (e.g., immunizations, use of condoms, use of sunscreen, use of medication, umbilical cord care)
- First aid (e.g., tic removal, bleeding)
- Safety (e.g., proper use of seat belts, helmets, walkers, water safety)

Health Restoration

- Information about tests, diagnoses, treatment, and medications
- Self-care skills or skills needed to care for a family member
- Resources within the healthcare setting and the community

Adaptation to Altered Health and Function

- Adaptation to changing health status
- Facilitation of strong self-image
- Grief and bereavement counseling
- Information about available treatments and likely outcomes
- Lifestyle adaptations
- Problem-solving skills
- Referrals to other healthcare facilities or services
- Strategies to deal with current problems (e.g., home IV skills, medications, diet, activity limits, prostheses)
- Strategies to deal with future problems (e.g., fear of pain with terminal cancer, future surgeries, treatments)

Source: Adapted from Berman et al. (2021).

TABLE 41.3 Comparison of the Teaching Process and the Nursing Process

Step	Teaching Process	Nursing Process
1	Collect data; analyze patient's learning strengths and deficits.	Collect data; analyze patient's strengths and deficits.
2	Make educational diagnoses.	Make nursing diagnoses.
3	Prepare teaching plan: ■ Write learning outcomes. ■ Select content and time frame. ■ Select teaching strategies.	Plan nursing goals/desired outcomes and select appropriate interventions.
4	Implement teaching plan.	Implement nursing strategies.
5	Evaluate patient learning based on achievement of learning outcomes.	Evaluate patient outcomes based on achievement of goal criteria.

Source: From Berman et al. (2021).

Teaching Individual Patients

The goal of health teaching is to improve the health of patients and their families. The nurse supports disease prevention and health promotion by implementing strategies that are founded on learning theories, exemplify the change process, and follow evidence-based learning approaches. The teaching process follows the steps of the nursing process to include assessment, planning, implementation, and evaluation. The teaching plan should be individualized to meet the needs of the patient and family. See **Table 41.3** » for a more detailed comparison of the teaching and nursing processes.

Patient teaching can occur in a variety of situations. The majority of teaching occurs with the patient while the nurse is providing direct care. An example of one-on-one teaching would be the nurse instructing a postoperative patient on wound care or discussing ways to control blood glucose level through diet and weight management with a patient being treated for type 2 diabetes. Family members or other patient support people may need to be instructed on providing care for vulnerable patients, such as caring for an infant whose mother requires surgery or hospital care or assisting a family member with care needs at home.

Because of shorter hospital stays, the time to provide patient education may be limited. Nurses must take care to provide education that will ensure for the patient's safety from one level of care to another, followed by plans to continue the teaching in the patient's home, if necessary. Any teaching provided should be documented on the patient's discharge information along with information that the patient requires to safely perform self-care in the home.

When educating patients, the nurse must ensure that the environment is conducive to learning and that both patient and nurse are adequately prepared for the teaching session. The following is a list of recommendations nurses should keep in mind when preparing the environment, the patient, and themselves for teaching:

- Coordinate a time with the patient to provide teaching,
- Create an environment that supports the patient's comfort and limits distractions.
- Provide the instructions in small segments, pausing periodically to assess the patient's response or need to alter the approach.
- Adapt the teaching plan based on the patient's reactions. If the patient seems confused, stop providing new material and address the area of confusion and ensure understanding before introducing new information.
- Expect to repeat the teaching. The patient may not remember the information, or the physical condition may prevent the patient from staying focused during the session.
- Evaluate the patient's (or family member/support person's) ability to perform a skill through **return demonstration**. Have the patient (or support person) "teach back" the skill to exhibit its mastery.

Teaching in the Community

Nurses may be asked to participate in community health education programs, either in response to a request by an organization or as an expectation of their employer. The types of community settings include schools, health departments, community recreation centers, and colleges or universities. Teaching in a community center provides an opportunity to share specific information to a large group of people. Topics that may be a part of community health education programs include cardiopulmonary resuscitation, nutrition, weight management, and a variety of safety programs. Patient teaching in the community can also be offered as small-group sessions with a targeted topic, such as preoperative education for a specific procedure, childbirth classes, and group sessions on infant care or caring for a loved one with dementia.

Clinical Example E

When providing teaching to groups, it may be necessary to alter the teaching to meet the needs of the members of specific groups. Consider the following example: During the fall sports season, three high school athletes develop staph infections. When planning education to address this situation, the school nurse identifies the groups who are the stakeholders in the health and well-being of the student-athletes: (1) the athletes themselves, (2) their parents and immediate family members, (3) the coaches, and (4) the teachers and other staff at the school.

The nurse reviews strategies that can be used to instruct these different groups. Providing each group with only a handout will be insufficient to meet the learning needs. Instead, the nurse decides to work with the school's athletic director and trainer to develop a teaching session for the coaches. This plan will reinforce individual hygiene and facility policies, as well as provide local and state regulations on preventing staph infections. In addition, the nurse plans to demonstrate proper disinfection of equipment such as wrestling mats.

In collaboration with the trainer, the nurse also develops and schedules a teaching session for the athletes and their families. Understanding the importance of peer influence in this group, the nurse obtains parental permission for one of the athletes who acquired the infection to speak to the others about what it was like to have the infection and to help persuade the other students to take steps to avoid contracting the infection.

Critical Thinking Questions

1. What are the primary takeaways from the teaching sessions for each stakeholder group?
2. How would the teaching methods used in the session for the coaches differ from those used in the session for athletes?
3. Discuss strategies that the nurse could use to promote individual hygiene among student-athletes.

Developing a Teaching Plan

Before creating a teaching plan, the nurse must assess the needs of the patient or group. For individual patients (and their families), the nurse should consider the patient's health history, physical and psychosocial assessment, and available support systems (e.g., caregivers or access to transportation). The nurse should also note various factors that influence the learning process, such as readiness and motivation to learn, reading and comprehension level, and mobility.

Using the Health History

The health history can be used as a starting point when identifying a patient's learning needs. Data within the health history that can be used include age and developmental level, patient's understanding of the health problem, health practices and beliefs, cultural needs, learning style, socioeconomic status (SES), and support systems. Some examples of interview questions that help elicit this information are provided in **Box 41.5** ».

Note that the same elements that affect an individual patient's learning needs also affect the needs of individuals in communities. For example, consider a nurse who is planning a teaching session on health promotion for individuals with high blood pressure. This session will be presented to residents at an independent living facility. Although the teaching plan for the group will be different from that for a single patient, the plan should still consider factors such as the residents' primary language, age and developmental level, and SES (e.g., access to transportation, health insurance coverage). The following sections take a closer look at these and other elements that influence patients' learning needs.

Box 41.5

Interview Questions That Help Reveal Patient Learning Needs

Questions About the Primary Health Problem

- Tell me what you know about your current health problem. What do you think caused it?
- What concerns do you have about your health problem?
- What do you or did you do at home to relieve the problem? How helpful was it?
- How has the problem affected what you can or cannot do during your usual activities (e.g., work, recreation, shopping, and housework)?
- Have the treatments you have started helped your problem? If so, how?
- What, if any, difficulties have the treatments caused you (e.g., inconvenience, cost, discomfort)?
- Tell me about the tests (surgery, treatments) you are going to have.

Questions About Health Beliefs

- How would you describe your health generally?
- What actions do you take to keep healthy?
- What potential health problems are of a concern to you because of family history, age, diet, occupation, inadequate exercise, or other habits, such as smoking?
- What changes would you be willing to make to decrease your risk for these problems or to improve your health (e.g., weight reduction, smoking cessation, reduction in alcohol intake)?

Questions About Cultural Factors

- What language do you use most often when speaking and writing?
- Are you seeking the advice of another health practitioner?
- Do you use herbs or other medications or treatments commonly used by members of your cultural group? Please tell me the names of these herbs/medications/treatments being used.
- Is your current primary care provider aware of you using these herbs/medications/treatments?
- Has your primary care provider given you any advice or treatments that conflict with values or beliefs you consider important?
- If a conflict with your primary care provider occurred about these herbs/medications/treatments, what did you do?

Questions About Learning Style

- Validate the patient's age and note the developmental level.
- What level of education have you achieved?
- Do you like to read?
- Where do you usually obtain health information (e.g., primary care provider, nurse, magazines, books, internet, pharmacist)?
- Do you like to learn new things to improve your health?
- How do you best learn new things?
  - By reading about them?
  - By talking about them?
  - By watching a movie or demonstration?
  - By using a computer?
  - By listening to a teacher?
  - By first being shown how something works, then doing it yourself?
  - On your own or in a group?

Questions About Support Systems

- Would you like a family member or friend to also learn about the things you must do to take care of yourself?
- Who do you think would be interested in learning with you?

Source: Adapted from Berman et al. (2021).

Age and Developmental Level

The patient's age is a starting point to identify the developmental level and serve as a guide for the type of health teaching required and the learning strategies to use. Determining the developmental level can be assessed by asking questions. For children, developmental level can be assessed by observing them during play and interactions with others. The developmental level of older adults may be determined through conversation and questioning. This approach may reveal cognitive ability, memory, and use of psychomotor skills. (See the Lifespan Considerations section for additional information.)

Understanding of the Health Problem

A starting point to determine patients' learning needs is to ask them to explain their current health problem and if they have any questions about the condition. From here the nurse can then ask if the health problem has had any effect on the patients' ability to perform routine activities and quality of life. At this time the nurse can suggest additional services that the patients might find beneficial to support them at home.

It can be challenging to learn individual patient health information in a group setting. To facilitate this, the nurse should make every effort to understand the patients' health issues in advance. Strategies to gain this information prior to a group teaching session include:

- Send each patient a brief survey in advance
- Survey the patients at the setting where teaching will be provided
- Conduct brief surveys as patients arrive for the teaching session.

For instance, in the situation with the students with the staph infection, the school nurse might ask the coaches to provide surveys to the athletes at the beginning of practice a week before the session. An alternative might be to hold a brief session with the team captains to learn the athletes' general habits, practices, and attitudes toward hygiene.

Health Beliefs and Practices

Health beliefs and practices impact how patients will receive health teaching and should be considered in any teaching plan. The health belief model described in Module 7, Health, Wellness, and Illness, provides a predictor of preventive health behavior. However, even if a patient's health beliefs should be changed, it is not the role of the nurse to do so and it may not be possible because of the interplaying factors involved in a health belief.

Cultural Factors

Many health beliefs and practices have cultural origins, some of which may influence diet, lifestyle, health, and illness. Cultural practices and values affect learning needs and should be incorporated into teaching plans. However, even after providing health information teaching, a patient may elect to follow cultural practices.

Economic Factors

The nurse should keep the patient's SES into consideration when planning and providing education. The patient may have limited financial resources to purchase syringes for insulin injections or strips to check capillary blood glucose levels. Because of this, the patient may not be able to comply with the teaching. When teaching a group of patients, the nurse must keep in mind the individual patient's economic situation, which can impact transportation, obtaining prescribed medications, or purchasing food.

Learning Styles

Despite the amount of research and study conducted to determine learning styles, assessing and identifying a patient's learning style may be challenging. Some patients are visual learners and prefer to observe instructions. Others prefer to read instructions and then ask questions. Another style of learner prefers to handle equipment to figure out how it works. Then there are patients who prefer to learn within a group setting since this offers them an opportunity to share and gain insight from others. And there are some other patients who learn best under stress. The fear of not following instruction or learning a skill promotes learning for these types of patients.

At times the nurse has limited time to assess the learning style of each patient and adapt the teaching before providing instructions. However, the nurse can ask how the patient has learned new information in the past and if it is the preferred method. One strategy that the nurse can use when it is challenging to prepare teaching based on a preferred learning style is to vary the methods used during the teaching. The nurse can begin with reviewing instructions or playing a short video, follow up with a demonstration of equipment, provide the patient with samples of the equipment to handle, and then return to additional verbal instructions. Varying the approaches helps address the different learning styles that the patient may prefer.

An additional challenge for the nurse would be preparing to teach a group of participants in a community setting. The nurse may not have the time to assess the learning style of each participant and is therefore planning an educational program without knowing if the strategy will be effective. In this situation, the nurse should use a variety of techniques in efforts to keep the participants engaged. The use of videos, question-and-answer sessions, demonstrations followed by return demonstrations, and small-group discussions are just a few suggestions that may be helpful when providing an educational program to the community.

Support Systems

Prior to instructing a patient, the nurse should learn if the patient has any family or support people that would benefit from learning the information. These additional individuals are there to support the patient by also learning any required skills or actions to take to support the changes the patient needs to make based on the health condition.

Using the Physical Examination

When working with individual patients, the nurse can use the general survey part of the physical examination to provide clues regarding the patient's learning needs. Specific areas of the examination that impact learning include cognitive status, mobility, nutritional level, and energy. The nurse can also use information gained from observing the patient perform self-care activities, ability to pay attention when receiving care, and willingness to participate in care activities.

Knowing the patient's sensory status is paramount because vision and hearing affect the type of content and approaches to use when teaching.

Determining Readiness to Learn

The nurse should not expect a patient to state the desire to learn specific information. Patients who are ready to learn may behave differently from those who are not. Evidence of readiness to learn includes seeking information from a variety of sources, talking to others, and showing an interest about learning more about the topic or issue. In contrast, the patient who is not ready to learn appears disinterested in the topic and may change the subject when an attempt at teaching is made. For example, if the nurse says, "I was wondering about a good time to show you how to change your dressing," a patient who is not ready to learn might respond "Oh, my wife will take care of everything." Observing the patient's reaction during a teaching moment provides additional information regarding the receptiveness of the patient to the teaching.

The nurse should consider specific characteristics when assessing a patient's readiness to learn, including:

- ***Physical readiness***. Can the patient focus on things other than physical status, or are pain, fatigue, and immobility consuming the individual's time and energy?
- ***Emotional readiness***. Is the patient able emotionally to learn self-care activities? A patient who is extremely anxious, depressed, or grieving over health status is not ready to learn.
- ***Cognitive readiness***. Can the patient think clearly? Is the patient under the influence of medications that alter cognition? Are the effects of anesthesia altering the patient's level of consciousness?

The nurse can promote readiness to learn by supporting the patient's physical and emotional status while recovering from an illness or surgery. As the patient's condition stabilizes or improves, opportunities to learn will become more evident.

For patients who attend educational programs in group settings, the attendance is voluntary and they are more motivated to learn new information. However, when attending a mandatory educational program in a group setting such as in school or an inpatient treatment program, patients may not be ready to learn. In these instances, it is especially important that nurses be able to manage problem behaviors, such as monopolizing. (See Module 38, Communication, for more information.)

Assessing Motivation

Motivation is a challenging characteristic. What might be viewed as motivating to one patient may not be to another. Motivation impacts a patient's desire to learn and is the greatest when the patient demonstrates readiness, the learning need is recognized, and the teaching is beneficial to the patient. It is not easy to assess motivation. Because of this, nurses should be alert for patient cues that indicate readiness to learn new information, such as "I'm ready to stop smoking." In contrast, the patient who demonstrates minimal interest in a topic, appears inattentive, and cancels scheduled appointments is not motivated to learn. See Module 35, Caring Interventions, for information on assessing patient readiness to change and motivational interviewing.

There are specific strategies that the nurse can use to increase patient motivation in both individual and group settings:

- Relate the learning to something the patient values as this will help the patient see the relevance of the learning.
- Make the learning situation pleasant and nonthreatening.
- Encourage self-direction and independence.
- Demonstrate a positive attitude about the patient's ability to learn.
- Provide ongoing support and encouragement as the patient attempts to learn (i.e., positive reinforcement).
- Create a learning situation in which the patient will experience success. (Succeeding in small tasks motivates the patient to continue learning.)
- Assist the patient to identify the benefits of changing a behavior.

Assessing Health Literacy

Literacy and *health literacy* are two closely related ideas. Literacy is a comprehensive measurement of an individual's mathematical, reading, writing, and language skills. A patient's literacy level affects the ability to understand and use information. **Health literacy** refers to the individual's ability to use literacy skills as a means of obtaining, understanding, and applying health information (CDC, 2020). Essentially, health literacy allows the patient to make sense of health information and use that information to make sound decisions about healthcare. The nurse must assess a patient's health literacy to create an effective teaching plan.

Health literacy is important because it impacts patient outcomes. Typically, patients with higher levels of health literacy have better outcomes. For example, patients with higher health literacy are more likely to read a prescription label accurately and take the correct number of pills at the correct times of day. Patients with low health literacy, on the other hand, are more likely to experience adverse events and hospitalization. Research suggests that 23.3% of the U.S. population has difficulty reading or understanding healthcare-related information (Knowles, 2018). **Box 41.6** » lists the groups at the greatest risk of low health literacy. The Focus on Diversity and Culture feature goes into further detail about health literacy in immigrant populations.

Box 41.6

Populations Most Likely to Experience Limited Health Literacy

- Adults older than 65 years of age
- Recent refugees and immigrants
- Individuals with less than a high school degree or GED
- Individuals with incomes at or below the poverty level
- Nonnative speakers of English (U.S. Department of Health and Human Services [DHHS], n.d.)

Focus on Diversity and Culture

Health Literacy in Immigrant Populations

Immigrants tend to have lower health literacy than nonimmigrants. Low health literacy is more responsible for a perceived lower quality of care in immigrants than many other factors, including education, income, and health insurance coverage (Baumeister et al., 2019). Public initiatives intended to improve health literacy do not always reach immigrants. This may be the result of SES, fear of discrimination or deportation, language and other social barriers, or a combination of factors. In addition, the combination of low health literacy and limited English proficiency cause immigrants to be at high risk for poor health (Feinberg, O'Connor, Owen-Smith, Ogrodnick, & Rothenberg, 2020). For the same reasons, health promotion and disease prevention services are often underused by immigrant populations (World Health Organization [WHO], 2019b).

Interventions that have been found effective for improving health literacy and access to services in immigrant populations include the use of informational pictograms and signs translated into multiple languages. Translated signs in particular are useful not only for helping patients learn but also for creating feelings of inclusion and belonging at the facility where they are used.

The use of cultural mediators may also be successful in improving health literacy and quality of care for immigrant patients. Cultural mediators are individuals with an understanding of patients' native cultures and their views of health, wellness, and medical interventions (WHO, 2019a). The cultural mediator may also be versed in the immigrant experience and may speak the patients' native language.

A key to improving immigrants' health literacy and access to healthcare initiatives is engaging them in the planning and implementation of strategies. The effectiveness of strategies should be evaluated regularly by immigrant patients, cultural mediators, and HCPs.

The large percentage of people with low health literacy is particularly worrisome in light of the increased availability of health information online. In order to address this concern, U.S. government health agencies have developed programs and initiatives designed to educate individuals and promote national and global health. In 2010, the DHHS released the *National Action Plan to Improve Health Literacy*. This plan is intended to help meet the goals and objectives outlined by *Healthy People*. The CDC (2020a) also developed a website for individuals, organizations, and HCPs that aims to improve health literacy and public health. This site is simply titled *Health Literacy* and can be accessed at http://www.cdc.gov/healthliteracy/.

Clinical Example F

David Rodriquez is a 28-year-old man who had an emergency appendectomy yesterday. He is to be discharged home later today. During discharge teaching, the nurse provides Mr. Rodriquez with handouts relating to wound care, medications, activity restrictions, and follow-up appointments. The nurse knows the handouts will fit Mr. Rodriquez's learning style because he said he likes to read; in fact, the nurse observed him reading a couple of times this morning.

Critical Thinking Questions

1. Should the nurse have used the handouts as a learning tool? Why or why not?
2. What strategies might patients use to avoid embarrassment by having to admit they cannot read?
3. What strategies might a nurse use to help a patient who cannot read learn about self-care?

Nurses play a major role in improving health literacy. An important first step for nurses is assessing a patient's general literacy. (See the Patient Teaching feature for information about patient behaviors that suggest a literacy deficit.) Once a patient's literacy level has been determined, the nurse should adjust written materials to the patient's level. In general, educational materials should be written at a fifth- or sixth-grade reading level. Materials should use the active voice rather than the passive voice and be written in the second person (*you*) rather than the third person (*the patient*). Priority information should appear first and be repeated several times. Sentences should be short and use easy, common one- or two-syllable words. For example, the word *use* should take the place of *utilize*, and the word *give* should be used rather than *administer*. Larger type size (14- to 16-point font) should be used, and important words should be boldfaced for emphasis. Simple pictures, drawings, or cartoons should also be used, if appropriate.

SAFETY ALERT Individuals with low reading skills may struggle not only with health teaching but with giving accurate informed consent for treatment. When working with these patients, review all components of the procedure and the consent document carefully, allowing time for the patient to ask questions.

Individuals with good reading skills are unlikely to be offended by simple reading material; in fact, they may prefer easy-to-read information. However, even the simplest written directions will not be helpful to patients with low or no reading skills. When working with these patients, the nurse should use multiple teaching methods, including pictures, role playing, and hands-on practice. The nurse can also read important information to patients, taking care to emphasize key points in simple terms. It may also be helpful to associate new information with information the patients already know or associate with their job or lifestyle.

Regardless of a patient's health literacy level, it is generally a good idea for the nurse to limit the amount of information presented in a single teaching session. Instead of one long session that provides a great deal of information, it is often better to provide more frequent sessions that focus on one or two major points. All teaching should involve the patient and use repetition to reinforce the information presented. Finally, the nurse should obtain feedback during the session by asking patients specific questions about the information presented or asking them to repeat what was learned in their own words.

SAFETY ALERT Highly technical language and nursing jargon are confusing to patients—even those with higher levels of health literacy. Confusing instructions may be ignored, placing the patients' health at risk. Verbal and written teaching must use simple, clear language that is readily understood by laypersons.

Patient Teaching
Identifying Low-Literacy Behaviors in Patients

Patients often will not admit to having difficulty reading because of the embarrassment it brings them, and many people at the lowest reading levels report that they "read well." A nurse who suspects a patient has difficulty reading may ask tactful questions, such as "Would you like me to go over it with you?"

It can be difficult to assess a patient's health literacy skills because the shame and stigma associated with limited literacy are major barriers. The following patient behaviors may cause a nurse to suspect a literacy problem:

- A pattern of nonadherence
- Insistence that the information is already known
- Reliance on friends or family members to read the document aloud
- A pattern of excuses for not reading the instructions (e.g., claiming that glasses are broken)

Identifying Learning Needs

The nursing diagnosis step in the nurse process for patients with learning needs can be addressed in two ways: (1) as the patient's primary concern or problem or (2) associated with the patient's response to health alterations or dysfunction.

Primary Concern or Problem

Learning needs based on a primary concern or problem are those that, when addressed, reduce or eliminate the issue. Examples of this would be a patient who needs to learn how to administer insulin to treat diabetes. Once the patient learns how to prepare the syringe, inject the medication, and dispose of the used supplies, the primary problem is solved. Additional steps for this situation would include storing the medication, obtaining the needed supplies, and evaluating the effectiveness of the medication through ongoing capillary blood glucose measurements.

The problem of a learning need as a primary concern can be identified as a(n):

- Educational requirement
- Educational need
- Need for teaching.

When working with patients who have insufficient knowledge, the nurse should provide information that has the potential to change the patient's behavior rather than focus on the behaviors caused by the patient's lack of knowledge.

Another type of statement that can be used to identify a learning need as a primary concern is "desire to learn." This statement indicates that the patient is seeking information or knowledge to address a particular problem or need.

Noncompliance or *nonadherence* is another term that may be appropriate when a learning need is the primary concern. This recognizes that the patient or caregiver may not always be able to follow the plan of care. Factors that influence a patient's compliance with health teaching include understanding or comprehending teaching, any negative side effects of the treatment, financial inability to carry out the treatment plan, language barriers, or poor teaching on the part of the healthcare team. The statement of noncompliance or nonadherence is not appropriate to use for the patient who is unable to follow instructions because of a cognitive deficit or for the patient who consciously decides to refuse recommended medical care.

Learning Need as a Response to Health Alteration

Another way to approach a patient's learning needs is to identify when teaching is required to address a problem that occurs as a response to a health alteration. The following are examples of statements that address this type of learning need:

- Potential for low fluid volume
- Inability to safely ambulate
- Difficulty providing self-care.

Establishing the Teaching Plan

The steps of the nursing process can serve as a guide for developing this plan. The teaching plan is best established with the participation of the patient as this will enhance the individual's motivation. The patient who assists in the development of the teaching plan is more likely to have successful outcomes.

Determining Teaching Priorities

After assessing the patient's learning needs, the next step when creating the teaching plan is to place the needs in order of priority. Priority should be determined by both the nurse and patient, with the patient's priorities being addressed first. Once this occurs, the patient is more motivated to continue with teaching to address any additional learning needs. For example, a patient who wants to know all about coronary artery disease may not be ready to learn how to make lifestyle changes until personal needs to learn more about the disease are met. Theoretical frameworks, such as Maslow's hierarchy of needs, can serve as a guide when establishing priorities.

Setting Learning Outcomes

Once the learning needs have been prioritized, the patient and nurse should collaborate to determine the desired learning outcomes. Learning outcomes are essentially the same as desired outcomes for nursing problems and are written in the same way. Characteristics of learning outcomes include:

- ***State the patient (learner) behavior or performance.*** For example, an appropriate learning outcome would be "Identify personal risk factors for heart disease" (patient behavior), *not* "Teach the patient about cardiac risk factors" (nurse behavior).
- ***Reflect an observable, measurable activity.*** The nurse must be able to evaluate whether the patient has mastered the learning through observing a change in patient behavior. Change may be visible (e.g., walking) or invisible (e.g., adding a column of figures). For example, an outcome might be written as "Selects low-fat foods from a menu"

Box 41.7

Examples of Verbs for Writing Learning Outcomes

Cognitive Domain	Affective Domain	Psychomotor Domain
Compares	Accepts	Assembles
Describes	Attends	Calculates
Evaluates	Chooses	Changes
Explains	Discusses	Demonstrates
Identifies	Displays	Measures
Labels	Initiates	Moves
Lists	Joins	Organizes
Names	Participates	Shows
Plans	Shares	Performs
Selects	Uses	
States		
Writes		

Source: From Berman et al. (2021).

(observable, measurable), *not* as "Understands low-fat diet" (unobservable and not measurable). Examples of measurable verbs that can be used in learning outcomes are shown in **Box 41.7** ». Avoid using words such as *knows*, *understands*, *believes*, and *appreciates* because they are neither observable nor measurable.

- ***May include conditions or modifiers as required to clarify or specify a change in behavior***. Examples include "Uses inhaler *independently* (condition) as taught" or "States *three* (modifier) factors that trigger asthma."
- ***Include criteria specifying the time in which learning should take place***. For example, "The patient will state three things that affect blood sugar level *by the end of the teaching session*."

Learning outcomes can be written to reflect the learner's command of simple to complex concepts. As an example, the learning outcome "The patient will list risk factors for type 2 diabetes" is a low-level knowledge outcome that requires the learner to identify all risk factors; it does not expect the patient to apply the information to a specific behavior. In comparison, the learning outcome "The patient will list personal risk factors for type 2 diabetes" requires that the learner understand risk factors in general but also identify personal behaviors that place the patient at risk for type 2 diabetes.

The learning outcomes should be written to address the specific type of behavior to affect and identify the specific domain (cognitive, psychomotor, or affective). In most cases, patients need to both learn new information and be able to apply that knowledge to change their personal behavior.

Choosing Content

The content of a teaching plan is the information that will be provided to the patient and is determined by the learning outcomes. If a patient's learning outcome is "Demonstrate walking with a cane after two sessions," the plan will include information about the appropriate use of the cane and the actions the patient will learn in order to safely walk with the device.

Many sources of information can be used when creating the content. These sources include books, nursing journals, the internet, and other nurses and primary care providers. Whatever sources that are used, the content should be:

- Accurate
- Current
- Based on learning outcomes
- Adjusted for the learner's age or developmental level, culture, and ability
- Consistent with information on the teaching plan
- Selected according to the amount time and resources available for teaching.

Selecting Teaching Strategies

Teaching strategies are approaches or methods used to provide information and facilitate learning. The nurse selects strategies based on the patient's preferences and the type of information to be shared. For example:

- Patients with minimal literacy need material presented through audio or visuals rather than reading
- Psychomotor skills require practice; discussion alone is insufficient to promote learning
- Group education sessions require a competent group leader.

Table 41.4 » lists some teaching strategies the nurse may find useful. Nurses should keep in mind both traditional methods of patient teaching (such as teach-back methods) and new strategies, such as group chats and smartphone apps (see the Evidence-Based Practice feature).

Organizing Learning Experiences

There are a variety of organizations that prepare generic teaching guides. These guides can be individualized to meet patients' needs while saving time necessary to create the plan. Advantages to using prepared plans include identifying standardized content and providing recommendations for methods to teach the content. Using these types of plans also ensures consistency of content for learners, which helps reduce confusion. For example, when teaching infant bathing, the nurse should be consistent about the types of soaps appropriate for the infant's bath and identify those that are not.

Whether implementing a plan devised by another person or developing an individualized teaching plan, the following guidelines can help the nurse sequence the learning experience:

- Begin with a topic of concern to the patient; for example, an adolescent newly diagnosed with asthma may not be interested in learning about triggers but may want to learn lifestyle changes necessary to continue to play soccer.

TABLE 41.4 Selected Teaching Strategies

Strategy	Major Type of Learning	Characteristics
Explanation or description (e.g., lecture)	Cognitive	Teacher controls content and pace. Learner is passive and therefore retains less information than when actively participating. Feedback is determined by teacher. May be given to individual or group.
One-to-one discussion	Affective, cognitive	Encourages participation by learner. Permits reinforcement and repetition at learner's level. Permits introduction of sensitive subjects.
Answering questions	Cognitive	Teacher controls most of content and pace. Learner may need to overcome cultural perception that asking questions is impolite and may embarrass the teacher. Can be used with individuals and groups. Teacher sometimes needs to confirm whether question has been answered by asking learner, for example, "Does that answer your question?"
Demonstration	Psychomotor	Often used with explanation. Can be used with individuals and small or large groups. Does not permit use of equipment by learner; learner is passive.
Discovery	Cognitive, affective	Teacher guides problem-solving situation. Learner is active participant; therefore, retention of information is high.
Group discussions	Affective, cognitive	Learner can obtain assistance from supportive group. Group members learn from one another. Teacher needs to keep the discussion focused and prevent monopolization by one or two learners.
Practice	Psychomotor	Allows repetition and immediate feedback. Permits hands-on experience.
Printed and audio-visual materials	Cognitive	Includes use of books, pamphlets, films, programmed instruction, and computer learning. Learners can proceed at their own speed. Nurse can act as resource person and need not be present during learning. Potentially ineffective if materials are written at too high a reading level. If English is the patient's second language, nurse should select materials that use the patient's preferred language (e.g., Spanish).
Role playing	Affective, cognitive	Permits expression of attitudes, values, and emotions. Can assist in development of communication skills. Involves active participation by learner. Teacher must create supportive, safe environment for learners to minimize anxiety.
Modeling	Affective, psychomotor	Nurse sets example by attitude, psychomotor skill.
Computer learning resources (e.g., group chats, video tutorials, smartphone apps)	All types of learning	Learner is active. Learner controls pace. Provides immediate reinforcement and review. Can be used with individuals or groups.

Source: From Berman et al. (2021).

- Assess what the patient already knows, then proceed to the unknown. This gives the patient confidence. Options for assessing knowledge before beginning teaching sessions include surveys or questionnaires completed online or in person before the session.
- Address any area that is causing the patient anxiety first. Reducing patient anxiety will improve concentration and retention of information. For example, a patient afraid of falling again may be fearful of learning to use a walker until the nurse explains how using the walker will reduce the risk of falling.
- Begin with the basics before proceeding to more complicated information or tasks. For example, when teaching a patient how to use a peak flow meter, teach the basics of using the meter and then teach the patient what to do if the individual's reading is in the yellow or red zone.
- Plan time to review the information and answer any questions the patient may have or to clarify information.
- If the patient does not have any questions, stating, "A few frequently asked questions are . . . " may be helpful.

Evidence-Based Practice

Finding Teaching Strategies That Help Patients Understand, Apply, and Retain Information

Problem

Patient teaching is a professional obligation of nurses but determining the most effective teaching strategy or strategies for each patient is challenging. The selected strategy must be appropriate for the patient's health literacy level and readiness to learn. It should help patients understand, apply, and retain the necessary information. With the many teaching methods available to nurses, identifying the ideal strategy for these outcomes can be difficult.

Evidence

Numerous studies have examined the effectiveness of various teaching methods on different patient populations. Chen et al. (2020) studied the use of social media to instruct patients with diabetes on glycemic control. The study included 2838 patients who received information via a group chat. The researchers found that, compared to typical face-to-face patient education, teaching delivered via or augmented with group chat was associated with significantly improved glucose management. The researchers also found that outcomes associated with education via group chat were sustained for up to 1 year.

Glenn, Wolfe, and Borgmann (2020) evaluated the effectiveness of preoperative video teaching about anxiety in pediatric patients between the ages of 7 and 14 scheduled for outpatient surgery. The participants were asked to complete an anxiety inventory for children before and after watching a preoperative teaching video. The results showed that 61% of the patients reported reduced preoperative anxiety after watching the video.

Talevski et al. (2020) reviewed studies conducted on the use of the teach-back method to instruct patients regarding self-care management, medication adherence, quality of life, health literacy, and adherence to dietary changes. (The teach-back method is explained in greater depth later in this exemplar.) Of the studies reviewed, 19 reported positive findings regarding disease knowledge, behavior change in self-care practices, and quality of life. Several studies reported improvement in medication adherence, diet changes, and self-care compared to control groups. One study showed an increase in health literacy scores after using this approach. From these studies, it was concluded that the teach-back method is effective across a wide range of settings, populations, and outcome measures.

Implications

Although each of these studies assesses different components of effectiveness, they all suggest that a variety of teaching methods can improve patient understanding, application, and retention of material.

Critical Thinking Application

1. Discuss the ways in which visual media might be used differently to teach pediatric patients and adolescents about leukemia.
2. How do patient goals dictate the way in which teaching strategies are used for patient teaching? Consider two diabetic patients, one who is learning to administer insulin and one who is struggling to stay active and lose weight. Assume both patients have similar health literacy and readiness to learn.
3. In what ways could visual media be adapted for teaching patients with visual impairment? What other strategies might be useful for teaching this patient population?

Showing Flexibility

Flexibility is essential when implementing any teaching plan because it may need to be revised. For example, the patient may become fatigued sooner than anticipated or receive too much information too quickly, the patient's needs may change, or external factors may intervene. An example of this would be the nurse planning to instruct a patient on wound care in the morning, but the patient requests another opportunity to observe the nurse before performing the task. In this situation, the teaching plan may need to be extended until the next day.

The nurse will also need to use teaching techniques that enhance learning and reduce or eliminate any barriers to learning, such as pain or fatigue. Teaching also occurs while providing patient care, such as when giving medications. Teaching provided during patient care should be documented in the patient's electronic health record.

Implementing the Teaching Plan

Knowledge alone is not enough to motivate individuals to change their behaviors. Rather, evidence indicates that patient engagement in the care plan promotes learning and improves care delivery (Bombard et al., 2018). Therefore, when implementing a teaching plan, the nurse must actively seek ways to get the patient interested and involved in not just the teaching process but the entire care process. This requires that the nurse reflect on the changes required as part of the care plan, the stages of the change process, the patient's desire to change, and anything that may hinder the change process. The teaching plan can be implemented once the patient decides it is time to change the behavior. When this occurs, the following guidelines may be helpful:

- Establish rapport with the patient before teaching. The nurse should know the patient's preferences and needs, factors that influence the individual's ability to learn, and the patient's capacity to be comfortable and trust the nurse.
- The nurse should build on the patient's previous knowledge and experiences to facilitate learning. For example, a patient who performed self-care on an abdominal wound will have experience before learning to change a dressing on a lower extremity.
- The length of time for each teaching session will vary and depends on the patient. When possible, consult with the patient about the best time for the session to occur. For example, some patients may prefer to learn new information in the morning when their spouse is at work or after having a nap when they feel refreshed. The nurse should be aware of patient cues that indicate a readiness to learn. For example, if a patient asks why a certain medication has been prescribed, the question provides an opportunity to explain the reason for the medication, evidence of effectiveness, any side effects, and if follow-up lab work is needed.

- When teaching, the nurse must communicate clearly and concisely. The words used when teaching need to have the same meaning to the patient and the nurse. For instance, a patient who is instructed to avoid placing water on a specific area of the skin needs to understand that that includes a wet or damp washcloth.
- The nurse should use the vocabulary of a layperson when teaching. Terms, abbreviations, and medical jargon can be confusing to a patient and should be avoided. Even words such as *void* or *feces* may be unfamiliar to a patient and abbreviations such as *SOB* (shortness of breath) can be misunderstood.
- The nurse needs to observe the patient during the teaching to ensure for the correct pace. If the pace is too fast, the individual might appear confused and become anxious. If the pace is too slow, the patient may appear bored and lose interest.
- The environment can detract from or assist learning. Noises or interruptions interfere with concentration, whereas a comfortable environment promotes learning. If possible, the patient should be out of bed during the teaching session. Most people associate a bed with rest and sleep, not with learning. Having the patient in a position and location associated with activity or learning helps facilitate learning. A patient who is watching a video in bed may be more likely to become drowsy during instruction than one who is sitting in a bedside chair.
- The nurse should use teaching aids that foster learning and help focus a learner's attention. The nurse should use the same equipment and supplies that the patient will use when performing the skill alone. All of the necessary equipment and visual aids should be assembled before the teaching session occurs. Audio-visual equipment should be checked for proper operation prior to the beginning of the session.
- Teaching that uses more than one sense enhances learning. For example, when changing a surgical dressing, the nurse can state the instructions (hearing), demonstrate changing the dressing (vision), and show how to use the equipment (touch).
- Ideally, learning is enhanced when the person discovers the information independently. However, this is not always appropriate or realistic in a hospital environment. What the nurse can do to enhance learning and stimulate motivation and self-direction includes providing specific, realistic, achievable outcomes; giving feedback; and helping the patient derive satisfaction from learning. Self-directed independent learning can also be enhanced by encouraging the patient to explore sources of information. If certain activities do not assist the patient to achieve identified outcomes, these activities need to be reassessed and possibly replaced. An explanation about a piece of equipment cannot replace providing the actual equipment for the patient to handle and use during a teaching session.
- Repetition reinforces learning. Summarizing content, rephrasing (using other words), and approaching the material from another point of view are ways of repeating and clarifying content. Recalling the famous quote by Edgar Dale might help: "We remember 10% of what we read, 20% of what we hear, 30% of what we see, 50% of what we see and hear . . . and 95% of what we teach" (Anderson, 1969).
- It might be helpful to use associations or "organizers" to introduce content during the teaching session. Organizers connect unknown information to known information in order to create a logical relationship. An example of an organizer would be: "You understand how urine flows down a catheter from the bladder. Now I will show you how to inject fluid so that it flows up the catheter into the bladder." The teaching that follows occurs within a known framework to the patient so that it adds meaning.
- The anticipated behavioral change that indicates learning has occurred must be realistic and congruent with the patient's lifestyle and resources. For example, it would be unrealistic to instruct a patient to soak in a tub of hot water two times a day if the patient does not have a bathtub at home or uses the stove to heat water.

Special Teaching Strategies

One-to-one discussion is the most common method of teaching used by nurses. However, there are a number of special teaching strategies that nurses can use to facilitate learning. These strategies include anticipatory guidance, patient contracting, group teaching, technology-assisted instruction, discovery/problem solving, behavior modification, the teach-back method, and transcultural teaching. The strategy selected must be appropriate for the patient and the learning objectives.

Anticipatory Guidance

Anticipatory guidance has been primarily associated with health promotion activities in pediatrics. In this context, nurses use anticipatory guidance to provide parents with information about developmental changes they can expect their child or children to exhibit as they grow and develop. However, anticipatory guidance can be used any time during the lifespan with the same focus: health promotion. For example, the nurse may provide anticipatory guidance to a family whose mother has Alzheimer disease to help them recognize safety concerns as the disease progresses. Anticipatory guidance may be provided to both individuals and groups. Nurses should consider several factors before providing anticipatory guidance, including the patient's age, developmental stage, health status, and health literacy level. See **Box 41.8** » for suggested anticipatory guidance topics.

Anticipatory guidance provided by healthcare professionals can help patients prevent health alterations or complications. Nurses can expect to use anticipatory guidance in the form of patient teaching in various settings, including:

- Prenatal visits
- Well-child/patient check-ups
- Annual medical/dental visits
- Community programs such as health screenings, health fairs, and safety programs.

Because the time for each visit is limited, nurses should build on a patient's current knowledge and care practices and start with a topic in which the patient expresses interest.

Box 41.8

Topics for Anticipatory Guidance

Children and Parents

- Growth and development
- Nutrition
- Risks of secondhand smoke
- Sleep safety and patterns

Adults

- UVA/UVB protection
- Responsible sexual behaviors
- Alcohol and drug use

Older Adults

- Fall prevention
- Medication use and side effects
- Advance directives

Additional topics about anticipatory guidance can be found in Exemplar 51.A, Health Promotion and Injury Prevention Across the Lifespan, in Module 51, Safety.

Source: Adapted from Berman et al. (2021).

Nursing using anticipatory guidance should reinforce what the patient and family are doing well and clear up any poorly understood concepts.

Nurses rely on resources in the community to enhance the guidance provided. For example, Bright Futures provides information for anticipatory guidance regarding children. State and local Safe Kids coalitions help inform families about injury prevention strategies. Schools provide health and safety programs throughout the year. Nurses need to be aware of the types of programs available in the community to reinforce concepts.

>> **Stay Current:** Visit Bright Futures at www.brightfutures.org and Safe Kids at www.safekids.org to enhance your teaching strategies for children.

Patient Contracting

Learning contracts are mutually developed verbal or written agreements between the teacher and the learner. Learning contracts encourage patient independence and control over personal health management and wellness. Essential elements include what the learner will learn, the way in which learning will be accomplished, resources for further learning, and rewards for consistent contract adherence and goal achievement (Berman et al., 2021). Use of a learning contract allows for freedom, mutual respect, and mutual responsibility.

Group Teaching

Teaching a group of patients is cost-effective and provides those in attendance an opportunity to share experiences and learn from others. A small group allows for discussion in which everyone can participate. A large group is less informal and requires the use of audio-visual aids such as films/videos, slides, or role-playing with the nurse.

All members involved in a particular group should have a common need (e.g., prenatal health or preoperative instruction). Sociocultural factors also should be considered when a group is being formed.

Technology-Assisted Instruction

Technology-assisted instruction (TAI) is the delivery of instruction or information through the use of technology. A variety of TAI options are available, ranging from live courses in which an instructor and learners can interact in the moment to asynchronous classes or instructional videos that learners can take at their convenience. TAI can offer a number of options. For example, learners may:

- Take a quiz after reading about a particular health problem.
- Learn psychomotor skills (e.g., identifying on the computer screen where to check the radial pulse).
- Practice complex problem-solving skills (e.g., calculating the amount of medication based on a capillary blood glucose level).

TAI can also be used in other ways. For example:

- Patients may use an application on an electronic device to learn about treatment for a health problem.
- Families or small groups of three to five patients may gather around one electronic device and take turns or work in teams while running a health-related program and answering questions together.
- Larger groups may view a display of a computer's monitor that is projected onto an overhead screen, while the teacher or learner manipulates the device to change the display on the screen.
- Individuals or small groups may use computers or other electronic devices through shared network platforms or through websites to attend a group training session.

Individuals using an electronic device are able to set the pace that meets their particular learning needs and, in some cases, even choose their preferred language. In group settings, the pace may be too slow for some learners and too fast for others. It is therefore helpful to group learners of similar needs and abilities together.

Many TAI programs offer the opportunity for immediate feedback. The correct answer is usually indicated by the use of colors, flashing signs, or written praise. When the learner selects an incorrect answer, the program may respond with an explanation of why that was not the best answer and encouragement to try again. Some programs feature simulated situations that allow learners to manipulate objects on the screen to learn psychomotor skills. When used to teach such skills, TAI must be followed up with practice on actual equipment supervised by the teacher.

Not every patient is comfortable with using electronic devices. Some may not have a computer or a smartphone due to financial considerations or lack of familiarity with current technology. Nurses should assess each patient's access and level of comfort with electronic devices before planning or recommending TAI to a patient.

Discovery/Problem Solving

Another teaching technique is the discovery/problem-solving method. When using this technique, the nurse presents some initial information. Then the nurse asks a question or presents a problem and asks the patient to apply the information learned. Sometimes referred to as **anticipatory problem solving**, this technique is particularly well suited to working with families and when helping patients learn important aspects of disease management. For example, the nurse might first provide information on asthma and how to prevent an asthma attack, and then ask family members what they can do to help their loved one stay healthy. This offers patients the opportunity to consider what they've learned and determine changes they can make themselves.

Behavior Modification

Based in behavioral theory, behavioral modification assumes that individual behaviors are learned and can be modified with instruction or training, especially when reinforcement is provided. When using this technique, desirable behavior is rewarded and undesirable behavior is ignored. For example, a patient participating in smoking cessation will receive praise for going without smoking, but any lapses will be ignored. For some patients and learning situations, a learning contract is combined with behavior modification. Essential elements of a learning contract using behavior modification include:

- The stated expectation that the patient will change behavior or master the task (i.e., quit smoking, take blood glucose level daily)
- Use of positive reinforcement when the patient exhibits desired behaviors with an agreement to ignore, rather than criticize, undesirable behavior.

Teach-Back Method

With the **teach-back method**, the nurse provides teaching on a particular topic, then asks the patient to describe the main points from that teaching using the patient's own words. This method is similar to return demonstration, except it requires the patient to show understanding through verbal communication instead of through actual physical performance of a task (Agency for Healthcare Research and Quality, 2018).

In order to successfully employ the teach-back method, the nurse should keep several points in mind. First and foremost, the nurse must provide all information in plain language that the patient can understand. The nurse should also pause periodically throughout the teaching session to check that the patient understands and remembers the material delivered so far. If the nurse asks for certain information but the patient cannot provide it or restates the information incorrectly, the nurse must clarify the areas of confusion before moving on to the next topic in the teaching session. Once the nurse has addressed all of the teaching topics, the nurse should once again ask the patient to explain major points not only from the most recent part of the session but also from earlier portions. To help increase and reinforce patient understanding throughout the session, the nurse may supplement the teach-back method with use of handouts and/or return demonstration (Yen & Leasure, 2019).

Although the teach-back method seems simple on its surface, it requires a great deal of preparation on the part of the nurse. Not only must the nurse plan the teaching session and select language and educational materials appropriate for each patient, but must also anticipate which topics are most likely to elicit confusion and necessitate further follow-up. The nurse must also practice use of this method so that it does not seem awkward or off-putting to patients or unnecessarily extend the length of the teaching session. Finally, the nurse should remember that the teach-back method is not a test of the patient's knowledge or learning capacity, but rather of how well the nurse explained the information (Yen & Leasure, 2019).

Transcultural Teaching

Transcultural teaching is an approach that takes into consideration barriers (such as language) that arise when the teacher and the learner come from different cultural backgrounds. Additional barriers include different concepts of time or space, patient preferences for traditional healing practices or culturally based beliefs that interfere with health teaching, and health conditions that can be changed with health promotion teaching. Prior to beginning any teaching, nurses should assess patients' cultural beliefs and practices to identify if there are any potential conflicts or other considerations that the nurse should incorporate into the teaching plan (see Module 24, Culture and Diversity, for information on assessment). To evaluate patient learning, use of the teach-back method has been found successful with patients from a variety of cultures (Purnell & Fenkl, 2019). Guidelines that nurses should consider when teaching patients from different cultural backgrounds include:

- Use teaching materials, pamphlets, and instructions in the patient's native language. Nurses who are unable to read the foreign language material should obtain the service of an interpreter to translate the learning material. Then the nurse can evaluate if the learning material is appropriate to meet the patient's learning needs.
- Use visual aids, such as pictures and diagrams, to communicate meaning. Purnell and Fenkl (2019) recommend these teaching aids be in the patient's native language. If this is not possible, the nurse should make arrangements for a professional interpreter to communicate the content to the patient.
- Use short sentences and simple language, focusing on one idea at a time. Avoid using medical jargon and abstract words that patients may not recognize or that may be easily misunderstood. Avoid using colloquialisms or slang, which can be misinterpreted easily.
- Allow time between teaching points for patients to retain information and ask questions.
- If the patient speaks in a low voice or has difficulty pronouncing words, the nurse should validate understanding to the greatest degree possible. This can be done by writing down what the patient said and asking the patient to read it back and verify accuracy or by confirming understanding with a caregiver.
- Be aware that nodding, maintaining eye contact, or smiling does not necessarily indicate understanding. These nonverbal actions may indicate a sign of respect. Patients from some cultures may feel that asking questions is a sign of disrespect or may embarrass the nurse or cause the nurse to "lose face."
- The nurse should invite and encourage the patient to ask questions during teaching. Explain to the patient that asking questions ensures that the information is understood. Negative questions should be avoided as these can be interpreted differently by the patient with English as a second language.

An example of a negative question might be, "You don't know when to take your medication?" Instead, this question should be presented as, "Tell me when you take your medication."

- Always offer to repeat the teaching. Some patients may believe that it is rude to ask to be shown something again or to express confusion.
- Should teaching about a procedure or function that relates to a personal body area be planned, it would be appropriate to have a nurse of the same sex provide the instructions. For teaching about personal care, birth control, sexually transmitted infections, and other potential private areas, a nurse of the same gender should provide the instruction. If possible, arrange for an interpreter of the same gender, if one is needed.
- Assess the need to involve family members in the teaching. Cultural preferences on this vary: in some cultures, this is not considered necessary. In others, the head of the family may be critical to patient teaching.
- Consider the patient's orientation to time. In present-oriented cultures, schedules are flexible and sleeping and eating patterns vary greatly. Instructing a patient to take a medication with a meal or at bedtime does not mean that these activities will occur at the same time every day. Because of this, assess the patient's daily routine before pairing an activity with a medication. The nurse should also ask if the patient has a clock or wristwatch and determine if the patient can tell time before instructing on a time to take a medication.
- When conflicts or incongruencies between the patient's cultural beliefs and practices and the information to be provided arise, the nurse should begin by focusing on health beliefs that are in agreement with the teaching, as this will integrate the instructions with a familiar health practice. Because the goal is to have a mutually agreeable plan, the nurse should decide which instructions support safety and then negotiate the less crucial traditional practices.

Evaluating Teaching and Learning

Nurses evaluate patient learning on an ongoing basis as instruction is provided as well as at the end to determine what has been learned.

Evaluating Learning

Evaluating learning is the same as evaluating outcomes for patient problems. The nurse determines the extent to which the patient achieves the outcomes identified during the planning phase of the teaching process. The outcomes serve two purposes: they direct the teaching plan and provide the criteria for evaluation. For example, the outcome "Selects foods that are low in carbohydrates" can be evaluated by asking the patient to name such foods or to select low-carbohydrate foods from a list.

Methods to evaluate learning depend on the content and type of instruction provided. The teach-back method has already been discussed. Other examples include:

- Return demonstration or direct observation of behavior (e.g., observing the patient demonstrate use of a capillary blood glucose monitor); this is the best method of evaluating teaching of psychomotor skills
- Use of post-tests or other written materials
- Oral questioning (e.g., asking the patient to restate information)
- Patient self-reporting
- The use of electronic monitoring devices. For example, some blood glucose monitors can provide printed readouts or even upload data directly to the HCP's database.

Confirming that cognitive learning has occurred does not ensure affective learning has taken place. For example, have parents learned to value health sufficiently to have their children wear protective gear when riding a bicycle? Do patients who state that they value health actually schedule routine examinations with a HCP or email their weekly blood pressure readings to their provider?

Depending on the outcome of the evaluation, the nurse might have to modify or repeat sections of the teaching plan if the outcomes have not been met or only partially met. This follow-up teaching may be accomplished during a home visit or over the telephone once the patient is discharged from a healthcare facility.

It is important to remember that behavior changes take time and practice. Some patients may have difficulty accepting the need to change behaviors, much less actually making a change. Some patients may desire to make a change but vacillate between the old and new behaviors. Nurses can assist patients by engaging in motivational interviewing to help determine the patient's stage of change and motivating factors (see Module 35, Caring Interventions). Nurses can help promote behavior change by providing understanding when patients vacillate and continuing to encourage patients to persist in making the necessary changes to improve their health and well-being.

Evaluating the Learning Experience

The process of teaching and the content of the teaching program should be evaluated by the nurse. This step of the process is similar to evaluating the effectiveness of nursing interventions to address patient problems. All factors, such as timing, teaching strategies, content, and patient achievement of outcomes, should be included in this evaluation. The patient's response (i.e., anxiety, boredom, interest) should be included in the evaluation. The patient should also evaluate the learning experience by providing feedback on what information, materials, approaches, and other elements were helpful, interesting, or confusing. To gather such information, the nurse might provide patients with a feedback questionnaire or perhaps even video learning sessions to see which aspects of the session seem to be most and least effective.

The nurse should expect the patient to forget some of the information provided. This is a normal occurrence that can be overcome by having the patient write down information, providing handouts, repeating important steps during the teaching, and engaging the patient in the learning process.

Documenting

As with any other intervention, the nurse documents the teaching provided because it serves as a legal record and communicates to other healthcare professionals that teaching occurred. Omitting documentation about teaching could be interpreted by others as the teaching did not occur.

Documentation should include the responses of the patient and support people to the instructions. What action did the patient or support person take that indicates learning occurred? Did the patient or support person say anything about the teaching activities? Was the patient able to perform the instructed skill or articulate specific knowledge? These observations need to be documented in the medical record as evidence that learning occurred. The following is a sample of documentation charting:

SAMPLE DOCUMENTATION

11/8/2021 1030 Learning to change a colostomy appliance after having a hemicolectomy 4 days ago. Patient hesitant to look at the stoma but handled the back plate and attached the collection bag with ease. Stated "I guess I will have to get used to seeing a part of my intestines every day." Will reinforce teaching and encourage more participation in the coming days. *C. Brown RN*

Some healthcare organizations and agencies use multiple-copy patient teaching forms that incorporate the medical and nursing problem list, the treatment plan, and the patient education. The patient and nurse sign the form after the teaching session is completed. One copy of the form is given to the patient as a record that the teaching was provided and can be used to reinforce any instructions. A second copy of the completed and signed form is placed in the patient's medical record. Areas to include when documenting teaching in the patient's medical record include:

- Identified learning needs
- Learning outcomes
- Content of instruction
- Patient outcomes
- Plan for additional teaching
- Patient response to/understanding of the teaching
- Resources used and provided.

The written teaching plan may be used as a resource to guide future teaching sessions and might also include:

- An outline or a list of actual information and skills taught
- List of teaching strategies used
- Time framework and content for each class
- Identified teaching outcomes and methods of evaluation.

Nursing Care Plan

A Patient Who Requires Teaching About Wound Care

Kevin McArthur is a 22-year-old male college student who received a laceration on his leg while playing in an intramural hockey game. During the game, Kevin became entangled with another player. He fell as a result of the encounter and landed on the other player's skate blade.

Kevin indicates that the injury occurred two hours ago and that it is barely bleeding. He tells you that he does not think the wound is a "big deal," but came to the health center after the game at his girlfriend's insistence.

ASSESSMENT	DIAGNOSES	PLANNING
Kevin is alert and oriented. He tells you he lives in a dormitory on campus and confirms that he is able to understand, read, and write English. He seems distracted, bored, and uninterested in performing wound self-care. You check his vitals and make the following assessments: T 38.7°C (101.6°F); P 66 beats/min; R 17/min; BP 115/74 mmHg. Kevin's weight is 85 kg (187.4 lb) and within normal limits for his height. Physical examination reveals a 7-cm (2.5-in.) laceration on the left lower anterior leg. There is redness and minor swelling around the laceration. You also note the presence of slight serosanguineous drainage.	▪ Lacerations ▪ Potential to develop a wound infection ▪ Teaching to care for the sutured wound	▪ The patient will describe normal wound healing. ▪ The patient will identify three main signs and symptoms of infection. ▪ The patient will identify supplies needed for wound care. ▪ The patient will correctly perform a return demonstration of wound cleansing and bandaging. ▪ The patient will describe appropriate action if questions or complications arise. ▪ The patient will identify date, time, and location of follow-up appointment for suture removal.

IMPLEMENTATION

- Assist the HCP with cleansing, suturing, and dressing the wound as ordered.
- Describe normal wound healing and provide written and visual instructions of the signs and symptoms of local infection and complications, including increased redness, swelling, purulent drainage, and pain at wound site. Discuss the symptoms of systemic infection, including fever and malaise.
- Identify and provide wound care supplies such as bandaging material (e.g., gauze wrap, nonadhesive pads, adhesive tape) and cleansing solution as prescribed by provider (e.g., mild soap and water, antimicrobial solution, triple-antibiotic ointment).
- Demonstrate wound cleansing and bandaging on the patient's wound. Remove wound dressings and have the patient perform return demonstration. Provide a written handout describing the procedure.
- Instruct on appropriate actions and follow-up if questions or complications occur. Provide written instructions listing available resources, clinic contact information, and treatment plan. Include the date, time, and location of next follow-up appointment in 10 days in written instructions.

(continued on next page)

Nursing Care Plan *(continued)*

EVALUATION

At the 10-day follow-up appointment, Kevin reports that he has forgotten to clean the wound and change the dressing "a few times." The dressing on his leg is clearly several days old and was haphazardly applied. His wound shows signs of local infection, including thick yellow discharge, redness, and swelling. Kevin's temperature is also elevated. The HCP diagnoses him with an abscess. His stitches are removed, and the wound is drained. Kevin is prescribed a 2-week course of antibiotics. He is also advised to soak the infected area with warm towels three times per day to aid the healing process.

CRITICAL THINKING

1. Discuss Kevin's readiness to learn at his initial appointment and describe indicators of his level of readiness. How might the nurse enhance his readiness to learn?
2. What are the priority learning outcomes for Kevin at his follow-up appointment? Which teaching methods might improve his compliance with the treatment regimen?
3. How would you handle the situation if Kevin continues to show a lack of interest in self–wound care in spite of the changes to your teaching methods?

REVIEW Patient/Consumer Education

RELATE Link the Concepts and Exemplars

Linking the exemplar of patient/consumer education with the concept of development:

1. How does the concept of development impact teaching and learning?
2. How should the nurse incorporate characteristics of each developmental stage when choosing teaching strategies?

Linking the exemplar of patient/consumer education with the concept of culture and diversity:

3. What aspects of culture should be considered before developing a teaching plan for a patient?
4. How should the nurse address teaching and learning when a patient's health beliefs and values differ from the nurse's own?

Linking the exemplar of patient/consumer education with the concept of cognition:

5. How should the nurse address teaching and learning for a patient with altered cognition?
6. How does the concept of cognition impact the nurse's teaching plan and the patient's learning?

REFER Go to Pearson MyLab Nursing and eText

REFLECT Apply Your Knowledge

Ms. Siminov is a 42-year-old computer programmer who is learning a new position after being unemployed for a year. She has been sitting for nearly 8 hours at work every day for the last 6 weeks and woke up one Saturday morning with both legs swollen from the knees to the ankles. She became concerned and went to the emergency department to be evaluated. After being admitted for a day for evaluation and diagnostic testing, she is diagnosed with statis lymphedema and preliminary signs of peripheral vascular disease.

As her nurse, you have been asked to teach Ms. Siminov about the disease process, diet, activity, skin care, and the use of compression stockings. As you begin teaching Ms. Siminov, you note that she is distracted and seems anxious to return home to go to work the next day.

1. How would you evaluate Ms. Siminov's readiness to learn?
2. Of what benefit would using technology-assisted instruction be when instructing this patient?
3. You recognize that you have a great deal of information to deliver to Ms. Siminov, and you are concerned that you will not be able to teach it all. What can you do to help her and still accomplish the learning outcomes?
4. How will you know if your teaching is effective?
5. How might your teaching differ if you were teaching Ms. Siminov at home rather than in a hospital or acute care setting?

References

Agency for Healthcare Research and Quality (AHRQ). (2018). *Health literacy toolkit*. https://psnet.ahrq.gov/issue/health-literacy-toolkit

American Nurses Association (ANA). (2015). Standard 12: Education. In *Nursing: Scope and standards of practice*. Author.

Anderson, H. M. (1969). *Dale's cone of experience*. https://www.queensu.ca/teachingandlearning/modules/active/documents/Dales_Cone_of_Experience_summary.pdf

Ball, J. W., Bindler, R. C., Cowen, K., & Shaw, M. (2022). *Principles of pediatric nursing: Caring for children* (8th ed.). Pearson.

Bastable, S. B. (2020). *Nurse as educator: Principles of teaching and learning for nursing practice* (5th ed.). Jones & Bartlett Learning.

Baumeister, A., Aldin, A., Chakraverty, D., Monsef, I., Jakob, T., Seven, U., et al. (2019). Interventions for improving health literacy in migrants. *Cochrane Database of Systematic Reviews*, Issue 4, Article No. CD013303. https://doi.org/10.1002/14651858.CD013303

Berman, A., Snyder, S. J., & Grandsen, G. (2021). *Kozier & Erb's fundamentals of nursing: concepts, process, and practice* (11th ed). Pearson.

Blais, K. K.., & Hayes, J. S. (2016). *Professional nursing practice: Concepts and perspectives* (7th ed.). Pearson.

Bloom, B. S. (Ed.). (1956). *Taxonomy of education objectives. Book 1: Cognitive domain*. Longman.

Bombard, Y., Baker, G. R., Orlando, E., Fancott, C., Bhatia, P., Casalino, S., et al. (2018). Engaging patients to improve quality of care: A systematic review. *Implementation Science, 13*(1), 98. https://doi.org/10.1186/s13012-018-0784-z

Bruner, J. (1966). *Toward a theory of instruction*. Harvard University Press.

Candela, L. (2012). From teaching to learning: Theoretical foundations. In D. M. Billings & J. A. Halstead (Eds.), *Teaching in nursing: A guide for faculty* (4th ed., pp. 202–243). Elsevier Saunders.

Centers for Disease Control and Prevention (CDC). (2020a). *Health literacy*. https://www.cdc.gov/healthliteracy/

Centers for Disease Control and Prevention (CDC). (2020b). *Learn about health literacy*. https://www.cdc.gov/healthliteracy/learn/

Chen, C., Wang, L, Chi, H., Chen, W., & Park. M. (2020). Comparative efficacy of social media delivered health education on glycemic control: A meta-analysis. *International Journal of Nursing Sciences, 7*(3), 359–368. https://doi.org/10.1016/j.ijnss.2020.04.010

De las Cuevas, C., de Leon, J., Peñate, W., & Betancourt, M. (2017). Factors influencing adherence to psychopharmacological medications in psychiatric patients: A structural equation modeling approach. *Patient Preference and Adherence, 11*, 681–690.

Döğer, E., Bozbulut, R., Soysal Acar, A. Ş., Ercan, Ş., Kılınç Uğurlu, A., Akbaş, E. D., et al. (2019). Effect of telehealth system on glycemic control in children and adolescents with type 1 diabetes. *Journal of Clinical Research in Pediatric Endocrinology, 11*(1), 70–75. https://doi.og/10.4274/jcrpe.galenos.2018.2018.0017

Erikson, K. (2018). *Mentorship in nursing: the case for inspiring and guiding the next generation of nurses*. https://www.rasmussen.edu/degrees/nursing/blog/mentorship-in-nursing/

Feinberg, I., O'Connor, M. H., Owen-Smith, A., Ogrodnick, M. M., & Rothenberg, R. (2020). The relationship between refugee health status and language, literacy, and time spent in the United States. *Health Literacy and Practice Research, 4*(4), e230–e236. https://doi.org/10.3928/24748307-20201109-01

Gardner, H. (1983). *Frames of mind: Theory of multiple intelligences*. Basic Books.

Glenn, J., Wolfe, K., & Borgmann, K. (2020). The evaluation of video teaching on preoperative anxiety in the outpatient pediatric surgical patients. *Journal of Perianesthesia Nursing, 35*(4). https://doi.org/10.1016/j.jopan.2020.06.008

Goleman, B. (2019). *Emotional intelligence for a better life*. Author.

Goleman, D. (1995). *Emotional intelligence*. Bantam Books.

Goodyear, C., & Goodyear, M. (2018a). Career development for nurse managers. *Nursing Management, 49*(3), 49–53. https://doi.org/10.1097/01.NUMA.0000530429.91645.e2

Goodyear, C., & Goodyear, M. (2018b). Supporting successful mentoring. *Nursing Management, 49*(4), 49–53. https://doi.org/10.1097/01.NUMA.0000531173.00718.06

Health on the Net Foundation. (n.d.). *A non for profit organization, promotes transparent and reliable health information online*. https://www.hon.ch/en/

Katzby, S. (2021). *Why the internet has become the most popular source for medical information*. https://www.pagerelease.com/why-the-internet-has-become-the-most-popular-source-for-medical-information/

Kim, J., Combs, K., Downs, J., & Tillman, F. (2018) Medication adherence: The elephant in the room. *U.S. Pharmacist, 43*(1), 30–34. https://www.uspharmacist.com/article/medication-adherence-the-elephant-in-the-room

Klaber, B. (2018). *Why collaboration is the key to the future of improvement*. Institute for Healthcare Improvement. http://www.ihi.org/communities/blogs/why-collaboration-is-the-key-to-the-future-of-improvement

Knowles, M. (2018). *Nearly one-fourth of US population has low health literacy: 5 findings*. Becker's Hospital Review. https://www.beckershospitalreview.com/patient-experience/nearly-one-fourth-of-us-population-has-low-health-literacy-5-findings.html

Knowles, M. S., Holton, E. F., & Swanson, R. A. (2005). *The adult learner* (6th ed.). Elsevier Butterworth-Heinemann. (Original work published 1973)

Lofland, J., Johnson, P. T., Ingham, M. P., Rosemas, S. C., White, J. C., & Ellis, L. (2017). Shared decision-making for biologic treatment of autoimmune disease: Influence on adherence, persistence, satisfaction, and health care costs. *Patient Preference and Adherence, 11*, 947–958.

Marenus, M. (2020). *Gardner's theory of multiple intelligences*. Simply Psychology. https://www.simplypsychology.org/multiple-intelligences.html

National Institute on Aging. (2018). *Online health information: Is it reliable?* https://www.nia.nih.gov/health/online-health-information-it-reliable

Phaneuf, A. (2020). *What is an EHR system? Definitions, benefits, problems and trends for electronic health records*. Business Insider. https://www.businessinsider.com/electronic-health-records-benefits-challenges

Purnell, L. D., & Fenkl, E. A. (2019). *Handbook for culturally competent care*. Springer.

Readability Formulas. (n.d.). *Automatic readability checker*. https://readabilityformulas.com/free-readability-formula-tests.php

Ross, S. M. (2018). *Medication adherence vs compliance: 4 ways they differ*. Comprehensive Medication Management. https://blog.cureatr.com/medication-adherence-vs-compliance-4-ways-they-differ

Talevski, J., Shee, A. W., Rasmussen, B., Kemp, G., & Beauchamp, A. (2020). Teach-back: A systematic review of implementation and impacts. *PLoS One, 15*(4). https://doi.org/10.1371/journal.pone.0231350

U.S. Department of Health and Human Services. (DHHS). (n.d.). *Quick guide to health literacy*. https://health.gov/our-work/health-literacy/health-literacy-online

U.S. Department of Health and Human Services (DHHS), Office of Disease Prevention and Health Promotion. (2010). *National action plan to improve health literacy*. Author. https://health.gov/sites/default/files/2019-09/Health_Literacy_Action_Plan.pdf

Welch, T. D., Strickland, H. P., & Sartain, A. (2019). Transition to nursing practice: A capstone simulation for the application of leadership skills in nursing practice. *Teaching and Learning in Nursing, 14*(4), 283–287. https://doi.org/10.1016/j.teln.2019.06.002

World Health Organization (WHO). (2019a). *What are the roles of intercultural mediators in health care and what is the evidence on their contributions and effectiveness in improving accessibility and quality of care for refugees and migrants in the WHO European Region?* https://www.ncbi.nlm.nih.gov/books/NBK550145/pdf/Bookshelf_NBK550145.pdf

World Health Organization (WHO). (2019b). *WHO European roadmap for implementation of health literacy initiatives through the life course*. https://www.euro.who.int/__data/assets/pdf_file/0003/409125/69wd14e_Rev1_RoadmapOn-HealthLiteracy_190323.pdf?ua=1

Yen, P. H., & Leasure, A. R. (2019). Use and effectiveness of the teach-back method in patient education and health outcomes. *Federal Practitioner, 36*(6), 36(6), 284–289.

Part V
Healthcare Domain

Part V consists of modules that outline and define principles related to the healthcare domain, including accountability, ethics, and quality improvement. Each module presents a concept that relates directly to professional nursing, its relationship to healthcare systems and policies, and how nursing within the healthcare system impacts patient health and well-being. Selected principles or topics of each concept are presented as exemplars. The exemplars in the module on safety, for example, cover health promotion and injury prevention across the lifespan, patient safety, nurse safety, and medication safety. Each module addresses the effect of that concept and the selected exemplars on the care of individuals across the lifespan, inclusive of their culture, their gender, and their developmental status.

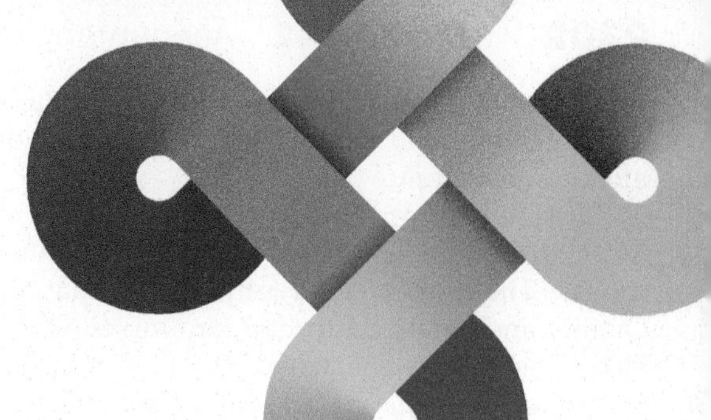

Module 42
Accountability

Module Outline and Learning Outcomes

The Concept of Accountability

Components of Accountability

42.1 Analyze how the nursing profession promotes accountability.

Concepts Related to Accountability

42.2 Outline the relationship between accountability and other concepts.

Socialization to Nursing

42.3 Analyze the process of socialization to nursing.

Factors Influencing Nursing Practice and Accountability

42.4 Differentiate factors that influence nursing practice and accountability.

Accountability Exemplars

Exemplar 42.A Competence

42.A Analyze competence as it relates to accountability.

The Concept of Accountability

Concept Key Terms

Accountability, **2701**
Autonomy, **2703**
Consumer, **2707**
Governance, **2703**
mHealth, **2708**
Patient Self-Determination Act (PSDA), **2708**
Responsibility, **2701**
Socialization, **2706**
Standards of care, **2701**
Standards of practice, **2701**
Telecommunication, **2708**
Telehealth, **2708**
Telenursing, **2708**

Accountability is one of the tenets of any professional practice. It implies a personal responsibility for one's actions and a commitment to improve practice. Accountability in nursing can be viewed as having professional, legal, and ethical components. To better understand accountability, nursing looks to professional organizations for clarity of what are acceptable standards of care. **Standards of care**, also known as **standards of practice**, are professional standards or guidelines used to describe a level of competency for practice; in other words, what a nurse should or should not do in practice. The standards are established by organizations such as The Joint Commission, the American Nurses Association (ANA), the National League for Nursing (NLN), and even the National Student Nurses' Association (NSNA). Each organization provides guidelines for acceptable practice. In general, The Joint Commission focuses on healthcare organizations, the ANA on nursing practice, the NLN on the education of nurses leading to practice, and the NSNA on the development of students as professionals. These organizations describe the responsibilities for which nurses are accountable, thereby setting desirable and achievable benchmarks against which the performance and care standards of individual nurses are measured.

Accountability and *responsibility* are words that are often used interchangeably. **Accountability** involves being answerable for the outcomes of an assignment or task, whether performed directly by the nurse or assigned to a subordinate. Nurses are responsible for the actions of subordinates or trainees. Nurses who assign tasks to others must be knowledgeable of the expertise of subordinates and must also clearly articulate the expectations of the assigned task. Subordinates are individuals who do not practice at the level of a Registered Nurse (RN). These individuals may include Licensed Professional Nurses (LPNs), nursing assistants or nurse aides, or medical assistants. **Responsibility** is the specific obligation associated with the performance of duties of a particular role. Nurses are responsible for performing their assigned tasks reliably, dependably, and to the best of their abilities. Nurses' sense of accountability guides their performance and ultimately leads to improved practice and better patient care.

The term *accountability* may also carry a negative connotation. When an error is made, the question "Who is accountable?" often translates into "Who is to blame?" The implication is that someone has failed. The negative image of accountability is what the public tends to see, especially since the release of *To Err Is Human* (1999), a landmark report by the Institute of Medicine (IOM). In the years since that report, organizations such as those mentioned earlier (The Joint Commission, NLN, ANA) have revised earlier practice statements and created newer standards for nurses to follow independently and jointly to ensure delivery of the safest, most competent care possible.

Attitudes toward incident reporting have shifted from individual blame to "what we can do to create a culture of safety." The Robert Wood Johnson Foundation sponsored Quality and Safety Education for Nurses (QSEN; 2014; see also Cronenwett, Sherwood, & Gelmon, 2009), an initiative to improve quality and safety in prelicensure nursing programs. QSEN addressed six competencies critical to the nursing role: patient-centered care, teamwork and collaboration, evidence-based practice, quality improvement, safety, and informatics. The initiative endorsed the idea that quality and safety education are core competencies that must be embedded in all programs that prepare nurses for basic practice. The practice of a *culture of safety* is promoted by a wide range of national and professional organizations, including the Agency for Healthcare Research and Quality (AHRQ; 2019). See Module 51, Safety, for more information on safety culture.

>> **Stay Current:** To learn more about the QSEN competencies, visit the QSEN Institute website at http://qsen.org.

National Guidance on Accountability

As outlined in the overview, guidance on accountability comes from national organizations in the form of benchmarks of patient care, standards of nursing practice, and codes of ethics.

The Joint Commission

The Joint Commission standards focus on healthcare organizations, whether they are inpatient, outpatient, or residential in focus. The Joint Commission's standards are considered the essential guidelines for acceptable performance in providing safe patient care.

For example, a standard of practice/care for medication administration set forth by The Joint Commission requires two patient identifiers prior to giving the prescribed dose. A nurse who chooses not to meet this requirement is failing to practice at the minimum standard acceptable to the profession and will be held accountable to the patient and the facility for which he or she works.

As another example, suppose a nurse has a patient who will need continued wound care for his left foot after discharge to home. The patient has said that he thinks he understands the procedure for changing his dressing and has promised to call if he needs any further teaching. The nurse knows that the standards of care dictate asking the patient to demonstrate how to change the dressing so that the nurse can evaluate the patient's understanding and ability to care for himself. The nurse must decide whether to allow the patient to go home without seeing him perform the dressing change or whether discharge needs to be delayed until the patient can demonstrate his understanding. In this scenario, the nurse is responsible for upholding the standards of care and is accountable for making the decision regarding discharge of this patient. More importantly, if the patient does not perform the dressing care properly at home and is readmitted for complications, the nurse will be responsible for that particular outcome and may be held accountable. As an alternative to the patient's demonstrating the dressing change, the nurse could opt for one of the following courses of action:

- Request an order for home healthcare to continue the teaching and follow up until the patient is comfortable on his own.
- Teach a family member to perform the dressing change in case the patient is not feeling well enough to do it on his own.
- Arrange for the patient to travel to an outpatient nursing facility for daily dressing changes.

Regardless of the chosen method, the nurse is accountable at discharge for ensuring that the patient can get his wound dressed as often as the order advises. The patient must rely on the nurse's judgment for the most favorable outcome.

ANA Standards of Nursing Practice

A professional organization's major functions include establishing and implementing standards of practice. The ANA's **standards of practice** are intended to describe the responsibilities for which nurses in the U.S. are accountable. The ANA uses the nursing process as a foundation to develop generic standards of nursing practice that apply regardless of area of specialization. Similarly, the ANA uses its Standards of Professional Performance to describe the expected behavior of professional nurses. Professional performance standards refer to enhancing general practice, ensuring appropriate education level, and maintaining successful working relationships with peers and collaborating with the healthcare team. An example related to general practice is that nurses must be careful not place any patient identifiers online or in any discussion format where the identity of the patient might be known. Patient identifiers do not have to be as specific as the patient's name, age, or diagnosis. They could be as vague as "the football player injured in yesterday's game is on our unit." Nurses must be acutely aware that any information, regardless of how subtle, might lead to the identity of the patient and violate the patient's right to privacy (ANA, 2015b).

Nurse Practice Acts

Nurse practice acts are legal acts that regulate the practice of nursing in the United States and Canada. Each state in the United States and each province in Canada has its own nurse practice act. While content may differ from jurisdiction to jurisdiction, the common purpose of all nurse practice acts is to protect the public. Nurses are responsible for knowing how their state's nurse practice act governs their practice. One example is that each state addresses how often nurses must renew their licenses, the minimum number of continuing credit education hours needed for renewal, and, more specifically, the minimum number of continuing education hours related to the state's legal requirements for safe practice. State nurse practice acts are an additional guide and address standards that promote patient safety such as performing duties and reporting errors or deviations from valid orders in a timely manner. Module 49, Legal Issues, discusses nurse practice acts in detail.

Codes of Ethics

Another important part of the nursing tradition is respect for the inherent worth and dignity of all people. To preserve this value, professionals in the nursing field must do what is considered right, even if doing so means they incur a personal cost. In other words, nurses must strive to maintain their integrity. As the needs and values of society change, so do its ethical codes. To promote accountability in the use of ethical behaviors, the nursing profession has developed its own codes of ethics specific to the aims of nursing and the problems that nurses typically face. These codes are discussed in detail in Module 44, Ethics.

» **Stay Current:** To learn more about your state's board of nursing and standards of practice, visit the National Council of State Boards of Nursing website at https://www.ncsbn.org/nurse-practice-act.htm.

Components of Accountability

Nursing as a profession embraces and promotes personal and professional accountability. Aspects of the profession that promote accountability include:

- Successful completion of a program providing the body of knowledge necessary for performance of the role
- A focus toward service, be it community or in an organizational capacity
- Allegiance to a code of ethics
- Autonomy of the role
- Membership in a professional organization.

These factors are described in greater detail in the sections that follow.

Education

Education is an important aspect of professional status. As such, nursing education requires study within a focused body of knowledge. Entry into registered nursing in the United States is open to any individual who successfully earns either a hospital diploma or an associate's, bachelor's, master's, or doctorate degree in nursing and subsequently passes the National Council Licensure Examination, or NCLEX. The vast majority of new RNs hold either an associate's or bachelor's degree in nursing (NLN, 2014). The ANA recommends a bachelor's degree to enter professional practice, and many magnet hospitals and academic health centers require that their RNs have at least a bachelor's degree. The landmark report *The Future of Nursing: Leading Change, Advancing Health* (IOM, 2010) provided recommendations for nurses leading to improved patient outcomes. Obtaining a bachelor's degree allows for nurses to practice to their fullest extent and has emerged as "top-of-license (TOL) practice." TOL practice identifies eight core nursing responsibilities, including outcomes-focused care and the facilitation of safe patient transitions; both require that nurses be accountable in practice (Buck et al., 2018; IOM, 2011; Loversidge et al., 2018). Many associate's-degree RNs later opt to pursue their bachelor's degree, typically through participation in an RN-to-BSN program that builds on existing knowledge and skills. Similarly, many bachelor's-degree RNs go on to earn a master's or doctorate degree in order to further advance in their careers (American Association of Colleges of Nursing, 2019a).

Body of Knowledge

As a profession, nursing has a well-defined body of knowledge and expertise that is always expanding. This knowledge base is the product of various conceptual nursing frameworks that inform practice, education, and ongoing research directed toward improving patient outcomes. The nursing profession continues to grow and develop its body of knowledge over time, utilizing an evidence-based practice approach that promotes accountability for safe nursing practice (see Module 45, Evidence-Based Practice, for more information).

Service Orientation

A service orientation means that nursing, unlike some occupations, is not primarily driven by considerations of profit. Rather, nursing emphasizes service to others as a matter of tradition and as a basis for accountability. Rules, policies, and codes of ethics guide and shape this tradition of service. Many, if not all, states have a Medical Reserve Corps consisting of all levels of medical professionals, including nurses, that volunteer to serve in times of a state or national crisis such as the coronavirus pandemic in 2020. During the pandemic, nurse members of the reserve corps were called upon to work with local public health departments to assist with collecting data, working phone banks, or dispensing information about treatment for concerned callers (Medical Reserve Corps, 2020). Nursing has been and continues to be an integral component of the healthcare delivery system.

Autonomy

Generally speaking, **autonomy** means independence or freedom; thus, a profession is autonomous if it is able to regulate itself and set standards of practice for its own members. One of the purposes of a professional association is to give its members autonomy. Professional status for nursing hinges to a large degree on the nursing profession's ability to function autonomously in how it formulates nursing policy and controls its own activity. Professional autonomy involves legal authority; a professional group is autonomous only if it possesses the legal authority to define its goals and responsibilities in how it delivers its services, describe its particular functions and roles, and determine its scope of practice. With respect to the autonomy of the nursing profession, state boards of nursing (detailed in Module 49, Legal Issues) hold this legal authority.

Autonomy for nurses on an individual level means professional responsibility, accountability for their actions, and the freedom to do their jobs as necessary while at work. As mentioned previously, TOL practice is an interprofessional approach for providing safe, evidence-based care in which nurses work to their fullest capacity. Nurses at all levels of practice take accountability for their actions when they advocate for their own autonomy and for that of their nurse colleagues.

Professional Organization

Professions are different from occupations in that they operate under the umbrella of a professional organization. This organizational structure provides **governance**, which establishes and maintains social, political, and economic arrangements that give professionals the means to control their professional affairs, including their practice, self-discipline, and working conditions. Module 47, Health Policy, fully describes the professional organizations that govern and differentiate the profession of nursing.

Concepts Related to Accountability

Because accountability is a key aspect of professional nursing, it affects all areas of nursing practice. On a basic level, nurses are answerable for ensuring that patients' essential health and wellness needs are addressed. This means the nurse is accountable for providing information about measures that protect and promote patients' physical health, such as preventive screenings, recommended immunizations, smoking cessation, adequate exercise, and a healthy diet. It also means that nurses must address the cognitive, psychologic, and spiritual dimensions of health, examples of which include teaching patients about stress management and making referrals to counselors, clergy, and similar resources as needed.

Beyond issues of health and wellness, nurses are also accountable for certain physical outcomes of patient care. These vary depending on setting, the patient's condition, state nurse practice acts, and healthcare providers' (HCPs') orders. Still, there are some things for which nurses are nearly always answerable. For example, in the hospital setting, nurses are typically accountable for ensuring that patients receive appropriate fluids and nutrition, have an environment that permits adequate rest and sleep, maintain appropriate oxygenation levels, and receive assistance with elimination, if necessary. Similarly, all nurses are accountable for promoting patient safety. This encompasses not just maintaining a safe physical environment within the healthcare setting, but also teaching patients about ways to reduce their risk of injury in various aspects of their daily lives. Helping patients maintain comfort (or at least achieve a manageable level of pain) is a related concern. Indeed, encouraging patients to give voice to any needs and providing appropriate comfort interventions are major accountability roles for nurses in their own right, and they also help promote a safer care environment.

Yet another key area of nursing accountability relates to trauma. Per both legal requirements and the ethical standards of the profession, nurses have a duty to report certain types of trauma to the proper authorities. This includes known and suspected abuse of children and older adults, as well as certain categories of violence-related injuries (e.g., gunshot wounds); exact requirements vary from state to state. Nurses must also continually remain aware of the potential for abuse of any vulnerable child or adult with whom they come into contact during their practice. Nurses are further accountable for preventing patients from engaging in self-directed violence, which means they must routinely assess patients for factors that may indicate an increased risk of self-harm, suicide, and suicidal ideation or intent.

Because teaching is a critical nursing function, it too is an important area of accountability—and one that extends to all patient care areas. As previously mentioned, nurses must provide patients with broad-based information about health, illness, and safety, but they are also accountable for educating patients about tests, procedures, diagnoses, treatments, and other self-care measures specific to their condition. In order to provide such teaching, nurses must first assess each patient's learning style and readiness to learn. Nurses are also accountable for their own ongoing education and professional development. This encompasses not just meeting state and institutional continuing education requirements, but also taking steps to apply what they have learned via evidence-based practice.

The coronavirus pandemic has made the public and particularly healthcare employees more vigilant than ever of the need for immunity and protection against infection. Nurses are usually on the front lines of patient care, be it in the community, the emergency department, or at the bedside. As such, nurses have a responsibility and obligation to protect their patients from disease transmission. On the frontlines, this may mean that nurses educate the public on the importance of immunizations or the spread of infection. At the bedside, this means that nurses have a knowledge of the spread of infection, healthcare-associated illnesses, and an awareness of self in the goal of protecting patients from exposure to whatever germs they might carry.

The Concepts Related to Accountability feature links some, but not all, of the concepts integral to accountability. They are presented in alphabetical order.

Case Study » Part 1

Jen Sturges is a new RN on the medical unit in a 245-bed hospital. During the evening shift, Jen starts her rounds with her five patients. One of her patients is a 45-year-old woman named Kathryn Miller, who has been admitted with a GI diagnosis and also has a history of back pain. During Jen's assessment of her pain level, Ms. Miller says she is "doing just fine," although she seems very anxious. As Jen reviews Ms. Miller's vital signs, which the CNA had recently taken, she notes a blood pressure much higher than usual. Jen comments that one of the symptoms of pain is elevated blood pressure. Ms. Miller describes trying to overrule her body by ignoring its signals and by having a dialogue between the "body me" and the "real me." Ms. Miller also states, "If I refuse to pay attention to my body, my pain will go away."

Jen realizes that Ms. Miller, although actually in pain, might not be allowing herself to pay attention. Jen asks her if she has discussed pain management with her primary HCP. Ms. Miller laughs and says, "My doctor tries to have me take narcotics, but I worry about those types of meds." As she speaks, Ms. Miller's hands are gripping the bed sheets and she is shaking. She says, "The pain is my enemy, and I don't talk to my enemies."

Jen knows that ignoring the body's signals of pain can cause serious consequences; for example, the patient's pain could intensify and the blood pressure could rise significantly. Jen also realizes that Ms. Miller needs to get appropriate treatment for her pain. After her assessment, Jen discusses her concerns about Ms. Miller with the unit charge nurse, including Ms. Miller's need for pain management and comfort.

Clinical Reasoning Questions Level I

1. Why is it important for Jen to complete her patient's assessment before leaving the room?
2. What further symptoms does Jen observe while she speaks with her patient?
3. What information should Jen share with the charge nurse to assist in meeting her patient's needs?

Clinical Reasoning Questions Level II

4. With what staff should Jen and the charge nurse plan to collaborate to find a better method for managing Ms. Miller's pain?
5. When a patient refuses pain management, why should the nurse pursue other solutions rather than simply acquiescing?

Concepts Related to Accountability

CONCEPT	RELATIONSHIP TO ACCOUNTABILITY	NURSING IMPLICATIONS
Comfort	The nurse is accountable for assessing the patient's level of comfort and providing effective interventions to promote or maintain patient comfort.	Assess patient's reported level of comfort at least once per shift, or more often as indicated by patient's condition. Report any deviations or changes in the level of comfort. Document patient's comfort level and any nursing interventions provided.
Evidence-Based Practice (EBP)	The nurse is accountable for practice within an EBP environment and for implementing evidence in own practice.	Conduct a literature search for current evidence and select appropriate nursing interventions based on the literature search.
Health, Wellness, Illness, and Injury	The nurse is accountable for assessing the patient's current level of health and wellness, then providing teaching, interventions, and referrals aimed at preserving and/or promoting health and preventing illness.	Assess patient's current overall health, including biophysical, cognitive, psychologic, and spiritual components. Provide teaching on general health promotion and illness prevention measures beneficial to all individuals (e.g., regular exercise, immunizations), as well as measures specific to the patient's risk factors and lifestyle (e.g., smoking cessation, heart-healthy diet). Refer patients to counselors, clergy, dietitians, physical therapists, support groups, and other outside resources as appropriate.
Infection	The nurse is accountable for protecting patients whose immune systems are compromised and subject to infection.	Assess patient's history for indications of a compromised immune system (e.g., autoimmune disorders, cancer or chemotherapy). Be aware of self and the need for personal protective equipment so as not to carry or transmit disease or infection. Be knowledgeable of disease transmission. Educate the public on the importance of immunizations and best practice for preventing disease transmission through safe hygiene practice.
Safety	The nurse is accountable for keeping patients safe within the healthcare environment, as well as for teaching patients ways to reduce the risk of illness and injury in their daily lives.	Identify and address safety hazards in the immediate healthcare environment. Assess patients' risk for various types of injury outside the healthcare environment. Report any concerns to the supervisor per unit/institution policy. Teach patients about actions that can reduce their risk of injury (e.g., helmet use when bicycling, proper use of child safety restraints).
Teaching and Learning	The nurse is accountable for patient education concerning all aspects of care. The nurse is accountable for staying up to date with the latest evidence for best practices. The nurse is accountable for providing current and accurate practice guidelines to subordinates, especially preceptors or mentors of new nurses or nursing students.	Assess patient and family learning needs. Assess readiness for learning. Design and implement educational interventions based on evidence of best practice. Read current journal articles and attend workshops or seminars that provide up-to-date information about procedures, medications, and other standards of practice. Stay up to date through continuing education.
Trauma	Patients may present with signs or symptoms of trauma and/or they may be at risk for abuse or violence. The nurse is accountable for taking action to prevent further harm; in some circumstances, the nurse may also have a legal duty to report.	Assess for signs of prior physical, emotional, or sexual abuse as part of the admission process. Assess for both risk of abuse and suicide risk as part of the admission process. Be aware of warning signs of abuse or suicide that may be demonstrated or verbalized by patients.

Socialization to Nursing

As previously mentioned, the members of a profession—and not outsiders—determine the standards of education and practice for that profession. Entering a profession is therefore similar to entering a new society, so it involves a complete socialization process far more extensive than what most non-professional occupations require. Socialization into a profession supports accountability because it has consequences for the nurse by instilling critical values and providing opportunities for interactions that support and promote accountability.

Socialization is the process by which individuals learn to become members of groups and society as well as learn the social rules defining the relationships into which they will enter. Professional socialization is a complex process. It requires an understanding of cultures that promote high performance and safe practice. An organization with a high-performance culture is dynamic and ever-changing as well as open to hearing about new ideas for improvement. Nurse managers establish clear expectations for behaviors that lead to zero patient harm (Cochrane, 2017). In order to know if the organization is a "fit" that focuses on accountability and promotes quality professional socialization, nurses need to understand the components of a dynamic learning culture. Namely, high-performance organizations promote accountability through transparency, the avoidance of blame, use of best-practice guidelines, and the input of staff. Individual perspectives are encouraged and supported (Persaud, 2019). Cultures in which fear and reprimand for reporting or criticism of mistakes are promoted over identifying paths to improvement are indicative of organizations that do not value accountable behavior (Yoo & Kim, 2017). Clear expectations, follow-through, and rewards or consequences are key components for successful socialization within an organization (Cox & Beeson, 2018).

Similarly, nursing education aids students in the development of individual professional values by helping them clarify and internalize these values. Faculty and/or staff nurses supervising students need to establish clear expectations for preparation and performance and help students understand their mistakes and patient consequences for such through reflective practice. The focus should also be on students' strengths so as involve them in the process of learning as a lifelong commitment to excellence in practice. The nursing code of ethics (described in Module 44, Ethics), standards of nursing practice, and the legal system itself (described in Module 49, Legal Issues) define specific values all professional nurses should share. The NSNA (2013) also adopted a code of academic and clinical conduct in 2001 (**Box 42.1** »)) that is an integral part of ethical practice. This code addresses students' responsibility in the academic environment and to society at large as they learn clinical skills in nursing care.

Box 42.1

National Student Nurses' Association Code of Academic and Clinical Conduct

Preamble

Students of nursing have a responsibility to society in learning the academic theory and clinical skills needed to provide nursing care. The clinical setting presents unique challenges and responsibilities while caring for human beings in a variety of healthcare environments.

The Code of Academic and Clinical Conduct is based on an understanding that to practice nursing as a student is an agreement to uphold the trust that society has placed in us. The statements of the code provide guidance for the nursing student in the personal development of an ethical foundation and need not be limited strictly to the academic or clinical environment but can assist in the holistic development of the individual.

A Code for Nursing Students

As students are involved in the clinical and academic environments, we believe that ethical principles are a necessary guide to professional development. Therefore, within these environments we:

1. Advocate for the rights of all clients.
2. Maintain client confidentiality.
3. Take appropriate action to ensure the safety of clients, self, and others.
4. Provide care for the client in a timely, compassionate and professional manner.
5. Communicate client care in a truthful, timely and accurate manner.
6. Actively promote the highest level of moral and ethical principles and accept responsibility for our actions.
7. Promote excellence in nursing by encouraging lifelong learning and professional development.
8. Treat others with respect and promote an environment that respects human rights, values, and choice of cultural and spiritual beliefs.
9. Collaborate in every reasonable manner with the academic faculty and clinical staff to ensure the highest quality of client care.
10. Use every opportunity to improve faculty and clinical staff understanding of the learning needs of nursing students.
11. Encourage faculty, clinical staff, and peers to mentor nursing students.
12. Refrain from performing any technique or procedure for which the student has not been adequately trained.
13. Refrain from any deliberate action or omission of care in the academic or clinical setting that creates unnecessary risk of injury to the client, self, or others.
14. Assist the staff nurse or preceptor in ensuring that there is full disclosure and that proper authorization is obtained from clients regarding any form of treatment or research.
15. Abstain from the use of alcoholic beverages or any substances in the academic and clinical setting that impair judgment.
16. Strive to achieve and maintain an optimal level of personal health.
17. Support access to treatment and rehabilitation for students who are experiencing impairments related to substance abuse and mental or physical health issues.
18. Uphold school policies and regulations related to academic and clinical performance, reserving the right to challenge and critique rules and regulations as per school grievance policy.

Note: This code was adopted by the NSNA House of Delegates, Nashville, Tennessee, on April 6, 2001. Reprinted with permission.

Case Study » Part 2

Jen Sturges meets with the charge nurse, Melinda Menendez, and briefly but clearly discusses her concerns about Ms. Miller's pain management and the objective signs she noted during her shift. Ms. Menendez asks Jen what she thinks is going on with Ms. Miller. Jen tells her that this is her first experience with a patient who has a history of pain but does not want to use any pain medications and ignores her apparent pain.

Ms. Menendez is concerned that Ms. Miller may be unable to participate in her care and other daily activities if she has uncontrolled pain during hospitalization. She asks Jen to join her while she speaks with Ms. Miller. After a few minutes of discussion, it becomes clear that Ms. Miller is afraid of the potential for narcotic abuse. It also appears that uncertainty about the meaning of her body's pain signals worries Ms. Miller about the safety of her physical activities at home and in the hospital. Ms. Menendez gently holds Ms. Miller's hand and tells her how important it is for her to take part in care activities and to allow the staff to manage pain and keep her as comfortable as possible. "To help you with this care," Ms. Menendez says, "I would like our social worker and clinical pharmacist to see you about your pain and other needs while you are here." Ms. Miller agrees with this plan.

Clinical Reasoning Question Level I

1. As the charge nurse, Ms. Menendez took an active role in further assessment of the patient's needs and communicated with Ms. Miller in a truthful and calm manner. Of what aspect of the ethical principles listed in the Code for Nursing Students is this an example?

Clinical Reasoning Question Level II

2. If Jen had delayed discussing her concerns with Ms. Menendez, would this have prevented further care and appropriate patient outcomes? Explain your answer.

Focus on Integrative Health

Integrative Health and Accountable Care Organizations

Integrative health strategies focus on the whole person, not just the disease, and emphasize preventive care, thus improving the health of the population. Integrative health techniques have a unique ability to improve the health of the population, enhance the patient experience of care, and reduce the per capita cost of care. According to the Centers for Medicare and Medicaid Services (CMS; 2020), accountable care organizations (ACOs) are groups of doctors, hospitals, and other HCPs that work to provide coordinated high-quality care to their Medicare patients. ACOs ensure that patients get timely, appropriate care while preventing medical errors and duplication of services (CMS, 2020). Community health centers (CHCs) and federally qualified health centers (FQHCs) provide primary, preventive, and nonmedical services to individuals regardless of their ability to pay. CHCs and FQHCs are usually found in areas where economic and environmental factors limit or prohibit access to preventive, behavioral, and/or social health services. Those services, along with access to nutritious food, safe and affordable housing, and access to health education, are among the social determinants of health (SDOH) that play an important role in the health of individuals and communities. Community health nurses and community health workers or navigators provide front-line support for those with limited abilities to navigate a complex health system. In some areas, ACOs and/or CHCs and FQHCs will collaborate with other organizations to sponsor or establish farmers' markets, healthcare screenings, and health education to reduce the impact of SDOH in their communities.

Factors Influencing Nursing Practice and Accountability

Various factors influence nursing as a profession, and because of the integral part nursing plays in the healthcare system as a whole, these factors typically also influence the entire healthcare system. Essentially, what affects the healthcare system will affect nursing as a profession, and the reverse is also true. Some of the most important factors affecting nursing practice include economics, consumer demand, science and technology, information availability and telecommunications, legislation, demographics, and the current nursing shortage.

Economics

In recent years, changes in public and private health insurance programs, particularly Medicare, have affected the demand for nursing care. Multiple and ongoing changes in the U.S. healthcare system present challenges to both nurses and the organizations in which they practice. For many years, the healthcare industry has been shifting its emphasis from inpatient to outpatient care with preadmission testing, increased outpatient same-day surgery, posthospitalization rehabilitation, home healthcare, health maintenance, physical fitness programs, and community health education programs. Acute care remains the primary nursing practice area, and patients are presenting with higher acuities and more complex needs. This necessitates hiring nurses with experience and advanced education and adjusting staffing ratios in order to provide safe care. In addition, with a shift from hospital-based care to outpatient settings, more nurses are being employed in community-based settings, such as home health agencies, hospices, and community clinics. These changes also affect the level of nursing education needed to safely and competently practice and meet the needs of the public within these settings.

As with acute care environments, the field of outpatient care has developed specialty areas to meet patient needs. For example, there are now outpatient facilities dedicated to such things as oncology symptom management, ostomy care, diabetes management, and palliative care for terminally ill patients. Various models of integrative care have also arisen in an attempt to better control rising healthcare costs, as described in the Focus on Integrative Health feature.

Consumer Demand

A **consumer** is any person or group that uses a service or commodity; thus, a consumer might be an individual, a group of individuals, or even an entire community. Because everyone has healthcare needs, the consumers of nursing services are the general public. Consumer needs are a driver for any market or service. For example, the drive for integrative healthcare services is motivated by more than the need to consolidate and lower the costs of healthcare; it is also motivated by consumer interest in the use of complementary health approaches. Another factor affecting consumer use of the healthcare system is that today's healthcare consumers are more knowledgeable and vocal about their needs and more invested in holding HCPs accountable for being responsive to their needs, in part due to the increasing amount of information available on the internet.

Science and Technology

Advances in science and technology greatly affect nursing practice, competence, and accountability. For example, recent progress in the field of molecular genetics has made it possible to identify individuals who are at elevated risk for a variety of hereditary diseases. However, the testing of healthy children for diseases that would develop only in adulthood raises many important ethical, legal, and social questions. These questions are further amplified by the fact that genetic testing is now available outside the traditional healthcare system, often without the mediation of physicians, nurses, or other healthcare professionals. Nurses therefore need to expand their knowledge base and technical skills as they adapt to meet new patient needs emerging out of the expanded use of technology.

Science and technology have affected other areas of nursing practice as well. Healthcare practitioners in most settings are now expected to learn how to use technologic advances such as sophisticated computerized equipment to monitor or treat patients. They are also expected to be able to use online electronic health report systems (CMS, 2020). In both acute inpatient settings and primary care practices, HCPs have integrated electronic health records (EHRs) successfully and have reported increased efficiency in retrieving medical records. However, patients frequently have the need to see more than a single primary HCP. Patients with high blood pressure, heart disease, diabetes, or cancer might simultaneously be seeing a cardiologist, endocrinologist, and oncologist. While the specialists all have EHRs, their different vendor systems might not connect or "talk" to each other. This can lead to fractured care and even pharmaceutical mismanagement. Caring for patients in a complex world requires systems where data can be safely shared, stored, protected, owned, and controlled in an ethical and responsible manner (Courbier, Dimond, &Bros-Facer, 2019).

Information Availability and Telecommunications

As the internet has evolved, so have various forms of **telecommunication**, or the means by which information is transferred from one site to another. Videoconferencing and virtual visits allow individuals and/or groups in two or more locations to communicate by simultaneous two-way video and audio transmissions. It is now even possible to monitor critical care patients in an ICU in a different city or rural area and to manage patient care from another part of the world. As technologies continue to change, nursing education must continue to evolve so that nurses have the knowledge and experience necessary to provide safe, effective care using these models.

Technology increases consumer access to health information. This requires that nurses be knowledgeable about accurate and reliable websites so that they can, in turn, teach patients about the importance of securing the best evidence-based information about their condition (Ngcobo, 2019). As the use of **telehealth**—the provision of long-distance healthcare through the use of technology such as videoconferencing, computers, or smartphones—continues to grow, **telenursing**—the provision of nursing care via telecommunication systems—will also continue to expand.

mHealth (mobile health) is increasing in popularity, and the need for such services became even more evident during the coronavirus pandemic. Mobile health, a category of telehealth, refers to healthcare services delivered via mobile devices such as smartphones and tablets. While telehealth is increasing in need and popularity, questions remain about access, accuracy, HIPAA privacy and security, and tracking and transmission of information with responsible parties. COVID-19 exposed the complexities of maintaining client privacy (HIPAA) while simultaneously needing to share information with multiple agencies outside of the patients' primary care providers (Lenert & Yeager McSwain, 2020; Odendaal et al., 2020).

Legislation

Changes in health legislation affect not just the nursing profession, but also consumers. The **Patient Self-Determination Act (PSDA)**, for example, requires that all competent adults be informed in writing upon admission to a healthcare institution about their rights to accept or refuse medical care and to use advance directives (American Bar Association, 2017). In many institutions, nurses are responsible for ensuring compliance with this law, as well as with similar regulatory requirements. In this way, legislative and other regulatory changes can directly affect the nurse's role in supporting patients and their families.

Nursing Workforce Capacity

Even though registered nurses make up the largest group of HCPs and even though the AACN (2019a) reported a 3.7% increase in enrollment at the baccalaureate level in 2018, for the foreseeable future, the nursing workforce is not projected to be sufficient to meet demand. Contributing factors (**Box 42.2** »)) include a shortage of nursing faculty, a significant segment of current nurses reaching retirement, changing demographics, an aging population, and high turnover rates.

Healthcare systems, policymakers, nursing educators, and professional organizations must work together to right-size the nursing workforce so that accountable, safe, quality care can be delivered. Some recommended actions for addressing this problem include the following:

- Giving nursing students the means to enter and progress through educational programs more rapidly and efficiently
- Stepping up efforts to recruit young people early in the course of their education (e.g., in middle and high school)
- Providing greater scheduling flexibility, better rewards for experienced nurses who serve as mentors, more adequate staffing, and increased salaries to improve nurses' work environment
- Increasing funding for nursing education.

Box 42.2

Factors Contributing to the Nursing Shortage

- Nursing school enrollment is not growing fast enough.
- According to a 2018 study conducted by the National Council of State Boards of Nursing (2015) and the Forum of State Nursing Workforce Centers, 50.9% of the RN workforce is age 50 or older. Furthermore, the Health Resources & Services Administration (HRSA; 2017b) predicts that in the next 10 to 15 years, more than 1 million RNs will reach retirement age and begin to withdraw from the workforce.
- New graduates are entering the workforce at an older age and will have fewer years to work.
- U.S. nursing schools turned away more than 75,000 qualified applicants in 2018 due to insufficient numbers of faculty, clinical placement sites, classroom space, preceptors, and also budget constraints.
- The number of individuals in the U.S. population age 65 and older is projected to be 83.7 million by 2050. This will result in an increased need for geriatric services, particularly for those individuals with comorbid conditions and chronic disease.
- Because of the increased acuity of hospital patients, demand for skilled and specialized nurses is rising. This is particularly important given the landmark study by Aiken et al. (2011), which found that a greater proportion of professional nurses at the bedside is directly associated with better patient and nurse outcomes.
- Inadequate wages and low nurse recruitment contribute to staffing shortages.
- Staffing shortages, including insufficient support staff, resulting in excessive workloads and greater reliance on overtime.
- Long hours and task overload cause high nurse turnover and vacancy rates, which have worsened as a result of the COVID-19 pandemic, with many nurses either leaving critical care or leaving the profession altogether.

Sources: Data from American Association of Colleges of Nursing (2019b); Cox, Willis, and Coustasse (2014); Health Resources & Services Administration (2017a); Phan (2021).

Case Study » Part 3

Lisa Rossi, the social worker, meets with Ms. Miller and learns that she is a single mother with a long history of back pain. Mrs. Miller appears dejected about the amount of time and effort she puts into being a mom. "I am not a person who gives in to things easily," Ms. Miller said. "That's why I think it is so unfair. Why me? There are so many things I should be able to do. And if I don't ignore my pain, it ruins so much in my life. I have been suffering through many snowboarding and camping trips with my children, but I don't want them to know that."

Ms. Rossi allows time for Ms. Miller to discuss her concerns and then briefly teaches her how to do slow yoga-type breathing to help her anxiety. After Ms. Miller practices the slower breathing, Ms. Rossi asks her whether she is ready to meet with the clinical pharmacist, who will work with her to find the best options for pain management both while she is in the hospital and after discharge. Ms. Miller agrees to the plan.

The information from the social worker helps Dan Kramer, the clinical pharmacist, plan appropriate interventions for Ms. Miller. Dr. Kramer is able to meet with her that evening, and afterward he discusses the medication plan with Jen Sturges and Ms. Menendez. The next day, after a dose of IV morphine along with oral acetaminophen, Ms. Miller is able to relax and take part in care activities. By the time the doctor discusses discharge plans with her, Ms. Miller describes how she had learned to recognize the pain not so much as an enemy, but rather as a signal to move or to calm down. She also learns that medication is not an enemy if it helps her with her daily life. In addition, she mentions that working with an occupational therapist has helped her understand how to calculate and plan all of her daily activities, physical and otherwise, to ensure her ability to participate in her usual social and occupational roles.

Clinical Reasoning Questions Level I

1. What role did technology play in the patient's care plan?
2. What information would you expect the social worker to share with Jen Sturges?

Clinical Reasoning Questions Level II

3. What role did the social worker take with Ms. Miller? How did the social worker's interview and discussion help with the patient's care and further activity?
4. Why was it important for the pharmacist to meet with the patient and then discuss the plans with Jen Sturges and Ms. Menendez?

REVIEW The Concept of Accountability

RELATE Link the Concepts

Linking the concept of accountability with the concept of legal issues:

1. What is the nurse's legal obligation to the patient related to accountability, and how is it regulated?
2. A nurse makes a medication error that results in harm to the patient. The nurse demonstrates accountability by immediately informing the physician and nursing supervisor when the error is recognized. How does the nurse's proper demonstration of accountability affect the nurse's legal responsibility?

Linking the concept of accountability with the concept of comfort:

3. What is the nurse's role in assessment and appropriate interventions to ensure comfort for the patient?
4. How does lack of patient comfort impede the patient's taking part in care plans and activities?

Linking the concept of accountability with the concept of ethics:

5. How does the nursing code of ethics reflect the expectation that the nurse is accountable when providing patient care?
6. A nurse believes that the physician has written orders that may endanger the patient. The nurse consults the physician, who refuses to alter the orders. What is the nurse's ethical obligation to the patient in order to demonstrate accountability?

REFER Go to Pearson MyLab Nursing and eText

REFLECT Apply Your Knowledge

Frank Epworth is a 78-year-old man who presents to the emergency department complaining of nausea and vomiting and severe pain in his left side and back, just below his ribs. Mr. Epworth states that these symptoms began suddenly. He also mentions that he is having difficulty passing urine; despite increased urge and several attempts to "go," he last urinated 2 hours ago, and at that time, he noted small amounts of blood in his urine. Based on these symptoms, the patient's reported medical history, and the physical examination, the physician suspects that Mr. Epworth has urolithiasis, or kidney stones. Imaging studies confirm the diagnosis. The physician has requested a urology consult. She has also ordered additional urinalysis and blood testing to learn more about Mr. Epworth's condition, but the results are still pending. In the meantime, you are the RN charged with Mr. Epworth's care.

As you review Mr. Epworth's chart, you note that the physician has authorized administration of Dilaudid 1 to 4 mg IV prn for pain management. The physician has also ordered you to push IV fluids at a rate of 500 mL/hour in hopes of helping Mr. Epworth pass the stone. Mr. Epworth's urine must also be collected, measured, and strained so that any stone fragments can be analyzed to determine their composition. After consulting the chart, you perform a brief nursing assessment during which Mr. Epworth rates his pain as 8 on a scale of 0 to 10. Therefore, after starting IV fluids as ordered, you administer 1 mg of Dilaudid. You also task the LPN involved in Mr. Epworth's care with urine collection responsibilities and helping Mr. Epworth remain as comfortable as possible.

1. Half an hour later, you speak with the LPN. He notes that Mr. Epworth passed 30 mL of urine about 5 minutes ago, which he noted in the patient's chart. He also states that he disposed of the urine without straining it for stones. As the RN, are you accountable for the LPN's error? Why or why not?
2. An hour after the initial administration of Dilaudid, you reassess Mr. Epworth's pain level. He says that the medication didn't seem to provide any relief, so you administer another 3 mg of Dilaudid per the doctor's order. Will you be accountable if this additional dose fails to control Mr. Epworth's pain? Why or why not?
3. Shortly after starting Mr. Epworth's IV, you recall reading recent clinical guidance advising that large fluid pushes are rarely effective in facilitating stone passage. In this scenario, how might the standards of nursing accountability affect your subsequent course of action?

Exemplar 42.A Competence

Exemplar Learning Outcomes

42.A Analyze competence as it relates to accountability.

- Describe the areas of competence.
- Explain the importance of lifelong competence for nurses.

Exemplar Key Terms

Competence, *2710*

Overview

In the past, nurses were considered competent, or able to do their job, if they could simply provide care and comfort. Today, **competence** implies that nurses practice to the fullest extent utilizing knowledge, skills, abilities, and judgment while enacting care. A competent nurse is one who uses critical-thinking, problem-solving, and ethical reasoning and decision-making skills in everyday practice (ANA, 2015b). This requires that nurses possess awareness of their own capabilities and be open to feedback and change.

Areas of Competence

Critical Thinking

In nursing, the process of learning to think critically in practice begins in school and, in particular, at the bedside. Clinical (or situational) learning helps students to connect classroom with practice. Because situational learning can never be perfectly replicated or repeated from one situation to another, students must learn how classroom material applies to individual patients, with differing circumstances, in a variety of settings. Situational learning is valuable in that it gives the student an opportunity to analyze, synthesize, and apply what is learned. Over time, the experiences provide a foundation from which judgments about future action are formed. Critical thinkers are open to the opinions of others yet rely on their knowledge to form a scientific basis for actions. Critical thinkers know themselves well and are willing to think, inquire, and investigate before making decisions (Ozcan & Elkoca, 2019; Von Colln-Appling & Giuliano, 2017). (More information on critical thinking can be found in Module 36, Clinical Decision Making.)

Problem Solving

Problem-solving is a core skill of competency for working with patients in complex environments (Mi Sook & Sue Kyung, 2019). It can be developed and enhanced over time through the use of evidence-based learning and practice. It also requires a knowledge of self, that is, the influence of one's emotions over practice choices. This is referred to as *emotional intelligence (EI)*. The nurse's ability to recognize, through emotional appraisal, when emotions rather than knowledge influence decisions is key to good problem-solving skills and promotes good working relationships with both patients and peers. (More information on problem solving can be found in Module 36, Clinical Decision Making.)

Ethical Reasoning and Decision Making

The Code of Ethics for Nurses (ANA, 2015) makes explicit the goals, values, and obligations of professional nurses. Ethical reasoning is based on an understanding of these. While student nurses may think that ethical reasoning is a skill that only nurses in critical care environments face, the truth is that nurses encounter the need for ethical reasoning across settings in everyday practice. Providing optimal care for patients requires ethical reasoning and decision making. Nurses must be mindful of each patient's preferences and circumstances as well as the nurses' own well-being. Coming to work in a physical and/or emotional compromised state as well as working in a demanding and stressful environment can endanger the welfare of the patient or, at the very least, can have an impact on the nurse's ability to deliver safe and competent care. (More information on ethical reasoning can be found in Module 44, Ethics.)

Competence for nurses is assurance for the public that they are getting the best care possible. While nurses are provided guidance through the Standards of Practice and Code of Ethics, each nurse is responsible for understanding one's own capabilities and limitations and the influence of one's emotions on patient care. In addition, nurses need to be cognizant of the influences of the environment in which they practice. Is it supportive, allowing for guidance, questioning, and openness to discussion? Is it safe, encouraging of error reporting? Is it inclusive, acknowledging the value of teamwork and collaboration? Is competence valued and continuing education a priority? Competence can be developed over time and is a foundational component of accountable care (Vernon, Chiarella, Papps, & Lark, 2019).

Promoting Lifelong Competence

Nurses gain competence gradually throughout nursing school until they reach a level at which they are judged safe and skillful enough to function as newly licensed nurses. Nurses continue to build competence throughout their career, with expertise coming from experience, gaining new knowledge, and improving performance of skills.

Maintaining and increasing competence in nursing require the nurse to continue learning. Professional development and continuing education opportunities come in a variety of forms, including seminars offered by colleges and professional organizations, professional and peer-reviewed journals, and hospital- or employer-sponsored classes on new equipment or procedures, as well as formal and informal discussions with peers and other members of the healthcare team. All nurses must continually assess their own level of knowledge and identify areas in which they need additional knowledge in order to provide appropriate patient care.

Even the most competent nurses sometimes encounter situations that make them question how best to respond. Luckily, nurses can collaborate with each other and with others on the interprofessional team, sharing opinions, ideas, and information. Although collaboration is helpful and even critical, each nurse is nevertheless accountable for one's own choices and must weigh all information and choose the best course of action. The nurse who recognizes that there will always be a need to collaborate with others maintains a safe practice.

Various models have been developed in an attempt to explain the process by which nurses attain competence. One classic model is that developed by Benner (2001), which describes five levels of proficiency in nursing: novice, advanced beginner, competent, proficient, and expert (**Box 42.3** »). Benner's model proposes that experience is essential for the development of professional expertise—and this idea has significant implications for teaching and learning.

Box 42.3

Benner's Stages of Nursing Expertise

Stage I: Novice

No experience (e.g., a nursing student). Performance is limited, inflexible, and governed by context-free rules and regulations rather than experience.

Stage II: Advanced Beginner

Demonstrates marginally acceptable performance.

Recognizes the meaningful aspects of a real situation. Has experienced enough real situations to make judgments about them.

Stage III: Competent

Has 2 or 3 years of experience. Demonstrates organizational and planning abilities. Differentiates important factors from less important aspects of care. Coordinates multiple complex care demands.

Stage IV: Proficient

Has 3 to 5 years of experience. Perceives situations as wholes rather than in terms of parts as in Stage II. Uses maxims as guides for what to consider in a situation. Has holistic understanding of the client, which improves decision making. Focuses on long-term goals.

Stage V: Expert

Performance is fluid, flexible, and highly proficient; no longer requires rules, guidelines, or maxims to connect an understanding of the situation to appropriate action. Demonstrates highly skilled intuitive and analytic ability in new situations. Is inclined to take a certain action because "it felt right."

Source: From Benner (2001). Pearson Education, Inc., New York, NY.

SAFETY ALERT As nurses pass through Benner's stages of nursing expertise, they gain not only knowledge and fluency but also a more intuitive sense of patient safety. By the expert level, medication doses and sterilization procedures that once required careful training and memorization become easy to perform. Even at the expert level, however, nurses are aware that double-checking their actions helps to ensure that patients' safety needs are always being met.

Regardless of their exact level of proficiency, all nurses must hold themselves accountable by frequently weighing and assessing their own competence. In all situations, nurses should understand that it is more honorable to say "I don't know" or ask "Would you help me?" than to say "I'm not sure but I think this is right" or "I'll figure it out as I go along." In fact, the first rule of competence in providing patient care is to ask for help whenever there is uncertainty about the safety of any given action. By doing so, nurses both invite opportunities to increase their own level of competence and hold themselves accountable for providing the highest quality of patient care.

Focus on Diversity and Culture

Teaching Cultural Competence

The population of the United States is rapidly changing, and it is estimated that, in the near future, minority and ethnic groups will constitute the majority of the population. As such, it is essential that nurses gain the skills necessary to communicate cross-culturally and be able to provide culturally sensitive care. The Institute of Medicine's (2002) report *Unequal Treatment* was foundational in that it exposed the disparities in healthcare when providers lack understanding of the cultures, values, and beliefs of individuals. More importantly, a generous body of evidence proves that, in the United States, people of color often have poorer health outcomes due to language barriers, low education, limited social support, a lack of insurance coverage, unequal access to healthy food and adequate housing, discriminatory attitudes from HCPs, and fear of healthcare systems (Mazanec, Verga, Foley, & Mehta, 2019; Spector, 2017). Healthcare organizations and programs of nursing must provide cultural competence training so that compassionate care can be delivered

Cultural competence training starts with a recognition of one's own values and beliefs and the impact they have on the care provided. It also requires great listening skills to have an understanding of the rites and traditions that impact care and influence outcomes. The nurse must be aware of treatment options that are discordant with the patients' values and beliefs and advocate for the patients' wishes, particularly if end-of-life or psychiatric care are needed. Lastly, nurses need to be aware of community resources that can provide the follow-up care necessary to prevent recurrence or readmission.

REVIEW Competence

RELATE Link the Concepts and Exemplars

Linking the exemplar on competence with the concept of legal issues:

1. What is the nurse's legal obligation to society and the profession to maintain competence?
2. How can nurses who lack competence in one area of nursing strengthen their knowledge and skills?

Linking the exemplar on competence with the concept of ethics:

3. What is the nurse's ethical obligation related to competence?
4. How does the nursing code of ethics address the issue of competence?

REFER Go to Pearson MyLab Nursing and eText

REFLECT Apply Your Knowledge

Tyree Campbell has worked in the labor and delivery unit of a large metropolitan hospital since graduating from nursing school 8 years ago. A new private hospital recently opened in town, and the census on Ms. Campbell's unit has been significantly lower. Tonight, Ms. Campbell reports to work and learns that more nurses are scheduled to work than there are patients. The decision has been made to float the excess staff to other units, and Ms. Campbell is asked to float to the neonatal intensive care unit (NICU). Her heart sinks, and she begins to feel the early signs of panic as she thinks, "How can I work in the NICU? I don't have any experience working there!"

1. What is Ms. Campbell's responsibility in this situation?
2. Can Ms. Campbell agree to float to the NICU if she is not competent to care for the patients on this unit? Explain your answer.
3. What should Ms. Campbell say to the nursing supervisor who has given her this assignment?

References

Agency for Healthcare Research and Quality (AHRQ). (2019). *Culture of safety*. https://psnet.ahrq.gov/primer/culture-safety

Aiken, L. H., Cimiotti, J. P., Sloane D. M., Smith, H. L., Flynn, L., & Neff, D. F. (2011). The effects of nurses staffing and nurse education on patient deaths in hospitals with different nurse work environments. *Medical Care, 49*(12), 1047–1053.

American Association of Colleges of Nursing (AACN). (2019a). *Degree completion programs for -registered nurses: RN to master's degree and RN to baccalaureate programs*. http://www.aacn.nche.edu/media-relations/fact-sheets/degree-completion-programs

American Association of Colleges of Nursing (AACN). (2019b). *Nursing shortage fact sheet*. http://www.aacn.nche.edu/media-relations/NrsgShortageFS.pdf

American Bar Association. (2017). *Law for older Americans*. https://www.-americanbar.org/groups/public_education/resources/law_issues_for_consumers/patient_self_determination_act.html

American Nurses Association (ANA). (2015a). *Code of ethics for nurses with interpretive statements* (3rd ed.). Author.

American Nurses Association (ANA). (2015b). *Nursing: Scope and standards of practice* (3rd ed.). Author.

Benner, P. (2001). *From novice to expert: Excellence and power in clinical nursing practice*. Pearson Education.

Buck, J., Loversidge, J., Chipps, E., Gallagher-Ford, L., Genter, L., & Yen, P-Y. (2018). Top-of-license nursing practice. Describing common nursing activities and nurses' experiences that hinder top-of license practice, Part 1. *Journal of Nursing Administration, 48*(5), 266–271.

Centers for Medicare and Medicaid Services (CMS). (modified 2020). *Accountable care organizations*. https://www.cms.gov/Medicare/Medicare-Fee-for-Service-Payment/ACO/

Cochrane, B. S. (2017). Leaders go first: creating and sustaining a culture of high performance. *Health Management Forum, 30*(5), 229–232.

Courbier, S., Dimond, R., & Bros-Facer, V. (2019). Share and protect our health data: An evidence based approach to rare disease patients' perspectives on data sharing and data protection-quantitative survey and recommendations. *Orphanet Journal of Rare Diseases, 14*(1), 175. https://doi.org/10.1186/s13023-019-1123-4

Cox, P., Willis, K., & Coustasse, A. (2014, March). *The American epidemic: The U.S. nursing shortage and turnover problem*. Paper presented at annual conference of the Business and Health Administration Association, Chicago.

Cox, S., & Beeson, G. (2018). Getting accountability right. *Nursing Management, 49*(9), 24–30. https://journals.lww.com/nursingmanagement/Fulltext/2018/09000/Getting_accountability_right.5.aspx

Cronenwett, L., Sherwood, G., & Gelmon, S. B. (2009). Improving quality and safety education: The QSEN learning collaborative. *Nursing Outlook, 57*, 304–312.

Health Resources & Services Administration. (2017a). *The future of the nursing workforce: National- and state-level projections, 2014–2030*. http://bhw.hrsa.gov/healthworkforce/index.html

Health Resources & Services Administration. (2017b). *Supply and demand projections of the nursing workforce 2014–2030*. http://bhw.hrsa.gov/healthworkforce/index.html

Institute of Medicine. (1999). *To err is human*. National Academies Press.

Institute of Medicine Committee on Understanding and Eliminating Racial and Ethnic Disparities in Health Care, Smedley, B. D., Stith, A. Y., & Nelson, A. R. (Eds.). (2003). *Unequal treatment: Confronting racial and ethnic disparities in health care*. National Academies Press.

Institute of Medicine. (2010). *The future of nursing: Leading change, advancing health*. http://www.iom.edu/Reports/2010/The-Future-of-Nursing-Leading-Change-Advancing-Health.aspx

The Joint Commission. (2020). *Hospital: 2020 National patient safety goals*. https://www.jointcommission.org/standards/national-patient-safety-goals/hospital-2020-national-patient-safety-goals/

Lenert, L., & Yeager McSwain, B., (2020). Balancing health privacy, health information exchange and research in the context of the COVID-19 pandemic. *Journal of American Medical Informatics Association, 27*(6), 963–966.

Loversidge, J., Yen, P.-Y., Chipps, E., Gallagher-Ford, L., Genter, L., & Buck, J. (2018). Top-of-license nursing practice, part 2: Differentiate BSN and ADN perceptions of top-of-license activities. *Journal of Nursing Administration, 48*(6), 329–334.

Mazanec, P., Verga, S., Foley, H., & Mehta, A. (2019). The need to cultural inclusivity in global palliative nursing. *Journal of Hospice and Palliative Care, 21*(6), E1–E8.

McCullough, L. B., Coverdale, J. H., & Chervenak, F. A. (2020). Trustworthiness and professionalism in academic medicine. *Academic Medicine, 95*(6), 828–832.

Medical Reserve Corps. (2019). *About volunteering*. https://mrc.hhs.gov/volunteerfldr/AboutVolunteering

Mi Sook, K., & Sue Kyung, S. (2019). Emotional intelligence, problem solving ability, self- efficacy, and clinical performance among nursing students: A structural equation model. *Korean Journal of Adult Nursing, 31*(4), 380–388.

National Council of State Boards of Nursing. (2015). *National nursing workforce study*. https://www.ncsbn.org/workforce.htm

National League for Nursing. (2014). *Number of basic RN programs, total and by program type: 2005 to 2014*. http://www.nln.org/docs/default-source/newsroom/nursing-education-statistics/number-of-basic-rn-programs-total-and-by-program-type-2005-to-2014.pdf

National Student Nurses' Association. (2013). *Code of ethics*. https://www.nsna.org/nsna-code-of-ethics.html

Ngcobo, S. (2019). The 4th industrial revolution; the impact on nursing. *Nursing Update*, pp. 22–24.

Odendaal, W., Watkins, J., Leon, N., Goudge, J., Griffits, F., Tomlinson, M., & Daniels, K. (2020). Health workers' perceptions and experiences of using mHealth technologies to deliver primary healthcare services: A qualitative evidence synthesis. *Cochrane Database of Systematic Reviews*, Issue 3, Article No. CD011942. https://doi.org/10.1002/14651858

Ozcan, H., & Elkoca, A. (2019). Critical thinking skills of nursing candidates. *International Journal of Caring Sciences, 12*(3), 600–606.

Persaud, D. (2019). Designing a performance measurement system for accountability, quality improvement, and innovation. *The Health Care Manager, 38*(1), 82–88.

Phan, S. (2021). *More nurses face burnout as COVID-19 pandemic exacerbates nursing shortage*. https://komonews.com/news/local/more-nurses-face-burnout-because-of-covid-19-pandemic-exacerbates-nursing-shortage

Quality and Safety Education for Nurses Institute. (2014). *Prelicensure KSAs*. http://qsen.org/competencies/pre-licensure-ksas/

Spector, R. (2017). *Cultural diversity in health and illness* (9th ed.). Pearson.

Storaker, A., Naden, D., & Saeteren, B. (2019). Hindrances to achieve professional confidence: the nurse's participation in ethical decision-making. *Nursing Ethics, 26*(3), 715–727.

Vernon, R., Chiarella, M., Papps, E., & Lark, A. (2019). Assuring competence or ensuring performance. *Collegian, 26*, 399–406.

Yoo, M. S., & Kim, K. J. (2017). Exploring the influence of nurse work environment and patient safety culture on attitudes toward incident reporting. *Journal of Nursing Administration, 47*(9), 434–440.

Module 43
Advocacy

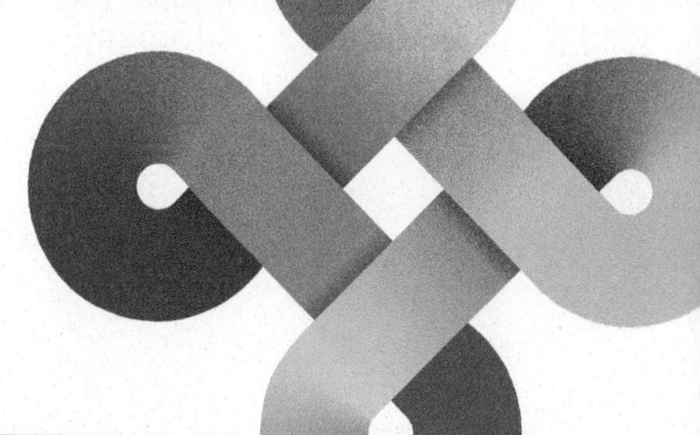

Module Outline and Learning Outcomes

The Concept of Advocacy

The Advocate's Role

43.1 Analyze the role of the advocate in the practice of nursing.

Advocacy Interventions

43.2 Summarize advocacy interventions used by nurses.

Concepts Related to Advocacy

43.3 Outline the relationship between advocacy and other concepts.

Unethical or Unsafe Practice or Unprofessional Conduct

43.4 Describe the nurse's role in reporting unprofessional actions.

Advocacy Exemplar

Exemplar 43.A Environmental Quality

43.A Analyze the health indicator of environmental quality as it relates to advocacy.

» The Concept of Advocacy

Concept Key Terms

Advocacy, **2715**
Patient advocacy, **2715**

Advocacy is a concept integral to both the International Council of Nurses' Code of Ethics for Nurses and the American Nurses Association (ANA) Code of Ethics for Nurses with Interpretive Statements (see Module 44, Ethics). Provision 3 of the ANA Code of Ethics (2015a) states that "the nurse promotes, advocates for, and protects the rights, health, and safety of the patient" (p. 9). **Advocacy** is generally defined as the act or process of supporting, defending, or assisting in another's cause. **Patient advocacy** has classically been defined as a process or strategy for acting on behalf of others (including patients, families, groups, or communities) to help them obtain services and rights that they might not otherwise receive but that they need to advance their well-being (Hanks, 2013; Jansson et al., 2014). The concept of advocacy in nursing has been recently analyzed, but no updated definition has emerged (Abbasini, Ahmadi, & Kazemnejad, 2020; Kalaitzidis & Jewell, 2020). Patient advocacy is a primary nursing role. The nurse may demonstrate advocacy by communicating the patient's needs to other health professionals; by facilitating, clarifying, or mediating communication between the patient and the healthcare provider (HCP); or by assisting patients to exercise their right to receive care that is consistent with their circumstances, values, beliefs, and preferences. Successful advocacy results in positive outcomes for patients. It also provides nurses with a sense of professional satisfaction, having met a duty to provide individualized, culturally sensitive, patient-centered care.

Nurses are ethically obligated to act as advocates for all patients, but particularly for those who cannot advocate for themselves. Advocacy can occur at any level, in any setting, from the bedside to the HCP's office, from advocating for the individual patient to advocating for an entire population through a call for changes in public policies and services.

Successful advocacy requires a balanced approach. It may not be possible to act on every patient request. Skilled nurse-advocates are able to explain the rationale for care limitations to the patient in plain language and also manage their own ability to cope with disappointing outcomes to prevent frustration and burnout.

Learning the patient advocate role begins during the nursing education experience. With time, the nurse will gain proficiency in this role and incorporate advocacy activities into daily professional practice.

The Advocate's Role

Navigating the healthcare system is a challenge for any patient. Advances in healthcare knowledge, technology, and system complexity have progressed exponentially in the 21st century. The result is that patients are rapidly moved through diagnosis and treatment in both inpatient and outpatient healthcare settings, often with little time for thoughts about self-determination or consideration of quality-of-life decisions. In addition, disparities in access and quality of healthcare, particularly for underserved and socioeconomically disadvantaged populations or those with poor literacy, are apparent in the U.S. healthcare system. These patients often have additional difficulty navigating the system, and th

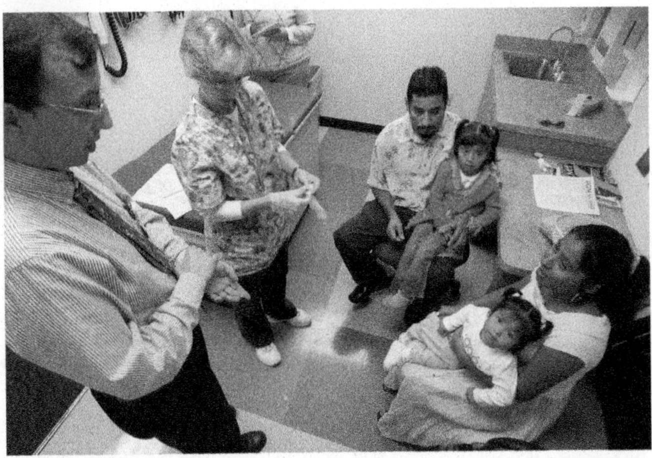

Figure 43.1 ›› At this clinic in Pittsburgh, Pennsylvania, patients not only receive healthcare, but also are helped to find a place to take English lessons, the closest Hispanic grocery store, and anything else they might need.
Source: Gene J. Puskar/AP Images.

may lack the resources to make quality decisions about their care. Even patients who are competent in English literacy, with advanced education, may have issues with healthcare literacy and a need for information provided in plain language. All of these patients, as well as their families and support systems, need assistance and empathy to help them manage information about their diagnosis, determine the best course through their treatment plan, and penetrate the layers of bureaucracy to access the required resources (**Figure 43-1** ››).

As an advocate, the nurse provides patients with much of the information they need to make informed healthcare decisions and supports patients' right to decide. Ideally, medical treatment decision making is shared between the patient and the HCP. When the patient makes decisions other than what is recommended by the HCP, the nurse can help mediate further conversation between the two and ensure that the patient is making an informed decision. The nurse advocates for the patient's right to make autonomous choices, even when those choices are incongruent with the nurse's own beliefs and values. The nurse-advocate must be careful to remain objective and respect the patient's choices without conveying approval or disapproval.

Attributes of the Nurse-Advocate

Although patient advocacy is considered to be an essential nursing function, supported and reinforced in contemporary nursing codes of conduct (American Nurses Association [ANA] Code of Ethics for Nurses with Interpretive Statements, 2015a; ANA Scope and Standards of Nursing Practice, 2015b; International Council of Nurses [ICN] Code of Ethics for Nurses, 2012), perspectives on how to approach patient advocacy and the boundaries of advocate roles are open to discourse. Questions have been raised historically (Cole, Wellard, & Mummery, 2014; Hyland, 2002; Schwartz, 2002) and continue to appear in current nursing and healthcare literature (Abbasini et al., 2020; Kalaitzidis & Jewell, 2020; Vitale, Germini, Massaro, & Fortunato, 2019), regarding the definition of patient advocacy and whether advocacy means supporting any healthcare decision the patient might make, regardless of its rationality or the extent of the resources available. Additional questions include the potential for advocacy to interfere with autonomous decision making, as well as whether nurses are the only healthcare professionals with a duty to safeguard patients' right to decide. Hyland's (2002) seminal discussion on advocacy asked the question, "Do nurses, in fact, have any right to assume a unique position as a patient advocate among a multitude of health professionals?" (p. 472). Bu and Jezewski's (2007) mid-range theory of patient advocacy has become the "gold standard" from the nursing point of view. This theory acknowledges the importance of patient advocacy as an essential nursing role and provides a clear definition. According to the authors, "patient advocacy is viewed as a process or strategy consisting of a series of specific actions for preserving, representing and/or safeguarding patients' rights, best interests and values in the healthcare system" (p. 104).

The overall goal of patient advocacy is to create an environment in which patients can exercise their right to decide and in which those rights can be protected, regardless of the environment or setting. Patient advocacy is complicated because of the complexity of the healthcare and legal systems and also because healthcare decision making is dependent on multiple patient-specific factors. Therefore, the nurse's actions to advocate for any patient must be individualized and depend on the clinical and situational context (Bu & Jezewski, 2007). Within each individual context, three broad core attributes of advocacy form the foundation for action (Bu & Jezewski, 2007):

1. Safeguarding patients' autonomy
2. Acting on behalf of patients
3. Championing social justice in the provision of healthcare.

Safeguarding Patients' Autonomy

Safeguarding patients' autonomy is the first core attribute. It requires respecting and promoting each patient's right to self-determination, except in those situations when the patient is incompetent to decide or does not wish to be involved in decision making (see Focus on Diversity and Culture: Patient Autonomy). Safeguarding the autonomy of a patient includes specific actions that both respect and promote the patient's ability to make healthcare decisions. For the patient to be able to exercise autonomy, two assumptions must be made. First, the patient holds primary responsibility for their own health and decision making and, second, the patient is legally competent to make healthcare decisions. The patient will likely need information to reach an informed decision; however, for this core attribute to apply, the patient's competency to decide cannot be in question (Bu & Jezewski, 2007). Examples of effective nursing actions that safeguard patients' autonomy include (Bu & Jezewski, 2007):

- Encouraging patients to share and document their goals, preferences, values, and beliefs
- Supporting patient values and choices even when they conflict with those of individual HCPs
- Providing patients with sufficient, timely information for making informed decisions about healthcare, ensuring a match between patients' health information literacy and the information provided.

Focus on Diversity and Culture

Patient Autonomy

Patient control over health decisions is a Western view that is not necessarily accepted in other cultures. In other societies, such as the Hmong population, health decisions may be made by the head of the family, a member of the community, or a religious leader. Some Hmong families traditionally make their healthcare decisions depending on how they classify their illness based on symptoms (for example, whether the cause is physical or spiritual) and their beliefs about the effectiveness of Western or traditional treatment for the problem (Lor et al., 2017). For women in traditional Vietnamese cultures, beliefs about susceptibility to breast cancer were found to depend on their beliefs about taking care of themselves, and beliefs about whether malignant breast lumps should be painful or actively growing was shown to affect the stage at which breast cancers in this population were identified (Kim, Hong, Lee, Ferrans, & Kim, 2019). The nurse must respect the patient's and family's views and honor their traditions regarding healthcare decision making. Even within the United States, a variety of cultures and traditions may practice healthcare customs that are unfamiliar to the nurse. In cultures such as Appalachia, fatalistic beliefs are common and affect the likelihood that people will receive preventive care. For example, there are complex factors contributing to why Appalachian women are less likely to complete a full human papillomavirus (HPV) vaccine series, or get them for their daughters, and therefore have higher rates of cervical cancer. These include low socioeconomic status and inadequate access to health care, inadequate social supports, and a variety of high-risk behaviors (Paskett et al., 2020). The ethics of advocacy require that the nurse honor the patient's and family's values, preferences, expressed needs, and right to self-determination.

Acting on Behalf of Patients

The second core attribute consists of acting on behalf of patients. When patients are unable to act on their own behalf, or do not wish to represent themselves in the decision-making process, a series of advocacy actions can both preserve and represent the patient's values, benefits, and rights. Examples of situations in which this core attribute applies includes periods during which patients are under anesthesia/sedation or when patients make a conscious choice to have an advocate act on their behalf. Acting on behalf of patients differs from safeguarding patient autonomy, and the two do not conflict because the nurse is advocating for patients who are in very different circumstances (Bu & Jezewski, 2007). If a patient lacks decision-making capacity (e.g., the patient with advanced dementia or the unconscious patient), is legally incompetent, or is a minor, a designated healthcare surrogate or legal guardian is usually appointed to act on the patient's behalf (see Module 49, Legal Issues, for more information).

Examples of advocacy interventions in which the nurse acts on behalf of patients include (Bu & Jezewski, 2007):

- Monitoring the quality and safety of healthcare delivered to the patient
- Taking action to intervene if the nurse has information that a treatment or intervention may violate the patient's wishes, directives, or best interests, when appropriate
- Expressing patients' wishes when they cannot do so for themselves (for example, during procedures requiring anesthesia/sedation)
- Ensuring that patients who are incompetent to make autonomous decisions have appropriate legal representation (for example, power of attorney or guardianship).

Championing Social Justice in Healthcare

Championing social justice in the provision of healthcare is the third core attribute of advocacy. This attribute is based on the ethics of justice (see Module 44, Ethics). Whereas the first two core attributes represent nursing advocacy at the microsocial level (i.e., working with individual patients), this core attribute represents nursing advocacy at the macrosocial level. This attribute calls for nurses to become involved in matters of health, education, and welfare related to the patients they serve in their organizations, community, or the larger society (Bu & Jezewski, 2007). This attribute could be actualized at the committee level in the nurse's organization, or the nurse might become active in a professional association, for example by serving on a legislative committee. Examples of advocacy actions related to championing social justice in healthcare include (Bu & Jezewski, 2007):

- Helping individual patients achieve healthcare goals by mobilizing resources available in the agency and/or community
- Acting on behalf of patients at policy and legislative levels, both within the agency and at the local, state, or federal level, or by advocating to eliminate disparities in any area of healthcare.

Empowering the Patient

The patient–HCP relationship has historically been characterized as paternalistic, with the physician or provider generally guiding decision making. However, the cultural ethic in Western healthcare has shifted toward patient-centered care. A patient-centered focus questions the effectiveness of a biomedical approach to care and links the concept of patient-centeredness to patient empowerment (Palumbo, 2019). As this shift has occurred, many definitions of patient empowerment have emerged. Palumbo (2019) synthesizes these perspectives, indicating that patient empowerment can be "understood as a relational—rather than an individual—construct . . . between the patients and the healthcare providers and relies on the commitment of both parties to implement a patient-centered approach to care" (p. 3). The advancement of patient empowerment is beneficial for patients, health professionals, and the healthcare system. Patient empowerment is particularly needed for patients with chronic disease because of the important links between self-management and integrated HCP support (European Patients Forum [EPF], 2017). The EPF created a framework called Empowering Patients in the Management of Chronic Diseases (EMPATHIE), which identifies five aspects of empowerment:

1. Self-efficacy
2. Self-awareness
3. Confidence
4. Coping skills
5. Health literacy.

The idea of patient partnership and empowerment is seen as a way to improve care and outcomes and reduce healthcare costs (EPF, 2017; Lian et al., 2018). For example, a long-term patient empowerment program for patients with type 2 diabetes projected healthcare cost savings over the long term (Lian et al., 2018). More importantly, self-management partnerships support patient confidence and self-efficacy, as well as daily life skills and improved healthcare outcomes. Tools and methods that support patient empowerment programs (Gomez-Velasco et al., 2019) include:

- *Booklets or manuals.* Printed and/or digital patient education materials focused on disease management.
- *Cell phone calls.* Direct communication or short text-messaging can facilitate patient care and monitoring and adherence to medication use, as well as to provide support and guidance.
- *Software.* Software programs have been developed that are specific for chronic disease monitoring using access to real-time information via the use of smartphones.
- *Mobile apps.* Clinical evaluation using apps for chronic disease self-care shows promise.
- *Telemedicine/telehealth.* Telehealth has been shown to help participants establish a self-care plan and set health goals.

These tools can help ensure that patients have the information they need and a connection to their HCPs. They are especially applicable to nursing because the nurse often has more opportunity to be present with patients when they need time, conversation, and empathy. An additional way for nurses to foster patient empowerment is by assisting patients to cultivate responsibility for their own health. Reminding patients that they are at the center of their own care may help them regain a sense of control. Educating patients about responsible and safe avenues for support can also promote patient empowerment; for example, an online support group for adolescents with cancer operated by a hospital may assist in promoting patient empowerment through social media. Using these strategies to empower patients to navigate healthcare decision making will help build a nurse–patient relationship of mutual respect, trust, and confidence.

Collaborating with Other Healthcare Providers

Given the complexity of healthcare systems, collaborating with other providers on the healthcare team as a way to advocate for patients' needs has developed on a global scale. In its seminal report *Framework for Action on Interprofessional Education and Collaborative Practice,* the World Health Organization (2010) discussed the countless benefits of collaborative practice, including greater collaborative decision making with patients. The Interprofessional Education Collaborative Expert Panel (2011) defines the concept of interprofessionality as "the process by which professionals reflect on and develop ways of practicing that provide an integrated and cohesive answer to the needs of the patient/population . . . . [I]t involves continuous interaction and knowledge sharing between professionals . . . to solve or explore a variety of . . . care issues all while seeking to optimize the patient's participation" (D'amour & Oandasan, 2005, p. 8). Interagency and interprofessional collaborations, as described in Module 37, Collaboration, are essential to making healthcare services work for patients. In some cases, collaboration with advocacy programs can result in additional avenues of instructional, emotional, and financial support for patients. For example, the National Alliance on Mental Illness (NAMI; www.nami.org) comprises hundreds of local affiliates and state organizations. NAMI (2020) provides support for individuals with mental illness and their families, including education, awareness, and advocacy, to promote solutions for the nation's mental health crisis and advances for mental health research.

Advocacy Programs

The federal government encourages states to develop advocacy programs to serve as a resource regarding the rights of those with mental illness or disability. Each state designates an agency or group to advocate for the rights of those with mental illness or disability and to investigate reported incidents involving neglect and abuse of these vulnerable patients in public or private mental health treatment settings, research facilities, and nursing homes. For example, Disability Rights North Carolina (www.disabilityrightsnc.org) is a federally mandated nonprofit organization charged with protecting the rights of children and adults with disabilities living in North Carolina. Another example, Disability Rights Ohio (www.disabilityrightsohio.org), a nonprofit corporation, is a federally mandated Protection and Advisory System for Individuals with Mental Illness (PAIMI).

The U.S. military has been faced with a number of health policy challenges and subsequently has instituted advocacy measures for veterans and active-duty personnel. Military personnel are at high risk for developing mental health conditions, including posttraumatic stress disorder (PTSD). Those at risk for PTSD include individuals who have experienced deployment for long periods of time associated with extreme combat conditions. The Psychological Health Center for Excellence (2007) developed baseline pre-deployment mental health standards for military personnel, and also post-deployment assessment screening standards, so persons at risk can be appropriately referred for treatment. These standards persist, and updated general recommendations for assessment of this complex health problem have been published as evidence emerges (Dutra, Hayes, & Keane, 2019). Nurses working with military personnel, veterans, or others at risk for PTSD should be aware of these standards and recommendations as well as other related standards, benefits, and interventions available to these patients.

>> **Stay Current:** The U.S. Department of Veterans Affairs and the Department of Defense publish clinical guidelines for the management of PTSD and acute stress reaction. These can be found at https://www.healthquality.va.gov/guidelines/MH/ptsd/.

Professional and Public Advocacy

Professional nursing organizations, such as the American Nurses Association, advocate at the state and national levels for the profession of nursing, for its members, and for those who benefit from the services nurses provide. Professional organizations are discussed in Module 47, Health Policy.

As advocates, nurses are in a position to promote and effect change. They need to understand the ethical issues in nursing and healthcare and to have an understanding of state and federal laws and regulations affecting nursing practice and the health of society.

Nurses may advocate as individuals speaking on their own behalf, or they may be asked to speak as a representative of their professional association. There are multiple and varied opportunities to speak publicly for the health, welfare, and safety of patients; to take steps to protect patient rights; to inform the public about issues and concerns by writing articles for the popular press; to lobby state legislators or congressional representatives on behalf of better healthcare for all people; and to run for political office. Gains made by nursing in developing and improving health policy at the organizational, institutional, and governmental levels help to achieve better healthcare for the public.

Advocating for Children and Families

To be an effective advocate for children and families, the nurse must be aware of the child's and family's needs, the family's resources, and the available healthcare options. The nurse should ensure that the family has adequate information about treatment options and that information is provided at a level matched with their health literacy and appropriate to the child's level of understanding. Treatment options should be in accord with the family's values and resources. Collaboration with other members of the healthcare team is essential, particularly if the family situation is complex, the healthcare issue has significant consequences, or the family's resources are minimal. If the nurse has the best information about these factors from the child/family point of view, communicating this information to the HCP and any other member of the healthcare team involved in the child's care is essential. The nurse can then play an important role in assisting the family and the child to make informed decisions and to act in the child's best interests. As an advocate for the child and family, the nurse must also intervene to prevent any potential or real harm during planning or treatment and must follow through in whatever way is most appropriate and matched to the situation.

Ensuring that the policies and resources of healthcare organizations meet the psychosocial needs of children and their families is also a part of nursing's role. For example, membership on a committee that develops policies or evidence-based practice guidelines, or a team planning modernization of the healthcare facility design, allows the nurse to contribute knowledge of the developmental and psychosocial needs of children that can help ensure that the organization addresses the needs of children and families (**Figure 43-2** »).

Table 43-1 » lists some examples of how nurses can advocate for children and families in their community.

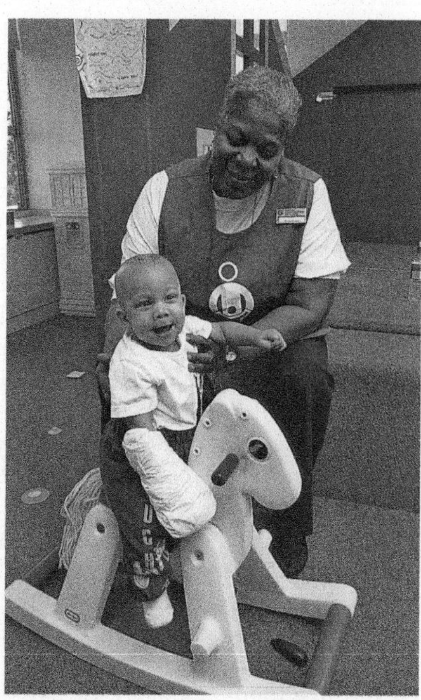

Figure 43.2 » Nurses must be aware of the needs of pediatric patients for play time and advocate for children to have play time as well as rest time and appropriate nutrition. Here, a volunteer grandmother plays with a young boy to provide stimulation and nurturing during his lengthy hospitalization.

Source: Pearson Education, Inc.

TABLE 43-1 Advocating for Children and Families

Health Need Example	Nurse Advocacy Actions
Members of the community need information about places to obtain immunizations.	■ Make a list of agencies that provide immunizations, including those with low-cost immunizations through the Vaccines for Children program. ■ Obtain financial assistance from a local foundation to print your findings. ■ Make copies available in child care centers and other community agencies.
A local homeless shelter has little in the way of self-care amenities for its clients.	■ Obtain donations of hotel-sized lotions, soaps, and shampoos from classmates and faculty that can be given to the shelter. ■ Visit several local hotels and ask if they will each donate a box of small toiletries for the residents. ■ Encourage volunteers to provide haircuts and styling or obtain donations to provide this service.
Your state has a law protecting the rights of any woman to bring her unwanted newborn baby to certain sites for the purpose of giving up her child without legal recriminations. Because many women do not know about the law, babies are abandoned in unsafe locations.	■ Find a local newspaper reporter who is willing to write an article about the law. ■ Run off copies of the article to distribute. ■ Make posters with necessary information for several community sites and the emergency department.

Source: Ball, J. W., Bindler, R. C., & Cowen, K. J. (2014). *Child health nursing: Partnering with children and families* (3rd ed.) (p. 336, Table 8–3). Prentice Hall. Pearson Education, Inc., Hoboken, NJ.

Advocating for Vulnerable Populations

Vulnerable populations generally include groups who are at greater risk for disease, disability, and reduced lifespan because of a lack of resources, risk factors, or a combination of these. These groups often include underserved populations, such as low-income seniors, younger persons with either physical or mental health–related disabilities, and individuals with limited English proficiency. Many older individuals in vulnerable groups are considered "dual eligible," in that they are enrolled in both Medicare and Medicaid programs. These individuals—who consist of the sickest and poorest patients, with higher rates of diabetes, pulmonary disease, stroke, mental health disorders, and Alzheimer disease—must navigate both government programs to access needed services. In fiscal year 2018, 12.2 million individuals were classified as "dual eligible" (Centers for Medicare and Medicaid Services, 2020). Strategies to ensure these vulnerable populations have access to healthcare services have been a concern of the American Hospital Association (2020) and a number of other organizations.

An additional category of vulnerable populations is patients who serve as research subjects. The National Institutes of Health (2019) has established vulnerable research subjects categories. These include pregnant women, human fetuses and neonates, children, and prisoners. Nurses are strong advocates for all vulnerable populations, both those in their care and those who are the subjects of healthcare research.

In the 21st century there is a need for new energy and political activism to ensure that the needs and the rights of individuals representing vulnerable populations are not overlooked. Advances in science, technology, and evidence-based practice continue to revolutionize how nurses practice (**Figure 43-3** »), and nurses must continue to advocate for fair and equitable access to high-quality care for all patients in a variety of settings, including acute care, free clinics, and primary care and specialty practices.

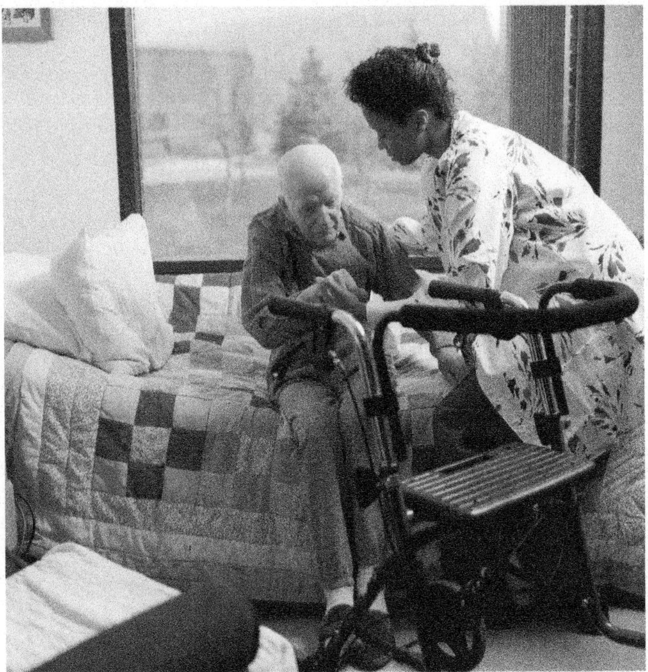

Figure 43.3 » Patients in long-term care facilities are often unable to advocate for themselves. Nurses should advocate for these individuals in many areas, including effective pain control.
Source: Stockbyte/Getty Images.

Clinical Example A

Lois Potter is a 78-year-old woman with hypertension and heart disease who is a longstanding patient at her primary care clinic. Today the nurse practitioner (NP) spoke with Mrs. Potter about her lab values. Her hemoglobin A_1c, which they have been monitoring over time with concern, shows that she has developed type 2 diabetes mellitus. The NP has prescribed miglitol, an alpha-glucosidase inhibitor. The nurse completing Mrs. Potter's discharge notes that Mrs. Potter is also taking digoxin to manage her heart disease and amlodipine for her hypertension. The nurse also notes that the NP has made no changes in her digoxin regimen. The NP has moved on to another patient's room and is unavailable for a consultation, and Mrs. Potter's cab has come to pick her up. The case management team will be meeting later this morning, and the nurse is a part of that interprofessional team meeting.

Critical Thinking Questions

1. What is the best first step for the nurse to take with regard to managing Mrs. Potter's medication regimen?
2. What information should the nurse communicate during the case management team meeting? How should she involve the NP? Which other team members should be a part of this collaborative conversation?
3. How can the nurse advocate for the patient in a way that ensures Mrs. Potter's medication safety? Can this be done using a collaborative, interprofessional team approach? How?

Two federal laws ensure the rights of individuals with disabilities. The Patient Self-Determination Act (PSDA) was enacted in 1991 to require healthcare institutions to inform patients of their healthcare decision-making rights and an institution's policies regarding recognition of advance directives. This law provided general protection rights to all patients, including those with disabilities (see Module 49, Legal Issues, for more information about the PSDA). Additionally, the Americans with Disabilities Act (ADA), first enacted in 1990, is a civil rights law that ensures people with disabilities have the same rights as everyone else. It prohibits discrimination against individuals by providing federal protection to those with physical and/or mental health disabilities in areas of public life such as employment, schools, transportation, and both public and private places open to the general public. The law was amended January 1, 2009, significantly updating the definition of "disability" (ADA National Network, 2020).

Clinical Example B

Ms. Donna Taylor is a 60-year-old woman who has a longstanding diagnosis of major depressive disorder. For the past few years, her depression has been well controlled on the antidepressant and dosage she takes now. One day at home, Ms. Taylor experiences confusion, is staring into space, is unable to answer questions or speak, and is making unusual movements. Her husband takes her to the emergency room, where it is determined she has had a seizure. The emergency department physician wants to rule out epilepsy. She will need a more extensive neurologic workup but pending that, the ED physician has written an order for Ms. Taylor to take antiseizure medication until she can meet with a neurologist. When he reviews her medication history, he sees that the antidepressant she has been taking will interact with the medication he is prescribing. The ED physician looks at Ms. Taylor and says, "You will need to discontinue your antidepressant so you can take this antiseizure medication." When the nurse enters to facilitate

Ms. Taylor's discharge, she tells the nurse about the instructions to discontinue her antidepressant, and while she is concerned about the seizure, she is even more concerned about any returning depression symptoms.

Critical Thinking Questions

1. How should the nurse respond to Ms. Taylor?
2. If you were Ms. Taylor's nurse, what would be the most appropriate way to advocate with the physician on her behalf? Explain your answer.
3. Who else on the healthcare team could you collaborate with to be sure Ms. Taylor gets the care she needs?

Nurses should be aware of the rights of individuals with disabilities: congenital, physical, and intellectual disabilities. The prevalence of individuals with disabilities is staggering, and it crosses the lifespan. Seventy percent of students in public schools who are secluded or physically restrained have disabilities, and 60% of individuals in jail have some type of mental disability. In addition, these individuals are socioeconomically disadvantaged; 48% have a personal annual income of $15,000 or less (American Civil Liberties Union, 2020).

Individuals with mental health issues are particularly vulnerable to abuse and neglect, either in their communities or in mental health settings that provide substandard care. The nurse's role is to advocate for the person's physical, sexual, and emotional safety, both in the community setting, during institutionalization, or during a short-stay admission or outpatient visit. Their personal rights include (Disability Rights of Ohio, 2020):

- The right to safety with people they know, including family, staff, and strangers.
- The right to be respected and treated with dignity.
- The right to have or not have a sexual relationship, including the right to permit or deny another person's touch.
- The right to control their money and possessions, such as cigarettes and clothing.
- The right to treatment in a place that respects their freedom and includes a current, written treatment plan that the patient participated in creating.
- The right to freedom from pharmacologic or physical restraint, seclusion, or isolation, except in an emergency.
- The right to refuse or accept a suggested medication. In most states, psychiatric facilities cannot force patients to take medication except in an emergency.
- The right to exercise these rights without punishment, withholding of treatment, loss of privileges, or physical/emotional abuse.

In addition:

- Institutionalization does not change a person's basic rights as a citizen under the U.S. Constitution. These include voting rights, free speech, and freedom from unreasonable search.
- The right to a living space that provides reasonable protection from harm, including physical or emotional abuse and the use of overmedication or excessive restraint.

Clinical Example C

Mr. William Johnson is a 53-year-old patient being seen in the outpatient clinic for treatment of an acute exacerbation of chronic bronchitis related to his chronic obstructive pulmonary disease (COPD). He is also being treated for schizophrenia. He takes the medication he receives from the clinic because he wants his symptoms to remain under control, but he doesn't like the side effects. Mr. Johnson has been a smoker for 40 years and has no intention of stopping. He is currently living with several other men in a supportive housing program, and he has an entry-level job at a local fast-food restaurant. Mr. Johnson has been disciplined by his generally understanding employer several times for behavior issues, but during his examination he tells you he fears being sent back to the mental health facility. On his last admission, the night staff who had treated him well during past admissions had been replaced by two new psychiatric technicians. When the nurse was on another unit, one of them restrained Mr. Johnson in his bed when he refused to share his cigarettes with him.

Critical Thinking Questions

1. How is this action by the psychiatric technician a violation of Mr. Johnson's rights?
2. What is the nurse's next step in advocating for Mr. Johnson?
3. Is this an example of advocacy at the level of the individual patient, at the community/policy level, or both?

Although laws protect basic healthcare rights and those of the disabled, miscommunication among providers and patients, as well as medical error, may still occur. Even when the letter of the law is followed, the spirit of the law may not be satisfied, particularly when working with patients with disabilities. For example, even if a patient reads and signs an informed consent document, comprehension of the information may be incomplete or absent. Nurses are often in a position to ensure that the procedures for procuring informed consent conform to both the letter and spirit of the law, particularly in the matter of patients with mental disabilities severe enough that capacity is questionable or incompetency has been determined. In these cases, the patient's guardian or an individual with durable power of attorney should be present and engaged in the informed consent process on the patient's behalf. Note that the nurse may not legally serve in that role; to do so would be considered a conflict of interest and could result in consequences for both the nurse and the organization. However, nurses are uniquely sensitive to the complex biopsychosocial issues involved in coping with disabilities and should be able to advocate for these patients as they navigate the healthcare system. If the nurse discovers that the patient is not competent to make healthcare decisions, and no durable power of attorney is on record, the nurse should contact the healthcare provider, as well as social services, to ensure that the appropriate next steps occur.

Advocacy Interventions

Novice nurses need to understand their employing organization's policies, appreciate the legal implications of their actions, and carefully consider options before advocating on behalf of patients. In addition, it is essential that nurses anticipate patients' advocacy needs. A rapid assessment can reveal the extent of patients' understanding of their health problem, plan of care, health literacy, support system, and coping ability *in that moment*. Then the nurse can plan initial advocacy interventions accordingly. Interventions must safeguard patients, but action must also be taken in context. In designing and conducting advocacy interventions, it is important to:

- Assess the patient's ability to cooperate and to make decisions.
- Assess the reliability of information provided *by the patient*, with regard to health history and family situation, especially if the patient exhibits impairment of cognitive function or mental instability. When necessary, engage family members as partners or, if appropriate, ensure the presence of the guardian or person with durable power of attorney.

Specific advocacy interventions may include:

- Educating patients and families about their legal rights regarding informed decision making
- Ensuring patients have a voice in their care and are intentionally engaged in shared decision making with all providers involved in their care
- Ensuring that patients have the necessary information to give informed consent
- Monitoring patients' care to safeguard patient rights
- Evaluating organizational policies and procedures to ensure protection of patient rights
- Intervening if other healthcare professionals provide care that does not consider the patient's stated preferences and values or does not engage the patient in decision making (if the patient is competent to decide).

Concepts Related to Advocacy

Nurses must take many other concepts into consideration when advocating for their patients. Examples include ethics, legal issues, professional behaviors, culture and diversity, and healthcare systems.

As stated earlier, the nurse's role as an advocate is based in nursing codes of ethics. Ethics and morals are related; morals are the principles on which judgments about right or wrong are based from a personal point of view. The role of the advocate is to uphold nursing's ethical principles.

Legal issues encompass the rights, responsibilities, and scope of nursing practice as expressed in national standards of care, state practice acts, and associated rules (regulations). All patients have the right to expect safe, effective, competent nursing practice.

Patients have the right to exercise their individual cultural beliefs and values and to have their unique health needs met. Nurses who advocate for culturally competent care, both in specific individual situations and in everyday practice, help ensure that patients' cultural beliefs, values, and needs are respected. In turn, this increases patient satisfaction with care and promotes the therapeutic relationship.

Access to healthcare remains challenging to millions of Americans. In many rural settings, for example, access to specialty care and quality mental healthcare is limited. Nurses who work in areas or with patient populations with limited access can advocate for their patients or region by seeking ways to collaborate with other agencies, advocating for increased funding from their local legislators, and advocating for affordable alternatives, such as telemedicine, as ways to improve and promote patient access to healthcare.

The nurse's duty to advocate on behalf of patients requires careful collaboration in the form of clear and continuous communication with the patient, family members, and other healthcare professionals on the decision-making team. It is important to remember to balance the role and duty of advocacy "watchdog" with an attitude of teamwork when it comes to working alongside other professionals on the healthcare team. For example, a busy consulting physician may engage a patient in a one-on-one discussion about a treatment option and obtain written informed consent, unaware that the patient was recently medicated with an opioid drug to manage pain and is having difficulty both concentrating and remembering. The nurse's role would be to inform the physician and together with the physician decide whether a family member of the patient's choice should be present for a rescheduled conversation, wait until such time as the effects of the opioid did not affect decision making, or both. Regardless, a time for the physician to repeat the conversation should be scheduled, and the consent form signed again. The nurse would document the facts in the patient's record. The duty of advocacy is then fulfilled, the patient's rights safeguarded, and a collaborative nurse–physician relationship established or advanced.

Patients with alterations in cellular regulation, especially any type of cancer, need strong advocates. At the microsocial level, nurses help ensure that patients have access to necessary treatments and services and that patients' holistic needs are met. For example, nurses working with children with cancer advocate that they have access to playtime and help their families find ways to continue their schooling. At the macrosocial level, nurses may find themselves advocating through professional organizations for increased funding or may advocate at their agency level for play areas that can accommodate pets.

Patients with alterations in mobility, particularly those who depend on the use of mobility assistive equipment, also need strong advocates. At the microsocial level, nurses ensure that patients have access to the equipment and devices they need, and accompanying treatments, services, and personnel who can assist them with activities of daily living, if necessary. Nurses can advocate for affiliate home healthcare agencies to ensure that the patient's home environment is safe relative to their mobility limitations. At the macrosocial level, nurses may advocate through their professional associations to increase funding for research and care for mobility-related health issues, or work with community organizations to ensure accessibility to public places is accommodated. The Concepts Related to Advocacy feature links some, but not all, of the concepts integral to advocacy. They are presented in alphabetical order.

Unethical or Unsafe Practice or Unprofessional Conduct

Nurses have a legal responsibility to intervene on behalf of any patient if they have reason to believe that another professional is engaging in practice that is unethical, unsafe, substandard, or unprofessional. State nurse practice acts

Concepts Related to Advocacy

CONCEPT	RELATIONSHIP TO ADVOCACY	NURSING IMPLICATIONS
Cellular Regulation	↑ Advocacy → ↑ awareness of individual and global needs as well as ↑ funding for research and treatment needs	■ Nurses advocate for system- and community-wide changes that address discriminatory practices in health care. They also advocate for programs that reduce social disparities of health (such as increased access to affordable, healthy foods) to reduce healthcare disparities and improve overall health of patients. ■ Nurses advocate for services for cancer patients or funding for cancer research.
Culture and Diversity	By advocating for patients' cultural and religious preferences, nurses ↑ patient satisfaction with care, promoting the therapeutic relationship.	■ The nurse practices culturally competent care by respecting each unique patient's values and advocating for patient rights to such care provided by healthcare organizations and providers. ■ Nursing advocates should respect the patient's diversity and promote equity of care.
Ethics	Ethics → advocacy, ↑ patient safety and autonomy	■ Nurses have an obligation to intervene and advocate when ethical dilemmas arise. The nurse should call ethical dilemmas to the attention of the HCP, the healthcare team, and the organization's ethics committee, as necessary and appropriate. ■ The nurse protects patients' right to make choices about care and to refuse treatment.
Healthcare Systems	Vulnerable patients experience ↑ barriers to access and ↑ challenges and discrimination.	■ The nurse should support patients by advocating for their right to access and receive equitable care in the healthcare system.
Legal Issues	Nurses who advocate ↑ patient safety and autonomy ↓ risk for negligence or error, ↑ trust in the profession.	■ The nurse-advocate should uphold the rights of patients in any situation and also monitor the care provided by other professionals caring for patients. The nurse is obligated to report any unethical or illegal behavior by another nurse, HCP, or other staff member.
Mobility	Advocacy is necessary to improve patient and caregiver understanding, ↓ risk for further injury or immobility, ↑ patient and caregiver quality of life.	■ Nurses advocate for patient access to appropriate care, mobility devices, and live in mobility-restricted safe environments. For example, the nurse may advocate for a person of short stature to receive an appropriately sized walker. ■ Nurses may advocate at the national, state, or community level for patients with mobility limitations (e.g., for research funding, public place accessibility).
Professional Behaviors	By acting professionally, nurses ↑ their credibility, thereby ↑ opportunities and chances for successful advocacy.	■ The nurse should continuously advocate for patients as a component of the professional scope of practice. ■ The nurse-advocate should act in accordance with professional and ethical standards.

include sections regulating the actions of the nurse in this regard, as well as reporting requirements. However, if the professional in question is not a nurse, the nurse should still intervene to safeguard the patient. The nurse who needs to intervene to protect a patient follows established agency or facility reporting procedures, but the first step is to notify the nurse's own direct supervisor—the person to whom the nurse reports directly. That individual can be essential in assisting the nurse who discovered the breach of conduct and in facilitating the reporting procedure. That person is also the nurse's resource if immediate assistance is needed to stop an unsafe practice before harm is done to the patient.

Common examples of unethical or unsafe conduct that requires nurses to advocate with one another or on behalf of a patient include boundary violations and nurses or team members working under the influence of drugs or alcohol. Boundary violations, such as engaging in an inappropriate relationship with a patient or coercing or restraining a patient to benefit the professional in some way (as in Clinical Example B in this module), are ethical issues that may be addressed by a state board of nursing. Both state nurse practice acts and the ANA Code of Ethics require nurses to report unethical nurse behaviors, including boundary violations.

Impairment of a coworker or team member is the most commonly encountered situation that combines unethical, unsafe, and unprofessional conduct. Impairment to practice may be the effect of a substance—legal, illegal, prescription, or over-the-counter. Impairment to practice safely may also result from extreme emotional distress (for example, a nurse who returns to work too soon following the death of a close family member). Because impairment has the potential to interfere with safe clinical practice, the nurse who observes or suspects impairment in any other health professional, nurse or non-nurse, is obligated to immediately report to a supervisor (ANA, 2015a). For more information, including warning signs that indicate impairment, please see the section Impaired Nurses in Module 22, Addiction.

A growing concern in healthcare regulation is the violation of a patient's privacy related to the inappropriate use of social and electronic media by HCPs. Nurses must consider confidentiality and privacy laws, patients' rights to be treated with dignity and respect, and trust as a foundation for nurse–patient relationships. Whether or not a post was an unintentional or nonmalicious act, posting confidential information about patients, including any health-related facts, conversations, or photographs, constitutes a breach of privacy. Such action may subject a nurse to disciplinary action by both the employing institution and the state board of nursing. In addition, the nurse may be subject to civil and criminal penalties (National Council of State Boards of Nursing, 2018). It is important that nurses work with their colleagues to keep one another attuned to the inappropriateness of using social media in this way; advocate for patient privacy and protection; if aware, report infractions; and always act in the best interest of the patient.

REVIEW The Concept of Advocacy

RELATE Link the Concepts

Linking the concept of advocacy with the concept of culture and diversity:

1. Consider each of the groups included within the description of vulnerable populations and provide examples of how the nurse can advocate for each.
2. Why might patients with values and beliefs that differ from the mainstream population require greater efforts with regard to advocacy?

Linking the concept of advocacy with the concept of ethics:

3. How does the ANA Code of Ethics (ANA, 2015a) address advocacy? Under what circumstances might a nurse experience conflict of interest when advocating for a patient? Is the nurse the sole HCP taking on the advocacy role, that is, how do nurses balance the unique contributions of the profession with the team approach?
4. Differentiate between the nurse's role of advocate for individuals who are temporarily unable to speak for themselves (such as persons who are intubated) versus the role of advocate for those who are competent to speak for themselves but, for whatever reason, do not.

Linking the concept of advocacy with the concept of legal issues:

5. What is the nurse's advocacy role when caring for a patient who is not competent to make healthcare decisions? Provide examples of other members of the healthcare team or organization who could be helpful in ensuring that the patient's advocacy needs are met.
6. How does the nurse practice act in your state address reporting of unethical or unsafe practice or boundary violations (such as posting patient healthcare information on social media). Is the reporting requirement for nurses, employers, or both?

REFER Go to Pearson MyLab Nursing and eText

REFLECT Apply Your Knowledge

Heather Adams is a neighbor in your apartment building. On weekends, you sometimes get together for morning coffee. Last weekend, Ms. Adams shared a concern that has been troubling her for a while. She is 31 years old and unmarried, and she lives alone. Her father is deceased, and her mother, who was diagnosed with Alzheimer disease several years ago, is now a resident in a long-term care facility for people with cognitive impairments. Ms. Adams is estranged from her only brother. When she was in her early 20s, she was hospitalized and treated for depression. Ms. Adams's fear is that, should she become incapacitated again with depression, the brother with whom she does not get along will make treatment decisions as her next of kin.

You have decided to invite Ms. Adams for coffee. Because Ms. Adams seems to be an individual who would benefit from a healthcare power of attorney, your intent is to have a conversation with her about her choices.

1. On what basis do you act as an advocate for Ms. Adams (i.e., as a neighbor/friend or as her nurse)?
2. Would it be ethical for you to serve as the surrogate decision maker? Explain your answer.
3. In your discussion with Ms. Adams, should you encourage her to see an attorney? Explain your answer.

» Exemplar 43.A Environmental Quality

Exemplar Learning Outcomes

43.A Analyze the health indicator of environmental quality as it relates to advocacy.

- Outline the components of environmental quality.
- Summarize the major impacts of environmental quality on public health.
- Describe community responses to alterations in environmental quality.
- Explain the nurse's role in advocating for patients affected by environmental quality.

Exemplar Key Terms

Environmental health hazards, *2725*
Environmental quality, *2725*

Overview

Environmental quality is one of the 12 leading health indicators published in *Healthy People 2020*. Its effect on health status is direct. For example, premature death, cancer, and long-term damage to respiratory and cardiovascular systems are all linked to poor air quality (Office of Disease Prevention and Health Promotion [ODPHP], 2020). **Environmental health hazards** include natural or human-made substances, states, or events that affect the natural environment, produce negative effects on the human ecosphere, and adversely affect health. Air and water pollution are two common environmental health issues; the data regarding exposure is staggering. *Healthy People 2020* reported that approximately 127 million people in the United States live in counties where air pollution exceeds national air quality standards (ODPHP, 2020). Furthermore, most recent data indicate that two out of every five children (approximately 40%) ages 3 to 11 living in the United States are exposed to secondhand smoke regularly (Centers for Disease Control and Prevention [CDC], 2018b). These issues and many others affect the health of citizens in the United States and globally; the actions of nurse-advocates focused on environmental quality can have profound effects.

Classification of Environmental Hazards

Both *Healthy People* and the CDC address environmental quality and its determinants differently; together, these topic categories provide an overview of the breadth of environmental factors that affect the nation's health. These lists are provided in **Table 43-2** ».

Two common environmental health hazards are air and water pollution (CDC, 2019a, 2019b). A key factor in air pollution is the level of ground-level ozone, which is a component of smog. Ground-level ozone is often responsible for increases in emergency department visits and hospitalizations for individuals with health problems associated with diminished lung function, such as asthma and COPD. Individuals at higher risk are those who live in geographic areas where ground-level ozone is likely to form at greater levels; contributing factors include heat, concentrations of precursor chemicals, methane emissions, wildfire emissions, and air stagnation (CDC, 2019a). Individuals at high risk in high-ozone geographic areas include those with diminished lung function who are also socioeconomically disadvantaged (e.g., those who lack air conditioning during high ground-level ozone times or who lack health insurance), older adults, children, or those with comorbidities.

TABLE 43-2 Selected Determinants of Environmental Quality and Environmental Health

Healthy People 2020 Determinants of Environmental Quality[1]	CDC National Center for Environmental Health: Environmental Health Topics (selected/combined)[2]
■ Improving air and water quality ■ Decreasing mental health stresses ■ Strengthening the social fabric of a community ■ Providing fair access to employment opportunities, education, and resources ■ Increasing options for physical activity and healthful diets ■ Decreasing injuries and accidents	■ Air quality, water quality, environmental chemical exposure ■ Carbon monoxide poisoning ■ Childhood lead poisoning prevention ■ Climate and health ■ Emergency response ■ Food safety; nutritional indicators ■ Laboratory quality assurance ■ Natural disasters ■ Newborn screening laboratory bulletin

[1] Based on HealthyPeople.gov. (2020). *Environmental quality.* https://www.healthypeople.gov/2020/leading-health-indicators/2020-lhi-topics/Environmental-Quality/determinants

[2] Adapted from Centers for Disease Control and Prevention (CDC). (2020). *National Center for Environmental Health.* https://www.cdc.gov/nceh/default.htm

Water pollution is also a concern. Local water supplies may be contaminated by environmental pollutants in water sources; healthy water may also be limited by drought and aquifer depletion, flooding events that overwhelm treatment plant capacity, natural disasters, and other factors (CDC, 2016).

The Effects of Environmental Quality on Public Health

A number of public health problems can be linked to exposure to environmental hazards, including asthma, congenital disabilities, heat stress illness, poor reproductive and birth outcomes, lead poisoning, heart disease, cancer, carbon monoxide poisoning, and developmental disabilities. Three of the most common health effects related to environmental hazards, and their associated environmental links, are shown in **Table 43-3** ».

Community Responses to Environmental Issues

A community's citizens are directly affected by local, national, and global environmental issues. One way for citizens to respond is to be empowered to make positive change and become active regarding one or more environmental issues that affect them directly. Communities can serve as activists locally in municipalities or join larger communities to make a larger impact. For example, the Natural Resources Defense Council (NRDC), a global group of more than 3 million online activists, including scientists, lawyers, and policy advocates, work to safeguard air, water, and natural systems. The NRDC helped pass the Clean Water Act in the 1970s. The organization identifies six priorities for keeping water clean, including (1) water pollution, (2) healthy rivers and ecosystems, (3) water-smart farms, (4) water-smart cities, (5) climate adaptation, and (6) safe drinking water. For the general public, they publish easy tricks that save water (NRDC, 2020b). These are steps that are possible for nurses working with community activist groups to actualize.

Advocating for Patients Affected by Their Environment

Nurses can intervene on behalf of patients affected by environmental quality in a number of ways across a variety of care settings. Nurses working in emergency departments, acute care, and primary care see the effects of environmental

TABLE 43-3 Select Health Effects and Related Environmental Hazards

Common Health Problems	Related Environmental Hazards
Asthma	■ Exposure to allergens and triggers, including tobacco smoke, dust mites, furry pets, mold, certain chemicals, and the particulate matter in outdoor air pollution ■ Particulate matter, which includes dust, dirt, soot, and smoke ■ When pollutants from vehicles, power plants, factories, and other sources come in contact with heat and sunlight, ground-level ozone forms, increasing risk for those with asthma who spend time outside
Birth defects	■ Environmental exposures to substances such as ionizing radiation, some endocrine-disrupting chemicals (e.g., polychlorinated biphenyls, or PCBs), dioxins, and pesticides have been linked to defects of the nervous system and developmental problems ■ Disinfection by-products in drinking water (e.g., trihalomethanes, or THMs) may increase risk for brain and spinal cord, urinary tract, and heart birth defects ■ Living near hazardous waste has been linked to birth defects, including spina bifida, cleft lip/palate, gastroschisis, and Down syndrome ■ More data are needed to make clear connections between environmental exposures and birth defects
Cancer	■ Exposure to ionizing radiation ■ Exposure to some industrial chemicals ■ Environmental tobacco smoke (secondhand smoke) ■ It may take up to 40 years of environmental exposure for a cancer to develop

Source: From Centers for Disease Control and Prevention (CDC). (2018a). *National Environmental Public Health Tracking: Health Effects.* https://ephtracking.cdc.gov/showHealthEffects.action

quality when they work with patients who experience health conditions affected by, or caused by, environmental hazards (**Figure 43-4** ›)). For example, nurses may care for individuals with asthma or COPD who are admitted with exacerbations during periods of poor air quality. Community/public health nurses are also well positioned to serve as advocates.

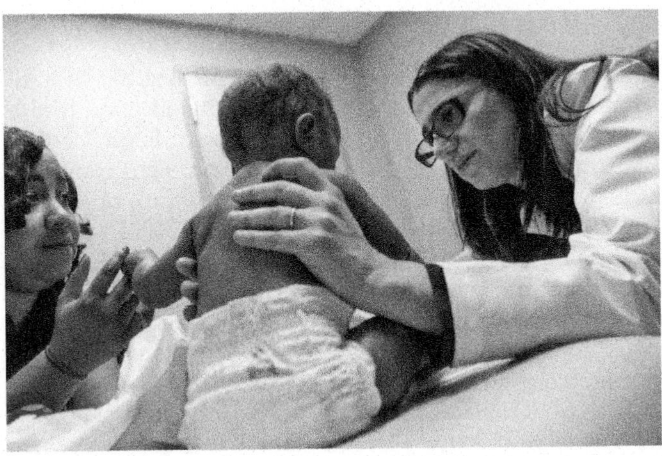

Figure 43.4 ›) Dr. Hanna-Attisha of Flint, Michigan, knew that an investigation of the water quality in Flint showed that it contained dangerous amounts of lead. She decided to conduct her own analysis using hospital records. She found that the number of Flint children with elevated levels of lead had doubled and tripled in some areas since the city had switched to a new water source 2 years earlier. Dr. Hanna-Attisha was so alarmed that she chose to hold a press conference rather than go through the months-long process of publishing her findings in a medical journal. She said she and her team had "an ethical, moral, professional responsibility to alert our community about this crisis."
Source: Detroit Free Press/ZUMA Press Inc/Alamy Stock Photo.

For example, underserved patients who live in substandard housing may have children at risk for lead poisoning from old peeling paint or old plumbing. Nurses can educate patients about environmental hazards and strategies to safeguard themselves or develop programs to educate the larger community. Nurses can act locally at the municipal, state, or national level to lobby government officials for change—for example, if community industries are known to be noncompliant with air pollution standards. Professional nursing associations generally identify legislative agendas focusing on state or federal legislation, depending on the scope of the association; as members, nurses can become involved on legislative committees and assist by providing data, or testimony, to support measures that safeguard the environment.

REVIEW Environmental Quality

RELATE Link the Concepts and Exemplars

Linking the exemplar of environmental quality with the concept of ethics:

1. Consider the air pollution exemplar and how different vulnerable populations, for example children with asthma, might be affected by living in areas prone to high summertime ground-level ozone measurements. What is the nurse's ethical responsibility to advocate for environmental quality that improves the health of vulnerable populations? Provide examples of how nurses could advocate for environmental quality improvement.

Linking the exemplar of environmental quality with the concept of healthcare systems:

2. Why might patients who experience health problems made worse by environmental hazards (such as lung or heart disease), and also represent vulnerable populations (for example, underserved populations or older adults), experience barriers to access to healthcare treatment for environmentally related health issues? Consider the Flint, Michigan, water crisis as an example (NRDC, 2020a). Why might these patients require greater advocacy?

Linking the exemplar of environmental quality with the concept of legal issues:

3. What is the nurse's role when advocating for the mother of a child with asthma who is living in substandard housing in poor condition with a leak in the roof?
4. What is the nurse's advocacy role when a patient presents with a health problem related to an unsafe work environment, such as constant exposure to toxic fumes?
5. What advantage does professional nursing hold when advocating, as a group, for environmental health and safety?
6. When nurses testify for an environmental quality issue, how do they represent themselves—as an individual citizen or as a member of the profession?

REFER Go to Pearson MyLab Nursing and eText

REFLECT Apply Your Knowledge

Jonathan Baker comes to the emergency department (ED) where you work complaining of difficulty breathing and shortness of breath. He has no other symptoms of upper respiratory disease, no history of chronic lung disease, and otherwise is in good health. As a part of your assessment you ask Mr. Baker about his living conditions, and he tells you that he lives in a subdivision very near the river that has flooded twice during the spring rainy season. The last flood was significant, and several weeks later, Jonathan and his wife are still working at cleaning up the aftermath. You ask him if he has noticed any musty, earthy smell or foul odor in the house, and he states that he has. He knows that there has been mold growth in the basement and first floor, but he has not had the time to deal with it or to call his insurance company.

You determine that Mr. Baker's respiratory problem is likely due to mold, and you immediately notify the HCP so the diagnosis can be confirmed and his condition appropriately treated.

1. What are your next steps advocating for Mr. Baker's health?
2. Is there any other role in which you might advocate for the health and well-being of other flood victims in your city/region?

References

Abbasini, M., Ahmadi, F., U & Kazemnejad, A. (2020). Patient advocacy in nursing: A concept analysis. *Nursing Ethics, 27*(1), 141–151. https://doi.org/10.1177/0969733019832950

ADA National Network. (2020). *What is the Americans with Disabilities Act (ADA)?* https://adata.org/learn-about-ada

American Civil Liberties Union. (2020). *Disability rights*. https://www.aclu.org/issues/disability-rights#current

American Hospital Association. (2020). *Ensuring access in vulnerable communities – Taskforce report and resources*. https://www.aha.org/issue-landing-page/2016-11-16-ensuring-access-vulnerable-communities-taskforce-report-and-resources

American Nurses Association. (ANA). (2015a). *Code of ethics for nurses and interpretive statements*. https://www.nursingworld.org/coe-view-only

American Nurses Association. (ANA). (2015b). *Nursing: Scope and standards of practice* (3rd ed.). Author.

Ball, J. W., Bindler, R. C., & Cowen, K. J. (2014). *Child health nursing: Partnering with children and families* (3rd ed.). Prentice Hall.

Bu, X., & Jezewski, M. A. (2007). Developing a mid-range theory of patient advocacy through concept analysis. *Journal of Advanced Nursing, 57*(1), 101–110.

Centers for Disease Control and Prevention (CDC). (2016). *Health studies – Promoting clean water for health*. https://www.cdc.gov/nceh/hsb/cwh/

Centers for Disease Control and Prevention (CDC). (2018a). *National Environmental Public Health Tracking Network: Health effects*. https://ephtracking.cdc.gov/showHealthEffects.action

Centers for Disease Control and Prevention (CDC). (2018b). *Secondhand smoke (SHS) facts*. https://www.cdc.gov/tobacco/data_statistics/fact_sheets/secondhand_smoke/general_facts/index.htm

Centers for Disease Control and Prevention (CDC). (2019a). *Air quality: Ozone and your health*. https://www.cdc.gov/air/ozone.html

Centers for Disease Control and Prevention (CDC). (2019b). *Climate and health: Climate effects on health—air pollution*. http://www.cdc.gov/climateandhealth/effects/air_pollution.htm

Centers for Disease Control and Prevention (CDC). (2020). *National Center for Environmental Health*. https://www.cdc.gov/nceh/default.htm

Centers for Medicare and Medicaid Services. (2020). *People dually eligible for Medicare and Medicaid*. https://www.cms.gov/Medicare-Medicaid-Coordination/Medicare-and-Medicaid-Coordination/Medicare-Medicaid-Coordination-Office/Downloads/MMCO_Factsheet.pdf

Cole, C., Wellard, S., & Mummery, J. (2014). Problematising autonomy and ethics in nursing. *Nursing Ethics, 21*(5), 576–582.

D'amour, D., & Oandasan, I. (2005). Interprofessionality as the field of Interprofessional practice and Interprofessional education: An emerging concept. *Journal of Interprofessional Care, 19*(Suppl. 1), 8–20.

Disability Rights of Ohio. (2020). *Abuse and neglect: awareness and reporting for individuals with mentally illness*. http://www.disabilityrightsohio.org/abuse-neglect-mi

Dutra, S., Hayes, J. P., & Keane, T. M. (2019). Issues in assessment of PTSD in military personnel. In B. A. Moore & W. E. Penk (Eds.), *Treating PTSD in military personnel: A clinical handbook* (pp. 22–45). Guilford Press.

European Patients Forum (EPF). (December, 2017). *Toolkit for patient organisations on patient empowerment*. https://www.eu-patient.eu/globalassets/library/publications/patient-empowerment---toolkit.pdf

Gomez-Valasco, D. V., Almeda-Valdes, P., Martagon, A. J., Galan-Ramirez, G. A., & Aguilar-Salinas, C. A. (2019). Empowerment of patients with type 2 diabetes: Current perspectives. *Diabetes, Metabolic Syndrome and Obesity: Targets and Therapy, 12*, 1311–1321. https://doi.org/10.2147/DMSO.S174910.

Hanks, R. G. (2013). Social advocacy: A call for nursing action. *Pastoral Psychology, 62*, 163–173. https://doi.org/10.1007/s11089-011-0404-1

HealthyPeople.gov. (2020). *Environmental quality*. https://www.healthypeople.gov/2020/leading-health-indicators/2020-lhi-topics/Environmental-Quality

Hyland, D. (2002). An exploration of the relationship between patient autonomy and patient advocacy: Implications for nursing practice. *Nursing Ethics, 9*(5), 472–482.

International Council of Nurses (ICN). (2012). *The ICN code of ethics for nurses*. https://www.icn.ch/sites/default/files/inline-files/2012_ICN_Codeofethicsfornurses_%20eng.pdf

Interprofessional Education Collaborative Expert Panel. (2011). *Core competencies for interprofessional collaborative practice: Report of an expert panel*. https://nebula.wsimg.com/3ee8a4b5b5f7ab794c742b14601d5f23?AccessKeyId=DC06780E69ED19E2B3A5&disposition=0&alloworigin=1

Jansson, B. S., Nyamathi, A., Duan, L., Kaplan, C., Heidemann, G., & Ananias, D. (2015). Validation of the patient advocacy engagement scale for health professionals. *Research in Nursing and Health, 38*(2), 162–172.

Kalaitzidis, E. & Jewell, P. (2020). The concept of advocacy in nursing: A critical analysis. *The Health Care Manager, 39*(2), 78–85. https://doi.org/10.1097/HCM.0000000000000292

Kim, J. G., Hong, H. C., Lee, H., Ferrans, C. E., & Kim, E. (2019). Cultural beliefs about breast cancer in Vietnamese women. *BMC Women's Health, 19*(74). https://doi.org/10.1186/s12905-019-0777-3

Lian, J., McGhee, S. M., So, C., Chau, J., Wong, C. K. H., Wong, W. C. W., & Lam, C. L. K. (2018). Long-term cost-effectiveness of a patient-empowerment programme for type 2 diabetes mellitus in primary care. *Diabetes, Obesity & Metabolism, 21*(1), 73–83. https://doi.org/10.1111/dom.13485

Lor, M., Xiong, P., Park, L., Schwei, R. J., & Jacobs, E. A. (2017). Western or traditional healers?: Understanding decision making in the Hmong population. *Western Journal of Nursing Research, 39*(3), 400–415. https://doi.org/10.1177/0193945916636484

National Alliance on Mental Illness. (2020). *About NAMI: What we do*. https://nami.org/About-NAMI/What-We-Do

National Council of State Boards of Nursing. (2018). *A nurse's guide to the use of social media*. https://www.ncsbn.org/3739.htm

National Institutes of Health, Office of Extramural Research. (2019). *Vulnerable and other populations requiring additional protections*. https://grants.nih.gov/policy/humansubjects/policies-and-regulations/vulnerable-populations.htm

Natural Resource Defense Council (NRDC) (2020a). *Flint water crisis: Everything you need to know*. https://www.nrdc.org/stories/flint-water-crisis-everything-you-need-know#sec-timeline

Natural Resource Defense Council (NRDC) (2020b). *Our work: Water*. https://www.nrdc.org/issues/water

Office of Disease Prevention and Health Promotion (ODPHP). (2020). *Healthy People 2020: Environmental quality*. https://www.healthypeople.gov/2020/leading-health-indicators/2020-lhi-topics/Environmental-Quality

Palumbo, R. (2017). *The bright side and the dark side of patient empowerment: Co-creation and co-destruction of value in the healthcare environment*. Springer.

Paskett, E. D., Pennell, M. L., Ruffin, M. T., Weghorst, C. M., Lu, B., Hade, Peng, J., Bernardo, B. M., & Wewers, M. E. (2020). A multi-level model to understand cervical cancer disparities in Appalachia. *Cancer Prevention Research, 13*, 223–228. https://doi.org/10.1158/1940-6207.CAPR-19-0239

Psychological Health Center for Excellence (PHCoE). (2007). *The Department of Defense plan to achieve the vision of the DoD Task Force on Mental Health*. https://www.pdhealth.mil/department-defense-plan-achieve-vision-dod-task-force-mental-health

Schwartz, L. (2002). Is there an advocate in the house?: The role of health care professionals in patient advocacy. *Journal of Medical Ethics, 28*, 37–40.

Vitale, E., Germini, F., Massaro, M. & Fortunato, R. S. (2019). How patients and nurses defined advocacy in nursing?: A review of the literature. *Journal of Health, Medicine and Nursing, 63*, 64–69. https://doi.org/10.7176/JHMN

World Health Organization (WHO). (2010). *Framework for action on interprofessional education and collaborative practice*. WHO Press. https://www.who.int/hrh/resources/framework_action/en/

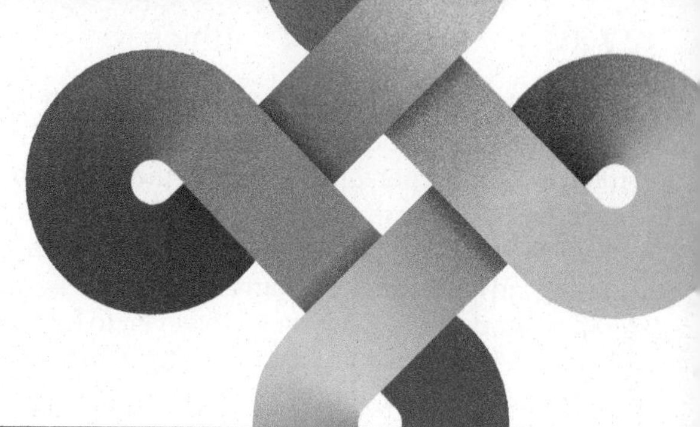

Module 44
Ethics

Module Outline and Learning Outcomes

The Concept of Ethics

Values

44.1 Analyze the relationship between values and ethics in nursing.

Concepts Related to Ethics

44.2 Outline the relationship between ethics and other concepts.

Nursing Codes of Ethics

44.3 Differentiate the various codes of ethics used in nursing.

Principles and Practices of Ethical Decision Making

44.4 Analyze the principles of ethical decision making.

Strategies to Enhance Ethical Decisions and Practice

44.5 Summarize strategies to enhance ethical decisions in practice.

Ethics Exemplars

Exemplar 44.A Morality

44.A Analyze morality as it relates to ethics.

Exemplar 44.B Ethical Dilemmas

44.B Analyze dilemmas related to ethics.

Exemplar 44.C Patient Rights

44.C Analyze patient rights as they relate to ethics.

›› The Concept of Ethics

Concept Key Terms

Advocate, **2730**
Altruism, **2730**
Autonomy, **2730**
Belief, **2730**
Beneficence, **2735**
Code of ethics, **2733**
Ethics, **2729**
Human dignity, **2730**
Integrity, **2730**
Justice, **2735**
Morality, **2729**
Nonmaleficence, **2735**
Social justice, **2730**
Values, **2730**
Values clarification, **2730**
Veracity, **2735**

Ethics, as applied in professional nursing, is defined as a system of moral principles or standards governing behaviors and relationships that is based on professional nursing beliefs and values. More broadly defined, ethics refers to the standards of right and wrong that influence human behavior, usually in terms of rights, obligations, benefits to society, fairness, or specific virtues. Ethical standards are based on the values of the group that holds to those standards, whether the group consists of individuals of the same religion, people from the same community, or individuals who share the same profession. Within the field of nursing, some of the most important ethical standards relate to the rights of patients and their families, such as the rights to privacy and self-determination.

The term *ethics* also refers to the study and development of the ethical standards of an individual, community, or profession. Nurses should constantly examine their personal ethical standards and understand how their personal ethics and morals compare to the ethical standards of the nursing profession.

Morality (or morals) is similar to ethics, and many people use the terms interchangeably. However, **morality** usually refers to private, personal standards of what is right and wrong in conduct, character, and attitude. Sometimes the first clue to the moral nature of a situation is the awareness of feelings such as guilt, hope, or shame. Another indicator is the tendency to respond to the situation with words such as *ought, should, right, wrong, good,* and *bad*. Moral issues are concerned with important social values and norms; they are not about trivial things.

Just as nurses should be able to distinguish between ethics and morality, they should be able to distinguish between morality and law. Laws reflect the moral values of a society and offer guidance in determining what is moral; however, an action can be legal but not moral. For example, an order for full resuscitation of a dying patient is legal, but one could still question whether the act is moral. Conversely, an action can be moral but illegal. For instance, if a child stops breathing at home, it is moral but not legal to exceed the speed limit when driving to the hospital. (Legal aspects of nursing practice are covered in depth in Module 49, Legal Issues.)

When people are ill, they may be unable to assert their rights as they would if they were healthy. When this happens, nurses have an ethical responsibility to advocate on behalf of the patient based on what the patient would want. An **advocate** is a person who expresses and defends the cause of another person. Therefore, the nurse advocates for the patient's best interest on the basis of the patient's values, not on the basis of the nurse's own ethical or moral values. Nursing advocacy takes many forms and is discussed in detail in Module 43, Advocacy. However, to function successfully in their capacity as advocates for patients, nurses need an understanding of ethical issues in nursing and healthcare.

Values

Values provide the foundation on which an individual's or group's ethical standards are built. Guido (2020) defines **values** as personal beliefs about what is true or right. A **belief** is an interpretation or conclusion that one accepts as true. Values can reflect both beliefs that are based on a particular tenet (doctrine) or body of tenets accepted by a group of individuals and beliefs that are based on a pattern of mental views established by cumulative prior experience. For example, many traditional Jewish beliefs are based on the tenets found in the Jewish Torah, but individual Jews may hold other or additional beliefs based on their own experiences. Personal values are developed through individual observation and experience and may be heavily influenced by social traditions and the cultural, ethnic, and religious norms experienced within a person's family and associated groups.

Nurses acquire professional values through socialization into the nursing profession by nursing school faculty and other nurses, through clinical and life experiences, and by following established professional codes of ethics. As part of this socialization, nurses develop insight into their own values and how their values influence their actions. One of the most helpful ways for nurses to develop such insight is through **values clarification**. Through this process of consciously identifying, examining, and developing individual values, nurses gain the ability to choose actions on the basis of deliberately adopted values.

Values clarification is important to both nurses and patients in supporting the provision of patient-centered care because it helps nurses learn how to identify patients' values and distinguish patients' values from their own. Values clarification is not a once-in-a-lifetime activity but an ongoing process of examining what one's values are and how these values inform or affect one's decisions and actions. Nursing students and professional nurses alike need to have a clear sense of their values specific to life, death, health, and illness. Values clarification exercises and real-life experience in carrying out treatment plans that contradict or challenge their beliefs about patients' best interests will assist nurses at all levels to develop expertise in responding to ethical issues.

Values Essential for the Professional Nurse

Although nurses ultimately have their own unique set of personal values, certain core values are shared by all members of the nursing profession. Nurses typically acquire these values through the process of socialization to the profession. According to the American Association of Colleges of Nursing (AACN; 2008), five values that are essential for all professional nurses are altruism, autonomy, human dignity, integrity, and social justice:

- **Altruism** is concern for the welfare and well-being of others. In practice, altruism is reflected in the nurse's concern for the welfare of patients, other nurses, and other healthcare providers (HCPs).
- **Autonomy** is the right to self-determination. Professional practice reflects autonomy when the nurse respects patients' rights to make decisions about their healthcare.
- **Human dignity** refers to the inherent worth and uniqueness of individuals and populations. The nurse who values and respects all patients and colleagues shows respect for human dignity.
- **Integrity** is acting in accordance with an appropriate code of ethics and accepted standards of practice. Integrity is reflected in professional practice when the nurse is honest and provides care based on an ethical framework that is accepted within the profession (e.g., the American Nurses Association [ANA] Code of Ethics).
- **Social justice** refers to the upholding of justice, or what is fair, on a social scale. Nurses act in accordance with social justice by treating all patients equally without regard to economic status, ethnicity, age, gender, religion, citizenship, disability, or sexual orientation.

Some professional behaviors associated with these five essential values include:

- Demonstrating professional standards of moral, ethical, and legal conduct
- Being accountable for personal and professional behaviors
- Maintaining professional communication and boundaries with patients, families, and colleagues
- Promoting safe, ethical care and acting to prevent unsafe, illegal, or unethical care
- Articulating the value of lifelong learning and pursuit of excellence as a professional.

Clarifying Patients' Values

The nurse must clarify a patient's values before preparing a care plan to best understand the impact these values may have on the patient's present condition and treatment plan. Values can affect patient preferences and priorities. For example, a patient who has had an amputation may place highest value on return to independent living while another patient facing lifelong disability may place greater value in engaging in social interaction. When a patient's values may conflict with healthcare needs, the nurse can use values clarification as an intervention. Behaviors that may indicate conflicting or unclear values include ignoring a HCP's recommendations, inconsistent communication or behaviors, repeated admissions to the healthcare facility for the same issue, and uncertainty about which course of action to take. Patients who exhibit any of these behaviors may benefit from values clarification or motivational interviewing to determine their readiness for change. Motivational interviewing and the stages of change are outlined in Module 35, Caring Interventions.

When assisting a patient with values clarification, it may be helpful to use the following seven-step-process (Al-Banna, 2017):

1. ***List alternatives***. Ask the patient to discuss other possible ways to address the issue at hand.
2. ***Examine possible consequences of choices***. After discussing all options, ask the patient to state what would possibly happen if a specific action is taken. For example, "How do you think that will be helpful?"
3. ***Choose freely***. As the patient discusses each possible option or action and potential consequences, ask the patient to determine how the choice is to be made and/or if the patient has a choice in the decision.
4. ***Feel good about the choice***. Once the patient has come to a decision, lead the patient through a discussion about its emotional impact. The nurse may say, "Tell me more about how this choice makes you feel."
5. ***Affirm the choice***. Once the patient has made a decision, discuss how the patient will communicate the decision to family and/or significant others.
6. ***Act on the choice***. Ask the patient to describe the plan for putting the decision in motion.
7. ***Act with a pattern***. It is important for the nurse to determine if this decision is a type of choice the patient would commonly make and if the patient can make similar actions consistently. The nurse could ask the patient if this decision resembles any other decision the patient has made or if the patient would make the choice again in the future.

When engaging in values clarification with a patient, nurses must guard against allowing their personal values to influence the discussion or alter the patient's ability to freely make a clear decision. If the patient requests information about the nurse's personal values, it is important for the nurse to clearly redirect the focus of the conversation to the patient.

Concepts Related to Ethics

Ethical patient care encompasses more than managing difficult care decisions or facing the moral issues surrounding a patient. Ethical care also involves appropriate completion of common care tasks, including pain control; providing adequate patient teaching; demonstrating respect for patients from diverse backgrounds; advocating for the rights of all patients, regardless of their level of development or cognition; ensuring confidentiality; advocating for patients' safety; and supporting patients' right to self-determination.

Society in the United States is increasingly diverse, and this diversity has ethical implications for nursing practice. In particular, nurses have a responsibility to show respect to all of their patients, regardless of gender, race, ethnicity, religion, disability, sexual orientation, or any other personal characteristic. This obligation is clearly stated in the ANA's *Code of Ethics for Nurses with Interpretive Statements* (2015a), which declares that nurses must respect the inherent dignity and rights of all patients, provide nursing services without bias or prejudice, work to eliminate disparities in care, and consider each patient's "culture, value systems, religious or spiritual beliefs, lifestyle, social support system, sexual orientation or gender expression, and primary language" when creating a plan of care (p. 1). In addition, ethical standards require that nurses neither project their own cultural preferences onto their patients nor view patients' cultural beliefs as inferior to or less valid than their own. For additional discussion of the intersection between diversity and nursing ethics, see the Focus on Diversity and Culture feature.

Of course, nurses have a responsibility to advocate for all patients, not just those who differ in terms of culture, cognition, or development. Part of the advocate role involves making sure that each patient's right to confidentiality is preserved. This requires the nurse to observe all laws and institutional policies meant to protect patient information. Ensuring confidentiality also means that the nurse must exercise good professional judgment when communicating with others, including the patient's family and other members of the healthcare team. Similarly, nurses must advocate for every patient's right to self-determination, including the right to establish advance directives and have them carried out according to the patient's wishes. Some, but not all, of the concepts integral to ethics are outlined in the Concepts Related to Ethics feature. They are listed in alphabetical order.

Concepts Related to Ethics

CONCEPT	RELATIONSHIP TO ETHICS	NURSING IMPLICATIONS
Advocacy	Nurses must ensure patients receive sufficient information on which to base consent for care and related treatment. Nurses must also provide an environment that allows patients to make their own care decisions, as appropriate.	■ Make sure medical staff clearly discuss all interventions with the patient and provide information sufficient to ensure informed consent. ■ Discuss the plan of care with the patient and allow self-determination as appropriate (e.g., allow the patient to try lifestyle modifications before medications). ■ Recognize the patient's right to refuse treatment and procedures.

(continued on next page)

Concepts Related to *(continued)*

CONCEPT	RELATIONSHIP TO ETHICS	NURSING IMPLICATIONS
Cognition and Development	Patients with developmental limitations or disorders that affect their cognitive function may not be able to understand the implications of a situation or may make important decisions on their own without adequate support. Nurses have a duty to advocate on behalf of these patients, not only to help preserve their rights to autonomy, dignity, and respect but also to help ensure that they do not experience abuse.	■ Understand state laws regarding the determination of incapacity and state and federal laws protecting the rights of disabled individuals. ■ Assume that patients have the capacity to make their own decisions unless there is clear evidence or documentation otherwise. ■ Understand the concept of guardianship, including when patients should be under the care of a guardian, as well as what limitations are placed on the guardian role. ■ Advocate for patients with limited cognition or intellectual ability when their rights appear to be in jeopardy or when others make decisions that may not be in their best interest.
Comfort	Chronic pain is a common problem in the United States, but many affected individuals lack access to healthcare resources that can help them adequately control their pain. Other people with chronic pain consume greater amounts of healthcare resources, causing shortages of these resources for other patients. Both sides of this situation raise ethical issues related to resource allocation and social justice and what constitutes an acceptable outcome of care for patients with chronic pain. The nurse also has an ethical obligation to collaborate with the patient and care team to manage the patient's pain in a way that minimizes the likelihood of medication abuse.	■ Become educated about chronic pain. ■ Engage with patients to develop a deeper understanding of the duration and severity of their pain. ■ Refer patients to pain management specialists as appropriate. ■ Help patients develop realistic expectations about the degree to which their pain can be alleviated. ■ Ask for support from supervisors or peers when advocating for appropriate patient care. ■ Recognize and set aside personal assumptions or biases surrounding opioid use. ■ Educate patients about and monitor for signs of opioid abuse or addiction.
Communication	Nurses are obligated to ensure the confidentiality of patient information during all care and in all care areas.	■ Ensure that access to patient information, such as online charting, is made available only to appropriate staff members. ■ Do not discuss a particular patient's situation with individuals who do not require this information as part of their job. ■ Observe all laws and institutional policies related to the confidentiality of patient information. ■ Inform the patient of policies and procedures that ensure confidentiality.
Legal Issues	The Health Insurance Portability and Accountability Act (HIPAA) sets forth specific guidelines nurses must follow to protect patient information. Thus, preserving patient confidentiality is both an ethical duty and a legal obligation. Nurses also help to protect patients' right to self-determination by ensuring that advance directives are in place and followed correctly.	■ Understand what constitutes "protected health information" under HIPAA's Privacy Rule. ■ Take appropriate measures to preserve the confidentiality of protected health information. ■ Discuss different types of advance directives with patients before surgery and other procedures that carry a degree of risk. ■ When patients are incapacitated, ensure that any advance directives are followed correctly and in the manner the patient intended.
Teaching and Learning	Because they are now sent home earlier than in years past, patients often require detailed instructions regarding critical aspects of their own care. The nurse has a professional obligation and an ethical duty to provide this teaching and to ensure that the patient understands the teaching and can properly carry out any self-care tasks.	■ Assess the patient's learning needs and abilities at the time of the initial encounter (whether in the emergency department [ED], operative unit, acute care unit, clinic, or home). ■ Plan teaching interventions for the patient using appropriate methods and materials. ■ Recognize and set aside personal assumptions and values about the best ways to receive care information. ■ Follow up to ensure that the patient understands the teaching and that the teaching furthers the patient's sense of autonomy and self-determination.

Focus on Diversity and Culture

Religion, Ethics, and Nursing Practice

For many people, including many nurses, the concepts of religion and ethics are intimately intertwined. For example, an individual's religion often informs beliefs about social justice, end-of-life issues, the nature of suffering, and the very meaning of human existence, to list just a few topics. When nurses encounter patients whose religious beliefs differ from their own, ethical conflicts may arise. Nurses can help to minimize the likelihood of such conflicts by keeping several principles in mind:

First, nurses should seek to identify any ethical common ground that exists between themselves and their patients. Despite the significant differences that exist between the world's many religions, most belief systems place some value on helping the less fortunate, taking responsibility for one's actions, and treating others as you wish to be treated, among other shared values. In many situations in which an ethical conflict initially seems to exist, the nurse and patient can reach a shared understanding of which course of action is most ethical by looking at the situation through the lens of these common beliefs.

Nurses should also recognize that not every person adheres to all of the beliefs typically associated with the person's religious background. For example, although official Roman Catholic teaching forbids the use of birth control and sets specific guidelines regarding end-of-life care, many Catholics find it morally and ethically acceptable to disregard these teachings. A thorough assessment of each patient's unique belief system can help the nurse to avoid assuming that religion-based ethical conflicts exist when they do not.

Above all, nurses must remember that they have an ethical obligation to respect the patient's beliefs and right to autonomy throughout the care process. The nurse should honor the patient's beliefs and decisions unless the patient's choices will cause the nurse to act in a way that violates the nurse's own deeply held beliefs. In such cases, the nurse should seek guidance from supervisors, ethics committees, and other resources as appropriate.

Case Study >> Part 1

June D'Angelo, a 49-year-old woman of Italian descent, presents to the emergency department (ED) late at night complaining of a severe migraine headache. Her vital signs show that her blood pressure is elevated at 210/104 mmHg. The ED physician discusses her history and finds that Ms. D'Angelo has been in the ED five times in the past year for the same problem. She was prescribed a daily blood pressure medication by her primary physician 3 weeks earlier; however, she says she is not taking the medication and has not even filled the prescription but instead has decided to take daily walks to manage her blood pressure.

The ED physician asks Ms. D'Angelo how recently her headaches began and how long each one typically lasts. She sighs and says that her migraines mostly never end and have gotten worse in the past 24 hours. When the physician leaves the bedside to call Ms. D'Angelo's HCP, he gives orders to the nurse for IV blood pressure medication for Ms. D'Angelo. As the nurse prepares to provide the IV medication, Ms. D'Angelo says, "I'll take this medication because I know it will make the pain go away. But I'm not taking that daily medication." The nurse then speaks with her to complete a brief nursing assessment to determine why she is reluctant to take the medication. Findings from the assessment indicate that Ms. D'Angelo relies on the ED to manage her pain and does not follow her primary HCP's instructions and that she feels exercise should be enough to manage her high blood pressure.

Critical Thinking Questions

1. What ethical issue is the nurse facing as she assesses this patient with frequent ED admissions?
2. What topics should be included in patient teaching for Ms. D'Angelo?
3. What further information should the nurse assess before planning patient teaching?
4. How can the nurse assist Ms. D'Angelo in planning how to manage her symptoms better?
5. Who should be involved in this patient's discharge planning and self-care? Explain.

Nursing Codes of Ethics

Ethical standards and behaviors are at the core of nursing practice. As a result, the nursing profession has developed formal codes of ethics to guide nurses in their work with patients and other healthcare professionals. A **code of ethics** is both a general guide for a profession's membership and a social contract with the public that the profession serves.

The Nightingale Pledge is considered the first code of nursing ethics used in the United States. Written in 1893 by Lystra Gretter, principal of the Farrand Training School for Nurses in Detroit, and patterned after the Hippocratic Oath for medicine, the Nightingale Pledge was named in honor of Florence Nightingale. The Nightingale Pledge is still used at many nursing schools' graduation ceremonies. It reads as follows:

> I solemnly pledge myself before God and in the presence of this assembly to pass my life in purity and to practice my profession faithfully. I will abstain from whatever is deleterious and mischievous, and will not take or knowingly administer any harmful drug. I will do all in my power to elevate the standard of my profession, and will hold in confidence all personal matters committed to my keeping, and all family affairs coming to my knowledge in the practice of my profession. With loyalty will I endeavor to aid the physician in his work and devote myself to the welfare of those committed to my care. (Gretter, 1910, p. 271)

Over the years, the Nightingale Pledge was modernized, then largely replaced by longer, more comprehensive codes of ethics. Today, the nursing profession depends primarily on two major codes of ethics: the International Council of Nurses (ICN) *Code of Ethics* and the ANA *Code of Ethics for Nurses*. These codes were initially adopted in the early 1950s and have undergone changes to reflect social and technologic change. The ICN code was most recently updated in 2012. The current version is presented in **Box 44.1** >>.

The latest version of the ANA *Code of Ethics for Nurses with Interpretive Statements* was released in 2015, after a 4-year period of input and revision. Within the United States, this code serves as a statement of nurses' ethical obligations and duties, as the profession's nonnegotiable ethical standard, and as the nursing profession's statement of commitment to society. All nurses should regularly refer to the ANA *Code of Ethics* to direct how they perform their duties in daily practice. The nine provisions of the ANA *Code of Ethics* appear in **Box 44.2** >>.

Box 44.1

The ICN Code of Ethics

1. Nurses and people
   - The nurse's primary professional responsibility is to people requiring nursing care.
   - In providing care, the nurse promotes an environment in which the human rights, values, customs and spiritual beliefs of the individual, family and community are respected.
   - The nurse ensures that the individual receives accurate, sufficient and timely information in a culturally appropriate manner on which to base consent for care and related treatment.
   - The nurse holds in confidence personal information and uses judgement in sharing this information.
   - The nurse shares with society the responsibility for initiating and supporting action to meet the health and social needs of the public, in particular those of vulnerable populations.
   - The nurse advocates for equity and social justice in resource allocation, access to health care and other social and economic services.
   - The nurse demonstrates professional values such as respectfulness, responsiveness, compassion, trustworthiness and integrity.
2. Nurses and practice
   - The nurse carries personal responsibility and accountability for nursing practice, and for maintaining competence by continual learning.
   - The nurse maintains a standard of personal health such that the ability to provide care is not compromised.
   - The nurse uses judgement regarding individual competence when accepting and delegating responsibility.
   - The nurse at all times maintains standards of personal conduct which reflect well on the profession and enhance its image and public confidence.
   - The nurse, in providing care, ensures that use of technology and scientific advances is compatible with the safety, dignity and rights of people.
   - The nurse strives to foster and maintain a practice culture promoting ethical behaviour and open dialogue.
3. Nurses and the profession
   - The nurse assumes the major role in determining and implementing acceptable standards of clinical nursing practice, management, research and education.
   - The nurse is active in developing a core of research-based professional knowledge that supports evidence-based practice.
   - The nurse is active in developing and sustaining a core of professional values.
   - The nurse, acting through the professional organisation, participates in creating a positive practice environment and maintaining safe, equitable social and economic working conditions in nursing.
   - The nurse practices to sustain and protect the natural environment and is aware of its consequences on health.
   - The nurse contributes to an ethical organisational environment and challenges unethical practices and settings.
4. Nurses and co-workers
   - The nurse sustains a collaborative and respectful relationship with co-workers in nursing and other fields.
   - The nurse takes appropriate action to safeguard individuals, families and communities when their health is endangered by a co-worker or any other person.
   - The nurse takes appropriate action to support and guide co-workers to advance ethical conduct.

Source: From International Council of Nurses (2012). Used by permission of the International Council of Nurses.

Box 44.2

The Provisions of the Code of Ethics for Nurses

Provision 1. The nurse practices with compassion and respect for the inherent dignity, worth, and unique attributes of every person.

Provision 2. The nurse's primary commitment is to the patient, whether an individual, family, group, community, or population.

Provision 3. The nurse promotes, advocates for, and protects the rights, health, and safety of the patient.

Provision 4. The nurse has authority, accountability, and responsibility for nursing practice; makes decisions; and takes action consistent with the obligation to promote health and to provide optimal care.

Provision 5. The nurse owes the same duties to self as to others, including the responsibility to promote health and safety, preserve wholeness of character and integrity, maintain competence, and continue personal and professional growth.

Provision 6. The nurse, through individual and collective effort, establishes, maintains, and improves the ethical environment of the work setting and conditions of employment that are conducive to safe, quality health care.

Provision 7. The nurse, in all roles and settings, advances the profession through research and scholarly inquiry, professional standards development, and the generation of both nursing and health policy.

Provision 8. The nurse collaborates with other health professionals and the public to protect human rights, promote health diplomacy, and reduce health disparities.

Provision 9. The profession of nursing, collectively through its professional organizations, must articulate nursing values, maintain the integrity of the profession, and integrate principles of social justice into nursing and health policy.

Source: From American Nursing Association (2015a), page v.

Using codes of ethics in everyday practice requires seeking knowledge and understanding of the patient's needs and preferences (whether the patient is a single individual, a family, a group, a community, or a population) as well as self-awareness on the part of the nurse. The following questions can help nurses apply Provision 2 to ethical problems (Kangasniemi & Haho, 2012; Lachman, 2012):

- What do I know about this patient's situation?
- What do I know about the patient's values and moral preferences?
- What assumptions am I making that require more data to clarify?
- What are my own feelings (and values) about the situation? How might they be influencing how I view and respond to the situation?
- Are my own values in conflict with those of the patient?
- What else do I need to know about this case, and where can I obtain this information?
- What can I never know about this case?
- Given my primary obligation to the patient, what should I do to be ethical?

SAFETY ALERT Although nurses have a duty to protect all research participants, they must pay special attention to research involving vulnerable populations, such as children, pregnant women, prisoners, older adults, and people with cognitive impairments. Because members of these groups often have limited autonomy, they are especially vulnerable to coercion, undue influence, and abuse.

Case Study » Part 2

After June D'Angelo receives her IV hypertension medication, she tells both her nurse and the physician that she feels much better, "just like last time." The ED physician asks the nurse to stay by the bedside as he tells Ms. D'Angelo about his phone conversation with her primary HCP. During the call, the physician learned about Ms. D'Angelo's tendency to miss appointments with her primary provider and her failure to fill prescriptions. The ED physician suggests that the best way for Ms. D'Angelo to avoid further ED visits is for her to collaborate with her primary provider to control her hypertension and headaches. The nurse then asks Ms. D'Angelo what barriers are preventing her from trusting and collaborating with her provider. She says that her main worry is that her blood pressure will be so high that she will miss work and need to see the physician too many times. The physician tells Ms. D'Angelo that he wants her to take responsibility for her own well-being, then asks a clinical nurse specialist to meet with Ms. D'Angelo to prepare an outpatient blood pressure management plan. Before Ms. D'Angelo is discharged from the ED, she is given a calendar listing her next two outpatient appointments and a prescription for a new blood pressure medication.

Critical Thinking Questions

1. Why was it important for the nurse to ask Ms. D'Angelo about barriers to outpatient care management?
2. How did the discussion at Ms. D'Angelo's bedside maximize her well-being?
3. How did the nurse and clinical nurse specialist assist the patient's need for autonomy?
4. Analyze how the bedside discussion was an example of collaborative practice in which nurses function effectively in cooperation with other healthcare professionals.

Principles and Practices of Ethical Decision Making

Individuals' personal, community, and professional values ultimately inform their decision-making processes. Each profession has its own set of values or principles that shape how its members approach ethical decisions. For professional nurses, the four primary principles that shape ethical decision making are autonomy, beneficence, justice, and veracity.

Autonomy

Autonomy is the right to self-determination. In the context of nursing, autonomy means that patients have the right to determine their own care. The nurse honors this principle by respecting the patient's decisions even if those decisions are in conflict with what the nurse believes is in the patient's best interest. The nurse violates the principle of autonomy by disregarding patient's choices, for example by medicating a patient even though the patient has refused the medication.

Beneficence

Beneficence requires that nurses take action to promote good because their basic obligation is to help others (Guido, 2020). For nurses, this obligation extends to include the related principle of **nonmaleficence**, which requires that nurses do no harm and instead safeguard their patients. Intentional harm is clearly not in keeping with this principle, but there can also be risk of harm in performing nursing interventions that are intended for good. Nonmaleficence does *not* mean that the nurse performs only actions that carry no risk to the patient. After all, many actions, such as administering medications, carry some degree of risk. In most cases, the risk of harm is weighed against the potential for benefit. Also, before the action is taken, the patient is given information about the potential benefits and risks, and the patient decides whether to accept the treatment. Consider the example of administering pain medication to a patient after an operation. The risks of discomfort from the injection and side effects from the medication are typically outweighed by the goal of relieving the patient's suffering.

Justice

Nurses must uphold the principle of justice in their practice. Here, **justice** means treating all patients fairly and in accordance with honor, standards, or law. This principle most commonly arises when decisions about the allocation of scarce resources must be made, as seen during the COVID-19 pandemic when many hospitals ran short on staff, personal protective equipment, and other resources. Nurses encounter the principle of justice any time they are challenged to give equal time and care to each patient.

Veracity

Individuals who always tell the truth reflect the principle of **veracity** (Guido, 2020). Veracity can be a particularly challenging principle for nurses, who may be faced with providing patients with complete information about their illness even though family members or significant others want the information withheld. Veracity is the principle that underlies the need for HCPs to give patients complete information before obtaining informed consent for any procedure.

Veracity is also one of several principles behind timely and accurate documentation of nursing interventions.

Applying the Principles

The ultimate goal of the ethical reasoning process should be to arrive at a decision that takes the patient's strengths and needs into account and provides the best evidence-based care for the patient while preserving the integrity of the patient, nurse, and other members of the healthcare team. A nurse's ethical obligations are divided among the patient, the HCP, the facility that employs the nurse, and the nurse's ethical values. An ethical decision requires addressing each obligation. For example, it is important that the nurse first consider the patient and what will best meet the patient's needs. This must be balanced with the patient's desires regarding healthcare and the desires of the patient's family members. The nurse must ensure that the patient is supported in all decisions and also support the family members in the relationship with the patient. While considering the patient's needs, the nurse must also follow all the policies of the agency that employs the nurse as well as the ANA standards of care.

Responsible ethical decision making is rational and systematic. It should be based on the ethical principles and codes described throughout this module and not on emotions, intuition, fixed policies, or precedent (i.e., an earlier similar occurrence). Frequently, the patient, family, and other members of the healthcare team all work together in reaching a decision (see **Figure 44.1** »). Sometimes families will seek help from a spiritual advisor, such as a minister, priest, imam, rabbi, or other trusted individual. Therefore, it is essential that nurses, other members of the healthcare team, and facility administration work to promote a more ethical practice environment through collaboration, communication, and compromise.

Dealing with ethical issues creates a great deal of stress; stress management becomes a valuable nursing skill. A nurse who works frequently with patients who are struggling with ethical issues requires a support system to assist in dealing with the ongoing stresses of the position. Regularly speaking with other healthcare professionals who are also involved in ethical issues can be helpful in providing the support the nurse needs.

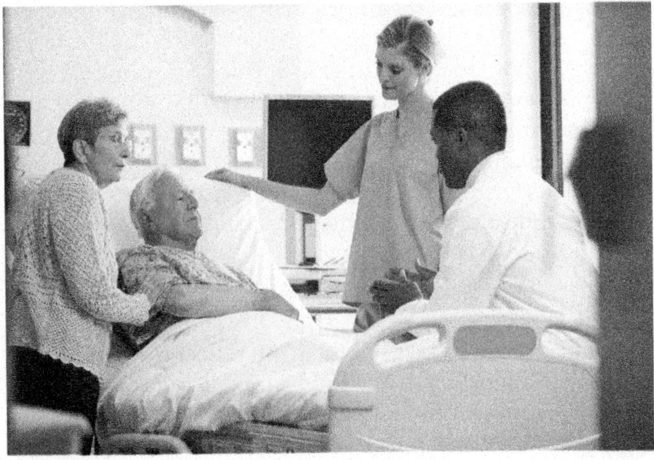

Figure 44.1 » When there is a need for ethical decisions with regard to patient advocacy, the patient, family, and healthcare team contribute to the final outcome.

Source: iStock/Getty Images.

Nurses encounter problems on a daily basis, but not all will be classified as either moral or ethical. It is important for the nurse to determine whether a *moral dilemma* exists before beginning the ethical decision-making process. Generally speaking, a moral dilemma is said to exist when the following criteria are satisfied:

- A situation presents potential solutions or actions that are in conflict with the needs of one or more individuals.
- There is one or more conflicting moral or ethical principles that can be applied to the situation.
- There is freedom to make a decision.
- The decision as to which course of action to take is influenced by personal feelings and by the situation itself.

When these conditions are met, the nurse should proceed with the ethical reasoning process. When they are not, the nurse should refer to professional standards of practice for guidance in determining the appropriate course of action.

Strategies to Enhance Ethical Decisions and Practice

Even when nurses do their best to adhere to the principles of their profession and engage in sound decision making, they still occasionally encounter organizational and social constraints that can hinder the ethical practice of nursing and create moral distress. Several strategies can help them overcome these hurdles. In particular, nurses can do the following:

- Be familiar with ethical principles and the ANA *Code of Ethics for Nurses.*
- Consider their own values and how they apply to ethical principles.
- Examine their own biases and provide nonjudgmental care to all patients.
- Seek continuing education related to ethical issues in nursing.
- Recognize that other healthcare professionals have differing values.
- Participate with others in discussing hypothetical ethical issues as a way of practicing the framework for ethical decision making.
- Be willing to serve on the agency ethics committee.
- Work with other healthcare professionals to ensure that nursing is included in policies related to ethical and moral issues.

Many organizations provide guidelines for evidence-based and ethical practice, some of which can be found online. For example, the Hartford Institute of Geriatric Nursing has developed a number of evidence-based nursing protocols for working with older patients. These protocols address topics such as advance directives, working with older adults with dementia, and discussing sexual health with older adults. The American College of Obstetrics and Gynecology and other professional nursing and medical organizations also make many of their guidelines for best practice available online.

Ethical dilemmas can occur during the normal provision of care. The frequency of ethical dilemmas was reported as being negatively correlated with the level of nursing skills (Dekeyser Ganz & Berkovitz, 2012). In effect, this study found that the less experienced nurses are, the more likely they are to encounter ethical dilemmas. Thus, for many nurses, seeking advice from a mentor or a more experienced peer is a strategy that can facilitate effective solutions and approaches to perceived ethical challenges. Organizational support for ethical decision making is another important factor (see the Evidence-Based Practice feature).

Another strategy that hospitals and other organizations have used to enhance ethical decision making is to implement an interdisciplinary ethics committee. The Joint Commission (2017) states that the culture of the healthcare facility must ensure that all care is given in an ethical manner. Healthcare facilities establish interdisciplinary committees to assist in making an ethical decision in the event the patient is not able to express personal wishes for care. These committees may also be used to determine the best ethical decision in the event that the patient and/or family is in conflict with the HCP or healthcare facility in regard to care.

Case Study » Part 3

Reread Parts 1 and 2 of the case study. Before the end of the shift, another staff member in the ED asks the nurse to pick up the phone. As soon as she says hello, a woman asks her, "Did June D'Angelo come to your department earlier today?" The nurse immediately realizes that this situation will become a HIPAA issue if she does not manage it carefully and correctly. She asks the woman, "Who is calling, please?" The woman groans loudly and says, "This is Mrs. Jones. I am June's supervisor where she works, and I need to know if she was there today." The nurse answers, "Mrs. Jones, I am sorry, but due to privacy rules, we cannot discuss any patient information or names on the phone and cannot confirm whether any patient was or was not in our department." Mrs. Jones becomes upset and states, "Then how can I know what is going on? June missed her shift today!" The nurse remains calm and replies, "My best suggestion is that you contact your employee directly yourself." At that point, Mrs. Jones hangs up.

Critical Thinking Questions

1. How did the nurse realize that this was a possible HIPAA issue?
2. What privacy and confidentiality rules and ethical guidelines was the nurse following?
3. Do you think the nurse managed the call correctly?

Evidence-Based Practice

Individual Ethical Decision Making, Knowledge of Ethics, and Organizational Support

Problem

Nurses are faced with ethical dilemmas every day, and these dilemmas often must be resolved quickly. Research suggests that nurses may feel vulnerable both before and after dealing with ethically volatile situations. In some cases, nurses do not feel sufficiently competent in their knowledge of ethics to be comfortable with their role in the decision-making process; in other cases, nurses do not feel that they receive adequate organizational support.

Evidence

Naseri-Salahshour and Sajadi (2020) explored newly licensed nurses' perception of ethics in the organizations in which they worked. In general, these nurses had a positive perception of the ethical climate; however, these positive perceptions were primarily reserved for patients, physicians, and fellow nurses. The organization itself and nurse managers were viewed less favorably. The nurses with the most positive perceptions of the ethical environment were those who self-identified as feeling very competent in their understanding of ethics.

Kim, Seo, and Kim (2018) assessed intensive care, medical–surgical, emergency, and oncology nurses on specific areas of difficulty in ethical decision making. Among the most significant difficulties, nurses identified a lack of education regarding ethics, a lack of organizational support for ethical decision making, and struggles to provide evidence-based care. However, the nurses' desire for organizational ethical support varied from department to department.

Jansen and Hanssen (2017) and Keresi, Carlsson, and Lindberg (2016) conducted similar research with psychiatric nurses. Their research suggested that nurses often felt squeezed between their own ethical values and the values of the organization as a whole. Nurses indicated that they often found themselves in the role of negotiator between the various stakeholder groups, which contributed to feelings of burnout and moral distress.

Implications

Nurses need organizational support in order to manage ethical dilemmas and cope with their role in the process. Kim et al. (2018) identify ethical counseling as a means of preventing fatigue in nurses' personal and professional lives. They also suggest that unit-specific in-house training be provided to improve nurses' feelings of ethical competence and aid in the development of practical solutions to ethical problems.

Poikkeus et al. (2020) suggest that nurse leaders take a greater role in orienting nurses to the ethical procedures and practices on their units and facilitate interprofessional discussions on ethics. They also support continuing ethics education for nurses.

Finally, Chooljian et al. (2016) encourage organizational ethics committees to serve in a supportive role for nurses. Typically, these committees are involved with nurses' ethical issues only when a dispute arises that requires committee attention. The researchers believe that organizations as a whole and nurses in particular could benefit from guidance and reassurance from the ethics committee throughout the decision-making process, even when the dilemmas involved do not require committee attention.

Critical Thinking Application

1. What conclusions can you draw about the way in which nurses build an ethical support network according to the research? In what ways do you think this type of support network is beneficial to nurses? In what way might it be detrimental to nurses?
2. In their research, Jansen and Hanssen and Keresi et al. describe that nurses feel conflicted between personal and organizational ethics. What does this suggest about the practicality of organizational ethics in clinical situations?
3. How would the increased involvement by organizational ethics committees suggested by Chooljian et al. improve the ethical climate of the organization? How would it help nurses avoid fatigue and burnout associated with ethical decision making?

REVIEW The Concept of Ethics

RELATE Link the Concepts

Linking the concept of ethics with the concept of addiction:

1. How does substance abuse affect people's ability to make ethical decisions based on their personal values and beliefs?
2. What parts of the ANA *Code of Ethics for Nurses* address impaired nurses?

Linking the concept of ethics with the concept of reproduction:

3. What are your personal beliefs regarding fertility treatments? How would you feel about a patient who has conceived multiple fetuses through fertility treatments and now wants to have selective reduction to reduce the number of fetuses she will carry to term?
4. As a nurse, what are your responsibilities to a teenager who is seeking information on birth control methods?

REFER Go to Pearson MyLab Nursing and eText

REFLECT Apply Your Knowledge

Keith Morgan, a 46-year-old man, fell and broke his leg several weeks ago. He is now receiving home healthcare. You are a home health nurse case manager, and you go to Mr. Morgan's home to assess his ability to ambulate. When you arrive, he is alert and oriented but continues to report a high pain level. During your assessment, he tells you that Tylenol just isn't effective in controlling his pain. When you ask Mr. Morgan about the effect of the narcotic that has been prescribed and documented as given by his primary nurse, he tells you that the nurse told him all he needed was Tylenol and that he has not taken any other pain medication.

1. How should you respond to Mr. Morgan?
2. What is your legal responsibility in this scenario? What is your ethical responsibility? What actions do you need to take?

>> Exemplar 44.A Morality

Exemplar Learning Outcomes

44.A Analyze morality as it relates to ethics.

- Explain the development of morality.
- Explain how moral theories can be used as a framework for examining ethical dilemmas.
- List three types of moral theories.
- Summarize moral principles.

Exemplar Key Terms

Accountability, *2739*
Consequence-based (teleologic) theories, *2738*
Fidelity, *2739*
Moral development, *2739*
Moral principles, *2739*
Moral rules, *2739*
Principles-based (deontologic) theories, *2738*
Relationship-based (caring) theories, *2739*
Responsibility, *2739*
Utilitarianism, *2738*
Utility, *2738*

Overview

Morality typically refers to an individual's private standards of what is right and wrong, not only in terms of conduct but also in terms of character and attitude. When the members of a group share many of these standards, morals may serve as the basis for the group's ethics, that is, its system of standards governing behaviors and relationships. Morals also help shape the laws of a society, although some actions may be legal but not moral, whereas others may be moral but illegal.

Just as people tend to confuse morality and ethics, they also tend to wrongly conflate morality and spirituality. Certainly, individuals' spiritual and/or religious beliefs may shape their ideas regarding right and wrong. For example, people may be morally opposed to blood transfusions, sterilization, abortion, contraception, or any number of medical interventions because their religion forbids these things. However, people need not hold any spiritual beliefs whatsoever to cultivate a clear sense of morality. (For more information, refer to Module 30, Spirituality.)

Theories of Morality and Moral Development

Because morality intersects with so many of humankind's "big questions" about life and death, it has long been a topic of philosophical interest and debate. Much of this interest has revolved around the theoretical basis of morality, while some of it has focused on formulating a clearer picture of the process by which a person's moral standards emerge.

Moral Frameworks

Nurses use moral theories or frameworks to understand their own and their patients' decisions concerning care. Developing a better understanding of these frameworks assists the nurse in recognizing ethical decisions and using the information to work with patients in clarifying their own situations. The most common moral theories are based on consequences, individual rights, and relationships.

- **Consequence-based (teleologic) theories** seek to determine if an action is good (right or wrong) based on the outcome of the action. In other words, was the action fair? Under the consequentialist theory known as **utilitarianism**, moral acts are those that work to ensure the most good is provided to the greatest number of people while causing harm to the least number of individuals; this is the principle of **utility**. This type of decision making may be used in situations where supplies of medications or treatments are limited.
- **Principles-based (deontologic) theories** are based on a belief that an individual action is determined by what is right and not by the result (consequence). Nurses may be

placed in a position to use this theory when the wishes of a family are not in alignment with what the nurse perceives as right or correct. For example, the nurse has a general obligation to be truthful with patients and may not want to lie to a patient who asks if he is dying even though the patient's spouse has given instructions not to tell the patient he is dying.

- **Relationship-based (caring) theories** emphasize characteristics such as courage, commitment, and generosity, viewing actions under a lens of caring and responsibility. Generally, relationship-based theories emphasize the welfare of the common good, in contrast to the individual rights promoted by principles-based theories.

Nurses use moral frameworks to assist in determining the best course of action for both the nurse and the patient. Although frameworks can assist in making moral decisions, they cannot guarantee or determine an outcome. For example, consider their use in the case of a 16-year-old who has relapsed for the third time with cancer. The healthcare team offers a possible treatment that has many side effects and has a very limited chance of producing another remission. The teen's parents want to begin the medication trial immediately, but the teen is refusing to take it. The nurses have worked with this young person for the last 6 years and support this teen's decision. Using consequences-based theory, the nurses approach the issue with the belief that the treatment will cause their patient more pain and has little probability of working. Furthermore, they believe there is a real possibility the parents will eventually feel guilty for making the teen take part in the treatment. Principles-based theories support the nurses' belief that the teen has the right to make his own decision about his treatment. Relationship-based theory suggests that the nurses help the parents understand what the teen is feeling and emphasize the desire the parents have to meet their child's needs, which the teen patient has expressed in a desire to refuse the treatment.

Moral Development

Moral development begins in infancy and continues throughout life. It is the process of learning the difference between right and wrong and informs each individual's determination of how to act in an ethical situation.

Lawrence Kohlberg and Carol Gilligan are two well-known theorists of moral development. Kohlberg's theory shows how morality develops as an individual moves from infancy to adulthood. Gilligan's theory focuses on women and emphasizes the roles of caring and justice in moral development. (Module 25, Development, provides a more complete discussion of these two theories.)

Moral Principles of Professional Nursing

Nursing is a profession that usually consists of different interactions with individuals who are dealing with health-related issues. Nurses utilize **moral principles**—broad philosophical concepts such as autonomy and beneficence—to assist in determining if an action is right or wrong. These principles are generally accepted by a group of persons to be useful for making decisions. Different moral values are held by individuals, which leads to the nurse facing ethical issues in the care of patients. These values then provide the nurse with guidelines, or **moral rules**, for deciding which action is best for the patient.

Like many professions, nursing is shaped by a set of guiding moral principles that shape how their members act. For nurses, the most important moral principles are autonomy, nonmaleficence, beneficence, justice, fidelity, veracity, responsibility, and accountability. Autonomy, beneficence, nonmaleficence, justice, and veracity were discussed earlier in this module.

Fidelity

The principle of **fidelity** is that the nurse is faithful and loyal in all actions with patients, colleagues, employers, and society, and also with themselves. Fidelity requires that the nurse recognize that any statement made to a patient must be upheld. For example, if the nurse tells the patient that a certain medication will be given the next time it is due, it is important for the nurse to deliver the medication at the prescribed time. Similarly, the nurse exhibits fidelity when following the HCP's order to administer medications at the prescribed times.

Accountability and Responsibility

Nurses must also have professional accountability and responsibility. **Accountability** involves being answerable for the outcomes of a task or assignment. Nurses are accountable for their own actions and behaviors, but they may also be accountable for the actions of others, such as subordinates or trainees. **Responsibility** is the specific obligation associated with the performance of duties of a particular role, and it belongs to the individual performing the duties. Thus, ethical nurses are able to explain the rationale behind every action and recognize the standards to which they will be held. (For more information, see Module 42, Accountability.)

NURSING PROCESS

Morality shapes the profession of nursing in many different ways. Not only do certain moral principles drive nursing theory, practice, and decision making but they also serve as the foundation for the professional codes of ethics described earlier in this module. Nonetheless, unethical or immoral behavior still occurs among nurses. Although only a very few individuals in the profession exhibit this behavior, all nurses must be able to identify, discourage, and report it. In fact, failure to report certain forms of immoral behavior by another healthcare professional is a violation of the ANA *Code of Ethics for Nurses* and the nurse–patient relationship.

SAFETY ALERT Nurses have both an ethical and a legal responsibility to report certain forms of abuse to the appropriate authorities. Depending on the state in which a nurse practices, mandatory reporting laws may include known and/or suspected child abuse and neglect, elder abuse and neglect, and/or domestic violence. Nurses must also take action to ensure the safety of suspected victims of abuse and neglect.

To guard against questionable and unethical practices, nurses must have a thorough understanding of their own morality and what constitutes right and wrong for them as individuals. They must also have a thorough understanding of their professional code of ethics and be able to identify when the ethics of another professional or agency are contrary to the *Code of Ethics for Nurses*. Furthermore, nurses must recognize that they will encounter patients at various stages of moral development, patients with questionable or confusing morals, and patients who are immoral. Nursing ethics and professional codes of conduct require nurses to deliver high-quality, professional care to all patients, regardless of the patients' morality. This can sometimes challenge even the most professional, experienced nurse. Examples of such challenges include the following:

- A patient with HIV is transferred to the intensive care unit (ICU) of a hospital from the prison infirmary. The patient has paraplegia with no ability to move his legs. He is serving a life sentence in prison for repeated child molestation and rape.
- A young woman comes to the local free health clinic with her boyfriend to get a pregnancy test. The test is positive. The boyfriend immediately starts talking to her about how she'll have to get an abortion.
- An older woman is brought to the ED by a friend who came to visit and found the woman lying in her own feces. She is weak and dehydrated. The friend says that the woman lives with her son and his wife.

To care for patients such as these, nurses must have an awareness of their own morality and ethics, a thorough understanding of the requirements they must follow under the professional code of ethics, and an understanding of the reporting requirements in their state and the procedures they must follow in their place of employment. Although a nurse's own personal beliefs, morality, and bias will influence how the nurse manages each situation, the nurse must ultimately remember the moral duty to provide the best possible care, no matter what the patient's morality or immorality may be. (See the Focus on Diversity and Culture feature for additional information.) The following sections take a closer look at how this duty comes into play during all stages of the nursing process.

Assessment

As with any patient, assessment of the patient who is immoral or who is exposed to immorality that involves abuse or mistreatment includes a nursing history and physical examination. Patients who are immoral may not be able or willing to participate in a trusting nurse–patient relationship and may not respond to attempts at therapeutic communication. In interviewing these patients, the nurse should maintain a calm, nonjudgmental manner and should ask open-ended questions in a matter-of-fact tone.

Diagnosis

Nursing diagnoses for an individual with moral dilemmas or distress or a patient with a family member or significant other with questionable morals will vary. For example, appropriate diagnoses in the scenarios mentioned earlier may include the following:

- The prisoner transferred to the ICU will have a number of diagnoses appropriate to his medical condition. In addition, the following nursing problems may be appropriate:
  - Moral conflict
  - Nonadherence
  - Social isolation.

  The young woman who has just found out she is pregnant may have the following problems:
  - Potential for situational low self-esteem
  - Vulnerability
  - Lack of knowledge about pregnancy.

  The older woman who was brought to the ED by a friend may have the following problems:
  - Impaired family functioning
  - Powerlessness
  - Social isolation.

Focus on Diversity and Culture

Cultural Relativism

Cultural relativism is the idea that people's morals are deeply rooted in the beliefs and behaviors of their particular culture. According to this principle, even though a person's moral principles may conflict with that of the nurse, the nurse should not automatically assume that these principles are indefensible or incorrect because they likely make sense when viewed through the lens of that person's culture (Butts & Rich, 2020).

Cultural relativism was first popularized by anthropologists and other social researchers who wanted to describe and compare cultures in a systematic manner that was free from bias. This concept has become increasingly widespread throughout the field of nursing as theorists and practitioners alike place greater emphasis on cross-cultural care. Nursing's embrace of this concept has helped to bring about a care environment in which many patients feel more autonomous, more respected, and more valued. However, cultural relativism also creates moral and ethical dilemmas for the nurse.

Consider, for example, the practice of female genital mutilation (FGM), sometimes also known as "female circumcision." Although FGM involves physical mutilation of underage girls, some African and Middle Eastern cultures view it as morally acceptable and an important rite of passage into adulthood. Most Western cultures, however—as well as the United Nations and the World Health Organization (WHO)—regard FGM as a clear violation of the rights to autonomy, consent, and freedom from harm. Cultural practices that raise similar concerns include child marriage and severe limitations on the rights of females. When nurses encounter situations like these, they must carefully evaluate what course of action will produce greater benefit and/or lesser harm to the patient. In some cases, as in the case of FGM, the nurse's duty to preserve the patient's rights to self-determination, consent, and freedom from harm far outweigh the nurse's duty to honor the cultural preferences of the patient and the patient's family. The nurse may also be legally required to act in a certain way. Because situations like these are fraught with potential moral, ethical, and legal implications, it is always wise for the nurse to seek the counsel of a mentor or supervisor before deciding on an appropriate course of action.

Planning

Individuals with moral dilemmas or distress may find it difficult to participate in the planning process; they may even show disdain for it. The nurse may try to obtain cooperation by capitalizing on needs the patient presents during the assessment. For example, the nurse might say, "You said you didn't want to be in pain anymore, so we need to run these tests to find out what is causing your pain so that we can treat it" or "I know you don't like the food here, but remember we discussed that to feel better, you have to get appropriate nutrition." Although outcomes for these patients will vary widely, a few frequently appropriate outcomes include the following:

- The patient will participate appropriately as able in the therapeutic regimen.
- The patient will refrain from causing disruptions that affect other patients and staff.
- The patient will be appropriately supervised during caring interventions, diagnostic procedures, and other activities. For example, a security staff member or member of law enforcement will be present during caring interventions for a patient with a history of assault.

Implementation

Caring for individuals with moral dilemmas or distress can be challenging, unpleasant, and time-consuming. Interventions that may be appropriate when working with these patients could include any of the following:

- Following procedures that ensure the safety of staff working with the patient and adding precautions or procedures as necessary to ensure safety of other patients and staff. Refer to the Safety Alert for additional information.

SAFETY ALERT When working with patients who are potentially dangerous, the nurse can help to ensure both personal safety and the safety of others by staying between the patient and the door and by notifying security to be present as necessary. Other appropriate measures may include restraining the patient, providing additional staff for interventions and procedures, and transporting the patient during times when hallways and other areas have the fewest people around.

- Encouraging patients to make informed decisions without pressure from others. In the earlier example of the young woman who learned that she was pregnant, her boyfriend was attempting to influence her decision. Although patients are free to seek advice from whomever they wish, the nurse must ensure that the patient makes a treatment decision free from coercion.
- Referring patients to spiritual leaders or mental health professionals as necessary. Consulting with these individuals may assist patients in the ethical decision-making process.

Evaluation

Treatment options that challenge individual morality and ethics, such as abortion and organ transplantation, often leave patients and family members second-guessing decisions after they have been made. Evaluation of patients who are faced with decisions that pose a challenge to their morality or of patients who lack morality should be based on the question "Is the patient satisfied that the best possible decision was made?" Nurses who work with patients in these situations should support autonomy; provide a listening, nonjudgmental ear; and continue to support the patient's decision after the conclusion of treatment.

Nursing Care Plan

A Patient Presenting with Morality Issues

Michael Dunham is a 50-year-old man with HIV who is also paraplegic. He is admitted to the intensive care unit (ICU) of the local hospital from the prison infirmary, where he has been for more than a month.

ASSESSMENT	DIAGNOSES	PLANNING
Mr. Dunham has a history of IV drug use and having sexual relations with female sex workers. He is on oxygen by nasal cannula. He is restrained to his bed. Almost every time members of the nursing staff work with him, he tries to spit on them in an effort to "give" them his disease. Upon arrival, the prison transport unit informs the head nurse that Mr. Dunham is serving a life sentence for molesting children and that he used his disability to trick preteen girls into coming close enough for him to handcuff them to his wheelchair so they could not escape his sexual abuse. Before releasing them, he would threaten to kill their parents if the girls told anyone what happened. Upon physical examination, the nurses working with Mr. Dunham find the following: ■ T 37.9°C oral (100.2°F), P 104 beats/min, R 32/min, BP 102/60 mmHg ■ Oxygen saturation 84%; breath sounds reveal coarse crackles in the left lower base	■ Moral conflict ■ Impaired social skills ■ Social isolation ■ Inadequate gas exchange	■ The patient will participate appropriately as able in the therapeutic regimen. ■ The patient will refrain from causing disruptions that affect other patients and staff. ■ The patient will be appropriately supervised during caring interventions, diagnostic procedures, and other activities. ■ Nursing staff will take appropriate precautions to prevent the spread of HIV.

Nursing Care Plan *(continued)*

ASSESSMENT	DIAGNOSES	PLANNING
■ Mild cyanosis of nail beds and mucous membranes ■ Use of accessory muscles to breathe with intercostal and suprasternal retractions ■ Flaccid paralysis of lower extremities since the patient was 8 years old ■ ECG shows two to three premature ventricular contractions per minute ■ HIV positive with CD4 T-cell count of 64; CBC showed WBC of 9.8, elevated lymphocyte, and low segs ■ Chest x-ray shows characteristic appearance of *Pneumocystis jirovecii*		

IMPLEMENTATION

- A correctional officer or member of the hospital security staff will be present during any intervention in which removing the restraints is necessary.
- Nurses will provide care in groups of two or more.
- The patient will be offered counseling and a referral to the hospital chaplain.
- The nurses caring for the patient will share their concerns with their supervisor or mentor.
- The patient will be consulted and asked to give permission for all treatments and therapies.
- Additional interventions will be used as warranted by medical condition and ordered by the attending physician.

EVALUATION

Mr. Dunham's condition continued to deteriorate, and he was placed on a mechanical ventilator. As it became increasingly difficult to meet his oxygenation needs, he was given paralytics. Mr. Dunham ultimately died of cardiorespiratory failure.

CRITICAL THINKING

1. Does a nurse who is assigned to care for this patient have the option of requesting a different assignment on the basis of feelings of revulsion, disgust, or anger at the patient's past history and behavior? Why or why not?
2. What interventions would be the most difficult for you to provide this patient? Explain your answer.
3. How would your moral beliefs regarding this patient's history and behavior affect your nursing care of the patient? Is it appropriate to reduce the quality of care you provide as a result? Explain your answer.

REVIEW Morality

RELATE Link the Concepts and Exemplars

Linking the exemplar of morality with the concept of development:

A mother brings her 13-year-old daughter to the gynecologist's office for the girl's first pelvic examination. The daughter is autistic and has a spoken vocabulary of fewer than 500 words. The mother tells the nurse that she wants to talk to the physician about getting her daughter's tubes tied or some other procedure that will keep her daughter from getting pregnant if anyone molests her.

1. How does the daughter's developmental level interfere with her ability to make autonomous decisions?
2. What ethical responsibilities do you have to the daughter in this situation?

Linking the exemplar of morality with the concept of comfort:

3. What moral or ethical issues are involved in patients' advance directives and do-not-resuscitate orders?
4. What are your feelings about the morality of do-not-resuscitate orders? How would you keep these feelings from influencing your discussions with a patient about do-not-resuscitate orders? Would your feelings change if the patient were a child or adolescent?

REFER Go to Pearson MyLab Nursing and eText

REFLECT Apply Your Knowledge

The nurse on the day shift at an inpatient rehabilitation center is making her morning rounds when she finds a young woman awake and crying in her bed. The woman has bruises on her wrists and forearms that were not there when the nurse last saw the patient the previous afternoon. When the nurse asks the patient what happened, the patient responds only by shaking her head, and she pulls away when the nurse reaches out to comfort her. The nurse checks the visitor logs and confirms that the patient had no visitors the night before.

1. What are the priorities of care for the patient at this moment?
2. What steps should the nurse take to try to determine what happened to this patient?
3. How should the nurse document her findings, and with whom should the nurse share these findings?
4. Does the nurse have an obligation to report these findings? If so, to whom must she report them?

» Exemplar 44.B Ethical Dilemmas

Exemplar Learning Outcomes

44.B Analyze dilemmas related to ethics.

- Propose solutions to ethical dilemmas based on an individual's problem and ethical principles.
- Analyze conflicts among nursing loyalties and obligations to patients, families, the multiprofessional team, and outside organizations.
- Critique the bioethical dilemmas that may arise during the care of patients and families.
- Explore the nurse's role in supporting patients' rights to information and counseling when making genetic testing decisions.
- Analyze the challenges and dilemmas patients and their families face when managing end-of-life care choices, advance directives, euthanasia, and the withdrawal of life support.
- Differentiate considerations related to ethical dilemmas for patients across the lifespan.

Exemplar Key Terms

Active euthanasia, *2747*
Assisted suicide, *2747*
Bioethical dilemma, *2745*
Ethical dilemma, *2743*
Euthanasia, *2747*
Withdrawing or withholding life-sustaining therapy (WWLST), *2748*

Overview

An **ethical dilemma** exists when two or more rights, values, obligations, or responsibilities come into conflict. Conflict may arise between the nurse's personal values and those of another individual or the organization. Conflict may also develop between the nurse's principles and the need to achieve a desired outcome. Conflict may occur between two or more individuals or groups to whom the nurse has an obligation, such as the patient, a colleague, the nursing profession, the nurse's employer, or society (Dekeyser Ganz & Berkovitz, 2012; Lachman, 2012).

A number of factors contribute to ethical dilemmas. Rapidly changing technology and conflicting societal and cultural values are among the most important factors today. Technology pervades most aspects of our lives, and today's nurses have grown up in a tech-driven society. The result is new ethical concerns that didn't exist 10—or even 5—years ago. Social change is also altering the way in which patients and nurses approach routine aspects of the healthcare experience. Nurses must be prepared to handle dilemmas related to these key drivers of change.

Other factors that contribute to ethical dilemmas include the development of conflicting loyalties and obligations among nurses. Competing allegiances to patients, families, colleagues, employers, and self can make it difficult for the nurse to determine the most ethical course of action. In addition, increasing pressure to contain healthcare costs at the organizational level may result in situations that give rise to ethical dilemmas.

No matter the contributing factors, the nurse must recognize ethical dilemmas and take appropriate action. Some dilemmas affect the care patients receive, and the nurse must be prepared to inform the patient and other staff members of these issues. Other dilemmas may involve an individual's nursing practice. When such issues arise, the nurse must act in a manner consistent with the ANA *Code of Ethics for Nurses*. No matter the dilemma a nurse faces, recognizing and managing ethical challenges—and evaluating the outcomes of interventions taken—promote ethical practice.

Factors Contributing to Ethical Dilemmas

Ethical dilemmas arise in many situations and touch many areas of nursing practice. In spite of the diverse nature of these dilemmas, they often start with common contributing factors. Technological change, social change, and conflicting loyalties are three such factors.

Technological Changes

Technological change creates new ethical dilemmas that did not previously exist. From the nursing perspective, there are two areas of technology that must be considered: medical technology and communications technology.

Medical technology continues to change as new treatments and devices revolutionize healthcare. Some devices, such as monitors, respirators, and feeding tubes, have been around for 50 to 100 years or more, but as they have become more sophisticated, they have presented more occasions for ethical dilemmas. For example, the decision of whether to provide life-sustaining measures to an 800-gram premature infant would not exist without modern technology.

Devices are not the only medical technology to radically change the healthcare landscape. Organ transplantation is another procedure that has experienced great advances and is also subject to ongoing ethical debate. These debates focus on both the donor and the recipient and concern the definitions of donor death in relation to organ viability and the proper procedure for selecting recipients on the basis of age, health factors, and time on the waiting list.

Communications technology is also of critical importance to nurses. Cell phones, tablets, and other "smart" devices have made people and organizations more connected. They have also changed the nature of what people share with one another. The downside of this connectedness is that it can be difficult to separate what is appropriate to share from what is inappropriate to share and when it is appropriate to do so. For example, an excited student nurse may snap a picture of herself and her preceptor on the first day of clinical education in the ED. If she posts the photo to her social media page, the confidentiality of any patients in the background has been compromised. In addition, taking the photograph and posting it during the time designated for clinical education is ethically questionable, as it takes the student's attention away from learning and from providing high-quality patient care, and it is probably also a violation of both school and facility policies.

In this situation, the student nurse also opens herself up to questions that may present an ethical dilemma. Suppose a friend's father was admitted to the ED that day and the friend saw the picture. The friend may ask the student nurse whether she saw his father, what his father's condition is, and whether his father is still in the ED. The student nurse is faced with the ethical dilemma of answering her friend's questions or maintaining his father's privacy.

Patients now have unprecedented access to medical information through their smart devices. Patients can search for information about their symptoms or condition and find numerous sources within seconds. Unfortunately, not all health information available on the internet is up to date, accurate, or trustworthy. This can create ethical issues for nurses. For instance, during a patient interview, a nurse may learn that a patient is treating her condition using a remedy she found online. The remedy is unlikely to cause harm to the patient but is also unlikely to provide any benefit. The nurse feels uncomfortable addressing the issue for fear of upsetting the patient. The nurse must decide whether it is ethically responsible to allow the patient to continue with a remedy that he knows will not do her any good. Often, situations such as these can be avoided if nurses proactively direct patients to reliable online sources of health information.

Medical and communications technology converge in some areas of nursing. Electronic health records (EHRs) are one example of this convergence. EHRs offer patients ready access to their own medical records via their devices and allow providers to quickly get a comprehensive view of a patient's history and care. In some organizations, care providers access EHRs on in-room computers or using tablet devices provided by the organization for that purpose. These records, although useful, present their own set of ethical dilemmas. For example, suppose a nurse knows that her brother is a patient at the clinic where she works. She suspects that he is ill, but when she asks him about it, he brushes her off. She may be able to review his EHR via the clinic's system, but from a professional standpoint, she should not do so unless she is providing care to him at the clinic, a situation that in itself presents an ethical dilemma. Other issues may arise if a nurse fails to log out of an EHR access device before taking a break or notices that another nurse has failed to log out. In addition, it may be tempting for nurses to use devices designated for EHR access for unauthorized personal purposes.

Social Changes

Social beliefs and ideas are constantly changing, in part because of the advances brought about by new technology. The increasing interconnectedness of people around the globe contributes to the pace at which these ideas are spread. These changes bring with them a variety of ethical dilemmas for all members of society. They have a particularly big impact on HCPs because they often affect how people choose to live and maintain their health.

One particularly important change relates to the way in which people define life. Some believe that life should be allowed to end naturally; others believe that everything possible should be done to preserve life. Modern medical technology has made it possible to preserve or extend life for individuals who are terminally ill or in a vegetative state. These patients may survive for weeks or months with medical assistance. This assistance is expensive and draws on scarce clinical resources. Patients or their families may feel strongly about maintaining life via this technology even if HCPs do not consider it appropriate. Conversely, the patient or family may be strongly opposed to such treatments even if care providers think that they are necessary. The nurse must be prepared to provide care in either of these scenarios. In addition, the nurse may be called on to participate in difficult conversations about these topics with patients, their families, and other HCPs.

Closely related to this is the issue of quality of life. Although life can be prolonged or maintained, it may not include the freedoms and experiences that are considered important by many people. For example, suppose a 14-year-old cancer patient has been given 2 months to live. A new treatment may extend his life an additional 2 months but is likely to be very painful. The patient and his family must weigh whether length of life or quality of life is more important to them. Another potentially complicating issue here is the patient's age; his parents may be in favor of the treatment while the patient himself may be against it. Unless the care is being provided in a state that recognizes the decision-making capabilities of mature minors, the patient cannot make this decision for himself. (See Module 49, Legal Issues, for more information about mature minors and minor consent.) This situation can be particularly challenging for the nurse who has strong personal opinions about the issues.

The way in which individuals define and pursue wellness is changing, too. One way this is evidenced is in the adoption of nontraditional diets and the growing popularity of complementary health approaches. For instance, gluten-free diets (in which only foods that do not contain gluten protein are consumed) have become much more popular. Some individuals adopt these diets because of celiac disease or gluten intolerance. For others, the diets are a conscious choice based on personal beliefs about health. Issues may arise, however, if patients' nutritional needs are not being met or if the patient chooses a nutritional complementary treatment approach that is either ineffective or has the potential for harm.

Another social change is the increasing public support of the use of medical marijuana—either whole, unprocessed plants or their extracts—to treat diseases or symptoms (National Center for Complementary and Integrative Health, 2019). Research suggests that the chemicals in marijuana can be useful for treating a variety of illnesses. Legal use of medical marijuana is regulated on the state level; the federal government does not recognize or approve medical use of the drug. Medical marijuana has the potential to create ethical dilemmas for the nurse. For example, the nurse may believe that it is a useful and appropriate treatment for a patient's condition, but the patient may be adamantly opposed to consumption of the drug. The converse may also occur: The nurse is opposed, but the patient is in favor.

Other social changes include increasing prevalence of mental health disorders and increasing awareness of the needs of transgender individuals. Providing nonjudgmental care that is free of stigma or bias regardless of the patient's health, mental health, sexuality, or gender is inherent in Provision 1 of the ANA Code of Ethics for Nurses.

Conflicting Loyalties and Obligations

According to the ANA *Code of Ethics for Nurses* (2015a), the nurse's primary commitment is to the patient. As part of that commitment, the nurse must engage the patient in care planning. In planning care with patients, it is not always easy to determine which actions best serve the patients' needs. For instance, the nurse may be aware that medical marijuana has been shown to be effective for a patient's condition. The patient has not responded to mainstream therapies, but medical marijuana is not legal in the state where the nurse and patient live. Although legal issues are involved, the nurse must determine whether, ethically, the patient should be made aware of this potentially effective alternative.

When planning and caring for a patient, the nurse must also consider the patient's family relationships. The nurse also has an obligation to the patient's family as well as the patient; however, it is important to remember that the nurse's first loyalty always lies with the patient. This is particularly important should conflicts arise between the patient and the family about care. Suppose a patient with necrotizing fasciitis of the foot has been presented with several care options by her physician, including amputation. The patient wants to pursue amputation, but her spouse would prefer that she receive a different treatment. The nurse may help the patient and her spouse reach an understanding but is ultimately obligated to ensure that the patient's wishes are met.

The nurse may also have loyalties to colleagues and the healthcare organization. For example, suppose a hospital denies a $2 per hour cost-of-living raise for the nursing staff. The staff as a whole chooses to strike, but each individual nurse must decide whether to honor the picket lines during the strike. The nurse may experience conflicting feelings about the need to support coworkers in their efforts to improve working conditions, the need to show loyalty to the organization, and the need to ensure that patients receive care and are not abandoned.

Ethical Dilemmas in Patient Care

Specific ethical issues related to human life or health often develop in the course of caring for patients. These issues are referred to as **bioethical dilemmas**. Bioethical dilemmas arise during the care of patients and families and often emerge from a combination of causative factors. HIV/AIDS, genetic testing, organ transplantation, and end-of-life decisions all present their own unique ethical dilemmas. For example, in 2020 and 2021, hospitals and healthcare systems in areas plagued by high numbers of people with severe COVID-19 symptoms faced numerous issues when patient need outweighed capacity (**Figure 44.2** »). These included sending patients out of area for treatment and rationing care provided by emergency medical services and hospitals.

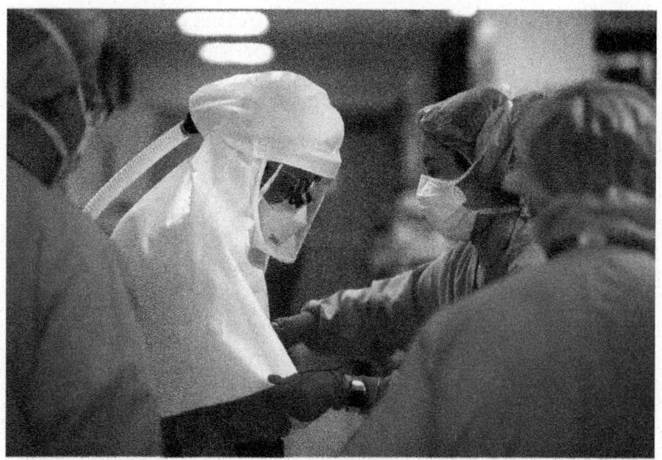

Figure 44.2 » From rationing treatment, vaccines, and PPE to the direct exposure of frontline workers, the COVID-19 pandemic presented a number of ethical dilemmas in healthcare.
Source: Justin Sullivan/Getty Images.

HIV and AIDS

HIV is a virus that attacks the immune system and may lead to AIDS. It is spread through contact with bodily fluids, including blood, breast milk, rectal fluids, semen, and vaginal fluids. Because contact with these fluids is often associated with sexual behavior and illicit drug use, HIV/AIDS bears a social stigma (Mahon, 2018). According to an ANA position statement on risk and responsibility in nursing, the nurse cannot set aside the moral obligation to care for the patient infected with HIV/AIDS unless the risk associated with providing that care exceeds the responsibility (ANA, 2015b). More information can be found in Exemplar 8.A, HIV/AIDS, in Module 8, Immunity.

There is no safe or effective cure for HIV/AIDS, which means that an individual who contracts the virus will have it for life. However, antiretroviral therapy (ART) can effectively control HIV as well as reduce the patient's risk of transmitting HIV.

Although ART is an important treatment that has changed the course of HIV infection for many patients, the combination of drugs involved is expensive. Private health insurance, Medicare, or Medicaid covers a portion of costs, but patients are responsible for deductibles and copayments, which may be costly. For patients without insurance, Medicare, or Medicaid coverage, the cost associated with ART may be prohibitive. This reality presents a number of ethical dilemmas, including whether it is ethical to allow a patient to endure a controllable condition because of inability to pay. Programs such as the Ryan White HIV/AIDS Program and the Health Center Program attempt to address these issues by providing care and medications to individuals who could not otherwise afford it. The Health Center Program in particular serves individuals in minority and traditionally underserved communities, which tend to have higher HIV infection rates (HIV.gov, 2020a, 2020b).

Patients have a duty to inform past and future sexual partners about their infection status. These conversations are difficult and have the potential to be confrontational; as a result, patients may avoid having them. The extended life expectancy and lowered risk of transmission associated with

ART may help patients feel justified in this decision. Such a choice presents an ethical dilemma for the nurse. The nurse has an obligation to the patient to maintain privacy, but the patient's partners also have a right to know they are at risk, to get testing, and to receive treatment, if necessary (Centers for Disease Control and Prevention, 2020).

Genetic Testing

Patients with genetic risk factors for chronic illness must make difficult decisions about genetic testing and test findings. For example, a patient with a family history of Huntington disease must decide whether to have predictive testing for the condition. If the test indicates that she will develop the condition, she must make decisions about the type of care she wants to receive in the future and whether to share information about her condition with others who may be affected by her diagnosis. Genetic testing can also present dilemmas for pregnant patients. If prenatal test results indicate a genetic condition, the pregnant patient must decide whether to undergo an elective abortion or deliver a child who may require medical and social support throughout life.

Working with individuals who are seeking information about genetic testing for themselves or for their children is a new and interesting ethical challenge for nurses. The increasing prominence of genetics in the media has contributed to growing awareness among families and patients about inherited conditions. As a result, patients are asking more questions of the nurses who care for them. The nursing code of ethics supports patients' rights to information and counseling in making genetic testing decisions. To provide the best information, nurses should know the legal requirements of their state related to genetic testing.

It is important that nurses understand the limitations of genetic testing and explain them to patients in an unbiased manner. Genetic tests typically provide information about the nature of the condition a patient has or may be at risk for developing. They do not, however, provide information about the severity of the condition or about the age or timing of occurrence (Centre for Genetics Education, 2020). Understanding these limitations can complicate the ethical dilemmas genetic testing presents to patients, including the decision about whether or not to be tested. For this reason, organizations that provide genetic testing also offer genetic counseling.

Genetic counseling may not be available to patients who use direct-to-consumer genetic tests rather than physician-ordered genetic tests. Direct-to-consumer tests can be purchased online for patients to collect a genetic sample at home and mail the sample to a laboratory. Results are sent to the consumer by mail or email. Some companies that provide these tests connect patients to counselors or physicians who can explain the results; some do not (National Human Genome Research Institute, 2020). One disadvantage is that patients may misinterpret their results and pursue treatment based on this misunderstanding. The nurse must decide whether to intervene and must be prepared to provide accurate information, support, and referrals as part of the intervention process.

Organ Transplantation

Organ transplantation is a sensitive issue in terms of both organ donation and organ allocation. In general, organs are procured from patients who are brain dead but whose hearts are still beating, though some organs may be recovered after circulatory death has occurred (Ball et al., 2020). Under the Uniform Anatomical Gift Act (UAGA), patients may elect to donate their organs after their death. Life support systems may be used around the time of death to maximize procurement of donor organs. According to provisions in the act, the need to use life support under UAGA overrides patient desires related to such measures in an advance directive. Although the intent of this provision is to prevent organ failure following brain death, it creates a clear ethical dilemma for HCPs, who may have to balance a patient's wish to donate her organs and her wish not to be placed on life support. Educating patients and their families about these issues when discussing organ donation and advance directives may reduce the occurrence of these dilemmas.

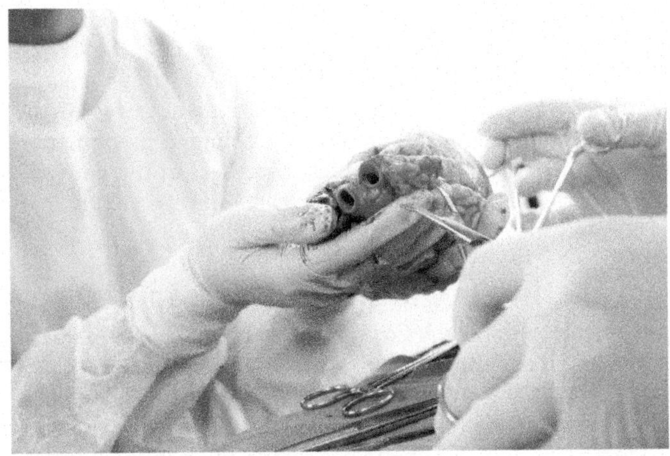

Figure 44.3 ››› Organ transplantation programs use formulas that balance utility, justice, and respect for persons to determine which patients receive organs.

Source: Fstop123/iStock/Getty Images.

Ethical issues also surround the allocation of donated organs, in part because there are many more patients in need of organs than there are organs available (**Figure 44.3 ›››**). Typically, beyond the more clear-cut issues of tissue or blood type compatibility, geography, and organ size is the more ambiguous issue of medical urgency (United Network for Organ Sharing, 2020). Organ transplantation programs use formulas that balance utility, justice, and respect for persons to determine which patients receive which organs and when they receive them. Utility weighs the good the transplant will do against the harm it may do. Justice explores whether distribution of the organ is fair. Respect for persons looks at the autonomy of the patients in decision making (Organ Procurement and Transplantation Network [OPTN], n.d.). These concepts are abstract, often in conflict with one another, and difficult to apply to individual human lives. Suppose, for example, that two patients are in need of a liver but only one liver is available. One patient is a 60-year-old with alcoholism and cirrhosis of the liver; the other is a 20-year-old with a hereditary condition who will die soon without a new liver. The 60-year-old is a brilliant scientist who conducts lifesaving research. The 20-year-old is young, with decades full of potential ahead. Determining which patient receives the organ is an ethical dilemma that is only somewhat simplified by the use of an allocation formula based on the principles of utility, justice, and respect for persons.

>> **Stay Current:** For more information on how donor kidneys from deceased individuals are allocated for transplant, visit the website of the United Network for Organ Sharing at https://unos.org/transplant/how-we-match-organs/.

End-of-Life Issues

Nurses may be faced with ethical dilemmas when caring for patients and/or families who have elected to stop medical treatments or who desire to withdraw life-sustaining therapies. It can be especially difficult when patients desire to end their life because of the perceived burden of the illness. It can also be challenging when cultural expectations about information sharing and end-of-life care differ from the nurse's expectations or even standard practice (see the Focus on Diversity feature).

In spite of increasing interest in and the urgent need for high-quality end-of-life care, there is no exact definition of the "end-of-life" interval or consensus about what constitutes end-of-life care. Many healthcare professionals use "end of life" to refer to the last few weeks before death occurs, although whether a patient is within weeks or even days of death can be difficult to predict.

Advance Directives

Many of the ethical dilemmas surrounding end-of-life care can be resolved if patients complete advance directives and ensure that they are available to HCPs. Advance directives are legal documents that provide written instructions to family and HCPs concerning therapies and treatments that may be allowed in the case of a life-threatening situation. These legal instructions may also include designation of a healthcare proxy, someone the patient designates to healthcare decisions for the patient in the event the individual is unable to do so (Guido, 2020). Examples of these instructions include what may or may not occur (ventilator support, chest compressions, emergency medications) if the patient stops breathing or the heart stops beating. It is important for the nurse to know if the patient has an advance directive in place and if the document is available to medical professionals caring for the patient. More information concerning advance directives can be found in Module 49, Legal Issues, and in Exemplar 3.B, End-of-Life Care, in Module 3, Comfort.

Euthanasia and Assisted Suicide

Euthanasia is an action (either active or passive) that leads to an individual's death prior to death by natural means. **Active euthanasia** occurs when a healthcare professional or the patient causes death to occur. *Passive euthanasia* occurs when an order is given to withhold life-sustaining treatment (Sarkar, 2018).

A variation of active euthanasia is **assisted suicide** (sometimes called "right to die"), in which patients are given the means to kill themselves if they request it. As of June 2020, nine states permitted provider-assisted suicide, in which patients with terminal conditions are allowed to request medication that will cause the end of the patient's life, although (at this time) no state permits HCPs to actively administer the medication (CNN Editorial Research, 2020). The ethics and morality of assisted suicide have been debated in the United States for a long time. For years, only Oregon, which passed the Death with Dignity Act in 1997, allowed physicians to provide lethal medications to qualifying patients who requested assistance. In January 2006, the U.S. Supreme Court upheld Oregon's assisted suicide regulations. This eventually paved the way for other states to pass similar legislation. Several other countries also have assisted suicide laws in place.

Right-to-die legislation is still controversial, and opposition to it by some cultural, religious, and other groups makes it an ethical issue that many nurses will be confronted wit'

Focus on Diversity and Culture

Variations in Autonomy and Information Sharing

In providing ethical care to patients, it is important to understand the key role that culture plays in healthcare and the ways in which different cultures view autonomy and information sharing. For example, in the United States, autonomous individual decision making is highly valued; as a result, respect for patient autonomy is central to healthcare in this country. Autonomy is not a universal cultural value, however, and some patients from Chinese, Korean, and Hispanic backgrounds may prefer to involve family members or tribal or spiritual leaders in their decision-making process (Smallwood, 2018). For example, in the Hmong culture, the head of the family may make the decision regarding whether or not an individual has surgery (Purnell & Fenkl, 2019).

It is also common for U.S. HCPs to disclose all information about a patient's condition to the patient, including whether the condition is life threatening. In some other cultures, it is common to withhold information about terminal prognoses from patients. The rationale for this approach is that it enables the patient to maintain hope.

In addition, cultural beliefs may require HCPs to carefully choose their language when disclosing information to patients and families. In some cultures, discussing the specifics of a patient's condition is seen as impolite and disrespectful; some groups may even consider it dangerous. For example, the Navajo culture traditionally believes that speaking about something can result in that thing taking place or that the nurse or provider may actually want the patient to die. Thus, discussing death can make it occur (Purnell & Fenkl, 2019). The underlying concern for this and other cultures with similar belief structures is that patients may become depressed, anxious, or hopeless as a result of a poor prognosis, and this can hasten their physical decline (Smallwood, 2018). Nurses working with patients from cultures with these belief structures should seek guidance on strategies for imparting negative information. Elders, spiritual leaders, and colleagues from these cultures may be the most appropriate sources of reliable information.

Nurses may fear ethical or even legal repercussions related to information sharing or withholding from patients with diverse cultural backgrounds. It is important for the nurse to develop a relationship with the patient and family and work with them to determine the best means of sharing essential information based on their beliefs and values (Purnell & Fenkl, 2019; Smallwood, 2018).

during their careers. The ANA's (2019a) position statement on assisted suicide states that performing active euthanasia and participating in assisted suicide violate the ANA *Code of Ethics for Nurses*. Nurses should understand the assisted suicide laws in their state so that they can adequately answer patients' questions; in doing so, they must be able to balance facts and patient concerns against their own personal biases and the ethics of their profession.

Withdrawing or Withholding Life-Sustaining Therapy

Withdrawing or withholding life-sustaining therapy (WWLST) is the removal or withholding of therapies that sustain life. Examples of life-sustaining therapies include respiratory (ventilator) and nutritional (parenteral feeding) support. WWLST is a complex process that can take several days to complete. During that time, nurses must be prepared to manage the process, the complex emotions experienced by the patient's family, and their own feelings about the process.

Patients may make the decision to terminate specific life-sustaining treatments or may decide that all present and future therapies will be discontinued or held and record their wishes in one or more advance directives. Healthcare professionals who are focused on curative treatments may find it difficult to accept a patient's wishes to discontinue specific treatments. It may be especially hard for nurses who have spent many hours caring for the patient. Nurses must realize that care of the patient continues, but the focus changes from curative to comfort. Palliative measures are instituted to ensure that the patient is comfortable and best able to spend quality time completing important tasks, such as saying goodbye to loved ones.

An important duty of the nurse is to make sure that patients understand that life-sustaining treatment may be resumed at any time. Nurses must also help patients and families know what treatments constitute life-sustaining treatments and what treatments are considered palliative, or comfort, measures.

Withdrawing or Withholding Nutrition and Fluids

It is generally accepted that providing nutrition and fluids is part of ordinary nursing practice and, therefore, a moral duty. However, for patients who are dying or who are unconscious and not expected to improve, provision of nutrition and fluids is considered a medical intervention rather than a comfort measure (Danis, 2018).

During the dying process, patients exhibit decreased oral intake, progressive fluid deficits, and progressive accumulation of drugs. These changes can worsen existing symptoms or create new ones; these, in turn, lead to further declines in oral intake. Research consistently suggests that, when this occurs, it is more harmful to administer nutrition and fluids to the patient than it is to withhold them (Danis, 2018). As a result, nurses in this situation are morally and professionally obligated to withhold nutrition and fluids—or any treatment.

The nurse must also honor competent and informed patients' refusal of nutrition and fluids, referred to as *voluntary cessation of intake*. The ANA *Code of Ethics for Nurses* (2015a) supports this position through the nurse's role as a patient advocate and through the moral principle of autonomy. Some religions oppose voluntary cessation on the grounds that it involves a decision that will lead to patient death; however, some groups consider voluntary cessation preferable to euthanasia or assisted suicide (Danis, 2018).

Families may view provision of nutrition and hydration as important care and comfort measures and may strongly oppose withdrawal or withholding. This can create ethical dilemmas for the nurse. The nurse must be prepared to explain the withdrawal and withholding process to the family and why doing so is important. In addition, nurses should be familiar with the laws in their state pertaining to voluntary cessation.

Clinical Example A

Conner Wolfe is a 14-year-old patient with cancer who is refusing chemotherapy after becoming very ill and weak after his first round of chemo. His oncologist has made it very clear that Conner has a 90% chance of being cured if he undergoes chemotherapy followed by radiation and an equal chance that he will die without it. Although Conner and his family do not follow any specific spiritual or cultural traditions, they believe in using "natural medicine" for curing illness. Conner is adamant that he does not want any more chemotherapy. His parents state that he was in "better health" before the first chemo treatment and that is proof that the chemo is bad for him. When asked what the parents intend to do if Conner's cancer metastasizes, the Wolfes say they will discuss that with Conner in the unlikely event that it occurs.

Critical Thinking Questions

1. What ethical dilemmas can you identify in this situation?
2. What is the nurse's responsibility regarding addressing these dilemmas?
3. What, if any, action should the hospital take regarding Conner's treatment? Why?

Ethical Issues in Nursing Practice

Ethics in nursing is not limited to bioethical dilemmas; it also includes nursing practice and the nurse's identity as a moral agent. This identity is shaped by contextual and organizational forces that impact the role, obligations, and duties of the nurse. These forces include corporate healthcare values and hierarchies and the growing demand for healthcare (Khoshmehr, Barkhordari-Sharifabad, Nasiriani, & Fallahzadeh, 2020).

Some everyday ethical challenges identified by nurses were categorized in a classic publication by Varcoe et al. (2004), who posited that nurses work as the "in-betweens." Specifically, nurses are caught in between various other players involved in healthcare, including HCPs and the patient and the patient and the family. Nurses are also caught between family members, between staff members, between managers, and between other colleagues. Within these relationships, nurses must constantly balance their loyalties.

Conflicts also arise from traditional power structures in healthcare. For example, nurses have expressed concern about being intimidated or dismissed by physicians when the nurses report observations that are not congruent with the proposed medical treatment plan. They have also voiced anxiety about being ignored by senior medical staff when they report concerns related to physician behavior or by administrators when they express concern over corporate values. In some cases, nurses may be threatened with job and license loss over such reports and concerns.

Additional conflicts arise as a result of staffing shortages and other situations in which the organization functions inefficiently (Burnell, 2019). When faced with inefficiencies, nurses must balance their limited time with the care that must be provided. In these situations, patient teaching, counseling, and support suffer as the nurse's focus moves to performance of physical tasks and functions.

The behavior of nurses is shaped by their organizational and professional roles and the settings in which they work. Their responses to ethical dilemmas are inseparable from the scenarios in which those dilemmas arise (Johansen & O'Brien, 2016). Therefore, clinical experiences are important for helping nurses develop ethical behaviors. In addition, supportive colleagues, educators, and approachable and responsible managers are important resources for ethical practice. In fact, nurses have reported that having the opportunity to discuss ethical concerns is both personally and professionally sustaining (Edmonson & Zelonka, 2019; Johnstone, 2012a).

Workplace Issues

A number of workplace issues outside of the bioethical realm affect nurses. Many of them are the result of financial constraints, personnel issues, and other organizational challenges. Two of the most common ethical dilemmas stemming from these factors involve limited resources and short staffing.

Allocation of Limited Health Resources

As healthcare costs continue to rise and more stringent cost containment strategies are implemented, allocation of limited supplies of healthcare goods and services has become an especially urgent issue. Examples of the goods and services affected include personal protective equipment, ventilators, organs suitable for transplantation, artificial joints, and specialist services.

The moral principle of autonomy cannot be observed when patients are unable to obtain the treatment they prefer either at the facility or by transfer (with patients' consent) to a facility that can provide the treatment. Certain treatments, such as organ transplantation, are limited in the number available, requiring healthcare professionals to apply the moral principle of justice to ensure that these limited resources are provided to patients who have the best chance of benefitting from that treatment. More information on allocation of resources is available in Module 46, Healthcare Systems.

Short Staffing

Because of a nationwide shortage of nurses, nursing care is becoming a limited health resource. Short staffing is a critical concern because a number of studies link staffing levels to safe patient care (AACN, 2020). Unfortunately, some facilities continue to staff nursing units with fewer registered nurses and more unlicensed caregivers. When this occurs, staffing may not be adequate to ensure patient safety or allow nurses to provide an appropriate level of care. California is the only state that has enacted legislation mandating specific nurse-to-patient ratios in hospitals and other healthcare settings (ANA, 2019b). Unfortunately, this is not the simple solution that it might seem. The need to maintain adequate staffing levels could force changes elsewhere in the organization that are detrimental to patient care. For example, the need to maintain adequate staffing may force an ED to limit the number of patients it can accept at one time. As a result, patients in need of emergency care might be turned away when that limit is reached.

Clinical Example B

The director of nursing is having difficulty staffing all the units adequately. Two units have already been closed. The director can either spread the available staff around the facility and keep the remaining units open, but with fewer nurses than is really safe, or close more units. The director needs to consider the welfare of the institution, the nursing staff, and the patients.

Critical Thinking Questions

1. How would you assess the ethical aspects of this issue?
2. What actions would you take? Why?
3. How does the ANA *Code of Ethics* inform the possible actions?

Working with Patients and Families

Working with patients and families is both rewarding and challenging. Clear communication and good clinical decision-making skills help the nurse develop positive relationships with these individuals. Ethical challenges may still arise, however; they include ensuring patient autonomy and maintaining patient privacy and confidentiality.

Patient Autonomy

Respect for patient autonomy is fundamental to nursing ethics, and nurses must recognize and defend the right of each patient to make decisions about healthcare. However, situations often arise in which patient autonomy is at risk. This risk may come in the form of a well-meaning family member who disagrees with the patient's decision or a physician or other HCP who either fails to hear the patient's concerns or disagrees with the patient's request or decision (Frellick, 2019). In these situations, the nurse is ethically obligated to advocate for the patient's right to make decisions.

Patient Privacy and Confidentiality

The Health Insurance Portability and Accountability Act of 1996 (HIPAA) requires that healthcare professionals keep private all information related to an individual's health and health-related decisions. Nurses or any healthcare professional who does not respect patient confidentiality may face large fines and the related agency will also incur large fines. Maintaining patient privacy and confidentiality is both a legal requirement and a cornerstone of the nurse–patient relationship. The patient must trust that conversations shared with the nurse will remain confidential. The nurse must inform the patient that certain information necessary for care will only be shared with those healthcare professionals directly involved in the patient's care. For further information, see Module 38, Communication, and Module 48, Informatics.

Academic Dishonesty

Ethical dilemmas are not just the concern of practicing nurses and are not limited to the workplace or to patient interactions; nursing students may find themselves facing ethical dilemmas in the classroom. Academic dishonesty is an important example of an ethical dilemma faced by nursing students. Examples of academic dishonesty include cheating, plagiarism, and failure to follow academic policies, such as the requirement to return examinations after test review sessions (Guerraro-Dib, Portales, & Heredia-Escorza, 2020).

Academic dishonesty affects student nurses in two primary ways. First, there is the temptation for the student nurse to personally engage in academic dishonesty. Busy schedules and the need to maintain grades at a certain level can make dishonesty appealing; however, engaging in dishonesty negatively affects learning and personal growth and, in turn, the student's future nursing practice. Second, student nurses may witness or be aware of friends engaging in academic dishonesty. In these situations, balancing friendship and ethics can be difficult.

The way student nurses approach academic dishonesty is important to their development of personal ethics. In personal ethics, individuals make decisions on the basis of their values and best interests (Lachman, 2012). Individuals are accountable for the consequences of their actions. This is in contrast to a professional ethical dilemma, in which the decision reflects the autonomy of the patient and the nurse is accountable to the patient's values and best interests. In spite of the differences between personal and professional ethics, personal ethics contribute to professional ethics. With increased experience and exposure on both personal and professional levels, students become better able to identify conflicting values and variables that affect the practicing nurse. See the clinical example that follows and **Box 44.3** ».

Box 44.3

An Exercise in Ethical Decision Making

When ethical dilemmas arise, the individual often has the choice of multiple courses of action. To determine the best course of action, you must consider the pros and cons of each and the consequences that may result. This can be difficult to do, especially for individuals who are new to the concept of ethical decision making.

For this exercise, refer to Clinical Example C of Elizabeth and Jasmine below. Then build your ethical decision-making skills by answering the following questions:

1. ***Identify a range of actions with potential outcomes.***
   What are the pros? What are the cons?
   If you choose to participate in the study group and then inform the instructor?
   If you choose to participate and not tell the instructor?
   If you choose not to participate and not tell the instructor?
   If you choose not to participate and to tell the instructor?
2. ***Decide on a course of action and carry it out.***
   What are you going to decide?
   On what do you base your decision?
   What does your decision tell others about you and your values?
   Does your decision predict future decisions/actions?
3. ***Evaluate/reevaluate the consequences of your decision/action.***
   What tools would you use to evaluate your decision/action after the fact?
   How would you determine what effect your decision/action had on others?

Clinical Example C

Elizabeth, a first-year nursing student, has obtained a copy of the first examination given last year in Nursing 110 from Jasmine, her assigned "Big Sister" from the second-year class. Jasmine emphasized that questions on nursing examinations are particularly hard to answer because they require application of information, not just recall. Elizabeth informs her selected study group that she has the exam and is willing to share it to help them focus their study time. You are a member of Elizabeth's study group.

Critical Thinking Questions

1. Will you participate? Why or why not?
2. Will you report Elizabeth to your instructor? Why or why not?
3. What ethical principle is involved in your decision process?
4. What conflicting values are involved in this scenario?
5. What additional information might help you make your decision? What difference does it make if you learn that Jasmine did not turn in the exam after a test review session?
6. What school policies are involved? What aspects of the ANA *Code of Ethics* apply?

Coping with Ethical Dilemmas

Ethical dilemmas occur frequently in everyday clinical practice. They require decision and action on the part of the nurse, and they have important implications for compassionate, high-quality patient care (Epstein & Turner, 2015; Song, 2018).

Nurses may be blindsided by ethical dilemmas and wonder why they did not recognize the potential for these dilemmas before they arose. Several ethical decision-making models have been proposed to assist nurses in these situations; however, these models may not always consider the underlying values of both the practitioner and the patient involved in the dilemma (Crowley & Gottlieb, 2012). The primary risk management model below is an example. It was designed to assist clinical staff in managing ethical decisions and it includes the following:

- ***Resource accumulation***. Acquisition of the requisite resources and skills before the occurrence of a stressor.
- ***Time***. Engagement in "free time" activities to relieve pressure and anxiety in order to better perceive the subtle cues that alert the practitioner to potential ethical dilemmas.
- ***Education***. Development of primary risk management skills through education and didactic training.
- ***Organization and planning***. Enhancement of organization and planning through teaching and modeling.
- ***Peer support and consultation***. Reliance on the practitioner's professional network, consisting of peers, supervisors, and colleagues, as a resource for primary prevention of ethical challenges (Crowley & Gottlieb, 2012, pp. 67–68).

Lifespan Considerations

When caring for patients at all stages of life, nurses may be faced with ethical dilemmas. Often, these dilemmas are specific to certain population groups; other times, they are related to bioethical issues common to patients of all ages. Regardless of the patient's age, the nurse must be prepared to handle these dilemmas in an ethically responsible manner.

Ethical Dilemmas Related to Infants and Children

Ethical dilemmas commonly arise in working with the pediatric population. This is in part because pediatric patients cannot make their own decisions. Parents or guardians have the authority to make healthcare decisions for their children. Dilemmas arise when parents or guardians and children do not agree on whether to go forward with a recommended treatment. In most cases, the nurse and other members of the healthcare team who have developed a therapeutic alliance with the child and family may be able to help them reach a joint decision by providing additional information and opportunity to discuss their concerns calmly and openly.

In some cases, the healthcare team may need to seek guidance from the organization's ethics committee related to parental decision making for a minor child. For example, when there is a potential conflict of interest—such as suspected child abuse and neglect—other measures may be necessary to provide appropriate care for the pediatric patient. In some cases, these measures may include involving the court system or the Department of Child Services.

In addition to these concerns, the bioethical issues discussed previously in this exemplar can take on different aspects when applied to the pediatric population. WWLST decisions can be especially difficult when the patient is an infant, child, or adolescent. In discussing the withdrawal or withholding of medical treatment for pediatric patients with their parents, it is critical to provide complete, clear information about the child's condition, prognosis, degree of pain and suffering, and potential for good quality of life (Hilton, 2019).

When facing these situations, HCPs must follow the requirements of the Child Abuse and Treatment Act of 1984, which deemed withholding of medically indicated treatment as child abuse except in cases in which providing care is futile, that is, cases in which the treatments will not provide any clear clinical benefit (Ball, Bindler, Cowen, & Shaw, 2017). Although it is rare for parents to refuse a medically indicated treatment that may benefit their child, the decision can be exceedingly difficult when the proposed treatment itself carries a high degree of risk, such as organ transplantation or major surgery.

There are particular issues involving children as organ transplant recipients. For instance, the Organ Transplant and Procurement Network prefers to allocate organs from child donors—rather than adult donors—to child recipients. This is due to the difference in size between child and adult organs and the fact that children often respond better to organs from child donors (OPTN, n.d.). OPTN also encourages the use of special considerations in allocating organs that gives pediatric patients priority in some situations. These include the prudential lifespan account, in which the unique quality of life benefits enjoyed by child recipients is considered; the fair innings principle, in which the ability to maximize the recipient's lifespan is considered; and the maximin principle, in which giving priority to the most disadvantaged individual or group is considered (OPTN, 2014). Taken together, these concepts present ethical dilemmas that affect both child and adult patients in need of organ transplantation.

Ethical Dilemmas Related to Adolescents

Ethical dilemmas involving the adolescent population tend to focus on issues of consent and confidentiality. Parents or guardians must consent to medical treatment for adolescents under the age of 18 unless the adolescent has been emancipated, resides in a state that recognizes mature minors, or is seeking specific types of treatment recognized by state law, such as birth control, prenatal care, and diagnosis and treatment of sexually transmitted infections. Minors may also be able to give consent for mental health counseling and substance abuse treatment (American Civil Liberties Union of Ohio, 2014; Guttmacher Institute, 2020).

Adolescent patients seeking care may wish to be examined without their parents being present; they may also prefer that their treatment remain confidential. Nurses should inform adolescent patients about mandatory reporting of imminent danger, evidence of abuse, and communicable diseases to the proper authorities (American Academy of Family Physicians [AAFP], 2019). Nurses should also notify adolescent patients that if the patient is covered under a parent's insurance, billing statements provided to that parent may include information about care. In addition, EHRs for minors are typically set up with parents as proxy. As a result, parents can read the information contained in the EHR unless the system is designed to restrict proxy access to confidential information (American College of Obstetricians and Gynecologists, 2020).

Nurses must be aware of state statutes related to adolescent care and confidentiality as well as their ethical obligations to their adolescent patients. Nurses may encourage adolescent patients to involve their parents or guardians in care decisions, but they must respect adolescent patients' right to autonomy in decision making. Failure to do so may give rise to patient concerns over confidentiality and result in patient refusal of treatment.

Ethical Dilemmas Related to Pregnant Women

Ethical issues related to pregnancy often focus on the delicate balance of maternal rights and fetal rights. For example, if a pregnant woman is in an accident that leaves her brain dead, it can be difficult to determine whether her life should be artificially sustained in order to deliver the child or whether life-sustaining technology should be discontinued. Two highly publicized cases occurred in 2014 and 2015. In one, the hospital attempted to keep the woman's body on life support against her wishes and those of her family (Goodwyn, 2014). In the other, the hospital and family collaborated to keep the woman's body alive for nearly 2 months, and her baby was born via cesarean section (Izadi, 2015). While the cases differed in many ways, they were similar in that the families and HCPs faced a dilemma with no clear ethical or legal solution.

Ethical issues can also arise in situations in which the mother's life is in danger. This may occur as a result of complications of pregnancy that threaten the mother's life or as a result of medical conditions unrelated to pregnancy, such as cancer. When these situations occur, the woman, family, and HCPs are faced with the difficult question of whether the mother's life or the child's life takes priority.

In these situations, personal opinions about abortion or the medical necessity of treatments that could harm the fetus complicate the decision-making process.

The discussion of maternal and fetal rights often stirs up complex emotions and strong opinions about the ethics and morality of pregnant patient care. Nurses should understand their state laws and organizational policies on these topics. They should also understand their rights and responsibilities related to conscientious objection (Lachman, 2014). See Module 49, Legal Issues, for more information.

Ethical Dilemmas Related to Older Adults

End-of-life issues are common sources of ethical dilemmas for nurses working with the older adult population. These may include issues associated with advance directives, assisted suicide, withdrawal or withholding of life-sustaining treatment, and withdrawal or withholding of nutrition and fluids.

Issues related to autonomy, competency, and decision making also commonly arise in the older adult population. Some older adults experience age-related cognitive impairments or untreated depression that may affect the decisions they make related to healthcare. In addition, family members or caregivers may have strong opinions about what the patient should or should not do and may question the patient's ability to make healthcare decisions (Martinez-Selles, Martinez-Selles, & Martinez-Selles, 2020). The combination of these factors can place the nurse in a difficult position. If the patient is competent to make her own medical decisions, the nurse must respect her autonomy in decision making. However, the nurse must consider the factors that may be at work and the risks and benefits associated with a treatment. In addition, the nurse must be prepared to face anger, disappointment, and questions from the patient's family. When these situations arise, it may be useful for the nurse to facilitate a discussion between the major stakeholders—including the physician, patient, and family—to ensure that everyone understands what the treatment entails and what its risks and benefits are and to help the patient reach a decision that affirms her autonomy while being acceptable to the other parties involved (Martinez-Selles et al., 2020).

Consent can also present issues with older adult patients who have been hospitalized. Typically, when patients are admitted to the hospital, they sign a blanket consent for treatment. By signing this form, the patient gives implicit consent for routine care. However, the patient can refuse or question any individual treatment. For example, the patient may refuse to allow the nurse to draw blood or administer a medication. When these situations arise, the nurse must respect the patient's autonomy, even if the nurse disagrees with the patient's decision. In many cases, these dilemmas can be worked through if the nurse explains the procedure and its purpose to the patient and asks about reasons for refusing it (Martinez-Selles et al., 2020).

SAFETY ALERT Forcing or coercing a patient to have a procedure that the patient has refused is unlawful and can result in legal consequences for the nurse.

REVIEW Ethical Dilemmas

RELATE Link the Concepts and Exemplars

Linking the exemplar of ethical dilemmas with the concept of legal issues:

1. What are your beliefs about advance directive planning for any patient who has a chronic illness, such as a cardiac illness, diabetes, or renal failure, regardless of the patient's age?
2. What is the nurse's role in discussing future care plans, such as end-of-life care, with chronically ill patients?

Linking the exemplar of ethical dilemmas with the concept of comfort:

3. What are your beliefs about ensuring comfort for patients with chronic pain?
4. Assess your understanding of pain management options to ensure comfort. What are your beliefs about the use of medications with a high potential of abuse for patients?

REFER Go to Pearson MyLab Nursing and eText

REFLECT Apply Your Knowledge

John Merchant is a 57-year-old man who was diagnosed with gastric cancer 3 years ago. At the time, surgeons performed a gastric resection followed by chemotherapy and radiation. He completed all treatments 2 years ago. Recently he began to notice that he was having some difficulty swallowing and he has just been diagnosed with an esophageal metastasis of the original cancer. The oncologist believes that it can be successfully treated with radiation, but that Mr. Merchant will be unable to swallow adequately to provide adequate nutrition during the treatment. The oncologist requested that Mr. Merchant have a jejunostomy tube surgically inserted to provide nutrition during treatment. Mr. Merchant is refusing this procedure and states that he completely understands the possible outcome, but he would prefer to take his chances. His family believes he does not understand that there is a good chance for a complete resolution of the cancer. The oncologist will not proceed with the radiation treatment unless the patient agrees to the feeding tube insertion. After consultation with the patient, family, and oncologist, the patient's primary nurse asks the ethics committee to assist in resolving this situation. After much discussion, Mr. Merchant agrees to the surgery to insert the feeding tube with the understanding that this could be discontinued at any time and the radiation therapy would still continue.

1. What ethical dilemmas did Mr. Merchant's primary nurse face in caring for this patient?
2. Why did the primary nurse choose the ethics committee to bring resolution to the situation?
3. How do you feel about Mr. Merchant's initial decision and his eventual agreement to the procedure? Why?
4. In what ways did the nurse working with Mr. Merchant advocate on his behalf? How is the nurse's role as an advocate related to nursing ethics?

» Exemplar 44.C Patient Rights

Exemplar Learning Outcomes

44.C Analyze patient rights as they relate to ethics.

- Examine the rights of patients in the healthcare system.
- Analyze support systems that exist for patients who feel that their rights have been violated by a healthcare agency or provider.
- Compare the contents of different documents or laws that address patient rights.
- Differentiate considerations related to patient rights across the lifespan.

Exemplar Key Terms

Patient responsibilities, *2754*
Patient rights, *2753*

Overview

All patients have rights when it comes to the healthcare they receive. Popularly called **patient rights**, these represent the fundamental care owed to patients by HCPs and the government (WHO, 2017). Some of these rights are guaranteed by federal law, such as the right to informed consent mandated in the Patient Self-Determination Act (see Module 49, Legal Issues). Other rights are governed by state laws. In addition, healthcare organizations often have a patient bill of rights, which details the rights the organization promises to uphold for its patients.

The importance of patient rights is evident in the American Nurses Association's Standards of Practice and Code of Ethics and the accreditation standards for various types of healthcare agencies set by The Joint Commission. The Joint Commission (2013b) also encourages patients to become more informed about their rights and more involved in their care through the Speak Up program. The essential points of this program are outlined in **Box 44.4** ».

Nurses should be aware of national and state laws pertaining to patient rights, as well as their employer's policies and procedures. Nurses should also be knowledgeable about the standards enacted by professional nursing bodies in an effort to protect patient rights and ensure nurse compliance with applicable laws.

Beyond laws, policies, and standards, nurses should understand their role in protecting patient rights. In addition, nurses should introduce patients to their patient rights and responsibilities and encourage them to engage as partners with their HCPs. Methods of doing so will vary depending on the patient's age and condition, but it is an important component of the nurse's role as a patient advocate.

Box 44.4

Patient Rights from The Joint Commission's Speak Up Campaign

Know Your Rights

- You have the right to be informed about the care you will receive.
- You have the right to get important information about your care in your preferred language.
- You have the right to get information in a manner that meets your needs if you have vision, speech, hearing, or mental impairments or a disability.
- You have the right to make decisions about your care.
- You have the right to refuse care.
- You have the right to know the names of the caregivers who treat you.
- You have the right to safe care.
- You have the right to have your pain addressed.
- You have the right to care that is free from discrimination. This means you should not be treated differently because of age, race, ethnicity, religion, culture, language, physical or mental disability, socioeconomic status, sex, sexual orientation, or gender identity or expression.
- You have the right to know when something goes wrong with your care.
- You have the right to get a list of all your current medications.
- You have the right to be listened to.
- You have the right to be treated with courtesy and respect.
- You have the right to have a personal representative, also called an advocate, with you during your care. Your advocate is a family member or friend of your choice.

Source: Adapted from The Joint Commission (2019).

Protecting Patients' Rights

In spite of the legal requirement and ethical duty to protect patient rights, many patients still experience violations of these rights as they navigate the healthcare system. Some of the most common violations involve confidentiality, privacy, informed consent, and nondiscrimination. Less commonly, violations may involve treatment that does not respect the dignity of the patient or that jeopardizes the patient's healthcare outcomes (Cohen & Ezer, 2013).

To protect patient rights, nurses must follow requirements related to informed consent. They must also be aware of the patient protection systems in place within their organizations and their state. In addition, they must recognize the importance of patient bills of rights and patient responsibilities in patient care.

Informed Consent

To ensure patient rights, the nurse must first identify the appropriate individual to provide informed consent for the patient (e.g., patient, parent, legal guardian). Also, it is vital to provide written materials in the patient's primary language. The nurse needs to understand and describe components of informed consent and how to participate in obtaining informed consent.

When obtaining informed consent, the nurse must understand how to verify that the patient comprehends and consents to care and procedures. In addition, the nurse must discuss various treatment options and decisions with the patient. Similarly, the nurse must educate patients and staff about patients' rights and responsibilities (e.g., ethical/legal issues) and know how to evaluate patient and staff understanding of patients' rights.

SAFETY ALERT When discussing informed consent with patients, the nurse should explain to patients their right to refuse a treatment or procedure.

Organizational and State Protections

Individual patients who feel that their rights are in danger or have been violated have a number of options. Many healthcare organizations have patient advocates who help them navigate the organizational system and intervene when necessary to ensure that the patient's rights are respected. This type of advocacy is particularly important for patients who require long-term care. In addition, many states have offices designated by the governor or secretary of health to assist patients with issues related to patient rights in long-term care.

The state department of health may also be able to help with patient rights issues. Nursing homes, homes for frail older adults, and licensed facilities for people with disabilities are regulated at the state level, and violations committed by these agencies may be reported for investigation (King, Harrington, Linedale, & Tanner, 2018). Legislatures in many states have also passed declarations of patients' rights that must be followed by nursing homes and other agencies that provide medical care and housing for patients.

Patient Bills of Rights

The first patient bill of rights was drafted by the American Hospital Association during the 1970s; since then, a number of different groups have created their own patient bills of rights (American Cancer Society, 2016). For example, in 1998, the President's Advisory Commission on Consumer Protection and Quality in the Health Care Industry adopted a bill of rights. This bill included, among other things, provisions about information disclosure, provider and plan choice, access to emergency services, participation in treatment decisions, nondiscrimination, and confidentiality. It also included information about filing complaints and appeals. The bill was intended to protect all consumers and was adopted by the federal government for employees covered under their insurance plans. A summary of this bill of rights is provided in **Box 44.5** ››.

The 1998 bill of rights served as the inspiration for a number of other patient bills of rights. Hospitals, patient organizations, government agencies, and insurance plans are among the different groups that have created patient bills of rights. Patient bills of rights have also been developed for hospice patients and patients with mental illness. Although these bills of rights differ from one another to some degree, most discuss privacy and confidentiality, nondiscrimination, language preferences, and patient involvement in treatment decisions.

Passage of the Affordable Care Act in 2010 was accompanied by a new patient bill of rights. This bill differs in content from other bills of rights in that it specifically addresses patient protections related to health insurance coverage. Areas discussed in this patient bill of rights include coverage for individuals with preexisting conditions, free preventive care, elimination of dollar limits, accountability for rate increases, and provider choice (HealthCare.gov, n.d.). The Affordable Care Act may be replaced in the coming years. Nurses should stay abreast of changes in healthcare laws and the ways in which they affect patients.

Box 44.5

A Summary of the Bill of Rights of the U.S. Advisory Commission on Consumer Protection and Quality in the Health Care Industry

- ***Information disclosure.*** You have the right to accurate and easily understood information about your health plan, healthcare professionals, and healthcare facilities. If you speak another language, have a physical or mental disability, or just don't understand something, help should be provided so you can make informed healthcare decisions.
- ***Choice of providers and plans.*** You have the right to a choice of HCPs who can give you high-quality healthcare when you need it.
- ***Access to emergency services.*** If you have severe pain, an injury, or sudden illness that makes you believe that your health is in serious danger, you have the right to be screened and stabilized using emergency services. These services should be provided whenever and wherever you need them, without the need to wait for authorization and without any financial penalty.
- ***Participation in treatment decisions.*** You have the right to know your treatment options and to take part in decisions about your care. Parents, guardians, family members, or others who you select can represent you if you cannot make your own decisions.
- ***Respect and nondiscrimination.*** You have a right to considerate, respectful care from your physicians, health plan representatives, and other HCPs that does not discriminate against you.
- ***Confidentiality of health information.*** You have the right to talk privately with HCPs and to have your healthcare information protected. You also have the right to read and copy your own medical records. You have the right to ask that your physician change your record if it is not accurate, relevant, or complete.
- ***Complaints and appeals.*** You have the right to a fair, fast, and objective review of any complaint you have against your health plan, physicians, hospitals, or other healthcare personnel. This includes complaints about waiting times, operating hours, the actions of healthcare personnel, and the adequacy of healthcare facilities.

Source: Based on President's Advisory Commission on Consumer Protection and Quality in the Health Care Industry (1998).

Patient Responsibilities

In addition to patient bills of rights, some organizations now publish lists of **patient responsibilities**. These lists emphasize that healthcare is a partnership between the patient and caregivers, that other patients have the right to be comfortable, and that there are consequences when patients do not comply with treatment plans. Common patient responsibilities include the following:

- Tell your healthcare team how you feel.
- Provide information about your health, past illnesses, and use of medications.

- Report accurate and complete information about your health to your healthcare team.
- Ask your healthcare team whether you need to change your medications before a procedure or test.
- Answer questions asked by your healthcare team.
- Cooperate with your healthcare team.
- Listen to instructions, read written material given to you, and ask questions if you do not understand something.
- Be considerate of the staff and other patients by limiting visitors, following smoking regulations, and using the telephone and television so as not to disturb others.
- Provide information about your health insurance, and work with the hospital to arrange for payment, if needed.
- Recognize the effects of your lifestyle on your health, and work with your hospital team to change your lifestyle as necessary.
- Follow the treatment plan recommended by your healthcare team.
- Accept the consequences if you fail to comply with instructions given to you.

Patient responsibilities lists are intended to encourage patients to take a more active role in their care and promote consideration of others within the healthcare environment. They are not intended to be a list of rules that patients must follow. In introducing patients to these responsibilities, it is important for nurses to make sure patients understand this difference.

Lifespan Considerations

At different points in the lifespan, patients experience different needs and concerns related to patient rights. In addition, some organizations have patient bills of rights that are specific to patients at different points in the lifespan. The nurse must ensure that the specific rights of these patients are respected.

Patient Rights Pertaining to Infants and Children

When working with pediatric patients, nurses are responsible for protecting the rights of both patients and their families. To support nurses in these efforts, the Association for the Care of Children's Health has developed the pediatric bill of rights, which outlines the need for family-centered care that provides developmentally appropriate psychosocial support. The Society of Pediatric Nurses (SPN) encourages hospitals and children's units across the country to adopt some version of this bill of rights (Mott, 2014). In doing so, the SPN hopes to better prepare families to understand the care that is being provided to their child and to create more positive healthcare experiences for pediatric patients and their loved ones.

A central theme in the pediatric bill of rights is allowing patients and families to remain together whenever possible during treatments and hospital stays. In some cases, this includes making arrangements for a family member to remain with the child overnight. Other supportive measures include allowing the child to have toys or clothes from home when possible and providing children with opportunities to play and engage in activities related to their personal interests. The goal of all these measures is to make patients and families comfortable and to maintain a sense of normalcy rather than emphasizing the child's illness (Mott, 2014).

The pediatric bill of rights includes many of the same provisions as other patient bills of rights with relation to privacy, information sharing, and respect for the individual. The primary difference is the focus on age-appropriate and developmentally appropriate applications of these concepts. Another difference is the application of these concepts to the family as a whole rather than to the patient as an individual.

Patient Rights Pertaining to Adolescents

Adolescent patients are also covered under the pediatric bill of rights. An important difference in caring for adolescents rather than young children is the role of family. As children reach adolescence, they may engage in behaviors or have care needs that they are embarrassed or worried about sharing with their families. In these situations, it is essential that nurses understand the state laws related to confidential care for adolescents and are prepared for the ethical dilemmas involved in providing this kind of care. (See Module 49, Legal Issues, and Exemplar 44.B, Ethical Dilemmas, in this module for more information.)

The pediatric bill of rights includes a privacy provision that is useful for working with adolescent patients. It states that patients have the right for their privacy to be honored as long as it is safe for the patient (Mott, 2014). Though the right of privacy must be honored, the AAFP (2019) encourages HCPs to make a reasonable effort to encourage adolescents to involve their family in their healthcare. This encouragement should be provided in a supportive manner with the clear understanding that involving parents or guardians in the decision-making process is not essential for the patient to receive care.

Another important consideration in caring for adolescent patients is their inclusion in nonconfidential healthcare decisions. For example, a teenage patient being treated for leukemia may have strong opinions about the types of treatment he would like to receive, even though his parents serve as his decision-making proxy. Adolescent patients have a right to have their opinions heard and considered by HCPs and family members (Campbell, 2019; Dikema, 2014). The nurse must facilitate conversations with family and other HCPs in these situations. See Exemplar 44.B, Ethical Dilemmas, in this module for more information on this topic.

Patient Rights Pertaining to Pregnant Women

Many pregnant patients may not be fully aware of their rights in regard to making healthcare decisions on behalf of themselves and their children and so may not exercise their rights. As a result, a major rights-related issue that nurses face with this population involves informing patients of their rights. Rights specific to the pregnant patient include the right to prenatal care, the right to choose a physician or midwife, and the right to give birth in the setting of her choice. In addition, the pregnant patient has the right to move freely during labor, to deliver in the position of her choice, and to have uninterrupted contact with her newborn provided that neither mother nor child experience a medical condition that prevents this (WHO, 2018).

Pregnant patients also have the right to culturally competent care, which has the added benefit of promoting patient trust in the healthcare team as well as promoting the overall health of mother and child. Provided the patient's cultural practices do not jeopardize the mother or the child, the nurse must respect the mother's wishes for culturally based practices. The nurse should also advocate with other HCPs for the patient's right to engage in these practices (Wint, Elias, Mendez, Mendez, & Gary-Webb, 2019).

A number of issues can develop that endanger a pregnant patient's rights. For example, the patient's right to prenatal care depends on the patient's access to care. As a result, patients without health insurance or in underserved communities may not be able to exercise this right. In addition, labor and delivery rights may be affected by organizational or unit regulations that limit patient movement, by HCPs who are unaware of the various rights of the pregnant patient, or by medical emergencies that necessitate that certain protocols be followed. The nurse should work with the patient and other providers to protect the patient's rights to the extent possible in a given situation.

Patient Rights Pertaining to Older Adults

One of the biggest patient rights issues for older patients involves long-term care provided in nursing homes and in skilled nursing facilities. Federal law requires that nursing homes protect and promote the rights of each resident. These include the rights of nondiscrimination, respect, freedom from abuse and neglect, and freedom from physical restraints. In addition, residents must be informed about fees and services in writing before admission, be allowed to manage their money as they see fit, be allowed to keep personal property in their rooms, and be able to see the HCP of their choice. Visitors must be allowed during reasonable hours, and necessary social services must be provided to residents. Residents must be able to file complaints without fear of reprisals and cannot be transferred or discharged unfairly (Medicare.gov, n.d.). Recently the Centers for Medicare and Medicaid Services (2020) issued a rule that bars nursing homes that receive federal funding from requiring that residents resolve disputes in arbitration instead of in court, making it easier for residents of nursing homes and their families to sue, if necessary, for claims such as elder abuse, sexual harassment, and wrongful death.

The rights of older patients may also be endangered in hospital settings, particularly if friends or family members are concerned about the patients' capacity for making their own medical decisions. In addition, the rights of patients who are no longer able to speak or make decisions for themselves may be at risk if the patients do not have advance directives in place. These issues are discussed in greater detail in Module 49, Legal Issues, and in Exemplar 44.B, Ethical Dilemmas, in this module.

REVIEW Patient Rights

RELATE Link the Concepts and Exemplars

Linking the exemplar of patient rights with the concept of healthcare systems:

1. Patients have the right to emergency care without bias. What are your beliefs about patients who use emergency care in place of primary care?
2. What are your beliefs about patient privacy when emergent or critical care is needed and patients cannot provide approval for their own care?

Linking the exemplar of patient rights with the concept of addiction:

3. Patients with persistent admissions for alcohol withdrawal therapy due to alcohol addiction need support to make the decision to get over this addiction. What are your beliefs about alcohol addiction and the nursing role in assisting a patient with these issues?
4. When adults who have had an extensive history of back pain with several narcotics taken each day need surgery, they often require a higher level of narcotics postoperatively. What is the nurse's role in supporting this type of patient in appropriate pain management?

REFER Go to Pearson MyLab Nursing and eText

REFLECT Apply Your Knowledge

James Casper is a 75-year-old widower who was admitted to the ED after a hit-and-run accident. Upon arrival, he was intubated, a chest tube was inserted, and he was rushed into surgery to repair damage to his spleen. After surgery, he was taken to the trauma unit to recover.

Mr. Casper has been on the trauma unit for 3 days now. He is awake and alert but still reports that he is experiencing pain. He has become increasingly agitated during his time on the unit. He has also complained repeatedly about nurses' "constant poking and prodding" of him. He has refused to see his daughter on several occasions when she has come to visit him.

Today, Candace Jones, the nurse assigned to Mr. Casper, has come to perform a venipuncture to get a blood sample for lab testing. He refuses to allow her to draw the blood. At first, Mr. Casper simply refuses to give her his arm; then, he began to yell at Ms. Jones and verbally berate her.

1. Upon admission into the ED, Mr. Casper signed a general consent for care form. Does this form supersede his right to refuse the venipuncture? Why or why not?
2. What is Ms. Jones' best means of proceeding in this situation without violating this patient's rights?
3. In what way has Mr. Casper violated his patient responsibilities in this scenario?

References

Al-Banna, D. A. (2017). Core professional and personal values of nurses about nursing in Erbil city hospitals: A profession, not just career. *Nurse Care Open Access Journal, 2*(6), 169–173.

American Academy of Family Physicians (AAFP). (2019). *Screening and counseling adolescents and young adults: A framework for comprehensive care*. https://www.aafp.org/afp/2020/0201/p147.html

American Association of Colleges of Nursing (AACN). (2008). *The essentials of baccalaureate education for professional nursing practice*. Author.

American Association of Colleges of Nursing (AACN). (2020). *Nursing shortage fact sheet*. https://www.aacnnursing.org/News-Information/Fact-Sheets/Nursing-Shortage

American Cancer Society. (2016). *Patient's bill of rights*. http://www.cancer.org/treatment/findingandpayingfortreatment/understandingfinancialandlegalmatters/patients-bill-of-rights

American Civil Liberties Union of Ohio. (2014). *Your health and the law: A guide for teens*. http://www.acluohio.org/wp-content/uploads/2014/06/TeenHealthGuide.pdf

American College of Obstetricians and Gynecologists (ACOG). (2020). *Confidentiality in adolescent health care*. ACOG Committee Opinion, Number 803. https://journals.lww.com/greenjournal/Fulltext/2020/04000/Confidentiality_in_Adolescent_Health_Care__ACOG.60.aspx

American Nurses Association (ANA). (2015a). *Code of ethics for nurses with interpretive statements*. http://nursingworld.org/Document-Vault/Ethics-1/Code-of-Ethics-for-Nurses.html

American Nurses Association (ANA). (2015b). *Position statement: Risk and responsibility in providing nursing care*. http://www.nursingworld.org/MainMenuCategories/EthicsStandards/Ethics-Position-Statements/Risk-and-Respons-ibility-in-Providing-Nursing-Care.html/Riskand-Responsibility PositionStatement2015.pdf

American Nurses Association (ANA). (2015c). *The year of ethics commences with first revision of code since 2001*. http://nursingworld.org/FunctionalMenuCategories/Media Resources/PressReleases/2015-NR/-The-Year-of-Ethics-Commences-with-First-Revision-of-Code-since-2001.html

American Nurses Association (ANA). (2019a). *ANA advises objectivity in new medical aid in dying position*. https://www.nursingworld.org/news/news-releases/2019-news-releases/ana-advises-objectivity-in-new-medical-aid-in-dying-position/

American Nurses Association (ANA). (2019b). *Nurse staffing crisis*. https://www.nursingworld.org/practice-policy/nurse-staffing/nurse-staffing-crisis/

Ball, I., Hornby, L., Rochwerg, B., Weiss, M., Gillrie, C., Chassé, M., et al. (2020). Management of the neurologically deceased organ donor: A Canadian clinical perspective guideline. *Canadian Medical Association Journal*, *192*(14), E361–E369.

Ball, J. W., Bindler, R. C., Cowen, K., & Shaw, M. (2017). *Principles of pediatric nursing: Caring for children* (7th ed.). Pearson.

Burnell, R. (2019). *How to resolve conflict as a nurse*. Nursing In Practice. https://www.nursinginpractice.com/professional/how-to-resolve-conflict-as-a-nurse/

Butts, J. B., & Rich, K. L. (2020). *Nursing ethics: Across the curriculum and into practice* (5th ed.). Jones & Bartlett.

Campbell, S. (2019). *At what age should kids be making their own medical decisions?* Healthline. https://www.healthline.com/health-news/at-what-age-should-children-be-allowed-to-make-their-own-medical-decisions

Centers for Disease Control and Protection (CDC). (2020). *HIV in the United States and dependent areas*. https://www.cdc.gov/hiv/statistics/overview/ataglance.html?CDC_AA_refVal=https%3A%2F%2Fwww.cdc.gov%2Fhiv%2Fstatistics%2Fbasics%2Fataglance.html

Centers for Medicare and Medicaid Services. (2020). *Revision history for LTC survey documents and files*. https://www.cms.gov/files/document/revision-history-ltc-survey-process-documents-and-files-updated-08312020.pdf

Centre for Genetics Education. (2020). *Fact sheet 15: Genetic and genomic testing*. https://www.genetics.edu.au/publications-and-resources/facts-sheets/fact-sheet-15-genetic-and-genomic-testing

Chooljian, D. M., Hallenbeck, J., Ezeji-Okoye, S. C., Sebesta, R., Iqbal, H., & Kuschner, W. G. (2016). Emotional support for health care professionals: A therapeutic role for the hospital ethics committee. *Journal of Social Work in End of Life and Palliative Care*, *12*(3), 277–288.

CNN Editorial Research. (2020). *Physician-assisted suicide fast facts*. https://www.cnn.com/2014/11/26/us/physician-assisted-suicide-fast-facts/index.html

Cohen, J., & Ezer, T. (2013). Human rights in patient care: A theoretical and practical framework. *Health and Human Rights Journal*, *15*(2). https://www.hhrjournal.org/2013/12/human-rights-in-patient-care-a-theoretical-and-practical-framework/

Crowley, J. D., & Gottlieb, M. C. (2012). Objects in the mirror are closer than they appear: A primary prevention model for ethical decision making. *Professional Psychology: Research and Practice*, *43*(1), 65–72.

Danis, M. (2018). *Stopping artificial nutrition and hydration at the end of life*. UpToDate. http://www.uptodate.com/contents/stopping-artificial-nutrition-and-hydration-at-the-end-of-life

Dekeyser Ganz, F., & Berkovitz, K. (2012). Surgical nurses' perceptions of ethical dilemmas, moral distress and quality of care. *Journal of Advanced Nursing* *68*(7), 1516–1525.

Dikema, D. S. (2014). *Parental decision making*. University of Washington. https://depts.washington.edu/bioethx/topics/parent.html

Edmondson, C., & Zelonka, C. (2019). Our own worst enemies: The nursing bullying epidemic. *Nursing Administration Quarterly*, *43*(3), 274–279.

Epstein, B., & Turner, M. (2015). The nursing code of ethics: Its value, its history. *Online Journal of Issues in Nursing*, *20*(2).

Frellick, M. (2019). *The ethics of advocacy*. American Nurses Association. https://www.nursingworld.org/practice-policy/nurse-staffing/nurse-staffing-crisis/

Goodwyn, W. (2014). *The strange case of Marlise Munoz and John Peter Smith Hospital*. http://www.npr.org/sections/health-shots/2014/01/28/267759687/the-strange-case-of-marlise-munoz-and-john-peter-smith-hospital

Gretter, L. (1910). Florence Nightingale pledge: Autograph manuscript dated 1893. *American Journal of Nursing*, *10*(4), 271.

Guerrero-Dib, J. G., Portales, L., & Heredia-Escorza, Y. (2020). Impact of academic integrity on workplace ethical behaviour. *International Journal for Educational Integrity*, *16*, 2.

Guido, G. W. (2020). *Legal and ethical issues in nursing* (7th ed.). Prentice Hall.

Guttmacher Institute. (2020). *An overview of consent to reproductive health services by young people*. Retrieved from https://www.guttmacher.org/state-policy/explore/overview-minors-consent-law

HealthCare.gov. (n.d.). *Health coverage rights and protections*. https://www.healthcare.gov/health-care-law-protections/rights-and-protections/

Hilton, L. (2019, April 1). Ethical practice when facing life-limiting disease. *Contemporary Pediatrics*. https://www.contemporarypediatrics.com/view/ethical-practice-when-facing-life-limiting-disease

HIV.gov. (2020a). *Paying for HIV care and treatment*. https://www.hiv.gov/hiv-basics/staying-in-hiv-care/hiv-treatment/paying-for-hiv-care-and-treatment

HIV.gov. (2020b). *U.S. statistics*. https://www.hiv.gov/hiv-basics/overview/data-and-trends/statistics

International Council of Nurses (ICN). (2012). *The ICN code of ethics for nurses*. https://www.icn.ch/sites/default/files/inline-files/2012_ICN_Codeofethicsfornurses_%20eng.pdf

Izadi, E. (2015, May 1). Woman delivers baby 54 days after being declared brain dead. *Washington Post*. https://www.washingtonpost.com/news/morning-mix/wp/2015/05/01/a-brain-dead-woman-was-kept-alive-for-54-days-to-deliver-her-baby/

Jansen, T. L., & Hanssen, I. (2017). Patient participation: Causing moral stress in psychiatric nursing? *Scandinavian Journal of Caring Science*, *31*(2), 388–394.

Johansen, M. L., & O'Brien, J. L. (2016). Decision making in nursing practice: A concept analysis. *Nursing Forum*, *51*(1), 40–48.

Johnstone, M. (2012). Workplace ethics and respect for colleagues. *Australian Nursing Journal*, *20*(2), 31.

Kangasniemi, M., & Haho, A. (2012). Human love—The inner essence of nursing ethics according to Estrid Rodhe: A study using the approach of history of ideas. *Scandinavian Journal of Caring Science*, *26*, 803–810.

Keresi, Z., Carlsson, G., & Lindberg, E. (2019). A caring relationship as a prerequisite for patient participation in a psychiatric care setting: A qualitative study from the nurses' perspective. *Nordic Journal of Nursing Research*, *39*(4), 218–225.

Khoshmehr, Z., Barkhordari-Sharifabad, M., Nasiriani, K., & Fallahzadeh, H. (2020). Moral courage and psychological empowerment among nurses. *BMC Nursing*, *19*, 43.

Kim, S., Seo, M., & Kim, D. R. (2018). Unmet needs for clinical ethics support services in nurse: Based on focus group interviews. *Nursing Ethics*, *25*(4), 505–519.

King, L., Harrington, A., Linedale, E., & Tanner, E. (2018). A mixed-methods thematic review: Health-related decision making by the older person. *Journal of Clinical Nursing*, *27*(7–8), e1327–e1343.

Lachman, V. D. (2012). Applying the ethics of care to your nursing practice. *MEDSURG Nursing*, *21*(2), 112–115.

Lachman, V. D. (2014). Conscientious objection in nursing: Definition and criteria for acceptance. *MEDSURG Nursing*, *23*(3), 196–198.

Mahon, C. (2018, September 28). *HIV and abortion—a human rights challenge*. Avert. https://www.avert.org/news/hiv-and-abortion-%E2%80%93-human-rights-challenge

Martinez-Selles, D., Martinez-Selles, M., & Martinez-Selles, H. (2020). Ethical issues in decision-making regarding the elderly affected by corona virus disease 2019: An expert opinion. *European Cardiology*, *15*, e48.

Medicare.gov. (n.d.). *What are your rights in a skilled nursing facility?* https://www.medicare.gov/what-medicare-covers/what-part-a-covers/skilled-nursing-facility-rights

Mott, S. (2014). The pediatric bill of rights. *Journal of Pediatric Nursing*, *29*(6), 709.

National Center for Complementary and Integrative Health (NCCIH). (2019). *Cannabis (marijuana) and cannabinoids: What you need to know*. https://www.nccih.nih.gov/health/cannabis-marijuana-and-cannabinoids-what-you-need-to-know

National Human Genome Research Institute. (2020). *Direct to consumer genomic testing*. Retrieved https://www.genome.gov/dna-day/15-ways/direct-to-consumer-genomic-testing

Naseri-Salahshour, V., & Sajadi, M. (2020). Ethical challenges of novice nurses in clinical practice: Iranian perspective. *International Nursing Review*, *67*(1), 76–83.

Organ Procurement and Transplantation Network (OPTN). (2014). *Ethical principles of pediatric organ allocation*. https://optn.transplant.hrsa.gov/resources/ethics/ethical-principles-of-pediatric-organ-allocation/

Organ Procurement and Transplantation Network (OPTN). (n.d.). *How organ allocation works*. https://optn.transplant.hrsa.gov/learn/about-transplantation/how-organ-allocation-works/

Poikkeus, T., Suhonen, R., Katajisto, J., & Leino-Kilpi, H. (2020). Relationships between organizational and individual support, nurses' ethical competence, ethical safety, and work satisfaction. *Health Care Management Review*, *45*(1), 83–93

President's Advisory Commission on Consumer Protection and Quality in the Health Care Industry. (1998). *Consumer bill of rights and responsibilities: Executive summary*. Agency for Healthcare Research and Quality. http://archive.ahrq.gov/hcqual/cborr/exsumm.html

Purnell, L. D., & Fenkl, E. A. (2019). *Handbook for culturally competent care*. Springer.

Sarkar, S. (2018, November 29). Euthanasia. *Law Times Journal*. https://lawtimesjournal.in/euthanasia/

Smallwood, R. (2018). *High costs of poor cultural competency in healthcare*. Relias. https://www.relias.com/blog/high-costs-of-poor-cultural-competency-in-healthcare

Song, J. (2018). Ethics education in nursing: Challenges for nurse educators. *Kai Tiaki Nursing Research*, *9*(1), 12–17.

The Joint Commission. (2013b). *Speak up: Know your rights*. http://www.jointcommission.org/assets/1/6/Know_Your_Rights_brochure.pdf

United Network for Organ Sharing. (2020). *How we match organs*. https://unos.org/transplant/how-we-match-organs/

Varcoe, C., Doane, G., Pauly, B., Rodney, P., Storch, J. L., Mahoney, K., et al. (2004). Ethical practice in nursing: Working the in-betweens. *Journal of Advanced Nursing*, *45*(3), 316–325.

Wint, K., Elias, T., Mendez, G., Mendez, D. D., & Gary-Webb, T. L. (2019). Experiences of community doulas working with low-income, African-American mothers. *Health Equity*, *3*(1), 109–116.

World Health Organization (WHO). (2017). *Human rights and health*. https://www.who.int/news-room/fact-sheets/detail/human-rights-and-health

World Health Organization (WHO). (2018). *Intrapartum care for a positive childbirth experience*. https://apps.who.int/iris/bitstream/handle/10665/272447/WHO-RHR-18.12-eng.pdf?ua=1

Module 45

Evidence-Based Practice

Module Outline and Learning Outcomes

The Concept of Evidence-Based Practice

Overview of Evidence-Based Practice

45.1 Summarize the evolution of evidence-based practice.

Concepts Related to Evidence-Based Practice

45.2 Outline the relationship between evidence-based practice and other concepts.

Nursing Clinical Research

45.3 Summarize the fundamentals of research methodology.

Developing Evidence-Based Practice

45.4 Analyze the four steps of developing evidence-based practice.

Strategies to Implement Evidence-Based Practice

45.5 Contrast differences between implementing individual and organizational evidence-based practice.

›› The Concept of Evidence-Based Practice

Concept Key Terms

Background questions, **2763**
Evidence, **2759**
Evidence-based nursing, **2759**
Evidence-based practice (EBP), **2759**
Foreground questions, **2764**
Informed consent, **2763**
Nursing clinical research, **2762**
Nursing research, **2762**
PICOT, **2764**
Qualitative research, **2762**
Quantitative research, **2762**
Research, **2759**
Research participants, **2762**
Translational research, **2760**

In 2001, the Institute of Medicine (IOM) published a report, *Crossing the Quality Chasm: A New Health System for the 21st Century*. This report addressed deficits in healthcare that caused preventable harm to patients and recommended implementing evidence-based practice (EBP) to reduce inappropriate variations in healthcare and facilitate the standardization of safe, quality patient care (Brittain, 2018). The IOM published another significant report in 2011, *The Future of Nursing: Leading Change, Advancing Health*. This report made recommendations including nursing academic changes for improved safe, quality, and best patient outcomes through care coordination, health promotion, quality improvement, and EBP (Sullivan, 2018).

Overview of Evidence-Based Practice

Evidence-based practice (EBP) provides a problem-solving blend of **research** (a formal, systematic way of answering a question or approaching a problem) and **evidence** (acquired nursing knowledge based on formal, systematic studies or expert opinion) with nursing experience (a progressive and continuous development of knowledge, skills, and behaviors to build proficiency in making clinical judgments about nursing care). Different professional organizations and healthcare agencies may vary slightly in their definitions of EBP. Generally, however, **evidence-based nursing** includes three components: (1) the best evidence from the most current research available, (2) the nurse's clinical expertise, and (3) the patient's preferences, which reflect values, needs, interests, and choices (see **Figure 45.1** ››). By integrating the three components of EBP into the clinical decision-making process, nurses can individualize patient care and provide best practice for patient-centered care (American Association of Nurse Practitioners, 2018; National Council of State Boards of Nursing, 2020; UNC Health Sciences Library, 2019).

Implementing research evidence is not a new concept. Florence Nightingale is often recognized as the first nurse theorist because of the methods process she used to develop evidence-based practice (Sher & Akhtar, 2018). During the Crimean War in the 1850s, Nightingale observed the sanitary conditions in military hospitals and the nurses providing care for the soldiers. She noticed a correlation between poor environmental sanitation in hospitals and increased death rates of wounded soldiers after being in hospitals. When Nightingale made sanitary improvements in hospitals, such as adding more lighting, better ventilation, and improved hygiene, diet, and cleanliness, she noted the soldiers had fewer infections and higher survival rates (Sher & Akhtar, 2018). Her process consisted of making observations, collecting data, analyzing

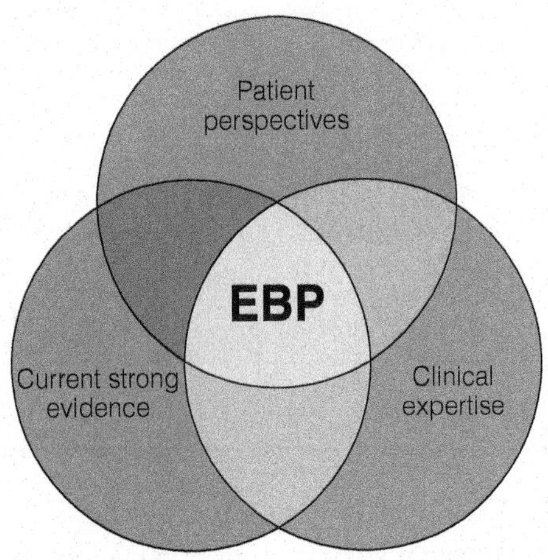

Figure 45.1 » These three components provide the framework for evidence-based practice that nurses use to provide optimized individual clinical care to patients.

the data, developing a hypothesis, testing the hypothesis with more data, determining a conclusion, summarizing her methods, and presenting the process to others.

Nightingale's actions were early rudiments of today's standards for EBP. She started with a question, "What was causing wounded soldiers to have high death rates while in the hospital?" She considered possibilities to explain the phenomenon. She made changes in the hospital environment and frequency of handwashing that positively affected soldier health outcomes. From these results, Nightingale developed a reasonable explanation supported by the data she had collected. Her theory of nursing focused on the environment and hygienic behaviors and how nurses can modify these conditions for best patient outcomes (Sher & Akhtar, 2018).

In 1971, Dr. Archie Cochrane criticized the lack of research evidence supporting many of the common healthcare interventions at that time. He argued for the need for more randomized controlled trials (RCTs) to gather reliable evidence for the determination of medical treatment options (Saint Thomas University [STU], 2019). Ten years later, Dr. David Sackett and a group of clinical epidemiologists started the evidence-based medicine (EBM) movement. They defined EBM as using current, best available medical evidence to make intentional, specific, and careful decisions about individual patient care that combines clinical expertise with clinical evidence from research (STU, 2019).

From these early efforts came **translational research**, a systematic approach of converting research knowledge into applications of healthcare for improved patient outcomes. The translation of scientific evidence into practical applications allows for enhanced human health, particularly when information flows back and forth between researchers and clinicians, allowing for further investigation of diseases and their effects on humans. The National Institutes of Health supports translational research through the Clinical and Translational Science Awards Consortium. The Centers for Disease Control and Prevention operates translational centers around the country.

Translational research has clear benefits for the continued development of EBP across nursing and other disciplines involved in healthcare systems. In particular, translational research may speed the process from discovery to application. This potential benefit also may carry risks for certain groups, depending on the research study. Researchers must adhere to the *Common Rule* regulations for involving human subject participants in research projects and studies (National Institutes of Health [NIH], 2019).

Currently with traditional research, there is a lag time of about 17 years from the time new evidence is identified to when it is actively used in practice (Luciano, 2019). This process includes many stages to disseminate the new evidence broadly and then to all individual healthcare systems, personnel and providers, leadership, and patients. Decisions are made about integrating or replacing current practice with the evidence. Any new evidence needs to be customized to become part of each clinical setting without weakening its effectiveness and benefits. The process usually requires much work and dedication among change agents, patient-care champions, staff educators, and patient educators. Even as healthcare professionals are embracing new evidenced-based practices, new research and evidence continue to become available.

Concepts Related to Evidence-Based Practice

EBP has widespread implications for all areas of nursing because it informs nursing procedures during the day-to-day care of patients. Part of the reason that EBP is so important is that it assists nurses in examining the *why* behind existing processes and procedures, encouraging nurses to advocate for patients by asking questions such as the following:

- Is this the best practice method available to support positive patient outcomes?
- Is there evidence supporting an improvement?

With the abundance of research available today, nurses are challenged to continuously evaluate and change their nursing practices based on current evidence. At the same time, as healthcare team members, nurses face the challenge of cost containment in managing care. Factors that influence decisions about potential interventions include availability of resources and requirements regarding reimbursement for services as stipulated by payment sources. Nurses must use best evidence related to finance and economics to develop a cost-conscious nursing practice (see Module 39, Managing Care, for additional information).

Patients' participation in decisions about care is based on their individual influences and preferences, including health beliefs, culture, spirituality, and traditions (see Module 24, Culture and Diversity, and Module 30, Spirituality, for more information). For example, patients can agree to a treatment such as supplemental oxygen, refuse a treatment such as a blood transfusion, ask for a second opinion from a specialist healthcare provider (HCP), and establish advance directives to ensure that they will be treated according to their preferences. Patients also may choose to incorporate integrative medicine into the plan of care (see Focus on Integrative Health). Many patients have access to resources that provide them with

Concepts Related to
Evidence-Based Practice

CONCEPT	RELATIONSHIP TO EVIDENCE-BASED PRACTICE	NURSING IMPLICATIONS
Accountability	Best practice standards of care, responsibility, and scope of nursing practice reflect EBP.	■ Nurses are responsible for providing the best, most current nursing care to their patients.
Clinical Decision Making	EBP provides scientific support for nurses in clinical thinking processes, making decisions, and using clinical judgment.	■ As problem solvers, nurses depend on current best practice to deliver high-quality care throughout the individual patient's nursing plan of care.
Health, Wellness, and Illness	Routine habits, including sleep patterns, hygiene practices, and exercise, impact an individual's current and future state of health and wellness.	■ Nurses are responsible for educating patients about evidence-based self-care practices that promote health and wellness and that reduce the risk for illness or injury.
Legal Issues	The evidence that supports EBP includes clinical knowledge, expert opinion, and information resulting from research. Evidence serves as an essential component of the foundation for professional nursing's scope and standards of practice.	■ Conduct that deviates from professional standards of practice constitutes malpractice.
Professional Behaviors	As a credible professional discipline, nursing has a responsibility to use EBP.	■ Best evidence needs to be integrated with the nurse's clinical experience and patient preferences.
Quality Improvement	Improving nursing care is a continuous process using current evidence to deliver safe and effective interventions resulting in best patient outcomes.	■ Improvement of the "why" "when," and "what" of nursing care is a dynamic process that can lead to changes in how nursing care is provided.

medical knowledge and clinical information through technology, including television and the internet, which can increase awareness of their condition and possible care options. Patients need to be a part of the process, and their preferences should be taken into consideration in clinical decisions about their care (see Module 36, Clinical Decision Making, for further information). The Concepts Related to Evidence-Based Practice feature outlines some, but not all, of the concepts that are integral to EBP. They are listed in alphabetical order.

Focus on Integrative Health
The Evidence for Integrative Medicine

Integrative medicine combines the principles of complementary health approaches (such as mindfulness or acupuncture) with conventional medical approaches. Integrative medicine emphasizes interprofessional collaboration among members of the healthcare team. Primary goals of integrative medicine include establishing best practices for promoting health and healing by way of combining evidence-based therapies with holistic approaches to healthcare. A study of nearly 500 patients with breast or gynecological cancer showed those undergoing integrative medicine more frequently had improved appetites, less fatigue, less anxiety and pain, slept better, and overall global health (Gannotta, 2018). Many integrative medicine centers associate with large teaching healthcare centers to be able to offer consultations, comprehensive care, or primary service.

Nursing Clinical Research

Nurses actively collaborate with other healthcare disciplines to provide high-quality patient care. They help patients navigate the healthcare environment and assume many roles, such as provider of care, advocate, teacher, and researcher (refer Module 42, Accountability, for additional information). Nurses help to ensure open and effective communication and continuity among all members of the healthcare team and patients and their families. Nurses who are actively involved in EBP access and use evidence from a variety of sources and disciplines to help guide their clinical practice and improve patient care. By using EBP, nurses also ensure the credibility of their profession and provide accountability for nursing care (**Box 45.1** »).

Box 45.1
An Example of Using EBP to Inform Practice

Traditionally, the hypoxic drive theory has held that patients with chronically elevated blood carbon dioxide levels, such as occurs with COPD, may experience respiratory failure if exposed to high levels of supplemental oxygen. The current evidence-based protocol recommends administering supplemental oxygen to patients with an oxygen saturation of ≤88% accompanied by frequent assessment of blood gases (Funk, 2019; Global Initiative for Chronic Obstructive Lung Disease [GOLD], 2020). Frequent blood gas measurements can help ensure adequate oxygenation and prevent increased CO_2 retention or worsening acidosis (GOLD, 2020).

Because evidence is a product of research, being familiar with the research process helps nurses to select and evaluate practices for best patient outcomes. In a very broad definition, *research* is obtaining information and objective facts to advance knowledge about a specific topic. **Nursing research** is the use of a systematic and strict scientific process to analyze phenomena of interest to all areas of nursing, including practice, education, and administration (Nieswiadomy, 2018). **Nursing clinical research** seeks answers to questions that will ultimately improve patient care, such as the following:

- What are the links between diet and the development of diabetes and cardiovascular disease?
- Is a new drug or medical device more effective than one already on the market?
- Do patients who undergo surgery at one medical center have a higher complication rate than those who are treated at another?
- Are patients satisfied with their care during hospitalization?

Familiarity with research methodology is becoming increasingly important to nursing practice. The ability to weigh the scientific merit of a research study is key to understanding the interpretation and implications of the research findings. Not all research findings have equal validity. One factor that influences the validity of a research study is the type of methodology that is used. The various methodologies used in clinical research include quantitative research and qualitative research.

Quantitative research uses precise measurement to collect data and analyze it statistically for a summary and a description of the resulting findings or to test relationships among variables. An example of a quantitative question is "Are there differences in skin breakdown between premature infants who are bathed with plain water and those who are bathed with bacteriostatic soap?"

Qualitative research investigates a question through narrative data that explores the subjective experiences of human beings and can provide nursing with a better understanding of the patient's perspective. Goals of qualitative research include the identification of patterns and themes. An example of a qualitative question is "What is the nature of coping and adjustment after a radical mastectomy?"

Today's nurses have a wealth of nursing research available that uses the scientific method to obtain evidence (**Box 45.2** »). Using this method limits subjective influences and bias and enhances the validity and reliability of the data.

Box 45.2

General Elements of the Scientific Method

- A question is asked about a phenomenon.
- A literature review is done to identify past research findings on the phenomenon.
- A hypothesis is proposed.
- A study, or experiment, is planned and executed.
- Data are collected, organized, and evaluated.
- A conclusion about the phenomenon is presented.

Funding

Funding from many sources is available to nurses who are interested in doing research to advance nursing science and generate evidence that supports improved patient care (Sigma Theta Tau International, 2020). This funding ranges from small research grants from local professional nursing chapters to larger grants awarded by state or national nursing organization foundations. Corporations, state agencies, and federal organizations also support nursing research grants. Awards are given in all areas of nursing, including gerontology, quality of life, health disparities, disease prevention, and nursing practice specialties. Examples of sources of awards and grants are Sigma Theta Tau International Honor Society of Nursing, Agency for Healthcare Research and Quality, National Institute of Nursing Research, National Council of State Boards of Nursing, Robert Wood Johnson Foundation, and the American Cancer Society.

Participants

All research studies require participants. Because each study targets a specific population (for example, women older than age 65 with a history of hypertension), researchers develop a list of criteria, which normally includes factors such as age, weight, gender, medical history, type and stage of a disease, and current medications. These qualifiers can be categorized as inclusion (acceptable) or exclusion (not acceptable) criteria. Inclusion and exclusion criteria are used to guide selection of participants that represent the target population while also ensuring protection of potential participants' physical safety and psychosocial well-being. Vulnerable populations that are subject to strict legal and ethical considerations include human fetuses, neonates, children, prisoners, educationally disadvantaged individuals, and individuals who are cognitively impaired (NIH, 2019). Even for individuals who are legally capable of consenting to participation in a research study, in some cases, safety concerns may prohibit participating. For example, particularly with medication-related research, individuals with certain medical diagnoses may be excluded from participating because of potential health risks. **Research participants** are defined as volunteers for a specific study project who meet all the inclusion criteria, have been informed of all aspects of the study, and have given informed consent.

Ethical and Legal Issues

Ethical principles used by nurses to protect patients receiving care are also used to protect participants in clinical research studies (see Module 44, Ethics, for further information). Ethical principles are at the core of such questions as "Did the researchers maintain the participants' confidentiality?" and "Did the participants experience physical harm or psychologic distress as a result of participating in the study?" Institutional review boards (IRBs) review research protocols and ensure that they adhere to ethical standards. As established by the 1979 landmark publication *The Belmont Report*, research must adhere to three main ethical principles: respect for persons, beneficence, and justice (Czubaruk, 2019).

Respect for persons comprises acknowledging and protecting the autonomy of all individuals, including individuals whose capacity to exercise autonomy is diminished because of disability, illness, circumstances that restrict liberty, or immaturity

(Czubaruk, 2019). Researchers must ensure that the volunteers are participating freely in a study, without coercion and after receiving full disclosure about the study and the potential risks involved. *Beneficence* requires that researchers protect participants from physical injury, psychologic harm, economic insult, and exploitation during or as a result of the study. It also addresses the requirement that the study be conducted for the benefit of others. *Justice* requires the fair treatment of all participants, including the right of participants to expect their personal information to be maintained under strict confidentiality and the protection of participant anonymity. The Health Insurance Portability and Accountability Act (HIPAA) includes a Privacy Rule, which creates a national standard for the disclosure of private health information.

Legal practices related to research studies include following criminal, civil, and tort laws. Study volunteers have a legal right to full disclosure of the study's purpose, required procedures, length, expectations, risks, and possible benefits before consenting to participate. **Informed consent** includes the right to receive this information as well as the right of participants to withdraw from the study at any time. Participants must give informed consent, usually in written form, before the study begins (refer to Module 49, Legal Issues, for information on informed consent).

Implications for Nursing Practice

The nursing profession includes both nurse clinicians and nurse researchers who are working to determine best evidence. Nursing clinical research is important to provide best evidence for EBP, to support nursing as a separate professional discipline, and to define current best practice standards of nursing care.

Providing Best Evidence for EBP

Best practices in nursing have continuously evolved as a result of research. In today's healthcare environment, it is especially crucial to participate in EBP. Practice based on the reasoning "we do it that way because we've always done it that way" is inadequate and fails to consider the research evidence supporting new and improved nursing practices. Integrating EBP is necessary to meet the current standards of high quality in nursing performance.

Supporting Nursing as a Professional Discipline

Simply stated, nurses want to be in control of nursing. Nursing history reflects its growth as a professional discipline and efforts to gain recognition as a profession in the eyes of the general public and in the eyes of members of the other healthcare professions.

The criteria for nursing to be recognized as a profession continue to evolve. They currently include the following:

- Specialized education requirements
- A body of well-defined knowledge and expertise
- Conducting ongoing research
- An orientation toward service to others
- Following a code of ethics
- Having autonomy as a profession
- Professional organization (see Module 40, Professionalism, and Module 42, Accountability, for additional information).

Note that the first two items in this list—specialized education requirements and a body of well-defined knowledge and expertise—both depend, in part, on nursing research.

Defining Current Best Practice Standards of Nursing Care

EBP supports changes in the responsibilities of nurses, including clinical decision making and clinical judgment, and the level and extent of nurses' accountability. Standards of nursing care are defined by the American Nurses Association, the National League for Nursing, and The Joint Commission (see Module 42, Accountability, for more information about standards of nursing care). These organizations periodically update standards to reflect current best evidence. Rights, responsibilities, and scopes of nursing practice are legally defined by state nurse practice acts from each state's Board of Nursing (see Module 40, Professionalism, and Module 49, Legal Issues, for additional information).

In addition to the standards set by professional organizations and state boards, each healthcare facility sets performance expectations for nursing care in its policies and procedures, in accordance with the state's nursing scope of practice. To protect themselves from liability, nurses need to follow policies and procedures as written. When practice evidence supporting better patient outcomes is discovered, the nurse becomes an advocate of that best evidence. Each facility has a process to follow in suggesting changes in policies and procedures; it may be a quality improvement committee, a policies and procedures committee, or a nursing unit's chain of command. There is room for any change that benefits staff and patients, and it is incumbent on nurses, as professionals, to advocate for changes that benefit their patients.

Developing Evidence-Based Practice

EBP is a combination of the knowledge that is generated from the clinician's experience, the research evidence, and the preferences of the patient. Nurses must commit to expanding the implementation of EBP within the nursing profession. Through such efforts, nurses continue their quest for the provision of safe, effective, high-quality patient care.

Step 1: Develop a Clinical Question

Formulating the clinical question is the first step in engaging in EBP (see **Figure 45.2** »). Clinical questions are generated in many ways but are usually encountered during patient care. A clinical question may be knowledge-based (a background question) or practice-based (a foreground question). The type of question developed helps determine how and where to search for an answer. **Background questions** are general questions that seek more information about a topic, such as diseases or medications. These questions serve to fill gaps in knowledge about a specific topic and take the form "What is . . . ?" or "What does . . . ?" The following are examples of background questions:

- Who is at risk for hypoglycemia?
- What are the side effects of a specific diuretic?

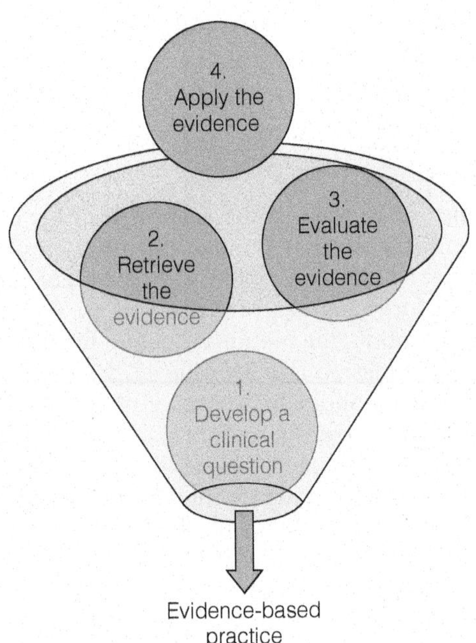

Figure 45.2 » The four steps in developing evidence-based practice funnel together to produce best nursing practice for safe, effective, high-quality patient care.

Answers to these questions can be found in textbooks, medical dictionaries, drug handbooks, and other educational materials.

Foreground questions are narrower in focus and are about a specific clinical issue. They are useful for finding nursing interventions that improve patient outcomes; in other words, they identify useful information about direct patient care. The following are examples of foreground questions:

- How does using an incentive spirometer (or not using one) affect the length of stay for a surgical patient?
- How does using a cooling blanket compare to using antipyretic medication as treatment for a patient with a high temperature?

Answers to these questions can be found in the studies conducted to elicit evidence. Types of research studies include the following:

- ***Meta-analysis.*** A group of studies on a given topic are examined, and their results are combined and analyzed as if they were from one large study.
- ***Case study.*** A case study is specific to one individual, issue, or event.
- ***Cohort study.*** A longitudinal study follows two groups and measures the outcomes of an exposure group with those of a group with no exposure.
- ***Case-control study.*** Individuals with and without a specific condition are compared to identify predictive variables.
- ***Randomized controlled trial (RCT).*** This is the strongest type of study in terms of validity. RCTs are designed to illustrate a cause-and-effect relationship by using a control group (participants who do not receive an intervention) and an experimental group (participants who do receive an intervention) (Duke University Medical Center Library, 2020).

Another consideration is determining the type of question that is of interest. This information helps to further narrow the clinical question. Types of questions are as follows:

- ***Diagnosis.*** How to select and interpret diagnostic tests and assess their accuracy, safety, and cost-effectiveness
- ***Therapy.*** How to select treatments that do more good than harm to patients and lead to the best outcomes
- ***Etiology.*** How to identify causes of a condition or disease
- ***Prognosis.*** How to predict a clinical course over time and possible complications related to a condition or disease process.

Clinicians commonly use the mnemonic PICOT (or, alternatively, PICO) to define and formulate a clinical question that will contribute to EBP. **PICOT** represents the elements of a clinical question (Nieswiadomy, 2018; Northern Arizona University, 2020):

Population (of patients) or **P**roblem of interest

Intervention, prognostic factor, or type of exposure

Comparison of interventions or main alternative to the intervention (including no intervention)

Outcome (desired effect)

Time frame (optional).

Both research studies and EBP projects use PICOT questions. PICOT develops foreground questions that apply EBP to clinical situations and problems (**Table 45.1** »).

Table 45.2 » shows an example of the following clinical question in PICOT format: Among postoperative orthopedic patients, does hourly rounding increase patient satisfaction ratings related to nursing care?

TABLE 45.1 PICOT

	Definition	Factors to Consider	Examples
Population or **P**roblem of interest	What is the common factor in the group of patients? Alternatively, what is the problem that will be addressed?	Characteristic(s) common to patients in the group.	A specific age, gender, health problem, or medication taken by all group members
Intervention	What will be done to the patients?	Activity shows the difference in the patient before and after the intervention.	A treatment, medication, therapy, test, or new routine of care

TABLE 45.1 PICOT *(continued)*

	Definition	Factors to Consider	Examples
Comparison group or comparing interventions	What is the difference (alternative) in the intervention being used when comparing two groups?	1. Can contrast an experimental group that receives an intervention with a control group that does not receive the intervention. 2. Can contrast an experimental group that receives the intervention of interest with a comparison group that receives a different intervention. 3. Can help establish a relationship, or the lack of a relationship, between an intervention and a predicted outcome.	1. Comparing two ways of doing something to find the best way. 2. Identifying the effect of taking medication A by comparing one group receiving medication A with a group receiving a placebo.
Outcome or desired effects	1. In response to the intervention, what is the desired effect for the patient? 2. In relationship to a selected problem, what is the desired improvement?	1. Desired effects of an intervention can be proved or disproved. 2. Improved outcomes can result from an intervention.	1. The desired effect is to minimize or eliminate a specific symptom. 2. An improved outcome is to reduce the time needed to accomplish a task.
Time frame (optional)	1. How long will the study last? 2. How long will it take to achieve the desired outcome?	Extent of time needed to study the impact of an intervention on a group may be brief or extended.	1. A brief time could be the first 12 hours after taking a medication. 2. An extended time could be 6 months following a treatment regimen.

TABLE 45.2 Example of Clinical Question in PICOT Format

Population	Intervention	Comparison	Outcome	Time
Postoperative orthopedic patients	Scheduled hourly rounding on a selected group of patients	No intervention/patients who are not subject to the hourly rounding protocol	Increased patient satisfaction ratings	Four weeks of implementation and data collection

Case Study » Part 1

Brent Calloway is the new nurse educator for a local hospital's medical–surgical unit. During the past few months, he has observed a high number of incident reports related to nursing procedures. He wonders whether there is something he can do to lower this number and improve patient safety in the unit. One of Brent's responsibilities is to organize a continuing education program for the annual review of competencies for the nurses. In past years, the nurses have had a mandatory annual meeting in which competencies were presented and demonstrated by the nurse educator while the nurses sat and watched. Brent is curious whether there is another, better approach to emphasize patient safety when the nurses review knowledge and skills for patient care.

Brent is aware that the staff development department uses computer technology for simulation scenarios during orientation for new nurses, and he wonders whether he could use that learning approach for continuing education programs in his division. Brent has helped with simulations in past employment and thinks that using this teaching strategy could support better patient safety. He questions whether changing the method of training could decrease the number of safety reports and improve patient outcomes.

Brent formulates the following PICOT elements:

P: Nursing staff

I: Simulation-based safety education

C: No intervention

O: Decreased incidence of procedural errors

T: 12 weeks for implementation of intervention and data collection.

On the basis of the identified PICOT elements, Brent formulates the following clinical question: "Among nursing staff, what is the effect of simulation-based safety education on the incidence of procedural errors?"

Before developing the EBP project, Brent plans to search for current research evidence related to the use of simulation-based education to promote safe nursing practice.

Clinical Reasoning Questions Level I

1. How does an EBP project differ from a research study? How would Brent's project development change if he were planning a research study instead of an EBP project?
2. What role did Brent's experience with computer-based simulation play in development of his clinical question?
3. Using the same PICOT elements, what are some other potential versions of the clinical question?
4. In Brent's clinical question, why is the target population stated as "nursing staff" instead of "medical–surgical patients"?

Clinical Reasoning Questions Level II

5. How important is it for Brent to have the support of his manager to be motivated to explore the potential of finding a better method of providing continuing education?
6. What is the value of nurses being inquisitive about the way things are done in their nursing practice?

TABLE 45.3 Order of Sections Typically Found in a Professional Research Article

Section	Function
Title	Gives the main topic of the research study.
Abstract	Provides a summary of the entire content of the journal article.
Introduction	Presents the question, or focus, of the investigative study; includes background of older research on same hypothesis.
Methods	Describes in detail all the aspects and methods of the study.
Results of study	Reports statistical data; may be in the form of charts or tables.
Conclusion	Summarizes and interprets the results of the study and statistical data in relation to the hypothesis; evaluates the findings of the study.
References	Lists the resources available for additional information.

Step 2: Retrieve the Evidence

Looking for clinical evidence from research sources usually includes a review of the relevant literature. When doing a literature review for evidence, nurses look for scientific elements in the journal article, including the abstract, or summary, of the article; an overview of the study conducted, including its methodology; a written conclusion based on the results of the study; and relevant references. The order of sections typically found in a professional research article is shown in **Table 45.3** ».

Nursing databases and resource links can yield a list of evidence articles related to the question at hand (**Table 45.4** »).

TABLE 45.4 Common Nursing Research Links

Name	Internet Website
Cochrane Review Database	http://www.cochrane.org
PubMed or MEDLINE Database (OVID) (includes international nursing index)	http://pubmed.gov
EBSCO Database a. DynaMed b. Cumulative Index to Nursing and Allied Health Literature (CINAHL) c. PsycINFO	a. ebscohost.com (through libraries and other institutions) b. mynursingkit.com (access EBSCO through Pearson Publishing, My Nursing Kit, My Search Lab)
Books and Articles Database	http://www.sciencedirect.com (Elsevier)
Agency for Healthcare Research and Quality (AHRQ)	https://www.ahrq.gov/cpi/about/otherwebsites/index.html http://guideline.gov http://www.qualitymeasures.ahrq.gov
Evidence-Based Nursing BMJ journals (Evidence-Based Nursing, 2020)	http://ebn.bmj.com
EBP Resources, Websites & Databases (Fuld Institute for EBP, 2019)	https://fuld.nursing.osu.edu/websites

Box 45.3

Nursing Journals

Examples of Research Journals in Nursing

Applied Nursing Research
Evidence-Based Nursing
International Journal of Nursing Studies
Journal of Nursing Scholarship
Nursing Research
Research in Nursing and Health
Scholarly Inquiry for Nursing Practice

Examples of Clinical and Specialty Nursing Journals That Publish Research

American Journal of Nursing
Journal of Emergency Nursing
Journal of Gerontologic Nursing
Journal of Nursing Administration
Journal of Nursing Education
Journal of Obstetric, Gynecologic and Neonatal Nursing
Journal of Pediatric Nursing
Journal of the American Psychiatric Nursing Association
MedSurg Nursing

Many databases have a tutorial available. Some databases offer only abstracts; others offer the full text of the article. All sources and sites should be judged on their degree of credibility. Research resources can be found in various ways. One is to use a review-of-literature article that presents studies relative to a topic and ends with an evaluative statement, or recommendation, regarding the studies described. Another way is to use a primary resource, which is the original published article. Secondary resources, when one author is writing about the original work of another author, can also be helpful. Focusing on the most recently published materials can help narrow the number of evidence resources.

The nurse who has difficulty accessing electronic databases from work or home should make use of local reference librarians and other available resources. Many libraries, particularly at colleges and universities, have access to nursing journals both online and in print (**Box 45.3** »). The nurse who cannot get support from employers and colleagues may want to do more networking with local chapters of professional organizations such as the American Nurses Association.

Case Study » Part 2

Recently, Brent Calloway read an article in his staff development journal about a research study that suggested that the use of simulation enhanced nursing competence and benefited patient safety. He wonders whether his unit could experience similar results. In the article, the nurses participating in the study reported high levels of satisfaction related to the use of simulation in a safety-controlled environment to support their learning. The results of the study also suggested that the incidence of nursing errors decreased by 30% following several sessions of simulation training.

By searching multiple databases, Brent finds several current, peer-reviewed resources, including research studies that suggest that there is a correlation between simulation-based safety training and a decreased incidence of nursing-related errors in patient care. Brent is excited about exploring the impact of implementing simulation-based education to improve nursing practice in his unit and, ultimately, to promote patient safety and improve patient outcomes.

Clinical Reasoning Questions Level I

1. Which search terms would be appropriate for Brent to use when searching an online database for scholarly resources related to his topic?
2. When seeking current scholarly resources, what limits should Brent place on the publication dates?

Clinical Reasoning Questions Level II

3. What are peer-reviewed resources? What is the rationale for Brent's inclusion of only peer-reviewed resources in the research review?
4. If Brent decided to search authoritative websites for information, what criteria would be most appropriate for use in the selection of the authoritative websites?

Step 3: Evaluate the Evidence

Evidence that is gathered must be critically appraised for validity (the degree to which the study measured what it intended to measure), reliability (the ability to produce consistent results with each use), and usefulness in applying the evidence in clinical practice. Nurses must be able to critique research articles to identify the strengths and weaknesses of the studies and their resulting evidence. By doing this, nurses can discard materials that do not meet the standards for application in patient care. Appraising clinical significance answers the question "Is the comparison difference significant enough to change nursing practice?" In other words, does the study yield information that is reliable and useful enough to warrant a change in practice? Unfortunately, it is sometimes difficult to know which evidence yields best nursing practice patient care.

To evaluate the significance of the information gathered, it is necessary to rate the strength of the evidence to determine its validity and its relevance to a given clinical situation (Oncology Nursing Society, 2020). Rating the strength of evidence helps to identify best choices to support greater effectiveness and positive outcomes in specific clinical situations. To categorize scientific data, various companies and organizations use different methods to illustrate the hierarchy or levels of evidence. Assigning levels of evidence can help nurses identify the strongest evidence available for use as best practice. There is general agreement that the highest level of research (research that is considered the most reliable and valid) includes large randomized controlled studies and meta-analyses of controlled studies (**Figure 45.3 ›**). Following this hierarchy, nurses can rate evidence strengths, compare the results, choose the strongest ones, and apply them to patient care for best results.

Many professional nursing organizations have developed guidelines to provide their members with evidence-based information they can use in the caring interventions of their nursing specialty. For example, the Institute for Emergency Nursing Research (IENR), which was launched by the Emergency Nurses Association (ENA; 2020), publishes Clinical Practice Guidelines (CPGs). Based on a comprehensive literature review and analysis, CPGs rate the strength of evidence and provide recommendation levels for practice: high, moderate, weak, and not recommended for practice (ENA, 2020).

Another example of rating the strength of evidence is called Putting Evidence into Practice (PEP) used by the Oncology Nursing Society (2020). PEP helps identify and qualify evidence-based interventions for patient care and teaching. The stoplight is used as an analogy to demonstrate the following categories of evidence strength:

Green light: Strong evidence supports interventions that are likely to be effective and helpful.

Yellow light: Not enough evidence is available to determine the effectiveness of the interventions as harmful or helpful.

Red light: Strong evidence indicates that interventions are likely to be ineffective or possibly harmful.

As nursing clinical research grows, so too does the amount of new published materials on nursing. Strategies that nurses can use to stay abreast of current information include participating in research committees, continuing education programs, and listservs or newsletters. Participation with other nurses in a research or journal club is an excellent way to maximize critical evaluation of current articles related to specific interests.

Hierarchy of Research						
Least powerful evidence	Somewhat stronger evidence	More compelling evidence comes from research studies				Gold standard
Opinions of reviewers that are based on their experience and knowledge	Opinions that come from well-known experts and respected authorities	Non-experimental studies: correlational, descriptive, qualitative	Quasi-experimental studies: time series, matched case-controls	Individual experimental studies	Meta-analysis of controlled studies	Large randomized controlled studies and meta-analyses of controlled studies

Figure 45.3 › Hierarchy of research.

Case Study » Part 3

When Brent Calloway discussed the use of evidence to make decisions about changing training methods to improve patient safety with the vice president of his division, she agreed that it was a good idea and was very excited about it. Brent has organized a team to help him explore the topic of using simulation for experiential learning, which could positively affect patient safety outcomes. The team includes a nurse from the staff development department who is familiar with using simulation training; two staff nurses and one nurse manager from the medical–surgical division, who would be directly affected by any changes that might be implemented; and a nurse from the quality improvement division who has experience in developing EBP.

At the first meeting, Brent explains the group's objective. He gives each member a copy of the journal article he had read previously, and he discusses his plan for the medical–surgical division. The group members decide on a course of action after discussing several possible ways to proceed. They decide to use the PICOT question Brent developed. Members of the team are asked to do a literature search for research evidence, critically appraise the evidence they find, and bring the highest-rated evidence to the next meeting for further evaluation by the team. The team will then evaluate the EBP outcomes and decide whether to change the current practice based on any new evidence found. Everyone is very enthusiastic, and they want to do all they can to help with this project.

Clinical Reasoning Questions Level I

1. Why would careful selection of members for this project team be important for the success of the project?
2. How would each team member evaluate the research evidence?
3. In the context of research findings, what is the difference between reliability and validity?

Clinical Reasoning Questions Level II

4. What other participants might Brent have asked to be on the project team to help during this EBP process?
5. What is the value of having all team members achieve consensus regarding the clinical question?

Step 4: Apply the Evidence

Once the evidence related to the clinical question has been collected and evaluated, the nurse is ready to integrate the best evidence with the nurse's own clinical experience and the patient's personal preferences. But that process in itself is not sufficient; once the nurse (or division or healthcare team) implements the change in practice, the change needs to be evaluated for its impact on patient outcomes. This process begins at implementation, with monitoring of the process to make sure the change is replicated as intended. Is it being done correctly? Does it yield the intended results? Were there any unexpected results? What areas need improvement? The nurse analyzes the data collected and decides to accept, reject, or modify the change for clinical practice. If the change shows benefits to the patient, the facility, through committee work, can choose to modify policies and procedures to reflect the new practice. The change then becomes a part of the nursing routine until it is fully integrated into the standards of care.

Individual nurses can follow this process to identify the best evidence for specific clinical questions they may have about delivering care to patients assigned to them. They can evaluate and change their routines of care to maximize positive patient outcomes, such as reducing the length of stay or promoting cost effectiveness. After evaluation and satisfaction with patient outcomes, nurses should expand the "EBP loop" by sharing the findings with other colleagues. The results can be disseminated in a variety of ways, both informally at the agency level and, more important, formally through presentations at national conferences and by submission of articles for publication in professional journals.

If this development process sounds familiar, it is probably because the steps are very similar to those of the nursing process of assessment, diagnosis, planning, implementing, and evaluation. Where the nursing process seeks to address the patient's holistic needs, the process of EBP deals with a specific clinical question that may be researched in an attempt to improve patient outcomes related to the clinical question.

The explosion of informatics in healthcare has also generated a need for a common language that individuals can use to access and share information. This common language allows nurses to code information to track nursing care processes and revise as necessary. Information technology involves more than providing or improving access to information; it also involves developing new ways for nurses to share information on best practice. Listservs, social media groups, blogs, and videoconferencing are just a few of the ways in which information may be shared through technology.

EBP is a continuing process because new evidence replaces older evidence; healthcare is not a static system; and over time, nurses advance their clinical expertise. What is known today may be changed tomorrow as science progresses. EBP gives a framework and set of tools that nurses can use systematically to improve as clinicians, using the best of its three components: patient preferences, clinical nursing experience, and current evidence (see Figure 45.1).

Case Study » Part 4

Evidence found by Brent Calloway's group demonstrated that simulation was an effective method of learning for nurses, as shown by several study outcomes brought before the group for discussion. The study outcomes the group included are:

- Decreased time required to implement interventions
- Improved organization and completion of simulated tasks
- Improved infection control
- Improved communication skills that supported quick, efficient actions
- Increased ability of nurses to anticipate needed patient interventions.

These results were very exciting to the team and reinforced the value of how changes in the delivery of continuing education can achieve a positive impact on patient safety.

After reflecting on all the evidence, the group decided on an educational plan for the nurses using a simulation teaching strategy. The medical–surgical division would be able to use the simulation unit in staff development for nurse competence. The two nurses and nurse manager would answer questions from nursing staff and would serve as the division champions for simulation. The nurse with additional training in EBP would continue to serve as a resource to staff.

In addition, Brent developed a schedule to visit all units in the division to discuss simulation, and the group posted flyers in the staff break rooms about simulation. The vice president of the medical–surgical division remained supportive of this EBP change process.

Two months after the first nurse competence simulation training was completed, Brent and the team reviewed safety reports related to nursing procedures. Initial results showed a 73% reduction in the number of safety problems. The nurses in the division reported an increased awareness of safety for patients because of the hands-on simulation training they had received. An increase in patient safety was demonstrated that supported better patient outcomes. As a result, other divisions in the hospital became interested in hearing more information about how the EBP change could enhance learning outcomes and positively affect patient safety in their divisions. A potential rollout for the whole hospital is on the agenda for discussion at the next quarterly management meeting.

Clinical Reasoning Questions Level I

1. Why was work done in advance to let the nurses know of an upcoming change in how things were being done?
2. What steps did Brent's team use to develop and implement the changes they sought?
3. Who ultimately benefited most from the EBP change in training? How?

Clinical Reasoning Questions Level II

4. For the EBP change in training to be successful, how important is "buy-in" from the nurses? From management? From the facility, as a whole, to support a general culture of EBP?
5. How could the project team integrate best evidence with nursing expertise and patient preferences in changing to an EBP method of training for the nurses?
6. In addition to improved patient safety outcomes, what benefits might result from implementation of EBP in this situation for the nurses? The facility?

Box 45.4
Barriers to Evidence-Based Practice

A barrier is anything that makes it difficult to progress or succeed in achieving an objective. Even though EBP can provide nurses with the satisfaction of knowing that they have given the best evidence-based care to their patients to promote high positive outcomes, some typical barriers challenge nurses in implementing EBP in their daily practice. Some common barriers nurses confront in using EBP are the following:

- Work schedule and workload demands
- Patient preferences that might conflict with best practice care
- Lack of access to technology to find evidence when needed
- Limited knowledge in skills for finding and evaluating evidence
- Lack of experience and confidence in developing strategies to promote evidence-based care
- Lack of support from supervisors or agency personnel
- Lack of access to continuing education programs (e.g., due to lack of time, lack of funding, distance from program site)
- Attitudes of individual nurses (including lack of confidence in using EBP, misperceptions about EBP, lack of motivation in integrating EBP into routines of patient care, and failure to understand the value of EBP)
- Resistance to change from traditional patient care routines.

By learning the skills of EBP and gaining confidence in it, nurses are in the best position to overcome such barriers.

Strategies to Implement Evidence-Based Practice

Because nurses represent the largest component of the healthcare workforce and are the primary providers of patient care, they play key roles as team members and leaders for an improved evidence-based, patient-centered healthcare system (Sullivan, 2018). One major strategy encouraged by professional nursing organizations and nurse educators is to include EBP knowledge, skills, and behaviors throughout all levels of nursing education programs. This supports development and clinical practice opportunities in providing best EBP and may inspire interest in continuing education to achieve nursing academic progression in preparation of a career in nursing research. From simple tasks, such as hand hygiene, to more complex tasks, such as medication administration, EBP is closely associated with all nursing standards of care and nursing procedures.

Individual Evidence-Based Practice

Some basic activities can provide a foundation for implementing EBP. These strategies can spark the necessary stimulus to engage in behaviors that encourage best practice. Participating in EBP contributes to the knowledge of nursing and patient care in today's healthcare systems and delivery of high-quality nursing care for best outcomes.

- Assess yourself to determine how much of your current nursing practice is evidence based. Make a list of actions you do in a clinical day. Beside each action, make a note whether it is evidence based, the routine everyone follows, a shortcut, or the way you learned it.
- Assess the obstacles that inhibit you from using EBP more frequently. These may include internal factors, such as beliefs or misconceptions, or external factors, such as lack of management support (**Box 45.4** »).
- Practice raising questions about current clinical practices and problem solving.
- Acquire more information to correct any misperceptions of EBP.
- If you only have limited time, focus on evidence content from high-yield sources—those that are current and are known for their high quality.
- Go to www.guideline.gov (AHRQ) for free collections of evidence reviews and practice guidelines published by a variety of groups on a wide range of topics, such as hearing screening, learning disorders screening, treatment, and prognosis.
- Learn how to rate evidence to determine the best evidence.
- Build awareness of how and why things are done to identify how much EBP is being used.
- Identify others interested in searching for evidence and evaluating it for collaborative opportunities such as a journal club.
- Volunteer to participate on an EBP committee.
- Participate in a research project.

» **Stay Current:** AHRQ sponsors evidence reports and technology assessments through systematic reviews for health literacy interventions and outcomes from their EBP Centers. Search for reports of interest to you at http://www.ahrq.gov/research/findings/evidence-based-reports/search.html.

Organizational Evidence-Based Practice

For new evidence to be disseminated to nurses providing patient care, a process needs to be in place to integrate EBP into clinical practice. Nurses can participate on evidence-based practice centers or committees (EPCs) developed by healthcare facilities to evaluate, distribute, pilot trials, and integrate evidence into institutional policies and procedures for quality improved patient care. There are also two initiatives that support nursing evidence-based research and practice for healthcare facilities. One initiative is accreditation through the Magnet Recognition Program® from the American Nurses' Credentialing Center (ANCC; 2020). The other is the Evidence-Based Practice Center Program with the AHRQ (2020).

The ANCC developed their Magnet program to recognize healthcare organizations that provide nursing excellence based on evidence and research in a professional practice environment. Magnet certification is the highest credential for nursing healthcare facilities in the United States. In 2019, there were 505 hospitals in the United States accredited as Magnet hospitals.

>> **Stay Current:** Go to https://www.nursingworld.org/organizational-programs/magnet/find-a-magnet-organization/ for a current list of Magnet facilities in the United States, listed by state.

Research institutions, medical centers, or universities in the United States and Canada can be awarded 5-year contracts to serve as EPCs in the Evidence-Based Practice Center Program. EPCs promote EBP across health systems through evidence reports, reviews, and assessments of technology and clinical practices relevant to health care, such as equipment, services, medications, cost effectiveness, and policies/procedures. Topics to research can be recommended by different professional organizations, patient groups, federal partners, and others. After conducting the research or collecting current research evidence, the EPC will write and distribute their analysis and report their results as evidence. Through their efforts, these centers can improve the quality and effectiveness of healthcare by reviewing all relevant scientific literature, synthesizing the evidence, and helping to translate the evidence-based research findings so they are more readily available to clinicians who are at the bedside providing care. In 2019, there were nine EPCs in the United States (AHRQ, 2020).

>> **Stay Current:** For more information on the nine EPCs, go to http://www.ahrq.gov/research/findings/evidence-based-reports/overview/index.html.

Clinical Practice Guidelines

Clinical practice guidelines are used by HCPs, nurses, and other medical professionals to assist them in making patient care decisions. The guidelines make recommendations for best patient care that are informed by evidence gathered from a systematic review of research. Clinical practice guidelines provide an assessment of the benefits and harms related to specific clinical options. **Table 45.5** >> provides

TABLE 45.5 Examples of Clinical Practice Guidelines

Children's Hospitals	
Best evidence statements	*Best evidence statements* are short, evidence-based clinical care recommendations about single topics derived from a blend of published evidence and precise reviews rather than on direct research. Each statement includes the following sections: Background, Clinical Question PICO, Target Population, Care Recommendations, Dimensions to Judge Evidence Strength, and Discussion of Evidence. These guidelines, protocols, and outcome data are intended to assist HCPs and nurses to make clinical decisions about the care of their patients (Cincinnati Children's Hospital Medical Center, 2020).
Clinical practice guidelines	*Clinical practice guidelines* are algorithms developed from systematic literature reviews of current care of pediatric patients or mutual agreement from subject-matter experts. These guidelines are intended to partner the judgment of HCPs with nurses and families to standardize patient care as appropriate for individual patients. Each algorithm guideline includes step-by-step risk and benefit assessments and alternative care options (Children's Mercy Hospital, 2020).
Specialty Nursing Organizations	
Current adult clinical nursing practice	Clinical nursing practice questions related to a specialty's patient care, nurse workforce, or legal-ethical responsibilities can be answered more quickly by having relevant current literature links and resources for EBP. Participation in an interactive online discussion board with others can also help answer clinical questions and questions about conducting research, funding, and studies (Academy of Medical-Surgical Nurses, 2020).
Professional Nursing Organizations	
Current clinical nursing resources	Peer-reviewed, evidence-based articles about current relevant nursing topics can be published in an organization's magazine to inform and educate nurses. Organizations can also function as a clearinghouse of up-to-date nursing practice resources for best patient outcomes through articles, web-based slide shows, and blogs (RCNi, 2020).
Health Specialty Organizations	
Current care during an active health crisis	Professionals unite together during a health crisis, such as a pandemic, in providing evidence-based, appropriate patient-centered care and support to patients and families. Best quality evidence practices are developed and communicated to all members to assist them as they make clinical decisions. For example: ■ The American College of Obstetrics and Gynecology (2020) provides information for patients about settings in which to give birth and health information about safety and risks for labor support, safe birth, and newborn care. ■ The American Academy of Allergy, Asthma, and Immunology (2020a, 2020b) provides resources for both clinicians and patients related to the prevention and treatment of COVID-19 in patients with asthma, allergic conditions, and immunodeficiencies.

examples of clinical practice guidelines from healthcare facilities (children's hospitals), a specialty nursing organization (Academy of Medical–Surgical Nurses), a professional nursing organization (Royal College of Nursing Publishing Company [RCNi]), and health specialty organizations (American College of Obstetricians and Gynecologists [ACOG] and American Academy of Allergy, Asthma, and Immunology [AAAAI]).

REVIEW The Concept of Evidence-Based Practice

RELATE Link the Concepts

Linking the concept of evidence-based practice with the concept of cellular regulation:

1. While caring for a pediatric patient with severe stomatitis secondary to chemotherapy, the nurse is concerned because the patient's mouth ulcers are not responding to current treatment. How can the nurse ensure that the HCP is using current EBP?
2. The nurse learns of a new treatment that has had great results with treatment-resistant stomatitis. What should the nurse do next?

Linking the concept of evidence-based practice with the concept of advocacy:

3. How can the nurse best advocate for a patient who is considering becoming a participant in a clinical trial?
4. The nurse is caring for a patient who is involved in a clinical research study. The patient says to the nurse, "I don't want to be a part of this study any longer. How do I get out of it?" What would be the nurse's therapeutic response to this patient?

REFER Go to Pearson MyLab Nursing and eText

- Additional review materials

REFLECT Apply Your Knowledge

You are caring for a patient with severe persistent asthma who requires daily doses of inhaled corticosteroids, with frequent use of oral steroids during periods of exacerbation. The patient has been invited to join a research study to determine the effects of a new medication for patients with severe persistent asthma. The lead researcher has provided the patient with the necessary information for informed consent. The patient has asked for time to think about it and discuss it with his spouse. When you enter the room, the patient asks, "What if I agree to participate and the medication doesn't work? Will that mean my asthma will get worse? Does that increase my chances of dying from an asthma attack?"

1. How can you best respond to the patient's questions?
2. How can you best advocate for this patient?
3. What are your ethical obligations to help this patient?

References

Academy of Medical-Surgical Nurses (AMSN). (2020). *Practice resources. Evidence-based practice.* https://www.amsn.org/practice-resources/evidence-based-practice

Agency for Healthcare Research and Quality (AHRQ). (2020). *Evidence-based practice center (EPC) program overview.* http://www.ahrq.gov/research/findings/evidence-based-reports/overview/index.html

American Academy of Allergy, Asthma, and Immunology (AAAAI). (2020a). *COVID-19 and asthma: What patients need to know.* https://www.aaaai.org/conditions-and-treatments/library/asthma-library/covid-asthma

American Academy of Allergy, Asthma, & Immunology (AAAAI). (2020b). *Resources for A/I clinicians during the COVID-19 pandemic.* https://education.aaaai.org/resources-for-a-i-clinicians/covid-19

American Association of Nurse Practitioners (AANP). (2018). *Why choose evidence-based practice?* https://www.aanp.org/news-feed/why-choose-evidence-based-practice

American College of Obstetricians and Gynecologists (ACOG). (2020). *Advocacy and health policy. Patient-centered care for pregnant patients during the COVID-19 pandemic.* https://www.acog.org/news/news-releases/2020/03/patient-centered-care-for-pregnant-patients-during-the-covid-19-pandemic

American Nurses Credentialing Center (ANCC). (2020). *ANCC Magnet Recognition Program®.* https://www.nursingworld.org/organizational-programs/magnet/

Brittain, M. (2018). *Across the chasm: Six aims for changing the health care system.* Institute for Healthcare Improvement. http://www.ihi.org/resources/Pages/ImprovementStories/Across-theChasmSixAimsforChangingtheHealthCareSystem.aspx

Children's Mercy Hospital (CMH). (2020). *Evidence-based practice, clinical practice guidelines.* https://www.childrensmercy.org/health-care-providers/evidence-based-practice/clinical-practice-guidelines/

Cincinnati Children's Hospital Medical Center (CCHMC). (2020). *Evidence-based care recommendations.* https://www.cincinnatichildrens.org/research/divisions/j/anderson-center/evidence-based-care/recommendations/topic

Czubaruk, K., (2019). *The Belmont Report: What is it and how does it relate to today's clinical trials?* Cancer Support Community. https://www.cancersupportcommunity.org/blog/2019/10/belmont-report-what-it-and-how-does-it-relate

Duke University Medical Center Library. (2020). *Introduction to evidence-based practice: Type of study.* http://guides.mclibrary.duke.edu/c.php?g=158201&p=1036068

Emergency Nurses Association (ENA). (2020). *ENA practice resources.* https://www.ena.org/practice-resources

Evidence-Based Nursing. (2020). *About evidence-based nursing.* http://ebn.bmj.com/site/about/

Fuld Institute for EBP, Ohio State University. (2019). *EBP Resources, Websites & Databases.* https://fuld.nursing.osu.edu/websites

Funk, G.-C. (2019). Oxygen titration in hypercapnic COPD exacerbation. *Central European Journal of Medicine, 131.* https://doi.org/10.1007/s00508-019-1472-y

Gannotta, R., (2018). Integrative medicine as a vital component of patient care. *Cureus, 10*(8), e3098. https://doi.org/10.7759/cureus.3098

Global Initiative for Chronic Obstructive Lung Disease (GOLD). (2020). *Global strategy for the diagnosis, management, and prevention of chronic obstructive pulmonary disease: 2020 report.* https://goldcopd.org/wp-content/uploads/2019/12/GOLD-2020-FINAL-ver1.2-03Dec19_WMV.pdf

Luciano, M. (2019). *4 ways to implement evidence-based practice at your hospital.* Advisory Board. https://www.advisory.com/daily-briefing/2019/09/10/evidence-based-practice

National Council of State Boards of Nursing (NCSBN). (2020). *Evidence-based regulation of nursing education.* https://www.ncsbn.org/668.htm

National Institutes of Health (NIH). (2019). *Policies & Regulations – Human subjects.* U.S. Department of Health and Human Services. https://grants.nih.gov/policy/humansubjects/policies-and-regulations.htm

Nieswiadomy, R. M. (2018). *Foundations of nursing research* (7th ed.). Pearson Education.

Northern Arizona University (NAU). (2020). *Evidence based practice.* https://libraryguides.nau.edu/c.php?g=665927&p=4682772

Oncology Nursing Society (ONS). (2020). *Symptom interventions overview.* https://www.ons.org/explore-resources/pep/pep-rating-system-overview

Royal College of Nursing Publishing Company (RCNi). *Nursing older people.* https://rcni.com/nursing-older-people/evidence-and-practice/clinical

Saint Thomas University (STU). (2019). *What you need to know about evidence-based practice in nursing.* https://online.stu.edu/articles/nursing/about-evidence-based-practice-in-nursing.aspx

Sher, A., & Akhtar, A. (2018). Clinical application of Nightingale's theory. *Journal of Clinical Research & Bioethics.* https://www.longdom.org/open-access/clinical-application-of-nightingales-theory-2155-9627-1000329.pdf

Sigma Theta Tau International. (2020). *Nursing research grants.* https://www.sigmanursing.org/advance-elevate/research/research-grants

Sullivan, T. (2018). Institute of Medicine report – The future of nursing: Leading change, advancing health. *Policy & Medicine.* https://www.policymed.com/2011/02/institute-of-medicine-report-the-future-of-nursing-leading-change-advancing-health.html

UNC Health Sciences Library. (2019). Evidence-based nursing introduction. http://guides.lib.unc.edu/c.php?g=8362&p=43029

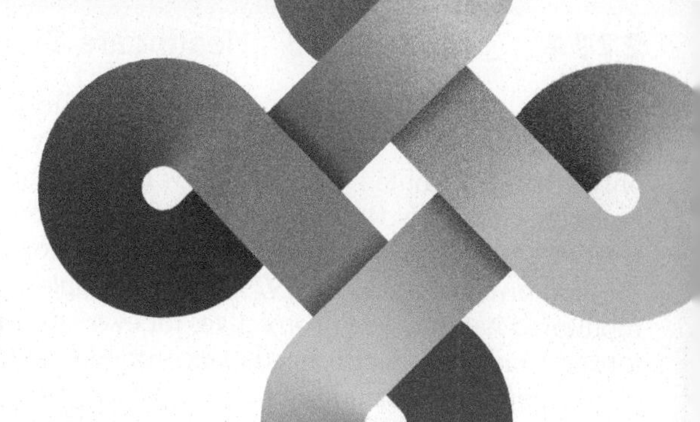

Module 46
Healthcare Systems

Module Outline and Learning Outcomes

The Concept of Healthcare Systems

Types of Healthcare Services and Settings

46.1 Differentiate the three levels of preventive healthcare systems.

Factors Affecting Delivery of Healthcare

46.2 Outline the factors affecting delivery of healthcare.

Frameworks for Providing Care

46.3 Differentiate the three common models of healthcare.

Access to Healthcare

46.4 Outline the factors that limit access to healthcare.

Nursing Care Delivery Systems

46.5 Differentiate the three models of nursing care delivery most frequently used.

Concepts Related to Healthcare Systems

46.6 Outline the relationship between healthcare systems and other concepts.

Need for Resource Allocation

46.7 Explain the issues with allocation of resources and the nurse's role in decision making.

Healthcare Systems Exemplar

Exemplar 46.A Emergency Preparedness

46. A Analyze emergency preparedness as it relates to healthcare systems.

>> The Concept of Healthcare Systems

Concept Key Terms

Adverse childhood experiences, 2776
Case management, 2777
Functional nursing, 2780
Health literacy, 2776
Health promotion, 2774
Managed care, 2777
Patient-focused care, 2777
Primary nursing, 2781
Primary prevention, 2773
Rationing, 2783
Resource allocation, 2783
Resiliency, 2776
Secondary prevention, 2773
Social determinants of health, 2776
Team nursing, 2780
Tertiary prevention, 2773
Underinsured, 2777
Uninsured, 2777
Unlicensed assistive personnel (UAP), 2780

The concept of healthcare systems relates to the methods of healthcare delivery and management, including financing and coordination of services. Particularly in the past two decades, new cost-containment strategies and advances in technology—both informatics and medical technology—have combined to significantly change healthcare systems in the United States.

Nurses must have a solid understanding of the different types of healthcare settings and frameworks used to provide care. Some agencies use a combination of models, and each agency has its own specific policies and procedures. Nurses must understand that the concept of healthcare systems impacts all other concepts. Nurses must know the requirements of the agency in which they practice.

In addition, nurses must understand the barriers patients face to accessing healthcare, the issues they themselves face when resources are insufficient to meet patients' needs, and their agency's and community's expectations for them when a disaster occurs.

Types of Healthcare Services and Settings

Healthcare delivery can be classified by the type of services offered. Today's healthcare systems tend to be oriented toward prevention. A **primary prevention** service focuses on health promotion and illness prevention. **Secondary prevention** services include the diagnosis and treatment of disease. **Tertiary prevention** consists of the restoration of health following an illness or accident and includes rehabilitation and palliative services.

Primary Prevention

Primary prevention attempts to promote healthy living and avoid development of disease as much as possible.

Until the 1980s, healthcare was actually illness/disease care. Individuals typically accessed the healthcare system only when confronted with an illness or accident. The 1979 Surgeon General's Report from the federal government's *Healthy People* program laid the foundation for a national prevention agenda. Since 1979, *Healthy People* has set and monitored national health objectives for every decade to meet a broad range of health needs, encouraged collaborations across communities and sectors, guided individuals toward making informed health decisions, and measured the impact of prevention activities. *Healthy People 2030* set 355 measurable objectives and identified a number of leading health indicators (discussed in Module 7, Health, Wellness, Illness, and Injury), which, if addressed, should result in an increase in the quality and length of life and the eradication of health disparities. Each iteration of *Healthy People* builds upon the visible and measurable results of national efforts to improve health; for example, significantly decreased smoking rates. Chosen topics range from health conditions, such as heart disease and stroke, to settings and systems—from global health to hospital and emergency services. Communities ranging in size from neighborhoods to municipalities may adapt their framework to set local goals and objectives or to set priorities for their geographical region or residents.

» **Stay Current:** For the framework of *Healthy People*, visit https://health.gov/healthypeople.

Health promotion efforts can choose to concentrate on improving individuals' health. The World Health Organization (WHO; 1998) defines **health promotion** as the process of enabling people to increase control over and to improve their health. While the primary purpose of health promotion is to improve an individual's quality of life, there are additional benefits. For example, preventing disease and using health promotion techniques to improve health are more cost effective than treating illness and disease; therefore, both approaches help to reduce healthcare expenses.

The nurse has an integral role in health promotion. The nurse's aim should be to teach patients how to remain healthy, thus preserving wellness. The overarching goal is to ensure that patients understand the importance of setting health goals for themselves and their children and that patients can assess, implement, and evaluate their personal health and wellness goals and modify them as their health needs change. Some examples of how nurses participate in health promotion include providing health education at windows of opportunity; evaluating and screening patients to identify prevention opportunities such as immunizations; and promoting wellness in the community by organizing and participating in local events such as health fairs.

Examples of current health promotion topics, identified both by *Healthy People 2030* and by individual states and communities, are nutrition and healthy eating, physical activity across the lifespan, sleep, tobacco use and smoking cessation, and preventive healthcare.

By implementing health promotion strategies, the nurse has an opportunity to step out of the secondary prevention area and into the primary prevention area. This shift increases nurses' workplace and career satisfaction because they have an opportunity to contribute to the health of all patients—not just those who are ill, but also those whose overall health status is free of illness, such as smokers who are disease free.

Secondary Prevention

Secondary prevention activities are aimed at early disease detection and treatment to prevent the progression of the disease and its associated symptoms. Screening is a means of early detection of diseases such as hypertension and vision or hearing problems. Screenings may be provided by primary healthcare providers (HCPs) and through health fairs. They may be offered to the general population or focused on groups at high risk.

Tertiary Prevention

Tertiary prevention involves restoring function and decreasing disease-related complications of an already established disease. When restoration to the previous level of functioning is not possible, clinical care is focused on controlling symptoms and promoting the highest quality of life. Tertiary prevention includes rehabilitation and palliative care.

The three levels of prevention are summarized in **Table 46.1** ».

Healthcare Settings

Primary care is delivered in a variety of settings, including physicians' offices, hospital-based clinics, community health centers, and public health service locations (**Figure 46.1** »). Primary care should not be confused with primary prevention, described in the previous section. Community health centers and public health organizations frequently offer health promotion activities at locations such as churches, shopping malls, and community cultural events.

In the context of managed care, the primary care setting is often the point of entry and the location of gatekeeping for all other medical care. Primary care involves the provision of health maintenance services such as routine physicals, immunizations, treatment of common acute illnesses, and support for psychosocial needs.

Secondary care is typically delivered in a hospital, outpatient surgical center, or specialist's office. The most cost-effective, efficient place of service should be selected as the optimal place of service. For example, a dermatologist may remove an adult's uncomplicated basal cell carcinoma in the office. In this instance, the office setting is the most appropriate, cost-effective place of service. Removal of this type of lesion involves only a minor surgical procedure under local anesthesia.

Tertiary care that involves complicated diagnostic or therapeutic procedures may be provided in a hospital, a rehabilitation center, or an extended care facility. Wherever a patient receives tertiary care, the nurse, as the patient's advocate, will coordinate the patient's care and treatment and ensure the patient's compliance with treatment.

Factors Affecting Delivery of Healthcare

A number of factors affect the ability of the nurse to deliver patient care, regardless of the competency or proficiency of the nurse or the level of care or the setting in which care is being delivered. These include changing demographics,

TABLE 46.1 Levels of Prevention

Level and Description	Examples
Primary Prevention	
Take action to prevent disease in generally healthy people and populations. Give people tools that empower them to improve their own health through positive actions such as smoking cessation and eating well.	■ Educate individuals, families, and populations on topics such as the importance of nutrition, exercise, dental hygiene, prenatal care, immunization, and smoking cessation. ■ Educate employers and employees about occupational safety as well as avoidance of occupational hazards. ■ Improve environmental sanitation and provide adequate housing and nutrition (e.g., removing lead from housing units, making fresh produce available in areas designated as food deserts).
Secondary Prevention	
Detect and then treat identified injuries and diseases early so that they can be cured or their associated symptoms and complications can be prevented or limited.	■ Perform risk assessments for healthy people who have risk factors for specific diseases such as coronary artery disease and diabetes; then work with each patient to develop and implement a risk reduction plan. ■ Encourage regular dental, vision, and medical screening examinations for children and adults (primary care providers should follow guidelines such as *Healthy People 2030* or the recommendations of the U.S. Preventive Services Task Force when evaluating patients' screening needs). ■ Teach patients to perform self-screening examinations such as testicular examinations and mole checks for possible melanoma. ■ In all settings, develop and implement care plans to treat patients' illnesses and injuries (e.g., administer medication and treatment regimens) and prevent complications (e.g., turn, position, and exercise patients to prevent pressure ulcers and deep venous thromboses); ensure adequate rest, food intake, and fluid intake to promote healing and promote fecal and urinary elimination.
Tertiary Prevention	
Begins after a condition is treated and stabilized or recognized as incurable. Includes the restoration of function and decrease of complications of an established disease. If restoration to the previous level of function is not possible, clinical care focuses on controlling symptoms and promoting the highest quality of life possible. Rehabilitation and palliative care are included in tertiary prevention.	■ Refer a patient with a new urostomy to an RN ostomy management specialist to learn how to care for and improve life with an ostomy. ■ Refer a patient with diabetes to a registered dietitian for education on how diet can affect the complications of diabetes. ■ Refer individuals with severe or chronic pain to a pain specialist to manage pain with an appropriate medication regimen and/or alternative treatment methods. ■ Refer individuals with mobility issues to physical therapy or rehabilitation services to promote mobility and prevent falls and other mobility-related complications.

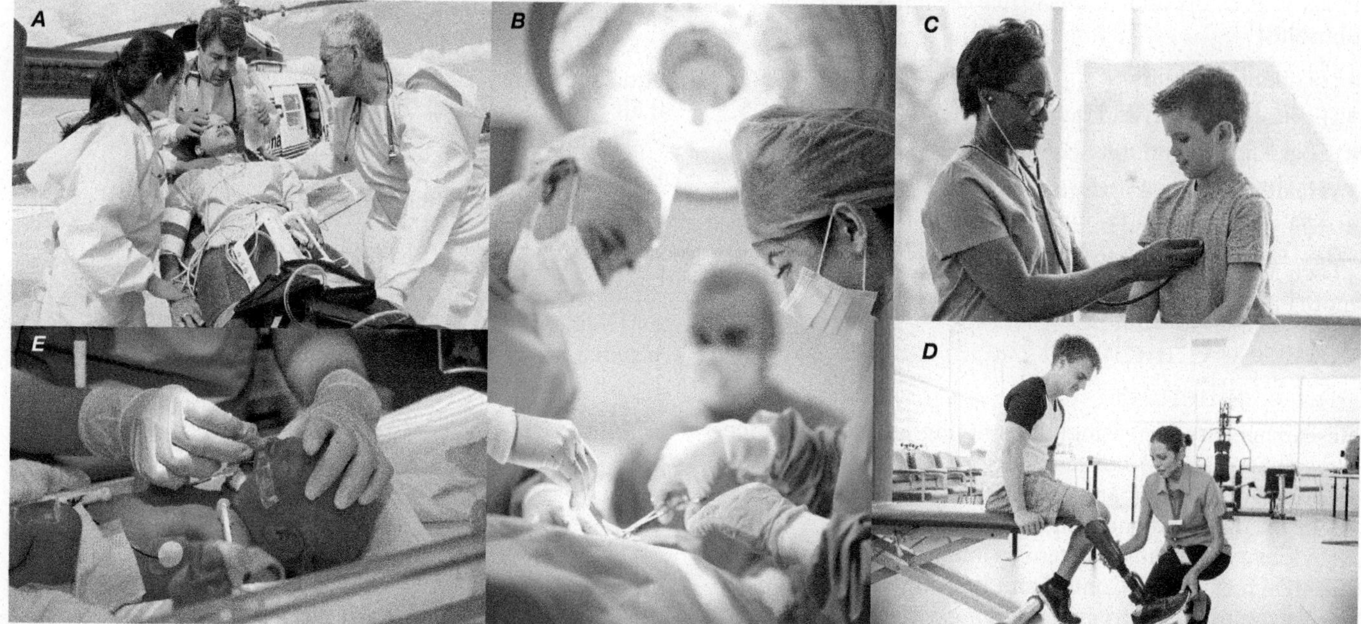

Figure 46.1 ›› Nurses practice in many healthcare settings. Clockwise from top left: ***A***, a nurse in an emergency department with a patient coming in from a medical flight; ***B***, a surgical nurse in an operating room; ***C***, a nurse in a pediatrician's office; ***D***, a nurse working in a rehabilitation hospital; and ***E***, a nurse in a neonatal intensive care unit. Other settings where nurses work include schools, public health departments, patients' homes, prisons, insurance companies, colleges and universities, and publishing companies.

Source: ***A***, Comstock/Stockbyte/Getty Images. ***B***, Sturti/iStock/Getty Images. ***C***, FatCamera/E+/Getty Images. ***D***, Johnny Greig/E+/Getty Images. ***E***, Pelicankate/iStock/Getty Images.

social determinants of health, advances in technology, and levels of health literacy of patients in the community.

Changing Demographics

Projecting the United States' population characteristics changes from 2020 to 2060, the U.S. Census Bureau (2020) predicted its residents will be more racially and ethnically diverse, as well as much older. Life expectancy is also expected to increase, leading to a graying nation. For example, the number of people age 85 and older will more than triple by 2060, from 6 million to 19 million.

Other major changes impacting healthcare delivery systems will be the drivers of mortality. A 2019 Harvard clinical study predicted that about half the adults in the United States will have obesity and about a quarter will have severe obesity by 2030. The researchers concluded that rising body mass index (BMI) rates will produce increased rates of chronic disease, medical spending, and mortality. The demographic characteristics of populations at highest risk for rising BMI rates include women, non-Hispanic Black adults, and those with annual incomes below $50,000 (Harvard School of Public Health, 2020a).

Social Determinants of Health

The *Healthy People* campaign defines **social determinants of health** (SDOH) as the environmental conditions in which people are active that affect their health, their functioning, and their quality-of-life outcomes and risks (Office of Disease Prevention and Health Promotion, 2020). These living conditions identify significant factors as to why some Americans are healthier than others and why a large number are not as healthy as they could be. This position is supported by health policy leaders such as the WHO and the National Partnership for Action to End Health Disparities. *Healthy People 2030*'s approach points to five key areas (determinants) of health:

- Economic stability
- Education access and quality
- Social and community context
- Healthcare access and quality
- Neighborhood and built environment.

See Module 7, Health, Wellness, Illness, and Injury, for more information on SDOH.

Adverse Childhood Experiences and Resiliency

Researchers are increasingly identifying **adverse childhood experiences** (ACEs) and **resiliency** as determinants of health in adulthood. ACEs are potentially traumatic events that occur in childhood and range from experiencing or witnessing violence to incarceration of an immediate family member (Centers for Disease Control and Prevention [CDC], 2020b). Approximately one in six children experience at least one traumatic event during childhood. ACEs increase risk for chronic disease, mental illness, sexually transmitted disease, and suicide (CDC, 2020b). Resiliency is an ability to withstand change or trauma with minimal long-term negative effects. To reduce the effects of childhood trauma, many communities are embracing efforts to build resiliency and improve access to supports for children at risk for ACEs.

Advances in Technology

Scientific knowledge related to healthcare continues to increase rapidly, leading to ever more sophisticated technology. Information management systems have been created and are continually being refined. Such systems support electronic health records, barcoding for medication administration, and use of online evidenced-based guidelines to provide appropriate care. Advances in laparoscopic surgical techniques have resulted in fewer hospitalizations for some surgeries because they can safely be performed at alternative sites such as surgical centers. Greater use of telemedicine visits has extended patient access to the clinical knowledge of specialists to remote geographical locations. Many advances in technology require specialized personnel, creating new opportunities for individuals seeking employment in the healthcare sector.

Health Literacy

The classic definition of **health literacy** is the capacity to obtain, communicate, process, and understand basic health information and services to make appropriate health decisions (Koh et al., 2012). For many tasks in healthcare systems, patients must employ print literacy (writing and reading), oral literacy (listening and speaking), numeracy (using and understanding numbers such as medication dosages), and technologic literacy (such as understanding online discharge instructions). A systematic review found that low levels of health literacy lead to a reduced ability to interpret health messages, a limited ability to take medications correctly, a lower likelihood of receiving preventive care, increased hospitalizations, and higher use of emergency care (Berkman, Sheridan, Donahue, Halpern, & Crotty, 2011). In the only population-level survey conducted by the National Center for Educational Statistics in 2003, researchers found that about half (53%) of adults had intermediate health literacy skills and 36% had a basic or below-basic level. Despite this educational shortcoming, our healthcare systems function as if all patients have literacy skills (Koh et al., 2012).

Healthcare illiteracy and ineffective communication place patients at risk for poor health outcomes. According to a Kaiser Family Foundation (2019b) research report, Black and Hispanic people as well as American Indians and Alaska Natives continue to experience striking health disparities, including high teen birth rates, increased infant mortality rates, and higher HIV or AIDS diagnoses and death rates. Providing health education programs for these populations is one of the key strategies for overcoming these health disparities.

Health literacy also involves policies and strategies at the organizational level. Agencies that strive to be health-literate organizations continuously work to improve verbal interactions, improve written communications, link to support systems, and engage patients and caregivers as partners in care and improvement efforts. Technology also plays a role. Many agencies offer virtual patient portals and websites that provide an array of evidence-based information and resources. Content ranges from topics such as how to prepare a child for surgery to tips on how to care for loved ones with chronic illnesses.

Frameworks for Providing Care

In the United States, the three common models of healthcare are managed care, case management, and patient-focused care. Sometimes the frameworks overlap (e.g., services may be coordinated through a case management model to patients whose health insurance plans use a managed care model).

Managed Care

Managed care, discussed in detail in Module 39, Managing Care, is a method of delivering cost-effective and high-quality care. Managed care is designed to improve outcomes for groups of patients; its framework can be adapted across all healthcare settings. The primary managed care models are health maintenance organizations (HMOs) and preferred provider organizations (PPOs). HMOs are more restrictive than PPOs and require that a patient select a primary care physician who manages the patient's secondary and tertiary services. Although a PPO is less restrictive, the direct costs to the patient are higher (e.g., higher premiums, copayments, and deductibles).

Case Management

The Case Management Society of America (2017) defines **case management** as "a collaborative process of assessment, planning, facilitation, care coordination, evaluation and advocacy for options and services to meet an individual's and family's comprehensive health needs through communication and available resources to promote patient safety, quality of care, and cost effective outcomes."

Interprofessional teams led by a case manager are at the heart of successful case management. Case management is essential when a patient has multiple care needs and requires the services of multiple providers. The goal of case management is to reach and then maintain the individual's optimal level of health, quality of life, and activities of daily living (ADLs) by ensuring that the individual's healthcare needs are met. The case manager may be a nurse, a social worker, or another healthcare team member. Case management enables patients to experience continuity of care, regardless of the location at which the care is provided. This activity on behalf of a patient may be limited to a hospitalization or may occur across settings in the community and/or at home.

Patient-focused Care

Patient-focused care is a delivery model that organizes healthcare around the expressed physical and emotional needs of the patient. Patient-focused care is generally understood to be an approach that considers patients and their families to be integral to decisions regarding healthcare delivery.

Access to Healthcare

For Americans who have healthcare coverage through an employer, high-quality healthcare is available without a long wait and at a reasonable cost. However, such healthcare is often beyond the reach of the many Americans who work for small employers, those who are unemployed and underemployed, the self-employed, and members of underserved populations. These groups face many challenges to accessing healthcare and, as a result, often have poorer health outcomes—in some cases worse than those of residents of developing countries. An annual report from the Agency for Healthcare Research and Quality (AHRQ), titled *National Healthcare Disparities Report*, has been published since 2003. The 2018 report confirms that people of racial and ethnic minority groups and those of low socioeconomic status have disproportionately more access problems than others. Inadequate access to healthcare has a large impact on society. For example, a failure to receive immunizations against or early treatment of contagious diseases can result in community outbreaks. The ACA healthcare reform act signed into law by President Barack Obama in 2010 was designed to remedy some disparities in access to health insurance coverage and other related problems. However, current data show that sizable disparities continue to provide obstacles to equitable healthcare for all Americans (see Focus on Diversity and Culture: COVID-19).

Uninsured individuals are those without any type of healthcare insurance coverage. Uninsured individuals do not qualify for public health insurance programs, such as Medicaid, and cannot buy group health insurance, usually because their employers do not offer health insurance benefits. Uninsured patients also include those who cannot afford to purchase group insurance through their employer because the insurance premiums are too expensive. During recent decades, even individuals who were self-employed had difficulty purchasing health insurance privately, either because the premiums were unaffordable or because they were denied coverage because of preexisting conditions. One of the most popular provisions of the ACA was that it prevented insurance companies from denying coverage based on preexisting conditions.

Underinsured individuals have healthcare insurance coverage that is insufficient to meet their needs. Examples include the child who is covered under a parent's company policy, but the policy does not include immunizations, and the patient with a chronic illness whose insurance does not include coverage for medications. Continued healthcare reform may resolve these gaps in coverage.

Access to healthcare means having "the timely use of personal health services to achieve the best health outcomes," as documented in the Institute of Medicine's 1993 report titled *Access to Healthcare in America*, a document that is still widely cited today. As noted in the report, accessing healthcare requires three discrete steps:

1. Gaining entry into the healthcare system
2. Getting access to sites of care where the patient can receive needed services
3. Finding providers with whom the patient can communicate, develop a trusting relationship, and have individual clinical needs met.

Lack of Health Insurance

The uninsured rate of Americans began to decrease with the enactment of the ACA in 2010. The rate reached its lowest point in 2016, had a modest increase in 2017, and officially increased in 2018. The uninsured rate is expected to continue to increase (Keith, 2019). The reasons include:

- Repeal of the ACA's mandate that individuals carry health insurance
- Expanded availability of non-ACA plans that do not cover preexisting conditions
- Rules about eligibility of noncitizens
- Lower enrollment in Medicaid coverage.

Focus on Diversity and Culture

COVID-19

As noted in the *National Healthcare Disparities Report*, access to healthcare goes beyond issues of healthcare insurance. Numerous factors can contribute to healthcare inequities. In May 2020, Doctors Without Borders, an international nonprofit emergency healthcare organization, dispatched a team to the Navajo Nation when it reported more cases of COVID-19 per capita than any U.S. state—even New York. Factors identified in the high rate of infection among the Navajo people included (Capatides, 2020; Navajo Department of Health, 2020):

- Lack of access to running water in reservation territory
- High rates of hypertension and diabetes among the Navajo people
- Many parts of the Navajo reservation are considered food deserts
- Lack of access to the internet, contributing to lack of access to information and telehealth services.

Across the United States, COVID-19 served to highlight not merely disparities in access to healthcare services but disparities of risk. Essential workers in low-paying jobs, individuals and families living or working in crowded conditions, workers who rely on public transportation, and people in nursing homes and jails or prisons were among those at greater risk of infection and death (Harvard School of Public Health, 2020b).

In 2018, more than half (55%) of those who did have insurance had employer-sponsored health insurance. Approximately 30% had insurance through Medicaid and/or Medicare, with 11% having individual coverage they obtained outside employment. Approximately 4% had military insurance.

In early 2019, 90.9% of people had health insurance, a sizable increase from 2010, but a rate less than the previous 2 years. An estimated 9.1% of people were uninsured in 2019 (Keith, 2019). Since the U.S. Census Bureau estimates the population of the United States to be 328.2 million for 2019, that would mean that about 30 million Americans did not have health insurance in that year.

The primary reason individuals are uninsured is that they cannot afford to be insured. Some 3 million poor uninsured adults earn too much money to qualify for Medicaid. People who are uninsured may delay treatment or opt not to receive it because they must choose to pay either for medical care or for basic necessities, such as food and housing. Most uninsured individuals do not receive healthcare services for free or at a reduced charge and are often billed at a higher rate. Nearly two-thirds (64%) of the uninsured people with medical bill problems are not able to make any payments. The outcomes of being uninsured include loss of savings, difficulty affording necessities, borrowing money, and facing persistent bill collection efforts (Kaiser Family Foundation, 2019a).

The need for health insurance is critical for the well-being of children. Children with health insurance are more likely to stay healthy, since they have access to needed services, such as well-child checkups and medications. They are more likely to have a usual source of healthcare. They are less likely to be absent from school due to untreated medical conditions such as asthma. As a result, they perform better in school, setting them on a long-term course for better health and better economic opportunities.

The ACA affected children favorably because it prevented insurance companies from denying coverage for preexisting conditions and from dropping insured individuals or their dependents because of the onset of serious illness. It also became increasingly perceived as affordable, so rates of insured children increased each year for the first half-dozen years after the passage of the ACA. However, recent data shows a negative turnaround in the number of insured children. Alker and Pham (2018) found that the rate of uninsured children was 4.7% in 2016 and 5% in 2017. They expect more children to lack insurance coverage in future years if no countermeasures are taken.

SAFETY ALERT In 1986, Congress enacted the Emergency Medical Treatment and Active Labor Act (EMTALA) to ensure public access to emergency services regardless of ability to pay. Prior to the enactment of this law, providers of emergency services often refused to treat patients who were uninsured and who could not afford to pay for services. Under Section 1867 of the Social Security Act, Medicare-participating hospitals that offer emergency services must provide a medical screening examination when a patient asks for examination for or treatment of an emergency medical condition (EMC), including active labor. The law requires that this service be provided regardless of an individual's ability to pay. Hospitals must also provide stabilizing treatment for patients with EMCs. If unable to stabilize a patient or if the patient requests it, the emergency care provider must arrange for an appropriate transfer (EMTALA, 2011).

Lack of a Usual Source of Care

According to the AHRQ (2020), individuals with a *usual source of care* (i.e., a facility where the individual regularly receives care) experience improved health outcomes, fewer health disparities, and lower costs. A usual source of care is sometimes referred to as a *medical home* or *healthcare home.*

If a patient has a primary care provider (i.e., a physician or nurse from whom the patient regularly receives care), trust and communication between the patient and provider are improved, resulting in the likelihood that the care provided to the patient will be appropriate and of high quality (AHRQ, 2020). A primary care provider who learns about the diverse needs of patients over time is better able to meet those needs. Despite this fact, over 40 million Americans do not receive regular care from a primary care provider.

The U.S. Department of Health and Human Services (DHHS), the American Academy of Pediatrics, and the American Medical Association developed national guidelines for preventive health services for infants, children, and adolescents (**Box 46.1** »). These guidelines are supported by the National Association of Pediatric Nurse Practitioners.

Children and families are better served when they have a usual source of healthcare that allows parents and caregivers

Box 46.1

National Guidelines for Health Promotion

- *Bright Futures*, American Academy of Pediatrics (original editions by Maternal and Child Health Bureau, Health Resources and Services Administration, DHHS), https://brightfutures.aap.org/Pages/default.aspx
- *Put Prevention Into Practice (PPIP)*, Agency for Healthcare Research and Quality, https://www.ahrq.gov/prevention/resources/chronic-care/marketing/pptools/index.html
- *Guide to Clinical Preventive Services, 2014*, U.S. Preventive Services Task Force, https://www.ahrq.gov/prevention/guidelines/guide/index.html
- *Guidelines for Adolescent Preventive Services* (American Medical Association, Elster, A. B.,& Kuznets, N. J.), book published in 1994 by William and Wilkins.

to forge an ongoing relationship and a high comfort level with their provider and increases the likelihood that they will seek healthcare for their children. Providers are able to give comprehensive, family-centered treatment because of their knowledge of the child and family, including the family's dynamics, possible risks, and need for protection. One source of such treatment is the patient-centered medical home, which is not a location but a standards-based approach to providing primary care in which the healthcare facility forges a partnership with the patient and the patient's family (**Box 46.2** »).

Perceptions of Need

Perceived need often affects an individual's decision to access the healthcare system. Patients may not always be able to accurately assess their own need for care. However, when they believe they need care for illness and injury and are unable to obtain it, they perceive that care is difficult to access. These perceived difficulties produce delays in getting appropriate care.

Clinical Example A

A nurse working for a large insurance company as a telephone triage nurse receives a call late at night from an enrolled member reporting that her 4-year-old daughter woke with ear pain that has not responded to acetaminophen administered by mouth 15 minutes ago. The mother reports that the child is crying in pain and requests authorization to go to the hospital emergency department (ED). The nurse provides strategies to treat the child's pain and explains that oral analgesics require as much as 30 minutes to begin taking effect. The nurse offers to make an appointment with the primary care provider in the morning. When the mother states that the child must be seen immediately, the nurse suggests that the mother take the child to a 24-hour urgent care center. The mother declines, insisting that the child be treated immediately at the ED.

Critical Thinking Questions

1. Does this nurse have the right to inform parents they cannot take the child to the ED because this is not an emergency?
2. How does the mother's perception of her child's medical needs affect her response?
3. What else might the nurse do to help the parent more accurately perceive the child's healthcare needs?

Box 46.2

Six Principles of a Patient-Centered Medical Home

The most standard definition of a patient-centered medical home is provided in the *Joint Principles of the Patient-Centered Medical Home*, adopted by the American Academy of Family Physicians, American Academy of Pediatrics, American College of Physicians, and American Osteopathic Association in 2007. This groundbreaking concept is still in use and forms the basis of a quality improvement curriculum in primary care education (Higgins, Schottenfeld, & Crosson, 2015). Since then, the model has evolved. Its vision and suggested methods have been adopted by the AHRQ (Primary Care Collaborative, 2020).

The AHRQ lists the following five features that characterize medical homes:

1. *Patient-centered:* Providers, patients, and their families form a partnership that respects patients' wants, needs, and preferences. Patients are educated and supported to make decisions, participating in their own care.
2. *Comprehensive:* Care is provided by a team that is accountable for patients' physical and mental health needs. This includes prevention and wellness activities, as well as acute and chronic care.
3. *Coordinated:* All elements of the entire healthcare system work together to provide care. This includes specialty care, hospitals, and home care community services and supports.
4. *Accessible:* Patients find care available to them through a variety of mechanisms: "after hours" care, 24/7 electronic or telephone access, and use of health IT innovations. The goal is to have shorter waiting times for care.
5. *Committed to quality and safety:* Patients and families are increasingly able to make informed decisions about their health, supported by quality improvement efforts of clinicians and staff.

Uneven Distribution of Services

The distribution of healthcare services in the United States is problematic because it is uneven. Many geographic areas and populations are medically underserved. Rural areas often lack medical resources. However, suburban and urban areas may also be underserved because of poverty as well as cultural and linguistic barriers to healthcare access. Another factor that causes a community or population to be underserved is a shortage of primary care professionals such as primary care physicians, nurse practitioners, nurses, and physician assistants. Availability varies from region to region, from state to state, and even within cities themselves, where the poorest communities may be underserved.

Data to support the description of an uneven distribution have been compiled by the U.S. Bureau of Labor Statistics. In general, the states with the highest number of registered nurses are found in the eastern half of the United States. The same pattern holds for nurse practitioners, who numbered 200,600 in 2019. Family medicine practitioners are only slightly more evenly distributed.

Approaches to Addressing Quality and Cost Issues

The ACA was created to ensure that all U.S. citizens have access to affordable, quality care and to curb the growth of healthcare costs. A health policy report by Blumenthal and Abrams (2020) looks at reasons why the ACA did not completely solve all the problems in the healthcare industry. They listed four possible reasons:

- Widespread uncertainty about the best path to take to improve health services.
- A great number of ACA initiatives and changes were launched at one time, and their introduction had to be absorbed by the existing health system.
- As a new undertaking with risks, the ACA would have naturally produced both successes and failures.
- Not all provisions of the ACA have received support from political leaders.

To understand the complexity of the situation, the role of the other nine concepts of the healthcare domain need to be considered. See the Concepts Related to Healthcare Systems section for an overview of each concept and its contribution to solutions for national healthcare quality and cost improvement.

>> **Stay Current:** Keep abreast of the changes in healthcare and insurance laws by visiting the U.S. Department of Health and Human Services at https://www.hhs.gov/healthcare/about-the-aca/index.html and Medicaid at https://www.medicaid.gov/medicaid/index.html.

Other, older programs include the following:

- Medicare for adults over age 65 or with qualifying diseases/disabilities
- Medicaid, which assists people with lower incomes and older adults who require services not covered by Medicare, such as nursing homes, as well as some people with disabilities
- The Children's Health Insurance Program (CHIP), which assists with coverage for children whose families earn too much income to qualify for Medicaid coverage but not enough income to afford private health insurance. In some states, CHIP insures pregnant women (HealthCare.gov, n.d.-a).

Local health departments and community health centers are sources of care for individuals without health insurance or who have gaps in their coverage. Community health centers offer primary and preventive care to millions of Americans for free or at a low cost. Anyone may obtain care from these clinics regardless of income. The cost of care is determined by using a sliding scale that is based on an individual's income (HealthCare.gov, n.d.-b). As illustrated in Clinical Example A, a patient's perceived need for healthcare services can be a barrier to access. It may cause patients to seek care that is unnecessary or care that is necessary but provided at an inappropriate and often more expensive place of service than needed. The nurse can change the patient's perception of need (thereby promoting appropriate and timely healthcare) by managing patient care; teaching adults about self-care and the care of their children; and teaching them when and how to access appropriate care.

Implementation of a team approach to healthcare favorably affects the availability and cost-effectiveness of primary care. As nonphysician members of the healthcare team manage the aspects of patient care that do not require a physician's expertise, physicians have more time available to devote to elements of care requiring their knowledge and skills.

Clinical Example B

Helena Alvarez is a pregnant 19-year-old woman who arrives at the ED of a small rural hospital with severe cramping pains and bleeding. She has no health insurance. No maternity services are available at this hospital, and no obstetricians are available in the community. There is a tertiary care facility about 100 miles away.

Critical Thinking Questions

1. How would you determine what options are available for providing care for Ms. Alvarez?
2. As a nurse, what are your obligations to Ms. Alvarez?

Nursing Care Delivery Systems

Three models of nursing care delivery are frequently used: functional nursing, team nursing, and primary nursing.

Functional Nursing

Functional nursing is a task-oriented approach to care delivery. Although it is not used routinely, it may be implemented when systems are stressed by factors such as inadequate staffing resulting from nursing shortages or significant weather events such as major snowstorms. In this approach, the head nurse delegates tasks to team members who complete these specific tasks rather than caring for specific patients. For example, one nurse is responsible for delivering medications and changing dressings, while another performs administrative functions such as monitoring orders and communicating with physicians and other departments to arrange for services. Functional nursing is an efficient approach because it enables the nursing team to complete many tasks in a short time. **Unlicensed assistive personnel (UAP)** are a critical component of functional nursing. They are paraprofessionals who are unlicensed but may be certified. The primary role of the UAP is to assist patient with ADLs and provide other types of basic care. UAP act under the direction of licensed professionals, such as registered nurses, who delegate activities to them. When UAP assist patients with activities such as feeding, bathing, and ambulating, registered nurses can focus on performing more complex tasks.

Because fewer nurses are needed, functional nursing is cost effective. However, depersonalization and fragmentation of care may result because there is limited opportunity for team members to view the patient holistically. Nurses often become dissatisfied with their role because it is limited to tasks. Patients also may be dissatisfied because they cannot identify "their nurse," that is, one individual who is responsible for their care.

Team Nursing

Team nursing is the delivery model most frequently used today. It is a means of providing individualized care. The approach was developed in response to the fragmentation

Evidence-Based Practice

Decentralized Workstations

Question

What is the evidence to support a team nursing concept of decentralized workstations, also known as pod nursing or care zones? In pod nursing, larger units are marked off into smaller areas. Teams of nurses and UAP work together in distinct geographical locations, where they have easier access to supplies and tools for documentation to keep them nearer to their patients.

Evidence

A study of a cardiovascular unit that changed from centralized to a decentralized arrangement found that the perceived benefit of the original centralization was more efficient patient care with a decrease in the amount that nurses had to walk to provide care. However, nurses reported satisfaction with proximity to patients and increased interaction with them (Fay, Carll-White, Schadler, Isaacs, & Real, 2017). Research based on surveys found that nurses were happier with centralized nursing stations; patients were more satisfied with decentralized arrangements (Real, Fay, Isaacs, Carll-White & Schadler, 2018). This conclusion was supported by a systematic review that found that satisfaction with decentralized nursing stations was positive for patients, but negative for nurses, who perceived less of a sense of teamwork (Jiminez, 2019).

Implications for Nursing Care

The implications for nursing care reinforce the fact that both nurses and their patients are sensitive to the environment in which care is provided. The research shows that both centralized and decentralized arrangements have their benefits and downsides. The priority that is valued by patients, interaction with caregivers, can be recognized and attended to, no matter the structure of the facility. The value that is prized by nurses, teamwork, can be achieved in ways other than close physical workplace proximity.

Critical Thinking Application

1. Discuss the impact of the environment in healthcare facilities that you have experienced. What factors made the setting more effectively a healing space? What would you change to promote a better environment?
2. How can nurses contribute to making positive changes in the design of healthcare workplaces?

of care inherent in the functional model. The registered nurse who serves as the team leader is accountable for the care provided to the patients assigned to the team. The team leader retains responsibility and authority for the patients' overall well-being but delegates some tasks to UAP. Team members are assigned tasks based on their ability to perform them. While this model frees the professional nurse to attend to more complex patient care tasks, frequent changes in assignments may lead to a lack of continuity of care for patients.

Primary Nursing

In the **primary nursing** model, one nurse has 24/7 authority and responsibility for the care of an assigned group of patients. The primary nurse (PN) cares for the assigned patients during her shift from the time of admission through discharge. Primary care nursing is a relationship-based model of care. The PN is responsible for assessing patients, developing care plans, and providing direct care. When the PN is absent, an associate nurse will provide care under the guidance of the care plan developed by the PN. In this model, UAP are actively involved in providing direct patient care and are assigned tasks by the PN or by the associate nurse in the PN's absence.

Concepts Related to Healthcare Systems

Healthcare systems refers to the broad array of people, institutions, and resources that provide care to people locally, within a state, across the nation, and internationally. Care is provided at many different places of service, and nurses must be prepared to function in each. Each component of the healthcare system faces its own ethical dilemmas, legal issues, managed care issues, and clinical decision-making challenges. While nurses may sometimes feel that their contributions to the system as a whole make little or no difference in the larger scheme of the healthcare system, that is not the case. Nurses play an important role in ensuring healthcare systems provide safe, ethical, evidence-based care to all patients. The Concepts Related to Healthcare Systems feature lists some, but not all, of the concepts integral to healthcare systems. They are listed in alphabetical order.

Need for Resource Allocation

Healthcare expenses in the United States rose by 3.9% in 2017. The per capita spending amounted to $10,739 (American Medical Association, 2020). The greatest portion of that expense is hospital care (**Figure 46.2** »). Many factors are responsible for the increasing cost of healthcare. These include greater longevity, increases in the prevalence of chronic diseases such as diabetes, continued medical advances (which may result in more accurate diagnoses and better treatment but are often more expensive than existing methods), technologic advances, consumer demand, and defensive medicine (ordering a test or procedure to avoid litigation). Inappropriate healthcare treatment choices by consumers have also contributed to increased healthcare costs. As discussed in Module 39, Managing Care, employees have enjoyed the benefits of employer-negotiated insurance plans, However, as patients, they have been insulated from and are often unaware of the cost of care. This lack of knowledge can result in uninformed decisions about the type and amount of healthcare needed. Mass advertising by pharmaceutical manufacturers and specialty treatment centers directed at consumers has also contributed to inappropriate treatment choices being made by the public.

Concepts Related to
Healthcare Systems

CONCEPT	RELATIONSHIP TO HEALTHCARE SYSTEMS	NURSING IMPLICATIONS
Accountability	All parties must be held responsible for their decisions and actions. This includes providers, patients, government agencies, insurance companies, and other businesses. Otherwise, patients may experience poor outcomes due to insufficient, improper, or inequitable care.	■ Recognize your responsibility to provide evidence-based care within your scope of practice. ■ Set a high standard for accountability to serve as an example for other providers.
Advocacy	Advocacy helps address inequities of care for people who are vulnerable, whether through disability, impairment, or socioeconomic inequities or other social determinants.	■ Consider yourself a permanent patient advocate. Be sensitive to evidence of inequalities of care in the populations you serve. ■ Be aware of the resources in your local area that assist vulnerable people get better access to higher-quality medical care and social welfare.
Ethics	Any changes or decisions made—from the sale of a hospital to life-or-death decisions in the ED—should consider the impact on people's lives. They should ensure consistency with high moral values and established codes of ethics and ethical norms.	■ Know what resources are available in your healthcare organization to address ethical concerns. ■ After decisions with ethical implications are implemented, spend some time reflecting on their impact on people's lives.
Evidence-Based Practice	Clinical activity should meet the National Academy of Sciences' 2009 goal of 90% of medical care supported by solid evidence of efficacy.	■ Commit to a regular program of completing professional development activities to know the latest best-practice findings. ■ Make sure that individuals ready for discharge are provided understandable directions for further self-care.
Health Policy	It is not enough to propose healthcare for all; it needs to be woven into the fabric of the U.S. healthcare standards in understandable documents and be evaluated for consistent outcomes.	■ Know what the rules and regulations are for healthcare standards in your healthcare organization. ■ Know where to report evidence of employees not following established policies and procedures.
Informatics	Technology must support a holistic approach to mental and physical health and wellness and provide personalized, effective healthcare.	■ Conduct a regular small self-audit of your documentation, to see if you are compliant with standards. ■ Be aware of how you can access statistics about your patient population.
Legal Issues	Issues of privacy, autonomy, fairness, and compliance to laws must be handled with sensitivity.	■ Be familiar with the state and federal laws that govern your nursing scope of practice. ■ Know how to contact the risk management staff of your organization, or staff who deal with liability issues.
Quality Improvement	Data on outcomes and satisfaction should be collected to provide a mirror of accomplishment.	■ Evaluate patients' input about their satisfaction with care, both verbal and written statements. ■ Celebrate wins of pleasing consumers of care with exceeding their expectations.
Safety	Patient-centered care will support the safety of all persons involved, not just patients but also families, providers, staff, and communities.	■ Assess patients' risk for injury in their homes or residential environments. ■ Teach basic safety practices to a wide range of individuals, patients, families, providers, staff, and communities.

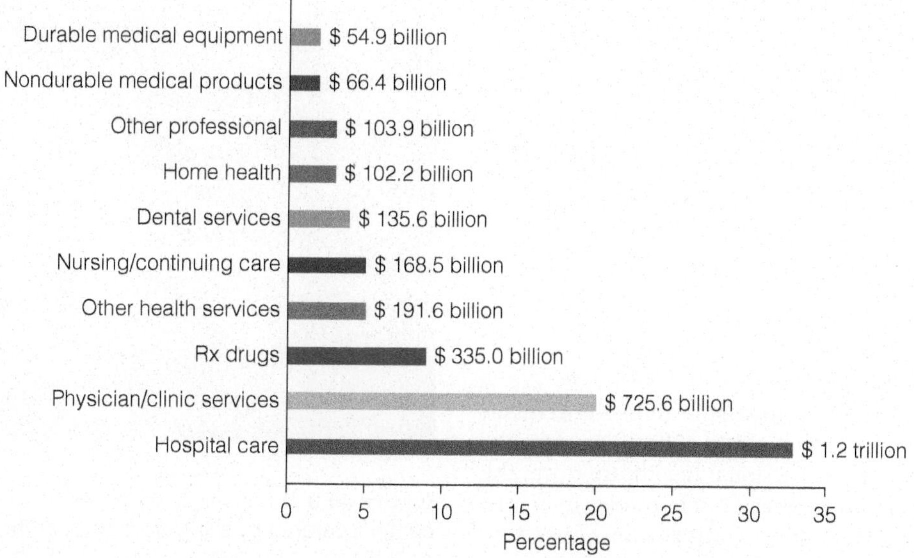

Figure 46.2 ›› A snapshot of U.S. healthcare expenditures in 2019.
Source: Centers for Medicare and Medicaid Services. (2019). National Health Expenditure Accounts. https://www.cms.gov.

Clinical Example C

An 8-year-old boy with a chronic blood disorder requires weekly blood transfusions. The hospital struggles to maintain a sufficient quantity of his rare blood type. The boy arrives at the ED at the same time as another patient who is bleeding profusely and has the same rare blood type. There is enough blood for only one of these patients.

Critical Thinking Questions

1. Which patient should receive the blood? Why?
2. What models or methods should be used to make the decision? Who should be responsible for making the decision?

As healthcare expenditures have increased, the need for **resource allocation**, the distribution of resources among competing groups of people or programs, has become increasingly recognized and, sometimes, controversial.

Examples of Resource Allocation

Rationing is a method of resource allocation used by individuals, insurance companies, and the government to prevent increases in the cost of healthcare or to reduce the cost of healthcare by limiting care provision. Bauchner (2019) describes four type of rationing:

- By access (type of insurance)
- By cost (out-of-pocket expenses)
- By restriction (the service is not available or paid for by a third party)
- By long waits (Canada and parts of the United States).

Individuals ration when they decide to provide self-care for an illness or injury, rather than seeking care from a HCP. Methods used by insurance companies to ration healthcare resources include limiting the number of HCPs from which patients can choose and denying coverage for services (e.g., services deemed to be experimental, those that are not supported by scientific evidence that prove their efficacy, or those for whom the patient has not used basic, less expensive initial level treatments). Insurance formularies limit the variety of medications that can be covered by insurance. The insurance company also can limit coverage to generic prescriptions.

The Organ Procurement and Transplantation Network

One of the best-known systems of allocating certain healthcare resources is the Organ Procurement and Transplantation Network (OPTN). The contribution of one organ donor can save up to eight lives (DHHS, n.d.). Currently almost 120,000 people await organ transplantation. Every 9 minutes another name is added to the waiting list. Unfortunately, there simply are not enough donated organs to meet the demand for transplants. As a result, approximately 17 people die daily without receiving a transplant (DHHS, n.d.). The OPTN, a contracted service of the DHHS, maintains the only national waiting list for organ transplantation. Multiple factors determine who receives a donor organ. Factors include blood and tissue type, medical urgency, organ size, time on the waiting list, and the geographic distance between the donor and the recipient (DHHS, n.d.). Preservation times also play a role. Common maximum organ preservation times are as follows (DHHS, n.d.):

- Heart, lung: 4 to 6 hours
- Liver: 8 to 12 hours
- Pancreas: 12 to 18 hours
- Kidney: 24 to 36 hours.

›› Stay Current: More information on organ donation and transplantation, including statistics and how to register as a donor, can be found at https://optn.transplant.hrsa.gov/learn/about-donation/.

COVID-19 Testing

In early 2020, there was an outbreak of a novel coronavirus, COVID-19. Initially, an adequate supply of diagnostic testing materials was not available. As the virus began to spread, the CDC realized that guidance had to be developed and implemented to ensure that individuals' clinical needs were evaluated before testing was ordered. The actual decisions about testing were made by state and local health departments and personal HCPs (CDC, 2020c). Initially, many health departments were forced to limit testing to HCPs, first responders, and hospitalized patients due to inadequate supplies of COVID-19 test kits (**Figure 46.3** »). Even as the supply chain improved, prescreening and referrals for testing continued to be required in most areas of the United States.

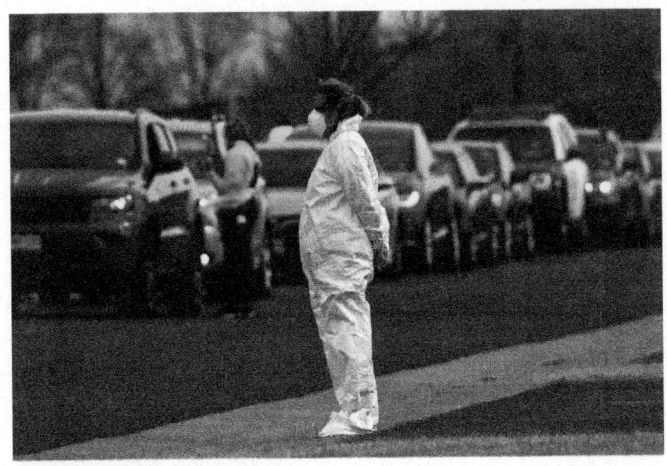

Figure 46.3 » Long lines for a drive-through COVID-19 testing center operated by the Colorado Department of Public Health.
Source: Michael Ciaglo/Getty Images.

Nurses and Allocation of Resources

The role of the nurse in the allocation of resources is a collaborative one. Nurses are the largest group of health professionals, and as part of the interprofessional healthcare team, the nurse participates in allocating healthcare resources. Thus, nurses develop a significant understanding of how appropriate allocation and misallocation of healthcare resources can affect patient needs and outcomes. Nurses must be aware of and participate in discussions that affect the allocation of healthcare resources in the workplace, in their communities, and at the federal level. Nurses are uniquely placed to advocate on behalf of patients when allocation of resources is being considered in their communities. They may advocate by talking with local legislators, writing to politicians, and engaging in discussions in their neighborhoods and social groups. As working professionals, nurses can participate in national discussions about resources through a number of professional organizations, such as the American Nurses Association.

REVIEW The Concept of Healthcare Systems

RELATE Link the Concepts

Linking the concept of healthcare systems with the concept of managing care:

You are a registered nurse leading a team that includes LPNs and UAP on a critical care unit of a hospital. You are planning care for a patient on a mechanical ventilator.

1. What aspects of this patient's care may be delegated to UAP?
2. What factors related to the delivery of healthcare may affect your ability to provide care for this patient, and what is their impact?

Linking the concept of healthcare systems with the concept of clinical decision making:

You are a registered nurse working in the ED of a rural hospital. Harvesting season has brought large numbers of Spanish-speaking families to the community. Almost all men and many women are migrant workers. A mother who speaks limited English brings her 5-year-old son to the ED. She says he has been vomiting for 2 days. He has a fever of 102°F. She says he does not have a regular HCP. He is not enrolled in any type of health insurance plan.

3. What factors will affect your ability to plan care for the child?
4. Which model of nursing care delivery would most benefit the child and his mother? Why?

Linking the concept of healthcare systems with the concept of reproduction:

5. What resources in your community are available to uninsured pregnant women?
6. Are the risks to the fetus any greater or any different when the pregnant mother is uninsured? Explain.

Linking the concept of healthcare systems with the concept of ethics:

7. What provisions of the ANA Code of Ethics address resource allocation?
8. What ethical considerations do you as an individual value that might affect how you would determine resource allocation?

REFER Go to Pearson MyLab Nursing and eText

REFLECT Apply Your Knowledge

Juan Santiago, 41 years old, makes an appointment with a HCP he has never seen before for an annual physical examination. During the nurse's initial assessment, the patient explains that he has never had a complete physical because he has always been healthy and hasn't had health insurance. After his recent college graduation, Mr. Santiago accepted a new job that offered full healthcare benefits, so he decided it was time to take care of his health. Although he appears anxious about what will happen during the exam, he does not ask any questions and avoids making eye contact with the nurse.

During the collection of his health history, Mr. Santiago reports smoking approximately 20 cigarettes per day, drinking 2 to 3 alcoholic beverages per week, and, until recently, working as a landscaper, a very physically demanding job. He describes the physical requirements of his new job as "a little bit of walking, but mostly desk work."

During the physical examination, the nurse notes a wound the size of a quarter on the anterior aspect of Mr. Santiago's left foot. It is erythematous and warm to the touch, and a small amount of purulent drainage seeps from the side of the wound. Mr. Santiago reports that the wound has been there for more than 6 weeks. He has applied over-the-counter antibiotic cream daily, but it still has not healed. The nurse asks Mr. Santiago about his weight; he admits losing about 10 pounds in the past month but denies changing his diet.

1. Describe primary, secondary, and tertiary care requirements for Mr. Santiago.
2. What referrals to other HCPs might be appropriate to assist in the treatment plan for this patient?
3. What type of assessment of health literacy would the nurse conduct with Mr. Santiago before providing written information?
4. What factors will influence care delivery to this patient? How will that alter the nurse's approach to providing care for him?

» Exemplar 46.A Emergency Preparedness

Exemplar Learning Outcomes

46.A Analyze emergency preparedness as it relates to healthcare systems.

- Describe the four phases of emergency management.
- Outline the organizations responsible for emergency management and response.
- Summarize the process of triage.
- Describe the safety zones used in site-specific disaster response.
- Summarize the methods used for handling bioterrorism disasters.
- Analyze the importance of collaboration during disaster response.
- Explain the role of nurses in emergency management and response.

Exemplar Key Terms

Bioterrorism, *2790*
Cold zone, *2790*
Community Emergency Response Team (CERT) program, *2787*
Disaster, *2785*
Emergency, *2785*
Emergency preparedness, *2785*
Emergency response, *2786*
Epidemic, *2785*
Federal Emergency Management Agency (FEMA), *2787*
Hot zone, *2790*
Local emergency management agency (LEMA), *2787*
Mass casualty incident (MCI), *2785*
Mitigation, *2785*
Pandemic, *2785*
Preparedness, *2785*
Recovery, *2787*
Reverse triage, *2787*
Supply chain, *2786*
Surge capacity, *2785*
Triage, *2787*
Warm zone, *2790*

Overview

An **emergency** is a sudden, often unforeseen event that threatens health or safety. A public emergency necessitating assistance from outside the affected community is a **disaster**. Disasters have three things in common: little or no warning before the event; available personnel and emergency services that are overwhelmed initially; and a serious threat to life, public health, and the environment. Infectious diseases may accompany disasters or can become disasters themselves. An **epidemic** is an infection that spreads rapidly in one or more specific locations. A **pandemic** is an infection that spreads rapidly around the world. A **mass casualty incident (MCI)** is an event that overwhelms the local healthcare system, where the number of casualties vastly exceeds the local resources and capabilities in a short period of time (DeNolf & Kahwaji, 2019).

Emergency preparedness is the act of making plans to prevent, respond to, and recover from emergencies. The CDC recommends an *all-hazards* approach to emergency preparedness. This approach provides for general preparation, including training, that can be applied in a wide variety of emergency situations. The impact on health and the healthcare system is similar regardless of the nature of the disaster. **Surge capacity** refers to a community's ability to rapidly meet the increased demand for qualified personnel and resources, including healthcare resources, in the event of a disaster.

The Four Phases of Emergency Management

Emergency management consists of four phases: mitigation, preparedness, response, and recovery.

Mitigation

The **mitigation** phase, which takes place both before and after an emergency occurs, consists of identifying potential hazards, taking action to reduce the likelihood of their occurrence, and minimizing the effects of those that cannot be prevented. An example of mitigation in an individual's disaster plan would be the purchase of flood insurance if they lived in a flood zone. Implementation of warning systems for tornadoes and tsunamis are examples of mitigation by local, state, or regional agencies. Installation of a warning system prior to an occurrence of a disaster is an example of excellent disaster planning. Installation after an event is an example of using lessons learned from a disaster to reduce the effect of future occurrences. Both are examples of mitigation.

Preparedness

The **preparedness** phase takes place before an emergency occurs. Risks are assessed and plans are developed to address them. Plans are designed to save lives and to assist first responders and rescue teams that are often overwhelmed by the initial demands of an emergency. Emergency plans are developed at the federal, regional, state, and local levels. The Federal Emergency Management Agency (FEMA), the Department of Homeland Security, and the CDC identify national threats, create plans at the national level, and coordinate planning efforts among many people, agencies, and levels of government. They provide guidance for the development of plans in local communities. For communities, the most critical task performed during the preparedness phase is the development of an emergency operations plan. These plans often include multiple components that address each of the many hazards and natural disasters that the community may face. They include identifying, organizing, and training emergency personnel; stockpiling equipment and supplies; implementing communication and warning systems; establishing emergency operations centers; and implementing response and evacuation plans. In all these activities, the emergency operations plan can include a description of the supply chain for obtaining equipment and supplies, as well as backup alternatives. The **supply chain** refers to a series of processes (from manufacturing to delivery) involved in the production and distribution of essential items (such as personal protective equipment). Any obstacle to ramping up the arrival of just-in-time items might prove critical in a disaster.

During the preparedness phase, individual nurses must gain an understanding of their expected roles in large-scale emergency situations and prepare for them. Because nurses will be required to allocate scarce resources and supplies and make critical and difficult patient care decisions, they must understand the ethics associated with their decisions. The American Nurses Association (ANA) is a good source of information to guide nurses' understanding of their roles and possible consequences.

Public health nurses have a specific role to play in the preparedness phase. They participate in community assessment of populations at risk during a disaster and develop care plans to address their functional needs. They also conduct training drills and evaluate operational plans and work with local stakeholders (ANA, 2017).

Nurses also must be aware of their employer's response plans and have a sense of how their state and local community will operate during an emergency. Nurses who choose to become disaster volunteers should register with an agency such as the American Red Cross to ensure they are properly trained and recognized as part of an organized system (ANA, n.d.).

During the preparedness phase, nurses must also develop an emergency plan for themselves and their immediate families. When this plan is complete, nurses can be confident that their families are prepared to weather an emergency in relative safety. With this assurance, nurses who choose to assist in a disaster or who are required to remain at the hospital during a disaster will be able to leave their families without delay and remain available until no longer needed.

The Federal Emergency Management Agency and the American Red Cross are two organizations that provide detailed information to assist individuals with the development of personal emergency plans. It is important for everyone to develop a plan for themselves and their families. They must ensure that not only the adults but also the children know what to do in an emergency.

Plans should address the basic emergency needs of any disaster. They should also include instructions for specific disasters, such as tornadoes, that may occur in the individual's location. Everyone should assemble a disaster kit that can be used in place or taken if evacuation is necessary. Escape routes for disasters that could occur within the home itself (e.g., gas leaks and fires) or for disasters that would require mass evacuation (e.g., floods and hurricanes) should be determined. Meeting places should be designated—someplace inside or outside the home where the family can unite. Family members should be provided contact information in case they are separated during a disaster. Someone outside of the immediate area should be identified as a central contact if family members are unable to reach each other locally. It is very important to shut off utilities as directed by emergency authorities or when forced to leave home. Insurance, medical, financial, and other vital records should be duplicated and stored in an off-site, safe location. Families should plan for special needs such as medications and medical equipment. Family members should be trained in first aid, including CPR. Review and update of the emergency plan on a regular basis are critical because someday someone's life may depend on it.

>> **Stay Current:** Visit https://www.fema.gov/pdf/areyouready/areyouready_full.pdffor FEMA's *Are You Ready? Guide—An In-Depth Guide to Citizen Preparedness*.

Emergency Response

The third phase, **emergency response**, is the implementation of emergency preparedness plans. These plans provide a means for responders to save lives, prevent additional property damage, and meet basic human needs. As soon as possible, those who are injured are triaged and given appropriate treatment. Other emergency activities include search-and-rescue operations, opening shelters to house survivors, and repairing utility infrastructure.

The emergency response plan is followed during and immediately after the emergency, simultaneously with the community's assessment of the disaster's immediate effects. Community agencies such as local law enforcement, paramedics, and ED personnel, as well as local governmental staff employed in the disaster response unit, are responsible for implementing the overall plan and its components.

Public health nurses are also part of this response effort. They ensure that logistics are in place to support community care and provide ongoing response planning during the crisis (ANA, 2017). Federal, state, and other outside resources support local efforts by providing first aid and other emergency medical assistance and by establishing or restoring communication and transportation. Public health nurses use population-based triage to assess communicable disease outbreak impact and needed response, assessing the probability of infectious diseases and addressing them, and identifying and providing support to individuals with mental health problems.

During the preparedness phase, nurses became familiar with the emergency plans of their employers and communities. They also familiarize themselves with the ANA's positions on nurses' emergency and disaster responsibilities. During the emergency response phase, nurses put the preparedness phase information to use. The responsibility of nurses during an emergency, like that of other first responders, is to do the greatest good for the greatest number of casualties. During an emergency, nurses will be asked to perform the fundamentals of nursing practice, but in a very stressful environment under extraordinary circumstances. They will be working under intense time constraints and must care for each victim quickly, then move on to the next one. They should not use their time to provide care that will be of minimal or questionable benefit. Nurses must observe both the physical and mental status of victims and ensure appropriate triage and treatment. Advanced practice nurses who have received training in emergency and trauma care will have significantly greater responsibilities than nurses with less training. During the crisis, nurses should be constantly aware of their defined scope of practice and must not exceed it.

Recovery

The **recovery** phase takes place after the emergency and is designed to restore the community to normal balance (restoration) or create a new, safer normal by updating the community's preparedness plan to address lessons learned during the emergency (mitigation). The recovery phase includes the reconstitution of government operations and services, if necessary, and includes the provision of public assistance by the private and public sectors. Other elements of the recovery phase may include rebuilding, reemployment, and the repair of essential infrastructure. During the recovery phase, each community must reassess risks and update plans to ensure that newly identified risks are addressed. Because of their education and experience, nurses are well qualified to participate in risk assessment and planning at the local, state, and national levels following a disaster. Nurses are also perfect candidates to educate their patients and communities about disaster preparation. In particular, public health nurses conduct rapid ongoing needs assessments at intervals to determine health and critical resource capacity after a natural disaster and work with community stakeholders to plan for any long-term health concerns following an incident. They also participate in the reconstruction of critical services and evaluate the long-term impact of the disaster consequences on the community (ANA, 2017).

Responsibility for Emergency Management and Response

State divisions of emergency management act as the **local emergency management agency (LEMA)** for each state. At the federal level, the **Federal Emergency Management Agency (FEMA)** is called upon to act and coordinate recovery efforts. Both are governmental agencies with expertise in public safety, emergency medical services, and management.

The U.S. Department of Homeland Security has created federal guidelines called the National Incident Management System that local governments must follow during an emergency or disaster (FEMA, 2020). Local governments have the primary responsibility for emergency management and response.

In the event of an emergency, first responders such as local fire departments and emergency medical technicians will be challenged to meet the needs of the public because of the sheer volume of assistance they will be asked to provide. In situations like this, citizen volunteers often act as extensions of the first responders. For this reason, it is beneficial for a community to develop a corps of trained citizens to provide such support.

In recognition of this, FEMA has developed the **Community Emergency Response Team (CERT) program** to prepare interested community members. Participants gain an understanding of their responsibility for preparing for a disaster, so they will be ready to safely assist themselves, their families, and their neighbors. The CERT program provides citizens with facts about what to expect following a major disaster in terms of immediate services; alerts citizens to their responsibility for mitigation and preparedness; trains citizens in needed lifesaving skills with an emphasis on decision-making skills, rescuer safety, and doing the greatest good for the most people; and organizing teams that act as an extension of first responder services, offering immediate help to victims until professional services are on site (U.S. Department of Homeland Security, 2020).

The CDC manages the Clinician Outreach Communication Activity (COCA) program to ensure that clinicians have up-to-date information. COCA is designed to provide two-way communication between clinicians and the CDC about emerging health threats such as pandemics, natural disasters, and terrorism. COCA keeps a list of emergency preparedness and training resources offered by federal agencies and COCA partners.

» **Stay Current:** Visit https://emergency.cdc.gov/coca/training.asp for COCA's list of conferences and training opportunities and to sign up for email updates from COCA.

Nursing Competencies for Emergency and Disaster Response

Nurses represent the largest pool of healthcare professionals and, for this reason, are called upon to assist in emergencies and disasters. MCIs are one example. Training in preparation for, recognition of, and response to MCIs will be beneficial to the nurse, the nurse's family, the nurse's employer, and the community. Some of the ways in which nurses have received training regarding MCIs include reading professional journal articles, participating in mock disaster drills, volunteering in community services, obtaining CERT certification, and actual nursing during an MCI. Emergency preparedness is a necessity, regardless of the nurse's educational preparation, area of expertise, or practice setting. For people affected by the emergency or disaster, mental health needs must be given equal priority with physical health needs in the preparedness phase.

» **Stay Current:** Visit the Multi-State Disaster Behavioral Health Consortium website at https://www.nasmhpd.org/content/multi-state-disaster-behavioral-health-consortium. The content on policy, publications, webinars, and training is sponsored by the National Association of State Mental Health Program Directors. The mission of the organization is to ensure that mental health needs are included in emergency preparedness planning efforts.

Triage

The process of **triage** involves prioritizing individuals for treatment based on severity of illness or injury and in light of the supplies and resources available. The objective of triage is to ensure early assessment and prioritize care based on severity of symptoms. Nurses perform triage every day in EDs. During an MCI, the demand on nurses' knowledge and skills will be even greater. No minimum number of casualties qualifies an event to be considered a MCI; it is the situation of possibly overwhelming the health system that determines a MCI.

Mass casualty incidents call for the implementation of **reverse triage**, in which the most severely injured or ill victims who require the greatest resources are treated last to allow the greatest number of victims to receive medical attention. A simple color classification system (START) is used to prioritize adult patients (**Figure 46.4** »). A separate algorithm, JumpSTART, has been developed for pediatric victims (**Figure 46.5** »). It is recommended that emergency medical personnel be assigned to triage. This frees physicians and nurses to provide needed care in a disaster.

During the pandemic of the infectious disease COVID-19, the broad scope of triage activity highlighted two functions: screening before any medical diagnosis or treatment was initiated and making decisions about ventilator use for severely respiratory-compromised patients. The CDC (2020a) designed a phone advice line tool for possible COVID-19 patients. In addition to a word-by-word verbal script for the nurse, it also contained a decision algorithm to help the nurse assess for the presence of life-threatening signs and symptoms (e.g., shallow breathing, cyanosis, level of consciousness) to determine the level of care required.

» **Stay Current:** To access the CDC's COVID-19 phone script or review the clinical decision algorithm, go to https://www.cdc.gov/coronavirus/2019-ncov/hcp/phone-guide/index.html.

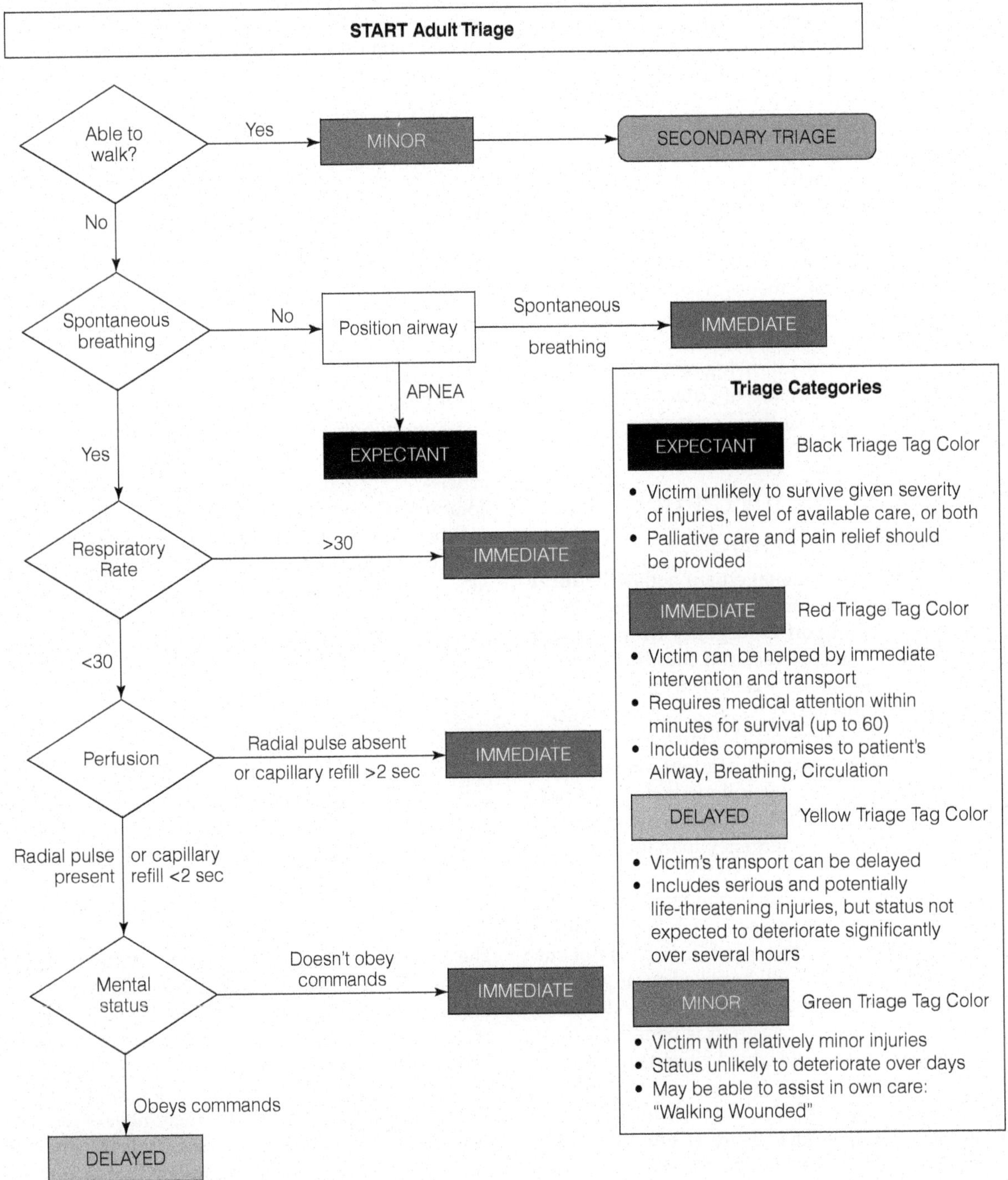

Figure 46.4 » START adult triage algorithm.

Source: U.S. Department of Health and Human Services (2020b).

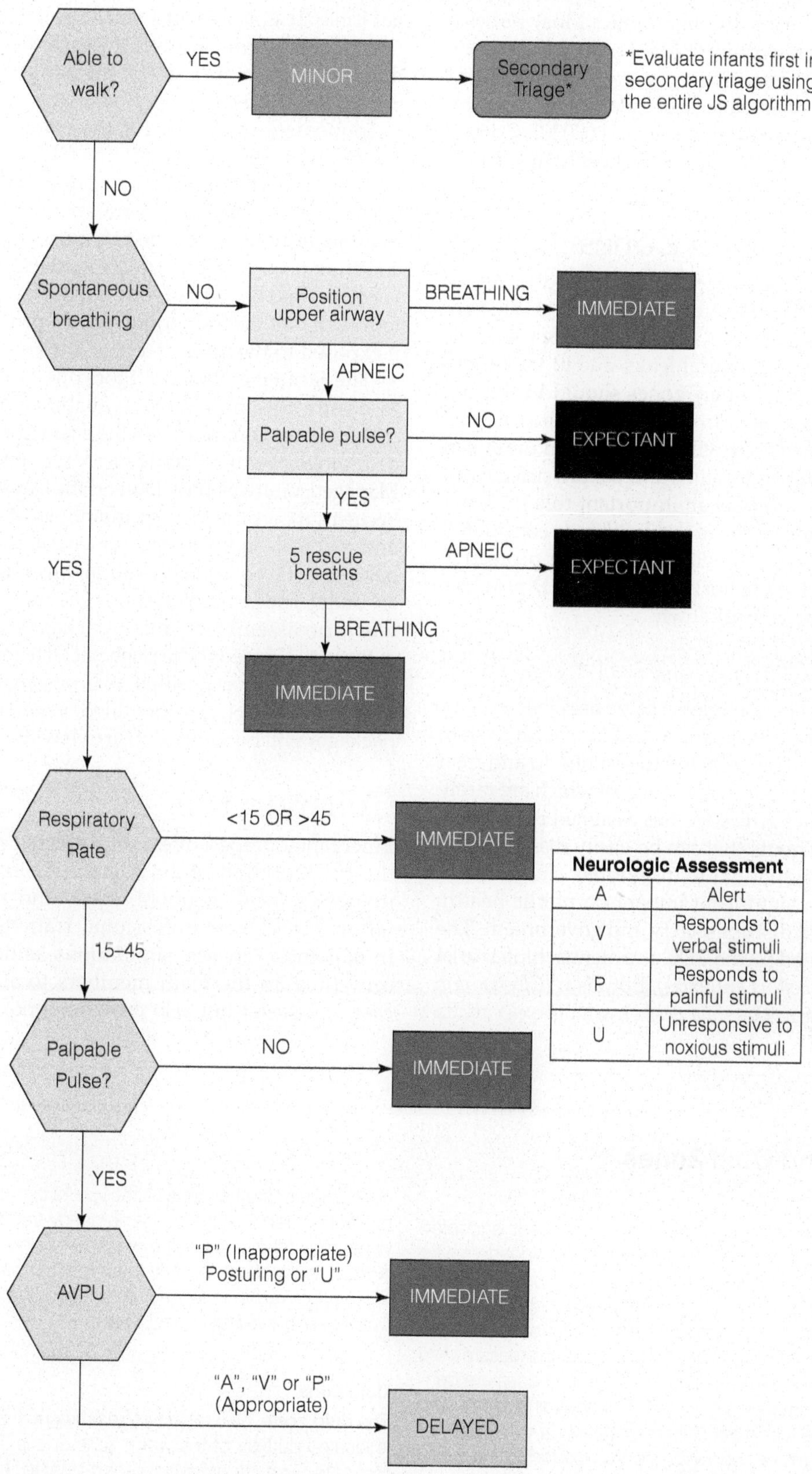

Neurologic Assessment	
A	Alert
V	Responds to verbal stimuli
P	Responds to painful stimuli
U	Unresponsive to noxious stimuli

Figure 46.5 ›› JumpSTART algorithm for pediatric victims.

Source: U.S. Department of Health and Human Services (2020a).

A 2020 article in the *Annals of Internal Medicine* reported results of a survey of facilities with 26 unique policies regarding ventilator triage during the pandemic. Most policies specified the triage team's composition. By profession, 89% required a physician, 70% required a nurse, and about a third called for the inclusion of an ethicist, chaplain, and/or respiratory therapist (Matheny Antommaria et al., 2020). Criteria for use of mechanical ventilators included benefit, need, age, and conservation of resources.

Site-Specific Disaster Zones

When a site-specific disaster occurs, access to the site of contamination is limited and safety zones are established. Examples of site-specific disasters are the release of weapons, such as bombs, and toxic chemical leaks due to tanker car derailment. The designated safety zones should be located uphill, upwind, and upstream from the site of the disaster. The configuration of each zone will vary based on the site of the occurrence. Topography, weather, and the physical layout (buildings, roads, etc.) will play an important role in designating the zones. The initial site of the incident is considered the hot zone. Only personnel with appropriate protective equipment are allowed in the hot zone. **Box 46.3** » provides more information on zone breakdown.

Bioterrorism

Bioterrorism is the deliberate release of viruses, bacteria, or other microbes as weapons. The U.S. public health system and primary HCPs must be prepared to respond to and treat the diseases caused by these agents, many of which are rarely seen in the United States. The CDC has assigned the highest priority to biological agents that can be easily disseminated or transmitted from individual to individual; cause a high mortality rate; have a significant impact on public health; cause public panic; and disrupt society and government. The primary agents identified by the CDC as potential bioterrorist threats are anthrax (*Bacillus anthracis*), botulism (*Clostridium botulinum* toxin), plague (*Yersinia pestis*), smallpox (variola major), tularemia (*Francisella tularensis*), and viral hemorrhagic fevers (filoviruses [e.g., Ebola and Marburg] and arenaviruses [e.g., Lassa and Machupo]) (CDC, 2018).

Nurses must be aware of the early signs and symptoms of these diseases as well as the methods of transmitting them. See **Table 46.2** ».

Immediate treatment for the primary biological agents used in terrorism is limited. The CDC has published guidelines for the treatment of inhaled anthrax with antibiotics and antitoxin (CDC, 2016a). There are no effective therapies for treating individuals infected by most of the other viruses that could be used in a bioterrorism attack. For some viruses, a vaccine could be created to stimulate the body's immune system such that the individual may be protected from infection if exposed to the virus at a later date.

The Strategic National Stockpile is a program designed to ensure the immediate availability of essential medical materials to a community in the event of a large-scale chemical or biological attack, as well as for use in other disasters. Managed jointly by the CDC and the Department of Homeland Security, it consists of large quantities of antibiotics; vaccines; and medical, surgical, and patient support supplies such as bandages, IV equipment, and airway supplies. In the case of an undetermined biological or chemical threat, the stockpile has a preassembled "push package" designed to meet a community's needs. The push packages are stored in locations that permit delivery within 12 hours after an attack. Once the threat has been clearly identified, vendor-managed inventory packages will be shipped to arrive within 24 to 36 hours.

Collaboration

Emergency preparedness and disaster response depend on the collaboration of an interprofessional healthcare team involving local, regional, state, and federal governmental agencies. Interprofessional training and participation in tabletop exercises, simulations, and mock incidents not only prepare the team members to assume their roles in case of disaster but also provide opportunities for frequent

Box 46.3

Hot, Warm, and Cold Zones

Hot Zone

The **hot zone** is the most dangerous zone because it is located immediately adjacent to the site of the disaster. All responders who enter the area must be protected by personal protective equipment (PPE) appropriate to the nature of the emergency. Because of the dangers inherent in this location, only the most basic services are performed: Victims are located; basic lifesaving measures are provided (e.g., airways are established and hemorrhages are controlled); antidotes are administered; and the dead and those who cannot be saved are identified. Decontamination of victims is not performed in the hot zone. Survivors are transported to the warm zone for decontamination. All contaminated supplies and equipment are left in the hot zone for collection and disposal at a later date.

Warm Zone

The **warm zone** (also referred to as the yellow, contamination, or contamination reduction zone) is located at least 300 feet from the outer edge of the hot zone. Although its primary purpose is decontamination, rapid triage and emergency treatment to stabilize survivors may take place in the warm zone. Individuals who have the highest levels of contamination are treated with the highest priority. PPE is required in this zone. After decontamination is completed, victims are moved to the cold zone.

Cold Zone

The **cold zone**, also referred to as the green zone or support zone, is located outside of the warm zone and is the site where decontaminated victims are triaged and treated. It is considered to be comparatively safe, although PPE is still required in case circumstances change (e.g., if wind direction shifts). The primary purpose of this zone is to provide medical services and to transport victims who require more than first aid to locations where they will be provided higher levels of service.

TABLE 46.2 Biological Pathogens of Highest Concern for Bioterrorism Attacks

Pathogen	Cause	Symptoms	Transmission
Anthrax	*Bacillus anthracis*, a spore-forming bacterium Three types: ■ Cutaneous ■ Respiratory ■ Gastrointestinal	■ Cutaneous: The first symptom is a small sore that becomes a blister, then progresses to a skin ulcer with a black spot in the center. All lesions are painless. ■ Respiratory: *Initially:* Sore throat, mild fever and muscle aches. *Later:* Respiratory symptoms, e.g., cough, chest discomfort, shortness of breath, tiredness and achy muscles. ■ Gastrointestinal: Nausea, loss of appetite, bloody diarrhea, and fever followed by bad stomach pain.	■ Cutaneous: Direct skin contact with spores; often result from handling products, such as wool, from infected animals ■ Respiratory: Inhalation of aerosolized spores (rare unless weaponized) ■ Gastrointestinal: Eating undercooked meat or dairy products from infected animals (rare)
Botulism	*Clostridium botulinum* toxin	Foodborne botulism symptoms: ■ Usually develop within 12–36 hours after exposure. ■ May include visual effects (e.g., double vision); neurologic symptoms, including slurred speech, dysphagia, and muscle weakness that begins in the shoulders and descends through the body to the calves; and paralysis of the breathing muscles, which, if left untreated, may result in death.	■ Foodborne: Individual ingests preformed toxin. ■ Infant: Occurs in small number of infants who harbor *C. botulinum* in their intestinal tract. ■ Wound botulism: Occurs when existing wounds are infected with the toxins of *C. botulinum*.
Plague	*Yersinia pestis*, a bacterium	■ Pneumonic plague develops within 1–6 days of exposure. ■ Fever, weakness, rapidly developing pneumonia with dyspnea, chest pain, cough, and sometimes bloody or watery sputum.	■ An old mnemonic is "The fleas and lice on rats and mice cause plague." ■ Bubonic plague is transmitted via an infected flea bite or exposure of broken skin to infected material. ■ Pneumonic plague is of particular interest as a biological weapon because it can be released via weaponized aerosol. It can also be transmitted from individual to individual.
Viral hemorrhagic fevers (VHF)	Several distinct families of zoonotic viruses that reside in an animal reservoir host (e.g., rodent) or arthropod vector (e.g., ticks and mosquitos)	Signs and symptoms, which develop after a 5- to 10-day incubation period, vary by the type of VHF. Early signs and symptoms often include marked fever, fatigue, dizziness, myalgia, weakness, exhaustion, and a rash on the trunk. Severe cases may be accompanied by bleeding under the skin, in internal organs, or from body orifices such as the mouth, eyes, or ears. Patients rarely die from this blood loss. Severe cases may cause shock, nervous system breakdowns, coma, delirium, and seizures. Renal failure may occur in some types of VHF.	■ VHFs are most commonly spread by exposure to an animal reservoir host or arthropod vector. Humans are not natural reservoirs for VHFs; however, some VHFs can be transmitted from individual to individual after an initial human has been infected.
Smallpox	Variola virus	■ During the incubation period (from 7 to 17 days), an infected individual has no symptoms and is not contagious. ■ Prodromal phase (2–4 days) symptoms include a fever of 101–104°F, head and body aches, and possibly vomiting. This phase may be contagious. ■ The early rash phase is the most contagious period. The rash first appears as spots on the tongue and in the mouth, which progress into sores that break open, allowing large amounts of virus to spread into the mouth and throat. Day 1: the rash, which begins on the face, spreads across the entire body. Day 3: raised bumps develop. Day 4: bumps fill with thick, opaque fluid with depression in the center that resembles a belly button—a distinguishing characteristic of smallpox. Fever increases again. ■ Pustular rash (duration of 5 days): Pustular bumps develop (they feel like BBs under the skin), then form a crust and scab over. The scabs fall off, leaving pitted scars. The individual is contagious until all the scabs have fallen off.	■ Direct and fairly long face-to-face exposure is usually necessary under normal circumstances; however, weaponized smallpox can be spread by aerosol. ■ Direct contact with body fluids or contaminated items such as clothing or bed linen could spread the disease. ■ Humans are the only natural host of variola.
Tularemia	*Francisella tularensis*	■ Sudden fever, chills, headache, diarrhea, muscle aches, joint pain, dry cough, and progressive weakness. ■ If *F. tularensis* was used as a biological weapon and made airborne for exposure by inhalation, the infected people would experience severe respiratory illness, including life-threatening pneumonia and systemic infection.	Spread by bacterium found in animals (especially rodents, rabbits, and hares). Means of spread include: ■ Being bitten by infected ticks, deerflies, other insects ■ Handling infected animal carcasses and skins ■ Eating or drinking contaminated food or water ■ Inhaling *F. tularensis*

Source: Based on Centers for Disease Control and Prevention (2018).

Box 46.4

The Emergency Medical Services System

The emergency medical services (EMS) system is a network of resources that provides emergency care and transportation, that is, prehospital care, to victims of illness, injury, or disaster. Trained and licensed EMS personnel work under the auspices of a medical director, usually a hospital-based physician, who is consulted as needed. There are four levels of EMS professionals.

EMRs and EMTs provide basic life support:

- *Emergency medical responders (EMRs)* provide initial emergency care, including assessment, opening airways, ventilating, controlling bleeding, performing CPR, stabilizing the spine and injured limbs, assisting with childbirth, and aiding other EMS personnel.
- *Emergency medical technicians (EMTs)* do everything EMRs do but have received additional training and certification. This permits them to assist patients with prescribed medications and give aspirins, NSAIDs, oral glucose, and other medications when indicated.

AEMTs and paramedics are qualified to provide advanced life support:

- *Advanced emergency medical technicians (AEMTs)* have received advanced emergency training so they may start and administer IV fluids; give medications; and assess the need for and provide advanced airway procedures.
- *Paramedics* receive the most training and are qualified to do more in-depth assessments of patients, including the assessment of abnormal heart rhythms, and to perform some invasive procedures.

evaluations of the plan. These evaluations lead to a more effective emergency plan and facilitate communications across the interprofessional team that is responsible for the development, implementation, and evaluation of an emergency response plan. Nurses often have contact with members of emergency medical services (EMS) in both EDs and disaster situations. A brief overview of the EMS system is presented in **Box 46.4** ».

Lifespan Considerations

Emergency Considerations for Children

In most cases, emergency planning, mitigation, and responses involving children include the parents or primary caregivers. The American Academy of Pediatrics sponsors an online information resource for parents in English and in Spanish called The AAP Parenting Website. Its mission includes developing policy, building coalitions, raising public awareness, and supporting training and professional education. In the case of the COVID-19 pandemic, the website featured a section about the coronavirus that described:

- Symptoms
- Risk factors
- Prevention measures
- Home care of infected individuals
- Dealing with school and childcare facility closures
- Talking to children about the virus and community responses (American Academy of Pediatrics, 2020).

Community and local emergency planning should take into consideration the needs of children. For example, even though parents are expected to provide formula and diapers for their own infants, planning for emergency shelters should include obtaining and providing infant formula and diapers. Likewise, trauma interventions for children, such as art and play therapies, should be included in any postevent plans intended to reduce the severity of acute mental health responses.

Emergency Considerations for Older Adults

Older adults are particularly vulnerable to disasters. They often have chronic diseases, which can worsen quickly due to lack of food, water, and extreme heat or cold. Older adults have a greater rate of reliance on medication, oxygen, or other treatments, some of which require electricity. Many older adults cannot survive long without certain medications or treatments. Older adults may also have limited mobility, diminished sensory awareness, inadequate thermoregulation mechanisms, and social and economic limitations that prevent adequate preparedness and limit their ability to manage during and/or after a disaster hits (CDC, 2016b).

Nursing Practice

The role of the nurse in a disaster or emergency will vary based on the type of disaster, its location, the number and condition of the victims, and the personnel (e.g., command staff, first responders, emergency medical technicians, police) and supplies that are available. Nurses may be called on to perform triage of patients, to perform first aid, or to stabilize patients in preparation for transfer to more advanced care.

Initially, the nurse must decide whether to assist during the disaster or not. This decision will be based on individual safety, family safety and needs, and the greater needs of the community at large. Nurses are never expected to jeopardize their own safety or the safety of their families or other rescuers by responding to a disaster. Nurses must also consider whether they have the appropriate skills to respond—that is, whether the skills of the nurse are adequate for the job or whether the job would be better left to individuals with advanced training in disaster response.

If the decision is made to participate, the nurse will follow the emergency preparedness plans created by the employing agency or within the community. The nurse must operate within the defined nursing scope of practice despite the temptation to step outside of those bounds when faced with critical care needs outside the nurse's scope of practice.

Individuals who choose to provide care during disasters must be aware of the ethics of doing so and the personal risk that may be involved. The American Nurses Association provides guidance in this area and is working to ensure that nurses who work within the framework suggested by ANA are protected from risks associated with providing care.

The injuries experienced during a disaster are specifically related to the type of disaster. For example, nurses working where an earthquake has occurred will treat multiple crush injuries. During the Boston Marathon on April 15, 2013, two explosions occurred. Nurses who had volunteered to provide medical services during the marathon suddenly found themselves in the unexpected position of caring for mass casualties who had sustained fractures, head trauma, severe abdominal injuries, and amputations (**Figure 46.6 ››**).

Nurses should assist their communities not only by providing emergency care during a disaster but also by becoming leaders as their communities prepare for potential disasters by creating or revising emergency preparedness and contingency plans.

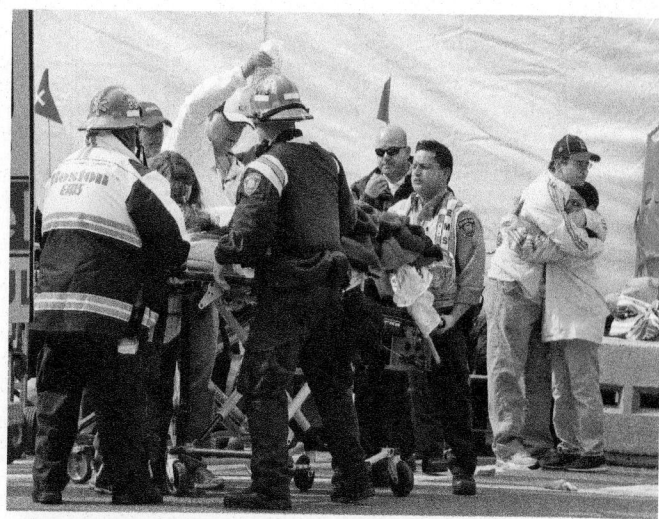

Figure 46.6 ›› EMS personnel and volunteer nurses helped care for hundreds of victims of the Boston Marathon bombings on April 15, 2013.

Source: Elise Amendola/AP Images.

REVIEW Emergency Preparedness

RELATE Link the Concepts and Exemplars

Linking the exemplar of emergency preparedness with the concept of professional behaviors:

1. What is the nurse's professional duty in a time of disaster?

Linking the exemplar of emergency preparedness with the concept of managing care:

2. Uninsured Americans are the most vulnerable individuals in the event of a pandemic event. How is early recognition related to access to care?

Linking the exemplar of emergency preparedness with the concept of ethics:

3. What ethical considerations are involved when allocating scarce resources, such as medication, equipment, and healthcare personnel, during a disaster?

REFER Go to Pearson MyLab Nursing and eText

REFLECT Apply Your Knowledge

Ed Jones is a 75-year-old retired cabinet maker who makes small toys in the basement of his home, located on the banks of the Deep River. He is independent and a widower. His primary care physician has prescribed antihypertensive medications and monitors his blood pressure regularly. When a week of heavy rainstorms flooded Mr. Jones's neighborhood, his home sustained much water damage and most of his equipment and wood were ruined. He waded through waist-deep water to reach a rescue boat, rather than waiting for it to pick him up. The EMTs who triage him decide to transfer him to the nearest ED.

You are the nurse assessing Mr. Jones. You observe that he has multiple cuts on his hands that are a result of woodworking and an ulcer on his right foot. He reports that the ulcer developed after a tool fell on his foot. He adds that he has not sought medical treatment for it. Mr. Jones's physical assessment findings reveal: T 100.7°F; P 96 beats/min, R 20 breaths/min, and BP 178/100 mmHg; his skin is cool and dry with multiple lesions on both hands and a stage II ulcer on his right dorsal foot with yellow-green exudate. His pain rated as 2 on a scale of 0 to 10. His lungs are clear, and his heart rate is regular. No edema is noted.

1. What actions did Mr. Jones take that probably exacerbated his skin lesions?
2. What additional information is needed so that you can form nursing diagnoses for Mr. Jones?
3. What nursing diagnoses do you believe would be appropriate?

References

Agency for Healthcare Research and Quality (AHRQ). (2020). *2018 national healthcare disparities report*. https://www.ahrq.gov/research/findings/nhqrdr/nhqdr18/index.html

Alker, J., & Pham, O. (2018). *Nation's progress on children's health coverage reverses course*. Georgetown University Health Policy Institute. https://ccf.georgetown.edu/wp-content/uploads/2018/11/UninsuredKids2018_Final_asof1128743pm.pdf

American Academy of Pediatrics (AAP). (2020). *The AAP parenting website*. https://healthychildren.org/English/Pages/default.aspx

American Medical Association (AMA). (2020). *Trends in health care spending*. https://www.ama-assn.org/about/research/trends-health-care-spending

American Nurses Association (ANA). (n.d.). *Disaster preparedness*. https://www.nursingworld.org/practice-policy/work-environment/health-safety/disaster-preparedness/

American Nurses Association (ANA). 2017. *Who will be there?: Ethics, the law, and a nurse's duty to respond in a disaster*. https://www.nursingworld.org/~4af058/globalassets/docs/ana/ethics/who-will-be-there_disaster-preparedness_2017.pdf

Bauchner, H. (2019). Rationing of health care in the United States: An inevitable consequence of increasing health care costs. *Journal of the American Medical Association, 321*(8), 751–752. https://doi.org/10.1001/jama.2019.1081

Berkman, N. D., Sheridan, S. L., Donahue, K. E., Halpern, D. J., & Crotty, K. (2011). Low health literacy and health outcomes: An updated systematic review. *Annals of Internal Medicine, 155*(2), 97–107.

Blumenthal, D., & Abrams, M. (2020). The Affordable Care Act at 10 years: Payment and delivery system reforms. *New England Journal of Medicine, 382*, 1057–1063. https://doi.org/10.1056/NEJMhpr1916092

Capatides, C. (2020). *Doctors Without Borders dispatches team to the Navajo Nation.* CBS News. https://www.cbsnews.com/news/doctors-without-borders-navajo-nation-coronavirus/

Case Management Society of America. (2017). *What is a case manager?* https://www.cmsa.org/who-we-are/what-is-a-case-manager/

Centers for Disease Control and Prevention (CDC). (2016a). *Anthrax: Treatment.* https://www.cdc.gov/anthrax/medical-care/treatment.html

Centers for Disease Control and Prevention (CDC). (2016b). *CDC's disaster planning goal: Protect vulnerable older adults.* https://www.cdc.gov/aging/pdf/disaster_planning_goal.pdf

Centers for Disease Control and Prevention (CDC). (2018). *Bioterrorism agents/diseases.* http://www.bt.cdc.gov/agent/agentlist-category.asp

Centers for Disease Control and Prevention (CDC). (2020a). *Phone advice line tool for possible COVID-19 patients.* https://www.cdc.gov/coronavirus/2019-ncov/hcp/phone-guide/index.html

Centers for Disease Control and Prevention (CDC). (2020b). *Preventing adverse childhood experiences.* https://www.cdc.gov/violenceprevention/childabuseandneglect/aces/fastfact.html

Centers for Disease Control and Prevention (CDC). (2020c). *Testing for COVID-19.* https://www.cdc.gov/coronavirus/2019-ncov/symptoms-testing/testing.html

DeNolf, R. L., & Kahwaji, C. I. (2019). *EMS, mass casualty management.* StatPearls. https://www.ncbi.nlm.nih.gov/books/NBK482373/

Emergency Medical Treatment and Active Labor Act (EMTALA). (2011). *Frequently asked questions on EMTALA.* http://www.emtala.com/faq.html

Fay, L., Carll-White, A., Schadler, A., Isaacs, K. B., & Real, K. (2017). Shifting landscapes: The impact of centralized and decentralized nursing station models on the efficiency of care. *HERD:Health Environments Research and Design Journal, 10*(5), 80–94. https://doi.org/10.1177/1937586717698812

Federal Emergency Management System (FEMA). (2020). *National Incident Management System.* https://www.fema.gov/emergency-managers/nims

Harvard School of Public Health. (2020a). *Close to half of U.S. population projected to have obesity by 2030.* https://www.hsph.harvard.edu/news/press-releases/half-of-us-to-have-obesity-by-2030/

Harvard School of Public Health. (2020b). *COVID-19 pandemic highlights longstanding health inequities in U.S.* https://www.hsph.harvard.edu/news/hsph-in-the-news/covid-19-pandemic-highlights-longstanding-health-inequities-in-u-s/

HealthCare.Gov. (n.d.-a). *The Children's Health Insurance Program (CHIP).* https://www.healthcare.gov/medicaid-chip/childrens-health-insurance-program/

HealthCare.Gov. (n.d.-b). *How to find low-cost health care in your community.* http://www.healthcare.gov/using-insurance/low-cost-care/community-health-centers

Higgins, T. C., Schottenfeld, L., & Crosson, J. (2015). *Primary care practice facilitation curriculum (Module 25)* (AHRQ Publication No. 15-0060-EF). Agency for Healthcare Research and Quality.

Institute of Medicine. (1993). *Access to healthcare in America.* National Academies Press.

Jimenez, F. E., Puumala, S. E., Apple, M., Bunker-Hellmich, L. A., Rich, R. K., & Brittin, J. (2019). Associations of patient and staff outcomes with inpatient unit designs incorporating decentralized caregiver workstations: A systematic review of empirical evidence. *HERD: Health Environments Research and Design Journal, 12*(1), 26–43. https://doi.org/10.1177/1937586718796590

Kaiser Family Foundation. (2019a). *Key facts about the uninsured population.* https://www.kff.org/uninsured/issue-brief/key-facts-about-the-uninsured-population/

Kaiser Family Foundation. (2019b). *Key facts on health and health care by race and ethnicity.* https://www.kff.org/disparities-policy/report/key-facts-on-health-and-health-care-by-race-and-ethnicity/

Keith, K. (2019) Uninsured rate rose in 2018, says Census Bureau report. *Health Affairs.* https://doi.org/10.1377/hblog20190911.805983

Koh, H. K., Berwick, D. M., Clancy, C. M., Baur, C., Brach, C., Harris, L. M., &Zerhusen, E. G. (2012). New federal policy initiatives to boost health literacy can help the nation move beyond the cycle of costly "crisis care." *Health Affairs, 31*(2), 434–443.

Matheny Antommaria, A. H., Gibb, T. S.McGuire, A. L., Root Wolpe, P., Wynia, M. K., Applewhite, et al. (2020). Ventilator triage policies during the COVID-19 pandemic at U.S. hospitals associated with members of the Association of Bioethics Program Directors. *Annals of Internal Medicine, 173*(3), 188–194. https://doi.org/10.7326/M20-1738

Navajo Department of Health. (2020). *COVID-19.* https://www.ndoh.navajo-nsn.gov/COVID-19

Office of Disease Prevention and Health Promotion. (2020). *Healthy People 2030 framework.* https://www.healthypeople.gov/2020/About-Healthy-People/Development-Healthy-People-2030/Framework

Primary Care Collaborative. (2020). *Defining the medical home.* https://www.pcpcc.org/about/medical-home

Real, K., Fay, L., Isaacs, K., Carll-White, A., & Schadler, A. (2018). Using systems theory to examine client and nurse structures, processes, and outcomes in centralized and decentralized units. *HERD:Health Environments Research and Design Journal, 11*(3), 22–37. https://doi.org/10.1177/1937586718763794

U.S. Census Bureau. (2020). *Demographic turning points for the United States: Population projections for 2020 to 2060.* https://www.census.gov/content/dam/Census/library/publications/2020/demo/p25-1144.pdf

U.S. Department of Health and Human Services (DHHS). (n.d.). *How organ allocation works.* Organ Procurement and Transplantation Network (OPTN). https://optn.transplant.hrsa.gov/learn/about-transplantation/how-organ-allocation-works/

U.S. Department of Health and Human Services. (2020a). *JumpSTART algorithm for pediatric victims.* https://chemm.nlm.nih.gov/startpediatric.htm

U.S. Department of Health and Human Services. (2020b).*START adult triage algorithm.* https://chemm.nlm.nih.gov/startadult.htm

U.S. Department of Homeland Security. (2020). *Community emergency response teams.* https://www.ready.gov/cert

World Health Organization (WHO). (1998). *Health promotion glossary.* http://whqlibdoc.who.int/hq/1998/WHO_HPR_HEP_98.1.pdf.

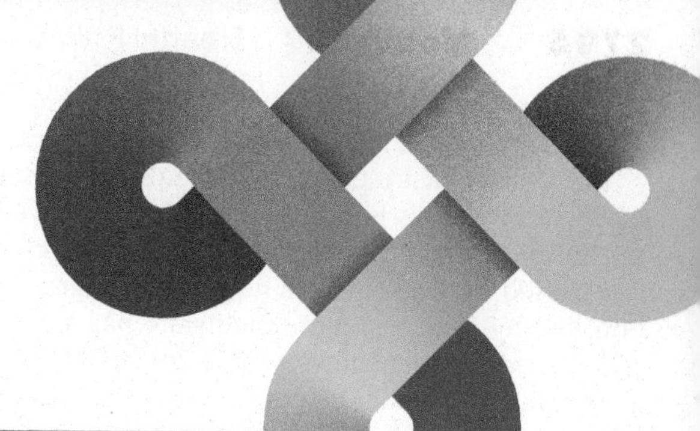

Module 47
Health Policy

Module Outline and Learning Outcomes

The Concept of Health Policy

Overview of Health Policy

47.1 Describe health policy, as an entity and as a process.

Developing Health Policies

47.2 Summarize the process of developing health policies.

Concepts Related to Health Policy

47.3 Outline the relationship between health policy and other concepts.

Federal, State, Local, and International Agencies

47.4 Outline the agencies or organizations involved in oversight or influence of health policy.

Accrediting Bodies

47.5 Analyze the role of accrediting organizations in the advancement of health policy.

Professional Associations

47.6 Analyze professional organizations' influences on health policy.

Healthcare Funding

47.7 Analyze types of health insurance and the health policies that regulate reimbursement.

›› The Concept of Health Policy

Concept Key Terms

Accreditation, **2800**
Children's Health Insurance Program (CHIP), **2804**
Consumer-driven healthcare plan (CDHP), **2803**
Co-payment, **2802**
Domestic partner, **2802**
Executive branch agency, **2796**
Health maintenance organization (HMO), **2803**
Health policy, **2795**
Indemnity, **2803**
Law, **2795**
Medicaid, **2803**
Medicare, **2803**
Medigap policy, **2803**
Point-of-service (POS) plan, **2803**
Preferred-provider organization (PPO), **2803**
Primary care provider (PCP), **2803**
Regulation, **2795**

Health policies drive the availability, safety, and quality of the healthcare provided in the United States. A poorly constructed policy or the absence of a needed policy can have a significant negative impact on the health and well-being of individuals or whole populations. Professional nurses must understand how healthcare policy affects patients, their own practice, and the organizations in which they work. Every day, nurses see the public's healthcare needs and can envision how new or revised health policies could improve the quality and safety of healthcare. Nurses can influence change by working with public officials at the local, community, state, and national levels as representatives of their professional association or as individual citizens.

Overview of Health Policy

The term **health policy** refers to actions taken by government bodies and other societal actors to attain specific health-related goals. Health policies include laws, regulations, government agency guidelines, position statements, resolutions, judicial decrees, and budget priorities.

Public health policy is established in **law** (statute) and **regulation** (rules) at the federal or state levels and is therefore enforceable by the government agency responsible for implementing the policy. Public health policy is subject to influence by nongovernmental healthcare organizations and health professions associations, education accreditation agencies, and private citizens. Public health policies have powerful effects on healthcare delivery systems, the health and well-being of U.S. citizens, and professional nursing issues ranging from scope of practice and safe staffing to nursing education funding and universal access to health insurance.

Private agencies may also develop health policy. Policies generated by private associations representing the interests of healthcare organizations, health professions, or health professions education associations are not established in law or regulation. However, they may have a significant influence, either directly or indirectly, on public policy in the areas of healthcare practice, access, research, funding, and education.

Public healthcare policy is generally first established in law. Lawmaking is the purview of the legislative branch of government. On the federal level, a bill becomes a law when it is passed by votes in both houses of Congress and signed into law by the president. Each state has a similar procedure for passing state laws, which are signed into law by the governor. Presidential vetoes, executive orders, and judicial interpretations of law also have the force of law; courts may determine the outcome of health policy if laws are vague or controversial (Milstead & Short, 2019).

Once a law has been passed, an **executive branch agency** of the federal or state government is responsible for administering it. The Centers for Disease Control and Prevention (CDC, 2020), for example, is an executive branch agency authorized to implement laws to protect the public against exposure and spread of highly communicable diseases. State executive branch agencies include state health departments and state boards of nursing. A state health department may have jurisdiction over local health departments and boards of health, sanitarians, and vital statistics, among other responsibilities. Boards of nursing are authorized to implement the nurse practice act in their state and license or discipline license holders to protect the public.

Laws provide broad mandates and are written somewhat generally to provide flexibility and so they can withstand the test of time. Therefore, the laws that create public health policy and the laws that create executive branch agencies also give the administering executive branch agencies the authority to write regulations. Regulations provide the detail that describes how the executive branch agency will carry out the law. A regulation must always refer directly to the law it seeks to amplify, and an agency cannot write rules that exceed its statutory authority; the original intent of the legislature that created the law must be honored (**Figure 47.1** »).

Developing Health Policies

Public healthcare policies are the product of both government processes and political forces. The process often begins when legislators or leaders in executive branch health agencies commit to solve a problem or bridge a gap in services. Sometimes constituents bring problems or gaps to their legislators' attention. In other cases, special interest groups, such as health professions associations, raise awareness and begin to lobby for a new health policy. Some initial questions precede construction of a bill's first draft, such as the following:

- What population of citizens will benefit? Is it large or small? Is it underserved and economically disadvantaged?
- What is the anticipated cost of implementing the policy? Do the benefits outweigh the cost of implementation?
- Who are the stakeholders? Is there support for the policy? If not, what issues are in question?
- Is there a body of scientific evidence to support the efficacy of the policy? Are there similar models that have been successful?

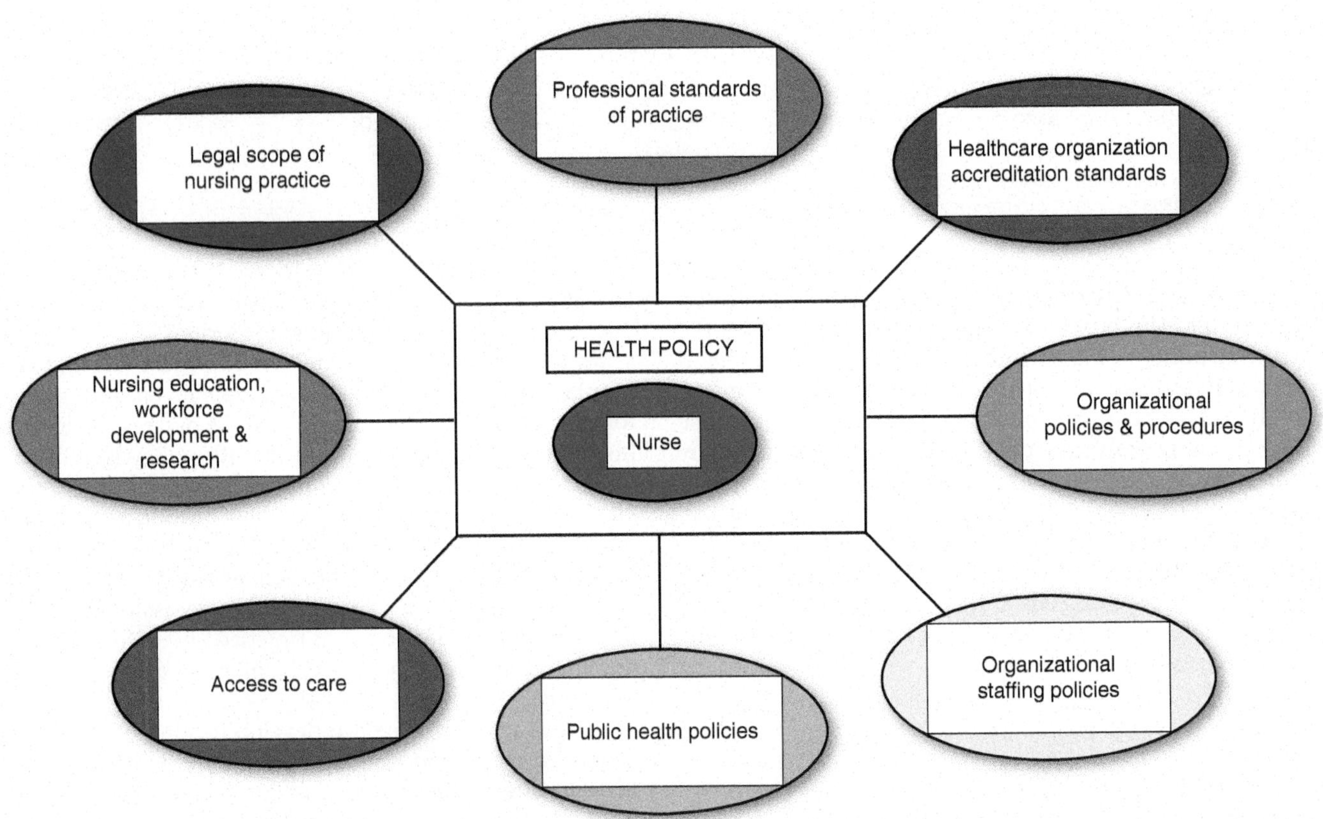

Figure 47.1 » Why is health policy relevant to nurses?

The four major stages in public policymaking are agenda setting, government response, implementation, and evaluation. In each stage, formal and informal relationships develop between stakeholders both inside and outside of government. Those serving in government positions can include legislators, bureaucrats such as regulatory officials, the president's or governor's staff, or the courts. Stakeholders outside government can include interested citizens who may or may not be constituents of specific legislators, institutions, and professional associations or other special interest groups.

How public policies are funded is also determined within a political framework. However, structured processes determine how money is allocated to fund governmental policies. For example, the federal budget process is formal and procedural, beginning with submission of a budget to Congress by the first Monday in February every year. Congress passes appropriations bills based on the president's recommendations and Congressional priorities, and if Congress does not pass all appropriations measures by the beginning of the fiscal year on October 1, it must enact a continuing resolution to keep the U.S. government running. The House and Senate Budget Committees have slightly different roles (U.S. Senate, n.d.); stakeholders may influence this process to attempt to gain funding for health policy agenda items as they would any other bill. An example of developing a health policy is described in **Box 47.1** ».

Concepts Related to Health Policy

A number of concepts in the Healthcare Domain relate to health policy. These include accountability, advocacy, ethics, healthcare systems, legal issues, quality improvement, and safety. A few of these integral to health policy are discussed in the Concepts Related to Health Policy feature. They are presented in alphabetical order.

Federal, State, Local, and International Agencies

Agencies with the authority to affect the health of citizens exist at the federal, state, local, and international levels. Their missions and scope of authority differ. Some have a broad scope of responsibility; others have very specific responsibilities. Some have extensive regulatory authority; others receive authority to enact programs from their parent departments.

Federal Agencies

Healthcare policies with direct effects on the nation's health are administered through the U.S. Department of Health and Human Services (DHHS) and the agencies it oversees. Other federal departments also administer policies that affect the nation's health. For example, the U.S. Department of Labor oversees policies that affect worker safety; these policies are administered through the Occupational Safety and Health Administration. The U.S. Environmental Protection Agency (2018) is responsible for protecting the environment; this also affects the nation's health.

U.S. Department of Health and Human Services

The DHHS is the principal federal health agency. It has 11 operating divisions (DHHS, 2015): Administration for Children and Families (ACF), Administration for Community Living (ACL), Agency for Healthcare Research and Quality (AHRQ), Agency for Toxic Substances and Disease Registry (ATSDR), Centers for Disease Control and Prevention (CDC), Centers for Medicare & Medicaid Services (CMS), U.S. Food and Drug Administration (FDA), Health Resources and Services Administration (HRSA), Indian Health Service (IHS), National Institutes of Health (NIH), and Substance Abuse and Mental Health Services Administration (SAMHSA).

Box 47.1

Developing an Evidence-Informed Health Policy: An Example

Evidence-based practice models provide processes to address clinical problems and improve healthcare outcomes. The same processes can be used to address health policy problems. For example, opioid and heroin abuse is a significant public health problem that has reached epidemic proportions in the United States. A specific issue is that individuals who overdose on opioids are often in respiratory and cardiac arrest when EMS arrives. EMS personnel administer naloxone (Narcan) onsite, but the time between the cardiopulmonary arrest and naloxone administration may be too long to ensure a positive outcome for the individual. The literature demonstrates:

1. Individuals with an opioid addiction are at particularly high risk for overdose immediately following rehabilitation, when their tolerance has been reduced.
2. Individuals who are most likely to be in the vicinity of the person who is overdosing are family or close friends, who may or may not have emergency medical training, supplies, or equipment.
3. The safety profile on naloxone suggests that it is about as safe for laypeople to administer as is epinephrine during anaphylaxis.

Using an evidence-informed health policy process, policymakers and stakeholders would examine the external evidence (including scientific evidence that naloxone is safe for administration by non-healthcare personnel), combine the evidence with their issue expertise (discussions with and testimony from stakeholders, professional experts, etc.), and combine that with lawmaker and stakeholder values and ethics (e.g., the value of making lifesaving naloxone available to those in a position to administer naloxone when it will be most effective: family and friends of individuals addicted to opioids) (Loversidge, 2016). This process can help to inform the dialogue necessary for the drafting of lifesaving legislation or other policies that will permit family and friends of persons addicted to opioids to have a dose of naloxone on hand, the training to administer the drug, and the education to understand the importance of follow-up by calling EMS. For example, in 2018, North Carolina's state health director issued a standing order permitting pharmacists in that state to dispense naloxone to individuals at risk for opiate-related overdose or their family members or friends upon request (North Carolina Department of Health and Human Services, 2020).

Concepts Related to Health Policy

CONCEPT	RELATIONSHIP TO HEALTH POLICY	NURSING IMPLICATIONS
Healthcare Systems	Access to healthcare is directly related to insurability. The Affordable Care Act changed the profile of insurability for millions of previously uninsured adults and children who would otherwise have been unable to afford healthcare insurance. Public health policies direct coding, billing, and reimbursement for care, which in turn may affect how care is provided and documented.	■ Nurses may find that insured individuals use primary care services more often. Continuity of care may improve for them, especially for individuals with chronic conditions. ■ Health policies related to managed care may have a variety of impacts on patients' healthcare. For example, one patient's health insurance plan may cover brand name (also called proprietary) prescription medication with a small co-payment. A patient on another plan might have a much higher co-payment for a brand name prescription; the nurse may need to work with the prescribing provider to ensure that the patient receives a prescription for the more cost-effective generic medication.
Legal Issues	The U.S. Constitution grants states the authority to govern selected professions such as nursing, medicine, and pharmacy. Authority to enforce the laws, known as practice acts, is granted to executive branch agencies, such as boards of nursing, or in some states, to an "umbrella board" that includes a division responsible for oversight of nursing.	■ Current licensure is required for practice as a nurse. Nurses are held accountable for knowing the legal nursing scope of practice in their state and what actions could place their licensure status in jeopardy. State boards of nursing also have authority to write regulations to amplify the practice act. Regulations typically address standards of safe and competent practice, delegation, and continuing education requirements. Nurses must know and comply with these regulations.
Quality Improvement	Some public health policies are enacted to advance science, translate science to practice, and support national health imperatives. The Agency for Healthcare Research and Quality (AHRQ), an agency of the Public Health Service in the U.S. Department of Health and Human Services, is responsible for improving the safety and quality of America's healthcare system. It develops knowledge, tools, and data needed to improve healthcare systems and help policymakers, healthcare professionals, and citizens make informed health decisions.	■ Nurses are accountable for competent, safe patient care. Part of that responsibility is becoming engaged in organizational quality improvement and quality management projects at the unit level or the organization committee level. Joint Commission–accredited hospitals typically use AHRQ quality indicators specific to their setting, which can provide helpful means to reach The Joint Commission National Patient Safety Goals and other quality improvement objectives.

The DHHS is a powerful agency that administers more grant dollars than all other federal agencies combined. The FY 2021 budget proposed $94.5 billion in discretionary budget authority and $1.3 trillion in mandatory funding, allocated to fund its 11 operating divisions and 8 agencies (DHHS, 2020).

» **Stay Current:** To learn more about the programs and services of the U.S. Department of Health and Human Services, go to http://www.hhs.gov/programs/index.html.

Occupational Safety and Health Administration

The Occupational Safety and Health Administration (OSHA), an agency of the U.S. Department of Labor, is tasked with ensuring the health and safety of Americans in the workplace. OSHA legislation covers most private-sector employers and their workers plus some employers and workers in the public sector. Part of OSHA's mission is to provide assistance to employers, who are responsible for providing a safe workplace and for reducing or eliminating workplace hazards. OSHA standards address a wide variety of hazards in industrial and healthcare workplaces (**Figure 47.2** »). One example is the availability of emergency eyewash stations (U.S. Department of Labor, n.d.).

» **Stay Current:** Go to www.osha.gov for the latest information from the Occupational Safety and Health Administration.

State Health Agencies

Each state mandates its own health policies and regulations in accord with federal policies and regulations. Each state has its own division or department of health and human services, with a scope of responsibility determined by that state. These departments generally report to the state's governor and are part of the executive branch of state government. State health departments are generally organized according to their core public health responsibilities, which include prevention

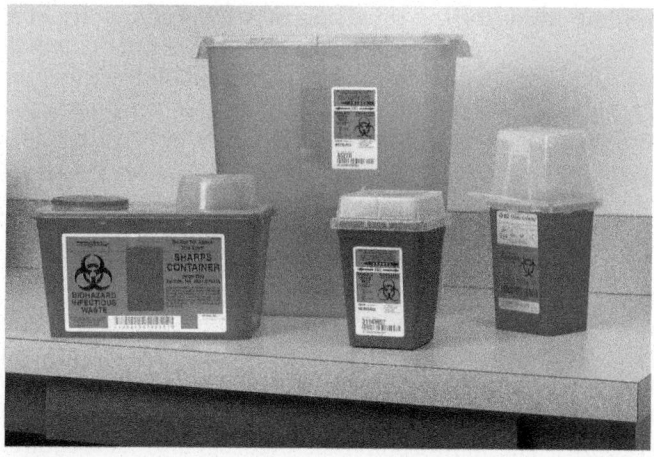

Figure 47.2 ⟫ OSHA regulations require use of sharps containers for discarding used needles.
Source: Michal Heron/Pearson Education, Inc.

and control of the spread of infectious disease, coordinating responses to events that threaten the public's health, building strong communities that can live disease and injury free, and addressing health inequities and disparities (Ohio Department of Health, n.d.). State health departments may also enforce county health department regulations and may license or register healthcare facilities such as hospitals and long-term care facilities, child care centers, clinical laboratories, and other service providers (such as portable x-ray suppliers). State health departments may also be responsible for overseeing the planning and construction of medical facilities and for receiving and resolving complaints about the facilities they regulate. They are often responsible for tracking state health data and statistics; maintaining birth, death, marriage, and divorce records; and enforcing statewide health laws, such as smoking bans. During disease outbreaks, they organize contact tracing efforts, and collect and analyze statewide tracking data.

State offices of emergency medical services (OEMSs) may be structurally connected to a larger state department, such as a state department of public safety. OEMSs are usually responsible for establishing training and certification standards for EMS personnel, accrediting training programs, overseeing the state's trauma system, and/or licensing medical transportation services. By ensuring that local EMS systems comply with the applicable regulations, OEMSs provide citizens access to high-quality emergency medical care.

Local Health Departments

At the county or municipal level, local departments of health administer health policies and offer many vital services to their communities. In counties that surround cities with large populations, both county and city health departments may exist, often with a division of responsibility. For example, the county health department may be responsible for regulating health issues with widespread effects, such as sanitation, retail food establishment safety, and waste disposal. City health departments may provide clinical, environmental, health promotion, and population-based services such as free clinics, sexual health, HIV/AIDs testing, and tuberculosis and dental clinics. City health departments are often responsible for developing and enforcing citywide health codes and for disease monitoring.

Local departments of health may oversee child care center sanitation and food safety and typically offer community-wide disease and injury prevention programs, which may be federally supported or arise in response to local issues. Such programs include injury prevention campaigns, lead poisoning prevention efforts, and making safety equipment such as smoke detectors, children's bicycle helmets, and infant car seats available to families at no cost. Local social services departments are typically responsible for administering Medicaid, the Child Health Insurance Program (CHIP), and the Women, Infants, and Children (WIC) supplemental nutrition program, which provides food assistance to pregnant women and children under age 5 who are at risk for malnutrition (**Figure 47.3** ⟫).

In the event of a disease outbreak, local health departments collect and analyze data to track and prevent infection spread. They may cooperate with the state health department to facilitate contact tracing. Surveillance and monitoring are essential tools that help health departments, both local and state, identify outbreaks and prevent greater numbers of the population from becoming infected.

Clinical Example A

Richard Taylor is a 46-year-old man who works as an assistant to social workers in a residential homeless shelter in an underserved area of the city. An increasing number of shelter residents have been showing symptoms of active tuberculosis (TB). Social workers have been sending these individuals to the free clinic associated with the shelter for treatment. Now Mr. Taylor and his coworkers have become concerned about their own risk, even though they have taken measures to quickly identify residents at risk and work appropriately with them. Mr. Taylor finds that his city health department does not conduct TB screening, so he seeks screening at a local drugstore with a nurse-managed clinic. He tests positive for TB.

Critical Thinking Questions

1. What information should the nurse practitioner have at hand to assist Mr. Taylor to access low-cost or free treatment?
2. What recommendations could the nurse make to Mr. Taylor to advocate for improved TB risk exposure prevention for employees and residents at the homeless shelter?

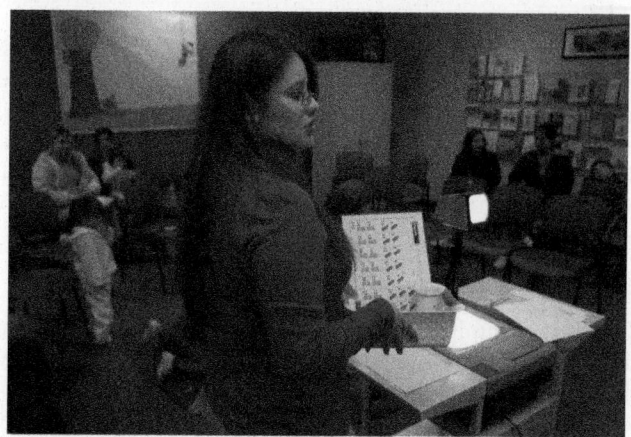

Figure 47.3 ⟫ An instructor uses a doll to demonstrate breastfeeding techniques to a group of women in a WIC program.
Source: The Sacramento Bee/Anne Chadwick Wil/ZUMA Press, Inc./Alamy Stock Photo.

International Health Agencies

International health organizations fall into three groups, depending on their funding sources and location: multilateral organizations, bilateral organizations, and nongovernmental organizations (NGOs). International health organizations typically provide support services and establish guiding policy. All the major multilateral organizations are part of the United Nations (UN). The premier international health organization is the World Health Organization, which is an intergovernmental agency related to the UN and is the only international health organization with legal authority. Bilateral agencies are governmental agencies with a home in a single country, such as the U.S. Agency for International Development (USAID). They provide aid to developing countries. NGOs, also known as private voluntary organizations (PVOs), are independent of any government. More than 1.5 million NGOs operate in the United States (U.S. Department of State, 2017). NGOs promote economic growth, human rights, social progress, and deliver assistance across the globe (USAID, 2019). Examples include Project Hope (2020), which provides essential medicine and supplies, volunteers, medical training, and disaster response; and World Central Kitchen (2020), which organizes emergency food relief in communities around the world.

Accrediting Bodies

Accreditation is a process of gaining recognition through a peer-review process that evaluates the quality of an organization based on the standards and criteria of the accreditation organization. Reputable accreditation organizations establish standards using a rigorous evidence-based process. Whereas state or federal licensing or certification is governmental, accreditation is private and voluntary; but achieving accreditation certifies that the organization meets quality criteria and is competent to provide the services or programs it offers. Accredited organizations must be reevaluated at intervals specified by the accrediting body. To achieve reaccreditation, an organization must provide evidence that it has continuously evaluated its own performance, has acted to correct deficiencies and continuously improved its performance, and continues to meet the accreditation standards.

The accreditation body conducts an on-site survey to validate the organization's self-assessment and performance and to determine whether the organization meets the required standards. This occurs at the initial accreditation visit and during periodic reaccreditation visits. Benefits of accreditation and the nurse's role in the process depend on the type of accreditation.

The Joint Commission

The Joint Commission is an independent, nonprofit organization that sets standards for and accredits healthcare provider (HCP) organizations, such as ambulatory care centers, behavioral HCPs, hospitals, and long-term care facilities. Its standards form the basis for the objective evaluation of healthcare organizations with the aim of measuring, assessing, and improving performance. Its standards focus on patient, individual, or resident care and organization functions that are important for the provision of safe, high-quality care (The Joint Commission, 2020a). Healthcare organizations are highly motivated to achieve accreditation by The Joint Commission, which brings not only greater consumer trust and respectability, but also credibility with private third-party payers, and helps organizations meet qualifications for Medicare and Medicaid reimbursement.

Although The Joint Commission is an independent, nongovernmental organization, its work significantly influences national quality and safety standards and the advancement of healthcare policy. For example, since 2003, The Joint Commission (2020b) has identified annual National Patient Safety Goals (NPSGs) (see Module 51, Safety) to help accredited organizations address specific patient safety concerns. The Joint Commission (2020c) also has requirements for reporting sentinel events (see Module 50, Quality Improvement). The NPSGs and the Sentinel Event reporting system provide benchmarks for quality improvement processes in healthcare organizations across the country.

A nurse's role in The Joint Commission accreditation process may include helping to develop, revise, or facilitate use of policies and procedures for nursing practice that are current and evidence based. The nurse may also participate in an organization's self-review activities. Nurses, especially those in management positions, may also be part of meetings with the accreditation survey team; survey teams are often interested in speaking with the HCPs who are most involved in maintaining standards at the point of care.

» **Stay Current:** Go to www.jointcommission.org for the latest information from The Joint Commission.

Clinical Example B

Darren Langdon is a 34-year-old staff RN on a medical–surgical unit in a hospital classified by The Joint Commission as a Critical Access Hospital. The nursing department has been preparing for The Joint Commission reaccreditation survey visit. Unrelated to the visit, Darren's unit has been concerned about the rate of catheter-associated urinary tract infections (CAUTIs). He has taken the lead in gathering data about the CAUTI rates on his unit compared to other units over the past 6 months, has done a review of the hospital's policies and procedures, has talked to the nurses on his unit about how they implement these, and has conducted a review of the current literature on CAUTIs. Having learned that the current hospital policy is outdated in comparison to what he found in the literature, Darren has been encouraged by the nurse manager, his fellow staff members, and nursing leadership to draft a new evidence-based policy to present to the hospital's policy and procedure committee.

The Joint Commission survey visitors come to Darren's unit during a reaccreditation survey visit. They have noticed the data on the CAUTI rates and are asking the nurse manager and staff to respond to questions about possible causes and actions. Darren's nurse manager asks him to meet with her and the visitors to discuss the unit's process and plan to address the CAUTI rates, at both the unit and organizational levels.

Critical Thinking Questions

1. What should Darren be aware of with regard to the National Patient Safety Goals? Is there a NPSG related to CAUTIs?
2. How should Darren explain to the survey visitors the process he used to address the CAUTI problem on his unit?

Nursing Education Program Accreditation

Although nursing program accreditation is considered voluntary, most graduate nursing programs and many RN-to-BSN programs require applicants to graduate from an accredited prelicensure/BSN program as a criterion for admission. The Commission on Collegiate Nursing Education (CCNE; 2020), an autonomous accrediting agency affiliated with the American Association of Colleges of Nursing (AACN; 2020), accredits baccalaureate and graduate education programs. The Accreditation Commission for Education in Nursing (ACEN) accredits all types of nursing education programs, including clinical doctorate, master's degree, baccalaureate degree, associate degree, diploma, and practical nursing education programs. The National League for Nursing Commission for Nursing Education Accreditation (NLN CNEA) was established in 2013. In the spring of 2016, the NLN CNEA issued standards of accreditation for practical nursing/vocational nursing, diploma, associate, bachelor, master's, and clinical doctorate degree programs. CNEA is an autonomous accreditation division of NLN (2020a).

National accreditation is separate from state board of nursing "approval," which is mandatory for prelicensure programs in every state. That is, nursing programs granting a degree that will qualify the graduate to take the NCLEX-RN or NCLEX-PN exam must have state board of nursing approval.

Professional Associations

Nursing associations exist to serve their specialized membership and advance the nursing profession. Professional nursing associations define standards of practice and professional behaviors, establish codes of ethics for their members, support nursing research, and participate in policy development at a level commensurate with the scope of their membership.

Examples of international and national professional associations can be found in **Table 47.1** ». Some national associations represent all registered nurses in the category they serve; others serve one of the many special-interest memberships. A number of national associations have state "branch" (sometimes called "state constituent") associations as well. The missions of these organizations include advocacy, education, provision of networking opportunities, and strengthening professional identities among members. Examples of specialty practice associations include the Academy of Medical-Surgical Nurses; the American Assisted Living Nurses Association; the American Association of Critical-Care Nurses; the National Association of Orthopaedic Nurses; and the Oncology Nursing Society. Professional associations for the four categories of advanced practice nurses (APRNs) also exist, such as the American Association of Nurse Practitioners, the National Association of Clinical Nurse Specialists, American College of Nurse-Midwives, and American Association of Nurse Anesthetists. Additionally, APRNs have access to professional associations specific to their subspecialties, for example, the National Association of Neonatal Nurse Practitioners.

TABLE 47.1 International and National Professional Associations

Professional Association	Membership and Focus Areas
International Council of Nurses (ICN)	■ Federation of more than 130 national nurses' associations ■ Represents nurses in more than 130 countries worldwide ■ World's oldest organization for health professionals ■ Has identified three key program areas: professional practice, regulation, and socioeconomic welfare (ICN, 2020)
Sigma Theta Tau International (STTI)	■ More than 135,000 active members in more than 100 countries and territories ■ Founded in 1922 by six nurses at Indiana University ■ Mission focused on developing nurse leaders anywhere to improve healthcare everywhere (STTI, 2020)
American Nurses Association (ANA)	■ Represents the more than 4 million registered nurses in the United States and U.S. territories ■ Exists to advance the nursing profession ■ The ANA establishes and publishes nursing standards of practice, the *Code of Ethics for Nurses*, and numerous other policies and guidelines related to nursing practice. ■ States have "branch" associations, affiliated with ANA (2020)
National Student Nurses Association (NSNA)	■ Mentors nursing students who are applying for initial licensure as registered nurses ■ Membership provides opportunities for workshop participation, networking, scholarships, and career planning (NSNA, 2020).
American Association of Colleges of Nursing (AACN)	■ "The national voice for America's baccalaureate and graduate nursing education" (AACN, 2020) ■ Membership consists of over 840 member schools of nursing (baccalaureate, graduate, and postgraduate programs) ■ Policy focus includes nursing education, research, and nursing workforce development
National League for Nursing (NLN)	■ First nursing organization in the United States ■ Membership consists of nursing education programs, nursing faculty, nursing students, and nursing leaders ■ Focused on building a strong and diverse nursing workforce ■ States have "branch" associations that are affiliated with NLN (2020b) ■ Public policy efforts focus on influencing policies that affect nursing workforce development, nursing education, and healthcare for underserved populations (NLN, 2019)

Several professional nursing associations exist to support and promote the interests of special nursing profession demographics. These include the Asian American/Pacific Islander Nurses Association, the American Assembly for Men in Nursing, the National Black Nurses Association, and the National Association of Hispanic Nurses.

Clinical Example C

Marsha Johnson, RN, BSN, graduated from a university college of nursing 10 years ago. Three years ago, she decided to continue her education and applied to an accredited certified registered nurse anesthetist (CRNA) program. She completed the program, passed the national certification exam, and was hired by a small-volume ambulatory surgery center. Ms. Johnson competently delivers care and enjoys her advanced practice role. She works with an anesthesiologist but is the only CRNA on staff. Ms. Johnson recently realized that as a nurse anesthetist, she has a limited number of professional contacts with other nurses employed at the center and that because the surgery center requires only one nurse anesthetist, she will not have many opportunities for interaction with peers or on-site educational opportunities specific to her role. She is starting to feel isolated.

Critical Thinking Questions

1. What professional association would you recommend to Ms. Johnson to fulfill her need for peers and CRNA-specific continuing education?
2. What networking and support are available from this association?
3. Where else could Ms. Johnson go for professional support?

Healthcare Funding

Perhaps the most important issue in health policy today is how healthcare is funded. Healthcare has historically been considered a market-based commodity in the United States. The sweeping social welfare legislation embodied in the Social Security Act of 1935 did not include healthcare coverage for all Americans. BlueCross BlueShield (2020), the earliest private insurance plans, were developed through the 1930s and 1940s and have grown from hospital and medical plans to encompass comprehensive coverage. With the advent of private insurance, the political pressure to enact government-operated health insurance was diffused. No progress was made on this issue until 1965, when the federal government entered healthcare financing with Medicare and Medicaid (Centers for Medicare & Medicaid Services, 2020). Despite innovative changes over time, the problem of uninsured Americans remains a persistent problem (Kaiser Family Foundation, 2019b).

Health insurance in the United States is available through private insurance companies and through government-funded programs for those who qualify. As part of the Affordable Care Act (ACA) passed by Congress in 2010, many individuals who did not qualify for Medicare or Medicaid and who would otherwise not have had access to health insurance gained improved access to health insurance coverage. Access to health insurance for individuals who do not qualify for Medicare or Medicaid or who do not have employer-based health insurance coverage varies from state to state and depends on policies enacted by state legislatures and Congress.

Private Healthcare System

Any health insurance not funded by government is private health insurance. Individuals purchase private health insurance plans to protect themselves from all or some of the medical, surgical, and preventive care expenses they would incur without coverage. The three basic private insurance plan types are employer-sponsored insurance, self-employment-based plans, and direct-purchase plans. There are also private insurance policies to supplement Medicare coverage.

Employment-sponsored insurance (ESI) is offered through an individual's employer or union. A recent study by the Commonwealth Fund found that 45% of adults ages 19 to 64 are inadequately insured, and that the greatest deterioration in both quality and comprehensiveness of coverage is related to changes in employer-sponsored plans (Collins, Bhupal, & Doty, 2019). Large employers usually purchase health insurance plans that offer healthcare coverage to eligible company employees. ESI coverage may be extended to include the spouse, dependents, or domestic partner of the employee. A **domestic partner** is an unmarried partner of the same or different sex. Group coverage may also be purchased through voluntary and membership associations, such as professional and trade groups, bar associations, local chambers of commerce, and AARP. Benefits of group health insurance, especially when provided by large employers, may include lower premium costs (the amount of money paid for insurance coverage) and better coverage for eligible employees and their families. The employer may pay nothing toward the premium or may make partial or full payment; the employee is responsible for the premium amount not paid by the employer. The insured may also be responsible for additional costs such as deductibles, coinsurance, and co-payments. A Kaiser Family Foundation (2019a) annual survey of employer-sponsored family coverage premiums discovered a 5% increase from 2018 to 2019, with average premiums reaching over $20,000 annually, of which employees paid (on average) $6,000. Premiums are different from **co-payments**, a set amount paid at the time of service (e.g., $20 for a primary-care physician office visit). Co-payments for specialty care are usually higher than those for primary care. An out-of-pocket maximum protects the patient from catastrophic healthcare costs; if medical expenses reach a certain amount during a 12-month period, the plan covers all usual and customary fees for the remainder of the year.

Self-employment-based health insurance coverage is available only to individuals who are self-employed, and only the policyholder is covered by the plan. Individuals who are self-employed and have chronic health conditions often experience difficulty trying to purchase health insurance through private insurers.

An individual who needs private health insurance and is ineligible for group coverage purchases an individual policy. The individual purchasing an individual plan is responsible for paying the premium as well as co-payments and deductibles. Individual health insurance policies are usually more expensive and coverage is more restricted than under group health coverage. A medical examination may be required to determine eligibility, and individuals with preexisting medical conditions may find it difficult to find a company that will provide health insurance.

Types of Private Health Insurance Plans

Health insurance plans offered in the United States range from health maintenance organizations, the most restrictive type, to indemnity plans (also known as "fee-for-service" plans), the least restrictive. Plans in the middle of the spectrum are point-of-service (POS) plans and preferred provider organizations (PPOs); both are considered managed-care plans and include features of both HMO and indemnity coverage. Usually, a greater selection of in-network providers is available in PPO and POS options than in HMOs.

Health maintenance organizations (HMOs) are insurance plans that limit coverage to care from physicians who contract with the specific HMO. Out-of-network care is not generally covered except in emergencies. HMOs may require that the person live or work in the service area. Participants must often select a **primary care provider (PCP)**, who serves as the gatekeeper to care and refers the patient to in-network hospitals and specialists when additional care is needed. HMOs typically provide a broad range of healthcare benefits; they often provide integrated care, covering preventive care and wellness.

A **preferred-provider organization (PPO)** does not require the insured to select a PCP. PPOs usually have larger networks of providers than HMOs and provide financial incentives that encourage insured persons to seek care from in-network providers. PPOs are less restrictive than HMOs but typically have higher co-payments.

A **point-of-service (POS) plan** is a hybrid of an HMO and a PPO. Each time insured individuals seek healthcare, they decide which option—HMO or PPO—to use. Members pay less if they use in-network physicians, hospitals, and other HCPs. If they opt to use out-of-network providers, they pay higher co-payments, coinsurance, and deductibles. The advantages of the POS plan are its flexibility and freedom of choice in comparison with a traditional HMO.

Indemnity plans allow the insured to self-select HCPs; that is, there is no network. These plans may use some managed-care techniques to control costs (e.g., preauthorization of MRIs).

The **consumer-driven healthcare plan (CDHP)** is a type of employer-sponsored coverage that combines a private insurance plan with a health savings account (HSA) or health reimbursement account (HRA). This type of plan typically has a higher deductible but lower monthly premiums. As part of the plan, the employer offers HSA or HRA accounts to all employees. Employees then save money in the HSA or HRA so that they can pay for deductibles and noncovered services. In some cases, the amount that goes into the HSA or HRA is provided by the employer as part of the employee benefits package.

Medigap Policies

A **Medigap policy** (i.e., Medicare supplemental insurance) is private health insurance designed to supplement Medicare coverage. These policies may pay co-payments, coinsurance, deductibles, and "gaps" in Medicare coverage (i.e., noncovered healthcare costs). If an individual has a Medigap policy, Medicare will pay its share first; then the Medigap policy will pay its share. Medigap policies are required to comply with federal and state laws and must be transparent in stating they are "Medicare Supplement Insurance." State laws designate the letters by which these policies can identify themselves.

Publicly Funded Healthcare

CMS is the federal agency and public funding system responsible for administering Medicare, Medicaid, and CHIP. Other public funding systems include the Veteran's Administration (VA); the Defense Health Program (TRICARE) for military personnel, their families, and military retirees; the Indian Health Service, which covers American Indians and Alaskan Natives; and the Federal Employees Health Benefits (FEHB) Program, which covers federal employees. Federally funded healthcare is subject to relevant federal legislation.

Medicare

Medicare is a federally funded health insurance program available to people age 65 and older who have worked in a Medicare-covered employment setting, younger people with disabilities, and people with end-stage renal disease or amyotrophic lateral sclerosis. Medicare covers 17.9% of Americans (U.S. Census Bureau, 2019). Four types of coverage are available through Medicare (**Box 47.2** »).

Medicare does not cover all medical expenses. Excluded services include long-term care, routine dental and eye care, hearing aids and the exams for fitting them, and cosmetic surgery. People often purchase Medigap policies from private companies to supplement or fill in the gaps in their Medicare coverage.

» **Stay Current:** For additional information about CMS and its programs, visit http://www.cms.hhs.gov.

Medicaid

Medicaid was established in 1965 under Title 19 of the Social Security Act. It is available to certain lower-income individuals and families, older adults, and people with disabilities who meet the eligibility requirements. Medicaid is jointly funded and administered by states and the federal government. Each state sets its own guidelines regarding eligibility and covered services, which are then matched by federal funding. Federal mandates require coverage of certain services (e.g., hospitalization, physician services, laboratory services, radiology studies, preventive services, prenatal care, nursing home and home health services, and medically necessary transportation). The federal match enables states to ensure comprehensive health coverage for as many of their residents as possible (Kaiser Family Foundation, 2020a). In 2014, the ACA changed the Medicaid eligibility requirements to allow more people to qualify. Also, the ACA offers additional community-based care programs as an alternative to nursing home care.

Supplemental Security Income

Supplemental Security Income (SSI) is a federal and state public assistance program funded by general taxes. SSI is designed to help older adults and people who are blind or disabled who have little or no income, including children who are blind and disabled. It provides cash for basic needs such as food, clothing, and housing.

Box 47.2

The Different Parts of Medicare

Medicare Part A (Hospital Insurance)

- Helps to cover inpatient care in hospitals.
- Helps to cover home healthcare and care in skilled nursing facilities and hospice.
- The covered individual must be age 65 or older, and either the individual or the individual's spouse must have been employed in a Medicare-covered employment setting and paid Medicare taxes for at least 10 years. Co-payments, coinsurance, or deductibles may apply.

Medicare Part B (Medical Insurance)

- Helps to cover medically necessary services provided by physicians and other HCPs, outpatient care, home healthcare, and durable medical equipment.
- Coverage includes partial payment for office visits to physicians and other HCPs; outpatient services, including screening exams such as mammograms and colonoscopies; and preventive services such as flu shots.
- All individuals covered by Medicare Part B pay an annual deductible and a 20% co-payment; the remaining covered costs are paid by Medicare.

Medicare Part C (Medicare Advantage Plans)

- A health coverage option run by private insurance companies approved by and under contract with Medicare.
- Includes all services covered under Parts A and B, usually includes Plan D prescription drug coverage, and may cover other services such as hearing and vision testing.
- Medicare pays the insurer for each individual enrolled in the plan. The insured must cover out-of-pocket expenses, including the Part B premium, an additional premium to the company providing the coverage, and applicable co-payments.

Medicare Part D (Medicare Prescription Drug Coverage)

- A prescription drug option run by private insurance companies, such as HMOs and PPOs, approved by and under contract with Medicare.
- May help lower prescription drug costs and help protect against higher costs in the future.

Source: Data from Centers for Medicare & Medicaid Services (n.d.).

Children's Health Insurance Program

Federal and matching state funding combine to provide the **Children's Health Insurance Program (CHIP)**, previously known as the State Child Health Insurance Program. CHIP provides health insurance coverage to children under the age of 19 whose families earn more than the Medicaid limits but cannot afford to purchase private healthcare coverage. Within broad federal guidelines, each state determines the design of its program, eligibility requirements, benefit packages, payment levels for coverage, and administrative and operating procedures. Federal requirements mandate that states include routine checkups, immunizations, dental and vision care, inpatient and outpatient hospital care, and laboratory and x-ray services in their benefits.

State-Funded Healthcare

State governments may administer programs targeting specific public health priorities, which are funded by either states or localities, frequently in combination with federal grants. Examples include maternal and child health, smoking cessation, obesity prevention, HIV/AIDS, substance abuse, and environmental health. In addition, state governments have a degree of responsibility for oversight related to the regulation of health insurance, HCPs, and public health activities.

Local-/County-Level Healthcare

In many states, local and county governments may fund public health initiatives or programs. Some local governments fund indigent care by subsidizing and running public hospitals and clinics. Two examples are New York City's Health and Hospital's Corporation and Chicago's Cook County Hospital. These hospitals, which serve individuals regardless of their ability to pay, also receive a large amount of operating money from Medicaid and Medicare. Therefore, health policy at the federal and local/county levels plays a part in shaping the funding models for these subsidized institutions.

The Affordable Care Act

The ACA included a number of provisions that reformed the health insurance market. These included measures to ensure that consumers receive value for the cost of their premiums, restricts insurers from charging unreasonable health insurance premiums, and holds insurance companies accountable for unjustified premium increases. In addition, the ACA banned annual dollar limits on essential coverage such as hospitals, physician, and pharmacy benefits; required that children of the insured be covered until they turn 26 years old; required new health plans to cover certain evidence-based preventive services and eliminate cost sharing for those services; and made it possible for Americans with preexisting conditions to gain and keep their coverage. The ACA included many additional provisions that benefit the consumer and requires health insurers to provide fair, equitable coverage and transparency of information.

From the beginning, the ACA met with controversy and experienced a troubled implementation period (see the Focus on Diversity and Culture feature). However, as of January 2017, more than 20 million previously uninsured individuals had gained healthcare insurance coverage through the provisions of the ACA (Greenberg, 2017; Levey, 2017). Since then, the ACA has faced a number of stumbling blocks as well as lawsuits challenging its validity. At the end of 2019, an estimated 11% of people in the United States (some 35 million Americans) still did not have health insurance (Cohen et al., 2020).

Focus on Diversity and Culture

The Affordable Care Act: Narrowing the Disparity Divide

The options afforded by the ACA provided an opportunity to narrow disparities in healthcare coverage that have long existed. Between the law's enactment in 2010 and 2016, coverage rates increased for all underserved racial and ethnic groups. The largest increases occurred following the 2014 implementation of the ACA Medicaid and Marketplace coverage expansions. The greatest impact in the uninsured rate was in the Hispanic population, which saw a reduction in the uninsured rate from 32.6% to 19.1% between the years 2010 and 2016. Other groups of color (including Black, Asian, and Native populations) experienced larger percentage point decreases in their uninsured rates as well, compared to white people over the same time period.

However, coverage gains stalled and started a reversal beginning in 2017 and continuing into 2018. As of 2018, most groups of color are still less likely to be insured compared to white people, with Hispanic populations 2.5 times more likely to be uninsured than white people during the period from 2010 to 2018. Furthermore, uninsured Black people are more likely to be affected by coverage gaps in states that have not expanded Medicaid. Additional disparities continue to persist, despite continuation of the ACA and the late adoption of Medicaid expansion by states such as Missouri (Artiga, Orgera, & Damico, 2020).

Since the ACA was enacted, several changes to the law have occurred. These include (1) the individual mandate requiring that all U.S. residents have health insurance or pay a penalty was eliminated; (2) payments from the federal government to insurers to motivate them to stay in the ACA insurance exchanges and help keep premiums down (called cost-sharing reduction subsidies) have ended; (3) access to short-term insurance "skinny" plans, which are less expansive but do not offer full protection, have expanded; and (4) employers and universities may now opt out of the ACA requirement to provide access to contraceptive care on the basis of religious or moral objections. (For more and current information on the ACA, see Kaiser Family Foundation, 2020b.)

REVIEW The Concept of Health Policy

RELATE Link the Concepts

Linking the concept of health policy with the concept of ethics:

1. How does enacting evidence-based policies or legislation align with ethical standards of nursing?
2. Which federal law protects patient privacy?

Linking the concept of health policy with the concept of legal issues:

3. Explore the board of nursing website in your state and find the section of law or rules related to the nurse's accountability for patient care and safety. What nursing actions or protective measures promote compliance with those sections of law or rule?

Linking the concept of health policy with the concept of safety:

4. Review The Joint Commission National Patient Safety Goals. Choose one that is relevant to a clinical area in which you have recently had experience. What nursing actions could you take to ensure that the NPSG is met?

REFER Go to Pearson MyLab Nursing and eText

REFLECT Apply Your Knowledge

Emma Jones is a 29-year-old woman who works for a small manufacturing firm. The demand for the firm's product has grown. To keep pace with the orders, the manufacturer bought some used equipment and hired more people, but the used equipment is noisier and less efficient than newer models. Ms. Jones visits the ear, nose, and throat clinic with a chief complaint of persistent ringing in her ears. As she provides her history, she and the nurse realize that the ringing began a week after the additional equipment was put into use. The ear protection that is available has to be shared because of the influx of new employees. This means that Ms. Jones and the other employees must rotate wearing ear protection. The supervisor has not yet purchased additional ear protection, and employees lack it for about one-quarter of their work shift.

1. What is the employer's responsibility for protecting the employees' hearing health?
2. What options does an employee have if the employer does not fulfill this responsibility?
3. As the nurse at the clinic, what could you do to advocate for a safer workplace for Ms. Jones and her fellow employees?

References

Accreditation Commission for Education in Nursing (ACEN). (2020). *Recognition as an accrediting agency.* https://www.acenursing.org/about/recognition/

American Association of Colleges of Nursing (AACN). (2020). *About AACN: Who we are.* http://www.aacn.nche.edu/about-aacn

American Nurses Association (ANA). (2020). *About ANA.* https://www.nursingworld.org/ana/about-ana/

Artiga, S., Orgera, S., & Damico, A. (2020). *Changes in health coverage by race and ethnicity since the ACA, 2010–2018.* https://www.kff.org/disparities-policy/issue-brief/changes-in-health-coverage-by-race-and-ethnicity-since-the-aca-2010-2018/

BlueCross BlueShield. (2020). *About us: An industry pioneer.* https://www.bcbs.com/about-us/industry-pioneer

Centers for Disease Control and Prevention (CDC). (2020). *Legal authorities for isolation and quarantine.* http://www.cdc.gov/quarantine/aboutlawsregulationsquarantineisolation.html

Centers for Medicare & Medicaid Services (n.d.). *Medicare and you.* https://www.medicare.gov/medicare-and-you

Centers for Medicare & Medicaid Services. (2020). *About CMS: History.* https://www.cms.gov/About-CMS/Agency-Information/History

Cohen, R. A., Cha, A. E., Martinez, M. E., & Terlizzi, E. P. (2020). *Health insurance coverage: Early release of estimates from the National Health Interview Survey, 2019.* National Center for Health Statistics. https://www.cdc.gov/nchs/data/nhis/earlyrelease/insur202009-508.pdf

Collins, S. R., Bhupal, H. K., & Doty, M. M. (2019). *Health insurance coverage eight years after the ACA.* The Commonwealth Fund. https://www.commonwealthfund.org/publications/issue-briefs/2019/feb/health-insurance-coverage-eight-years-after-aca

Commission on Collegiate Nursing Education. (2020). *Who we are.* https://www.aacnnursing.org/CCNE-Accreditation/Who-We-Are

Greenberg, J. (2017). *Medicaid expansion drove health insurance coverage under health law, Rand Paul says.* Politifact. http://www.politifact.com/truth-o-meter/statements/2017/jan/15/rand-paul/medicaid-expansion-drove-health-insurance-coverage/

International Council of Nurses (ICN). (2020). *International Council of Nurses.* https://www.who.int/workforcealliance/members_partners/member_list/icn/en/

Kaiser Family Foundation. (2019a). *2019 employer health benefits survey.* https://www.kff.org/health-costs/report/2019-employer-health-benefits-survey/

Kaiser Family Foundation. (2019b). *Key facts about the uninsured population.* http://kff.org/uninsured/fact-sheet/key-facts-about-the-uninsured-population/

Kaiser Family Foundation. (2020a). *Featured affordable care act resources.* https://www.kff.org/tag/affordable-care-act/

Kaiser Family Foundation (2020b) *Medicaid financing: How does it work and what are the implications?* https://www.kff.org/medicaid/issue-brief/medicaid-financing-how-does-it-work-and-what-are-the-implications/

Levey, N. M. (2017, March 15). Obamacare enrollment drops, to 12.2 million, as Congress debates repeal. *Los Angeles Times.* http://www.latimes.com/nation/nationnow/la-na-pol-obamacare-sign-up-20170315-story.html

Loversidge, J. M. (2016). An evidence-informed health policy model: adapting evidence-based practice for nursing education and regulation. *Journal of Nursing Regulation, 7*(2), 27–33.

Milstead, J. A., & Short, N. M. (2019). Informing public policy: An important role for registered nurses. In J. A. Milstead & N. M. Short (Eds.), *Health policy and politics: A nurse's guide* (6th ed., pp. 1–15). Jones & Bartlett.

National League for Nursing (NLN). (2019). *Public policy agenda 2019–2020.* http://www.nln.org/docs/default-source/advocacy-public-policy/public-policy-agenda-pdf49b8c85c78366c709642ff00005f0421.pdf?sfvrsn=2

National League for Nursing (NLN). (2020a). *CNEA mission and values.* http://www.nln.org/accreditation-services/the-nln-commission-for-nursing-education-accreditation-(cnea)

National League for Nursing (NLN). (2020b). *NLN: About.* http://www.nln.org/about

National Student Nurses Association (NSNA). (2020). *About NSNA.* https://www.nsna.org/about-nsna.html

North Carolina Department of Health and Human Services. (2020). *Naloxone saves: A harm reduction resource for North Carolina.* http://www.naloxonesaves.org/for-pharmacists/north-carolinas-standing-order-for-naloxone/

Ohio Department of Health. (n.d.). *Who we are/about us: Welcome to the Ohio Department of Health.* https://odh.ohio.gov/wps/portal/gov/odh/about-us

Project Hope. (2020). *Project Hope: About us.* https://www.projecthope.org/about-us/

Sigma Theta Tau International (STTI). (2020). *STTI organizational fact sheet.* http://www.nursingsociety.org/why-stti/about-stti/sigma-theta-tau-international-organizational-fact-sheet

The Joint Commission. (2020a). *About our standards.* https://www.jointcommission.org/standards/about-our-standards/

The Joint Commission. (2020b). *National patient safety goals.* https://www.jointcommission.org/standards/national-patient-safety-goals/

The Joint Commission. (2020c). *Sentinel event.* https://www.jointcommission.org/resources/patient-safety-topics/sentinel-event/

U.S. Agency for International Development. (2019). *Non-governmental organizations (NGOs).* https://www.usaid.gov/partnership-opportunities/ngo

U.S. Census Bureau. (2019). *Health insurance coverage in the United States: 2018.* https://www.census.gov/library/publications/2019/demo/p60-267.html

U.S. Department of Health and Human Services (DHHS). (2015). *HHS agencies & offices.* http://www.hhs.gov/about/agencies/hhs-agencies-and-offices/index.html#

U.S. Department of Health and Human Services (DHHS). (2020) *HHS FY 2021 Budget in brief.* https://www.hhs.gov/about/budget/fy2021/index.html

U.S. Department of Labor. (n.d.). *OSHA: About OSHA.* https://www.osha.gov/about.html

U.S. Department of State. (2017). *Non-governmental organizations (NGOs) in the United States: Fact sheet.* https://www.state.gov/non-governmental-organizations-ngos-in-the-united-states/

U.S. Environmental Protection Agency. (2018). *Our mission and what we do.* https://www.epa.gov/aboutepa/our-mission-and-what-we-do

U. S. Senate. (n.d.) *Budget.* https://www.senate.gov/reference/reference_index_subjects/Budget_vrd.htm

World Central Kitchen. (2020). *Chef relief team.* wck.org/chef-relief-team

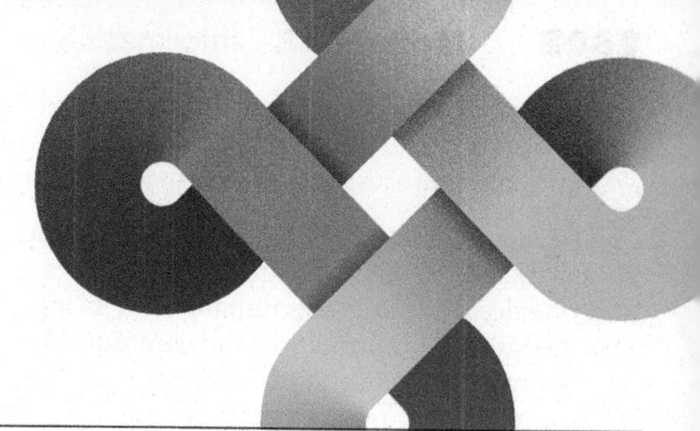

Module 48
Informatics

Module Outline and Learning Outcomes

The Concept of Informatics

Nursing Informatics

48.1 Analyze informatics as a key component of nursing practice.

Concepts Related to Informatics

48.2 Outline the relationship between informatics and other concepts.

Healthcare Information Systems

48.3 Explain the use of informatics in healthcare.

Computerized Medical Records

48.4 Analyze the uses of computerized medical records.

Telehealth

48.5 Analyze the use of informatics for telehealth.

Geographic Information Systems

48.6 Explain the use of geographic information systems.

Patient Education and E-Health

48.7 Analyze the use of the internet for patient education and e-health.

Ergonomic Considerations

48.8 Differentiate good ergonomics from poor ergonomics.

Informatics Exemplars

Exemplar 48.A Clinical Decision Support Systems

48.A Analyze clinical decision support systems as they relate to informatics.

Exemplar 48.B Individual Information at Point of Care

48.B Analyze individual information at point of care as it relates to informatics.

» The Concept of Informatics

Concept Key Terms

Biomedical informatics, **2807**
Clinical decision support system, **2812**
Clinical information system, **2809**
Computer vision syndrome, **2817**
Device integration, **2812**
E-health, **2814**
Electronic health record (EHR), **2808**
Electronic medical record (EMR), **2808**
Ergonomics, **2815**
Geographic information system (GIS), **2814**
Health Level 7 (HL7), **2811**
Nursing informatics (NI), **2807**
Repetitive strain injury, **2816**
Telehealth, **2813**

Today's healthcare professionals handle extraordinary amounts of information. At the bedside and in the examination room, nurses and other clinicians assess patients' health status and prioritize and provide care. Each action creates new data that must be recorded and used at different points of service from direct care to billing related to the cost of that care. In today's clinical environment, that information is created, stored, and accessed with the help of technology.

Biomedical informatics applies the principles of computer and information science to the advancement of health professions education, public health, and patient care. It is interprofessional and involves the computer, cognitive, and social sciences (American Medical Informatics Association [AMIA], 2011).

Nursing Informatics

The relationship between nursing and informatics is so critical that the American Nurses Association (ANA) recognized nursing informatics as a specialty in 1992, and the American Nurses Credentialing Center began offering board certification for nursing informatics in 1995. The ANA (n.d.) defines **nursing informatics (NI)** as

> the specialty that integrates nursing science with multiple information management and analytical sciences to identify, define, manage, and communicate data, information, knowledge, and wisdom in nursing practice. NI supports nurses, consumers, patients, the interprofessional healthcare team, and other stakeholders in their decision-making in all roles and settings

to achieve desired outcomes. This support is accomplished through the use of information structures, information processes, and information technology.

The nursing section of the American Medical Informatics Association (2020) defines nursing informatics as the science and practice that integrates nursing, and its information and knowledge, with information and communication technologies to promote the health of people, families, and communities worldwide.

Even in the few settings that do not yet use electronic health records (EHRs) (**Box 48.1** »), nurses use technology every day: Cardiac monitors, mechanical ventilators, and many blood pressure cuffs use computer technology, as do most telephone systems. Informatics is an everyday occurrence in the practice of nursing.

Informatics and Health Policy

Both professional organizations and government entities recognize and support the careful, purposeful implementation of informatics in healthcare environments. The Healthcare Information and Management Systems Society (HIMSS) works to improve healthcare quality, safety, and outcomes through improving the use of information technology (IT) and systems. HIMSS is a nonprofit organization with both individual and corporate members. AMIA is another organization dedicated to the development and application of health informatics to support patient care and teaching. The Alliance for Nursing Informatics (ANI) works to support and advance the areas of informatics leadership, practice, education, policy, and research. It works closely with other organizations such as HIMSS and AMIA. These groups promote the use of health IT and sponsor conferences as well as policy development. The Technology Informatics Guiding Educational Reform (TIGER) initiative focuses on integrating technology and informatics competencies into nursing education as well as practice. The TIGER initiative is currently integrated into the HIMSS network.

» **Stay Current:** For more information about the TIGER initiative, visit http://www.himss.org/professionaldevelopment/tiger-initiative.

The administrations of both President George W. Bush and President Barack Obama contributed to the use of informatics in the delivery of healthcare across the United States. Electronic medical documentation is thought to help reduce errors, reduce healthcare costs, and improve the quality of care delivered to patients. The Bush administration introduced a policy that, over the course of 10 years, would encourage the use of electronic documentation of the healthcare record. The Obama administration took this policy further with the introduction of the American Recovery and Reinvestment Act of 2009, which provided $27 billion worth of incentives to HCPs to promote the use of electronic medical records. Through the Health Information Technology for Economic and Clinical Health Act (HITECH), the funding is directed toward EHRs. The Centers for Medicare and Medicaid Services (CMS) and the Office of the National Coordinator for Health Information Technology (ONC) are charged with the oversight of health information technology efforts. ONC is overseeing the achievement of meaningful use objectives, which are reported back to CMS to authorize financial reimbursement. Meaningful use is built on the five pillars of health outcomes (CMS, 2019):

- Improving care coordination
- Improving quality, safety, and efficiency and reducing health disparities
- Ensure adequate privacy and security protection for personal health information
- Engaging patients and their families in their health
- Improving population and public health.

Informatics and Service Delivery

Informatics has broad implications for service delivery. For example, addiction and overdoses of prescription opioids are an increasing problem in the United States. Reports of overdoses have increased more than threefold since the 1990s. In 2016, overdose deaths among those who used or misused opioids was 42,000 (Substance Abuse and Mental Health Services Administration, 2018). Efforts are being made to

Box 48.1

EMR versus EHR

A nurse will hear many different terms to describe a computerized medical record, and the list will probably continue to change. The two most commonly used terms are electronic medical records and EHRs.

Electronic medical records (EMRs) are similar to an electronic chart used in a clinician's office. Their focus is on diagnosis and treatment. They can help track information over time (e.g., weight, blood pressure, cholesterol readings) and identify when patients are due for routine preventive health maintenance such as vaccines and mammograms. A disadvantage of these systems is that most of them are designed to stay within a clinical setting and are not meant to travel beyond it. A patient who needs to see a specialist may need a paper printout of the EMR to take to the specialty appointment.

Electronic health records (EHRs) give a broader view of the patient's health. They are designed so that multiple clinicians from multiple disciplines (e.g., family practice, nursing, pharmacy, specialists) can all have simultaneous access to the patient's health information. This access provides patients with more comprehensive management of their health and is designed to improve the quality of care they receive. EHRs enhance communication with other clinicians, they provide easy access to patient information, they can provide automated formulary checks by health plans to avoid problems with prescriptions, and they can link to public health systems such as registries and communicable disease data banks (HealthIT.gov, 2018). One significant advantage is e-prescribing, in which healthcare providers (HCPs) can communicate directly with the pharmacy to order prescriptions. This can reduce errors, lower costs, and improve care (HealthIT.gov, 2019a).

This text uses *EHR* when discussing documentation, as it is the broader, more encompassing term.

enhance tracking of prescriptions of opioids through electronic tracking at the state level. In addition, the Centers for Disease Control and Prevention (CDC; 2019) works with healthcare agencies to track prescriptions and emergency department visits for overdoses in an attempt to identify people who are or have been abusers. The ability to link computerized written orders with patient EHRs on regional and national levels can help identify and monitor individuals who are at risk and make it easier to identify people who engage in "doctor shopping" to obtain narcotics for abuse or illegal sale. Tracking mechanisms can also help identify HCPs who write bogus opioid prescriptions and receive a financial kickback from sellers.

One of the often-cited benefits of EHRs is improved quality of care delivered to patients. Formerly known as Meaningful Use, Promoting Interoperability is a rebranding of the CMS EHR incentive program (Bresnick, 2018). Under this new program CMS (2020c) encourages eligible professionals and hospitals to "adopt, implement, upgrade and demonstrate the meaningful use of certified health record technology (CEHRT)." As of October 2018, approximately 546,000 HCPs participated in the Promoting Interoperability Program (CMS, 2020a).

Concepts Related to Informatics

The use of informatics has created many challenges for nurses. Patients have increasing access to a variety of health-related information, such as recommendations for diet and monitoring weight. Nurses must be attentive to ensure that their patients are getting good-quality information and using it appropriately. It is also important to recognize that some patients will be unable or unwilling to use electronic means to access health information. Nurses are in a good position to help patients find the most appropriate means of getting and using healthcare information.

Protecting health information is also important, and vigilance is necessary to protect patient information and to ensure that protected information is not released inadvertently. The rise of social media has created ethical challenges, especially when nurses and patients know each other socially from events or activities outside the workplace. Despite the great possibilities for improving patient care through quality improvement efforts and tracking patient use of medications, nurses must take care to use informatics within established guidelines consistent with the scope of nursing practice and professional, ethical, and legal requirements. Some, but not all, of the concepts integral to informatics are outlined in the Concepts Related to Informatics feature. They are presented in alphabetical order.

Healthcare Information Systems

The increasing use of technology by healthcare facilities requires that nurses have a basic knowledge of the types of information systems used, the purposes and abilities of these systems to support patient care, and the nurse's responsibilities related to using these systems.

In the days of paper charts, only one individual at a time could access a patient's chart and add information to it. A **clinical information system** allows multiple disciplines to simultaneously access the patient's chart and record data that can be viewed and analyzed by a number of HCPs in real time, providing the most accurate and current information about the patient so that the best decisions about the care of that patient can be made.

A clinical information system must give the nurse the ability to access patient information and provide data necessary to execute the nursing process of assessing, diagnosing, planning, implementing, and evaluating the care of the patient. When the system is used at the point of care, the nurse can immediately record patient information based on assessment of the patient's current condition. The nurse should also have access to diagnostic data (e.g., laboratory values), diagnoses, assessments, plans, and evaluations of the patient from the viewpoint of other healthcare professionals (e.g., physicians, physical therapists). Pharmacy information, such as medication, route, dose, and time, should be available in the patient's chart in real time. The chart should also include safety features, such as warnings for drug interactions or incorrect dosages. Most clinical information systems also contain clinical decision support, which is discussed later in this module. The system should also allow the nurse to print discharge instructions to review with the patient.

Computerized Medical Records

On the surface, a computerized medical record may appear to be nothing more than a digital form of a patient's paper chart. Many systems start out that way. However, rapid technologic advances have transformed these static charts into dynamic systems.

Purpose

The purpose of a computerized medical record is to unify a patient's entire health history into one single source of information about the patient's health, including the patient's medical and surgical histories, diagnostic tests and treatments, medications, and therapies. It is meant to be multidisciplinary and multispecialty in nature. It is meant not to simply record the past but to aid clinicians in the patient's future healthcare, improve quality of care, lower costs of care, and facilitate research. It is meant to be portable, so that if a patient lives in New York but requires emergency care in Los Angeles, all of the patient's medical information is available to help the HCPs in Los Angeles make the best possible decisions about the care of the patient. A meta-analysis of EHRs found their use impacts the quality of healthcare, increases guideline adherence, and is also effective in reducing medication errors. Furthermore, EHRs with decision support systems show better outcomes than those without (Campanella et al., 2016).

To deliver the best quality of care, promote safety, maintain efficiency, and prevent nurse and clinician burnout, computerized health records should contain the following functionality (Ommaya et al., 2018).

- ***Patient support.*** Patients should be able to access their health records. Patients can take a more active role in their care if they have the ability to track appointments and health maintenance, monitor their weight and laboratory results, and access educational materials related to their health condition.

Concepts Related to
Informatics

CONCEPT	RELATIONSHIP TO INFORMATICS	NURSING IMPLICATIONS
Addiction	EHRs give HCPs, including nurses, access to the patient's entire health history, not just information from this particular encounter at this particular facility. Linking of EHR information may help identify individuals who are at risk for opioid addiction and who are engaged in obtaining these drugs illegally.	■ Assess appropriate use of addictive medications; many patients have legitimate need for prescription opioids. ■ Be alert for duplicate opioid prescriptions within a patient's record, especially from multiple providers.
Ethics	With social media, lines between patients and providers can be blurred.	■ Nurses must be aware that employers have developed social media policies to address how employees should interact in the social media space. Items covered in this policy may include cautions against sharing confidential patient information, use of your employee email to sign up, and reminders that your posts should not appear as if you are speaking for the hospital or clinical area of employment. ■ Nurses must weigh the implications of "friending" patients that they care for (especially in areas with long-term interaction). ■ Anticipate how to handle patients who attempt to cross boundaries by using social media.
Legal Issues	It is necessary to keep protected health information confidential and to ensure that the information entered in a patient's health record is accurate.	■ Nurses must be aware of HIPAA and HITECH rules. Among the most critical activities: — Keep passwords private. — Do not leave screens containing protected health information unattended. — Access charts only of patients to whom you are assigned. — Always verify that you are charting on the correct patient's chart and that the information is recorded accurately.
Nutrition	Smartphone applications allow patients to determine and track the nutritional value of foods they eat.	■ Use of these applications may increase ease of tracking nutritional intake for the purposes of dietary recall and weight monitoring. ■ Anticipate that some patients may not have smartphones or may have minimal data plans that limit their ability to use this technology. Work with patients to establish other, convenient means to track dietary intake.
Quality Improvement	With many EHRs, quality metrics can be easily tracked for improvement within a department or hospital system. Tracking information to use for quality improvement initiatives requires users to understand how to use technology correctly. Nurses must be at the table as new systems are evaluated and put in place, and they must advocate to ensure that they will receive adequate training to implement the system safely and accurately.	■ Assess your own comfort and ability level related to use of electronic/computer equipment. Attend training sessions; seek follow-up help as necessary. ■ Be alert for the possibility for error; enter information accurately every time.
Safety	EHRs can provide tools to improve patient safety, such as reminders. Clinical Decision Support Systems are also used to ensure that appropriate protocols are used when patients meet certain criteria.	■ Nurses benefit from electronic reminders to assist them when they are busy to ensure that key assessments such as neurologic assessments in stroke patients are done in a timely manner. ■ Flags in the system alert nurses to complete screening tools such as fall risk or pressure ulcer screening. HCPs can access evidence-based practice care bundles for patients who meet criteria for sepsis and other diagnoses.

- ***Health information and data.*** Important data, such as chronic and acute medical and psychiatric diagnoses, medications, allergies, and diagnostic tests, can help those professionals caring for the patient to make rapid decisions, if necessary.
- ***Administrative processes.*** The ability to manage schedules, insurance information, and inventory can help healthcare facilities focus on patient-centered care.
- ***Results management.*** Access to past and current diagnostic tests can help nurses and other clinicians recognize changes in a patient's state of health faster.
- ***Reporting.*** Healthcare facilities can comply more easily with regulatory requests and help report disease surveillance and patient safety matters such as medical device recalls.
- ***Secure electronic communication and connectivity.*** Secure and accurate communication between medical providers at different facilities that are caring for the same patient helps with continuity of care and timely diagnoses.
- ***Order management.*** Computerized physician order entry (CPOE) helps with accuracy and decreases times from order to treatment. CPOE should be available for pharmacy, laboratory, radiologic tests, and ancillary services such as physical and occupational therapy.
- ***Decision support.*** The care of the patient can be enhanced through the use of a clinical decision support system. These systems can display best practice standards, notifications for preventive screenings, and alerts for drug interactions.

Components

Real-time documentation of patient data can help all clinicians care for the patient. The nurse should be given the tools to record assessments, nursing diagnoses, plans, interventions, and evaluations. The work that nurses have done in caring for the patient has traditionally been invisible to other disciplines, so the ability to carry the nursing process over into electronic records will help promote the work that nurses do in caring for the patient. *Uniform language* is the consistent use of the same terminology among providers, facilities, institutions, and organizations when describing all patient data, including that pertaining to assessment and treatment. Uniform language (discussed further in Exemplar 48.A, Clinical Decision Support Systems, in this module) is vital for communicating to other nurses and health professionals the value that nurses provide in the care of the patient.

NANDA International (NANDA-I) has been involved in developing uniform language for nursing since the 1970s. NANDA-I diagnoses are available in many electronic health systems. The Nursing Interventions Classifications (NIC) include both physiologic and psychologic interventions that nurses perform with patients and their families. Nurses use both NANDA-I and NIC to formulate care plans for the patient in the EHR. The Nursing Outcomes Classification (NOC) is designed to assess the outcomes of patients based on the nursing interventions performed. Both NIC and NOC have been approved for use in **Health Level 7 (HL7)** terminology, which provides a framework and composes standards "for the exchange, integration, sharing, and retrieval of electronic health information that supports clinical practice and the management, delivery and evaluation of health services" (Health Level Seven International, n.d.).

Health Insurance Portability and Accountability Act of 1996

A major concern for both patients and HCPs is the protection of private health information. Private health information includes any details that could identify a particular patient, such as name, phone number, hospital medical record number, diagnosis, or Social Security number. The Health Insurance Portability and Accountability Act of 1996, commonly referred to as HIPAA, limits who may have access to a patient's health information, whether that information is in written, oral, or electronic form. It also gives patients the right to view their own health records, make corrections to their records, and receive notification of how their information may be used or shared (e.g., for research or marketing purposes; U.S. Department of Health and Human Services [DHHS], n.d.). HITECH added more strength to the existing HIPAA protection of patients' medical information (DHHS, 2017).

Nurses should use many of the same rules for protecting patient privacy that were practiced before the advent of electronic records. Information about a patient should not be discussed in public areas, such as hospital cafeterias or elevators. Any paper documents that may contain protected health information should be placed in designated shred bins. Technology-related considerations for nurses include not sharing passwords, not leaving a computer screen with protected health information unattended, and not posting any patient information on public social networks such as Facebook, Instagram, or Twitter (see **Box 48.2** ›› and **Figure 48.1** ››). Commonsense habits related to confidentiality must be practiced. In the days of paper charts, it may have been possible to obtain unauthorized access to a neighbor's or celebrity's chart without being detected. Now it is very easy to ascertain electronically each time a patient's chart is accessed and by whom. A nurse who improperly accesses a patient's chart could face loss of employment and possible fine, loss of licensure, and/or legal action.

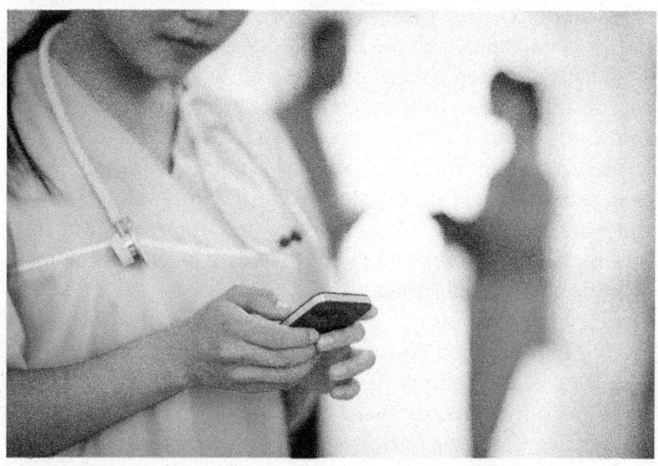

Figure 48.1 ›› Do not post any information at all on any social media about any patient in your facility.
Source: Wavebreakmedia/iStock/Getty Images.

Box 48.2

Social Media and the Workplace

In the United States, over 99% of all hospitals have a Facebook page and many use Twitter, Instagram, or other platforms (Evariant, 2019). It has become necessary to do this to communicate and engage with patients. This has become increasingly important since a 2018 study found 80% of those who use the internet search for healthcare information (Chen, Li, Liang, & Tsai, 2018). Because so much of the communication is now through social media platforms, HIPAA has released guidelines to help healthcare providers and systems. These guidelines include recommendations such as (DHHS, 2018):

- Don't talk about patients but do talk about conditions.
- Don't be anonymous.
- Don't mix personal and professional lives.

The American Nurses Association (ANA) has developed a set of media guidelines for nurses. They caution that inappropriate posts by nurses to social media can result in licensure and legal repercussions. Sharing any information at all about patients with your friends on social media is inappropriate and violates HIPAA and the Nursing Code of Ethics (ANA, 2018).

» **Stay Current:** Visit the American Nurses Association's Healthy Nurse, Healthy Nation website (https://www.healthynursehealthynation.org) to read more about guidelines for use of social media.

Despite the move to EHRs, medical fraud still occurs. In 2019, CMS enacted a rule that will ensure they have more control over payment for services by allowing them to block certain providers from payment if those providers are doing business with organizations who have had their enrollment status revoked (Advisory Board, 2019).

Quality Assurance

On the surface, the implementation of EHRs would seem likely to automatically improve the quality of patient care. It has the potential to do that, but an EHR is just a tool, and outcomes of care depend, in part, on how this tool is used.

Accuracy

Recording accurate patient health information is vital, whether the nurse is using a paper or an electronic system. First encounters with an electronic charting system involve a learning curve that increases the chance of errors in recording data that will be left in a patient's chart. For example, someone who is new to the system may not know how to remove a blood pressure reading that was 225/124 because the arterial line transducer was on the floor or how to mark that reading as faulty data. In many charting systems, more than one chart may be open at the same time, so entering information on the wrong chart may be easy. An accidental click of a mouse on the wrong medication can cause the provider who is not paying attention to order or give the wrong medication. **Device integration**, which automatically enters patient vital signs into the EHR, is possible in some systems. This has increased in use and is found not only in intensive care units but also in telemetry, obstetrics, and even general care units. Device integration allows real-time accurate data to be recorded in the patient's chart directly from the device (e.g., a blood pressure monitor or cardiac monitor). It allows the nurse to more quickly analyze and interpret that data and make adjustments to the plan of care based on the most current information (Dusseux, 2020).

Some EHR systems use templates and cut-and-paste functions designed to promote efficiency. For example, a pediatric clinic seeing 10 otherwise healthy children who have ear infections can use a template or cut/copy function to forward the information that is within normal limits and just focus on the infection, saving precious time that would otherwise be spent manually clicking boxes for negative or normal findings. However, overuse of these functions can result in inaccurate data being recorded in a patient's chart, risking future decisions about medical care based on faulty information. For example, if there has been a significant change in the patient's condition and a practitioner uses a "copy forward" or "copy paste" function to duplicate the previous day's progress notes, then care of the patient can be seriously compromised. A systematic review found that 66–90% of clinicians use this function regularly (Tsou et al., 2017). A patient's medical record is only as valuable as the information that is entered in it, and *nurses have a duty to ensure that they enter only timely and accurate information*. Risk management, insurance companies, and regulatory bodies as well as other clinicians will be looking at the data in the patient's record, so it is imperative that nurses take the time to learn proper documentation within the electronic system that their employer adopts.

Critical Thinking

The fact that the EHR is merely a tool cannot be overemphasized. As with paper charting, the patient and not the record should have first priority in the nurse's attention. Although it may be difficult when electronic records are used, nurses must learn to focus their attention on the patient and not the computer. Employers should give nurses adequate training on the use of their electronic system and regularly monitor documentation (Tsou et al., 2017).

Clinical decision support systems are a type of artificial intelligence that analyzes data and provides information about evidenced-based practices. These systems can help improve patient safety and quality of care. However, they cannot take the place of sound nursing judgment. The use of clinical decision support systems in nursing practice is described further in the exemplar on Clinical Decision Support Systems in this module.

Uniform Language

For greater efficiency, nurses should use uniform language in their documentation. Uniform nursing diagnoses, along with uniform descriptors of nursing interventions and outcomes, can help clarify care of the patient not only to other nurses but to other disciplines as well. Some documentation within an electronic record may have only standardized descriptors available for the end user. The use of uniform language also aids nursing research.

Clinical Example A

Mary Wilson is a 19-year-old with a history of grand mal seizures. She takes two antiepileptic medications: phenytoin and topiramate. Her seizures are fairly well controlled, and she has an average of three seizures per year. Ms. Wilson is getting ready to go out of state to college and visits her primary care provider for a physical before she leaves. The office has just installed a new EHR system. Because of an early regional outbreak of influenza, the office is overbooked with appointments. The practitioner that Ms. Wilson usually sees is on vacation. The other practitioner rushes through Ms. Wilson's appointment and does not take a thorough history or discuss medications that she is taking. Ms. Wilson presents as a healthy 19-year-old, so the practitioner uses the "copy and paste healthy adult" format for her chart.

Ms. Wilson goes out of state to school. After class one day, she decides to go for a run to relieve the stress of her classes. While she is on her run, she experiences a grand mal seizure. A motorist finds her unconscious in a postictal state and calls for emergency services. Ms. Wilson is transported to the hospital, which happens to be on the same EHR system as her primary care provider. She is still not conscious when she is examined, but she has identification with her name and birthdate on it. The emergency department staff looks at Ms. Wilson's EHR, but there is no mention of her seizure disorder. She is sent for emergency CT scans and an MRI of her brain.

Critical Thinking Questions

1. What mistakes did the provider at Ms. Wilson's primary care office make with her record?
2. How did the omission of information affect the care that Ms. Wilson received at the hospital?
3. What complications regarding health insurance might arise if she is at an out-of-state school?

Telehealth

Telehealth uses telecommunications technologies (e.g., videoconferencing, streaming media, store and forward imaging, and land-based and wireless communications) to allow patients access to care that they might not otherwise be able to obtain. The terms *telehealth* and *telemedicine* are often used interchangeably, but according to the Health Resources Administration, *telehealth* is much broader and can encompass health-related education, public health, and health administration (HealthIT.gov, 2019b). Telehealth is not meant to replace all provider face-to-face visits, but it can be used to help manage patients with chronic physical and mental disorders, particularly those who live in rural areas where access to specialists is limited or requires travel. In many states, reimbursement for telehealth visits is the same as that for in-person visits. This makes telehealth an attractive and cost-effective option for both patients and providers (HealthIT.gov, 2019c). The coronavirus pandemic that began in 2019 had a significant impact on telehealth use and the willingness of insurance companies and CMS to pay for telehealth visits not normally covered (Clason, 2020).

Research on the effectiveness of telehealth has found evidence to support its use in patients with chronic conditions and with those receiving psychotherapy as part of behavioral health. In particular, improvement in outcomes such as mortality, quality of life, and reductions in admissions have been noted in patients with chronic diseases (Agency for Healthcare Research and Quality [AHRQ], 2019).

Benefits of telehealth include:

- ***Access to healthcare is increased.*** Patients in rural areas can reduce the need to travel, and they receive access to specialists that may not be available in their community.
- ***Health outcomes are improved.*** Increased access to care can reduce complications and increase diagnostic and treatment options from specialists.
- ***Healthcare costs can be reduced.*** The expenses involved in frequent long-distance travel are reduced or eliminated, and home monitoring of chronic conditions can help reduce hospital admissions.
- ***Telehealth may help with shortages of HCPs.*** Many HCPs are not willing to move to rural communities. Telehealth can give patients access to primary care providers and specialists from other areas.

In 2020 the Federal Communications Commission launched a $200 million COVID-19 telehealth program to support the expansion of telehealth and remote monitoring. This was funded as part of the CARES Act and will likely have a significant impact on the adoption of telehealth (American Telemedicine, 2020)

>> **Stay Current:** Visit the website of the American Telehealth Organization for updates on current policies, including the latest on CMS reimbursement and support for telehealth: http://www.americantelemed.org/home.

Barriers to Patient Participation

Some patients may be reluctant to use telehealth services if they lack understanding of or experience with technology. The lack of availability of broadband internet service throughout the country also limits participation. In addition, many patients are not aware that these services exist or that their HCP is willing to participate in this type of interaction. On the provider side, reimbursement challenges still exist and vary from state to state. Obtaining a license to practice across state lines varies by state. Some offer a special telehealth license, and some allow providers to practice in bordering states (Center for Connected Health Policy, n.d.). The COVID-19 pandemic has imposed temporary exceptions to this; however, it is not known at this time how things will change moving forward.

Clinical Example B

Jack Anderson is an 85-year-old retired machinist. He has an eighth-grade education and lives on a fixed income in a rural community 100 miles from a major city. He has congestive heart failure (CHF) and takes a loop diuretic (furosemide) and digoxin for his condition, both of which he gets through a mail-order pharmacy. Mr. Anderson has Medicare but tries to limit his doctor visits because he doesn't like to drive to the city and the cost of gas puts a strain on his monthly budget. His community has high-speed internet, but Mr. Anderson has not installed it because "he moved to the country to get away from everyone."

Critical Thinking Questions

1. Discuss several factors that would make Mr. Anderson an ideal candidate for telehealth.
2. When Mr. Anderson comes in for an appointment, what could the nurse say to encourage him to participate in telehealth to manage his CHF?
3. If Mr. Anderson agrees to participate in telehealth, what should the practitioner assess in each of the telehealth sessions with him?

Geographic Information Systems

A **geographic information system (GIS)** uses location to capture, manage, and analyze data. This technology has been used both inside and outside of healthcare. It relies on satellite imaging and the global positioning system (GPS) to capture geographic data. Those data are then managed and stored on a database. Healthcare policymakers, researchers, and public health professionals use GIS to understand a health problem. GIS is being used to:

- ***Identify health trends.*** This combines individuals' health data from electronic records, data from wearables (such as Fitbits), and data from their environment to determine if there are clusters of cancer in an area or obesity related to certain areas or climates.
- ***Track the spread of infectious diseases.*** Data is used to map where diseases are most likely to spread next and gain an understanding of vaccination rates.
- ***Use personal technology.*** Data from wearable technologies has the ability to determine trends in heart rate and sleeping patterns of individuals and to determine if that varies in different geographic areas.
- ***Incorporate social media.*** Through the use of social media, researchers are able to query posts or tweets for keywords such as *flu* or *influenza* to create a visual map of where the flu outbreaks are geographically located.

Public health nurses and administrators can use GIS to track where chronic disease programs should be placed, to monitor the effectiveness of these programs, to plan new treatment facilities, and to track acute health problems, among many other uses. GIS gives HCPs the tools to show where services are provided and where health services are needed (Dempsey, 2019). During pandemics or infectious disease outbreaks, GIS can be used to track and monitor cases (Dempsey, 2020).

Patient Education and E-Health

Besides changing the ways in which HCPs handle and use information, informatics is changing the way patients view their health. Some studies have indicated that when patients have access to their EHRs, they feel more knowledgeable about their health and disease processes, are more engaged during visits with their primary care provider, and feel more empowered to participate in disease management and wellness activities (HealthIT.gov, 2020). Smartphone technology offers many add-on utilities and applications. Individuals can read and monitor their blood pressure or track their blood glucose levels using smartphones. Many fitness training applications allow users to share their successes on social media sites. Other applications are available for tracking calories in certain food items, recording caloric intake for the day, and tracking weight loss.

Wearable technologies such as fitness bands (Fitbit, Garmin, Apple Watch) have become popular. Many people use them to track steps, count calories, track quality of sleep, and set fitness goals. The devices also allow HCPs to track data and make more informed healthcare decisions with their patients. They can monitor blood pressure and blood oxygenation in addition to activity (Steger, 2020). Nurses need to understand a patient's level of e-health literacy as more people turn to online sources of health information and patient portals are increasingly being used for patient information (Levin-Zamir & Bertschi, 2018).

Online Consumer Medical Information

E-health is defined as, "the use of information and communications technologies for health" (World Health Organization, 2020). *Mobile health* (m-health) is a subset of e-health and includes the use of mobile technologies for health. The new umbrella term, *digital health*, encompasses e-health, m-health, and emerging areas in data science, genomics, and artificial intelligence.

Many healthcare consumers seek information from the internet on various healthcare conditions, symptoms, diseases, drugs, nutrition, and fitness (AHRQ, 2017). The amount continues to increase; therefore, it is important to make sure consumers get the best information and understand how to evaluate different web-based sources.

Box 48.3 » provides some information on evaluating health-related websites that is useful for both patients and nurses who want to stay current.

Online Patient Portals

Many health facilities are using the internet to give patients access to and control over their own health records. Some of these sites are called *patient portals*. Online registration is required, and a user identification and password are needed for each visit. Through many of these portals, patients can schedule routine appointments and request prescription refills from their primary care office (**Figure 48.2** »). Patients also can communicate electronically with their HCP, although some portals are not yet encrypted to allow secure transmission of protected health information. Hospitals are using the internet to schedule some radiology procedures such as mammograms online. Some EHRs allow patients to access parts of their health records. Information such as laboratory and pathology reports, medication records, and due dates for routine screenings and immunizations may be available. The use of these services leads to improved patient engagement, improved adherence to medication, and facilitation of patient–provider communication. Concerns about privacy still remain and some patients still see some of the portal functions as inadequate (Dendere et al., 2019).

Online Administrative Tools

Patient portals can also perform administrative functions. Patients are able to view and verify their demographic and insurance information. Many providers are placing their new patient paperwork online for patients to complete before

Box 48.3

Evaluating Web-Based Health Information

When looking online for medical information, ask yourself the following questions:

- *Where does the information come from?* Reliable websites clearly indicate the source of the information. They often provide additional sources of information.
- *Who hosts the site?* Websites that end in *.gov* are government-sponsored, *.org* indicates a noncommercial sponsor, and *.edu* identifies an academic or university sponsor. These are usually reliable sources of information. Websites that end in *.com* indicate commercial sponsorship and may or may not provide accurate information.
- *What type of information is presented?* Is the information authored by a health professional or scientist? Is the information evidenced based? Does it contain research information?
- *Is the information current?* Review dates should be clearly posted. The most current information should be used, as practices in some areas change rapidly.
- *Is the website trying to sell a product?* Websites that are promoting a product or supplement probably do not contain accurate information and should be avoided.
- *Is your privacy being protected?* Read the website's privacy policy. Do not provide personal information unless you are comfortable with how the website will handle that information.

Sources: National Institutes of Health (2011); National Network of Libraries of Medicine (2020).

their first appointment. Some systems send automated text or voice-message reminders for upcoming appointments. Other systems may send automated messages to a group of patients, such as reminders for influenza vaccinations. The patient often has the ability to view any outstanding balances and make payments online.

Patient portals can also be used by patients to fill out previsit questionnaires and to electronically check in for their upcoming appointments. Health insurance companies give providers online access to information about the patient's insurance coverage, including information on providers and hospitals in the insurance company's network. Providers often can see the dates of coverage and co-pays and deductibles paid to date and, in some cases, they can obtain instant online authorization of procedures such as MRIs.

Some websites allow patients to compare health professionals based on specialty, languages spoken, and clinical training. Hospitals and nursing homes can be compared based on quality measures and demographics (e.g., location, size). Websites vary: Some use only patients' ratings, and others use less subjective data.

Ergonomic Considerations

Use of technology can impact both workflow and body mechanics. The addition of computers in healthcare may seem innocent enough, but without proper planning and implementation, it can lead to serious injuries to the user. The risk of injury increases with professions that require pushing, pulling, frequent or heavy lifting, prolonged awkward positions, or repetitive, forceful, or prolonged exertion of the hands (Occupational Safety and Health Administration [OSHA], n.d.-a).

Ergonomics is "the science of fitting workplace conditions and job demands to the capabilities of the working population" (OSHA, n.d.-a). Ergonomics examines the type of work being done, the tools being used, and the body mechanics of both the work and the tools, and then suggests the best way to do that work with those tools to limit overuse and harm (U.S. National Library of Medicine, n.d.).

For working on a computer, the goal of ergonomics is to set up a workstation that allows a neutral body position (**Figure 48.3** ≫). The head, neck, and torso should be

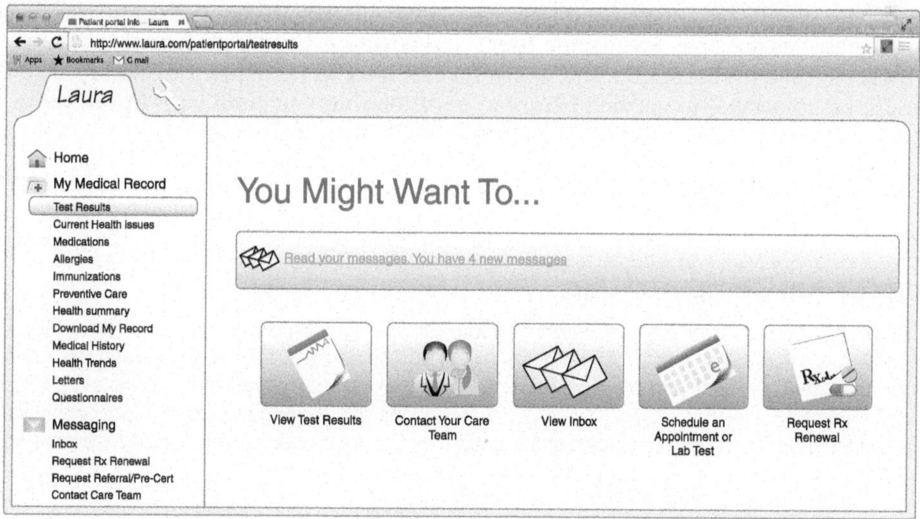

Figure 48.2 ≫ Patients can use their patient portal to send and receive messages, view test results, schedule an appointment, and order prescription refills.

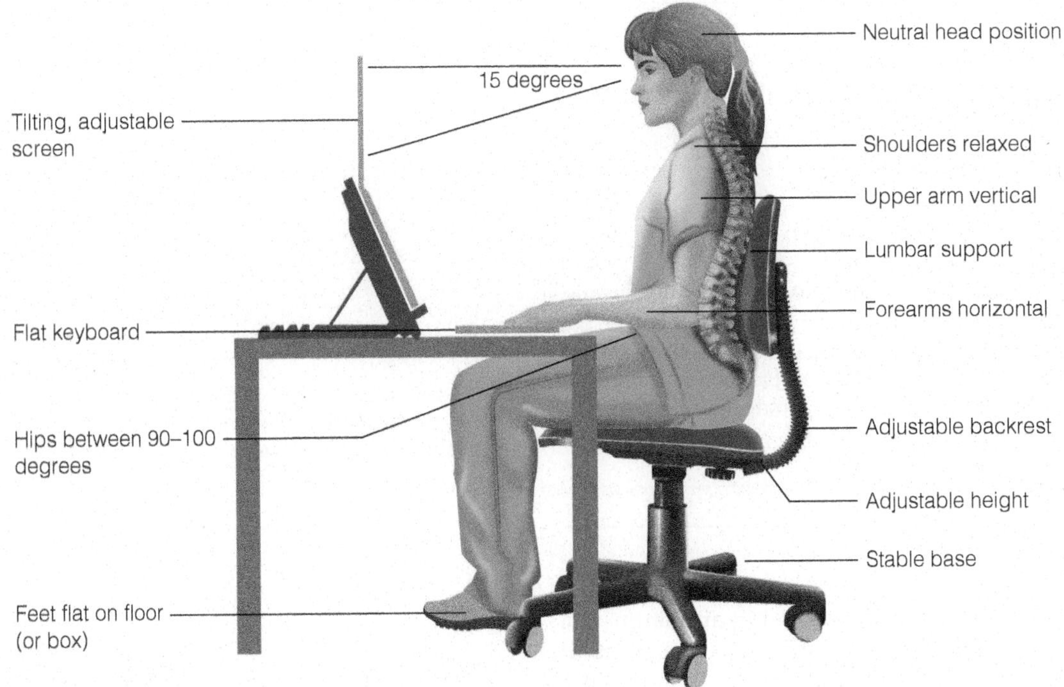

Figure 48.3 » Maintaining neutral position while working at a computer will help prevent the development of repetitive strain injuries.

in alignment. Shoulders and upper arms should be perpendicular to the floor and relaxed. The upper arms and elbows should be close to the body. Forearms, wrists, and hands should be straight and in line. When the worker is sitting, the thighs should be parallel to the floor and the feet should rest flat on the floor or be supported by a footrest (OSHA, n.d.-a).

» **Stay Current:** A checklist that looks at each component of the computer system (keyboard, monitor, chair, and work surfaces) is available online at www.osha.gov/SLTC/etools/computerworkstations/checklist.html.

Workstations on wheels (WOWs) require the user to pull or push them to different locations for use. The position of the monitor, keyboard, or mouse on the WOW can also lead to bad posture and injury. These carts should be as lightweight and maneuverable as possible. Ideally, the user should be able to tilt the screen at different angles, and workstation platforms should be adjustable to varying heights. See **Box 48.4** » for ways to incorporate good ergonomics in computer use.

Improper workstation setup or improper body mechanics can lead to injury. Common complaints after prolonged computer use include fatigue or pain in the neck, shoulders, back, arms, wrists, and hands. Some of these symptoms can be alleviated by proper ergonomics or breaks from the computer when possible. Sometimes simple aches and pains can lead to more serious injuries that cause disability. The two most common injuries are repetitive strain injury and computer vision syndrome (Princeton University, 2017).

Repetitive strain injury, or repetitive motion disorder, occurs when the limbs are subjected to repetitive use, awkward positions, or forced positions. These injuries can affect nerves, tendons, and muscles. Tendinitis is a common occurrence, but carpal tunnel syndrome is more serious and can lead to permanent disability if not treated. Symptoms of tendinitis include pain in the wrist, elbow, shoulder, or

Box 48.4

Good Ergonomics for Computer Use

- Maintain good posture whether sitting or standing, aligning your ears, shoulders, and hips.
- Avoid overreaching. Keep the keyboard and mouse within easy reach.
- Keep your wrists in a straight position and your elbows at a slightly open angle.
- Position the monitor so that you can see the screen without tilting your neck up or down or turning your head.
- Use light force when typing on the keyboard.
- Customize font sizes and screen resolution to maximize comfort.
- Take frequent breaks. Eye breaks are important as well as stretching and moving around at regular intervals.
- Ensure proper lighting and reduce glare from the screen.

If you experience numbness, weakness, or pain, seek medical attention.

Sources: Princeton University (2017); University of Michigan (2017).

neck; numbness or tingling in the fingers; difficulty grasping objects; and a decrease in the size of the affected hand. Treatment should not be delayed and can include changes in posture, stretching, muscle strengthening, and rest. Rest is a key component; treatment and healing require time. Carpal tunnel syndrome is a more serious repetitive strain injury caused by repeated bending or use of the fingers or wrists that results in median nerve compression. Pain, numbness, and tingling in the palm of the hand and in the thumb and index fingers or the middle fingers are common symptoms. Surgery may be required if the injury is severe enough or does not respond to conservative treatment. If left untreated, carpal tunnel syndrome can lead to muscle wasting, decreased sensation, and permanent disability (Princeton University, 2017).

Computer vision syndrome, or eyestrain, is the most common sequela of computer use. Using the computer for more than 3 hours a day puts one at risk, so many individuals are affected. Symptoms include eye fatigue, headaches, blurred vision, dry eyes, and changes in color perception. If left untreated, computer vision syndrome can lead to a decrease in work efficiency, general fatigue, and increased myopia. It can be caused by monitor glare, monitor position (too close or incorrect angle), or quick eye movements while typing and looking at a source document. Correct monitor position, antiglare screen covers, correct lighting, and proper document placement can all help reduce the effects of computer vision syndrome. It is also important to take breaks and to blink (Princeton University, 2017).

REVIEW The Concept of Informatics

RELATE Link the Concepts

Linking the concept of informatics with the concept of legal issues:

1. Name three ways in which a nurse can keep protected health information secure.
2. What are some ramifications of looking up information in a local celebrity's chart if you are not taking care of that individual?

Linking the concept of informatics with the concept of addiction:

3. You are a nurse at a busy inner-city emergency department. It is 3:00 a.m. on a Saturday when a patient comes in asking for a narcotic prescription. She reports that she usually gets her prescription from her primary care provider for ankle pain from an old injury, but she forgot to call during the week. Describe how an EHR can assist you in caring for this patient.
4. What type of questionnaire tools could be built into an EHR to assist with screening patients for chemical dependency?

REFER Go to Pearson MyLab Nursing and eText

REFLECT Apply Your Knowledge

Susan Johnson is a 45-year-old RN who works in a busy medical–surgical unit. Her hospital just installed an EHR system, and because of the layout of the unit, it was decided that the nurses would chart using workstations on wheels. Susan is excited about the new computerized system and has adapted to it quickly. She usually works three 12-hour shifts a week, but a few nurses are out on maternity leave, so she has been picking up extra hours. She has been noticing some tension and pain in her neck and shoulders, especially after her shifts.

1. What are some factors that may be contributing to the tension and pain in Susan's neck and shoulders?
2. What are some things that Susan could try to alleviate these symptoms?
3. What are some advantages to using WOWs for patient documentation?

» Exemplar 48.A Clinical Decision Support Systems

Exemplar Learning Outcomes

48.A Analyze clinical decision support systems as they relate to informatics.

- Describe the role of uniform languages in clinical decision support systems.
- Describe the use of computers in nursing research.
- Describe the use of computers in nursing administration.

Exemplar Key Terms

Clinical decision support systems, *2817*
Dashboard, *2818*

Overview

Clinical decision support systems (CDSSs) are an important addition to EHRs. A CDSS can be a general system that is used as developed by the vendor, or it can be customized by the organization. A CDSS uses a knowledge base and programmed rules, protocols, and evidence-based guidelines to match against patient data in the EHR and deliver alerts or recommendations to the provider. A CDSS can improve patient care by reducing medication errors, increasing adherence to best-practice protocols, and decreasing costs. However, a CDSS can be challenging: If it is not set up correctly, too difficult to navigate, or creates too many alerts (leading to alert fatigue), users will become frustrated, and this can negatively impact patient care.

Nurses' Use of Clinical Decision Support Systems

EHRs and CDSSs are designed to provide nurses with alerts, reminders, and recommendations to guide best practice and support clinical decision making. Lopez et al. (2017) conducted an integrative review of research on clinical support systems for nurses. Conclusions indicated nurses' use of CDSSs included nursing diagnostic support, medication management, improving situational awareness, supporting guideline adherence, and triage. They also found that CDSSs that direct bedside RN decision making show promise for improving quality of care.

Using Research

The use of EHRs that contain clinical decision support systems should help promote best practices through nursing research and make it easier to use current nursing research at the point of care (Lopez et al., 2017). More high-quality research is needed to evaluate the impact of nurse-focused CDSSs. Research in the area of adoption of CDSS is helpful in understanding the barriers to using those best practices (Sutton et al., 2020).

Computers in Nursing Research

With the introduction of the EHR, computers will be available to nurses in all practice settings. Research environments will be no different. Conducting nursing research should be easier with the use of uniform language and the ability to query EHRs. The steps of the nursing research process should remain the same. Technology can assist nurses in many ways to gain additional information: The nurse can use the EHR to research the patient's medical history to determine if the patient has been prescribed a particular drug and what responses the patient experienced following administration. The nurse can use the internet to conduct a literature search to determine if there is more information on use of that drug in certain populations or to get additional information related to potential side effects. For a detailed discussion of nursing research, including a list of nursing research databases, see Module 45, Evidence-Based Practice.

Computers in Nursing Administration

Many EHRs give administrators tools to manage budgets, staffing, quality initiatives, and productivity information. The use of dashboards puts all of this information at the administrator's fingertips. A **dashboard** presents information about a healthcare facility's key performance indicators and displays the information in an easy-to-read format, often with charts or graphs. Some information can be displayed in real time. EHRs can create reports that track data over short-term periods (the past week) or long-term periods (the past year).

Human Resources

Human resource departments and payroll departments can benefit from computerization by tracking personnel within the healthcare system. Professional licenses and credentials expire and must be renewed. It would be a daunting task to keep track of this information manually for a large facility that employs thousands of healthcare professionals. A computerized system can monitor license expiration and when recredentialing of a provider is required. Mandatory hospital education, employee attendance, and performance reviews can all be tracked. When government regulatory agencies make their visits, all of this information is easier to obtain and review. Payroll systems are more accurate with a computerized system. Employees can have access to their available hours of vacation and sick time and may be able to view their paycheck online a few days before they are paid.

Medical Records Management

Much of medical records management revolves around finances. The process begins when a patient schedules an appointment or enters the system on an emergency basis. An informatics system can help schedule the appointment, verify insurance coverage and co-pay information, collect the patient's demographic information, and collect any outstanding payments or co-pays. If the patient is being admitted to the hospital, the system can help with obtaining insurance authorization and assigning a room and bed that have been marked clean and available by the system (and a roommate of the same gender if it is not a private room). The patients' condition can be coded for payment based on their code (HIMSS, 2016). International Classification of Diseases (ICD) codes are used to report inpatient procedures and medical diagnoses (Center for Medicare and Medicaid Services [CMS], 2020b). Current procedural terminology (CPT) describes surgical, medical, and diagnostic services; hearing and vision services; occupational and physical therapy services; and transportation. The Healthcare Common Procedure Coding System (HCPCS) contains two levels: Level I is the CPT coding and Level II codes a wide array of services, such as durable medical equipment, outpatient chemotherapy drugs, medical supplies, orthotics, and prosthetics (CMS 2020b).

Facilities Management

Another system that most nurses are unfamiliar with is materials management and supply chain. When a patient needs a surgical dressing changed, the nurse goes to the supply room and grabs a new dressing without much thought about how it got there. As in many areas of healthcare, the materials management and supply chain community pushed for standardization for efficiency and cost savings. The first standard is that each institution has a Global Location Number (GLN) instead of an account number to make location of the institution easier. The second standard is that each product used in a facility has a Global Trade Item Number (GTIN) instead of a custom item number. It is thought that these standards will help by reducing errors in shipments, streamlining recall processes, enabling facilities to negotiate better contract pricing, and improving the supplier's ability to meet contract requirements. Electronic systems, with or without barcode scanning, can help make equipment use and tracking more efficient and help reduce costs. These systems also make it easier to keep track of supplies on hand and assist with ordering supplies or materials as they are used.

Budget and Finance

Before the patient's chart can be finalized and closed, it is reviewed to make sure all coding is correct so that proper information is sent to the billing department. Some facilities do their own billing; others hire separate companies for this. If a patient is receiving care in the hospital, there are usually two separate billing processes. One is professional billing, which covers fees for services provided by surgeons, radiologists, and anesthesiologists. The other is hospital billing, which covers room and board and supplies. Incorrect billing can result in a claim being denied by a patient's insurance company. This denial could leave either the patient or the hospital responsible for the bill, so there is usually a process for billers to submit appeals or resolve claim denials. It is a very complicated system that can be made easier through an electronic administration system.

Reimbursement rates for procedures and diagnoses change regularly, and a computerized contract management system helps facilities track rates of reimbursement and real-time changes in policies for different health insurance plans. Pay-for-performance systems will drive areas of reimbursement such as chronic disease management and care for acute disease without causing unnecessary harm (NEJM Catalyst, 2018). Financial systems within healthcare facilities can benefit greatly from use of an electronic system. They are responsible for sharing information between billing systems, materials management, and staffing/human resources in order to determine the financial health of the facility. The data provided is crucial for making strategic decisions about a healthcare institution and in planning organizational budgets. Executives and managers can view financial information over both short- and long-term time frames and adjust their resources and fiscal planning appropriately.

Quality Assurance and Utilization Reviews

Computerized systems facilitate the tracking of patient outcomes. Unexpected or poor patient outcomes can be tracked by risk management (the legal department of a health system). Quality outcomes information can also be easily tracked. Outcome tracking helps identify faulty processes and assists in modifying policies and procedures to improve patient outcomes for a particular diagnosis or department within a health organization. Using CDSS and quality improvement efforts, health centers can build in best practice protocols to improve patient care and outcomes (NEJM Catalyst, 2018).

Accreditation

The availability of quality metrics will make it easier to meet and document the requirements of regulatory agencies. Agencies such as the Centers for Medicare and Medicaid Services and The Joint Commission implement policies that health facilities must follow in order to receive reimbursement by many health insurance plans. There are also smaller yet still important standards that must be maintained for certification, such as trauma status from the American College of Surgeons or stroke center status from The Joint Commission. EHRs simplify the data-gathering process when each of these agencies reviews a facility for accreditation.

REVIEW Clinical Decision Support Systems

RELATE Link the Concepts and Exemplars

Linking the exemplar of clinical decision support systems to the concept of cellular regulation:

1. Discuss how clinical decision support systems could improve outcomes for patients with cancer.
2. Name three cancer screening tools that could be built into an EHR.
3. Discuss the benefits of making reminders for cancer screenings available to HCPs and to patients.

Linking the exemplar of clinical decision support systems to the concept of health policy:

4. You are working in the operating room, and your supervisor always requires that the employees in the department enter a higher level-of-diagnosis code on each trauma patient's chart. What are some ramifications?
5. What impact does a change in a federal or state health policy have on clinical decision support systems?

REFER Go to Pearson MyLab Nursing and eText

REFLECT Apply Your Knowledge

You are the nurse manager for an orthopedic unit that has just installed an EHR system with an administrative system. You have been short-staffed for several months.

1. How can an administrative system help get more nursing positions approved for your unit?
2. What other features of an administrative system do you think will have the greatest impact on your unit and why?

Exemplar 48.B Individual Information at Point of Care

Exemplar Learning Outcomes

48.B Analyze individual information at point of care as it relates to informatics.

- Summarize the advantages of point-of-care service delivery.
- Outline uses of computer-based patient records in community and hospital settings.

Exemplar Key Terms

Case managers, *2820*
Point of care, *2820*

Overview

Studies indicate that the more direct nursing care a patient receives, the better the quality and safety of the care that is delivered and the more satisfied both nurse and patient are with the care. Nurses have reported that documenting is an activity that consumes much of their time and takes time away from the bedside. The ability to enter data into a patient's chart while at the patient's bedside seems like a valid compromise. Most EHRs allow recording of vital signs, medication documentation, assessment notes, and responses to nursing intervention (**Figure 48.4** ⟫). One of the selling points of an EHR is that charting at point of care is possible and that it helps to increase efficiency. Interventions at **point of care** refers to interventions or testing that takes place using transportable, portable, or hand-held devices near the patient (Clifford, 2018). This setup provides on-the-spot information about the patient rather than having to wait for the results from blood or urine samples sent to the laboratory.

Computer-Based Patient Records

Although the EHR has the potential to forever change how healthcare is delivered in the United States, it is important to understand that, in many instances, the electronic record cannot and should not replace real-time (face-to-face or telephone) communication with peers, other health professionals, and especially the patient. An acute change in the patient's condition still requires a phone call to the HCP. News of pathology reports that indicate cancer should still be delivered in person by the provider and not discovered by the patient online. As systems become more advanced and interfaces more integrated, nurses must not lose sight of the human element in the delivery of care.

Patient Monitoring and Computerized Diagnostics

Advances in electronic systems are changing monitoring and tracking of patient care. Many facilities now use systems that allow electronic transmission of information, such as the weight from the scale on the bed, intravenous pump rates, barcode scanning of medications that are administered, vital sign information, barcode scanning of blood administration, and ventilator settings. Many departments within a hospital or other facility may enter data about the patient into the record so that all practitioners have the information easily available rather than having to flip through a paper chart. Some examples are laboratory diagnostics and many radiologic exams, such as MRI and CT scans (**Figure 48.5** ⟫). With some systems, the radiologic image as well as the radiologist's report are available at the bedside. The patient's medication administration record also may be viewed by all providers involved in care of the patient (**Figure 48.6** ⟫).

Community and Home Health

Each year, more than 4 million people are admitted to or reside in nursing homes and skilled nursing facilities; another 1 million reside in assisted living communities (Centers for Disease Control and Prevention [CDC], 2016). In 2015 (the most recent year for which data were available at the time of this writing), nearly 5 million patients received some degree of home healthcare (CDC, 2016). Nurses are the main providers of this care to patients, many of whom are receiving home healthcare for a chronic disease such as diabetes or congestive heart failure. It is difficult sometimes to stay current with the management of complex medical issues that home healthcare nurses are facing. The incorporation of current evidence-based clinical practice guidelines into the EHR system that is used by the home healthcare agency can improve the quality of care that these patients receive.

Case Management

Case managers help manage the care of certain patient populations, including patients with chronic medical conditions, such as diabetes; patients recovering from acute conditions, such as those receiving joint replacement; and patients with psychiatric disorders. EHRs can assist the case manager by allowing trending of patient progress, documentation of patient education, and observation of quality metrics to help decrease readmission rates for these populations. EHRs also allow improved coordination of care among providers because they are all working off of one chart.

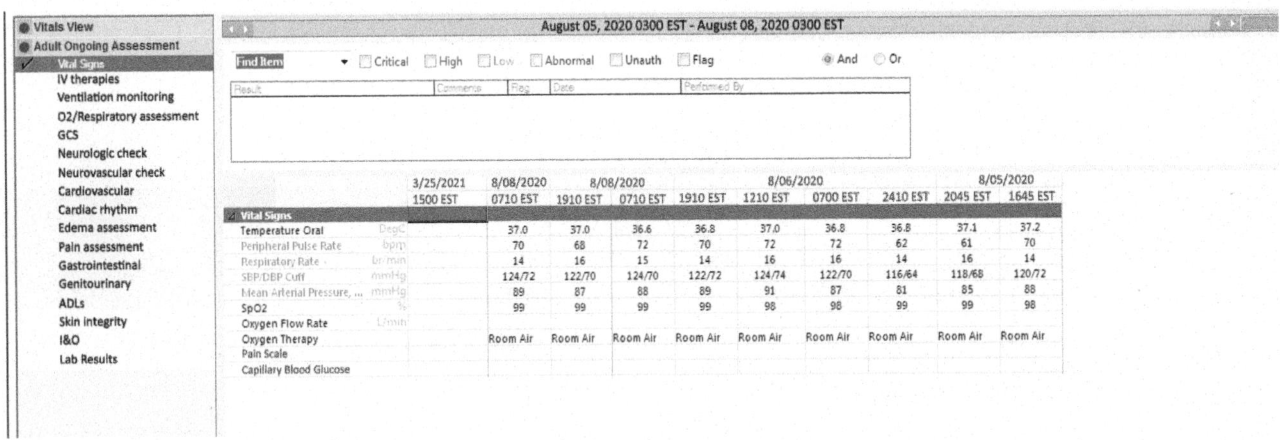

Figure 48.4 ⟫ This EHR screen displays the patient's vital signs. They can be entered by the nurse (or anyone with security rights to do so) at the bedside and they can be displayed wherever needed.

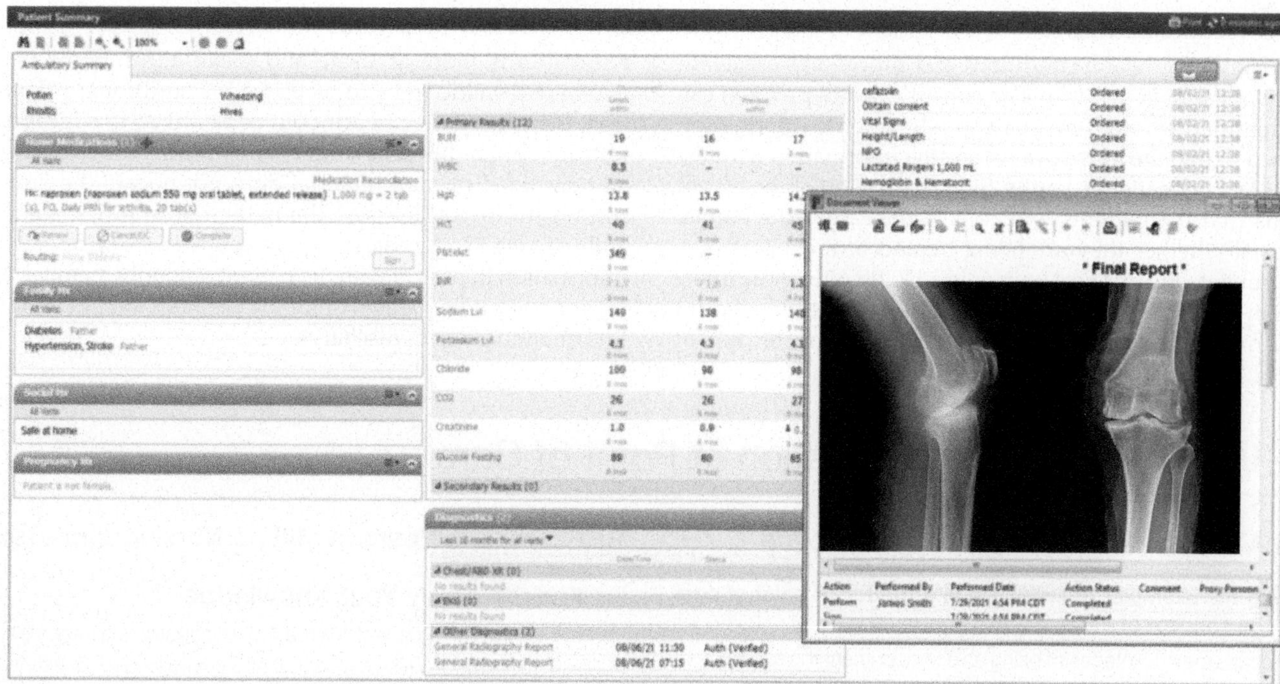

Figure 48.5 ›› This EHR screen displays a summary view of all available laboratory results and diagnostic imaging for a particular patient. Summary information is reported first so that the user gets the overview and can then “drill down” to see the details.

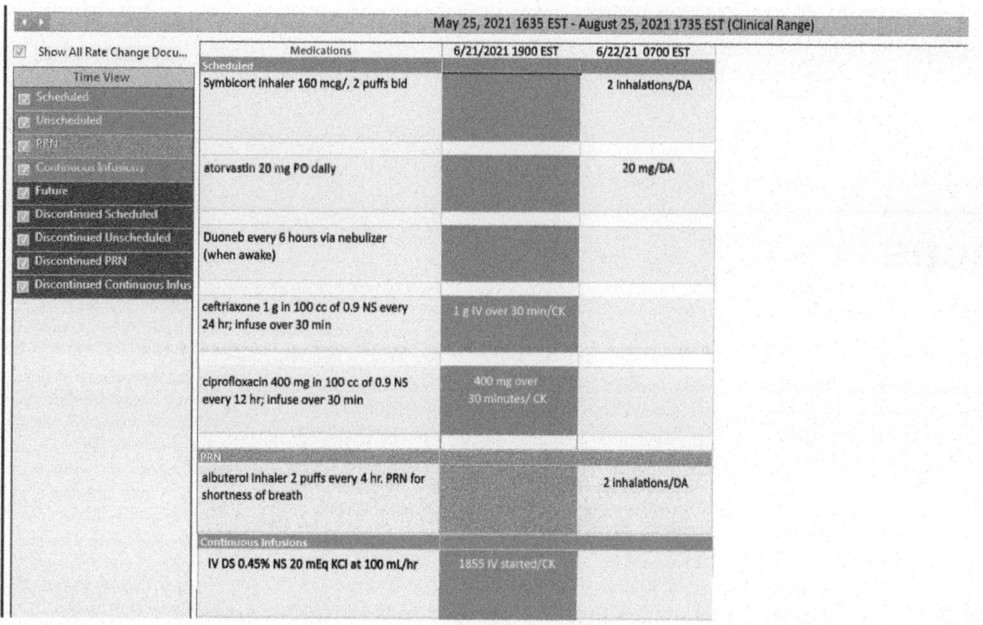

Figure 48.6 ›› This EHR screen shows a medication administration record for several regularly scheduled medications. The worksheet displays the next time the medications are scheduled to be administered.

Patient Education

Instructions for health conditions and procedures are available in most EHR systems. The patient's health problem can be identified through menus and educational information printed so that the nurse can review the information with the patient or the patient's family. Standardization of the record means that the patients will receive the same educational material whether they are being treated in the emergency department, on a surgical unit, or in a HCP's office. The information contained within the educational material should be current and evidence based, so that the task of patient education is more accurate and meaningful. Some material may provide links to websites for additional information. Many systems can print out or be linked to educational information in different languages as well. (Note that use of standardized printed material does not negate the nurse's responsibility to (1) assess the patient or family member's ability to read and understand the information, (2) review the information in person with the patient or family member, and (3) ensure that the patient or family member understands the information prior to discharge.

REVIEW Individual Information at Point of Care

RELATE Link the Concepts and Exemplars

Linking the exemplar of individual information at point of care with the concept of assessment:

1. Discuss the advantages of being able to document the assessment of your patient at the point of care with an electronic record rather than a centralized charting location.
2. Explain how point-of-care documentation of your patient assessment can be used as an opportunity for patient teaching.

Linking the exemplar of individual information at point of care with the concept of oxygenation:

3. What point-of-care information can you obtain from an electronic medical record about the patient's past and present oxygenation status that may influence immediate nursing interventions?
4. How might point-of-care recording of pulse oximeter values have an advantage over recording them from a centralized monitoring station in the intensive care unit?

REFER Go to Pearson MyLab Nursing and eText

REFLECT Apply Your Knowledge

You are caring for a patient from another country who just had his appendix removed. You log into your health system's electronic record to obtain discharge information. The patient and the family speak limited English. Their language of origin is not listed among the languages for which there are materials for appendectomy discharge instructions.

1. What are some options that you can use to try to educate the patient on taking care of his incision site?
2. How would you document your interventions in the electronic record?

References

Advisory Board. (2019). *CMS has a new plan to combat health care fraud.* https://www.advisory.com/daily-briefing/2019/09/10/fraud

Agency for Healthcare Research and Quality (AHRQ). (2017). *The CAHPS ambulatory care improvement guide.* https://www.ahrq.gov/sites/default/files/wysiwyg/cahps/quality-improvement/improvement-guide/6-strategies-for-improving/access/cahps-strategy-6d.pdf

Agency for Healthcare Research and Quality (AHRQ). (2019). *Telehealth for acute and chronic conditions.* https://effectivehealthcare.ahrq.gov/products/telehealth-acute-chronic/research

American Nurses Association (ANA). (n.d.). *Nursing informatics: Scope and standards of practice* (2nd ed.). Author.

American Nurses Association (ANA). (2018). *Social media dos and don'ts for nurses.* https://engage.healthynursehealthynation.org/blogs/8/1507

American Telemedicine. (2020). *FCC Covid-19 telehealth program application guidance.* https://www.americantelemed.org/policies/fcc-covid-19-telehealth-program-application-guidance/

American Medical Informatics Association (AMIA). (2011). *What is biomedical and health informatics?* https://www.amia.org/sites/default/files/What-is-Informatics-Fact-Sheet-040811.pdf

American Medical Informatics Association (AMIA). (2020). *Nursing informatics.* https://www.amia.org/programs/working-groups/nursing-informatics.

Beck, M. (2016, June 26). How telemedicine is transforming health care. *Wall Street Journal.* http://www.wsj.com/articles/how-telemedicine-is-transforming-health-care-1466993402

Bresnick, J. (2018). *CMS renames meaningful use to highlight interoperability goals.* Health IT Analytics. https://healthitanalytics.com/news/cms-renames-meaningful-use-to-highlight-interoperability-goals

Campanella, P., Lovato, E., Marone, C., Fallacara, L., Mancuso, A., Ricciardi, W., & Specchia, M. L. (2016). The impact of electronic health records on healthcare quality: A systematic review and meta-analysis. *European Journal of Public Health, 26*(1), 60–64.

Center for Connected Health Policy. (n.d.). *State telehealth laws and reimbursement policies.* https://www.cchpca.org/telehealth-policy/state-telehealth-laws-and-reimbursement-policies-report

Centers for Disease Control and Prevention (CDC). (2016). *Home healthcare.* https://www.cdc.gov/nchs/fastats/home-health-care.htm

Centers for Disease Control and Prevention (CDC). (2019). *State information.* https://www.cdc.gov/drugoverdose/states/index.html

Centers for Medicare and Medicaid Services (CMS). (2019). *Meaningful use.* http://www.cdc.gov/ehrmeaningfuluse/introduction.html.

Centers for Medicare and Medicaid Services (CMS). (2020a). *Data and program reports.* https://www.cms.gov/regulations-and-guidance/legislation/ehrincentiveprograms/dataandreports.html

Centers for Medicare and Medicaid Services (CMS). (2020b). HCPCS coding questions. https://www.cms.gov/Medicare/Coding/MedHCPCSGenInfo/HCPCS_Coding_Questions

Centers for Medicare and Medicaid Services (CMS). (2020c). *Promoting interoperability program.* https://www.cms.gov/Regulations-and-Guidance/Legislation/EHRIncentivePrograms/index?redirect=/EHRIncentivePrograms

Chen, Y. Y., Li, C. M., Liang, J. C., & Tsai, C. C. (2018). Health information obtained from the internet and changes in medical decision making: questionnaire development and cross-sectional survey. *Journal of Medical Internet Research, 20*(2), e47.

Clauson, L. (2020). *Telehealth visits surge along with coronavirus cases.* Roll Call. https://www.rollcall.com/2020/03/24/telehealth-visits-balloon-along-with-coronavirus-cases/

Clifford, J. (2018). *The pros and cons of point of care testing vs laboratory testing.* MLO. https://www.mlo-online.com/continuing-education/article/13017084/the-pros-and-cons-of-pointofcare-testing-vs-laboratory-testing

Dempsey, C. (2019). *What is GIS?* GIS Lounge. https://www.gislounge.com/what-is-gis/

Dempsey, C. (2020). *This map is tracking the coronavirus (covid-19) in near-realtime.* GIS Lounge. https://www.gislounge.com/this-map-is-tracking-the-novel-coronavirus-in-near-realtime/

Dendere, R., Slade, C., Burton-Jones, A., Sullivan, C., Staib, A., & Janda, M. (2019). Patient portals facilitating engagement with inpatient electronic medical records: a systematic review. *Journal of Medical Internet Research, 21*(4), e12779.

Dusseux, E. (2020). *IoT and medical device integration: How we get there.* Healthcare Business & Technology. http://www.healthcarebusinesstech.com/iot-and-medical-device-integration-how-we-get-there/

Evariant. (2019). *The role of social media in healthcare: Benefits & challenges.* https://www.evariant.com/blog/the-evolving-role-of-social-media-in-healthcare?origin=Blog&origin=%20HIPPA%20Compliance%20Social%20Media%202015%2009%2010blog_20150910hippacompliancesocialmedia

HealthIT.gov. (2018). *Medical practice efficiencies and cost savings.* https://www.healthit.gov/providers-professionals/medical-practice-efficiencies-cost-savings

HealthIT.gov (2019a). *What is electronic prescribing.* https://www.healthit.gov/faq/what-electronic-prescribing

HealthIT.gov. (2019b). *What is telehealth? How is it different from telemedicine?* https://www.healthit.gov/providers-professionals/faqs/what-telehealth-how-telehealth-different-telemedicine

HealthIT.gov (2019c). *Why is telehealth important to rural providers?* https://www.healthit.gov/faq/why-telehealth-important-rural-providers

HealthIT.gov (2020). *Patient engagement.* https://www.healthit.gov/playbook/patient-engagement/

Health Level Seven International. (n.d.). *About HL7.* http://www.hl7.org/about/index.cfm?ref=nav.

Levin-Zamir, D., & Bertschi, I. (2018). Media health literacy, ehealth literacy, and the role of the social environment in context. *International Journal of Environmental Research and Public Health, 15*(8), 1643.

Lopez, K. D., Gephart, S. M., Raszewski, R., Sousa, V., Shehorn, L. E., & Abraham, J. (2017). Integrative review of clinical decision support for registered nurses in acute care settings. *Journal of the American Medical Informatics Association, 24*(2), 441–450.

National Institutes of Health. (2011). *How to evaluate health information on the internet: Questions and answers.* https://ods.od.nih.gov/Health_Information/How_To_Evaluate_Health_Information_on_the_Internet_Questions_and_Answers.aspx

National Network of Libraries of Medicine. (2020). *Evaluating health websites.* https://nnlm.gov/professional-development/topics/health-websites.

NEJM Catalyst. (2018). *What is pay for performance in health care.* https://catalyst.nejm.org/doi/full/10.1056/CAT.18.0245

Occupational Safety and Health Administration (OSHA). (n.d.-a). *Prevention of musculoskeletal disorders in the workplace: Ergonomics.* http://www.osha.gov/SLTC/ergonomics

Occupational Safety and Health Administration (OSHA). (n.d.-b). *Computer workstations: Checklist.* http://www.osha.gov/SLTC/etools/computerworkstations/checklist.html

Ommaya, A. K., Cipriano, P. F., Hoyt, D. B., Horvath, K. A., Tang, P., Paz, H. L., et al. (2018). Care-centered clinical documentation in the digital environment: Solutions to alleviate burnout. *NAM Perspectives.* https://doi.org/10.31478/201801c

Princeton University, University Health Services. (2017). *Ergonomics and computer use.* http://www.princeton.edu/uhs/healthy-living/hot-topics/ergonomics

Steger, A. (2020, April 17). Weighing the pros and cons of wearable health technology. *HealthTech.* https://healthtechmagazine.net/article/2020/04/weighing-pros-and-cons-wearable-health-technology-perfcon

Substance Abuse and Mental Health Services Administration. (2018). *Opioid overdose prevention toolkit.* https://store.samhsa.gov/product/Opioid-Overdose-Prevention-Toolkit/SMA18-4742

Sutton, R. T., Pincock, D., Baumgart, D. C., Sadowski, D. C., Fedorak, R. N., & Kroeker, K. I. (2020). An overview of clinical decision support systems: benefits, risks, and strategies for success. *NPJ Digital Medicine, 3*(1), 1–10.

Tsou, A. Y., Lehmann, C. U., Michel, J., Solomon, R., Possanza, L., & Gandhi, T. (2017). Safe practices for copy and paste in the EHR. *Applied Clinical Informatics, 26*(1), 12–34.

University of Michigan, University Health Service. (2017). *Computer ergonomics: How to protect yourself from strain and pain.* https://www.uhs.umich.edu/computerergonomics

U.S. Department of Health and Human Services (DHHS). (n.d.). *Your rights under HIPAA.* www.hhs.gov/hipaa/for-individuals/guidance-materials-for-consumers/index.html

U.S. Department of Health and Human Services (DHHS). (2017). *HITECH act: Enforcement of the clinical rule.* https://www.hhs.gov/hipaa/for-professionals/special-topics/hitech-act-enforcement-interim-final-rule/index.html

U.S. Department of Health and Human Services (DHHS). (2018). *Social media.* https://www.hhs.gov/web/social-media/index.html

U.S. National Library of Medicine, National Institutes of Health. (n.d.). *Ergonomics.* http://www.nlm.nih.gov/medlineplus/ergonomics.html

World Health Organization. (2020). *eHealth at WHO.* https://www.who.int/ehealth/en/

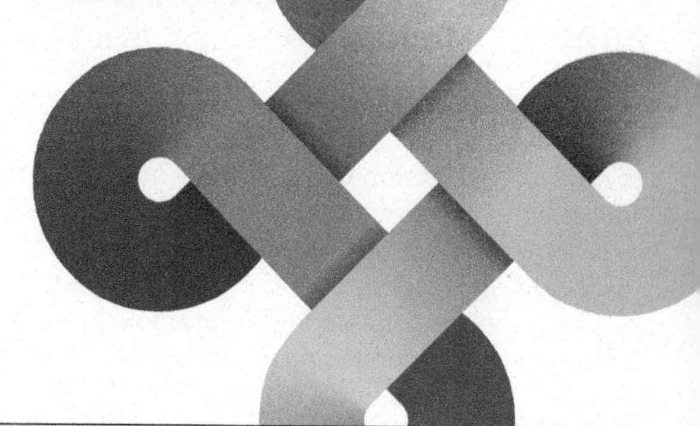

Module 49
Legal Issues

Module Outline and Learning Outcomes

The Concept of Legal Issues

Sources and Types of Laws

49.1 Analyze the sources of laws and types of laws.

Tort Law

49.2 Analyze tort law and its implication for nursing.

Concepts Related to Legal Issues

49.3 Outline the relationship between legal issues and other concepts.

Strategies to Prevent Incidents of Professional Negligence

49.4 Outline strategies to prevent incidents of professional negligence.

The Standard of Care

49.5 Analyze the impact of the standard of care on legal issues.

Selected Laws That Affect Nursing Practice

49.6 Outline laws that affect nursing practice.

Lifespan Considerations

49.7 Differentiate considerations related to legal issues throughout the lifespan.

Legal Issues Exemplars

Exemplar 49.A Nurse Practice Acts

49.A Analyze nurse practice acts as they relate to legal issues.

Exemplar 49.B Advance Directives

49.B Analyze advance directives as they relate to legal issues.

Exemplar 49.C Health Insurance Portability and Accountability Act

49.C Analyze HIPAA as it relates to legal issues.

Exemplar 49.D Mandatory Reporting

49.D Analyze mandatory reporting as it relates to legal issues.

Exemplar 49.E Risk Management

49.E Analyze risk management as it relates to legal issues.

›› The Concept of Legal Issues

Concept Key Terms

Administrative laws, **2826**
Assault, **2828**
Battery, **2828**
Breach of duty, **2828**
Causation, **2828**
Civil law, **2827**
Competency, **2832**
Controlled Substances Act (CSA), **2832**
Crime, **2826**
Criminal law, **2826**
Damages, **2828**
Duty, **2828**
Expressed consent, **2831**
False imprisonment, **2828**
Foreseeability, **2828**
Good Samaritan laws, **2833**
Implied consent, **2831**
Informed consent, **2831**
Injury or harm, **2828**
Law, **2826**
Liability, **2828**
Malpractice, **2825**
Negligence, **2827**
Standards of care, **2828**
Statute of limitations, **2828**
Statutory laws, **2826**
Tort, **2827**
Whistleblower, **2833**
Whistleblowing, **2833**

Legal issues in nursing encompass the rights, responsibilities, and scope of nursing practice as defined by state nurse practice acts and as legislated through criminal and civil laws. All patients have a privilege, demand, or claim by virtue of law or *right* (that which is proper or just) to expect competent nursing services. The nursing student must be equipped to provide safe nursing care consistent with legal requirements and to gain an awareness of ways to minimize the risks of errors due to accident, carelessness, system failures, or malpractice.

Malpractice is conduct that deviates from the standard of practice dictated by a profession. According to the National Practitioner Data Bank, professional nurses were responsible for 795 of 11,810 malpractice payments paid in 2018. That is just under 7% of malpractice payments made during that year (Singh, 2020). The number of nursing malpractice cases is associated with both the liability risks of nursing practice and an increasingly well-informed patient base.

›› **Stay Current:** The National Practitioner Data Bank is an excellent source of research and information on healthcare and nursing topics. Visit their website at www.npdb.hrsa.gov for more information.

Providing safe care requires the nurse to have more than just a knowledge of anatomy and physiology, pathophysiology, and medications and therapies. It also requires knowledge of the regulations of healthcare providers (HCPs), institutions, payment systems, and federal and state laws that are interconnected within the domain of the healthcare system. Upon enrollment, the nursing student begins learning about laws and regulations that affect nursing practice. Legal and professional regulations address both nursing practice and the practices of healthcare organizations that serve as workplaces for nurses at all levels of practice. Many healthcare agency policies and procedures exist to ensure that relevant laws are followed (1) to promote patient safety and reduce the risk for errors resulting in adverse events and (2) to protect both healthcare staff and healthcare agencies as a whole. For example, policies regarding identifying and managing patient valuables help ensure that patients' belongings are cared for and respected and also act to prevent theft or accidental loss.

To provide safe, effective care and maintain personal protection from liability, nurses must be aware of the applicable regulations they must follow in every nursing encounter. Awareness begins with understanding general legal concepts and continues as the nursing student starts to learn about the laws and regulations that directly affect the daily activities of nursing.

Sources and Types of Laws

Guido (2020) defines **law** as the "sum total of the rules and regulations by which a society is governed." Law is made at the federal, state, and local levels to reflect the ever-changing needs and expectations of a society. **Statutory laws** are made by the legislative branches of the government, including the U.S. Congress, state legislatures, and city and county governments. The U.S. Constitution grants the federal government power to make laws; the states have inherent power to act to maintain health, public order, safety, and welfare except where the Constitution restricts their ability to do so.

Nursing laws are examples of state statutory laws. Each state has a nurse practice act that contains the laws pertaining to nursing practice in that state. Nurse practice acts are discussed in detail in Exemplar 49.A in this module. Other statutory laws that affect the practice of nursing include statutes of limitation, protection and reporting laws, natural death acts, and informed consent laws.

A legislative body, through statutory law, delegates the responsibility for the administration and enforcement of those laws to administrative agencies. Administrative agencies may be granted additional power to interpret those laws and enact policies or procedures by which those laws will be implemented and enforced. These policies or procedures are often referred to as **administrative laws**. State boards of nursing are examples of administrative agencies that are delegated the power to interpret and enforce law by the legislatures that govern them.

An overview of the sources of law is shown in **Figure 49.1 ››**. Selected categories of law that may affect nurses are shown in **Table 49.1 ››**.

Both criminal and civil laws have implications for the practicing nurse. **Criminal law** defines conduct that is harmful to another individual or to society as a whole and that may be punishable by fines or imprisonment. A **crime** is an act prohibited by statute or by common-law principles. Crimes are considered to be committed against the state rather than the individual. Examples of crimes include homicide, theft, and manslaughter. Crimes are classified by severity, more serious crimes being classified as *felonies* and lesser offenses

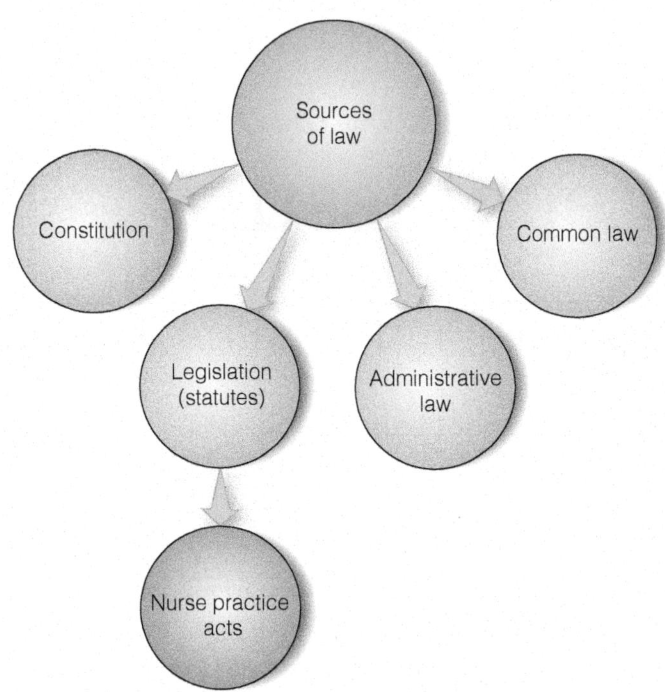

Figure 49.1 ›› Overview of the sources of law.

TABLE 49.1 Selected Categories of Laws Affecting Nurses

Category	Examples
Constitutional	Due process Equal protection
Statutory (legislative)	Nurse practice acts Good Samaritan acts Child and adult abuse laws Advance directives Sexual harassment laws Americans with Disabilities Act
Criminal (public)	Homicide, manslaughter Theft Arson Active euthanasia Sexual assault Illegal possession of controlled drugs
Contracts (private/civil)	Nurse and patient Nurse and employer Nurse and insurance provider Patient and agency
Torts (private/civil)	Negligence/malpractice Libel and slander Invasion of privacy Assault and battery False imprisonment Abandonment

Source: From Berman, Snyder, and Frandsen (2021). Pearson Education, Inc., Hoboken, NJ.

being termed *misdemeanors*. Criminal laws are enforced by law enforcement and government prosecutors.

Civil law deals with the rights and duties of private individuals or citizens and is most often enforced through lawsuits. A **tort** is a civil wrong committed against an individual or an individual's property. An individual who violates tort law may be sued and compensation awarded to those wrongfully injured by those violations. Torts may be intentional or unintentional.

Tort Law

Tort law defines and addresses unintentional and intentional actions or omissions that result in harm to another person or persons or harm to another's personal property. Unintentional torts discussed here include negligence and malpractice. Intentional torts include assault, battery, false imprisonment, and invasion of privacy.

Unintentional Torts

It is especially important for nurses and other HCPs to understand negligence and malpractice.

Negligence

Negligence is conduct that deviates from what a reasonable person would do in a particular circumstance. The "reasonable person" standard describes an individual in society who exercises average care, skill, and judgment in conduct as a comparative standard for determining liability. According to this standard, an individual who undertakes a particular activity is ordinarily considered to have the knowledge common to others who engage in that activity; for example, a motorist must know the rules of the road. A negligent act occurs when an individual damages the person or property of another without any intent to injure. This damage may be due to carelessness on the part of the individual who committed the act. For example, a driver who is talking on a cell phone or otherwise not paying attention and causes an automobile crash by failing to stop at a stop sign may be considered negligent and would be liable for any damages to any person or property.

In a legal action to establish negligence, the injured party needs to prove that the other party had a *duty of reasonable care*, that the other party *did not maintain reasonable care*, and that the failure to maintain such reasonable care *caused* (resulted in) *injuries* to the aggrieved party. In the example of the automobile crash, all drivers have the duty to operate their vehicles safely and follow traffic laws. If a driver fails to do so and this failure results in injury to any other person or damage to property, that driver would meet all of the criteria to be held negligent and would therefore be accountable for paying damages to the injured party.

Malpractice

When discussing negligence, it is important to note that the standard of a "reasonable person" is different for individuals in specific professional occupations. If an individual engages in an activity that requires special skills, education, training, or licensure—such as piloting a plane or providing professional nursing care—the standard by which that person's conduct is measured is the conduct of a reasonably skilled, competent, and experienced individual who is a qualified member of the group that is authorized to engage in that activity (**Box 49.1** »). Should an individual fail to meet the standard of conduct for their profession, this failure may be considered an instance of *professional negligence,* also known as *malpractice*.

Malpractice includes acts and omissions committed by a professional in the course of performing professional duties. Malpractice is one of the most important areas of the law for nurses because any negligent act or omission, however unintentional, may rise to the standard of malpractice and may jeopardize the professional nurse's license and, more

---

Box 49.1

Categories and Examples of Negligence That Result in Malpractice

Failure to Follow Standards of Care

Failure to:

- Perform a complete admission assessment or design a plan of care.
- Adhere to standardized protocols or institutional policies and procedures (e.g., using an improper injection site).
- Follow a provider or prescriber's verbal or written orders, if appropriate.
- Provide an environment that promotes safety.
- Adequately monitor the patient's condition and take appropriate action to protect the patient.
- Notify the provider or prescriber of any changes in the patient's condition.

Failure to Communicate and Document Accurately

Failure to:

- Understand and use informatics to properly communicate knowledge of the patient's condition.
- Document and communicate assessment findings, laboratory values, or any changes in patient status to the provider and the healthcare team.

Failure to Act as a Patient Advocate

Failure to:

- Question orders when a patient's condition warrants it.
- Question incomplete or illegible medical orders.
- Report unsafe practice to the proper persons.

Failure to Supervise Adequately

Failure to:

- Know the skill levels of supervised personnel
- Adequately monitor supervised personnel

Sources: Based on Berman et al. (2021); Guido (2020).

importantly, patient safety. It is also important to remember that anyone who performs the special skills associated with a particular profession, whether qualified or not, is held to the standards of conduct of those who are properly qualified to do so because the public relies on the special expertise of those who engage in such activities. Thus, a nursing student is held to the same standard of conduct as an experienced, licensed professional nurse.

Elements of Professional Negligence or Malpractice

Six elements of professional negligence or malpractice are required to establish **liability**, which is defined as the state of being legally obligated and responsible:

- The patient must be owed a **duty**, a legally enforceable obligation to adhere to a particular standard of care (Guido, 2020). The formation of a provider–patient relationship is the basis for finding that the HCP owes a duty to the patient. A nurse–patient relationship begins when the nurse accepts responsibility for providing nursing care to a patient (North Carolina Board of Nursing, 2020).
- A deviation from the standard of care owed to the patient, called a **breach of duty**, must occur by either commission or omission. For example, the nurse has a duty to correctly administer medication to a patient. Giving the patient the wrong dose of medication would be a breach of duty.
- The element of **foreseeability** (certain events may reasonably be expected to cause specific results) must be present. The nurse should know in advance, or reasonably anticipate, that damage or injury will probably ensue from acts or omissions.
- The injury must have resulted as a direct result of the professional's breach of duty, called **causation**. Typically, a patient cannot successfully make a claim for malpractice on acquiring a healthcare-associated infection. Only if the patient could show that a specific nurse did not follow the standard of aseptic technique would the standard of causation be met.
- The plaintiff must demonstrate that some type of physical, financial, or emotional **injury or harm** resulted from the breach of owed duty. If the nurse gave the wrong medication but no harm occurred, the elements are not present for malpractice.

SAFETY ALERT Nurses administering medications must know why the patient is receiving the medication, the acceptable dosage range, possible adverse effects, toxicity levels, and contraindications.

- The basic purpose of a malpractice lawsuit is to award damages sufficient to restore the plaintiff's original position, as far as is financially possible. The amount of the **damages**, or compensation, for the plaintiff's loss or injury may include enough money to pay for any medical fees associated with the injury. If the plaintiff lost the ability to work as a result of the injury, damages could include compensation for lost wages as well as for medical fees. With evidence of apparent physical harm, the court may order compensation for emotional damages (pain and suffering) as well. Punitive damages may be awarded as punishment if the nurse's misconduct is deemed malicious, willful, or wanton (Guido, 2020).

Related Doctrines

Several legal doctrines, or principles, are related to negligence and malpractice. One such doctrine is *respondeat superior* ("let the master answer"). A lawsuit for a negligent act or omission performed by a nurse generally will also name the nurse's employer. Employers may also be held liable for negligence if they fail to provide adequate human and material resources for nursing care, fail to properly educate nurses on the use of new equipment or procedures, or fail to orient nurses to the facility. Another doctrine is *res ipsa loquitur* ("the thing speaks for itself"). In some cases, the harm cannot be traced to a specific HCP or standard but does not normally occur unless there has been some type of negligence. An example is harm that results when a surgical instrument is inadvertently left in a patient during surgery.

Statute of Limitations

There is a limit to the amount of time that can pass between recognition of harm and bringing a suit. This is referred to as the **statute of limitations**. The exact time limitation varies by type of suit and state, but plaintiffs typically have 1 to 2 years from the time that they knew of the injury or had reason to believe that an injury was sustained to file a malpractice lawsuit. Statutes of limitations applying to minors vary from state to state; some states identify specific variances such as extended time limits for specific types of injuries.

Intentional Torts

A number of intentional torts—actions taken by an individual with the intent to perform the action—have a bearing on nursing practice. The willful nature of these actions and the intent behind them separate intentional torts from negligence and malpractice.

Assault, Battery, and False Imprisonment

Assault is the action of creating an apprehension of offensive, insulting, or physically injurious touching. Assault can occur without an individual's actually being touched. Threatening a patient who refuses to agree with starting an intravenous line is assault. **Battery**, on the other hand, is defined as willful touching of another individual (or the individual's clothes or even something the individual is carrying) that is unwanted, embarrassing, or unwarranted, such as touching done without permission or giving an injection without a patient's consent. Even the simple act of ambulation requires the patient's consent. Forcing a patient to ambulate against their will may be considered battery (Guido, 2020).

Guido (2020) defines **false imprisonment** as the "unjustifiable detention of a person without legal warrant to confine the person." False imprisonment includes confining the patient to the room or restraining the patient to the bed with the intent to restrict or prevent the individual's freedom. Detaining a patient who wishes to leave against medical advice is generally considered false imprisonment.

Because **standards of care** (the skills and learning common to their profession, including the nursing process) prohibit nurses from forcing patients to participate in treatment or to engage in any action against the patient's will, assault, battery, and false imprisonment are actions that violate standards of care and may rise to the level of civil or criminal action against the nurse.

Invasion of Privacy

According to the Fourth Amendment to the U.S. Constitution, individuals have the right to privacy. Information concerning patients is confidential and may not be disclosed without authorization. The patient's right to privacy extends to use of the patient's name as well as photographic or videographic representations of the patient (e.g., the patient's picture may not be used without proper authorization). This right extends to control of the patient's personal belongings, personal space, and immediate territory. The nurse–patient relationship is based on trust. Searching a patient's room, touching personal belongings without first requesting permission, and entering a patient's room without knocking are behaviors that potentially violate this trust. Most healthcare agencies have policies and procedures that specify to whom and under what circumstances patient information can be released, and they have appropriate procedures for managing patient environments and personal property within the agency. Failure to follow these policies could lead to a claim of invasion of privacy.

Nurses are bound by the Privacy Rule of the Health Insurance Portability and Accountability Act (HIPAA) to protect the privacy of the patient's protected health information. This includes information related to mental and physical conditions, healthcare services provided, and payment for services rendered. It also includes name, address, birth date, and Social Security number (Tariq & Hackert, 2020). HIPAA protections represent the minimum requirements for privacy. State law and professional codes may afford additional protections, in which case the stricter law is enforced. HIPAA and the Privacy Rule are discussed in more detail in Exemplar 49.C in this module.

Concepts Related to Legal Issues

Safety and legal issues are closely connected. Ensuring patient safety and preventing care errors have important legal implications for nurses, as well as implications for the health of their patients. As many as 1 in 10 patients experience adverse events during hospital stays; a large number of these events involve medication errors (World Health Organization, 2019). Prevention measures are essential for reducing these events; equally important is properly reporting any errors that do occur. Proper reporting can minimize the impact errors have on patients and help organizations and individuals gain valuable insight into the causes of errors. Unfortunately, nurses sometimes do not report errors. If uncovered later on, these errors and the subsequent failure to report could have professional and legal ramifications.

Issues of consent are important for all nurses but present special considerations in managing care. Nurse managers must adhere to legal requirements related to safety, communication, and many other areas; they must also ensure that other members of the care team follow these requirements. When requirements are not followed by team members, the nurse manager must identify and correct the situation. In addition, managers must ensure that patient care tasks are delegated appropriately to licensed and unlicensed staff and that these tasks are carried out correctly and completely according to state nurse practice acts and facility policy.

The Concepts Related to Legal Issues feature outlines some of the many ways in which legal issues intersect with other concepts. The concepts are presented in alphabetical order.

Strategies to Prevent Incidents of Professional Negligence

Situations may arise in nursing practice that can lead to reported negligence or malpractice cases. A continuing issue in nursing is medication errors, which must be clearly documented and discussed with the patient (Institute for Safe Medication Practice [ISMP], 2020). Other situations in which problems may arise include communicating care concerns and key information about the patient's condition; ensuring that providers' orders are clear; understanding how to use equipment in practice; and providing appropriate mentoring, assessment, and care plans for patients (Lum & Lau, 2018; Wojciechowski, 2019).

Maintaining Patient Safety

The nurse must always be aware of any safety issues related to a patient. Older and hospitalized patients may become confused by procedures, medications, and the change in environment. The nurse is responsible for implementing appropriate safety measures at patient admission following facility protocols and best practice. The nurse is also responsible for educating the patient and caregivers about safety measures and reasons for their use.

SAFETY ALERT Patient falls are a common cause of injury to the patient and may result in legal action against the nurse and/or the healthcare facility for possible negligence. The nurse must carefully assess for fall risk and document all measures taken in relation to that assessment.

The nurse must be aware of and attend to all patient issues to prevent a charge of malpractice by a patient or family based on the nurse's failure to observe and act. Any patient issue that is not addressed by the nurse could ultimately result in a complaint of negligence. For example, the nurse who ignores a patient's complaint of sudden head pain may be accused of malpractice if the patient then loses consciousness due to brain bleed. Consistent patient assessment and documentation will assist the nurse in being aware of and addressing patient needs.

Another issue that may be a cause of malpractice is incorrect identification of a patient. The nurse must always check the patient's identification during each patient encounter to ensure that the correct patient is receiving the correct care.

Using Effective Communication

Nurses interact with patients and families during the provision of care. Poor communication skills may cause the patient or family to view the nurse as less than competent. Poor communication coupled with a negative outcome can increase the chance of a malpractice claim. Clear communication and attentive listening regarding the patient's healthcare and patient education can help decrease the risk of bad outcomes and demonstrate an element of caring. Accurate documentation and reporting (see Exemplar 38.C, Documentation, in

Concepts Related to
Legal Issues

CONCEPT	RELATIONSHIP TO LEGAL ISSUES	NURSING IMPLICATIONS
Cognition	Patients demonstrate the capacity to understand the benefits, risks, and alternatives for care. If this capacity exists, consent must be given voluntarily.	■ Provide information about procedures and conditions appropriate to the patient's cognitive level. ■ Work with the care team to assess the patient's capacity to give consent. ■ Assist the patient with consent forms and answer any questions the patient may have. ■ Work with the surrogate decision maker if the patient lacks the capacity to provide consent.
Comfort	Patients have the legal right to receive appropriate end-of-life (EOL) care. All hospitals receiving Medicare and Medicaid funds are legally responsible to provide advance directive information and support patients' advance directive needs.	■ Assess own assumptions or biases surrounding EOL care. ■ Assess your knowledge of appropriate EOL care options in your practice area. ■ Ask for support from supervisor or peers to assist in advocating for appropriate EOL care. ■ Anticipate further assessment of information patients and family members may need. ■ Be aware that advance directives improve the EOL planning process by giving patients peace of mind and easing family conflict during health crises.
Communication	Nurses must ensure the privacy of all patient information during all care and in all care areas and must follow HIPAA regulations.	■ Ensure that patient information, such as electronic records, is accessible only for appropriate use by appropriate staff members. ■ Discuss with your patients how you ensure privacy. ■ Ensure that patient care is discussed only with appropriate individuals and not outside the care unit.

Module 38, Communication) provide a source of information that will either support or refute allegations of malpractice. Nursing documentation should be completed according to policy and should clearly depict the timeline of care, including assessments, interventions, the patient's response to interventions, and notification of information outside treatment protocol (e.g., abnormal lab values, changes in patient assessment). Remember that this document serves as the legal record of what occurred, so nurses should document defensively, be inclusive, and not rely on their own or the patient's memories of the details of care.

Minimizing the Risk of Medication Errors

Administration of medications has been identified as a high-risk activity for error. Prevention of medication errors requires a systems approach involving all interprofessional healthcare personnel. Information on reducing medication errors is provided in Exemplar 51.D, Medication Safety, in Module 51, Safety.

Obtaining Professional Liability Insurance

Nurses, like physicians, should carry professional liability insurance to manage their personal financial risk. Occurrence-based coverage covers incidents that occurred during the time period the policy was in effect, regardless of whether the policy was still in effect when the claim was made. Claims-made policies provide coverage only if the incident occurred and the claim was reported during the active policy period. Policies should identify limits of liability, declarations, deductibles, exclusions, reservation of rights, covered injuries, defense costs, coverage conditions, and supplementary payments.

Policies may be individual, group, or employer sponsored. Individual coverage provides the broadest coverage to the policyholder. This type of policy covers the named policyholder on a 24-hour basis as long as the individual's actions fall within the scope of practice. Employer-sponsored coverage provides the narrowest coverage for the individual nurse; the policy covers only actions performed during work as an employee of the institution. Nursing students are generally required to carry liability insurance for the duration of the education program, although some programs insure students under a broad institutional policy.

The Standard of Care

The applicable state nurse practice act and administrative rules form the basis of the standard of care to which each nurse is held. They define professional conduct and the scope of practice for the licensed nurse and identify activities for all levels of personnel providing nursing care. These laws are not static, and every nurse needs to be aware of any changes.

The nurse's specific job description will contribute to defining the standard of care. Employers can limit but not expand the scope of practice, and the nurse is held to functioning within the scope of employment.

Although agency policies and procedures may seem to contain overwhelming amounts of information, they serve to define the standard of care. The prudent nurse reviews and implements the policies and procedures relevant to practice. If there is a conflict between current practice and policy, the nurse should be proactive in resolving the conflict through quality improvement processes (see Module 50, Quality Improvement).

A primary source for defining the standard of care is the prevailing national nursing standards. These include the American Nurses Association (ANA) Standards of Practice as well as specialty practice standards appropriate to a nurse's practice (e.g., standards for critical care nurses). Nurses who follow these standards will provide their patients with the best care possible and minimize the likelihood of committing any unintentional act that may rise to the level of malpractice.

Selected Laws That Affect Nursing Practice

In addition to tort laws, a number of other laws affect nursing practice. These include laws related to informed consent and competency, as well as laws regarding the Controlled Substance Act and the Good Samaritan Act. Because states have the freedom to enact additional legislation that may further define or restrict aspects addressed by federal law, all nurses should be aware of the laws that govern or affect nursing practice in their own states.

Informed Consent

Informed consent refers to the patient's legal and ethical rights to be informed of, and give or refuse permission for, any healthcare procedure or treatment. The healthcare provider has the duty to disclose information about proposed treatment in terms the patient can reasonably understand. The healthcare provider must also disclose information about available alternatives, the risks and benefits of each treatment option, and the patient's right to refuse treatment.

Informed consent should contain the following elements:

- The reason the patient requires treatment (presenting problem or diagnosis)
- The reason the specific procedure or treatment is needed
- How the procedure or treatment will help or benefit the patient and what the patient can experience during or as a result of the intervention
- Possible negative side effects or negative outcomes of the procedure or treatment
- Alternatives to the recommended procedure or treatment, including the possibility of declining treatment. Advantages and disadvantages of all alternatives should be presented.

Informed consent must be given voluntarily without the patient experiencing any pressure or fear. The HCP must be careful to present the information to the patient in an impartial manner to prevent undue influence on the patient.

Healthcare professionals must be careful to use words that a patient can understand when engaging in the informed consent process. Assessment of the patient's ability to see, hear, and read must be completed to ensure the patient has full understanding of the issue being discussed. It may be necessary to read the consent to the patient or provide an interpreter prior to the patient signing the consent. Use of a family member as an interpreter should be avoided to ensure patient privacy and accuracy of the information being presented. The nurse should also consider the patient's cultural and spiritual preferences when asking a patient to make decisions about a procedure or treatment. Some religions and some cultures have specific practices that affect healthcare, although patients may or may not follow them (Colwell, 2019).

The nurse should follow the employing agency's specific protocols regarding informed consent. Obtaining informed consent for specific medical and surgical treatments is the responsibility of the individual who will perform the procedure. Consent must be obtained for all procedures and treatments, including nursing care. However, this does not require written consent before each occurrence. Most nurses rely on **expressed consent** (an oral or written agreement) or **implied consent** based on a patient's action. The patient either verbally indicates participation in the care or nonverbally takes actions that are consistent with the care. For example, patients who position their bodies for an injection or cooperate with the taking of vital signs are expressing implied consent. While state laws generally hold the physician or provider liable for failure to obtain informed consent, nurses need to understand implied versus obtained consent.

Focus on Diversity and Culture

Cognitive Impairment and Informed Consent

Cognitively impaired adult patients present special particular concerns when it comes to informed consent. The presence of cognitive impairment does not automatically preclude a patient from giving consent, although some patients who have been declared legally incompetent by a court will have a legal guardian who must give consent. In determining whether a patient without a legal guardian is able to give informed consent, the patient's capacity to understand the benefits, risks, and alternatives for care and to make and communicate a decision must be considered (Vanderbilt Kennedy Center, 2020). This capacity can change over time and may be affected by the nature and complexity of the decision involved; therefore, the patient's capacity should be assessed and documented for each treatment. If a patient does not have the capacity to consent or it is unclear whether the patient has the capacity, decision making should be delegated to a surrogate, following agency procedure. Consent is required for elective and therapeutic surgeries, diagnostic procedures, and procedures that involve sedation or anesthesia. Consent is not required for time-sensitive, lifesaving emergency procedures (Vanderbilt Kennedy Center, 2020).

Competency for Consent

Competency is a legal presumption applied to individuals when they become adults. Competency gives adults the right to negotiate certain legal activities, such as making a will or entering into a contract. In most states, an individual is considered to be competent at 18 years of age unless some evidence to the contrary persuades a court to declare that individual incompetent.

Adults who have been declared legally incompetent through a court order are provided a legal guardian. The legal guardian should give HCPs a copy of the court order granting the authority to make healthcare decisions on the other adult's behalf. Examples of adults who may be legally incompetent include those who have sustained a debilitating brain injury as a result of a motor-vehicle crash and those who have profound intellectual disability.

An adult may be rendered temporarily incompetent by narcotic medication or a serious fall or may gradually be rendered incompetent as a result of dementia. The nurse who has concerns about a patient's level of competency should alert the primary care provider. If the primary care provider determines that the patient is not competent for the purposes of informed consent, the provider will determine whether the emergency doctrine applies (see the Consent in an Emergency section below) or whether someone else can validly make healthcare decisions on the patient's behalf. State laws regarding consent for adults who are rendered temporarily incompetent vary. Courts generally presume continuing competency of adults unless the healthcare facility can show that the patient is unable to understand the consequences of their actions (Guido, 2020). All healthcare staff, including nurses, should be familiar with their state's laws and with the policies and procedures of their employing agency. Nurses should recognize the effect of issues related to competency on providing nursing care because patients have the right to decline nursing care as well as medical procedures. The Focus on Diversity and Culture feature discusses how a patient's cognitive impairment may affect the process of obtaining informed consent.

Consent in an Emergency

In most states, the law assumes an individual's consent to medical treatment when the individual is in imminent danger of loss of life or limb and unable to give informed consent. In other words, the emergency doctrine assumes that the individual would reasonably consent to treatment if able to do so. This doctrine serves as a guiding principle that permits HCPs to perform potentially lifesaving procedures under circumstances that make it impossible or impractical to obtain consent. The emergency doctrine may not always apply. For example, it does not extend to allowing HCPs to implement a treatment or procedure to which the patient would not reasonably consent if the patient were able to do so. It also does not permit HCPs to provide a treatment or procedure that the patient previously refused. For example, if a patient has previously refused a procedure on religious grounds, HCPs may not implement the procedure if the patient becomes unconscious.

Child Participation in Healthcare Decisions

For a minor child (under age 18), a parent or guardian must give informed consent for medical treatment. Specific legal exceptions do exist, however, including situations when:

- The emergency doctrine applies
- The child is an *emancipated minor* (one who is no longer under parental control and manages their own financial affairs)
- The child is a resident of a state that allows a *mature minor* to give valid consent (for example, 14- and 15-year-old adolescents who are able to understand treatment risks)
- A court order to proceed with treatment exists
- The law recognizes the minor as having the ability to consent to a specific treatment.

In the majority of states, a minor who is the parent of a child may give informed consent for healthcare treatment of the child. Some states also permit teenagers of a certain age who are seeking certain types of care to do so without parental consent. Types of care that may not require parental permission, depending on state law, include contraceptive services, prenatal care, mental health counseling, diagnosis and treatment of sexually transmitted infections, and treatment of substance abuse (American Civil Liberties Union of Ohio, 2014; Keller, 2020).

In some states, mature minors are permitted to give consent for treatment or to refuse treatment. In some cases, minors must convince a judge that they are mature enough to make an independent judgment about consent for treatment. Nurses need to know the state and federal laws regarding consent as well as the agency's policies and procedures regarding informed consent (Nurse Journal, 2020). North Carolina law, for example, provides for all minors over the age of 12 to consent for contraceptive services, treatment of sexually transmitted infections, and prenatal care (Keller, 2020). For an overview of minor consent laws in the United States, see **Box 49.2** ».

Clinical Example A

Marvin Martinice, a 15-year-old boy with acute myelocytic leukemia, has come out of his second remission with an acute onset of fever, joint pain, and petechiae. A bone marrow transplant is one of the few remaining therapeutic options. Although Marvin has agreed to a transplantation if a suitable donor is found, he does not want to be resuscitated and placed on life-support equipment should he go into a cardiac arrest. Marvin has talked extensively with the hospital chaplain and social worker and feels comfortable with his decision. His parents want an all-out effort to sustain his life until a donor is located.

Critical Thinking Questions

1. In general, what happens when parents and children have conflicting opinions about treatment?
2. Assume you are a nurse involved in Marvin's care. What is your role, if any, in addressing the difference of opinion between Marvin and his parents regarding available treatment options?

Controlled Substances Act

The **Controlled Substances Act (CSA)** is a federal law that requires drugs to be classified on the basis of the substance's medical use, potential for abuse, and safety risks. The classifications are referred to as schedules and are numbered from I to V; Schedules I and II have the highest potential for

Box 49.2

Overview of Minor Consent Laws

Contraceptive Services

Twenty-seven states and the District of Columbia allow minors (beginning at either age 12 or 14 depending on the state) to consent to contraceptive services. Nineteen states allow only certain categories of minors to consent to contraceptive services. Four states have no specific law related to consent of minors to contraceptive services.

Sexually Transmitted Infections Services

Forty-five states and the District of Columbia allow all minors age 12 and older to consent to services for sexually transmitted infections. Hawaii, New Hampshire, North Dakota, and Idaho allow consent beginning at age 14. South Carolina allows consent beginning at age 16.

Prenatal Care

Thirty-three states and the District of Columbia explicitly allow all minors to consent to prenatal care. Fourteen of these states permit the provider to inform the minor's parents if the provider deems it in the patient's interest to do so.

Adoption

Twenty-eight states and the District of Columbia allow all minor parents to choose to place their child for adoption.

Medical Care for a Child

Thirty states and the District of Columbia allow all minor parents to consent to medical care for their child. The remaining 20 states have no relevant explicit policy or case law.

Abortion

Two states and the District of Columbia explicitly allow all minors to consent to abortion services. Twenty-one states require that at least one parent consent to a minor's abortion, while 10 states require prior notification of at least one parent. State laws regarding abortion may change; be sure to know the laws in your state.

Sources: Data from Centers for Disease Control and Prevention (2021); Guttmacher Institute (2020a, 2020c).

abuse (**Table 49.2** »). The CSA is enforced by the U.S. Drug Enforcement Agency, which regulates a closed system of distribution. This system provides for registration with unique identifiers for legitimate handlers of controlled substances and required record keeping that traces the flow of any drug from the time it is first imported or manufactured, through the distribution level, to the pharmacy or hospital that dispenses it, and then to the patient who receives it. Each state has its own requirements for prescribers. Nurses must abide by the rules and regulations of their state.

» **Stay Current:** For more information about the Controlled Substance Act, visit the Office of Diversion Control's website at www.deadiversion.usdoj.gov/21cfr/21usc.

Good Samaritan Laws

Most states have **Good Samaritan laws** that encourage HCPs to help victims in an emergency. These laws are designed to protect healthcare workers from potential liability when volunteering their skills outside of an employment contract (**Figure 49.2** »). To be protected by Good Samaritan laws, a nurse must adhere to the standard of nursing care during all volunteer activities. Nurses should provide only care that is consistent with their level of training and licensure. Once having made the decision to render emergency care, the nurse is responsible for following through by providing the necessary care or safely placing the victim in the care of someone who can provide the appropriate care (Matt, 2018). Before volunteering their skills, nurses should review the nurse practice act and the Good Samaritan law in the state in which they work.

Whistleblowing Laws

Whistleblowing is the disclosure of an employer's unsafe or illegal practices and/or polices by an employee (Guido, 2020). The employee who reports such practices or policies is called a **whistleblower**. The Whistleblower Protection Act of 1989 establishes certain protections for individuals who report gross misconduct on the part of their employers to federal authorities; additional protections may vary by state. To qualify for

TABLE 49.2 U.S. Drug Schedules and Examples

		Dependency Potential			
Drug Schedule	Abuse Potential	Physical Dependence	Psychologic Dependence	Examples	Therapeutic Use
I	Highest	High	High	Heroin, peyote, marijuana, MDMA ("ecstasy")	Medical use of marijuana/cannabis limited to specific states
II	High	High	High	Morphine, opium, cocaine, oxycodone, fentanyl, methadone, amphetamine, pentobarbital	Current accepted medical use in the United States with severe restrictions; prescription required
III	Moderate	Moderate	High	Tylenol with codeine, anabolic steroids, buprenorphine, ketamine	Current accepted medical use in the United States; prescription required
IV	Lower	Lower	Lower	Alprazolam, clonazepam, lorazepam, midazolam, diazepam	Current accepted medical use in the United States; prescription required
V	Lowest	Lowest	Lowest	Cough medicine containing codeine, ezogabine	Current accepted medical use in the United States; no prescription required

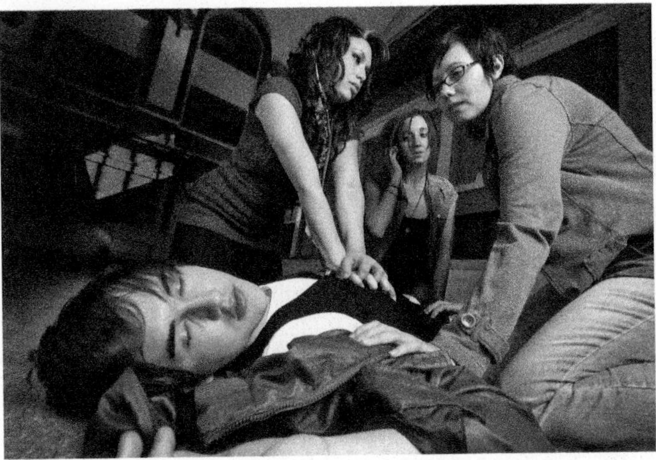

Figure 49.2 » Good Samaritan laws protect healthcare workers from liability when they volunteer their services in an emergency.
Source: Jsteck/E+/Getty Images.

protection under the federal act, the employee must make every effort to resolve the issue via the employer's internal reporting procedures before going outside of the organization. In addition, an employee does not qualify for protection under the act unless the employer has threatened or engaged in retaliation against the employee as a result of the employee's complaint.

Simple error or misconduct on the part of the employer does not qualify under the Whistleblower Protection Act. Typically, the activity or policy in question must violate a state or federal law or rule, and the employer must be aware that the activity or policy is a violation. Examples include billing fraud, failure to maintain safety equipment, and chronic insufficient staffing. The employee making the complaint must give the employer written notice and an appropriate amount of time to correct the issue. To be considered a whistleblower, the employee must also make or threaten to make a report to the appropriate state or federal agency.

Whistleblower laws exist to prevent retaliation by the employer against reasonable, good faith reporting of illegal, unethical, or unsafe conduct in order to provide a safe environment for patients. However, the nurse who makes a report outside of the employing agency should be prepared for the possibility of negative consequences. These may include personal consequences such as losing the support or friendship of coworkers. They may also include retaliatory or discriminatory actions, including dismissal, demotion, discipline, or intimidation. These actions are prohibited by the Occupational Safety and Health Act. To prevail in a discrimination claim, an employee must report discriminatory actions to the Occupational Safety and Health Administration before resigning from the place of employment.

Lifespan Considerations

Nurses should be aware of how legal issues may affect patients of different age groups and must understand their responsibilities for protecting their patients and themselves when these issues arise. No matter the age or condition of the patients with whom the nurse works, failure to keep up with changes in laws or regulations can endanger patients and place the nurse at risk for liability.

Legal Issues Pertaining to Infants and Children

Nurses are mandated reporters of child abuse or suspected child abuse, including physical, emotional, and sexual maltreatment. Although statutes related to reporting vary from state to state, nurses who fail to report abuse may face civil charges. Reports should be complete and accurate and should be made according to the policy of the organization for which the nurse works. In addition to reporting the abuse within the organizational framework, the nurse should personally report the abuse to the proper authorities. When abuse is reported, all pertinent information in the patient's medical record is required by law to be disclosed to the reporting agency. As such, reporting abuse or suspected abuse represents an exception to patient confidentiality rules (CDC, 2020).

Nurses should be aware of common signs of abuse in both infants and children. For example, bruising in infants can indicate physical abuse; vomiting, irritability, and lethargy may indicate head injury. Older children may exhibit unexplained injuries or bruises, injuries that do not match the explanations given, and untreated medical problems. Children and adolescents who report sexual abuse may exhibit no abnormal physical findings in an exam, though cultures may indicate the presence of sexually transmitted infections. If the parent or guardian of a child is responsible for the abuse, health history and interview information provided by that individual may be vague or intentionally misleading (Herendeen, Blevins, Anson, & Smith, 2014).

Accurate reporting of abuse and suspected abuse is essential for protecting the child and safeguarding the nurse both professionally and personally. The nurse is required to report the facts or circumstances that led to the belief that abuse occurred but does not have the burden of proof. Reports must be made in good faith and without malicious intent. Most states allow reports to be made anonymously but may encourage the reporter to provide identifying and contact information to aid in the investigation. In most states, if the reporter's identity is known, it is not disclosed to the individual suspected of committing the abuse (Child Welfare Information Gateway, 2019). Mandatory reporting is discussed further in Exemplar 49.D in this module.

» **Stay Current:** Nurses should be familiar with the child abuse reporting statutes in their state. Search by state and topic at the U.S. Department of Health and Human Services' Child Welfare Information Gateway at https://www.childwelfare.gov/topics/systemwide/laws-policies/statutes/manda/.

Legal Issues Pertaining to Adolescents

Confidentiality is a concern for some adolescents seeking care, particularly care related to contraception, sexual health, substance abuse, or mental health. Nurses should be familiar with federal and state laws related to adolescent confidentiality. Trust and honesty are essential. Nurses should ensure that patients understand that confidentiality will be maintained when possible, but that it cannot be guaranteed in some circumstances. For example, if the patient is covered under a parent's or guardian's insurance, billing and benefits statements provided to the parent or guardian may include information about care. It is also important that patients understand that the authorities must be contacted if a patient is in imminent danger, if there is evidence of abuse, or if the patient has certain communicable diseases (American Academy of Family Physicians, 2019).

Adolescent patients may wish to be examined or receive counseling separately from their parents or guardians. The nurse should make every effort to honor this request, though doing so may lead to confrontation with the parents or guardians. Understanding state statutes and organizational policy related to adolescent confidentially is essential when situations such as this arise.

The use of electronic health records (EHRs) presents additional concerns about confidentiality for adolescents. In general, child and adolescent EHRs are set up with parents or guardians as proxy. As a result, these individuals are able to view information contained in the EHR. Some EHR systems offer customizable modules that can be configured to restrict the proxy's access to confidential or sensitive information; some systems do not. Certain information gathered during general exams—such as social or sexual history—may be accessible to parents or guardians via the EHR unless it is included with the restricted information. If the system does not allow for customization to restrict information, patients should be informed that parents or guardians can access these records (American College of Obstetricians and Gynecologists, 2020).

When providing confidential care to adolescents, the nurse should encourage adolescents to consider involving parents or guardians in their decision making. The nurse should make it clear that this is a suggestion and not a requirement for receiving care. Patients who feel pressured to involve parents or guardians or who fear that their confidentiality may be breached may refuse treatment and may not receive the care they need.

Legal Issues Pertaining to Pregnant Women

Legal rights of pregnant women in the United States have been a subject of debate for many years. Perhaps the most famous example of this surrounds the Supreme Court's 1973 ruling in *Roe v. Wade*. In this ruling, the court deemed it unconstitutional for states to outlaw abortion during the first trimester of pregnancy and placed restrictions on states' ability to regulate abortion during the second and third trimesters. Since the ruling, abortion has remained a contentious issue in the United States. Statutes related to abortion vary from state to state and include regulations related to gestational limits, insurance coverage for procedures, and mandated counseling (Guttmacher Institute, 2020b).

In addition to statutes related directly to abortion, a number of states have passed fetal protection laws. The intent of these laws is to protect both mothers and fetuses and punish individuals who harm them. In some cases, however, these laws have raised questions about a woman's right to refuse certain tests or treatments during pregnancy (Law Teacher, 2019).

Abortion and fetal protection laws may create ethical or moral dilemmas for nurses. It is of the utmost importance that nurses know their state's statutes and their organization's policies on these matters. In addition, nurses should understand their rights of conscientious objection and their responsibilities in the event that they choose to be a conscientious objector. Conscientious objection is the refusal by the nurse to engage in a procedure because doing so would violate the nurse's moral or ethical principles (Ko, Koh, & Lee, 2020). Abortion, sterilization, and contraception are reproduction-related procedures that may give rise to conscientious objection. Currently, 45 states allow individual HCPs to refuse to participate in abortions, and 42 states allow institutions to refuse to provide them (Guttmacher Institute, 2020b). Nurses who choose to be conscientious objectors should make their refusal known in advance of the procedure to allow for necessary staffing adjustments. If advance notice is not possible, the nurse is duty bound to remain with the patient until another nurse can take over the patient's care. Failure to do so may be considered patient abandonment (Ko et al., 2020).

Legal Issues Pertaining to Older Adults

In many states, nurses are mandatory reporters of elder mistreatment, which encompasses elder abuse, neglect, and exploitation. Medicare requires that nursing facilities monitor patients for signs of mistreatment. Specific types of elder mistreatment include physical, emotional, verbal, and sexual abuse, as well as neglect and financial abuse. Signs of possible elder abuse include bruises, lacerations, fractures, open wounds, and untreated injuries in various stages of healing. Dehydration, malnutrition, and poor personal hygiene may signal elder neglect. Agitation, withdrawal, and sudden changes in behavior or financial situation may be indicative of other types of mistreatment (National Center on Elder Abuse [NCEA], n.d.). It is the nurses' responsibility to understand the reporting laws in their state and to report mistreatment or suspected mistreatment to the appropriate authorities. Failure to do so may result in civil or criminal penalties (Myhre, Saga, Malmedal, Ostaszkiewicz, & Nakrem, 2020). Even if state law does not identify them as mandatory reporters, it is advisable for nurses to report mistreatment or suspected mistreatment.

Screening and assessment are essential for identifying elder mistreatment. Patient interviews are commonly included in the assessment process, but age-related cognitive impairments can limit their effectiveness. Patients may also be hesitant to disclose mistreatment in an interview for fear that the abuse will worsen if they do so (Myhre et al., 2020). Elder mistreatment can be a difficult topic to broach with patients and family members or care providers who may be involved in the mistreatment. In addition, some signs of elder mistreatment are similar to signs associated with normal age-related changes and conditions. To help nurses better address and identify elder mistreatment, many state and national resources exist. State boards of nursing and the NCEA offer useful information on this topic.

>> **Stay Current:** The website of the National Center on Elder Abuse can be found at https://ncea.acl.gov.

End-of-life care is another important consideration for nurses working with older adults. EOL encompasses both planning and delivery of care. When an advance directive (AD) exists, the nurse is bound to provide care in accordance with the patient's wishes and organizational policy. When no AD exists, patients with the capacity to make EOL decisions for themselves may work with the nurse to determine the type of care they prefer (American Cancer Society, 2019). Advance directives are discussed in more detail in Exemplar 49.B in this module. For more on EOL care, see Exemplar 3.B, End-of-Life Care, in Module 3, Comfort.

REVIEW The Concept of Legal Issues

RELATE Link the Concepts

Linking the concept of legal issues with the concept of clinical decision making:

1. How does the nursing process support nurses in maintaining appropriate standards of care?
2. What type of consent is necessary for the nurse to take a patient's temperature and vital signs? For the patient to undergo an x-ray if a broken leg is suspected?

Linking the concept of legal issues with the concept of communication:

3. How does a change-of-shift report minimize the nurse's risk for professional negligence or malpractice?
4. What types of communication result in the best quality of patient care and are therefore most likely to prevent the nurse from being accused of malpractice?

REFER Go to Pearson MyLab Nursing and eText

REFLECT Apply Your Knowledge

Joanne Otunde, a coworker who is a registered nurse (RN) on your surgical unit, returned to work about 6 weeks ago following back surgery. Since her return, you have noticed that she is frequently and uncharacteristically late for work and has called in sick six times. Twice you have witnessed Joanne treating a nurse's aide harshly. Ms. Glancy, a patient who is 2 days postoperative, puts her light on and tells you that she is in severe pain and that the pain medication she received did not have any effect on the pain level. She states, "It's the strangest thing. The pill never seems to work in the evenings the way it does in the daytime and at night." You report Ms. Glancy's pain to Joanne, who is her primary nurse. At the end of the shift, you and an oncoming nurse are doing the narcotic count and notice that Joanne has given six doses of the same narcotic during the shift and one dose is documented as having been given at 8:00 p.m. to a patient who had been discharged at 5:00 p.m.

1. What are your responsibilities? Should you take any action? If so, why? If not, why not?
2. What laws do you need to review? What policies?

Exemplar 49.A Nurse Practice Acts

Exemplar Learning Outcomes

49.A Analyze nurse practice acts as they relate to legal issues.

- Explain how boards of nursing oversee licensure.
- Describe the National Council of State Boards of Nursing.
- Outline the Nurse Licensure Compact.
- Differentiate credentialing and certification.
- Explain the duties and responsibilities of nursing students.

Exemplar Key Terms

Certification, *2838*
Credentialing, *2838*
Mutual recognition model, *2838*
Nolo contendere, *2837*
Nurse practice act (NPA), *2836*
Responsibility, *2839*

Overview

The practice of nursing is regulated at the state level through a **nurse practice act (NPA)**. An NPA is a series of state statutes that define the scope of practice, standards for education programs, licensure requirements, and grounds for disciplinary actions. The law provides a framework for establishing nursing actions in the care of patients (**Box 49.3**). Laws set the boundaries for and maintain a standard of nursing practice (**Figure 49.3**). The nurse is held accountable to the specific standards for licensure and grounds for revocation in the state of employment. For the RN, the provisions of NPAs are quite similar from state to state. Greater variation exists in the scope of practice for the licensed practical nurse (LPN) and licensed vocational nurse (LVN).

Box 49.3
Anatomy of a Nurse Practice Act

Typically, the following components are addressed in an NPA. Nursing students and practicing nurses should understand the NPA for the state in which they are working and how each component of the NPA affects practice. Components of an NPA include the following:

- Definition of nursing
- Requirements for licensure
- Penalty for practicing without a license
- Exemptions from licensure
- Licensure across jurisdictions.

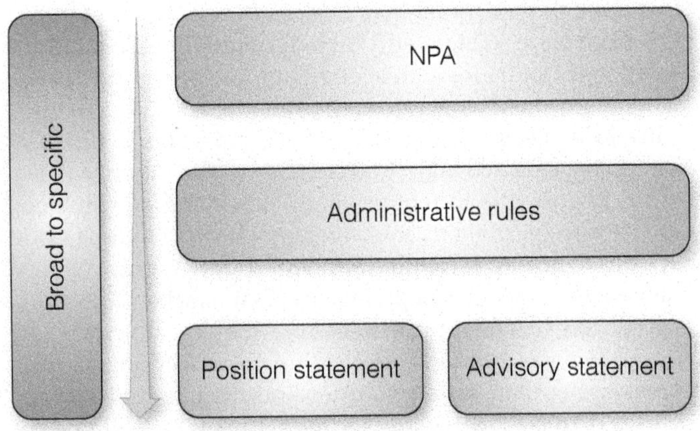

Figure 49.3 Relationship among nurse practice acts, administrative rules, and position/advisory statements.

Each state's NPA is enforced and administered by a state board of nursing (BON), though some states use other titles for this regulatory board. BONs were established some 100 years ago to standardize the education of nurses, establish standards for safe nursing practice, and issue licenses to protect the public from unprepared, unsafe practitioners. Over the years, BONs have expanded their scope. Programs for impaired nurses, remediation of practice issues, and participation in multistate licensure compacts are all part of BONs today. BONs also act as a forum for citizens to report and discuss concerns regarding nursing services they have received. In this way, BONs continue to work toward their goal of protecting the public health.

The state's NPA dictates the membership of the state's BON, which usually includes a mix of RNs, LPNs/LVNs, advanced practice registered nurses (APRNs), and consumers. The members of the BON are appointed according to the regulations in each state, with the exception of North Carolina. North Carolina is the only state in which licensed nurses serving on the board are elected by other licensed nurses and members of the public who serve are appointed.

Licensure

Licensure allows a nurse the legal privilege to practice nursing as defined in the state's NPA. Through the process of licensure, the BON ensures the provision of safe nursing care to the public. Typically, BONs oversee licensure through the following activities:

- Establishing and monitoring educational standards for nursing education programs
- Defining professional standards
- Examining and renewing the licenses of duly qualified applicants
- Investigating violations of the NPA
- Sanctioning (to the point of initiating prosecution against) those who violate the NPA
- Holding disciplinary hearings for possible suspension or revocation of a license
- Establishing and overseeing diversity programs in some states. The Focus on Diversity and Culture feature looks at efforts to increase diversity in the nursing workforce.

Each BON oversees the administration of a licensure examination that measures the competencies needed to perform safely and effectively as a newly licensed, entry-level nurse. The National Council of State Boards of Nursing (NCSBN) has developed two licensure examinations, the National Council Licensure Examination for Registered Nurses (NCLEX-RN®) and the National Council Licensure Examination for Practical Nurses (NCLEX-PN®), for state and territory BONs to implement as part of their requirements for licensure. The NCSBN also offers two additional examinations: the National Nurse Aide Assessment Program and the Medication Aide Certification Examination (NCSBN, 2020).

Licenses are issued by the state or territory in which the applicant nurse wishes to practice. For licensed nurses at all levels of practice, the BON monitors compliance with state laws, including maintaining continued competency and annual renewal of licensure. To maintain the privilege to practice afforded by the license, the individual nurse is required to demonstrate awareness and application of standards of nursing care and meet their responsibilities to both patients and the healthcare system. The board is also responsible for taking action against nurses who have exhibited unsafe nursing practice or otherwise engaged in professional misconduct or who fail to meet requirements for licensure renewal.

Each BON details what charges of professional misconduct may result in the revocation or suspension of a nurse's license. Most BONs will take action against the nurse who is found guilty of charges such as:

- Giving false information or withholding material information from the board in procuring or attempting to procure a license to practice nursing.
- Being convicted of or pleading either guilty or *nolo contendere* to any crime that indicates the nurse is unfit or incompetent to practice or has deceived or defrauded the public. In pleading ***nolo contendere***, the individual neither admits nor denies committing the crime but agree[illegible]

Focus on Diversity and Culture

Diversity and the Nursing Workforce

Since 2004, the Institute of Medicine (IOM) has emphasized the connection between a diverse nursing workforce and culturally competent nursing care. The IOM and many professional nursing organizations argue that diversity among nurses will improve access to care for minority patients and will result in greater patient satisfaction (American Association of Colleges of Nursing [AACN], 2019, 2020).

A diverse workforce begins by increasing the number of students of color enrolled in nursing programs, as well as increasing the number of men entering nursing. The AACN (2020) reports that the number of students of color in nursing programs has steadily increased since 2011, up to just over one-third of students at all levels. The number of male students in nursing programs has remained fairly steady at around 12–13% (AACN, 2019).

Federal government involvement has been an important factor in these increases, supporting a number of initiatives, some through collaboration with the AACN. Through the Nursing Workforce Diversity program, the Health Resources and Services Administration is striving to increase educational opportunities for groups that are underrepresented in the RN population (AACN, 2019). The program provides grants to schools of nursing that are committed to increasing the number of minority graduates. Recipient organizations can use funds for scholarships, stipends, and advanced education preparation. The AACN also collaborates with other professional nursing organizations to advocate for increased federal funding for Nursing Workforce Diversity Grants, which provide financial support to students from disadvantaged backgrounds.

A number of other professional nursing organizations offer programs to promote diversity at all levels of nursing programs. One example is the National Black Nurses Association's mentorship program, which seeks to support NBNA member nurses as they begin their careers or transition into new nursing roles or nursing leadership roles.

to a punishment (usually a fine or jail time) as if guilty. Usually, this type of plea is entered because it cannot be used as an admission of guilt if a civil lawsuit is initiated following the conclusion of a criminal trial.

- Engaging in conduct that endangers the public health.
- Being unfit or incompetent to practice by reason of deliberate or negligent acts or omissions, regardless of whether actual injury to the patient is established.
- Engaging in conduct that deceives, defrauds, or harms the public in the course of professional activities or services.

National Council of State Boards of Nursing

The NCSBN provides leadership to advance regulatory excellence for public protection. The membership of the NCSBN includes BONs in the 50 states, the District of Columbia, and four U.S. territories (Guam, Virgin Islands, American Samoa, and the Northern Mariana Islands). Four states (California, Georgia, Louisiana, and West Virginia) have separate BONs for RNs and LPNs/LVNs.

The NCSBN offers a number of services that support member BONs. It is responsible for developing the licensure and assessment exams mentioned earlier. In addition, the NCSBN offers continuing education opportunities via its e-learning community.

The NCSBN also serves as an important source of data and research about nursing practice (**Box 49.4** ⟫). It maintains a central nursing database called Nursys that coordinates nurse licensure information for the United States. It also works with BONs to promote uniform regulation of nursing practice. The Nurse Licensure Compact is an important outcome of these activities.

⟫ **Stay Current:** Contact information for state boards of nursing and information about licensure and NCSBN research can be found at https://www.ncsbn.org/boards.htm.

Nurse Licensure Compact

The **mutual recognition model** of nurse licensure allows a nurse to have a single license that confers the privilege to practice in other states that are part of the Nurse Licensure Compact (**Box 49.5** ⟫). Monitoring the nurse's license and taking any needed disciplinary actions are the responsibilities of the state that issues the license. It is similar to the driver's license model: A single license to drive is issued in the individual's state of primary residency, but this license also gives the individual the privilege to drive in other Drivers' License Compact states.

SAFETY ALERT When practicing in a mutual recognition state, nurses are held accountable for following the laws and rules of the state in which they are practicing, not the state that issued the license.

To achieve mutual recognition, each state must enact legislation or regulations authorizing the Nurse Licensure Compact. States that enter the compact also adopt administrative rules and regulations for implementation of the compact. More than 30 states are currently part of the compact.

⟫ **Stay Current:** For information on states participating in the compact, go to https://www.ncsbn.org/nurse-licensure-compact.htm.

Credentialing

Although a nursing license grants the legal privilege to practice, **credentialing** is the formal identification of professionals who meet predetermined standards of professional skill or competence. The federal government has used the term **certification** to define the credentialing process by which a nongovernmental agency or association recognizes the professional competence of an individual who has met certain predetermined qualifications specified by the agency or association. The American Nurses Credentialing Center (ANCC), a subsidiary of the ANA, provides credentialing

Box 49.4

NCSBN Research in 2021

Assessing the Impact of COVID-19 on Nursing Education

- Impact of rapid changes in nursing education caused by the COVID-19 pandemic

Global Regulatory Atlas Waiver Study

- Determination of regulatory changes made in response to the COVID-19 pandemic

Board of Nursing Pilot Study Regarding Resolution of Discipline Cases

- Study with 10 state boards of nursing to determine the best timing and practices in disciplinary actions

Economic Impact of Nurse Licensure Compact on Newly Adopting States

- Study to determine increased costs, revenue losses, and increased workloads to the boards of nursing

2010–2020 NURSYS Discipline Case Review

- Study focusing on trends in disciplinary action and any changes in board action in the last 10 years

Evaluation of the Effectiveness of the eNLC Information Campaign

- Study to determine if educational materials sent to newly adopting states was effective in understanding the implications of the enhanced nurse compact license

Source: National Council of State Board of Nursing (2021b).

Box 49.5

Mutual Recognition Model

- Each state has to enter into an interstate compact, called the Nurse Licensure Compact (NLC), that allows nurses to practice in more than one state.
- Multistate licensure privilege means the nurse has the authority to practice nursing in another state that has signed an interstate compact. It is not an additional license.
- Nurses must have a license in their primary state of legal residency if that state is an NLC state.
- The states continue to have authority in determining licensure requirements and disciplinary actions.
- The nurse is held accountable for knowing and practicing the nursing practice laws and regulations in the state where the patient is located.
- Enactment does not change a state's nurse practice act.
- Complaints and/or violations are addressed by the home state (place of residence) and the remote state (place of practice).
- RNs and LPNs/LVNs are included in the interstate compact or NLC. There is a separate APRN Compact. A state must be a member of the NLC for RNs and LPNs before entering into an APRN Compact. A state must adopt both compacts to cover LPNs/RNs and APRNs for mutual recognition.
- The COVID-19 pandemic created a need for emergency action by certain states in order to meet nursing needs. Emergency licensing waivers and applicable statutory provisions were made available at the NCBSN's website.

Source: National Council of State Boards of Nursing (2021a).

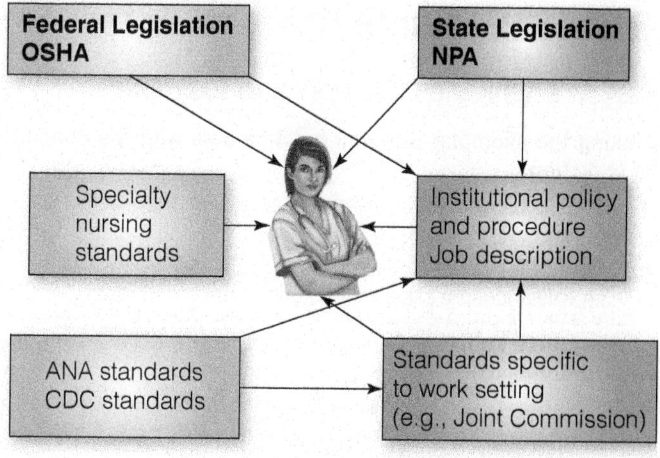

Figure 49.4 » Impact of laws and standards on nurses.

programs to certify nurses in specialty practice areas, recognizes healthcare organizations for nursing excellence through the Magnet Recognition Program, and accredits providers of continuing nursing education and nursing specialty organizations.

Federal organizations, such as The Joint Commission and the Centers for Medicare and Medicaid Services, and federal guidelines affect the standards of care the nurse is held accountable for practicing. Individual healthcare agencies must implement policies, procedures, and job descriptions to ensure that the nurses they employ follow all applicable regulations and guidelines. The nurse needs to know the employing institution's policies and procedures and the specific job descriptions of the licensed and unlicensed nursing personnel. The purpose of knowing the standards of care is to protect both the patient and the nurse.

The impact of laws and standards on nurses is profound (**Figure 49.4 »**). The professional nurse is held accountable for many standards and statutes. Knowledge of the laws that regulate and affect nursing practice enables the nurse to practice within current legal principles and be aware of their legal obligations and responsibilities.

Nursing Students

Each NPA addresses the duties and responsibilities of nursing students in that state. Typically, this includes language that allows nursing students the privilege to practice nursing without a license while engaged in the clinical practicum of an approved nursing education program under the supervision of qualified faculty. Nursing students have the ultimate **responsibility** (accountability for their actions that includes the obligation to answer for an act done and to repair any injury one may have caused) for their own actions. Guidelines for clinical performance for nursing students typically include:

1. Provide safe nursing care.
2. Understand program and facility policies and procedures before undertaking any clinical assignment.
3. Demonstrate knowledge about the patient's condition, interventions, medications, and treatments.
4. Perform care only to the highest level of nursing knowledge; if you are unprepared for a clinical assignment, inform your instructor.
5. Seek help before beginning a procedure about which you are unsure; if the instructor is not readily available, allow the staff nurse to perform the intervention.

Nursing students are held accountable to the same standard of care as licensed nurses. Nursing faculty members are held accountable for appropriate assignment and supervision of students.

SAFETY ALERT Student nurses do not practice on a faculty member's license. The only individual who can legally practice on a license is the individual whose name appears on the license.

Standards of Practice

Nursing, as a profession, has a responsibility to self-regulate by defining the practice of nursing, researching and developing the practice, establishing standards of practice, and providing for the education and credentialing of nurses. The ANA, the largest professional nursing organization, has established Standards of Clinical Nursing Practice, which address both standards for nursing care and standards for professional performance. Standards of practice are also available for various nursing specialties, including pediatric nursing, nurse anesthesia practice, critical care nursing, and psychiatric nursing.

REVIEW Nurse Practice Acts

RELATE Link the Concepts and Exemplars

Linking the exemplar of nurse practice acts with the concept of addiction:

1. What resources does your state's board of nursing offer for nurses who are struggling with substance abuse?
2. What would you do if you realized that a nurse you were working with was under the influence of drugs or alcohol? Explain.

Linking the exemplar of nurse practice acts with the concept of accountability:

3. What does your state's NPA say about the accountability of nursing students? How is that different from what the NPA says about the accountability of registered nurses?
4. How does your state's board of nursing support or assist nurses in their professional development?

REFER Go to Pearson MyLab Nursing and eText

REFLECT Apply Your Knowledge

Sarah Coulton is a RN who works with you in a primary care clinic. Her husband has been notified that his employer is transferring him to another state, and Sarah and her family will be moving in a couple of months.

1. Where will Sarah be able to find information on which states have mutual recognition with your state?
2. What steps might Sarah need to take if she learns that she is moving to a state that is not part of the Nurse Licensure Compact?

» Exemplar 49.B Advance Directives

Exemplar Learning Outcomes

49.B Analyze advance directives as they relate to legal issues.

- Describe types of healthcare advance directives.
- Outline elements of advance directives.
- Explain the role of the nurse in assisting families with advance directives.

Exemplar Key Terms

Durable power of attorney, *2840*
Healthcare advance directive, *2840*
Living will, *2840*
Patient Self-Determination Act (PSDA), *2840*

Overview

A **healthcare advance directive** (sometimes referred to as an AD) is a legal document executed by an individual that expresses that individual's desires regarding medical treatment that may be used if and when the individual is no longer able to communicate preferences directly (Kim, 2019). The patient's right to use ADs is guaranteed in the Patient Self-Determination Act. The **Patient Self-Determination Act (PSDA)** is a federal law requiring healthcare institutions that receive federal funding (but not individual HCPs) to do the following:

1. At the time of admission, give patients a written summary of:
   - Healthcare decision-making rights. (Each state has developed such a summary for hospitals, nursing homes, and home health agencies to use.)
   - The facility's policies with respect to recognizing ADs.
2. Ask patients whether they have an AD and document the AD's existence in the medical record. (It is up to the patient to provide a copy of the AD.)
3. Educate staff and community about ADs.
4. Ensure that the individuals know that the facility never discriminates on the basis of whether or not the individual has an AD.

Competent patients may execute ADs at any time. ADs are formal, written documents that typically outline the patient's desires related to:

- Use or withholding of hydration and/or total parenteral nutrition
- Resuscitation or intubation in the event of a life-threatening emergency (Do-not-resuscitate and do-not-intubate orders are discussed in Exemplar 3.B, End-of-Life Care, in Module 3, Comfort.)
- The individual with the authority to make decisions on the patient's behalf in the event the patient is unable to do so (referred to as a *healthcare surrogate*).

Types of ADs include the **living will** and the **durable power of attorney**. A living will provides instructions to HCPs and family members about what medical treatments will be allowed or disallowed during a life-threatening event. The individual may also appoint a specific person to make healthcare decisions in the event the patient is unable to make these decisions. This document is known as a *durable power of attorney for health care* and the individual appointed by the patient is known as the *healthcare surrogate* or *proxy*. These documents are usually put together into one legal form. See the Focus on Diversity and Culture feature for information on the use of ADs by different populations.

» **Stay Current:** Information about advance directives can be found at the Health in Aging Organization website at https://www.nia.nih.gov/health/publication/end-life-helping-comfort-and-care/planning-end-life-care-decisions.

Focus on Diversity and Culture

Advance Directives

A majority of people living in the United States feel that individuals have the right to direct what sort of medical treatment they receive at the end of life. Despite this widespread belief, fewer than one-third of Americans have established ADs—and this percentage is even lower among people of color. As a result, people of color are significantly less likely than white people to have their final wishes followed (American Psychological Association, 2019; Hope Health, 2019).

There are multiple reasons why people of color are less likely to have ADs than their white counterparts. These may include (American Psychological Association, 2019; Vilpert, Borrat-Besson, Maurer, & Borasio, 2018):

- Language barriers that make it difficult for those who don't speak English to understand the forms and terminology used by healthcare professionals
- Distrust in the healthcare system based on previous discrimination
- Inaccurate perceptions of the purpose of ADs
- Desire for more aggressive treatment and a perception that an AD may prevent that type of treatment
- Reluctance to discuss their diagnosis outside the family and therefore to engage in advance care planning
- Provider bias resulting in failure to offer options for advance care planning
- Reduced access to care.

In some cultures, such as in some Japanese traditions, it is considered inappropriate to talk about serious illness and death openly, which can create a barrier to advance care planning (American Psychological Association, 2019; Purnell & Fenkl, 2019).

Nurses are in an ideal position to help all patients and their families to better understand the value of ADs and establish these documents as needed. One key step is to encourage patients to discuss EOL issues with their loved ones; here, the nurse should emphasize the importance of the discussion itself rather than the need to obtain a signed AD. To foster such discussions, nurses should approach the topic in a manner that is appropriate to each patient's cultural, religious, and personal preferences. This requires that nurses be knowledgeable about other cultures and try to consider the situation from their patients' point of view. It is often useful to frame ADs as positive devices that clarify what care measures an individual wants, rather than what measures they wish to avoid. Patients may also find reassurance in the idea that ADs relieve their loved ones of the burden of making life-or-death decisions on their behalf. Nurses should be sure to explain any unclear or culturally sensitive terminology used in AD documents. In addition, nurses can further promote AD adoption by encouraging their employers and other healthcare organizations to use EOL planning documents that are simple to read and understand, as well as culturally and linguistically appropriate to various communities (American Psychological Association, 2019).

Clinical Example B

Gary Casper, a 65-year-old man, has been in the hospital several times in the past year with a deteriorating diagnosis. After Shondra Lewis, the patient's RN, completes her assessment of Mr. Casper's current condition and his concerns, she contacts the case management department for assistance with his concerns regarding his end-of-life care choices. Ms. Lewis tells the case manager that the patient's wife will not allow him to prepare an AD, which Mr. Casper wants to do, since he decided to be DNR on this current admission. The next day, the case manager meets with Mr. Casper separately from his wife to discuss his right for self-determination and how to prepare an AD form. Mr. Casper is relieved that he can complete the form in the hospital, but he is concerned that his wife will still be able to prevent this, as he does not want her to have a power of attorney for him. Plans are put in process for Mr. Casper to complete the AD with appropriate staff and another family member while the provider speaks with Mrs. Casper in a conference room.

Critical Thinking Questions

1. How did the staff support this patient's right to self-determination?
2. Did the provider violate the wife's right to be with her spouse in this case? Explain.
3. How can nursing staff further assist Mr. Casper in facing end-of-life care choices?
4. How can the staff support Mrs. Casper as she faces the end of her husband's life?

Elements of an Advance Directive

A broadly drafted AD usually gives an agent or surrogate decision maker authority to:

- Consent to or refuse any medical treatment or diagnostic procedure relating to the individual's physical or mental health, including artificial nutrition and hydration.
- Hire or discharge medical providers and authorize admission to medical and long-term care facilities.
- Consent to measures for comfort care and pain relief.
- Have access to all medical records.
- Take whatever measures are necessary to carry out wishes, including granting releases or waivers to medical facilities and seeking judicial remedies if problems arise.

Each individual state determines what may be included in a healthcare AD. Once the document is executed, the patient's signature must be witnessed by two witnesses who are not members of the patient's immediate family. In some states, the patient has the option to limit the authority of the healthcare agent as desired. Nurses working with a patient who has an AD should ensure that they understand what the patient's AD includes and should know the laws in the state related to self-determination as well as the employing agency's policies and procedures for following ADs.

>> **Stay Current:** Samples of state-specific forms can be obtained from the National Hospice and Palliative Care Organization at https://www.nhpco.org/patients-and-caregivers/advance-care-planning/advance-directives.

One popular AD is Five Wishes. This form was developed to simplify the process of drafting an AD and is specifically designed to address not only the healthcare aspects of EOL, but the emotional and spiritual issues as well (Aging with Dignity, 2020). The form is easy to use and addresses five areas:

1. The person who will make care decisions when the patient cannot
2. The kinds of medical treatment the patient does and does not want
3. The level of comfort the patient would prefer
4. The way the patient would prefer to be treated by others
5. The information the patient would like loved ones to know.

Five Wishes is widely used and is legally valid for use by patients age 18 and older in most states, although in some states it may need to be appended to a state-required form. Five Wishes is available in many languages, including braille (Aging with Dignity, 2020).

Role of the Nurse

End-of-life decisions are often very difficult for both patients and their families. The nurse assists them to understand that an AD provides instructions for care but that these instructions can be changed at any time. This reassurance can be especially helpful if the patient's condition has the potential to improve.

SAFETY ALERT Patients should provide copies of their AD to all HCPs and facilities. They should also give a copy of the AD to family members to present to first responders and emergency departments to ensure the patient's wishes are followed.

The nurse needs to assess whether the patient and family have an accurate understanding of life-sustaining measures. Patients and families may misunderstand what actions may sustain life and base their decisions on these misconceptions. The nurse needs to incorporate teaching in this area and continue to be supportive of patients' decisions. The Evidence-Based Practice feature looks at additional aspects that may affect a patient's likelihood to have an AD.

For patients without an AD who no longer have the capacity to make decisions, a surrogate may be selected. Nurses may be involved in assessing a patient's capacity, but selection of a surrogate is typically dictated by the state. Generally, the spouse is the first choice as surrogate, followed by an adult child, a parent, and an adult sibling. Decision making by the surrogate is generally governed by one of two criteria. The first is the substituted judgment standard. With this standard, the surrogate infers the choice the patient would make on the basis of past conversations with the patient or knowledge of the patient's beliefs and values. The second is the best interest standard. With this standard, the surrogate weighs the benefits and risks of treatment options and selects the one that they believe will be most beneficial for the patient.

Evidence-Based Practice

End-of-Life Care

Problem

When working with patients diagnosed with serious and complicated illness, nurses must be prepared to discuss ADs. Studies indicate a number of barriers to completion of ADs. At the organizational level, these include provider discomfort with discussing do-not-resuscitate and other advance care options (Bular & Goldim, 2019). Patient-related factors include literacy level, level of understanding of illness, level of trust or distrust in the healthcare system, and caregiver agreement or disagreement with the patient's illness or desire for implementing ADs (American Psychological Association, 2019; Bular & Goldim, 2019). Without ADs in place, HCPs and families may be faced with making decisions without knowing the patient's personal preferences.

Evidence

In a study of 2748 patient encounters in Oklahoma, researchers compared the use of the state of Oklahoma's AD form versus the use of Five Wishes (mentioned earlier). Fifty-four percent of those offered the state's form accepted its use, compared to 82% of those offered the Five Wishes form. Researchers' analysis indicated a clear preference for Five Wishes among both patients and providers, finding that it was easier to read and understand and more clearly captured preferences for end-of-life care (Wickersham, Gowin, Deen, & Nagykaldi, 2019).

The need for reducing patient barriers to completing ADs and ensuring patient autonomy in healthcare decisions accelerated with the COVID-19 pandemic. With family members and caregivers unable to be present with patients in the hospital, some facilities began instituting a somewhat controversial DNR protocol, with providers placing a DNR order in the records of patients unlikely to survive the illness (Curtis, Kross, & Stapleton, 2020).

Implications

The Oklahoma study and the harrowing experiences of the pandemic emphasize the need for discussions about future health decisions to be made early during an illness or injury that is likely to cause significant patient decline or death, including the need to use forms that facilitate patient understanding and discussion between providers and patients and their families.

Critical Thinking Application

1. In what ways can healthcare forms and terminology impede patient and provider use of DNRs and other AD forms?
2. Why is family support for creation of a DNR order important in working with a terminally ill patient? How can the nurse leverage this support?

REVIEW Advance Directives

RELATE Link the Concepts and Exemplars

Linking the exemplar of advance directives with the concept of cognition:

1. Why might it be advisable to discuss development of ADs with a patient who is in the early stages of Alzheimer disease?
2. How might a patient with schizophrenia benefit from an AD that includes instructions related to psychiatric care and treatment?

Linking the exemplar of advance directives with the concept of communication:

3. What communication strategies would you use to address the need to develop ADs with a patient? With the patient's family members?
4. What communication strategies would you use to help a family member understand that his mother is no longer able to make her own decisions and it is time to review and follow the ADs that she put in place?

REFER Go to Pearson MyLab Nursing and eText

REFLECT Apply Your Knowledge

Heather King is a 53-year-old woman who is hospitalized with a newly diagnosed malignant brain tumor. She has signed an AD that indicates she does not want any extraordinary measures to keep her alive if she has an incurable or irreversible condition that will result in her death within a relatively short period of time. The neurosurgeon has presented her with treatment options. Ms. King refuses treatment for the tumor, requesting only palliative care "until the time comes." Her husband speaks to the neurosurgeon outside of Ms. King's room, stating, "I want everything possible done! The children and I have discussed this, and we don't agree with not treating the tumor."

1. What should happen with Ms. King's treatment? Why?
2. How may the family's reaction affect implementation of the AD?
3. In what circumstances could the patient's family member refuse or consent to treatment for the patient?
4. What law, rule, or policy describes the nurse's responsibility?

» Exemplar 49.C Health Insurance Portability and Accountability Act

Exemplar Learning Outcomes

49.C Analyze the Health Insurance Portability and Accountability Act (HIPAA) as it relates to legal issues.

- Explain the purpose of HIPAA.
- Explain how the Privacy Rule covers protected health information.
- Differentiate privacy and confidentiality.

Exemplar Key Terms

Confidentiality, *2844*
Health Insurance Portability and Accountability Act (HIPAA), *2843*
Privacy, *2844*
Protected health information, *2843*

Overview

The **Health Insurance Portability and Accountability Act (HIPAA)** of 1996 was enacted by Congress to:

- Minimize the exclusion of preexisting conditions as a barrier to healthcare insurance
- Designate special rights for individuals who lose their health coverage
- Eliminate medical underwriting in group plans
- Establish the Privacy Rule, which created a national standard for the disclosure of private health information. This rule affects all HCPs as well as health insurance plan providers (Tariq & Hackert, 2020).

Protected Health Information

The Privacy Rule protects all "individually identifiable health information" held or transmitted in any form or medium, whether electronic, paper, or oral. The rule calls this information **protected health information** and delineates it further to include information that identifies the individual (e.g., name, address, birth date, and Social Security number) or for which a reasonable basis exists to believe the information can be used to identify the individual as it relates to the following:

- The individual's past, present, or future physical or mental health or condition
- The provision of healthcare to the individual
- The past, present, or future payment for the provision of healthcare to the individual.

HIPAA also includes provisions regarding access to medical records, requires notice of privacy practices and opportunity for confidential communications, limits use of medical information beyond the sharing among HCPs directly involved in providing care, and prohibits of the use of personal information for marketing.

In the event that a patient feels a healthcare plan or provider has violated their rights according to HIPAA, the patient may file a formal complaint either directly to the entity that committed the violation or to the office for Civil Rights of the U.S. Department of Health and Human Services. Information about how to file a complaint should be included in each entity's notice of privacy practices. Willful violation of the Privacy Rule can result in civil or criminal penalties for the individuals involved. In most cases, violations th are corrected within 30 days are not subject to civil penalties (American Medical Association, 2016).

Nurses must maintain an understanding of current law in order to protect the patient's privacy and to avoid civil punitive damage suits and possible criminal charges. Nurses should be familiar with the particular policies of their employers.

Clinical Example C

D'Alice Jones and Otis Harvey are RNs in the oncology unit at Mercy Hospital. They are standing behind the nurse's station having a whispered conversation about Sandy Wagner, a 60-year-old female patient with terminal cancer.

"She didn't do well with today's treatment. She's been vomiting at least twice an hour for the last three hours," D'Alice says.

"Poor Mrs. Wagner. I wish there was more we could do to make her feel better. But she's refused all pain and antinausea medication," Otis replies.

"I know. She told me today that she's about ready to give up on treatments and just let whatever happens happen," D'Alice responds.

Just then, D'Alice and Otis notice Mrs. Wagner's son standing a few feet from the nurses' station with a horrified look on his face. When he sees them looking at him, he quickly turns and walks away.

Critical Thinking Questions

1. Assuming that the patient's son overheard their conversation, are the two nurses in violation of the Privacy Rule? Why or why not?
2. What additional precautions could the nurses have taken to avoid their conversation being overheard?

In spite of the extensive efforts of the healthcare industry, the general population remains confused about their actual rights, and some healthcare workers remain unclear about what is and is not allowed under HIPAA (Tariq & Hackert, 2020). Ultimately, maintaining the security of protected health information provides for the protection of the most vulnerable populations, and personnel in covered entities will need to continue to learn and implement the HIPAA standards.

SAFETY ALERT Patient information belongs to the patient and may only be shared with individuals who have a documented need to know. Nurses must avoid all situations where confidential patient information may be shared inadvertently. For example, nurses should only discuss patient information in secure areas where conversations cannot be overheard by nonhealthcare personnel.

Privacy versus Confidentiality

Privacy includes the right of individuals to keep their personal information from being disclosed. Individuals decide when, where, and with whom to share their health information. **Confidentiality** refers to the assurance the patient has that private information will not be disclosed without the patient's consent. Confidentiality applies both to the nature of the information the nurse obtains from the patient and to how the nurse treats patient information once it has been disclosed to the nurse (ANA, 2015):

- ***Obtaining information.*** Nurses should request and record only information pertinent to the health status of patients to whom they are assigned. If the nurse runs into a neighbor in the emergency department (ED) waiting room, for example, it would be inappropriate for the nurse to ask the neighbor, "What are you doing here?" This would inadvertently invite protected information that this nurse does not need for provision of healthcare.
- ***Disclosing information.*** Information obtained from the patient should be disclosed only to individuals who are directly involved in providing that patient's healthcare. Even the presence of the individual in the healthcare setting is protected information. It would be a breach of confidentiality, for example, for the nurse to go home and tell their own family that a state senator or representative, the family's pastor, a neighbor, or anyone else was a patient. Protection of patient information, once disclosed, is one tenet of the nurse's responsibility as the patient's advocate, and challenges to patient privacy can include other members of the interprofessional team.
- ***Advocating for confidentiality.*** Nurses are professionally obligated not only to avoid participating in discussions of patients outside communications directly related to providing care but also to curb others from participation. Gossiping at work is common in many organizations, but it has no place in the healthcare setting. Celebrity status, notoriety, and an unusual medical condition all add to the potential risks to confidentiality. If the nurse is in a coffee shop and hears another nurse or HCP discussing a patient, the nurse is expected to redirect those professionals to maintain patient privacy.

In addition to the actions and behaviors described here, nurses should be familiar with the specific policies and procedures for protecting patient privacy and confidentiality for the healthcare agency in which they work.

Disclosure

A patient's protected health information can be disclosed under certain conditions without express permission from the patient. These disclosures include providing information to the patient, to other providers who are treating the patient, and to individuals involved in payment processing and other healthcare operations. Information must also be disclosed where required by law or court order, where necessary to protect public health, and when abuse or neglect are suspected. When such disclosure occurs, information should be limited to the minimum necessary for the situation. Providing information beyond what is required is a breach of the Privacy Rule. Informal patient permission may be sufficient for providing information to the patient's family, friends, or other individuals identified by the patient (Tariq & Hackert, 2020). In general, when circumstances give the patient the opportunity to agree or object, the nurse should ask for the patient's permission to disclose information.

Incidental disclosure of patient information may occur in some circumstances. For example, conversations with patients or colleagues about patient care may be overheard by others. The Privacy Rule permits some incidental disclosure of this sort, provided that appropriate safeguards are in place. In this case, reasonable safeguards would include holding such conversations in private locations, if possible; if this is not possible, the nurse should try to speak quietly (Tariq & Hackert, 2020).

REVIEW Health Insurance Portability and Accountability Act

RELATE Link the Concepts and Exemplars

Linking the exemplar of Health Insurance Portability and Accountability Act with the concept of trauma:

1. When and how is it appropriate to break the confidentiality of patients who threaten harm to themselves or others?
2. What additional considerations are involved when it comes to protecting the confidentiality of victims of domestic violence? Of child abuse?

Linking the exemplar of Health Insurance Portability and Accountability Act with the concept of reproduction:

You are the nurse at a local high school. A 16-year-old student has been in the bathroom off and on all morning. She is very nauseated but has been adamant about staying at school. You sit down to talk with her and learn that she thinks she is pregnant. She says, "I don't know what to do. I don't want my parents to know."

3. What are your responsibilities to this patient regarding her privacy and confidentiality?
4. What are the laws in your state that relate to the ability of minors to make independent decisions regarding their own pregnancies?

REFER Go to Pearson MyLab Nursing and eText

REFLECT Apply Your Knowledge

Michael Nguyen is a nurse on the medical–surgical unit of a busy suburban hospital. Approximately 20 minutes ago, the nursing unit was notified that seven patients who were involved in a motor-vehicle crash and are receiving treatment in the ED are expected to be admitted to the med–surg unit in varying conditions. Carole Fulton, another nurse working on the unit, has been liaising with the ED staff about the situation. Michael goes to answer a patient call bell. When he returns to the nursing desk, he overhears Carole on her cell phone saying, "Yes, that accident on Highway 40. Yeah, apparently it's really bad. I saw Reverend Mitchell downstairs. Yeah. No. His daughter was a passenger. OK. Bye." Carole hangs up the phone and puts it in her purse, saying, "My mom. She called to tell me she got home safely from work." Thirty minutes later, Michael receives a report on a patient named Elizabeth Mitchell who is being transported up from the ED.

1. What concerns might Michael have about the content of Carole's phone call with her mother? How might Carole have violated Ms. Mitchell's privacy or confidentiality?
2. If you had been Michael, what responsibility would you have to address your concerns?

Exemplar 49.D Mandatory Reporting

Exemplar Learning Outcomes

49.D Analyze mandatory reporting as it relates to legal issues.

- Describe the legalities of mandatory reporting.
- Outline situations that require mandatory reporting.
- Differentiate considerations related to mandatory reporting across the lifespan.

Exemplar Key Terms

Good faith immunity, *2846*
Mandatory reporting, *2845*

Overview

The term **mandatory reporting** refers to the legal requirement to report an act, event, or situation that is designated by state or local law as a reportable event (Fischer-Owens, Lukehahr, & Tate, 2017). Disclosure statutes mandate the reporting of certain types of health information, and all states mandate the reporting of certain vital statistics, including births and deaths. Many states also require HCPs to report abortions and neonatal deaths. Federal and state laws mandate the reporting of communicable diseases, including sexually transmitted infections. This exemplar discusses the nurse's responsibilities related to mandatory reporting as well as the types of acts, events, and situations that are reportable.

Legal Requirements for Mandatory Reporting

In most states, nurses are required to report abuse or suspected abuse, certain types of injuries and illness, and crimes involving minors. Nurses have a legal obligation to report conduct that is incompetent, unethical, and illegal. This may include reporting violence, abuse, or neglect toward patients or other nurses and extends to reporting conduct involving third parties, including family members and other HCPs. Each state's NPA includes requirements for reporting nurses who are in violation of the act.

As a general rule, when reporting situations involving patients, the nurse reports the required information through the administrative chain of the institution, beginning with the nurse's immediate supervisor and the primary HCP. All information reported is documented in the patient record. When reporting nurses who are in violation of the NPA, the nurse may be required to report the relevant facts to both the institution and the state BON.

Regardless of the situation, the nurse is not required to conduct any type of investigation or otherwise confirm that the suspected act or incident has, in fact, occurred. The nurse is required only to have a good faith suspicion based on information disclosed by a patient, physical symptoms observed in a patient, or the nurse's personal observations of behavior on the part of a patient, colleague, or third party. The reporting nurse may be granted immunity from liability unless the nurse knows that the report is false or acts with reckless disregard, without concern for the validity of the allegations made.

Good Faith Immunity

In every state, healthcare workers are protected from civil or criminal liabilities when they report suspected child abuse

Box 49.6

Guidelines Regarding Disclosure of Health Information

Depending on the setting, the nurse may be the only professional with firsthand information necessary for making an accurate report. General guidelines that nurses should follow regarding reporting health-related information include the following:

- Know the federal and state laws concerning duty to report.
- Report the required information to the appropriate governmental agency promptly.
- Comply with reporting laws in good faith.
- Follow agency policy carefully when making a report.
- Avoid a breach of confidentiality and report only the information required.

Source: Based on Guido (2020).

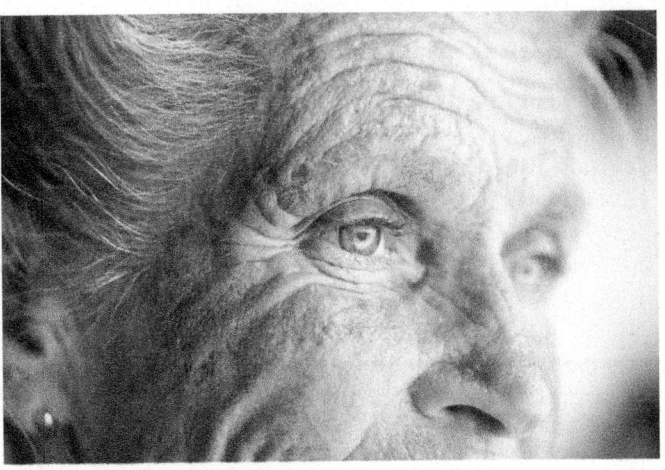

Figure 49.5 »» Elder mistreatment includes physical, emotional, verbal, and sexual abuse and neglect.
Source: Jodi Jacobson/E+/Getty Images.

in good faith, even if the subsequent investigation does not make a determination of abuse. This is called **good faith immunity**. Good faith immunity also typically applies to reports of elder mistreatment, particular illnesses or injuries, and crimes involving minors.

When reporting incidents subject to good faith immunity, the nurse or HCP may be required to disclose protected health information. This includes patient name, age, gender, race, residence, or present location as well as the nature and extent of the abuse, injury, or illness. Disclosure of this information under these circumstances is not considered a violation of the HIPAA Privacy Rule. Guidelines regarding disclosure of health information as a mandatory reporter are presented in **Box 49.6** »».

SAFETY ALERT Good faith immunity applies only to required information that is reported to the appropriate agency or office. Information reported above and beyond that which is mandated may not be protected under good faith immunity.

Mandatory Reporting of Abuse or Neglect of Minors and Older Adults

The circumstances in which a nurse must report child abuse vary among states. In most states, a report must be made when the nurse has reason to believe abuse has occurred because of things that are seen or heard in the work environment. In addition, nurses may be required to report knowledge or observation of a child being subjected to conditions that are likely to result in harm. Mandatory reporters must cite the facts or circumstances that led to their suspicions of abuse, but do not have the burden of proof (Child Welfare Information Gateway, 2019).

States also have specific laws pertaining to the mistreatment of adults and older adults (**Figure 49.5** »»). These laws may be similar to those that govern the abuse and neglect of children. For example, many states generally offer good faith immunity to individuals who report suspected abuse or neglect of an older adult or an adult with a disability. Nurses should know the laws of their individual states and their agency's policies for reporting suspected mistreatment of an adult or older adult (Myhre et al., 2020). Additional information on this topic can be found in Module 32, Trauma.

Mandatory Reporting of Certain Injuries and Illnesses

Primary HCPs are mandated to report certain types of injuries and illnesses to the appropriate authorities. Injuries and illnesses that typically fall under the reporting laws include the following:

- Bullet wounds, gunshot wounds, powder burns, or any other injuries arising or suspected of arising from the discharge of a gun or firearm
- Illnesses that appear to be caused by poisoning
- Injuries caused by, or appearing to be caused by, a knife or other sharp or pointed instrument if the provider or surgeon treating the individual suspects that a criminal act may have been involved
- Any wound, injury, or illness resulting in bodily harm as a result of a suspected criminal act or act of violence
- Infectious diseases, such as tuberculosis and *Escherichia coli* infection.

Most agencies have a policy and procedure in place for routine reporting of these injuries and illnesses. For example, injuries that are or appear to be due to violence are typically first seen in the ED; therefore, organizations typically designate the ED to report these injuries. A diagnosis of an infectious disease, on the other hand, may occur at any point in the healthcare interaction, so the nurse needs to be familiar with the agency policy for reporting infectious diseases and ensure that the report is made when warranted. As with abuse situations, good faith immunity typically applies.

Mandatory reporting of infectious conditions is a cornerstone of maintaining public health. Since 1878, the U.S. Public Health System has been collecting information on infectious conditions for the purpose of early identification and control of massive outbreaks, including, when necessary, instituting quarantines. High-profile diseases, such as COVID-19, and threats of bioterrorism have brought renewed attention to this system of ongoing monitoring. The Centers for Disease Control and Prevention's National Notifiable Diseases Surveillance System (NNDSS) has identified more than 50 infectious diseases in the United States that must be reported. Among these are anthrax, botulism, cholera, hepatitis, HIV, and syphilis.

Data are reported at the county level, with providers reporting these diseases and conditions to local health departments. For diseases and conditions that must be reported within 24 hours, the initial report is made by telephone to the health department, and the written report is made within 7 days. Each county health department reports to the state's department of health, where data are managed and maintained. Data on many diseases and conditions are provided from the state level to the Centers for Disease Control and Prevention, which publishes the *Morbidity and Mortality Weekly Report*. Although the law targets physician reporting, nurses need to be aware of the policies and procedures for reporting within their place of employment, especially nurses who are employed directly by their local health department.

>> **Stay Current:** Visit the National Diseases Surveillance System website at https://wwwn.cdc.gov/nndss for more information. A complete list of event codes of the NNDSS can be found at https://wwwn.cdc.gov/nndss/case-notification/related-documentation.html#event-code-lists.

Clinical Example D

Randy Wallace is a 6-year-old boy who is a first grader at Park Hills Elementary school, where Maya Anderson is the school nurse. One afternoon, Randy's teacher brings him to Miss Anderson's office because of an injury he sustained during recess. While tending to Randy's injury, Miss Anderson notices a number of bruises on Randy's arms in various states of healing. After dressing his injury and sending him back out on the playground, she asks Randy's teacher about his bruises. He laughs and says, "Randy? He's my little daredevil. I can't turn my back on him for a second or I find him climbing up on desks, dancing across the radiator, or otherwise risking his life. His mom says he is the same way at home."

Critical Thinking Questions

1. Are Randy's injuries sufficient to produce good faith suspicion of child abuse? If not, what additional information might be necessary to produce good faith suspicion?
2. In what ways might the teacher's attitude about Randy's injuries suggest negligence as a mandatory reporter?

Mandatory Reporting of Nurses Who Are in Violation of the Nurse Practice Act

Not all instances of mandatory reporting by nurses involve patients; nurses must also report other nurses who are in violation of their state's NPA. Violations of the NPA and proper reporting procedures for violations are governed by the state BON. For example, North Carolina's General Statutes (NCGS § 90-171.47) mandate that any individual who has reasonable cause to suspect that a nurse is in violation of the NPA has the duty to report the relevant facts to the BON. BONs take these reports very seriously; as a result, their websites generally make reporting forms readily available. Employers typically use a different reporting form than that used by members of the general public.

The NPA spells out any formal action the board may take, and it usually requires clear and convincing evidence that the nurse has violated state nursing laws or rules. The nature of alleged violations varies widely, and cases are decided on their own merits. Many complaints are resolved through informal processes, though in some instances, a formal administrative hearing is held.

BONs are required to respect each nurse's right to due process. This ensures that the nurse is informed of any allegations regarding their practice, that the nurse has an opportunity to respond to and defend against the allegations, and that the matter is heard by a fair and impartial body.

REVIEW Mandatory Reporting

RELATE Link the Concepts and Exemplars

Linking the exemplar of mandatory reporting with the concept of trauma:

1. Why do you think nurses and HCPs have a duty to report injuries sustained during or as a result of a criminal act?
2. Why do you think mandatory reporting laws include the requirement to report injuries resulting from the discharge of a firearm?

Linking the exemplar of mandatory reporting with the concept of infection:

3. How do requirements and procedures for reporting HIV infection in your state or agency differ from requirements and procedures for reporting anthrax?
4. How do requirements and procedures for reporting shigellosis in your state or agency differ from requirements and procedures for reporting meningococcal disease?

REFER Go to Pearson MyLab Nursing and eText

REFLECT Apply Your Knowledge

Jenny Erickson, an 85-year-old woman who is a widow, came into the ED after she apparently fell at home. Her neighbor and friend, Elinor Jones, was waiting for Mrs. Erickson to go to lunch with her and tried calling her several times. After getting no response for more than an hour, Mrs. Jones called the police, who found Mrs. Erickson on the kitchen floor. During the ED assessment, the nurse, Lynn Gutierrez, noted multiple bruises on Mrs. Erickson's legs, her upper arms, and both sides of her rib cage. When she asked her about the bruises, she said that she has been "falling a lot." The bruises were in several different stages of healing and coloring.

When Lynn asked whether she lived alone, Mrs. Erickson began crying and shivering. Mrs. Jones heard her friend crying and asked to speak with the nurse. Lynn spoke with Mrs. Jones away from the ED bedside. "I don't mean to get anyone in trouble, but Jenny has been living with her daughter and son-in-law for the past two years. I'm worried that they are upset having her there." Lynn realized that Mrs. Jones might have information that could explain why Mrs. Erickson had so many bruises. "Has Mrs. Erickson complained at all? I mean, has her family hurt her?" Mrs. Jones nodded her head. "I think so. I've heard her son-in-law yelling at her before, and Jenny had a big bruise on her forehead a month ago right after that."

1. What does the nurse need to do next?
2. How can the ED staff support Mrs. Erickson and ensure her safety while she is in the ED?
3. How can the nursing staff further assist Mrs. Erickson with the possible abuse?
4. What report must be done for this patient, and by whom?

Exemplar 49.E Risk Management

Exemplar Learning Outcomes

49.E Analyze risk management as it relates to legal issues.

- Explain the concept of risk management.
- Outline strategies for risk management.
- Explain the use of incident reports.

Exemplar Key Terms

Discovery, *2849*
Incident report, *2849*
Risk management, *2848*
Variances, *2849*

Overview

Risk management focuses on limiting a healthcare agency's financial and legal risk associated with the delivery of care, particularly in terms of lawsuits, ideally before incidents occur. Risk management is a process that identifies, analyzes, and treats potential hazards within a setting for the purpose of identifying and rectifying the hazards, thus preventing harm. Nurses play an important role in risk management because they are responsible for both patient safety and high-quality care.

Risk management focuses on areas at high risk for incidents, such as overall patient safety, medication administration, assessment and communication of allergies, and falls. The use of equipment and technology—including assessment of the functioning of equipment prior to use—also falls under the risk management umbrella.

Strategies for Risk Management

A facility may have an individual or a team dedicated to risk management. In most cases, there will be a designated risk manager whose overall role is to collaborate with the interprofessional healthcare team to maintain a safe and effective healthcare environment and prevent or reduce financial and legal risk to the organization.

Healthcare organizations can use several strategies to minimize risk. One of the most basic strategies is protecting against financial risk by purchasing insurance or by self-insuring. Other strategies involve identifying the areas in which incidents commonly occur and implementing practices to minimize the likelihood of incidents in these areas. Data collection, incident report systems, and staff education related to risk and documentation are all important for identifying and protecting against these types of risks. Strategies related to three common incident areas—implementing physician's orders, providing competent nursing care, and reducing pediatric medical errors—are discussed later in this section.

No matter how well an organization manages risk, incidents do still occur. Organizations should develop an investigation and reporting protocol for incidents that have the potential to result in lawsuits. When such incidents occur, an investigation should begin as soon as possible after the incident.

Risk management strategies, reporting systems, and investigation practices should be regularly monitored and updated as needed. In addition, information gathered by reporting systems and via investigation should be used to educate staff in preparation for future incidents. For more information on how to prevent risk, see Module 50, Quality Improvement, and Module 51, Safety.

SAFETY ALERT In addition to patient safety, healthcare organizations must consider risks to nonpatient visitors. These include community members and patients' family and friends. The organization can be found liable for falls and other accidents that occur on its property and should have proper protocols and risk management strategies in place for these occurrences.

Implementing Provider Orders

Prior to beginning any procedure or medication administration, the nurse must ensure there is nothing that could possibly put the patient at risk. For example, the nurse must determine if a specific medication is within the safe dosage range and contact the HCP for clarification if the ordered dose is not within a safe range. Once the nurse determines it is safe to administer the medication or complete the procedure, it must be completed in a safe manner.

Following are examples of issues that may arise that should cause the nurse to do a thorough investigation prior to proceeding:

- The nurse should question any order that the patient questions. It may be as simple as a patient wondering why the medication being administered is only one tablet when the patient takes two tablets of the medication at home. The nurse must stop at this point and make sure the order and medication are correct.
- The nurse should question any order that is continued once a patient's condition has changed. For example, the

patient receives blood pressure medication every morning at 9:00 a.m. Prior to giving the medication, the patient's blood pressure is found to be 92/50 mmHg. The nurse must withhold the medication and notify the HCP to prevent any injury to the patient.

- The nurse must verify any verbal or telephone order received. To avoid any error occurring, the nurse must read the order back to the HCP and then document the confirmation with date, time, and circumstances of the order.
- The nurse must make sure that all orders are written in the proper manner, which includes the medication name, dosage, timing of administration, and type of administration (po, IM, IV). The nurse also ensures that the order is able to be easily read and may be safely performed.

Providing Competent Nursing Care

Providing competent and caring patient care is the basis for ensuring the patient is treated safely. The nurse must be very familiar with the state scope of practice and also the specific policies of the healthcare facilities. It is also important the nurse fully understands the scope of practice of all of the personnel at the healthcare facility. If the nurse feels that their knowledge is inadequate, the supervisor or manager should be alerted.

SAFETY ALERT The nurse's first encounter with a patient should include a thorough assessment of the patient's environment. This provides the nurse with possible risks that the patient could encounter and actions to take to limit these risks.

Following the nursing process is essential to minimizing patient risk of injury. Beginning with assessment and proceeding through evaluation, the nurse is alert to any areas of potential risk for harm. It is important to remember that communication helps prevent patient injury by ensuring the patient and family fully understand the treatment plan.

Reducing Pediatric Medical Errors

Children are at a higher risk for medical errors than other patients and may also be more vulnerable to harm from errors because of their immature physiology (ISMP, 2020). Reasons for increased medical errors among children include the following (ISMP, 2020; Mangus & Mahajan, 2019):

- Dosage calculations for children are more complicated, often requiring calculation based on weight or body surface area.
- Some medications require dilution to be administered to infants and young children; failure to dilute a medication properly can result in an adverse or sentinel event.
- Very young and nonverbal children may be unable to communicate that they are having a reaction to the medication.

Incident Reports

As part of risk management, each healthcare organization has an incident reporting system. Nurses participate in this process by completing the required forms when they are involved in an incident and by following policies and procedures.

An **incident report** is an agency record of an accident or incident that occurred within the agency. It is designed to collect adequate information to assist personnel in preventing future incidents or occurrences. Incident reports are also called *variance reports* or *unusual occurrence reports*. Examples of occurrences that would be reported include medication administration **variances** (e.g., wrong medication, wrong dose, wrong route, wrong time, or omissions) and a patient or visitor falling.

In some jurisdictions, incident reports may be used in discovery. **Discovery** is the legal process of obtaining information before a trial. Although most incidents do not result in lawsuits, a nurse completing an incident report should always fill out the report as though it is discoverable. No language regarding liability should be included. The report should completely and accurately document the facts without assumptions, conclusions, or blame. The report should include the patient's account of the incident in direct quotes and should identify all witnesses to the incident. Incident reports generally include the following:

- Names and identifying information of any patients and healthcare personnel involved in the incident as well as information on witnesses (if any)
- The location, time, and date of the incident
- Equipment or medication involved (if medication, state the medication's name and dosage).

Although the event that prompted the incident report is noted in the patient's chart, there should be no entry in the patient's chart to indicate that an incident report was completed. For example, if the patient was given the wrong medication, the actual administration of the medication will be noted in the patient's chart. If the patient required any treatment as a result of the event, that also is noted in the patient's chart (Guido, 2020).

Nurses engage in risk management by following ANA standards of care and practice, by following their employing agency's policies and procedures, and by working collaboratively to ensure that patient safety is maintained at all times. Risk management is required of every nurse every day in the course of practicing nursing.

REVIEW Risk Management

RELATE Link the Concepts and Exemplars

Linking the exemplar of risk management with the concept of assessment:

1. How does a thorough assessment of a patient contribute to risk management?
2. Nurses are required to do their own assessment of a patient after receiving a report during shift change or patient transfer. How might failure to conduct this assessment or failure to do it in a timely manner affect the patient's risk for adverse outcomes?

Linking the exemplar of risk management with the concept of communication:

3. How does a change-of-shift report minimize the nurse's risk for professional negligence or malpractice?
4. How does accuracy in documentation contribute to risk management?

REFER Go to Pearson MyLab Nursing and eText

REFLECT Apply Your Knowledge

Three nurses were getting ready for the shift change report outside the room of an older adult patient. Kim Nelson whispered to the other two nurses, "The doctor ordered the wrong dosage for Mr. Stivers. It took more than an hour to get in contact with her to clarify the order."

Randy Carson shook his head, knowing that this had become a common problem on their unit. "So, Kim, did she finally fix the order?"

Kim sighed and said, "Yes, but it didn't end there. Shortly after I gave Mr. Stivers the medication, he had difficulty breathing."

Pam Troy felt worried about this. She had been a nurse for only 2 years, but she knew that any problems when a medication is given are of critical concern. "Well, was it still the wrong dosage?"

Kim avoided looking at the other two nurses. "I need to get ready for report."

Randy was also concerned. "Wait, Kim. What happened?"

"Okay, so then I found out he's allergic to the medication I gave him."

Pam spoke up again. "Are you going to do an incident report?"

Kim shook her head. "No, I don't want to be sued or lose my job."

1. Is this case an example of nursing negligence? Explain.
2. What is the evidence that this issue may need an incident report?
3. What further information should the nurse seek before reporting an error?
4. Who else needs to know that there was a medication error with the patient?

References

Aging with Dignity. (2020). *Five Wishes*. https://fivewishes.org

American Academy of Family Physicians (AAFP). (2019). *Screening and counseling adolescents and young adults: A framework for comprehensive care*. https://www.aafp.org/afp/2020/0201/p147.html

American Association of Colleges of Nursing (AACN). (2019). *Enhancing diversity in the workforce*. https://www.aacnnursing.org/News-Information/Fact-Sheets/Enhancing-Diversity

American Association of Colleges of Nursing (AACN). (2020). *Latest data on diversity*. https://www.aacnnursing.org/Diversity-Inclusion/Latest-Data

American Cancer Society (ACS). (2019). *Advance directives*. https://www.cancer.org/content/dam/CRC/PDF/Public/6045.00.pdf

American Civil Liberties Union (ACLU) of Ohio. (2014). *Your health and the law: A guide for teens*. http://www.acluohio.org/-wp-content/uploads/2014/06/TeenHealthGuide.pdf

American College of Obstetricians and Gynecologists (ACOG). (2020). *Committee opinion: Confidentiality in adolescent health care* (ACOG Committee Opinion No. 803). *Obstetrics & Gynecology*, 135(4), e171–177. https://journals.lww.com/greenjournal/Fulltext/2020/04000/Confidentiality_in_Adolescent_Health_Care__ACOG.60

American Medical Association (AMA). (2016). *HIPAA violations and enforcement*. https://www.ama-assn.org/practice-management/hipaa/hipaa-violations-enforcement

American Nurses Association (ANA). (2015). *American Nurses Association position statement on privacy and confidentiality*. https://www.nursingworld.org/practice-policy/nursing-excellence/official-position-statements/id/privacy-and-confidentiality/

American Psychological Association. (2019). *Culturally diverse communities and palliative and end-of-life care*. https://www.apa.org/pi/aging/programs/eol/end-of-life-diversity.pdf

Berman, A., Snyder, S., & Frandsen, G. (2021). *Kozier & Erb's fundamentals of nursing: Concepts, process, and practice* (11th ed.). Pearson.

Bular, P. G., & Goldim, J. R. (2019). Barriers to the composition and implementation of advance directives in oncology: A literature review. *Ecancermedicalscience*, 13, 974.

Centers for Disease Control and Protection (CDC). (2020). *The public health approach to violence prevention*. https://www.cdc.gov/violenceprevention/publichealthissue/publichealthapproach.html

Centers for Disease Control and Prevention (CDC). (2021). *State laws that enable a minor to provide informed consent to receive HIV and STD services*. https://www.cdc.gov/hiv/policies/law/states/minors.html.

Child Welfare Information Gateway. (2019). *Mandatory reporters of child abuse and neglect*. U.S. Department of Health and Human Services, Children's Bureau. https://www.childwelfare.gov/topics/systemwide/laws-policies/statutes/manda/

Colwell, J. (2019). *Respecting religion in the hospital*. ACP Hospitalist. https://www.acphospitalist.org/archives/2019/10/respecting-religion-in-the-hospital.htm

Curtis, J. R., Kross, E. K., & Stapleton, R. D. (2020). The importance of addressing advance care planning and decisions about do-not-resuscitate orders during novel coronavirus 2019 (COVID-19). *Journal of the American Medical Association*, 323(18), 1771–1772. https://doi.org/10.1001/jama.2020.4894

Fischer-Owens, S., Lukefahr, J., & Tate, A. (2017). Oral and dental aspects of child abuse and neglect. *Pediatric Dentistry*, 39(4), 278–283.

Guido, G. W. (2020). *Legal and ethical issues in nursing* (7th ed.). Pearson.

Guttmacher Institute. (2020a). *Minors' access to contraceptive services*. https://www.guttmacher.org/state-policy/explore/minors-access-contraceptive-services

Guttmacher Institute. (2020b). *An overview of abortion laws*. https://www.guttmacher.org/state-policy/explore/overview-abortion-laws

Guttmacher Institute. (2020c). *An overview of consent to reproductive health services by young people*. https://www.guttmacher.org/state-policy/explore/overview-minors-consent-law

Herendeen, P. A., Blevins, R., Anson, E., & Smith, J. (2014). Barriers to and consequences of mandated reporting of child abuse by nurse -practitioners. *Journal of Pediatric Health Care*, *28(1)*: e1–e7. https://doi.org/10.1016/j.pedhc.2013.06.004.

Hope Health. (2019). *Advance directives: Making your end-of-life wishes known*. https://www.hopehealthco.org/blog/advance-directives-make-your-end-of-life-wishes-known/

Institute for Safe Medication Practice (ISMP). (2020). *ISMP publishes top 10 list of medication errors and hazards covered in newsletter*. https://www.ismp.org/news/ismp-publishes-top-10-list-medication-errors-and-hazards-covered-newsletter

Keller, L. (2020). Reducing STI cases: Young people deserve better sexual health information and services. *Guttmacher Policy Review*, 23. https://www.guttmacher.org/gpr/2020/04/reducing-sti-cases-young-people-deserve-better-sexual-health-information-and-services

Kim, H. (2019). Factors influencing attitudes toward advance directive in nursing students. *Journal of Korean Academic Society of Nursing Education*, 25(2), 227–237.

Ko, C. M., Koh, C. K., & Lee, Y. S. (2020). An ethical issue: Nurses' conscientious objection regarding induced abortion in South Korea. *BMC Medical Ethics*, 21, 106. https://doi.org/10.1186/s12910-020-00552-9

Law Teacher. (2019). *Rights of fetus and mother in the abortion debate*. https://www.lawteacher.net/free-law-essays/medical-law/rights-of-fetus-and-mother-law-essays.php

Lum, K., & Lau, A. (2018). *Healthcare service failure: How dissatisfied patients respond to poor quality service. International Journal of Operations & Production Management*, 38(5), 1245–1270. https://doi.org/10.1108/IJOPM-11-2016-0669

Mangus, C., & Mahajan, P. (2019). Common medical errors in pediatric emergency medicine. *Clinical Pediatric Emergency Medicine*, 20(3), 100714. https://doi.org/10.1016/j.cpem.2019.100714

Matt, S. (2018). Good Samaritan laws: Will I be protected if I help? *The Nurse Practitioner*, 43(3), 52–54. https://doi.org/10.1097/01.NPR.0000530216.62772.19

Myhre, J., Saga, S., Malmedal, W., Ostaszkiewicz, J., & Nakrem, S. (2020). Elder abuse and neglect: An overlooked patient safety issue. A focus group study of nursing home leaders' perceptions of elder abuse and neglect. *BMC Health Services Research*, 20, 199. https://doi.org/10.1186/s12913-020-5047-4

National Center on Elder Abuse (NCEA). (n.d.). *Red flags of abuse*. https://ncea.acl.gov/NCEA/media/docs/Red-Flags-of-Elder-Abuse-English.pdf

National Council of State Boards of Nursing (NCSBN). (2020). *NCLEX & other exams*. https://www.ncsbn.org/NCLEX.htm

National Council of State Boards of Nursing (NCSBN). (2021a). *Nurse licensure compact (NLC)*. Retrieved from https://www.ncsbn.org/nurse-licensure-compact.htm

National Council of State Boards of Nursing (NCSBN). (2021b). *Ongoing research*. https://ncsbn.org/ongoing-research.htm

North Carolina Board of Nursing. (2020). *Nursing practice*. https://www.ncbon.com/practice-registered-nurse

Nurse Journal. (2020). *Codes of practice and informed consent*. https://nursejournal.org/community/codes-of-practice-and-informed-consent/

Purnell, L. D., & Fenkl, E. A. (2019). *Handbook for culturally competent care*. Springer.

Tariq, R., & Hackert, P. (2020). *Patient confidentiality*. StatPearls. https://pubmed.ncbi.nlm.nih.gov/30137825/

Singh, H. (2020). *National Practitioner Data Bank: Adverse action and medical malpractice reports*. https://www.npdb.hrsa.gov/analysistool.

Wickersham, E., Gowin, M., Deen, M. H., & Nagykaldi, Z. (2019). Improving the adoption of advance directives in primary care practices. *Journal of the American Board of Family Medicine*, 32(3), 168–179.

World Health Organization (WHO). (2019). *Patient safety*. https://www.who.int/news-room/facts-in-pictures/detail/patient-safety

Vanderbilt Kennedy Center. (2020). *Health care for adults with intellectual and developmental disabilities: Toolkit for primary care providers*. https://iddtoolkit.vkcsites.org

Vilpert, S., Borrat-Besson, C., Maurer, J., & Borasio, D. (2018). Awareness, approval and completion of advance directives in older adults in Switzerland. *Swiss Medical Weekly*, 148, w14642. https://doi.org/10.4414/smw.2018.14642

Wojciechowski, M. (2019). *What's the difference between employer provided malpractice insurance and individual professional liability insurance?* DailyNurse. https://dailynurse.com/whats-the-difference-between-employer-provided-malpractice-insurance-and-individual-professional-liability-insurance/

Module 50

Quality Improvement

Module Outline and Learning Outcomes

The Concept of Quality Improvement

Improving the Quality of Healthcare

50.1 Summarize the need for improving the quality of healthcare.

National Initiatives

50.2 Summarize federal, state, and local initiatives to improve healthcare.

Concepts Related to Quality Improvement

50.3 Outline the relationship between quality improvement and other concepts.

The Quality Improvement Process

50.4 Outline the quality improvement process.

Quality Management Programs

50.5 Differentiate commonly used quality management programs.

» The Concept of Quality Improvement

Concept Key Terms

Audit, **2854**
Benchmarking, **2853**
Blame-free environment, **2858**
Breach of care, **2856**
Breach of duty, **2856**
Concurrent audit, **2854**
Continuous quality improvement (CQI), **2860**
Indicator, **2855**
Intraprofessional assessment, **2853**
Just culture, **2858**
Lean Six Sigma, **2861**
Outcome standards, **2855**
Outcomes management, **2854**
Peer review, **2853**
Performance improvement, **2853**
Plan–Do–Study–Act (PDSA), **2860**
Process standards, **2855**
Quality, **2851**
Quality assurance, **2860**
Quality improvement, **2851**
Quality management, **2851**
Retrospective audit, **2854**
Risk management, **2856**
Root cause analysis, **2856**
Sentinel event, **2856**
Six Sigma, **2861**
Standards, **2855**
Structure standards, **2855**
Total quality management (TQM), **2860**
Utilization review, **2855**

The Institute of Medicine (IOM; 2001), which is now part of The National Academies, has defined **quality** as "the degree to which health services for individuals and populations increase the likelihood of desired health outcomes and are consistent with current professional knowledge." In addition, high-quality care involves "providing patients with appropriate services in a technically competent manner, with good communication, shared decision making, and cultural sensitivity."

Improving the Quality of Healthcare

One way in which nurses can provide high-quality care is participating in quality improvement and quality management. **Quality improvement** consists of "systematic and continuous actions that lead to measurable improvement in healthcare services and the health status of targeted patient groups" (Health Resources and Services Administration, 2011). **Quality management** includes evaluation of medical and nursing processes for quality and effectiveness compared to accepted standards in order to correct problems before they harm patients and to prevent errors in treatment. Quality management also aims to provide cost-effective care by preventing overuse, misuse, and underuse of medical resources.

In its report *To Err Is Human: Building a Safer Health System*, the IOM (2000) stated that medical errors account for approximately 98,000 deaths per year. Since the report's release, multiple studies have investigated the incidence of preventable medical errors. A study conducted by Johns Hopkins University calculated that medical errors result in more than 250,000 deaths per year in the United States (Makary & Daniel, 2016). This indicates that medical errors are a leading cause of death in the United States. Medication errors alone are often studied; a systematic review found that overall medication error rates occur at a median rate of 19.6–25.6% (Keers, Williams, Cooke, & Ashcroft, 2013).

In 2001, the IOM released a follow-up report titled *Crossing the Quality Chasm: A New Health System for the 21st Century*. This report concluded that the current healthcare system was too disorganized to adequately care for individuals with multiple chronic illnesses. The report suggested that a new

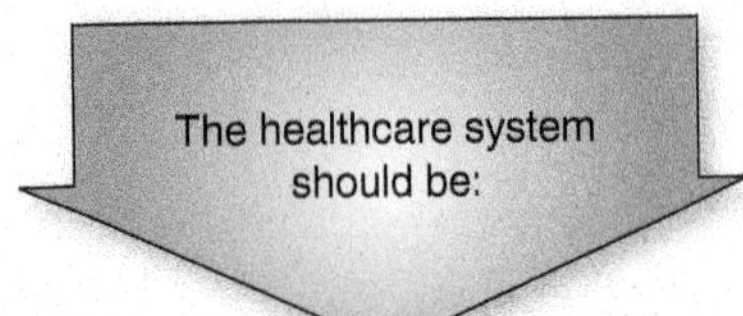

Safe—avoiding injuries to patients from the care that is intended to help them

Effective—providing services based on scientific knowledge to all who could benefit and refraining from providing services to those not likely to benefit (avoiding underuse and overuse, respectively)

Patient-centered—providing care that is respectful of and responsive to individual patient preferences, needs and values and ensuring that patient values guide all clinical decisions

Timely—reducing wait time that may result in harmful delays for both those who receive and those who give care

Efficient—avoiding waste, including waste of equipment, supplies, ideas, and energy

Equitable—providing care that does not vary in quality because of personal characteristics such as gender, ethnicity, or geographic location

Figure 50.1 »» Six aims for improving the healthcare system.

healthcare system should be developed that improves care, partly through the use of rapidly advancing technology. In an effort to improve the healthcare system, *Crossing the Quality Chasm* proposed six aims for improvement: The healthcare system should be safe, effective, patient-centered, timely, efficient, and equitable (**Figure 50.1** »»). These aims remain relevant today.

National Initiatives

Following the IOM reports, the healthcare industry began to embrace quality improvement. The need to improve patient safety and health outcomes and to implement changes to support these improvements was obvious to individuals working at every level of healthcare. State and federal governments have also contributed to initiatives aimed at improving the quality of healthcare.

Federal Initiatives

Governmental agencies such as the U.S. Department of Health and Human Services (DHHS), physicians' groups such as the American Medical Association, and professional nursing organizations such as the American Nurses Association (ANA) have developed indicators of high-quality care and measures to document the quality of care. Three important efforts are the development of the National Database of Nursing Quality Indicators (NDNQI), the publication of *Patient Safety and Quality: An Evidence-Based Handbook for Nurses*, and the development of National Patient Safety Goals by The Joint Commission (n.d.-b). These programs and documents aim to collect and provide data that identify areas for improvement and encourage facilities to meet quality goals.

More recently, the Patient Protection and Affordable Care Act, commonly known as the *Affordable Care Act (ACA)*, was enacted in 2010 in an attempt to make healthcare affordable for all Americans. Some of these changes included expanding and reforming Medicaid and Medicare; incentives to reduce 30-day readmission rates; and incentives to reduce wasteful spending by healthcare facilities. Changes to the healthcare system that are detailed in the ACA began implementation in 2010 and have continued as healthcare laws are constantly changing.

»» **Stay Current:** Keep abreast of the changes in healthcare and insurance laws by visiting the U.S. Department of Health and Human Services at https://www.hhs.gov/healthcare/about-the-aca/index.html and Medicaid.gov at https://www.cms.gov/cciio/index.

To improve the health of the population, the Agency for Healthcare Research and Quality (AHRQ, 2015a) developed the National Quality Strategy, which contains three broad aims:

- ***Better Care:*** Improve the overall quality by making healthcare more patient-centered, reliable, accessible, and safe.
- ***Healthy People/Healthy Communities:*** Improve the health of the U.S. population by supporting proven interventions to address behavioral, social, and environmental determinants of health in addition to delivering higher-quality care.
- ***Affordable Care:*** Reduce the cost of quality healthcare for individuals, families, employers, and government.

To achieve these aims, the National Quality Strategy will focus on six priorities (**Box 50.1** »»).

Box 50.1

Six Priorities for High-Quality Care

1. ***Patient Safety:*** Making care safer by reducing harm caused in the delivery of care.
2. ***Person- and Family-Centered Care:*** Ensuring that each person and family is engaged as partners in their care.
3. ***Care Coordination:*** Promoting effective communication and coordination of care.
4. ***Effective Prevention and Treatment:*** Promoting the most effective prevention and treatment practices for the leading causes of mortality, starting with cardiovascular disease.
5. ***Healthy Living:*** Working with communities to promote wide use of best practices to enable healthy living.
6. ***Affordability:*** Making quality care more affordable for individuals, families, employers, and governments by developing and spreading new healthcare delivery models.

Source: From Agency for Healthcare Research and Quality (2018).

State and Local Initiatives

Even with the advent of the ACA, states are partially responsible for providing state health insurance programs for low-income individuals and families. Recent years have seen an increase in the number of insurers entering the healthcare marketplace and expanding their service areas (Henry J. Kaiser Family Foundation, 2020). However, insurer participation is still variable within states and rural areas. In 2021, 78% of marketplace enrollees will have three or more insurers to select from.

The ACA offers states the option of implementing a basic health program (BHP) for low-income adults and legal immigrants. Under the BHP, states contract with health plans and providers to provide at least the minimum essential benefits under the ACA, and the federal government helps to subsidize the program (Medicaid, n.d.).

Quality Initiatives

A review of the first 5 years of the ACA found some improvements in the quality of healthcare, although it is too early to determine whether the trends will continue and whether the improvements are related to the new laws or to other initiatives that were already ongoing. This is, in part, because it can take up to 12 months after patient discharge for the reporting and collection of data to agencies such as the Centers for Medicaid and Medicare Services (CMS) and The Joint Commission (Austin & Kachalia, 2020). Despite this lag, available data indicate that 30-day readmission rates for Medicare patients have declined by over 1%, and the incidence of healthcare-associated complications is also declining. Many healthcare organizations have signed up for bundled payment options, with some reports indicating bundled payments reduce costs, especially for orthopedic procedures (Freeman, Coyne, & Kingsdale, 2020; Navathe, Troxel, Liao et al., 2017).

With the arrival of the COVID-19 pandemic, it quickly became apparent that organizations were going to be challenged to maintain, collect, and report quality measures. In early 2020, federal agencies began pausing requirements for hospitals and healthcare organizations to collect and report data related to quality of care. At that time, CMS announced that it would pause the use of data from healthcare organizations as a requirement for payment (Austin & Kachalia, 2020).

Concepts Related to Quality Improvement

Some ways in which healthcare quality can be improved include properly using advance directives, following privacy laws, and striving to reduce errors. Quality improvement uses a variety of methods to improve care, including the use of evidence-based practices and quality improvement methods adopted from industry. Quality management programs track overall patient progress on certain key indicators (such as infection rates, fall rates, and incidence of pressure injuries) to determine how well patients are cared for and what measures need to be taken to improve care on the unit. If new devices are used on the unit for the prevention of pressure injuries, they are tracked by the quality department to determine whether pressure injury rates decline. Patients' records are also used to track quality measures called core measures. Certain key measures are tracked to make sure patients are being discharged with the appropriate medications and follow-up for conditions such as stroke and myocardial infarction.

Safety culture is important to monitor. Many health systems use the AHRQ's Patient Safety Culture Survey to monitor the safety culture to evaluate how staff perceive the environment and if they are comfortable reporting errors so improvements can be made. Patient-centered care is also an important safety issue. Including patients' preferences is an important area to support high-quality care. Selected concepts integral to quality improvement are outlined in the Concepts Related to Quality Improvement feature. They are presented in alphabetical order.

The Quality Improvement Process

Quality improvement is a continuous multistep, multilevel process that identifies areas for improvement based on performance and industry standards. Quality improvement involves analyzing current protocols of care and their associated outcomes and comparing those outcomes to those of leaders in high-quality care (called **benchmarking**). Quality improvement also involves identifying areas for improvement, researching factors that contribute to better outcomes, and implementing changes to improve outcomes. Patient outcomes must then be analyzed to determine the effectiveness of the changes and identify areas for further improvement. In addition, if a facility consistently provides a better quality of care than similar facilities do, the facility that is demonstrating excellence is responsible for documenting its methods to help improve care at other facilities. When quality improvement is directly linked to the performance of an individual, team, unit, or organization, it is called **performance improvement**.

Analysis of Current Protocols and Outcomes

To begin quality improvement, an individual, unit, or facility must understand its baseline performance records. Performance can be assessed on an intraprofessional level or an interprofessional level. In addition, it can focus on patient outcomes, cost effectiveness, resource utilization, or the integration of these aspects of care.

Intraprofessional Assessment

Intraprofessional assessment occurs within a group of individuals who have similar positions within a healthcare system, such as a group of nurses or a group of surgeons. Such an assessment is important for identifying areas of improvement at each level of care. Intraprofessional assessment includes peer reviews, audits, and outcomes management.

Peer Reviews

A **peer review** is used to professionally critique a colleague's work on the basis of predetermined standards. This allows nurses to assess other nurses in a safe, nonpunitive environment. Using this process, nurses work together to analyze complicated cases and determine the standards by which they will collectively be held accountable. It also allows

Concepts Related to
Quality Improvement

CONCEPT	RELATIONSHIP TO QUALITY IMPROVEMENT	NURSING IMPLICATIONS
Ethics	Patients have the right to the best quality of care.	■ Anticipate the need to provide high-quality care to all individuals, regardless of race, gender, sexual orientation, or ability to pay for services. ■ Be aware of disparities in treatment among population groups; advocate for high-quality care for all individuals. ■ Consult with patients to determine their preferences for care; provide culturally competent care. ■ Be aware of patient preferences that are not ethical, such as refusal of lifesaving blood transfusions for a child.
Informatics	Electronic health records can be used at the point of care and can be easily transmitted to collaborating healthcare workers to improve continuity of care.	■ Accurately record a patient's medical history and results of diagnostic tests for current and future use and to share patient information with relevant healthcare providers (HCPs). ■ Realize the importance of keeping all electronic and paper records up to date. ■ Provide education on the use of electronic records at the point of care. ■ Use informatics to identify areas for improvement, such as tracking healthcare-associated infections or identifying geographic locations that are without adequate healthcare resources.
Legal Issues	Consistently following federal and state laws will improve the quality of patient care.	■ Be alert to potential abusive situations; quality of care can be improved by preventing future abuse. ■ Be alert to behavior of healthcare workers (including one's self) that could increase risk of harm to patients or violate any patient's privacy; seek to counsel individuals performing reckless acts. ■ Anticipate asking patients or family members about legal documents such as living wills, healthcare proxy, and preference for do not resuscitate (DNR) orders. ■ Avoid blaming healthcare workers for inadvertent mistakes that result in patient harm; instead, debrief the individual and provide education on how to avoid future errors. ■ Participate in efforts to improve laws and healthcare protocols and treatments.

issues to be discussed by those with firsthand knowledge and produces recommendations that the nursing staff will understand and accept.

Audits

An **audit** is an examination of records to verify accuracy and proper use. An audit usually examines financial or medical records and can be for a single patient, a group of similar patients, an individual clinician, a unit, or a whole facility. If the audit is focused on one discipline (such as nursing), it is an intraprofessional assessment. If the audit is focused on multiple disciplines (e.g., both nurses and physicians), it becomes an interprofessional assessment.

In nursing, most audits are either retrospective or concurrent. A **retrospective audit** is performed after a patient's discharge. It compares care provided to one patient with care provided to patients with similar conditions, and recommendations are made to change procedures, if needed. A **concurrent audit** is performed while the patient is still undergoing care at the healthcare facility. It is used to evaluate the adequacy of the nursing care the patient is receiving and to determine whether desired outcomes are being met. This allows changes to be made, if needed, to prevent adverse events or to improve the patient's care.

Outcomes Management

Outcomes management uses patient experiences to guide improvement in all areas of healthcare by providing a link between medical interventions and health outcomes and between health outcomes and cost of care. An outcomes management system focuses on the results healthcare practitioners would like to achieve (ReportingMD, n.d.). Outcomes management can be used both to discover areas for improvement and to analyze areas of excellence to determine factors that contribute to success or failure. In 2004, the National Institutes of Health (n.d.) began an outcomes management program called PROMIS (Patient Reported Outcomes Measurement Information System). PROMIS collects information from patients to measure their health status in the areas of physical, mental, and social well-being.

This program continues to provide clinicians with access to patient-reported information about the effectiveness of treatments and the symptoms that patients experience to help improve communication, manage chronic diseases, and design treatment plans.

Interprofessional Assessment

Patient care involves collaboration among providers in multiple disciplines. For example, a patient with obesity and type 2 diabetes who is recovering from bariatric surgery may require care from a surgeon, a physician, a nurse, and a dietitian. To collaborate effectively, these individuals must have efficient communication, coordination, and integration of care. An interprofessional assessment (or interdisciplinary assessment) involves more than one discipline such as nursing and physical therapy.

In addition to peer reviews, audits, and outcomes management, interprofessional assessments include utilization reviews. A **utilization review** analyzes the use of resources to identify areas of overuse, misuse, and underuse. This protects the facility from unnecessary and inappropriate use of resources. Utilization review is required by Medicaid for specific services and by The Joint Commission for facility accreditation. A utilization review may identify areas in which resources are being overused, such as urinary catheterization for incontinent patients who are ambulatory or areas in which resources are lacking, such as inadequate staffing.

Clinical Example A

Ruth Davison is a 74-year-old woman who has been admitted to the same-day surgery center for elective right carpal tunnel repair (CTR). One hour before surgery, Mrs. Davison receives cefazolin (Ancef) 1 g IV as a prophylactic antibiotic. Anesthesia for the procedure consists of injection of local anesthetic at the surgical site with no administration of sedation.

After completion of the CTR, Mrs. Davison is stable, awake, and alert. She is monitored in the postanesthesia care unit (PACU) for 1 hour. Once she meets all discharge criteria, she is prepared for discharge to her home. Mrs. Davison's discharge instructions include keeping her surgical dressing in place for 2 days, after which time she may remove the dressing. She is further instructed to keep the dressing clean and dry while it is in place and to immediately report any drainage noted on the dressing. Mrs. Davison also is instructed to immediately report any redness, drainage, or swelling noted at her incision site following dressing removal. She is further advised that her sutures are absorbable and, thus, do not need to be removed. After verbalizing understanding of her discharge instructions and signing the discharge record, Mrs. Davison is transported to her home by her daughter.

The following morning, the same-day surgery center receives a phone call from Mrs. Davison, who reports that she has removed her dressing and now notes "a little" bleeding and redness at her incision site. After reviewing Mrs. Davison's discharge record, the nurse reminds her that her instructions included leaving her dressing in place for 2 days. Mrs. Davison states that she does not recall being told to leave her dressing intact for 2 days and asks, "How was I supposed to be able to tell if the wound looked okay with the dressing covering it?" She further notes that she is concerned that her surgical wound may be infected.

Mrs. Davison is scheduled for a follow-up appointment with her surgeon that afternoon. At her follow-up appointment, Mrs. Davison's wound is evaluated and cleansed and a dressing is reapplied. Her surgeon instructs Mrs. Davison to return to his office in 3 days, at which time her dressing will be removed and her wound will be reevaluated for signs and symptoms of infection.

As a result of Mrs. Davison's apparent misunderstanding of her discharge instructions and subsequent need for two additional appointments with her physician, an intraprofessional assessment is initiated. Two registered nurses who provided care to Mrs. Davison, two additional registered nurses, and the nurse manager review her case. They compare Mrs. Davison's case to the cases of patients of similar age, cultural background, and surgical procedure. The nurse manager also follows up with Mrs. Davison to hear her perspective on the care she received, her understanding of the discharge instructions, the symptoms she experienced, and her overall satisfaction with her care.

Critical Thinking Questions

1. Identify the portions of the intraprofessional assessment that reflect peer review, auditing, and outcomes management.
2. Why is it important to compare Mrs. Davison's care with care received by other patients who correctly followed discharge instructions?
3. Describe the impact that a patient's perspective can have on quality improvement.

Benchmarking

Benchmarking is a method that is used to compare the performance of an individual or organization to industry standards. **Standards** of care are based on established models of high-quality performance and may reflect the performance of industry leaders, scientific or clinical research, or recommendations of professional organizations such as the ANA. These standards are continually being updated, so nurses must use research and other reliable sources of information to stay up to date on current recommendations and standards.

The Donabedian model of quality improvement (originally developed by physician and researcher Avedis Donabedian) states that standards usually relate to three dimensions of high-quality care: structure, process, and outcome. **Structure standards** relate to material resources, human resources, and general organizational structure. They focus on the organization's capacity and systems for providing care. **Process standards** focus on the steps used to lead to a particular outcome. They are used to determine whether a set of steps exists and whether those steps are being followed. **Outcome standards** focus on the performance of a process, such as the number of bedridden patients who develop a pressure injury (AHRQ, 2015b).

Benchmarking uses **indicators**, or statistics, that reflect the organization's performance in a specific area to compare the quality of care within the organization to industry standards. Indicators must be measurable, objective, and sensitive to changes in performance. Indicators can include generic or specific standards of care as stated by the ANA, specialty organizations, or the organization or unit implementing quality improvement strategies.

For example, a nursing unit decides to evaluate the quality of the care provided to newly admitted patients. The unit determines that the indicators for the study will be a completed initial assessment within 1 hour of admission, a documented and accurate nursing plan of care by the end of the shift, and accurate implementation of providers' orders. The indicators are then compared against each newly admitted patient's medical records to benchmark the frequency with which the indicators were met. The nurses on the unit will be informed if the study indicates whether or not nursing care provided complies with the standards for the unit.

Targeting Areas for Improvement

Once the current level of performance has been compared with industry standards, areas that need improvement can be identified. On the basis of the policies and procedures already in place, each healthcare facility will have different areas in need of improvement. These may reflect general practices (such as use of a specific ointment for wounds) or specific practices (such as frequency of checking vital signs on older patients after pacemaker implantation). They may be identified on the basis of a bad outcome for one patient or a trend of poor outcomes for multiple patients. Some areas needing improvement are identified as a result of a required investigation after adverse events. For example, a sentinel event or breach of care will always prompt a required investigation. Risk management can also be used to identify risk factors and develop associated protocols for reducing or preventing adverse events.

Sentinel Events

The Joint Commission (n.d.-a) has defined a **sentinel event** as "an unexpected occurrence involving death or serious physical or psychologic injury, or the risk thereof. Serious injury specifically includes loss of limb or function. The phrase 'the risk thereof' includes any process variation for which a recurrence would carry a significant chance of a serious adverse outcome." Sentinel events require immediate investigation and response.

In an effort to continuously improve the safety and quality of healthcare provided to the public, The Joint Commission reviews a facility's response to sentinel events as part of its accreditation process. The goals of the sentinel event policy are to have a positive impact on patient care, prevent sentinel events, understand the factors that contributed to the event, increase the general knowledge about sentinel events, and maintain the confidence of the public in accredited organizations.

If a sentinel event occurs, accredited organizations are expected to respond appropriately, including conducting a credible **root cause analysis** called RCA2 (problem solving to identify the root cause of faults), developing a plan to reduce future risk of sentinel events, implementing improvements, and monitoring the effectiveness of improvements (The Joint Commission, n.d.-a). In addition, The Joint Commission conducts reviews for a specific subset of sentinel events, including the following:

- Unanticipated death or major permanent loss not associated with the patient's original illness
- Invasive procedures on the wrong patient, at the wrong site, or with the wrong procedure
- Unintended retention of a foreign object in a patient after surgery
- Radiation overdose or delivery of radiation to the wrong body region
- Administration of an incompatible blood transfusion
- Abduction, rape, assault, homicide, or suicide of any patient or staff member while at the healthcare facility or suicide within 72 hours of discharge
- Severe neonatal hyperbilirubinemia
- Any elopement of a patient from a staffed around-the-clock setting leading to death, permanent harm, or severe temporary harm.

>> **Stay Current:** The National Council of State Boards of Nursing offers a video and guide to conducting root cause analyses. For more information, go to ncsbn.org.

Breach of Care

A **breach of care** or **breach of duty** occurs when a nurse deviates from the standard of care. This deviation will depend on the relevant statutes, rules, and regulations that govern practice (HG.org, n.d.). A benchmarking report by CRICO, the risk management arm of the Harvard Medical Institutions, conducted in 2018 found nurses are often involved in cases around bedside care (medication administration and monitoring, IVs, catheters, wound care) and clinical assessment and monitoring activities (falls, pressure injuries). Nurses are also involved in cases with other healthcare team members that involve communication breakdowns (Hoffman, 2019).

Quality improvement efforts seek to determine weaknesses in procedures and processes as well as organizational issues that can affect nurses' ability to provide nursing care consistent with established professional standards of care. Nurses can reduce the risk of committing a breach of care by reporting problems to nursing supervisors, remaining current in their skills and education, basing all care on the nursing process model, and documenting care provided as well as the patient's response to interventions. Following these procedures reduces the risk of an adverse event and resulting malpractice suit.

Risk Management

Risk management is " . . . the clinical and administrative systems, processes, and reports employed to detect, monitor, assess, mitigate, and prevent risks" (NEJM Catalyst, 2018). Risk management includes both proactive components to prevent adverse events and reactive components to minimize damage from adverse events. Risk assessment must occur daily, and all individuals must be dedicated to keeping patients safe from harm.

The risk management process:

- Identifies risks that may lead to patient or staff injury or financial loss
- Reviews systems that monitor risks, such as patient questionnaires or incident reports
- Analyzes the frequency, severity, and cause of past adverse events
- Analyzes new procedures with potential risk to patients
- Stays up to date on current laws pertaining to healthcare
- Identifies the need for patient and staff education.

Using this information, the risk management team can identify areas of risk and implement strategies to reduce risk as much as possible.

Because of their close contact with patients, nurses are perfectly positioned to analyze patient satisfaction, identify specific patient risks, and implement strategies at the bedside to reduce patient risk of an adverse event. Patient satisfaction is a key factor in risk management. A dissatisfied patient presents a higher risk for liability than a satisfied patient. A nurse who becomes aware of patient dissatisfaction should take steps to communicate with the patient to clarify misunderstandings, advocate for the patient to receive better care, and notify a supervisor about potential problems. Personal care by a nurse and a nurse manager can calm a patient or the patient's family, identify problems before they become an emergency, and improve the quality of care. (For more information, see Exemplar 49.E, Risk Management, in Module 49, Legal Issues.)

Clinical Example B

At an extended care facility, Reuben Meyers, an 84-year-old man with Alzheimer disease, was discovered to be missing from his bed at 2:15 a.m. A search resulted in finding Mr. Meyers lying in the street, the victim of a hit-and-run motor-vehicle accident. He was unconscious when he was found. A physical assessment identified a right hip injury, which later was revealed to be a fractured right hip. He also had a 2-inch-long open gash in the right temporal region of his head. After closure of his head wound and surgical repair of his hip, Mr. Meyers remained unconscious until his death 12 days later. An investigation found that security cameras had recorded Mr. Meyers wandering from the extended care facility at 1:30 a.m. Traffic cameras recorded the hit-and-run accident at 2:08 a.m.

Critical Thinking Questions

1. On the basis of the limited description of this sentinel event, what standards of nursing care may have been breached?
2. What potential legal ramifications may this event have for the nurses who were caring for Mr. Meyers and for the nursing home facility?
3. Develop a risk management program to identify risks for similar sentinel events and propose strategies to improve the quality of care and reduce the risk of wandering outdoors for patients with Alzheimer disease.

Identifying Factors That Promote Better Outcomes

Identification of problem areas or adverse events demands intervention to improve patient safety. This involves a planning process that identifies the cause of adverse events through a root cause analysis and researches the literature for methods of improvement. Nurses can participate with a team of other clinicians to plan the changes needed to improve the quality of care. Organizations such as The Joint Commission identify patient safety goals every year for organizations to focus on. The 2021 goals for hospitals include ensuring patients are identified safely (e.g., right patient; see Exemplar 51.D, Medication Safety, in Module 51, Safety), improving staff communication (see Module 38, Communication), using alarms safely, and preventing infections (see Module 9, Infection) (The Joint Commission, n.d.). Nursing has a role in impacting all of these goals to promote better patient outcomes. Additional factors that promote better outcomes are summarized next.

Root Cause Analysis

A root cause analysis is required by The Joint Commission for sentinel events and is recommended for any adverse event. The goals of the root cause analysis are to identify the reasons for failures or problems and to develop an action plan for improvement to decrease the likelihood of future adverse events. The root cause analysis is now referred to as RCA2: Improving Root Cause Analysis and Actions to Prevent Harm. This expanded process was developed to ensure the identification and implementation of sustained systems-based improvement to work toward making healthcare safer (Institute for Healthcare Improvement [IHI], 2020). This analysis focuses on systems and processes, not on individual performance, and it analyzes both special causes (factors that cause variation beyond what is normal) and common causes (factors that occur because of normal variation in the system). The action plan should include identification of who is responsible for implementing and overseeing improvements, pilot testing to ensure the success of the changes, timelines for implementing changes, and strategies for measuring the effectiveness of changes (IHI, 2020).

Reducing Medication Errors

The National Coordinating Council for Medication Error Reporting and Prevention (n.d.) defines a medication error as "any preventable event that may cause or lead to inappropriate medication use or patient harm while the medication is in the control of the healthcare professional, patient, or consumer." An adverse drug event (ADE) is defined as harm experienced by a patient as a result of exposure to a medication. Not all ADEs are the result of a medication error, but many are preventable. One of the highest-risk drugs used in the inpatient setting is anticoagulant intravenous heparin. The Institute for Safe Medication Practice maintains a list of high-alert medications such as look-alike, sound-alike medications to assist clinicians with identifying medications that can either look similar or have similar names, but that have very different chemical properties that can cause harm to the patient if they are mixed up. Another group of high-alert medications are those that can cause problems in older adults. The American Geriatrics Society publishes a set of guidelines (the Beers Criteria® for Potentially Inappropriate Medication Use in Older Adults) to help improve the care of adults age 65 and older. The Beers Criteria includes medications (such as benzodiazepines) that should be eliminated or carefully managed to avoid complications (Fixen, 2019).

Several national- and facility-implemented interventions have been designed to decrease medication errors. These include barcoding both patients' identification bands and medications, regulating similar names of drugs that may cause confusion, implementing a pharmacy first-dose review, and using a computerized physician order entry system.

Staffing Practices in Nursing

Multiple studies have established a link between decreased nurse staffing and adverse patient outcomes. One consideration of nurse staffing is the nursing skills mix (proportion of total hours provided by registered nurses). One systematic review found that an increased number of nursing hours was associated with improved outcomes. These improved outcomes included reductions in ulcer, gastritis, acute myocardial infarction, restraint use, failure-to-rescue, pneumonia, sepsis, urinary tract infection, 30-day mortality, pressure injury, infections, and shock/cardiac arrest/heart failure (Twigg et al., 2019). Nursing-sensitive indicators are measured by many healthcare systems as part of the NDNQI, established by the ANA in 2007 to evaluate linkages between staffing and quality of care, now administered by Press Ganey. Currently Press Ganey (n.d.) has combined the NDNQI with patient experience and nurse engagement to provide nursing and other leaders with a comprehensive set of quality data. This information helps nurse leaders and nursing teams to gain insights into where there are areas that need improvement and where things are going well. The NDNQI indicators are listed in **Box 50.2** ».

Resource Utilization

The value of healthcare can be increased by reducing costs while maintaining or improving the quality of care. This can be accomplished by implementing measures to reduce waste that may result from unnecessary or inefficient services, prices that are too high, excess administrative costs, missed prevention opportunities, and medical fraud (IOM, 2010). Examples of waste that are directly applicable to nurses include medical errors that result in prolonged inpatient days, scheduling an additional visit for patient education only, and lost time because of unorganized supplies, poorly maintained equipment, or inadequate documentation.

Blame-free Environment

According to the IOM's report *To Err Is Human* (2000), most errors in healthcare are a result of the healthcare system and not the fault of any single individual. If a nurse or another member of the healthcare team is afraid to report errors for fear of punishment or because reporting does not result in positive change, then problems within the system cannot be identified and addressed. Therefore, a key component in quality improvement is establishing a **blame-free environment** in which HCPs can report errors or near misses without the fear of punishment (AHRQ, 2019). This helps identify problems so corrections can be made and future adverse events can be prevented. The Evidence-Based Practice feature discusses methods for reducing errors and increasing the reporting of errors.

Just Culture

One difficulty in establishing a blame-free environment is that although many errors are a result of the healthcare system, some errors are the result of personal mistakes and demand accountability. **Just culture** attempts to balance the blame-free environment with appropriate accountability by focusing on correcting problems that lead individuals to engage in unsafe behavior while maintaining individual accountability by establishing zero tolerance for reckless behavior (AHRQ, 2019). Just culture differentiates among human error, at-risk behavior, and reckless behavior, in contrast to the "no blame" approach of the blame-free environment. Just culture is based on the understanding that errors are often the result of system failures rather than human failures. It recognizes that an atmosphere of punishment impedes error prevention by promoting intimidation and secrecy rather than shared accountability. Just culture focuses on the system rather than the individual while still maintaining an environment of individual accountability for both front-line staff and leaders and managers. This is critical: When front-line staff fail to report safety errors because of a fear of suspension or termination,

Box 50.2

Nursing-Sensitive Indicators

Nursing-sensitive indicators reflect the quantity and quality of nursing care in the areas of structure, process, and outcome (Press Ganey, n.d.).

STRUCTURE	PROCESS	OUTCOME
Nursing turnover	Pediatric pain assessment, intervention, reassessment (AIR) cycles completed	Catheter-associated urinary tract infections (CAUTI)
RN education/certification	Care coordination	Central line catheter-associated blood stream infections (CLABSI)
Nursing skill mix	Device utilization	Hospital readmissions
Admissions/discharge/transfer	Pain impairing function*	Multiresistant organisms
Emergency department throughput	Patient falls*	*C-difficile* and MRSA infections
Workforce characteristics	Pressure injuries*	Ventilator-associated events (VAE)
Patient contacts	Restraints	Ventilator-associated pneumonia (VAP)
Patient volume and flow		Unplanned postoperative transfers/admissions
		Pediatric peripheral intravenous infiltrations
		Patient burns
		Surgical errors
		Assaults by psychiatric patient
		Assaults on nursing personnel

Measured as both a process and an outcome.

Evidence-Based Practice

Methods to Reduce Errors

Problem

The most effective way to identify and correct problems in healthcare is by consistently reporting errors and potential errors/near misses so that the healthcare team can learn from them. However, studies indicate that safety climate and safety culture and clinician willingness to report errors are linked (Weaver et al., 2013).

Evidence

One method to reduce medical errors is to eliminate barriers to error reporting. Fear of social and professional consequences is a significant barrier to medication error reporting (Yang et al., 2020). A study looking at medication error reporting found that nurses were not as likely to report errors that they themselves made as they were to report errors made by others (Jember, Hailu, Messele, Demeke, & Hassen, 2018). Another study found that nurses who scored high on a systems thinking scale were more likely to report medical errors (Hwang & Park, 2017). In addition, many nurses and clinicians do not realize that near misses and errors that do not cause harm should also be reported.

Another method to reduce medical errors is to improve the nurses' work environment. The American Association of Critical Care Nurses (n.d.) has established six standards for a healthy work environment: skilled communication, true collaboration, effective decision making, appropriate staffing, meaningful recognition, and authentic leadership. In addition, fostering a safety culture can lead to decreased errors and increased reporting. A systematic review of interventions to promote safety cultures found that a combination of interventions such as patient safety rounds, implementation of best care practices, teamwork interventions, and continuous learning improves patient safety and quality (Weaver et al., 2013).

Implications

Eliminating barriers to error reporting and establishing a healthy work environment can lead to reduced errors and increased reporting of errors. However, changing from a culture of blame to a safety culture requires time and dedication from the entire organization. As individuals on the front line of patient care, nurses play a critical role in the establishment of a safety culture by helping to identify problems and by working to implement changes to practice that will reduce errors. Education about a blame-free environment and taking personal responsibility to report errors are two ways in which nurses can contribute to quality improvement in healthcare.

Critical Thinking Application

1. Consider situations in which you, a fellow nurse, or a physician makes medication errors that do not result in patient harm. In which situations would you complete an error report? Why?
2. Identify personal barriers that would prevent you from reporting a medical error caused by the system, a coworker, or yourself.
3. Research the current error reporting systems in place at a local hospital, nursing home, and primary care clinic.

healthcare managers may develop an inaccurate understanding of the care provided by the organization. This hampers ongoing quality improvement efforts, further risking patient safety (Dekker & Breakey, 2016). Successfully establishing an environment of just culture requires that leadership encourage proactive system management as well as individual accountability. It also requires that employees consider themselves stakeholders and act to establish and maintain the just culture environment. Just culture does not, however, accept or tolerate gross misconduct (e.g., employees working under the influence of alcohol or narcotics) or conscious disregard of patient and staff safety.

In a just culture environment, each member has the responsibility to take action to prevent and respond to errors. A just culture environment recognizes that errors are more often the result of system failures than individual error. When individual error does occur, it is more likely to be accidental than willful or neglectful. For example, if the hospital pharmacy dispenses the wrong medication or if the department in charge of stocking supplies for a unit orders an inadequate amount of supplies, those errors may result from inadequate systems as much as from individual carelessness.

As more organizations begin to embrace just culture, front-line staff are likely to feel more support from management in critical areas, including staffing. From time to time, however, nurses and other front-line staff may find themselves in situations in which management is unresponsive to suggestions for improvement or reporting of critical shortages or potential for errors related to patient safety. In these cases, staff may find themselves in the awkward position of needing to report these problems outside the agency.

Personal Responsibility

All nurses must be involved in quality improvement. Nursing students demonstrate concern for quality by making a commitment never to perform an act that they are uncertain how to perform, by showing accountability for their actions, and by admitting to errors if they occur. Each nurse, whether a nursing student or a practicing nurse, has the responsibility to know the policies and procedures in the facility where clinical training is performed and to follow them exactly. In addition, nurses are responsible for understanding how to report errors, including paperwork that should be completed and individuals to whom errors should be reported.

Implementing New Protocols

When a problem is identified and a plan put in place to improve the quality of care, that plan must be implemented. The most important step in implementing new procedures is educating nurses and other clinicians about the importance of the new process, the steps involved, and associated reporting procedures. Education can take place in large or small groups, as a self-study, or during orientation. Each individual must then take personal responsibility to implement the needed changes to improve the quality of care.

Evaluating Efficacy of New Protocols

Finally, the implemented changes must be evaluated to assess their impact on patient care, patient outcomes, patient and clinician satisfaction, and resource utilization. Data related to the original problem must be collected and are then analyzed on the basis of the benchmark standards to determine whether standards are being met. This process is called **quality assurance**. If standards are not met, the quality improvement is continued with the goal of achieving the desired goals.

Quality Management Programs

The process of quality improvement is accomplished through use of a quality management program. A quality management program must include both information about current practices and outcomes and accountability for the individuals who oversee and perform patient care. Advances in technology are vital to quality management because clinical information systems can be used to track patient outcomes and actions that led to patient harm (see Module 48, Informatics). For example, data from a clinical information system can be used to track the occurrence of healthcare-associated infections, including the location of the infection (e.g., urinary system, respiratory system, and skin), frequency of patient assessment, materials used to treat the patient, and other relevant factors. Changes in hand hygiene protocols, equipment and medical supplies used, wound care protocols, and patient placement can then be implemented to reduce the incidence of healthcare-associated infections. To be successful, these changes must then be accepted and used by the entire staff.

Healthcare organizations use different quality management programs depending on their clientele and specialty area. Commonly used quality management programs include total quality management, continuous quality improvement, Six Sigma, and Lean Six Sigma. Each of these programs includes a comprehensive quality management plan.

Comprehensive Quality Management

A quality management plan is used to help healthcare facilities integrate new programs, models, and technologies with the primary care services that are already in place. The plan should address needs of engagement (improving the experience of care), population health, and value (per capita costs). The plan should be comprehensive, looking at quality and safety in clinical, managerial, administrative, and facility-related aspects of the organization. It should design, implement, monitor, and improve methods to increase the quality of care in keeping with the organization's mission and core values. Most organizations will develop quality management plans that require cooperation between departments as well as unit-specific plans.

Quality management plans should be patient focused, collecting and evaluating data for improvement of patient outcomes, expectations, and satisfaction. Patient satisfaction surveys can be used to track the effectiveness of changes from the patient's perspective. Nurses often perform this follow-up through personal visits, forms, or phone calls. If any problems are noted, the nurse can then report back to the HCP or nurse manager to help improve patient care.

Total Quality Management

Total quality management (TQM), a comprehensive management philosophy that was invented by Walter Shewhart and made famous by W. Edwards Deming, is used to improve quality and productivity by using data and statistics to improve systems processes. The hallmark of TQM is that it relies on teamwork throughout the organization, involving all departments and employees and including both suppliers and customers. Its essential elements include communication, feedback, fact-based decision making, and a focus on continual improvement.

A system of quality improvement most often associated with TQM is Deming's **Plan–Do–Study–Act (PDSA)** (**Figure 50.2** »), which was modified from Shewhart's Plan–Do–Check–Act or Plan–Do–Check–Adjust. During planning, individuals on the TQM team define the goal, collect data, and outline a strategy to reach the goal. In the Do phase, the plan is implemented on a small scale to determine whether it will be effective. This is followed by the Study phase, in which the outcomes of the Do phase are analyzed and compared to the expected outcomes. In the Act phase, the team must decide whether the goal was met, plan further changes, and decide whether the original goal is attainable based on the results of the previous interventions. If the goal was met, then the team must decide whether the changes should be implemented throughout the organization.

Continuous Quality Improvement

In healthcare, **continuous quality improvement (CQI)** is defined "a process of progressive incremental improvement of processes, safety and patient care" (O'Donnell & Gupta, 2020). CQI can be applied to a specific problem, development and implementation of policies and procedures, resource utilization, or implementation of evidence-based practices.

CQI is a customer-driven process. In healthcare, the customer can be internal or external to the system. Internal customers include employees of a healthcare organization, such as nurses, physicians, therapists, medical record staff, billing specialists, and other employees. External customers include

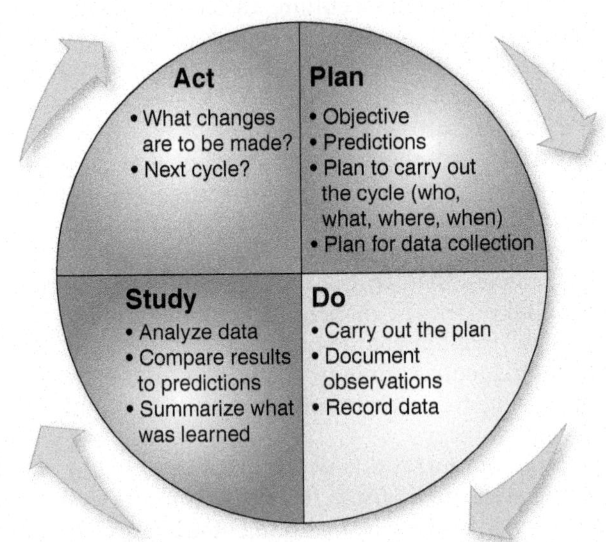

Figure 50.2 » PDSA cycle.

the individuals who seek healthcare as well as their family members and significant others. External customers also include other individuals and entities with whom internal patients interact, such as insurance companies, managed care organizations, equipment or material suppliers, social service agencies, and law enforcement officials. Customer satisfaction is the end goal of CQI. CQI is also system focused, emphasizing system errors rather than individual errors. Therefore, CQI requires involvement by everyone with knowledge of the system, from senior management to individuals providing everyday care to patients (Skochelak, 2020).

Clinical Example C

An unidentified middle-aged woman is transported to the emergency department (ED) by two law enforcement officers. The officers report that the individual was observed "wandering around on a highway" and that complaints were received from passing motorists about the woman's behavior. The officers also report that, upon their arrival, the woman was unable to provide any identification, nor was she verbally responsive to their questions. She did, however, willingly seat herself in their squad car upon request. The officers state that the woman is being transferred to the ED for evaluation, as they are uncertain about the etiology of her behaviors.

Lynne Bryten, RN, is the ED triage nurse. The unidentified woman, who is clutching a doll, appears to be awake and alert. She is clean and dressed appropriately, and her tennis shoes appear to be relatively new. Ms. Bryten attempts to perform an initial interview, but the woman does not respond to her questions. She permits Ms. Bryten to assess her vital signs, all of which are within normal limits. She exhibits no apparent indications of traumatic injury, and her pupils are equal and responsive to light. Although the woman is not verbally responsive to Ms. Bryten's questions, she appears to follow directions during the assessment. The woman is admitted to the ED as an unidentified patient. Ms. Bryten escorts the patient and the law enforcement officers into the ED and notifies the ED physician of their arrival.

Dr. Terrence Garvinner, the attending ED physician, receives Ms. Bryten's report. Upon entering the patient's room, he introduces himself and performs a brief patient assessment. The patient remains verbally unresponsive, but she follows Dr. Garvinner's directions. Afterward, Dr. Garvinner asks the law enforcement officers to speak with him privately. They accompany him to an empty ED room.

Dr. Garvinner informs the law enforcement officers that the patient does not appear to have any physical injury; rather, she may be developmentally delayed. He suggests that the officers check missing person reports and contact residential treatment centers to determine whether or not the patient may have wandered away from one of the local residential care centers. Dr. Garvinner questions the officers as to why they did not use this approach initially. One of the officers responds, "We have no way of knowing if she has a medical problem. That's why we brought her here. Plus, we have other calls coming in—we're swamped." Dr. Garvinner responds, "We have no way of identifying this woman. She appears to be a vulnerable adult who may be lost. We have a full waiting room, and we don't have staff available to serve as detectives. I believe you have an entire department dedicated to performing detective work."

Critical Thinking Questions

1. Identify the internal and external customers in this scenario.
2. Summarize the conflict between the law enforcement officers and the ED physician. Is either argument correct? Why or why not?
3. In the context of healthcare, how can internal and external conflict affect the patient who is seeking treatment or in need of assistance?
4. What additional external resources may be helpful in identifying the patient and assisting with her safe return to her residence?
5. How might the process of quality management be applied to address and manage future situations such as the one described in the scenario?

Six Sigma

Six Sigma is a quality improvement program that was originally implemented by Motorola and General Electric to reduce variation within a process to produce a near-perfect product. Sigma is a Greek letter often used to measure deviation from a standard; to receive a sigma level of 6, only 3.4 products per million are allowed to be defective. In this system, a defect is defined as anything that could lead to patient dissatisfaction. Defects in healthcare could range from relatively minor problems such as providing the wrong size gown to a patient to major problems such as performing an amputation on the wrong limb. Six Sigma primarily uses the **DMAIC** system to improve outcomes (Mason, Nicolay, & Darzi, 2015):

Define the problem, determine a goal, and form a team to address the problem.

Measure: Obtain data related to the current process, the problem, and the desired goal.

Analyze: Look at the data to determine cause-and-effect relationships related to the problem.

Improve: Develop solutions to problems and implement those solutions.

Control: Implement measures to sustain positive changes and continuously monitor the process to ensure goals are being met.

Six Sigma may also use the DMADV methodology: Define, Measure, Analyze, Design, and Verify.

Six Sigma uses teams of individuals with intimate knowledge of the problem and training in Six Sigma principles. Master Black Belts are experts in Six Sigma who can assist in data calculations and function as a resource for the team. The team is led by a Black Belt with extensive knowledge of Six Sigma. Green Belts are team members with some experience with Six Sigma, and Yellow and White Belts are relatively new to the Six Sigma system. Six Sigma is most successful when the entire organization, including both administrators and clinicians, is involved in planning and implementing changes.

Lean Six Sigma

Lean Six Sigma combines the strategies of Six Sigma, described above, with the Lean system. The objective of the Lean system is to eliminate waste to maximize value. Waste is defined as anything that does not bring value to the customer. Therefore, Lean Six Sigma is a methodology used to reduce waste and provide consistency in the quality of care. It primarily uses the DMAIC system that is used in Six Sigma. Studies conducted using the Lean Six Sigma focus on single case studies and a recent systemic review found there is an increase in the number of empirical research being published (Henrique & Godinho Filho, 2020).

>> **Stay Current:** Six Sigma and Lean Six Sigma training and certification are available from a number of organizations. For an example, visit https://www.purdue.edu/leansixsigmaonline/blog/healthcare-advancement-with-lean-six-sigma/.

REVIEW The Concept of Quality Improvement

RELATE Link the Concepts

Linking the concept of quality improvement with the concept of collaboration:

1. How can the nurse use conflict management skills to resolve patient or family member dissatisfaction with care?
2. How does strong interprofessional team communication improve the outcomes of total quality management?

Linking the concept of quality improvement with the concept of managing care:

3. How does an effective quality improvement process reduce the cost of care?
4. How does proper care coordination improve the quality of care provided to patients?

REFER Go to Pearson MyLab Nursing and eText

REFLECT Apply Your Knowledge

Jose Hernandez is a newly licensed nurse who has accepted a job working on a busy genitourinary unit in the local community hospital. During orientation, he is working the evening shift with a preceptor. On this particular evening, the unit has been very busy, and the charge nurse asks Jose's preceptor, Fred McFarlane, to take a few patients in addition to acting as a preceptor for Jose with his assigned patients. Fred agrees and instructs Jose to seek him out if he needs help or has any questions.

Quite by chance, Jose notices that Fred makes a medication error when he fails to administer an ordered medication at an appropriate time to one of Fred's assigned patients. Jose doesn't say anything because Fred acknowledges the error independently, but Jose isn't sure what to do at the end of the shift when he realizes that Fred is not going to fill out an incident report.

1. Should an incident report be filled out regarding Fred's late administration of a medication to the patient if no harm resulted? Explain the rationale for your answer.
2. Who is responsible for completing an incident report if one is required? Explain.
3. What is Jose's responsibility related to the error if he had no care responsibility related to the patient who received the medication later than ordered?
4. How would you handle this situation if you were Jose?

References

Agency for Healthcare Research and Quality (AHRQ). (2015a). *About the National Quality Strategy*. https://www.ahrq.gov/workingforquality/about/index.html#aims

Agency for Healthcare Research and Quality (AHRQ). (2015b). *Medication errors*. https://psnet.ahrq.gov/primers/primer/23/-medication-errors

Agency for Healthcare Research and Quality (AHRQ). (2018). *2018 national healthcare quality and disparities report*. https://www.ahrq.gov/research/findings/nhqrdr/nhqdr18/index.html

Agency for Healthcare Research and Quality (AHRQ). (2019). *Safety culture*. http://psnet.ahrq.gov/primer.aspx?primerID=5

American Association of Critical Care Nurses (AACN). (n.d.). *Is your work environment healthy?* https://www.aacn.org/nursing-excellence/healthy-work-environments

Austin, J. M., & Kachalia, A. (2020). The state of healthcare quality measurement in the era of COVID-19: The importance of doing better. *Journal of the American Medical Association, 324*(4), 333–334. https://doi.org/10.1001/jama.2020.11461

Dekker, S. W., & Breakey, H. (2016). "Just culture": Improving safety by achieving substantive, procedural and restorative justice. *Safety Science, 85*, 187–193. https://doi.org/10.1016/j.ssci.2016.01.018

Freeman, R., Coyne, J., & Kingsdale, J. (2020). Successes and failures with bundled payments in the commercial market. *The American Journal of Managed Care, 26*(20), e300–e304.

Fixen, D. R. (2019). 2019 AGS Beers Criteria for older adults. *Pharmacy Today, 25*(11), 42–54.

Health Resources and Services Administration (HRSA). (2011). *Quality improvement*. http://www.hrsa.gov/quality/toolbox/508pdfs/qualityimprovement.pdf

Henry J. Kaiser Family Foundation. (2020). *For 3rd year in a row, more insurers are entering the ACA marketplaces, creating more options for customers*. https://www.kff.org/private-insurance/press-release/for-3rd-year-in-a-row-more-insurers-are-entering-the-aca-marketplaces-creating-more-options-for-consumers/

HG.org. (n.d.). *Negligence & breach of duty of care*. https://www.hg.org/legal-articles/negligence-and-breach-of-duty-of-care-20316

Hoffman, J. (2019, April). *Taking a second look at nursing malpractice cases*. CRICO. https://www.rmf.harvard.edu/Clinician-Resources/Newsletter-and-Publication/2019/SPS-April-Nursing

Henrique, D. B., & Godinho Filho, M. (2020). A systematic literature review of empirical research in Lean and Six Sigma in healthcare. *Total Quality Management and Business Excellence, 31*(3–4), 429–449.

Hwang, J. I., & Park, H. A. (2017). Nurses' systems thinking competency, medical error reporting, and the occurrence of adverse events: A cross-sectional study. *Contemporary Nurse, 53*(6), 622–632. https://doi.org/10.1080/10376178.2017.1409081

Institute for Healthcare Improvement (IHI). (2020). *RCA2: Improving root cause analyses and actions to prevent harm*. http://www.ihi.org/resources/Pages/Tools/RCA2-Improving-Root-Cause-Analyses-and-Actions-to-Prevent-Harm.aspx

Institute of Medicine (IOM). (2000). *To err is human: Building a safer health system*. National Academies Press.

Institute of Medicine (IOM). (2001). *Crossing the quality chasm: A new health system for the 21st -century*. National Academies Press.

Institute of Medicine (IOM). (2010). *The healthcare imperative: Lowering costs and improving outcomes*. National Academies Press.

Jember, A., Hailu, M., Messele, A., Demeke, T., & Hassen, M. (2018). Proportion of medication error reporting and associated factors among nurses: A cross sectional study. *BMC Nursing, 17*(1), 9. https://doi.org/10.1186/s12912-018-0280-4

Keers, R. N., Williams, S. D., Cooke, J., & Ashcroft, D. M. (2013). Prevalence and nature of medication administration errors in health care settings: A systematic review of direct observational evidence. *Annals of Pharmacotherapy, 47*(2), 237–256. https://doi.org/10.1345/aph.1R147

Makary, M. A., & Daniel, M. (2016). Medical error—the third leading cause of death in the US. *British Medical Journal, 353*, i2139. https://doi.org/10.1136/bmj.i2139.

Mason, S. E., Nicolay, C. R., & Darzi, A. (2015). The use of Lean and Six Sigma methodologies in surgery: A systematic review. *The Surgeon, 13*(2), 91–100. https://doi.org/10.1016/j.surge.2014.08.002

Medicaid (n.d.). *Basic health program*. https://www.medicaid.gov/basic-health-program/index.html

National Coordinating Council for Medication Error Reporting and Prevention. (n.d.). *About -medication errors*. https://www.nccmerp.org/about-medication-errors

National Institutes of Health. (n.d.). *PROMIS overview*. https://www.healthmeasures.net/explore-measurement-systems/promis

Navathe, A. S., Troxel, A. B., Liao, J. M., Nan, N., Zhu, J., Zhong, W., & Emanuel, E. J. (2017). Cost of joint replacement using bundled payment models. *JAMA Internal Medicine, 177*(2), 214–222.

NEJM Catalyst. (2018, April 25). *What is risk management in healthcare?* https://catalyst.nejm.org/doi/full/10.1056/CAT.18.0197

O'Donnell, B., & Gupta, V. (2020). *Continuous quality improvement*. StatPearls. https://www.ncbi.nlm.nih.gov/books/NBK559239/

Press Ganey. (n.d.). *Turn nursing quality insights into improved patient experiences*. https://www.pressganey.com/resources/program-summary/ndnqi-solution-summary

ReportingMD. (n.d.). *Outcomes management*. https://reportingmd.com/outcomes-management/

Skochelak, S. E. (Ed.). (2020). *Health systems science e-book*. Elsevier.

The Joint Commission. (n.d.-a). *Sentinel event policy and procedures*. http://www.jointcommission.org/Sentinel_Event_Policy_and_Procedures

The Joint Commission. (n.d.-b). *2021 National patient safety goals*. https://www.jointcommission.org/standards/national-patient-safety-goals/

Twigg, D. E., Kutzer, Y., Jacob, E., & Seaman, K. (2019). A quantitative systematic review of the association between nurse skill mix and nursing-sensitive patient outcomes in the acute care setting. *Journal of Advanced Nursing, 75*(12), 3404–3423. https://doi.org/10.1111/jan.14194

Weaver, S. J., Lubomksi, L. H., Wilson, R. F., Pfoh, E. R., Martinez, K. A., & Dy, S. M. (2013). Promoting a culture of safety as a patient safety strategy: A systematic review. *Annals of Internal Medicine, 158*(5, Pt. 2), 369–374. https://doi.org/10.7326/0003-4819-158-5-201303051-00002

Yang, R., Pepper, G. A., Wang, H., Liu, T., Wu, D., & Jiang, Y. (2020). The mediating role of power distance and face-saving on nurses' fear of medication error reporting: A cross-sectional survey. *International Journal of Nursing Studies, 105*, 103494. yhttps://doi.org/10.1016/j.ijnurstu.2019.103494

Module 51
Safety

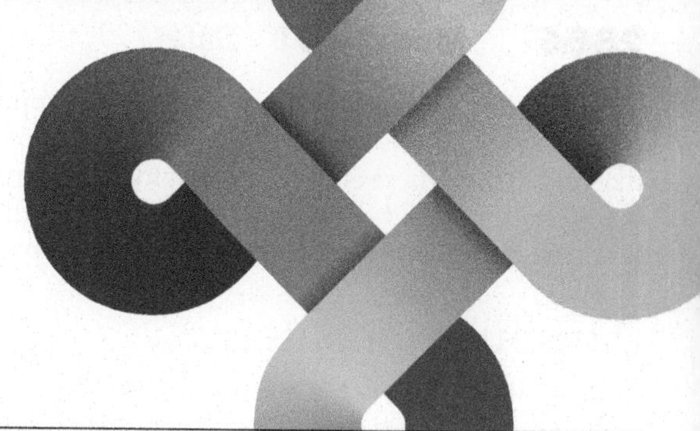

Module Outline and Learning Outcomes

The Concept of Safety

Attributes of Safety

51.1 Analyze the attributes of safety.

Alterations to Safety

51.2 Differentiate common alterations of safety.

Concepts Related to Safety

51.3 Summarize the relationship between safety and other concepts.

Health Promotion

51.4 Explain the promotion of health safety.

Nursing Assessment

51.5 Differentiate common assessment data used to examine safety.

Independent Interventions

51.6 Explain independent interventions that can be implemented for the patient's safety.

Collaborative Efforts

51.7 Summarize collaborative efforts used by interprofessional teams and patients for safety in healthcare settings.

Safety Exemplars

Exemplar 51.A Health Promotion and Injury Prevention Across the Lifespan

51.A Analyze health promotion and injury prevention across the lifespan as they relate to safety.

Exemplar 51.B Patient Safety

51.B Analyze safety as it relates to patients in home care and healthcare settings.

Exemplar 51.C Nurse Safety

51.C Analyze safety as it relates to being a nurse.

Exemplar 51.D Medication Safety

51.D Analyze safety of management and administration of medications across the lifespan.

» The Concept of Safety

Concept Key Terms

Attributes of safety, **2864**
National Patient Safety Goals (NPSGs), **2871**
Never event, **2864**
Quality, **2864**
Quality and Safety Education for Nurses (QSEN), **2871**
Safety, **2864**
Safety culture, **2868**
Standard precautions, **2868**

How important is the quality of safety in healthcare settings? Is it only essential in an acute healthcare facility? Or extended healthcare facility? What about healthcare at a community setting? Or in a patient's home? When quality and safety are not priorities in healthcare settings, safety records reflect increases in accidents, errors, injuries, and infections. Statistics about patients in healthcare settings reflect that every year, one in 25 patients acquires a healthcare-associated infection; a patient on Medicare has a one in four chance of experiencing harm, injury, or death when admitted to a hospital; and as many as 440,000 patients die every year as a result of preventable hospital errors (Hospital Safety Score, 2019). Many of these adverse occurrences could have been prevented.

Is safety limited to patients, or does it also include the healthcare workforce? It is a safety issue when the patient is left in a tightly tied wrist restraint throughout the night shift without being checked and complains of tingling and numbness below the restraint. But what about the patient with congestive heart failure who is on a salt-free diet but who is being given packs of salt from staff? Don't accidents just happen sometimes? As in the example of an elderly patient who was told not to get out of bed without help, but who does, and then trips over a towel left on the floor, falls, and fractures a hip. Or the nurse in a hurry who forgets to perform hand hygiene after changing a patient's IV dressing and before moving to the next patient who needs a Foley catheter inserted. What about chemical exposure, attacks of violence, needlesticks, and musculoskeletal injuries nurses may receive? Who is responsible to be alert for safety hazards like these, and where is the safety net to avoid errors, prevent infections, and stop accidents? Are they all from faulty systems or conditions, or are people a part of the problem, too?

Attributes of Safety

Unsafe situations related to the quality of safety can occur in healthcare facilities, homes of patients, and community settings. **Safety** refers to decreasing risks of dangers or hazards to prevent actual or potential bodily harm. **Quality** measures the care provided to promote best outcomes within the management of healthcare systems (Agency for Healthcare Research and Quality [AHRQ], 2020a). It requires everyone in a healthcare facility to engage in safe behaviors and be aware of surroundings to protect against unsafe situations and prevent safety hazards.

Attributes of safety are the qualities or properties of remaining safe. They are the precautions individuals take to be safe and prevent adverse occurrences. Examples of attributes or precautions healthcare facilities can implement to improve quality and safety include the following (Occupational Safety and Health Administration [OSHA], 2020b):

1. Schedule and analyze hazard surveys and safety/health inspections in all areas.
2. Implement an effective hazard reporting system available to employees.
3. Investigate all safety incidents for root causes.
4. Keep safety, health rules, and work practices readily available.
5. Have applicable OSHA-mandated safety programs in place.
6. Make sure personal protective equipment is being used effectively.
7. Confirm the facility has disaster plans for internal and external emergency situations.
8. Provide safety and health training for all levels of employees at least annually.

Active partnership between healthcare staff and patients is an effective way to maximize the quality of safety and minimize risks of hazards and errors resulting in accidents and injuries. Everyone positively or negatively impacts safety and quality in the healthcare environment, including patients. Nurses need to encourage patients to:

- Be assertive to actively speak up and ask questions about medications, therapies, tests, and procedures to know the "what" and "why" of these and anticipated results.
- Be knowledgeable about their condition or illness and be aware of how to prevent complications while in a healthcare facility.
- Have a support person to assist in these areas and be vigilant about the safety of care for the patient.
- Practice safe behaviors such as washing hands appropriately, asking for help when needed, eating appropriate foods on their prescribed diet, and reporting any mistakes noticed to the nurse or another staff member.

Healthcare employees need to be competent in and willing to use a range of safety skills. They also need to have the ability to identify safety hazards, take responsibility for correcting them, and be part of the solution to prevent them from happening again. Quality improvement and risk management of health services within healthcare concentrate on identifying and making changes to improve quality and safety for everyone (see Module 50, Quality Improvement, for more information).

Alterations to Safety

Nurses play a major role in ensuring patient safety, but even still, sometimes adverse events happen, assessments may be incomplete, or a step or two during a procedure may be skipped. Even unintentional mistakes may result in longer hospital stays, accidents, injuries, infections, functional decline, or death. **Figure 51.1** ›› illustrates how sometimes decisions made may seem to make sense at the time, but later can negatively impact patient safety.

In some cases, catastrophic adverse events serve as motivators for prevention, spurring healthcare facilities, advocacy organizations, and even families to act to try to prevent tragic events from happening to others. Small safety initiatives may grow into national initiatives using public service announcements, social media, and other forms of media communication. This can help build awareness of how routine procedures can quickly become life-threatening safety hazards within healthcare facilities. The Patient Safety Movement, for example, promotes patient safety and quality of care to help prevent healthcare-associated deaths, as well as **never events**, which are preventable hazards that can result in injury or death and that should never happen to patients. A checklist may give information about a given topic, such as pressure injuries or falls, what to do to avoid complications, how to notice something is wrong, how to talk with the healthcare provider (HCP), when to notify a nurse for help, and how to ask appropriate questions. See Module 50, Quality Improvement for a discussion of sentinel events.

›› **Stay Current:** Visit the website of the Patient Safety Movement to see the patient safety checklists at https://patientsafetymovement.org.

Another national initiative from the Centers for Disease Control and Prevention (CDC) and the Safe Injection Practices Coalition began after an investigation was completed on multiple cases of hepatitis exposure. Evidence showed that the problem stemmed from basic infection control inconsistencies involving the unsafe medication administration practice of reusing syringes, which caused contamination of medication vials used on subsequent patients. The coalition developed an initiative called *One Needle, One Syringe at One Time,* whose goal is to eliminate adverse events resulting from unsafe injection practices. Since its inception, this initiative has notified nearly 200,000 patients of potential exposure to hepatitis or HIV related to unsafe medication administration (CDC, 2019e).

›› **Stay Current:** Visit the One and Only website at https://www.cdc.gov/injectionsafety/one-and-only.html to learn more about this campaign.

Healthcare facilities can maintain quality and safety to help decrease hazards, accidents, and adverse events by combining the efforts of three groups: the healthcare organization, its employees, and the patients.

Three Nurses Making Decisions about a Patient's Safety

First: Read about Tammy, our patient.

Tammy Odom is a 6-year-old patient with a history of bronchial asthma. Tammy is 40 inches tall, weighs 42 pounds, and is allergic to peanuts. She was admitted through the emergency department at 0200 this morning with acute exacerbation/bronchitis. Tammy's mother, Mrs. Odom, told the nurse that Tammy had a cold a few days ago. She also said that Tammy had been at her friend's house spending the night. At approximately 1900, the friend's mother called her and told her that Tammy had to use her rescue inhaler and still was having a hard time breathing. At that time, she found out the friend's father smokes in the house. Mrs. Odom said the recent drop in temperature may also have contributed to Tammy's breathing problems and reported that Tammy is allergic to peanuts and shellfish.

The nurse making rounds before breakfast notes the following assessment data: temperature 99.2°F (o), pulse 112, respirations 26, blood pressure 112/52, O_2 saturation 95% on room air, minimal wheezing bilateral lower lobes, no retractions or use of accessory muscles for respirations, and speaking in whole sentences. Tammy tells the nurse about the bag of candy her friend gave her the night before. When looking at the candy, the nurse notes some peanut butter cups and explains to Tammy she should not eat them because of her allergy to peanuts. Tammy says she is saving those for her mother who likes them, but that she has not eaten any of them. The nurse notes an empty wrapper in the candy bag. An unlicensed assistive personnel (UAP) is assigned to help Tammy and her mother as needed.

Answer the following questions:

1. What else do you want to assess about Tammy's situation and physical condition?
2. What do you suspect as the trigger of her asthma exacerbation? Why?
3. What is your priority intervention at this time?

Second: Read about nurses A, B, and C.

Nurse A

The nurse thinks Tammy looks better now, safe in the hospital, so she thinks about her other patients that need her help.

The nurse tells Tammy's mother to call her if Tammy needs anything.

Nurse B

The nurse thinks Tammy ate a peanut butter cup causing her asthma problem, so she takes the bag of candy away so she won't eat any more of them.

The nurse thinks Tammy is safe now and just needs to rest, so busies herself caring for her other patients.

Nurses A and B

Throughout the morning, Tammy had episodes of increased wheezing, dyspnea, and respirations, lasting about 10 minutes each time. She is having more distress, speaking in broken sentences, and working harder to breathe with increased wheezing in all lung fields in the afternoon. Vital signs are temperature 99.6 (o), pulse 118, respirations 34, blood pressure 118/62, and O_2 saturation 92% room air. While Tammy is trying to play a game with the UAP, her dyspnea worsens and her mother puts the call light on for help.

Nurse A: The nurse walks in the room, and quickly notices the respiratory distress Tammy is having. She tells Tammy's mother she was sorry but thought Tammy was better because she hadn't heard from her. She tells Tammy's mother she needs to call the physician and leaves the room.

Nurse B: When the nurse finally gets to Tammy's room about 15 minutes later, she can't understand what happened and becomes very anxious because she thought she had taken care of the problem when she took the bag of candy away. She calls for help, raises the HOB, starts Tammy on oxygen, and has someone call the physician.

Nurse C

The nurse thinks about what might be triggering Tammy's asthma and discusses this with her mother—her recent cold, the change in weather, the smoker's home, the peanut butter cups.

The nurse plans to keep close check on Tammy and asks other team members caring for her to keep an eye on her also.

While checking on Tammy at 1000, the UAP was cleaning up Tammy's bedside table. The nurse observed Tammy was having trouble breathing and coughing. She heard Tammy tell the UAP that she smelled funny. The nurse smelled the UAP and smelled tobacco smoke on the clothing. She pulled the UAP outside the door and discovered the UAP was a smoker. The nurse determined every time the UAP had gone into Tammy's room during the morning, it was triggering Tammy's asthma and she would begin having more breathing difficulty. The UAP was unaware that the smoke smell would cause Tammy a breathing problem. The nurse immediately reassigned this UAP to another patient and had a nonsmoker UAP assigned to Tammy. Within an hour Tammy was breathing in a more relaxed way and resting comfortably with minimal wheezing heard.

Answer the following questions:

4. At what point do you consider Tammy safe from respiratory distress from her asthma? Explain.
5. What was the faulty thinking from Nurse A? Nurse B?
6. Nurse C used reasoning based on significant cues to make a clinical judgment about what was triggering Tammy's respiratory distress. Can you follow her critical thinking process?
7. What should Nurse C say to the UAP with smoke in her clothing?
8. Can you identify eight mistakes in thinking or lack of knowledge in this scenario? How would they have been avoided?
9. What were the consequences for Tammy due to decisions by Nurse A and Nurse B?
10. What were the benefits for Tammy due to decisions by Nurse C?

Figure 51.1 ›› Three nurses making decisions about a patient's safety. This is a scenario looking at perspectives of three different nurses based on decisions they make about the same situation. Follow the directions and answer the questions.

1. Organizational support for promoting a safety culture encourages all employees to intentionally and actively make safe choices in what they do and how they do it as they keep a mindset for quality and safe practices for patients and others. Consumers of healthcare are encouraged to consider safety when selecting a healthcare facility for procedures, surgeries, and hospitalizations, which can serve as an incentive for healthcare facilities to make safety more of a priority.
2. Involvement by healthcare employees to consistently follow and promote health safety rules and standards for the environment and patient care and to be safety advocates for others. Healthcare employees are essential to maintaining the safe environment and care within a facility.
3. Encouraging patients to engage in every aspect of their care throughout their course of stay. They need to ask questions about the quality and safety of procedures performed, medications administered, or other care provided to them.

>> **Stay Current:** Visit http://www.hospitalsafetyscore.org/what-is-patient- for an example of 28 measures to find the safety score of your local hospital.

Concepts Related to Safety

Every area of nursing is related to safety. Many nursing actions, such as hand hygiene and patient identification validation, promote well-being and safety for patients and others. As partners in their own plans of care, patients can participate in safety behaviors such as infection control, fall precautions, and accident prevention. Nurses also ensure their own safety by following policies and procedures, by engaging in therapeutic communication that promotes patient self-esteem and reduces patient anxiety, and by using critical thinking to prioritize patient care. The Concepts Related to Safety feature links some, but not all, of the concepts integral to safety. They are presented in alphabetical order.

Health Promotion

In the United States, there is a collaborative effort of several federal agencies to improve the nation's health. Workplace promotion programs are offered to employees at many companies and organizations that include wellness programs about nutrition, smoking cessation, stress management, and safety. Individuals can select from a variety of wellness, exercise, weight management, and stress management programs available to meet their own needs. Strategies for promoting health across the lifespan are discussed in Exemplar 51.A.

>> **Stay Current:** Follow individual state laws on child passenger safety seats for infants and children at http://www.ghsa.org/html/stateinfo/laws/childsafety_laws.html.

Nursing Assessment

Patients admitted to healthcare facilities initially undergo a comprehensive nursing assessment, including observation, an interview, and a physical examination. As a proactive measure, this initial assessment includes specific age-appropriate questions and observations that focus on safety needs. Each healthcare setting has its own safety checklists based on recommendations of healthcare organizations such as The Joint Commission. Risk-based assessment data help to identify patients who may require special precautions to prevent harm and minimize consequences from debilitation or exacerbation of a preexisting risk while in healthcare settings. This assessment process can further be divided into three levels of safety risk based on patient responses: low, medium, or high.

Observation and Patient Interview

During initial interviews with patients, nurses may use checklists to quickly identify physical, psychologic, and emotional areas to further explore for potential safety issues or health promotion needs. For example, if the patient is asked, "Have you ever noticed blood in your stool?" and the patient responds, "Yes," the nurse should then explore this with the patient. If the patient responds, "Yes, sometimes" to the question, "Have you ever thought about hurting yourself?" the nurse takes this seriously and assesses the patient's current risk for suicide or self-harm.

In addition to gathering assessment data through the interview, nurses are constantly observing patients for age-appropriate assessment data such as communication and speech patterns, mobility, eye contact, general appearance, balance, and other cues. Information relevant to risk for safety includes data related to:

- Ability to communicate
- Ability to provide self-care
- Cognitive or memory impairments; visual or other sensory deficits
- Bowel and bladder elimination and control
- Susceptibility to falls or any other safety risks
- Mobility impairments; use of assistive devices
- Presence of Foley catheter, PEG tube, colostomy, or tracheostomy
- Skin integrity
- Nutritional status.

Teaching patients measures to reduce their vulnerability for safety issues in a healthcare facility, community setting (such as at school), or home can help keep patients engaged in their nursing plan of care. See the feature Patient Teaching: Patient Practices That Promote Safety in Healthcare Settings.

Physical Examination

Nurses are continuously observing patients, monitoring for unsafe changes in conditions, and making decisions about appropriate responses. For example, a nurse walks into a patient's room and assesses a patient with diabetes. The patient is confused, agitated, and has a respiratory rate of 28 with a sweet odor to the breath. The nurse notices several candy wrappers on the bedside table. Based on this assessment data, the nurse quickly performs a blood glucose reading using a glucometer, which indicates a blood glucose level of 308 after two checks. The patient has changed from a safe blood glucose level to an unsafe increased level outside of normal range for this patient. Intervention is required.

Concepts Related to Safety

CONCEPT	RELATIONSHIP TO SAFETY	NURSING IMPLICATIONS
Accountability	■ Unsafe nursing practice, behaviors, and thinking could cause harm to patients and others, and if not addressed, will continue to occur.	■ Unsafe nursing practice should be reported and addressed. ■ Competency in providing quality safe nursing care develops when following standards of care.
Advocacy	■ Vulnerable populations may unintentionally make unsafe decisions about their healthcare. ■ Sometimes unethical, immoral, or illegal actions result in unsafe treatments and behaviors by professionals.	■ Nurses can support patients in making safe appropriate decisions by providing accurate and complete information using patients' primary language to help them understand the decision to be made. ■ Nurses can uphold the rights of patients, including the right to have quality safe treatment in a safe environment.
Assessment	■ Data are used to monitor for changes in conditions of patients. ■ Data can show numerical values indicating safe or unsafe parameters for patients' body systems.	■ Nurses continuously collect assessment data, interpret it, and intervene as appropriate for quality and safety of patient care. ■ Data can change, and nurses need to monitor these changes to help prevent unsafe physical, emotional, or psychologic conditions for patients.
Clinical Decision Making	■ Nurses consider safety (both the patient's safety and the safety of other healthcare workers) in all phases of the nursing process and while prioritizing patient needs.	■ Assess patients for safety risks, factors that impact risks for falls, and ability to perform activities of daily living (ADLs) such as vision, hearing, mobility, and balance, and risk for or presence of abuse or neglect. ■ Provide patient teaching regarding safety measures as appropriate based on assessment and evaluation of interventions.
Evidence-Based Practice	■ Evidence supports that many errors occurring in the healthcare setting can be avoided with improved performance of healthcare workers. ■ Evidence supports that everyone in the healthcare environment, including patients, can improve quality and safety.	■ Nurses can form partnerships with patients to work together for quality and safety of care. ■ Evidence provides best practices for safety in nursing interventions. ■ Improvements in quality and safety of patient-centered care contribute to best patient outcomes.
Quality Improvement	■ Improving quality of care for all patients involves ensuring and considering the safety of patients at all times when providing nursing care.	■ Ensure a high quality of care in all interactions with patients. ■ Resolve any safety concerns in the patient's immediate bed area. ■ Ensure that the correct patient is receiving the correct type and amount of medication. ■ Follow safety and procedural guidelines for patient care.

Patient Teaching

Patient Practices That Promote Safety in Healthcare Settings

Patients are at a higher risk for acquiring a healthcare-associated infection or injury because of the quality of safety in some healthcare settings. By following the steps below, patients can help make healthcare safer and help prevent healthcare-associated infections and injuries.

1. Keep your hands clean and use frequent hand hygiene to remove microorganisms.
2. Only take antibiotics prescribed by your HCP.
3. Receive age-related vaccinations to avoid infections such as influenza and pneumonia.
4. Report any signs or symptoms of infection to your HCP within a short time.
5. Remind healthcare personnel, family, and visitors to clean their hands before touching you or preparing meals for you.
6. Let your HCP know if you have recently had an infection.
7. Healthcare personnel may need to wear special gowns and gloves when providing your care.
8. When housekeeping employees want to clean your hospital room, let them.
9. If having surgery, ask your HCP how to help avoid postsurgery infections.
10. Your HCP may order lab tests if you have been exposed to pathogens.

Source: From Centers for Disease Control and Prevention (2019d).

There are four acute changes in condition that nurses must investigate to determine appropriate interventions and urgency in responding to them:

- ***Cognitive changes***, such as decreased level of consciousness, change in memory, change in mood, difficulty thinking, and acute confusion.
- ***Physical changes***, such as changes in vital signs, change in oxygen saturation, change in skin color, change in appearance of an incision, onset of diaphoresis, seizure activity, and an onset of pain.
- ***Functional changes***, such as respiratory distress, change in mobility, onset of slurred speech, weakness of an extremity, numbness of an extremity, and acute function deficit.
- ***Behavioral changes***, such as inappropriate movements, disorientation to time and place, hallucinating, depression, and wandering (AHRQ, 2018).

For example, changes in sputum color from clear to yellow, consistency from watery to tenacious, and amount from small to copious will influence the quality and safety of the patient's airway, so intervention is needed. Another example would be the older adult who develops acute slurring of speech, inability to move an arm, drooling, and inability to talk coherently and has facial drooping on one side of the face, indicating a neurologic situation that needs immediate intervention for the safety of the patient.

Independent Interventions

Everyone, including healthcare workers, patients, families, and visitors, must assertively perform safety behaviors to prevent injuries, accidents, infections, and errors in all healthcare environments. In all settings, policies and procedures such as standard precautions assist nurses and other HCPs in ensuring the safety of the environment. The COVID-19 pandemic reinforced both the evidence and need for frequent hand hygiene (see Evidence-Based Practice: Effective Hand Hygiene as a Defense Against Infectious Disease).

Standard Precautions

Standard precautions incorporate those guidelines previously referred to as universal precautions and body substance isolation (BSI). Standard precautions include measures such as the use of proper hand hygiene, protective equipment, and safe injection practices and the effective management of potentially contaminated surfaces or equipment. The transfer of infectious agents between nurses and patients is a serious safety concern to be addressed (see Module 9, Infection, for further information).

Latex Exposure

Latex precautions are of particular importance to nurses because products containing latex are common in the healthcare industry. Latex gloves, blood pressure cuffs, IV tubes, bandages, syringes, and catheters are among some of the common devices found in medical settings that can contain latex. Exposure to latex can trigger a latex allergy, which can become a serious problem for nurses, patients, and others. Symptoms may begin as itching, burning, redness, and swelling of the hands and fingers when latex gloves are worn or contact with other latex equipment or supplies occurs. Symptoms may become more severe, leading to asthma or anaphylaxis. Over a period of time, exposure to latex can develop into occupational asthma (American Academy of Allergy, Asthma & Immunology, 2020).

A number of precautions can be employed to avoid latex exposure for both healthcare workers and patients. Hypoallergenic (and specifically latex-free) and powderless gloves are helpful in preventing exposure. Not all hypoallergenic gloves are latex-free, so this should be ensured if an allergy or sensitivity is indicated. The powder from gloves can absorb the latex and then spread it when the gloves are removed; this can then release the allergen into the air, potentially affecting those with a severe sensitivity. Hand hygiene after taking off gloves is extremely important in preventing exposure to others.

Chemical Exposure

Exposure to hazardous and toxic substances is of paramount concern in the healthcare environment. Many chemicals found in this setting can be dangerous, including cleaning supplies, disinfectants, paints, and certain forms of air pollutants. To reduce hazardous exposures, healthcare facilities are using safer alternatives that are now available. Product solutions can not only be safe in the work environment, but also support a safer environment. One method to reduce environmental hazards for hospitals is by "going green," to dispose of medical waste in an environmentally friendly way following regulations developed by OSHA. Many hospitals are currently taking steps to reduce medical waste and energy consumption (Becker's Hospital Review, 2018).

>> **Stay Current:** For more information on hospitals going green, visit http://www.healthcarebusinesstech.com/going-green-hospital/.

Collaborative Efforts

Many local organizations in addition to international, federal, and state agencies collaborate to support quality health, safety, and cost-efficiency initiatives in healthcare. Collaborative community initiatives may be started by community members in response to a serious, community-wide health issue. They may start through state-funded or federally funded initiatives that begin in response to larger statewide or nationally recognized health issues and that provide funding at the community level to address these issues. Although national healthcare safety initiatives vary in approach, in general they support collaboration of government agencies, healthcare facilities, and people who work in healthcare to have safe, healthy work environments and to provide patients safe quality care for best patient outcomes. **Table 51.1** >> lists a number of current safety initiatives.

Safety Culture

Even with safety initiatives in place, injuries, accidents, and errors can still happen in healthcare facilities, homes, and communities. Initiatives, policies, and mandates need to include the "people factor" to be successful. Everyone in healthcare wants to have a safe and healthy environment, and it takes everyone to make it happen by creating a culture of safety. A **safety culture** is a general feeling of shared

Evidence-Based Practice

Effective Hand Hygiene as a Defense Against Infectious Disease

Background

The World Health Organization (WHO) works with countries around the world when an infectious disease has been identified or a new pathogen has been discovered. An infectious disease can progress quickly from a localized outbreak, to an epidemic, and finally to a worldwide pandemic, threatening the lives and health of large numbers of people. To stop infectious disease from spreading, the first recommended prevention step by the WHO is effective handwashing. The Centers for Disease Control and Prevention (CDC) considers hand hygiene as the most efficient and cost-effective way to limit disease dissemination. In one research project, researchers focused on the global transmission of respiratory viruses during air travel and in airports. Using epidemiological modeling and simulations, researchers concluded that hand hygiene inside airports could potentially inhibit a pandemic by 24 to 69% (Cohut, 2020; Nicolaides et al., 2020).

Problem

Over the past 100 years, the United States has been one of many countries affected by periodic worldwide viral infectious disease outbreaks, epidemics, and pandemics from novel influenza viruses and novel coronaviruses such as:

- Spanish influenza (H1N1), 1918 pandemic
- Asian flu (Influenza A, H2N2), 1956 pandemic
- Hong Kong flu (Influenza A, H3N2), 1968 pandemic
- Severe acute respiratory syndrome (SARS), 2003 epidemic
- Zika virus, 2014 epidemic
- Ebola virus, 2014 outbreak
- Novel coronavirus (COVID-19), declared a pandemic by the World Health Organization in 2020

The emergence of any new infectious disease prompts research on etiology, prevention, mitigation, treatment, and response. Across decades, countries, and diseases, one evidence-based practice continues to be essential to reducing disease transmission: *hand hygiene*. Correctly done, hand hygiene remains an essential, cost-effective safety practice in the prevention and control of infectious diseases spread through person-to-person transmission (**Figure 51.2** »).

Many materials and tools developed by the WHO were used in the response and recovery of the areas involved in these outbreaks and pandemics. The WHO works with public health agencies and governments around the world to ensure essential information on disease prevention, including the value of hand hygiene, is made available in numerous languages and formats.

The CDC uses a scientific approach to protect the United States from infectious disease threats through research and evidence-based prevention and control policies and programs. Data are collected by monitoring, assessing, and surveillance in support of the country's preparedness and response capacity. In 2020, the CDC developed two national handwashing campaigns called *Clean Hands Save Lives* and *Life is Better with Clean Hands* to reduce the spread of infectious respiratory illness, promote healthiness, and raise awareness about the importance of hand hygiene. The campaigns focused on the five steps people should take to effectively wash their hands and how to use an alcohol-based hand sanitizer containing at least 60% alcohol. Campaign materials included videos, posters, and public service announcements.

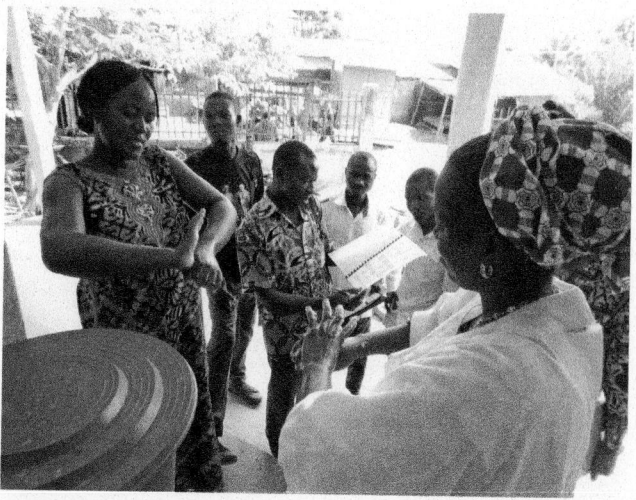

Figure 51.2 » Hand hygiene plays an important role in controlling the spread of infectious diseases. People have to be taught proper hand hygiene techniques to help them prevent contracting an infectious disease.

Source: Centers for Disease Control and Prevention (2020a).

Implications

- Nurses in all settings can help reduce the spread of any infectious illness by teaching and modeling good hand hygiene.
- Effective handwashing continues to be an important evidence-based standard transmission-based precaution to prevent transmission of infectious disease, along with:
  - Maintaining social distancing
  - Not touching the eyes, nose, and mouth
  - Covering the mouth and nose or using tissues when coughing or sneezing

Critical Thinking Application

1. To reinforce the importance of hand hygiene to others, what can nurses do?
2. How can hand hygiene compliance affect the number of healthcare-associated infections that occur? Who needs to participate in this safety prevention behavior?

Sources: Centers for Disease Control and Prevention (2020a, 2020c); Cohut (2020); MPHonline (2020); Nicolaides et al., 2020; World Health Organization (2020a, 2020b).

attitudes, values, practices, and beliefs that result in behaviors and feelings of responsibility for safety in all daily routines (AHRQ, 2019a). Safety awareness is heightened throughout all areas.

Organizations and employees working together can build and maintain a safety culture, resulting in improved safety and quality of care for patients and fewer unsafe and unhealthy conditions for themselves. This means anyone can

TABLE 51.1 Safety Initiatives

Organization	Intent	Contributions
Agency for Healthcare Research and Quality, U.S. Department of Health and Human Services	Produce evidence that supports healthcare safety, make it more available, cost-effective, equitable, and higher quality while reducing medical errors and improving patient safety.	■ *Patient Safety Primer, Patient Safety 101* (2019c), https://psnet.ahrq.gov/primer/patient-safety-101 ■ For other AHRQ publications and products, go to http://www.ahrq.gov/research/publications/index.html
Centers for Disease Control and Prevention	Engages in health research, surveillance, promotion, and response to promote and increase the health security of the United States.	■ A list of some of the CDC's numerous national health and safety initiatives, strategies, and plans of action that provide leadership to public health efforts across the United States can be found on their website at https://www.cdc.gov/publichealthgateway/strategy/index.html
National Institute of Medicine (NAM)	Provides reliable evidence to the government and the private sector to support informed health decisions about assessment and improvement of healthcare systems and policies.	■ *To Err Is Human: The Next 20 Years* (2019), https://www.jointcommission.org/en/resources/news-and-multimedia/blogs/high-reliability-healthcare/2019/11/to-err-is-human-the-next-20-years/ ■ *Crossing the Quality Chasm: A New Health System for the 21st Century* (2001) ■ *Keeping Patients Safe: Transforming the Work Environment of Nurses* (2004) ■ *Envisioning the Future of Health Professional Education* (2015), http://www.nationalacademies.org/hmd/Global/News%20Announcements/Crossing-the-Quality-Chasm-The-IOM-Health-Care-Quality-Initiative.aspx ■ For more IOM studies and activities, go to http://www.nationalacademies.org/hmd/
The Joint Commission	Promotes quality and safety through accreditation and certification of healthcare facilities representing high quality, safety, and value for patients.	■ *National Patient Safety Goals* (2020a), https://www.hfmmagazine.com/articles/3821-joint-commission-releases-2020-national-patient-safety-goals ■ SpeakUp initiative (2020b), https://www.griffinhealth.org/griffin-hospital/patient-safety/speak-up-initiative
National Institute for Occupational Safety and Health (NIOSH)	A federal agency that provides evidence-supported recommendations on the prevention of worker injuries and illnesses to preserve human resources.	■ Develops and enforces workplace safety and health regulations https://www.cdc.gov/niosh/about/default.html ■ Provides multiple training programs and educational publications/products https://www.cdc.gov/niosh/pubs/default.html
Occupational Safety and Health Administration, U.S. Department of Labor	A national public health regulatory agency that protects workers against safety and health hazards in the work environment by enforcing compliance with health and safety standards.	■ Occupational Safety and Health Act (OSH Act; 1970), https://www.epa.gov/laws-regulations/summary-occupational-safety-and-health-act ■ Enforcement inspections https://www.osha.gov/OshDoc/data_General_Facts/factsheet-inspections.pdf ■ Worker, environmental, and nuclear safety laws enforced https://www.osha.gov/Publications/3439at-a-glance.pdf ■ Worker's rights laws https://www.osha.gov/workers/
Quality and Safety Education for Nurses (QSEN)	Designed to prepare nursing students with knowledge, skills, and attitudes (KSAs) needed to improve quality and safety of patient care using systems thinking.	■ QSEN Competencies https://qsen.org/competencies/ ■ KSAs for undergraduate prelicensure nursing programs http://qsen.org/competencies/pre-licensure-ksas/ ■ KSAs for graduate education nursing programs http://qsen.org/competencies/graduate-ksas/
World Health Organization	International authority to direct and coordinate health within the United Nations' system.	■ International preparedness, surveillance, and response to health emergencies threatening human health security https://www.who.int/activities/rapidly-detecting-and-responding-to-health-emergencies ■ Multiple WHO patient safety training programs and activities http://www.who.int/patientsafety/education/en/

report unsafe conditions or behaviors and help find solutions to correct them.

A safety culture is a blame-free environment. With a focus on systems, individuals can report errors or near misses without fearing reprimand or punishment. Some healthcare facilities have created a *just culture* that looks not only at systems but also at how they may have contributed to an individual's unsafe action (see Module 50, Quality Improvement, for further information). Everyone in a healthcare safety culture is aware of the importance of their work and is determined to consistently do their work correctly and safely. Everyone is involved with the planning, implementation, and evaluation of initiatives for safety and health concerns, actively working together to find methods for quality improvement.

Some things healthcare facilities can do to support safety initiatives are to:

1. Make necessary resources available
2. Include all levels of employees in decision making about safety initiatives
3. Celebrate improvements when quality programs are implemented
4. Conduct management walk-arounds to support staff
5. Offer periodic safety training
6. Share successes in improved patient outcomes and safety goals attained.

Benefits of creating a safety culture include improved job satisfaction for staff, fewer safety and health hazards that

TABLE 51.2 QSEN Nursing Competencies

QSEN Competency	Definition
Patient-Centered Care	Blends patient, family, and community in patient care decisions. Values, preferences, beliefs, and culture are taken into consideration during the patient's care.
Quality Improvement	Participates in root cause analysis of sentinel adverse events to identify what can be learned from them that can be used in future similar situations to improve quality, safety, and outcomes.
Evidence-Based Practice	Combines evidence from research, clinical expertise and experience, and patient/family preferences and values for best patient-centered interventions and care.
Teamwork and Collaboration	Because treatment sometimes involves multiple departments and 24-hour care, intra- and interprofessional teamwork and collaboration during shifts is necessary for optimal care.
Informatics	Stay current in technology knowledge and skills needed to support quality of patient care and maintain the safety of patient information.
Safety	Activities such as knowledge sharing and error reporting are used to create a culture of safety.

Source: Based on QSEN Institute. (2020). QSEN Competencies. Retrieved from https://qsen.org/competencies/.

affect both patients and employees, and a decrease in injuries, accidents, illnesses, and errors.

Quality and Safety Education for Nurses

In 2005, the Robert Wood Johnson Foundation funded a group of distinguished nursing leaders and faculty to use the Institute of Medicine's healthcare clinician competencies from the *Crossing the Quality Chasm: A New Health System for the 21st Century* report. These nursing competencies, called **Quality and Safety Education for Nurses (QSEN)**, help prepare nursing students with practical experience in providing safer, more effective care. They are further defined with the specific knowledge, skills, and attitudes (KSAs) necessary to provide better quality and safety in healthcare settings (see **Table 51.2** »).

National Patient Safety Goals

The Joint Commission began its **National Patient Safety Goals (NPSG)** program in 2002 to help accredited organizations deal with specific topics on patient safety. NPSGs are developed and revised with input from healthcare professionals, providers, consumers, subject-matter experts, risk managers, engineers, and government agencies such as the Centers for Medicare & Medicaid Services. Goals are determined by analyzing safety and quality concerns and evaluating which ones will have the maximum impact and usefulness in providing safe and quality care for the minimum cost. NPSGs are updated annually. Each goal is accompanied by elements of performance that The Joint Commission identifies as necessary to meet the goal. For example, among the NPSGs required for hospital accreditation in 2020 is the *goal* that agencies identify patients correctly, which is accompanied by two *elements of performance*, which relate to (1) consistently using two methods of identifying the patient and (2) ensuring that patients receiving blood transfusions are correctly identified prior to transfusion.

» **Stay Current:** For the most current National Patient Safety Goals, go to the website of The Joint Commission at https://www.jointcommission.org/standards/national-patient-safety-goals/.

REVIEW The Concept of Safety

RELATE Link the Concepts

Linking the concept of safety with the concept of tissue integrity:

1. Describe safety precautions that can be taken to prevent skin breakdown.
2. The nurse is caring for a patient with third-degree burns over 50% of their body. Identify three nursing interventions that promote safety while also facilitating the patient's healing and providing comfort.

Linking the concept of safety with the concept of ethics:

3. Explain the ethical considerations in a scenario in which a patient has been given the wrong medication, but with no adverse effects. Discuss the patient's right to be informed about the mistake. How should the nurse who committed the error handle this situation?
4. A surgeon nearly performed the wrong surgery on a patient, but the mistake was caught before a surgical incision was made. The correct surgery was performed, but the surgeon has not reported the original error. Does this scenario require submitting a report? Describe the dilemma faced by the surgical team in this scenario.

Linking the concept of safety with the concept of oxygenation:

5. What are some teaching points the nurse should discuss with a patient with chronic obstructive pulmonary disease who keeps changing their oxygen settings?
6. Describe safety considerations when beginning supplemental oxygen on a patient with asthma.

READY Go to Volume 3: Clinical Nursing Skills

REFER Go to Pearson MyLab Nursing and eText

REFLECT Apply Your Knowledge

A 72-year-old patient is admitted to the hospital for treatment of severe dehydration secondary to an advanced and untreated urinary tract infection. She is normally very independent and does not often like to ask for help, particularly when she needs to use the bathroom. The patient's nurse recognizes the patient's desire for independence, but also realizes that she is at a heightened risk for falling because of the infection and corresponding dehydration-related signs and symptoms, including weakness and dizziness. The nurse talks to the patient about the risk of falling, as well as the possible injuries that could occur if she were to fall. He does not want the patient to lose her sense of independence, so he rearranges the chairs in the room so she has a clear line from the bed to the bathroom. The nurse then discusses the need for the patient to wear socks and/or slippers with gripper bottoms when she walks to the bathroom to further prevent falling. Together the nurse and patient develop a plan of care that respects the patient's needs and also works to ensure her overall safety.

1. Describe three reasons why the patient's situation represents an advanced risk for falling.
2. Explain the nurse's approach to the situation described above. What communication and collaboration efforts does he employ?
3. Evaluate the nurse's recommendations for the patient. Are these recommendations appropriate? Why or why not?
4. Would the situation above be any different if the patient were 30 years old? If so, how? Explain your answer.

Exemplar 51.A Health Promotion and Injury Prevention Across the Lifespan

Exemplar Learning Outcomes

51.A Analyze health promotion and injury prevention across the lifespan as they relate to safety.

- Summarize the risks for injury, health promotion, and injury prevention in the prenatal period and for newborns and infants.
- Outline the risks for injury, health promotion, and injury prevention for toddlers and preschoolers.
- Contrast safety considerations in healthcare settings for school-age and adolescent patients.
- Summarize the risks for injury, health promotion, and injury prevention for young and middle-aged adults.
- Outline the risks for injury, health promotion, and injury prevention for older adults.
- Plan nursing interventions for health promotion and injury prevention for individuals with disabilities.

Exemplar Key Terms

Congenital anomaly, *2873*
Functional decline, *2878*

Overview

Health promotion includes activities that increase well-being and enhance health, such as appropriate nutrition, oral health, physical activity, and mental health. To be more effective, nurses can build partnerships with families so healthcare visits include all family members present to participate in discussions about questions or health topics they may have, support family strengths, improve communication, and work together as a team. These family-centered visits also provide opportunities for nurses to observe each family member; note family dynamics; assess nutrition, growth and development, and mental and spiritual health; and promote injury prevention strategies for everyone.

Illness prevention strategies focus mainly on the prevention of disease. Screening tests are procedures used to detect the possible presence of health conditions before symptoms are apparent. Vision and hearing screening tests are frequently conducted when children begin attending school. Most screening tests are not diagnostic by themselves but are followed by further diagnostic tests if the screening result is positive. Once a screening test identifies the existence of a health condition, intervention can begin.

Health promotion and safety needs vary across the lifespan, with parents taking care of the needs of infants and young children, school-age children and adolescents accepting more responsibility for their health, adults bearing complete responsibility for their health, and older adults often sharing responsibility with their adult children.

Safety in the Prenatal Period and for Newborns and Infants

The Prenatal Period

The prenatal or gestational period is the developmental period between conception and birth.

Early and regular prenatal care can result in having a healthy pregnancy, which promotes a healthy birth. Some women will make changes in their health routines before they become pregnant to further promote a healthy pregnancy. Examples of changes to health routines may include quitting smoking, attaining a healthy weight, or learning about familial health conditions. Genetic counseling can help people learn more about genetic health conditions and the chances of having a child with a gene-related condition.

Prenatal care can help prevent complications and provide women with information about how to protect the fetus and ensure fetal health and development. The HCP can monitor the mother's health and development of the fetus during the pregnancy. Some prenatal risks are controllable, such as cessation of smoking, drinking alcohol, or taking certain medications during pregnancy, and some are not, such as first-time pregnancy after the age of 35 or occurrence of a familial physical abnormality. Cardiovascular disease, preeclampsia, and obstetric hemorrhage also increase the risk for poor maternal peripartum (the time immediately before or just after birth) outcomes (California Maternal Quality Care Collaborative, 2020).

Fetal mortality is the intrauterine death of a fetus at any gestational age. The majority of fetal deaths occur early in pregnancy. The following risk factors for peripartum mortality have been identified: maternal obesity, smoking during pregnancy, severe hypertension or diabetes, congenital anomalies, infections, placental and cord problems, and intrauterine growth retardation (CDC, 2019a).

Prenatal care by a HCP as soon as pregnancy is determined can help increase incidence of having a healthy baby. See the exemplar on Antepartum Care in Module 33, Reproduction, for more information.

Newborns and Infants

In the United States, one in every 33 babies born is affected by congenital anomalies each year (CDC, 2019c). **Congenital anomalies** are changes in physical structure present at birth that can affect many parts of the body, such as the heart, foot, or palate. Depending on the severity and location of the anomaly, expected lifespan may or may not be affected (CDC, 2019c). Examples include congenital heart defects, Down syndrome, spina bifida, and lower-limb reduction defects. Birth weight is a good predictor of the survival and healthy development of a newborn. Newborns are screened while still in the hospital for critical congenital anomalies that are not visible, such as hearing loss, heart defects, hemoglobin disorders, hormonal insufficiency, cystic fibrosis, or inability to process certain nutrients. Types of screening and how many conditions to look for are determined by each state. See Exemplar 33.D, Newborn Care, in Module 33, Reproduction, for more information.

Congenital anomalies and short gestation continue to be common causes of mortality as the neonate, or newborn, matures into an infant. Sudden infant death syndrome is the leading cause of death among infants between ages 1 and 12 months (U.S. National Library of Medicine, 2020). Complications during delivery and unintentional injuries also can result in infant death, with the most common unintentional injuries resulting from suffocation, often as a result of co-sleeping (CDC, 2018b). See Exemplar 15.F, Unexpected Sudden Infant Death, in Module 15, Oxygenation, for more information.

Falls are the number one cause of unintentional, nonfatal injuries occurring in childhood (CDC, 2019l). Because of their immature musculoskeletal systems and relative immobility, infants are susceptible to falls; and because of their soft heads, infants are particularly susceptible to traumatic brain injury. Parents and caregivers can be instrumental in preventing falls and other accidental injuries. Nurses can assist in prevention by teaching parents to use safety devices, such as stair gates and guard rails, to help prevent falls by infants and small children learning how to move about and walk.

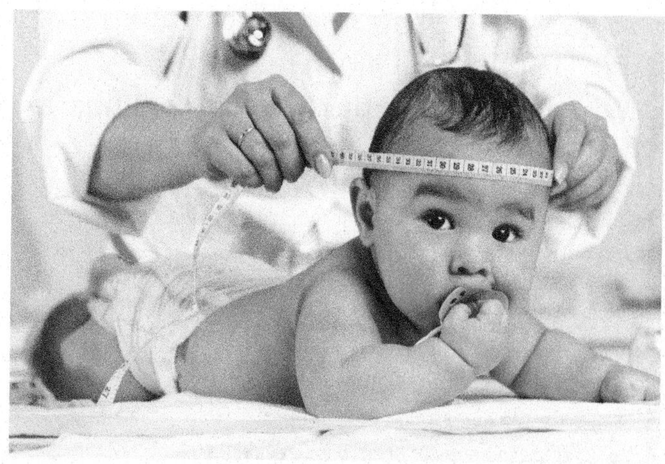

Figure 51.3 » An infant's head circumference is measured at every well-child visit.

Source: ArtMarie/iStock/Getty Images.

Nursing Implications

Newborns and infants are measured for growth and developmental trends at each visit to the HCP. Measurements of their length, weight, and head circumference can be compared with weight gain and growth percentile ranges (**Figure 51.3** »). Observing the newborn and infant for developmental milestones such as lifting the head, smiling, rolling front to back, sitting without support, playing with toys, and imitating sounds readily provides assessment data for trending as the infant grows older. First-time parents may need more teaching and demonstrations of newborn care to be comfortable and safe in caring for their new infant at home. See **Table 51.3** » for strategies for promoting infant safety. Teach parents and caregivers when to contact the infant's HCP as outlined in the Patient Teaching feature.

TABLE 51.3 Strategies for Promoting Infant Safety

Strategies for Injury Prevention	Strategies for Disease Prevention
▪ Swaddle newborns so they feel secure; allow free movement of arms and hands ▪ Position infants on the back during sleep periods; put infants to sleep in warm clothing on a firm mattress in a crib or bassinet; do not place blankets, bumpers, pillows, or toys in the crib ▪ Position infant on the abdomen during supervised play periods ▪ Encourage appropriate toys such as crib mobile, soft toys, musical toys ▪ Create an environment that is infant centered, allowing for learning, thinking, responding, and solving problems ▪ Know choking and CPR procedures for an infant	▪ Other considerations: motor-vehicle safety restraints, shaken baby syndrome, bed-sharing, drowning, suffocation, burns, falls, pet safety, fire safety, poisoning, and gun safety ▪ Avoid secondhand smoke exposure ▪ Reduce risks for sudden infant death syndrome ▪ Use proper hand hygiene before handling infant ▪ Limit exposure to large crowds, especially in cold season ▪ Begin oral care by gently wiping gums with soft gauze 1–2 times a day ▪ Vaccinate infant with routine immunizations such as hepatitis B, DTP, *Haemophilus influenzae* type b, inactivated poliovirus, pneumococcus, influenza, and rotavirus

Sources: Ball, Bindler, Cowen, and Shaw (2020); Centers for Disease Control and Prevention (2019i, 2019l); National Institute of Child Health and Human Development (2020).

Patient Teaching

When to Contact the Infant's Healthcare Provider

Encourage parents and caregivers to call the HCP any time they have a question. Teach them to call the pediatrician's office for the following situations:

- Seizure activity
- Rectal temperature of 100.4°F or above
- Change in skin color and presence of petechiae or skin rash
- Refusal to eat or drink
- Change in behavior or activity unusual for infant
- Repeated or projectile vomiting; frequent diarrhea
- Any trauma or injury; high-pitched cry for more than 1 hour
- No wet diaper for 8 hours
- Labored breathing, wheezing, or grunting

Sources: Children's Hospital of St. Louis (2020); KidsHealth (2018).

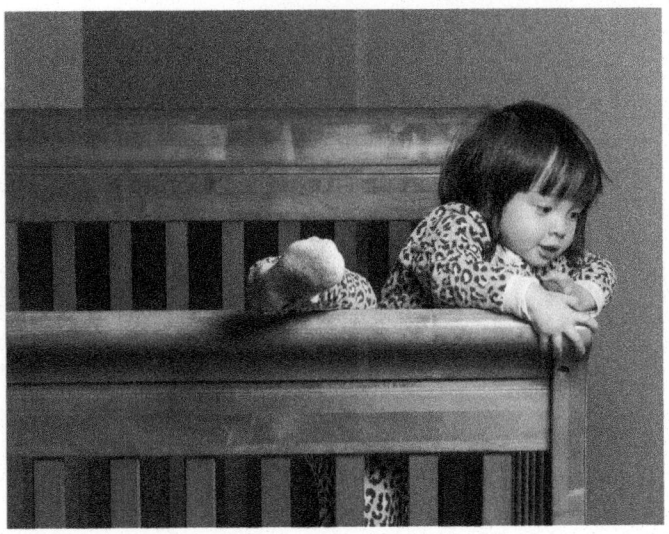

Figure 51.4 » Toddlers are vulnerable to accidents as they try new skills and explore the world.

Source: Michael Pettigrew/Shutterstock.

» **Stay Current:** The CDC provides information for current recommended immunization schedules for children age 0 through 18 years old: http://www.cdc.gov/vaccines/schedules/downloads/child/0-18yrs-child-combined-schedule.pdf.

Safety for Toddlers and Preschoolers

Among all ages of children, unintentional injuries are the leading cause of death. Risks related to unintentional injury vary by age; for example, the toddler's mobility increases their risk for drowning in a swimming pool, whereas the infant is more likely to drown in the bathtub or a bucket, and bicycle accidents are more common among school-age children. Note that the risk for ingesting chemicals or medications is highest among toddlers, preschoolers, and school-age children. Patient education for parents and caregivers of children in these age groups includes keeping all medications and chemicals out of reach.

Toddlers

Toddlers begin walking, exploring the world around them, testing limits, and playing with anything in reach (**Figure 51.4 »**). Their small size and developing bones make them particularly vulnerable during motor-vehicle crashes or when hit, pushed, or shaken. Drowning is of particular concern, particularly around swimming pools. The leading causes of death for this age group are accidents with unintentional injuries, congenital malformations, malignant cancers, and homicide (CDC, 2019l). Toddlers also are at risk for injury or death due to fires or burns and suffocation. Another cause of death for young children occurs when they are left locked in parked motor vehicles.

SAFETY ALERT Even on a mild day (72°F), the temperature inside a closed car can escalate 30–40°F in an hour. Heat stroke may occur when the body temperature exceeds 104°F. Each year, an average of 39 children die in hot cars in the United States (Kids and Cars, 2019).

» **Stay Current:** For a list of safety tips and strategies parents and caregivers can use to prevent children from getting locked in vehicles, visit the Kids and Cars website at http://www.kidsandcars.org/heat-stroke.html.

Preschoolers

Preschool-age children are more mobile and coordinated than toddlers, yet not fully aware of the dangers that surround them. Although the number of injuries and fatalities are reduced compared to toddlers, the most common causes of injury and fatality in preschoolers are generally the same. The leading cause of death for this age group is accidents with unintentional injuries. Motor-vehicle crashes are the leading cause of child deaths (Advisory Board, 2018). Researchers note that firearm-related injuries among young children is the second highest cause of child deaths, and the third highest cause of death is malignant cancers (Advisory Board, 2018).

Nursing Implications

Toddlers and preschoolers continue to be measured for growth and developmental trends. Measurements of their standing height, weight, and body mass index (BMI) are done and compared with height and weight percentile ranges. Children are monitored for development of fine and gross motor abilities; social behaviors and socialization with others; language development; and temperament. Observing the toddler and preschooler for developmental milestones

TABLE 51.4 Strategies for Promoting Safety for Toddlers and Preschoolers

Strategies for Injury Prevention	Strategies for Disease Prevention
■ Help with food choices and eating patterns; eat fewer fast foods and more fruits and vegetables ■ Provide physical activities that use large muscle groups ■ Help child learn about what is right and wrong and rules that guide behaviors ■ Discipline the child for undesirable behaviors ■ Prevent exposure to environmental toxins ■ Prevent lead exposure in the home ■ Use appropriate harness straps or lap and shoulder belts for car safety ■ Other considerations: falls, drowning, poisoning, burns, motor-vehicle crashes, and pedestrian accidents	■ Avoid secondhand smoke exposure ■ Teach child to brush teeth; have scheduled dentist visits ■ Encourage adequate sleep and rest ■ Teach child safety around strangers ■ Be alert for electrical cords hanging down, water temperature higher than 120°F, sun exposure, and playing unsupervised ■ Teach child about hand hygiene and calling for help using the telephone ■ Vaccinate child with routine immunizations such as hepatitis A and B series, DTP, *Haemophilus influenzae* type b, inactivated poliovirus, pneumococcal, influenza, measles–mumps–rubella, and varicella ■ Teach children about crossing streets, riding bicycles, playing in water safety, and avoiding fire hazards ■ Know choking and CPR procedures for a child

Sources: Ball et al. (2020); Centers for Disease Control and Prevention (2019i, 2019l).

such as walking, drinking from a cup, feeding self, kicking a ball, drawing lines on paper, stating name, and building a tower of blocks provides assessment data for trending as the child grows older. Screen children for anemia, number and condition of teeth, signs of possible abuse such as bruising, and skin or gait problems. Teaching parents and caregivers about risk factors associated with these age groups can help reduce the incidence of unintentional injuries. See **Table 51.4** » for strategies for promoting safety for toddlers and preschoolers.

Safety for School-Age Children and Adolescents

School-Age Children

School-age children (those 5 to 12 years old) are much more active than younger children and can play farther from home with less supervision. They are less dependent on parents and caregivers than younger children and move faster on foot and on bicycles, leading to more falls, accidents, and playground injuries. Unintentional injuries account for almost one-third of deaths in this age group, most of which are caused by motor-vehicle crashes. Nonfatal injuries mainly come from unintentional falls. In line with the increased activity of children this age, overexertion and bicycle accidents both contribute to injuries (CDC, 2019l).

Adolescents

Adolescents (between 12 and 18 years old) are exposed to a number of new risks. They are trying to develop their own identities apart from parents and caregivers, facing increasing peer pressure from all directions, receiving driver's licenses, and playing contact sports. They are most likely to start experimenting with drugs and alcohol in this age range. They are also experiencing emotional turmoil, leading to outward aggression and fighting or internalizing and suicide. Now competing more seriously in sports and play, adolescents age 12 to 15 have the highest rate of injury during sports and play (**Figure 51.5** »).

Most deaths for this age group are due to unintentional injuries from motor-vehicle crashes, malignant cancers, and heart disease. Suicides, which do not qualify as unintentional, but which are preventable, account for a high percentage of adolescent deaths. Unintentional nonfatal injuries most often result from being struck by or against something, falling,

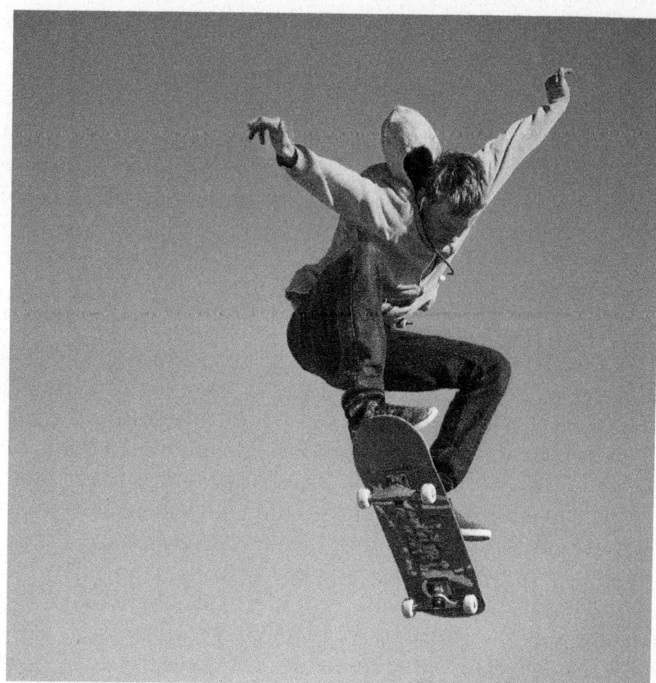

Figure 51.5 » This teenage skateboarder is at risk for fractures and head injury because he is not wearing protective equipment.
Source: yanik88/Shutterstock.

TABLE 51.5 Strategies for Promoting Safety in School-Age Children

Strategies to Prevent Injury	Strategies to Prevent Disease
■ Latchkey children who come home to an empty house after school need encouragement to remain safe, responsible, and have feelings of security ■ Teach children about fire, firearms, water, and other safety hazards and what to do in emergencies ■ Teach children about safety around interacting with strangers—accepting rides from them, chatting with them online, or talking with them on the phone ■ Promote healthy sleep behaviors ■ Use proper safety equipment to avoid sports injuries, especially from sports such as skateboarding, football, soccer, skiing, rollerblading, and motorcycle and ATV riding ■ Teach children safe resources such as teachers, school counselors, and police or security ■ Watch for signs of risky behaviors such as substance abuse, smoking, aggression and violence, eating disorders, and anxiety ■ Other considerations: pedestrian or biking accidents, handling firearms unsupervised, burns from experiments with flames or toxic substances, assault from a stranger, and what to do when scared and alone in a public or private area	■ Encourage independent food choices, including fruits and vegetables; suggest frequent snacks of nonfat and nonsugar choices ■ Continue oral health with brushing, flossing, and dentist visits ■ Teach children how to prevent diseases by washing their hands, avoiding respiratory infections, and avoiding causes of gastrointestinal illness ■ Connect health with risk behaviors such as smoking, poor oral hygiene, low physical activity, having above-normal weight, and skin problems ■ Limit television and video-game time ■ Continue with immunizations as needed

Sources: Ball et al. (2020); Centers for Disease Control and Prevention (2019i, 2019l).

overexertion, and poisoning (with 80% of these due to drug exposure of some kind) (CDC, 2019l).

Nursing Implications

School-age children continue to have their height, weight, and BMI monitored. Their bodies are refining muscular strength and coordination. They need encouragement to establish good health habits for nutrition, physical activity, and mental health and to avoid tobacco, alcohol, and drugs. Children are learning decision-making and problem-solving skills and refining skills for sports such as eye–hand coordination, agility, and speed. Their deciduous teeth are being replaced by permanent teeth. They are increasingly more active in afterschool activities such as sports and clubs.

Continue observation for developmental milestones such as independence in bathroom and dressing activities, reading, developing hobbies, playing a musical instrument, writing well, using a computer, developing self-esteem with feelings of self-worth related to physical appearance and social interactions, developing a positive body image, having prepuberty changes (girls may begin to menstruate), and building relationships outside of family. Also observe for common mental disorders involving anxiety, worry, fears, stress, sleep disorders, and depression. These observations provide assessment data for trending as the child grows older. Screen for blood pressure, bruising, repeated infections, changes in school performance or behavior, medications being taken, and any integrative therapies used.

Parents and caregivers need to adapt discipline methods to actions such as withholding privileges and using time-out; spanking and yelling should be avoided. School-age children can be taught risk factors and how to help reduce the incidence of unintentional injuries, such as by wearing a helmet when riding a bicycle. See **Table 51.5** » for strategies for promoting safety for school-age children; also see the Patient Teaching feature on the use of bicycle helmets.

When caring for adolescents, continue to monitor height, weight, and BMI. Observing the adolescent for developmental milestones provides assessment data for trending as the individual grows older. Self-concept continues to evolve; body changes may lead to decisions about sexual behaviors. Older adolescents should be asked if they are having sexual intercourse and, if so, if they are using protection against pregnancy and sexually transmitted infections. Ask about confusion with sexuality, sexual practices, and gay, lesbian, or bisexual activities. Their relationships and friends are very important, and they will test limits of parents and engage in conflicts with them. School offers peer support and meaningful activities but also causes stress, worry about grades, and violent or unsupportive school situations. Injuries are a major health hazard for this age group, so caregivers need to be made aware of risk factors and how to reduce the incidence of unintentional injuries to prevent them. See **Table 51.6** » for strategies that parents and caregivers can use to promote safety in adolescents.

Safety for Adults

Young Adults

Young adults, ages 18 to 40 years, are generally striking out on their own, getting jobs, being educated, getting married, and having kids. However, this independent living means making their own choices and mistakes, some of which can lead to life-altering changes. Young adults die from

TABLE 51.6 Strategies for Promoting Safety in Adolescents

Strategies to Prevent Injury	Strategies to Prevent Disease
■ Encourage consumption of nutritional foods to support immune system, physical activity, and metabolism ■ Encourage adequate sleep ■ Encourage regular physical activity and use of appropriate sports safety equipment ■ Avoid high noise levels, such as when listening to music through earbuds or headphones ■ Encourage oral health behaviors; be alert for ulcers or unusual growths in mouth from self-induced vomiting or chewing tobacco ■ Observe for signs of depression such as changes in behavior, school performance, sleep, and appetite; sadness; poor concentration; feelings of worthlessness; thoughts of death or suicide ■ Observe for signs of substance abuse such as changes in behavior, school performance, sleep, and appetite; lack of responsibility; inability to set goals; hopelessness; multiple accidents ■ Teach and encourage safe driving behaviors ■ Other considerations: safety with four-wheelers, boats, jet skis, farm machinery, tools, drowning, sun exposure, fires, firearms, hearing problems from loud music, abuse	■ Seek medical attention for acne and skin infections ■ Seek medical treatment for anemia, monitor dietary choices, encourage rest periods ■ Discuss bowel and bladder patterns and teach dietary choices and importance of fluid intake ■ Discuss aseptic technique needed for body piercing and tattooing to avoid infection ■ Discuss wellness habits such as healthy eating, exercise activity, amount of sleep, and emotional support ■ Use sunscreen to avoid sunburn and risk for later skin lesions ■ Discuss and provide information about sexually transmitted infections such as HIV, syphilis, hepatitis A, genital warts, and herpes that can be spread through unprotected sexual contact; provide protection options against acquiring these diseases ■ Discuss physical and emotional complications of eating disorders and obtain counseling if needed ■ Discuss safety and protection if being abused or bullied by another individual, observe for signs of abuse, provide information about strategies to remain calm and protect oneself from altercations, provide safe adults to go to when needing assistance ■ Observe for signs and symptoms of substance abuse and provide medical help as needed, monitor for any drug paraphernalia or drugs, discuss addiction and safety implications of certain drugs in the body ■ Stress importance of cessation of smoking, vaping, and use of nicotine products to avoid addiction and chronic health conditions ■ Common immunizations recommended: TD if last one >10 years ago, second measles–mumps–rubella, meningococcal vaccine recommended, human papillomavirus vaccine (three-dose series), annual influenza vaccine

Sources: Ball et al. (2020); Centers for Disease Control and Prevention (2019i, 2019l).

Patient Teaching

Bicycle and Skateboard Safety

Children ages 5 to 14 years have a high rate of nonfatal bicycle-related injuries. Children ages 13 to 16 years have a high rate of nonfatal skateboard-related injuries. Helmets can reduce the number of head and brain injuries if worn correctly (**Figure 51.6** »); unfortunately, they often are either not worn or worn incorrectly (too far back on the head) (CDC, 2020b).

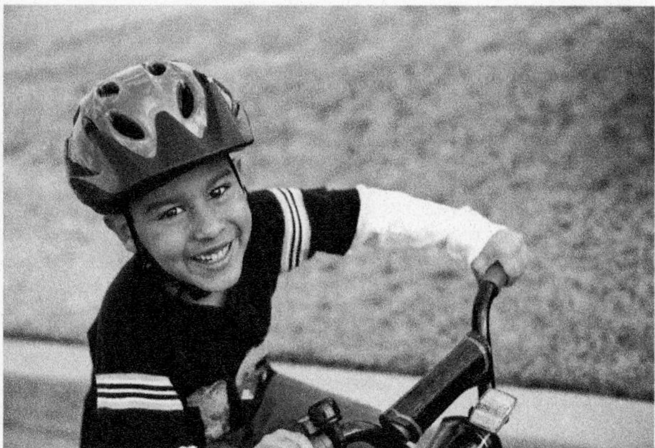

Figure 51.6 » Wearing an age-appropriate, well-fitting helmet helps reduce the risk of head and brain injuries.
Source: Marilyn Nieves/iStock/Getty Images.

Suggested interventions for reducing injuries and fatalities to bicyclists and skateboarders include:

- Wearing fluorescent clothing (to be more visible from farther away)
- Wearing retro-reflective clothing (to be more visible at night)
- Wearing age-appropriate helmets that are well maintained
- Adding lights on the bicycle (or bicyclist) such as front white lights and rear red lights
- Wearing wrist guards, elbow and knee pads, and appropriate shoes
- Making sure the helmet is fitting properly; it should fit snugly all around with no spaces between the foam and the user's head
- Wearing the helmet correctly: (1) the bottom of the pad inside the front of the helmet is one or two finger widths above the eyebrows, (2) the back of the helmet should not touch the top of the neck, (3) side straps should form a "V" shape under and slightly in front of the ears, (4) the chin strap should be centered under the chin and fit snugly, not moving in any direction.

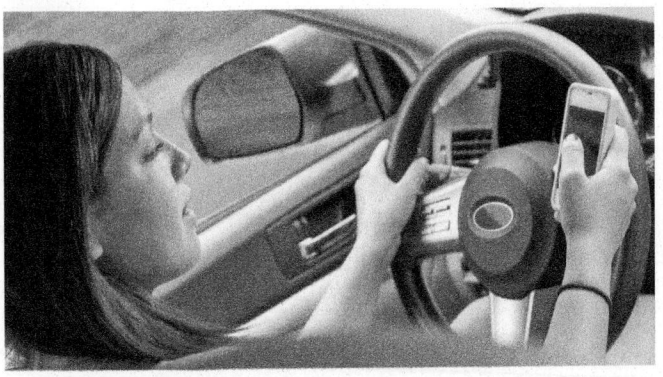

Figure 51.7 ›› Individuals who text while driving are more likely to be in a crash than those who do not.

Source: Nycshooter/iStock/Getty Images.

unintentional injuries resulting from poisoning (mostly by drugs, narcotics, medicines, or biological agents); motor-vehicle crashes; malignant cancers; heart disease; suicide; and homicides (**Figure 51.7** ››) (CDC, 2019l). Sources of nonfatal injuries include unintentional falls, inadvertent overexertion, and being accidentally struck by or against something (CDC, 2019l). Overexertion can be a particular concern among recreational athletes, who may be at greater risk for dehydration, exposure-related illness, or sports-related injury.

Middle Adults

Middle adults, ages 40 to 65 years, are beginning to look toward retirement. Middle adults have started to slow down, probably becoming less active and developing some chronic health problems as the healing process slows. For the first time, unintentional injuries are not the leading cause of death. Instead, malignant cancers account for one-third of deaths. Heart disease is the second leading cause of death, due to age and obesity. Unintentional injuries that result in death are caused by poisoning, mostly from drugs, narcotics, medicines, or biological agents. A little over one-quarter of fatalities are due to motor-vehicle traffic and falls. Suicides in this age group represent a small percentage of deaths. For the middle adults who experience injuries that do not end in fatality, the majority of these injuries are due to unintentional falls and the others due to overexertion, accidental injury by being hit by or against something, and motor-vehicle crashes (CDC, 2019i).

Strategies for promoting safety for adults are shown in **Table 51.7** ››.

›› **Stay Current:** The CDC provides information for current recommended immunization schedules for adults: http://www.cdc.gov/vaccines/schedules/downloads/adult/adult-schedule-easy-read.pdf.

Safety for Older Adults

About 63% of older adults retire between the ages of 57 and 66 years. Many continue to work well into older adulthood, some at second or part-time jobs after they retire from careers (DQYDJ, 2019).

Data show that more retired healthy individuals remain in the workforce until reaching the age of 70 (DQYDJ, 2019). As older adults continue to age, living independently can become challenging for those experiencing chronic illnesses that impact cognition or mobility. Chronic diseases such as heart disease, malignant cancers, cerebrovascular illness (stroke), chronic respiratory disease, Alzheimer disease, and diabetes are common causes of fatality in this age group. The highest cause of death from unintentional injury is falls, followed by motor-vehicle crashes, suffocation, poisoning, and fire (CDC, 2019l).

Older adults in assisted living facilities or living in their own homes need to take steps to actively prevent functional decline. **Functional decline** is a reduction in the quality of or ability for physical or cognitive function. It may only take a couple of days for it to manifest through changes such as diminished ability to complete ADLs, impaired mobility, decreased musculoskeletal strength, and reduced physical endurance (Government of South Australia, 2019).

By reducing the risk of functional decline, nurses and independent older adults can help prevent related complications,

TABLE 51.7 Strategies for Promoting Safety in Adults

Strategies to Prevent Injury	Strategies to Prevent Disease
■ Do not be distracted when driving a motor vehicle, such as texting, talking on cell phone, eating, drinking, looking at a GPS device, or adjusting the radio ■ Do appropriate exercise activities, check with HCP before beginning new physical activities ■ Seek medical help if at-home care does not improve an injury ■ Avoid stressing back when lifting or moving heavy objects ■ Stay alert and use caution when using equipment and household appliances ■ Stay alert and use caution to avoid tripping on objects and falling ■ Use ergonomic aids when using a computer ■ Use safety seat belt when driving or riding in a motor vehicle ■ Keep a simple first aid kit at home and in motor vehicle in case of accidents ■ Use integrative health therapies such as herbs, green tea, massage, and yoga to relax the body and mind	■ Do basic medical screening for conditions that may lead to chronic medical illness or disease ■ Have annual health checkups ■ Maintain healthy weight by eating nutritious foods ■ Practice health behaviors such as hand hygiene ■ Follow a prudent lifestyle and take medications as prescribed to control chronic conditions such as hypertension and diabetes ■ Avoid exposure to infectious conditions such as crowds in cold season ■ Use sunscreen to avoid sunburn and risk for later skin lesions ■ Follow immunization guidelines appropriate for adults such as annual flu vaccine, Tdap every 10 years, shingles zoster vaccine, and pneumococcal vaccine ■ Omit lifestyle risks such as smoking, drinking alcohol, abusing drugs, and engaging in unprotected sexual intercourse with many partners

Sources: Centers for Disease Control and Prevention (2019l, 2020e).

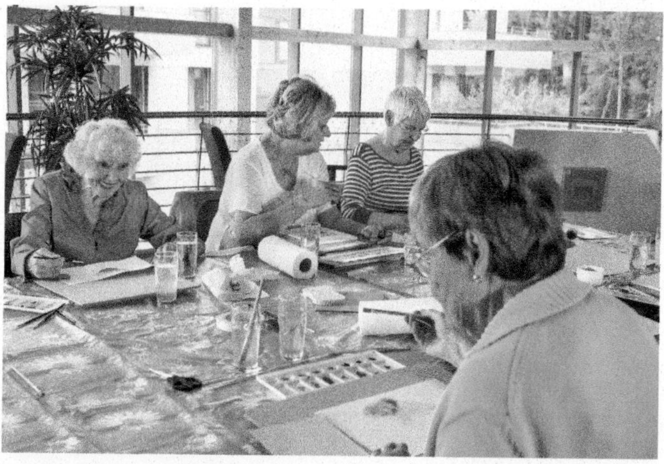

Figure 51.8 ⟫ Senior centers offer companionship and activities for older adults.

Source: Horsche/iStock/Getty Images.

such as pressure injuries, delirium and depression, decreased mobility, loss of independence, and incontinence. Strategies to reduce functional decline including encouraging older adults to keep mobile, active, and engaged in ADLs as physically and cognitively able. Precautionary measures need to be implemented to prevent injury in the elderly with impaired mobility or altered cognitive function. Reorientation to the patient's room, how to get to a restroom, and how to call for help will also help reduce functional decline when in an assisted living facility.

Some communities have daycare centers with staff trained to work with older adults. Some offer senior centers that provide a variety of activities for the elderly to participate in and socialize with others their age (**Figure 51.8 ⟫**). There are also many federal, state, local, and private advocacy organizations dedicated to providing services for the elderly, such as Meals on Wheels, which delivers lunch to qualifying older adults in their homes. Oral care remains important to prevent periodontal diseases such as oral and pharyngeal cancers. See the Patient Teaching feature for factors affecting oral health and **Table 51.8 ⟫** for strategies to promote safety in older adults who live in the community.

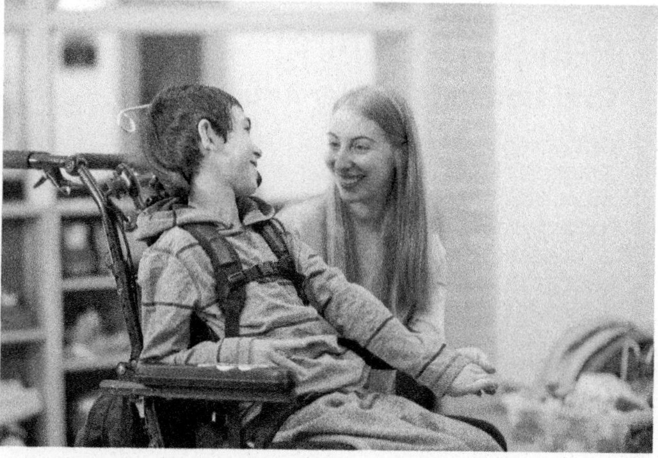

Figure 51.9 ⟫ Because of the Individuals with Disabilities Education Act, all students are guaranteed a free and appropriate education. Here a boy with cerebral palsy works with his aide in the classroom.

Source: FatCamera/E+/Getty Images.

Safety for Individuals with Disabilities

Safety is focused on the developmental level and physical capabilities of individuals. Strategies to prevent unintentional injuries can be adapted for those with disabilities. *Individuals with disabilities* refers to individuals with mental, emotional, or physical disabilities who may require special care or assistance to communicate, ambulate, perform self-care activities, or make decisions. This may include people with autism, Down syndrome, speech and language impairments, mobility impairments, reading and learning disabilities, and cerebral palsy. Individuals with conditions that affect attention, memory, or communication, such as Alzheimer disease and attention-deficit/hyperactivity disorder, may also be included in this category.

Individuals with moderate and significant disabilities require assistance or accommodation in all settings (**Figure 51.9 ⟫**). For example, parents and care providers can create a safe home environment by using safety equipment,

TABLE 51.8 Strategies for Promoting Safety in Community-Dwelling Older Adults

Strategies to Prevent Injury	Strategies to Prevent Disease
■ Maintain mobility, activity, and function as tolerated and able to do ■ Have safety supports in the home for mobility, such as handrails, shower seats, chairs with adjustable heights, adequate lighting, and low beds ■ Seek help when needed for household upkeep, yard maintenance, repair work, and so on ■ Minimize clutter in the home ■ Wear footwear with skid-resistant soles ■ Keep assistive devices such as canes, walkers, glasses, and hearing aids, close and accessible to use ■ Know about prescribed medications and their side effects ■ Be aware of physical limitations to avoid injuries and accidents ■ Socialize with others for psychosocial healthiness as desired	■ Schedule an annual comprehensive assessment of physical, cognitive, emotional, and functional status ■ Maintain appropriate body weight by eating a variety of fruits, vegetables, and proteins ■ Drink adequate fluids to stay hydrated ■ Exercise joints and muscles to maintain mobility and flexibility ■ Do assessment self-checks for changes to skin integrity, respiratory status, musculoskeletal movements, and routine body functions ■ Be actively engaged in health safety behaviors such as frequent hand hygiene ■ Be aware of surroundings and alert for safety hazards to avoid ■ Avoid temperature extremes

Sources: Centers for Disease Control and Prevention (2019b, 2020d, 2020f).

Patient Teaching

Oral Health for Older Adults

Older adults are at risk for poor oral health for a number of reasons. Almost one in five adults 65 years or older have lost some of their natural teeth, which may lead them to choose soft, easily chewed foods and avoid fresh fruits and vegetables (CDC, 2019g). Older adults face an increasing risk of acquiring periodontal disease. Oral and pharyngeal cancers, primarily diagnosed in older adults, have poor prognoses. Those with the poorest oral health are those who are socioeconomically disadvantaged, do not have dental insurance, and are members of ethnic minorities. Those who are disabled, unable to leave bed or home, or institutionalized have higher risk of poor oral health (CDC, 2019g).

Another factor that contributes to poor oral health is the high number of prescription and over-the-counter (OTC) drugs older adults take that cause a dry mouth. Saliva contains antimicrobial components as well as minerals that help rebuild tooth enamel attacked by decay-causing bacteria, so when saliva production is decreased, the risk for oral disease is increased. There are also chronic neurologic or musculoskeletal conditions such as Alzheimer disease and stroke that limit the ability of older adults to perform oral health self-care.

Nurses should encourage older adults and/or those assisting them to:

- Periodically assess the mouth for changes in appearance, tenderness of gums, sensitivity of teeth, presence of saliva, cracked skin areas, ulcerations, or pain and report anything unusual to their HCP.
- Observe for bleeding gums when brushing natural teeth, red swollen gums, and chronic bad taste or bad breath, as these may indicate gum disease.
- Remember to stay hydrated to maintain good salivary flow. Dry mouth may occur as a side effect of certain medications prescribed.
- Notice if the corners of the mouth and the lips are dry and cracked. A lubricant can be applied as needed to prevent problems with skin integrity.
- Clean any dentures daily and rinse them after every meal. Ensure food particles and other debris are removed after each meal.
- Brush teeth every day, as able, and after every meal, or have assistance with oral care.
- Have oral hygiene materials available, such as toothbrushes, toothpaste, denture cleaning products, and mouthwash.
- Prevent aspiration with positioning and assistance as needed during mouth care.
- Schedule annual appointments with the dentist.

Source: Based on Centers for Disease Control and Prevention (2019h).

such as smoke alarms that signal with a light, handrails to prevent falls, and life jackets for water safety that are specially fitted to the individual. If the individual tends to wander, family can talk with neighbors and ask for their help keeping watch and to contact them if they see the individual unsupervised. As appropriate, individuals with disabilities can wear a bracelet or some other kind of identification. Special locks or alarms on exit doors may be necessary to alert caregivers that the individual is trying to leave the building.

Here are suggested questions to address for safety and injury prevention:

1. Can the individual move about, handle things, and explore?
2. Is there any safety equipment or modifications that are appropriate for the individual?
3. Does the individual have difficulty talking or understanding?
4. Does the individual have difficulty making decisions? (CDC, 2019j)

Many individuals with disabilities depend on others to help ensure their safety and security. Parents and other family members may need assistance to locate community resources to help provide appropriate care and respite care. Nurses can assess what needs the individual has that will require assistance from others and discuss resources with the family. Nurses can provide support and encouragement for the individuals and their families. Teaching is important to show family members how equipment, supplies, and procedures are used or performed. A team of caregivers may be essential to provide supervision and care. This also can provide a variety of relationships with caregivers and the individual. Family members may need encouragement and support to accept respite care as a time of refreshing and reenergizing without feelings of guilt. Strategies for promoting safety for individuals with disabilities are outlined in **Table 51.9** ».

NURSING PROCESS

Individualized patient care includes appropriate developmental and chronologic health promotion and injury prevention considerations. Safety is often a priority. Nurses need to take into account safety hazards that may result in injuries associated with all age groups across the lifespan, such as accidental poisoning for small children or falls for older adults.

Assessment

Both objective and subjective data are used to assess the need for maintaining the current level of health or readiness to improve it:

- ***Observation and patient interview.*** History of lifestyle risk behaviors, frequency of injuries from chronic conditions, developmental challenges, sensory and motor deficits, change in sustainability of current health status, changes in family dynamics, ability to live independently, and so on.
- ***Physical examination.*** Vital signs, heart and lung sounds, mobility, sensory and motor disabilities, changes due to lifestyle risk behaviors, cognition abilities, current injuries noted, and so on.

TABLE 51.9 Strategies for Promoting Safety for Individuals with Disabilities

Strategies to Prevent Injury	Strategies to Prevent Disease
■ Adapt safety restraints and seats in motor vehicles as appropriate to keep individual safe ■ Advocate to have neighborhood audible crosswalk signals installed ■ Have safety evacuation plans at home for fire, include flashing lights for hearing impaired and special equipment as appropriate ■ Install soft surfaces in outside play areas ■ Match sports activities to individual's abilities ■ Provide special equipment or protection for individuals needing assistive devices ■ Match toys, games, and hobbies to individual's developmental level ■ Dress appropriately for the weather ■ Be alert for home safety issues: electrical outlets, electrical cords, climbing on furniture, hot water temperature; knowing where to find bathroom, bedroom, dining room	■ Avoid secondhand smoke exposure ■ Teach individual to brush teeth, have scheduled dentist visits ■ Encourage adequate sleep and rest ■ Teach individual safety around strangers ■ Maintain airway with suctioning as needed or, if able, effective coughing ■ Teach individual about hand hygiene and using a telephone to call for help ■ Schedule routine immunizations for age group ■ Provide oxygen therapy as prescribed

Source: Center for Children with Special Needs (2018); Centers for Disease Control and Prevention (2019j, 2019n).

Diagnosis

There are many nursing diagnoses about promoting health and preventing injuries for all ages of patients. Promoting health can focus on psychologic, emotional, physical, and spiritual health, and preventing injuries can address environmental conditions, the patient's current state of well-being, or the patient's homeostasis status. Here are a few common examples of safety and health promotion nursing diagnoses:

- Inadequate protection
- Risky health behavior
- Inadequate health maintenance
- Ready to learn about self-care.

Planning

Goals for improved health reflect the nursing diagnosis and include input from the patient, such as:

- The patient will assess his skin for lesions every month.
- The patient will verbalize three ways to be physically active each day.
- The patient will actively participate in a community-based smoking-cessation program.
- The patient will be able to correctly demonstrate how to empty his colostomy bag by discharge.

Implementation

There are many nursing actions that help patients improve their health while in a healthcare setting (acute care facility, extended care facility, community facility, or home setting). There are many opportunities for nurses to teach patients about being more active in safe self-care behaviors to prevent injuries. All interventions need to be prioritized to best meet patient needs. Some intervention examples are:

- Demonstrate to patient how to use a mirror to assess for skin lesions on the back.
- Assist patient in finding a smoking-cessation program in their community.
- Encourage patient to observe and then participate in emptying their colostomy bag.
- Collaborate with the physical therapist to teach patient appropriate physical exercises.

Evaluation

Expected outcomes may include the following:

- The patient is able to correctly empty their colostomy bag when needed.
- The patient attends a smoking-cessation program in the community.
- The patient is able to verbalize how to assess for lesions on their back using a mirror.
- The patient is able to demonstrate three physical activities that can be done during the day.

The safety and health conditions of a patient can change quickly. Because of this, the nurse needs to continuously monitor the patient's health status by observing for cues indicating a difference between previous and current assessment data. Promoting safety and well-being for the patient needs to be a priority during every nurse–patient interaction.

REVIEW Health Promotion and Injury Prevention Across the Lifespan

RELATE Link the Concepts and Exemplars

Linking the exemplar on health promotion and injury prevention across the lifespan with the concept of culture and diversity:

1. Discuss how an individual's culture may impact their environmental exposures and lifestyle choices.
2. How might the nurse integrate cultural considerations in an assessment of an individual's safety throughout the lifespan?

Linking the exemplar of health promotion and injury prevention across the lifespan with the concept of communication:

3. Differentiate ways of teaching an adult, a school-age child, and a toddler about hand hygiene safety.
4. Contrast safety considerations when providing care to a primary English-speaking patient and to a patient who speaks English as a second language.

READY Go to Volume 3: Clinical Nursing Skills

REFER Go to Pearson MyLab Nursing and eText

REFLECT Apply Your Knowledge

An older adult patient was admitted to the hospital 3 days ago subsequent to a fall. They sustained a right hip fracture and a mild concussion. The patient had been outside gardening on an afternoon where the temperature reached a high of 92 degrees. When the patient stood up to walk into the house, they experienced vertigo and fell to the ground. After the patient recovers from surgical repair of their hip fracture, they will be transferred to a rehabilitation facility.

1. How might age-related physiologic changes have contributed to the patient's fall and subsequent injuries?
2. Why is the patient being transferred to a rehabilitation facility, as opposed to being discharged to home?
3. Develop a nursing plan of care for the patient.

Exemplar 51.B Patient Safety

Exemplar Learning Outcomes

51.B Analyze safety as it relates to patients in home care and healthcare settings.

- Evaluate the quality of safety in home care settings.
- Write safety nursing interventions for patients in healthcare settings.
- Contrast lifespan considerations for safety in healthcare settings.
- Plan nursing interventions for quality, safety, and best patient outcomes.

Exemplar Key Terms

Chemical restraints, *2884*
Elder abuse, *2882*
Handoff reporting, *2883*
Healthcare-associated infections (HAIs), *2884*
Never events, *2885*
Physical restraints, *2884*
SBAR, *2883*
Seclusion, *2884*
Sentinel events, *2885*
Wrong-site surgery (WSS), *2885*

Overview

Individualized patient care incorporates numerous developmental considerations. Patients who present with illness or injuries are assessed not only in terms of their developmental age group, but also about safety concerns for the age group. Nurses need to take into account common injuries and safety hazards associated with all age groups across the lifespan. These considerations for safety should take place in all healthcare settings, including acute care facilities, extended care facilities, community settings, and home settings. In addition, nurses play an essential role in empowering patients to speak up on their own behalf.

Many healthcare facilities have adopted a patient safety educational program called SPEAK UP, launched by The Joint Commission (Griffin Hospital, 2020). This safety program helps individuals in healthcare and home settings be more aware of safety hazards that can cause injuries and accidents. The initiative educates patients and empowers them to be an active partner in their care. SPEAK UP stands for (Griffin Hospital, 2020):

Speak up if you have questions or concerns

Pay attention when you receive care (medications, treatments, therapies)

Educate yourself about your illness, medical history, and diagnoses

Ask a trusted friend or family member to advocate for you

Know what medications you take and why you take them

Use healthcare facilities that you have checked out

Participate actively in decisions made about your care and therapies.

Safety in Home Care Settings

Home healthcare has become an established regulated program of care and services that older adults are using more now that they are living longer. A variety of medical, therapeutic, and nonmedical services, such as wound care, dietary counseling, physical therapy, skilled nursing services, occupational therapy, and homemaker services, are now available in private homes from healthcare professionals. Data from the Administration for Community Living show that one out of six noninstitutionalized older adults are in fair or poor health, so many need some level of assistance in the home. The home health industry and government agencies are responding to these needs (Robertson, 2019).

As the older adult population continues to grow, so does the suspected number of unreported elder abuse cases (National Adult Protective Services Association [NAPSA], 2020). **Elder abuse** is defined as intentional actions by a family member, caregiver, or other that inflicts harm or puts the older adult at risk for harm, including failure to meet basic needs or protect the older adult from harm. In a national study, it was reported that approximately 90% of abusers were family members (NAPSA, 2020).

Older adults over the age of 65 with disabilities are more vulnerable to abuse that puts their health, safety, well-being, and ability to take care of themselves at risk. Another high-risk group for abuse is those with dementia. Victims of elder abuse and neglect have additional health conditions, such as digestive problems, depression, anxiety, chronic pain, and heart problems. Many older adults on fixed incomes also experience financial exploitation with very damaging losses affecting their lifestyles and ability to take care of themselves (NAPSA, 2020). See Exemplar 32.A, Abuse, in Module 32, Trauma, for further information.

Stay Current: Learn more about federal and state policies on elder abuse at https://ncea.acl.gov/What-We-Do/Policy.aspx.

There are many environmental improvements that address safety risk measures in home settings. Examples of environmental safety improvements are:

- Installing handrails along walls and grab bars in bathrooms
- Designing wider hallways and doorways for using walkers and wheelchairs
- Installing easy-grip door handles, water faucets, and cabinets
- Removing scatter rugs or adding nonslip padding underneath
- Ensuring that a bell or way to call for help is easily accessible
- Providing adequate lighting
- Giving the patient the ability to control room temperatures for comfort
- Ensuring that fire and disaster plans are available.

Older adults with one or more chronic illnesses may be taking medications that can increase risk for confusion or compromise mobility. Nurses working with patients from this population assess for risks to safety related to both prescribed and OTC medications and supplements (see Exemplar 51.D).

Safety in Healthcare Settings

Because patient care can be very complicated in the healthcare setting, there is a need for coordination, flexibility, and adjustments made among HCPs. Treatment protocols can be complicated and time-sensitive; HCPs can modify their prescribed orders by changing them, adding new ones, or stopping old ones by telephone, face-to-face, or in writing. Keeping quality and safety priorities for everyone is a continuous challenge.

Communication of patient information, called **handoff reporting**, between nursing units, shifts, other departments, staff, and HCPs is critical. Unfortunately, it is also a common cause of error if not all patient information is given or if there is not enough time to give complete information and information about the patient is fragmented (Shahid & Thomas, 2018). To organize necessary patient information and standardize handoff communication, many healthcare facilities are using a communication tool called SBAR, which stands for:

Situation
Background
Assessment
Recommendations

For further information, go to Module 38, Communication, and see **Figure 51.10** ».

For these reasons, and despite the best intentions of nurses and other providers, adverse events and medical errors occur frequently. Healthcare staff constantly strive to keep these adverse events to a minimum, targeting common clinical occurrences such as adverse drug events, falls, healthcare-associated infections, improper use of restraints, and wrong-site surgery. Unfortunately, in some healthcare facilities safety may not be a high priority, leading to complacency and tolerance of low performance, which can contribute to poor quality and patterns of unsafe behaviors and uncaring attitudes.

SBAR Report	
Report given by:	Time :______
Report received by:	Phone:______
S	**Situation:** Patient name Age Location Code status Current vital signs and O_2 saturation Patient's current status
B	**Background:** Admitting date and diagnosis Allergies Diagnostic tests pending Patient's physical/mental status Oxygen in use or not
A	**Assessment:** Lungs, heart, neurologic status IV sites/fluids/rates Diet and intake/output Active precautions Isolation precautions Special care—tubes, wounds
R	**Recommendations:** Suggestions for diagnostic tests Treatments Transfer to critical care Come to see patient

Figure 51.10 » Information included in an SBAR handoff report.

Falls

Falls are very common in healthcare facilities and homes and are a special risk for those ages 65 and older. Thirty percent of older adults report falling each year (CDC, 2019b). Falls among older adults result in 3 million emergency department visits every year, making falls the most common cause of nonfatal injuries and the leading cause of injury-related death in older adults (CDC, 2019b). In nursing homes, 50–75% of residents fall each year, with an average of 2.6 falls per person per year (Nursing Home Abuse Center, 2020).

Falls can cause numerous injuries, including fractured bones, excessive bleeding, traumatic brain injury, and death. Patients who display memory impairment and muscle weakness, as well as those individuals who require assistive devices such as canes or walkers for ambulation, are especially at risk. Numerous prescription and OTC medications also increase the risk of falls (CDC, 2020e).

In a clinical setting, numerous strategies can be implemented to reduce the risk of falls. Examples of nursing interventions that may be applicable to the care of the patient who is at risk for falling may include the following:

- Remove obstacles from walking paths, including patient rooms, corridors, and stairwells.
- Keep frequently used items within easy reach.
- Ensure that patient rooms are well lit.

- Make sure patients wear shoes with soles that provide adequate traction, as opposed to wearing slippers or going barefoot.
- Assess the patient's vision and make sure they are using any prescribed eyewear, because poor and blurry vision increases the risk of falling.
- Use side rails on patient beds to prevent falls while the patient is sleeping.
- Be aware of each patient's medication regimen, including side effects and interactions, because side effects such as dizziness or drowsiness can substantially increase the risk of a fall. Request that an HCP or pharmacist review patient medications when necessary (CDC, 2020e).

Healthcare-Associated Infections

Healthcare-associated infections (HAIs) are infections that occur while a patient is being treated for another condition. The CDC (2018a) estimates that one in 31 hospitalized patients contract an HAI during their hospital stay for medical treatment. HAIs can be very serious because hospitalized patients are usually weaker or immunocompromised because of the injury or illness that hospitalized them in the first place. Common HAIs and pathogens that are frequently associated with HAIs are discussed in Module 9, Infection.

Patients can help prevent infection through becoming knowledgeable about their treatment and recovery plan, being proactive about blood sugar control, losing weight prior to surgery, and quitting smoking. Nurses are also vital in preventing HAIs and must take appropriate measures to ensure that they are not unknowingly spreading illness between patients. Among other safety measures, appropriate hand hygiene and disinfectant techniques are particularly important.

Restraints and Safety Devices

A number of restraints and safety devices are available to partially or fully limit the patient's mobility. They are applied only when absolutely necessary to protect the patient from injuring self or others and only with a HCP's order.

Chemical restraints are pharmacologic agents, such as sedatives, hypnotics, neuroleptics, and antianxiety medications, that are administered to agitated patients to control unsafe physical movements and behaviors. **Seclusion** is confining a patient to a room involuntarily and preventing the patient from leaving. Typically, acute care units do not have space for a seclusion room, so this category is more appropriate for emergency departments and psychiatric units than acute care settings. Other devices that may be considered forms of restraints include wheelchairs with stationary lap trays, bed rails, and geri chairs. Generally, if the patient can release or remove the device without assistance, the device is not considered to be a restraint. Infant and child restraints include crib nets, elbow restraints, and mummy restraints.

Physical restraints are wrapped, buckled, or tied to a patient's arms, legs, or trunk of the body to limit or restrict movement. They cannot be used as a form of punishment, a convenience measure, or to prevent a patient from leaving a given setting. Regulations stipulate the following conditions for restraints: (1) a HCP must order specific restraints, physical or chemical, to be applied to the patient; (2) the order for restraints cannot be a standing order or prn order; and (3) when there is an urgency to protect the patient and others, restraints can be applied and then the HCP can be notified as soon as possible for an order. Legally, a competent patient who simply does not comply with their care cannot be restrained; this may be construed as assault and battery or false imprisonment.

Restraint alternatives and least restrictive forms of restraint must be tried first. If they are unsuccessful, then chemical or physical restraints can be implemented as a last resort for the safety of the patient and others. There must be documented evidence of less restrictive measures that were tried without success, including interventions to modify the patient's behavior or the environment. Safety devices such as bed alarms and portable location trackers can help prevent falls or wandering among patients who need assistance to move about safely. Examples of alternatives to help control the patient's behaviors and avoid restraints include (Burke, 2020):

- Having a family member or sitter stay with the patient
- Using distractions and diversional activities
- Using a calm voice and soothing tone
- Limiting the number of staff working with the patient
- Using deescalation strategies
- Reorienting the confused patient
- Assessing/addressing problems causing agitation, such as wanting to get up and go to the bathroom
- Offering therapeutic reassurance.

Although restraints are intended to protect the patient, their use also may result in injury or even death. Psychosocial effects are also a concern: Adult patients who are restrained may experience depression as well as a sense of dehumanization, and pediatric patients may feel they are being punished. Whenever restraints are used, the nurse must follow strict guidelines to ensure the patient's safety. These guidelines include:

- Assessment at least every 2 hours that includes skin and circulation status, patient's response, and effect of restraints
- New verbal order every 24 hours if there is not a written order
- Periodic removal of restraints so the patient can freely move the affected body part, range-of-motion (ROM) exercises can be performed, and the patient can be repositioned
- Offering fluid, foods, and toileting periodically
- Evaluation to determine if continued restraint is needed
- Appropriate and complete documentation of the restraint intervention.

Commonly used restraints include limb, soft belt, safety strap, or vest immobilizers or mitt, elbow, or hand restraints (**Figure 51.11** »). Limb restraints and mitts, which are typically made of cloth, may be used when limb immobilization is needed for therapeutic purposes—for example, to prevent dislodgment of an intravenous infusion device or removal of dressings. To ensure the safety of patients who

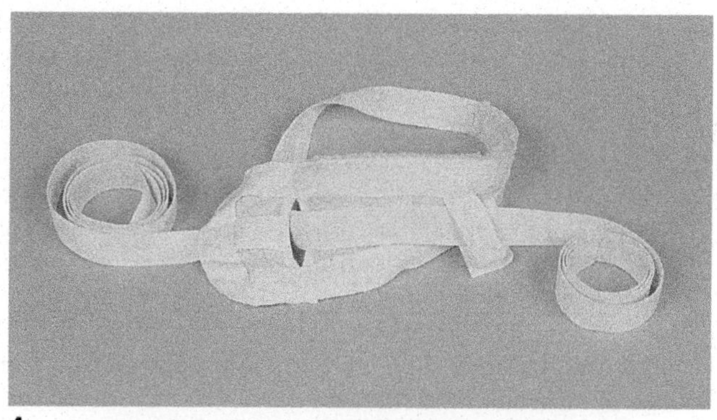

A

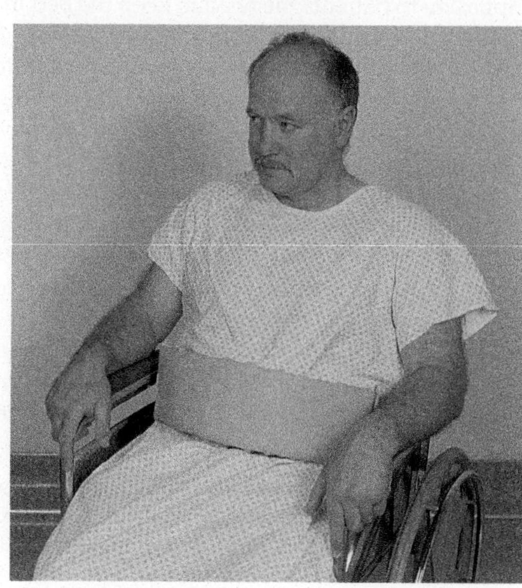

B

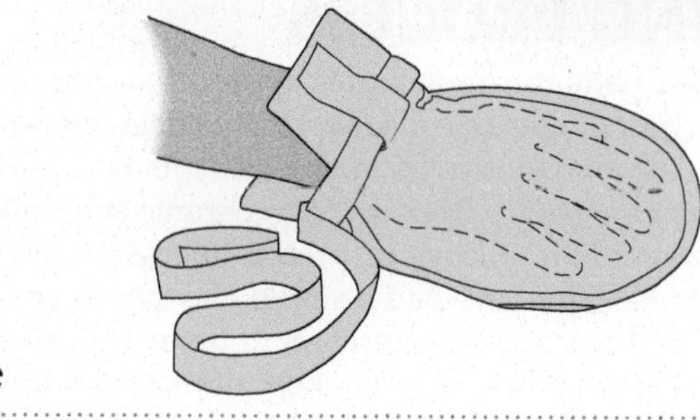

C

Figure 51.11 » Various types of restraints. ***A***, Limb restraint. ***B***, Belt restraint. ***C***, Mitt restraint.
Source: ***A*** & ***B***, Pearson Education, Inc.

are transported by wheelchair or gurney, soft belt restraints, safety strap body restraints, or vest restraints are used. Soft belt restraints and immobilizers may be used to protect patients who are confined to a chair or a bed. To protect confused patients or very small children from scratching and injuring their skin, mitt restraints, mittens, or hand restraints may be used.

Communicating with Parents of Pediatric Patients

Working Phase

Parents and caregivers of pediatric patients often have questions about the child's care. Give them opportunities to ask questions and respond honestly and at a vocabulary level they will understand. Be friendly, relaxed, and genuine in responses.

- Hello, Mrs. Rodriguez, remember me? I'm Peter, the nurse taking care of your son today. I was told you had a question about how he tried to climb out of his crib.
- Hi, Mrs. Rodriguez, it's good to see you again. I was just getting your son back in his crib. Could you help me with his other arm?
- Good morning, Mrs. Rodriguez, did you want to see me about your son crying when you had to leave yesterday?

Wrong-Site Surgery

Wrong-site surgery (WSS), or *wrong-site, wrong-procedure, wrong-patient surgery*, are errors that should not occur and have been designated as **sentinel events** or **never events** by the National Quality Forum. *Wrong-site* refers to surgery performed on an incorrect body site or to surgery performed on the wrong side of the correct body site: for example, removing the right upper lung lobe instead of the left upper lung lobe or removing the right side of the right upper lung lobe instead of removing the left side of the right upper lung lobe. *Wrong procedure* refers to the right patient undergoing an incorrect surgical procedure. *Wrong-patient* refers to the patient undergoing a surgical procedure intended for another patient. WSSs are fairly rare and happen approximately one in every 112,000 surgical procedures, averaging one such error every 5 to 10 years in a given healthcare facility (AHRQ, 2019b). Some factors are:

- Inadequate patient assessment
- Inadequate safety culture
- Communication failure
- Inadequate medical record review
- Multiple procedures on multiple parts of a patient performed during a single operation
- Failure to include the patient and family when identifying the correct operation site
- Failure to clearly mark the correct operation site
- Failure to recheck information before starting the operation.

WSS is a serious patient risk because it subjects a patient to severe and unnecessary trauma. Surgery teams also feel the effects because they can be subjected to negative morale, insurers that will not pay for WSS, malpractice claims, and disciplinary actions by licensing boards. To prevent WSS, The Joint Commission developed a universal protocol that has been adopted by numerous medical and professional organizations (AHRQ, 2019d). The universal protocol is outlined in Module 17, Perioperative Care.

Lifespan Considerations in Healthcare Settings

Healthcare facilities are strange environments, full of strange new sounds, people, equipment, and activity. Preparing for this experience can help reduce patient anxiety and promote patient comfort and satisfaction with care. In general, giving patients honest information at a level they can understand, answering any questions they may have, and providing them support and encouragement will help them be more at ease. The following sections present some common safety considerations for children, older adults, and pregnant patients.

Safety Considerations for Children

1. Very young children learn about their world by touching and playing with objects around them, so keep medications, sharp objects, and equipment out of reach.
2. Suggest families bring in a few comfort items the child is familiar with, such as photos, a favorite blanket, or a favorite small toy.
3. Maintain the child's daily routines and habits as much as appropriate.
4. Suggest that families help their child stay busy with age-appropriate activities they like to do.
5. Encourage family members to respect safety signs such as washing hands, keeping a security door closed, and not allowing the pediatric patient to run down the hallways or be out of their sight at any time.
6. Be aware when parents or caregivers leave the child alone.
7. Remember that children and infants can move very quickly and fall from a crib or bed.
8. Communicate with children using language that is appropriate for their developmental level.
9. Infant and child patients must wear proper identification at all times.

Safety Considerations for Pregnant Patients

1. Patients need to continue to follow prenatal care guidelines as approved by their HCP.
2. Nurses can reduce risk for maternal complications and morbidity by assessing for chronic conditions such as asthma, diabetes, and cardiovascular disease. Timely assessment, follow-up, and patient teaching about medications and treatments can reduce both maternal and fetal risk for complications.
3. Patients should be screened for peripartum depression at least once during the pregnancy.
4. Patients need to know how medications, procedures, and treatments could affect their pregnancy or their child. Nurses can reinforce information provided by the patient's treating HCP.
5. Nurses can encourage pregnant patients to avoid risks of infection or injury.

Safety considerations for the newborn include teaching the mother and other family members to never leave the baby alone in the mother's room, only give the baby to personnel with appropriate photo identification name badges, always use an infant crib when transporting the baby, always leave the baby on the postpartum unit, and never give interested strangers on the unit personal information about themselves or the baby.

Safety Considerations for Older Adults

1. Encourage patients to have a family member or someone they trust to advocate for them while they are in the hospital.
2. Encourage patients to have someone bring their prescription and OTC medications, herbs, and dietary supplements to the hospital to review and include in their admission information.
3. If a patient has any known allergies to medicines, materials, foods, soaps, and so on, this information needs to be posted in appropriate places such as on the medical record, the medication administration record, and as hospital policy dictates.
4. Emphasize to patients the importance of using the call button to ask for help getting up to use the restroom or walking around the hallway.
5. Emphasize to patients the need to keep the bed in a low and locked position with upper side rails raised.
6. Emphasize the importance of wearing an identification band while in the hospital and encourage patients to make sure it is checked before receiving medications or treatments.
7. Discuss routines of mealtimes, bathing, procedures, treatments, and other care with patients and, as appropriate, accommodate any cultural, spiritual, or personal rituals, habits, or activities patients would like to continue doing while in the hospital.
8. Communicate with patients in their language and at their developmental level for understanding. Provide orientation to day, place, and name to patients as needed.

>> Stay Current: The STEADI initiative focuses on reducing falls among older adults. STEADI consists of three elements: screening, assessment, and intervention to reduce fall risk. For more information and materials for HCPs, go to https://www.cdc.gov/steadi/materials.html.

NURSING PROCESS

Individualized patient care includes appropriate developmental and chronologic age-specific safety considerations. Safety is a common priority for many patients because of motor or sensory changes from acute or chronic conditions inhibiting functional abilities to protect themselves. For example, patients who have had a stroke may not independently be able to reposition themselves to protect the integrity of their skin from breakdown, and children with cystic fibrosis may not be able to cough up and remove their secretions in order to protect their airways and keep them open for air exchange.

Assessment

Both objective and subjective data are used to assess the safety needs of patients:

- ***Observation and patient interview.*** History of falls, balance issues, medications that may cause orthostatic hypotension, chronic conditions, mobility deficits, sensory deficits, and so on
- ***Physical examination.*** Vital signs, ROM, skin assessment, hearing or visual difficulties, heart and lung sounds, tremors, impaired balance, and so on

Diagnosis

Because of the nature and large number of safety hazards in healthcare settings, there are many nursing diagnoses appropriate for patients focused on safety. Safety can include elements in the environment, the patient's situation, or the patient's homeostasis status. Here are a few examples:

- Lack of knowledge about . . .
- Impaired skin integrity
- Impaired airway clearance
- Poor thermoregulation
- Risk of infection

Planning

Safety goals are decided on by the patient and the nurse and would reflect the nursing diagnosis label, such as:

- The patient will have clear breath sounds by discharge.
- The patient will be able to correctly demonstrate walking with a cane 25 feet by (date).
- The patient will remain free from infection, bleeding, falls, injury, poisoning, and suicide.
- The patient will verbalize three things to do to safely get up out of the bed and sit in a chair by (date).

Implementation

There are many nursing actions that can be done to keep patients safe while in a healthcare setting (acute care facility, extended care facility, community facility, or home setting). There are many opportunities for nurses to teach patients about using safety behaviors to prevent accidents. All interventions need to be prioritized to best meet the safety needs for the patient. Some intervention examples are:

- Assess patient's feet for cracking and dryness and apply lotion after bathing time.
- Collaborate with the physical therapist to teach patient correct cane walking.
- Encourage the patient to use the incentive spirometer every hour while awake as tolerated.
- Staff will promptly respond when patient's call light is activated for assistance to get up to use the restroom.

Evaluation

Expected outcomes may include the following:

- The patient has clear breath sounds at time of discharge.
- The patient is able to correctly demonstrate walking with a cane for 25 feet.
- The patient remains free from infection, bleeding, falls, injury, poisoning, suicide, and so on.
- The patient is able to verbalize three things to do to safely get up out of the bed and sit in a chair.

The nursing plan of care follows a sequence of actions that have a causal relationship. Clustering assessment data results in the identification of the nursing diagnosis; the nursing diagnosis informs goal setting; goals stimulate decisions regarding what interventions will help the patient reach the goal; and evaluation is completed to determine if the interventions were successful in supporting the goal to be obtained. If the goal is not reached, the whole process is reevaluated to determine if the goal and interventions were appropriate for the assessment data and nursing diagnosis. Changes in the goal or interventions may be necessary to individualize them for best patient outcomes.

REVIEW Patient Safety

RELATE Link the Concepts and Exemplars

Linking the exemplar of patient safety with the concept of perioperative care:

1. The nurse notices that a child patient waiting to go to surgery is drinking a glass of milk. What are the priority safety actions for the nurse? Why?
2. Immediate postoperative assessment of a patient postanesthesia would include which priority safety data?

Linking the exemplar of patient safety with the concept of mood and affect:

3. Sometimes patients who are in the manic phase of bipolar disorder are placed in seclusion for a period of time. What are the safety concerns of the staff for making this decision?
4. Is it a potential safety problem when a depressed patient begins putting their affairs in order? Why or why not?

Linking the exemplar of patient safety with the concept of acid–base balance:

5. When a diabetic patient has hyperglycemia, the blood pH goes down, indicating metabolic acidosis. How will the body attempt to correct the metabolic acidosis and return to a pH within normal range?
6. When a patient overuses bicarbonate of soda for an indigestion problem, what safety problem might this cause for the patient's acid–base balance? What needs to be done to correct it?

READY Go to Volume 3: Clinical Nursing Skills

REFER Go to Pearson MyLab Nursing and eText

REFLECT Apply Your Knowledge

A 9-year-old patient is admitted for observation to the medical unit with closed head trauma after falling off his bicycle and hitting his head; he was not wearing his safety helmet. He is drowsy, crying at times, and complaining of a headache. He had two episodes of vomiting while in the emergency department. Last set of vital signs were T 98.8°F, P 102, R 16, B/P 108/72, O_2 saturation 96% room air. His pupils are slightly sluggish but PERRLA. The provider has ordered HOB elevated 30 degrees, phenytoin 125 mg IV BID, and acetaminophen 480 mg PO every 6 hours prn headache. Orders also include NPO status and neuro checks every 2 hours using the Glasgow Coma Scale.

1. What are priority safety considerations with this patient?
2. What might be the reason the patient is receiving phenytoin? What might be the reason he is NPO? What might be the reason to elevate the head of the bed 30 degrees?
3. What priority teaching should the nurse identify at this time to do when the patient is more alert and awake and the parents are present before discharge?

Exemplar 51.C Nurse Safety

Exemplar Learning Outcomes

51.C Analyze safety as it relates to being a nurse.

- Outline the agencies that regulate workplace safety for nurses.
- Describe the etiology and prevalence of injuries to nurses.
- Summarize strategies to prevent injury in nursing practice.

Exemplar Key Terms

Burnout, 2892
Compassion fatigue, 2892
National Institute for Occupational Safety and Health (NIOSH), 2888
Nurse Practice Act (NPA), 2888
Occupational Safety and Health Administration (OSHA), 2888
Scoop method, 2890
Workplace violence, 2891

Overview

Work-related risks, such as bloodborne pathogens, needlesticks, latex allergies, musculoskeletal injuries, mental stress, and violence from patients, are inherent among all healthcare occupations. According to the results of the survey by the Bureau of Labor Statistics, in 2019 healthcare and social assistance occupations had the highest number of nonfatal job-related injuries and illnesses of all occupations, reporting 544,800 injuries and 32,700 workplace illnesses annually (Fabian, 2020). (It should be noted that these are pre-COVID-19 figures.)

Safety in the workplace is critical to job satisfaction and employee retention rates. In nursing, protocols for safety promotion and injury prevention have become more prevalent over the years. These protocols are designed to protect members of the healthcare team and patients.

Regulation of Workplace Safety

The Occupational Safety and Health Act of 1970 created both the **Occupational Safety and Health Administration (OSHA)** and the **National Institute for Occupational Safety and Health (NIOSH)**. OSHA is part of the U.S. Department of Labor. It is a national public health agency to protect workers from safety hazards and health risks in the workplace. NIOSH is part of the Centers for Disease Control and Prevention in the U.S. Department of Health and Human Services. It is a federal agency that conducts research and produces evidence used to find solutions and interventions to protect the safety and health of workers (CDC, 2018c).

Occupational Safety and Health Administration

OSHA enforces the guidelines presented in the OSHA Act of 1970, requiring its covered employees to report specific incidents and illnesses in a timely manner. OSHA developed standards, enforcement actions, compliance assistance, and cooperative programs to prevent injuries and illnesses. OSHA enforces the rights of workers to have a safe work environment. Workers can file a complaint about unsafe work conditions through their whistleblower program asking for an on-site inspection of the situation from OSHA and will be protected from employer retaliation (OSHA, 2020c).

One of the primary functions of OSHA includes consulting with both employees and employers regarding prevention methods for the injuries and illnesses that are most prevalent in each particular work environment. For example, OSHA's involvement with those in the nursing sector includes preventive measures against needlesticks, bloodborne pathogens, and aggression from patients. Inspections of the workplace are conducted by OSHA employees to ensure that individuals are complying with standards. In the healthcare setting, for example, hand hygiene procedures, the use of gloves when working with patients, or the availability of puncture-resistant sharps containers could be monitored.

National Institute for Occupational Safety and Health

According to the CDC (2018c), "the mission of NIOSH is to generate new knowledge in the field of occupational safety and health and to transfer that knowledge into practice for the betterment of workers." NIOSH conducts scientific research to provide advances in safety both in the workplace and for the population at large. In addition to research, NIOSH also develops recommendations for safety procedures, distributes information, provides training videos, and evaluates workplace health hazards.

Research conducted by NIOSH focuses on numerous topics relating to different sectors of the workforce. For example, NIOSH compiles research on the effects of stress in the workplace, which is particularly common in the healthcare community because of the nature of the work being performed. NIOSH can evaluate work environments for health hazards and recommend ways to reduce or eliminate them through its *Health Hazard Evaluation Program.*

Boards of Nursing

In order to protect the public's health and welfare from nurses who are not prepared or competent to provide safe nursing care, state governments used their police powers to enact laws to protect citizens and minimize harm of unsafe nursing practice. These laws are included in the **Nurse Practice Act (NPA)** of each state and authorized by the state's legislature. The guidelines in the NPA focus on safety parameters for nurses to provide safe and effective nursing care for public protection (National Council of State Boards of Nursing [NCSBN], 2020).

Boards of Nursing act to ensure safety by establishing academic requirements for nursing prelicensure programs, identifying standards for all areas from clinical learning experiences to faculty qualifications. Boards of Nursing also establish requirements for licensure, including taking the National Council Licensure Examination for Registered Nurse (NCLEX-RN) and continuing education requirements (NCSBN, 2020). Equally as important, Boards of Nursing establish procedures for reporting errors and violations made by licensed nurses and act to investigate such reports.

Employers, coworkers, the public, healthcare facilities, and others can send anonymous complaints to the Board of Nursing. Complaints about conduct include sexual misconduct, stealing, fraud, confidentiality issues, boundary violations, impairment while working, and drug diversion. Unsafe nurse practice includes inappropriate delegation, abandonment, neglect, exceeding scope of practice, and documentation issues (NCSBN, 2020). See Exemplar 49.A, Nurse Practice Acts, in Module 49, Legal Issues, for more information.

In 2020, the NCSBN responded quickly to the COVID-19 pandemic with changes in NCLEX testing policies and support for states in verifying licensure for nurses returning to work from retirement. Along with the National League for Nursing, NCSBN called for healthcare facilities to continue to offer clinical education to students (National League for Nursing, 2020).

Etiology of Injury and Illness

Injuries and illnesses in the workplace occur in almost every profession. Causes of workplace illness and injury vary by profession. Nurses working in a variety of industries face workplace hazards when performing routine nursing responsibilities. While providing patient care, overexertion and body movements can make them vulnerable to slips, trips, falls, and back injuries. Nurses can come in contact with potentially harmful and hazardous substances. These include radiation, drugs, cleaning chemicals, and unintentional needlesticks that can result in exposure-related injuries and illnesses. Exposure to and transmission of infectious pathogens through contact (such as methicillin-resistant *Staphylococcus aureus*), droplets (such as COVID-19), or air (such as tuberculosis) can result in harmful and serious illnesses for nurses. It is projected that between 2018 and 2028 there will be an increase of 12% in the hiring of registered nurses, above the average for all other occupations (Bureau of Labor Statistics [BLS], 2020).

Prevalence

In 2016, nurses experienced 19,790 nonfatal injuries and illnesses resulting from workplace hazards in private industries (BLS, 2018). Most of these injuries (74.1%) occurred in hospital settings, which reflects a higher incidence than in all other areas in which nurses work, including long-term care facilities (BLS, 2018). Musculoskeletal disorder injuries (such as sprains and tears) requiring time away from work accounted for 51% of all reported injuries and illnesses to RNs in 2016. Of these, some 5,490 cases involved injuries to the back, requiring an average recovery time of 7 days (BLS, 2018).

Most occupational injuries reported by nurses were among those over the age of 45. Nurses ages 35 to 44 accounted for 23.3% of the total, those ages 45 to 54 accounted for 27%, and those ages 55 to 64 accounted for 24.7% (BLS, 2018). Older RNs experienced more severe injuries and illnesses than younger RNs.

Three observations can be made about the occurrence of nonfatal occupational injuries and illnesses involving nurses in 2016 from the above data (BLS, 2018):

- The majority of nurse nonfatal injuries and illnesses resulted from workplace hazards in a hospital setting.
- Nurses experienced more occurrences of musculoskeletal disorders than experienced in other occupations.

All occupational injuries and illnesses have social and economic implications for the workers and their families, ranging from medical costs to loss of quality of life to pain and suffering. Employers and society also share the burden for consequences of occupational safety and health hazards in the workplace. Data collection is dependent on national surveillance systems to record new cases and provide information that can be used to reduce occupational hazards and health issues to prevent injuries, illnesses, and death among healthcare personnel.

Nurses are at high risk for musculoskeletal system and connective tissue injuries because of their work patterns, the increased acuity of patients, the need to keep patients mobile, and the increase in numbers of obese patients. Resources such as training, lifting devices, and lift teams can potentially reduce the number of occupational injuries of healthcare workers. Healthcare facilities can establish and support a safety culture among their employees. Emphasis on occupational safety and health practices can promote a safer work environment and support patient safety. While nurses in all settings have understood this as a critical issue for decades, the onset of the COVID-19 pandemic in 2020 and the lack of personal protective equipment (PPE) available to healthcare workers brought this issue to national awareness. NIOSH can help healthcare facilities identify hazards of safety and health and provide them with a variety of tools and materials to improve employee safety and health (CDC, 2018c).

Illness and Injury Prevention in Nursing Practice

Nurses experience both physical and psychologic demands throughout their shifts. Pressures can come from workforce downsizing, working more hours, the work pace, increased acuity levels of patients, the escalating number of older patients, the complexity of the environment, extended workloads, an older nurse workforce, and the potential for violence and chemical exposures. These factors can contribute to acute or long-term health problems, such as musculoskeletal injuries and disorders, infections, mental health changes, insufficient sleep patterns, and chronic exhaustion (AHRQ, 2020b).

There are many occupational hazards for nurses and other healthcare workers found in all healthcare settings, including acute care, extended-care, and community-based facilities and the home environment. These hazards put healthcare workers at risk for a variety of safety concerns, including exposure to infectious diseases, such as blood and body fluid pathogens, and injuries or accidents. In 2018, healthcare and social assistance workers accounted for 577,500 cases of nonfatal occupational injuries and illnesses (BLS, 2019). To create a safer work environment and prevent illness and injury in nursing practice, the focus needs to be on building an awareness of potential safety hazards and finding solutions to prevent them. For example, exposure to many illnesses can be minimized with simple measures such as hand hygiene and sanitation protocols.

Nurses provide care for patients with diagnosed and sometimes undiagnosed infectious diseases such as influenza, norovirus, methicillin-resistant *Staphylococcus aureus* tuberculosis, HIV, and COVID-19 (RegisteredNursing.org, 2019). Vaccines are available to protect against some pathogens, and healthcare employees are encouraged to take advantage of employer-provided vaccination programs.

>> **Stay Current:** Visit http://www.cdc.gov/vaccines/adults/rec-vac/hcw.html for current CDC recommended vaccines and changes in immunizations for nurses and other healthcare workers.

The CDC has developed comprehensive infection control recommendations that include standard, contact, and airborne precautions for all settings of patient care. Healthcare facilities and organizations that provide home healthcare services have policies and procedures that address safety infection control measures. Guidelines for preventing the transmission of infectious pathogens through use of PPE are available. The proper use of respirators by nurses and other healthcare workers is another preventive practice. Nurses can implement the following strategies to prevent illness:

- Perform frequent and complete hand hygiene
- Don PPE following CDC guidelines *every time*
- If working with a patient on isolation precautions, call for assistance as needed
- Avoid touching the nose, eye areas, and mouth on one's own face
- Engage in self-care to keep the immune system healthy: appropriate diet, sleep, relaxation, and activity
- If beginning to feel sick at work, go home as soon as appropriate
- If feeling sick at home, don't go to work; stay at home.

Nurses must be vigilant in the prevention of injuries and illness in their workplace environment, in their nursing practice, and for their own personal safety. Healthcare facilities have policies for preventing injuries and maintaining a safe work environment. Safe practice and protocols can be implemented to sustain a nurse's well-being when working with infectious (or potentially infectious) agents, needles, latex, chemical exposure, and patient handling.

Needlestick Injuries

Needlestick and sharps injuries are a large and growing problem in the healthcare industry. Some 600 exposures occur every day in U.S. hospitals. Approximately 60 pathogens (i.e., viruses, bacteria, fungi, or parasites) can be transmitted by needles (Grimmond, 2020). The CDC believes that over half of all sharps injuries are not reported as required, including those that happen to HCPs, laboratory personnel, and housekeeping staff. Sharps injuries are very serious and can result in numerous illnesses. The *STOP STICKS* campaign, initiated by NIOSH, works to raise awareness of the risks associated with bloodborne pathogens most commonly associated with sharps injuries, such as HIV and hepatitis B and C. Although this campaign was originally developed for emergency departments and operating rooms, the ideas extend to all other healthcare fields that use sharps. The *STOP STICKS* campaign provides resources for exposure prevention methods and equipment evaluations and the requirements for sharps disposal containers (CDC, 2019k).

In 2018, nurses incurred 38.9% of injuries from reported needlesticks (Grimmond, 2020). When working with used or contaminated sharps, nurses should employ extra precautions to avoid unnecessary injuries. Needles that have been used are almost never recapped (unless this is necessary because of protocol) and are disposed of in an appropriate sharps container. Approved disposal containers should be present wherever sharps are used and must be both puncture resistant and leakproof on the bottom and all sides. If sharps do need to be recapped, this should be done with the use of another device (such as a hemostat), or with the **scoop method**. In the scoop method, the cap is placed on a table or hard surface and the tip of the needle is guided into the cap; to ensure the cap is on tight, it can be pressed against a hard surface such as a table or wall. Nurses should *never* hold the cap in one hand while trying to guide the tip of the needle into the cap with the other—this method substantially increases the risk of a sharps-related injury. Needlestick and sharps injuries arise from a number of different situations, such as not implementing proper disposal techniques, failure to recap the needle, bumping into an uncapped and used needle, or contact with a used scalpel (CDC, 2019k).

>> **Stay Current:** Visit https://www.cdc.gov/nora/councils/hcsa/stopsticks/default.html for more information on the STOP STICKS campaign.

Chemical Exposure

Nurses can be exposed to a high level of chemicals used in sterilizing and pest control, volatile organic compounds such as formaldehyde, and pharmaceuticals such as antineoplastics. These products come in a variety of forms, including gas, aerosol, and skin contaminants, so they can be absorbed through the lungs or skin. Exposure may be a one-time occurrence, but it can also occur over time. Some chemicals are regulated in terms of exposure, requiring employees to take more precautionary measures when handling these substances. However, many common chemicals and compounds can cause both injury and illness if they are accidentally spilled or ignited (OSHA, 2020a).

Safe Patient Handling

The Nurse and Healthcare Worker Protection Act of 2015 was proposed in an effort to prevent injuries to nurses, healthcare workers, and patients. The act discusses the large number of musculoskeletal disorders and injuries that affect nurses that are often the result of helping to move, lift, or reposition patients. The safe patient handling and injury prevention standard within the act requires the use of mechanical devices to lift or move patients, unless the use of these devices proves to be unsafe or is contraindicated for the patient for some reason. Using mechanical devices to help move patients aids in avoiding unnecessary musculoskeletal injuries for both nurses and other healthcare workers (**Figure 51.12** >>). The act also establishes extensive training in safe patient handling methods for all nurses on The Association of Safe Patient Handling Professionals website at www.asphp.org.

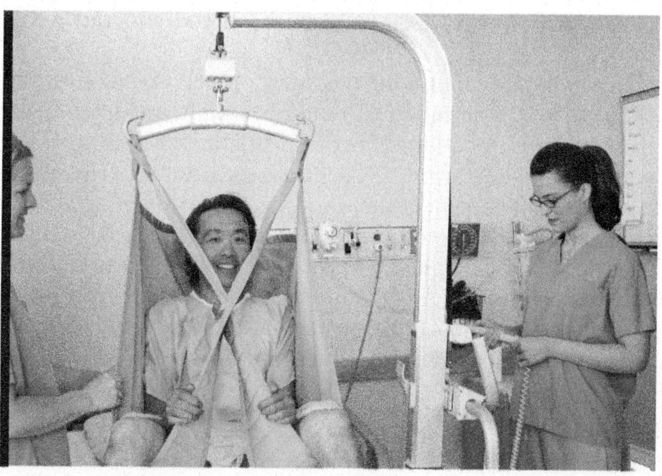

Figure 51.12 » Nurses using a floor-mounted mechanical lift to move a patient.

Source: Trish233/iStock/Getty Images.

Effective and safe patient handling helps to promote patient safety as well as nurse safety. Patient handling can be done more safely by using height-adjustable electric beds, mobile mechanical and ceiling-mounted patient lifts, antifriction devices, band transfer aids, and bed or chair repositioning.

Workplace Violence Protection

Workplace violence is defined by NIOSH as "any physical assault, threatening behavior or verbal abuse occurring in the work setting" (CDC, 2019f). Nurses and other healthcare workers are at particular risk of violence in the workplace. Violence can come from patients, their families, or visitors because of inadequate workplace security, unrestricted movement by visitors around the healthcare facility, personal relationship altercations in the workplace, or a healthcare worker bullying another worker. Although routinely there are higher risks of injuries from assaults by patients or their families in an emergency department or mental health nursing unit, no department in a healthcare facility is immune from workplace violence. Potential injuries include nurses being scratched, hit, kicked, beat, bitten, and sometimes threatened with weapons such as knives or guns.

Some strategies to prevent workplace violence are keep hair tucked away, use breakaway lanyards, be aware of and note any change in surroundings, and note verbal and nonverbal cues that signal increasing patient agitation or anger, inappropriate abusive language or behaviors from coworkers, and signs that someone may be acutely emotionally upset to the degree that they are unable to think clearly with a change in rational behaviors. Some healthcare facilities offer employees training in managing aggressive behaviors (**Figure 51.13 »**).

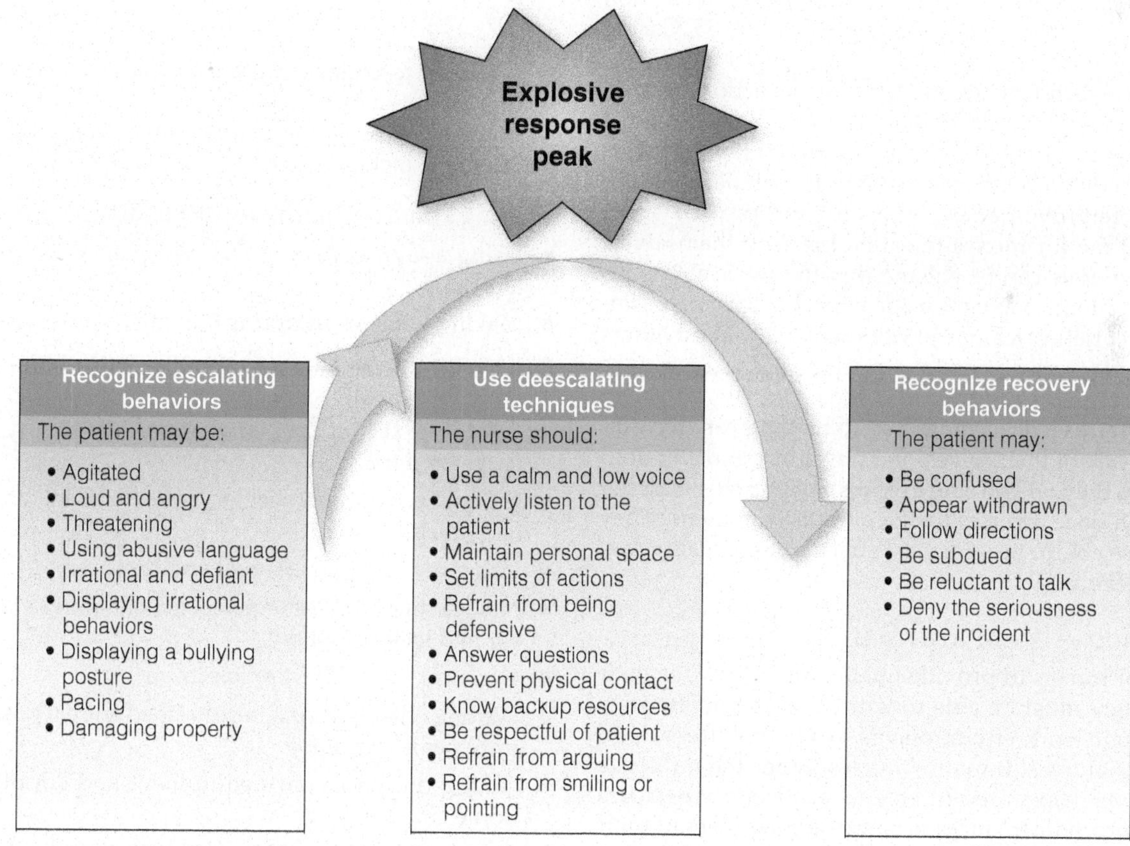

Figure 51.13 » The process of deescalating aggressive behaviors includes three stages: recognizing escalating behaviors, using deescalating techniques, and recognizing recovery behaviors.

Many states have enacted legislation to address violence in the workplace by increasing punishments for those who attack nurses and by requiring employers to provide training on workplace violence. NIOSH collects data on reports of violence against nurses in order to aid in further prevention efforts and to develop training programs and new policies aimed at increasing safety measures for nurses and other healthcare workers (CDC, 2019f).

Mental Health Safety

Caring for others is a hallmark of the nursing profession. As a helping profession, nursing involves significant responsibility for the well-being of others on many levels in addition to working in a highly stressful environment. Prolonged response to the many nursing work stressors mentioned at the beginning of this exemplar can lead not only to fatigue and distress but also to physical, mental, and emotional depletion, often referred to as **burnout** or **compassion fatigue**. Nurses who experience compassion fatigue also experience less satisfaction from their work and are less engaged with their patients. The quality of their performance and interactions is affected.

It is essential for nurses to take care of their own physical and emotional selves so they can be physically, mentally, and emotionally prepared to care for their patients. Nurses need to look at themselves and recognize where stressors are coming from and think about what they can do to reduce stress and strain. These include maintaining a healthy lifestyle, engaging in healthy coping mechanisms and support systems, and learning to say "no" when appropriate to limit extra demands on their time. Additional information on self-care in nursing can be found in Module 35, Caring Interventions.

Healthcare facilities can and should take actions to support their nursing workforce. For example, they can invest in reduced nurse–patient ratios to lessen nurse work pressures. This would give nurses more time with patients and potentially improve patient outcomes and provide short periods of time for nurses to eat and refresh themselves. Workplace morale can be enhanced with appreciation and incentives for improvements made in patient safety and satisfaction. Debriefing teams can work with nurses and others after psychologically stressful situations occur. Employee assistance programs can address compassion fatigue. When nurses are refreshed, recommitted to helping care for others, taking care of themselves, and physically and emotionally healthy, they will be able to withstand the challenges of nursing and once again enjoy helping their patients. They will again be able to provide safe, effective, and quality care for their patients.

Substance Abuse and Safety

In order for nurses to provide quality and safety for their patients, they must be able to withstand the many pressures of their work environments as well as stressors in their personal lives. Impaired nurses under the influence of alcohol or drugs are not able to proficiently perform necessary procedures, make accurate decisions about their nursing responsibilities, or make necessary critical clinical judgments about patient care. Impairment in the clinical environment increases risks to both patient and nurse safety.

Every Board of Nursing has substance abuse policies, procedures, and expectation guidelines about treatment, nursing license status, rehabilitation, peer nurse support groups, and conditions of returning to the nursing workforce. There may be legal involvement of federal drug enforcement agencies if controlled narcotic substances have been diverted, used, or sold to others. Employee assistance programs can support recovering nurses. Addiction is treatable, recovery is difficult but possible, and relapse can happen (for more information about substance abuse among nurses, see Module 22, Addiction).

Home Healthcare Nurses and Injuries

Providing home health nursing care can be just as challenging and rewarding as providing care in a healthcare facility. Unfortunately, it also can have many of the same safety hazards—for example, bloodborne and infectious pathogens, needlesticks, latex, chemical exposure, and patient handling. In addition to these, home healthcare nurses may also contend with hostile animals, unhygienic and dangerous surroundings, and road travel to patients' homes. OSHA has many materials on safety available for healthcare workers on their website.

Safety measures for the home health nurse begin with an assessment of the patient's home and neighborhood to identify potential risks. This assessment can be a part of the discharge planning and patient/family education to help create a safe environment for everyone. Ongoing safety training for nurses should include personal protection maneuvers, prevention of infectious disease, needlestick safety, minimizing latex allergic reactions, avoiding chemical exposure, and prevention of musculoskeletal injuries.

Common steps to follow to maintain safety for the home health nurse include:

- Being aware of immediate surroundings
- Using a GPS system or detailed map to know address locations
- Making home visits during daylight hours, if possible
- Parking the car in a lighted area with minimal shrubs close by
- Avoiding setting personal items or supply bags on carpeted floor
- Using mechanical devices to assist in lifting and moving as available
- Using nonlatex gloves and hand sanitizer
- Not leaving supplies or personal belongings visible in the car and locking doors
- Carrying extra PPE supplies in car
- Waiting outside door if unrestrained animal poses a threat until pet is restrained
- Taking only necessary equipment and supplies inside home
- Anticipating homes that may not be cooled or heated and wearing appropriate clothing.

REVIEW Nurse Safety

RELATE Link the Concepts and Exemplars

Linking the exemplar on nurse safety with the concept of mobility:

1. Describe methods of helping a patient with multiple sclerosis to reposition without compromising the nurse's own musculoskeletal health.
2. Among nurses, what are some common causes of back injury in the workplace? What are some methods for decreasing the incidence of these injuries?

Linking the exemplar on nurse safety with the concept of communication:

3. During a home visit, a patient becomes verbally aggressive toward the nurse. What communication techniques should the nurse employ with this patient? Explain your answer.

Linking the exemplar on nurse safety with the concept of reproduction:

4. The new mother is trying to hold her newborn while eating breakfast. What are some potential safety problems with this situation? What should the nurse do?
5. A nurse making rounds notices that a newborn is being carried by the mother, who is taking a short walk down the hallway. Is this a safety concern? Why or why not?

READY Go to Volume 3: Clinical Nursing Skills

REFER Go to Pearson MyLab Nursing and eText

REFLECT Apply Your Knowledge

The nurse is inserting an intravenous (IV) access device into a patient's arm. The patient has advanced hepatitis C and has been admitted to the hospital because of hepatitis-induced liver failure. After inserting the IV device, the nurse places the needle portion on the patient's bed so he can quickly secure infusion tubing to the IV port. When the patient moves her arm, the needle falls to the floor. Upon retrieving the needle, the nurse accidentally punctures himself. Once the needle has punctured his skin, he immediately stops what he is doing and washes the injury site thoroughly with warm, soapy water.

1. After cleansing the injury site, what should be the nurse's next action?
2. Could the nurse have done anything differently in this situation to avoid the injury? Explain your answer.
3. Explain the postexposure follow-up guidelines for individuals who sustain needlestick injuries.

» Exemplar 51.D Medication Safety

Exemplar Learning Outcomes

51.D Analyze medication administration as it relates to safety.

- Differentiate among pharmacokinetics, pharmacodynamics, and pharmacotherapy.
- Analyze strategies nurses use to promote safe medication administration across care settings and for patients taking medications at home.
- Examine current considerations in the nursing care of diverse groups of patients in need of pharmacotherapy.
- Describe strategies for ensuring safe medication use by patients across the lifespan.

Exemplar Key Terms

Adverse drug event, *2895*
Efficacy, *2895*
Medication reconciliation, *2897*
Pharmacodynamics, *2894*
Pharmacogenetics, *2898*
Pharmacokinetics, *2894*
Pharmacology, *2893*
Pharmacotherapy, *2894*
Polypharmacy, *2901*
Rights of administration, *2896*
Target effects, *2894*

Pharmacology Overview

Pharmacologic practices have been recorded in ancient civilizations throughout the world for centuries. Earliest records list various medicinal plants and herbs, animal products, and compound mixtures being used to treat pain, fever, and an assortment of bodily ailments. Today, **pharmacology** is the science of how drugs influence body systems and how the body responds to them. The practice of nursing requires a basic comprehension of anatomy and physiology, pathophysiology, chemistry, and microbiology to understand the chemical interactions and biological effects of medications. This information is valuable to promoting best patient outcomes for patients receiving *pharmacotherapy*, or therapeutic drug treatment.

Medication competencies for nurses include:

- Accurate dose calculations
- Safe drug administration
- Familiarity with drug and food actions and interactions that can affect a change in body systems and the patient's well-being.

In the United States, all drugs that are developed are tested before approval for safe, effective use. It is through the process of discovery, development, testing, and approval that drugs acquire their names. When a new drug is discovered, it receives a chemical name based on its chemical composition and molecular structure. After several years of further development, required testing, regulatory approval from the U.S.

Food and Drug Administration (FDA) and clinical trials, the drug receives a generic name from the U.S. Adopted Name (USAN), which identifies the drug's active ingredient. The drug company then gives the drug a trade, or brand, name and can market the new medication. For example:

- Chemical Name: N-acetyl-p-aminophenol
- Generic Name: acetaminophen
- Brand Name: Tylenol

In 2019, the FDA approved more than 20,000 new prescription drugs for marketing in the United States.

Pharmacokinetics

Pharmacokinetics relates to the four processes used to move drugs through the body: absorption, distribution, metabolism, and excretion. *Absorption* refers to the movement of drugs from the administration site into the bloodstream.

In the bloodstream, drugs move throughout the body to reach and bind to their target cells at specific receptor sites. This is the *distribution* process. At different points in the distribution process, a drug may encounter one or more barriers. Examples of barriers include capillary wall membranes, intercellular fluids, the blood–brain barrier, and the placental barrier. As a drug travels through the bloodstream, it can negatively affect tissues or organs that are not target receptor sites.

Once a drug is distributed to receptors, *metabolism* occurs. During metabolism, the drug is broken down through hydration, hydrolysis, oxidization, or reduction. Most metabolism takes place in the liver, where enzymes reduce drug molecules into metabolites. The metabolites are then *excreted* as waste, mostly through urine and feces. However, drugs may also be excreted in saliva, sweat, exhaled air, or breast milk.

Because drugs go to several areas of the body at the same time, measuring the blood level of a drug is usually the most accurate way to measure a drug's concentration in the body when assessing its effect on the patient. This can be especially important when working with younger and older patients, whose age can influence pharmacokinetic processes (see Focus on Diversity and Culture: Age and Pharmacokinetics).

Pharmacodynamics

Pharmacodynamics studies how the body reacts to the composition of drugs, such as the drug's molecular, biochemical, and physiologic effects. These effects can be classified as immediate or delayed and as direct or indirect. How the body reacts to drugs can be affected by body changes due to aging, genetic factors, disease processes, body mass, or interactions with other drugs. The pharmacologic effect on the body can be affected by how well the drug binds with the target receptor site and its concentration at the target receptor site. As nurses manage drug therapeutic treatments, they can observe for changes in the effectiveness of body systems, assess for potential adverse drug effects caused by medications, and better understand how body organs can work more efficiently with appropriate drug therapy (**Box 51.1** »).

Pharmacotherapy

Pharmacotherapy is the treatment of diseases and medical conditions using pharmaceutical drugs. Medication therapy may be used to prevent or cure an illness, minimize/relieve symptoms, or promote health. For example, an antibiotic is given to cure infection and an antipyretic is given to lower fever. Studies show that some medications intended for treating one medical condition have been found to have unexpected benefits and additional uses in promoting health by minimizing other medical conditions not previously diagnosed. For example, one study concluded that losartan, an antihypertensive medication, also was effective in treating hyperuricemia. Losartan lowers serum uric acid by increasing uric acid excretion, which reduces the formation of uric acid crystals and lowers the risk for incident gout (Paauw, 2018).

Therapeutic use of medications takes into account both a drug's action as well as potential reactions. The drug's **target effect** is the expected action the drug will have on the patient. Potential reactions include:

- ***Side effects.*** Wanted or unwanted secondary effects that occur when taking medications. They vary for each individual and can occur when a patient first starts taking

Focus on Diversity and Culture

Age and Pharmacokinetics

As people age, the pharmacokinetic processes of absorption, distribution, metabolism, and excretion of drugs change. Young children, with their immature systems and healthy livers, may experience greater side effects and require age- or size-related dosages. However, they also metabolize drugs faster than adults and their bodies also tend to excrete medications faster (Potter & Moller, 2020).

In contrast, older adults tend to metabolize and excrete (or clear) drugs at a much slower rate. This has two important implications for nurses. The first is that an older adult who has taken the same medication for a chronic condition for many years may begin to exhibit symptoms of drug toxicity. This can occur if the patient is not metabolizing and excreting the drug quickly enough, causing increased concentration (or a buildup) of the drug in the bloodstream. This may occur over a period of weeks, making it difficult to identify drug toxicity until adverse effects develop. The second consideration is that the older adult patient may need a lower starting dose of a medication and perhaps a longer trial before determining if the dosage needs to be increased.

There are other age-related considerations. Small-bowel surface areas decrease as people age, which can lead to increased constipation and decreased calcium absorption, although it usually doesn't affect absorption for most drugs. Another consideration is that body fat usually increases with age, and total body weight lessens. In turn, this increases the distribution volume of high lipoid drugs such as diazepam. As serum albumin decreases, risk for toxic effects from drugs such as phenytoin and warfarin increases. Aging kidneys may not be able to eliminate drugs as well as they used to. Because blood creatinine levels may remain normal, the creatinine clearance level is used to guide dosing for drugs eliminated by the kidneys (Ruscin & Linnebur, 2019).

Box 51.1

Adverse Drug Events

An **adverse drug event** (ADE) occurs when an individual patient is harmed by a medication. This occurs when a medication fails to achieve the expected therapeutic response and, instead, causes a harmful response, *or* when a patient receives an incorrect medication or dosage in error that results in harm to the patient. Injuries from medication administration can affect the liver, skin, kidney, heart, or muscle or cause general hypersensitivity reactions (AHRQ, 2019b). ADEs are defined according to their degree of injury and impact on the body:

- *Suspected Adverse Reaction:* Implies a reasonable possibility that an ADE was caused by a drug.
- *Adverse Reaction:* Implies an ADE was caused by a drug.
- *Adverse Event of Special Interest:* Implies ADE was caused by a drug and requires continued monitoring.
- *Unexpected ADE:* Implies the ADE was not suspected or included with risk information or that it is more severe than expected.
- *Serious ADE:* Implies hospitalization or extended care needed or may be disabling or result in significant incapacity of doing everyday functions.
- *Life-Threatening ADE:* Implies an immediate risk of death (Institute for Clinical and Translational Science, 2019).

Adverse drug events can occur anywhere throughout the medication administration process, from order to administration. ADEs can occur in any healthcare setting, including at home. They can involve health professionals who prescribe, prepare, and administer medications and patients who receive them.

Approximately 5% of hospitalized patients experience ADEs. Each year, ADEs cause approximately 700,000 emergency department visits and about 100,000 hospital admissions. Transitions in care settings are also sources of preventable medication-related harm (AHRQ, 2019c). The majority of ADEs are preventable. High-alert medications, such as insulin, anticoagulants, and opioids, have the highest risk of causing harm and thus require special alertness to safety guidelines when administering them.

a medication, when dosage changes are made, or when a patient stops taking a medication. A wanted side effect example is the benefit of induced drowsiness when a patient needs to rest. Nausea, headache, constipation, dryness of mouth, and skin rash are examples of unwanted side effects.

- ***Adverse effects.*** Undesirable, harmful effects of a medication. Examples include anaphylaxis, lowered blood pressure, toxicity, stomach irritation with bleeding, and anemia. See Box 51.1 for more information on adverse drug events.
- ***Teratogenic effects.*** Teratogenic medications affect development of the embryo or fetus during pregnancy. Teratogenic effects are physical or functional malformations such as cleft palate, heart defects, and spina bifida. They can also cause spontaneous abortions, miscarriages, and preterm labor. Examples of teratogenic medications include aminopterin, phenytoin, valproic acid, warfarin, and angiotensin-converting enzyme (ACE) inhibitors.
- ***Drug–drug interactions.*** Reactions between two or more drugs that can decrease the efficacy of a drug, enhance the action of a drug, or result in undesirable side effects. In some cases, mild interactions are predictable and therefore may be manageable. However, some drug–drug interactions are known to be dangerous and should be avoided. Examples of serious drug–drug interactions are warfarin and erythromycin, digoxin and quinidine, and theophylline and ciprofloxacin.
- ***Drug–food interactions.*** Reactions between drugs and foods, beverages, or dietary supplements may cause unwanted or unexpected results. Drug effects can be increased, decreased, change the body's ability to use the drug, or cause a serious side effect. Examples of drug–food interactions are verapamil and grapefruit juice, diphenhydramine and alcohol, and levothyroxine and any food or beverage.

When an HCP determines that medication needs to be prescribed, the provider will select a drug for its features—targeted effect or action, route of administration, and dosage—and safety considerations. Safety considerations may include side effects, cost, and overall therapeutic efficacy. **Efficacy** refers to a medication's ability to achieve the intended response.

In addition, the prescribing provider will carefully evaluate the risks and benefits of using the drug. The patient's medical history is also taken into consideration. Effective drug treatments can improve patient outcomes by relieving symptoms, improving function, maintaining mobility, or prolonging life. Drug treatments with low efficacy can cause ADEs such as discomfort, disability, or in rare cases, death.

Pharmacotherapy is often used along with other treatments or therapies. For example, a patient receiving chemotherapy drugs can be prescribed antinausea or antiemetic medications or a combination of the two to prevent, minimize, or relieve nausea and vomiting associated with chemotherapy.

Medication Administration and Management

Nurses are responsible and accountable for following nursing standards for their scope of practice in using knowledge and skills to provide safe, effective, and appropriate drug therapy. Using the nursing process helps nurses in managing medication administration, patient monitoring, and patient education to protect patients and limit risks of harm from ADEs.

Mistakes can occur at any of six stages when medications are:

- Ordered
- Transcribed
- Dispensed
- Administered
- Monitored
- Documented.

Almost 50% of medication errors occur when the provider creates the medication order. Examples of errors include wrong medication, wrong route, wrong dose, and wrong frequency. Data indicate that between 30 and 70% of these errors are recognized, questioned, and stopped by nurses, pharmacists, or electronic safeguards before medications are administered to patients (Tariq & Scherbak, 2019).

Because nurses are most involved with administering medications to patients, they need to be competent and alert for potentially unsafe medications or errors in medication orders before administering them to patients. Nurses are responsible for clarifying erroneous, unusual, or conflicting medical orders. This is essential to prevent harm to the patient resulting from a medication error.

Following the six core **rights of administration** (right patient, right drug, right dose, right time, right route, and right documentation) provides a safety check for nurses administering medications.

Medication Orders and Schedules

Before administering medication(s) to patients, nurses check provider orders in patient medical records to verify that medication orders have all required elements present (**Table 51.10** »).

Each healthcare facility has policies and procedures for safe medication administration. These policies can define types of orders, routine times of frequency, and guidelines as to when nurses can receive medication orders orally.

After administering any medication, nurses document on patient medication administration records (MAR) the name of medications, dosages, routes, forms, sites (if appropriate), and times medications were administered and their initials or name and title within a short amount of time. PRN medications ordered may require notations in the nurse's notes section of patient medical records in addition to MAR to explain why they were given. Following medication administration, the nurse should evaluate and record the patient's response according to the facility's policies and procedures.

Some orders for PRN medications (as well as some standing orders) require that the nurse follow established *parameters* for administration. Parameters provide measurable safety guidelines to help prevent drug adverse events. Insulin sliding scales (which specify dosing depending on the patient's blood glucose level) are a type of parameter for drug administration. Another example might be an order that includes administration of a second dose if the patient fails to achieve adequate response as identified by the prescribing provider.

Communicating with Healthcare Providers

Clarifying Medication Orders

Healthcare providers may unintentionally select the wrong dosage or medication name when entering a medication order in the patient's electronic medical record. Be professional and concise when clarifying medication orders with providers over the telephone.

"Hi Dr. Stanford, this is Sally Green, the nurse taking care of your patient, Mr. Keys, who was admitted with hematuria to the med-surg floor at Grady Hospital.

- I am calling to check with you about the order you entered this morning for Mr. Keys. Did you mean to order Lasix 400 mg PO every morning? Is this correct?"
- I'm calling about the Lasix order you entered for Mr. Keys this morning that reads, 'Lasix 400 mg PO every morning.'"
- Would you please clarify the dosage of Lasix you want Mr. Keys to have every morning in the order you entered in his EMR?"

Medication Administration

Nurses need to be familiar with policies and procedures for medication administration in healthcare facilities or organizations where they are employed. Before administering any medications, nurses should be familiar with actions, dose ranges, correct dose calculations, route procedures, possible interactions, side effects, and adverse effects of the medications.

Nurses should assess patients before and after medication administration. They should provide patient teaching about the medication(s) before administration and perform documentation done quickly after medication administration, including all appropriate information following facility policy. Nurses can provide safe medication administration

TABLE 51.10 Medication Orders

Required Elements and Types of Orders	
■ Patient's name and date of birth ■ Date and time order created, signature of HCP who ordered the medication ■ Name of the drug (generic and/or brand), dosage, route, frequency, duration, reason for the medication, and any special instructions	
Types of Orders	
Standing Order	■ An order dependent upon the presence of specific clinical criteria ■ All patients meeting the specific clinical criteria for the order receive the same medication or treatment
Single Order	■ Administer a single dose at a specific time ■ Example: oxycodone one 5-mg tablet PO at 0700 one time today
PRN order	■ Administer as needed for a specified time interval between doses for a specific symptom or cluster of symptoms ■ Example: acetaminophen 325 mg PO every 6 hr PRN for headache
STAT order	■ Administer one time, immediately ■ Example: furosemide 20 mg IV push STAT

by following the six core rights of medication administration listed below:

1. Right patient	Two identifiers needed to verify patient's identity
2. Right drug	The medication label matches the HCP's order and is appropriate to treat the patient
3. Right dose	The strength and dose on label match the order or requires cutting tablet in half or giving multiple tablets for ordered dose
4. Right time	Scheduled time matches ordered time interval for doses
5. Right route	Route matches ordered route to administer medication
6. Right documentation	Documentation is done right after medication is administered

By ensuring that the right medication at the right dose is being given to the right patient at the right time and by the right route, the nurse's actions help to ensure quality and safety for the patient, protecting the patient against a possible adverse reaction or an overdose. In addition, by correctly documenting when and how the medication was administered (as well as which medication and dosage), the nurse prevents anyone else from accidentally duplicating administration of the medication order.

>> **Skills:** See Skill 2.11, Medication Administration Systems, in Volume 3. Routes of medication administration are also covered in Volume 3.

Nurses working in settings with older adults should be aware of the American Geriatrics Society 2019 Beers Criteria for Potentially Inappropriate Medication Use in Older Adults (American Geriatric Society, 2019; Greenberg, 2019). The Beers Criteria provide evidence-based lists of medications that are potentially inappropriate for HCPs to prescribe for older adults. The drugs listed are updated by an interprofessional expert group that reviews published evidence every 3 years. Healthcare providers use this information in addition to their own clinical judgment and common sense to identify appropriate medications and dosages for individual patients. The goal is to improve safety, have quality patient outcomes, and prevent ADEs. Examples of medications identified in the Beers Criteria include anticholinergics, such as oral diphenhydramine, and many benzodiazepines, such as diazepam and lorazepam. Benzodiazepines, for example, are associated with increased risk for falls among older adults (Díaz-Gutiérrez et al., 2017).

>> **Stay Current:** The complete Beers Criteria list can be found at https://www.americangeriatrics.org/media-center/news/older-people-medications-are-common-updated-ags-beers-criteriar-aims-make-sure.

Medication Monitoring

Nurses work with HCPs and pharmacists to maintain safety of continuum of care when patients move from nursing unit to nursing unit or from one healthcare facility to another facility or home. Each year, The Joint Commission disseminates National Patient Safety Goals that provide specific guidelines for accredited healthcare facilities to follow to prevent medication mistakes such as the need to label medications appropriately, take precautions for administering anticoagulant therapy, and follow guidelines for conducting medication reconciliations. **Medication reconciliation** is the action of checking any new medication prescribed against a patient's current medications and reconciling or addressing any potential problems. This comparison helps to identify any duplications, potential drug–drug interactions, and forgotten drugs so that only current medications needed by patients will be continued.

Nurses coordinate the continuum of pharmacotherapy through communication between the sending nurse and the receiving nurse when patients move between nursing units and healthcare facilities. Nurses also communicate with families of patients when they are discharged home in an attempt to ensure continued safety in medication administration. For example, a follow-up call a day or two after discharge provides an opportunity for patients or their family members to ask questions or report any side effects.

Patient Education

Nurses can help prevent medication errors in a number of ways, including by engaging patients in discussions about their medication(s). Medication teaching begins with assessment of current medications prescribed as well as the patient's use of OTC medications and supplements. Medication teaching includes:

- The names and purposes of all medications
- How to read labels on medication containers
- When and how medications should be taken
- Common side effects and how to address them
- ADEs that should be reported to HCPs
- Possible drug interactions with other drugs, food, and diseases
- How to check expiration dates on medication containers at scheduled intervals
- How to dispose of medications as recommended by the pharmacy or HCP's office
- Not mixing medications in one medicine container
- Keeping medications at the correct temperature in the refrigerator and separate from foods
- Not skipping doses of medication
- Not sharing personal prescription medications with others and not taking prescription medications that do not have one's name on the label.

Additional information related to patient teaching can be found in the Lifespan Considerations section.

The World Health Organization (2020c) has identified *five moments* that nurses can teach patients to help them recognize an opportunity to ensure their own safety:

- At the time the medication is prescribed and the patient *starts* taking the medication.
- When the patient gets home and is *taking* the medication and may forget the instructions or begin to experience side effects.

- When a new medication is *added*, and interactions may occur
- When *reviewing* medications at the next appointment
- And when the patient *stops* taking a medication.

Nurses can help patients understand how they can promote their own safety in these situations. For example, by encouraging patients to call the provider or the pharmacist if they have any questions once they get home.

Issues with Patient Self-Administration

Patients with alterations in cognition or memory, vision, or physical dexterity are at increased risk for overdosing or underdosing when taking medications at home. One assessment tool frequently used with older patients to determine functional ability in activities of daily living, including self-administration of medications, is the Lawton Instrumental Activities of Daily Living Scale (IADL) (Coyne, 2019). Use of the IADL can help nurses determine if patients are capable of safely maintaining medication adherence by assessing:

- Patient health literacy and level of knowledge about prescribed medications, including potential side effects and when to seek medical help
- Any hurdles to medication adherence specific to the patient.

Use of the IADL can help the nurse determine if a patient needs supportive assistance when developing treatment plans. For example, patients in the early stages of dementia or patients with mild intellectual disability may need visual cues (such as a chart with photos) or other reminders to help them maintain treatment adherence (**Figure 51.14** »). The nurse may help the patient program their smartphone to alert them to when it's time to take a medication or suggest a smartphone equipped with telehealth services, including medication reminders.

For patients who are disabled, a nurse case manager or social worker may be able to arrange for assistance with medication adherence if family members are not able to provide support. Some home health assistance may be available for short periods of time depending on the patient's acuity. In other instances, nurses may have to help patients find alternative solutions. For example, what if a patient with hand tremors is prescribed an injectable medication, and the patient's health insurance will only cover the medication if the patient self-administers at home? The nurse may have to arrange to teach a family member how to administer the medication or find another alternative, such as advocating for a different medication that can be administered orally or advocating for the patient to receive the medication at the provider's office at no charge. Patients are discouraged from self-administration or using their own medications while in a healthcare facility as doing so may interfere with patients receiving correct medications ordered in the right dose and at the right time. Some facilities may secure home medications and return them to patients at discharge, or they may ask a family member or friend to take any medications brought from home with them.

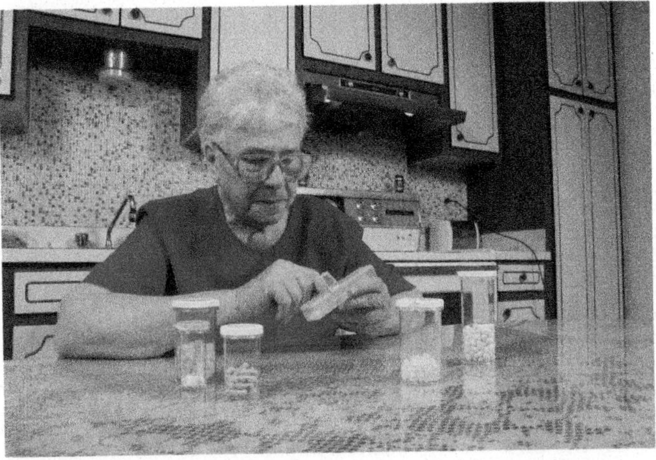

Figure 51.14 » Pill boxes that identify the day and/or time medications should be taken can help prevent patients from missing doses.

Source: Pinkcandy/Shutterstock.

» **Stay Current:** Visit https://consultgeri.org/try-this/general-assessment/issue-23.pdf to review the IADL tool used with older adults to assess functional ability in activities of daily living.

Care Considerations

Cultural, biological, environmental, and social factors can influence not only patient health, but also risk for diseases, medical conditions, and increased stress. All of these factors can be incorporated when nurses are assessing, planning, providing, and evaluating care for patients. Nurses being culturally sensitive can help meet the challenges of accommodating each individual's cultural differences.

Genetic and Cultural Variations

Pharmacogenetics is the study of how genetics can influence a drug response. Evidence indicates that a dosage of a medication that works for one ethnic group may not work as well for another group of people because of differences in genetics and diet (Caffrey, 2019). In other words, ethnic origin can be a factor in metabolism. For example, Kim et al. (2004) are one of many groups of researchers to recognize that people of East Asian ancestry metabolize certain drugs at a slower rate than Caucasians. Rajman et al. (2017) noted that there is greater genetic diversity among people of African descent and that there may be regional differences in drug responses and reactions.

Although individual practices and responses vary, an understanding of cultural differences can help nurses in the assessment of patients and assist in the exploration of best treatments and potential drug–drug interactions. Being familiar with the patient's diet, use of tobacco and alcohol, herbal supplements, or alternative remedies are important considerations. For example, a patient may take garlic as an herbal supplement, not realizing that it can lower blood pressure, which could be dangerous if the patient is also taking antihypertensive medication. Another patient may avoid taking pain medication in fear of becoming addicted to it. Nurses need to be culturally sensitive when taking care of patients with cultural differences and remain nonjudgmental of behaviors and responses from patients. For further information about developing cultural competence as a nurse, see Module 24, Culture and Diversity.

Environment

The environment in which individuals live can influence their behaviors, health, nutrition, relationships, intellect, and lifestyles. Living environments are becoming less traditional because of educational, situational, financial, substance abuse, mental illness, and criminal circumstances. Nurses today work in settings such as community clinics, jails, prisons, shelters, and colleges, among others. In these diverse settings, nurses provide medical education programs, treatments, care planning, and medication monitoring and management.

Students attending college often live away from home in a dormitory or apartment. Without direct parental supervision and support, some students begin to experiment by using medications to stay up late to study, reduce anxiety, or achieve euphoria. Students may misuse prescription medications by taking a higher dose than prescribed or by trying another student's medication, both of which are illegal. Equally as dangerous, students with chronic illness may have difficulty following their medication schedules without parental reminders or when daily routines fluctuate due to variable work and class schedules. Educating young adults before they leave home for college or move out to live on their own can help prevent inappropriate medication use that may lead to accidental harm.

Each night in the United States, more than 500,000 people experience homelessness (National Alliance to End Homelessness, 2020). A variety of factors lead to homelessness, but the most common are lack of affordable housing in a community, loss of employment, and loss of support systems (Jackson & Winegarden, 2019). People who lack stable, safe housing usually also lack health insurance and access to healthcare and therefore experience discontinuities in care and may not have access to the routines and other supports to take medication safely and consistently.

When people are admitted to correctional institutions and report they are taking medications currently or bring their medications with them, they can continue their medications unless there is a reason to discontinue them. Medications are reviewed and should follow the medication schedule the inmate followed before admission. If medications brought in are not labeled or not in the original pharmacy packaging, they cannot be accepted. Continuity of care is important to help prevent ADRs. Medication management is provided in a manner equal to community practice (National Commission on Correctional Health Care, 2020). Some facilities offer medication-assisted treatment (MAT) for inmates who report opioid addiction. MAT uses drugs to minimize withdrawal symptoms and can assist in promoting recovery and reducing relapse rates.

Communicating with Patients

Working Phase

Patients who live in homeless shelters, in transitional housing, or on the streets can be distrustful of others. Be friendly and relaxed, and use open-ended questions, even when you think patients may not remember you.

- Hi, Mary, my name is Sally. I'm the nurse that gave you your medication 3 weeks ago. How are you feeling since you've been on the medication?
- Tell me more about why you stopped taking the medication.

Addiction

Addiction is characterized by uncontrollable substance use despite harmful consequences. In 2018, about one in five people ages 12 and older in the United States used illicit drugs such as marijuana, cocaine, and heroin. Of this group of people, 43.5 million were marijuana users. Another 10.3 million people misused opioids in 2018, which includes heroin or misused prescriptions of pain relievers (Substance Abuse and Mental Health Services Administration [SAMHSA], 2019a).

Established, daily substance abuse can damage organs, leading to chronic disease. For example, long-term alcohol abuse is associated with liver cirrhosis and chronic nicotine use is associated with a number of cancers. For some individuals, chronic illness can lead to substance abuse if long-term use of a medication for physical conditions leads to addiction. For example, chronic back pain treated with narcotic medications can lead to dependence on and abuse of pain-relieving medications. Furthermore, having a chronic condition increases a patient's risk for anxiety and depression (Desert Hope, 2019; National Institute of Mental Health, 2020), which in turn may cause a patient to use or misuse substances in an effort to relieve psychologic symptoms.

In some cases, medications may be prescribed to help patients stop misusing drugs, remain in treatment, and avoid relapse. Treatment medications can help reduce symptoms of anxiety, restlessness, sleeplessness, muscle aches, seizures, and depression when patients first stop using drugs and are going through withdrawal (National Institute on Drug Abuse, 2018). See Module 22, Addiction, for more information.

Ethical Issues

Nurses are responsible for following ethical standards for the nursing profession when providing patient care. Ethical practice and conduct focus on relationships of nurses to patients and their families, with nurses and other healthcare professionals, and with society at large. Ethical dilemmas are situations that nurses can encounter that cause moral distress to take action and "right the wrong." Three examples of ethical issues related to medication administration are childhood immunizations, paying for prescriptions, and nurses self-reporting medication errors.

Childhood Immunizations

In the United States, each state has legislation that requires school-age students to have specified vaccines. Every state allows exemptions to immunization laws for medical reasons. There are two other types of exemptions that vary from state to state: religious exemption and philosophical exemption. *Religious exemption* permits parents to exempt their children from vaccination when it challenges their spiritual or religious beliefs. Philosophical exemption means children may be exempted from vaccination because of parents' personal philosophical, moral, or conscientious beliefs. At the time of this writing, 47 states and Washington, D.C. grant religious exemptions for those with religious objections to immunizations and 17 states allow exemptions for those with philosophical objections (National Conference of State Legislatures, 2020).

When parents choose not to have their children immunized, this can result in a public health threat in the school environment and community. Nurses can explore wh parents do not want their children to be immunized, including answering any questions about false information the parents have received. Nurses can provide parents with accurate data about immunizations and the importance of having their children vaccinated. See Module 8, Immunity, for more information about vaccinations.

Costs of Prescriptions

The most recent survey from the National Center for Health Statistics found that about 46% of people in the United States use at least one prescription drug (Martin, Hales, Gu, & Ogden, 2019). Of this number, the most commonly used drugs over the lifespan were:

- Asthma drugs in young children
- Stimulants to treat attention-deficit disorder in adolescents
- Antidepressants in young and middle-aged adults
- Drugs to treat diabetes and high cholesterol in older adults.

Older adults had the highest percentage of pharmacotherapy use, at 85% (Martin et al., 2019).

The cost for some prescriptions has risen so high that even people with health insurance coverage for medications are having trouble paying for them. For example, in 2019, regular insulin cost as much as $185 per 10 mL vial (Lee, 2019).

What happens when people cannot afford their medications? Some may borrow money, use money from their savings accounts, buy less food, ration their medications (e.g., by taking their medication only every other day), or go without their medications altogether. This can become a situational crisis for many people, especially older adults who live on fixed incomes.

Nurses can take time to listen to patients struggling with the high cost of medication with compassion and understanding. Nurses can assist patients by suggesting that they let their HCPs know they are not able to buy their prescriptions and ask if changing to generic drugs is possible.

Nurses should be aware of nonprofit, public, and private assistance programs in their communities that help qualifying patients receive prescriptions free or at a lower cost. In addition, many pharmaceutical companies offer co-pay assistance to patients, although often these are not available to patients on Medicaid or Medicare. There are government programs at the local, state, and national levels to help pay for prescriptions for qualifying patients. These include Medicare Part D, RX Hope, RX Assist, Needy Meds, The Partnership for Prescription Assistance, Together Rx Access, and Extra Help (Mental Health America, 2020). If transportation is a barrier, nurses can suggest using a reputable online pharmacy or arranging for medications to be delivered via mail order, which is available through a number of popular pharmacy chains.

SAFETY ALERT Caution patients against ordering medications from outside the United States. Not only is this illegal, but medications from other countries may have dangerous additives or even be counterfeit. Many pharmacy chains now offer mail-order programs, and the nurse or pharmacist may be able to assist patients with how to order medications delivered by mail.

Nurses Self-Reporting Medication Errors

Nurses can make medication administration errors at any point during administration, including during documentation. Mistakes may occur if a nurse fails to pay attention, hurries to give a medication, is unfamiliar with a medication, forgets to administer a scheduled medication, or is careless or fatigued. Mistakes can also result from a systemwide problem such as understaffing.

Nurses are ethically responsible to self-report medication errors as soon as possible to immediate supervisors, such as charge nurses or nurse managers. If the medication error affected the patient (e.g., a medication was not administered or the wrong medication or dose was administered), the nurse must report the error to the patient's HCP. Notifications need to be documented in the patient's medical records. Nurses who make medication errors are responsible for completing medication error incident forms according to facility policy. This form is then sent to the Quality Assurance or Risk Management Department for review, analysis, recommendations of safety changes, trending, follow-up, and filing. Nurses may receive consequences or be required to participate in safe medication administration education programs by the nurse manager of the unit.

Lifespan Considerations

The potential for medication misuse—intentionally or by accident—exists in every home and healthcare setting, regardless of the patient's age. For all patients, assess patient and family use of supplements or practices that are culturally based to prevent unpleasant or dangerous interactions with any medications recommended by the HCP.

Children and Adolescents

A common-sense safety guideline for parents and caregivers is to refrain from giving a baby less than 2 months old any medication that has not been prescribed or recommended by their HCPs. This includes OTC medications. Nurses can also encourage parents and caregivers to either designate one person to give the medications or to come up with a system to track medication administration. This will help prevent miscommunication and guard against accidentally giving the child a double dose of medication.

Additional information to include in patient teaching for parents and caregivers can be found in **Box 51.2** », Guidelines for Medication Safety at Home

One of the major safety concerns impacting adolescents in the United States is the misuse and abuse of prescription and OTC drugs, either by taking medications without a prescription or by incorrectly following directions on medication labels. Each drug used inappropriately can have short- and long-range consequences that can harm an adolescent's developing brain.

Pregnant Women

Many women who are pregnant take medications before and during pregnancy to treat medical conditions. Research shows 70% of women take a minimum of one prescription medication, and approximately 90% of pregnant women take a minimum of one medication during pregnancy (CDC, 2019m). While many drugs can be used safely during

Box 51.2

Guidelines for Medication Safety at Home

Regardless of age, educate all patients on the need to store medications securely in a cool, dry place. If a patient requires injections at home, additional teaching and return demonstration are necessary prior to discharge. Homes with children should use the child-lock feature on medication bottles. Parents or caregivers should put medicines away each time they give a medication. If antibiotics are prescribed, specify the need to take the medication as prescribed until finished, even if the patient is feeling better.

Infants and Toddlers

- Give medications only after checking first with the child's healthcare provider.
- Do not use medications intended for older children or adults on infants and younger children.
- Do not share one child's medication with other children without consulting the healthcare provider.
- Follow directions on the label.
- If possible, give medications to infants when they are sitting up.
- If the infant cannot sit up, hold the baby at a slight angle with the head higher than the feet, aim a dropper toward the baby's cheek, and release the medication. Avoid pointing the dropper toward the back of the baby's mouth to prevent gagging or choking.
- To avoid choking, do not hold the baby's nares or hold the head back when giving oral medications

Preschool and School-Age Children

- Avoid calling medications "candy" or anything similar to prevent confusion in young children.
- Do not allow children to take medication unsupervised.
- Ask visitors if they carry medication and, if so, ask them to store it out of the reach of children.
- Do not substitute a kitchen spoon for the dosing device or spoon that comes with a medication.
- Post the Poison Control Hotline number by the phone or store it in your smartphone: **1-800-222-1222**.
- For children prescribed tablets or capsules, assess the child's ability to swallow prior to discharge. For children who have difficulty swallowing, suggest parents give tablets or capsules in some pudding or applesauce. Clarify prior to discharge whether or not the medication can be crushed.

Adolescents

- Monitor the number of tablets or capsules in containers.
- If a medication is discontinued, dispose of the remaining doses safely. Ask your pharmacist how to do this.
- Teach adolescents to treat both prescription and OTC medications with caution.

Pregnant Women

- Discuss all medications, including OTC supplements, with your healthcare provider.
- Drug labels and information sheets provide information on how medications may affect women who are pregnant or breastfeeding.
- No drug is guaranteed to be 100% safe for use during pregnancy.
- Do not stop taking prescription medications without speaking to your healthcare provider. Some medications need to be tapered off slowly.

Older Adults

- Use a single pharmacy to help prevent accidentally taking medications that are incompatible with each other.
- Take medications as directed.
- Establish a routine for taking medications to help prevent forgetting to take them or accidentally taking a medication twice.
- Use visual cues or smartphone reminders as needed.
- Contact your healthcare provider if you experience any unpleasant side effects or have any questions.

Sources: Adams, Holland, and Urban (2020); CDC (2020g); Medstar Visiting Nursing Association (2020); Tabloski (2019).

pregnancy, there are some medications that may cause congenital anomalies, miscarriages, prematurity, or developmental disabilities mainly during the first and third trimesters. There are a few drugs that pregnant women should not take because of risk for harm to the developing fetus. One example is angiotensin-converting enzyme inhibitors. When taken in the first and last trimester, they can cause miscarriage, low amniotic fluid levels, or deformity in the baby. Nonsteroidal anti-inflammatory drugs taken in the third trimester can increase the risk of injury to the baby's heart (Anderson, 2019).

Nurses can help educate pregnant women about prescription and OTC medications and encourage women to ask questions, use appropriate online websites for information, read labels, and report any concerns to their HCPs.

Nurses can provide emotional support and educational information about benefits and risks of medications for pregnant women and their babies, how to find creditable online resources for more medication information, the importance of taking prenatal vitamins, and the impact of using illegal drugs, alcohol, or tobacco products. Pharmacists are also good resources for questions about medication safety.

Older Adults

Older adults taking prescription or OTC medications are at high risk for drug-related side effects, ADEs, toxicity, and overdose because of age-related body changes. Age-related changes include an increased amount of fat distribution from increased body fat compared to muscle mass, decreased drug excretion from diminished renal function, increased concentration in the blood due to slow clearance from extended drug half-lives, and ADEs from decreased liver function (Tabloski, 2019).

Polypharmacy, the use of two or more medications concurrently, increases the older adult's risk for adverse effects. Encourage patients to use a single pharmacy so that the pharmacist can help patients guard against multiple HCPs accidentally prescribing drugs that are incompatible with each other. Teach older adult patients and the families to bring a current list of all medications to each healthcare appointment. This assists the nurse in assessing patients' use of medications to determine if they are taking medications according to directions and if they have added or discontinued taking any medications. This also provides the opportunity to ensure that older adults are not taking any medications that may increase their risk for falls or other injuries. Because of the many risk factors related to medication use in older adults, nurses must be cautious in administering medications and continuously monitor for effectiveness of drugs when providing pharmacotherapy to older adult patients.

REVIEW Medication Safety

RELATE Link the Concepts and Exemplars

Linking the exemplar on medication safety with the concept of teaching and learning:

1. A patient's daughter will be helping the patient care for a burn on his arm. What information should the nurse include when demonstrating how to safely apply a topical medication to the patient's daughter?
2. What are some common safety guidelines the nurse can discuss with parents of a preschool child when the child is started on an antibiotic for a 10-day course?

Linking the exemplar on medication safety with the concept of advocacy:

3. A patient lets the nurse know he is retired and on a limited income so is unable to buy the HCP's prescribed medications. What suggestions can the nurse make to the patient?
4. The nurse observes an assigned older adult patient having difficulty maintaining her balance while walking down the hallway using a cane. What can the nurse do to help the patient in this situation?

Linking the exemplar on medication safety with the concept of perfusion:

5. During the admission assessment, the nurse observes the patient has one large medication container with a variety of different medications in it. When asked about it, the patient smiles and says, "That's so I keep them all in one place." Is this safe? Why or why not? And what should the nurse do?
6. The patient tells the office nurse that he ran out of his medication 2 days ago, so he has been taking his spouse's cardiac medication. What should the nurse do?

READY Go to Volume 3: Clinical Nursing Skills

REFER Go to Pearson MyLab Nursing and eText

REFLECT Apply Your Knowledge

The nurse at a skilled nursing facility is preparing a medication at the medication cart when a family member stops at the cart and begins asking questions about her father, who is a patient on the floor. After talking with the family member, the nurse grabs the medication she had prepared and quickly goes into the patient's room but forgets to bring the patient's MAR into the room. The nurse identifies the patient, gives the medication, and leaves the room. When back at the med cart, the nurse realizes she administered another patient's medication instead of the ordered medication. The nurse is upset but feels no one will ever know what happened and doesn't take any action.

1. What should the nurse have done after realizing she gave the wrong medication to the patient in this scenario? What could happen to the patient?

References

Adams, M., Holland, L. N., & Urban, C Q, (2020). *Pharmacology for nurses: A pathophysiologic approach* (6th ed.). Pearson.

Advisory Board. (2018). *The 10 leading causes of death for US children, charted.* https://www.advisory.com/daily-briefing/2018/12/21/child-death

Agency for Healthcare Research and Quality (AHRQ). (2018). *Improving patient safety in long-term care facilities. Module 1. Detecting change in a resident's condition.* https://www.ahrq.gov/patient-safety/settings/long-term-care/resource/facilities/ltc/gdmod1.html on 2/29/2020.

Agency for Healthcare Research and Quality (AHRQ). (2019a). *Culture of safety.* from https://psnet.ahrq.gov/primer/culture-safety

Agency for Healthcare Research and Quality (AHRQ), (2019b). *Medication errors and adverse drug events.* https://psnet.ahrq.gov/primer/medication-errors-and-adverse-drug-events

Agency for Healthcare Research and Quality (AHRQ). (2019c). *Patient safety primer, patient safety 101.* https://psnet.ahrq.gov/primer/patient-safety-101

Agency for Healthcare Research and Quality (AHRQ). (2019d). *Patient safety primer, wrong-site, wrong-procedure, and wrong-patient surgery.* https://psnet.ahrq.gov/primer/wrong-site-wrong-procedure-and-wrong-patient-surgery

Agency for Healthcare Research and Quality (AHRQ). (2020a). *AHRQ's quality & patient safety programs by setting: Hospital.* https://www.ahrq.gov/patient-safety/settings/hospital/index.html

Agency for Healthcare Research and Quality (AHRQ). (2020b). *What's new.* https://www.ahrq.gov/evidencenow/whatsnew/index.html

American Academy of Allergy, Asthma & Immunology (AAAAI). (2020). *Latex allergy.* https://www.aaaai.org/conditions-and-treatments/library/allergy-library/latex-allergy

American Geriatrics Society (AGS). (2019). *For older people, medications are common; Updated AGS BEERS Criteria aims to make sure they're appropriate, too.* https://www.americangeriatrics.org/media-center/news/older-people-medications-are-common-updated-ags-beers-criteriar-aims-make-sure

Anderson, L. (2019). *OTC medication use in pregnancy: Wise or worrisome?* Drugs.com. https://www.drugs.com/slideshow/otc-medication-use-during-pregnancy-1046

Ball, J. W., Bindler, R. C., Cowen, K., & Shaw, M. (2020). *Principles of pediatric nursing: Caring for children* (7th ed.). Pearson.

Becker's Hospital Review. (2018). *68 of the greenest hospitals in America – 2018.* https://www.beckershospitalreview.com/lists/68-of-the-greenest-hospitals-in-america-2018.html

Bureau of Labor Statistics (BLS). (2018). *Occupational injuries and illnesses among registered nurses.* U.S. Department of Labor. https://www.bls.gov/opub/mlr/2018/article/occupational-injuries-and-illnesses-among-registered-nurses.htm

Bureau of Labor Statistics (BLS). (2019). *TED: The Economics Daily, 2.8 million nonfatal workplace injuries and illnesses occurred in 2018.* U.S. Department of Labor. https://www.bls.gov/opub/ted/2019/2-point-8-million-nonfatal-workplace-injuries-and-illnesses-occurred-in-2018.htm

Bureau of Labor Statistics (BLS). (2020). *Occupational outlook handbook, registered nurses.* U.S. Department of Labor. https://www.bls.gov/ooh/healthcare/registered-nurses.htm

Burke, A. (2020). *Use of restraints and safety devices: NCLEX-RN.* RegisteredNursing.org. https://www.registerednursing.org/nclex/use-restraints-safety-devices/

Caffrey, M. (2019, May 22). Where culture and science collide: How ethnic, social factors affect response to psychotropic drugs. *American Journal of Managed Care.* https://www.ajmc.com/conferences/apa-2019/where-culture-and-science-collide-how-ethnic-social-factors-affect-response-to-psychotropic-drugs

California Maternal Quality Care Collaborative. (2020). *QI initiatives.* https://www.cmqcc.org/qi-initiatives

Center for Children with Special Needs (CCSN). (2018). *Playground safety for your child with special needs.* https://cshcn.org/resources-contacts/safety-tips/playground-safety-for-your-child-with-special-needs/

Centers for Disease Control and Prevention (CDC). (2018a). *Healthcare-associated infections (HAI) data.* https://www.cdc.gov/hai/data/index.html?CDC_AA_refVal=https%3A%2F%2Fwww.cdc.gov%2Fhai%2Fsurveillance%2Findex.html

Centers for Disease Control and Prevention (CDC). (2018b). *Lack of change in perinatal mortality in the United States, 2014–2016.* https://www.cdc.gov/nchs/data/databriefs/db316.pdf

Centers for Disease Control and Prevention (CDC). (2018c). *The National Institute for Occupational Safety and Health (NIOSH).* https://www.cdc.gov/niosh/about/default.html

Centers for Disease Control and Prevention (CDC). (2019a). *About infant mortality.* https://www.cdc.gov/reproductivehealth/maternalinfanthealth/infantmortality.htm

Centers for Disease Control and Prevention (CDC). (2019b). *Coordinated care plan to prevent older adult falls.* https://www.cdc.gov/steadi/pdf/Steadi-Coordinated-Care-Final-4_24_19.pdf

Centers for Disease Control and Prevention (CDC). (2019c). *Data & statistics on birth defects.* https://www.cdc.gov/ncbddd/birthdefects/data.html

Centers for Disease Control and Prevention (CDC). (2019d). *Healthcare-associated infections, patient safety.* https://www.cdc.gov/HAI/patientSafety/patient-safety.html

Centers for Disease Control and Prevention (CDC). (2019e). *Injection safety: One & Only Campaign.* https://www.cdc.gov/injectionsafety/one-and-only.html

Centers for Disease Control and Prevention (CDC). (2019f). *Occupational violence: Workplace violence prevention for nurses* (CDC Course No. WB2908–NIOSH Pub. No. 2013-155). http://www.cdc.gov/niosh/topics/violence/training_nurses.html

Centers for Disease Control and Prevention (CDC). (2019g). *Oral health for older Americans: Facts about older adult oral health.* https://www.cdc.gov/oralhealth/basics/adult-oral-health/adult_older.htm

Centers for Disease Control and Prevention (CDC). (2019h). *Oral health tips: What can adults do to maintain good oral health?* https://www.cdc.gov/oralhealth/basics/adult-oral-health/tips.html

Centers for Disease Control and Prevention (CDC). (2019i). *Protect the ones you love: Child injuries are preventable.* https://www.cdc.gov/safechild/index.html

Centers for Disease Control and Prevention (CDC). (2019j). *Safety and children with disabilities.* http://www.cdc.gov/ncbddd/disabilityandsafety/child-safety.html

Centers for Disease Control and Prevention (CDC). (2019k). *Stop Sticks campaign.* https://www.cdc.gov/nora/councils/hcsa/stopsticks/default.html

Centers for Disease Control and Prevention (CDC). (2019l). *Ten leading causes of death and injury.* https://www.cdc.gov/injury/wisqars/LeadingCauses_images.html

Centers for Disease Control and Prevention (CDC). (2019m). *Treating for two: Medicine and pregnancy.* https://www.cdc.gov/pregnancy/meds/treatingfortwo/

Centers for Disease Control and Prevention (CDC). (2019n). *What are child abuse and neglect?* https://www.cdc.gov/violenceprevention/childabuseandneglect/fastfact.html

Centers for Disease Control and Prevention (CDC). (2020a). *Coronavirus (COVID-19).* https://www.cdc.gov/coronavirus/2019-ncov/index.html

Centers for Disease Control and Prevention (CDC). (2020b). *Get a heads up on bike helmet safety.* https://www.cdc.gov/headsup/pdfs/helmets/HeadsUp_HelmetFactSheet_Bike_508.pdf

Centers for Disease Control and Prevention (CDC). (2020c). *Handwashing: Clean hands save lives.* https://www.cdc.gov/handwashing/index.html

Centers for Disease Control and Prevention (CDC). (2020d). *Home and recreational safety: Publications and resources.* https://www.cdc.gov/homeandrecreationalsafety/falls/pubs.html

Centers for Disease Control and Prevention (CDC). (2020e). *Injury prevention & control: WISQARS injury data.* https://www.cdc.gov/injury/wisqars/index.html

Centers for Disease Control and Prevention (CDC). (2020f). *Move Your Way campaign.* https://health.gov/our-work/physical-activity/move-your-way-campaign

Centers for Disease Control and Prevention (CDC). (2020g). *Put your medicines up and away and out of sight.* https://www.cdc.gov/features/medicationstorage/index.html

Children's Hospital of St. Louis. (2020). *A parent's guide to calling the doctor.* Retrieved from https://www.stlouischildrens.org/health-resources/pulse/parents-guide-calling-doctor

Cohut, M. (2020). *Why hand washing really could slow down an epidemic.* Medical News Today. https://www.medicalnewstoday.com/articles/why-hand-washing-really-could-slow-down-an-epidemic

Coyne, R. (2019). *The Lawton Instrumental Activities of Daily Living (IADL) Scale.* Hartford Institute for Geriatric Nursing. Retrieved from https://consultgeri.org/try-this/general-assessment/issue-23.pdf

Desert Hope. (2019). *Treating comorbid substance abuse and chronic disease.* https://deserthopetreatment.com/co-occurring-disorders/comorbid-chronic-disease/

Díaz-Gutiérrez, M. J., Martinez-Cengotitabengoa, M., Saez de Adana, E., Cano, A. I., Martinez-Cengotitabengoa, M. T., Besga, A., Segarra, R., & González-Pinto, A. (2017). Relationship between the use of benzodiazepines and falls in older adults: A systematic review. *Maturitas, 101,* 17–22.

DQYDJ. (2019). *Average retirement age in the United States.* https://dqydj.com/average-retirement-age-in-the-united-states/

Fabian, J. (2020). *Workplace injury statistics – 2019 year-end data for workplace accidents, injuries, and deaths.* Workplace Injury Source. https://workinjurysource.com/workplace-injury-statistics-2019/

Government of South Australia. (2019). *What is functional decline?* SA Health. https://www.sahealth.sa.gov.au/wps/wcm/connect/public+content/sa+health+internet/clinical+resources/clinical+topics/older+people/care+of+older+people+toolkit/what+is+functional+decline+-+the+toolkit

Greenberg, S. (2019). *The 2019 American Geriatrics Society updated Beers Criteria® for potentially inappropriate medication use in older adults.* Hartford Institute for Geriatric Nursing. https://consultgeri.org/try-this/general-assessment/issue-16

Griffin Hospital. (2020). *Speak Up Initiative.* https://www.griffinhealth.org/griffin-hospital/patient-safety/speak-up-initiative

Grimmond, T. (2020). *Sharps injuries: Emotional, statistical challenges.* Relias Media. https://www.reliasmedia.com/articles/145445-sharps-injuries-emotional-statistical-challenges

Hospital Safety Score. (2019). *What is patient safety?: Errors, injuries, accidents, infections.* http://www.hospitalsafetyscore.org/what-is-patient-safety_m#errors

Institute for Clinical and Translational Science (ICTS). (2019). *Safety of the subject* [PowerPoint presentation]. University of Iowa. https://icts.uiowa.edu/sites/icts . . . /Safety%20of%20the%20Subject.pptx

Jackson, K., & Winegarden, W. (2019). *San Francisco's homeless crisis: How policy reforms and private charities can move more people to self-sufficiency.* Pacific Research Institute.

Kids and Cars. (2019). *Heat stroke.* https://www.kidsandcars.org/heatstroke-day/

KidsHealth. (2018). *Fevers.* https://kidshealth.org/en/parents/fever.html

Kim, K., Johnson, J. A., & Derendorf, H. (2004). Differences in drug pharmacokinetics between east Asians and Caucasians and the role of genetic polymorphisms. *Journal of Clinical Pharmacology, 44*(10)1083–104.

Lee, B. (2019). *How much does insulin cost?: Here's how 23 brands compare.* GoodRx. https://www.goodrx.com/blog/how-much-does-insulin-cost-compare-brands/

Martin, C. B., Hales, C. M., Gu, Q. & Ogden, C. L. (2019). *Prescription drug use in the United States, 2015–2016* (NHCS Data Brief No. 334). Centers for Disease Control and Prevention. https://www.cdc.gov/nchs/data/databriefs/db334-h.pdf

MedStar Visiting Nurse Association. (2020). *Home health care: Medication management.* https://www.medstarvna.org/home-health-care/medication-management/

Mental Health America (MHA). (2020). *How can I get help paying for my prescriptions?* https://www.mhanational.org/how-can-i-get-help-paying-my-prescriptions

National Commission on Correctional Health Care (NCCHC). (2020). *Medication services.* https://www.ncchc.org/spotlight-on-the-standards-23-2

MPHonline. (2020). *Outbreak: 10 of the worst pandemics in history.* https://www.mphonline.org/worst-pandemics-in-history/

National Adult Protective Services Association (NAPSA). (2020). *Get informed.* https://www.napsa-now.org/get-informed/

National Alliance to End Homelessness. (2020). *State of homelessness in America.* https://endhomelessness.org/homelessness-in-america/homelessness-statistics/state-of-homelessness-report/

National Conference of State Legislatures (NCSL). (2020). *States with religious and philosophical exemptions from school immunization requirements.* https://www.ncsl.org/research/health/school-immunization-exemption-state-laws.aspx

National Council of State Boards of Nursing (NCSBN). (2020). *Nurse Practice Act toolkit.* https://www.ncsbn.org/npa-toolkit.htm

National Institute of Child Health and Human Development. (2020). *About SIDS and safe infant sleep.* https://safetosleep.nichd.nih.gov/safesleepbasics/about

National Institute on Drug Abuse. (2018). *Drugs, brains, and behavior: The science of addiction. treatment and recovery.* https://www.drugabuse.gov/publications/drugs-brains-behavior-science-addiction/treatment-recovery

National Institute of Mental Health. (2020). *Chronic illness and mental health.* https://www.nimh.nih.gov/health/publications/chronic-illness-mental-health/index.shtml

National League for Nursing. (2020). *Nursing leaders call for flexibility in the path to graduation to ensure greater numbers of new nurses.* http://www.nln.org/newsroom/news-releases/news-release/2020/03/24/nursing-leaders-call-for-flexibility-in-the-path-to-graduation-to-ensure-greater-numbers-of-new-nurses

Nicolaides, C., Avraam, D., Cueto-Felgueroso, L., Gonzalez, M. C., & Juanes, R. (2020). Hand-hygiene mitigation strategies against global disease spreading through the air transportation network. *Risk Analysis, 40*(4), 723–740.

Nursing Home Abuse Center. (2020). *Signs of neglect.* https://www.nursinghomeabusecenter.org/signs-of-neglect/

Occupational Safety and Health Administration (OSHA). (2020a). *Chemical hazards and toxic substances: Controlling exposure.* https://www.osha.gov/SLTC/hazardoustoxicsubstances/control.html

Occupational Safety and Health Administration (OSHA). (2020b). *Healthcare.* https://www.osha.gov/SLTC/healthcarefacilities/index.html

Occupational Safety and Health Administration (OSHA). (2020c). *How to file a whistleblower complaint.* https://www.whistleblowers.gov/complaint_page

Paauw, D. (2018). *10 little known uses for common, everyday drugs.* Medscape. https://www.medscape.com/slideshow/little-known-uses-common-drugs-6010993#3

Potter, M. L., & Moller, M. D. (2020). *Psychiatric–mental health nursing: From suffering to hope* (2nd ed.). Pearson.

QSEN Institute. (2020). *QSEN competencies.* https://qsen.org/competencies/pre-licensure-ksas/

Rajman, I., Knapp, L., Morgan, T., & Masimirembwa, C. (2017). African genetic diversity: Implications for cytochrome P450-mediated drug metabolism and drug development. *EBioMedicine, 17,* 67–74.

RegisteredNursing.org. (2019). How do nurses protect themselves from highly infectious patients? https://www.registerednursing.org/how-nurses-protect-from-highly-infectious-patients/

Robertson, L. (2019). *Testimony from Lance Robertson on Older Americans Act: Protecting and supporting seniors as they age before Special Committee on Aging.* U.S. Department of Health and Human Services. https://www.hhs.gov/about/agencies/asl/testimony/2019-05/older-americans-act-protecting-and-supporting-seniors-as-they-age.html

Ruscin, J. M., & Linnebur, S. A. (2019). *Pharmacokinetics in older adults.* Merck Manual Professional Version.

https://www.merckmanuals.com/professional/geriatrics/drug-therapy-in-older-adults/pharmacokinetics-in-older-adults

Shahid, S., & Thomas, S. (2018). *Situation, Background, Assessment, Recommendation (SBAR) communication tool for handoff in health care – A narrative review.* Safety in Health. https://safetyinhealth.biomedcentral.com/track/pdf/10.1186/s40886-018-0073-1

Substance Abuse and Mental Health Services Administration (SAMHSA). (2019a). *Key substance use and mental health indicators in the United States: Results from the 2018 National Survey on Drug Use and Health.* https://www.samhsa.gov/data/sites/default/files/cbhsq-reports/NSDUHNationalFindingsReport2018/NSDUHNationalFindingsReport2018.pdf

Tabloski, P. A. (2019). *Gerontological nursing: The essential guide to clinical practice* (4th ed.). Pearson.

Tariq, R. A., & Scherbak, Y. (2019). *Medication errors.* StatPearls. https://www.ncbi.nlm.nih.gov/books/NBK519065/

The Joint Commission. (2020a). *National Patient Safety Goals.* https://www.jointcommission.org/en/standards/national-patient-safety-goals/

The Joint Commission. (2020b). *Speak Up campaigns.* https://www.jointcommission.org/resources/for-consumers/speak-up-campaigns/

U.S. National Library of Medicine. (2020). *Sudden infant death syndrome.* https://medlineplus.gov/suddeninfantdeathsyndrome.html

World Health Organization (WHO). (2020a). *Coronavirus.* https://www.who.int/health-topics/coronavirus

World Health Organization (WHO). (2020b). *Coronavirus disease 2019 (COVID-19).* https://www.who.int/docs/default-source/coronaviruse/situation-reports/20200311-sitrep-51-covid-19.pdf?sfvrsn=1ba62e57_10

World Health Organization (WHO). (2020c). *Patient safety: 5 moments for medication safety.* https://www.who.int/patientsafety/medication-safety/5moments/en/

Glossary

ABC The essential functions of airway, breathing, and circulation.

ABCD An enhancement of the **ABC** mnemonic, with the **D** representing one of four indicators depending on agency use: defibrillation, deficiency, deadly bleeding, or disability.

ABCDE A mnemonic that helps identify the highest-priority concerns when caring for trauma patients: Airway, Breathing and ventilation, Circulation and hemorrhage control, Disability and neurologic assessment, and Exposure and environmental control.

Abnormal uterine bleeding (AUB) Vaginal bleeding that is usually painless but is abnormal in amount, duration, or time of occurrence.

Abortion Spontaneous loss or termination of pregnancy that occurs before the end of 20 weeks' gestation or the birth of a fetus/newborn who weighs less than 500 g. Also called *miscarriage*.

Absence seizures Also called *petit mal seizures*, absence seizures involve both hemispheres of the brain as well as deeper structures such as the thalamus, basal ganglia, and upper brainstem. They are considered a type of generalized seizure.

Absorption The process of moving nutrients and fluid from the external environment of the gastrointestinal tract to the internal environment. May also refer to the intake of any specific nutrient.

Abstinence Voluntarily going without alcohol, drugs, or other pleasurable substances or activities.

Abuse of power An attempt by individuals to use their position or authority in a manner that shames, controls, demeans, humiliates, or denigrates another individual to gain emotional, psychologic, or physical advantage over that individual.

Acanthosis nigricans A condition associated with type 2 diabetes in which the skin appears dark and thick, which is a marker of insulin resistance.

Accelerations A transient increase in the fetal heart rate normally caused by fetal movement.

Accommodation 1. The ability of the eye to adjust to variations in distance. 2. The process of a change whereby cognitive processes mature sufficiently to allow an individual to solve problems that were unsolvable before.

Accountability The ability and willingness of individuals to assume responsibility for their actions and to accept the consequences of their behavior.

Accreditation A peer-review process that evaluates and certifies the quality of an organization.

Acculturation The process of adapting to the majority culture and accepting it as one's own.

Acid indigestion A condition in which an individual can taste the stomach acid when it flows back into the esophagus.

Acidosis The condition that results when hydrogen ion concentration increases above normal, causing the pH to drop below 7.35.

Acids Substances that release hydrogen ions in solution.

Acquired aplastic anemia A rare condition in which the bone marrow fails to produce all three types of blood cells, leading to pancytopenia, a deficiency in both RBCs and WBCs. Normal bone marrow is replaced by fat.

Acquired brain injury An assault that occurs to the brain that includes nontraumatic injury, such as from a stroke or infectious disease, and trauma to the brain, such as a concussion or more severe traumatic brain injury.

Acquired immunity Immunity developed after exposure to a pathogen.

Acquired immunodeficiency syndrome (AIDS) An immune system deficit induced by infection with the human immunodeficiency virus (HIV). AIDS is characterized by opportunistic infections.

Acrocyanosis A bluish discoloration of the hands and feet.

Acrosomal reaction One of the processes a sperm must undergo before fertilization can occur. The acrosomes of the sperm surrounding the ovum release their enzymes and thus break down the hyaluronic acid in the ovum's corona radiata.

Actinic keratosis An epidermal skin lesion directly related to chronic sun exposure and photodamage. Also called *senile keratosis* or *solar keratosis*.

Action potential The electrical activity produced by movement of ions across cell membranes that stimulates muscle contraction.

Active acquired immunity Antibodies formed in response to an illness or an immunization while a woman is pregnant.

Active euthanasia Actions to bring about a patient's death directly, with or without patient consent.

Active immunity Production of antibodies or development of immune lymphocytes against specific antigens.

Active listening Fully concentrating on both the content and emotion of a person's message, rather than just passively hearing the words a person says.

Active transport A method that requires additional energy (in the form of adenosine triphosphate) to move substances against the concentration gradient (from low concentration to high concentration).

Activities of daily living (ADLs) Activities used routinely in daily life, such as grooming, eating, bathing, and dressing.

Activity tolerance The type and amount of exercise or daily living activities that an individual is able to perform without experiencing adverse effects.

Actual loss A change in or unavailability of something or someone of value that can be recognized by others.

Acupuncture A form of alternative treatment that involves inserting thin needles through a person's skin at specific points on the body, to various depths. It can help with pain relief and various other symptoms.

Acute coronary syndrome (ACS) Any condition that develops due to sudden, reduced blood flow to the heart.

Acute fatigue A sudden onset of physical and mental exhaustion or weariness, particularly after a period of mental or physical stress.

Acute illness An alteration in health or functioning characterized by severe symptoms of relatively short duration.

Acute infection An infection that appears suddenly and lasts for a short time.

Acute kidney injury (AKI) Proposed as a more accurate term for *acute renal failure*, it is defined as a sudden decline in kidney function that causes disturbances in fluid, electrolyte, and acid–base balances.

Acute lymphocytic leukemia (ALL) The most common type of leukemia in children and adolescents, marked by the proliferation of malignant cells that resemble immature lymphocytes.

Acute myeloid leukemia (AML) A disorder characterized by uncontrolled proliferation of myeloblasts and hyperplasia of the bone marrow and spleen.

Acute myocardial infarction (AMI) A life-threatening condition that occurs when blood flow to a portion of the cardiac muscle is blocked. If circulation to the affected myocardium is not promptly restored, loss of functional myocardium affects the heart's ability to maintain an effective cardiac output, ultimately leading to cardiogenic shock and death.

Acute otitis media (AOM) Usually referred to as an "ear infection," it is a sudden inflammation of the middle ear caused by an infection.

Acute pain Temporary, localized, and sudden pain that lasts for less than 6 months and has an identifiable cause, such as trauma, surgery, or inflammation.

Acute pancreatitis An inflammatory disorder that involves self-destruction of the pancreas by its own enzymes through autodigestion.

Acute postinfectious glomerulonephritis (APIGN) Inflammation of the glomerular capillary membrane that is most often seen in children as a response to a group A beta-hemolytic streptococcal infection of the skin or pharynx or as a result of infection by *Staphylococcus*, *Pneumococcus*, or Coxsackie virus.

Acute renal failure (ARF) A rapid decline in renal function with azotemia, fluid, and electrolyte imbalances. It may be reversed with prompt intervention.

Acute respiratory distress syndrome (ARDS) A disorder with rapid onset characterized by noncardiac pulmonary edema and progressive refractory hypoxemia. It is a life-threatening emergency.

Acute stress disorder A condition that may occur following an individual experiencing, learning of, or witnessing an extremely stressful event that involves the threat of death, actual or threatened serious injury, or actual or threatened physical or sexual violation.

Acute tubular necrosis (ATN) The destruction of tubular epithelial cells, which causes an abrupt and progressive decline of renal function.

Adaptation 1. The use of physiologic and psychologic processes to come to terms with the implications and outcomes of stressors. Also called *coping behavior*. 2. The return to normal functioning, even when homeostasis cannot be regained.

Adaptation phase The phase during a crisis in which the individual meets the challenges presented and uses resources to successfully resolve the crisis.

Adaptive behavior Everyday skills, including conceptual skills, social skills, and practical skills.

Addiction A psychologic or physical need for a substance (such as alcohol) or process (such as gambling) to the extent that the individual will risk negative consequences in an attempt to meet the need.

Addictive behaviors Compulsive, problematic patterns of action resulting in psychologic and/or physiologic dependence.

Addison disease A disorder that results from adrenal insufficiency, particularly a cortisol deficiency.

Adherence Attachment to a regimen. Also called *compliance*.

Adhesions Fibrous bands of scar tissue.

Adjustment disorder with depressed mood A maladaptive reaction to an identifiable psychosocial stressor or stressors that occurs within 3 months after the onset of the stressor and has persisted for no longer than 6 months. Also called *adjustment disorder* or *situational depression*.

Adjustment phase Initial phase experienced in response to crisis, characterized by disorganization and unsuccessful attempts to meet the crisis.

Administrative laws Responsibilities that may be interpreted and enforced by an agency that has been delegated the power of oversight by the governing legislation.

Adolescent family A family in which one or more parents are adolescents.

Adult learning theory A theory that suggests that adult learners differ from child learners in fundamental ways: they need to know why they should learn something, prefer that others treat them as capable of self-direction, have life experiences that enhance their current learning, and are ready to learn what must be known in order to care for themselves.

Advance directives Legal documents that express an individual's desires regarding healthcare and/or financial affairs in the event of incapacity. Also called *healthcare advance directives*.

Adverse childhood experiences (ACEs) Traumatic events occurring in childhood that are linked to chronic health problems, mental illness, and substance abuse in adulthood.

Adverse drug event Injury that results from a medication-related intervention.

Advocacy Protecting individuals by expressing and defending their cause on their behalf.

Advocate An individual who expresses and defends the cause of another.

Aerobic exercise An activity during which the amount of oxygen taken into the body is greater than that used to perform the activity.

Afebrile Without fever.

Affect The immediate and observable emotional expression of mood, which people communicate verbally and nonverbally; the outward manifestation of what the individual is feeling.

Affective commitment An attachment to a profession that includes identification with and involvement in the profession.

Afterload The force that ventricles must overcome to eject their blood volume.

Afterpains Cramplike pains caused by intermittent contractions of the uterus that occur after childbirth.

Age-related cataracts An eye condition in which the lens fibers and proteins change and degenerate. The proteins clump, clouding the lens and reducing light transmission to the retina. This process generally begins at the periphery of the lens; it gradually spreads to involve the central portion. The entire lens may eventually become opaque.

Age-related macular degeneration (AMD) A gradual degeneration in the macular area of the retina that is the leading cause of blindness in people over age 65.

Ageism A deep and profound prejudice in American society against older adults.

Aggravated assault An unlawful attack by one individual on another for the purpose of inflicting severe or aggravated bodily injury. This type of assault usually is accompanied by the use of a weapon or by means likely to produce death or great bodily harm.

Aggression Any form of behavior directed toward the goal of harming or injuring another living being.

Aggressive behavior Behavior directed toward getting what one wants without considering the feelings of others.

Aggressive communicators Individuals who tend to focus on their own needs and become impatient when these needs are not met.

Agnosia The inability to recognize one or more objects that previously were familiar.

Agoraphobia A condition that is characterized by anxiety associated with two or more of the following situations: being in enclosed spaces, being in open spaces, using public transportation, being in a crowd or standing in a line of people, or being alone outside the home environment.

AIDS dementia complex The most common cause of mental status changes for patients with HIV infection. This dementia results from a direct effect of the virus on the brain and affects cognitive, motor, and behavioral functioning. Fluctuating memory loss, confusion, difficulty concentrating, lethargy, and diminished motor speed are typical manifestations.

Air trapping Decreased airflow with exhalation caused by edema of the air passages.

Airborne precautions Used for patients who are known to have or suspected of having serious illnesses transmitted by airborne droplet nuclei smaller than 5 microns, such as tuberculosis.

Airway clearance techniques (ACTs) Nonpharmacologic strategies for clearing the airway. Examples include coughing, huffing, and **chest physical therapy**.

Airway remodeling Structural changes of the airway caused by a disease, such as asthma, resulting in progressive or permanent loss of lung function.

Airway resistance The effort or force needed to move oxygen through the trachea to the lungs.

Akathisia Restlessness.

Alcohol dependence A primary, chronic disease characterized by use or abuse of alcohol; genetic, psychosocial, and environmental factors influence its development and manifestations. Also called *alcoholism*.

Alcohol intoxication The presence of clinically significant behavioral or psychologic changes due to alcohol use. Changes may include any combination of inappropriate sexual or aggressive behavior, mood lability, impaired judgment, and impaired social or occupational functioning.

Alcohol overdose A toxic condition that results from excessive consumption of large amounts of alcohol in a very short period of time.

Alcohol use disorder Also called *alcoholism* or *alcohol abuse*, it is chronic disease characterized by inability to control the primary addictive behavior (drinking), fixation with and continued use of alcohol regardless of consequences, and impaired thought processes.

Alcohol withdrawal delirium A medical emergency usually occurring 3 to 5 days following alcohol withdrawal and lasting 2 to 3 days. Characterized by paranoia, disorientation, delusions, visual hallucinations, elevated vital signs, vomiting, diarrhea, and diaphoresis. Also known as *delirium tremens (DTs)*.

Alcohol withdrawal syndrome Condition that typically begins about 6 to 8 hours after an individual with alcoholism takes his or her last drink. Early symptoms include irritability, anxiety, insomnia, tremors, sweating, and a mild tachycardia.

Alcoholic cirrhosis A progressive, irreversible liver disorder resulting from excessive consumption of alcohol. Also called *Laënnec cirrhosis*.

Alcoholism A primary, chronic disease characterized by use or abuse of alcohol; genetic, psychosocial, and environmental factors influence its development and manifestations. Also called *alcohol dependence*.

Alkalosis The condition that results when hydrogen ion concentration falls below normal and the pH level rises above 7.45.

Allen test A measurement of radial or ulnar artery patency; either the radial or ulnar artery is digitally compressed by the examiner after blood has been forced out of the hand by clenching it into a fist.

Allergen An environmental or exogenous antigen that provokes a hypersensitivity response.

Allergic contact dermatitis A cell-mediated or delayed hypersensitivity to a wide variety of allergens.

Allergy A hypersensitivity response to environmental or exogenous antigens.

Allogeneic blood transfusion A transfusion using blood that has been donated by the community.

Allogeneic bone marrow transplant A transplant using bone marrow from a matched donor.

Allografts Grafts between members of the same species who have different genotypes and HLA antigens. Human skin that has been harvested from cadavers is usually used. Also called *homograft*.

Alloimmunization The reaction of the immune system to donated tissue.

Allostasis Necessary changes that must occur to achieve the characteristic stability of homeostasis.

Allostatic load The physical cost of adaptation to physiologic or psychosocial stressors.

Alogia Limited or impoverished speech.

Alopecia Hair loss.

Alternative healthcare Treatments or therapies that are not part of standard medical practice, such as acupuncture or a special diet.

Alternative therapies Also referred to as *alternative medicine*, a term used to describe use of these diverse therapies *instead of* conventional therapies, including acupuncture; cultural practices related to food preparation or practices at specific times of the day or during the week.

Altruism A concern for the welfare and well-being of others.

Alveoli Terminal structures of the respiratory system where gas exchange occurs.

Alzheimer disease (AD) The most common kind of dementia, Alzheimer disease involves progressive dementia, memory loss, and the inability to participate in activities of daily living and self-care.

Ambulation The ability to walk from place to place independently with or without an assistive device.

Amblyopia Lazy eye; one eye has reduced vision even with no identifiable cause, and the reduced vision is not correctable by corrective lenses.

Amenorrhea The absence of menstruation.

Amnesia Loss of recent or remote memory.

Amniocentesis A procedure used to obtain amniotic fluid for genetic testing to determine fetal abnormalities or fetal lung maturity in the third trimester of pregnancy.

Amnion A thin protective membrane that contains amniotic fluid.

Amniotic fluid The liquid surrounding the fetus in utero. It absorbs shocks, permits fetal movement, and prevents heat loss.

Amphetamine A powerful stimulant that, when used improperly or abused, poses a severe health risk due to its devastating physical and neurologic consequences, including amphetamine-induced mental disorders.

Amputation Partial or total removal of an extremity or body part.

Amyloid plaques Seen in Alzheimer disease and formed when groups of nerve cells degenerate and clump around the amyloid core in the spaces between the neurons in the brain. They consist primarily of insoluble deposits of beta-amyloid, a protein fragment from a larger protein called amyloid precursor protein, mixed with other neurons and non-nerve cells.

Anaerobic exercise Activity in which the muscles cannot draw out enough oxygen from the bloodstream, and anaerobic pathways are used to provide additional energy for storing for a short time.

Anal stimulation The stimulation of the anus with the fingers, mouth, or sex toys for sexual pleasure.

Anaphylactic shock Shock resulting from a widespread hypersensitivity reaction. Also called *anaphylaxis*.

Anaphylaxis An acute systemic type I hypersensitivity (allergic) response that may result in shock and death. It occurs in highly sensitive persons following exposure to a specific antigen, usually through injection or ingestion.

Anaplasia The regression of a cell to an immature or undifferentiated cell type.

Anasarca Severe, generalized edema.

Androgen A hormone that stimulates the development and maintenance of male sex characteristics.

Anemia An abnormally low number of circulating RBCs, low hemoglobin concentration, or both.

Anergic Unable to react to common antigens.

Aneurysm A weakened arterial wall that creates a bulge, or distention, of the artery. If it ruptures, it can result in internal bleeding or stroke and can sometimes be fatal.

Anger A subjective sense of intense displeasure, irritation, or animosity.

Angina pectoris Chest pain resulting from reduced coronary blood flow caused by a temporary imbalance between myocardial blood supply and demand. Also called *angina*.

Angiotensin-converting enzyme (ACE) Located on the inner surface of all blood vessels, it is a central component of the renin–angiotensin–aldosterone system, which controls blood pressure by regulating the volume of fluids in the body. It converts the hormone angiotensin I to the active vasoconstrictor angiotensin II.

Angle-closure glaucoma A type of glaucoma that results from a narrowing of the anterior chamber angle due to corneal flattening or bulging of the iris into the anterior chamber. Also called *narrow-angle* or *closed-angle glaucoma*.

Anhedonia The inability to feel pleasure.

Anion Ion that carries a negative charge.

Anomia Difficulty naming people and things.

Anorexia Loss of appetite.

Anorexia nervosa (AN) A potentially life-threatening disorder characterized by extreme perfectionism, weight fear, significant weight loss, body image disturbances, strenuous exercising, peculiar food-handling patterns, and reductions in heart rate, blood pressure, metabolic rate, and the production of estrogen or testosterone.

Antepartum Time between conception and the onset of labor; usually used to describe the period during which a woman is pregnant.

Anthropometric measurements Measurements that can help identify individuals who are at risk for undernutrition or overnutrition. Specific measurements include height, length (in babies), weight, body mass index, waist-to-hip circumference, and skinfold thickness.

Antibodies Proteins that work against antigens.

Antibody-mediated cytotoxic hypersensitivity (type II) A type of allergic reaction that involves the rupture of cells targeted by the immune response that may affect a variety of organs and tissues.

Antibody-mediated (humoral) immune response Activation of B cells to produce antibodies to respond to antigens such as bacteria, bacterial toxins, and free viruses.

Anticipatory grief Grief experienced in advance of a loss, such as the wife who grieves before her ailing husband dies.

Anticipatory guidance Information about developmental changes that can be expected in the future.

Anticipatory loss A loss that is experienced before the loss actually occurs. For example, the gradual decline and eventual death of a family member who has Alzheimer disease.

Anticipatory problem solving Initial information is presented to a patient or learner, who is then asked a question or presented with a problem and then is asked to apply the information learned.

Antidiuretic hormone Hormone that regulates water excretion from the kidneys.

Antigen Foreign substance that triggers the immune response.

Antigenic drift Describes small changes that occur continuously as a virus makes copies of itself.

Antigenic shift When two different strains of a virus infect the same cell and exchange genetic material to create a new subtype of the virus.

Antiretroviral therapy (ART) Pharmacologic therapy that stops or suppresses the activity of a retrovirus, preventing further weakening of the immune system and thereby minimizing opportunistic infections.

Antiseptics Agents that inhibit the growth of some microorganisms.

Antisocial personality disorder (ASPD) One of several types of personality disorders defined by the DSM-5, it is characterized by a pattern of disregard for and violation of the rights of others.

Anuria The failure of the kidneys to produce urine, resulting in a total lack of urination or output of less than 100 mL/day in an adult.

Anxiety A stress response characterized by feelings of apprehension, dread, mental uneasiness, and a sense of helplessness in response to an actual or perceived threat to the well-being of oneself or others.

Anxious distress A combination of symptoms often associated with anxiety, including restlessness, impaired concentration due to worry, fear of something awful happening, and fear of losing control. Anxious distress often manifests in patients with depression and bipolar disorders and is associated with an increased risk for suicide.

Aortic stenosis (AS) Narrowing of the aortic valve that obstructs blood flow to systemic circulation.

Aortocaval compression Also referred to as *supine hypotensive syndrome* or *vena caval syndrome*, it is a condition in pregnancy when the enlarging uterus presses on the vena cava and aorta and its collateral circulation.

Apathy A lack of interest or enthusiasm.

Apgar score A physical assessment of a newborn at 1 minute and 5 minutes after birth on a scale from 1 to 10 that includes heart rate, respiratory effort, muscle tone, reflex irritability, and skin color.

Aphakia Absence of the lens of the eye (e.g., after surgical removal of a cataract).

Aphasia Defective or absent language function.

Apical-radial pulse A comparison of the apical and radial pulses, which are normally identical. A pulse deficit can indicate certain cardiovascular disorders.

Apnea Absence of breathing.

Apnea of prematurity Absence of breathing for 20 seconds or longer, or for less than 20 seconds when associated with cyanosis, pallor, and bradycardia. A common problem in a preterm infant of less than 36 weeks' gestation, usually presenting between day 2 and day 7 of life.

Appendectomy Surgical removal of the appendix.

Appendicitis Inflammation of the vermiform appendix.

Approach coping The use of confrontation to change the stressor by taking direct action.

Approximated Term describing successful closure of a wound with little or no tissue loss.

Apraxia The inability to perform purposeful movements and use objects correctly.

Arousal Alertness regulated in the brain by the **reticular activating system.**

Arrogance Excessive pride and a feeling of superiority.

Arrhythmogenic right-ventricular dysplasia (ARVD) A condition that results when the body progressively replaces the muscle of the right ventricle with fatty and fibrous tissue.

Arterial blood gas (ABG) A laboratory test used to evaluate oxygen and carbon dioxide exchange and the acid–base balance within the blood.

Arterial blood pressure A measure of the pressure exerted by the blood as it flows through the arteries.

Arteriosclerosis An arterial disorder characterized by thickening, loss of elasticity, and calcification of arterial walls.

Arteriovenous (AV) fistula An artificial connection between a vein and an artery created for long-term vascular access.

Arthrodesis A procedure that permanently fuses two or more bones together at a joint using pins, plates, screws, and rods. Also called *joint fusion*.

Arthroplasty Total joint replacement.

Arthroscopy A surgical procedure in which a thin, lighted tube with a camera in one end is inserted into a joint in order to allow a surgeon to visualize joint structure more easily.

Artificial disk surgery Surgery to replace a herniated disk with an artificial disk in order to maintain flexibility of the spinal joint.

Artificial rupture of membranes A process of rupturing of the membranes by the certified nurse-midwife or physician using an instrument called an amniohook. Completed if spontaneous rupture of membranes does not occur.

ASA Physical Status Classification System A physical risk classification category that determines the type and dosage of sedation a patient can receive.

Ascites Excess fluid in the peritoneal cavity.

Asepsis The absence of disease-causing organisms.

Assault The action of creating an apprehension of offensive, insulting, or physically injurious touching.

Assertive behavior Behavior that consists of expressing one's wishes and opinions, or taking care of oneself, but not at the expense of others.

Assertive communicators Individuals who tend to declare and affirm their opinions. In doing this, however, they respect the rights of others to communicate in the same fashion.

Assertive community treatment (ACT) A therapeutic regimen for individuals with moderate to severe mental illness that provides patients with individually tailored services within their communities.

Assessment The systematic and continuous collection of data about a patient for the purpose of determining the patient's current and ongoing health status, predicting the patient's health risks, and identifying appropriate health-promoting activities.

Assignment The transfer of responsibility to accomplish a task, without the transfer of authority.

Assimilation 1. The process of adapting to and integrating characteristics of the dominant culture as one's own. 2. The process by which humans encounter and react to new situations by using the mechanisms they already possess.

Assisted reproductive technology (ART) Fertility treatments in which either eggs or embryos are handled.

Assisted suicide Self-administration of a lethal dose of medication provided by a physician or healthcare provider in order to intentionally end a patient's life with the goal of relieving pain and suffering.

Associative play A stage of play in which children play together or share tasks during play.

Astereognosis The inability to identify objects by touch.

Asthma A chronic inflammatory disease of the lungs characterized by recurrent episodes of wheezing, breathlessness, chest tightness, and coughing.

Asynclitism A condition that occurs when the sagittal suture is directed toward either the symphysis pubis or the sacral promontory and is felt to be misaligned.

Asystole Cardiac standstill.

Ataxia Lack of muscle coordination.

Atelectasis Collapse of lung tissue following obstruction of the bronchus or bronchioles.

Atherectomy A procedure to remove plaque from a lesion, specifically an **atheroma**.

Atheroma Complex lesion consisting of lipids, fibrous tissue, collagen, calcium, cellular debris, and capillaries. The formation of atheromas is the final stage of **atherosclerosis**.

Atherosclerosis A form of arteriosclerosis in which deposits of fat and fibrin obstruct and harden the arteries.

Atrial gallop (S_4) A heart sound produced by atrial contraction and ejection of blood into the ventricle during late diastole. Also called the *fourth heart sound*.

Atrial kick An extra bolus of blood delivered to the ventricles before they contract.

Atrial natriuretic factor (ANF) A peptide hormone released from cells in the atrium of the heart in response to excess blood volume and stretching of the atrial walls.

Atrial septal defect (ASD) An opening in the atrial septum that permits left-to-right shunting of blood.

Atrioventricular (AV) canal defect A combination of defects in the atrial and ventricular septa and portions of tricuspid and mitral valves. A complete AV canal defect allows blood to travel freely among all four chambers of the heart. Also called *endocardial cushion defect*.

Atrophy The wasting-away or decrease in size of an organ, muscle, or tissue.

Attention-deficit disorder (ADD) A variation in central nervous system processing characterized by developmentally inappropriate behaviors involving inattention.

Attention-deficit/hyperactivity disorder (ADHD) A variation in central nervous system processing characterized by developmentally inappropriate behaviors involving inattention, hyperactivity, and impulsivity.

Attentive listening The process of listening actively, using all the senses. Also called *mindful listening*.

Attributes of safety The quality or properties of remaining safe.

Audiologist A healthcare professional specializing in identifying, diagnosing, treating, and monitoring disorders of the auditory and vestibular portions of the ear.

Audit An examination of records to verify accuracy and proper use.

Auditory Of or relating to hearing.

Aura An olfactory or visual sensory sensation that may provide an early warning sign of a seizure.

Aural pressure Congestion in the ear.

Auscultation Listening to the sounds produced within the body. Auscultation can be direct using the unaided ear or indirect using a stethoscope or other listening device.

Authority 1. The power to command other individuals and direct their activities. 2. The right to act or to accomplish a task.

Autism spectrum disorder (ASD) A developmental disorder in which individuals have persistent deficits in social communication and social interaction and restricted, repetitive patterns of behavior, interests, or activities.

Autoantibodies Antibodies that react to an individual's own tissues.

Autocratic (authoritarian) leader A leader who makes decisions for the group based on the belief that individuals are externally motivated and are incapable of independent decision making.

Autografting A procedure performed in the surgical suite in which part of a patient's healthy skin is removed and used to effect permanent skin coverage over a wound area.

Autoimmune disorder Failure of immune system to recognize itself, resulting in normal host tissue being targeted by immune defenses.

Autologous blood transfusion A blood transfusion using a patient's own blood.

Autologous bone marrow transplant Bone marrow transplant using a patient's own bone marrow.

Automaticity The ability to generate an electrical impulse.

Automatism A repetitive reaction that occurs automatically, without conscious thought. Examples include lip smacking, eyelid fluttering, aimless walking, picking at clothing, and swallowing.

Autonomic dysreflexia An abrupt onset of excessively high blood pressure as the result of an overactive autonomic nervous system. An exaggerated sympathetic response that occurs in patients with spinal cord injuries at or above the T6 level. Also called *autonomic hyperreflexia*.

Autonomy 1. The state of being independent and self-directed without outside control. 2. The right to make one's own decisions.

Autoregulation The control of cerebral blood flow by vasoconstricting or vasodilating the cerebral vessels, thus regulating the amount of blood that reaches the brain.

Autosome A single chromosome from any one of the 22 pairs of chromosomes not involved in sex determination (X or Y); humans have 22 pairs of autosomes.

Avascular necrosis The death of bone tissue due to lack of blood supply. Also called *osteonecrosis*.

Avoidance coping The use of both behaviors and cognitive processes to avoid a stressor.

Avoidant personality disorder (APD) One of several types of personality disorders recognized by the DSM-5, APD is characterized by a pattern of social withdrawal along with a sense of inadequacy, fear, and hypersensitivity to potential rejection or shame.

Avolition The inability to persist in goal-directed activities.

Awareness The ability to perceive environmental stimuli and body reactions and to respond appropriately through thought and action.

Axon A nerve fiber.

Azotemia Increased levels of nitrogenous wastes in the blood.

B lymphocytes (B cells) Integral to specific immune response, they are activated and mature into either plasma cells, which secrete antibodies, or memory cells.

B-type natriuretic peptide (BNP) Functions as both a vasodilator and a regulator of sodium and water excretion.

Babinski reflex The fanning and extension of the toes or flexion of the toes due to gentle stroking on the sole of the foot. Also called the *Babinski response.*

Bacilli Rod-shaped bacteria.

Background questions General questions asked of a patient that seek more information about a topic, such as diseases and medications.

Bacteremia The presence of bacteria in the blood.

Bacteria The most common category of infection-causing microorganisms.

Bactericidal agent Destroys bacteria.

Bacteriostatic agent Prevents the growth and reproduction of some bacteria.

Balance State of equilibrium that is vital for movement, body positioning, and coordination.

Balanitis Inflammation of the glans.

Balloon tamponade The inflation of the balloon tip of a multiple-lumen nasogastric tube to control bleeding.

Ballottement The passive fetal movement elicited when the examiner inserts two gloved fingers into the vagina and pushes against the cervix.

Barlow maneuver A procedure used to evaluate an infant for hip dislocation or instability in which the healthcare provider grasps and adducts the infant's thigh and then applies gentle downward pressure.

Barotrauma Lung injury caused by alveolar overdistention. Also called *volutrauma.*

Barrel chest An increase in the anteroposterior chest diameter resulting from air trapping and hyperinflation.

Basal cell cancer An epithelial tumor believed to originate either from the basal layer of the epidermis or from cells in the surrounding dermal structures. Also called *basal cell carcinoma.*

Basal metabolic rate (BMR) The amount of energy expended by the body at rest.

Base excess (BE) A calculated value also known as *buffer base capacity.* The BE measures substances that can accept or combine with hydrogen ions. It reflects the degree of acid–base imbalance by indicating the status of the body's total buffering capacity.

Baseline fetal heart rate The average fetal heart rate rounded to increments of 5 bpm observed during a 10-minute period of monitoring. This excludes periodic or episodic changes, periods of marked variability, and segments of the baseline that differ by more than 25 bpm.

Baseline fetal heart rate variability Fluctuation in the fetal heart rate baseline of 2 cycles per minute or greater, with irregular amplitude and inconstant frequency.

Bases Substances that accept hydrogen ions in solution. Also called *alkalis.*

Basic needs The physical needs of an individual, such as eating, sleeping, resting, self-care, and physical stability.

Battery The willful touching of another individual, an individual's clothes, or even something the individual is carrying that is unwanted, embarrassing, or unwarranted.

Behavioral therapy A form of therapy in which patients learn techniques to modify or change maladaptive behaviors.

Behaviorist theory A theory that suggests that learning takes place when an individual's reaction to a stimulus is either positively or negatively reinforced.

Belief An interpretation or conclusion that one accepts as true.

Benchmark Used to compare the performance of an individual or organization to industry standards.

Beneficence The act of doing good or beneficial actions.

Benign Referring to a growth or tumor that does not endanger life or health and tends to not recur after treatment.

Benign prostatic hyperplasia (BPH) Nonmalignant enlargement of the prostate gland commonly seen in the aging man.

Bereavement The subjective response experienced by the surviving loved ones after the death of an individual with whom they have shared a significant relationship.

Bias The favoring of a group or individual over another.

Bicarbonate (HCO_3^-) A chemical buffer that keeps blood pH from becoming too acidic or too alkalotic.

Bicarbonate buffer system An acid–base homeostatic mechanism involving the balance of carbonic acid, bicarbonate ion, and carbon dioxide in order to maintain pH in the blood and duodenum, among other tissues, to support proper metabolic function.

Bilevel positive airway pressure (BiPAP) Mechanical ventilation that provides inspiratory positive airway pressure as well as airway support during expiration.

Binge drinking The consumption of five or more drinks containing alcohol in a single session.

Binge eating The ingestion of huge amounts of food (about 3,500 kcal) within a short time (about 1 hour).

Binge-eating disorder (BED) An eating disorder characterized by recurring episodes of binge eating, a sense of lack of control, and negative feelings about oneself, but without intervening periods of behavior such as self-induced vomiting, purging by laxatives, fasting, or prolonged exercise.

Binuclear family A postdivorce family in which the biologic children are members of two nuclear households—that of the father and that of the mother—and the children alternate between the two homes.

Bioethical dilemma Ethical dilemma of human life or health that arises in the care of patients and families; often emerges from a combination of causative factors.

Biological rhythm A cyclical event or function that consists of repeated occurrences and repeated, regular intervals between occurrences. Biological rhythms can refer to both physical and psychologic patterns.

Biomedical informatics The interprofessional science that deals with biomedical information's structure, acquisition, and use.

Bioterrorism The deliberate release of viruses, bacteria, or other microbes as weapons.

Bipolar disorder A mood disorder characterized by alternating depression and elation, with periods of normal mood in between. Formerly called *manic–depressive disorder.*

Birth equity Describes optimal maternal and child outcomes for pregnant and postpartum women and their babies. Recognized as a risk category as a result of the additional risk for morbidity and mortality that Black women face during the peripartum and postpartum periods.

Bisphosphonates Drugs used to treat osteoporosis that inhibit bone reabsorption by suppressing osteoclast activity.

Blackouts A form of amnesia about events that occurred during a drinking period. This is often seen in the early stages of alcoholism.

Bladder training Gradually increases the bladder capacity by increasing the intervals between voidings and resisting the urge to void.

Blame-free environment An environment in which healthcare providers can report errors or near misses without the fear of punishment.

Blastocyst A structure formed in early pregnancy. It possesses an inner cell mass that subsequently forms the embryo.

Blended family A family formed after the death or divorce of a parent; may include stepparents on both sides, stepchildren, and half-siblings.

Blepharism Spasms that cause the eye to blink continuously.

Blood flow The volume of blood transported in a vessel, in an organ, or throughout the entire circulation over a given period of time.

Blood pressure The force that blood exerts against the walls of the arteries as it is pumped from the heart.

Blood urea nitrogen (BUN) A measure of blood level of urea, the end product of protein metabolism.

Bloodborne pathogens Microorganisms carried in blood and body fluids that are capable of infecting other individuals with serious and difficult-to-treat viral infections.

Bloody show The pink-tinged secretions resulting from a small amount of blood loss from the exposed cervical capillaries during pregnancy.

Blunt trauma Trauma that occurs without any communication between the damaged tissues and the outside environment.

Body image The mental image of the physical self.

Body mass index (BMI) A method of comparing weight to height as an indirect measure of body fat.

Body substance isolation (BSI) System that employs generic infection control precautions for all patients, except those with the few airborne diseases.

Body surface area (BSA) The relationship between height and weight measured in square meters.

Bone marrow transplant (BMT) The treatment of disease by infusing patients with their own bone marrow or that of a healthy donor.

Bone mineral density Amount of minerals in bone.

Borborygmus Hyperactive, high-pitched, tinkling, rushing, or growling bowel sounds heard in diarrhea or at the onset of bowel obstruction.

Borderline personality disorder (BPD) One of several personality disorders defined in the DSM-5, it is marked by unstable interpersonal relationships, self-image, affect, and impulsiveness.

Boundaries The invisible lines that define the amount and kind of contact allowable among members of a family and between the family and outside systems.

Boutonnière deformity A flexion deformity of the proximal interphalangeal joints with extension of the distal interphalangeal joint.

Bowel incontinence The inability to voluntarily control the passage of fecal contents and intestinal gas through the anal sphincter. Also called *fecal incontinence*.

Brachytherapy Radiation treatment given by placing radioactive material directly in or near the target, which is often a tumor.

Bradycardia A heart rate in an adult of less than 60 bpm.

Bradykinesia Slowed movements due to muscle rigidity.

Bradypnea A respiratory rate of less than 10 breaths per minute in adults.

Brain death The cessation and irreversibility of all brain functions, including those of the brainstem.

Brainstem Contains the midbrain, pons, and medulla oblongata. Located between the cerebrum and spinal cord, it connects pathways between the higher and lower structures, and where 10 of the 12 pairs of cranial nerves originate.

Braxton Hicks contractions Intermittent painless uterine contractions that may occur every 10 to 20 minutes and occur more frequently near the end of pregnancy.

Brazelton Neonatal Behavioral Assessment Scale A scale developed to assess a newborn's state changes, temperament, and individual behavioral patterns.

Breach of care A deviation from the standard of care owed a patient. Also called *breach of duty*.

Breach of duty A deviation from the standard of care owed a patient. Also called *breach of care*.

Breakthrough pain A sudden flare-up or increase in pain despite comfort with or without baseline analgesia.

Breast cancer The unregulated growth of abnormal cells in breast tissue.

Breast-concerning surgery (BCS) Excision of the primary cancerous tumor and adjacent tissue in the breast followed by radiation therapy.

Breathing exercises Techniques used to slow the breathing rate by focusing on taking regular and deep breaths from the diaphragm.

Brief strategic family therapy (BSFT) A family systems approach to addiction treatment in which one member's problem behaviors appear to stem from unhealthy family interactions.

Bronchial sounds Loud, high-pitched sounds heard over the trachea that are longer on exhalation than inhalation.

Bronchiectasis Chronic dilation of the bronchi and bronchioles.

Bronchiolitis A lower respiratory tract illness that occurs when an infecting agent (virus or bacterium) causes inflammation and obstruction of the small airways.

Bronchitis Inflammation of the mucous membranes of the bronchial tubes.

Bronchogenic carcinomas Tumors of the airway epithelium.

Bronchoscopy A procedure that allows direct visualization of the lungs by inserting a bronchoscope orally into the trachea and advancing it to the bronchi bifurcation.

Bronchovesicular sound The sound created as air moves within the bronchial tree.

Brown adipose tissue (BAT) A specific store of fat in newborn infants that appears dark brown due to enriched blood supply, dense cellular content, and abundant nerve endings.

Bruits Blowing sound sometimes heard due to restriction of blood flow through the vessels.

Buffers Substances that prevent major changes in pH by releasing hydrogen ions.

Bulimia nervosa (BN) A type of eating disorder characterized by an obsessive focus on weight and body size and cycles of binge eating followed by purging.

Bullying Aggressive or intimidating behavior committed against another who is not a sibling or dating partner.

Bureaucratic leader A leader who relies on the organization's rules, policies, and procedures to direct the group's work efforts.

Burn An injury resulting from exposure to heat, chemicals, radiation, or electric current.

Burn shock Hypovolemic shock resulting from the shift of a massive amount of fluid from the intracellular and intravascular compartments into the interstitium following burn injury. Also called *hypovolemic shock*.

Burnout Stress related to caregiving duties that has adverse emotional and physical effects on the nurse and is also associated with reduced quality of care and decreased patient satisfaction with nursing care.

C-type natriuretic peptide (CNP) Functions as both a vasodilator and a regulator of sodium and water excretion.

Cachexia Physical wasting from weight loss and loss of muscle mass due to the rapid growth and reproduction of cancer cells and their need for increased nutrients.

Caffeine A stimulant that increases the heart rate and acts as a diuretic.

Calcium oxalate A chemical compound from which kidney stones may form.

Calcium phosphate A chemical compound from which kidney stones may form.

Calculi Renal stones.

Call-out One of the standardized communication strategies developed to facilitate interprofessional communication and reduce errors, it is used to report critical information to all members of the team at the same time.

Cancer A family of complex diseases with manifestations that vary according to body system and type of tumor cells.

Candidiasis A common, opportunistic fungal infection in patients with AIDS.

Cannabis sativa The plant source of marijuana.

Capacitation One of the processes a sperm must undergo before fertilization can occur. It involves the removal of the plasma membrane overlying the spermatozoa's acrosomal area and the loss of seminal plasma proteins.

Caput succedaneum A localized, easily identifiable, soft area of the scalp, generally resulting from a long and difficult labor or vacuum extraction.

Carbohydrate One of the three major macronutrients primarily derived from plant foods. These foods contain simple and complex sugars and starches.

Carcinogen A substance that causes cancer.

Carcinogenesis The production or origin of cancer.

Cardiac arrest The cessation of heart function that precedes biologic death.

Cardiac cycle One contraction and relaxation of the heart; a single heartbeat.

Cardiac index (CI) The cardiac output adjusted for the patient's body size or body surface area.

Cardiac markers Proteins released from necrotic heart muscle.

Cardiac muscle troponins A group of proteins found in heart muscle fibers that regulate muscular contraction.

Cardiac output (CO) The amount of blood pumped by the ventricles into the pulmonary and systemic circulations in 1 minute.

Cardiac rehabilitation A medically supervised program designed to aid people with their recovery from heart attack, heart surgery, and percutaneous coronary intervention.

Cardiac reserve The heart's ability to respond to the body's changing need for cardiac output.

Cardiac tamponade Compression of the heart caused by collected blood or fluid in the pericardium.

Cardinal movements A series of changes in position that allow the fetus to move through the birth canal. Also called *mechanisms of labor.*

Cardiogenic shock Shock that occurs when the heart's pumping ability is compromised to the point that it cannot maintain cardiac output and adequate tissue perfusion.

Cardiomyopathy Disease that affects the heart muscle's ability to pump effectively. Primary abnormality of the heart muscle that affects its structural or functional characteristics.

Cardiopulmonary resuscitation (CPR) A mechanical attempt to maintain tissue perfusion and oxygenation using oral resuscitation and external cardiac compressions.

Care coordination The means by which an interprofessional team works with a patient to ensure that the care received across the healthcare continuum meets the patient's needs.

Care map Expected outcomes and care strategies developed through collaboration by the healthcare team. Also called a *critical pathway.*

Caregiver burden The psychologic, physical, and financial cost of caring for an individual with a chronic physical or mental illness.

Caring In the context of the nursing profession, caring encompasses various intentions and actions; for example, recognizing and responding to patient status and behaviors, attending to the patient and the family, engaging with the healthcare team, and maintaining a positive attitude.

Caring for the dying The act of helping patients live as comfortably as possible until death and helping the patient's support individuals cope with death.

Carpal spasm Involuntary contraction of the hand and fingers due to decreased calcium levels.

Carphologia Involuntary, repeated lint picking.

Carrier Human or animal reservoir of a specific infectious agent that usually does not manifest any clinical signs of the disease.

Cartilage A type of flexible connective tissue found throughout the body.

Case management (CM) The coordination of patient care over time using the combination of health and social services necessary to meet the individual patient's needs.

Case managers Individuals who help manage the care of certain patient populations, including patients with chronic medical conditions, such as diabetes; patients recovering from acute conditions, such as those receiving joint replacement; and patients managing psychiatric disorders.

Case method A patient-centered method of managing care in which one nurse is assigned to, and is responsible for, the comprehensive care of a group of patients during an 8- or 12-hour shift.

Caseation necrosis A process in which tissue infected with *Mycobacterium tuberculosis* dies and forms a cheeselike center in the infectious bacilli.

Cast A rigid device applied to immobilize injured bones and promote healing.

Cataract An opacification (clouding) of the lens of the eye due to a breakdown of proteins within the lens.

Catatonia Unresponsiveness to the environment or others.

Catheter-associated urinary tract infection (CAUTI) Results when bacteria enter the catheter system at the connection between the catheter and the drainage system or through the emptying tube of the drainage bag.

Cation Ion that carries a positive charge.

Cauda equina syndrome (CES) A condition that occurs when the nerve roots of the cauda equine are compressed. It may result in permanent neurologic impairment, including urinary incontinence and paralysis.

Causation To make a successful claim for malpractice, an injury must have occurred as a direct consequence of a nurse's or other healthcare professional's breach of duty.

Celiac disease A chronic immune-mediated disorder of the small intestine in which the absorption of nutrients, particularly fats, is impaired. Also known as *celiac sprue* or *nontropical sprue.*

Cell cycle The four phases of cell growth and development.

Cell-mediated (cellular) immune response Direct or indirect inactivation of antigen by lymphocytes.

Cellular immune response Disordered T-cell function.

Cellulitis An acute bacterial infection of the dermis and underlying connective tissue. It is characterized by red or lilac, tender, warm, edematous skin that may have an ill-defined, nonelevated border.

Central nervous system (CNS) One of two principal parts of the neurologic system, it consists of the brain and the spinal cord.

Central nervous system depressants A type of drug that acts to slow brain function, decreasing levels of alertness and awareness. They include barbiturates, benzodiazepines, paraldehyde, meprobamate, and chloral hydrate.

Central pain 1. A type of pain related to a lesion in the brain that may spontaneously produce high-frequency bursts of impulses that are perceived as pain. 2. A type of pain caused by damage to the central nervous system that may manifest in constant pain, pain paroxysms, evoked pain, or allodynia. Patients may describe their pain as "pins and needles," aching, or lacerating.

Centration Focusing only on one particular aspect of a situation or the ability to concentrate.

Cephalocaudal The head-to-toe direction of growth and development.

Cephalohematoma A collection of blood resulting from ruptured blood vessels between the surface of a cranial bone and the periosteal membrane. Also called an *entrapped hemorrhage.*

Cerebellum Located below the cerebrum and behind the brainstem, it coordinates stimuli from the cerebral cortex to provide precise timing for skeletal muscle coordination and smooth movements.

Cerebral palsy (CP) A group of chronic conditions affecting body movement, coordination, and posture that results from a nonprogressive abnormality of the immature brain.

Cerebral perfusion pressure (CPP) The pressure it takes for the heart to provide the brain with blood. It is calculated by finding the difference between arterial pressure and intracranial pressure. Normal CPP is 0 to 95 mmHg.

Cerebrospinal fluid (CSF) Located in the subarachnoid space, between the arachnoid mater and the pia mater, it cushions the brain and spinal cord and helps prevent injury to these tissues.

Cerebrum The largest portion of the brain, it is composed of gray matter and has two hemispheres divided into four regions or lobes.

Certification The credentialing process by which a nongovernmental agency or association recognizes the professional competence of an individual who has met the predetermined qualifications specified by the agency or association.

Cerumen Earwax.

Cervical cap A latex cup-shaped contraceptive device, used with spermicidal cream or jelly, that fits snugly over the cervix and is held in place by suction.

Cervical collar A device that stabilizes and maintains neutral alignment of the cervical spine; it is used with patients with potential or suspected cervical spine injury. Also called *C-collar*.

Cervical ripening The softening and effacing of the cervix.

Cesarean birth The birth of an infant through an abdominal and uterine incision.

CFTR modulators A treatment for **cystic fibrosis** that attacks the cause of the problem—issues with the CFTR protein—rather than just CF's clinical manifestations.

Chadwick sign Blue-purple discoloration of the cervix.

Chain of command The hierarchy of authority and responsibility within an organization.

Chancre A painless ulceration formed during the first stage of syphilis.

Change-of-shift report A type of handoff communication given to all nurses on the next shift.

Charcot-Marie-Tooth (CMT) disease The most common inherited form of **peripheral neuropathy**, it is characterized by a slowly progressive degeneration of the muscles of the foot, lower leg, hand, and forearm. Symptoms usually present between adolescence and young adulthood.

Charismatic leader A rare type of leader who is characterized by a strong, emotional relationship between the leader and the group members.

Chart A formal, legal document that provides evidence of a patient's care. Also called a *patient record* or a *clinical record*.

Charting The process of making an entry on a patient record. Also called *recording* or *documenting*.

Charting by exception (CBE) A documentation system in which only abnormal or significant findings or exceptions to norms are recorded.

Cheilosis Cracking of lips.

Chemical conjunctivitis An irritation of the conjunctiva by chemicals used to treat the eyes.

Chemical restraints Pharmacologic agents administered for the purpose of controlling hyperactive behavior in agitated patients.

Chemotaxis The movement of cells in response to a chemical stimulus.

Chemotherapy Cancer treatment involving the use of cytotoxic medications to decrease tumor size, adjunctive to surgery or radiation therapy, or to prevent or treat suspected metastases.

Chest physical therapy An **airway clearance technique** that involves clapping and **percussion**.

Chest x-ray (CXR) Allows for two-dimensional visualization of the contents of the thoracic cavity.

Child abuse Any act or failure to act on the part of a parent or caretaker that results in the death, serious physical or emotional harm, sexual abuse, or exploitation of a child.

Childfree family A family without children.

Childhood traumatic grief A grief reaction that occurs when an important person in a child's life dies as the result of a traumatic event or circumstances the child views as traumatic.

Children's Health Insurance Program (CHIP) State- and federal-funded healthcare coverage for children under the age of 19 whose families earn more than the Medicaid limits but cannot afford to purchase private healthcare coverage.

Chlamydia A group of sexually transmitted infections caused by *Chlamydia trachomatis*.

Chloasma Brownish pigmentation over the bridge of the nose and the cheeks during pregnancy and in some women who are taking oral contraceptives. Also called *melasma gravidarum* or *mask of pregnancy*.

Cholangitis Duct inflammation.

Cholecystitis Inflammation of the gallbladder.

Cholelithiasis The formation of stones (*calculi* or *gallstones*) in the gallbladder or biliary duct system.

Chorion The first and outmost embryonic membrane to form, the chorion has many fingerlike projections called chorionic membranes on its surface.

Chromosomes Tightly coiled strands of DNA within the nucleus that contain genetic information.

Chronic bronchitis A disorder of excessive bronchial mucous secretion.

Chronic fatigue Profound fatigue of long duration that is not improved by rest.

Chronic fatigue syndrome A complex disorder in which the patient experiences unrelenting fatigue and associated symptoms that are not alleviated by substantial rest and that cannot be otherwise explained for a period of 6 months or longer. Also called *myalgic encephalomyelitis*.

Chronic hypertension Hypertensive disorder of pregnancy based on a known history prior to pregnancy, that is discovered during the pregnancy prior to 20 weeks' gestation, or that persists for more than 12 weeks postpartum.

Chronic illness An alteration in health or function that lasts for an extended period of time, usually 6 months or longer, and often for the duration of the individual's life.

Chronic infection An infection that develops slowly and persists for months or sometimes years.

Chronic kidney disease (CKD) A type of renal failure that progresses slowly with few symptoms until the kidneys are severely damaged and unable to meet the excretory needs of the body. Also called *chronic renal failure*.

Chronic lymphocytic leukemia (CLL) A disorder characterized by the proliferation and accumulation of small, abnormal, mature lymphocytes in the bone marrow, peripheral blood, and body tissues.

Chronic myeloid leukemia (CML) A disorder characterized by abnormal proliferation of all bone marrow elements.

Chronic obstructive pulmonary disease (COPD) A specific progressive disorder that slowly alters the structures of the respiratory system over time, irreversibly affecting lung function.

Chronic pain Prolonged pain, usually lasting longer than 6 months. It is not always associated with an identifiable cause and is often unresponsive to conventional medical treatment.

Chronic pancreatitis An irreversible process characterized by chronic inflammation, fibrosis, and gradual destruction of functional pancreatic tissue.

Chronic traumatic encephalopathy (CTE) A form of dementia associated with a history of multiple concussions.

Chronic venous insufficiency (CVI) A disorder of inadequate venous return over a prolonged period of time.

Chvostek sign Facial grimacing caused by repeated contractions of the facial muscle. A test used to check for hypocalcemia.

Circadian rhythms Regular fluctuations in the body's physiologic processes occurring in a 24-hour cycle.

Circumcision A surgical procedure in which the prepuce, an epithelial layer covering the penis, is separated from the glans penis and excised. This procedure permits exposure of the glans for easier cleaning.

Cirrhosis The end stage of chronic liver disease. It is a progressive, irreversible disorder, eventually leading to liver failure.

Civil law The area of law that deals with the rights and duties of private persons or citizens and is most often enforced through the awarding of damages or compensation.

CK-MB A subset of CK enzyme specific to cardiac muscle. Elevated CK-MB is an indicator of myocardial infarction. Also called *MB-bands*.

Classism The oppression of groups of people based on their socioeconomic status.

Clean A state of medical asepsis in which almost all microorganisms are absent.

Clinical database The full extent of information about a patient, including the nursing health history, physical assessment, primary care provider's history and physical examination, results of laboratory and diagnostic tests, and material contributed by other health personnel.

Clinical decision making A process nurses use in the clinical setting to evaluate and select the best actions to meet desired goals.

Clinical decision support system A system that analyzes data and provides information about evidence-based practices. These systems can help improve patient safety and quality of care when used with sound nursing and medical judgment.

Clinical information system A software-based system that allows multiple disciplines to simultaneously access a patient's chart and record data that can be viewed and analyzed by a number of healthcare providers in real time. These systems are designed to provide the most accurate and current information about a patient so that the best decisions concerning the care of that patient can be made.

Clinical judgment A highly complex cognitive process through which nurses solve problems by applying clinical reasoning, critical thinking, and decision-making skills.

Clinical pathway A standardized, evidence-based, multidisciplinary plan that outlines the expected care required for patients with common, predictable—usually medical—conditions.

Clinical reasoning The use of careful reasoning by nurses in the clinical setting to improve patient care. It requires critical thinking and the ability to reflect on previous situations and decisions and evaluate their effectiveness.

Clonic phase Typically the second phase in a generalized or tonic–clonic seizure, characterized by alternating muscular contraction and relaxation.

Closed fracture A bone fracture in which the skin remains intact. Also called a *simple fracture*.

Closed questions Restrictive questions in an interview that require only a "yes" or "no" or short, specific answer.

Clotting Also known as **coagulation**, the process by which blood changes from liquid into a gel-like substance in order to stop bleeding from a damaged vessel.

Clotting factor Multiple plasma proteins involved in coagulation.

Coagulation Also known as **clotting**, the process by which blood changes from liquid into a gel-like substance for the purpose of forming a clot to stop bleeding from a damaged vessel.

Coagulation cascade A process that activates clotting factors, plasma proteins used in the formation of blood clots.

Coanalgesics Drugs that have analgesic properties, potentiate the effects of pain medications, relieve other discomforts, or reduce the side effects of analgesic drugs. Coanalgesics are especially effective at reducing neuropathic pain.

Coarctation of the aorta (COA) Narrowing or constriction in the descending aorta, often near the ductus arteriosus or left subclavian artery, which obstructs the systemic blood outflow.

Cobb angle A technique to estimate the degree of curvature of the spine using lines drawn from the vertebrae at the upper and lower limits of the curve that tilt most dramatically toward the apex of the curve.

Cocaine A powerful stimulant of natural origin that acts at the nerve terminals to prevent the reuptake of dopamine and norepinephrine, which in turn results in vasoconstriction, tachycardia, and hypertension.

Code of ethics A general guide for a profession's membership and a social contract with the public that it serves.

Codependence A cluster of maladaptive behaviors exhibited by significant others of a substance-abusing individual that serves to enable and protect the abuse at the expense of living a full and satisfying life.

Cognition The complex set of mental activities through which individuals acquire, process, store, retrieve, and apply information.

Cognitive appraisal The process of appraising, sorting, assessing, categorizing, evaluating, and framing the significance of an event or stressor with respect to an individual's own well-being.

Cognitive-behavioral therapy (CBT) The use of cognitive techniques and behavior modification to change detrimental beliefs and thought patterns.

Cognitive deficits Inclusive term to describe any characteristic that impairs the cognition process.

Cognitive development The manner in which people learn to think, reason, and use language.

Cognitive domain The learning domain that includes the six intellectual abilities and thinking processes: knowing, comprehending, applying, analysis, synthesis, and evaluation. Also called the *thinking domain*.

Cognitive skills Intellectual skills or thought processes that include problem solving, decision making, critical thinking, and creativity.

Cognitive symptoms Cognitive symptoms of schizophrenia include deficits in memory, attention, language, visual-spatial awareness, social and emotional perception, and intellectual and executive function.

Cognitive theory A learning theory that recognizes the developmental level of learners and the social, emotional, and physical contexts in which learning takes place. Also called *cognitivism*.

Cohesiveness The attachment that group members feel toward each other, the group, or the group's purpose.

Coitus interruptus A method of contraception in which the man withdraws from the woman's vagina when he feels that ejaculation is impending.

Cold zone When a disaster occurs, this zone, located outside the warm zone, is where decontaminated victims are triaged and treated. Also called the *green zone* or the *support zone*.

Colectomy Surgical resection and removal of the colon.

Collaboration Two or more people working toward a common goal.

Collaborative intervention The actions a nurse carries out in collaboration with other healthcare team members, such as physical therapists, social workers, dietitians, and physicians.

Collagen A whitish protein substance that adds tensile strength to a wound.

Colon cancer Cancer of the third segment of the large bowel that may or may not include the anus.

Colonization The process by which strains of microorganisms become resident flora, capable of growing and multiplying.

Color blindness Deficient color vision that occurs when one or more pigments are missing within the cones in the retina.

Colorectal cancer Cancer of both the colon and rectum.

Colostomy A surgical opening into the colon.

Colostrum The initial milk that begins to be secreted during midpregnancy and that is immediately available to the baby at birth.

Column plan A nursing care plan that uses columns to categorize data for each phase of the nursing process. This type of care plan may include four columns: (1) nursing diagnoses, (2) goals/desired outcomes, (3) nursing interventions, and (4) evaluation. Some include only three columns.

Combined oral contraceptives (COCs) A safe, highly effective contraceptive pill combining estrogen and progestin. Also called *birth control pills.*

Comfort To ease the grief or trouble of others; to give hope.

Commanding The supervision of work to communicate and achieve goals.

Commitment The state or an instance of being obligated or emotionally impelled.

Communicable disease An illness that is transmitted directly from one person or animal to another by contact with body fluids or that is indirectly transmitted by contact with contaminated objects or vectors.

Communication The exchange of information, feelings, thoughts, and ideals through verbal or other techniques.

Community Emergency Response Team (CERT) program A Federal Emergency Management Agency–organized program that prepares participants to safely assist themselves, their families, and their neighbors in case of a disaster.

Community violence Violent acts perpetrated in public areas by individuals who are not intimately related to their victims, such as shootings, gang violence, bullying, hate crimes, and social unrest.

Comorbidity The presence of two or more disease processes.

Compartment syndrome A condition in which the tissue pressure in a muscle compartment exceeds the microvascular pressure, interrupting cellular perfusion.

Compassion An awareness of and concern for other individuals' suffering.

Compassion fatigue The fatigue, distress, and physical, mental, and emotional depletion experienced by nurses (or other healthcare professionals or caregivers) in reaction to prolonged stress.

Competence Possessing the knowledge and skills necessary to perform one's job appropriately and safely.

Competency A legal presumption of ability to negotiate activities and make decisions on one's own behalf.

Complementary healthcare Also referred to as *alternative therapies,* any of the diverse array of practices, therapies, and supplements that are not considered part of conventional or traditional medicine that are used in addition to conventional treatments.

Complete spinal cord injury An injury that involves a total loss of all sensory and motor function below the level of the injury; usually the damage is irreversible.

Complex trauma Exposure to multiple traumatic events or an accumulation of traumatic events throughout a lifetime.

Compliance 1. The relationship between the volume of the intracranial components and intracranial pressure. 2. The amount of distention or expansion the ventricles can achieve to increase stroke volume. 3. The extent to which an individual's behavior coincides with medical or health advice.

Compression A condition that occurs when a vertical force is applied to the spinal column, such as occurs by falling and landing on the feet or buttocks or diving into shallow water.

Compromised host An individual who is at increased risk of infection.

Compulsion A repetitive behavior or mental activity (such as counting) used in an attempt to mitigate the obsessive thoughts and reduce feelings of anxiety.

Computer vision syndrome The most common sequela of computer use. Symptoms include eye fatigue, headaches, blurred vision, dry eyes, and changes in color perception. Also called *eye strain.*

Concentration gradient Difference in solute concentration.

Concept map A visual representation of a nursing plan of care in a patterned diagram with data and ideas. Various shapes and colors are used to show relationships and connections in combination with lines or arrows.

Concrete thinking A type of thinking characterized by a focus on facts and details coupled with an inability to generalize or think abstractly.

Concurrent audit An evaluation of the adequacy of the nursing care a patient is receiving and a determination of whether desired outcomes are being met while the individual is still undergoing care at the healthcare facility.

Concussion Mild **traumatic brain injury**.

Condom A sheath of synthetic material that covers the penis to prevent conception or disease.

Confabulation Making up information to fill memory gaps; used as a defensive mechanism for a person's attempt to protect self-esteem when confronted with memory loss.

Confidentiality The assurance a patient has that private information will not be disclosed without the patient's consent.

Conflict When there is disagreement or discord among individuals, groups, or organizations that prevents problem solving and interferes with effective communication.

Conflict competence Purposeful development of cognitive, behavioral, and emotional skills that assist individuals in preventing and reducing conflict.

Confusion An alteration in cognition that makes it difficult to think clearly, focus attention, or make decisions.

Confusion Assessment Method (CAM) A two-part test that differentiates between delirium and dementia. It is specifically designed to account for and control ageism.

Congenital cataracts A type of cataract that may appear in a child at birth or in childhood, usually in both eyes.

Congenital dermal melanocytosis Sometimes called **Mongolian spots**, it is a bluish-black or gray-blue pigmentation on the dorsal area and the buttocks of newborns.

Congenital glaucoma A primary form of **glaucoma** caused by an abnormal development in the ocular drainage system that is sometimes diagnosed at birth but is usually diagnosed within the first year. When diagnosed within the first year, it is often referred to as **infantile glaucoma**. When diagnosed after age 3, it may be referred to as **juvenile glaucoma**.

Congenital heart defect A defect of the heart or great vessels that is present at birth.

Congruent communication Communication in which the verbal and nonverbal aspects of the message match.

Conjunctiva The thin, transparent membrane that covers the anterior surface of the eye and lines the inner surfaces of the eyelids.

Conjunctivitis Inflammation of the conjunctiva. The most common eye disease, it is usually caused by a bacterial or viral infection.

Connective tissue Tissue made of fiber that forms the framework for support of the body's tissue and organs.

Consciousness A condition in which an individual is aware of self and environment and is able to respond appropriately to stimuli. Full consciousness requires both normal arousal and full cognition.

Consequence-based (teleologic) theories Theories that look to the outcomes (consequences) of an action in judging whether that action is right or wrong.

Conservation The concept that matter is not changed when its form is altered.

Consolidation Solidification of damaged cells and tissue during immune response to inflammation, specifically in the lungs.

Constipation Fewer than three bowel movements per week or the difficult passage of stools.

Constructivist theory Learning is a developmental process constructed from individual experiences. Knowledge acquisition is the ongoing assimilation and accommodation of new experiences and interpretations.

Consumer An individual, a group of people, or a community that uses a service or commodity.

Consumer-driven healthcare plan (CDHP) A type of employer-sponsored coverage that combines a private insurance plan with a Health Savings Account (HSA) or Health Reimbursement Account (HRA).

Contact dermatitis An inflammation of the skin that occurs in response to direct contact with an allergen or irritant.

Contact precautions Used for patients who are known to have or suspected of having serious illnesses that are easily transmitted by direct contact with the patient or by contact with items in the environment, such as *Shigella*.

Contingency plan A plan identifying and managing unplanned and unexpected events that interfere with getting work done efficiently and effectively and in a timely manner.

Continuance commitment The awareness of the costs associated with leaving a profession that inhibits an individual from doing so. Considered the weakest type of commitment to a profession.

Continuous bladder irrigation (CBI) A method used to prevent the formation of blood clots.

Continuous positive airway pressure (CPAP) Mechanical ventilation that applies positive pressure to the airways of a patient who is breathing spontaneously. Breathing is patient triggered and pressure controlled. It is used to help maintain open airways and alveoli, decreasing the work of breathing.

Continuous quality improvement (CQI) A structured organizational process for involving personnel in planning and executing a continuous flow of improvements to provide quality healthcare that meets or exceeds expectations.

Continuous renal replacement therapy (CRRT) A form of dialysis in which blood is continuously circulated through a highly porous hemofilter from artery to vein or vein to vein.

Contractility The inherent capability of the cardiac muscle fibers to shorten.

Contraction stress test (CST) A method of evaluating the respiratory function (oxygen and carbon dioxide exchange) of a placenta.

Contracture Permanent shortening of connective tissue.

Contralateral deficit Loss or impairment of sensorimotor functions on the side of the body opposite the side of the brain that is damaged by stroke.

Contrecoup injury This injury occurs when the brain strikes the side of the skull opposite to the side of impact.

Controlled Substance Act (CSA) A federal law that requires drugs to be classified based on the substance's medical use, potential for abuse, and safety risks.

Controlling (monitoring) The managerial process of comparing actual results with projected results, similar to the evaluation step in the nursing process. Controlling includes establishing performance standards, determining how to measure performance and creating the tools that will permit consistent measurement, evaluating performance, and providing feedback.

Contusion A bruise on the brain.

Convection The process of heat transfer through the fluid motion of air or water across the skin.

Convergence The medial rotation of the eyeballs so that each is directed toward the viewed object.

Co-occurring disorder Comorbid or concurrent diagnosis of a substance use disorder and a psychiatric disorder. One disorder can precede and cause the other, such as the theorized relationship between alcoholism and depression.

Cooperative play The stage of play in which children work together to contribute to a unified whole, such as forming a sports team or dancing in an ensemble.

Coordinating (directing) The managerial process of effectively motivating, communicating, and delegating tasks in order to complete an organization's work.

Co-payment The set payment owed by an insured individual at the time a covered service is rendered.

Coping A dynamic process through which an individual applies cognitive and behavioral measures to handle internal and external demands that are perceived by the individual as exceeding available resources.

Corneal abrasion Disruption of the superficial epithelium of the cornea.

Corneal reflex Closure of eyelids (blinking) due to corneal irritation.

Coronary artery bypass grafting (CABG) A procedure in which a section of a vein or artery is used to create a connection, or bypass, between the aorta and the blocked coronary artery beyond the obstruction.

Coronary artery disease (CAD) The most common type of heart disease, it is caused by impaired blood flow to the myocardium.

Coronary circulation A network of vessels that supply the heart muscle.

Corpus luteum A small yellow body that develops within a ruptured ovarian follicle.

Corrective action The steps taken to overcome a job performance problem.

Coryza Inflammation of the mucous membranes lining the nose, usually associated with nasal discharge.

Cotyledons Subdivisions of the placenta made up of anchoring villi and decidual tissue.

Countershock phase The second part of an alarm reaction during which the sympathetic nervous system stimulation triggers the body's defenses.

Coup injury An injury that occurs when the brain strikes the same side of the skull as the side of impact.

Coup-contrecoup injury In this type of injury, the brain strikes the coup side, then bounces back and strikes the contrecoup side, resulting in contusions on both sides of the brain.

Couplet Two premature ventricular contractions in a row.

Covert conflict Conflict that is not obvious or may be underlying, expressed in reactive or avoidant behaviors.

Crackles High-pitched popping sounds heard on inspiration due to fluid associated with or resulting from inflammation, or exudates, within the lung fields, or localized atelectasis.

Craving A clinical manifestation of alcohol abuse in which the individual has a compelling urge to consume alcohol.

Creatine kinase (CK) An enzyme important for cellular function that is found principally in cardiac and skeletal muscle and the brain.

Creatinine clearance A test that uses 24-hour urine and serum creatinine levels to determine the glomerular filtration rate; a sensitive indicator of renal function.

Creativity The ability to find or create a unique solution to a unique problem when traditional interventions are not effective.

Creativity techniques Strategies, such as brainstorming sessions, that use the creative potential of the group to generate a large number of possible options quickly.

Credentialing The formal identification of professionals who meet predetermined standards of professional skill or competence.

Credibility The quality of being truthful, trustworthy, and reliable.

Crepitation A grating or cracking sound.

Crime An act prohibited by statute or by common law principles.

Criminal law The area of law that deals with conduct that is harmful to another individual or to society as a whole and that may be punishable by fines or imprisonment.

Crisis Any acute incident that can evolve from a situation or event and that overwhelms an individual's normal coping process.

Crisis counseling A meeting that focuses on brief solutions, focused interventions, and supportive care during or after a crisis. It also considers the individual's physical vulnerability and degree of emotional stability.

Crisis intervention An emergent approach to care that is intended to assist patients with recognizing a crisis situation and identifying and implementing an immediate, short-term solution.

Crisis intervention centers Organizations that provide telephone consultation for patients in crisis. Some also offer consultation through email and online chatting or texts.

Critical pathway Expected outcomes and care strategies developed through collaboration by the healthcare team. Also called a *case map*.

Critical thinking All or part of the process of questioning, analysis, synthesis, interpretation, inference, inductive and deductive reasoning, intuition, application, and creativity.

Crohn disease A chronic, relapsing inflammatory bowel disorder affecting the gastrointestinal tract. Also known as *regional enteritis*.

Crowning During birth, the appearance of the newborn's head or presenting fetal part at the vaginal orifice.

Cryptorchidism Failure of one or both testes to descend into the scrotum.

Cues Signs and symptoms of physical or mental illness or injury, health behaviors, and risk and protective factors.

Cultural competence The ability to apply the knowledge and skills needed to provide high-quality, evidence-based care to patients of diverse backgrounds and beliefs to overcome barriers and access resources promoting health and wellness.

Cultural groups Racial, ethnic, religious, or social groups with specific group behaviors and characteristics that are learned and shared, including language, customs, beliefs, and values.

Cultural humility The recognition that a healthcare provider's personal cultural values are not superior to the cultural values of others, thus preventing an abuse of power.

Cultural values Preferred ways of behaving or thinking that are sustained over time and used to govern a cultural group's actions and decisions.

Culture The patterns of behavior and thinking that people living in social groups learn, develop, and share.

Curling ulcers Acute ulcerations of the stomach or duodenum that form following a burn injury.

Cushing syndrome A disorder resulting from too much cortisol in the body. It can develop in individuals who take too much exogenous glucocorticosteroid for asthma or other disorders, or it can develop as a result of the overproduction of endogenous cortisol due to a pituitary or adrenal tumor.

Cyanosis Gray to blue or purple skin color caused by deoxygenated hemoglobin.

Cyber-bullying Aggression or bullying that occurs through the use of technology (e.g., social media, texting, or email).

Cycle of violence Violence that occurs with a patterned frequency, usually in three phases: initial tension due to communication failures, an abusive incident, and a honeymoon stage in which the aggressor may show love and affection. It may also refer to violence that spans multiple generations in a family.

Cyclothymic disorder A type of bipolar disorder characterized by chronic, fluctuating mood disturbances involving numerous periods of hypomanic symptoms and numerous periods of depressive symptoms.

Cystic fibrosis (CF) An inherited disorder that affects the secretory glands, particularly the glands that are responsible for secreting mucus, digestive enzymes, and sweat.

Cystic fibrosis transmembrane conductance regulator (CFTR) protein A protein that is central to the movement of chloride into and out of the body cells.

Cystitis Inflammation of the urinary bladder.

Cystoscopy Endoscopy of the urinary tract. Also called *catheterization*.

Cytokines Proteins that carry messages for immune system function.

Daily hassles The individual day-to-day tensions/stressors that people face.

Daily Nutritional Goals The essential dietary components recommended by the federal government for pregnant and lactating women.

Damages Compensation sufficient to restore plaintiffs to their original position, so far as is financially possible.

Dashboard An interface that gathers, organizes, and displays a healthcare facility's key performance indicators in an easy-to-read format, often with charts or graphs.

Dawn phenomenon A rise in blood glucose between 4:00 a.m. and 8:00 a.m. that is not a response to hypoglycemia.

Dead space Areas of the lung that are ventilated but not perfused.

Death anxiety Worry or fear related to death or dying.

Debridement The process of removing painful or necrotic material, including all loose tissue, wound debris, and dead tissue, from a wound.

Decelerations The periodic decreases in fetal heart rate from the normal baseline.

Decerebrate posturing An abnormal posture adopted by an unconscious individual that indicates deteriorating brain function. It is characterized by an extended neck; clenched jaw; arms pronated, extended, and close to the sides; legs extended and feet plantar flexed.

Decibels (dB) Units of loudness.

Decision tree A graphic model that visually represents the choices, outcomes, and risks to be anticipated.

Decompensation Loss of effective compensation.

Decorticate posturing An abnormal posture adopted by an unconscious individual that indicates deteriorating brain function. It is characterized by the upper arms kept close to the sides; the elbows, wrists, and fingers flexed; the legs extended and internally rotated; and the feet plantar flexed.

Deductive reasoning A "top-down" method of logical thinking that starts with a conclusion and analyzes the situation for valid, significant cues. One of two methods of logical thinking that are used to determine if decisions are reasonable.

Deep brain stimulation (DBS) A procedure in which a neurostimulator is implanted into an individual to send electrical signals to one of three brain regions—the subthalamic nucleus, the globus pallidus, or the thalamus—in order to reduce symptoms of Parkinson disease.

Deep venous thrombosis (DVT) A blood clot that forms along the intimal lining of a large vein, usually in a leg.

Defecation The expulsion of feces from the anus and rectum.

Defense mechanism Unconscious psychologic processes developed for the purpose of defending the personality. Also called *ego defense mechanisms*.

Defibrillation An emergency procedure that delivers an electrical shock to stop ventricular fibrillation and return to a rhythm that promotes cardiac output sufficient to sustain life.

Defining characteristics The cluster of signs and symptoms that indicate the presence of a particular diagnostic label.

Dehiscence An unintended separation of wound margins due to incomplete healing.

Dehydration A condition that occurs when a body does not take in as much water as it loses or lacks sufficient reserves to maintain proper function.

Delayed ejaculation Once called *male orgasmic disorder*, involves extreme difficulty ejaculating, despite the ability to maintain an erection for long periods (in some cases, an hour or more).

Delayed hypersensitivity (type IV) A type of allergic reaction that involves an exaggerated interaction between an antigen and normal cell-mediated mechanisms. It develops 1 to 2 days after exposure to an antigen.

Delayed union The delayed healing of bones beyond the expected time period.

Delegate An individual who assumes responsibility for the actual performance of an assigned task or procedure.

Delegation The transfer of responsibility and authority for completing an activity to a qualified individual.

Delegator An individual who assigns a task to another individual to perform but retains accountability for the outcome.

Delirium An acute cognitive disorder that affects functional independence.

Delirium tremens (DTs) A medical emergency usually occurring 3 to 5 days following alcohol withdrawal and lasting 2 t 3 days. Characterized by paranoia, disorientation, delusions, visual hallucinations, elevated vital signs, vomiting, diarrhea, and diaphoresis. Also known as *alcohol withdrawal delirium*.

Delusions False ideas or beliefs not based in reality.

Dementia A progressive, irreversible loss of cognitive function, often manifesting in early stages as memory loss.

Democratic leader A leader who assumes that individuals are internally motivated, are capable of making decisions, and value independence. They typically provide constructive feedback, offer information, make suggestions, and ask questions to gain information or to help group members grow in their ability to make decisions.

Demyelination A condition in which cells of the immune system, such as lymphocytes and macrophages, cross the blood–brain barrier and attack and destroy the myelin sheath.

Dental caries Cavities.

Dentifrice A commercial cleaning compound for teeth.

Deoxyribonucleic acid (DNA) One of two types of nucleic acid made by cells, DNA contains the genetic instructions for the development and functioning of human beings.

Dependence A physiologic need for a substance that the patient cannot control, and that results in withdrawal symptoms if the substance is withheld.

Dependent edema Fluid that accumulates in gravity-dependent areas of the body.

Dependent intervention Activities carried out under a physician's orders or supervision, or according to specified routines or protocols.

Dependent personality disorder (DPD) One of several personality disorders defined in the DSM-5, it is marked by a pervasive, excessive, and unrealistic need to be cared for; fear of separation; lack of self-confidence; an inability to make decisions; and an inability to function independently.

Depersonalization A feeling of strangeness or unreality about the physical self.

Depolarization 1. The rapid inflow of sodium ions, causing an electrical change in which the inside of a cell becomes positive in relation to the outside. 2. The phase in which the heart contracts as a result of ion channel functions.

Depression A persistent, abnormally low mood characterized by feelings of emptiness, hopelessness, sadness, or despair often accompanied by a loss of interest in activities, including those related to daily living.

Depressive disorder with peripartum onset See **Postpartum depression**.

Dermatome An area of skin innervated by the cutaneous branch of one spinal nerve.

Dermis The second layer of skin, which is made of a flexible connective tissue. It is richly supplied with blood cells, nerve fibers, and lymphatic vessels, as well as most of the hair follicles, sebaceous glands, and sweat glands.

Desaturated blood Blood that is low in oxygen as a result of oxygenated and deoxygenated blood mixing due to a congenital heart defect.

Detrusor muscle The smooth muscle layers of the bladder wall, the muscle allows the bladder to expand as it fills with urine and contract as it releases urine during voiding.

Development An increase in the complexity and function of skill progression, the individual's capacity and skill to adapt to the environment. Related to growth.

Developmental disability Any of a variety of chronic conditions characterized by mental and/or physical impairment.

Developmental milestones A set of functional skills or age-specific tasks that most children can do by a certain age.

Developmental stage A level of achievement for a particular segment of an individual's life.

Developmental task A skill or behavior pattern learned during stages of development.

Device integration Real-time, accurate data is recorded in the patient's chart directly from a device (e.g., blood pressure monitor). It allows the nurse to more quickly analyze and interpret that data and make adjustments to the plan of care based on the most current information.

Diabetes insipidus (DI) A rare disorder that occurs when the kidneys pass an abnormally large volume of urine that is dilute and odorless.

Diabetes mellitus Group of chronic disorders of the endocrine pancreas, all categorized under a broad diagnostic label. The condition is characterized by inappropriate hyperglycemia caused by a relative or absolute deficiency of insulin or by a cellular resistance to the action of insulin. Also called *diabetes*.

Diabetic ketoacidosis (DKA) A form of metabolic acidosis that develops when there is an absolute deficiency of insulin and an increase in the insulin counterregulatory hormones. It may also be induced by stress in an individual with type 1 diabetes.

Diabetic nephropathy Disease of the kidneys in patients with diabetes that is characterized by the presence of albumin in the urine, hypertension, edema, and progressive renal insufficiency.

Diabetic neuropathies Disorders of the peripheral nerves and the autonomic nervous system in patients with diabetes, which manifest in one or more of the following: sensory and motor impairment, muscle weakness and pain, cranial nerve disorders, impaired vasomotor function, impaired gastrointestinal function, and impaired genitourinary function.

Diabetic retinopathy The collective name for the changes in the retina that occur in the person with diabetes. The retinal capillary structure undergoes alterations in blood flow, leading to retinal ischemia and a breakdown in the blood–retinal barrier.

Diagnosis-related groups (DRGs) A system of price control regulation that classifies patient illnesses based on diagnoses and pays hospitals a predetermined sum for each specific diagnosis regardless of the actual cost of services, the length of stay, or the acuity or complexity of the patient's illness.

Diagnostic label Standardized NANDA-I names for nursing diagnoses.

Dialectical behavior therapy (DBT) In this variant of cognitive-behavioral therapy, patients are taught how to regulate destructive emotions, practice mindfulness, and better tolerate distress.

Dialysate Dialysis solution.

Dialysis A process by which fluids and molecules pass through a semipermeable membrane from an area of higher solute concentration to one of lower solute concentration according to the rules of osmosis. It is used to remove excess fluid and metabolic waste products in renal failure.

Diaphragm A flexible disk that covers the cervix to prevent conception.

Diaphragmatic breathing Deep-breathing exercises beneficial in reducing respiratory rate, oxygen demand, and work of breathing.

Diarrhea The passage of liquid feces and an increased frequency of defecation.

Diastasis recti In pregnancy, a vertical bulge caused by separation of the rectus abdominis muscle due to pressure of the enlarging uterus.

Diastasis recti abdominis A separation of the abdominal muscle.

Diastole The phase of ventricular relaxation between heartbeats.

Diastolic blood pressure The minimum pressure within the arteries during diastole.

Diencephalon Area of the brain consisting of the thalamus (sometimes called the *dorsal thalamus*), hypothalamus, epithalamus, and subthalamus.

Diet recall Patient history of intake over a specified period of time.

Dietary fiber A polysaccharide carbohydrate that contributes to disease prevention, especially in the gastrointestinal tract and the cardiovascular system.

Dietary Reference Intakes (DRIs) A standardized, recommended nutrient intake to support a healthy diet often provided by health organizations.

Dietitian Also called a *nutritionist*, a professional who provides expertise in the use of nutrition to treat disease.

Differentiated practice A system in which each nurse's educational preparation and skill sets are evaluated and used to determine how they will best be used.

Differentiation A process occurring over many cell cycles that allows cells to specialize in certain tasks.

Diffuse axonal injury An injury that occurs because of a rotational deceleration that is dramatic enough to cause damage to the brain's white matter in the form of widespread disruption of axon fibers and myelin sheaths.

Diffusion The continual intermingling of molecules in liquids, gases, or solids brought about by the random movement of the molecules.

Digestion The conversion of food by means of its mechanical and chemical breakdown into absorbable substances in the gastrointestinal tract.

Digital rectal examination (DRE) An examination to detect for abnormalities in the rectum that can be detected through palpation.

Dihydrotestosterone (DHT) The androgen that mediates prostatic growth at all ages; formed in the prostate from testosterone.

Dilated cardiomyopathy The most common form of cardiomyopathy, it is characterized by the dilation of the heart chambers and impaired ventricular contraction.

Directive interview A highly structured interview that elicits specific health information.

Dirty In medical asepsis, a term used to indicate that microorganisms are likely to be present.

Disability A physical or mental health impairment that restricts a person's function.

Disaster An event that occurs with little or no warning in which available personnel and emergency services are initially overwhelmed and a serious threat to life, public health, and the environment is posed.

Discharge planning A plan of care that prepares a patient for discharge, including training in any necessary health skills.

Discipline A method of teaching children the rules for how to behave in society and what is expected in different circumstances.

Discoid lesions Raised, scaly, circular lesions with an erythematous rim.

Discovery The legal process of obtaining information before a trial.

Discrimination The differential treatment of individuals or groups, based on categories such as race, age, weight, gender, or social class, that occurs when an individual acts on prejudice and denies other people one or more of their fundamental rights.

Discussion An informal oral consideration of a subject by two or more healthcare personnel to identify a problem or establish strategies to resolve a problem.

Disease A detectable alteration in body function resulting from infection by microorganisms that causes a reduction of capacities or a shortening of the normal lifespan. Also called *pathogenesis*.

Disease surveillance Monitoring patterns of disease occurrence from cases of infections and communicable diseases reported by healthcare workers to state officials.

Diseases of adaptation Stress-related illnesses, such as peptic ulcers and hypertension.

Disenfranchised grief Grief that occurs when an individual is unable to acknowledge a loss to other persons. Also called *ambiguous loss*.

Disinfectants Agents that destroy pathogens other than spores.

Disinhibition One of the six trait domains associated with personality disorders that is noted for the presence of irresponsibility, impulsivity, and risk taking.

Diskectomy The removal of all or part of the nucleus pulposus of an intervertebral disk.

Dismissal Termination of employment.

Disorganized thinking Difficulty logically connecting thoughts, leading to garbled speech.

Disseminated intravascular coagulation (DIC) A disruption of hemostasis characterized by widespread intravascular clotting and bleeding. It may be acute and life-threatening or it may be relatively mild.

Distracted driving The act of driving a motor vehicle while doing any activity that takes attention away from the road. Activities include texting, talking on the phone, eating, drinking, reading a map, talking to passengers, looking at a GPS, and adjusting the radio.

Distress A stress that is associated with inadequacy, insecurity, and loss.

Distributive shock Shock that results from widespread vasodilation and decreased peripheral resistance. Also called *vasogenic shock*.

Diuresis The production and excretion of abnormally large amounts of urine. Also called *polyuria*.

Diuretics Pharmacologic agents that increase urine formation and secretion.

Diversity The unique variations among and between individuals that are informed by genetics and cultural background, but that are refined by experience and personal choice.

Diverticula Saclike projections of mucosa through the muscular layer of the wall of a canal or organ (e.g., the bladder wall, colon, or large intestine).

Diverticulitis Inflamed diverticula, which cause obstruction, perforation, and bleeding.

Diverticulosis A condition that occurs when diverticula develop in the large intestine.

Documenting The process of making an entry on a patient record. Also called *recording* or *charting*.

Doll's-eye reflex An oculomotor response in which the eyes move in the opposite direction as the head turns to the side. Also called the *oculocephalic reflex*.

Domestic partner An unmarried partner of the same or opposite sex.

Do-not-intubate (DNI) order Usually written by a physician for a patient who has a terminal illness or is near death, this order is usually based on the wishes of the patient and family that no lifesaving measures be provided once the patient stops breathing.

Do-not-resuscitate (DNR) order Usually written by a physician for a patient who has a terminal illness or is near death, this order is usually based on the wishes of the patient and family that no cardiopulmonary resuscitation be performed for respiratory or cardiac arrest. Also called a *no-code order*.

Dopamine A brain neurotransmitter that regulates voluntary movement, reward-seeking behavior, memory and learning, attention, sleep, affect, and many other functions.

Dormant Temporarily inactive but not dead.

Doula A paid caregiver who has typically received special training and may even be certified in caring for laboring women.

Down syndrome A developmental disorder that occurs when an individual is born with an extra full or partial chromosome. It is associated with intellectual disability and a wide variety of physical impairments that can range from mild to severe.

Dramatic play The stage of play in which individuals use props to act out the drama of human life.

Dressler syndrome A symptom complex characterized by fever and chest pain that may develop days to weeks after an acute myocardial infarction. It is thought to be a hypersensitivity response to necrotic tissue or an autoimmune disorder.

Droplet nuclei Residue of evaporated droplets emitted by an infected host; can remain in the air for long periods of time.

Droplet precautions Used for patients who are known to have or suspected of having serious illnesses transmitted by particle droplets larger than 5 microns, such as pertussis or pneumonia.

Drusen Deposits that accumulate beneath the pigment epithelium of the retina of the eye.

Dubowitz tool A tool for assessing newborns that includes neuromuscular tone assessments, such as head lag, ventral suspension, and leg recoil.

Ductus arteriosus Fetal artery connecting the aorta and the pulmonary artery. It allows blood to detour away from the lungs before birth.

Ductus venosus Fetal vessel that shunts a portion of umbilical vein blood flow directly to the inferior vena cava. It allows oxygenated blood from the placenta to bypass the liver.

Dullness A thudlike sound produced by dense tissue such as the liver, spleen, or heart.

Duodenal ulcer A peptic ulcer occurring in the duodenum.

Durable power of attorney A legal designation of another individual, usually a family member, significant other, or close personal friend, to make healthcare or other decisions on an individual's behalf.

Duration 1. The length of a sound. 2. The length of time from the beginning of a contraction to the completion of that same contraction.

Duty A legally enforceable obligation to conform to a particular standard of conduct that is owed to a patient.

Dysarthria Any disturbance in muscular control of speech.

Dysfunctional uterine bleeding (DUB) Irregular uterine bleeding most commonly caused by lack of egg production, usually occurring in adolescence and in perimenopause.

Dysmenorrhea Painful menstruation.

Dyspareunia Painful intercourse.

Dysphagia Difficulty swallowing.

Dysplasia A loss of DNA control over differentiation occurring in response to adverse conditions.

Dyspnea Shortness of breath or difficulty breathing that is uncomfortable or painful, or when breathing is insufficient to meet oxygen demand.

Dyspraxia Difficulty with the acquisition of motor learning and coordination through the process of growth and development.

Dysrhythmia Abnormal heart rate or rhythm. Also called *arrhythmia*.

Dysthymia A chronic depressive disorder with symptoms that are less severe than those of major depressive disorder. Also called *persistent depressive disorder* or *dysthymic disorder*.

Dystonia Severe muscle spasms, particularly of the back, neck, tongue, and face.

Dysuria Difficult or painful urination.

Early deceleration During birth, a condition that occurs when the fetal head is compressed and cerebral blood flow decreases, causing central vagal stimulation. Usually associated with the onset of uterine contractions.

Early (primary) postpartum hemorrhage Hemorrhage that occurs in the first 24 hours after childbirth.

Eating disorder A chronic disturbance in eating or eating-related practices usually characterized by obsessions with food and weight, often to the extent that daily functioning is impaired and physical and psychologic health are threatened.

Echolalia The compulsive parroting of a word or phrase just spoken by another.

Echopraxia The compulsive imitation of the movements of another.

Eclampsia A major complication of pregnancy characterized by hypertension, albuminuria, oliguria, tonic and clonic convulsions, and coma.

Ecologic theory A theory of development that emphasizes the presence of mutual interactions between an individual and all of life's settings.

Ecomap Visual representation of how the family unit interacts with the external community environment, including schools, religious institutions, occupational duties, and recreational pursuits.

Ectopic beats Impulses originating outside normal conduction pathways of the heart that interrupt the normal conduction sequence and may not initiate a normal muscle contraction.

Edema Swelling caused by excess fluid trapped in body tissue.

Effacement The drawing-up of the internal os and the cervical canal into the uterine side walls.

Effectiveness In healthcare, providing services based on scientific knowledge to all who could benefit and refraining from providing services to those not likely to benefit.

Efficacy A medication's ability to achieve the intended response.

Efficiency In healthcare, avoiding waste of equipment, supplies, ideas, and energy.

Ego defense mechanisms Unconscious psychologic processes developed for the purpose of defending the personality. Also called *defense mechanisms*.

Ego-syntonic The perception that one's behaviors and beliefs are normal and any difficulties with other people are external to oneself.

Egocentrism Ability to see things only from one's own point of view.

E-health Healthcare resources accessible to patients via electronic media.

Ejection fraction (EF) The fraction or percentage of the diastolic volume that is ejected from the heart during systole.

Elder abuse The intentional physical, emotional, or sexual mistreatment or neglect of an individual 65 years of age and older.

Elderspeak A speech style similar to baby talk that communicates a message of dependence and incompetence to older adults.

Electrocardiogram (ECG) A graphic record of the heart's activity.

Electrocardiography A diagnostic test of cardiac function.

Electroconvulsive therapy (ECT) A treatment procedure during which an electric current is passed through the brain. It is useful to patients with severe depression, acute mania, some psychotic conditions, and those who are acutely suicidal.

Electroencephalogram (EEG) Measures and records the brain's electrical activity.

Electrolyte A charged ion capable of conducting electricity.

Electromyogram A diagnostic technique that measures the electrical activity of the muscles at rest and during contraction.

Electronic communication Transmitting information though email, social networking, text messaging, and other electronic means.

Electronic fetal monitoring The measurement and tracing of the fetal heart rate, which allows many of its characteristics to be visually assessed.

Electronic health record (EHR) A health record system that is designed so that multiple clinicians from multiple disciplines (e.g., family practice, nursing, pharmacy, specialists) can all have simultaneous access to a patient's health information.

Electronic medical record (EMR) A system focused on diagnosis and treatment. It tracks information over time (weight, blood pressure, cholesterol readings) and identifies when a patient is due for routine preventive health maintenance such as vaccines and mammograms.

Elimination The secretion and excretion of body wastes from the kidneys and intestines.

Embolus A particle or aggregate of blood, fat, or pathogens or a bubble of air that obstructs a blood vessel.

Embryo The early stage of development of the young of any organism. In humans the embryonic period is from about 2 to 8 weeks' gestation and is characterized by cellular differentiation and predominantly hyperplastic growth.

Embryonic membranes The amnion and chorion.

Emergency A sudden, often unforeseen event that threatens health or safety.

Emergency contraception Contraception that is used after sexual activity.

Emergency preparedness The act of making plans to prevent, respond to, and recover from emergencies.

Emergency response The implementation of emergency preparedness plans.

Emesis The act of vomiting; occurs when inspiratory muscles of the thorax (including the diaphragm) and abdomen contract, increasing intrathoracic and intra-abdominal pressures.

Emotion-focused coping The regulation of emotional responses to distress when the stressor is perceived to be beyond an individual's control.

Emotional intelligence Measurement of individuals' abilities to differentiate between their own thoughts and feelings, recognize the thoughts and feelings of others, and show discernment when using emotions to influence decisions.

Emotions Feeling responses to a wide variety of emotional stimuli.

Emphysema A progressive pulmonary disease characterized by destruction of the walls of the alveoli, with resulting enlargement of abnormal air spaces.

Empowerment A process whereby patients take a lead role, as opposed to a passive role, in managing their health.

Empyema Accumulation of purulent (infected) exudate in a space (e.g., the pleural cavity or gallbladder).

Enabling behavior Any action by an individual that consciously or unconsciously facilitates substance dependence.

Enamel A hard substance that encapsulates the crown, the uppermost part of the tooth.

Encapsulated Enclosed.

Encopresis Abnormal elimination pattern characterized by recurrent soiling or passage of stool at inappropriate times.

Enculturation The process by which children learn culture from adults. Also called *cultural transmission*.

End-of-dose medication failure Pain experienced at the end of one dose of medication before the next dose is scheduled.

End of life The final weeks of life when death is imminent.

End-of-life care The nursing care provided to a patient who is dying or who is near death.

End-stage renal disease (ESRD) The final stage of chronic kidney disease, when the kidneys are unable to excrete metabolic wastes and regulate fluid and electrolyte balance adequately.

Endocardial cushion defect A combination of defects in the atrial and ventricular septa and portions of the tricuspid and mitral valves. A complete AV canal defect allows blood to travel freely among all four chambers of the heart. Also called *atrioventricular (AV) canal defect*.

Endogenous Developing from within.

Endogenous insulin Insulin that is produced by an individual's own body.

Endolymph fluid Found deep in the inner ear within the **membranous labyrinth**, it bathes the sensory cells for balance and hearing in the inner ear, allowing them to function normally.

Endometriosis A condition that occurs when endometrial tissue implants on organs outside the uterus, causing pain, fibrosis, and adhesions.

Endometritis Inflammation of the endometrium within 6 weeks after delivery.

Endotoxins Found in the cell wall of gram-negative bacteria, they are released only when the cell is disrupted. They act as activators of many human regulatory systems, producing fever, inflammation, and potentially clotting, bleeding, or hypotension when released in large quantities.

Endurance training Aerobic activities that increase heart rate, respiratory rate, and metabolism, such as distance running, cycling, swimming, and hiking.

Engagement The passing of the fetus into the pelvic inlet in preparation for birth.

Enophthalmos Sunken appearance of the eyes.

Enteral nutrition Tube feeding used to meet calorie and protein requirements in patients who are unable to consume enough food on their own.

Entropion Inversion of the eyelid.

Enuresis Involuntary passing of urine in children after bladder control is achieved.

Environmental health hazards Factors that impede individual and community health and include natural or human-made substances, states, or events that affect the natural environment, produce negative effects on the human ecosphere, and adversely affect health.

Environmental quality One of the 12 leading health indicators identified by *Healthy People 2030*, environmental quality refers to the ability of the environment to promote and sustain individual and community health.

Enzymes Chemicals that induce a chemical reaction in order to assist in the breakdown of nutrients.

Eosinophil A type of leukocyte found in large numbers in the respiratory and gastrointestinal tracts. Eosinophils are thought to be responsible for protecting the body from parasitic worms. They also play a role in the hypersensitivity response by inactivating some of the inflammatory chemicals released during the inflammatory response.

Epidemic Widespread outbreak of infectious disease with many infected people.

Epidermis The surface or outermost part of the skin consisting of four to five layers of epithelial cells.

Epidural Type of anesthesia commonly used to provide pain relief for the laboring woman.

Epigenetic External influences or effects on gene expression.

Epilepsy A chronic disorder characterized by recurrent, unprovoked seizures secondary to a central nervous system disorder.

Epiphyseal plate Cartilage between the epiphysis and diaphysis found in the long bones of children.

Episiotomy A surgical incision of the perineal body to enlarge the outlet.

Epispadias Congenital abnormality in which the meatus is located on the upper side of the glans.

Epstein pearls Small, glistening, white specks that feel hard to the touch on the hard palate and gum margins.

Erb-Duchenne paralysis (Erb palsy) Damage affecting the upper arm between the fifth and sixth cervical nerves, causing paralysis.

Erectile disorder Term used to describe **erectile dysfunction** when the cause of the disorder is unrelated to physical causes (e.g., it results as a side effect of a substance or medication).

Erectile dysfunction (ED) The inability of a man to attain and maintain an erection sufficient to permit satisfactory sexual intercourse.

Ergonomics The science of fitting workplace conditions and job demands to the capabilities of the working population.

Erythema A reddening of the skin.

Erythema toxicum neonatorum An eruption of lesions in the area surrounding a hair follicle that are firm, vary in size from 1 to 3 mm, and consist of a white or pale yellow papule or pustule with an erythematous base. Also called *newborn rash* or *flea bite dermatitis*.

Erythropoietin Produced by the kidneys, hormone that controls RBC production.

Eschar Hard, leathery crust that covers a burn wound and harbors necrotic tissue.

Escharotomy Surgical removal of eschar from the torso or extremity to prevent circumferential constriction.

Essential nutrients The macro- and micronutrients needed for the body's survival.

Essential tremors Tremors that are not associated with another condition and may be genetic in origin.

Estimated date of birth (EDB) The approximated date of childbirth. Also called *estimated date of delivery*.

Estrogen The primary hormone responsible for female sex characteristics.

Ethical dilemma A state of conflict that occurs when two or more rights, values, obligations, or responsibilities come into conflict.

Ethics The rules or principles that govern right or moral conduct.

Ethnic group Group of individuals who have common racial characteristics and share a cultural heritage.

Etiology A causal relationship between a problem and its related or risk factors.

Eupnea Breathing within the expected respiratory rates.

Eustachian tube Connects the middle ear with the nasopharynx to help equalize the pressure in the middle ear with the atmospheric pressure.

Eustress Good stress that is associated with accomplishment and victory.

Euthanasia From the Greek for *painless*, *easy*, *gentle*, or *good death*, now commonly used to signify a killing prompted by a humanitarian motive.

Euthymia Stable or normal mood.

Euthyroid A normal thyroid state.

Evaluation Reassessment of a patient following nursing or medical intervention or therapy.

Evaluation statement A written comment on the care plan or in the nurse's notes about progress following an evaluation. An evaluation statement must contain the date and time evaluation was done; a conclusion statement determining goal met, partially met, or not met; and a supporting statement giving the results of how the patient did or did not achieve the goal.

Evidence Clinical knowledge, expert opinion, or information resulting from research.

Evidence-based nursing An integration of the best evidence available, nursing expertise, and the values and preferences of the individuals, families, and communities who are served.

Evidence-based practice (EBP) The application of research in areas that are of interest to nursing and in the actual practice of nursing.

Evisceration Protrusion of internal viscera through a wound.

Exacerbation A reappearance of symptoms of a chronic illness. Also called a *flare-up*.

Excitement phase This second phase of the sexual response cycle is marked by an increase in blood flow to various body parts, resulting in erection of the penis and clitoris and swelling of the labia, testes, and breasts.

Excoriation Area of loss of the superficial layers of the skin. Also called *denuded area*.

Executive branch agency Part of the federal or state government responsible for administering laws; for example, the Centers for Disease Control and Prevention is authorized to implement laws to protect the public against exposure and spread of highly communicable diseases.

Executive function The mental skills involved in planning and executing complex tasks.

Exercise Physical activity that is planned and structured and involves repetitive body movements; the goal is to improve or maintain one or more components of physical fitness.

Exercise intolerance Decreased ability to participate in activities using large skeletal muscles because of fatigue or dyspnea.

Exogenous Developing from outside sources.

Exogenous insulin Insulin from a source outside the body.

Exophthalmos Protruding eyes.

Exotoxins Soluble proteins that microorganisms secrete into surrounding tissue. They are highly poisonous, causing cell death or dysfunction.

Expectorate To expel or spit out.

Expiration The act of exhaling air in respiration.

Expressed consent An oral or written agreement.

Expressive jargon Using unintelligible words with normal speech intonations as if truly communicating in words.

Expressive speech The ability to speak and be understood by others.

Extended family The relatives of nuclear families, such as grandparents, aunts, and uncles.

Extended-kin network family A form of extended family in which two nuclear families of primary or unmarried kin live in proximity to each other and share a social support network, goods, and services.

Extension to deep tissue Previously called a *fourth-degree burn*, it is a deep and potentially life-threatening burn, causing damage that extends through all skin layers into underlying soft tissue and involving muscle as well as bone.

External environmental stressors Triggers outside of an individual that demand change or disrupt homeostasis.

External locus of control An individual's believe that outside powers, such as luck or fate, determine life events.

Extracapsular extraction A surgical treatment for cataracts in which the anterior capsule, nucleus, and cortex of the lens are removed, leaving the posterior capsule intact.

Extracapsular hip fracture A fracture involving the trochanteric region between the neck and diaphysis of the femur.

Extracellular fluid (ECF) Fluid found outside the cells. It accounts for about one-third of total body fluid and is subdivided into compartments. The two main compartments are intravascular and interstitial.

Extracorporeal shock wave lithotripsy (ESWL) A noninvasive technique for fragmenting kidney stones using shock waves generated outside the body.

Extrapyramidal symptoms (EPS) A particularly serious set of adverse reactions to antipsychotic drugs, including acute dystonia, akathisia, parkinsonism, and tardive dyskinesia.

Extrinsic pathway During coagulation, this pathway is initiated when blood leaks out of a vessel and into the tissue spaces.

Extubation The process of withdrawing a breathing tube on completion of anesthesia and the surgical case.

Exudate Material, such as fluid and cells, that has escaped from blood vessels during the inflammatory process and is deposited in tissue or on tissue surfaces.

Exudative macular degeneration A form of macular degeneration characterized by the formation of new, weak blood vessels in the potential space between the choroid and the retina. Also referred to as the *wet form of macular degeneration*.

Eye movement desensitization and reprocessing (EMDR) A form of psychotherapy that contains elements of a number of types of therapy, including cognitive-behavioral therapy and body-centered therapy.

Failure to thrive (FTT) 1. Inability to meet or maintain developmental milestones related to physical growth due to undernutrition. 2. A syndrome in which an infant falls below the fifth percentile for weight and height on a standard growth chart or is falling in percentiles on a growth chart.

Faith To believe in or be committed to something or someone.

Faith community nurse A nurse who works in a church, social service agency, or nonprofit organization, or independently, providing holistic nursing care, healing, and spiritual care to members of a community.

False imprisonment The unjustifiable detention of an individual without legal warrant to confine the person.

False pelvis The portion of the pelvis above the linea terminalis that supports the enlarged pregnant uterus.

Family Individuals who are joined together by marriage, blood, adoption, or residence in the same household.

Family behavior therapy (FBT) Type of therapy in which a patient and at least one significant other, such as a cohabiting partner or a parent, try to apply the behavioral strategies taught in sessions and acquire new skills to improve the home environment.

Family-centered care A model of healthcare service that is provided in partnership with the patient and family.

Family cohesion The emotional bonding between family members.

Family communication Includes listening, speaking, self-disclosure, and tracking abilities of the family as a group.

Family coping mechanisms The behaviors families use to deal with stress or changes imposed from either within or outside the family.

Family development The growth or progress of communication patterns, roles, and interactions within a family.

Family therapy A form of therapy in which the family system is treated as a unit and the focus is on family dynamics.

Fasciculation An irregular movement or a twitch.

Fasciectomy Excising a wound to the level of fascia. Also called *fascial excision*.

Fat embolism syndrome (FES) Occurs when fat globules lodge in the pulmonary vascular bed or peripheral circulation.

Fatigue A condition characterized by a lack of energy and motivation that may or may not be accompanied by drowsiness.

Fear A sense of apprehension triggered by a perceived threat to safety or well-being, including a painful stimulus or dangerous event.

Febrile Having a fever.

Febrile seizures Generalized seizures that usually occur in children as the result of rapid temperature rise above 39°C (102°F), usually in association with an acute illness. No evidence of intracranial infection or other defined cause is found in relation.

Fecal impaction A mass or collection of hardened feces in the folds of the rectum.

Fecal incontinence The loss of voluntary ability to control fecal and gaseous discharges through the anal sphincter. Also called *bowel incontinence*.

Fecalith A hard mass of feces.

Feces Body wastes and undigested food eliminated from the bowel. Also called *stool*.

Federal Emergency Management Agency (FEMA) Government agency with expertise in public safety, emergency medical services, and management called upon to act and coordinate recovery efforts after a disaster.

Feedback Determination of whether the information met the patient's goals or to evaluate the effectiveness of the instruction provided.

Feeding and eating disorders Chronic disturbances in eating or eating-related practices that result in impairment in food consumption or absorption to the extent that daily functioning is affected and physical and psychologic health are significantly impaired.

Female orgasmic disorder The persistent delay or absence of orgasm following a phase of normal sexual excitement.

Female reproductive cycle The monthly rhythmic changes in sexually mature women; composed of the ovarian cycle, during which ovulation occurs, and the uterine cycle, during which menstruation occurs.

Female sexual interest/arousal disorder Persistent decreased or absent sexual thoughts, interest in sexual activity, mental or physical feelings of arousal, and/or pleasurable sensation during sexual activity.

Fertility awareness–based (FAB) methods Contraception based on an understanding of the changes that occur throughout a woman's ovulatory cycle. Also called *natural family planning*.

Fertilization The process by which a sperm fuses with an ovum to form a new diploid cell, or zygote.

Festination Rapid, small steps, as if an individual is trying to run.

Fetal alcohol spectrum disorder See **Fetal alcohol syndrome (FAS)**.

Fetal alcohol syndrome (FAS) A developmental disorder that occurs when a developing fetus is exposed to ethyl alcohol. It is associated with physical, intellectual, behavioral, and/or learning disabilities. Also called *fetal alcohol spectrum disorder*.

Fetal attitude The flexion or extension of the fetal body and extremities.

Fetal bradycardia A fetal heart rate of less than 110 bpm during a 10-minute period or longer.

Fetal demise Death of a fetus that occurs after 20 weeks' gestation. Also called a *stillbirth* or *intrauterine fetal death (IUFD)*.

Fetal heart rate (FHR) The number of times the fetal heart beats per minute; normal range is 110 to 160.

Fetal lie The relationship of the cephalocaudal axis, or spinal column, of the fetus to the cephalocaudal axis, or spinal column, of the woman. The fetus may be in a longitudinal or transverse lie.

Fetal movement record A noninvasive technique that enables the pregnant woman to monitor and record movements easily and without expense.

Fetal position The relationship of the landmark on the presenting fetal part to the front, sides, or back of the maternal pelvis.

Fetal presentation The body part of the fetus entering the pelvis in a single or multiple pregnancy.

Fetal tachycardia A fetal heart rate of 161 bpm or more during a 10-minute period of continuous monitoring or longer.

Fetus The child in utero from about the seventh to ninth week of gestation until birth.

Fever A protective immune response to foreign antigens within the body that increases the cellular metabolic rate, thus increasing the body's temperature.

Fever of unknown origin A temperature above 100.9°F (38.3°C) that occurs on several occasions within a short time span, lasts for more than 3 weeks, and does not have a definitive cause after 1 week of clinical investigation.

Fiber A polysaccharide that contributes to disease prevention, especially in the gastrointestinal tract and the cardiovascular system.

Fibrin Connective tissue.

Fibrin degradation products Potent anticoagulants.

Fibrinogen Protein, specifically a clotting factor (factor I), that is essential for proper blood clot formation.

Fibrinolysis The enzymatic breakdown of fibrin in blood clots.

Fibromyalgia A chronic disorder characterized by widespread musculoskeletal pain, fatigue, and multiple tender points.

Fidelity A moral principle that obligates an individual to be faithful to agreements and responsibilities they have undertaken.

Filtration A process whereby fluid and solutes move together across a membrane from a compartment with higher pressure to a compartment with lower pressure.

First heart sound (S_1) The heart sound produced by the closure of the AV valve; characterized by the syllable "lub."

5 Ps neurovascular assessment An assessment checklist for pain, pulse, pallor, paralysis/paresis, and paresthesia.

Flaccidity Absence of muscle tone. Also called *hypotonia.*

Flashbacks The recurrence of images, sounds, smells, or feelings from a traumatic event; often triggered by daily events, such as a car backfiring on the street or the smell of a perpetrator's cologne.

Flat affect Minimal facial expression and movement, sometimes monotonic speech patterns.

Flatness An extremely dull sound produced by very dense tissue, such as muscle or bone.

Flatulence The presence of excessive amounts of gas in the stomach or intestines.

Flatus Gas or air normally present in the stomach or intestines.

Flexibility training Exercises intended to improve muscle elasticity and length, joint structure, and balance, including yoga, Pilates, t'ai chi, and stretching.

Flight of ideas Rapidly changing, fragmentary thoughts.

Flow sheet A specific assessment criteria in a particular format, such as human needs or functional health patterns.

Fluid resuscitation The administration of intravenous fluids to restore circulating blood volume during an acute period of increasing capillary permeability.

Fluid volume deficit (FVD) Substantial loss of both water and electrolytes in similar proportions from the extracellular fluid. Also called *hypovolemia.*

Fluid volume excess (FVE) Excessive fluid retained by the body. The retention of both water and sodium in similar proportions to normal extracellular fluid. Also called *hypervolemia.*

Fluoroscope A scope used to project visual examination images on a fluorescent screen.

Focal seizures Seizures that are caused by abnormal electrical activity in one hemisphere or in a specific area of the cerebral cortex, most often the temporal, frontal, or parietal lobe. The seizure may spread regionally, and the symptoms are related to the region of the cortex that is affected. Also known as *partial seizures.*

Focus charting Date and time, focus, and progress notes are recorded for a specific condition, nursing diagnosis, and behavior to make the patient and the patient's concerns and strengths the focus of care.

Folic acid A vitamin that is required for normal growth, reproduction, and lactation and that prevents the macrocytic, megaloblastic anemia of pregnancy.

Follicle-stimulating hormone (FSH) Hormone produced by the anterior pituitary during the first half of the menstrual cycle, stimulating development of the graafian follicle.

Fontanels The intersections of membranous spaces between the cranial bones of a fetus.

Food allergy An immune system overreaction to the proteins in selected foods.

Food choice An individual's decision of what and how much to eat of a specific food. This decision can be influenced by a number of conscious and unconscious factors such as taste, preparation, smell, habits, convenience, availability, and cost.

Food desert Any area of population where it is difficult to find good-quality, affordable fresh fruits, vegetables, and whole grains.

Food insecurity Results when one or more members of a household must reduce their eating patterns due to a lack of money or lack of resources to access appropriate amounts and varieties of food.

Food intolerance Also called *food sensitivity*, occurs when an individual has trouble digesting a particular food.

Foramen ovale An opening between the atria of the fetal heart.

Forced expiratory volume in 1 second (FEV_1) The amount of air that can be exhaled in 1 second as measured by a spirometer.

Forceps-assisted birth The use of forceps to assist the birth of a fetus by providing traction or by providing the means to rotate the fetal head to an occiput-anterior position. Also called an *instrumental delivery, operative delivery*, or *operative vaginal delivery.*

Forceps marks Reddened areas over the cheeks and jaws on an infant caused by a difficult forceps birth.

Foreground question Questions that are narrow in focus about a specific clinical issue.

Foreseeability The ability to foresee events that reasonably may be expected to cause specific results.

Formal group A group with formalized goals, designated management, and only partly voluntary membership.

Formal leader A leader who is selected by an organization and given official authority to make decisions and act.

Formation The process that facilitates the transformation of an individual from a layperson to a professional nurse.

Foster family A family consisting of one or more adults caring for one or more children from other families when the children can no longer live with their birth parents.

Fourth heart sound (S_4) A heart sound produced by atrial contraction and ejection of blood into the ventricle during late diastole. Also called *atrial gallop.*

Fracture A break in the continuity of a bone.

Fragile X syndrome A developmental disorder caused by a single recessive gene abnormality on the X chromosome. It is associated most notably with intellectual disability, often accompanied by attention-deficit/hyperactivity disorder and other behavioral problems.

Frank–Starling mechanism An increase in venous return that increases ventricular filling and myocardial stretch, which increases the force of contraction.

Free-floating anxiety Excessive worry about everyday events; worry that is hard to control and the focus of which may shift from moment to moment.

Freezing A condition in which one's feet feel as if stuck to the floor.

Frequency The time between the beginning of one contraction and the beginning of the next contraction.

Frostbite An injury of the skin resulting from freezing.

Full-thickness burn A burn that involves all layers of the skin, including the epidermis, the dermis, and the epidermal appendages.

Fulminant colitis An acute form of ulcerative colitis that involves the entire colon; manifestations include severe bloody diarrhea, acute abdominal pain, and fever.

Functional decline A reduction in the quality of physical or cognitive function.

Functional family therapy (FFT) Family-based treatment that combines a family systems view of family functioning with behavioral techniques to improve communication, problem-solving, conflict-resolution, and parenting skills.

Functional method A method of coordinating care that focuses on the jobs to be completed as part of patient care (e.g., bed making and temperature measurement). In this task-oriented approach, personnel with less educational preparation than the professional nurse (e.g., unlicensed assistive personnel) perform aspects of care with less complex requirements.

Functional nursing A task-oriented approach to care delivery used in situations of inadequate staffing or nursing shortages.

Functional status The ability to safely perform activities of daily living.

Functional strength The body's ability to perform work.

Fundus The rounded, uppermost portion of the uterus.

Fungi A type of microorganism capable of producing infection. Yeasts and molds are common types.

Gambling disorder An **addiction** to gambling despite the risk of losing something of value (e.g., a home) and an inability to stop gambling.

Gamete Female or male germ cell; contains a haploid number of chromosomes.

Gametogenesis The process by which germ cells are produced.

Gastric lavage Irrigation of the stomach with large quantities of normal saline.

Gastric outlet obstruction Obstruction of the pyloric region of the stomach and duodenum that impairs gastric outflow; a potential complication of peptic ulcer disease.

Gastric ulcer A peptic ulcer that occurs in the stomach.

Gastrocolic reflex The increased peristalsis of the colon after food has entered the stomach.

Gastroenteritis An inflammation of the lining of the intestines caused by a virus, bacteria, or parasites.

Gastroesophageal reflux disease (GERD) A disease in which stomach contents flow back up into the esophagus.

Gate control theory Melzack and Wall's 1965 theory stating that the perception of pain is controlled by the overall activity of small-diameter (pain) fibers versus large-diameter (heat, cold, mechanical) fibers.

Gender Also termed *sex*, the cultural and social behaviors, characteristics, and identities associated with being female, male, and in some cultures, a third gender (neither male or female or a combination of both male and female).

Gender dysphoria Having strong and persistent feelings of discomfort with one's assigned gender.

Gender identity One's self-image as a female or male.

Gender-role behavior The outward expression of an individual's sense of maleness or femaleness as well as the expression of what is perceived as gender-appropriate behavior.

General adaptation syndrome (GAS) A three-stage chain of events in an individual's stress response.

Generalized anxiety disorder (GAD) A condition that occurs when an individual experiences intense tension and worry, even if no external stressors are present.

Generalized edema Fluid that has a more uniform distribution in interstitial spaces throughout the body.

Generalized seizures The result of diffuse electrical activity that often begins in both hemispheres of the brain simultaneously, then spreads throughout the cortex into the brainstem. As a result, movements and spasms displayed by the patient are bilateral and symmetric.

Generational cohort Individuals born in the same general time span who share key life experiences, including historical events, public heroes, pastimes, and early work experiences.

Genital herpes A sexually transmitted infection caused by the herpes simplex virus.

Genital intercourse Penetration of the vagina by the penis. Also called *coitus*.

Genital warts A sexually transmitted infection caused by the human papillomavirus.

Genito-pelvic pain/penetration disorder Persistent or recurrent dyspareunia (pain) or fear of pain before or during vaginal penetration.

Genogram Visual representation of sex showing lines of birth descent through the generations.

Genome All of the DNA in a human cell, or the complete set of inheritance for an individual.

Genotype The pattern of genes on chromosomes.

Geographic information system (GIS) A system that relies on satellite imaging and global positioning systems to capture, manage, and analyze geographical data.

Geriatric failure to thrive (GFTT) A condition in which older patients experience a multidimensional decline in physical functioning that is characterized by weight loss of more than 5% of baseline body weight, decreased appetite, undernutrition, dehydration, depression, and cognitive and immune impairment.

Gestation Period of intrauterine development from conception through birth; pregnancy.

Gestational age assessment tools Methods to determine an infant's age at birth assessing external physical characteristics and neurologic or neuromuscular development.

Gestational diabetes mellitus (GDM) A carbohydrate intolerance of variable severity with onset or first recognition during pregnancy.

Gestational hypertension Occurring in the second half of pregnancy in a previously normotensive mother, it is diagnosed is when the BP is greater than or equal to 140/90 mmHg on at least two occasions that are at least 6 hours apart.

Gingiva The gums.

Gingivitis Red, swollen gingiva.

Glaucoma A condition characterized by optic neuropathy with gradual loss of peripheral vision and, usually, increased intraocular pressure of the eye.

Global evaluative dimension of the self Degree to which an individual likes themself, as a whole being.

Global self-esteem See **Global evaluative dimension of the self.**

Glomerular filtration rate (GFR) The rate at which fluid is filtered through the kidneys.

Glomerulonephritis Inflammation of the glomerular capillary membrane.

Glucagon Produced by alpha cells, glucagon is a hormone that decreases glucose oxidation and promotes an increase in the blood glucose level by signaling the liver to release glucose from glycogen stores. In addition to stimulating the breakdown of glycogen in the liver, glucagon stimulates the formation of carbohydrates in the liver and the breakdown of lipids in both the liver and adipose tissue.

Gluconeogenesis The formation of glucose from fats and proteins.

Glucosuria The excretion of glucose in the urine.

Glycogen The stored form of glucose found predominantly in the liver and skeletal muscles.

Glycogenolysis The breakdown of liver glycogen.

Glycosuria The excretion of carbohydrates into the urine.

Goal Broad statement about something patients strive to achieve and indicates progress toward desired patient behaviors or actions.

Goiter An enlarged thyroid gland

Gonadotropin-releasing hormone (GnRH) A hormone secreted by the hypothalamus that stimulates the anterior pituitary to secrete follicle-stimulating hormone and luteinizing hormone.

Gonadotropins Hormones that stimulate the gonads, or sex glands, to carry out their reproductive or endocrine functions.

Gonorrhea A sexually transmitted infection caused by *Neisseria gonorrhoeae.*

Good faith immunity Law or laws that protect healthcare workers from civil or criminal liabilities when they report suspected child abuse in good faith, even if the subsequent investigation does not make a determination of abuse.

Good Samaritan laws Specific laws designed to protect healthcare workers from potential liability when volunteering their skills outside of an employment contract.

Goodell sign Softening of the cervix.

Governance The establishment and maintenance of social, political, and economic arrangements by which professionals control their practice, their self-discipline, their working conditions, and their professional affairs.

Graafian follicle The ovarian cyst containing the ripe ovum, which secretes estrogens.

Grading A standardized method of judging a tumor's aggressiveness based on the level of differentiation and mitotic rate, where the least malignant cells are classified grade 1 and the most aggressive malignant cells are classified grade 4.

Graft-versus-host disease A series of immunologic reactions in response to transplanted cells.

Gram stain A diagnostic test conducted to identify infecting organisms in urine by shape and characteristic.

Granulation tissue Young connective tissue with new capillaries formed in the healing process.

Graves disease An autoimmune disorder marked by an enlarged thyroid and signs of hyperthyroidism.

Grief The total psychologic, biological, and behavioral response to the emotional experience related to loss.

Grooming The psychologic and emotional manipulation of a child or adolescent with the goal to exploit or abuse.

Group Three or more individuals who have a common purpose, interact with each other, influence each other, and are interdependent.

Group therapy A form of therapy that allows group members to help each other with psychologic, cognitive, behavioral, and spiritual dysfunctions through a process of change, aided by a professional group therapist.

Groupthink A type of decision making characterized by a group's failure to critically examine their own processes and practices or to recognize and respond to change.

Growth Physical change and increase in size.

Guillain-Barré syndrome (GBS) An acute inflammatory demyelinating disorder of the peripheral nervous system characterized by an acute onset of motor paralysis (usually ascending).

Gustatory Of or relating to taste.

Gynecomastia Abnormal enlargement of the breast(s) in men.

H_1 receptors Cellular histamine receptors that are present in the smooth muscle of the vascular system, the bronchial tree, and the digestive tract. Stimulation of these receptors results in itching, pain, edema, bronchoconstriction, and other characteristic symptoms of inflammation and allergy.

H_2 receptors Cellular histamine receptors present primarily in the stomach; their stimulation results in the secretion of large amounts of hydrochloric acid.

H_4 receptors Located in peripheral WBCs and mast cells, they are involved in immune responses.

Habit training Attempts to keep patients dry by having them void at regular intervals.

Habituation The newborn's ability to process and respond to complex stimulations.

Halitosis Bad breath.

Hallucination The perception of seeing, hearing, or feeling something that is not present in reality.

Hallucinogens Type of drugs that induce the same thoughts, perceptions, and feelings that occur in dreams. They include phencyclidine (PCP), 3,4-methylenedioxymethamphetamine (MDMA or ecstasy), D-lysergic acid diethylamide (LSD), mescaline, dimethyltryptamine (DMT), and psilocin.

Handoff The transfer and acceptance of patient care responsibility from one nurse to another, such as at the end of a shift.

Handoff communication A verbal or written exchange of information. It encompasses the nursing team and all other members of the healthcare team who care for a patient at any given time.

Harlequin sign A reddening of the skin on one side of an infant's body while the other side remains pale. Also called *clown color change*.

Hashimoto thyroiditis An autoimmune disorder in which antibodies destroy thyroid tissue.

Health A state of complete physical, mental, and social well-being.

Health assessment A systematic process through which the nurse collects data about a patient to create a holistic plan of care, including an interview to determine health history and a patient's current presenting problem and a physical assessment.

Health beliefs Concepts about health that an individual believes are true, regardless of whether or not they are founded in fact.

Health disparity A difference in a measurement of access to or quality of healthcare services between an individual or group possessing a defined characteristic when other variables have been controlled, such as individual health choices, disease courses, and other variations from the normative measure.

Health Insurance Portability and Accountability Act (HIPAA) Legislation enacted by Congress to minimize the exclusion of preexisting conditions as a barrier to healthcare insurance, designate special rights for those who lose other health coverage, and eliminate medical underwriting in group plans. The act includes the Privacy Rule, which creates a national standard for the disclosure of private health information.

Health Level 7 (HL7) A framework designed for the exchange, integration, sharing, and retrieval of electronic health information that supports clinical practice and the management, delivery, and evaluation of health services.

Health literacy An individual's ability to use literacy skills as a means of obtaining, understanding, and applying health information.

Health maintenance organization (HMO) The most restrictive type of private health insurance plan. Participants must select a primary care provider who provides basic medical services and, as the gatekeeper to care, refers the patient to in-network hospitals and specialists when additional care is needed.

Health policy The actions and decisions by government bodies and professional organizations that affect whether or not healthcare organizations and individuals working within the healthcare system can achieve their healthcare goals.

Health promotion A way of thinking and acting in order to increase individuals' overall health and well-being regardless of their health and illness status or age.

Health promotion diagnosis A patient's readiness to improve an aspect of health.

Health restoration Care focusing on the ill patient that extends from early detection of disease through helping the patient during the recovery period.

Healthcare advance directive Legal document that allows an individual to plan for healthcare and/or financial affairs in the event of incapacity. Also called *advance directive* or *advance healthcare directive*.

Healthcare-associated infection (HAI) Infections associated with the delivery of healthcare services in a facility such as a hospital or nursing home. Also called a *nosocomial infection*.

Healthcare proxy An individual selected to speak to physicians and other healthcare providers on behalf of a patient to determine the best course of treatment.

Healthy lifestyle behaviors Activities that can improve an individual's health and well-being and lower the risk of disease, such as physical exercise.

Heart block A block in the normal electrical conduction of the heart.

Heart failure (HF) The inability of the heart to pump adequate blood to meet the metabolic demands of the body.

Heart murmur Harsh, blowing sounds caused by disruption of blood flow into the heart, between the chambers of the heart, or from the heart into the pulmonary or aortic systems.

Heartburn A burning sensation in the chest or throat. Also called *pyrosis*.

Heat balance When the amount of heat produced by the body equals the amount of heat lost.

Heat exhaustion Excessive heat exposure and dehydration that causes paleness, dizziness, nausea, vomiting, fainting, and a moderately increased temperature (38.3 to 38.9°C [101 to 102°F]).

Heat stroke A serious form of heat exhaustion that can be life-threatening, generally caused by exercising in hot weather. Patients will have warm, flushed skin, often do not sweat, and have a temperature of 41°C (106°F) or higher. A patient may be also delirious, unconscious, or having seizures.

Heaving Lifting of the chest wall during contraction.

Hegar sign One of the physical changes detectable during the first 3 months of pregnancy, it is a softening of the isthmus of the uterus, the area between the cervix and the body of the uterus.

Helper T cells Cells that play a vital role in normal immune system function, recognizing foreign antigens and infected cells and activating antibody-producing B cells. They are the primary cells infected by the human immunodeficiency virus.

HELPP syndrome A cluster of changes, including hemolysis, elevated liver enzymes, and low platelet count, sometimes associated with preeclampsia.

Hematochezia Bright blood in the stool.

Hematocrit The proportion of cells and plasma in blood. Also refers to the laboratory test that measures the hematocrit. This test can also be used to detect severe dehydration or overhydration.

Hematoma A localized collection of blood underneath the skin that may appear as a bruise.

Hematuria The presence of blood in the urine.

Hemianopia The loss of half of the visual field of one or both eyes.

Hemiarthroplasty Hip replacement that involves replacement of the ball, the head, or the femur.

Hemiparesis Weakness of the left or right half of the body.

Hemiplegia Paralysis of the left or right half of the body.

Hemodialysis A process by which a patient's blood flows through vascular catheters, passes by the dialysate in an external machine, and then returns to the patient.

Hemodynamics The study of forces involved in blood circulation.

Hemoglobin The oxygen-carrying molecule within RBCs; a laboratory test to measure the amount of hemoglobin.

Hemoglobin A1C Commonly used to diagnose prediabetes and diabetes, it is a simple blood test that measures average blood sugar levels over the past 3 months.

Hemoglobinopathy A disorder of hemoglobin.

Hemolysis The destruction of RBCs; releases hemoglobin into the circulation.

Hemolytic anemia A disorder that results from the premature destruction of RBCs.

Hemoptysis Bloody sputum.

Hemorrhage Rapid or excessive bleeding.

Hemorrhagic stroke Occurs when vascular rupture spills blood into surrounding space, damaging neurons, resulting in blood flow loss and brain cell death.

Hemosiderosis The storage of excessive iron in tissues and organs.

Hemostasis The cessation of bleeding.

Hemotympanum Bleeding into or behind the tympanic membrane.

Hepatitis The inflammation of the liver triggered by a virus, alcohol, medications, toxins, autoimmune disorder, or other pathogens.

Hernia A protrusion in the intestine through the inguinal wall or canal.

Herniated intervertebral disk A rupture of the cartilage surrounding the intervertebral disk with protrusion of the nucleus pulposus. Also called a *ruptured disk, slipped disk,* or *herniated nucleus pulposus*.

Heroin An illicit central nervous system depressant narcotic that alters perception and produces euphoria.

Heterograft Skin used for transplantation that was obtained from an animal, usually a pig. Also called a *xenograft*.

Heterosexism The view that heterosexuality is the only correct sexual orientation.

Hip fracture A fracture of the femur at the head, neck, or trochanteric regions.

Hippocampus A small, curved body in the brain. Part of the limbic system, it plays a major role in memory formation.

Hirsutism An increased growth of coarse hair on the face and trunk.

Histamine A key chemical mediator of inflammation.

Histrionic personality disorder (HPD) One of several personality disorders defined in the DSM-5, it is characterized by a lifelong tendency for dramatic, egocentric, attention-seeking response patterns.

Holistic health A clinical mindset that considers more than the physiologic health status of an individual.

Holistic nursing Form of whole-health nursing that involves providing individualized care for the whole patient, including the mind, body, and spirit, and not just care for the patient's presenting symptoms or medical diagnosis.

Holosystolic Term used to describe the sounds heard during the entire phase of systole.

Homeostasis The body's ability to maintain a stable, balanced internal environment despite the constant challenges posed by external influences.

Homograft Grafts between members of the same species who have different genotypes and HLA antigens. Usually human skin that has been harvested from cadavers. Also called an *allograft*.

Homologous chromosomes The two paired chromosomes that are inherited, one from each parent.

Homophobia The fear, hatred, or mistrust of people who are gay and lesbian, often expressed in overt displays of discrimination.

Horizontal violence Aggressive acts committed against a nurse by one or more nursing colleagues.

Hormone replacement therapy (HRT) Administration of hormones, usually estrogen and a progestin, to alleviate the symptoms of menopause.

Hormone therapy Type of therapy often used in the treatment of individuals with breast cancer.

Hormones Chemical messengers secreted by various glands that exert controlling effects on the cells of the body.

Hospice An organization that provides end-of-life care for patients either in their homes or in a hospital setting.

Hospice care The support and care for persons in the last phase of an incurable disease so that they may live as fully and comfortably as possible until their death.

Hot zone When a disaster occurs, the hot zone is the most dangerous zone because it is located immediately adjacent to the site of the disaster. All responders who enter the area must be protected by personal protective equipment.

Human chorionic gonadotropin (HCG) A hormone produced by the chorionic villi that is found in the urine of pregnant women. Also called *prolan*.

Human dignity The inherent worth and uniqueness of individuals and populations.

Human immunodeficiency virus (HIV) A primary immunodeficiency disorder that is spread primarily through sexual contact with an infected person. It is the virus that causes acquired immunodeficiency syndrome (AIDS).

Human leukocyte antigen (HLA) The major histocompatibility complex gene.

Humoral immune response Hyperreactive response of B cells characteristic of systemic lupus erythematosus (SLE).

Hunger The feeling that makes individuals think of food and encourages them to satisfy this feeling by eating.

Hydrocephalus A condition characterized by enlargement of the head caused by inadequate drainage of cerebrospinal fluid.

Hydronephrosis An accumulation of urine in the renal pelvis as a result of obstructed outflow.

Hydrostatic pressure The pressure a fluid exerts within a closed system on the walls of its container. The hydrostatic pressure of blood is the force blood exerts against the vascular walls (e.g., the artery walls). The principle involved in hydrostatic pressure is that fluids move from an area of greater pressure to an area of lesser pressure.

Hydroureter Distention of the ureter with urine.

Hypercalcemia Elevated blood levels of calcium.

Hypercapnia A condition marked by a $PaCO_2$ level above 45 mmHg. Also known as **hypercarbia**.

Hypercarbia See **Hypercapnia**.

Hyperchloremia Elevated chloride levels in the blood.

Hypercyanotic episode A potentially life-threatening episode of hypoxia. Also called a *tet episode*.

Hyperemia Increased blood flow to an area.

Hyperextension Forcible backward bending.

Hyperflexion Forcible forward bending.

Hyperglycemia Elevated glucose levels.

Hyperkalemia Elevated potassium levels in the blood.

Hypermagnesemia Elevated magnesium levels in the blood.

Hypernatremia Elevated sodium levels in the blood.

Hyperopia Farsightedness.

Hyperosmolar hyperglycemic state (HHS) A disorder characterized by a plasma osmolarity of 340 mOsm/L or greater, elevated blood glucose levels, and altered levels of consciousness. It occurs in individuals who have type 2 diabetes mellitus.

Hyperplasia An increase in the number or density of normal cells.

Hyperresonance An abnormal, booming sound that can be heard over an emphysematous lung.

Hyperresponsiveness An exaggerated response, as with bronchoconstriction in asthma.

Hypersensitivity An overreaction of the immune system to an antigen or antigens.

Hypersomnia The inability to stay awake during the day, despite obtaining sufficient sleep at night.

Hypertension (HTN) Excess pressure in the arterial portion of the circulatory system, specifically a systolic blood pressure of 140 mmHg or higher or a diastolic blood pressure of 90 mmHg or higher.

Hypertensive crisis A systolic blood pressure greater than 180 mmHg and diastolic blood pressure higher than 120 mmHg. Also called *malignant hypertension* or **hypertensive emergency**.

Hypertensive emergency A systolic blood pressure greater than 180 mmHg and diastolic blood pressure higher than 120 mmHg. Also called *malignant hypertension* or **hypertensive crisis**.

Hypertensive encephalopathy A syndrome characterized by extremely high blood pressure, altered level of consciousness, increased intracranial pressure, papilledema, and seizures.

Hyperthermia A condition that occurs when a body produces more heat than is lost.

Hyperthermia blanket An electronically controlled blanket that provides a specified temperature

Hyperthermic A body temperature above 37.8°C (100°F).

Hyperthyroidism A disorder caused by excessive delivery of thyroid hormone to the peripheral tissues. Also called *thyrotoxicosis*.

Hypertonic Refers to solutions that have a higher osmolality than body fluids; 3% sodium chloride is a hypertonic solution.

Hypertrophic cardiomyopathy A disorder characterized by decreased compliance of the left ventricle and hypertrophy of the ventricular muscle mass.

Hypertrophic scar An overgrowth of dermal tissue that remains within the boundaries of the wound.

Hypertrophy An enlargement of glandular cells or muscles.

Hyperventilation Unusually fast respirations or overbreathing causing an imbalance of oxygen and carbon dioxide.

Hypervolemia The excessive retention of both water and sodium in similar proportions to normal extracellular fluid. Also called *fluid volume excess*.

Hyphema Bleeding into the anterior chamber of the eye.

Hypocalcemia Decreased blood levels of calcium.

Hypocapnia A condition that results when $PaCO_2$ falls below 35 mmHg. Also called **hypocarbia**.

Hypocarbia See **Hypocapnia**.

Hypochloremia Decreased blood levels of chloride.

Hypodermis The layer of loose connective tissue and fat cells that lies below the dermis. Also called *subcutaneous tissue*.

Hypodermoclysis Fluid administered subcutaneously.

Hypoglycemia Diminished glucose levels.

Hypokalemia Decreased blood levels of potassium.

Hypomagnesemia Decreased blood levels of magnesium.

Hypomania A less extreme form of mania that is not severe enough to markedly impair functioning or require hospitalization.

Hyponatremia Decreased blood levels of sodium.

Hypoperfusion Decreased blood flow.

Hypophonia A lowered voice volume.

Hypophosphatemia Decreased blood levels of phosphate.

Hypoplastic left heart syndrome (HLHS) One of the most severe congenital heart defects, characterized by absence or stenosis of mitral and aortic valves, an abnormally small left ventricle, a small aorta, and aortic or mitral stenosis or atresia.

Hypotension A below-normal blood pressure reading between 85 and 110 mmHg.

Hypothalamic–pituitary axis In the brain, responsible for the regulation of endocrine glands and, consequently, hormones.

Hypothermia A condition that occurs when a body loses more heat than it produces.

Hypothermic A body temperature below 36°C (97°F).

Hypothyroidism A disorder resulting when the thyroid gland produces an insufficient amount of thyroid hormone.

Hypotonic Refers to solutions that have a lower osmolality than body fluids, such as one-half normal saline.

Hypoventilation An abnormally slow respiratory rate that leads to inadequate oxygen delivery to the lungs as well as an increase in retention of carbon dioxide.

Hypovolemia Loss of both water and electrolytes in similar proportions from extracellular fluid. Also called *fluid volume deficit.*

Hypovolemic shock Shock caused by a decrease in intravascular volume of 15% or more.

Hypoxemia Decreased oxygen levels in the blood that result when PaO_2 falls below 80 mmHg.

Hypoxia Decreased delivery of oxygen to the tissues.

Iatrogenic A condition induced by the effects of treatment.

Iatrogenic infection A type of infection that results directly from diagnostic or therapeutic procedures.

Ideal body image A mental representation of what individuals believe their body should look like.

Ideal self How individuals think they should be or would prefer to be.

Idiopathic pain A type of pain that occurs unpredictably and is not associated with any known cause, making it difficult to treat.

IgE-mediated hypersensitivity (type I) Allergic reactions, such as allergic asthma, hay fever, allergic conjunctivitis, hives, and anaphylactic shock, which can occur through ingestion of a food or medication, injection of a medication, inhalation of a triggering substance, or absorption via skin contact.

Ileostomy A surgical opening made in the ileum of the small intestine.

Ileus A condition that causes a temporary cessation of the passage of material through the intestines, usually lasting 24 to 48 hours.

Illness A state in which an individual's physical, emotional, intellectual, social, developmental, or spiritual functioning is diminished.

Illness behavior A coping mechanism that includes the ways in which an individual describes, monitors, and interprets symptoms and the individual's ability to take remedial action and use the healthcare system.

Illness prevention Healthcare focusing on maintaining optimal health by preventing disease through programs on immunizations, prenatal and infant care, and prevention of sexually transmitted infections.

Imagery A relaxation technique in which the patient focuses on pleasant images such as a beach or a garden to replace negative images such as pain and darkness. Also called *guided imagery.*

Immobility A reduction in the amount and control of one's movement.

Immune complex–mediated hypersensitivity (type III) Reactions that are characterized by tissue damage caused by the activation of complement in response to antigen–antibody immune complexes that are deposited in tissues.

Immunity The body's natural or induced response to infection and the conditions associated with its response.

Immunization Vaccine that introduces an antigen into the body, allowing immunity against a disease to develop naturally.

Immunocompetent Term used to describe patients who have an immune system that identifies antigens and effectively destroys or removes them.

Immunodeficiency A condition that develops when the immune system is incompetent or unable to respond effectively.

Immunoglobulin (Ig) A protein that functions as an antibody.

Immunosuppression Inability of the immune system to respond to an antigen. Occurs in response to disease or medications; may be intentional to prevent rejection of transplants or a side effect of some medications.

Impaired control A pattern of symptoms of substance use disorder, which include taking a substance in larger amounts over a longer period of time; wanting to reduce use and reporting multiple unsuccessful attempts to cut down or quit; spending a lot of time obtaining, using, or recovering from the effects of the substance; and having daily activities that revolve around the substance.

Implementation The action phase of the nursing process in which nurses take all acquired data and determine interventions that would be most appropriate to help the patient reach the stated goal.

Implied consent Nonverbal consent indicated by a patient's cooperative actions.

Impotence Inability to achieve or maintain an erection.

Impulse conduction The transmission of an impulse along the nerve pathways to the spinal cord and directly to the brain.

Impulsiveness Acting without considering the consequences of one's behavior. Also called *impulsivity.*

In vitro fertilization (IVF) A process in which a woman's eggs are collected from her ovaries, fertilized in the laboratory, and then placed into her uterus after normal embryo development has begun.

Incentive spirometry A breathing exercise using an incentive spirometer that helps patients breathe deeply to expand the lungs. This process can help patients clear mucus secretions and increase the amount of oxygen delivered to the bronchi and alveoli.

Incident pain A type of breakthrough pain that is predictable because it is precipitated by an event or activity such as coughing or changing position.

Incident report An agency record of an accident or incident occurring within the agency. This record is designed to collect adequate information to assist personnel in preventing future incidents or occurrences. Also called *variance reports* or *unusual occurrence reports.*

Incivility Rude and disruptive behaviors that can progress to aggression, bullying, and violence.

Incomplete spinal cord injury An injury that involves only a partial loss of sensory and motor function below the level of the injury.

Increased intracranial pressure Sustained, elevated pressure (15 mmHg or higher in adults) in the cranial cavity.

Indemnity A type of health insurance program that allows the insured to self-select healthcare providers and has no predefined network.

Independent intervention The activities that nurses are licensed to do within their scope of practice; in other words, areas of healthcare that are unique to nursing and separate and distinct from medical management.

Indicator A statistic that reflects the organization's performance in a specific area.

Individualized education plan A school-based intervention for children who need educational support to address their developmental needs.

Individualized family service plan An early childhood intervention that identifies the child and family's strengths and weaknesses and designs activities and goals to help the child meet developmental milestones.

Inductive reasoning A "bottom-up" method of logical thinking that starts with putting significant cues together in order to reach a conclusion. It is a method of logical thinking that is used to determine if decisions are reasonable.

Infantile glaucoma **Congenital glaucoma** diagnosed within the first year of life.

Infection An invasion of the body tissue by microorganisms with the potential to cause illness or disease.

Infectious disease Any communicable disease that is caused by microorganisms that are commonly transmitted from one person to another or from an animal to an individual.

Infertility A lack of conception despite unprotected sexual intercourse for at least 12 months.

Inflammation An adaptive response to what the body sees as harmful, such as an allergen, illness, or injury. Inflammation is typically characterized by pain, heat, redness, and swelling. Also called *inflammatory response.*

Inflammatory bowel disease (IBD) Chronic inflammation of the bowel common to a group of conditions that includes Crohn disease and ulcerative colitis.

Inflammatory response A fundamental type of response by the body to disease and injury; a response characterized by the classical signs of pain, heat, redness, and swelling.

Influenza A highly contagious viral respiratory disease characterized by coryza (inflammation of the mucous membranes lining the nose usually associated with nasal discharge), fever, cough, and systemic symptoms such as headache and malaise (vague feeling of physical discomfort).

Informal groups A type of group that functions with much less structure than a formal or semiformal group. Characteristics of informal groups include easily recognized, basic objectives; rotational leadership; and no set of written rules or regulations.

Informal leader A leader who is not officially appointed to direct the activities of others but, because of seniority, age, or special abilities, is recognized by the group as a leader and plays an important role in influencing colleagues, coworkers, or other group members to achieve the group's goals.

Informed consent 1. A patient's legal and ethical rights to be informed of and give permission for any healthcare procedure or treatment. 2. A study volunteer's legal right to be informed with full disclosure of the study's purpose, required procedures, length of the study, expectations, risks, and possible benefits before consenting to participate. Also includes the right to withdraw from the study at any time.

Inhalant A substance inhaled to produce euphoria. Categorized into three types: anesthetics, volatile nitrites, and organic solvents.

Injury or harm An act or event that causes damage, harm, or loss to a body's functioning.

Inquiry A search for knowledge or facts in order to gain clarification and find solutions to problems.

Insomnia The inability to fall asleep or remain asleep.

Inspection A visual, auditory, and olfactory examination or assessment of a patient to note health condition.

Inspiration The act of inhaling air in respiration.

Instrumental activities of daily living Activities that relate to independent living, such as shopping, cooking, managing medications, driving, and using the phone or computer.

Insubordination Defiance of authority, such as the refusal to complete a task as assigned.

Insulin A hormone that facilitates the uptake and use of glucose by cells and prevents an excessive breakdown of glycogen in the liver and muscle. In doing so, insulin acts to decrease blood glucose levels.

Integrative healthcare The process of incorporating **complementary healthcare** into mainstream Western healthcare.

Integrity Adherence to a strict moral or ethical code.

Integumentary system The body's system that includes skin, hair, and nails and the sebaceous, sweat, and mammary glands.

Intellect The ability to learn and understand knowledge; the capacity for thinking and reasoning intelligently.

Intellectual disability Significant limitations in intellectual functioning and adaptive behavior prior to the age of 18. Previously called *mental retardation*.

Intellectual functioning General intelligence or mental capacity, including an individual's abilities to learn, use logic, and solve problems.

Intensity 1. The amplitude of a sound produced. 2. The strength of the contraction during acme, the peak of a uterine contraction during the birth process.

Interdisciplinary Referring to professionals or paraprofessionals from various disciplines.

Intergenerational family A family in which more than two generations live together.

Intergroup conflict Conflict that occurs between teams that are in competition or opposition to one another.

Intermittent claudication A cramping or aching pain in the calves of the legs, the thighs, and the buttocks that occurs with a predictable level of activity.

Internal environment The physical, spiritual, cognitive, emotional, and psychologic well-being of an individual that depends on the satisfaction of these basic human needs.

Internal locus of control An individual's belief that their actions, choices, and behaviors can impact life events.

Internet gaming disorder The persistent use of the internet to engage in games, often with other players, leading to clinically significant impairment or distress. May also be referred to as *internet gaming addiction*.

Interorganizational conflict Usually conflict that occurs between two organizations that exist within one market.

Interpersonal conflict Conflict that occurs between two or more individuals due to differences, competition, or concern about territory, control, or loss.

Interpersonal skills Critical to nursing communication, the competent nurse in this area is self-aware, reflective, respectful, and genuinely interested in the lifestyles, beliefs, values, and cultural and ethnic differences among fellow healthcare professionals and patient populations.

Interpersonal violence Violence that occurs within relationships, between family members, intimate partners, acquaintances, or strangers that does not aim to further the goals of a formal group or cause.

Interprofessional Referring to professionals from multiple or various disciplines.

Intersex A general term used to describe a variety of conditions in which reproductive or sexual anatomy does not fit the typical definitions of male or female.

Interstitial fluid Accounts for approximately 75% of extracellular fluid; surrounds the cells.

Interval training Alternating short bursts of higher-intensity activity into a sustained aerobic workout, which can be incorporated when using stationary bikes, ellipticals, and other low-impact exercise machines.

Intervention Activities conducted or attempts made by the nurse to influence a positive change in a patient's health status or behavior; a personalized confrontation that prevents an addict from denying the addiction problem and forces them to face the negative aspects of their behavior and enroll in treatment.

Interview Verbal communication that the nurse plans with a definite purpose, which can be to get information or give education, identify issues of mutual concern, use criteria to evaluate the healing process, or provide support in the form of counseling or therapy.

Intimacy A relationship that entails commitment, companionship, affective intimacy, social support, physical closeness, and mutuality.

Intimate distance Communication that is characterized by body contact, heightened sensations of body heat and smell, and vocalizations that are low.

Intimate partner violence (IPV) The act of inflicting sexual, emotional, or physical harm on a current or previous partner or spouse.

Intra-aortic balloon pump (IABP) Also called *intra-aortic balloon counterpulsation*, it is a mechanical circulatory support device that may be used after cardiac surgery or to treat cardiogenic shock following acute myocardial infarction. It temporarily supports cardiac function, allowing the heart to recover gradually by decreasing myocardial workload and oxygen demand and increasing perfusion of the coronary arteries.

Intracapsular hip fracture A hip fracture involving the head or neck of the femur.

Intracellular fluid (ICF) Fluid found within the body cells that contains solute vital to the metabolic processes of the cells. Also called *cellular fluid*.

Intracranial compliance Shifting of venous blood or cerebrospinal fluid out of the cranium and into the spinal column in an effort to maintain a near constant intracranial pressure.

Intracranial hypertension A sustained state of increased intracranial pressure that is potentially life-threatening.

Intracranial regulation The processes that affect intracranial compensation and adaptive neurologic function.

Intractable seizures Seizures that continue to occur even with optimal medical management.

Intradiskal electrothermal therapy (IDET) The use of thermal energy to treat pain from a bulging spinal disk.

Intraocular pressure A force within the eye that causes tissue damage.

Intraoperative The phase of an operative process in which the surgical procedure actually takes place.

Intrapartum The time from the onset of true labor until the birth of the infant and expulsion of the placenta.

Intrapersonal conflict Conflict that occurs within an individual, arising from stress or tension that results from real or perceived pressure generated by incompatible expectations or goals.

Intraprofessional assessment An evaluation that occurs within a group of individuals with a similar position in the healthcare system, such as a group of nurses or a group of surgeons, to identify areas of improvement at each level of care.

Intrathecal pump A small medical device that delivers pain medication directly to the spinal cord.

Intrauterine contraception (IUC) A safe, effective method of reversible contraception that is designed to be inserted into the uterus by a qualified healthcare provider and left in place for an extended period, providing continuous contraceptive protection.

Intrauterine fetal death (IUFD) Death of a fetus that occurs after 20 weeks' gestation. Often referred to as *stillbirth* or *fetal demise*.

Intrauterine pressure catheter A device that measures the pressure in the uterine cavity.

Intravascular fluid Accounts for approximately 20% of the extracellular fluid and is found within the vascular system. Also called *plasma*.

Intravenous pyelography (IVP) A diagnostic test used to evaluate the structure and excretory function of the kidneys, ureters, and bladder.

Intrinsic pathway During coagulation, this pathway is initiated when exposed collagen in the wall of the damaged blood vessel triggers a series of reactions.

Introspection The personal exploration and evaluation of one's own thoughts, emotions, behaviors, and values incorporating both verbal and nonverbal feedback from others.

Intubation The process of inserting a breathing tube.

Intuition The use of nursing knowledge, experience, and expertise for understanding without the conscious use of reasoning.

Invasion Occurs when cancerous cells overtake adjacent tissues.

Involuntary admission The detention of a patient in a psychiatric or medical facility against the patient's will, normally reserved for cases in which the individual is a danger to self or others.

Involution The rapid reduction in size of the uterus and the return of the uterus to a nonpregnant state.

Ions Electrically charged particles.

Iron deficiency anemia A disorder that results when the supply of iron in the body is insufficient for the formation of RBCs.

Irritant contact dermatitis An inflammation of the skin from irritants; it is not a hypersensitivity response.

Ischemia Insufficient blood supply.

Ischemic Deprived of oxygen.

Ischemic stroke Type of stroke that occurs when a blood clot, circulating foreign matter, or vascular narrowing interrupts the blood supply.

Isoelectric line A straight line on an electrocardiograph that indicates the absence of electrical activity.

Isokinetic exercises Resistive exercises that involve muscle contraction or tension against resistance; can be either isotonic or isometric.

Isolation Measures designed to prevent the spread of infection to health personnel, patients, and visitors.

Isometric exercises Static or sitting exercises in which muscles contract without moving the joint.

Isotonic A solution that has the same osmolality as body fluids. Normal saline, 0.9% sodium chloride, is an isotonic solution.

Isotonic exercises Dynamic exercises in which the muscle shortens to produce muscle contractions and active movement.

Isotonic fluid volume deficit A type of fluid imbalance that occurs when electrolytes are lost along with fluid.

Jaundice A yellow pigmentation of body tissues caused by the presence of bile pigments.

Joint arthroplasty The reconstruction or replacement of a joint.

Joint custody Occurs when two parents who are not married have equal responsibility and legal rights for their shared children.

Joint fusion A procedure that permanently fuses two or more bones together at a joint using pins, plates, screws, and rods. Also called *arthrodesis*.

Joint irrigation A fluid injected into the joint to allow the surgeon to visualize joint structures more easily and to help remove debris and infection in the joint.

Joint resurfacing A procedure in which a little bone is removed at the articulating surface of the joint and a metal replacement is fitted over the end of the bone.

Just culture An attempt to balance a blame-free environment with appropriate accountability by focusing on correcting problems that lead individuals to engage in unsafe behavior while maintaining individual accountability by establishing zero tolerance for reckless behavior.

Justice Fairness.

Juvenile glaucoma **Congenital glaucoma** diagnosed after age 3.

Juvenile macular degeneration A pediatric form of **age-related macular degeneration** that is inherited rather than acquired.

Juvenile rheumatoid arthritis (JRA) A chronic inflammatory autoimmune disease diagnosed in children that is characterized by joint inflammation resulting in decreased mobility, swelling, and pain.

Kaposi sarcoma (KS) Often the presenting symptom of AIDS, it remains the most common cancer associated with the disease. It is caused by a virus called the Kaposi sarcoma–associated herpes virus, also known as human herpes virus 8.

Karyotype A pictorial analysis of chromosomes.

Kcalorie See **Kilocalories.**

Kegel exercises The act of tightening the perineal muscle in order to strengthen the pubococcygeus muscle and increase its elasticity.

Keloid A scar that extends beyond the boundaries of the original wound.

Keratin A fibrous, water-repellent protein that gives the epidermis its tough, protective quality.

Keratotic basal cell carcinoma Type of skin cancer appearing on the ears that contains basal cells and squamoid-appearing cells that keratinize.

Ketonuria The presence of ketones in the urine.

Ketosis An accumulation of ketone bodies produced during oxidation of fatty acids.

Kilocalories A term used to identify the energy-producing ability of nutrients. Also called *Kcalories* or *kcal*.

Kindling Long-term changes in brain neurotransmission that occur after repeated detoxifications.

Kinesthesia The ability to perceive movement and sense of position.

Kinesthetic A term referring to awareness of the position and movement of body parts.

Korotkoff sounds The series of sounds identified while taking a blood pressure using a stethoscope.

Kosher Acceptable to or prepared according to Jewish law.

Kussmaul respirations Deep, rapid respirations associated with compensatory mechanisms.

Kyphosis A convex curvature of the spine that may decrease mobility.

Labor induction The stimulation of uterine contractions before the spontaneous onset of labor, with or without ruptured fetal membranes, for the purpose of accomplishing birth.

Labyrinthitis Inflammation of the inner ear. Also called *otitis interna*.

Laceration Disruption of the brain tissue caused by the entrance of a foreign object such as a bullet, knife, or skull fragment.

Lactase deficiency An individual's inability to digest lactose because of a deficiency of lactase, the enzyme that breaks down lactose into monosaccharides. Also called *lactose intolerance*.

Lactation consultant A specially trained individual who provides breastfeeding support and care to mothers, infants, children, families, and communities.

Lacto-ovo-vegetarians Vegetarians who include milk, dairy products, and eggs in their diets.

Lactose intolerance An individual's inability to digest lactose because of a deficiency of lactase, the enzyme that breaks down lactose into monosaccharides. Also called *lactose deficiency*.

Lactovegetarians Vegetarians who include dairy products but no eggs in their diets.

Laissez-faire leader A leader who recognizes a group's need for autonomy and self-regulation. The leader assumes a "hands-off" approach, being less directive and more permissive than other types of leaders.

Laminectomy The surgical removal of the vertebral lamina.

Laminotomy The surgical removal of part of the vertebral lamina.

Lanugo A large quantity of fine hair found on some newborns.

Late deceleration A condition caused by uteroplacental insufficiency resulting from decreased blood flow and oxygen transfer to the fetus through the intervillous spaces during uterine contractions.

Late (secondary) postpartum hemorrhage Postpartum hemorrhage that occurs from 24 hours to 6 weeks after birth.

Law The sum total of the rules and regulations by which a society is governed.

Laxatives Medications that stimulate bowel activity and assist in fecal elimination.

Lead (electrocardiographic) An insulated wire that connects an electrocardiograph to the electrodes attached to a patient.

Leader An individual with the ability to rule, guide, or inspire others to think or act as that individual recommends.

Leading question A closed question that gives the patient an opportunity to decide whether the answer is true or not.

Lean Six Sigma A methodology used to reduce waste and provide consistency in the quality of care.

Learned helplessness A sense of helplessness that nothing the individual does can change an aspect of a situation or stressor; often reinforced by repeated failures, it is common in individuals with major depressive disorder.

Learning An outcome that occurs after being exposed to information that adds to knowledge and skill.

Learning disabilities Disorders that impair an individual's ability to receive and process information, causing reduced functioning in verbal, linguistic, reasoning, and academic skills; neurologic conditions in which the brain cannot receive or process information normally.

Learning need An identified deficit in knowledge, information, or skills needed to achieve a particular goal.

Leopold maneuvers A systematic way to evaluate the maternal abdomen.

Lesion An observable change in skin structure that may indicate disorders in other systems and organs.

Leukemia A group of chronic malignant disorders of WBCs and WBC precursors.

Leukocytes The primary cells involved in both nonspecific and specific immune system responses. Also known as *white blood cells (WBCs)*.

Leukocytosis An increase in the number of leukocytes in the blood (above 10,000/mm^3), in response to infection or inflammation.

Leukopenia A decrease in the number of circulating leukocytes.

Level of injury The vertical location of an injury along the spinal column.

Lewy bodies Abnormal aggregates of proteins, including alpha-synuclein.

LGBTQ family A family headed by lesbian, gay, bisexual, transgender, or queer/questioning partners.

Liability The state of being legally obliged and responsible.

Libido Sexual desire.

Licensed practical nurses (LPNs) Members of a nursing team who provide direct patient care under the direction of a registered nurse, physician, or other licensed practitioner.

Lichenification The thickening of the skin.

Lightening The effects that occur when the fetus begins to settle into the pelvic inlet.

Limbic system A set of structures located deep inside the brain; includes the hippocampus.

Limit setting Establishing clear and consistent rules or guidelines for child or patient behavior.

Line authority The power to direct the activities of subordinates within an organization.

Lipids The macronutrient that provides most of the body's energy at 9 kcal/g. There are three categories of lipids: triglycerides, phospholipids, and sterols. Also called *fats*.

Lithiasis Stone formation.

Lithotripsy The preferred treatment for urinary calculi; uses sound or shock waves to crush a stone.

Living will A document that provides written directions about life-prolonging procedures to provide instructions when an individual can no longer communicate in a life-threatening situation.

Lobes Specialized cognitive regions in the hemispheres of the brain.

Local adaptation syndrome (LAS) A stress response that affects only one organ or body system.

Local emergency management agency (LEMA) A governmental agency with expertise in public safety, emergency medical services, and management.

Local infection Invasion by a microorganism that is limited to the specific part of the body where the microorganism remains.

Localized responses Common manifestations of type I hypersensitivity, they are typically atopic responses; that is, they have a strong genetic predisposition. Atopic reactions are the result of localized, rather than systemic, IgE-mediated responses to an allergen. They are prompted by contact of the allergen with IgE in the bronchial tree, nasal mucosa, and conjunctival tissues.

Lochia The discharge through which the uterus rids itself of the debris remaining after birth. The discharge should change appearance and contents as healing commences.

Lochia alba The final discharge as the uterus completes healing; composed primarily of leukocytes, decidual cells, epithelial cells, fat, cervical mucus, cholesterol crystals, and bacteria.

Lochia rubra The dark red initial discharge as the uterus eliminates epithelial cells, erythrocytes, leukocytes, shreds of decidua, and occasionally fetal meconium, lanugo, and vernix in the first 1 to 2 days following birth.

Lochia serosa A light pink discharge of serous exudate, shreds of degenerating decidua, erythrocytes, leukocytes, cervical mucus, and numerous microorganisms from the uterus 3 to 10 days following birth.

Locked-in syndrome A state of consciousness in which the patient is alert and fully aware of the environment and has intact cognitive abilities but is unable to communicate through speech or movement because of blocked efferent pathways from the brain. Motor paralysis affects all voluntary muscles, although the upper cranial nerves (I through IV) may remain intact, allowing the patient to communicate through eye movements and blinking.

Locus of control The extent to which patients believe their health status is under their own or others' control.

Long-term memory The final process or destination for information to be stored indefinitely.

Loose association An indication of disordered thinking characterized by the shifting of verbal ideas from one topic to another, with no apparent relationship between thoughts, and the person speaking being unaware that the topics are unconnected. Commonly seen in schizophrenia.

Lordosis A concave curvature of the spine that may decrease mobility.

Loss A situation in which someone or something that is valued becomes altered or no longer available.

Lower body obesity Identified by a waist-to-hip ratio of less than 0.8; more commonly seen in women. Also called *peripheral obesity*.

Lung abscess A local area of necrosis and pus formation within the lung.

Lupus nephritis Inflammation of the kidneys resulting from systemic lupus erythematosus.

Luteinizing hormone (LH) Anterior pituitary hormone responsible for stimulating ovulation and for development of the corpus luteum.

Lymphadenopathy The enlargement of lymph nodes with or without tenderness. It may be caused by inflammation, infection, or malignancy of the nodes or the regions drained by the nodes.

Lymphangitis Inflammation of a lymph vessel.

Lymphedema Accumulation of fluid in the soft tissues of the arm caused by removal of lymph channels.

Lyse Disintegrate.

Maceration Tissues softened by prolonged wetting or soaking.

Macronutrients Essential nutrients needed by the body in large amounts to survive: carbohydrates, proteins, and fats.

Macrophages Large phagocytes that are important in the body's defense against chronic infections.

Macular degeneration A progressive disorder involving loss of central vision due to damage to the retina.

Magical thinking Believing that events occur because of one's thoughts or actions.

Major depressive disorder (MDD) A mood disorder characterized by loss of interest in life and unresponsiveness, moving from mild to severe, with severe symptoms lasting at least 2 weeks. Also called *unipolar depression*.

Major depressive episode Characterized by a change in several aspects of an individual's emotional state and functioning consistently over a period of 14 days or longer.

Major trauma A serious single-system injury (such as the amputation of a leg) or multiple-system injuries (simultaneous injuries such as a punctured lung, traumatic brain injury, and crushed bones in the arms and legs). Also called *multisystem trauma*.

Malabsorption A condition in which the intestinal mucosa is unable to absorb nutrients, resulting in nutrients being excreted in the stool.

Malaise Vague feeling of physical discomfort.

Maldigestion A condition in which there is inadequate preparation of chyme for absorption of nutrients; can also result in malabsorption.

Male hypoactive sexual desire disorder A deficiency in or absence of sexual fantasies and persistently low interest or a total lack of interest in sexual activity.

Malignant Term used to refer to a cell or growth that, if not treated, will recur, continue to grow, and spread to other sites in the body, ending in death.

Malignant hyperthermia A musculoskeletal disorder resulting from an inherited cellular deficit that places the patient in a hypermetabolic state.

Malnutrition Health effects due to insufficient nutrient intake or stores. Also called *undernutrition*.

Malpractice Conduct deviating from the standard of practice dictated by a profession.

Malpresentation A condition that occurs when a fetus passes into the pelvic inlet with a breech or shoulder presentation. These presentations are associated with difficulties during labor.

Malunion The healing of bones in an anatomically incorrect position. Surgical correction may be needed.

Managed care A healthcare delivery system designed to provide cost-effective, high-quality care for groups of patients from the time of their initial contact with the health system through the conclusion of their health problem.

Manager An individual employed by an organization and granted the required authority, responsibility, accountability, and power to accomplish the organization's goals.

Mandatory health insurance Health insurance is provided by large, nonprofit health organizations centered around large employers or work-based associations or else is provided by government-sponsored programs. Everyone belongs to one of these two types of insurance plans, thus ensuring universal coverage.

Mandatory reporting A legal requirement to report an act, event, or situation that is designated by state or local law as a reportable event.

Mania An abnormal and persistently elevated, expansive, or irritable mood lasting at least 1 week, significantly impairing social or occupational functioning and generally requiring hospitalization.

Manipulation Controlling behavior used to exploit others for personal gain.

Margination The accumulation of leukocytes along the inner surface of blood vessels. Occurs as part of the inflammatory process.

Maslow's hierarchy of needs A concept proposed by Abraham Maslow in which he proposed the existence of levels of human needs that could be organized into five categories: physiologic, safety, love and belonging, esteem, and self-actualization.

Mass-casualty incident (MCI) An event that overwhelms the local healthcare system, where the number of casualties vastly exceeds the local resources and capabilities in a short period of time.

Massage therapy The scientific manipulation of the soft tissues of the body for the purposes of promoting healing and wellness.

Massive transfusion A series of blood parcels, including packed RBCs, fresh frozen plasma, cryo units, and platelet pheresis administered to a patient who has lost a substantial amount of blood.

Mast cells Leukocytes that detect foreign agents or injury and respond by releasing histamine, thereby activating the inflammatory process.

Masturbation The self-stimulation of one's genitals for sexual pleasure.

Maternal role attainment (MRA) The process by which a woman learns mothering behaviors and becomes comfortable with her identity as a mother.

Maturational crisis A crisis that occurs normally as an individual progresses through the life cycle.

Mature milk A white or slightly blue-tinged color milk that presents by 2 weeks postpartum and continues thereafter until lactation ceases.

McDonald sign A probable sign of pregnancy characterized by an ease in flexing the body of the uterus against the cervix.

Mean arterial pressure (MAP) The average pressure in the arterial circulation throughout the cardiac cycle.

Meaning-focused coping The use of revaluation to reduce the appraisal of a threat.

Meatus A body passage or opening.

Meconium The first fecal material passed by a newborn, normally within 8 to 24 hours after birth.

Medicaid A state-administered health insurance program available to certain lower-income individuals and families, older adults, and people with disabilities.

Medical asepsis All practices intended to confine a specific microorganism to a specific area, thus limiting the number, growth, and transmission of the microorganism.

Medicare A federally funded health insurance program available to people age 65 and older, younger people with disabilities, and people with end-stage renal disease.

Medication reconciliation The action of checking any new medication prescribed against a patient's current medications, which helps to identify any duplications, potential drug–drug interactions, and forgotten drugs so that only current medications needed by patients are continued.

Medigap policy A private health insurance plan designed to supplement Medicare coverage. It may pay copayments, coinsurance, deductibles, and "gaps" in Medicare coverage (i.e., noncovered healthcare costs). Also called *Medicare supplemental insurance.*

Meditation The act of focusing one's thoughts or engaging in self-reflection or contemplation.

Meiosis A reductive division of sex cells, producing ova or sperm with a half set (haploid) of chromosomes.

Melanin A shield that protects the keratinocytes and the nerve endings in the dermis from the damaging effects of ultraviolet light.

Melanoma A type of malignant skin cancer that arises from melanocytes.

Melasma gravidarum See **Chloasma**.

Menarche First menses.

Membranous labyrinth A collection of fluid-filled tubes and chambers in the inner ear that contain the receptors for the senses of equilibrium and hearing.

Mendelian (single-gene) inheritance Traits that are passed on by a single gene. Also called *single-gene inheritance.*

Ménière disease Also called *idiopathic endolymphatic hydrops*, it is a disorder of the inner ear that causes **tinnitus**, **vertigo**, imbalance, hearing loss, and **aural pressure**.

Meninges Three connective tissue membranes that cover, protect, and nourish the central nervous system.

Menometrorrhagia Irregular, excessive, prolonged menstruation.

Menopause The permanent cessation of menses.

Menorrhagia Excessive or prolonged menstruation that occurs at regular intervals.

Menstrual cycle The cyclic phases of menstruation that normally occur about every 28 days.

Menstruation The periodic shedding of the uterine lining in a woman of childbearing age who is not pregnant.

Mental health A state of well-being in which individuals are able to work productively, cope with change and adversity, engage in meaningful relationships, and realize their own potential.

Mental illness A condition that affects emotions, thinking, behavior, or any combination of the three; mental illness is characterized by symptoms that are severe enough to impair functioning.

Mental retardation See **Intellectual disability**.

Mentor Experienced nurses who coach, advise, and support the personal and professional growth of a less-experienced or novice mentee or protégé in a professional relationship by discussing mutual goals and providing accountability.

Metabolic acidosis This bicarbonate deficit is characterized by a low pH (<7.35), low bicarbonate (<24 mEq/L), and $PaCO_2$ less than 38 mmHg. It may be caused by excess acid in the body or loss of bicarbonate from the body.

Metabolic alkalosis This bicarbonate excess is characterized by a high pH (>7.45), a high bicarbonate (>28 mEq/L), and $PaCO_2$ higher than 45 mmHg. It may be caused by loss of acid or excess bicarbonate in the body.

Metabolic syndrome A disorder characterized by the presence of three or more of the following: increased waist circumference, hypertension, elevated blood triglycerides and fasting blood glucose, and low HDL cholesterol.

Metabolism The complex process of biochemical reactions occurring in the body's cells necessary to produce energy, repair cells, and sustain life.

Metaplasia A change in the normal pattern of differentiation such that dividing cells differentiate into cell types not normally found at that location in the body.

Metastasis The process by which spreading of malignant neoplasms occurs; the transfer of disease from one organ or part to another.

Metrorrhagia Bleeding between menstrual periods.

mHealth Short for mobile health, it refers to healthcare services delivered via mobile devices such as smartphones and tablets.

Micronutrients Essential nutrients needed by the body in small quantities, such as vitamins and minerals.

Microstaging The assessment of the level of invasion of a malignant melanoma and the maximum tumor thickness.

Micturition Releasing urine from the urinary bladder. Also called *voiding* or *urination*.

Middle ear effusion Results when negative pressure in the middle ear causes sterile serous fluid to move from the capillaries into the space.

Milia Exposed sebaceous glands that appear as raised white spots on the face, especially across the nose on infants within the first month after birth.

Milieu therapy A therapeutic recovery environment that supports behavior changes, teaches new coping skills, and helps the patient move from addiction to sobriety.

Milliequivalent (mEq) The chemical combining power of the ion, or the capacity of cations to combine with anions to form molecules.

Mindfulness A cognitive method of paying attention and building awareness of thoughts, emotions, and actions in the present moment.

Minerals Salts dissolved in water that carry electrical charge and work with other nutrients to maintain fluid balance throughout the body. Also called *electrolytes*.

Minimal enteral nutrition Small-volume feedings of formula or human milk (usually $<24\ \text{mL} \cdot \text{kg}^{-1} \cdot \text{day}^{-1}$) designed to "prime" the premature infant's intestinal tract and stimulate many of its hormonal and enzymatic functions.

Minor trauma Trauma that affects a single part or system of the body and is usually treated in a physician's office or in a hospital's emergency department.

Minority Refers to an individual or group of individuals who are outside the dominant group.

Miscarriage The loss of a fetus prior to 20 weeks' gestation. Also called a *spontaneous abortion*.

Mitigation A phase that takes place before and after an emergency that consists of identifying potential hazards, minimizing effects, and reducing the likelihood of their occurrence.

Mitosis The process of cell division.

Modeling Observing the behavior of people who have successfully achieved a goal that they have set for themselves and, through observing, acquiring ideas for behavior and coping strategies.

Modified radical mastectomy The removal of the breast tissue and lymph nodes under the arm, leaving the chest wall muscles intact.

Modifiers Words used in nursing diagnoses to indicate the direction, intensity, or severity of the problem.

Molding The asymmetrical appearance of an infant's head caused by overlapping of the cranial bones during labor and birth.

Mongolian spots Macular areas of bluish-black or gray-blue pigmentation on the dorsal area and the buttocks; common in newborns of Asian, Hispanic, and African descent and in newborns of other dark-skinned races.

Monitoring Type of assessment that compares a patient's current status to baseline data previously obtained.

Monoamine oxidase inhibitor (MAOI) A drug that inhibits monoamine oxidase, an enzyme that terminates the actions of neurotransmitters such as dopamine, norepinephrine, epinephrine, and serotonin. These drugs are used to treat individuals who have not responded to typical treatments for depression.

Mononeuropathies Isolated peripheral neuropathies that affect a single nerve.

Monophasic A term used to describe rheumatoid arthritis when it occurs for a limited time and then improves.

Monopolizing The domination of a discussion by one member of a group.

Monro-Kellie hypothesis A hypothesis that states if the volume of any of the three intracranial components (the brain, cerebrospinal fluid, and blood) increases, the volume of the others must decrease to maintain normal pressures in the cranial cavity.

Mood An individual's internal, subjective, sustained emotional state.

Mood stabilizers Drugs used for treatment of bipolar disorder because they moderate extreme shifts in emotions between mania and depression.

Moral behavior The way in which an individual perceives and responds to society's requirements.

Moral development 1. The process of learning to tell the difference between right and wrong and of learning what ought and ought not to be done. 2. The pattern of change in moral behavior that occurs with age.

Moral principles Statements about broad, general, philosophical concepts such as autonomy and justice.

Moral rules Specific prescriptions for actions.

Morality Private, personal standards of what is right and wrong in conduct, character, and attitude; the requirements necessary for people to live together in society.

Morals A code of acceptable behavior, a sense of right and wrong, what a person ought to do.

Morbid obesity A condition in which an individual weighs more than 200% of ideal body weight or has a BMI >40.

Morning sickness A term that refers to the nausea and vomiting that a woman may experience in early pregnancy. This lay term is sometimes used because these symptoms frequently occur in the early part of the day and disappear within a few hours.

Moro reflex In response to being lifted, then suddenly lowered or surprised by a loud noise, a newborn will straighten the arms and hands outward while the knees flex. Slowly, the arms return to the chest, as in an embrace. The fingers spread, forming a "C," and the newborn may cry.

Morpheaform basal cell carcinoma Rarest form of basal cell carcinoma, which forms finger-like projections.

Morula Developmental stage of the fertilized ovum in which there is a solid mass of cells.

Mosaicism The expression of two cell lines, each with a different chromosomal number, in an individual.

Motility The process of moving food and fluid through the gastrointestinal tract from the mouth to the anus.

Motivational interviewing A technique frequently used in addictions counseling to explore any ambivalence that exists about a behavior change. It uses four key elements: avoiding the righting reflex, listening with empathy, exploring intrinsic motivations, and encouraging patient self-efficacy.

Motor-vehicle crash (MVC) The unintentional collision of one or more motor vehicles with another vehicle or object.

Mottling A lacy pattern of dilated blood vessels under the skin.

Mourning The behavioral process through which grief is eventually resolved or altered; it is often influenced by culture, spiritual beliefs, and custom.

Movement technique A relaxation technique, such as yoga or t'ai chi, designed to improve strength, balance, and mental calmness.

Mucolytics Medications that help break up thick mucus secretions in the airways.

Multiculturalism Characterized by many subcultures coexisting within a given society in which no one culture dominates.

Multidrug-resistant (MDR) Acquired nonsusceptibility to at least one agent in three or more antimicrobial categories.

Multifocal A term used to describe premature ventricular contractions that arise from different ectopic sites and appear distinct on an electrocardiogram.

Multigravida Term used to describe a woman who has been pregnant more than once.

Multipara Term used to describe a woman who has had more than one pregnancy in which the fetus was viable.

Multiple sclerosis (MS) A chronic demyelinating neurologic disease of the central nervous system associated with an abnormal immune response to an environmental factor.

Multisystem trauma Serious single-system injury (such as the amputation of a leg) or multiple-system injuries (simultaneous injuries such as a punctured lung, traumatic brain injury, and crushed bones in the arms and legs). Also called **major trauma**.

Murmur An unusual whooshing or swishing sound heard on auscultation.

Muscle relaxation A relaxation technique that involves consciously tightening and then relaxing each muscle progressively from either head to toe or toe to head.

Mutual recognition model A licensing system that allows a nurse to have a single license that confers the privilege to practice in other states that are part of the Nurse Licensure Compact.

Mutual respect When members of an interprofessional team value the contributions and knowledge of each team member and treat all members as equals.

Mycobacterium tuberculosis The bacterium that causes tuberculosis.

Mydriasis Abnormal or excessive dilation of the pupil of the eye, usually caused by a disease or drug.

Myelin The fatty, segmented wrappings that normally protect and insulate nerves. Also called *myelin sheath*.

Myelogram A diagnostic technique in which dye is injected into the spinal fluid and visualized by x-ray in order to identify areas of pressure on the spinal cord or nerves due to herniated disks.

Myocardial hypertrophy An increase in the size of muscle cells of the myocardium.

Myopia Nearsightedness.

Myringotomy A surgical incision of the tympanic membrane.

Myxedema The hypothyroid state with characteristic accumulation of nonpitting edema in the connective tissues throughout the body.

Myxedema coma A life-threatening complication of long-standing, untreated hypothyroidism, usually triggered by an acute illness or trauma.

Nägele rule A common method of determining the estimated date of birth using the first day of the last menstrual period, subtracting 3 months, adding 7 days, and adding 1 year.

NANDA-I The acronym for North American Nursing Diagnosis Association.

Narcissism Self-centered behavior in which individuals feel entitled to special favors due to a mistaken perception that they are superior to others.

Narcissistic personality disorder (NPD) One of several personality disorders defined in the DSM-5, it is marked by in a pattern of grandiosity, difficulty regulating self-esteem, and the need for admiration and attention from others.

Narcolepsy A disorder characterized by daytime sleep attacks or excessive daytime sleepiness.

Narcotics See **Opioids.**

National Institute for Occupational Safety and Health (NIOSH) An organization that focuses on generating new knowledge in the field of occupational safety and health and transferring that knowledge into practice for the betterment of workers.

National Patient Safety Goals (NPSGs) Formulated goals to assist accredited organizations with specific topics about patient safety.

Natural killer (NK) cells Large, granular cells found in the spleen, lymph nodes, bone marrow, and blood. They provide immune surveillance and resistance to infection, and they play an important role in the destruction of early malignant cells.

Nature The genetic or hereditary capability of the individual.

Nausea A vague, but unpleasant, subjective sensation of sickness or queasiness.

Necrosis Dead tissue.

Negative airflow room A room where airflow is controlled to prevent the air from circulating into the hallway or other rooms. Multiple fresh-air exchanges dilute the concentration of droplet nuclei in a negative airflow room. Also called *negative flow room.*

Negative pressure ventilators A device that creates negative pressure externally to draw the chest outward and air into the lungs, mimicking spontaneous breathing.

Negative symptoms Loss or absence of a normal function seen in mentally healthy adults, such as the ability to care for oneself; commonly seen in schizophrenia.

Neglect According to the Child Abuse Prevention and Treatment Act, defined as "any recent act or failure to act on the part of a parent or caretaker which results in death, serious physical or emotional harm, sexual abuse or exploitation" of a child or "an act or failure to act which presents an imminent risk of serious harm" to a child.

Neglect syndrome A disorder of attention that can result from stroke, which is characterized by the inability to integrate and use perceptions from the affected side. Also called *unilateral neglect.*

Negligence Any conduct that deviates from what a reasonable person would do in a particular circumstance.

Neologisms Use of meaningless words that only have meaning to the individual using them.

Neonatal abstinence syndrome (NAS) A combination of neonatal signs and symptoms caused by withdrawal of gestational opioid exposure. Also called **neonatal opioid withdrawal syndrome (NOWS).**

Neonatal anemia A disorder caused by blood loss, hemolysis, and impaired RBC production related to birth.

Neonatal mortality risk An infant's chance of death within the first 28 days of life.

Neonatal opioid withdrawal syndrome (NOWS) A combination of neonatal signs and symptoms caused by withdrawal of gestational opioid exposure. Also called **neonatal abstinence syndrome (NAS).**

Neonatal transition The first few hours after birth, in which a newborn's body systems adapt to extrauterine life.

Neonatology The field of medicine providing care for sick and premature infants.

Neoplasm A mass of new tissue that grows independently of its surrounding structures and has no physiologic purpose.

Nephrectomy Removal of a kidney.

Nephritis Inflammation of the kidneys.

Nephrolithiasis The formation of stones in the kidney.

Nephrolithotomy A procedure for removal of a staghorn calculus that invades the calyces and renal parenchyma.

Nephrotoxins Substances that damage nerves or nerve tissue.

Nerve block A chemical interruption of a nerve pathway, effected by injecting a local anesthetic into the nerve.

Networking The act of developing and maintaining relationships with others within and outside of the nursing profession and affiliated organizations to improve nursing practice, advance career goals, offer support, share information, and provide advice.

Neurofibrillary tangles Seen in patients with Alzheimer disease, they are thick, insoluble clots of protein inside the damaged brain cells or neurons.

Neurogenic bladder Interference with the normal mechanisms of urine elimination in which the patient does not perceive bladder fullness and is unable to control the urinary sphincters; usually the result of impaired neurologic function.

Neurogenic shock The result of an imbalance between parasympathetic and sympathetic stimulation of vascular smooth muscle.

Neuroleptic malignant syndrome (NMS) A potentially fatal condition caused by antipsychotic medications that block dopamine receptors. It is characterized by fever, rigidity, and increased prolactin levels.

Neuron The basic or specialized cell of the nervous system that carries electrical impulses throughout the body.

Neuropathic pain A type of pain experienced by people who have damaged or malfunctioning nerves.

Neurotransmitters Chemical messengers that carry information between neurons.

Neutral question An open-ended question the patient can answer without direction or pressure.

Neutral thermal environment (NTE) A specific environmental temperature range in which the rates of oxygen consumption and metabolism are minimal and the internal body temperature is maintained because of thermal balance.

Never events Preventable hazards that can result in injury or death and that should never happen to patients.

Nevi Moles.

Nevus flammeus (port-wine stain) A capillary angioma directly below the epidermis. It is a nonelevated, sharply demarcated, red-to-purple area of dense capillaries. In infants of African descent, it may appear as a purple-black stain.

Nevus vasculosus (strawberry mark) A capillary hemangioma consisting of newly formed and enlarged capillaries in the dermal and subdermal layers. It is a raised, clearly delineated, dark red, rough-surfaced birthmark commonly found in the head region.

New Ballard score Specific criteria designed for accurate assessment of the gestational age of newborns between 20 and 28 weeks of gestation and weighing less than 1500 g.

Newborn Infant from birth through the first 28 days of life.

Nicotine A highly addictive chemical that is found in tobacco and enters the body via the lungs (cigarettes, pipes, and cigars) and oral mucous membranes (chewing tobacco as well as smoking).

Nicotine replacement therapy (NRT) A pharmacologic therapy designed to relieve some of the physiologic effects of withdrawal, including cravings, for patients trying to quit smoking or using tobacco. NRT transdermal patches and gums are available over the counter; nicotine inhalers and nasal sprays are available by prescription only.

Nociceptive pain A type of pain resulting from external stimuli on an uninjured, fully functional nervous system.

Nociceptors The nerve receptors for pain.

Nocturia Voiding two or more times at night.

Nocturnal emissions Orgasm and emission of semen during sleep. Also called *wet dreams*.

Nocturnal enuresis Involuntary urination at night after bladder control has been achieved. Also called *bedwetting*.

Nodular basal cell carcinoma Most common type of basal cell cancer, usually appearing on face, neck, and head.

Noise-induced hearing loss (NIHL) A condition associated with prolonged exposure to sound of greater than or equal to 85 dB.

Nolo contendere A term used when an individual neither admits to nor denies committing a crime but agrees to a punishment as if guilty.

Nondirective interview An unstructured interview in which the nurse allows the patient to control the purpose, subject matter, and pacing.

Nonexudative macular degeneration The most common form of macular degeneration, it is characterized by the accumulation of deposits beneath the pigment epithelium of the retina, causing the pigment epithelium to detach and interfere with the sensory function of the macula. Also referred to as the dry form of macular degeneration.

Noninvasive positive pressure ventilatoin (NIPPV) Ventilator support using a tight-fitting face mask, thus avoiding intubation.

Nonmaleficence The duty to do no harm.

Non-Mendelian (multifactorial) inheritance Traits that are passed on by the influence of multiple genes.

Nonpenetrating injury Also called a closed injury, this type is associated with blunt-force injuries that do not result in the entrance of a foreign object into the body.

Non-small-cell carcinoma Lung cancers other than small-cell carcinoma.

Nonstress test (NST) A widely used method of evaluating fetal status; may be used alone or as part of a more comprehensive diagnostic assessment called a biophysical profile.

Nonsuicidal self-injury behaviors (NSSI) Intentional self-inflicted acts of harm to body tissue without the intent of suicide.

Nonunion Failure of the ends of a fracture to heal together after at least 3 months.

Nonverbal communication Transmitting information through gestures, facial expressions, or touch.

Nonvolatile acid An acid produced in the body from sources other than carbon dioxide and not excreted by the lungs.

Normal sinus rhythm (NSR) The normal heart rhythm, in which impulses originate in the sinus node and travel through all normal conduction pathways without delay.

Normative commitment A feeling of obligation to continue in a profession due to benefits or positive experiences derived from it.

Normothermia Normal body temperature.

NREM (non–REM) sleep Non-rapid-eye-movement sleep occurs when activity in the *reticular activating system* is inhibited.

Nuclear family A family structure consisting of a husband and wife and their biological children.

Nucleation The formation of a crystal from a liquid.

Nulligravida Term used to describe a woman who has never been pregnant.

Nullipara Term used to describe a woman who has not given birth to a viable fetus.

Nurse practice act (NPA) State-level statutes that define and regulate nursing practices.

Nursing clinical research Research that seeks to answer questions that ultimately will improve patient care.

Nursing diagnosis A clinical judgment about individual, family, or community responses to actual and potential health problems/life processes.

Nursing informatics (NI) A specialty that integrates nursing science, computer science, and information science to manage and communicate data, information, knowledge, and wisdom in nursing practice.

Nursing plan of care A written or electronic guideline that organizes information about an individual patient's or family's care.

Nursing process The process used to identify a patient's health status and actual or potential healthcare problems or needs, to establish plans to meet the identified needs, to deliver specific nursing interventions to meet those needs, and to evaluate the success of those interventions.

Nursing research A systematic and strict scientific process that tests hypotheses about health-related illness and conditions and processes of nursing care practices.

Nursing transactional model The relationship among the nurse, the patient, and the environment in which they interact.

Nurture The effects of the environment on an individual's performance.

Nutrient density The ratio of good nutrients to calories a food contains.

Nutrients Substances found in food used by the body to promote growth, maintenance, and repair.

Nutrition The process by which the body ingests, absorbs, transports, uses, and eliminates nutrients in food.

Nutritionist Also called a *dietitian*, a professional who provides expertise in the use of nutrition to treat disease.

Nystagmus Involuntary rapid eye movement.

Obesity An excess of adipose tissue.

Object permanence The ability to understand that when something is out of sight it still exists.

Objective data Information that is detectable by an observer or can be measured or tested against an accepted standard. Also called *overt data* or *signs*.

Obligatory urine output The minimum amount of urine per day needed to excrete toxic waste products, which is 400 to 600 mL.

Observational learning The process of acquiring new skills or altering old behaviors by watching other people.

Obsession A recurrent, unwanted, and often distressing thought or image that leads to feelings of fear and anxiety.

Obsessive–compulsive disorder (OCD) A disabling condition characterized by obsessive thoughts and compulsive, repetitive behaviors that dominate an individual's life.

Obsessive–compulsive personality disorder (OCPD) One of several personality disorders defined in the DSM-5, it is marked by fear and anxiety concerning loss of control over situations, objects, or people.

Obstructive shock Shock caused by an obstruction in the heart or great vessels that either impedes venous return or prevents effective cardiac pumping action.

Occult blood Blood in stool that cannot be seen with the naked eye.

Occupational exposure Skin, eye, mucous membrane, or parenteral contact with blood or other potentially infectious materials that may result from the performance of an employee's duties.

Occupational Safety and Health Administration (OSHA) An organization that enforces the guidelines presented in the OSHA Act of 1970, requiring its covered employees to report specific incidents and illnesses in a timely manner.

Oculocephalic reflex An oculomotor response in which the eyes move in the opposite direction as the head turns to the side. Also called **doll's-eye reflex**.

Olfactory Of or relating to smell.

Oligomenorrhea Light or infrequent menstruation and occurs when cycles are longer than 6 to 7 weeks. Usually related to hormonal imbalances such as those seen in polycystic ovary syndrome.

Oliguria The production of abnormally small amounts of urine by the kidney.

"On–off" effect A sudden lack of symptom control and unexpected dyskinesias appearing as drug effectiveness diminishes.

Oncogenes Genes that promote cell proliferation and are capable of triggering cancerous characteristics.

Oncology The study of cancer.

Oncotic pressure A pulling force exerted by colloids that helps maintain the water content of blood by pulling water from the interstitial space into the vascular compartment. Also called *colloid osmotic pressure.*

Online enticement When an individual communicates, via the internet, with someone believed to be a child with the intent to commit a sexual offense or abduction.

Online shopping addiction Excessive online shopping, often associated with overspending and aided by the internet, characterized by compulsive and addictive forms of consumption and buying behavior.

Oogenesis The process that produces the female gamete, called an ovum (egg).

Open-angle glaucoma The most common form of glaucoma, it is a chronic, gradually progressive disease that typically affects both eyes.

Open-ended question A question that allows patients to discover, explore, elaborate, clarify, or illustrate their thoughts or feelings.

Open fracture A fracture in which the skin integrity is disrupted. Also called a *compound fracture.*

Open reduction and internal fixation (ORIF) The surgical insertion of nails, screws, plates, or pins to hold fractured bones in place.

Operative sterilization A surgical procedure that permanently prevents pregnancy.

Opiates A type of drug derived from natural or synthetic opiates that is used as a pain reliever. They include morphine, meperidine, codeine, hydrocodone, and oxycodone.

Opioids Drugs that act on one or more of three opioid receptors: mu, delta, and kappa. They are controlled substances due to their potential for abuse. Also called *narcotics.*

Opportunistic infection An invasion of the body tissue by microorganisms appearing in an individual with immunodeficiency that would normally not affect a person with an intact immune system.

Opportunistic pathogen A microorganism that causes disease only in susceptible individuals.

Optimism A feeling that things will turn out for the best.

Oral–genital sex Kissing, licking, or sucking of the genitals for sexual pleasure.

Oral rehydration solution (ORS) A specially created solution that contains a mixture of water, glucose, sodium, potassium, and other electrolytes that helps replace lost fluids and nutrients that the body needs to work properly.

Orchiectomy Surgical removal of the testes.

Organizational chart A chart that depicts the formal hierarchical structure and related responsibilities within a traditional organization.

Organizational commitment The relative strength of an individual's relationship and sense of belonging to an organization.

Organizing The process of coordinating the work to be done. Formally, it involves identifying the work of the organization, dividing the labor, developing the chain of command, and assigning authority.

Orgasmic phase The phase of the sexual response cycle that is marked by the involuntary release of sexual tension accompanied by physiologic and psychologic release.

Orientation 1. A structured program of activities to help new employees adapt to their new workplace; it is geared toward helping newly employed nurses to be successful. 2. A newborn's ability to be alert to, follow, and fixate on appealing and attractive, complex visual stimuli. 3. A component of normal perception that includes four basic elements: person, place, time, and situation.

Orthopnea Difficulty breathing when supine.

Orthopneic position A body position with the head and arms supported on the overbed table to facilitate breathing.

Orthostatic hypotension Blood pressure that falls when a patient sits up (from a lying position) or stands, often causing the individual to feel light-headed or faint.

Orthotic devices Orthopedic devices that may include splints or braces applied to reduce strain on a joint.

Ortolani maneuver A procedure used to evaluate an infant for developmental dysplastic hip.

Osmolality A measure of the concentration of solutes in body fluids. It is determined by the total solute concentration within a fluid compartment and is measured as parts of solute per kilogram of water.

Osmolarity A measure of the total milliosmoles per liter of solution, or the concentration of molecules per volume of solution.

Osmoreceptor A sensory receptor that detects changes in osmotic pressure and is primarily found in the hypothalamus.

Osmosis The movement of water across cell membranes, from a less concentrated solution to a more concentrated solution.

Osmotic pressure The power of a solution to draw water across a semipermeable membrane.

Osteoarthritis (OA) The most common form of arthritis in older adults. It is caused by chronic degenerative changes in the cartilage and synovial membranes of the joints.

Osteoblasts Cells that form bone.

Osteoclasts Cells that resorb bone.

Osteoporosis A metabolic bone disorder characterized by loss of bone mass, increased bone fragility, and increased risk of fractures.

Osteotomy 1. Surgical removal of a wedge of bones above or below a joint to realign the joint and shift weight away from the damaged portion of a joint. 2. An incision into or transection of the bone.

Otitis externa Inflammation of the ear canal. It is often called *swimmer's ear* because it is most frequently found in people who spend significant time in the water.

Otitis interna An inflammation of the inner ear. Also called *labyrinthitis.*

Otitis media Inflammation of the middle ear.

Otoscope A hand-held instrument with a light and a cone-shaped attachment; known as an *ear speculum.*

Outcome The specific, observable criteria used to evaluate whether goals have been met and the effectiveness of nursing actions.

Outcome standards Standards that focus on the performance of a process, such as the number of bedridden patients who develop a pressure injury.

Outcomes management Management process that uses patient experiences to guide improvement in all areas of healthcare by providing a link between medical interventions and health outcomes and between health outcomes and cost of care.

Ovaries Female sex glands in which the ova are formed and in which estrogen and progesterone are produced. Normally, a woman has two ovaries.

Overnutrition Health effects caused by excessive or accelerated nutrient intake or stores, such as obesity, hypertension, hypercholesterolemia, or toxic levels of stored vitamins or minerals.

Overt conflict Conflict that occurs when people or groups openly disagree.

Ovulation Normal process of discharging a mature ovum from an ovary approximately 14 days before the onset of menses.

Oxygenation The mechanism that facilitates or impairs the body's ability to supply oxygen to all cells of the body.

Pacemaker An external or implanted pulse generator used to provide an electrical stimulus to the heart when the heart fails to generate or conduct its own stimulus at a rate that maintains the cardiac output.

$PaCO_2$ A measure of the pressure exerted by dissolved carbon dioxide in the blood; it reflects the respiratory component of acid–base regulation and balance because it is regulated by the lungs.

Pain An unpleasant sensory and emotional experience associated with actual or potential tissue damage.

Pain threshold The point at which pain is initially perceived.

Pain tolerance The duration of time or intensity of pain an individual will endure before demonstrating pain responses.

Palliative care Nursing care that improves the quality of life of patients and their families facing life-threatening illness by preventing, assessing, and treating pain and other physical, psychosocial, and spiritual problems.

Palpation A method of assessment that involves touching the areas related to the body system to determine symmetry, equality of the size, shape, or condition of opposite sides of the body.

Pancreatitis Inflammation of the pancreas that occurs when pancreatic enzymes are released into the pancreas itself, causing autodigestion of pancreatic tissues.

Pandemic Widespread global outbreak of an infectious disease.

Panic disorder A sudden attack of terror, sometimes accompanied by a pounding heart, sweating, fainting, or dizziness.

Pannus An abnormal tissue layer that includes newly formed blood vessels. Pannus leads to scar tissue formation that immobilizes joints.

PaO_2 A measure of the pressure exerted by oxygen that is dissolved in the plasma.

Para Term used to describe a woman who has borne offspring who reached the age of viability.

Paracentesis Aspiration of fluid from the peritoneal cavity.

Parallel play A stage of play in which toddlers play side by side with similar objects, but do not play together.

Paranoia Feelings of extreme suspicion that others are following or attempting to harm oneself; experienced by some individuals with psychosis.

Paranoid personality disorder (PPD) One of several personality disorders defined in the DSM-5, it is characterized by the inability to trust others, hypervigilance, pathologic jealousy, and prejudicial and judgmental tendencies.

Paraphimosis Condition in which the retracted foreskin becomes trapped over the glans and tightens on the penis, causing painful swelling.

Paraplegia Paralysis of all or part of the lower portion of the body.

Parasite One of the four categories of microorganisms, parasites live on other organisms.

Parasomnias Abnormal behaviors that may interfere with sleep and may occur during sleep.

Paresis Weakness.

Paresthesia Sensation of prickling, tingling, or numbing.

Parkinson disease (PD) A degenerative disorder of the central nervous system resulting from the death of neurons that produce the brain neurotransmitter dopamine.

Parkinsonian gait Altered gait characterized by small, shuffling steps, as well as bradykinesia or festination.

Parkinsonism The motor symptoms of Parkinson disease: tremors, muscle rigidity, postural instability, and bradykinesia.

Paroxysmal Occurring in bursts with an abrupt onset and termination.

Paroxysmal nocturnal dyspnea A sudden episode of shortness of breath occurring at night during sleep.

Partial-thickness burns Burns that involve the entire dermis and the papillae of the dermis (superficial partial-thickness burns) or extend into the hair follicles (deep partial-thickness burns).

Passive acquired immunity A condition that occurs when a pregnant woman passes IgG antibodies to a fetus in utero.

Passive behavior Behavior that seeks to avoid conflict at any cost, even at the expense of one's own happiness.

Passive communicators Individuals who focus on the needs of others. They often deny themselves any sort of power, which causes them to become frustrated.

Passive immunity Temporary protection—provided by antibodies produced by other people or animals—against disease-producing antigens. Protection is gradually lost when these acquired antibodies are used up either by natural degradation or by combining with the antigen.

Patch testing A test used to identify allergens causing dermatitis. An adhesive patch with common allergens is placed on the back between the scapulae. The patch is generally removed after several days; if there is no reaction to a particular allergen, that allergen is eliminated as a possible cause of dermatitis.

Patent airway An airway that is open and free of obstruction.

Patent ductus arteriosus (PDA) A congenital connection between the great vessels that normally closes after birth, allowing blood from the right and left side of the heart to mix.

Pathogen A microorganism that causes disease.

Pathogenicity The ability to produce disease.

Patient advocacy Process or strategy for acting on behalf of others, including patients, families, groups, or communities, to help them obtain services and rights that they might not otherwise receive but that they need to advance their well-being.

Patient-centered medical home (PCMH) A model of care in which a patient's primary care provider works with the patient and family to develop a personalized plan that addresses the patient's physical and mental health needs across the lifespan.

Patient-focused care A delivery model that organizes healthcare around the expressed physical and emotional needs of the patient.

Patient record A formal, legal document that provides evidence of a patient's care. Also called a *chart* or a *clinical record*.

Patient responsibilities Emphasize that healthcare is a partnership between the patient and caregivers, that other patients have the right to be comfortable, and that there are consequences when patients do not comply with treatment plans.

Patient rights The fundamental care owed to patients by healthcare providers and the government.

Patient Self-Determination Act (PSDA) A federal law that requires every competent adult to be informed in writing on admission to a healthcare institution about their rights to accept or refuse medical care and to use advance directives.

Pauciarticular arthritis A form of juvenile rheumatoid arthritis that primarily affects the knees, ankles, and elbows; it occurs more frequently in females.

Peak expiratory flow rate (PEFR) A measurement used to monitor the ability of an individual to exhale a specific volume of air related to the individual's age, sex, height, and weight.

Peer review A method to professionally critique a colleague's work based on predetermined standards.

Pelvic inlet Upper border of the true pelvis.

Pelvic outlet Lower border of the true pelvis.

Pelvic tilt An exercise that helps prevent or reduce back strain as it strengthens abdominal muscles. Also called *pelvic rocking*.

Penetrating injury Also called an *open injury*, it causes an open wound with focal damage around the site of the injury. When referring to eye injuries specifically, in a penetrating injury, the layers of the eye spontaneously reapproximate after entry of a sharp-pointed object or small missile (e.g., a BB) into the globe.

Penetrating trauma Trauma that occurs when a foreign object enters the body, causing damage to body structures.

Penta screen Maternal screening that measures five indicators whose presence may suggest fetal complications: AFP, beta hCG, unconjugated estriol, inhibin A, and invasive trophoblast antigen.

Peptic ulcer A break in the mucosal lining of the gastrointestinal tract exposed to acid-pepsin secretions, including the esophagus, stomach, and duodenum.

Peptic ulcer disease (PUD) A break in the mucous lining of the gastrointestinal tract where it comes in contact with gastric juice.

Perceived loss A loss that is experienced by one person but cannot be verified by others.

Perception Awareness and interpretation of stimuli; the ability of the individual to interpret the environment.

Percussion A method of tapping the chest or back to assess underlying structures. More forceful striking of the skin with cupped hands is sometimes called *clapping*.

Percutaneous coronary revascularization (PCR) A procedure used to restore blood flow to the ischemic myocardium in patients with coronary artery disease.

Percutaneous transluminal coronary angioplasty (PTCA) A type of PCR (see above entry) in which a balloon-tipped catheter is threaded over a guidewire, with the balloon positioned across the area of narrowing.

Perforating injury A type of eye injury in which the layers of the eye do not spontaneously reapproximate after the entry of a sharp-pointed object or small missile (e.g., a BB) into the globe, which results in rupture of the globe and potential loss of ocular contents.

Perforation Rupture, as in the penetration of ulcer through mucosal wall.

Performance improvement Quality of care improvement that is linked directly linked to the performance of an individual, team, unit, or organization.

Pericarditis Inflammation of the pericardial tissue surrounding the heart.

Pericardium A double layer of fibroserous membrane that encases and anchors the heart.

Perimenopause A period of hormonal change during which the body gradually transitions toward permanent infertility.

Perinatal loss Death of a fetus or infant that occurs between the time of conception and the end of the newborn period 28 days after birth.

Periodic breathing A breathing pattern characterized by pauses lasting 5 to 15 seconds.

Periodontal disease Gum disease.

Perioperative The three phases of a surgical procedure: the preoperative phase, intraoperative phase, and postoperative phase.

Perioperative nursing care Nursing care provided during any or all of the three phases of surgery: preoperative, intraoperative, and postoperative.

Peripartum cardiomyopathy A rare but serious dysfunction of the left ventricle that occurs in the last month of pregnancy or the first 5 months postpartum in a woman with no previous history of heart disease.

Peripheral nervous system (PNS) One of two principal parts of the neurologic system, it consists of the cranial nerves and the spinal nerves.

Peripheral neuropathy A condition that results when trauma or a disease process interferes with innervation of peripheral nerves.

Peripheral pulse A pulse located away from the heart, in the foot or the wrist.

Peripheral vascular disease (PVD) A disorder in which arteriosclerosis and atherosclerosis affect circulation to peripheral tissues, particularly the lower extremities.

Peripheral vascular resistance The opposing forces or impedance to blood flow as the arterial channels become more and more distant from the heart.

Peristalsis The process of wavelike muscular contractions that propel food and digestive products through the digestive tract.

Peritoneal dialysis The process by which dialysate is instilled into the abdominal cavity through a catheter, allowed to rest there while fluids and molecules exchange, and then removed through the catheter.

Peritonitis Inflammation and bacterial infection of the abdominal area.

Pernicious anemia A disorder that results from a failure to absorb dietary vitamin B_{12}.

Persistent bacteriuria The reappearance of bacteria in urine due to a persistent source of infection causing repeated infection after the initial cure.

Persistent depressive disorder Chronic depression that affects an individual for the majority of most days for at least 2 years (1 year for children and adolescents). May be interrupted by periods of normal mood that do not exceed 2 months over the course of the 2 years. Also called *dysthymic disorder*.

Persistent vegetative state A permanent condition of complete unawareness of self and the environment and loss of all cognitive functions. Also called *irreversible coma*.

Personal distance Communication characterized by moderate voice tones and less noticeable body heat and smell. Physical contact such as a handshake or touching a shoulder is possible.

Personal identity The conscious sense of individuality and uniqueness that is continually evolving throughout life.

Personal space The distance people prefer in interactions with others.

Personality The individual qualities, including habitual behavior patterns, that make a person unique; the outward expression of the inner self.

Personality disorder (PD) Rigid, stereotyped behavioral patterns that deviate markedly from the norm of an individual's culture and persist throughout the person's life. They are characterized by a lifelong maladaptive pattern of perceiving, thinking, and relating that impairs social or occupational functioning.

Personality traits The elements and patterns that make up an individual's personality.

Pescatarian Similar to a vegetarian but includes fish in the diet.

Pessimism A feeling that a situation is always bad and may become worse.

pH A measurement of the hydrogen ion concentration of a solution.

Phagocytosis A process by which a foreign agent or target cell is engulfed, destroyed, and digested. Neutrophils and macrophages, known as phagocytes, are the primary cells involved in phagocytosis.

Phantom pain A confusing pain syndrome that occurs following surgical or traumatic amputation of a limb. The patient experiences pain in the missing body part even though there is complete mental awareness that the limb is gone. Also called *phantom limb syndrome*.

Pharmacodynamics Study of how the body reacts to the composition of drugs, such as the drug's molecular, biochemical, and physiologic effects.

Pharmacogenetics Study of how genetics can influence response to a drug.

Pharmacology Science of how drugs influence body systems and how the body responds to them.

Pharmacokinetics Related to the four processes used to move drugs through the body: absorption, distribution, metabolism, and excretion.

Phase of mutual regulation Time period during which a mother and her infant seek to determine the degree of control each partner in their relationship will exert. In this phase of adjustment, a balance is sought between the needs of the mother and the needs of the infant.

Phenotype The observable expression of genetic traits.

Philadelphia chromosome The balanced translocation of chromosome 22 to chromosome 9; associated with chronic myeloid leukemia.

Phimosis Tightness of the prepuce that prevents retraction of the foreskin.

Phobia An individual's experience of intense, persistent fear or anxiety associated with a particular object or situation, or **stressor**, and tendency to avoid that stressor at all costs.

Photophobia Sensitivity to light.

Physical abuse Unexplained injuries, bruising, and fractures, as well as multiple injuries in different stages of healing.

Physical activity Body movement produced by skeletal muscle contraction that increases energy expenditure.

Physical attending The conveyed act of being with another individual through physical posturing.

Physical fitness The ability to carry out tasks with vigor and alertness and without fatigue, while still maintaining enough energy for other tasks.

Physical restraint Any manual method, material, device, or equipment that is attached to the patient's body with the intention of limiting or restricting free movement of the head, arms, legs, or body.

Physiologic anemia of the newborn A type of anemia that occurs as a result of the normal, gradual drop in hemoglobin for the first 6 to 12 weeks of life.

Physiologic anemia of pregnancy Apparent anemia that results during pregnancy because the plasma volume increases more than the erythrocytes increase. Also called *pseudoanemia.*

Physiologic jaundice A yellow discoloration of the skin caused by accelerated destruction of fetal RBCs, impaired conjugation of bilirubin, and increased bilirubin reabsorption from the intestinal tract.

Physiologic tremors Tremors that occur normally as a result of physiologic exhaustion or emotional stress.

Pica The craving for and persistent eating of non-nutritive substances not ordinarily considered to be edible or nutritionally valuable, such as soil, clay, and soap.

PICOT A mnemonic method used by clinicians to define and formulate a clinical question driving the search for evidence-based practice. PICOT stands for Population of a group, Intervention or activity focus, Comparison group, Outcome(s) or desired effects, and Time frame.

PIE documentation model A simplified approach to problem-oriented documentation that focuses on the nursing process and is an acronym for Problems, Interventions, and Evaluation of nursing care.

Pigmented basal cell carcinoma Less common skin cancer found on the head, neck, and face.

Pill-rolling Rubbing of the thumb and fingers together accompanying other tremors.

Pilot projects Limited trials to determine problems with problem-solving alternatives. Their strategies may resemble research projects and may be linked to quality improvement initiatives.

Pitfall A hidden trap that catches people unaware and undermines their plans.

Placenta A flat, disk-shaped organ that is highly vascular and normally forms in the upper segment of the endometrium of the uterus; exchanges nutrients and gases between the fetus and the mother.

Placenta previa Occurs when the placenta partially or totally covers the mother's cervix; can result in severe bleeding before or during delivery.

Placental abruption A condition that occurs when the placenta detaches from the uterine wall before delivery. May or may not result in fetal demise, but a fetus's survival depends on the stage of development and prompt medical treatment.

Plan–do–study–act (PDSA) A system of quality improvement most often associated with total quality management.

Plan of care Written by a member of the healthcare team and listed in a patient's progress notes, it identifies the problem and generates the plan for addressing that problem.

Planning The four-stage managerial process that establishes objectives, evaluates the present situation in order to predict future trends and events, formulates a planning statement, and converts the plan into an action statement.

Plaque 1. An invisible soft film that adheres to the enamel surface of teeth. Consists of bacteria, saliva molecules, and remnants of epithelial cells and leukocytes. 2. Scar tissue on myelin sheath due to repeated attacks by the immune system.

Plasmapheresis Removal of a harmful component from plasma. Also called *plasma exchange therapy.*

Plasmin An important enzyme present in blood that degrades many blood plasma proteins, including fibrin clots.

Plasminogen The inactive precursor of plasmin.

Plateau phase A phase of the **sexual response cycle** during which individuals experience strong, prolonged sexual arousal. It is typically maintained by physical stimulation.

Play therapist A therapist who designs and provides recreational activities to promote emotional and/or physical healing and wellness.

Pleural effusion Accumulation of excess fluid in the pleural cavity.

Pleural friction rub Associated with pleural inflammation, it occurs when inflamed pleural surfaces slide across one another. This low-pitched, crackling sound is typically present during both inspiration and expiration.

Pleural space The region between the visceral and parietal pleura.

Pleuritic pain Sharp localized chest pain that increases with breathing and coughing.

Pleuritis Local extension of an infection to involve the pleura.

Pleximeter The middle finger of the nondominant hand. Often used in indirect percussion techniques.

Plexor The middle finger of the dominant hand. Often used in indirect percussion techniques.

***Pneumocystis jirovecii* pneumonia (PJP)** An opportunistic infection that is not pathogenic in those with intact immune systems.

Pneumonia Inflammation of the lung parenchyma (the respiratory bronchioles and alveoli).

Pneumothorax A partial lung collapse due to air or gas collecting in the lung or in the pleural space that surrounds the lungs.

Point of care Interventions or testing that provides on-the-spot information about the patient rather than having to send blood or urine samples down to a laboratory and wait for results to be returned.

Point of maximal impulse (PMI) A pulse located at the apex of the heart. Also called the *apical pulse.*

Point-of-service (POS) plan An insurance plan that allows participants to choose between a health maintenance organization or a preferred provider organization each time they seek healthcare.

Polyarticular arthritis A form of juvenile rheumatoid arthritis that involves many joints (five or more), particularly the small joints of the hands and fingers. It may also affect the hips, knees, feet, ankles, and neck.

Polycythemia An increase in the production of RBCs.

Polydipsia Excessive thirst.

Polyneuropathies Bilateral sensory disorders; they are the most common types of neuropathy associated with diabetes.

Polyp A small vascular growth on the surface of any mucous membrane.

Polyphagia Excessive hunger.

Polypharmacy Use of multiple drugs to treat one or more conditions.

Polysomnography (PSG) A recording of the biophysical changes that a patient experiences during sleep.

Polysubstance abuse The simultaneous abuse of many substances.

Polyuria The production of abnormally large amounts of urine. Also called *diuresis*.

Pop-ups Unexpected things or events occurring during the day that require time and attention in addition to the regular plan for the day.

Positive end-expiratory pressure (PEEP) Mechanical ventilation in which a positive pressure is maintained in the airways during exhalation and between breaths to help keep alveoli open.

Positive pressure ventilator A mechanical device that pushes air into the lungs through an invasive device such as an endotracheal tube or tracheostomy tube, rather than drawing air in by negative pressure.

Positive reinforcement Giving rewards such as praise or encouragement for a learner's achievements.

Positive symptoms Excessive or added behaviors that are not normally seen in healthy adults, such as delusions; commonly seen in schizophrenia.

Postanesthesia care unit (PACU) Designated unit for postoperative recovery of patients who do not require intensive care following a surgical procedure with anesthesia.

Postconception age The fertilization age of the fetus.

Postconcussion syndrome A series of concussion-like symptoms that occur 7 to 10 days after a concussion. Manifestations include nausea, headache, dizziness, fatigue, memory problems, difficulty concentrating, insomnia, light and noise sensitivity, and/or personality changes.

Postictal period A period of varying lengths immediately following seizure activity in which level of consciousness is decreased.

Postmenopausal bleeding Bleeding that occurs after menopause has occurred; may be caused by endometrial polyps, endometrial hyperplasia, or uterine cancer.

Postmenopause Beyond 1 year after the last menstrual period.

Postoperative The third phase of an operative process in which recovery occurs.

Postpartum hemorrhage A loss of blood equal to or greater than 1000 mL along with symptoms of hypovolemia following birth. The hemorrhage is classified as *early* if it occurs within the first 24 hours and *late* if it occurs after the first 24 hours.

Postpartum After childbirth.

Postpartum blues A maternal adjustment reaction occurring in the first few postpartum days, characterized by mild depression, tearfulness, anxiety, headache, and irritability.

Postpartum depression A severe form of depression that affects new mothers, often beginning within 3 months of delivery but that may strike at any time during the first year after having a child. Also called *depressive disorder with peripartum onset*.

Postpartum endometritis (metritis) An inflammation of the endometrium portion of the uterine lining occurring anytime up to 6 weeks postpartum.

Postpartum psychosis Severe psychosis occurring within the first 3 months after birth that usually requires hospitalization.

Postterm labor Labor that occurs after 42 weeks' gestation.

Postterm newborn Any infant born after 42 weeks' gestation.

Postterm pregnancy Pregnancy that lasts beyond 42 weeks' gestation.

Posttraumatic stress disorder (PTSD) A trauma- and stressor-related disorder that can evolve after exposure to a traumatic or overwhelming event in which an individual's physical health was endangered.

Postural drainage The drainage by gravity of secretions from various lung segments.

Postural instability A stooped posture that leads to balance problems and falls.

Poverty A lack of income to meet basic needs that include food and nutrition, education and other basic services, productive resources for income, and healthcare.

PPD Tuberculin skin test. See **Purified protein derivative.**

Prader-Willi syndrome (PWS) A congenital disorder of the 15th chromosome that causes an unrelenting feeling of hunger, but also low muscle tone, short stature, incomplete sexual development, mild to severe intellectual disability, and behavioral problems.

Praxis The ability to control movement in a deliberate, smooth, and coordinated fashion.

Precipitating factor A practice, behavior, or environmental factor that gives rise to a specific incident of violence.

Prediabetes Individuals who are at increased risk of developing type 2 diabetes.

Predisposing factor A practice, behavior, or environmental factor that increases the potential of an individual's risk of violent victimization or perpetration of violence.

Preeclampsia An increase in blood pressure after 20 weeks of gestation accompanied by proteinuria. May also be accompanied by albuminuria and edema. Also called *toxemia of pregnancy*.

Preferred provider organization (PPO) A type of health insurance program that does not require its participants to select a primary care provider. They usually have larger networks of providers than health maintenance organizations (HMOs) and provide financial incentives that encourage participants to seek care from in-network providers. They are less restrictive than HMOs but typically have higher co-payments.

Prejudice A negative belief or preference that is generalized about a group that leads to prejudgment.

Preload The amount of cardiac muscle fiber tension, or stretch, that exists at the end of diastole.

Premature ejaculation Ejaculation that occurs consistently before or shortly after penetration (i.e., before both partners are able to achieve satisfaction).

Premature junctional contractions Heartbeats that occur before the next expected beat of the underlying rhythm.

Premature rupture of membranes (PROM) Spontaneous rupture of membranes and leakage of amniotic fluid before the onset of labor at any gestational age.

Prenatal education Programs offered to expectant families, adolescents, women, or partners to provide education regarding the pregnancy, labor, and birth experience.

Preoperative The first phase of an operative process in which the patient is identified as a candidate for surgical intervention, assessed, and prepared for surgery.

Preparedness The phase that takes place before an emergency occurs during which risks are assessed and plans are developed to address them.

Preprocedure verification process A standardized process used to verify that the correct procedure is being implemented on the correct patient at the correct site and that all items necessary for the procedure are available.

Presbycusis Age-related loss of the ability to hear high-frequency sounds; may occur because of cochlear hair cell degeneration or loss of auditory neurons in the organ of Corti.

Presbyopia Impaired near vision resulting from a loss of elasticity of the lens related to aging.

Presencing Being present with a patient and being open, receptive, and available at all levels without judging or labeling.

Presenting part The first part of the fetus to enter and settle in the pelvic inlet during fetal presentation.

Pressure injury Ischemic lesions of the skin and underlying tissue caused by external pressure that impairs the flow of blood and lymph.

Preterm newborn An infant born at less than 37 completed weeks of gestation.

Preterm premature rupture of the membranes (PPROM) A condition that occurs when membranes rupture and amniotic fluid leaks from the vagina before 37 weeks of gestation.

Priapism Persistent, painful erection of the penis.

Primary appraisal The evaluation of an event or circumstance in terms of its potential to harm, benefit, threaten, or challenge an individual.

Primary care provider (PCP) A healthcare provider who provides basic medical service and acts as a gatekeeper to more specialized care, referring patients to in-network hospitals and specialists.

Primary group A small, intimate group in which the relationships among members are personal, spontaneous, sentimental, cooperative, and inclusive.

Primary hypertension A persistently elevated systemic blood pressure. Also called *essential hypertension.*

Primary immune response When an individual is exposed to an antigen, the B-lymphocyte system produces antibodies that react specifically with that antigen over the first 3 days.

Primary intention healing Healing that occurs where the tissue surfaces have been closed and there is minimal or no tissue loss. It is characterized by the formation of minimal granulation tissue and scarring. Also called *primary union* or *first intention healing.*

Primary nursing A model in which one nurse has 24/7 authority and responsibility for the care of an assigned group of patients.

Primary prevention Methods designed to focus on health promotion and illness prevention.

Primary sex characteristics The reproductive organs.

Primigravida A woman who is pregnant for the first time.

Primipara Term used to describe a woman who has given birth to her first child (past the point of viability), whether or not that child is living or was alive at birth.

Principles-based (deontologic) theories Theories that involve logical and formal processes and emphasize individual rights, duties, and obligations.

Prioritizing care A process that helps nurses manage time and establish an order for completing responsibilities and care interventions for a single patient or for a group of patients.

Priority Something given or meriting attention before competing alternatives.

Privacy The right of individuals to keep their personal information from being disclosed.

Private insurance Health insurance provided by private or publicly owned companies such as Blue Cross Blue Shield, Kaiser, or Aetna.

Probiotics Microorganisms that aid in digestion and help to protect the body from harmful bacteria.

Problem-focused coping Managing or altering a stressor, event, or circumstance in response to distress.

Problem-focused diagnosis A prioritized diagnosis made when recognizing and analyzing cues during patient assessment.

Problem-oriented medical record (POMR) A recording system in which data are arranged according to the problems the patient has rather than the source of the information. Also called *problem-oriented record (POR).*

Problem-oriented record (POR) See **Problem-oriented medical record (POMR).**

Problem solving Evaluating a challenging situation, identifying potential steps to resolve the situation, and then implementing those steps.

Process addictions Compulsive behaviors that serve to reduce anxiety such as workaholism, gambling, shopping, cutting, pornography, spending and indebtedness, internet surfing or gaming, eating disorders, and sexual addictions.

Process standards Standards that focus on the steps used to lead to a particular outcome. It is used to determine if a set of steps exists and if those steps are being followed.

Productivity The performance measure of both the effectiveness and efficiency of nursing care.

Profession An occupation that requires extensive education or a calling that requires special knowledge, skill, and preparation.

Professional development The process of continually seeking to develop competence as a nurse, through continuing education and planned activities to enhance role performance.

Professionalism Acting with the knowledge, skill, and preparation of a professional.

Progesterone Hormone produced by the corpus luteum, adrenal cortex, and placenta whose function is to stimulate proliferation of the endometrium to facilitate growth of the embryo.

Projectile vomiting Vomiting in which emesis may be spewed up to 2 to 3 feet out of a baby's mouth. A major symptom of pyloric stenosis.

Prolonged grief disorder When a person persistently mourns a loss longer than 6 months.

Prone Face-down position.

Proprioception The body's sense of its position.

Proprioceptive Sensations that contribute to motor function and spatial awareness.

Prospective payment system (PPS) A system in which hospitals determine the amount to be billed to an insurance company before the patient is ever admitted to the hospital.

Prostate-specific antigen (PSA) A protein produced in the cells of the prostate gland.

Prostatectomy Surgical removal of part or all of the prostate gland.

Prostatitis An inflammation of the prostate gland.

Prostatodynia A condition in which the patient experiences the symptoms of prostatitis, but shows no evidence of inflammation or infection.

Protected health information Personal information or healthcare data that could identify an individual. This information is protected and defined by HIPAA's Privacy Rule.

Protective factor 1. A practice, behavior, or environmental factor that provides strength and assistance to children and families in dealing with crises and risk factors. 2. A practice, behavior, or environmental factor that decreases the potential of an individual to perpetuate violence or victimization.

Protein A macronutrient that contains nitrogen and is a critical component of all tissues in the human body, including muscle, bone, and blood.

Proteinuria Excess protein in urine.

Prothrombin A protein produced by the liver that helps in blood clotting.

Proxemics The study of distance between people in their interactions.

Proximodistal Growth that proceeds from the center of the body outward.

Pruritus Itching of the skin.

Pseudoexacerbation A temporary aggravation of symptoms that is directly related to a trigger and subsides as soon as the trigger is removed.

Pseudomenstruation Blood or whitish discharge that may occasionally be observed on the diapers of female newborns caused by the withdrawal of maternal hormones.

Psychoanalytic theory A framework for personality development that emphasizes the presence of unconscious impulses and their influence on behaviors and the formation of self; developed by Sigmund Freud (1856–1939).

Psychogenic pain Pain that is experienced in the absence of any diagnosed physiologic cause or event.

Psychologic abuse Belittling an individual's sense of self-worth and self-love, sometimes to the point of feeling it is impossible to do anything correctly.

Psychomotor retardation A state in which thinking and body movements are noticeably slower than normal and speech is slowed or absent.

Psychosis A mental health condition characterized by delusions, hallucinations, illusions, disorganized behavior, and a difficulty relating to others. Also called *psychotic disorder.*

Psychostimulants Stimulants that have a high potential for abuse. They include cocaine and amphetamines.

Ptosis Drooping of the eyelid.

Puberty The stage during which an individual reaches sexual maturity.

Public distance Communication that requires loud, clear vocalizations with careful enunciation.

Public insurance Health insurance financed by the government.

Public self How an individual wishes to be perceived by others.

Puerperium The time immediately following childbirth during which physiologic changes that occurred during pregnancy begin to return to normal. Also called *postpartum period.*

Pulmonary circulation Circulation through the right side of the heart, the pulmonary artery, the pulmonary capillaries, and the pulmonary vein.

Pulmonary embolism (PE) The obstruction of blood flow in part of the pulmonary vascular system by an embolus. Also called *pulmonary thromboembolism.*

Pulmonary function test (PFT) A test designed to provide information about ventilation airflow, lung volume, and the capacity and diffusion of gas.

Pulmonary vascular resistance The force or resistance of the blood in the pulmonary circulation.

Pulse A wave of blood created by the contraction of the left ventricle of the heart.

Pulse deficit When the radial pulse falls behind the apical rate, indicating weak, ineffective contractions of the left ventricle.

Pulse oximetry A noninvasive method of assessing arterial blood oxygenation.

Pulse pressure The difference between the systolic and diastolic pressure.

Pulse rhythm The pattern of the beats and the intervals between the beats.

Pulse volume Also called the *pulse strength* or *amplitude,* it is the force of blood with each heartbeat.

Punctual On time.

Punishment Action taken to enforce rules when a child misbehaves.

Purging Self-induced vomiting or misuse of laxatives, diuretics, or enemas.

Purified protein derivative (PPD) Used to screen for tuberculosis in a tuberculin test. A small amount of the PPD is injected and the body's response interpreted.

Pursed-lip breathing Exhaling through a narrow opening between the lips to prolong the expiratory phase in an effort to promote more alveolar emptying while maintaining open alveoli.

Purulent exudate A large quantity of cells and necrotic debris that form an opaque or milky discharge that is thicker than serous exudate. Also called *pus* or *suppuration.*

Pus The common name for *purulent exudate.*

Pyelolithotomy An incision into and removal of a stone from the kidney pelvis.

Pyelonephritis Inflammation of the renal pelvis and parenchyma, the functional kidney tissue.

Pyloric stenosis A thickening of the pyloric muscle resulting in a narrowing of the pyloric sphincter between the stomach and small intestine.

Pyogenic bacteria Bacteria that produces purulent exudate or pus.

Pyorrhea Advanced periodontal disease.

Pyuria Cloudy or pus-filled urine.

Quadriplegia Complete loss of function of the upper and lower body, including the arms, trunk, legs, and pelvic organs. Also called *tetraplegia.*

Quadruple screen The most widely used test to screen for Down syndrome (trisomy 21), trisomy 18, and neural tube defects.

Qualitative research Investigates a question through narrative data from interviews, storytelling, and description of observation to provide a better understanding of a patient's perspective.

Quality 1. A subjective description of a sound, for example: whistling, gurgling, or snapping. 2. The degree to which health services for individuals and populations increase the likelihood of desired health outcomes and are consistent with current professional knowledge.

Quality and Safety Education for Nurses (QSEN) A program designed to identify and standardize the six core competencies of nursing: patient-centered care, teamwork and collaboration, evidence-based practice, quality improvement, safety, and informatics.

Quality assurance The process of collecting data related to a problem and then analyzing the data based on benchmark standards to determine if standards are being met.

Quality improvement The process of using systematic and continuous actions that lead to measurable improvement in healthcare services and the health status of targeted patient groups.

Quality management The evaluation of medical and nursing processes for quality and effectiveness compared to accepted standards in order to correct problems before they harm patients and to prevent errors in treatment.

Quantitative research Uses precise measurements for data collection and employs statistical analysis to provide specific and objective data about a topic.

Quantum leadership Type of leadership that examines the context of the leader, the group, and the task to be accomplished or problem to be solved.

Quickening The mother's perception of fetal movement.

Race A term used to describe socially defined populations that share genetically transmitted physical characteristics, such as skin color and bone structure.

Racism The oppression of a group of people based on their perceived race.

Radiation The process of heat transfer with no physical contact.

Radiation cataracts A type of cataract that may result from long-term exposure to radiation.

Radical mastectomy The removal of an entire affected breast, its underlying chest muscles, and the lymph nodes under the arms. Compare with **Simple mastectomy**.

Radiofrequency ablation Also called *rhizotomy,* it is a nonsurgical, minimally invasive procedure that uses heat to reduce or stop the transmission of pain.

Range of motion (ROM) The degree to which a joint can be moved; a measurement of flexion and extension.

Range-of-motion (ROM) exercises Exercises designed to take each joint through all possible movements to maintain flexibility and movement in the joint.

Rape Any penetration, no matter how slight, of the vagina or anus with any body part or object, or oral penetration by a sex organ of another person, without the consent of the victim.

Rapport An understanding between two or more people.

Rational emotive behavior therapy (REBT) An active, solution-oriented therapy that focuses on resolving emotional, cognitive, and behavioral problems resulting from faulty evaluation of negative life events.

Rationing A method of resource allocation used by individuals, insurance companies, and the government to prevent increases in the cost of healthcare or to reduce the cost of healthcare by limiting care provision.

Readiness to learn The demonstration of behaviors or cues that reflect a learner's motivation to learn at a specific time.

Real self The perceived true self.

Reappraisal Following attempts to cope with a stressor, an individual evaluates which coping mechanisms were successful and which were not and, ideally, begins another attempt to respond to the stressor and return to homeostasis.

Receptive speech The ability to understand the spoken word.

Receptor A nerve cell that converts a stimulus to a nerve impulse. Most receptors are specific, that is, sensitive to only one type of stimulus.

Record A formal, legal document that provides evidence of a patient's care. Also called a *patient record* or a *clinical chart*.

Recording The process of making an entry on a patient record. Also called *charting* or *documenting*.

Recovery 1. Return to (or exceed) preillness levels of functioning. 2. A continued state of voluntary sobriety in which an individual maintains personal health and functions normally. 3. A phase of mental illness in which symptoms of the disorder are present but under control.

Red blood cells (RBCs) Blood cells shaped like biconcave disks that contain the hemoglobin required for oxygen transport to body tissues; the most common type of blood cell. Also called *erythrocytes*.

Reduction Surgical placement of a broken bone in the correct alignment.

Referred pain Pain that is perceived in an area distant from the site of the stimulus.

Reflection The action of making sense of occurrences, situations, or decisions by carefully considering the totality of the experience: what worked or did not work, what could have been done differently to achieve better outcomes, what was done well, what necessary resources were available, and so on.

Reflexes The rapid, involuntary, predictable motor responses to a stimulus.

Reflux A backward flow of acidic secretions into the lower esophagus.

Refraction The bending of light rays as they pass from one medium to another medium of different optical density.

Refractory hypoxemia The decrease of particle arterial oxygen despite administration of oxygen at high flow rates.

Refractory period A phase during which myocardial cells resist stimulation.

Regeneration The replacement or renewal of destroyed tissue cells by cells that are identical or similar in structure and function.

Registered nurses (RNs) The members of a nursing team who are specially licensed and trained to deliver direct patient care, including patient assessment, identification of health problems, and development and coordination of care.

Regulation A rule.

Regurgitation The backflow of blood into the atria during systole.

Rehabilitation A level of wellness in which symptoms of the condition are under control to the extent that the affected individual can engage in goal-directed activities.

Reinfection The development of a new infection with a different pathogen following successful treatment.

Reinforcement Consequences that lead to an increase in a particular behavior.

Relapse Return of an acute phase of illness after recovery.

Relationship-based (caring) theories Theories that stress courage, generosity, commitment, and the need to nurture and maintain relationships.

Religion A set of doctrines accepted by a group of people who gather together regularly to worship that offers a means to relate to God or a higher power; an organized system of beliefs and practices.

Relocation syndrome Decline in functioning associated with the stress of moving to another environment.

REM sleep Rapid-eye-movement sleep that occurs during sleep about every 90 minutes and lasts 5 to 30 minutes. The brain is highly active in this phase, and most dreams will take place during REM sleep.

Remission 1. A period during a chronic illness in which the symptoms of the illness disappear. 2. A sustained recovery lasting 8 weeks or more.

Remodeling Bone synthesis and breakdown.

Remyelination Repair of the damaged myelin sheath by oligodendrocytes.

Renal colic Acute, severe flank pain on an affected side that develops when a stone obstructs the ureter, causing ureteral spasm.

Renal failure A condition in which the kidneys are unable to remove accumulated metabolites from the blood or produce urine, resulting in altered fluid, electrolyte, and acid–base balance.

Renal insufficiency Decrease in the kidneys' ability to conserve sodium and concentrate the urine.

Renin–angiotensin–aldosterone system System initiated by specialized receptors in the juxtaglomerular cells of the kidney nephrons that respond to changes in renal perfusion.

Repetitive strain injury A nerve, tendon, or muscle condition that occurs when the limbs are subjected to repetitive use, awkward positions, or forced positions. Also called *repetitive motion disorder*.

Repolarization The process that returns the cell to its resting, polarized state.

Report An oral, written, or electronic communication intended to convey information to others.

Reporting The communication of specific information to a designated individual or group.

Reproduction Fertilization resulting from sexual intercourse between a man and a woman.

Research A formal, systematic way of answering a question or approaching a problem.

Research participants Volunteers for a specific study project who meet all the inclusion criteria, have been informed of all aspects of the study, and have signed informed consent forms.

Reservoir A source of microorganisms.

Residual urine Urine that remains in the bladder after voiding.

Resilience/resiliency The way in which an individual adapts successfully to crisis events to develop positive outcomes, involving numerous biological, psychologic, social, and cultural factors and determinants.

Resolution phase The fourth and final phase of the sexual response cycle marked by a return to an unaroused state.

Resonance A hollow sound, such as the sound produced by lungs filled with air.

Resource An asset that helps nurses meet patient needs.

Resource allocation The distribution of resources among competing groups of people or programs.

Respiration The act of inhaling (inspiration) and exhaling (expiration) air to transport oxygen to the alveoli so that oxygen is exchanged for carbon dioxide and the carbon dioxide expelled from the body.

Respiratory acidosis A condition that is caused by an excess of dissolved carbon dioxide, or carbonic acid. It is characterized by a pH of less than 7.35 and a $PaCO_2$ greater than 45 mmHg. It may be caused by hypoventilation.

Respiratory alkalosis A condition that results when pH rises above 7.45 and $PaCO_2$ falls below 35 mmHg. It is caused by hyperventilation (unusually fast respiration, or overbreathing), leading to a carbon dioxide deficit.

Respiratory depression A decrease in the depth and rate of breathing.

Respiratory syncytial virus (RSV) A highly contagious respiratory infection that affects almost all children before 2 years of age.

Responsibility The specific accountability or liability associated with the performance of duties of a particular role.

Rest pain Cramping or aching pain in the calves of the legs, the thighs, and the buttocks that occurs while at rest.

Restless legs syndrome (RLS) A neurologic sensorimotor disorder that is characterized by an overwhelming urge to move the legs when at rest.

Restraints Any devices or medications intended to protect the patient from injuring self or others through partially or fully limiting the patient's mobility.

Restrictive cardiomyopathy A disorder characterized by rigid ventricular walls that impair diastolic filling.

Reticular activating system (RAS) Modulation of sleep–wake transitions that occurs when the reticular formation, a network of ascending nerves, relays information about alertness and arousal to the cerebral cortex and directs the brain's attention to sensory events.

Retinal detachment Separation of the retina or sensory portion of the eye from the choroid.

Retractions Visible sinking of the chest wall, or sunken areas seen between the ribs during inspiration.

Retrograde conduction Cardiac conduction against the normal flow or pattern.

Retrograde ejaculation Ejaculation that occurs with fluid traveling into the bladder instead of out through the urethra.

Retropulsion The tendency to topple backward when bumped or when rising, standing, or turning.

Retrospective audit An evaluation performed after a patient's discharge comparing the care provided to the patient with care provided to patients with similar conditions.

Return demonstration Having a patient (or support person) "teach back" a skill to exhibit its mastery.

Reverse triage A method in which the most severely injured or ill victims who require the greatest resources are treated last to allow the greatest number of victims to receive medical attention.

Revision Modifications to initial desired outcomes or interventions.

Revision surgery The replacement of an artificial joint after 10 years or more.

Rh disease A rare condition where the mother is Rh negative while the child is Rh positive. If this condition arises, the mother's body will see the Rh-positive cells in the fetus as foreign and will then produce antibodies to fight off the Rh-positive cells. May result in fetal demise in extreme cases.

Rheumatoid arthritis (RA) A chronic systemic autoimmune disease that causes inflammation of connective tissue, primarily in the joints.

Rhinorrhea Drainage of mucus from the nose. Commonly known as a runny nose.

Rhonchi A long, low-pitched sound that continues throughout inspiration, suggesting a blockage of large airway passages.

Ribonucleic acid (RNA) One of two types of nucleic acid made by cells. It is made up of ribose rather than deoxyribose and contains information that has been copied from DNA (the other type of nucleic acid).

Rights of administration A safety check for nurses administering medications following six core rights: right patient, right drug, right dose, right time, right route, and right documentation.

Rigidity Resistance to movement because of the involuntary contraction of all skeletal muscles.

Risk factor A practice, behavior, or environmental factor that increases the potential of negative effects on an individual's health.

Risk management Preventive policies and processes that focus on limiting a healthcare agency's financial and legal risk associated with the delivery of care, particularly in terms of lawsuits.

Risk nursing diagnosis Anticipation of a problem that has not yet occurred or a condition that has not yet been diagnosed but is within the realm of probability for a patient.

Risky use Repeated use of substances in situations in which it is physically hazardous and despite knowledge that the individual has a persistent physical or psychologic problem caused or worsened by substance use.

Role ambiguity Occurs when expectations are unclear and when people do not know how to perform their roles and/or are unable to predict the reactions of others to their behavior.

Role conflict Emotional conflict arising when competing demands are made on an individual in the fulfillment of his or her multiple social roles.

Role development Teaching and modeling the behaviors needed to successfully assume a particular role.

Role mastery Occurs when an individual's behaviors meet or exceed social expectations.

Role performance The demonstration of behaviors or actions associated with a given role.

Role strain The stress or strain experienced by an individual when incompatible behavior, expectations, or obligations are associated with a single social role.

Root cause analysis An evaluation required by The Joint Commission that is focused on identifying areas of improvement that would decrease the likelihood of future adverse events and developing an action plan for improvement.

Rooting reflex In response to a light touch of a finger on an infant's cheek close to the mouth, the infant's head will rotate toward the stimulation and attempt to suck the finger.

Rotational injury An injury caused by lateral flexion or twisting of the head and neck.

Rupture of membranes The rupturing of amniotic membranes before the onset of labor.

Safety Decreasing risks of dangers or hazards to prevent accidents, injuries, mistakes, and harm.

Safety culture A general feeling of shared attitudes, values, practices, and beliefs which result in behaviors and feelings of responsibility for safety in all daily routines.

Salient cue The leading, most noticeable, or most important information about a patient's health status.

Saline An isotonic solution of 0.9% sodium chloride.

Sanguineous exudate A large amount of RBCs that form a bright or dark red discharge indicating new or old damage to capillaries. Also called *hemorrhagic exudate*.

Sarcopenia The process of atrophy due to age.

Satiety The sensation of fullness and satisfaction that should inhibit eating until the next meal.

Saturated fat A triglyceride fat that contains all of the hydrogen ions it is capable of holding.

SBAR A tool to communicate critical information about a patient in the following order: Situation, Background, Assessment, and Recommendation.

SBIRT A method of screening for substance use and abuse. Screening to assess severity and appropriate level of treatment; Brief Intervention to increase insight and awareness and motivate patients toward behavioral change; and Referral to Treatment as appropriate.

Scaling The rating of the severity of symptoms or problems.

Scapegoat An individual who has been selected to take the blame for another individual or for a group.

Scenario planning A group process strategy that encourages members of a group to create hypothetical or "possible future" situations.

Scheduled toileting Toileting at regular intervals.

Schistocytes Fragmented RBCs.

Schizoaffective disorder A psychotic disorder with features of both schizophrenia and mood disorders.

Schizoid personality disorder (SPD) One of several personality disorders defined in the DSM-5, it is characterized by a lifelong pattern of indifference to others, absence of humor, and social isolation.

Schizophrenia The most common psychotic disorder, schizophrenia is a combination of disordered thinking, perceptual disturbances, behavioral abnormalities, affective disruptions, and impaired social competency.

Schizophreniform disorder A disorder with rapid onset of psychotic symptoms, very similar to schizophrenia, lasting less than 6 months.

Schizotypal personality disorder One of several personality disorders defined in the DSM-5, it is characterized by a pattern of disturbed interpersonal relationships, thought patterns, appearance, and behavior.

Sciatica Lumbar back pain that radiates down the posterior leg to the ankle due to irritation or compression of all or part of the sciatic nerve.

Scoliometer A diagnostic test used to measure a patient's rib hump when in the Adam position.

Scoliosis A lateral, or sideways, curvature of the spine.

Scoop method A safe method of recapping sharps in which the cap is placed on a needle or a hard surface and the needle is guided into the cap.

Seasonal affective disorder (SAD) A mood disorder typically characterized by depression during fall and winter and normal mood or hypomania during spring and summer.

Seclusion Involuntary confinement of a patient to a room.

Second heart sound (S_2) The heart sound produced by closure of the semilunar valves; characterized by the syllable "dub."

Second impact syndrome (SIS) A constellation of clinical manifestations that can occur when an individual receives a second concussion before the initial concussion is completely healed.

Secondary appraisal When an individual attempts to predict the impact, intensity, and duration of the coping behavior necessary to respond to the stressor.

Secondary cataracts A type of cataract that may form after surgery to treat another eye disorder, such as glaucoma, or as an effect of medication or another primary disorder.

Secondary group A group that is larger, more impersonal, and less sentimental than a primary group.

Secondary hypertension Elevated blood pressure resulting from an identifiable underlying process.

Secondary immune response Subsequent encounters with an antigen following the primary immune response that result in triggering memory cells.

Secondary infertility The inability to conceive after one or more successful pregnancies, or the inability to sustain a pregnancy.

Secondary intention healing Healing that occurs when a wound's edges cannot or should not close. Repair time is typically longer, scarring is greater, and susceptibility to infection is greater.

Secondary prevention Methods that focus on the diagnosis and treatment of disease.

Secondary sex characteristics Bodily traits that develop over time and are influenced by a person's sex but not directly involved in reproduction.

Segmental mastectomy See **Lumpectomy**.

Seizures Periods of abnormal electrical discharges in the brain that cause involuntary movement as well as behavior and sensory alterations.

Selective serotonin reuptake inhibitor (SSRI) A drug that selectively inhibits the reuptake of serotonin into nerve terminals; used mostly for depression.

Self The entirety of an individual's being, including body, sensations, emotions, and thoughts, as well as a conscious awareness of one's own being.

Self-awareness The relationship between individuals' perception of themselves and others' perceptions of them.

Self-concept The personal perception of the self formed in response to interactions with others and the environment throughout the course of an individual's lifetime.

Self-efficacy The expectation that someone can produce a desired outcome.

Self-esteem One's judgment of one's own worth.

Self-help group A group of individuals who come together to face a common problem or difficulty.

Self-quieting ability The ability of newborns to use their own resources to quiet and comfort themselves.

Semen Sperm mixed with seminal fluid, ejaculated during sexual activity.

Semiformal group A group with formalized structure, delineated hierarchy, and voluntary, but selective, membership.

Sensitization An increased reaction to pain over time, or a reduced threshold for reaction to painful stimuli.

Sensory memory The earliest stage of memory in which visual input and auditory information are retained for less than a few seconds.

Sensory perception The conscious organization and translation of external data or stimuli into meaningful information.

Sensory reception The process of receiving external stimuli or data. External stimuli are visual (sight), auditory (hearing), olfactory (smell), tactile (touch), and gustatory (taste).

Sentinel event An unexpected occurrence involving death or serious physical or psychologic injury, or the risk thereof.

Sepsis 1. A whole-body inflammatory process resulting in acute illness. 2. A state of infection.

Septal defect A congenital heart defect that connects the right and left side of the heart.

Septic shock Altered perfusion resulting from a systemic infection that manifests with hypotension, delayed capillary refill, and inadequate perfusion and oxygenation of vital body tissues. Also called *septicemia.*

Septicemia See **Septic shock**.

Serious mental illness Mental illness that is severe enough to impair daily functioning and the ability to achieve life goals.

Seroconversion Antibody response to a disease or vaccine.

Serosanguineous exudate A clear or blood-tinged discharge commonly seen in surgical incisions.

Serotonin syndrome A condition that may occur in individuals taking two or more medications that increase serotonin levels. Symptoms include hypertension or hypotension, agitation, shivering, changes in mental status, symptoms of gastrointestinal distress, restlessness, tremor, muscle rigidity, unreactive pupils, and tachypnea.

Serous exudate A watery, clear or straw-colored discharge that accompanies mild inflammation.

Serum bicarbonate (HCO_3) A value that reflects the renal regulation of acid–base balance. The normal HCO_3 value is 24 to 28 mEq/L.

Serum sickness A systemic type III hypersensitivity response, usually in response to a drug such as penicillin or a sulfonamide.

Servant leadership A theory of leadership rooted in the belief that the most effective leaders are those who are motivated primarily by a desire to serve, rather than a desire to lead.

Seven Rights Right person, right assessment, right drug, right dose, right route, right time, right documentation.

Sex 1. The act of reproduction. 2. The biological characteristics—physical, anatomical, and chromosomal—that traditionally define male and female.

Sex addiction Persistent, excessive sexual behaviors.

Sex chromosomes The 23rd pair of chromosomes found in a cell's nucleus; it determines an individual's sex.

Sexism When male values, beliefs, or activities are preferred over female ones.

Sexual abuse Any sexual act that is perpetrated against someone's will including rape, attempted sexual acts, unwanted sexual contact, voyeurism, and sexual harassment. Also called *sexual violence*.

Sexual dysfunction Any persistent disturbance in an individual's sexual response.

Sexual health A state of physical, emotional, mental, and social well-being in relation to sexuality, not merely the absence of disease, dysfunction, or infirmity. It requires a positive and respectful approach to sexuality and sexual relationships.

Sexual orientation The sexual attraction of an individual to the same sex, the opposite sex, or both sexes.

Sexual response cycle The cycle of sexual arousal and orgasm.

Sex trafficking A form of human trafficking that organizes the movement of people between and within countries by use of force, fraud, or coercion for the purpose of sexual exploitation or commercial sex acts.

Sexual assault Sexual contact or behavior that occurs without explicit consent of the victim.

Sexual violence Any sexual act, attempt to obtain a sexual act, unwanted sexual comments or advances, or acts to traffic, or otherwise directed against a person's sexuality using coercion regardless of the relationship to the victim or the setting.

Sexuality An individually expressed and highly personal phenomenon, and its meaning evolves from life experiences, encompassing sexual preferences and orientation, sex drive, and sexual feelings.

Sexually transmitted diseases (STDs) Diseases caused by viruses or retroviruses that cannot be cured, such as human papillomavirus, herpes simplex virus, and human immunodeficiency virus.

Sexually transmitted infections (STIs) Infections transmitted by vaginal, oral, and anal intimate contact and intercourse.

SHARE A method of handoff reporting: Standardize critical content; Hardwire within your system; Allow opportunity to ask questions; Reinforce quality and measurement; Educate and coach.

Shared governance A method that aims to distribute decision making among a group of people.

Shared leadership The concept that a professional workplace is made up of many leaders.

Shearing force A condition that results when one tissue layer slides over another.

Shock A clinical syndrome characterized by a systemic imbalance between oxygen supply and demand.

Shock phase The initial part of an alarm reaction during which the sympathetic nervous system is suppressed and an individual may experience manifestations such as hypotension, decreased body temperature, and decreased muscle tone.

Short bowel syndrome A condition in which the transit time of ingested foods and fluids is reduced and digestive processes are impaired because of a resection of significant portions of the small intestine.

Short-term memory Information held in the brain for immediate use; what an individual has in mind at a given moment.

Shunt A natural or artificially created tunnel or passage that allows blood to flow through an area.

Sickle cell anemia An inherited chronic hemolytic anemia, it is the most common form of sickle cell disease.

Sickle cell crisis Severe episodes of fever and intense pain that are the hallmark of sickle cell disease. Also called *vaso-occlusive crisis*.

Sickle cell disease (SCD) A hereditary hemoglobinopathy characterized by replacement of normal hemoglobin with abnormal hemoglobin S (Hgb S) in RBCs.

Sickle cell trait Carrying one copy of the defective sickle cell gene, which can be passed on to children but does not usually cause the illness.

Sickling A process in which RBCs take on the characteristic sickle shape following deoxygenation in patients who have sickle cell disease.

Signs See **Objective data**.

Simple assault An unlawful physical attack by one person upon another in which neither the offender displays a weapon nor the victim suffers any obvious severe or aggravated bodily injury involving apparent broken bones, loss of teeth, possible internal injury, severe laceration, or loss of consciousness.

Simple mastectomy The removal of a complete breast only. Compare with **Radical mastectomy**.

Single-parent family A family in which only one parent resides in the home and is the primary caretaker and provider for the family.

Situational crisis A crisis that involves an unexpected stressor or circumstance that occurs in the course of daily living.

Situational depression A maladaptive reaction to an identifiable psychosocial stressor or stressors that occurs within 3 months after the onset of the stressor and has persisted for no longer than 6 months. Also called *adjustment disorder with depressed mood*.

Situational leader A leader who is flexible in task and relationship behaviors, considers the staff members' abilities, knows the nature of the task to be done, and is sensitive to the context or environment in which the task takes place.

Six Sigma A quality improvement program originally implemented by Motorola and General Electric that focuses on reducing variation within a process to produce a near-perfect product.

Skin turgor The elasticity of skin.

Sleep An altered state of consciousness in which an individual's perception and reaction to the environment are decreased.

Sleep apnea A disorder characterized by frequent short breathing pauses during sleep.

Sleep hygiene Interventions used to promote quality sleep at night.

Sleep loss A duration of sleep shorter than the recommended 7 to 8 hours a night for an adult.

Small-cell carcinoma A highly malignant cancer usually associated with the lung.

SMART An acronym to provide assistance in writing a patient-centered goal statement that means Single action (choose a specific, single action to focus on), Measurable result (observable or measurable result), Attainable (level appropriate), Relevant (customized specifically for patient's needs), and Time-limited (specific time frame for goal to be completed).

SOAP An acronym for collective data in a progress note; it stands for subjective data, objective data, assessment, and planning.

SOAPIER Short for subjective data, objective data, assessment, plan of care, intervention, evaluation, and revision.

Sobriety A state of habitually refraining from using alcohol or drugs.

Social cognition The ability to process and apply social information accurately and effectively.

Social determinants of health The environmental conditions in which people are active that affect their health, their functioning, and their quality-of-life outcomes and risks.

Social distance Communication characterized by a clear visual perception of the whole person. Body heat and odor are imperceptible, eye contact is increased, and vocalizations are loud enough to be overheard by others.

Social impairment Dysfunction due to substance use that may exhibit, for example, as failure to fulfill major roles at work, school, or home.

Social justice A framework in which to explore the complexities surrounding the variety of factors that impact diverse and vulnerable populations.

Social learning theory Learning (the acquiring of new skills or altering of old behaviors) that primarily results from watching and interacting with others.

Socialization The process by which individuals learn to become members of groups and society and learn the social rules defining relationships into which they will enter.

Socialized insurance A system in which all medically necessary services are covered, including physician care, hospital services, and to some extent, prescription drugs.

Socialized medicine State government-owned and controlled healthcare services.

Solitary play A stage of play in which an infant still plays primarily alone but enjoys the presence of others.

Solute Substance that dissolves in liquid.

Solvent The component of a solution that can dissolve a solute.

Somatic cells Cells that make up the tissue of the body, with a full complement (diploid) of chromosomes, as opposed to sex cells.

Somatic pain Pain arising from nerve receptors originating in the skin or close to the surface of the body.

Somatization The process by which psychologic distress is experienced and communicated in the form of somatic symptoms.

Somogyi phenomenon A combination of hypoglycemia during the night with a rebound, morning rise in blood glucose to hyperglycemic levels.

Spasticity Increased muscle tone, usually with some degree of weakness.

Specific defenses Immune system responses directed against identifiable bacteria, viruses, fungi, or other infectious agents.

Specific gravity An indicator of urine concentration that can be performed quickly and easily by nursing personnel.

Specific phobia An intense or extreme fear with regard to a particular object or situation.

Specific self-esteem How much one approves of certain parts of oneself.

Spermarche Onset of sperm production.

Spermatogenesis The process by which mature spermatozoa are formed.

Spermicide A cream, jelly, foam, vaginal film, or suppository that is inserted into the vagina before intercourse to destroy sperm and prevent conception.

Spinal concussion A temporary and mild spinal injury with various degrees of sensory impairment or motor weakness.

Spinal cord A continuation of the medulla oblongata, it has the ability to transmit impulses to and from the brain via the ascending and descending pathways.

Spinal cord injury (SCI) Trauma to the spinal cord that results from excessive force to the spinal column.

Spinal cord stimulation A form of therapy used with persistent pain that has not been controlled with less invasive therapies. It involves the insertion of an electrode (a single channel or multichannel device) adjacent to the spinal cord in the epidural space. The electrode(s) is attached to an impulse-generator (external or implanted) that sends electric impulses to the spinal cord to control pain.

Spinal fusion The insertion of a wedge-shaped piece of bone or bone chips between the vertebrae to stabilize them and reduce pain.

Spinal shock A condition that is characterized by spinal cord swelling, decreased blood flow and blood pressure, and complete loss of motor function, spinal reflexes, and autonomic function below the level of injury.

Spiritual care actions Interventions that support spiritual wellness, such as a sense of humor, which can promote a connection between the nurse and patient through laughter.

Spiritual distress/discomfort A challenge to the spiritual well-being or to the belief system that provides strength, hope, and meaning to life; a feeling of being separated from interconnectedness with others or with a higher power.

Spiritual health The overall feeling of strength, hope, and fulfillment that encourages people to find life-sustaining and enriching opportunities.

Spiritual wellness A feeling of inner peace and of being generally alive, purposeful, and fulfilled; the feeling is rooted in spiritual values and/or specific religious beliefs.

Spirituality The part of being human that seeks meaningfulness through personal connection, which may include belief in or relationship with some higher power, creative force, driving being, or infinite source of energy.

Spirometry A means of measuring inhalation and exhalation, although the key measurements are forced expiratory volume over 1 second (FEV_1) and the ratio of FEV_1 to forced vital capacity (FEV_1/FVC). In other words, how much and how quickly an individual exhales air as measured by spirometry is an indicator of the degree of pulmonary function deficit.

Splint An easily adjustable device that stabilizes injuries, usually before swelling has subsided or after the reparative phase of healing.

Splitting 1. The inability to integrate contradictory experiences. 2. The inclination to perceive people or situations as one extreme or the other.

Spontaneous abortion The loss of a fetus prior to 20 weeks of gestation. Also called *miscarriage*.

Spontaneous rupture of membranes (SROM) The rupturing of membranes during the height of an intense contraction with a gush of fluid out of the vagina.

Sporadic AD One of the two basic types of Alzheimer disease, it shows no clear pattern of inheritance, although genetic factors may contribute to the disorder. It typically does not develop until after the age of 65. Also called *late-onset Alzheimer disease*.

Sprain A stretching or tearing of ligaments.

Sputum Mucus or mucopurulent matter expectorated from the lungs.

Squamous cell carcinoma A malignant tumor of the squamous epithelium of the skin or mucous membranes.

Staff authority The power to provide advice and support to employees or departments but not to assign tasks.

Stage of exhaustion Stage in which the body ceases to maintain its adaptation to a stressor; the stressor overwhelms the individual's ability to cope or mount a continued defense, resulting in the depletion of energy and resources.

Stage of resistance Stage in which the body attempts to move toward restoration of homeostasis while continuing to respond to the stressor.

Staghorn calculi A type of calculi associated with a urinary tract infection caused by urease-producing bacteria such as *Proteus*. These stones can grow to become very large, filling the renal pelvis and calyces. Also called *struvite calculi*.

Staging A system of classifying cancer according to the size of the tumor, involvement of lymph nodes, and metastasis to distant sites.

Standard precautions Safety guidelines, such as proper hand hygiene, use of proper protective equipment, safe injection practices, and effective management of potentially contaminated surfaces or equipment, that are designed to decrease the risk of transmitting unidentified pathogens. Also called *universal precautions* and *body substance isolation (BSI)*.

Standardized plan A nursing care plan that specifies the nursing care for groups of patients with common needs (e.g., all patients with myocardial infarction).

Standards Models of high-quality performance that may reflect the performance of industry leaders, scientific or clinical research, or recommendations of professional organizations such as the American Nurses Association.

Standards of care Guidelines used to determine what a nurse should or should not do and may be defined as a benchmark of achievement based on a desired level of excellence.

Standards of practice A standardized description of nurses' responsibilities.

Standards of professional performance The behaviors expected in the professional nursing role by the American Nurses Association.

Station The location of the fetal presenting part in the maternal pelvis in relation to the ischial spine.

Status asthmaticus A severe, prolonged form of asthma that is difficult to treat.

Status epilepticus A continuous seizure that lasts for more than 30 minutes or a series of seizures during which time consciousness is not regained.

Statute of limitations The limit to the amount of time that can pass between recognition of harm and bringing a suit.

Statutory laws Laws made by any legislative branch of the government, including the U.S. Congress, state legislatures, and city and county governments.

Steatorrhea Fatty, frothy, foul-smelling stools caused by a decrease in pancreatic enzyme secretion.

Stem cell transplantation (SCT) The infusion of immature stem cells to replenish a patient's blood cell lines; used as an alternative to bone marrow transplantation.

Stenosis Narrowing of the valve, valve area, or great artery above the valve.

Stent A short, narrow tube inserted into the lumen of a vessel (e.g., artery) to relieve blockage.

Step-down therapy A gradual reduction in the dosage and number of drugs used in a therapeutic regimen.

Stereognosis The ability to perceive and understand an object through touch.

Stereotyping The act of generalizing that all people in a group are the same.

Stereotypy Rigid and obsessive behavior.

Sterile field An area free of microorganisms.

Sterile technique Practices that keep an area or object free of all microorganisms. Also known as *surgical asepsis*.

Sterilization 1. A process that destroys all microorganisms, including spores and viruses. 2. An inclusive term that refers to surgical procedures that permanently prevent pregnancy.

Stigma A collection of negative attitudes and beliefs that lead people to fear, reject, avoid, and discriminate against people with mental illness.

Stillbirth Death of a fetus that occurs after 20 weeks of gestation. Also called *fetal demise* or *intrauterine fetal death (IUFD)*.

Stimulus The agent or act that stimulates a nerve receptor.

Stimulus-based stress model A model that defines stress as being a life event that requires change or adaptation on the part of the individual who is experiencing the life event.

Stoma An artificial opening in the abdominal wall; it may be permanent or temporary.

Stool Body wastes and undigested food eliminated from the bowel. Also called *feces*.

Strabismus Misalignment of the eyes.

Strain A stretching or tearing of a muscle or tendon.

Strategic plan A plan of continual assessment, planning, and evaluation to guide future decisions and developments.

Strength training Exercises that use resistance to strengthen muscle groups, which include use of elastic resistance bands, lifting weights, or body-weight resistance exercises, such as push-ups, planks, pull-ups, and squats.

Stress The body's general, nonspecific response to the demands placed on it by a stressor.

Stress fracture A fracture that results from disease that has weakened the bone.

Stress mediators Hormonal triggers that are intended to promote adaptation through mechanisms such as triggering a necessary increase in heart rate and blood pressure when faced with physical danger.

Stress response Physiologic changes triggered by stress; includes activation of the neural, neuroendocrine, and endocrine systems, as well as activation of target organs.

Stressor An external influence that threatens to disrupt the equilibrium that is needed to maintain homeostasis.

Striae Whitish-silver stretch marks seen in obesity and during or after pregnancy.

Stridor A high-pitched sound within the trachea and larynx that suggests narrowing of the tracheal passage.

Stroke A condition in which neurologic deficits result from a sudden decrease in blood flow to a localized area of the brain. Also called *cerebrovascular accident* or *brain attack*.

Stroke volume (SV) The amount of blood pumped into the aorta with each contraction of the left ventricle that is measured by the difference between the end-diastolic volume and the end-systolic volume.

Structural-functional theory Focuses on family structure and function, examining family relationships and how they affect the functions of the family and relationships with other systems.

Structure standards Standards related to material resources, human resources, and general organizational structure.

Struvite calculi A type of calculi associated with a urinary tract infection caused by urease-producing bacteria such as *Proteus*. These stones can grow to become very large, filling the renal pelvis and calyces. Also called *staghorn stones*.

Subconjunctival hemorrhage Temporary, nonpathogenic hemorrhages that are caused by the changes in vascular tension or ocular pressure during birth.

Subculture Minority groups characterized by specific norms, beliefs, and values that coexist with a dominant culture.

Subcutaneous tissue The layer of loose connective tissue and fat cells that lies below the dermis. Also called *hypodermis*.

Subinvolution A slowing of the descent of the uterus during the postpregnancy healing process.

Subjective data Information that is apparent to only the patient affected and can be described or verified by only that patient. Also called *symptoms* or *covert data*.

Substance abuse The use of any chemical in a fashion inconsistent with medical or culturally defined social norms despite physical, psychologic, or social adverse effects.

Substance use disorder (SUD) The actual addictive process to a substance, such as alcohol or opiates.

Sucking reflex Occurs in response to a finger or nipple inserted into an infant's mouth; the infant responds by beginning to rhythmically suck on the finger.

Suctioning Aspirating secretions through a catheter connected to a suction machine or wall suction outlet.

Sudden cardiac death (SCD) Unexpected death occurring within 1 hour of the onset of cardiovascular symptoms.

Sudden infant death syndrome (SIDS) The sudden death of an apparently healthy infant that remains unexplained after other possible causes have been ruled out through autopsy, death scene investigation, and review of the medical history.

Sudden unexpected death in epilepsy (SUDEP) Sudden and unexpected death in an individual diagnosed with epilepsy.

Sudden unexpected infant death (SUID) A term used to describe the sudden and unexpected death, often happening during sleep, of a baby less than 1 year old in which the cause was not obvious before investigation.

Suicidal ideation A case of an individual constantly considering, planning, or thinking about suicide.

Suicide An act of an individual inflicting self-harm resulting in death.

Suicide attempt An act of an individual inflicting self-harm with the intent to cause death that is not successful.

Sundowning A behavioral change commonly seen in patients with dementia, characterized by increased agitation, time disorientation, and wandering behaviors during afternoon and evening hours; it is accelerated on overcast days.

Superficial burn A burn that involves only the epidermal layer of the skin.

Superficial thrombophlebitis A blood clot blocking one or more veins near the skin's surface.

Superimposed preeclampsia Occurs when a woman previously diagnosed with chronic hypertension develops hypertension-related end-organ dysfunction in pregnancy or worsening hypertension that is resistant to treatment.

Supine On the back.

Supine hypotensive syndrome Also referred to as *aortocaval compression* or *vena caval syndrome*, it is a condition in pregnancy when the enlarging uterus presses on the vena cava and aorta and its collateral circulation.

Supply chain A series of processes (from manufacturing to delivery) involved in the production and distribution of essential items.

Suppuration A large quantity of cells and necrotic debris that form an opaque or milky discharge that is thicker than serous exudate. Also called *pus* or *purulent exudate*.

Surfactant Specialized cells that control surface tension and keep alveoli from collapsing and sticking to themselves.

Surge capacity A community's ability to rapidly meet the increased demand for qualified personnel and resources, including healthcare resources, in the event of a disaster.

Surgical asepsis Practices that keep an area or object free of all microorganisms. Also called *sterile technique*.

Surgical debridement The process of excising a wound to the level of fascia or sequentially removing thin slices of a burn wound to the level of viable tissue.

Sutures The membranous spaces between the cranial bones of a fetus.

Swan-neck deformity Caused by rheumatoid arthritis, it is characterized by hyperextension of the proximal interphalangeal joints with compensatory flexion of the distal interphalangeal joints.

Sweat test Typically administered twice, it measures the amount of salt in the baby's sweat and is most effective for a cystic fibrosis diagnosis; a high level of salt confirms the diagnosis.

Symptom See **Subjective data**.

Synchronized cardioversion Delivery of direct electrical current synchronized with the patient's heart rhythm.

Synclitism A condition that occurs when the sagittal suture is midway between the symphysis pubis and the sacral promontory and is felt to be aligned.

Syncope Transient loss of consciousness and muscle tone after exercise or activity.

Syndrome diagnosis A cluster of nursing diagnoses that occur together and may result in best patient outcomes if addressed at the same time.

Syndrome of inappropriate antidiuretic hormone secretion (SIADH) A condition in which the body makes too much antidiuretic hormone, which helps the kidneys control the amount of water the body loses through the urine. It causes the body to retain too much water.

Synovectomy Excision of synovial membrane; this procedure is used as a treatment for rheumatoid arthritis.

Synovitis Inflammation of the synovial membrane lining the articular capsule of a joint.

Syphilis A complex systemic sexually transmitted infection caused by the spirochete *Treponema pallidum*.

Systemic arthritis A form of juvenile rheumatoid arthritis that is characteristically manifested by high fever, polyarthritis, and rheumatoid rash. Systemic arthritis also affects internal organs and joints.

Systemic circulation Circulation through the left side of the heart, the aorta and its branches, the capillaries that supply the brain and peripheral tissues, the systemic venous system, and the vena cava.

Systemic lupus erythematosus (SLE) A chronic, inflammatory connective tissue disease.

Systemic response Results because of a widespread antibody–antigen reaction. Systemic responses include anaphylaxis, urticaria, or angioedema.

Systemic vascular resistance (SVR) The force or resistance of the blood in the body's blood vessels that helps return blood to the heart.

Systems theory The study of how a system operates, including how it interacts with other systems and how its components interact with each other within the system itself.

Systole The phase of ventricular contraction.

Systolic blood pressure The maximum pressure exerted within the arteries when the heart compresses.

T lymphocyte (T cells) A type of leukocyte that matures in the thymus gland and is integral to the specific immune response.

Tachycardia An excessively fast heart rate greater than 100 bpm in an adult.

Tachypnea A respiratory rate greater than 20 bpm in adults.

Tactile Of or relating to touch.

Tanner stages Stages of physical growth of the breasts and pubic hair in girls and the genitalia and pubic hair in boys.

Tardive dyskinesia A condition characterized by repetitive, involuntary body movement of varying severity that may not cease after medication cessation; includes unusual tongue and face movements such as lip smacking and wormlike motions of the tongue.

Target effects The expected action a drug will have on a patient.

Tartar A visible, hard deposit of plaque and dead bacteria that forms at the gumlines. Also called *dental calculus*.

Teach-back method A patient teaching strategy in which the nurse provides information to a patient and asks the individual to restate the information to ensure that the patient understands it correctly.

Teaching A process that uses planned strategies and approaches with the goal of changing behavior.

Team Two or more individuals who agree to work in tandem to accomplish a common goal.

Team nursing The delivery of individualized nursing care to a group of patients by a team led by a professional nurse.

Technical skills Also called *procedural* or *psychomotor skills*, they are the practice-oriented, tactile skills performed in patient care, which include dressing changes, equipment use, venous access initiation, sterile procedures, and other direct patient-care interventions.

Telangiectatic nevi (storkbites) Pale pink or red spots frequently found on the eyelids, nose, lower occipital bone, and nape of the neck of young children. These areas have no clinical significance and usually fade by the second birthday.

Telecommunication The transmission of information from one site to another, using equipment to send information in the form of signs, signals, words, or pictures by cable, radio, or other systems.

Telehealth A system that employs the use of telecommunications technologies (e.g., videoconferencing, streaming media, real-time forwarding imaging, and land-based and wireless communications) to allow patients access to care that they might not otherwise be able to obtain. Also called *telemedicine* or *remote patient monitoring*.

Telenursing The provision of nursing care via **telecommunication**.

Temperament The combination of biological and physical characteristics that influence personality and behavior specific to each individual.

Tendinitis Inflammation of a tendon.

Teratogen Any substance that adversely affects the normal growth and development of the fetus.

Terminal weaning The gradual withdrawal of mechanical ventilation when survival without assisted ventilation is not expected.

Territoriality A concept of the space and things that an individual considers as belonging to the self.

Tertiary intention healing Healing that occurs after closing a wound that has been left open for 3 to 5 days to allow edema or infection to resolve. Also called *delayed primary intention*.

Tertiary prevention Methods that focus on the restoration of health following an illness or accident and include rehabilitation and palliative services.

Testosterone The primary male sex hormone produced by the testes.

Tetany Tonic muscle spasms.

Tetralogy of Fallot A rare disease that consists of four defects: pulmonic stenosis, right-ventricular hypertrophy, ventricular-septal defect, and an overriding aorta.

Tetraplegia Complete loss of function of the upper and lower body, including the arms, trunk, legs, and pelvic organs. Also called *quadriplegia*.

Thalassemia Inherited disorder of hemoglobin synthesis in which either the alpha or beta chains of the hemoglobin molecule are missing or defective.

Thelarche The beginning of breast development in females.

Theory of multiple intelligences Theory that describes the different types of intelligences as posited by researcher Howard Gardner.

Therapeutic communication An interactive process between a nurse and a patient that helps the patient to overcome temporary stress, to get along with other people, to adjust to situations that cannot be altered, and to overcome any psychologic blocks that may stand in the way of self-realizations.

Therapeutic insemination The process of depositing semen at the cervical os or in the uterus by mechanical means.

Therapeutic relationship Nurse–patient relationship that is focused on helping patients manage problems and become better at helping themselves.

Thermoregulation The body process that balances heat production and heat loss to maintain the body's temperature.

Third heart sound (S_3) Heart sound that is sometimes heard after the second heart sound in children, young adults, and pregnant women during the third trimester. Also called a *ventricular gallop*.

Third spacing A shift of fluid from the vascular space into an area where it is not available to support normal physiologic processes.

Thoracentesis Needle insertion into the pleural space to remove fluid accumulation.

Thoracolumbar sacral orthosis (TLSO) A brace contoured to conform to the body and support the spine. Also called an *underarm brace* or *Boston brace*.

Thought blocking Speech stopped in midsentence as if the thought disappeared from the individual's head.

Thought disorders Disorders associated with schizophrenia that involve an abnormal way of thinking, such as disorganized thinking, sensory overload, thought blocking, neologisms, loose association, clang, and perseveration.

Threshold potential The point at which an action potential is capable of being generated.

Thrill A palpable vibration over the precordium or an artery.

Thrombin An enzyme in blood plasma that causes the clotting of blood by converting fibrinogen to fibrin.

Thromboemboli Emboli created by a blood clot.

Thrombophlebitis Sometimes called *phlebitis*, condition in which a blood clot forms and blocks one or more veins. Clots typically form in the legs but can form in the arms and neck in rare instances.

Thrush White patches that look like milk curds that adhere to the mucous membranes usually caused by an infected vaginal tract during birth, antibiotic use, or poor hand hygiene. Bleeding may occur if patches are removed.

Thyroid crisis See **Thyroid storm**.

Thyroid storm An extreme state of hyperthyroidism. Now extremely rare due to improved diagnosis and treatment methods. Also called *thyroid crisis*.

Thyroidectomy Surgical removal of all or part of the thyroid gland.

Thyroiditis Inflammation of the thyroid gland.

Thyrotoxicosis A disorder caused by excessive delivery of thyroid hormone to the peripheral tissues. Also called *hyperthyroidism*.

Tics Semi-involuntary movements that are sudden, repetitive, and nonrhythmic. They may involve muscle groups or vocalizations (motor or phonic).

Time constraints Deadlines for completion.

Time-out A preprocedure verification to ensure the correct procedure is being performed at the right site on the right patient.

Time priority A time constraint to complete an action.

Tinea pedis Fungal infection of the feet. Also called *athlete's foot*.

Tinnitus The perception of sound or noise in the ears without stimulus from the environment.

Tissue factor (TF) A protein found on the surface of some body cells.

Tolerance State in which a particular dose elicits a smaller response than it formerly did. With increased tolerance, the individual needs higher and higher doses to obtain the desired response.

Tone 1. The amount of tension or resistance to movement in a muscle. 2. The ability of vessels to constrict or dilate to maintain normal pressure.

Tonic phase Initial phase of a generalized seizure, manifested by unconsciousness and continuous muscular contraction.

Torsades de pointes A type of ventricular tachycardia associated with a prolongation of the QT interval.

Tort A civil wrong committed against an individual or an individual's property.

Total parenteral nutrition (TPN) The intravenous administration of amino acids, often with added carbohydrates, fats, electrolytes, vitamins, and minerals.

Total quality management (TQM) A comprehensive management philosophy that improves quality and productivity by using data and statistics to improve system processes.

Toxic multinodular goiter A tumor characterized by small, discrete, independently functioning nodules in the thyroid gland tissue that secrete excessive amounts of thyroid hormone.

Toxoplasmosis Space-occupying lesions common in patients with AIDS that may cause headache, altered mental status, and neurologic deficits.

Tracheostomy An artificial airway in the neck for long-term ventilatory support.

Trachoma A chronic conjunctivitis caused by *Chlamydia trachomatis*. It is a significant preventable cause of blindness worldwide.

Traction The application of a straightening or pulling force to return or maintain fractured bones in their normal anatomic position.

Transactional leader A leader who has a relationship with followers based on an exchange of some resource valued by the follower.

Transductive reasoning Connecting two events in a cause-and-effect relationship simply because they occur together in time.

Transection An injury that occurs when an individual is injured by a gunshot, stabbing, or similar force, which may partially or completely sever the spinal cord.

Transference The transfer of feelings that were originally evoked by one's parents or significant others to people in the present setting.

Transformational leader A leader who fosters creativity, risk taking, commitment, and collaboration by empowering a group to share in an organization's vision. The leader inspires others with a clear, attractive, and attainable goal and enlists them to participate in attaining the goal.

Transfusion reaction A type II or cytotoxic hypersensitivity reaction to blood of an incompatible type.

Transgender Gradations of human characteristics running from female to male; more commonly, an individual who expresses a gender identity different from that with which the person was born.

Transient ischemic attack (TIA) A brief period of localized cerebral ischemia that causes neurologic deficits lasting for less than 24 hours. Also called a *mini-stroke.*

Transitional milk A light yellow milk that is more copious than colostrum and contains more fat, lactose, water-soluble vitamins, and calories; it usually presents between the second and fifth day following birth.

Transjugular intrahepatic portosystemic shunt (TIPS) An expandable metal stent inserted through a transcutaneous needle to channel blood from the portal vein into the hepatic vein, bypassing the cirrhotic liver.

Translational research A systematic approach of converting research knowledge into applications of healthcare for improved patient outcomes.

Transmigrate To move or pass from one place to another.

Transplacental immunity Passive immunity transferred from mother to infant.

Transposition of the great arteries (TGA) A congenital heart defect in which the pulmonary artery, the outflow tract for the left ventricle, and the aorta, the outflow tract for the right ventricle, are transposed.

Transthyretin amyloid cardiomyopathy (ATTR-CM) Amyloid deposits in the myocardium that cause progressive heart failure.

Transurethral resection of the prostate (TURP) A procedure that removes obstructing prostate tissue using the wire loop of a resectoscope and electrocautery inserted through the urethra.

Transverse diameter The largest diameter of the pelvic inlet; helps determine its shape.

Trauma An injury to human tissues and organs resulting from the transfer of energy from an external environmental source, such as a motor vehicle, a fire, or a sharp object.

Trauma-informed care A framework for recognizing and responding to trauma and its effects and preventing retraumatization, emphasizing the need to understand the impact of trauma and provide physical and psychological safety for both the patient and the healthcare provider.

Traumatic brain injury (TBI) An injury resulting from an external physical force, such as a blow or jolt to the head, that causes displacement of the brain within the skull and disruption of normal brain function.

Traumatic cataracts A type of cataract that may result from an injury to the eye.

Tremors Rhythmic, involuntary movements or twitching of the extremities.

Triage The process of identifying priorities for implementing care.

Trial and error A group decision strategy in which the most viable solution is attempted.

Tricyclic antidepressant (TCA) A class of drugs that inhibit the reuptake of both norepinephrine and serotonin into presynaptic nerve terminals. They are primarily used in the pharmacotherapy of depression.

Triglycerides Substances converted from dietary fats and carbohydrates to store energy in fat cells.

Triplet Three premature ventricular contractions in a row.

Tripod position A position of sitting and leaning forward; often used by patients who are having difficulty breathing.

Trisomies The result of a normal gamete (egg or sperm) uniting with a gamete that contains an extra chromosome.

Trisomy 21 A condition that occurs when an individual born with Down syndrome has an additional full chromosome present.

Trophoblast A layer of tissue in the female uterus, supplying the embryo with nourishment and later forming the major part of the placenta.

Trousseau sign Spasmodic contraction of the hand and fingers in response to occlusion of the blood supply by a blood pressure cuff; caused by decreased blood calcium levels. A test used to check for hypocalcemia.

True pelvis The portion that lies below the linea terminalis; made up of the inlet, cavity, and outlet.

Tubal ligation A surgical procedure to clip, tie off, band, or plug the fallopian tubes to sterilize a female patient.

Tubercle A granulomatous lesion (a sealed-off colony of bacilli) formed from *Mycobacterium tuberculosis.*

Tuberculosis (TB) A chronic, recurrent infectious disease caused by *Mycobacterium tuberculosis*. It usually affects the lungs, but any organ can be affected.

Tumor marker A protein molecule detectable in serum or other body fluids that is used to highlight suspicious regions for follow-up.

TURP syndrome A condition that is characterized by hyponatremia, decreased hematocrit, hypertension, bradycardia, nausea, and confusion.

Two-career family A family in which both partners are employed by choice or necessity. A two-career family may or may not have children.

Tympanic membrane A thin, tense membrane that separates the middle ear from the external auditory canal, protecting the middle ear from the external environment.

Tympanocentesis A surgical incision of the tympanic membrane. Also called *myringotomy.*

Tympanogram A test that provides a graph of the middle ear's ability to transmit sound.

Tympanostomy tubes Pressuring-equalizing tubes inserted to provide the middle ear with ventilation and drainage during healing.

Tympany A musical or drumlike sound produced from an air-filled stomach.

Type 1 diabetes (T1D) An absolute deficiency of insulin related to pancreatic beta cell destruction that results in severe hyperglycemia and diabetic ketoacidosis, among other symptoms.

Type 2 diabetes (T2D) A relative deficiency of insulin, which may be related to insulin resistance and inadequate secretion of insulin to meet body needs. Both of these components are usually present at time of diagnosis.

Ulcer A break in the GI mucosa that develops when the mucosal barrier is unable to protect the mucosa from damage by hydrochloric acid and pepsin, the gastric digestive juices.

Ulcerative colitis A chronic inflammatory bowel disorder that affects the mucosa and submucosa of the colon and rectum.

Ultrafiltration Removal of excess body water using a hydrostatic pressure gradient.

Ultrasound A test using intermittent ultrasonic waves transmitted by an alternating current to a transducer and applied to the abdomen.

Umbilical cord A cord that connects the fetus to the placenta of the mother for the purpose of carrying nourishment from the mother to the fetus and passing waste back from the fetus to the mother.

Underinsured Individuals whose healthcare coverage is insufficient to meet their needs.

Undernutrition Health effects due to insufficient or diminished nutrient intake or stores. Also known as *malnutrition.*

Unifocal When a ventricular impulse arises from one ectopic site.

Uninsured Individuals who are without any type of healthcare coverage.

Unipolar depression A mood disorder characterized by loss of interest in life and unresponsiveness, moving from mild to severe, with severe symptoms lasting at least 2 weeks. Also called *major depressive disorder (MDD).*

Universal precautions (UP) Safety guidelines, such as proper hand hygiene, use of proper protective equipment, safe injection practices, and effective management of potentially contaminated surfaces or equipment, that are designed to decrease the risk of transmitting unidentified pathogens. Also called *standard precautions* and *body substance isolation (BSI).*

Universal Protocol Established guidelines for healthcare professionals to prevent errors during surgical procedures, including wrong-site surgery.

Unlicensed assistive personnel (UAP) Members of a nursing team who assume delegated aspects of basic patient care such as bathing, assisting with feeding, and collecting specimens. Include certified nurse assistants, hospital attendants, nurse technicians, and orderlies.

Unresolved bacteriuria The presence of bacteria in urine that fails to resolve with treatment.

Unsaturated fat A triglyceride fat that does not contain all of the hydrogen ions it is capable of holding.

Upper body obesity Identified by a waist-to-hip ratio of greater than 1 in men or 0.8 in women. Also called *central obesity.*

Uremia Excessive amounts of urea in the blood.

Uremic fetor A urine-like breath odor often associated with a metallic taste in the mouth.

Uremic frost Crystallized deposits of urea on the skin.

Ureteral stent A thin catheter inserted into the ureter to provide for urine flow and ureteral support.

Ureterolithotomy An incision in the affected ureter to remove a calculus.

Ureteroplasty The surgical repair of a ureter.

Urgency The sudden, strong desire to void.

Urgency factor A way to illustrate how much time can safely lapse before doing interventions without compromising patient outcomes.

Uric acid stones Develop when the urine concentration of uric acid is high.

Urinary calculi Stones in the urinary tract.

Urinary drainage system Those organs required to drain urine from the kidneys, including the ureters, urinary bladder, and urethra.

Urinary frequency The need to urinate often, specifically more than four to six times a day.

Urinary hesitancy A delay and difficulty in initiating voiding; often associated with dysuria.

Urinary incontinence Involuntary urination due to the temporary or permanent inability of the external sphincter muscles to control the flow of urine from the bladder. Also called *involuntary urination.*

Urinary retention The accumulation of urine in the bladder and inability of the bladder to empty itself, resulting in overdistention of the bladder.

Urinary tract infection (UTI) An infection in any part of your urinary system, which includes the kidneys, ureters, bladder, and urethra.

Urination Releasing urine from the urinary bladder. Also called *voiding* or *micturition.*

Urine specific gravity (SG) A measure of the concentration of solutes in the urine.

Urolithiasis The formation of stones in the urinary tract.

Urticaria Patches of pale, itchy wheals in an erythematous area. Also known as *hives.*

Uterine atony The relaxation of uterine muscle tone.

Uterus The hollow muscular organ in which the fertilized ovum is implanted and in which the developing fetus is nourished until birth.

Utilitarianism A form of consequentialist theory that views a good act as one that brings the most good and the least harm for the greatest number of people. This is called the *principle of utility.*

Utility See **Utilitarianism.**

Utilization review An evaluation of the use of resources to identify areas of overuse, misuse, and underuse.

Uveitis Inflammation of the middle layer of the eye called the uvea.

Vaccine Suspensions of whole or fractionated bacteria or viruses that have been treated to make them nonpathogenic; introduced by immunization to provoke active immunity.

Vacuum extraction An obstetric procedure used by healthcare providers to assist the birth of a fetus by applying suction to the fetal head.

Vagina The muscular and membranous tube that connects the external genitals with the uterus.

Vaginal birth after cesarean (VBAC) An option for a mother to choose a trial of labor and vaginal birth after having a cesarean for a previous child, provided the previous cesarean was required due to a nonrecurring indication and the mother meets the guidelines established by the American College of Obstetricians and Gynecologists.

Vaginismus The involuntary spasm of the outer one-third of the vaginal muscles, making penetration of the vagina painful and sometimes impossible.

Validation The act of verifying the accuracy and factuality of data.

Valsalva maneuver Forced exhalation against a closed glottis.

Values Personal beliefs about truth and the worth of behaviors or objects; standards that influence behavior.

Values clarification A process of consciously identifying, examining, and developing individual values that helps nurses gain the ability to choose actions on the basis of deliberately adopted values.

Variable decelerations A condition that occurs if the umbilical cord becomes compressed, reducing blood flow between the placenta and fetus. Fetal hypertension stimulates the baroreceptors in the aortic arch and carotid sinuses, slowing the fetal heart rate.

Variance 1. An unmet goal. 2. An incident or accident that affects a patient or a visitor in a healthcare facility.

Vasectomy A procedure to surgically sever the vas deferens on both sides of the scrotum to sterilize a male patient.

Vaso-occlusive crisis See **Sickle cell crisis.**

Vegan A type of vegetarian diet that excludes all animal and fish products, including dairy, meat, eggs, and honey.

Vena caval syndrome Occurs when the gravid uterus compresses the vena cava of a supine woman, reducing blood flow to the woman's heart. This may cause maternal hypotension. May also be referred to as *supine hypotensive syndrome* or *aortocaval compression.*

Venous stasis The collection and stagnation of blood in the lower extremities.

Venous thrombectomy Surgical removal of a blood clot from the femoral vein to prevent pulmonary embolism or gangrene.

Venous thrombosis A condition in which a blood clot (thrombus) forms on the wall of a vein, accompanied by inflammation of the vein wall and some degree of obstructed venous blood flow. Also called *thrombophlebitis.*

Ventilation The exchange of oxygen and carbon dioxide.

Ventilation-perfusion (V-Q) The movement of oxygen across the alveolar–capillary membrane into a well-perfusing capillary.

Ventricular aneurysm An outpouching of the ventricular wall that does not contract during systole, causing stroke volume to decrease.

Ventricular assist device (VAD) A device that temporarily takes partial or complete control of cardiac function, such as for a heart transplant.

Ventricular bigeminy A premature ventricular contraction following each normal beat.

Ventricular gallop (S_3) Heart sound sometimes heard after the second heart sound in children, young adults, and pregnant women during the third trimester. Also called the *third heart sound*.

Ventricular septal defect (VSD) An opening in the ventricular septum that causes increased pulmonary blood flow.

Ventricular trigeminy A premature ventricular contraction every third beat.

Veracity A moral principle that holds that an individual should tell the truth and not lie.

Verbal abuse Malicious, repeated, harmful mistreatment of an individual with whom one works, regardless of whether that individual is an equal, a superior, or a subordinate.

Verbal communication Transmitting information through the spoken or written word.

Vernix caseosa A whitish, cheeselike substance that covers a fetus while in utero.

Vertical rotation The degree of rotation of the vertebrae.

Vertical transmission Perinatal transmission of an infection, such as the human immunodeficiency virus, from mother to infant.

Vertigo A sensation of whirling or rotation.

Very-low-calorie diets A program providing a protein-sparing modified fast (400 to 800 kcal/day or less) under close medical supervision.

Vesicoureteral reflux A condition in which urine moves from the bladder back toward the kidney. A common risk factor in children who develop pyelonephritis that may also be seen in adults whose bladder outflow is obstructed.

Vesicular sounds The soft and breezy sounds of air moving in and out of the lobes at the alveolar level.

Vestibulo-ocular reflex Eye movement that functions to stabilize gaze by countering movement of the head.

Vibration A series of vigorous quiverings produced by hands that are placed flat against the patient's chest wall.

Vicarious trauma Risk of healthcare providers from exposure to and caring for survivors of firsthand trauma.

Violence The use of excessive force against other individuals or oneself, often resulting in physical or psychologic injuries or death.

Virchow triad Three factors associated with thrombophlebitis: stasis of blood, vessel damage, and increased blood coagulability.

Virulence The ability of a microorganism to produce disease.

Virus A type of microorganism that must enter living cells in order to reproduce.

Visceral Of or relating to any large organ in the body.

Visceral pain Pain arising from body organs. It is dull and poorly localized because of the low number of nociceptors.

Viscosupplementation A treatment for osteoarthritis of the knee that involves injecting lubricating substances directly into the knee.

Visual Of or relating to sight.

Vitamins Micronutrient compounds that are involved in regulating body functioning. Most vitamins, with the exceptions of vitamins D and K, cannot be manufactured within the body and must be consumed through dietary intake.

Vitiligo An autoimmune disorder that results in loss of melanin in patches of the face, hands, or groin.

Voiding Releasing urine from the urinary bladder. Also called *urination* or *micturition*.

Voiding cystourethrography Use of a contrast medium and x-rays to assess the bladder and urethra when filled and during voiding.

Volatile acid Acids eliminated from the body as a gas.

Voluntary admission The detention of a patient in a psychiatric or medical facility at the patient's request.

Voluntary insurance Healthcare insurance that provides no guarantee of universality because coverage may be expensive and difficult to purchase.

Vomiting The forceful expulsion of the contents of the upper gastrointestinal tract resulting from contraction of muscles in the gut and abdominal wall.

Vulnerability An individual's susceptibility to react to a specific stressor.

Vulnerability factors A practice, behavior, or environmental factor that increases the potential of an individual becoming a victim of violence.

Vulnerable populations Social groups with inadequate access to healthcare because they lack resources and are exposed to more risk factors.

Vulva The external female genitals.

Warm zone When a disaster occurs, this zone, located at least 300 feet from the outer edge of a hot zone, is where decontamination occurs and rapid triage and emergency treatment are given to stabilize victims. Also called the *yellow zone*, *contamination zone*, or *contamination reduction zone*.

Water deficit A value greater than 295 mOsm/kg, indicating the concentration of solute is too great or the water content is too little in the body.

Water excess A value less than 275 mOsm/kg, indicating too little solute for the amount of water or too much water for the amount of the solute in the body.

Weaning 1. The process of removing ventilator support and reestablishing spontaneous, independent respirations. 2. The process of discontinuing breastfeeding and transitioning an infant to another feeding method.

Well-being A subjective perception of feeling well that can be described objectively and measured.

Wellness A state of well-being that encompasses self-responsibility, dynamic growth, nutrition, physical fitness, emotional health, preventive healthcare, and the whole being of the individual.

Wernicke encephalopathy A condition typically seen in people with alcohol use disorder that is characterized by ataxia (lack of coordination), abnormal eye movements, and confusion.

Wharton jelly Specialized connective tissue that surrounds the blood vessels in the umbilical cord.

Wheezing A high-pitched whistling sound most often heard on expiration and caused by the narrowing of bronchi; can also be heard on inspiration.

Whiplash An injury that results from sudden impact to a motor vehicle that causes an individual's head and neck to be forcibly contorted, resulting in injury to the spine.

Whistleblower A nurse or other individual who goes outside of an organization for the public's best interest when the organization fails to follow procedures regarding safety and patient care.

Whistleblowing The act of going outside of an organization for the public's best interest when an organization fails to follow procedures regarding safety and patient care.

White blood cells (WBCs) See **Leukocytes**.

Withdrawal Abstinence from substances.

Withdrawing or withholding life-sustaining therapy (WWLST) The withdrawal of extraordinary means of life support, such as removing a ventilator or withholding special attempts to revive a patient, and allowing the patient to die of the underlying medical condition.

Work ethic A belief in the importance and moral worth of work.

Work of breathing (WOB) The amount of energy or oxygen consumption needed by the respiratory muscles to produce enough ventilation and respiration to meet the metabolic demands of the body.

Workplace bullying Verbal attacks, refusal to help or assist others, speaking negatively, or taunting that can cause physical and psychologic stress to the victim, adversely affect patient safety and outcomes, and create a negative work environment.

Workplace violence Any physical assault, threatening behavior, or verbal abuse occurring in the workplace.

Worldview The way in which people in a culture perceive ideas and attitudes about the world, other people, and life in general.

Worst-case scenario Technique designed to help groups make decisions that involve risk. The worst-case outcome is outlined for each alternative, and then the scenario with the comparatively best outcome is selected as the preferred outcome. This technique helps ensure that the "least of all evils" is selected.

Wrong-site surgery (WSS) A surgical operation that is performed at the wrong location on a patient's body due to error.

Xenograft Skin used for transplantation that was obtained from an animal, usually a pig. Also called *heterograft*.

Xerostomia Dry mouth that occurs when an individual's supply of saliva is reduced.

Youth violence An adverse childhood experience that occurs in minors and may continue into young adulthood that includes being a victim of violence, a violent offender, or a witness to violence.

Zollinger-Ellison syndrome A form of peptic ulcer disease caused by a gastrinoma, or gastrin-secreting tumor of the pancreas, stomach, or intestines.

Zygote A fertilized egg.

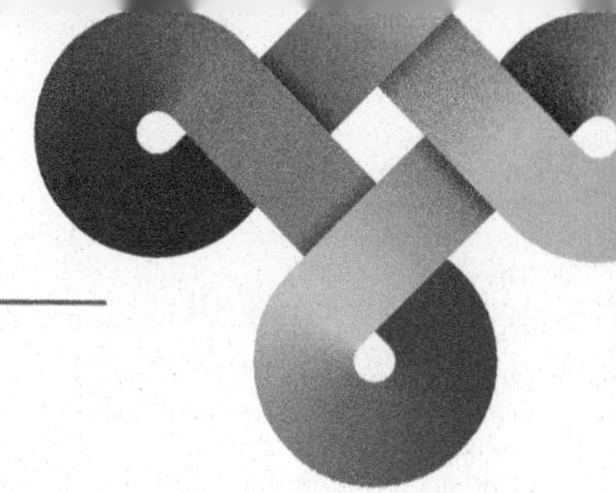

Index

Contains entries for Volumes 1 and 2.
Red type indicates a concept.
Bold type indicates an exemplar.
f indicates an entry from a figure.
t indicates an entry from a table or box.

C

D

E

J

K

L

M

N

P

Q

R

T

U

V

W

X

Y

Z